OPERATIVE MICROSURGERY

NOTICE

OPERATIVE MICROSURGERY

J. Brian Boyd, MD
Professor and Chief of Plastic Surgery
Harbor-UCLA Medical Center
Torrance, California

Neil F. Jones, MD
Chief of Hand Surgery
Professor of Plastic and Reconstructive Surgery
Professor of Orthopedic Surgery
University of California
Irvine, California

Mc Graw Hill Education

New York Chicago San Francisco Athens London Madrid Mexico City
Milan New Delhi Singapore Sydney Toronto

Operative Microsurgery

1 2 3 4 5 6 7 8 9 0 CTP/CTP 18 17 16 15 14

ISBN 978-0-07-174558-1
MHID 0-07-174558-0

This book was set in Adobe Garamond by Cenveo® Publisher Services.
The editors were Brian Belval and Brian Kearns.
The production supervisor was Catherine Saggese.
Project management was provided by Vastavikta Sharma, Cenveo Publisher Services.
The cover designer was Anthony Landi.
China Translation and Printing Services, Inc. was the printer and binder.

This book is printed on acid-free paper.

Library of Congress Cataloging-in-Publication Data

Operative microsurgery / [edited by] John Brian Boyd, Neil F. Jones.
p. ; cm.
Includes bibliographical references.
ISBN 978-0-07-174558-1 (hardcover : alk. paper)—ISBN 0-07-174558-0 (hardcover : alk. paper)
I. Boyd, John Brian, editor. II. Jones, Neil Ford, editor.
[DNLM: 1. Microsurgery—methods. WO 512]
RD33.6
617′.05—dc23 2014022184

CONTENTS

SECTION 1

INTRODUCTION: FLAP ANATOMY, EXPOSURE, AND ELEVATION

SECTION 2

HEAD AND NECK

SECTION 3

THE TRUNK

SECTION 4

UPPER LIMB

SECTION 5

LOWER LIMB

CONTRIBUTORS

Christina Y. Ahn, MD, FACS
Associate Professor of Surgery (Plastic)
Department of Plastic and Reconstructive Surgery
New York University
Langone Medical Center
New York, New York

Robert J. Allen, Sr., MD
Institute of Reconstructive Plastic Surgery
New York University
Center for Microsurgical Breast Reconstruction
New York Eye and Ear Infirmary
New York, New York

Claudio Angrigiani, MD
Chief, Division of Plastic Surgery
Hospital Santojanni
Buenos Aires, Argentina

Mark W. Ashton, MBBS, MD, FRACS
The Jack Brockhoff Reconstructive Plastic Surgery Research Unit
Department of Anatomy and Cell Biology
University of Melbourne
Melbourne, Victoria, Australia

Carla Baldrighi, MD
Department of Reconstructive Microsurgery
Ospedale CTO
Azienda Ospedaliero-Universitaria Careggi
Florence, Italy

Jacques Baudet, MD
Pole Ouest Centre Hospitalo Universitaire Pellegrin
Université Bordeaux 2
France

Elisabeth K. Beahm, MD, FACS
Professor, Department of Plastic Surgery
University of Texas MD Anderson Cancer Center
Houston, Texas

Giles W. Becker, MA, MB, BChir, FRCS (Tr and Orth)
Assistant Professor of Surgery
Reconstructive and Plastic Surgery
University of Arizona
Tucson, Arizona

Zoubir Belkheyar
Clinique Paris-Montmartre
Marcadet, Paris

R Ravindra Bharathi, MS, MCh, DNB
Senior Consultant Plastic Surgeon
Ganga Hospital
Coimbatore, India

Waseem Bhat
Department of Plastic and Reconstructive Surgery
Leeds General Infirmary
Leeds Teaching Hospitals NHS Trust
Leeds, United Kingdom

Rolfe Birch, MChir, FRCP&S (Glas), FRCS (Edin and Eng)
Emeritus Professor of Orthopaedics
University College London;
Professor in Neurological Orthopedic Surgery
University College London;
Visiting Professor, Department of Academic Neurology
Imperial College London;
Honorary Orthopaedic Consultant
Hospital for Sick Children
London, United Kingdom

Allen T. Bishop, MD
Professor of Orthopedic Surgery
Mayo Clinic College of Medicine
Consultant, Division of Hand Surgery
Department of Orthopedic Surgery
Mayo Clinic
Rochester, Minnesota

Anders Björkman, MD, PhD
Associate Professor
Department of Handsurgery
Skane University Hospital
Malmö, Sweden

Carrie Black, MD
Fellow, Plastic Surgery
Department of Surgery
University of Minnesota
Minneapolis, Minnesota

Phillip Blondeel, MD, PhD, FCCP
Department of Plastic and Reconstructive Surgery
University Hospital Gent
Gent, Belgium

Branko Bojovic, MD
Assistant Professor
Plastic, Reconstructive and Maxillofacial Surgery
R Adams Cowley Shock Trauma Center
University of Maryland School of Medicine
Baltimore, Maryland
Assistant Professor
Department of Plastic Surgery
Johns Hopkins School of Medicine
Baltimore, Maryland

Gregory H. Borschel, MD
Division of Plastic Surgery
The Hospital for Sick Children
Toronto, Ontario, Canada

Vaughan Bowen, MD
Division of Orthopaedic Surgery
Foothills Medical Centre
Alberta, Canada

J. Brian Boyd, MD, FRCS, FRCSC, FACS
Professor and Chief of Plastic Surgery
Harbor-UCLA Medical Center
Torrance, California

Warren C. Breidenbach III, MD
Division of Reconstructive & Plastic Surgery
Department of Surgery
University of Arizona College of Medicine
Tucson, Arizona

P. Niclas Broer, MD
Institute of Reconstructive Plastic Surgery
New York University
New York, New York

Giorgio Brunelli, MD
School of Medicine
University of Brescia
Italy

Edward W. Buchel, MD, BSc, FACS
Associate Professor
Department of Surgery
Section of Plastic Surgery
Head, Section of Plastic Surgery
University of Manitoba
Health Sciences Center
Winnipeg, Manitoba

Gregory M. Buncke, MD
Director
The Buncke Medical Clinic
Chairman of Plastic Surgery
California Pacific Medical Center
San Francisco, California

Rudolf Buntic, MD
Program Director
The Buncke Clinic
Chief of Microsurgery
California Pacific Medical Center
San Francisco, California

Charles E. Butler, MD, FACS
Professor and Chairman
Department of Plastic Surgery
The University of Texas MD Anderson Cancer Center
Houston, Texas

Vincent Casoli, MD
Pole Ouest Centre Hospitalo Universitaire Pellegrin
Université Bordeaux 2
France

Paul S. Cederna, MD, FACS
Professor, Section of Plastic Surgery
Associate Chair, Department of Surgery
Associate Chief of Staff, University of Michigan Health Systems
Ann Arbor, Michigan

Rodney K. Chan, MD, FACS, FRCSC
Chief, Plastic and Reconstructive Surgery
Clinical Division and Burn Center
United States Army Institute of Surgical Research
San Antonio Military Medical Center
Fort Sam Houston, Texas
Associate Professor of Surgery
Normal M. Rich Department of Surgery
Uniformed Services University
Bethesda, Maryland

David W. Chang, MD, FACS
Department of Plastic Surgery
The University of Texas MD Anderson Cancer Center
Houston, Texas

Johnny T. Chang, MD
The Buncke Clinic
California Pacific Medical Center
San Francisco, California

Albert H. Chao, MD
Assistant Professor of Clinical Surgery
The Ohio State University
Department of Plastic Surgery
Columbus, Ohio

Fuguo Chen, MD, PhD
Professor
Division of Reconstructive Microsurgery
Department of Plastic and Reconstructive Surgery
Shanghai Ninth People's Hospital
Shanghai JiaoTong University, School of Medicine
Shanghai, China

Hung Chi Chen, MD, MHA, FACS
Professor, Department of Plastic Surgery
China Medical University Hospital
Taiwan

Kaixiang Cheng, MD
Professor
Division of Reconstructive Microsurgery
Department of Plastic and Reconstructive Surgery
Shanghai Ninth People's Hospital
Shanghai JiaoTong University, School of Medicine
Shanghai, China

Ming-Huei Cheng, MD, MBA, FACS
Professor, Division of Reconstructive Microsurgery
Department of Plastic and Reconstructive Surgery
Chang Gung Memorial Hospital
Taoyuan, Taiwan

David T. W. Chiu, MD, FACS
Professor of Plastic Surgery and Neurosurgery
Chief of Hand Surgery
Director of New York Nerve Center
Institute of Reconstructive Plastic Surgery
Department of Plastic Surgery
New York University
New York, New York

David Chwei-Chin Chuang, MD
Professor
Department of Plastic Surgery
Chang Gung Memorial Hospital
Chang Gung University
Taipei-Linkou, Taiwan

Howard M. Clarke, MD, PhD, FRCS (C), FACS, FAAP
Professor of Surgery
Department of Surgery
University of Toronto
Active Staff Surgeon
Division of Plastic Surgery
Hospital for Sick Children
Toronto, Ontario

Russell J. Corlett, MBBS, FRACS
The Jack Brockhoff Reconstructive Plastic Surgery Research Unit
Department of Anatomy and Cell Biology
University of Melbourne
Melbourne, Victoria, Australia

A. Lee Dellon, MD, PhD
Professor of Plastic Surgery and Professor of Neurosurgery
Johns Hopkins University;
Director of the Dellon Institutes for Peripheral Nerve Surgery
Baltimore, Maryland

Risal Djohan, MD
Section Head for Breast Surgery for Dept Plastic Surgery
Program Director of Microsurgery Fellowship Program
Cleveland Clinic
Cleveland, Ohio

Kazuteru Doi, MD, PhD
President
Ogori Daiichi General Hospital
Director
Department of Orthopedic Surgery
Ogori Daiichi General Hospital
Ogori, Yamaguchi, Japan
Clinical Professor
Department of Orthopedic Surgery
Yamaguchi University School of Medicine
Ube, Yamaguchi, Japan

Amir H. Dorafshar, MBChB, FAAP, FACS
Assistant Professor
Department of Plastic and Reconstructive Surgery
Johns Hopkins School of Medicine
Baltimore, Maryland

David Elliot, MA(Oxon), FRCS
Hand Surgeon
St Andrew's Centre for Plastic Surgery
Broomfield Hospital
Chelmsford, Essex, United Kingdom

Adel Fattah, PhD, FRCS (Plast)
Consultant Plastic and Microsurgeon
Department of Plastic Surgery
Alder Hey Children's NHS Foundation Trust
Liverpool, United Kingdom

Joshua Fosnot, MD
Assistant Professor of Surgery
Division of Plastic Surgery
The University of Pennsylvania Health System
Philadelphia, Pennsylvania

Jennifer L. Giuffre, MD, FRCSC
Assistant Professor
Plastic Surgery
University of Manitoba
Section of Plastic Surgery
Department of Surgery
Winnipeg, Manitoba, Canada

Lawrence J. Gottlieb, MD, FACS
Professor of Surgery
Director of Burn & Complex Wound Center
Director of Reconstructive Microsurgery Fellowship
Section of Plastic and Reconstructive Surgery
The University of Chicago Medicine & Biological Sciences
Chicago, Illinois

David Todd Greenspun, MD
Center for Microsurgical Breast Reconstruction
New York Eye and Ear Infirmary
New York, New York

Matthew M. Hanasono, MD
Associate Professor
Department of Plastic Surgery
The University of Texas MD Anderson Cancer Center
Houston, Texas

Douglas P. Hanel, MD
Professor
Section of Hand and Microvascular Surgery
Director of Orthopaedic Education
Department of Orthopaedics and Sports Medicine
University of Washington
Seattle, Washington

Summer E. Hanson, MD, PhD
Division of Plastic and Reconstructive Surgery
University of Wisconsin
School of Medicine and Public Health
Madison, Wisconsin

Isaac Harvey, MD
Women's and Children's Hospital
Department of Plastic and Reconstructive Surgery
North Adelaide, Adelaide
South Australia, Australia

Thomas Hayakawa, BSc, MD, FRCS(C)
Assistant Professor
Department of Surgery
Section of Plastic Surgery
Director of Microsurgery
University of Manitoba, Health Sciences Center
Winnipeg, Manitoba

Piet Hoebeke, MD, PhD, FEBU, FEAPU
Head of Department of Urology
Professor of Paediatric Urology & Urogenital Reconstruction
Ghent University Hospital
Gent, Belgium

Stefan O.P. Hofer, MD, PhD, FRCS(C)
Wharton Chair in Reconstructive Plastic Surgery
Professor of Surgery, University of Toronto
Chief, Division of Plastic Surgery at the Department of Surgery and Department of Surgical Oncology, University Health Network
Toronto, Ontario, Canada

Jung-Ju Huang, MD
Assistant Professor
Division of Reconstructive Microsurgery
Department of Plastic and Reconstructive Surgery
Chang Gung Memorial Hospital
Taoyuan, Taiwan

Georg M. Huemer, MSc, MBA
Section of Plastic and Reconstructive Surgery
General Hospital Linz
Linz, Austria

Marco Innocenti, MD
Director, Reconstructive Microsurgery
Careggi University Hospital
Florence, Italy

Andrew Ives, MBBS, FRACS
Taylor Lab
Department of Anatomy and Neuroscience
University of Melbourne
Melbourne, Victoria, Australia

Reza Jarrahy, MD
Associate Professor
Division of Plastic and Reconstructive Surgery
University of California
Los Angeles, California

Neil F. Jones, MD
Chief of Hand Surgery
Professor of Plastic and Reconstructive Surgery
Professor of Orthopedic Surgery
University of California
Irvine, California
Formerly, Professor and Chief of Hand Surgery
University of California
Los Angeles, California

Bruce Kaplan, MD
Professor of Medicine and Pharmacology
University of Kansas
Lawrence, Kansas

Simon P.J. Kay, FRCS, FRCS(Plas), FRCSE(Hon)
Professor of Hand Surgery and Consultant Plastic Surgeon
University of Leeds
Leeds Teaching Hospitals NHS Trust
Leeds, United Kingdom

Kazuki Kikuchi, MD
Department of Plastic and Reconstructive Surgery
Graduate School of Medicine
The University of Tokyo
Tokyo, Japan

Jason H. Ko, MD
Assistant Professor
Section of Hand and Microvascular Surgery
Division of Plastic Surgery
Department of Orthopaedics and Sports Medicine
University of Washington
Seattle, Washington

L. Andrew Koman, MD
Professor and Chair
Department of Orthopaedic Surgery
Wake Forest School of Medicine
Executive Director, Musculoskeletal Service Line
Wake Forest Baptist Health
Winston-Salem, North Carolina

Isao Koshima, MD
Professor and Chief
Plastic and Reconstructive Surgery
Graduate School of Medicine
The University of Tokyo
Hongo, Bunkyo-ku, Tokyo

Mauricio Kuri, MD
Microsurgical and Hand Fellow
The Buncke Clinic
San Francisco, California

Wee-Leon Lam, MBChB, FRCS(Plast)
Consultant Plastic and Hand Surgeon
Royal Hospital for Sick Children, Edinburgh
Honorary Clinical Senior Lecturer
University of Edinburgh
United Kingdom

Maria M. LoTempio, MD, FACS
Assistant Professor
Department of Surgery-Divison of Plastic Surgery
Medical University of South Carolina
Charleston, South Carolina;
Clinical Assistant Professor of Surgery at Weill Cornell Medical College
Department of Surgery-Division of Plastic Surgery
New York, New York

Steven M. Levine, MD
Institute of Reconstructive Plastic Surgery
New York University
New York, New York

Joshua Louis Levine, MD
Center for Microsurgical Breast Reconstruction
New York Eye and Ear Infirmary
New York, New York

Zhongyu Li, MD, PhD
Associate Professor
Department of Orthopaedic Surgery
Wake Forest School of Medicine
Wake Forest Baptist Medical Center
Winston-Salem, North Carolina

Chih-Hung Lin, MD
Department of Plastic and Reconstructive Surgery
Chang Gung Memorial Hospital and College of Medicine
Linkou, Taiwan

Andrew Lindford, MBBS, MRCS
Department of Plastic Surgery
Helsinki University Hospital
Helsinki, Finland

William Lineaweaver, MD, FACS
Medical Director
JMS Burn and Reconstruction Center
Central Mississippi Medical Center
Jackson, Mississippi

Joan E. Lipa, MD, MSc, FRCS(C), FACS
Associate Professor
Department of Surgery, Division of Plastic Surgery
University of Toronto
Toronto, Ontario, Canada

Steven Lo, MA, BMBCh, MSc, MRCS, FRCS (Plast)
Locum Consultant in Plastic Surgery
Queen Victoria Hospital, East Grinstead
Sussex, United Kingdom

Robert Lohman, MD
Cleveland Clinic
Plastic Surgery Department
Cleveland, Ohio

Maria M. LoTempio, FACS
Assistant Professor
Department of Surgery-Divison of Plastic Surgery
Medical University of South Carolina
Charleston, South Carolina
Clinical Assistant Professor of Surgery at Weill Cornell Medical College
Department of Surgery-Division of Plastic Surgery
New York, New York

Göran Lundborg, MD, PhD
Professor of Hand Surgery
Hand Surgery, Department of Clinical Sciences
Lund University
Skåne University Hospital
Malmö, Sweden

Eldon Mah, MBBS, FRACS
Division of Plastic & Reconstructive Surgery
Toronto General Hospital
Toronto, Ontario

Ajay L. Mahajan, FRCSI, MMedSc, MD, FRCS (Plast)
Akademikliniken
Stockholm, Sweden

Yutaka Maki, MD, PhD
Chairman of the Board of Directors
Niigata Hand Surgery Foundation
Chuo-Ku, Niigata-Shi, Japan

Ralph T. Manktelow, MD, FRCS(C), Retired
Professor of Surgery
University of Toronto
Toronto, Ontario

Hani S. Matloub, MD
Professor of Plastic Surgery
Medical College of Wisconsin
Milwaukee, Wisconsin

Babak J. Mehrara, MD, FACS
Associate Attending Surgeon, Plastic and Reconstructive Surgery Section, Department of Surgery
Memorial Sloan-Kettering Cancer Center
New York, New York;
Associate Professor of Surgery
Division of Plastic & Reconstructive Surgery
University of Toronto,
Toronto, Ontario

Emmanuel G. Melissinos, MD, FACS
Clinical Professor of Surgery
Division of Plastic and Reconstructive Surgery and
Department of Orthopedic Surgery
University of Texas
Houston, Texas

Makoto Mihara, MD
Department of Plastic and Reconstructive Surgery
Graduate School of Medicine
The University of Tokyo
Tokyo, Japan

Michael J. Miller, MD
Professor of Plastic Surgery
Chair, Department of Plastic Surgery
The Ohio State University
Columbus, Ohio

Stan J. Monstrey, MD, PhD
Professor and Chairman
Department of Plastic Surgery
University Hospital
Ghent, Belgium

Wayne A. Morrison
St Vincent's Hospital, Melbourne
Melbourne, Australia

Christine A. Muhleman, OTR/L, CHT
Hand Therapist
University of Arizona Health Network
Therapy Services
Tucson, Arizona

Mitsunaga Narushima, MD
Department of Plastic and Reconstructive Surgery
Graduate School of Medicine
The University of Tokyo
Tokyo, Japan

Dung H. Nguyen, MD, PharmD
Clinical Assistant Professor
Division of Plastic and Reconstructive Surgery Stanford University
Palo Alto, California

Christine B. Novak, PT, PhD
Associate Professor of Surgery
Division of Plastic & Reconstructive Surgery
University of Toronto
Toronto, Ontario

Christophe Oberlin
Hôpital Bichat
Paris, France

Fusa Ogata, MD
Department of Plastic and Reconstructive Surgery
Graduate School of Medicine
The University of Tokyo
Tokyo, Japan

Can Ozturk, MD
Academic Clinical Associate
Department of Head and Neck Surgery/Plastic and Reconstructive Surgery
Roswell Park Cancer Institute
Buffalo, New York

Cemile Nurdan Ozturk, MD
Cleveland Clinic Foundation
Plastic Surgery Department
Cleveland, Ohio

William C. Pederson, MD, FACS
Fellowship Director
The Hand Center of San Antonio
Adjunct Professor of Surgery
The University of Texas Health Science Center
San Antonio, Texas

Philippe Pelissier, MD
Pole Ouest Centre Hospitalo Universitaire Pellegrin
Université Bordeaux 2
France

Aaron T. Pelletier, MD
Plastic and Reconstructive Surgery
Director of Reconstructive Microsurgery
Midwestern Regional Medical Center
Cancer Treatment Centers of America®
Zion, Illinois

Vincent Pinsolle, MD
Pole Ouest Centre Hospitalo Universitaire Pellegrin
Université Bordeaux 2
France

Julian J. Pribaz, MD
Division of Plastic Surgery
Brigham and Women's Hospital
Boston, Massachusetts

Marc J. Richard, MD
Associate Professor
Department of Orthopaedic Surgery
Duke University Medical Center
Durham, North Carolina

Eduardo D. Rodriguez, MD
Division of Plastic Surgery
R Adams Cowley Shock Trauma Center
University of Maryland Medical Center
Baltimore, Maryland

S. Raja Sabapathy, MS, MCh (Plast), DNB (Plast), FRCS (Edin)
Chairman
Department of Plastic and Hand Surgery
Ganga Hospital
Coimbatore, India

Bauback Safa, MD, MBA
Attending Surgeon
The Buncke Clinic
San Francisco, California

James Robert Sanger, MD, FACS
Professor of Plastic Surgery
Department of Plastic Surgery
Medical College of Wisconsin
Chief of Plastic and Reconstructive Surgery
Clement Zablocki Veterans Administration Hospital
Milwaukee, Wisconsin

Thomas Sarlikiotis, MD
Fellow
Hand/Upper Extremity Service
Department of Orthopaedic Surgery
Wake Forest University School of Medicine
Winston-Salem, North Carolina

Christiana Savvidou, MD, PhD
Senior Fellow in Hand and Microsurgery
University of Louisville School of Medicine
Louisville, Kentucky

Naoya Sawamoto, MD
Lecturers in Plastic and Reconstructive Surgery
University of Tokyo
Tokyo, Japan

Luis R. Scheker, MD
Associate Clinical Professor of Plastic and Reconstructive Surgery
University of Louisville School of Medicine
Louisville, Kentucky

Dennis T. Schmahl, OTR/L
Hand Therapist
St. Mary's Hospital
Out-patient Therapy Department
Tucson, Arizona

Thomas Schoeller, MSc
Chief, Department of Plastic and Reconstructive Surgery
Marien Hospital
Stuttgart, Germany

Yukio Seki, MD
Department of Plastic and Reconstructive Surgery
Graduate School of Medicine
The University of Tokyo
Tokyo, Japan

Joseph M. Serletti, MD, FACS
Division of Plastic Surgery
The University of Pennsylvania Health System
Philadelphia, Pennsylvania

Randy Sherman, MD
Vice Chair – Department of Surgery
Cedars Sinai Medical Center
Clinical Professor of Surgery
Keck School of Medicine
University of Southern California
Los Angeles, California

Minoru Shibata, MD, PhD
Professor and Chief
Division of Plastic and Reconstructive Surgery
Niigata University Graduate School of Medical and Dental Sciences
Niigata, Japan

Alexander Y. Shin, MD
Professor, Orthopedic Surgery
Mayo Clinic
Department of Orthopedic Surgery
Division of Hand and Microvascular Surgery
Rochester, Minnesota

David E. Sieber, MD
Fellow Plastic Surgery
Department of Surgery
University of Minnesota
Minneapolis, Minnesota

John W. Siebert, MD
Professor of Surgery
Division of Plastic and Reconstructive Surgery
University of Wisconsin – Madison, School of Medicine and Public Health
Madison, Wisconsin

Maria Siemionow, MD, PHD, DSc
Professor of Orthopaedics
Department of Orthopaedics
University of Illinois at Chicago
Chicago, Illinois

Roman J. Skoracki, MD
Professor, Plastic Surgery
The Ohio State University
Columbus, Ohio

Beth Paterson Smith, PhD
Professor
Department of Orthopaedic Surgery
Wake Forest School of Medicine
Winston-Salem, North Carolina

Hooman Soltanian, MD, FACS
Vice Chair, Department of Plastic Surgery
Residency Program Director
Associate Professor
Case Medical Center
Cleveland, Ohio

Robert J. Spinner, MD
Departments of Neurologic Surgery and Orthopedics
Mayo Clinic
Rochester, Minnesota

William Swartz, MD
Clinical Professor of Plastic Surgery
University of Pittsburgh Medical School
Pittsburgh, Pennsylvania

Neil Tanna, MD, MBA
Institute of Reconstructive Plastic Surgery
New York University
New York, New York

G. Ian Taylor, AO, MBBS, MD, FRACS
Taylor Lab
Department of Anatomy and Neuroscience
University of Melbourne
Melbourne, Australia

Charles Y. Tseng, MD
Assistant Clinical Professor
David Geffen School of Medicine
Division of Plastic and Reconstructive Surgery
University of California
Los Angeles, California

Erkki Tukiainen, MD, PhD
Department of Plastic Surgery
Helsinki University Hospital
Helsinki, Finland

Tolga Turker, MD
Assistant Professor of Surgery
Reconstructive and Plastic Surgery
University of Arizona
Tucson, Arizona

Joseph Upton, MD
Clinical Professor of Surgery
Beth Israel Deaconess Medical Center
Boston, Massachusetts

James R. Urbaniak, MD
Virginia Flowers Baker Professor of Orthopaedic Surgery
Duke University Medical Center
Durham, North Carolina

Allen L. Van Beek, MD, FACS
Adjunct Professor
Department of Surgery
University of Minnesota
Minneapolis, Minnesota

Julie Vanille Vasile, MD
Center for Microsurgical Breast Reconstruction
New York Eye and Ear Infirmary
New York, New York;
Stamford Hospital
Stamford, Connecticut

Hari Venkatramani, MCh (Plast), DNB (Plast), EDHS
Senior Consultant
Trauma Reconstructive Surgery
Ganga Hospital
Coimbatore, India

Fausto Viterbo, MD, MS, PhD
Associate Professor and Head of Plastic Surgery Division
Botucatu School of Medicine
UNESP, Brazil

Robert L. Walton, MD, FACS
Professor of Surgery
Division of Plastic Surgery
Northwestern University
Feinberg School of Medicine
Chicago, Illinois

Fu-Chan Wei, MD, FACS
Professor and Chancellor
Department of Plastic Surgery
College of Medicine, Chang Gung University
Chang Gung Memorial Hospital
Taoyuan, Taiwan

Iain S. Whitaker, BA (Hons), MBBChir, MA Cantab, PhD, FRCS (Plast)
The Jack Brockhoff Reconstructive Plastic Surgery Research Unit
Department of Anatomy and Cell Biology
University of Melbourne
Melbourne, Victoria, Australia;
Swansea University College of Medicine
Swansea University
Swansea, Wales, United Kingdom

Thomas Willson, MD
Chief Resident in Surgery
Saint Joseph Hospital
Chicago, Illinois

Robert I.S. Winterton, MBBS, MRCS (Eng), FRCS (Plast)
Department of Plastic and Reconstructive Surgery
Leeds General Infirmary
Leeds Teaching Hospitals NHS Trust
Leeds, United Kingdom

Sang-Hyun Woo
President, Cheon & Woo's Institute for Hand & Reconstructive Microsurgery
W Hospital
Daegu, Korea

Michael B. Wood, MD
Professor, Orthopedic Surgery
Mayo Clinic College of Medicine
Rochester, Minnesota

Peirong Yu, MD
Professor
Department of Plastic Surgery
University of Texas MD Anderson Cancer Center
Houston, Texas

Yixin Zhang, MD, PhD
Professor, Chief of Division of Reconstructive Microsurgery
Assistant Chief of Department of Plastic and Reconstructive Surgery
Shanghai Ninth People's Hospital
Shanghai JiaoTong University, School of Medcine
Shanghai, China

Toni Zhong, MD, MSc, FRCS(C)
Division of Plastic & Reconstructive Surgery
Toronto General Hospital
Toronto, Ontario

Ronald M. Zuker, MD, FRCSC, FACS, FAAP, FRCSEd (Hon)
Consultant Surgeon
Division of Plastic and Reconstructive Surgery
The Hospital for Sick Children
Professor of Surgery
The University of Toronto
Toronto, Canada

PREFACE

We stand at a crossroads in the development of reconstructive microsurgery. Having almost exhausted the finite anatomy of the human body in the quest for new donor sites, we have entered the realm of *supermicrosurgery* and *free-style* free flaps, where practically any tissue may be harvested or replanted to reconstruct our patients. In other words, we have passed from the definite to the infinite. Indeed, the possibilities now exceed our capacity for classification, whereas before they were limited by incomplete anatomical knowledge as well as our technical inability to perform the surgery. Having defined the anatomic microcirculation of the skin, muscles, and bone, for which we owe Professor G. Ian Taylor and his coworkers an enormous debt of gratitude; it is likely that in the future we will look to composite tissue allotransplantation (CTA) to reconstruct complex defects poorly reconstructed by "conventional" microsurgical techniques, although the huge problems of rejection and chronic immunosuppression still remain.

Now is also the time when most of the first generation of reconstructive microsurgeons are retiring; have retired; or, alas, passed away. This textbook is therefore a tribute to those microsurgeons; some of whom have emerged from the Elysian fields of retirement, from their farms, golf courses, trout streams and duck blinds, or merely from the contemplation of lives well spent; to contribute their valuable and perhaps historic experience to this textbook before it is lost forever. Their passing from active practice may mark the end of an era—but surely the beginning of a new one, for we stand on the shoulders of these giants—and constitutes another justification for the timing of this work.

We have tried to eliminate duplication and padding by assuming a certain level of microsurgical expertise or at least knowledge in our readers. There are no introductory chapters on how to perform a microvascular anastomosis or a microneural repair. These techniques are exhaustively showcased elsewhere and best learned in vivo—preferably in an animal model. The reader will not find any account of the history of microsurgery or microsurgical instruments, apart from that pertaining to some of the procedures outlined in the various chapters. The anatomy of the human body is described in anatomical tomes and will not be repeated here except as it applies to specific operative procedures.

The book is essentially divided into two parts—firstly, descriptions of specific operative techniques, each of which should serve as a recipe for the average microsurgeon to perform the procedure independently; and secondly, chapters on problem-based clinical applications in each of the anatomical areas—the head and neck, trunk, upper and lower limbs. There is inevitably some overlap for the purposes of continuity, and some specific chapters simply stand alone. We have made no attempt to make this an encyclopedic work—there are several flaps that the reader will not find here: our purpose has been to describe flaps in reasonably common usage, so there will be inevitable omissions. If glaring, these will of course be corrected in any future editions. The fact that the book has had a somewhat prolonged gestation may mean that the very latest reference may not be cited—perhaps a future online version will permit frequent updates to be made. Alas, most textbooks face the same problem!

When planning this book, we contemplated who the target audience would be. The answer is embodied in the title. The text is aimed at reconstructive microsurgeons across the entire spectrum of surgical specialties. These include Plastic Surgeons, Orthopedic Surgeons, Hand Surgeons, Head and Neck Surgeons, Oral-Maxillofacial Surgeons, and Urologists. We feel that this book will be extremely useful to residents, fellows, and younger surgeons starting to practice reconstructive microsurgery in any of these fields, and will hopefully find a place in the libraries of their training programs.

We would like to heartily thank all the authors of the various chapters, for it is largely upon their efforts that the impact of this book will rest. They all accepted their tasks willingly and dedicated a significant amount of their valuable time, distilling their unique knowledge, and putting pen to paper or, rather, fingers to keyboard. We would particularly like to thank those contributors whose native language is not English and therefore their effort much greater.

Our thanks are also due to the staff at McGraw-Hill who have consistently held our feet to the fire, yet maintained their support throughout. These include Brian Kearns and Brian Belval as well as our copy editor, Sylvia Rebert. Her quiet persistence and thoroughness has been a great asset in the project and it is to her that we owe a profound debt of gratitude.

Finally, we would be remiss if we did not acknowledge the support of our wives, Jeanette and Barbara, who suffered through long evenings, weekends, and vacations where the need for internet service was paramount and the usual amusements took second place to long spells on the laptop computer, midnight texting to contributors, a constant torrent of e-mails, and the inevitable conference calls. Without their unstinting support, this book would not have been possible.

JBB, NFJ, 2014

SECTION 1

INTRODUCTION: FLAP ANATOMY, EXPOSURE AND ELEVATION

CHAPTER 1

The Microvascular Anastomosis

Russell J. Corlett, Iain S. Whitaker, and Mark W. Ashton

THE MICROVASCULAR ANASTOMOSIS

In 1902, French vascular surgeon Alexis Carrel challenged the widely held belief that vascular anastomosis was not possible (1). He pioneered new techniques such as the triangulation of vessels; the use of sharp, round-bodied needles to minimize intimal damage; and irrigation with crystalloid to perform the first successful anastomosis. Many of his ideas are still used today. Carrel won a Nobel Prize in recognition of his work in 1912. Microvascular surgery as we understand it today—the anastomosis of vessels a few millimeters in diameter using microscopic assistance—was born in 1960 when Jules Jacobson, at the University of Vermont, carried out the first microanastomosis, coupling vessels as small as 1.4 mm diameter. Innovations in reconstructive microsurgery followed swiftly during the 1960s and 1970s. The first publication by Buncke and Schulz (2) in 1966 reported a successful rabbit ear replantation, requiring union of vessels 1 mm in size. In 1968, Cobbett performed the first human microsurgical transplantation of the great toe to the thumb (3). The published 30-year follow-up (4) shows the impact of these early procedures on the standard of life of patients for the long term.

Microsurgery moved from experimental to mainstream with the development of specialized microsurgical instruments by individuals such as Acland (5). These included fine-tipped toothed forceps designed to produce minimal intimal damage to vessels, accurate sharp microsurgical scissors, fine vessel dilators, and an array of micro-clamps available in single and double configurations. Recently, the microsurgeons' tray has been supplemented with microvessel clips, venous couplers, and suction pads. The goal of faster, more stable microvascular anastomoses continues to drive innovation and scientific progress in the field of microsurgery.

Before performing the microvascular anastomoses, it is vital to set the stage. I am reminded of when I was a trainee doing a stint in orthopedics when one of the surgeons regularly could insert a closed Kuntscher nail in a fractured femur in 6 minutes skin to skin. He did this not by cutting corners or rushing but because he spent time getting the patient in exactly the right position on the orthopedic table and virtually reducing the fracture before starting to scrub. The same principle applies with microvascular surgery. As Acland preached on his microsurgery course at Louisville for many years, "Preparation is the only shortcut you need to take."

Patient Positioning

For both surgeon and assistant, the ideal position for a microanastomosis is on the surface, not in a deep hole or under a bony shelf. It may necessitate putting a sandbag under a shoulder, extending the neck, flexing the knees, or abducting the hips, and this needs to be organized preoperatively. Careful use of self-retaining retractors or sutures to hold back the skin edge will further refine anastomotic exposure and access.

The Pedicle

The recipient vessels should be as long as possible to permit them to reach closer to the surface and to allow adequate exposure, access, and vessel rotation. The worst possible recipient is a short stump of vessel coming directly out of the depths of the wound that will not tolerate rotation. The diameter of the donor and recipient vessels should ideally match in size, and the recipient artery and vein should be able to be approximated without kinking or the need to dissect a long way into the pedicle. A vein graft should be planned if the pedicle is likely to be too short, and another team is organized to harvest it simultaneously with flap elevation.

The Surgical Area

The surgeon and assistant should position themselves opposite each other, ideally sitting on height-adjustable stools, with their hands comfortably supported on sterile towels or packs if necessary. Although experienced microsurgeons can do the anastomoses standing up without hand support, it is not ideal and is especially difficult if the surgeon is tired after a long procedure. The nurse and instruments should be in easy reach without the need to turn around, and the microscope and its controls should be readily accessible to the surgeon.

Hemostasis is important because it is undesirable to have the anastomoses or the vein graft disappear up the assistant's suction cannula. The new "background" material incorporating suction may help solve this potential problem. An alternative is a "wrung-out" saline-soaked gauze. The flap vessels are checked for length to see that they will comfortably reach the recipients and that they are not twisted or kinked around a tight band or projection. They are positioned so that they lie in a gentle curve. The recipient vessels' adventitia should be trimmed and the artery checked for a spurt to see that there is sufficient flow. The microvascular clamp is also loosened to ensure that the vessels are not being held in a rotated position that will kink the anastomoses when released later.

The Anastomoses

The ideal position for a right-handed surgeon is for the vessels to be positioned in a 2 to 8 o'clock orientation (10 to 4 o'clock for a left-handed surgeon) because this results in a natural hand movement for suturing. On many occasions, this is not possible. The deepest or the most difficult anastomoses should be done first.

End-to-End Artery Anastomosis

The vessels should preferably be close to the same diameter. The smaller vessel can be enlarged by cutting obliquely (spatulation) but should not exceed around 20 degrees because it will kink the anastomosis. The recipient vessels are dissected to provide sufficient length to apply a microvascular clamp well away from the anastomoses and to allow the vessel to be rotated. Depending on the surgeon's preference, either two single clamps or a double approximating clamp is used. The vessels are flushed with heparinized saline to remove any adherent clot, and a cuff of loose adventitial tissue excised. Sutures are placed in the 3 and 9 o'clock positions with the end left long as a stay suture, the vessel rotated, and the back wall sutured. On completion, the vessel is returned to the front and checked to make sure that the first row of sutures has not caught the front wall, and then the front wall is sutured from one side to the other. The penultimate and final sutures are passed through both walls but left untied while the lumen is inspected before proceeding to tie them. This technique allows a clear view of both the last sutures to ensure that the back wall has not been caught.

An approximating double clamp makes rotation of the vessel easier, but sometimes there is insufficient room to apply it. The job of the assistant is to hold the anastomoses in the optimal position, to cut the sutures, and very occasionally retrieve a loose end. He or she must resist the temptation to help with the suturing because it inevitably creates a moving target. When not actively involved, the assistant must keep his or her instruments out of the field to prevent them from obstructing the surgeon's view or constituting a distraction.

An alternative method is to place the first suture in the middle of the back wall and progressively suture forward from this on either side. This is sometimes necessary in a difficult situation, but it is technically more demanding to take even bites of both vessels so as not to end up with a discrepancy on the front wall.

Vein

It is common to have a degree of mismatch with the diameter of the veins; however, a moderate degree is well tolerated. The vessels are triangulated with three stay sutures, each placed one third of the way around the circumference of the anastomosis. Usually, only two or three sutures are placed between them, and because of the low pressure, any leakage readily stops. One good vein is usually sufficient in the head and neck, but in the limbs, where venous spasm is common, a larger superficial vein is often added (where feasible) to a vena comitans anastomosis. When suturing to a large vein such as the internal jugular, then an end-to-side anastomosis is appropriate.

End-to-Side Anastomosis

This is a useful technique for both arteries and veins when the recipient vessel is large and there is significant vessel diameter discrepancy. It is often mandated for the artery in limb salvage when dealing with a "one-vessel" leg.

The flap vessel is cut a little obliquely so that when joined, it is angled in the direction of flow. An incision is made in the donor vessel to correspond with the diameter of the flap vessel. We do not recommended the excision of a portion of the donor vessel because it is usually unnecessary and all too easy to excise too much of the wall, especially if there is a degree of vessel spasm. However, others perform an arteriotomy by excising an oval section of vessel wall either with microscissors or by using an arteriotomy device.

A continuous suture technique may be used in most cases. The first suture is placed in the heel position with both the tail and suture left long. A second suture is similarly placed in the toe position and both ends also left long. Ideally, these sutures should be short (5–6 cm long) to prevent snagging. The heel suture is taken and passed from outside to inside the lumen and the back wall sutured from the inside tying eventually to the tail of the toe suture. The spacing of the sutures should be closer at the heel and toe positions where leaks are more common. The loops of the suture need to be snugged after each bite and any looseness eliminated before the final tie. Care needs to be taken to ensure that the instruments do not have sharp edges that would risk cutting the continuous suture. The heel suture is then taken and used to suture the front wall from the outside tying at the end to the tail of the heel suture. If the assistant is right handed, the front wall is in a natural position for him or her to suture. This anastomoses is very quick and is best done with either 7-0 or 8-0 nylon.

Smaller vessels may require an interrupted technique. The principles are the same, but the back wall is usually sutured under direct vision, requiring some vessel rotation (Figure 1-1).

Vein Grafts

The need for a vein graft can and should be anticipated. For example, in the case of flaps with short pedicles (DCIA, fibula) or where there is an extensive zone of injury, radiation, or previous resection of vessels from neck dissection. A suitable vein is marked out and then dissected, taking care to tie off each tributary in turn. An ink line is marked along the side to ensure that there are no twists when inserted. When both the artery and vein need to be lengthened, then a vein graft (Corlett) loop is used (6). This may be attached to either the artery and vein of the flap or to those of the recipient vessels (in an orthodromic manner) depending on suitability. If the pedicle is to be tunneled and the anastomoses will be under the tunnel, then it is attached to the flap pedicle. This has the advantage that it can

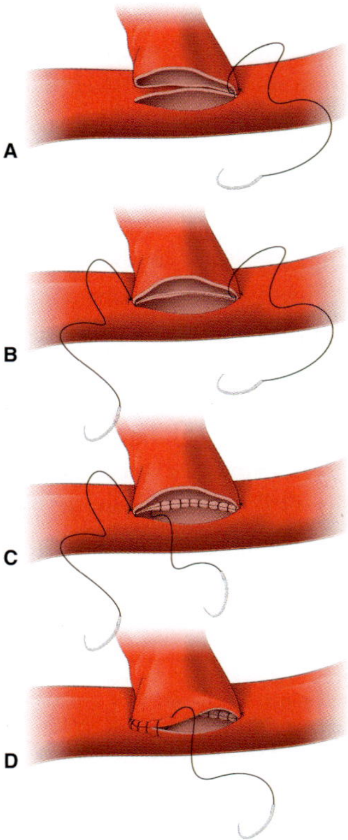

FIGURE 1-1 (**A**) Suture in the toe of end to side with the tail of the suture left long and the rest of the suture left intact. (**B**) Heel suture inserted and both the suture and tail placed to one side. Back wall repair commenced by passing tail suture into the lumen close to the tail suture, and the back wall repaired from inside the lumen. (**C**) Back wall repair taking care to ensure that loops are tight before tying the back wall suture to the loose end of the heel suture. (**D**) Front wall repair from outside the lumen using the heel suture and tying to the loose end of the toe suture. (This suture is most easily done by the co-surgeon if he or she is right handed.)

be done on a side table under ideal conditions. If the recipient vessels are deep and awkward to reach, then the loop is sutured to them first because the loop can be easily moved from side to side without a bulky flap in the way and the second set of anastomoses comfortably done on the surface. This works well for recipient vessels behind the knee or in the axilla. It is important to orient the graft in the right direction with the distal end of the vein graft sutured to the artery (orthodromic). The loop needs to be longer than required to allow for errors in judgment and so that it may be trimmed to fit. A variation of this is to take a long superficial vein when using a radial forearm flap and to form a loop by attaching the proximal end to the artery. The loop may be divided at a convenient point to facilitate flap transfer, thus lengthening both artery and vein with only one extra anastomosis. When a second flap is required (a skin flap and a bone flap), one can use a radial forearm flap to provide the skin and attach the bone flap (DCIA or fibula) to the distal end of the radial vessels (Figure 1-2).

Zone of Injury

Vascular complications are significantly higher if the anastomoses are carried out in the zone of injury. This can be avoided by either choosing a flap with a pedicle long enough to reach normal vessels or by using vein grafts.

Irradiated vessels present a different challenge because they are friable, and the intima tends to be pushed away from the media by the needle. To overcome this, they are sutured from the inside, thus tending to push the intima onto the rest of the vessel wall. This is done by passing the needle through the donor vessel first.

Instruments and Sutures

Except for vessels smaller than 1 mm, 9-0 nylon is used for nearly all tissue transfers, with 8-0 nylon for the larger veins and end-to-side anastomoses. Some digital replants and free tissue transfers in children may require use of 10-0 nylon.

The needle should be noncutting. A good needle holder, spring scissors with straight blades, two pairs of vessel dilating forceps, and a selection of microvascular clamps (including an approximating double clamp) are sufficient for most situations. The clamps should be tested to ensure that they are not too tight and likely to damage the vessel intima.

Traditional Suture Technique

The needle is curved and designed to be inserted in a rotational movement, thereby avoiding the tendency to scythe through the vessel wall. This is particularly important in a soft-walled or irradiated vessel. The suture placement is the minimum that will prevent the vessel from leaking, and in the case of arteries, they are positioned the same distance apart as the thickness of the bite in the vessel wall. In the case of a vein, the distance is less. The sutures should be tied snuggly but not enough to deform the vessel wall. The vessel dilator is introduced into the lumen to separate the vessel walls while the needle is passed to avoid damage to the intima from grasping the whole vessel wall. If there is a clear view of the vessel walls on both sides, it is permissible to suture both with one passage; otherwise, separate bites of each vessel should be taken. Before tying the last suture, the vessel is

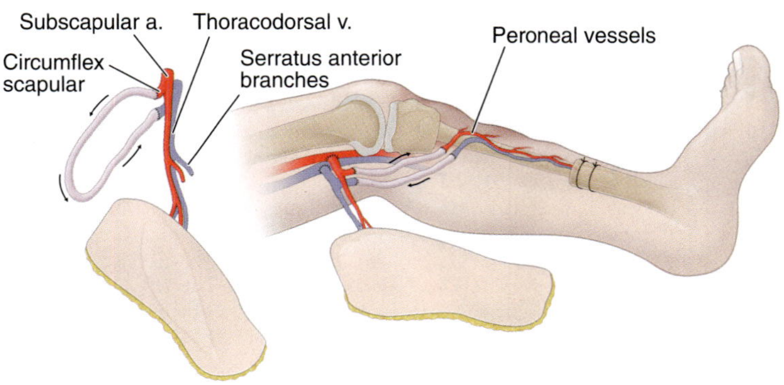

FIGURE 1-2 The "Corlett loop" drawing is an illustration of a patient with a complex injury to the upper tibia and extensive soft tissue loss. The patient had languished in Tasmania for some months before being referred, so the repair was done in one stage as a last-ditch stand with a latissimus dorsi and fibula. The subscapular vessels were joined to the popliteal, and the fibula was joined via the loop to the circumflex scapular vessels with the anastomoses done on the surface.

flushed with heparinized saline. The clamps are taken off in sequence. The arterial clamps should be removed first and those on the vein removed *after* it has filled with blood to confirm the presence of flow through the flap. To deal with moderate bleeding from the artery, the anastomoses may be wrapped in a piece of plastic background material and a cottonoid and 5 minutes allowed to elapse, by which time most will have stopped. Rushing in to place extra sutures can sometimes cause more problems; however, copious bleeding will certainly require an extra suture.

Nonsuture Anastomosis

Although a meticulously sutured microvascular anastomosis remains standard practice, there is a growing body of evidence supporting the use of coupling and clipping devices. Several units worldwide have adopted the use of these devices and report advantages in terms of speed and ease of use over traditional anastomoses. Innovators in the field have shown potential use in arterial anastomoses, end-to-side anastomoses and even irradiated tissue. Detractors of these devices cite the need for training microsurgeons to develop the necessary skills to perform difficult anastomoses when devices cannot be used. As the cost of couplers and clipping systems falls, the cost savings associated with shorter operating times may make these more commonplace. Currently, the evidence supporting the use of both the Unilink Coupler and the VCS clip applicator has achieved level 2b as defined by the Oxford Centre for Evidence Based Medicine (7). Currently, there is little evidence beyond small series supporting glues and laser-assisted bonding in microsurgery (8). Recent interest in robotics in other branches of surgery has spilled over into microsurgery with proof of concept papers reporting successful use of robots in experimental microsurgical models (9,10). Bioabsorbable stents and glues are also currently being investigated (11).

Closure

Before closing the wound, it is important to check to ensure that there is no twist or kink in the pedicle following inflow and vessel dilation. Meticulous hemostasis is mandatory, and a drain tube should be placed under direct vision away from the pedicle, loosely sutured in place. It is useful to place a suture in the skin over the pedicle to mark a point that may be monitored postoperatively with a handheld Doppler. It is vital to ensure that there are no tight bandages or tapes crossing the path of venous drainage from the flap. A good example is the unfortunate use of tracheostomy tapes around the neck or tight bandages around the limbs. It always helps to elevate the part to aid venous drainage.

Postoperative Monitoring

Accurate assessment of the perfusion of free tissue transfers has always been a challenge for surgeons undertaking microvascular reconstructive procedures. Microvascular free tissue transfer today has a high success rate, which is partly due to the effective monitoring of flap circulation after surgery. Recent advances in technology and improvements in surgical technique have led to reported success rates of between 95% and 98% (12). The aim of postoperative surveillance is the early recognition of flap compromise to improve chances of flap salvage and lower morbidity and mortality rates. In many cases, the complexities of flap microcirculation are difficult to assess despite all the subjective and objective examination techniques available today. This is more difficult when the free tissue transfer is not visible for monitoring. Routine monitoring of free flaps is often undertaken by nursing staff on the ward, and it is mandatory that one spends necessary time in educating these staff members and giving them the appropriate instruction as well as monitoring their experience. Junior medical staff often have little experience of such monitoring, especially in the current training system with ever-diminishing working hours and shorter rotations. Clinical tests and simple adjunctive methods such as the handheld Doppler are the most commonly used monitoring tools (13, 14). There are proponents of techniques such as the implantable Doppler probe (15), laser Doppler flowmeter (16), microdialysis (17), near-infrared spectroscopy (18), and color duplex sonography (19). Nevertheless, it has been shown in large series that our current practice of monitoring flaps using simple clinical tests and handheld Doppler is effective (20).

REFERENCES

1. Carrel A. La technique operatoire des anastomoses vasculaires et la transplantation des visceres. *Lyon Med* 1964;212:1561–1568.
2. Buncke HJ, Schulz WP. Total ear reimplantation in the rabbit utilising microminiature vascular anastomoses. *Br J Plast Surg* 1966;19(1):15–22.
3. Cobbett JR. Free digital transfer. Report of a case of transfer of a great toe to replace an amputated thumb. *J Bone Joint Surg Br* 1969;51(4):677–679.
4. Whitworthm IH, Pickford MA. The first toe-to-hand transfer: a thirty-year follow-up. *J Hand Surg Br* 2000;25(6):608–610.
5. Acland RD. Modified needle holder for microsurgery. *Br Med J* 1969;1(5644):635.
6. Taylor GI, Townsend PL, Corlett RJ. Superiority of the deep circumflex iliac vessels as the supply for free groin flap. *Plast Reconstr Surg* 1979;54:745.
7. Pratt GF, Rozen WM, Chubb D, et al. Modern adjuncts and technologies in microsurgery: an historical and evidence-based review. *Microsurgery* 2010;30(8):657–666.
8. Cho AB, Wei TH, Torres LR, et al. Fibrin glue application in microvascular anastomosis: comparative study of two free flaps series. *Microsurgery* 2009;29(1):24–28.
9. Katz RD, Rosson GD, Taylor JA, Singh NK. Robotics in microsurgery: use of a surgical robot to perform a free flap in a pig. *Microsurgery* 2005;25(7):566–569.
10. Taleb C, Nectoux E, Liverneaux P. Limb replantation with two robots: a feasibility study in a pig model. *Microsurgery* 2009;29(3):232–235.
11. Ueda K, Mukai T, Ichinose S, et al. Bioabsorbable device for small-caliber vessel anastomosis. *Microsurgery* 2010;30(6):494–501.
12. Whitaker I, Karoo R, Oliver D, et al. Current techniques in the post-operative monitoring of microvascular free-tissue transfers. *Eur J Plast Surg* 2005;27:315–321.
13. Whitaker IS, Gulati V, Ross GL, et al. Variations in the postoperative management of free tissue transfers to the head and neck in the United Kingdom. *Br J Oral Maxillofac Surg* 2007;45(1):16–18.
14. Whitaker IS, Oliver DW, Ganchi PA. Postoperative monitoring of microvascular tissue transfers: current practice in the United kingdom and Ireland. *Plast Reconstr Surg* 2003;111(6):2118–2119.
15. Smit JM, Whitaker IS, Liss AG, et al. Postoperative monitoring of microvascular breast reconstructions using the implantable Cook-Swartz Doppler system: a study of 145 probes & technical discussion. *J Plast Reconstr Aesthet Surg* 2009;62(10):1286–1292.
16. Yuen JC, Feng Z. Monitoring free flaps using the laser Doppler flowmeter: five-year experience. *Plast Reconstr Surg* 2000;105(1):55–61.
17. Nielsen HT, Gutberg N, Birke-Sorensen H. Monitoring of intraoral free flaps with microdialysis. *Br J Oral Maxillofac Surg* 2011;49(7):521–526.
18. Thorniley MS, Sinclair JS, Barnett NJ, et al. The use of near-infrared spectroscopy for assessing flap viability during reconstructive surgery. *Br J Plast Surg* 1998;51(3):218–226.
19. Seres L, Makula E, Morvay Z, Borbely L. Color Doppler ultrasound for monitoring free flaps in the head and neck region. *J Craniofac Surg* 2002;13(1):75–78.
20. Chubb D, Rozen WM, Whitaker IS, et al. The efficacy of clinical assessment in the postoperative monitoring of free flaps: a review of 1140 consecutive cases. *Plast Reconstr Surg* 2010;125(4):1157–1166.

CHAPTER 2

The Angiosome Concept

G. Ian Taylor and Andrew Ives

Flap surgery has evolved over the years, but the vascular anatomy of the body, obvious in the pure anatomical setting, has been known for generations. Its clinical relevance and application to flap success or failure has been, however, only a relatively recent discovery.

Detailed studies of the vascular tree have been performed over the past 150 years by Manchot (1889) (1,2) (Figure 2-1), Spalteholz (1893) (3), Pieri (1918) (4), Esser (1929) (5), and Salmon (1936) (6,7), to name but a few. These foreign language accounts went largely unnoticed in the English-speaking surgical world, where flaps were being designed randomly and assigned empirical length–breadth ratios that by experience ensured success.

Free flaps (8,9) heralded a renaissance in the study of vascular anatomy. With the introduction of musculocutaneous flaps (10), fasciocutaneous flaps (11,12), tissue expansion (13), flap delay (14), and latterly perforator flaps (15–18), surgeons have been seen returning to the dissecting rooms to define the detailed vascular architecture of these flaps and to look for others. Furthermore, the static anatomy of the deceased has given way to the dynamic anatomy of the living subject and the injured patient.

BACKGROUND

Before looking at the angiosome concept and its clinical applications, it is important to understand how it evolved from its initial origins into the concept that it is today. As with most discoveries, the answer was hidden in plain sight; it only took unusual clinical problems and detective work to bring it into the light of day, or more accurately, into the light of the dissecting room!

It began in the early 1970s with McGregor and Morgan (19) differentiating between flaps based on a known axial supply and those based randomly on vessels in the area. In 1973, Taylor and Daniel (8,9) raised a free flap of cutaneous tissue on its source artery, and McCraw (20–22) and Mathes and Nahai (23) revived the musculocutaneous flap concept. These procedures demanded a detailed knowledge of the cutaneous vasculature. In an evolving process, the senior author and colleagues have dissected and injected lead oxide into the arterial tree (Figure 2-2) of more than 1000 fresh cadavers, including 25 total-body studies (50 sides) and more than 3000 individual muscle studies. Following the success of "the free flap" (8,9), their initial studies focused on donor sites for single tissue transfer—the skin (24), the muscles (24), the nerves (25), and the tendons (26). Next followed a search for composite flaps, supplied by a single vascular pedicle, to repair compound defects in one stage. These combinations included skin and tendon (26); skin and muscle (25–27); and skin, muscle, and bone (28–30). Success of these composite free flaps reinforced an evolving concept that frequently single-source vessels supplied multiple tissues in a specific region. Consequently, the search led to the examination of various regions (31–34), which were ultimately tied together in total-body studies of fresh cadavers. It was through the synthesis of these studies that the angiosome concept was born (35).

As a logical extension of these studies, focus was later directed toward the venous side (Figure 2-3) of the vasculature. Studies of the venous territories of the body highlighted and reinforced the angiosome concept, revealing that it applied not only to arteries but to the veins as well (33). Hence, each angiosome consisted of an arteriosome and its corresponding venosome (36). A search for functional (neurosensory and neuromotor) free flaps led to studies of the peripheral nerves, the muscles, and their relationships to the vasculature of the body, thus creating the "functional angiosome" (37).

Eventually, with a nod to Darwin's *Origin of the Species*, a study of the comparative anatomy of humans, mammals, and other vertebrates showed that the angiosome concept crossed evolutionary boundaries (38), and subsequent embryologic studies in quail (39,40) revealed its development in utero (Figure 2-4).

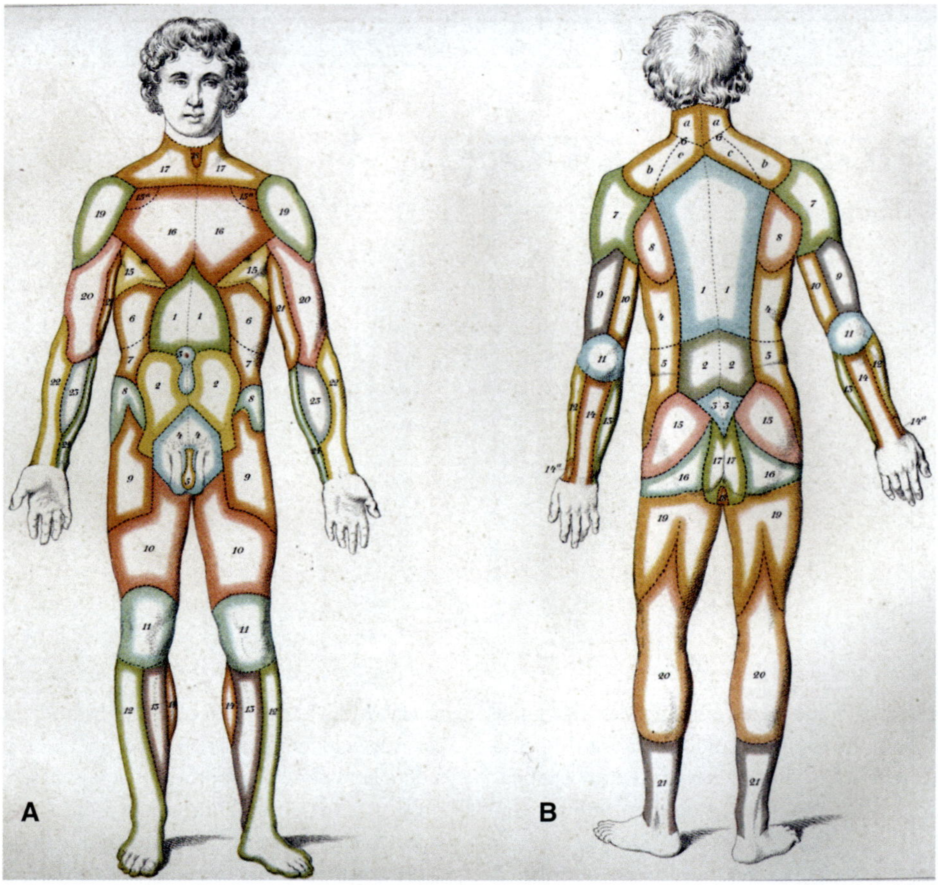

FIGURE 2-1 (**A**) Cutaneous vascular territories, ventral surface: 1, superficial superior epigastric artery; 2, superficial inferior epigastric artery; 3, superior and inferior epigastric arteries; 4, external pudendal arteries; 5, dorsal penile arteries; 6, perforating branches from the intercostal arteries; 7, perforation branches from the lumbar arteries; 8, superficial circumflex iliac artery; 9, profunda femoris artery (circumflex femoral arteries); 10, femoral artery; 11, superficial genicular artery; 12, anterior tibial artery; 13, posterior tibial artery; 14, popliteal artery (sural arteries); 15, thoracic arteries; 15a, thoracoacromial artery; 16, perforating branches of the internal mammary artery; 17, thyrocervical trunk; 18, superior thyroid artery; 19, subcutaneous anterior deltoid artery; 20, brachial artery; 21, superior ulnar collateral artery; 22, radial artery; 23, median artery; and 24, ulnar artery. (**B**) Cutaneous vascular territories, dorsal surface: 1, dorsal branches from the intercostal arteries: 2, dorsal branches of the lumbar arteries; 3, dorsal branches from the sacral arteries; 4, posterior perforating branches of the intercostal arteries; 5, posterior perforating branches of the lumbar arteries; 6, thyrocervical trunk (a, of the superficial artery; b, of the transverse scapular artery; c, of the transverse cervical artery); 7, subcutaneous posterior deltoid artery; 8, superficial circumflex scapular artery; 9, inferior radial collateral artery; 10, superior ulnar collateral artery; 11, cubital rete; 12, radial artery; 13, ulnar artery; 14, external and internal interosseous arteries; 15, superior gluteal artery; 16, inferior gluteal artery; 17, internal pudendal artery; 18, obturator artery; 19, perforating branches of the profunda femoris arteries; 20, popliteal artery; and 21, anterior and posterior tibial arteries.

The final piece of the puzzle is the lymphatic system. Initial studies (41) showed that whereas the dominant lymphatic channels follow the primary venous system (Figure 2-5), smaller secondary lymphatic perforators follow the secondary venous system in keeping with the angiosome concept.

THE ANGIOSOME CONCEPT

Before examining the angiosome concept, it is important to understand and appreciate the relationship of the vessels, their territories, and their nomenclature.

Definitions

Source Arteries

These are segmental or distributing vessels that supply a particular body region.

Cutaneous Perforator

A cutaneous perforator is any vessel that pierces the outer layer of the deep fascia to supply the skin. These arise *directly* from the underlying source arteries or *indirectly* from branches of the source vessel after it enters and supplies the deep tissues—in particular, the muscles—but also other tissues such as nerve, tendon, bone, or glands (Figures 2-6 to 2-8).

Direct Cutaneous Perforator Arteries

Direct cutaneous perforator arteries arise from the source artery or one of its branches en route to the deep tissues, especially the muscles. They pass in the intermuscular septa *between* muscles and other deep structures to pierce the deep fascia and reach the skin. Usually large and spaced apart, they provide branches to the deep structures such as muscles and tendons as they pass toward the surface (see Figures 2-6 and 2-8).

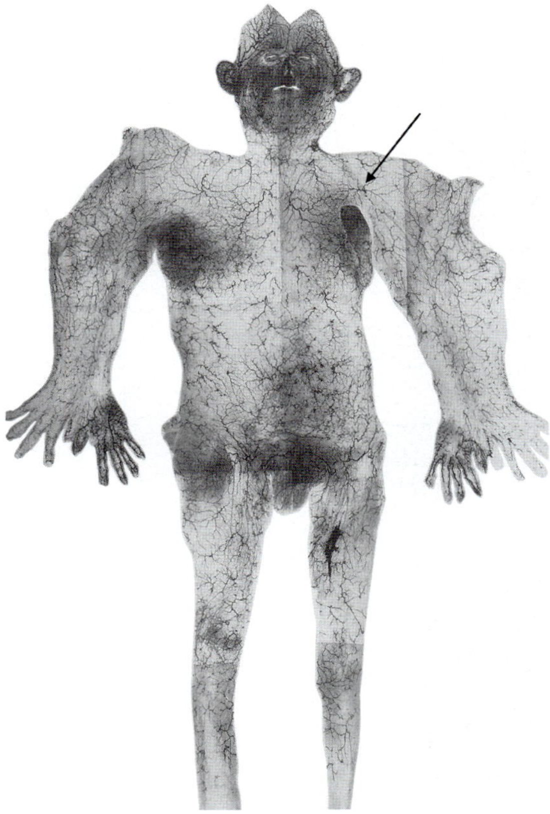

FIGURE 2-2 Montage of the cutaneous arteries of the body. The arrow highlights the acromiothoracic perforator enlarged in Figure 2–10A. (Reproduced with permission from Taylor GI, Palmer JH. The vascular territories (angiosomes) of the body: experimental study and clinical applications. *Br J Plast Surg* 1987;40:113.)

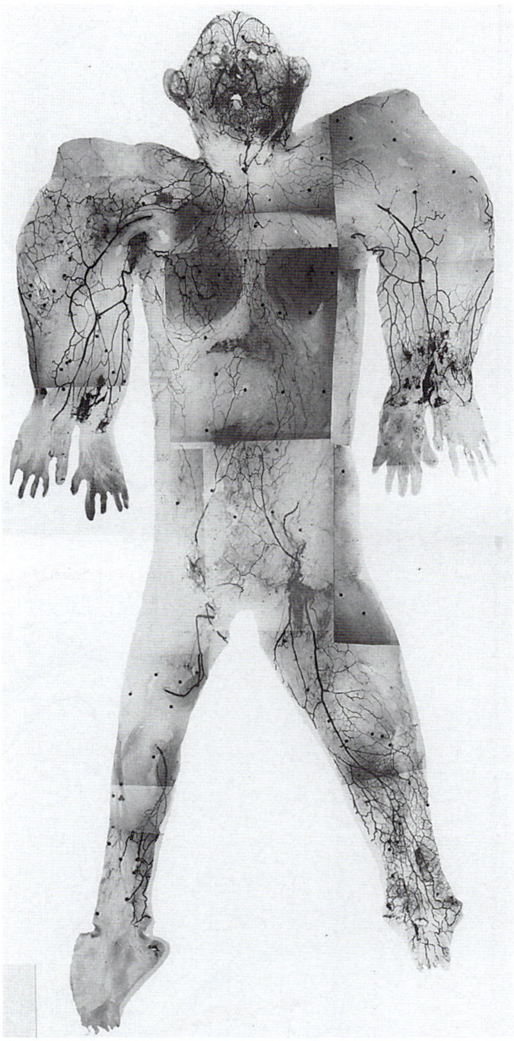

FIGURE 2-3 The venous network of the integument of a female subject. (Reproduced with permission from Taylor GI, Caddy CM, Watterson PA, Crock JG. The venous territories (venosomes) of the human body: experimental study and clinical implications. *Plast Reconstr Surg* 1990;86:185.)

Indirect Cutaneous Perforator Arteries

Indirect cutaneous perforator arteries arise from branches of the source arteries after they supply the deep tissues and emerge from that deep tissue, usually muscle, *before* they pierce the deep fascia. They are often large and well developed such as the internal thoracic and deep inferior epigastric musculocutaneous perforators or small terminal branches providing a supplementary supply to the skin (see Figures 2-6 and 2-8). The indirect cutaneous perforators are the basis of the musculocutaneous perforator flaps.

Arteriosome

This is a three-dimensional anatomical territory of tissue including bone, muscle, tendon, and integument supplied by a source artery and with its boundary defined by a perimeter of either "true" or "choke" anastomotic vessels (see Figures 2-4, 2-6, and 2-8). It can be subdivided further as the artery branches into smaller composite units. In the skin, the final angiosome module is supplied by the cutaneous perforator (Figures 2-9 and 2-10).

Venosome

A venosome is a venous territory drained by the same source vein that accompanies the source artery and its branches (see Figures 2-4 and 2-7). Note the similarity between Figures 2-6 and 2-7.

Choke Vessels

Choke vessels are reduced caliber anastomotic vessels that link adjacent arterial territories (see Figures 2-10A and 2-10C). Plentiful in the integument, they play an important part in regulating and distributing blood flow to the skin and consequently play an important role in skin flap survival (see later discussion of the delay phenomenon).

True Anastomoses

True anastomoses consist of vessels that link adjacent arterial territories without reduction in caliber (see Figures 2-10B and 2-10C); this is seen most commonly within muscles or accompanying cutaneous nerves.

The Concept

As a result of the total-body studies of the blood supply to the skin and underlying deep tissues, combined with extensive

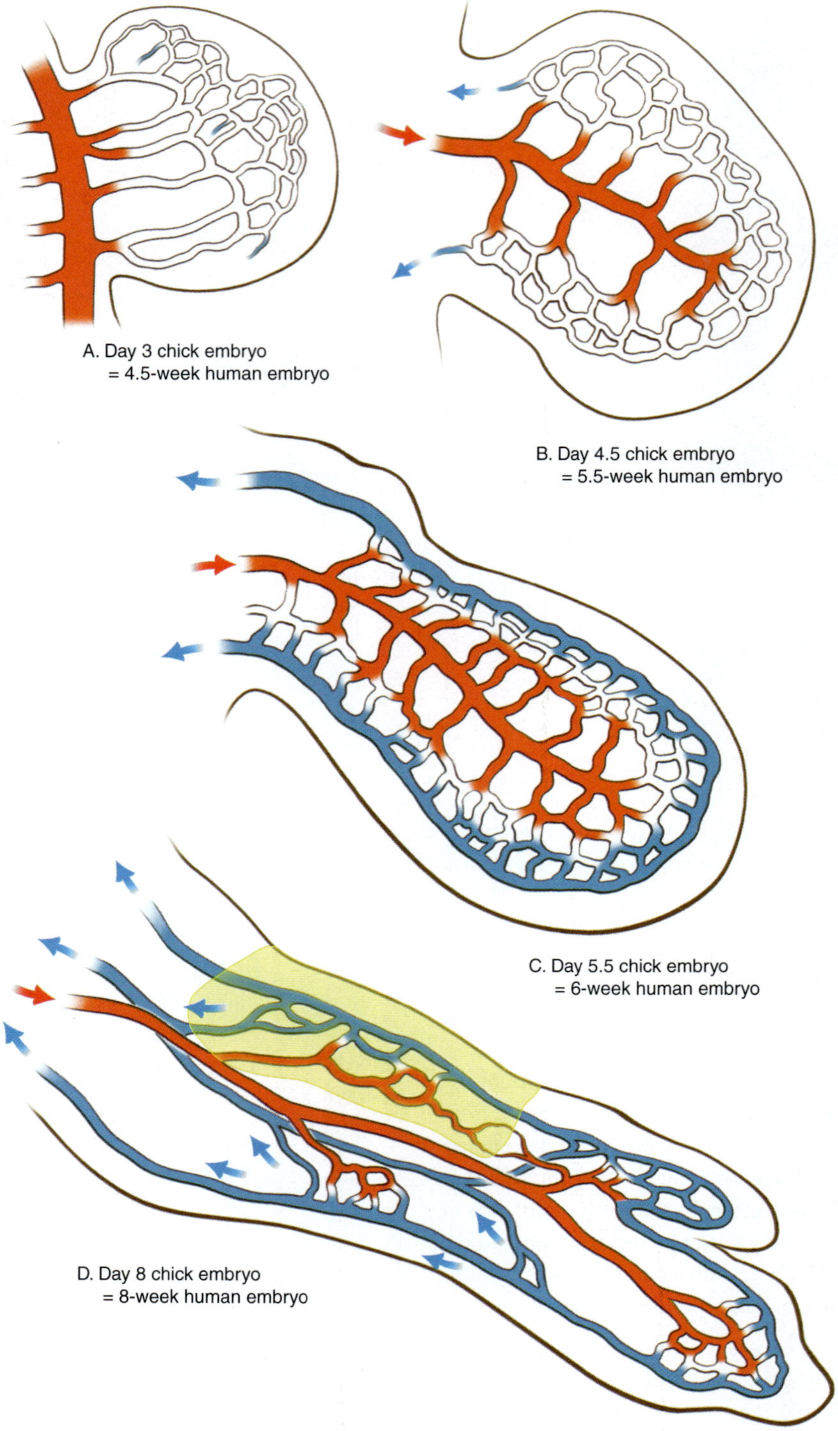

FIGURE 2-4 Diagram of developing arteries and veins in the forelimb of one of our quail embryos where approximately 1 day in the quail equates to 1 week in the human embryo. Note that whereas the *primary* venous system, which develops first, drains the ectoderm (later the dermis) and the deep tissues along the surface of the embryo, the *secondary* venous system develops centrally, connects with the primary system, and drains areas of the ectoderm (dermis) radially and then axially along the limb in company with the arteries showing the development of the basic angiosome module (yellow). Compare with Figure 2–32. (Reproduced with permission from G. Ian Taylor, "The Angiosome Concept and Tissue Transfer." CRC Press, Nov. 8, 2013.)

reviews of previous works, especially those by Manchot (1,2) and Salmon (6,7), it has been possible to divide the body into three-dimensional anatomical vascular territories (35). These three-dimensional composite blocks of tissue, supplied by a source artery and its accompanying vein that span between skin and bone, are defined as *angiosomes* (Figures 2-2, 2-3, 2-6, 2-7, and 2-9 to 2-13). Each angiosome can be divided into matching arteriosomes and venosomes (35,36).

These composite blocks fit together as a three-dimensional jigsaw (see Figure 2-13), with some having large cutaneous components overlying a smaller deep component and vice versa. Some have no cutaneous components at all, and this is

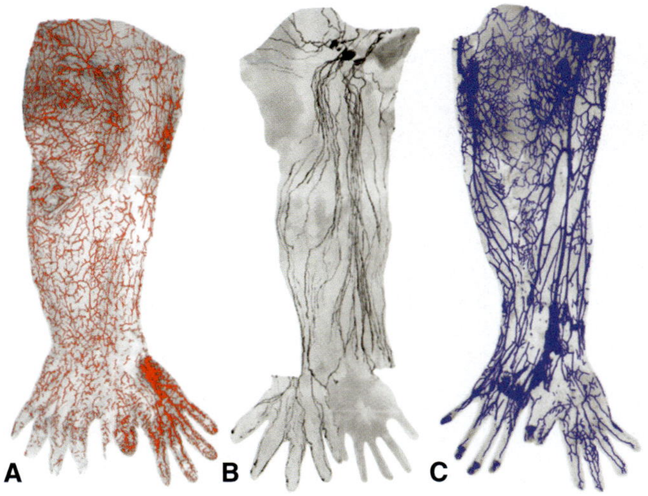

FIGURE 2-5 Comparison of the arterial (**A**), lymphatic (**B**), and venous (**C**) networks in three separate cadaver studies. The radiographs have been colored subsequently in A and C for easy comparison. (From Suami H, Taylor GI, Pan WR. The lymphatic territories of the upper limb: anatomical study and clinical implications. *Plast Reconstr Surg* 2007;119(6):1813–1822.)

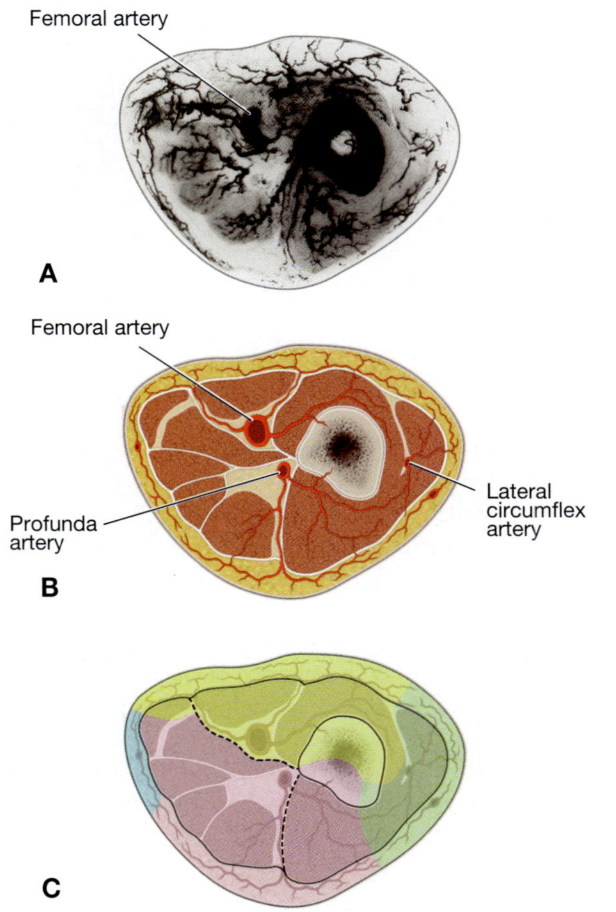

FIGURE 2-6 Cross-sectional studies to illustrate the origin and course of the cutaneous perforators from their source arteries in the deep tissues. Radiographic lead oxide study (**A**) at mid-thigh level. Schematic diagrams, with vessels added following the connective tissue framework in (**B**) and the corresponding angiosomes supplied by each of the source vessels (**C**). Note that the territories span from the bone to the skin and that the boundaries between territories lie between or within muscles and bone.

seen especially in the head and neck (42). Forty source artery angiosomes that supply 376 cutaneous perforators (Figures 2-11 and 2-12) of 0.5 mm or greater diameter (35) link together over the entire body similar to a patchwork quilt (Figure 2-13). Each angiosome can be subdivided further—for example, the lumbar and intercostal angiosomes—and this concept can be traced down to the final branches in the vascular tree, which in the skin are the cutaneous perforators (see Figures 2-8 to 2-10) (35,43).

We can therefore define the *cutaneous perforator angiosome* as a territory of skin supplied anatomically by a perforating artery that emerges from the *outer layer* of the deep fascia and is accompanied by venae comitantes (single or double).

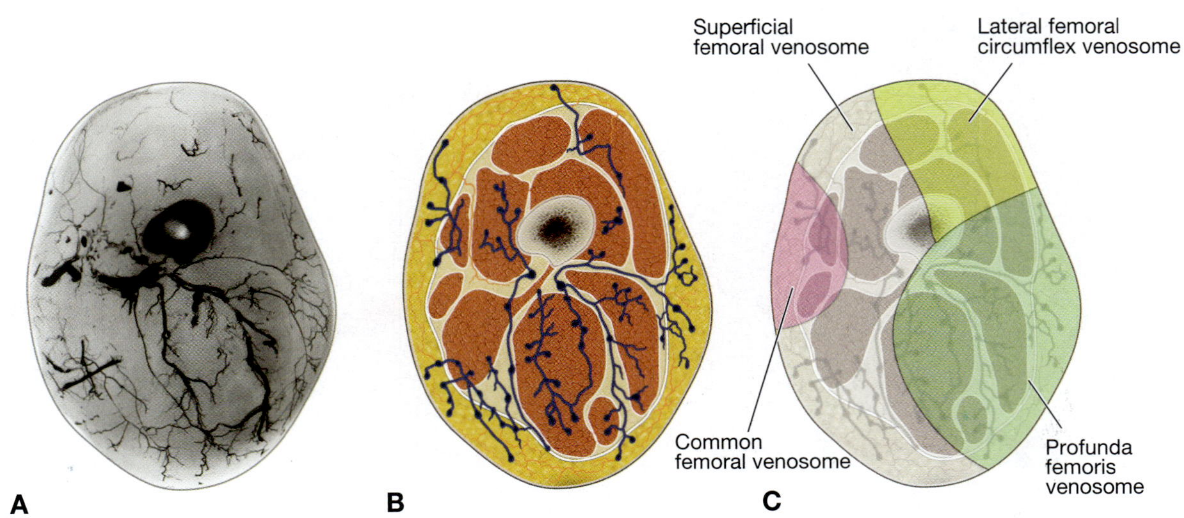

FIGURE 2-7 Cross-sectional lead oxide study (**A**) of the venous drainage of the thigh and schematic diagrams showing the perforators lying within the intermuscular and intramuscular septa (**B**) and corresponding venosomes (**C**). Note also that similar to the angiosomes, the territories of the venosomes span from bone to skin, that their boundaries lie between or within muscles, and that these junctions are often represented by oscillating zones in the soft tissues.

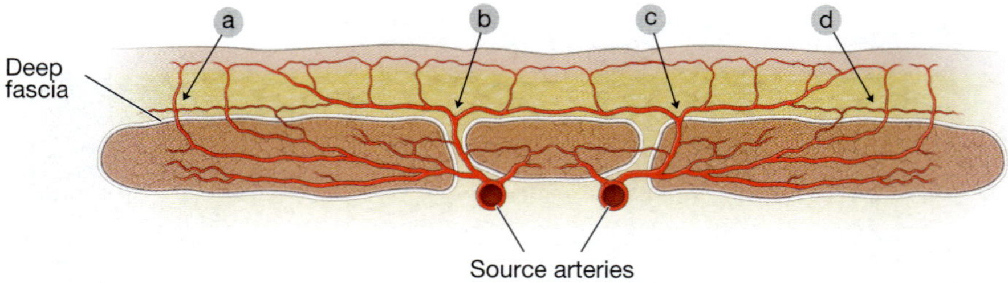

FIGURE 2-8 A schematic diagram shows a single direct septocutaneous perforator (b) and various indirect musculocutaneous perforators of varying sizes that pierce the muscle (or other specialized deep tissues) early (c) or late (a and d) to supply the overlying integument. In each case, the perforator supplies all adjacent tissues between the source artery and the skin.

The boundary of this cutaneous angiosome is defined by a perimeter of anastomotic arteries, which may be of reduced (choke) or similar (true) caliber (see Figure 2-10). A similar pattern with bidirectional communicating veins (devoid of valves) defines the venosome boundary of the venous perforator (Figures 2-14 and 2-15).

In some source artery angiosomes, the cutaneous perforators are multiple (e.g., the internal thoracic artery), but in other angiosomes, the source artery has just one large cutaneous perforator (e.g., the superficial inferior epigastric artery) (Figure 2-16). The same pattern of supply applies to the deep tissues, especially the muscles (e.g., the latissimus dorsi, where the source artery may supply one or several muscle branches).

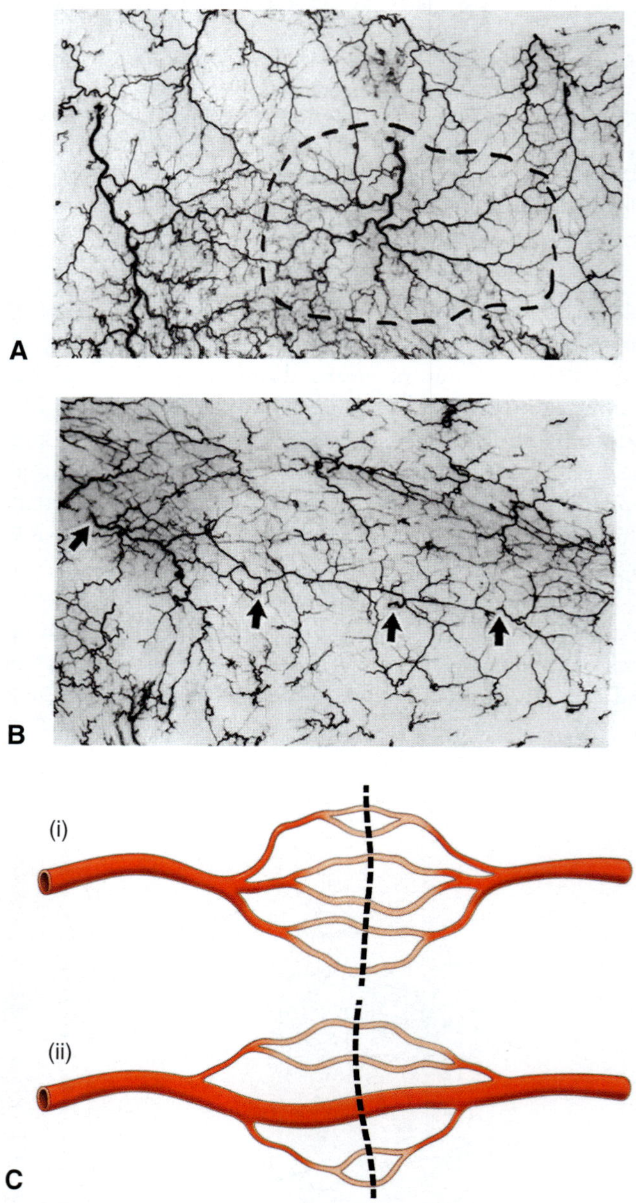

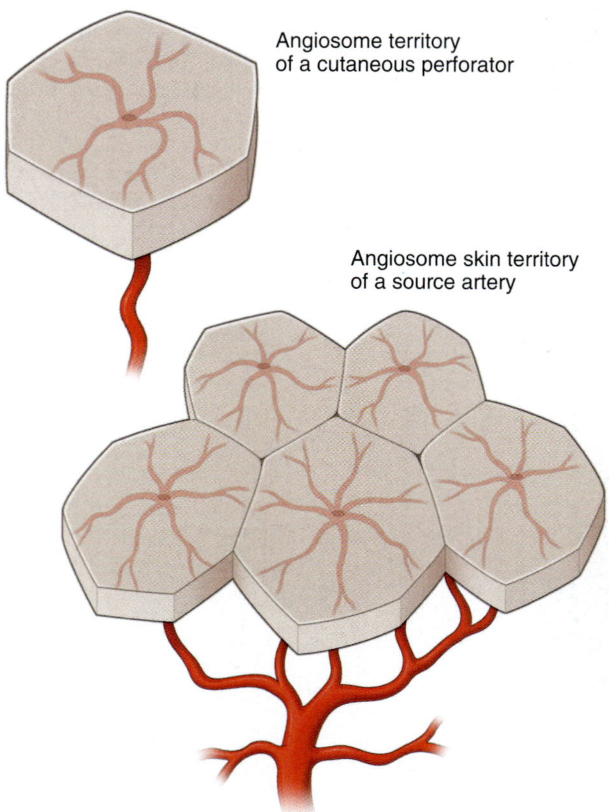

FIGURE 2-9 Schematic representation of the cutaneous perforator angiosomes showing the basic skin module (left) and several modules of different sizes combined to represent the cutaneous territory of a source artery (right).

FIGURE 2-10 (**A**) The anatomical territory of an acromiothoracic cutaneous perforator defined by a line drawn through its perimeter of anastomotic vessels. (**B**) The chain-linked system of skin perforators (arrows) connected by true anastomoses without a change in caliber accompanying a cutaneous nerve in the arm. (**C**) Schematic representations of choke anastomoses (i) and true anastomoses (ii) between adjacent arteries.

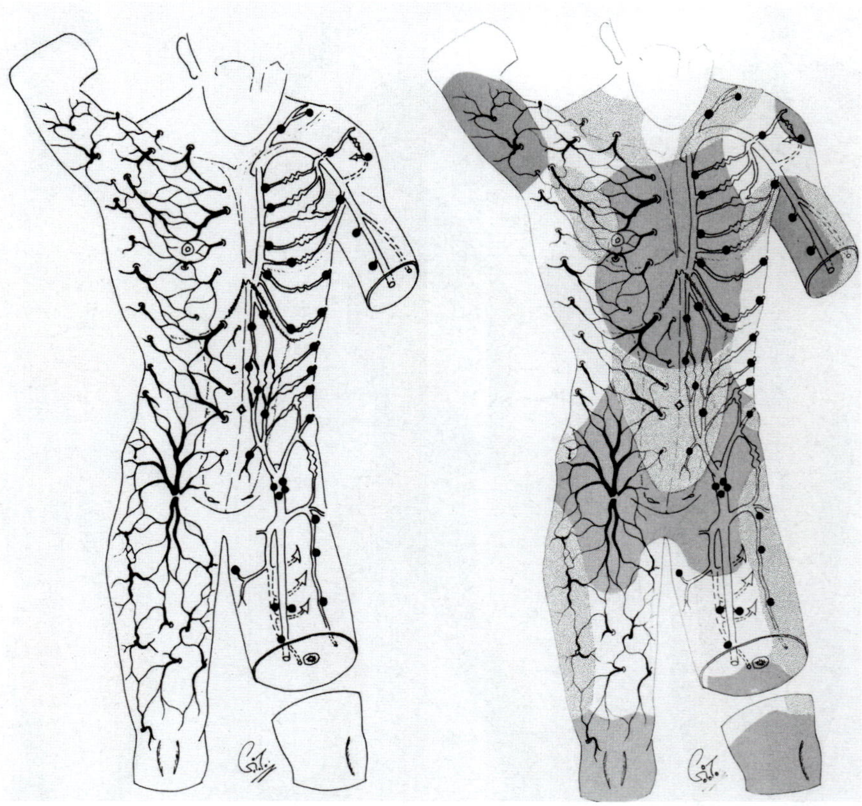

FIGURE 2-11 Schematic diagrams showing how we defined the angiosomes. (**A**) The cutaneous perforators with their choke connections are depicted on the left of the diagram. The origin of these perforators from their underlying source arteries and their muscular branches are shown on the right. (**B**) The vascular territories of each source artery are illustrated in the integument (left) and deep tissues (right) by lines drawn through the choke connecting vessels. Note that the territories correspond in these two layers and how they appear as sectors in the limbs.

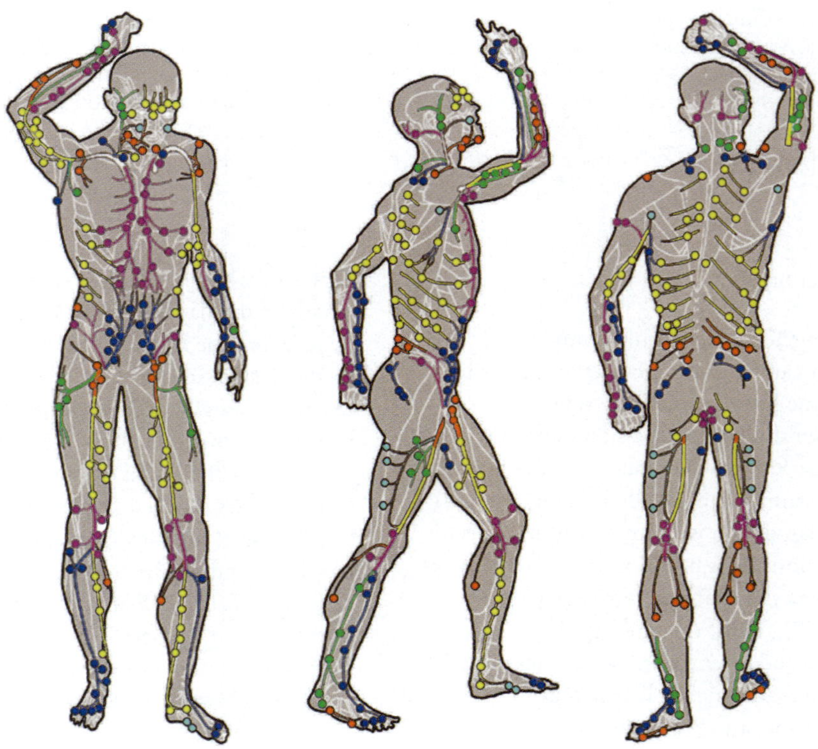

FIGURE 2-12 The sites of emergence of an average of 376 direct and indirect cutaneous arterial perforators of 0.5 mm or greater averaged from all studies. Note their concentration near the dorsal and ventral midlines, around the base of the skull, and over or near the intermuscular septa. Whereas direct perforators are more common in the limbs, indirect perforators predominate in the torso. The vessels were color coded to match their underlying source arteries and to correlate with the angiosomes of the body. Compares with Figures 2-11 and 2-13. (Reproduced with permission from Taylor GI, Palmer JH. The vascular territories (angiosomes) of the body: experimental study and clinical applications. *Br J Plast Surg* 1987;40:113).

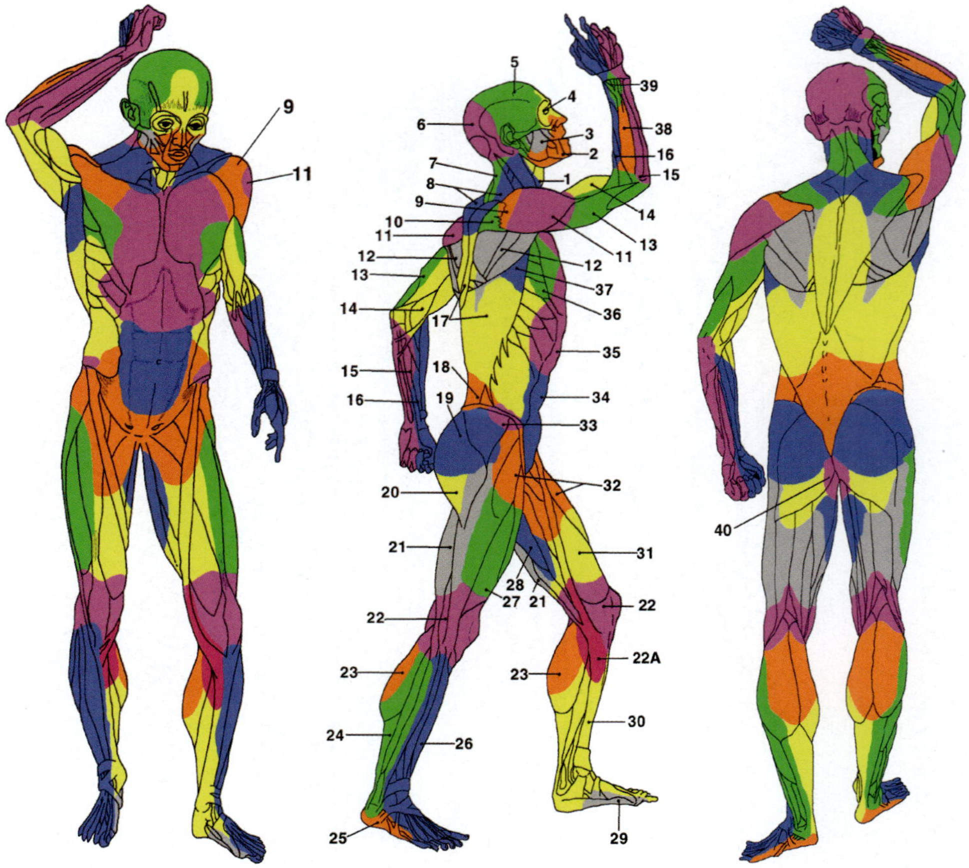

FIGURE 2-13 The three-dimensional vascular territories—angiosomes—encompassing all tissues between skin and bone from the (1) thyroid, (2) facial, (3) buccal (internal maxillary), (4) ophthalmic, (5) superficial temporal, (6) occipital, (7) deep cervical, (8) transverse cervical, (9) acromiothoracic, (10) suprascapular, (11) posterior circumflex humeral, (12) circumflex scapular, (13) profunda brachii, (14) brachial, (15) ulnar, (16), radial, (17) intercostals, (18) lumbar, (19) superior gluteal, (20) inferior gluteal, (21) profunda femoris, (22) popliteal, (22a) descending geniculate (saphenous), (23) sural, (24) peroneal, (25) lateral plantar, (26) anterior tibial, (27) lateral femoral circumflex, (28) adductor (profunda), (29) medial plantar, (30) posterior tibial, (31) superficial femoral, (32) common femoral, (33) deep circumflex iliac, (34) deep inferior epigastric, (35) internal thoracic, (36) lateral thoracic, (37) thoraco-dorsal, (38) posterior interosseous, (39) anterior interosseous, and (40) internal pudendal source territories. (Reproduced with permission from Taylor GI, Palmer JH. The vascular territories (angiosomes) of the body: experimental study and clinical applications. *Br J Plast Surg* 1987;40:113.)

This has several implications:

1. Each angiosome defines the safe anatomic boundary of tissue in each layer that can be transferred separately or in combination on the same source artery and vein. Furthermore, it has been shown that if a skin flap is raised on a single cutaneous perforator, the tissue in any adjacent cutaneous angiosome territory can usually be captured and incorporated into the flap design without fear of necrosis (14,8,4–46). When necrosis does occur, it does so usually in the *choke zone* between the captured territory and the one beyond (Figure 2-17). Thus, the safe length of a skin flap depends on the size and orientation of the anatomical territory of the perforator on which it is based, as well as those of adjacent perforators around its perimeter. This corresponds to the reliable *clinical* territory of a cutaneous perforator at the flap base where the anastomotic connections are by choke vessels. If these connections are by "true" anastomoses seen often accompanying cutaneous nerves or where the skin is very mobile, then the survival length of the flap will be of similar length to that achieved by delaying the flap (14,18,44–46).
2. In the deep tissues, the junction between angiosome territories usually occurs *within* muscles rather than between them. These muscles therefore provide a vital "detour" for the blood supply in case the source artery or vein becomes blocked (Figure 2-18).
3. Because most muscles span one or more angiosome territories and receive a blood supply from each territory they cross, it is possible to capture a skin island in one territory via the muscle supply in the adjacent territory. This is why many musculocutaneous flaps are successful (e.g., the pectoralis major, latissimus dorsi, and rectus abdominis flaps).

A clinical demonstration of the anatomical and clinical relevance of the angiosome theory can be seen in cases of fulminant meningococcal septicemia. Although the areas of

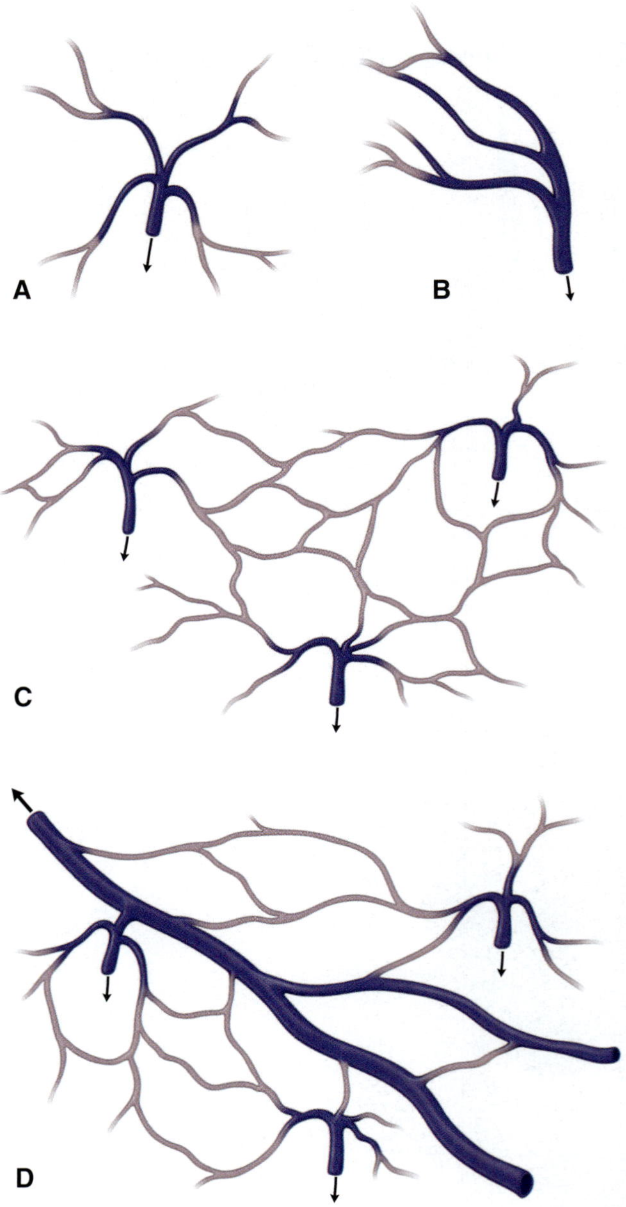

FIGURE 2-14 Schematic diagrams of the basic venous module (**A**), its modified arrangement in different areas (**B**), and how these modules interconnect to form a continuous network (**C**). In the integument, this network of venous perforators of the secondary venous system is connected in the subdermal plexus with the longitudinal channels of the primary venous system (**D**). The valved segments (blue) and the avalvular bidirectional oscillating veins (yellow) are highlighted.

skin necrosis appear to occur randomly, they tend to correspond to angiosome skin territories, the toxins being prevented from spreading and affecting adjacent skin territories by the spasm they elicit in the choke vessels. Similarly, a whole source artery angiosome can be afflicted with loss of blocks of tissue from the bone to the integument, corresponding to the anatomical boundaries of the source artery angiosome (Figures 2-19 and 2-20).

THE LEGACY

Anatomical Concepts

1. Vessels follow the connective tissue framework of the body.

This is fundamental to the design of *all* flaps but particularly to fasciocutaneous and septocutaneous flaps. The vascular system develops in the mesoderm of an embryo as a continuous meshwork of vessels. Specialized tissues develop within the interstices of this network, and as the tissues develop, the vessels become encased within them. Because it is a continuous network, these encased vessels remain in continuity with the vessels that travel between the tissues, and these latter vessels enlarge and are reorganized into vascular pedicles, probably by a process that includes apoptosis.

It is important to remember that the connective tissue of the body consists of two systems of fascia, the superficial and the deep. The superficial fascia lies between the dermis of the skin and the outer layer of the deep fascia. It houses the subcutaneous fat, breast tissue, and remnants of the panniculus carnosis such as the platysma and muscles of facial expression. The deep fascia, on the other hand, is much more rigid than the superficial fascia. It has a tough outer layer that sometimes anchors the origin of muscles. From this outer layer, often incorrectly called the deep fascia, tough *intermuscular* septa radiate deeply to become continuous with the periosteum of the underlying bone. Rigid in some areas and loose in others, these septa anchor the outer sheath to the underlying skeleton. From these septa and from the periosteum, the deep fascia continues into the muscles as *intramuscular* septa (see Figure 2-6).

Cutaneous perforators arise from a source artery or one of its muscular branches, either before or after entering a muscle, and then follow the intermuscular or intramuscular connective tissue of the deep fascia. Whereas those coursing between the muscles are the *direct* cutaneous perforators, those passing through the muscles are *indirect* cutaneous perforators (see Figure 2-8). They then pierce the outer layer of the deep fascia and traverse the superficial fascia to the dermis of the skin. Their trajectory and size depends on skin mobility (Figure 2-21).

The importance of the relationship of the vessels to the different types of connective tissue is evident when the surgeon raises a cutaneous flap including the outer layer of the deep fascia (fasciocutaneous) or when it includes the intermuscular or intramuscular septa (septocutaneous). The surgeon needs to be aware of the variability of the anatomy that can occur. For example, the cutaneous perforators of the peroneal artery in the calf may be either direct or indirect. If one is raising a compound skin and bone flap in this area, the cutaneous perforators may travel beside the lateral intermuscular septum and pass directly to the skin, especially in the distal leg. However, they can arise from the muscular branches to the soleus muscle as indirect perforators at a considerable distance from the intermuscular septum. This will necessitate a difficult intramuscular dissection of the perforators as seen in the proximal calf.

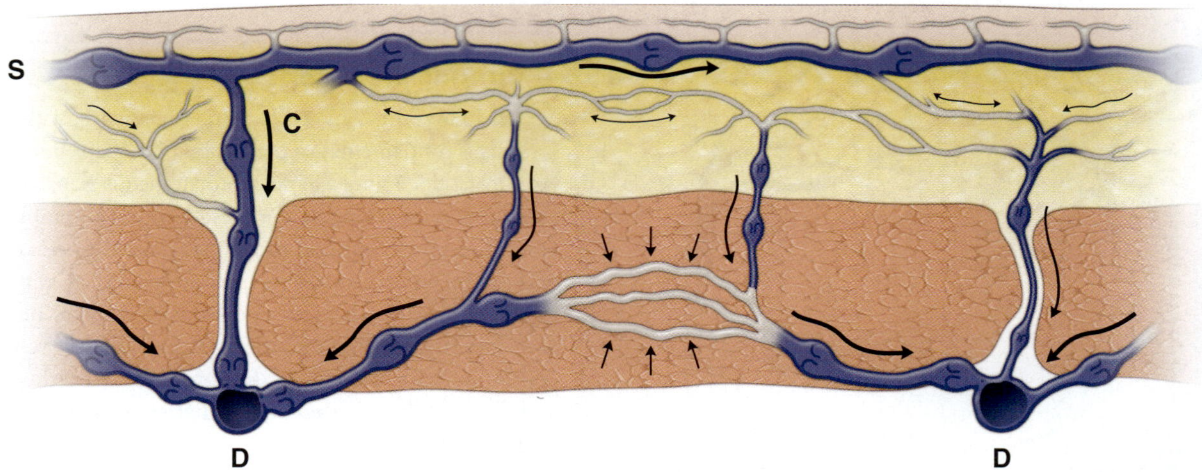

FIGURE 2-15 Composite diagram of the integument and underlying muscle (shaded) illustrating the primary superficial (S) and secondary deep (D) venous systems with their interconnections in the superficial and the deep tissues. A large vena communicans (C) connects these systems, and the alternative pathways of four venae comitantes of the perforating arteries are shown. Note the bidirectional system of veins (yellow) within the superficial fascia and the muscle (small arrows) and the diverging direction of flow of the muscle veins as determined by the orientation of their valves.

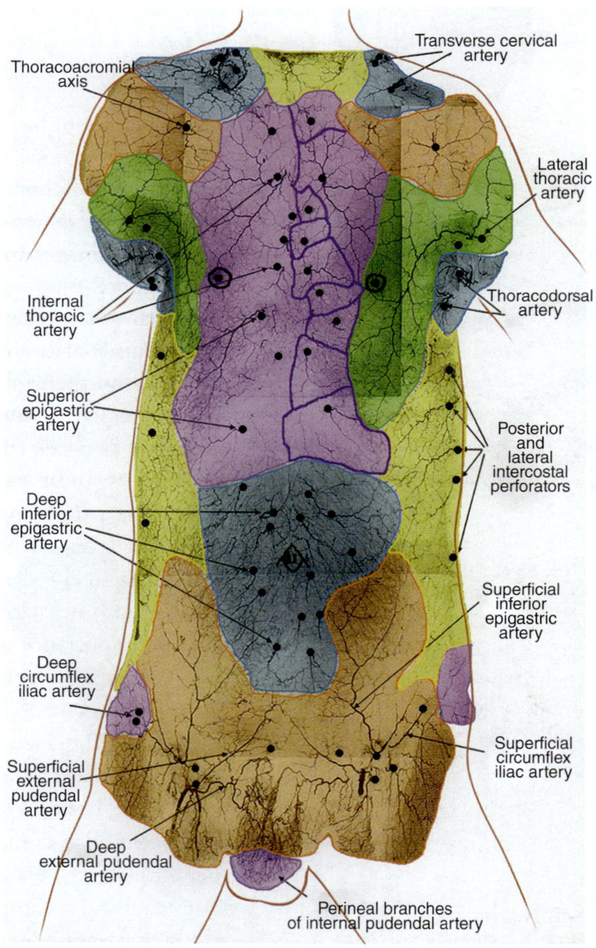

FIGURE 2-16 The angiosome territories of the anterior chest and abdominal regions of the torso with each territory mapped to match the underlying source arteries with lines drawn through the perimeter of usually choke anastomotic arteries. Note that the superficial inferior epigastric artery (SIEA) and the lateral thoracic angiosomes are supplied by a single large cutaneous perforator compared, for example, with the internal thoracic, lateral intercostal and deep inferior epigastric artery (DIEA) angiosomes that have multiple cutaneous perforators, each of which could be subdivided further into individual cutaneous (angiosome) territories. This has been done on one side of the internal thoracic–superior epigastric territory to illustrate this point. The nipple areolar complex and umbilicus are indicated. (Reproduced with permission from Taylor GI, Colett RJ, Dhar S, and Ashton MW. The anatomical (angiosome) and clinical territories of the cutaneous perforating arteries: what goes around comes around. *Plast Reconstr Surg* 2011;127(4):1447–1459.)

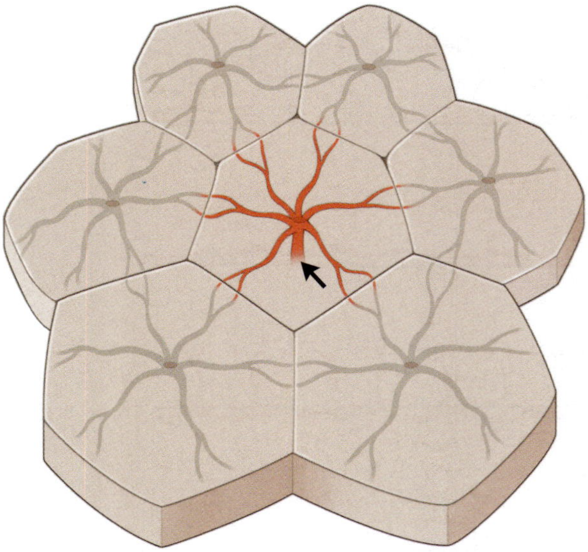

FIGURE 2-17 Schematic representation of the safe *clinical* territory of a cutaneous perforator (arrow) where anatomical territories of adjacent perforators are captured radially. Note beyond the captured perforators, the irregular circumference of the necrosis line (dotted).

2. Vessels interconnect to form a continuous three-dimensional network of vascular arcades.

   The blood supply consists of a three-dimensional network of vessels similar to the highways and roads of a national road system connecting cities and homes. It has developed this way to bring blood to the capillary bed and to deliver and remove it at a constant pressure.

   This meshwork of linked vascular territories that supply the skin are fed and drained by arteries and veins that pierce the outer layer of the deep fascia at fixed skin points.

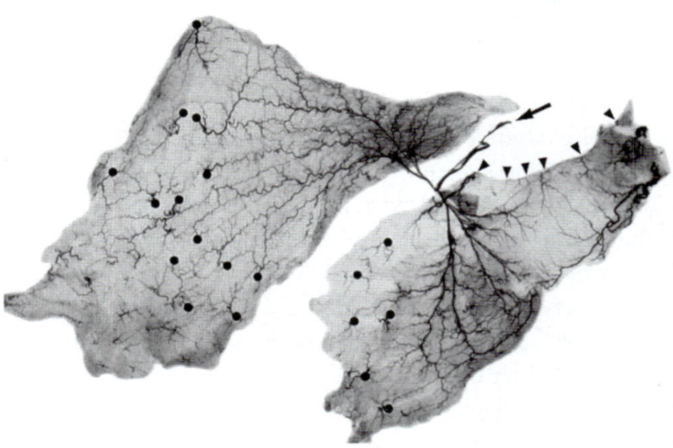

FIGURE 2-18 Radiologic study of the latissimus dorsi (left) and the serratus anterior (right) muscles after total body injection with lead oxide. Dots highlight perforators from the intercostals and lumbar arteries providing bypass routes from the aorta. Note the connections between these muscles from branches of the thoracodorsal artery (large arrow) that provide a bypass shunt to either muscle if the thoracodorsal artery is damaged proximally or to the upper limb via the axillary artery if the subclavian artery is interrupted.

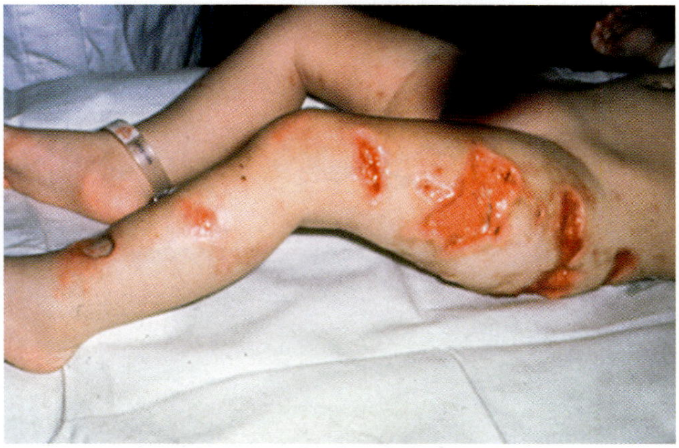

FIGURE 2-19 Meningococcal septicemia with patches of skin and subcutaneous tissue necrosis matching cutaneous artery perforator angiosome territories in the thigh.

If a "roadblock" occurs in a significant vessel, the presence of choke or true arterial anastomoses and avalvular vein segments exist to allow blood to flow either into or out of the area by an alternative bypass route, thereby maintaining an equal pressure at the capillary beds.

This three-dimensional concept was first published by John Hunter in 1794 (47). He demonstrated that the arcades in the hands and the feet became smaller and increased in frequency as the arteries became more distal (Figure 2-22). In general, the largest arcades are formed by the segmental or source arteries of the angiosomes as they course between tissues. The branches to the deep tissues and the cutaneous perforators (both direct and indirect) form the smaller arcades that in turn link arteries to arterioles and thence to capillaries at the tissue interface.

Although these arcades are modified in an embryo by tissue growth and differentiation, the basic pattern remains. Even in one of the most basic tissues, granulation tissue, the vascular pattern of arcades is faithfully reproduced.

There are no end arteries. Their branches are linked to each other and to the branches of their neighbors in arcades. The "keystone" of the arch is either by similar caliber true

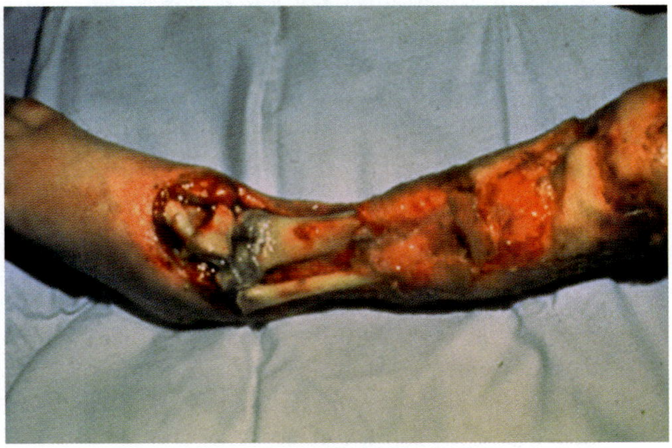

FIGURE 2-20 Meningococcal septicemia with necrosis matching the source artery angiosome of the anterior tibial artery.

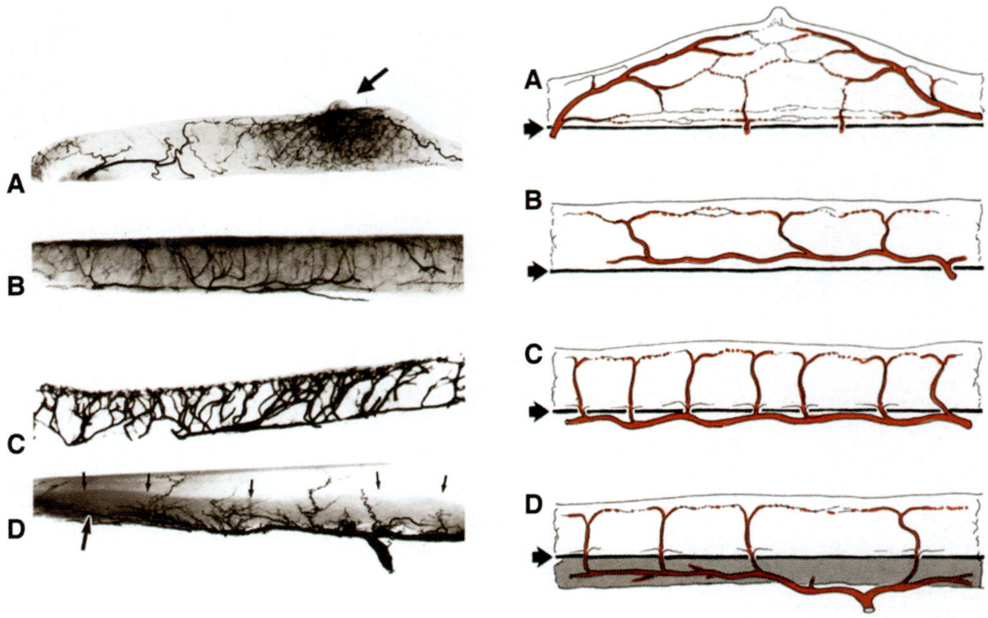

FIGURE 2-21 Sectional strip radiographic studies of the breast (**A**), thigh (**B**), sole of the foot (**C**), and buttock (**D**). D includes the underlying gluteus maximus muscle. The schematic diagram illustrates the dominant horizontal axis of *direct* cutaneous vessels in A, B, and C and the *indirect* perforators in D that provide the primary supply to the skin in each case and their relationship to the deep fascia (arrow). In A, they predominate in the subdermal plexus. Note from left to right the internal thoracic perforator and lateral thoracic artery converging on the nipple in the radiograph of this loose skin region of the torso. In B, they are seen coursing on the surface of the deep fascia in this relatively fixed skin area. In C, the source artery itself is the dominant horizontal vessel supplying the skin, coursing beneath the deep fascia in this rigidly fixed skin region. In D, small arrows define the deep fascia, and the large arrow indicates the large fasciocutaneous branch of the gluteal artery, which descends with the posterior cutaneous nerve of the thigh. (From Taylor GI, Palmer JH. The vascular territories (angiosomes) of the body: experimental study and clinical applications. *Br J Plast Surg* 1987;40:113.)

anastomoses or more commonly by reduced caliber choke vessels. It is this perimeter of keystone vessels that determines the vascular territory of each artery (see Figure 2-10) and has implications in the delay phenomenon (see later discussion).

The venous system has a similar arrangement but in reverse (see Figures 2-14 and 2-15). However, it is important to appreciate that the venous system is in fact two separate systems that develop separately in an embryo at different times and that they interconnect (see Figure 2-4). The *primary* system of veins develops first at about 5 weeks in the subectodermal region of an embryo and is represented by the large caliber horizontal vessels that course long distances above the deep fascia accompanied usually by cutaneous nerves. Examples include the basilic, saphenous, and external jugular veins. The *secondary* system develops about 1 week later. This network consists of central axial source veins that accompany axial source arteries and receive perforating veins from the subectodermal region. They pierce the deep fascia and accompany the developing cutaneous arteries as venae comitantes (see Figure 2-4).

Commencing in the dermal and subdermal plexi, avalvular collecting veins either converge on valved venous perforators of the secondary venous system that pierce the deep fascia or they drain to the primary longitudinal subdermal system of large valved veins. The perforating veins interconnect via avalvular channels to allow equilibrium of flow and pressure between them. Within the integument, this network of venous perforators of the secondary venous system is connected with the large-bore horizontal longitudinal channels of the primary venous system (see Figures 2-4, 2-14, and 2-15). It is for this reason that, for example, the radial forearm free flap can be transferred and drained successfully on either the radial venae comitantes of the secondary venous system or the primary cephalic or basilic veins.

3. Vessel size and orientation are the product of tissue growth and differentiation.

John Hunter (47) suggested more than 200 years ago that at some stage of fetal development (and certainly at birth), there are a fixed number of arteries in the human body and that these then undergo modification because of growth and differentiation. This explains why, for example, long vessels converge on the nipple from the periphery as the breast develops and why vessels radiate from the groin as a curled fetus extends and the lower limb grows distally (Figures 2-16 and 2-23).

This has clinical relevance in tissue expansion where the existing vessels in the skin and subcutaneous tissue hypertrophy and elongate as the expander is filled. Hence, an expander should be preferentially placed in an area between fixed skin sites and beneath mobile skin.

Similarly, the size and orientation of vessels can be modified by pathological processes. For example, an expanding tumor may compress adjacent vessels while developing a circulation of its own, obstruction of a main vessel pathway

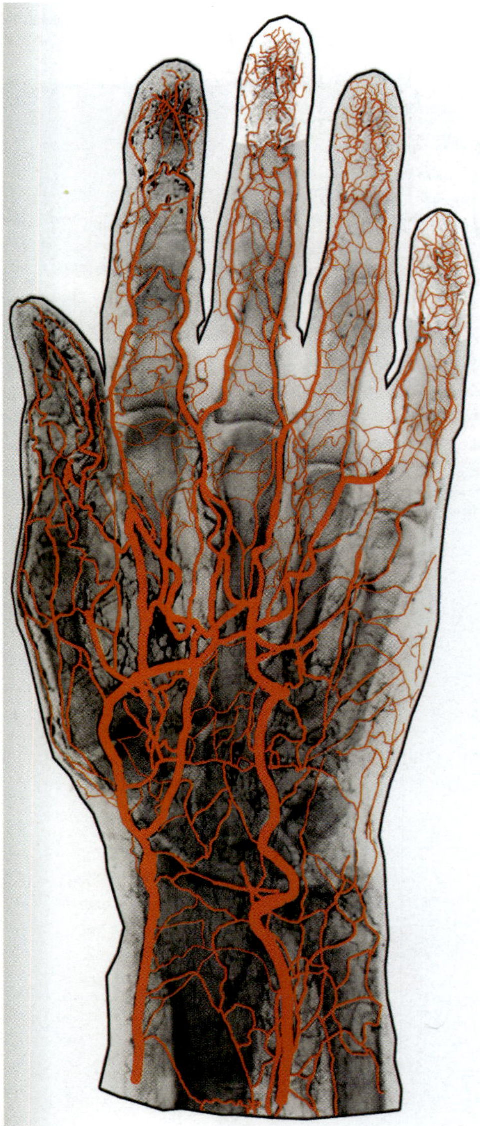

FIGURE 2-22 Vascular arcades in the hand traced over a lead oxide radiograph showing that these arcades get progressively smaller and more numerous as they approach the capillary bed of the fingers and palm.

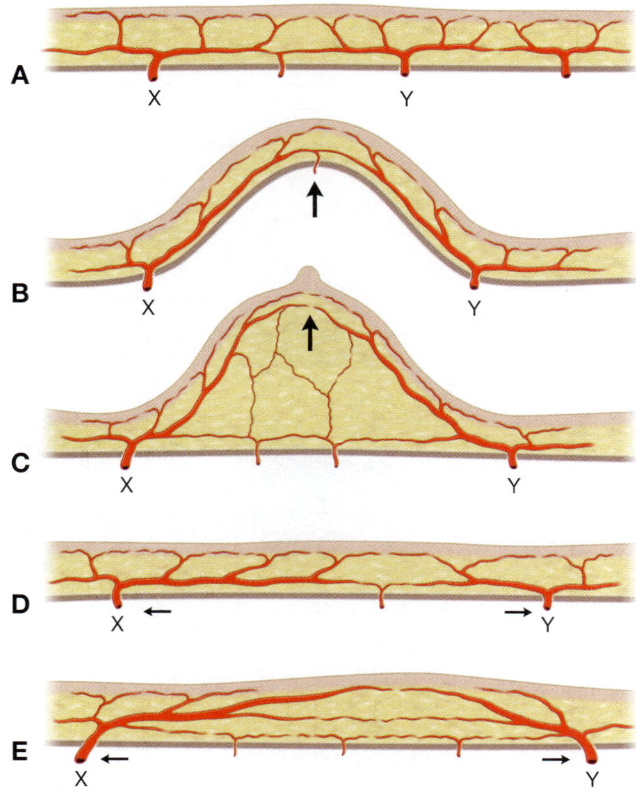

FIGURE 2-23 Schematic diagram to illustrate John Hunter's hypothesis of a fixed number of cutaneous arteries in a fetus and how growth and differentiation of the tissues could modify the definitive size and relationship of the arteries X and Y in different regions of the body after they pierce the deep fascia. (**A**) The "resting state." (**B**) The vessels are stretched by expansion of structures beneath the deep fascia, for example, the skull and brain. (**C**) The vessels are stretched and compressed toward the dermis by the developing breast above the deep fascia. (**D**) The vessels are stretched apart by the developing long bones but still retain a dominant relationship to the deep fascia. (**E**) Growth again stretches the vessels apart, but this time a gliding plane develops between the deep fascia and the subcutaneous fat in this loose skin area, for example, the iliac fossa.

such as in coarctation of the aorta results in hypertrophy of bypass collaterals, and even pregnancy or obesity result in enlargement of the existing vasculature of the abdominal wall integument.

In the animal world, there are excellent examples where, for example, the basic blueprint of the blood supply to the scalp has been modified by the different size of the brain in different species, as it has by differing functional demands of the nose and ears (Figure 2-24) (48). Similarly, the angiosomes of the torso have been modified as different animals developed with different functional requirements (Figure 2-25).

4. Whereas arteries radiate from fixed to mobile areas, veins converge from mobile to fixed.

The dominant cutaneous vessels perforate the outer layer of the deep fascia at fixed sites where it is anchored. The overlying integument is also fixed at these sites and is seen easily in a well-muscled person. This is apparent around or through the attached perimeter of muscles such as the pectoralis major, in the groin and axilla, in skin creases, and over intermuscular and large intramuscular septa. From their point of emergence from the deep fascia, they travel for variable distances depending on skin mobility. The more mobile the skin, the longer the vessels (see Figures 2-21 and 2-23).

It follows that where tissue is mobile over a long distance, large flaps are available for transfer and should generally be based at the fixed margin or end of that tissue where the axial vessel is likely to enter. Examples are the large axial skin flaps based in the groin and parasternal areas (see Figure 2-16).

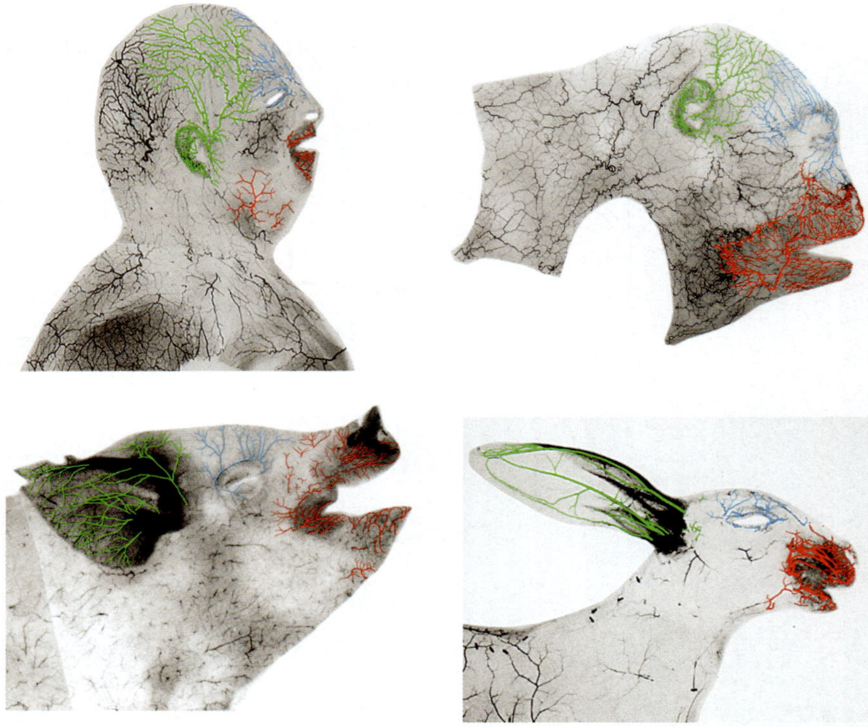

FIGURE 2-24 The cutaneous angiosomes of the superficial temporal (green), ophthalmic (blue), and facial (red) arteries in a human matched to a monkey, pig, and rabbit showing that the basic blueprint is the same but has been modified by growth and development in each species.

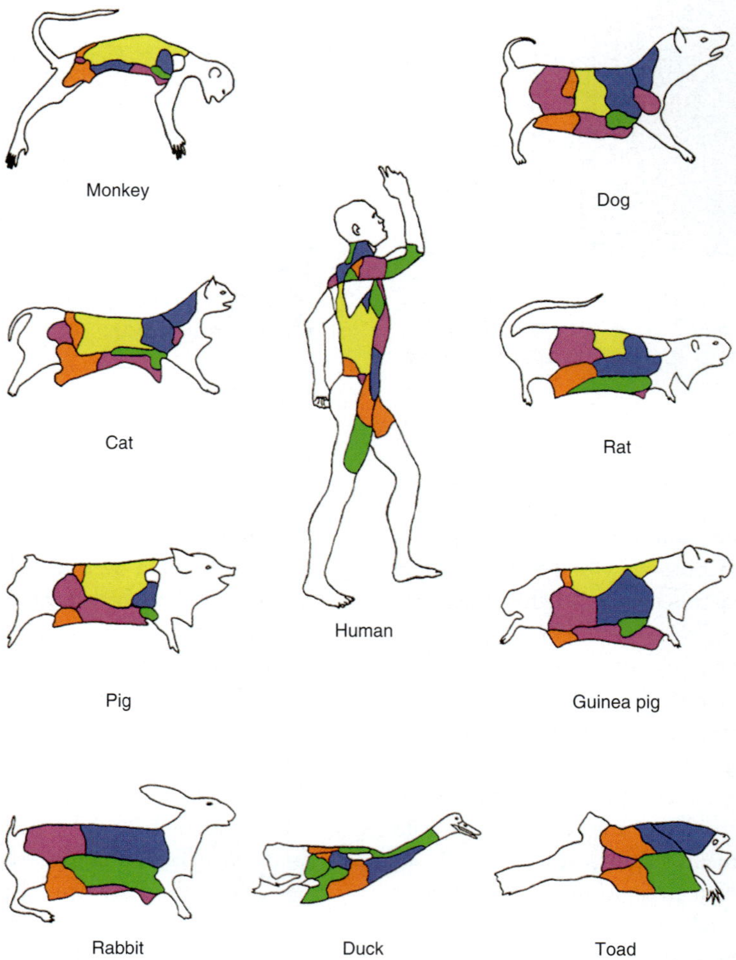

FIGURE 2-25 Angiosomes of various vertebrates colored to compare with the human. Compare with Figure 2-13 for identification

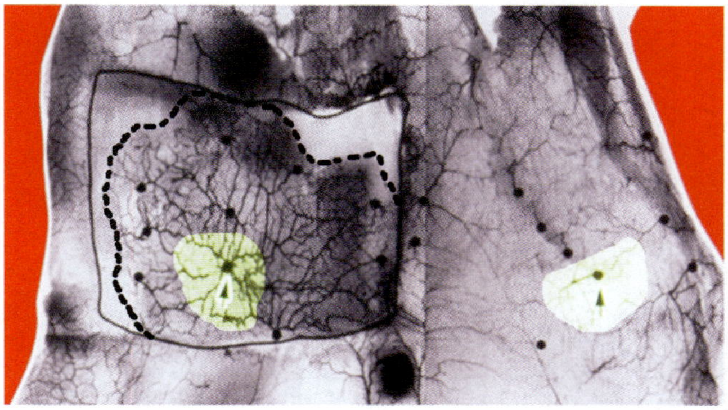

FIGURE 2-26 Skin from the torso of a dog that was removed by midline dorsal incision after the raising of a large island flap on one side (outlined) 1 week previously on a single arteriovenous pedicel (arrow). Comparable vessels are identified with dots and arrows on each side of the ventral midline. Note the anatomical territory of this perforator (shaded yellow) and that (1) the choke vessels have enlarged to the size of true anastomoses within the flap, (2) the scalloped necrosis border is evident inside the flap margins (dotted), and (3) at least one adjacent vascular territory has been captured radially on the artery in the flap pedicle to define the clinical territory of this perforator. Note also the different size of each perforator that varies with skin mobility and that *all* vessels in the flap have enlarged. (Reproduced with permission from Callegari PR, Taylor GI, Caddy CM, Minabe T. An anatomical review of the delay phenomenon: 1. Experimental studies. *Plast Reconstr Surg* 1992;89:39.)

The farther the distance between fixed points, the longer the safe dimensions of the flap. The reliability of the flap length can be assessed with the use of a Doppler probe (16) to locate the precise position of the perforators as they emerge from the deep fascia. More recently, the use of computed tomography angiography (CTA) (49) to identify adjacent cutaneous perforators and then connecting them together in the flap axis has met with demonstrable success (18,48). This proves that one adjacent vascular territory can be captured with safety in any direction around the primary angiosome and has been verified in our animal experiments (Figure 2-26) (14,18,44–46).

5. Vessels obey the law of equilibrium.

This law of equilibrium, as described by Debreuil-Chambardel, states that "the anatomical territories of adjacent arteries bear an inverse relationship to each other yet combine to supply the same region." If one vessel is small, then its partner will be large and vice versa. The deltopectoral flap of Bakamjian is an excellent example of this law.

The deltopectoral flap is based medially over the second to fourth intercostal spaces to capture the internal thoracic perforators. The dissection commences laterally over the shoulder tip and proceeds medially. If small perforators are noted over the deltoid muscle, especially in the deltopectoral groove, the dissection is continued medially on the assumption that the internal thoracic perforators will be large. If, however, there is a large perforator seen laterally in the deltopectoral groove, then the perforator is ligated, and further flap dissection delayed for 1 week because the internal thoracic perforators will more than likely be small.

This is demonstrated in Figure 2-16 showing the angiosomes of the anterior chest and the abdominal regions of the torso. If we look at the lateral thoracic territories (shaded green on both sides), we see that the territory on the left side is much larger than that on the subject's right, and in each case, the internal thoracic territory is either smaller or larger from the midline to compensate. This reciprocal relationship can be followed into the abdomen where, for example, the territories of the deep (blue) and superficial (orange) inferior epigastric territories are compared across the midline.

6. Vessels have a relatively constant destination but may have a variable origin.

This is typical of the vessels in the groin that supply the skin of the lower abdomen and upper thigh. The superficial inferior epigastric and superficial circumflex iliac arteries may arise separately from the common femoral artery as a combined trunk or from one of its branches (24). Whatever the case, their destination is always the same (Figure 2-27).

This may not be of particular importance in the raising of pedicled flaps where the vessels are not dissected to their origin but is very significant in cases when the flap is to be isolated on its feeding vessels for microvascular transfer.

CTA is being used increasingly more often to locate the origin of these vessels before surgery and is replacing Doppler probes in some institutions (Figure 2-28) (49).

7. Vessels hitchhike with nerves.

There is an intimate relationship between nerves and vessels, not only in the deep tissues but in all areas of the body, including the skin and subcutaneous tissue (37). The cutaneous nerves are usually accompanied by arteries and veins that are often the dominant supply to that region of the body. For example, the basilic vein and a chain linked system of cutaneous arteries course with branches of the medial cutaneous nerve of the forearm (Figure 2-29A). The long and short neurovascular systems in the lower limb and the intercostal systems in the torso (Figure 2-29B) are other examples.

Where the cutaneous arteries exist as a chain linked system of perforators to accompany the nerve, they are joined in series by *true* anastomoses with no change in vessel caliber, thereby providing the basis for long flaps in the region. When the nerve crosses a fixed skin site, it often picks up its next vascular companion, seen in the groin where the lateral cutaneous nerve of the thigh crosses or is crossed by the superficial circumflex iliac artery (see Figure 2-29B).

No matter what the relationship of the vessels and nerve to each other as they pierce the deep fascia, the main trunk of the vessel or some of its branches will peel off and course parallel to the nerve. This relationship between the vessels and the nerves again presents a basis for long flaps but with the added potential for providing sensation at the repair site.

8. Venous networks consist of linked valvular and avalvular channels that allow equilibrium of flow and pressure.

Veins are usually thought of as large channels in the subcutaneous and deep tissues with valves that direct flow towards the heart. Although this is true to some degree,

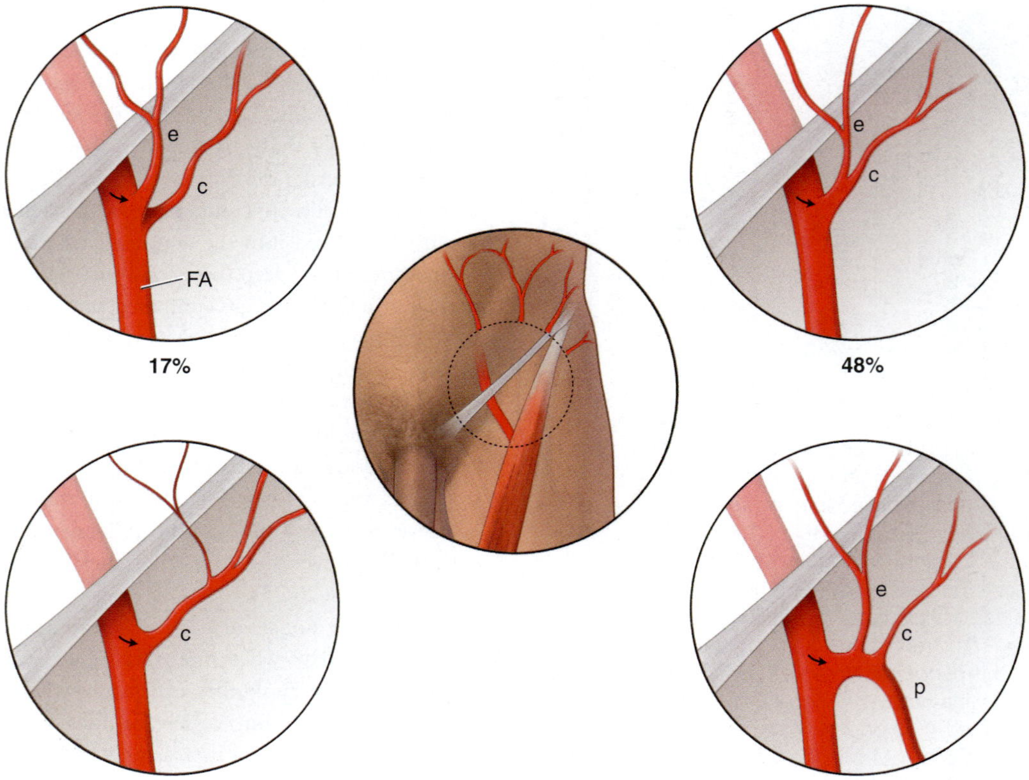

FIGURE 2-27 The variations in origin of the superficial inferior epigastric artery (SIEA) (e) and the superficial circumflex iliac artery (SCIA) (c) from the femoral artery (FA) or its profunda branch (P) in 100 dissections.

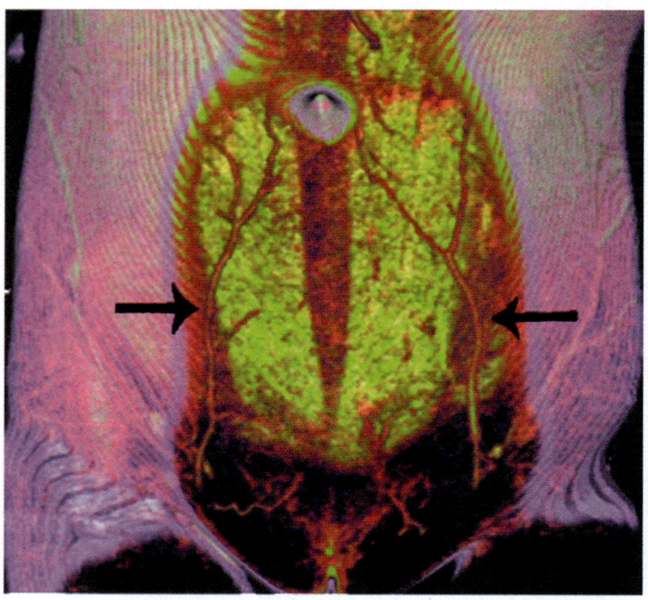

FIGURE 2-28 Computed tomography angiogram (CTA) of the abdominal wall vasculature with an axial maximum intensity projection (MIP) image demonstrating the superficial inferior epigastric arteries (SIEAs) (black arrows) and a number of deep inferior epigastric artery (DIEA) perforators emerging from the rectus muscles. Note the divarication of the recti in this study.

there are numerous venous channels, both small and large, that are free of valves. These avalvular (oscillating) vessels allow bidirectional flow between venous territories whose valves may be orientated in opposite directions, thus allowing for the equilibration of flow and pressure (36).

The valved component of the venous network exists either as longitudinal channels in the subcutaneous or deep tissues or in the collecting veins as they converge on the pedicle of the venous perforator (see Figures 2-14 and 2-15).

The avalvular component can reach significant dimensions. These veins allow free flow between the valved channels of adjacent territories, territories whose valves are orientated in the opposite direction seen especially in muscles with more than one territory (Figure 2-30). They are also found between the valved channels of the same system, and similar to the choke arteries, they define the boundaries of the venosomes.

If the venous pathway is traced from the capillary bed to the cutaneous perforator or to the pedicle draining a muscle, there is an interesting sequence of valvular and avalvular segments that make up this pathway. This combination of segments can make it difficult to perfuse the venous system in a retrograde manner or to attempt to arterialize a venous free flap (Figure 2-31).

9. The nervous and vascular systems develop embryologically in harmony.

As mentioned earlier, the anatomical patterns of nerves and vessels are closely matched in the periphery. Previous

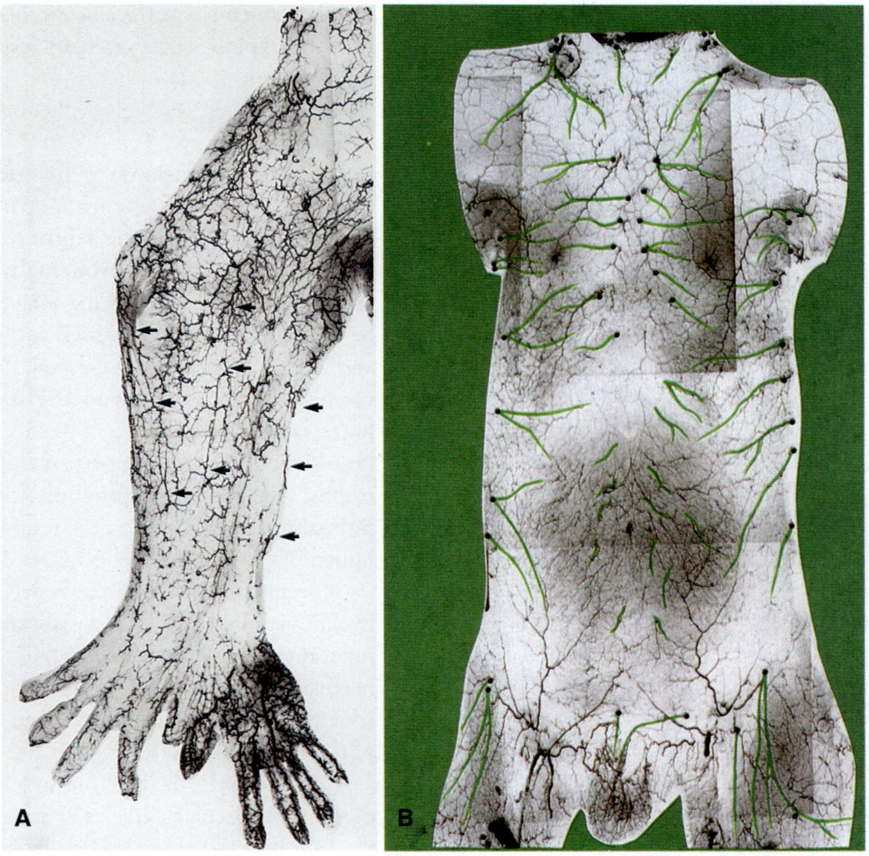

FIGURE 2-29 Arterial injection studies of the right upper limb and torso. Note the chain-linked systems of arteries (arrows) that course with the cutaneous nerves in the upper limb. On the torso, the nerves are marked green on the arterial study. They course with the cutaneous arteries, cross them at angles and collect arterial branches, or approach the arteries from opposite directions (arrows). (Reproduced with permission from Taylor GI, Gianoutsos MP, Morris SF. The neurovascular territories of the skin and muscles: anatomic study and clinical implications. *Plast Reconstr Surg* 1994;94:1.)

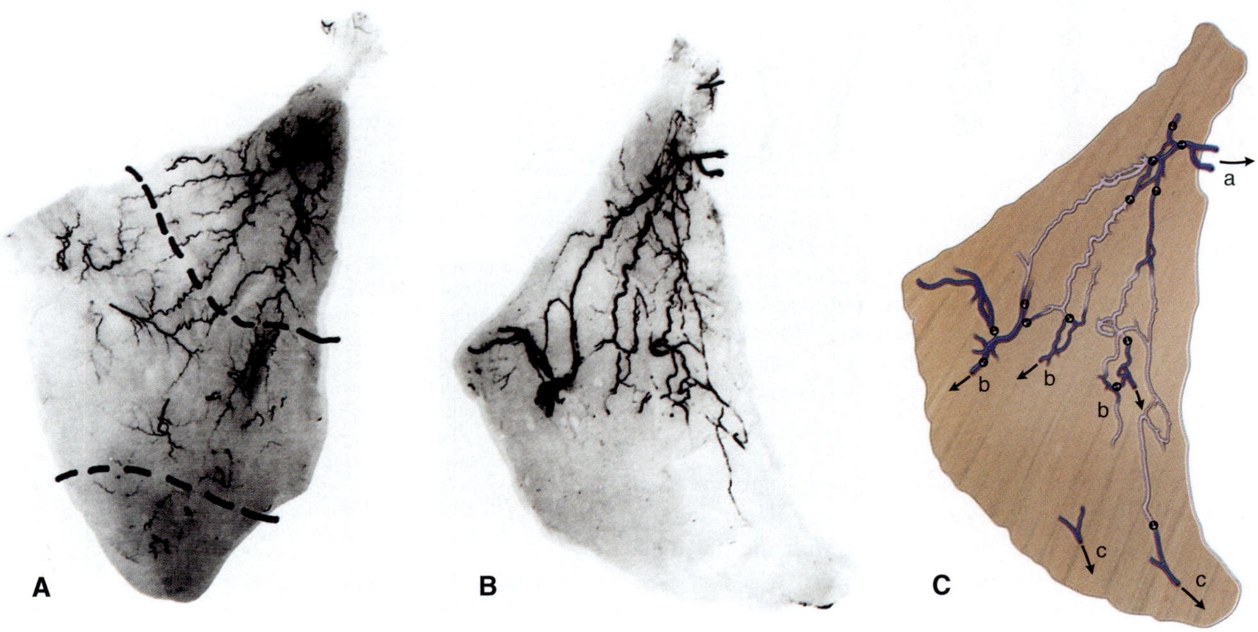

FIGURE 2-30 Comparative arteriogram (**A**), venogram (**B**), and venous tracing (**C**) of the latissimus dorsi muscle. The arteriogram has heavy dotted lines drawn through the choke vessels to segregate the muscle into appropriate angiosomes. In the venous tracing, the valvular segments (which correspond to the arterial territories) are colored blue, and the avalvular oscillating vein segments (which correspond to the choke arteries in the arteriogram) are colored yellow. The pedicles drain the latissimus dorsi to (a) the subscapular vein (b) the posterior intercostal veins and (c) the lumbar veins.

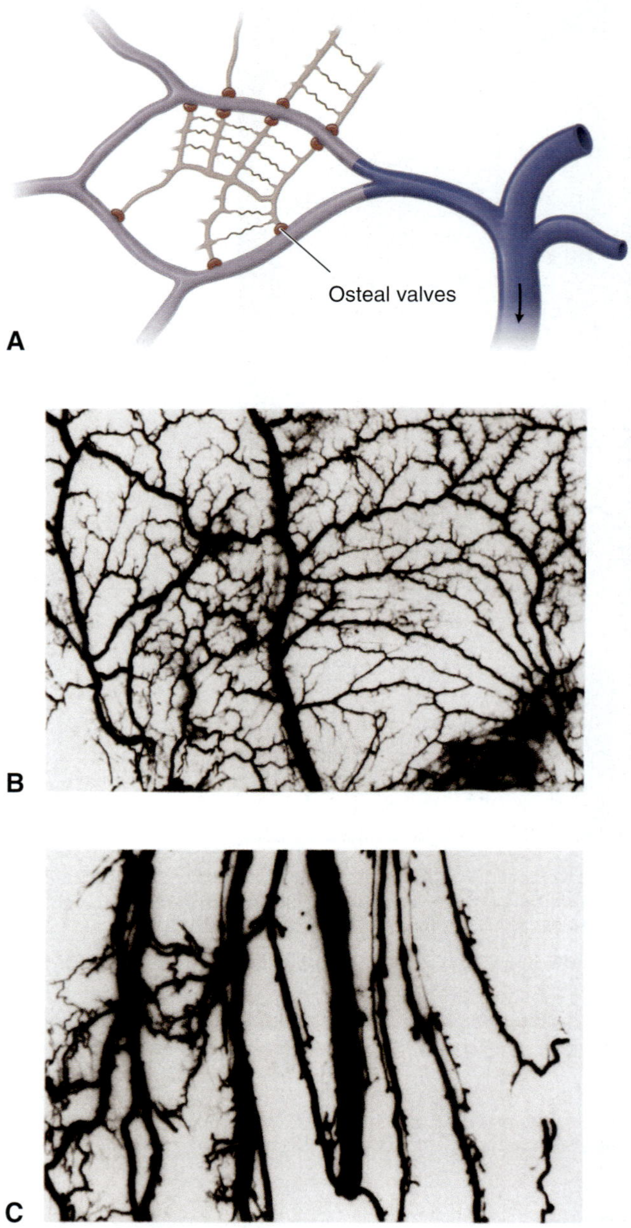

FIGURE 2-31 (Above) Schematic representation of a venous perforator showing the primary, secondary, and tertiary venous arcades. Note the osteal valves that guard the entry of the secondary tier veins (small arrows). (Center) A close-up study of the venous network of the scalp showing the preceding features except that these veins are devoid of valves. (Below) The osteal valves have arrested the radiopaque mixture in this muscle study and appear as small diverticular-like projections on the side of the veins.

hypotheses have assumed that either the peripheral nerves determine the characteristic vascular pattern—the neurogenic theory—or that the reverse is true with the blood supply leading the way—the angiogenic theory.

However, research (39,40) in quail embryos has shown that despite a close spatial relationship, neither peripheral nerves nor blood vessels determined the anatomical pattern of the other. Neurovascular congruency appears to be determined by a shared molecular patterning mechanism involving Sema3A and NRP1 (50). Peripheral nerves, however, do travel on the outer surface of the vascular platform to establish the typical neurovascular relationship seen in adult limbs (Figure 2-32).

10. The extent of the delay phenomenon is explained by angiosome theory

Skin flap dimensions can be extended by incorporating a "delay" procedure (Figure 2-33). When they are raised, existing arteries along the axis of the flap enlarge. This has been demonstrated experimentally in the animal model (Figures 2-26 and 2-34). One adjacent vascular territory can be captured safely on the vessels at the flap base (Figures 2-17 and 2-26). When a flap is delayed, the choke vessels between vascular territories dilate to the size of true anastomoses; however, this takes between 48 to 72 hours to occur. It has been shown that this is a permanent event because of hypertrophy, elongation, and multiplication of cells in the vessel intima, media, and adventitia, resulting in an increase in the lumen of the choke vessel (Figures 2-26 and 2-35).

It seems that these choke vessels play an important role in flap viability because necrosis takes place usually in this junctional zone between arterial territories and that the necrosis line takes 3 to 4 days to declare, about the same time the maximal changes are seen occurring in the lumen of the choke vessels (see Figures 2-26 and 2-34).

Flap survival can therefore be extended by the strategic division of vascular pedicles at various time intervals along the length of the proposed flap. For example, the survival of the skin paddle of the transverse rectus abdominis myocutaneous (TRAM) flap of Hartrampf can be extended by a previous division of the superficial inferior epigastric arteries (SIEAs) and the deep inferior epigastric arteries (DIEAs) at the lower border of the proposed skin paddle (18), seen also in our animal studies (Figures 2-35 and 2-36) (14).

REFERENCES

1. Manchot C. Die Hautarterien des Menschlichen Korpers. Leipzig: F.C.W. Vogel, 1889.
2. Manchot C. The Cutaneous Arteries of the Human Body. New York: Springer-Verlag, 1983.
3. Spalteholz W. Die Vertheilung der Blutgefasse in der Haut. *Arch Anat* 1893.
4. Pieri G. La Circolazione Cutanea Degli Arti e del Tronco in Rapporto alla Tecnica della Chirurgia e Plastica Cinematica. *Chir Organi Mov* 1918;2:37.
5. Esser JFS. Artery Flaps. Antwerp: De Vos-van Kleef, 1929.
6. Salmon M. Arteres de la Peau. Paris: Masson, 1936.
7. Salmon M, Taylor GI, Tempest M (eds). Arteries of the Skin. (eds). London: Churchill-Livingstone, 1988.
8. Taylor GI, Daniel RK. The free flap: composite tissue transfer by vascular anastomosis. *Aust N Z J Surg* 1973;43:1
9. Daniel RK, Taylor GI. Distant transfer of an island flap by microvascular anastomoses. *Plast Reconstr Surg* 1973;52:111.
10. McCraw JB, Dibbell DG, Carraway JH. Clinical definition of independent myocutaneous vascular territories. *Plast Reconstr Surg* 1977;60:341.
11. Cormack GC, Lamberty BGH. The Arterial Anatomy of Skin Flaps. Edinburgh: Churchill-Livingstone, 1986.
12. Ponten B. The fasciocutaneous flap: its use in soft tissue defects of the lower leg. *Br J Plast Surg* 1982;34:215.
13. Radovan C. Breast reconstruction after mastectomy using the temporary expander. *Plast Reconstr Surg* 1982;69:195.
14. Dhar SC, Taylor GI. The delay phenomenon: the story unfolds. *Plast Reconstr Surg* 1999;104(7):2079–2091.
15. Hallock GG. Direct and indirect perforator flaps: the history and the controversy. *Plast Reconstr Surg* 2003;111:855.

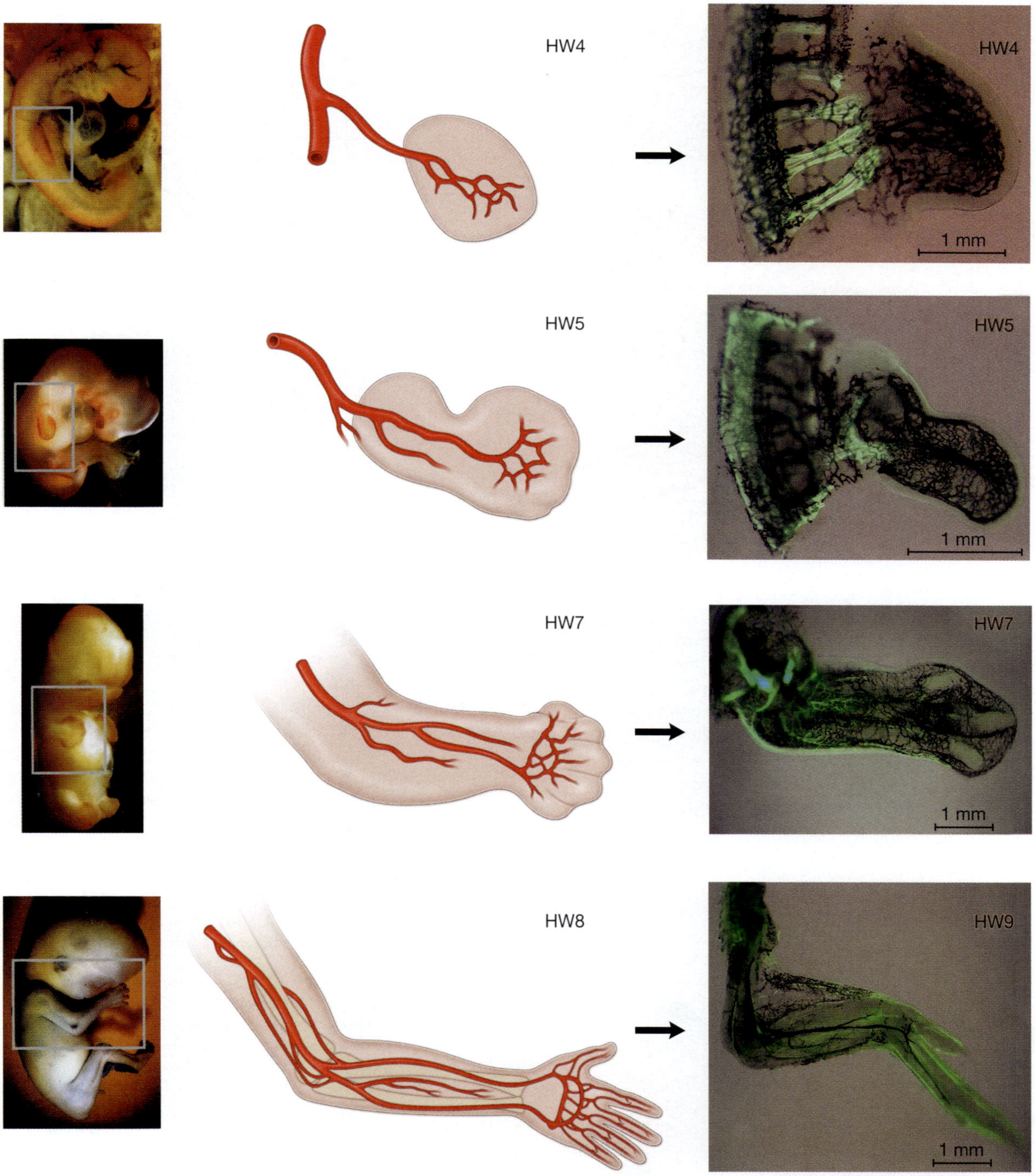

FIGURE 2-32 Homology of vertebrate upper limb development. Comparison of human (left and middle columns) and quail (right hand column) upper limb development. In terms of their respective developmental stages (size, shape, and structures), a 4-day-old quail embryo (E4) upper limb is equivalent to a 4-week-old human embryo upper limb (HW4). Similarly, an E8 quail upper limb is equivalent to an HW8 human upper limb. The correlation on 1 day of quail embryonic development with 1 week of human embryonic development can only be easily applied between E4 and E8 (HW4-HW8). Blood vessels (black) are perfused with India ink, and the nerves (green) are labeled with immunofluorescent antibodies. In E7 and E9, the ectoderm fluoresces green as well in some areas.

16. Taylor GI, McCarten G, Doyle M. The use of the Doppler probe for planning flaps: anatomical study and clinical applications. *Br J Plast Surg* 1990;43:1.
17. Taylor GI. The angiosomes of the body and their supply to perforator flaps. *Clin Plastic Surg* 2003;30:331–342.
18. Taylor GI, Corlett RJ, Dhar SC, Ashton MW. The anatomical (angiosome) and clinical territories of the cutaneous perforating arteries: what goes around comes around. *Plast Reconstr Surg* 2011;127(4):1447–1459.
19. McGregor IA, Morgan G. Axial and random pattern flaps. *Br J Plast Surg* 1973;26:202.
20. McCraw JB, Dibbell DG, Carraway JH. Clinical definition of independent myocutaneous vascular territories. *Plast Reconstr Surg* 1977;60:341.
21. McCraw JB. The recent history of myocutaneous flaps. *Clin Plast Surg* 1980;7:3.
22. McCraw JB, Dibbell DG. Experimental definition of independent myocutaneous vascular territories. *Plast Reconstr Surg* 1977;60:212.
23. Mathes SJ, Nahai F. Clinical Atlas of Muscle and Musculocutaneous Flaps. St. Louis: Mosby, 1979.
24. Taylor GI, Daniel RK. The anatomy of several free flap donor sites. *Plast Reconstr Surg* 1975;56:243.

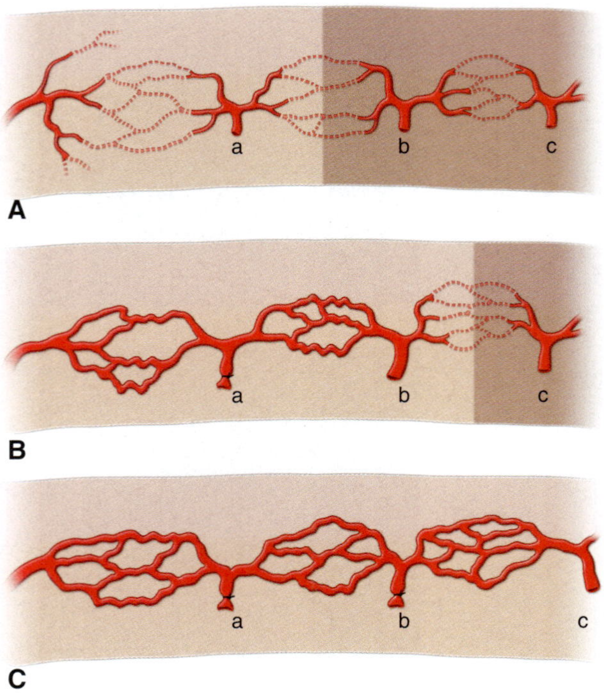

FIGURE 2-33 Diagrammatic representation of the same flap raised with and without a surgical delay to illustrate the necrosis line and the changes in the choke vessels. In X, the adjacent territory a is captured with safety, and the necrosis line occurs at the choke–vessel interface with vessel b or the one beyond. In Y, vessel a has been delayed. Note the effect on the choke vessels and the site of necrosis line. In Z, vessels a and b have been delayed. Vessel c is divided at the tip of this bipedicled flap at a second stage to provide the longest flap, the situation that exists in the stages of the tube pedicle transfer of Gillies.

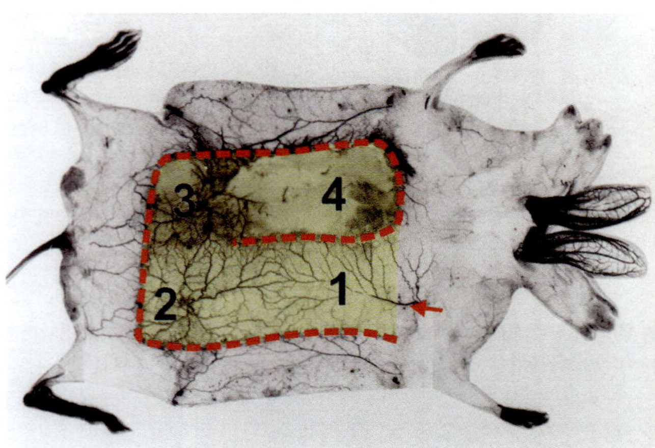

FIGURE 2-34 Radiograph showing a four-territory U-shaped rabbit skin flap raised without a delay procedure at 1 week (red dots). Note that the blood supply from the vascular pedicle (arrows) is not able to keep territories 3 and 4 alive. The rabbit has been split down the ventral midline. (Reproduced from Taylor GI, Corlett RJ, Dhar S, Ashton MW. The anatomical (angiosome) and clinical territories of the cutaneous perforating arteries: what goes around comes around. *Plast Reconstr Surg* 2011;127(4):1447–1459.)

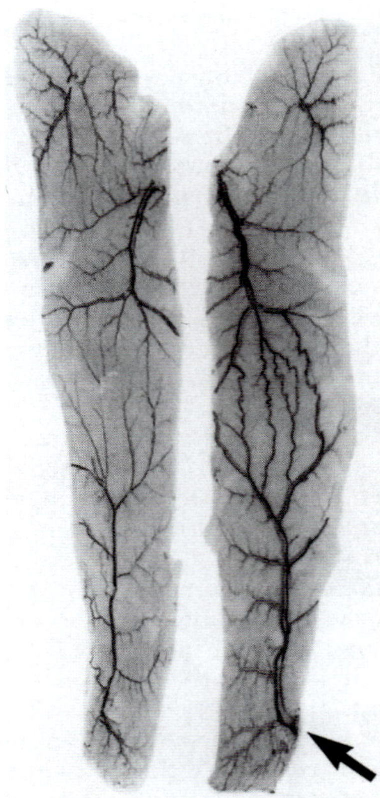

FIGURE 2-35 Arteriogram of control (left) and delayed (right) rectus abdominis muscles of a dog 7 days after surgery. Note the dilated choke vessels in the delayed flap by ligation of the deep inferior epigastric artery (arrow). (From Dhar SC, Taylor GI. The delay phenomenon: the story unfolds. *Plast Reconstr Surg* 1999;104:2079.)

25. Taylor GI, Ham FJ. The free vascularised nerve graft. *Plast Reconstr Surg* 1976;57:413.
26. Taylor GI, Townsend PL, Corlett RJ. Composite free flap and tendon transfer: an anatomical study and a clinical technique. *Br J Plast Surg* 1979;32:170.
27. Taylor GI, Corlett RJ, Boyd JB. The extended deep inferior epigastric flap: a clinical technique. *Plast Reconstr Surg* 1983;72:751–761.
28. Taylor GI, Watson N. One stage repair of compound leg defects with revascularised flaps of groin skin and iliac bone. *Plast Reconstr Surg* 1978;61:494.
29. Taylor GI, Townsend PL, Corlett RJ. Superiority of the deep circumflex iliac vessels as the supply for free groin flaps: experimental work. *Plast Reconstr Surg* 1979;64:595.
30. Taylor GI, Townsend PL, Corlett RJ. Superiority of the deep circumflex iliac vessels as the supply for free groin flaps: clinical work. *Plast Reconstr Surg* 1979;64:745.
31. Palmar JH, Taylor GI. The vascular territories of the anterior chest wall. *Br J Plast Surg* 1986;38:287–299.
32. Reid CD, Taylor GI. The vascular territory of the acromiothoracic axis. *Br J Plast Surg* 1984;37:194–212.
33. Boyd JB, Taylor GI, Corlett RJ. The vascular territories of the superior epigastric and deep inferior epigastric systems. *Plast Reconstr Surg* 1984;73:1–16.
34. Moon HK, Taylor GI. The vascular anatomy of rectus abdominis musculocutaneous flaps based on the deep superior epigastric system. *Plast Reconstr Surg* 1988;82:815–832.
35. Taylor GI, Palmer JH. The vascular territories (angiosomes) of the body: experimental study and clinical applications. *Br Plast Surg* 1987;40:113.
36. Taylor GI, Caddy CM, Watterson PA, Crock JG. The venous territories (venosomes) of the human body: experimental study and clinical implications. *Plast Reconstr Surg* 1990;86:85.
37. Taylor GI, Gianoutsos MP, Morris SF. The neurovascular territories of the skin and muscles: anatomic study and clinical implications. *Plast Reconstr Surg* 1994;94:1.

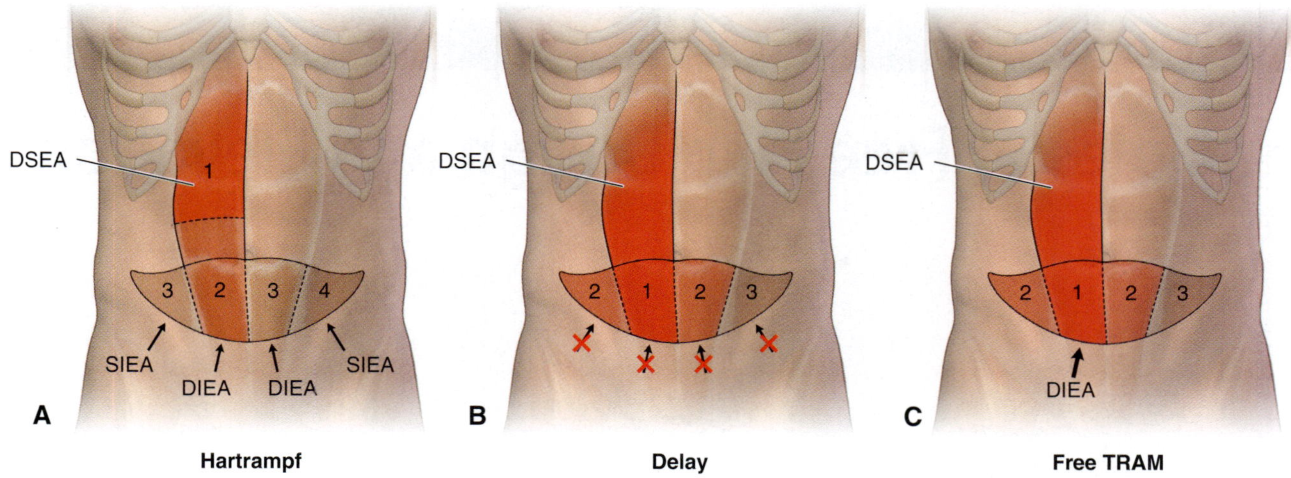

FIGURE 2-36 Schematic representation of the sequential vascular territories captured on the deep superior epigastric artery (DSEA) above in **A** and **B** and on the DIEA in C. In B, vascular anastomoses have opened up in the rectus muscle so that the DSEA and deep inferior epigastric artery (DIEA) coalesce into one vascular territory. Now the blood supply to this delayed skin flap in B is similar to that of the free flap based on the DIEA. TRAM, transverse rectus abdominis myocutaneous.

38. Taylor GI, Minabe T. The angiosomes of the mammals and other vertebrates. *Plast Reconstr Surg* 1992;89:181.
39. Taylor GI, Bates D, Newgreen DF. The developing neurovascular anatomy of the embryo: a technique of simultaneous evaluation using fluorescent labeling, confocal microscopy and three-dimensional reconstruction. *Plast Reconstr Surg* 2001;108:597.
40. Bates D, Taylor GI, Newgreen D. The pattern of neurovascular development in the forelimb of the quail embryo. *Dev Biol* 2002;249:300–320.
41. Suami H, Taylor GI, Pan WR. The lymphatic territories of the upper limb: anatomical study and clinical implications. *Plast Reconstr Surg* 2007;119:1813.
42. Houseman ND, Taylor GI, Pan W-R. The angiosomes of the head and neck; anatomic study and clinical applications. *Plast Reconstr Surg* 2000; 105(7):2287–2313.
43. Taylor GI, Palmer JH, McManammy D. The vascular territories of the body (angiosomes) and their clinical applications. In McCarthy (ed). Plastic Surgery, vol. 1. Philadelphia: Saunders, 1990.
44. Morris SF, Taylor GI. The time sequence of the delay phenomenon: when is a surgical delay effective? An experimental study. *Plast Reconstr Surg* 1995;95:526.
45. Taylor GI, Corlett RJ, Caddy C, Zelt RG. An anatomical review of the delay phenomenon: II. Clinical applications. *Plast Reconstr Surg* 1992; 89:408.
46. Callegari PR, Taylor GI, Caddy CM, Minabe T. An anatomical review of the delay phenomenon: 1. Experimental studies. *Plast Reconstr Surg* 1992;89:397.
47. Hunter JA. Treatise on the Blood, Inflammation and Gunshot Wounds. London: John Richardson, 1994.
48. Rozen WM, Ashton MW, Le Roux CM, et al The perforator angiosome: a new concept in the design of deep inferior epigastric artery perforator flaps for breast reconstruction. *Microsurgery* 2010;30:1–7.
49. Rozen WM, Palmer KP, Suami H, et al. The DIEA branching pattern and its relationship to perforators: the importance of preoperative CT angiography for DIEA perforator flaps. *Plast Reconstr Surg* 2008;121(2): 367–373.
50. Bates D, Taylor GI, Minichiello J, et al. Neurovascular congruence results from a shared patterning mechanism that utilises Semaphorin 3A and Neuropilin-1. *Dev Biol* 2003;255:77–98.

CHAPTER 3

Principles of Free Flap Design and Elevation

Phillip Blondeel

HISTORY OF FLAP DESIGN

In the history of surgical reconstruction, our common goal has been to move a flap of tissue to the area of need and ensure that this tissue stays viable. Over the years, this has been achieved in various ways. The perfusion to the skin was described as early as 1628 by William Harvey (1). But it was not until 1889, when Carl Manchot described the principals of perforator vessels systematically and in great detail (2), that skin perfusion was better understood. Cutaneous arterial territories were further elaborated by Salmon in 1936 (3), but it was later in the 1970s when Taylor and Daniel described specific vascular anatomy of various free flap donor sites (4). Subsequently, Palmer and Taylor did extensive work on establishing the angiosomes of the body (5), which contributed immensely toward planning and designing free flaps. Recent dynamic vascular studies investigating "perforasomes" in the body have further enriched our knowledge about the vascular supply to the integument by perforator vessels (6).

Initial concepts of flap design, with variable success, involved the planning of random pattern flaps such that the length to breadth ratio was confined to 2:1, allowing perfusion of the skin mainly by subdermal vascular plexus (7) or including the plexus above and below the fascia to design the "super flaps" described by Ponten (8). However, flaps did not need to be based on the subdermal vascular plexuses as was shown by Esser (9), who designed flaps on blood vessels directly perfusing an area without the need to retain the overlying skin. This was further reiterated by the fact that Antia and Buch replanted a dermofat flap by anastomosing the perfusing blood vessels (10). Microvascular transfer of flaps eventually became popular after Taylor and Daniel first described free tissue transfer (11). Taylor has continued to investigate the vascular trees of the body in order to design new free and pedicled skin flaps. Subsequently, various flaps were described for use as free microsurgical transfer of tissue. However, most of these were designed such that the skin paddle was perfused by perforator vessels from the underlying muscle (12). The skin paddle was designed either directly over the muscle (13) or over its fascial extension (14), requiring the sacrifice of these structures for the sake of harvesting the skin. Direct dissection and exposure of the perforators was then regarded as unnecessarily dangerous. Eventually, Koshima and Soeda (15) developed the concept of perforator flap surgery, which was later popularized by Allen (16) and Blondeel (17). The evolution of perforator flap surgery resulted in a departure from the concept of a need for an intact interface between muscle and overlying soft tissues for the skin paddle to survive. Over the years, we have further refined our technical skills and have now entered the era of supermicrosurgery (18) when we cannot only harvest perforator flaps based on very small caliber blood vessels, but we are also in a position to anastomose these flaps to equally fine perforating vessels in the recipient area. This has widened our choice of donor areas for harvesting free flaps and has contributed immensely to the reduction in donor site morbidity.

TYPES OF FREE FLAPS

Based on Composition

- **Single-component flap:** Any tissue can be transferred as a free flap based on its blood supply. This can involve individual transfer of skin and subcutaneous tissue, fat, fascia, muscle, bone, nerve, or tendon (Figure 3-1A). Some of these flaps can also be used as *flow-through flaps* in *which the flap not* only provides soft tissue reconstruction but the vessels in the flap may also help in restoring vascular continuity in limb or digit injuries.
- **Multiple-component "composite tissue" flap:** These are flaps in which different tissues are transferred en bloc: the flap includes multiple components sharing the same blood supply in a single flap (Figure 3-1B).

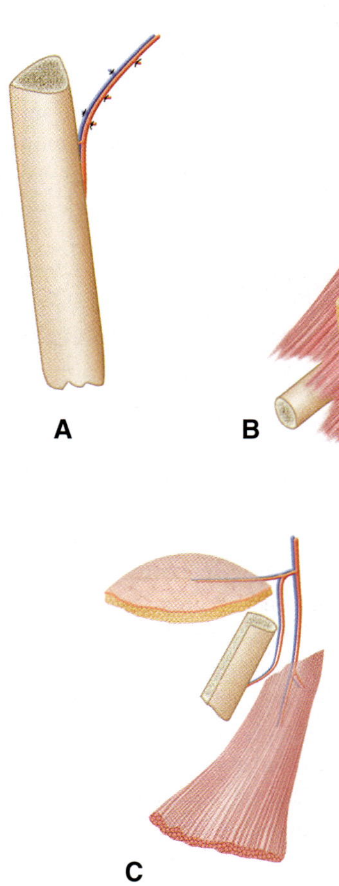

FIGURE 3-1 (**A**) Single-component flap consisting of a vascularized free fibula that can be used in defects where only bone needs to be reconstructed. (**B**) Multiple-component "composite sandwich" flap consisting of bone, muscle, and overlying skin and subcutaneous tissue conjoined together. This flap can be used in reconstruction of composite defects when all of these tissues need to be replaced en bloc. (**C**) Multiple-component "composite vascular tree" flap consisting of bone (scapula), muscle (latissimus dorsi), skin, and subcutaneous tissue (scapular) on their individual vascular supply from a common source vessel (subscapular vessels). This flap can be used in reconstruction of multiple defects of different tissues in close proximity.

- **Multiple-component "composite vascular tree" flap:** These are flaps in which the different components of tissue are based on different branches of the pedicle vessels (Figure 3-1C) These flaps are useful in cases when there are multiple defects of different tissues in close proximity to one another. *Monitoring flaps* are examples of these and are useful for *the surveillance* of buried flaps that cannot be observed directly for viability (e.g., jejunal transfers in pharyngeal reconstruction). In these cases, a segment of the jejunum is exteriorized on its individual vascular branch and excised in a few days when the free tissue transfer has been successful.

Based on Source of Blood Supply

- **"Designated" free flaps:** These are based on particular source vessels. Dissection in these flaps progresses antegrade from the "trunk to the leaves." These flaps are based on the angiosome concept described by Taylor.
- **"Free-style" free flaps:** These are designed around perforators found in the donor area. As stated by Wei, any region of the body can be chosen as a donor site as long as there is an audible pulsatile Doppler signal suggesting the presence of a perforator vessel of significant caliber (19). Dissection in these flaps proceeds retrograde from the "foliage to the roots." It should, however, be noted that the course of the perforator may be unpredictable, thus rendering dissection difficult, especially in case of small and long perforators. Microvascular anastomosis in small-caliber perforators may also prove to be challenging. Moreover, the skin territory and intraoperative flap thinning should be more conservative compared with conventional flaps.
- **Conjoined free flaps:** A large single flap consisting of multiple flap territories, each supplied by their own blood vessels, can be used as a conjoined flap. Intraflap anastomosis may have to be carried out between the blood vessels of the adjacent territories. If the blood vessels supplying these different territories arise from the same perforator vessels, then these are described as branch-based conjoined perforator flaps (20).
- **Venous flaps:** Venous flaps can be harvested from practically anywhere based on the superficial venous system, not having to rely on and sacrifice any arteries. However, the survival of these flaps has not always been reliable. Arterialized venous flaps have a better survival rate because high-flow arterial blood is diverted into the venous system. These flaps can be further optimized by using a small-caliber vein for inflow and a larger caliber vein for outflow, preferably two or more veins for outflow (21). Choosing two veins that are spaced well apart with a good venous plexus between them can increase area of flap. Venous flaps are discussed in detail elsewhere in this text.

Based on Level of Dissection

Donor site morbidity increases with increased dissection and sacrifice of tissue. Over the years, the sacrifice of tissue has been progressively reduced to address this.

- **Musculocutaneous flaps:** These have been workhorse flaps for years and are composite blocks of muscle, overlying skin, and subcutaneous tissue based on the blood supply of the muscle. However, sacrifice of a muscle can result in significant donor site morbidity.
- **Muscle-sparing fasciocutaneous flaps:** In an attempt to reduce the donor site morbidity, muscle-sparing flaps are designed such that a part of the muscle essential for conducting the blood supply to its overlying skin and subcutaneous tissue is harvested in the flap. Although this reduces the donor site morbidity to some extent, it still involves sacrifice of some of the muscle with resultant functional significance.
- **Perforator flaps:** These flaps are based on the perforator vessels directly perfusing the skin and subcutaneous tissue without including any muscle. The dissection of the pedicle in these flaps is either intermuscular (septocutaneous

perforators) or intramuscular (musculocutaneous perforators). Because muscle is not sacrificed in these flaps, donor site morbidity is significantly reduced.
- **Super microsurgical perforator flaps:** Although the muscle is not harvested in a perforator flap, dissection of flaps in which the perforator vessel has an intramuscular course results in disruption of the muscle with an associated increase in recovery time after the surgery. Super microsurgical perforator flaps are based on superficial small-caliber perforator vessels without extensively dissecting the vessels to their origin through deeper tissues. Donor site morbidity in these flaps is minimal, but supermicrosurgery on small-caliber vessels can be technically challenging.
- **Thin flaps, super thin flaps, and microdissected flaps:** Even perforator flaps consisting of only skin and subcutaneous tissue can at times be bulky and pose an aesthetic concern, necessitating debulking at a second stage. This can be avoided by thinning the flaps at the first stage, where the subcutaneous tissue is dissected off the flaps to varying degree to conform to varying thickness of the defect. Kimura et al. have taken this to the extreme by microdissecting the branches of the perforator vessels to tailor the flap to reconstruct complex defects (22).

Perforator Flap Classifications

As described by Hallock, any vessel that enters the superficial plane through a defined fenestration in the deep fascia is a perforator vessel. Over the past few years, a plethora of flaps based on perforator vessels have been described. The Gent consensus on perforator flaps has attempted to clarify the basic concepts of perforator flaps so that surgeons may share a common platform while describing various flaps (23). The definitions stated below are a result of this consensus.

- **Definition 1:** A perforator flap is a flap consisting of skin, subcutaneous fat, or both. The vessels that supply blood to the flap are isolated perforator(s). These perforators may pass either through or in between the deep tissues (mostly muscle).
- **Definition 2:** A muscle perforator is a blood vessel that traverses through muscle to supply the overlying skin.
- **Definition 3:** A septal perforator is a blood vessel that traverses only through septum to supply the overlying skin.
- **Definition 4:** A flap that is vascularized by a muscle perforator is called a muscle perforator flap.
- **Definition 5:** A flap vascularized by a septal perforator is called a septal perforator flap.
- **Definition 6:** A perforator flap should be named after the nutrient artery or vessels and not after the underlying muscle. If there is a potential to harvest multiple perforator flaps from one vessel, the name of each flap should be based on its anatomical region or muscle.

In an attempt to further standardize the description of perforator flaps, we have recently described the key elements that should be stated when describing a perforator flap (24). Aspects of the perforator flap such as the vessel of origin, the type of vascular dissection, the muscle involved, and finally the type of perforator vessel all contribute to easier understanding of the described flap, not only from an anatomical viewpoint but also in relation to the surgical approach to the flap. These terms provide clarity and will give surgeons a precise idea of a given perforator and the level of surgical difficulty.

PLANNING A FREE FLAP

Assessing the Reconstructive Need

The defect to be reconstructed needs to be assessed for the structures that need to be reconstructed. Ideally, “like” tissues should be used to replace the lost tissue. Reconstructive needs vary widely and may be for restoration of form, function, or both. For instance, whereas reconstruction of the breast is essentially carried out for restoring the form (with obvious psychological benefits), a free vascularized nerve graft is carried out to restore function, and a composite free tissue transfer composed of bone and soft tissue will need to be carried out to restore form and function in reconstruction of the mandible and its overlying soft tissue. Hence, the defect needs to be analyzed for its size, shape, location, and composition. It should be emphasized that after the tissue contracture surrounding the defect is released, the final defect can be significantly larger than the apparent defect. The cause of the defect might have an impact on the reconstruction and should be investigated. It is sensible to use the traditional reconstructive ladder approach of starting out with simple direct closure of the defect and progressing up the reconstructive ladder to complex microsurgical tissue transfer as necessary. However, as aptly suggested by Mathes and Nahai (25), it is often more practical to use the reconstructive technique best suited for the defect even though this may be more complex. Moreover, nowadays, technical refinements and surgical training have contributed toward making microsurgical transfers far less complex.

Assessing the Recipient Area

The planning of a free flap is dictated by the indication for reconstruction and the reconstructive needs. The indication for reconstruction might be for trauma; after oncologic resection, or for congenital or acquired deformities. When carrying out free tissue reconstruction in an area affected by trauma, consideration should be given to the effect of trauma in the surrounding tissues and the state of the potential recipient vessels. Because these vessels may have sustained intimal injury and have the potential to thrombose, the microvascular anastomosis needs to be performed well outside the zone of trauma. To achieve this, a flap with a long pedicle will have to be planned. It may even be necessary to use a Corlett loop of vein to help lengthen the pedicle (26). For reconstructions carried out for oncologic resections, the possibility of adjuvant radiotherapy should be considered. If this has been given before the reconstruction, recipient vessels may be fragile and encased in scar tissue. When reconstruction is carried out for congenital deformities, the vascular anatomy in the recipient area might be altered, and this should be anticipated.

Assessing the Patient

Several factors affect the success of the microsurgical procedure and wound healing. These should be taken into consideration when carrying out free tissue transfer and appropriate measures, as stated below, should be taken to optimize the patient for the operation.

Geriatric Patients

Free tissue transfer in an elderly patient can be daunting, but age alone should not be a contraindication to surgery. In patients older than 65 years of age, cardiac output is only 70% of that at the age of 30 years, and renal function is reduced by 50%. Hypertension is present in more than 40% of this population and is the most common factor for morbidity and mortality resulting from surgery and anesthesia. However, on correction of preexisting medical conditions, there is no significant difference between elderly patients in comparison with younger patients, and free tissue transfer can be carried out successfully in this group of patients without significant complications (27). However, medical morbidity increases with increasing American Society of Anesthesiology status, and surgical morbidity increases with increasing operating time (28). In view of this, any preexisting illness should be evaluated and the patient optimized using a multidisciplinary approach among the internist, anesthesiologist, and surgeon. Also, convalescence from an operation takes longer in this group of patients, thus prolonging hospital stays.

Pediatric Patients

Although free flap transfer is technically more challenging in children, there is a high success rate because children generally do not have associated comorbidities and recover well from prolonged anesthesia (29). Pediatric patients have pristine anatomy that has not been altered by systemic disease, and they usually heal well, especially with good reinnervation after sensory or motor nerve coaptation. It is particularly important not to sacrifice muscle flaps in this group of patients. We have always aimed to attain reconstruction with minimal donor site morbidity, and we have successfully achieved this by using perforator flaps even when the patient has been as young as 28 weeks of age (30)!

Smoking

Patients who are active smokers and those who have smoked up to within 4 weeks of the operation are at increased risk of flap and donor site complications. Cigarette smoking increases platelet aggregation and the risk of thrombosis. Also, nicotine causes cutaneous vasoconstriction by activating the sympathetic nervous system and reduces the capillary blood flow. In addition, carbon monoxide binds to hemoglobin and contributes to tissue hypoxia. Smokers have a higher incidence of delayed wound healing (27) and infection (31). There is also an increased incidence of marginal necrosis and partial flap loss in actively smoking patients (27). If the patient has quit smoking in the recent past, it may be worthwhile to make sure that the patient is not using nicotine patches!

Diabetes

In a patient with diabetes, there can be risks of abnormalities in endothelial and red blood cell function and platelet function, altered blood viscosity, and abnormal intimal repair. But with good glycemic control, the incidence of flap and donor site complications does not differ significantly among patients with type 1 diabetes or type 2 diabetes and those without diabetes (32).

Hypertension

Hypertension may be associated with other comorbidities in the patient, and the blood vessels may be affected by atherosclerosis. This has obvious thrombogenic implications in microsurgical transfers. Therefore, there is an increased incidence of flap complications in patients with hypertension (33), and this needs to be considered when planning free flaps in these patients.

Obesity

Obese patients (body mass index >30) not only pose anesthetic risks, but the outcome of free flap surgery in these patients is also compromised. There is a significant rate of marginal necrosis, loss of flap, and seroma formation in the donor site (27). These factors need to be considered when planning a microsurgical transfer in these patients.

Hematologic Disorders

In patients with hematologic disorders, the surgeon needs to liaise with the patient's hematologist and be familiar with the preoperative medical condition of the patient and potential postoperative complications. The medical condition of the patient should be closely monitored before and after the surgery. Patients with hemophilia with deficient factor VIII are prone to bleeding and hematoma. These patients should receive recombinant factor VIII to prevent complications (34). On the other hand, patients can have hypercoagulable states as a result of genetic mutations of coagulation factors or because of acquired causes such as malignancy and certain autoimmune or endocrine disorders (35). The patient should be optimized, and appropriate perioperative anticoagulation therapy should be considered.

Deep Vein Thrombosis

Patients for free flap surgery are at risk for developing deep vein thrombosis (DVT) because some of these procedures can be prolonged. These patients should be commenced on subcutaneous heparin before surgery or low-molecular-weight heparin a few hours after. Either should be continued at least until discharge. Graduated compressions stockings are applied on admission and intermittent pneumatic compression during and after the operative procedure. Investigation of the venous systems is particularly important in patients undergoing lower extremity free tissue transfer who are at high risk of DVT or when there is a clinical suspicion of DVT (36).

Peripheral Vascular Disease

Although free flap reconstruction of the lower extremity in the presence of peripheral vascular disease has been debatable, free tissue transfer has been shown to have a good success rate even in these patients (37). Flap loss is low, and limb salvage, ambulation, and long-term survival rates in these patients are excellent. Hence, it is worthwhile to carry out reconstructive procedures in these patients after optimizing circulation to the limb as much as possible rather than amputating their limbs.

Adjuvant Chemotherapy

Chemotherapy induces immunosuppression, resulting in an increased susceptibility of the host to opportunistic pathogens or malignancies. Although there have been concerns about reconstructions being carried out after neoadjuvant chemotherapy, this has not been the case, and chemotherapy does not appear to increase the risk of major surgical complications (38).

Adjuvant Radiotherapy

Preoperative radiotherapy increases the risk of vascular complications during the performance of the microvascular anastomosis (39). Tissues that have been exposed to radiotherapy pose a technical challenge because the vessels tend to be thin walled, friable, and encased in scar tissue. However, this does not have any effect on delayed complications with the vascular anastomosis, flap loss, fat necrosis, infection, skin flap necrosis, hematoma, and seroma. Although the dose of the radiation does not seem to affect the postoperative complications, the incidence of complications has been noted to increase with increasing interval between the radiotherapy and surgery. In the head and neck, it has been recommended to plan surgery within 6 weeks of adjuvant radiotherapy to minimize complications (40). However, there are conflicting data on the subject, with other authors suggesting that autogenous breast reconstruction be delayed for as long as 12 months (41). It should also be noted that radiotherapy after the reconstruction can also lead to significant complications and can affect the aesthetic outcome of the reconstruction, especially if it has been carried out for reconstructing aesthetically sensitive areas such as the breast.

Trauma

If the free flap reconstruction is being carried out for reconstruction of a defect as a result of trauma, it is essential that the "zone of injury" be assessed. This zone refers to the inflammatory response of the soft tissues to trauma and extends beyond the actual wound (42). Although tissue is viable in this area, the blood vessels tend to suffer from microvascular injury and are thereby prone to thrombosis. This combined with the perivascular changes results in failure of microvascular anastomosis if the anastomosis has not been carried out beyond the "zone of trauma." Also, it has been shown in the lower limb that venous insufficiency and partial flap loss are greater when the superficial venous system is used instead of the deep venous system (43). It is important to evaluate the residual vascular supply of the leg by angiography so that ideal recipient vessels can be selected without compromising the circulation to the foot.

Pregnancy

Prolonged procedures such as free tissue transfers tend to be avoided in pregnant patients because they may not be safe for the patient and the fetus. However, when faced with an emergency, it may be necessary to do so. In these cases, it should be noted that pregnancy renders the patient hypercoagulable; and free tissue transfers may fail as a result of thrombosis of the microvascular anastomosis. It may be essential to treat these patients with heparin to avoid such complications (44).

Evaluating Available Options

Depending on the reconstructive needs, a flap best suitable for the defect is selected. In an *emergency procedure,* such as reconstruction in lower limb trauma, the surgeon uses what is available. Special considerations with regard to trauma, as stated previously, need to be taken into account. It should be remembered that amputated parts that are not suitable for replanting should still be considered for their value as a "fillet" flap (the bone is removed, and the resulting "fillet" is used as a soft tissue free flap simply for wound closure) rather than sacrificing a donor area.

However, in an *elective procedure,* the surgeon has the opportunity to plan and design the most appropriate flap and if necessary prefabricate and tailor a flap to suit the defect to be reconstructed. In pondering the options, one needs to consider the general condition of the patient, the composition of the flap needed to replace like tissue with like, and the expected donor site morbidity.

DESIGNING A FREE FLAP

Flaps should be designed according to the reconstructive needs of the defect in addition to restoring the aesthetic form of the injured part. Reconstruction in the limbs may need the transfer of tendons or muscle as functional components of the flap. If muscle is transferred as a functional component, its motor nerve will also need to be harvested along with the muscle and coapted to a recipient motor nerve at the recipient site. Functional reconstruction of the lower lip and the oral sphincter may require reconstruction with a composite transfer of radial forearm flap along with the palmaris longus tendon. Reconstruction of areas such as the lower face, involving the mandible or maxilla, requires the transfer of bone as a component of a composite flap. Flaps may need to include sensory nerves to provide protective sensation in the reconstructed area. This is particularly important in reconstructions of the sole of the foot and that of an amputation stump. Irrespective of the method of reconstruction chosen, it is a good idea to have a backup option in case the operation does not go according to plan. Although this is often not necessary if proper planning has been done, it does help take out the stress of planning when the surgeon finds him- or herself in a difficult situation.

Various preoperative investigative techniques are useful for identifying the vascular architecture and planning a flap. Although the handheld Doppler is cheap and easy to use, it has its limitations. Color duplex ultrasound scans have been shown to be of value not only in identifying perforator vessels (45) but have also incidentally revealed silent infrainguinal claudication that would have rendered harvest of an anterolateral thigh (ALT) flap unsafe (46). In our practice, the use contrast enhanced computed tomography angiography (CTA) has helped us to not only identify the dominant perforators but has also given us detailed information about the course of the vessels and their perfusion pattern in the skin and subcutaneous tissue (47). This has obvious advantages in harvesting a well-perfused flap and reducing the incidence of partial necrosis or fat necrosis within it. Also, a perforator that has a course that is easier to dissect with minimal trauma to the muscle can be selected as the feeder vessel for the flap. Knowing exactly where these perforator vessels are located helps save operative time.

Occasionally, incidental pathology is found in the abdomen while performing a scan for a deep inferior epigastric perforator (DIEP) flap. However, a CT scan does involve exposing the patient to radiation, and modalities such as Magnetic resonance angiography (MRA) have been used in an attempt to avoid this. Septocutaneous perforators appear to be better identified with bolus chase MRA (48), but newer generation MR imaging has been shown to be effective in analysis of the vascular architecture without the need for contrast (49). These techniques help to analyze small vessel architecture. However, we must not forget that vascular flow is dynamic and in addition to assessing the vascular network, it would also be helpful to know about the small vessel flow characteristics. This can be achieved by either assessing transit time flow volume (TTFV) (50) or by four-dimensional CTA (6). This might further aid in reducing incidence of partial necrosis of flaps.

Depending on the reconstructive needs, the flap can be designed either based on named pedicle vessels, as a *designated* free flap, or the flap can be designed on perforator vessels identified by Doppler or preoperative CTA, as a *free-style* free flap. When choosing a flap, one should select a flap in which the pedicle vessels are long enough to reach the recipient vessels and match them in caliber. This is particularly important in cases of trauma in which the anastomosis will need to be performed outside the zone of trauma. Vein grafts may be necessary and have been used successfully in such cases (51). Alternatively, a Corlett loop consisting of a temporary arteriovenous fistula may be used.

Consideration should be given to matching the color and texture of donor skin to that of the recipient area. This is often an issue in head and neck reconstruction in which the patient ends up having a pale patch of skin occupying the reconstructed area. There have been some promising results to address this by resurfacing the flap with a split-thickness skin graft harvested from the scalp (52). But ideally, a flap that matches color and texture of the recipient area should be selected if possible.

One should consider components of the flap necessary for reconstructing the defect. A multiple-component flap may be necessary, such as harvesting the ALT flap along with its underlying fascia lata for reconstruction of both the Achilles tendon and skin cover. Skin along with its underlying cartilage may need to be harvested as a free flap from the root of the auricular helix to reconstruct the nasal ala. When the recipient bed is heavily scarred or a nerve gap is exceptionally long, a vascularized nerve graft may transferred as a free flap. Like for like tissues should be replaced as far as possible, a unique example of this being reconstruction of a tubular structure such as the urethra with a free vascularized appendix transfer (53)!

Free tissue transfers are relatively long procedures, and every attempt must be made to reduce operating time as much as possible. Proper preoperatively planning helps reduce time wasted on planning in the operating room (OR). It is important to have OR staff who are familiar with the procedure and are involved in it on a regular basis. All necessary equipment and instruments should be at hand. The conditions in the OR should allow the procedure to flow seamlessly. Selecting a flap that can be harvested without the need for a change in position of the patient during the surgery and one that allows for a two-team approach also saves time.

Tailoring Flaps to Specific Defects

Defects in Need of Specialized Tissue

For defects requiring reconstruction with multiple components of tissue, flaps can be *prefabricated* to include cartilage or bone as required along with skin and subcutaneous tissue. Prefabrication can also be combined with tissue engineering and skin substitutes such as Integra can be prefabricated and transferred as part of free flaps (54). Similarly, flaps can be *prelaminated*. For example, a radial forearm flap can be prelaminated with a skin graft and used to provide skin and mucosal lining for extensive cheek defects.

Defects with a Large Surface Area

From time to time, we are faced with situations in which a large surface area needs to be reconstructed. In such a situation, one of the following options may be considered.

- **Preexpansion:** When a flap with a large area of skin needs to be harvested, preexpansion may be considered to obtain a large flap as well as to reduce the donor site morbidity after flap harvest. This may also be done by dissecting out the perforator vessel perfusing the skin paddle first and then expanding it, rather than carrying out random expansion (55).
- **Multiple** or **conjoined flaps:** These flaps can be inset adjacent to each other, similar to a mosaic, to reconstruct the defect. These would, however, involve harvesting more than one flap with the consequences of increased operating time.
- **Supercharging flaps:** The main issue with a single flap of large surface area is the unreliable vascularity of the part of the flap that is most distal to the pedicle vessels. Performing an additional microsurgical anastomosis between vessels in this area and another set of recipient vessels, thereby "supercharging" the flap, can augment perfusion to this part of the flap (56).
- **Bipedicle flaps:** In flaps of large surface area, distal part of the flap can also be perfused by performing an intraflap anastomosis, such that vessels perfusing the distal part of the flap are anastomosed to branches of the main pedicle vessels (57). In these cases, only one set of recipient vessels is required.

Defects with Large Volume Deficit

Large flaps may also be required to fill up a defect where volume is more important than surface area. These defects can be addressed by one of the following options.

- **Deepithelialized and folded in:** Excess parts of a large flap can be deepithelialized and folded under the flap so as to add volume to the flap. In bilateral breast reconstructions in which each DIEP flap is half the donor area, volume is created in the inferior pole using this technique (58).
- **Double stacked flaps:** Volume can also be created by using two flaps, one above the other, when the bottom flap has been deepithelialized (59). This, however, necessitates two sets of microvascular anastomoses and prolongs the operating time.
- **"Vascular matrix" flaps:** This is a concept that is currently gaining favor. In patients who do not have a perforator flap of adequate volume, we tend to transfer the flap as a vascular matrix and then augment the volume of the flap by performing fat transfer into the flap (60). This not only helps in reducing donor site morbidity by harvesting a perforator flap but also relieves the patient of fat in undesired areas.

Donor Site Factors

Aesthetic Morbidity

When planning a free flap, one should aim to close the donor site directly with minimal aesthetic morbidity. As stated earlier, for a flap of very large surface area, expansion of the flap should be considered to facilitate direct closure. Donor area for a flap should be carefully selected such that the resultant scar is in a concealed area. An abdominoplasty scar after a DIEP flap harvest is a very good example of this. Not only is the scar well concealed, but harvesting the flap from this area also improves the abdominal contour of patients who have a redundant abdominal apron. There should be no distortion of the contour in the donor area. Although the superior gluteal artery perforator (SGAP) flap has been used for breast reconstruction, the conventional SGAP flap distorts one aesthetic area in an attempt to restore aesthetics in another. The modified SGAP flap, which is harvested more cranially, helps to address this issue (61).

Functional Morbidity

Harvest of muscle flaps has its associated morbidity, and when possible, perforator flaps should be harvested instead. The anterolateral thigh flap has gained in popularity for these very reasons; and a good guide for direct closure of the donor site is to harvest flaps that have a width of less than 16% of the thigh circumference (62). In other donor areas such as the abdominal wall, an attempt to reduce functional morbidity has been made by preserving most of the muscle while harvesting the transverse rectus abdominis musculocutaneous (TRAM) flap. Although there have been claims that there is no significant difference in donor site morbidity after harvest of such muscle-sparing flaps such as the MS-2 TRAM flap, studies have shown that muscle-sparing TRAM flaps result in a decline in abdominal strength in the upper abdominal area (63). Detailed studies looking at the isometric, concentric, and eccentric muscle strengths after harvest of a flap from the abdominal wall show that eccentric muscle strength is greater after harvest of a DIEP flap compared with a MS-2 TRAM flap harvest (64,65). Muscle flaps may need to be used for a functional transfer. In these cases, a relatively expendable muscle, such as the gracilis, should be used.

Designing a Flap in Presence of Donor Site Scars

Preexisting scars in the donor area are not necessarily a contraindication to harvesting flaps from these areas. However, preoperative investigations may need to be carried out to confirm the presence of the pedicle vessels of the flap. In the presence of scars in the donor area, it is important to design the flap with care. Peripheral areas distal to scars in a flap tend to have compromised circulation and should be avoided. Existing scars should be included in incisions at the edge of the flap. If this is not possible and an incision parallel to the old scar has to be made, then care should be taken not to undermine the area between the old scar and the new incision to avoid wound breakdown or delayed wound healing in the donor area. It should also be borne in mind that pedicle dissection in a previous operated area may be tedious because of dissection through scarred tissue.

ELEVATING THE FREE FLAP

Preoperative Markings

Donor Area

The boundaries of the flap should be marked, including the position of the pedicle. If underlying bone is to be included in the flap, then its position in relation to the flap should be marked. The dimensions of the flap should be in accordance with the requirements of the defect. In delayed reconstructions, it should be noted that after release of all of the scar tissue, the resulting defect is often larger than initially apparent. In perforator flaps, the perforator vessels should be identified with the aid of preoperative investigations and marked on the flap. As mentioned earlier, our investigation of choice is CTA. The DIEP flap is the one most commonly subjected to CTA in our practice. The perforator vessels are marked along the x- and y-axes, with the umbilicus as a fixed landmark, at zero (Figure 3-2). This contributes immensely to effortless identification and dissection of perforators while elevating the flap.

Recipient Area

Normal anatomy around the recipient area should be marked to help achieve symmetry in reconstruction. The area to be reconstructed is marked. If there is an apparent wound that needs to be reconstructed, then the boundaries of the defect are evident. But in delayed reconstructions, the area to be reconstructed needs to be assessed and marked. This corresponds to the "footprint" in breast reconstructions, which is essentially the outline of the base of the breast to be reconstructed (Figure 3-3) (58).

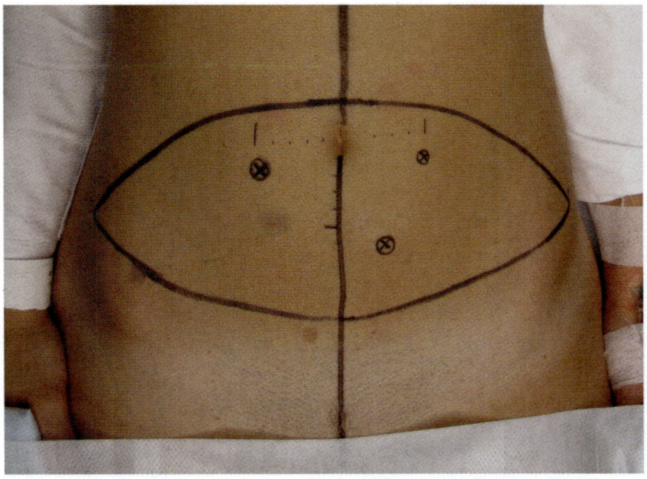

FIGURE 3-2 Donor area of a deep inferior epigastric perforator flap where the perforator vessels have been marked based on the findings of the computed tomography angiogram. With the umbilicus as zero, the perforator vessels are marked around it on the x- and y-axes. The dominant ones have been marked as a cross in a circle.

Preparing the Patient

Positioning the Patient

Ideally, the patient should be positioned such that both the recipient and donor sites are accessible to facilitate a two-team approach. Pressure areas should be carefully padded to protect them, and care should be taken to prevent peripheral nerve and ocular injury. Unexposed parts of the patient should be covered with a warming blanket to prevent hypothermia.

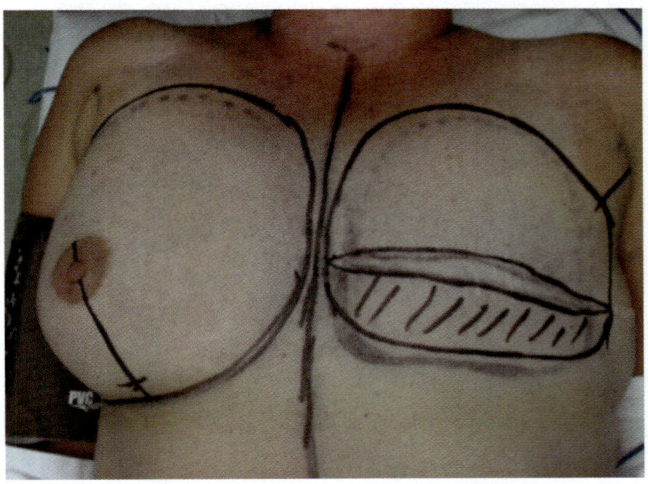

FIGURE 3-3 The recipient area of a patient who is about to undergo a secondary breast reconstruction of the left and risk reducing immediate reconstruction on the right side. The "footprint" of the breast has been marked on the left side in accordance with her right breast, but do note that the inframammary line appears to be more cranial on the left side. This is because the line has been marked after pulling down on the abdominal skin as would happen after harvest of the abdominal skin and direct closure of the donor area. Also, the inframammary line will have a tendency to shift more caudally after the scar has been excised and the contracted tissue is released.

Optimal Anesthesia

The anesthesiologist is an important individual in maximizing the success of microsurgery by controlling the hemodynamics and the regional blood flow (66). The basic goal of the anesthesia is to maintain an optimal blood flow for the vascularized free flap. This can be achieved by increasing the circulatory blood flow; maintaining a normal body temperature to avoid peripheral vasoconstriction; reducing vasoconstriction resulting from pain, anxiety, hyperventilation, or drugs; and treating hypotension caused by extensive sympathetic block and low cardiac output. A hyperdynamic circulation can be obtained by hypervolemic or normovolemic hemodilution and by a decrease in systemic vascular resistance. It is important to adequately replace volume loss. General anesthesia combined with various types of regional anesthesia is largely preferred for microvascular surgery. Homeostasis should be maintained through avoidance of hypoxia, hypocapnia, and hypovolemia (all factors that can decrease cardiac output and induce local vasoconstriction).

General anesthesia induces hypotension, but surgeons have been reluctant to allow the use of vasopressor agents because the concomitant vasoconstriction may lead to difficulty in identifying perforator vessels, increasing operating time, and potentially affecting flap survival. However, it now seems that vasopressors do not seem to increase the above risks in microsurgery (67).

Operative Dissection

The following operative technique is for harvesting a perforator flap in a retrograde manner ("foliage to roots"). This can be applied both for "designated" and "free-style" perforator free flaps. The later part of the description (submuscular dissection) applies to harvest of a muscle flap.

Supramuscular Dissection

After incision along the margins of the flap, the incision is progressively deepened while the surgeon looks out for any large superficial veins leading away from the flap. It is worthwhile to preserve any large veins that are encountered. This is particularly useful when elevating large flaps such as the DIEP flap, where preservation the superficial inferior epigastric vein, especially if it found to be large, can be a useful "lifeboat" in cases of venous insufficiency (68). If there is an issue with perfusion of the flap, often this is due to venous congestion, and it is useful to be able to relieve this by using the preserved vein. However, it is not advisable to perform more than one venous anastomosis of the same venous system (e.g., both venae comitantes) because it has been shown that venous blood flow is faster in a single vein anastomosis and slows down when an additional vein is anastomosed (69). This increases the risk for venous thrombosis and flap failure (43). In free-style perforator flaps, only on one margin of the flap should be incised to look for underlying perforators. If suitable perforators are not found in the area, then the wound can be closed without sacrificing the donor area.

In a designated perforator flap, the flap should be elevated in a subfacial plane with the aid of a Colorado needle mounted on a monopolar diathermy in the cutting mode (Figure 3-4). We use the Valley Lab Force FX at the 35/35 setting for coagulation/cutting modes. When near the area of the perforator vessels,

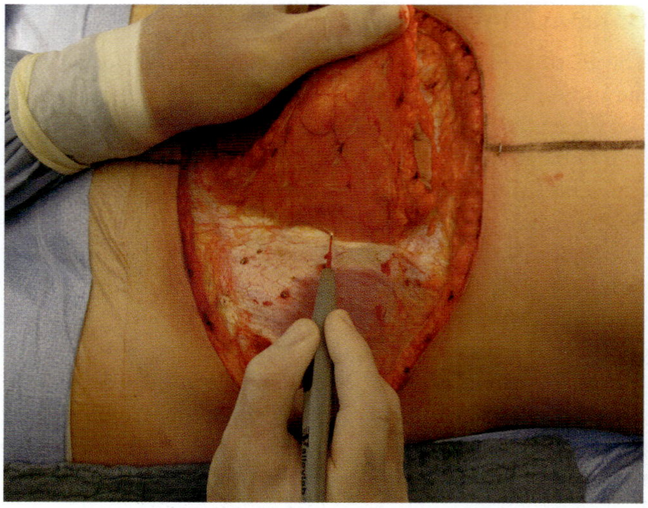

FIGURE 3-4 Swift elevation of the lateral parts of the deep inferior epigastric perforator flap is carried out with the aid of a sharp-tipped Colorado needle mounted on a monopolar diathermy at a high setting.

we change the pinpoint to a flat tip and step down the setting of the machine to 18/18. This allows for a safe and dry dissection plane until the perforator vessels are found (Figure 3-5). After the perforator vessels have been identified, dissection around them is carried out with the help of Blondeel micro-scissors (Figure 3-6). These are microscissors with a ring handle to them that allow for fine dissection around the perforator vessels. The perforator vessels are then followed down through the perforation in the aponeurosis into the muscle.

Intramuscular Dissection

The muscle fibers overlying the perforator vessels are gently split with the aid of a micro bipolar diathermy forceps with the

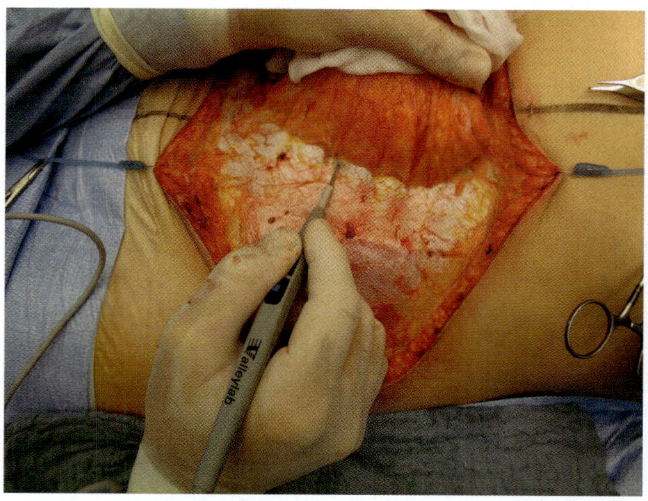

FIGURE 3-5 The sharp-pointed Colorado tip is replaced with a flat tip at a low diathermy setting to allow careful and bloodless dissection of the area bearing the perforator vessels. This gently dissects through the tissues surrounding the perforator vessels and helps in locating them but at the same time avoids any damage to them. Without electric current, the blade can be used for blunt dissection.

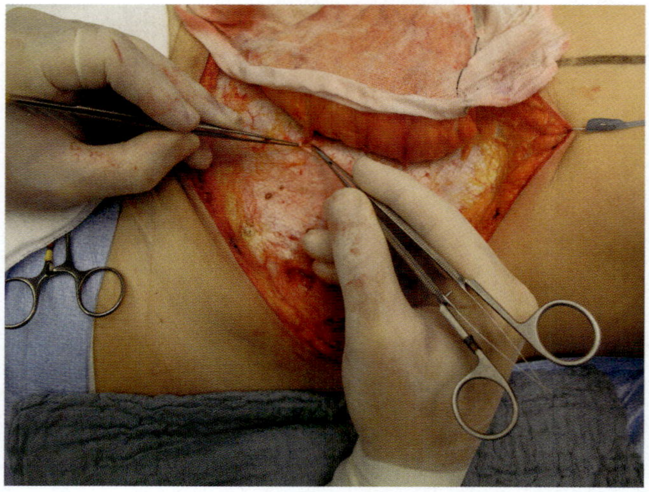

A

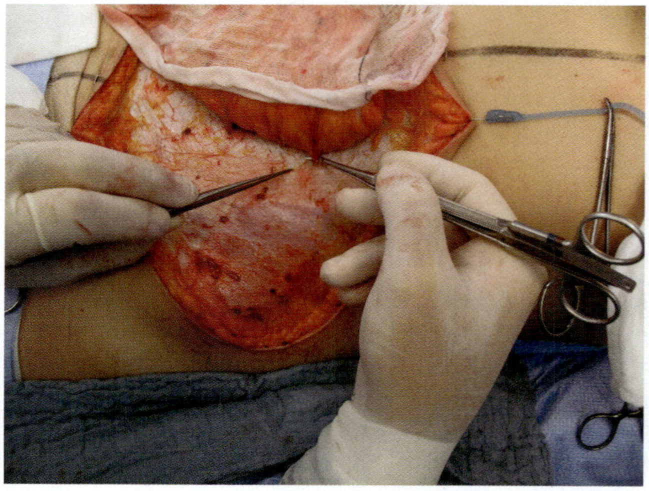

B

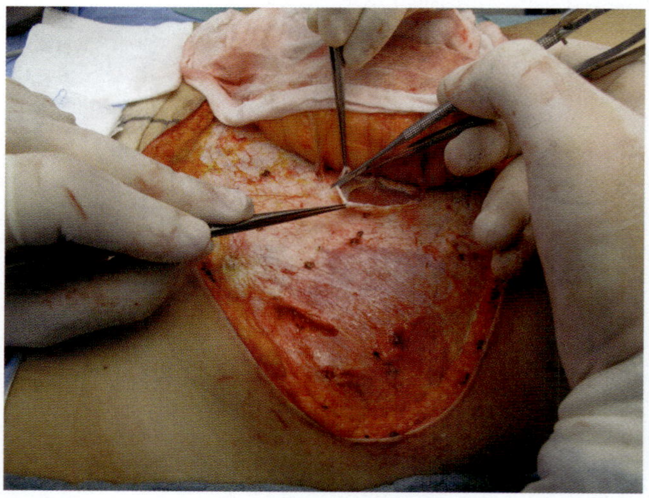

C

FIGURE 3-6 (**A**) After the perforator vessels have been identified, dissection is carried out with a sharp Blondeel microsurgical scissors to help dissect around the perforator vessel and free them up. (**B**) In a first step, all surrounding tissues 360 degrees around the perforator are lifted off the deep fascia over a short distance. (**C**) Starting from the border of the gap in the deep fascia through which the perforator pierces, the fascia is opened up cranially and distally.

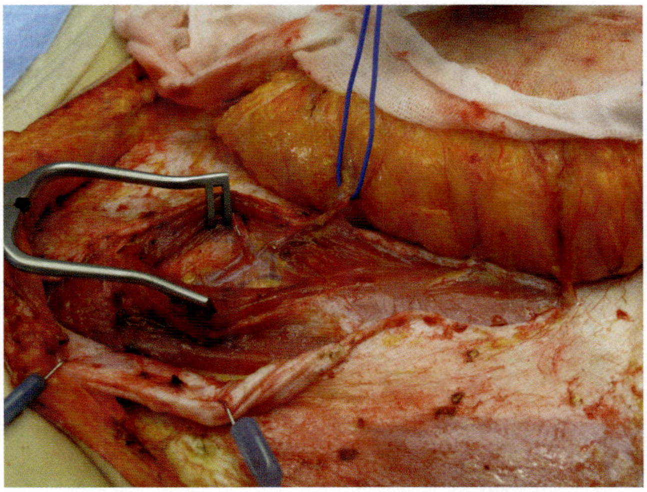

FIGURE 3-7 A vascular loop is passed around the perforator. This can then be used to gently manipulate the pedicle around without having to grasp the pedicle directly, thus avoiding any trauma to it. This mainly helps in dissecting the pedicle in its intramuscular part.

diathermy machine set at 11. Branches from the perforator vessels into the muscle are gently dissected, and micro Ligaclips are applied before their division. Care should be taken not to diathermy these vessels because heat can be transmitted to the perforator vessels, injuring them. One should also look for motor nerves that often accompany these muscular branches and safeguard them. Vascular loops are used around the pedicle vessels to gently handle them during the intramuscular dissection (Figure 3-7). The pedicle should be handled delicately to avoid spasm of the vessels. It is important, however, to remove the vascular loop as soon as the dissection has been completed to avoid accidental avulsion of the pedicle!

Submuscular Dissection

The pedicle vessels are then traced to the under surface of the muscle, the muscle retracted, and the vessels followed to their point of origin from the main vessels. Any side branches are ligated and divided along the way, taking care to preserve any motor nerve branches. The pedicle is dissected until vessels of adequate length and caliber have been exposed. At this point, the vessels are ligated and divided when the recipient site and the recipient vessels have been prepared. We tend to mark the artery with a Ligaclip and leave the vein free to drain the flap. It may be worthwhile to mark one side of the pedicle vessels with indelible ink to prevent twisting on transfer of the flap. If a musculocutaneous flap is being raised, it is useful to secure the fascia to the muscle to avoid shearing of the perforator vessels.

After harvest of the flap, it is transferred to the recipient area, anastomosed to the recipient vessels, and inset to give a satisfactory reconstruction (Figure 3-8). The principles necessary to achieve a successful microsurgical transfer of the flap are described later in this book.

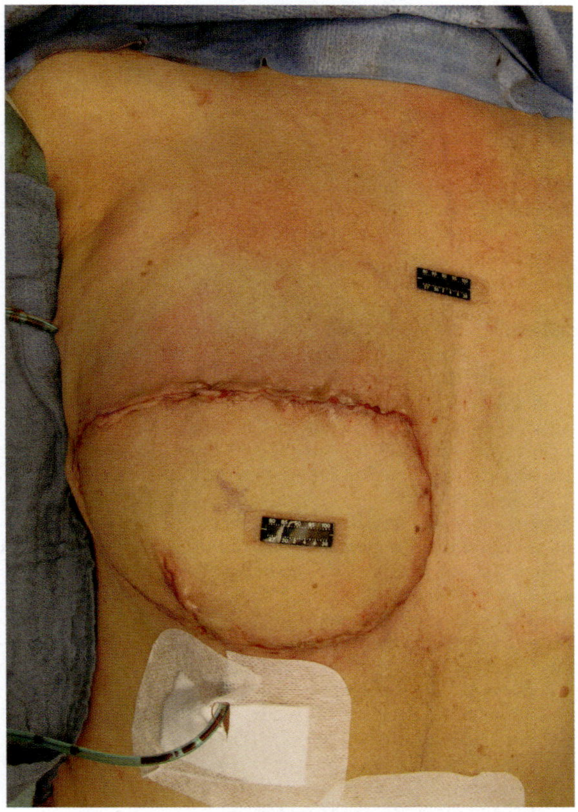

FIGURE 3-8 A deep inferior epigastric artery perforator flap has been transferred from the abdominal area to the chest. This free flap has been used to reconstruct the right breast, resulting in a satisfactory outcome. Temperature strips are placed to compare the skin temperature of the flap and surrounding skin.

REFERENCES

1. Harvey W. An anatomical disputation concerning the movement of the heart and blood in living creatures. Oxford: Blackwell Scientific, 1976.
2. Manchot C. Die Hautarterien des Menschlichen Korpers. Leipzig: FCW Vogel, 1889.
3. Salmon M. Arteres de la Peau. Paris: Mason et Cie, 1936.
4. Taylor GI, Daniel RK. The anatomy of several free flap donor sites. *Plast Reconstr Surg* 1975;56(3):243–253.
5. Taylor GI, Palmer JH. The vascular territories (angiosomes) of the body: experimental study and clinical applications. *Br J Plast Surg* 1987;40(2):113–141.
6. Saint-Cyr M, Wong C, Schaverien M, et al. The perforasome theory: vascular anatomy and clinical implications. *Plast Reconstr Surg* 2009;124(5):1529–1544.
7. Pearl RM, Johnson D. The vascular supply to the skin: an anatomical and physiological reappraisal—part II. *Ann Plast Surg* 1983;11(3):196–205.
8. Ponten B. The fasciocutaneous flap: its use in soft tissue defects of the lower leg. *Br J Plast Surg* 1981;34(2):215–220.
9. Esser J. General rules used in simple plastic work on Austrian war-wounded soldiers. *Surg Gynecol Obstet* 1917:34.
10. Antia NH, Buch VI. Transfer of an abdominal dermo-fat graft by direct anastomosis of blood vessels. *Br J Plast Surg* 1971;24(1):15–19.
11. Taylor GI, Daniel RK. The free flap: composite tissue transfer by vascular anastomosis. *Aust N Z J Surg* 1973;43(1):1–3.
12. McCraw JB. The recent history of myocutaneous flaps. *Clin Plast Surg* 1980;7(1):3–7.
13. Tanzini I. Sopra il mio nuovo processo di amputazione dell mammella. (Coverage of the anterior chest wall following mastectomy). *Gazz Med Ital* 1906:57.
14. Pittet B, Mahajan AL, Alizadeh N, et al. The free serratus anterior flap and its cutaneous component for reconstruction of the face: a series of 27 cases. *Plast Reconstr Surg* 2006;117(4):1277–1288.
15. Koshima I, Soeda S. Inferior epigastric artery skin flaps without rectus abdominis muscle. *Br J Plast Surg* 1989;42(6):645–648.
16. Allen RJ, Treece P. Deep inferior epigastric perforator flap for breast reconstruction. *Ann Plast Surg* 1994;32(1):32–38.
17. Blondeel PN. One hundred free DIEP flap breast reconstructions: a personal experience. *Br J Plast Surg* 1999;52(2):104–111.

18. Koshima I, Yamamoto T, Narushima M, et al. Perforator flaps and supermicrosurgery. *Clin Plast Surg* 2010;37(4):683–689,vii–iii.
19. Wei FC, Mardini S. Free-style free flaps. *Plast Reconstr Surg* 2004;114(4):910–916.
20. Hallock GG. Branch-based conjoined perforator flaps. *Plast Reconstr Surg* 2008;121(5):1642–1649.
21. Pittet B, Quinodoz P, Alizadeh N, et al. Optimizing the arterialized venous flap. *Plast Reconstr Surg* 2008;122(6):1681–1689.
22. Kimura N, Saitoh M, Okamura T, et al. Concept and anatomical basis of microdissected tailoring method for free flap transfer. *Plast Reconstr Surg* 2009;123(1):152–162.
23. Blondeel PN, Van Landuyt KH, Monstrey SJ, et al. The "Gent" consensus on perforator flap terminology: preliminary definitions. *Plast Reconstr Surg* 2003;112(5):1378–1383; quiz 1383, 1516; discussion 1384–1387.
24. Sinna R, Boloorchi A, Mahajan AL, et al. What should define a "perforator flap"? *Plast Reconstr Surg* 2010;126(6):2258–2263.
25. Mathes SJ, Nahai F. Reconstructive Surgery: Principles, Anatomy, and Technique. San Francisco: Churchill Livingstone, 1997.
26. Ethunandan M, Cole R, Flood TR. Corlett loop for microvascular reconstruction in a neck depleted of vessels. *Br J Oral Maxillofac Surg* 2007;45(6):493–495.
27. Seidenstuecker K, Mahajan MB, Richrath AL, et al. Morbidity of microsurgical breast reconstruction in patients with comorbid conditions. In Annual Conference of the German Society for Plastic, Reconstructive, and Aesthetic Surgery, Hannover, 2009.
28. Serletti JM, Higgins JP, Moran S, Orlando GS. Factors affecting outcome in free-tissue transfer in the elderly. *Plast Reconstr Surg* 2000;106(1):66–70.
29. Upton J, Guo L. Pediatric free tissue transfer: a 29-year experience with 433 transfers. *Plast Reconstr Surg* 2008;121(5):1725–1737.
30. Van Landuyt K, Hamdi M, Blondeel P, et al. Free perforator flaps in children. *Plast Reconstr Surg* 2005;116(1):159–169.
31. Spear SL, Ducic I, Cuoco F, Hannan C. The effect of smoking on flap and donor-site complications in pedicled TRAM breast reconstruction. *Plast Reconstr Surg* 2005;116(7):1873–1880.
32. Miller RB, Reece G, Kroll SS, et al. Microvascular breast reconstruction in the diabetic patient. *Plast Reconstr Surg* 2007;119(1):38–45; discussion 46–48.
33. Gill PS, Hunt JP, Guerra AB, et al. A 10-year retrospective review of 758 DIEP flaps for breast reconstruction. *Plast Reconstr Surg* 2004;113(4): 1153–1160.
34. Drimmer MA, Demas C, Saidi P, Kim HC. Reconstructive plastic surgery in hemophiliacs. *Plast Reconstr Surg* 1988;81(1):91–93.
35. Davison SP, Kessler CM, Al-Attar A. Microvascular free flap failure caused by unrecognized hypercoagulability. *Plast Reconstr Surg* 2009;124(2):490–495.
36. Murray DJ, Neligan PC, Novak CB, et al. Free tissue transfer and deep vein thrombosis. *J Plast Reconstr Aesthet Surg* 2008;61(6):687–692.
37. Moran SL, Illig KA, Green RM, Serletti JM. Free-tissue transfer in patients with peripheral vascular disease: a 10-year experience. *Plast Reconstr Surg* 2002;109(3):999–1006.
38. Azzawi K, Ismail A, Earl H, et al. Influence of neoadjuvant chemotherapy on outcomes of immediate breast reconstruction. *Plast Reconstr Surg* 2010;126(1):1–11.
39. Fosnot J, Fischer JP, Smartt JM Jr, et al. Does previous chest wall irradiation increase vascular complications in free autologous breast reconstruction? *Plast Reconstr Surg* 2011;127(2):496–504.
40. Halle M, Bodin I, Tornvall P, et al. Timing of radiotherapy in head and neck free flap reconstruction—a study of postoperative complications. *J Plast Reconstr Aesthet Surg* 2009;62(7):889–895.
41. Baumann DP, Crosby MA, Selber JC, et al. Optimal timing of delayed free lower abdominal flap breast reconstruction after postmastectomy radiation therapy. *Plast Reconstr Surg* 2011;127(3):1100–1116.
42. Isenberg JS, Sherman R. Zone of injury: a valid concept in microvascular reconstruction of the traumatized lower limb? *Ann Plast Surg* 1996;36(3):270–272.
43. Lorenzo AR, Lin CH, Lin CH, et al. Selection of the recipient vein in microvascular flap reconstruction of the lower extremity: analysis of 362 free-tissue transfers. *J Plast Reconstr Aesthet Surg* 2011;64(5):649–655.
44. Leong M, Granick MS. Microvascular tissue transfer in a pregnant patient. *J Reconstr Microsurg* 1998;14(6):411–415.
45. Seidenstucker K, Munder B, Richrath P, et al. A prospective study using color flow duplex ultrasonography for abdominal perforator mapping in microvascular breast reconstruction. *Med Sci Monit* 2010;16(8): MT65–MT70.
46. Patel RS, Higgins KM, Enepekides DJ, Hamilton PA. Clinical utility of colour flow Doppler ultrasonography in planning anterolateral thigh flap harvest. *J Otolaryngol Head Neck Surg* 2010;39(5):566–571.
47. Uppal RS, Casaer B, Van Landuyt K, Blondeel P. The efficacy of preoperative mapping of perforators in reducing operative times and complications in perforator flap breast reconstruction. *J Plast Reconstr Aesthet Surg* 2009;62(7):859–864.
48. Sandhu GS, Rezaee RP, Wright K, et al. Time-resolved and bolus-chase MR angiography of the leg: branching pattern analysis and identification of septocutaneous perforators. *AJR Am J Roentgenol* 2010;195(4): 858–864.
49. Masia J, Kosutic D, Cervelli D, et al. In search of the ideal method in perforator mapping: noncontrast magnetic resonance imaging. *J Reconstr Microsurg* 2010;26(1):29–35.
50. Visscher K, Boyd K, Ross DC, et al. Refining perforator selection for DIEP breast reconstruction using transit time flow volume measurements. *J Reconstr Microsurg* 2010;26(5):285–290.
51. Germann G, Steinau HU. The clinical reliability of vein grafts in free-flap transfer. *J Reconstr Microsurg* 1996;12(1):11–17.
52. Lannon DA, Novak CB, Neligan PC. Resurfacing of colour-mismatched free flaps on the face with split-thickness skin grafts from the scalp. *J Plast Reconstr Aesthet Surg* 2009;62(11):1363–1366.
53. Koshima I, Inagawa K, Okuyama N, Moriguchi T. Free vascularized appendix transfer for reconstruction of penile urethras with severe fibrosis. *Plast Reconstr Surg* 1999;103(3):964–969.
54. Houle JM, Neumeister MW. A prefabricated, tissue-engineered Integra free flap. *Plast Reconstr Surg* 2007;120(5):1322–1325.
55. Tsai FC. A new method: perforator-based tissue expansion for a preexpanded free cutaneous perforator flap. *Burns* 2003;29(8):845–848.
56. Van Landuyt K, Blondeel P, Hamdi M, et al. The versatile DIEP flap: its use in lower extremity reconstruction. *Br J Plast Surg* 2005;58(1):2–13.
57. Mahajan AL, Cadeneli PF, Van Waes C, et al. Bipedicled DIEP flaps for reconstruction of soft-tissue deficiencies in male patients. In British Association of Plastic, Reconstructive and Aesthetic Surgeons meeting, Sheffield, UK, 2010.
58. Blondeel PN, Hijjawi J, Depypere H, et al. Shaping the breast in aesthetic and reconstructive breast surgery: an easy three-step principle. Part II—breast reconstruction after total mastectomy. *Plast Reconstr Surg* 2009;123(3): 794–805.
59. Ali RS, Garrido A, Ramakrishnan V. Stacked free hemi-DIEP flaps: a method of autologous breast reconstruction in a patient with midline abdominal scarring. *Br J Plast Surg* 2002;55(4):351–353.
60. Blondeel PN. Aesthetic breast reconstruction; state of the art of perforator flaps. In Second Italian Meeting on Perforator Flaps and Aesthetic Refinements, Bologna, Italy, 2010.
61. Mahajan AL, Sinna R, Van Landuy K. Improving outcome in SGAP flap breast reconstruction. In British Association of Plastic, Reconstructive and Aesthetic Surgeons meeting, Sheffield, UK, 2010.
62. Boca R, Kuo YR, Hsieh CH, et al. A reliable parameter for primary closure of the free anterolateral thigh flap donor site. *Plast Reconstr Surg* 2010;126(5):1558–1562.
63. Selber JC, Nelson J, Fosnot J, et al. A prospective study comparing the functional impact of SIEA, DIEP, and muscle-sparing free TRAM flaps on the abdominal wall: part I. unilateral reconstruction. *Plast Reconstr Surg* 2010;126(4):1142–1153.
64. Blondeel N, Vanderstraeten GG, Monstrey SJ, et al. The donor site morbidity of free DIEP flaps and free TRAM flaps for breast reconstruction. *Br J Plast Surg* 1997;50(5):322–330.
65. Bonde CT, Lund H, Fridberg M, et al. Abdominal strength after breast reconstruction using a free abdominal flap. *J Plast Reconstr Aesthet Surg* 2007;60(5):519–523.
66. Hagau N, Longrois D. Anesthesia for free vascularized tissue transfer. *Microsurgery* 2009;29(2):161–167.
67. Chen C, Nguyen MD, Bar-Meir E, et al. Effects of vasopressor administration on the outcomes of microsurgical breast reconstruction. *Ann Plast Surg* 2010; 65(1):28–31.
68. Blondeel PN, Arnstein M, Verstraete K, et al. Venous congestion and blood flow in free transverse rectus abdominis myocutaneous and deep inferior epigastric perforator flaps. *Plast Reconstr Surg* 2000;106(6): 1295–1299.
69. Hanasono MM, Kocak E, Ogunleye O, et al. One versus two venous anastomoses in microvascular free flap surgery. *Plast Reconstr Surg* 2010; 126(5):1548–1557.

CHAPTER 4

Exposure of Nerves and Vessels

Matthew M. Hanasono

The availability of recipient arteries and veins with sufficient caliber and blood flow within the vicinity of the defect site is paramount to success in microvascular free flap surgery. Dissection of recipient vessels as well as nerves for sensory and motor reinnervation may be difficult given the high density of critical structures within some regions, especially in the face of prior surgery or radiation. Knowledge of regional anatomy is essential to avoiding complications. Additionally, in some cases, adequate local vessels are not available or cannot be dissected without a significant risk for injury to nerves, blood vessels, and vital organs. In these cases, it is necessary to be prepared for the use of alternative vessels in adjacent regions. It is also wise to give some consideration to preserving additional vessels during recipient vessel preparation in case a second free flap is needed at a later date.

HEAD AND NECK

Blood Vessel Anatomy

The branches of the external carotid artery (ECA), from proximal to distal, are the superior thyroid, ascending pharyngeal, lingual, facial, occipital, posterior auricular, superficial temporal, and (internal) maxillary arteries (Figure 4-1). Most commonly, either the superior thyroid artery or the facial artery is selected as the recipient artery when free tissue transfer is performed in the lower two thirds of the head and neck (1,2). The superior thyroid artery arises anteriorly just superior to the carotid bulb. The facial artery arises just after or from a common trunk with the lingual artery and passes beneath the hypoglossal nerve and digastric muscle tendon. From there, it passes behind or through the submandibular gland before it becomes more superficial and ascends the medial cheek. The occipital artery is occasionally useful as a recipient vessel, particularly for occipital scalp and posterior neck reconstructions. It crosses superficial to the internal carotid artery, internal jugular vein (IJV), vagus nerve, and spinal accessory nerve. The ascending pharyngeal artery is not commonly used because it comes off the ECA medially and is usually of very small caliber, as is the posterior auricular artery. The superficial temporal artery is located most cephalad and is often used in reconstruction of the upper third of the face and scalp. The ECA itself may serve as a recipient artery. When possible, this vessel is used as a recipient artery distal to its lower branches to preserve vascularity to the head and neck as well as to save other vessels for future free flaps should they be required.

Venous anatomy in the neck is more variable (Figure 4-2). The IJV originates from the jugular foramen as a continuation of the sigmoid sinus at the skull base and travels medial to the sternocleidomastoid muscle, eventually draining into the subclavian vein. The IJV usually receives multiple branches, including the retromandibular vein, common facial vein, lingual vein, pharyngeal vein, superior thyroid vein, middle thyroid vein, and occipital vein. Many of these branches may share a common origin (3). The external jugular vein (EJV) lies deep to the platysma muscle but superficial to the sternocleidomastoid muscle. It is formed by the junction of a branch of the retromandibular vein and the posterior auricular vein. Use of the anterior jugular vein, which empties into either the EJV or subclavian vein, as a recipient vessel has not been well documented, most likely because of its frequent ligation in neck dissection, low flow, proximity to the tracheostomy site, and susceptibility to flow interruption by compression. Recently, use of the posterolateral cervical vein, which runs beneath the anterior border of the trapezius and drains into the subclavian vein, as a recipient vein has been reported (Figure 4-3) (4).

Nerve Anatomy

The facial nerve exits the intracranial cavity via the stylomastoid foramen. The styloid process, which is palpable inferior to the earlobe, lies posterior and deep to the foramen. After giving

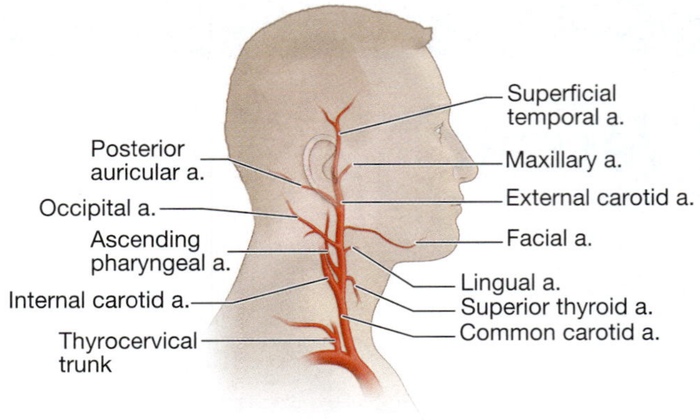

FIGURE 4-1 Head and neck arterial anatomy. Asc ph A, ascending pharyngeal artery; CCA, common carotid artery; ECA, external carotid artery; FA, facial artery; ICA, internal carotid artery; IMA, internal maxillary artery; LA, lingual artery; OA, occipital artery; post auric A, posterior auricular artery; sup temp A, superficial temporal artery; sup thy A, superior thyroid artery; TCA, transverse cervical artery.

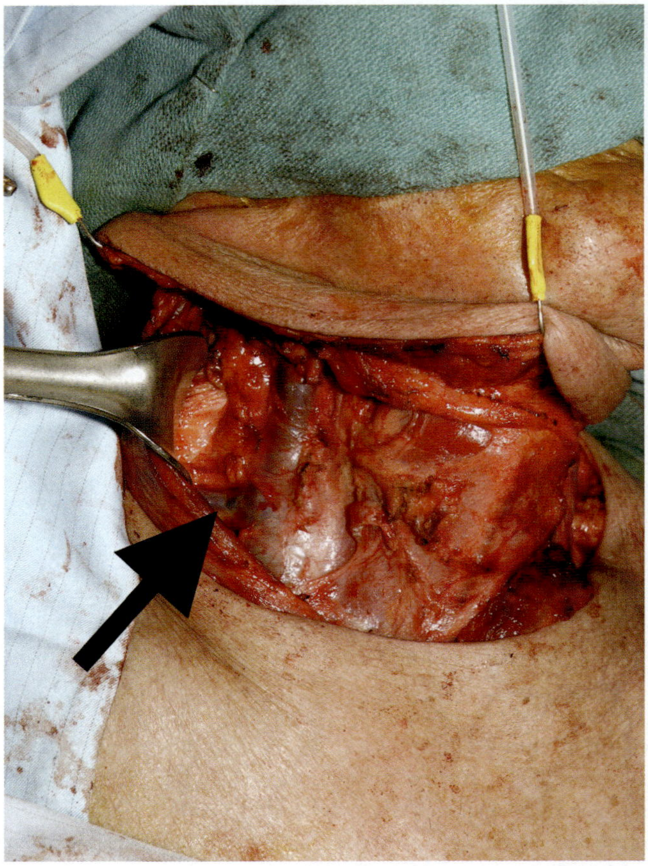

FIGURE 4-3 The posterolateral cervical vein (arrow) arising from the internal jugular vein and lying beneath the trapezius muscle.

off a postauricular motor branch and a motor branch to the posterior body of the digastric muscle, the nerve enters the parenchyma of the parotid gland, where it divides into a superior temporozygomatic division and an inferior cervicofacial division, both of which, in turn, branch multiple times. Although the zygomatic and buccal branches are usually highly redundant and interconnected, the temporal, marginal mandibular, and cervical branches are less so. The branches of the facial nerve innervate 14 of the 17 muscles of facial expression on their deep surface. The three muscles that are supplied on their superficial surfaces are the buccinator, levator anguli oris, and mentalis muscles. The temporal branch (or branches) of the facial nerve is usually identified along an imaginary line connecting a point 0.5 cm inferior to the tragus to a point 1.5 cm above the lateral brow (Pitanguy's line). Most of the temporal branch lies within the superficial temporal fascia. The marginal mandibular branch lies at or below the inferior border of the mandible, deep to the platysma muscle (until it becomes more superficial in the region of the oral commissure) and lies superficial to the facial artery and vein.

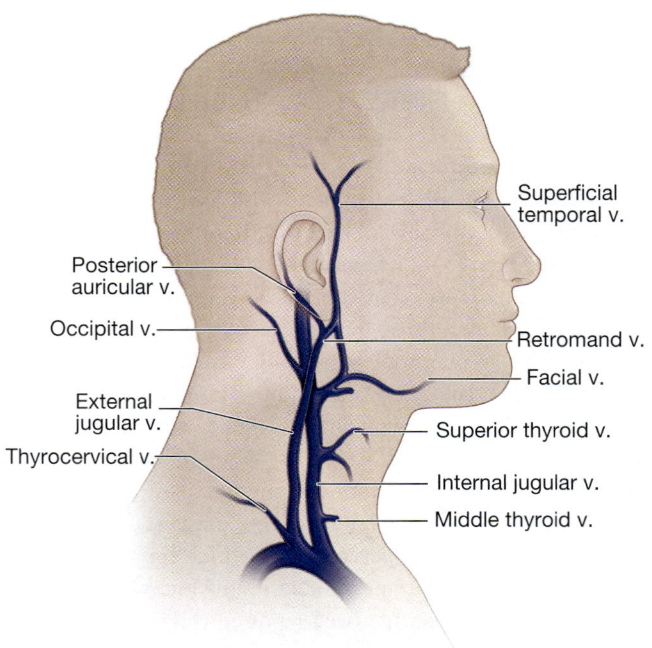

FIGURE 4-2 Head and neck venous anatomy. EJV, external jugular vein; FV, facial vein; IJV, internal jugular vein; mid thy V, middle thyroid vein; OV, occipital vein; post auric V, posterior auricular vein; retromand V, retromandibular vein; sup temp V, superficial temporal vein; sup thy V, superior thyroid vein; TCV, transverse cervical vein.

Blood Vessel Dissection

Recipient vessels are generally well exposed after neck dissection. The facial artery is normally ligated just above the digastric tendon after the submandibular gland has been removed as part of the neck dissection and is usually usable as a recipient artery. It may need to be dissected and transposed from under the digastric muscle and hypoglossal nerve to achieve adequate length and larger caliber. The lingual artery may be another good option for use as a recipient artery, provided the contralateral lingual artery has not been ligated so that adequate blood supply is maintained to the tongue.

The common facial vein is usually ligated and may be available for use as a recipient vein using an end-to-end anastomosis. The EJV is frequently ligated during neck dissections, but the

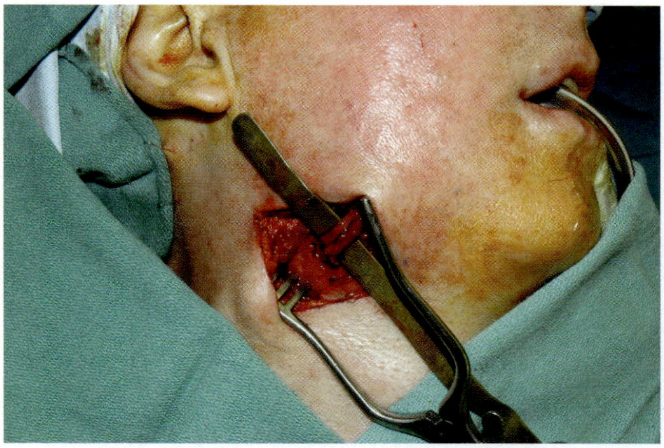

FIGURE 4-4 Exposure of the facial artery and vein at the inferior border of the mandible.

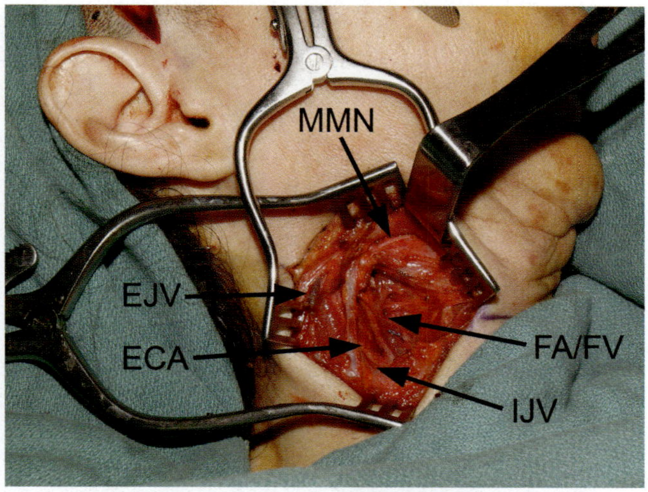

FIGURE 4-5 Cervical exposure demonstrating the external carotid artery (ECA), external jugular vein (EJV), marginal mandibular nerve (MMN), facial artery and vein (FA/FV), and internal jugular vein (IJV).

remnant may also be satisfactory for use as a recipient vein. When the IJV has been ligated, it may still be possible to perform an end-to-end anastomosis to the remaining vein, if the size mismatch is not too great or an end-to-side microvascular anastomosis to the stump if the mismatch is significant (5).

When a concurrent neck dissection has not been performed, a limited access incision just below the inferior border of the mandible over the palpable pulsations of the facial artery may be made and result in exposing the facial artery and vein above the submandibular gland (Figure 4-4). Typically used for midfacial reconstructions, this exposure allows the anastomosis to be performed without need for further dissection of the neck, although the caliber of the facial blood vessels may be small at this level. These vessels lie deep to the platysma muscle, which must be divided. The marginal mandibular nerve is identified crossing the facial vein superficially at a right angle in this region within the superficial layer of the deep cervical fascia and is elevated from the vein and gently retracted out of the way.

For access to the ECA, IJV, and the EJV, a wider transverse incision is made approximately two fingerbreadths below the inferior border of the mandibular body, within a skin crease, if possible (Figure 4-5). Subplatysmal flaps then are elevated. Care is taken to not injure the EJV, which may also be used as a recipient vessel, posteriorly. The common facial vein is identified superficial to the submandibular gland, which is a lobular structure located partially below the lower border of the mandibular body. Again, care is taken to protect the marginal mandibular branch of the facial nerve. The facial artery can be identified above or below the submandibular gland and dissected from the gland to gain length, taking care to control small branches and the associated venous plexus that surrounds the artery in this region. The facial artery and vein may also be used to identify the ECA and IJV by tracing them proximally.

Alternately, the carotid artery and IJV may be directly exposed by retraction of the sternocleidomastoid muscle posteriorly. The spinal accessory nerve will be encountered entering the sternocleidomastoid muscle on its medial surface, superiorly. The IJV is located posterior and lateral within the carotid sheath. The common carotid artery, carotid bulb, and ECA can be identified medial and anterior to the IJV. The vagus nerve, which lies between the IJV and the carotid artery, is carefully preserved. Additionally, the ansa cervicalis, which is a loop of nerves that arise from the hypoglossal nerve anteriorly and the cervical spinal nerves (C2 and C3) posteriorly and supply the strap muscles, should be spared if possible. The ansa cervicalis lies on the superficial surface of the IJV and carotid artery.

For reconstructions of the upper third of the face or the scalp, the superficial temporal vessels are accessed through a separate incision in the preauricular area. This incision is usually zigzagged so that it lies within the preauricular skin crease to minimize visibility of the postoperative scar (Figure 4-6). The pulsations of the superficial temporal artery are usually palpable just anterior to the upper margin of the auricular helix. Careful, atraumatic dissection is important because the superficial temporal vein is thin walled and can easily be damaged. The superficial temporal vessels are usually of small caliber unless they are dissected proximally, into the parenchyma of the parotid gland. Dissection is usually terminated at the level of the tragus to avoid injury to the facial nerve. At this level, the vessels are usually of satisfactory caliber for microvascular anastomosis, averaging 1.8 to 2.7 mm for the artery and 2.1 to 3.3 mm for the vein (6).

Alternative Recipient Vessels

Microvascular reconstruction of head and neck defects is often significantly more challenging in patients who have previously undergone neck dissection or radiation therapy to the neck (7–10). A history of neck dissection or preoperative radiation therapy to the neck may result in the paucity of recipient blood vessels adequate for successful free tissue transfer. Fibrosis and scarring may also make dissection tedious, obliterating tissue planes and increasing the friability of blood vessels. In these cases, dissection of recipient vessels in the contralateral neck or outside the head and neck area may be the safest or the only option.

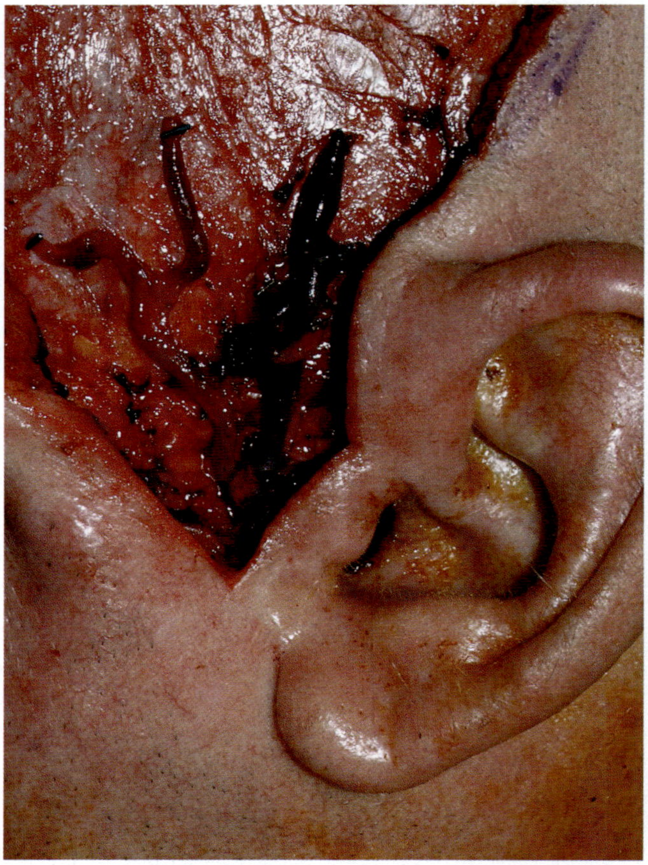

FIGURE 4-6 Exposure of the superficial temporal artery and vein through a preauricular incision.

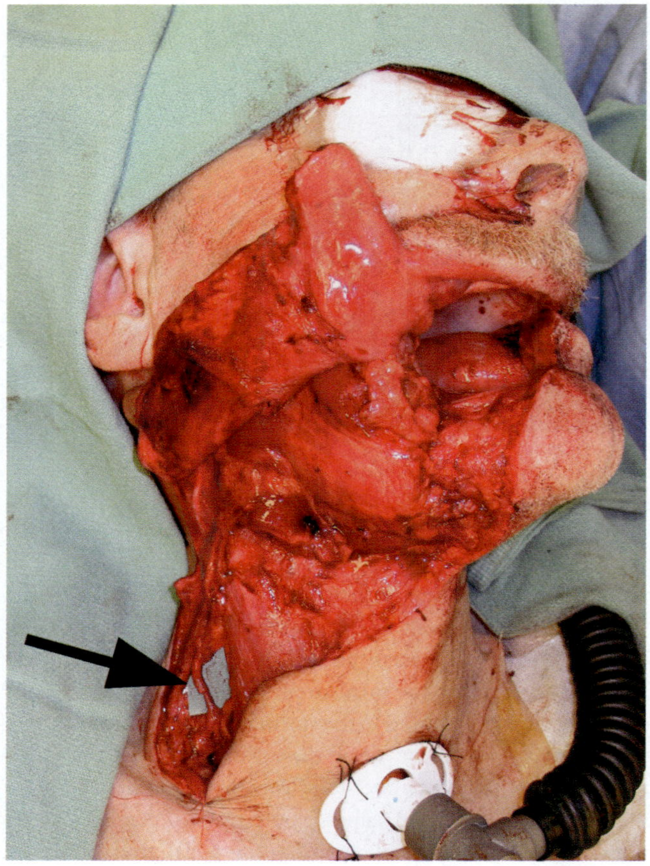

FIGURE 4-7 Use of the transverse cervical artery and vein as recipient vessels.

The use of the transverse cervical artery and vein has proven to be a valuable strategy when the upper cervical vessels cannot be used. The transverse cervical artery arises medially in the neck from the thyrocervical trunk. The transverse cervical artery travels from medial to lateral and then turns inferiorly to supply the trapezius muscle from its deep surface. The transverse cervical vein accompanies the transverse cervical artery and is usually superficial and slightly superior to the artery. The transverse cervical vein drains into the EJV or the subclavian vein. The cervical incision is usually extended with a downward incision in the direction of the ipsilateral acromial process, or a separate supraclavicular incision can be made (Figure 4-7). The omohyoid muscle, which is identified lateral to the posterior border of the sternocleidomastoid muscle and about 2 cm superior to the clavicle, is a surgical landmark for the transverse cervical artery and vein, which lie deep to the muscle within the supraclavicular fatty tissue (11).

The cephalic vein can be a very useful alternative source of venous drainage in head and neck microvascular surgery. Advantages of the cephalic vein are that it requires only a single venous anastomosis (as opposed two anastomoses for an interposition vein graft), provides a long pedicle, lies outside the zone of radiation or prior surgery, and is associated with a generous diameter for microvascular anastomosis (12). The cephalic vein usually identified in the deltopectoral groove and traced distally, anterior to the lateral bicipital groove (Figure 4-8) (12,13).

Use of the internal mammary vessels for head and neck surgery has not commonly been reported but is well-known in breast reconstruction with autologous free tissue transfer (see later discussion) (14). The internal mammary vessels are usually located by removal of the second or third costal cartilage after division of the overlying pectoralis muscle. Inferior to the third rib, the caliber of the vein diminishes significantly and is usually less than 1.5 mm (15).

The thoracoacromial artery and its accompanying vein have also been described as a potential source for recipient vessels in head and neck reconstruction (16,17). The thoracoacromial artery arises from the axillary artery and divides into acromial, deltoid, clavicular, and pectoral branches. The pectoral branch, which lies beneath the pectoralis major muscle within a perivascular fat pad, is most commonly used as a recipient vessel. It lies along a line that is perpendicular to the midpoint of a line connecting the suprasternal notch to the nipple. Use of the pectoral branch of the thoracoacromial trunk for end-to-end anastomoses prevents use of the pedicled pectoralis major flap. However, when the pectoralis major muscle flap has already been transferred and adequate healing has taken place, division and use of the pectoral branches, which remain well preserved within the perivascular fat pad, as recipient vessels is possible (17).

Nerve Dissection

Dissection of the contralateral facial nerve when performing cross-facial nerve grafting before facial reanimation with a neurotized muscle free flap is accomplished through a facelift incision or modified Blair incision (a preauricular incision that

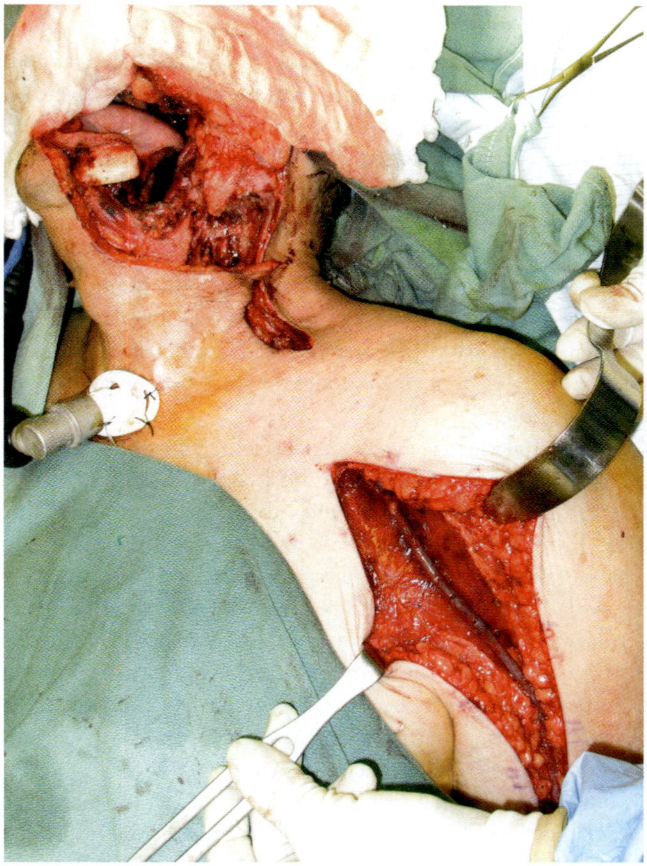

FIGURE 4-8 Harvest of a cephalic vein for recipient vessel anastomosis. The vein is transposed to the neck with care taken not to kink or twist the vessel.

curves anteriorly inferior to the angle of the mandible to lie within a transverse neck crease). The skin is elevated in a plane beneath the superficial musculoaponeurotic system (SMAS), immediately above the parotid fascia. Multiple branches of the facial nerve will be seen arising from the parotid gland. The zygomatic and buccal nerve branches communicate with each other via internuncial branches as they arborize and supply various muscles of facial expression. Therefore, one of the distal branches can be sacrificed after verifying redundant muscle innervation by an adjacent branch with a nerve stimulator. A buccal branch can also be dissected through an intraoral incision or a facial incision in the vicinity of the melolabial crease. More than one branch is identified before transection to ensure redundant innervation of the contralateral facial muscles. The surgeon should also verify that the selected branch results in levator anguli oris muscle movement when stimulated.

When the main trunk of the paralyzed facial nerve must be dissected, the proximal facial nerve is found in the triangle formed by the tragal cartilage (tragal pointer), posterior belly of the digastric muscle, and sternocleidomastoid muscle. The nerve is located about 1 cm inferior and medial to the tragal cartilaginous pointer. The nerve is usually dissected anteriorly to where the temporozygomatic and cervicofacial branches separate from each other by dividing the parotid gland superficial to them, essentially performing a superficial parotidectomy.

When the ipsilateral trigeminal motor nerve is used as the donor nerve for facial reanimation, the branch to the masseter muscle is selected. It is found by retraction of the posterior border of the masseter muscle with selective lysis of muscle fibers. The nerve is seen entering the deep surface of the muscle and travels obliquely toward the oral commissure.

The hypoglossal nerve lies deep and nearly parallel to the posterior belly of the digastric muscle. It crosses lateral to the internal and external carotid arteries, superior to the carotid bulb. Dissection is performed by superior retraction of the submandibular gland. The descendens hypoglossi nerve, which joins cervical fibers to become the ansa cervicalis, can be seen branching from the hypoglossal nerve. Nerve crossover procedures to the facial nerve are performed in an end-to-side or an end-to-end fashion, preserving a portion of the hypoglossal nerve so that tongue motor innervation is maintained.

Potential Complications

Nerve injury to the marginal mandibular branch of the facial nerve, the great auricular or other cervicospinal sensory nerves, the hypoglossal nerve, the ansa cervicalis, the spinal accessory nerve, and the vagus nerves are all potential complications of neck recipient vessel preparation. The spinal accessory nerve originates posterior to the jugular vein, enters the medial surface of the sternocleidomastoid muscle, and exits its posterior border just superior to the great auricular nerve after giving off motor branches to the muscle. Sacrifice of the spinal accessory nerve is debilitating, resulting in shoulder drop, pain in the glenohumeral joint, and weakness with limited movement in the shoulder caused by loss of trapezius muscle function.

The possibility of a chyle leak from either the thoracic duct in the left neck or the accessory thoracic duct in the right neck also exists, particularly when performing dissection of the transverse cervical artery and vein within the supraclavicular region of the neck. If a chyle leak is identified, an attempt may be made to repair it with microvascular suture. Otherwise, the duct is ligated. When a chyle leak is recognized after surgery as an accumulation of milky fluid beneath the skin flap, an attempt may be made to treat it conservatively with closed suction drainage and dietary modifications (a medium-chain triglyceride diet should decrease the volume of chyle) (18). If conservative management is unsuccessful, operative reexploration is indicated.

Care must also be exercised in dissecting the IJV. A large inadvertent venotomy may not only result in severe hemorrhage but also a life-threatening air embolism. Similarly, a gentle technique is required when manipulating the carotid artery. In patients with atherosclerosis, there is risk for dislodging atheromatous plaques, resulting in cerebrovascular insult. Pressure on the carotid bulb may also result in bradycardia or even asystole. Bradycardia usually ceases when manipulation of the carotid bulb stops but can also be remedied by periadventitial injection of 2% lidocaine (19). Finally, although the blood supply to the head and neck is rich and there are multiple interconnections between blood vessels, acute ligation of several branches can result in tissue devascularization, such as bilateral lingual artery ligation resulting in tongue necrosis.

BREAST

Blood Vessel Anatomy

In most centers, the internal mammary blood vessels are the preferred recipient vessels for microvascular breast reconstruction. The internal mammary artery (IMA) arises from the subclavian artery, although it occasionally has a common origin with the thyrocervical trunk, scapular artery, dorsal scapular artery, thyroid artery, or costocervical trunk. It courses caudally under the brachiocephalic vein, lying on the surface of the pleura, and gives off branches at each intercostal space. At the level of the sixth intercostal space or the seventh costal cartilage, the IMA divides into the superior epigastric and musculophrenic arteries. The IMA is usually located 11 to 13 mm from the lateral border of the sternum (20, 21). In the vicinity of the second or third costal cartilage, the internal mammary veins coalesce into a single vein. When two veins are present, the medial vein is usually larger. When accessed at a level where the two veins have come together, the single vein usually lies medial to the artery and is usually larger on the right side of the chest. Below the sixth intercostal space or seventh costal cartilage, the internal mammary vein may exist as a venous plexus.

The thoracodorsal and circumflex scapular arteries arise from the subscapular artery, which in turn arises from the axillary artery. The circumflex scapular artery travels through the triangular space formed by the long head of the triceps, teres major, and teres minor muscles and ultimately becomes a cutaneous blood vessel. The thoracodorsal artery divides into a serratus anterior branch (or branches) and a latissimus dorsi branch. The serratus anterior branch of the thoracodorsal artery lies on the superficial surface of the serratus anterior muscle and supplies the lower four to six slips of the muscle. The latissimus dorsi branch of the thoracodorsal artery enters the latissimus dorsi muscle on its deep surface.

Nerve Anatomy

Nerves in the chest region available for creating sensate breast reconstructions include the intercostobrachial nerve, lateral cutaneous branches of the intercostal nerves, and anterior cutaneous branches of the intercostal nerves (22,23). The intercostobrachial nerve arises laterally from the second intercostal nerve. Unlike the subsequent lateral cutaneous branches, it does not divide into anterior and posterior branches but instead crosses the axilla to the medial side of the arm, receiving fibers from the medial brachial cutaneous nerve, and supplies the skin of the upper half of the medial and posterior part of the arm, communicating also with the posterior brachial cutaneous branch of the radial nerve. The other intercostal nerves send anterior and posterior lateral cutaneous branches that arise from the intercostal space just beneath each rib in the anterior axillary line, usually between the serratus anterior muscle insertions onto the ribs. They are accompanied by posterior intercostal arteries and veins. The parasternal anterior cutaneous nerves penetrate the intercostal muscles just lateral to the internal mammary vessel perforators.

Blood Vessel Exposure

To expose the internal mammary blood vessels, pectoralis major muscle fibers are divided over the third costal cartilage. The perichondrium of the third rib is incised along its superficial surface and separated from the costal cartilage using a periosteal elevator. The cartilage is then detached from the rib and sternum using rongeurs. The deep perichondrium is then elevated from lateral to medial, taking care not to avulse vascular branches arising from or draining into the internal mammary vessels (Figure 4-9). Because of the delicate nature of the internal mammary vessels and their side branches, this dissection should be performed under loupe or even microscope magnification.

The costal cartilage may also be left in position, and the internal mammary vessels may be isolated in the interspace between the second and third ribs or the third and fourth ribs (24). In this case, the pectoralis major muscle is split in the region of the selected interspace, and the intercostal muscles are exposed. The intercostal muscles are dissected from the costal cartilages and elevated from lateral to medial, beginning about 2 to 3 cm from the lateral border of the sternum. Dissection must be done with care because there are usually more branches arising from the internal mammary vessels in the interspace than underneath the costal cartilage.

Finally, the internal mammary perforators, which pierce the medial portion of the pectoralis major muscle to supply the chest skin, may also be used as recipient blood vessels. The internal mammary perforator arteries are smaller in diameter (mean, 1.9 mm) than the internal mammary arteries (mean, 2.6 mm), but the internal mammary perforator veins are similar in diameter to the internal mammary vein (25). Perforators in the second or third intercostal space are most frequently used for breast reconstruction. The perforator vessels may be dissected intramuscularly to obtain greater length and may be of larger caliber more proximal to the main internal mammary blood vessels themselves.

Following an axillary dissection, the thoracodorsal vessels are usually exposed and require little additional dissection. The thoracodorsal nerve usually runs anterior to the blood vessels

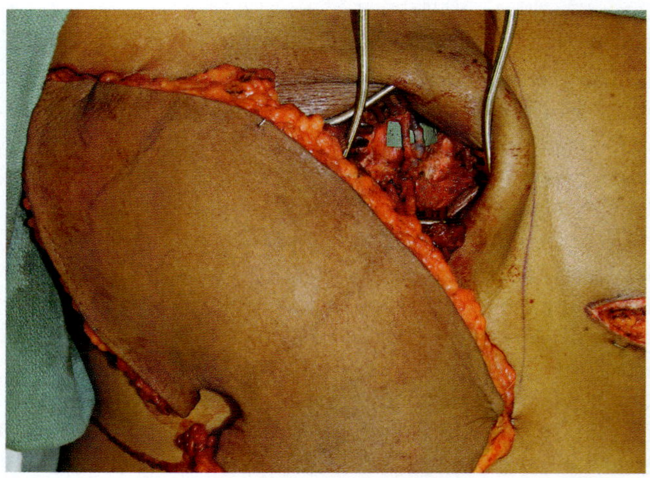

FIGURE 4-9 Internal mammary artery and vein as recipient blood vessels for breast reconstruction with a microvascular free flap.

and should be carefully preserved. If an axillary dissection has not been performed, the axillary fat is dissected off the chest wall, beginning immediately posterior to the lateral border of the pectoralis major muscle. The lateral thoracic vein is usually encountered within the axillary fat and can be traced proximally to the axillary vein. Dissection within the axillary fat posterior to the origin of the lateral thoracic vein usually reveals the proximal portion of the thoracodorsal artery and vein, as well as the thoracodorsal nerve. Self-retaining retractors can be helpful in the deep portion of the axilla. The thoracodorsal vessels are traced along the deep surface of the latissimus dorsi muscle. Intramuscular dissection can be performed to increase pedicle length. Occasionally, the serratus branch of the thoracodorsal artery is sufficiently large for microvascular anastomosis. Using this vessel has the potential of leaving the thoracodorsal artery intact in case a pedicled latissimus flap becomes necessary later—the latissimus "lifeboat." Another way of preserving this option is by dividing the thoracodorsal vessels proximal to the take-off of the serratus branch and performing the anastomoses there. This leaves intact the communication between the serratus branch and the thoracodorsal artery distal to its division and thus offers the prospect of elevating the latissimus flap based on retrograde flow from the serratus branch (26).

Alternative Recipient Vessels

When the internal mammary vessels and the thoracodorsal vessels are not options as recipient vessels or additional vessels are needed for a second flap or secondary pedicle, several options exist. Both the lateral thoracic vessels and the thoracoacromial vessels can be used as additional sources of blood supply. As mentioned, the lateral thoracic vessels lie against the chest wall, proximally beneath the lateral portion of the pectoralis major muscle. The lateral thoracic artery is a direct branch off the axillary artery and runs alongside the long thoracic nerve. There is an accompanying lateral thoracic vein that empties into the axillary vein. The lateral thoracic artery is of smaller caliber than the thoracodorsal artery; the lateral thoracic vein is usually of larger caliber than the thoracodorsal vein. The location of the thoracoacromial vessels is as described earlier for head and neck reconstruction. In terms of an additional source of venous drainage alone, the cephalic vein can also be used, as in the head and neck. The vein is most easily identified by making an incision in the region of the anterior axillary fold and locating the vein within the deltopectoral groove. After sufficient length has been obtained, the vessel is transposed into the breast pocket and the axillary incision closed. Finally, the distal IMA has been used clinically and appears to supply adequate flow in the retrograde direction to satisfactorily perfuse a free flap. The internal mammary vein can also accommodate retrograde flow via the distal vein (27).

Nerve Exposure

The intercostobrachial nerve is identified in the axilla. It courses transversely in the superficial portion of the axillary fibrofatty tissue, superficial to the thoracodorsal vessels and nerve. There are several branches of this nerve, and any of these branches may be used for sensory coaptation. The lateral cutaneous nerves are segmental nerves arising from each intercostal space, with the exception of the second intercostal space, from which the intercostobrachial nerve arises. They are branches of the intercostal nerves, which run inferior to each rib, and pierce the chest wall musculature in the region of the midaxillary line. The anterior cutaneous nerves are also branches of the intercostal nerves and pierce the chest wall musculature lateral to the sternal border and the internal mammary perforating blood vessels (26,27).

Potential Complications

Pneumothorax is a potential complication of internal mammary vessel harvest. A small tear in the pleura can sometimes be repaired directly with sutures. Before tying the sutures, a small flexible catheter (e.g., "red rubber" urinary catheter) is inserted through the tear and placed under suction to evacuate air from the pleural space and withdrawn as the sutures are tightened. More significant pleural injuries may require placement of a chest tube.

UPPER LIMB

Blood Vessel Anatomy

The brachial artery is a continuation of the axillary artery beyond the lower margin of the teres minor muscle. The brachial artery courses medially in a midaxial position adjacent to the humerus in the anterior compartment of the upper arm (Figure 4-10). The profunda brachii artery arises from the posterior surface of the brachial artery. It splits into the radial collateral artery and the middle collateral artery, which course anterior and posterior to the medial humeral epicondyle, respectively. The radial collateral artery anastomoses with the radial recurrent artery, arising from the radial artery in the forearm. The middle collateral artery anastomoses with the interosseous recurrent artery, arising from the common interosseous artery. The brachial artery also gives off the superior ulnar collateral and, more distally, the inferior ulnar collateral artery, which anastomose with the posterior and anterior recurrent ulnar arteries, respectively. Along with the distal branches of the profunda brachii artery, these vessels form a rich anastomotic network of small vessels anterior and posterior to the elbow joint. Distal to the elbow, the brachial artery bifurcates into the radial and ulnar arteries.

The radial and ulnar arteries lie on the anterior surface of the forearm, laterally and medially, respectively. The radial artery lies between the brachioradialis and flexor pollicis longus muscles. The artery winds laterally around the wrist, passing through the anatomic snuffbox and between the heads of the first dorsal interosseous muscle. It passes anteriorly between the heads of the adductor pollicis muscle and joins the deep branch of the ulnar artery to form the deep palmar arch. The ulnar artery reaches the medial side of the forearm about halfway between the elbow and the wrist. It courses between the flexor carpi ulnaris and the flexor digitorum profundus and superficialis muscles. It then crosses the transverse carpal ligament on

CHAPTER 4

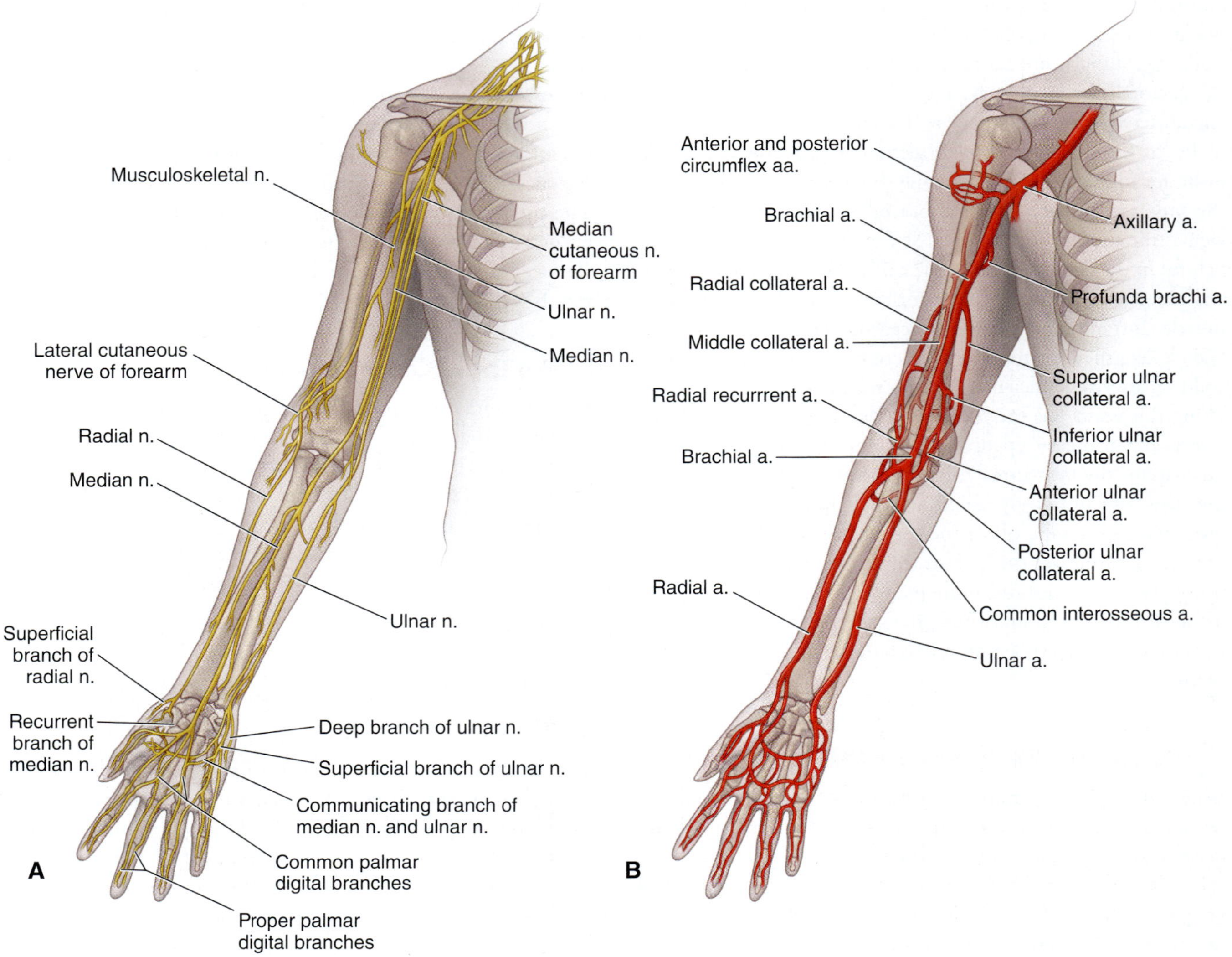

FIGURE 4-10 Arteries and nerves of the upper extremity. a, artery; n, nerve.

the radial side of the pisiform bone in the wrist and divides into the ulnar portions of the superficial and deep palmar arches.

The common interosseous artery arises from the proximal ulnar artery. It immediately divides into anterior and posterior interosseous arteries, which travel in the extensor and flexor compartments of the forearm, respectively. A third branch of the common interosseous artery, the recurrent interosseous artery, anastomoses with the profunda brachii artery in the upper arm, as mentioned earlier.

The arteries of the upper extremity are accompanied by venae comitantes, which ultimately drain into the brachial vein. In addition to the venae comitantes, there is a system of veins that lie superficial to the deep fascia. The two main veins of this superficial system are the cephalic and basilic veins. The cephalic vein originates at the level of the anatomic snuffbox in the wrist, travels along the radial dorsal border of the forearm and the anterolateral surface of the biceps brachii muscle into the deltopectoral groove of the shoulder, and ultimately empties into the axillary vein. The basilic vein originates on the ulnar side of the dorsal venous network of the hand and travels along the medial surface of the forearm and arm until it pierces the deep fascia, about halfway between the elbow and shoulder, to join with the anterior and posterior circumflex humeral veins before joining the brachial vein to form the axillary vein. The cephalic and basilic veins communicate in the region of the cubital fossa via the median cubital vein.

Nerve Anatomy

The median nerve is formed by contributions from the lateral and medial cords of the brachial plexus in the axilla and travels within the anterior compartment of the arm. Proximally, the median nerve lies lateral to the brachial artery. Distally, the median nerve crosses anterior to the brachial artery and assumes a position medial to it. As it approaches the cubital fossa, the median nerve is covered by the lacertus fibrosis (bicipital aponeurosis) (28,29). The nerve passes out of the cubital fossa between the humeral and ulnar heads of the pronator teres muscle. The median nerve does not give off branches within the arm.

In the forearm, the median nerve gives off the anterior interosseous nerve (AIN) just after it exits between the heads of the pronator teres muscle. The AIN supplies the flexor pollicis longus, the lateral half of the flexor digitorum profundus, and the pronator quadratus muscles as well as sending articular branches to the wrist and carpal joints. The median nerve then passes behind the flexor superficialis arch and comes to lie deep on the volar surface of the forearm between the flexor digitorum superficialis and flexor digitorum profundus muscles. About 5 cm proximal to the transverse carpal ligament, the median nerve becomes superficial to the flexor digitorum superficialis muscle bellies and lies between the flexor digitorum superficialis and flexor carpi radialis muscle tendons. The median nerve then passes into the carpal tunnel after which it divides into a number of branches that supply sensation and motor function to the hand.

The ulnar nerve is a terminal branch of the medial cord of the brachial plexus. It enters the arm on the medial side of the brachial artery but leaves the flexor compartment about halfway down the upper arm by piercing the medial intermuscular septum. Similar to the median nerve, the ulnar nerve has no motor branches in the upper arm. Continuing between the septum and the medial head of the triceps muscle, it enters the cubital tunnel, which lies along the groove on the posterior aspect of the medial epicondyle of the humerus. The floor of the tunnel is made up of the ulnar collateral ligament of the elbow and the roof of the tunnel is Osborne's ligament, an aponeurotic band that spans the medial humeral epicondyle and the olecranon (30).

After exiting the cubital tunnel, the ulnar nerve enters the forearm between the humeral and ulnar heads of the flexor carpi ulnaris muscle. Similar to Osborne's ligament, the arcuate ligament, which connects the two heads of the flexor carpi ulnaris muscle, is a potential site of ulnar nerve compression. The nerve is joined in the forearm by the ulnar artery. Within the forearm, the ulnar nerve sends motor branches to the flexor carpi ulnaris and the medial half of the flexor digitorum profundus muscles, as well as gives rise to a palmar cutaneous branch that then supplies the medial palm, and a dorsal branch that passes medially, deep to the flexor carpi ulnaris muscle to reach the dorsal aspect of the hand. At the wrist, the ulnar nerve enters Guyon's canal, which is a depression between the pisiform bone and the hook of the hamate that is covered by the volar carpal ligament and the pisohamate ligament (31). Within Guyon's canal, the ulnar nerve divides into deep and superficial branches, which supply sensory and motor innervation to the hand.

The radial nerve is a terminal branch of the posterior cord of the brachial plexus. Initially lying on the posterior wall of the axilla, the radial nerve travels under the lower border of the teres major muscle through the triangular interval, which is formed by this muscle, the long head of the triceps muscle, and the shaft of the humerus. The radial nerve travels posteriorly around the humerus in a spiral groove between the attachments of the lateral and medial heads of the triceps muscle. It is in this region that the radial nerve is susceptible to injury when a humeral fracture occurs. The radial nerve is first joined by the profunda brachii artery after the triangular interval and then by the radial collateral artery in the spiral groove. About two-thirds of the way down the arm, the radial nerve reaches the lateral side of the humerus and pierces the lateral intermuscular septum, entering the anterior compartment of the arm. Within the arm, the radial nerve supplies the triceps and anconeus muscles via proximal medial muscular branches and the brachioradialis and extensor carpi radialis longus muscles via distal lateral muscular branches.

The radial nerve enters the flexor compartment in the lower part of the arm and passes into the forearm beneath the brachioradialis muscle. After it enters the forearm, the radial nerve immediately divides into a superficial and a deep branch. The deep branch passes laterally around the radius between the fibers of the supinator and reaches the extensor compartment where it becomes the posterior interosseous nerve (PIN), which gives off numerous motor branches to supply all of the muscles on the radial and dorsal surface of the forearm, except the anconeus, brachioradialis, and extensor carpi radialis longus muscles, and then terminates at the dorsal wrist (32). The superficial branch continues deep to the brachioradialis muscle and is joined on its medial side by the radial artery at the junction of the upper and middle thirds of the forearm (33). In the lower third of the forearm, it passes through the brachioradialis muscle and supplies sensation to the wrist and dorsal hand. The radial nerve gives off several other sensory branches, including the posterior cutaneous nerve of the arm, the lateral cutaneous nerve of the arm, and posterior cutaneous nerve of the forearm.

Blood Vessel Dissection

In the upper arm, the brachial artery and vein are usually the simplest choices for recipient vessels. They are exposed by simply making a longitudinal incision in the medial arm between the biceps and triceps brachii muscles (Figure 4-11).

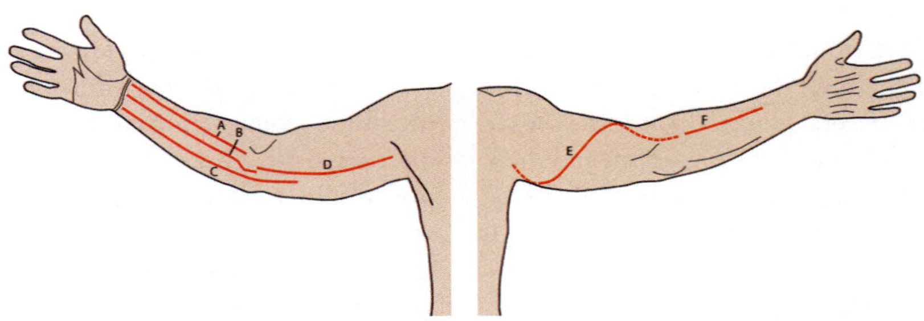

FIGURE 4-11 Incisions for upper extremity vessels and nerves. (**A**) Radial artery and radial nerve in the forearm. (**B**) Median nerve and anterior interosseous nerve in the forearm. (**C**) Ulnar artery and nerve at the elbow and forearm. (**D**) Brachial artery and vein and median and ulnar nerves. (**E**) Radial nerve in the arm. (**F**) Radial nerve in the forearm.

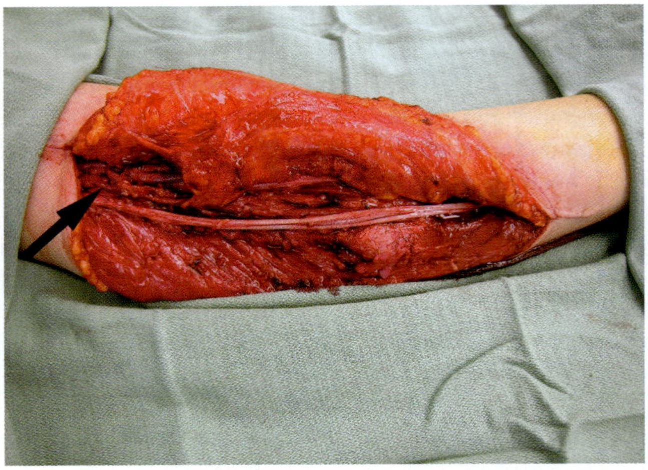

FIGURE 4-12 Brachial artery and vein as recipient blood vessels using an end-to-side anastomosis (arrow) for free flap reconstruction of a medial arm wound.

Distally, the brachial artery is located anterior to the elbow and medial to the biceps tendon, where its pulse is easily palpated. The vein lies medial and posterior to the artery. Because the brachial artery is the major blood supply to the arm, a branch must be used or an end-to-side anastomosis must be performed (Figure 4-12).

The collateral arteries may be used end to end but are often of small caliber and may not be accompanied by suitable venae comitantes for microvascular anastomosis. If the collateral vessels are used, it is often simplest to use one of the superficial veins for the venous anastomosis. The superior ulnar collateral artery lies medially in the posterior compartment. The radial collateral artery, which lies in the lateral arm, may be useful for lateral defects.

The posterior circumflex humeral artery, a branch of the axillary artery, is also a useful recipient vessel. Sacrifice of this vessel does not compromise limb perfusion. The posterior circumflex humeral artery travels through the quadrangular space with the axillary nerve between the teres minor and major superiorly and inferiorly, respectively, and the lateral head of the triceps and the medial humeral border medially and laterally, respectively. Although the posterior circumflex humeral artery is deep, it is readily identified and large in caliber. The anterior circumflex humeral artery tends to be of small caliber and must be tediously dissected beneath the coracobrachialis and biceps muscles.

Both the radial and ulnar arteries are palpable in the wrist and can be traced backward from there toward the medial elbow where they originate from the brachial artery. The radial artery runs deep to the brachioradialis muscle proximally for about two thirds the length of the forearm and then becomes more superficial, lying just deep to the fascia between the brachioradialis and flexor carpi radialis tendons distally. The radial artery can be exposed by making an incision of the appropriate length along a line that connects the midpoint of the cubital fossa to the palpable radial pulse at the wrist.

In the proximal half of the forearm, the ulnar artery is deeply seated, being covered by the pronator teres, flexor carpi radialis, palmaris longus, and flexor digitorum superficialis muscles, but lies above the brachialis and flexor digitorum profundus muscles. In the distal half of the forearm, the ulnar artery lies between the flexor carpi ulnaris and flexor digitorum superficialis muscles and their tendons. The ulnar artery can be exposed by making an incision of the appropriate length along a line that connects the medial epicondyle to the pisiform bone. Care must be taken during ulnar artery dissection not to injure the ulnar nerve.

The radial or ulnar artery is most commonly used as a recipient vessel in the forearm. An end-to-end anastomosis is acceptable provided the palmar arches are patent as evidenced by a normal Allen's test result or angiography when physical findings are equivocal. The venae comitantes of the radial or ulnar arteries can be used as recipient veins. If larger caliber veins are needed, the cephalic or basilic veins can be located through the same incision used to expose the radial or ulnar arteries, respectively. The cephalic vein usually lies lateral to the radial artery, and the basilic vein usually lies medial to the ulnar artery, both within the superficial subcutaneous fat, above the deep fascia of the forearm.

Nerve Dissection

The median nerve is closely associated with the brachial artery in the arm. It can be exposed through an incision along the medial aspect of the upper arm within the bicipital groove, as can the ulnar nerve, musculocutaneous nerve, and the brachial artery and vein. Distally, the median nerve crosses anterior to the brachial artery and comes to lie on its medial side anterior to the elbow joint.

The operative approach to the median nerve in the forearm is a longitudinal incision along the medial border of the biceps brachii muscle in the distal upper arm, curving transversely at the elbow flexion crease, then along the distal medial border of the pronator teres muscle, continuing to the wrist crease. Distally, the incision can be extended obliquely toward the ring finger. The safe side of the median nerve in the proximal forearm is the radial side because its branches come off the ulnar side. The median nerve is often best identified proximal to the lacertus fibrosis and then traced distally through the region of the pronator teres muscle and the superficial flexor arch.

The approach to the ulnar nerve at the elbow is through a posteromedial longitudinal incision, which may be curved or zigzagged. The ulnar nerve should be freed for at least 8 cm proximal to the medial epicondyle to ensure release from the arcade of Struthers, which is a thin aponeurotic band extending from the medial head of the triceps to the medial intermuscular septum, if it is to be transposed or otherwise placed under tension to prevent nerve compression by this structure. The ulnar collateral artery accompanies the ulnar nerve in the condylar groove. Exposure in the forearm is via a straight or "lazy S" incision along the line connecting the pisiform to the medial epicondyle. Throughout the forearm, the ulnar nerve travels beneath the flexor carpi ulnaris muscle. Exposure is achieved by separating the flexor carpi ulnaris from the flexor digitorum superficialis muscle. The ulnar artery lies directly medial to the nerve in the lower two thirds of the forearm.

To prevent contractures, exposure of the median and ulnar nerves in the wrist and palm should not cross the flexor crease at 90 degrees. Proximal and distal to the wrist crease, longitudinal incisions should be used to avoid injury to the cutaneous nerve branches. The carpal tunnel ligament should be opened on the ulnar side, radial to the hook of the hamate, to avoid injury to the motor branch of the median nerve, which comes off the radial side. Entry to Guyon's canal is also via this exposure. If the motor branch to the median nerve is transligamentous, it must be released to prevent traction palsy.

The radial nerve is exposed by separating the long and lateral heads of the triceps. By moving the muscle bellies from side to side, the entire course of the radial nerve can be visualized. The radial nerve stays in close proximity to the humerus as it travels on top of the spiral groove. Distally in the arm, it pierces an intermuscular septum between the brachioradialis and brachialis muscles.

In the lower arm and forearm, the radial nerve can be exposed through an incision that begins between the brachialis and the brachioradialis muscles and extends dorsally into the forearm between the extensor carpi radialis brevis and the extensor digitorum communis muscles, which are most easily identified distally initially, and then dissected from each other proximally. Reflection of the brachioradialis muscle laterally allows identification of the radial nerve deep to the muscle. Care must be taken to minimize lateral muscle dissection, which could injure the motor branches to the muscle. Multiple motor branches and the posterior antebrachial cutaneous nerve branch from the radial nerve can be visualized through this exposure. The PIN is usually located on the proximal side of the supinator muscle about 5 cm distal to the tip of the lateral condyle of the humerus, although its location is variable. The PIN enters the supinator through a fibrous arch formed by the thickened edge of the proximal superficial head of the supinator, termed the *arcade of Frohse*.

Potential Complications

In the case of both the upper and lower extremities, distal vascular compromise secondary to surgical manipulation of critical blood vessels for microvascular anastomoses is the primary concern. Preoperative angiography should strongly be considered in the presence of abnormal physical findings (e.g., abnormal or equivocal Allen's test) or a history of trauma or prior surgery. Whenever possible, expendable blood vessels should be used as recipient vessels, or an end-to-side anastomosis should be performed. If an end-to-side anastomosis is not feasible, use of a "flow-through" free flap may be another way of maintaining adequate distal perfusion. Also, in the setting of prior trauma, delayed thrombosis caused by previously undetected vessel injury may occur. Resecting the recipient blood vessel beyond the zone of injury or use of alternative recipient vessels outside the zone of injury should be performed. In some cases, the extent of injury is difficult to judge even with preoperative angiography. Use of a "backup" venous anastomosis to a separate recipient vein is one way to help ensure against venous compromise. For example, anastomosis of one of the free flap pedicle vena comitans to the vena comitans of the recipient artery and anastomosis of the other free flap pedicle vena comitans to a superficial vein might be performed to decrease the likelihood of flap failure caused by gradual venous thrombosis secondary to undetected recipient vessel damage by blunt force trauma.

LOWER LIMB

Blood Vessel Anatomy

The external iliac artery becomes the common femoral artery (CFA) at the inguinal ligament. It usually divides into the superficial femoral artery (SFA) and the profunda femoris artery several centimeters distal to the inguinal ligament, although it may occasionally divide proximal to the ligament (Figure 4-13). The SFA passes through the femoral triangle; courses through the subsartorial (Hunter's) canal; and ends at the adductor magnus hiatus, where it becomes the popliteal artery. The lateral femoral circumflex artery (LCFA) arises laterally from the profunda femoris artery about 1.5 cm distal to the branching point of the SFA and the profunda femoris artery and further divides in to ascending, transverse, and descending branches. The medial femoral circumflex artery (MCFA) arises posterolaterally from the profunda femoris artery at about the same level as the LCFA. Rarely, the LCFA and MCFA may arise directly from the CFA. The profunda femoris artery also gives off four branches that perforate the adductor magnus muscle.

The popliteal artery runs through the popliteal fossa, a diamond-shaped space bounded superiorly by the semitendinosus and semimembranosus muscles (medial) and biceps femoris muscle (lateral) and inferiorly by the two heads of the gastrocnemius muscle and the plantaris muscle. The popliteal artery gives off multiple branches, including the sural arteries, which supply the gastrocnemius muscle, and the two superior, one middle, and two inferior genicular arteries. At the inferior border of the popliteal fossa, the popliteal artery divides into the anterior and posterior tibial arteries. The posterior tibial artery, also called the tibioperoneal trunk at this point, then gives rise to the peroneal artery.

The anterior tibial artery lies within the anterior compartment of the lower leg, between the extensor hallucis longus (lateral) and tibialis anterior muscle (medial), just anterior to the interosseous membrane between the tibia and fibula bones. At the ankle, it passes deep to the extensor retinaculum midway between the medial and lateral malleoli. The anterior tibial artery then becomes the dorsalis pedis artery and runs lateral to the tendon of the extensor hallucis longus muscle.

The posterior tibial and peroneal arteries are located within the posterior compartment of the lower leg. The posterior tibial artery lies anterior to the soleus muscle and posterior to the tibialis posterior muscle. Distally, it lies medial to the Achilles tendon and can be palpated posterior to the medial malleolus. The medial and lateral plantar arteries arise from the posterior

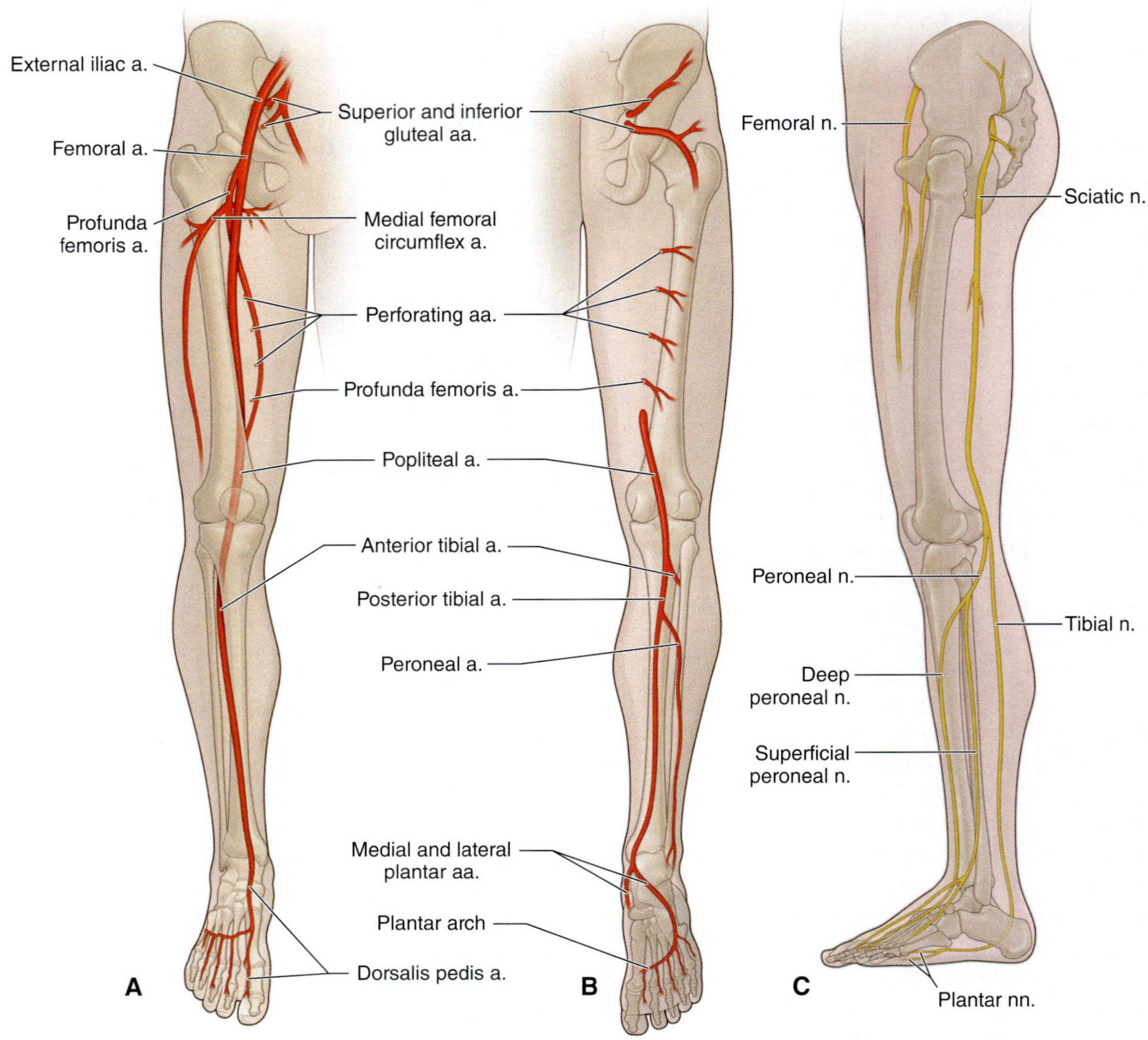

FIGURE 4-13 Arteries and nerves of the lower extremity. a, artery; n, nerve.

tibial artery in the foot. The peroneal artery runs medial to the fibula bone. The peroneal artery becomes the lateral calcaneal artery when it reaches the lateral surface of the calcaneus. The peroneal artery is the sole or dominant blood supply to the foot up to 5% of the time, in which case it is called the peronea magna artery (34).

A deep venous system parallels the lower extremity arterial system as venae comitantes of the major arteries. Analogous to the upper extremity, a superficial venous system runs above the deep fascia of the lower extremity in the subcutaneous tissue. The superficial system drains into the deep system via perforating veins or into the lesser and greater saphenous veins. The lesser saphenous vein drains the lateral side of the dorsal venous arch of the foot and runs posterior to the lateral malleolus and anterior to the Achilles tendon at the ankle. It then moves toward the posterior midline of the leg. It drains into the popliteal vein, either by penetrating the deep fascia in the upper third of the leg or in the popliteal fossa. The greater saphenous vein drains the medial side of the dorsal venous arch of the foot and runs anterior to the medial malleolus, medial to the tibia, passes posterior the medial femoral condyle, and eventually passes through an opening in the fascia lata of the anterior thigh emptying into the femoral vein.

Nerve Anatomy

The femoral nerve is the largest branch of the lumbar plexus and arises from the dorsal divisions of the ventral rami of the second, third, and fourth lumbar nerves. It emerges from beneath the inguinal ligament, lateral to the CFA, which is lateral to the common femoral vein (CFV), and splits into anterior and posterior divisions. The anterior division gives off anterior cutaneous and muscular branches to the pectineus and sartorius muscles. The posterior division gives off the long saphenous nerve, which supplies sensation to the medial leg, muscular branches to the quadriceps muscle, and articular branches to the knee joint. The long saphenous nerve travels lateral to the greater saphenous vein in the leg.

The sciatic nerve is the largest nerve in the body and arises from spinal nerves L4 to S3. It gives off articular branches to the hip joint and muscular branches to the biceps femoris, semitendinosus, semimembranosus, and adductor magnus muscles in the thigh. The muscular branch continues in the lower leg as the tibial nerve and common peroneal nerve. The sciatic nerve leaves the pelvis through the greater sciatic notch, inferior to the piriformis muscle, and is accompanied by the inferior gluteal artery. It is covered superficially by the gluteus maximus and crosses the hip joint.

Before entering the popliteal fossa, the common peroneal nerve branches from the tibial nerve, which begins lateral but comes to lie on top of (posterior to) the popliteal artery and vein. The tibial nerve then travels anterior to the soleus and comes to lie alongside the posterior tibial artery and veins. Eventually, the tibial nerve exits from beneath the arch of the soleus muscle and moves medially to pass behind the medial malleolus posterior to the posterior tibial vessels. The tibial nerve supplies the gastrocnemius, popliteus, soleus, and plantaris muscles; provides an articular branch to the knee; and forms the medial sural cutaneous nerve, which also receives some fibers from the common peroneal nerve to become the sural nerve. Below the soleus muscle, the nerve supplies the tibialis posterior, flexor digitorum longus, and flexor hallucis longus muscles. The tibial nerve divides into the medial and lateral plantar nerves, which supply various muscles of the foot as well as cutaneous sensation.

The common peroneal nerve is found beneath the lateral border of the popliteal fossa, where it gives off the lateral sural cutaneous nerve to the skin of the calf and a communicating branch to the medial sural cutaneous nerve, as well as articular branches. It follows the biceps femoris toward the head of the fibula, which it winds around obliquely. Beneath the peroneus longus muscle, it divides into the superficial peroneal nerve and the deep peroneal nerve. The superficial peroneal nerve innervates the peroneus longus and brevis muscles and supplies sensation to the dorsum of the foot. The deep peroneal nerve innervates the muscles of the anterior compartment, including the tibialis anterior muscle and the toe extensors.

As mentioned, the sural nerve results from the junction of fibers from the tibial and common peroneal nerves via the medial and lateral sural cutaneous nerves, respectively. It travels superficial to the deep fascia of the leg along the lateral border of the Achilles tendon. At the ankle, it lies in the groove between the lateral malleolus and the calcaneus. It continues in the foot as the lateral dorsal cutaneous nerve. It is responsible for sensory innervation of the lateral leg and dorsal lateral foot and ankle, including the dorsum of the fifth digit.

Blood Vessel Exposure

For reconstruction of the thigh, the common and superficial femoral, profunda femoris, lateral or medial circumflex femoral vessels, and their branches are all potential recipients. The CFA can be palpated below the inguinal ligament halfway between the anterior superior iliac spine and the pubic symphysis. The CFV is medial to the CFA, and the femoral nerve is lateral. The saphenous vein drains into the CFV medially. These vessels are exposed by making a direct incision in the groin and thigh where the pulse is palpated. The SFA and superficial femoral vein (SFV) are extensions of the CFA and CFV, lying deep to the sartorius muscle until they pass into the adductor canal. The SFA and SFV can be exposed by making an incision over the sartorius muscle (Figure 4-14).

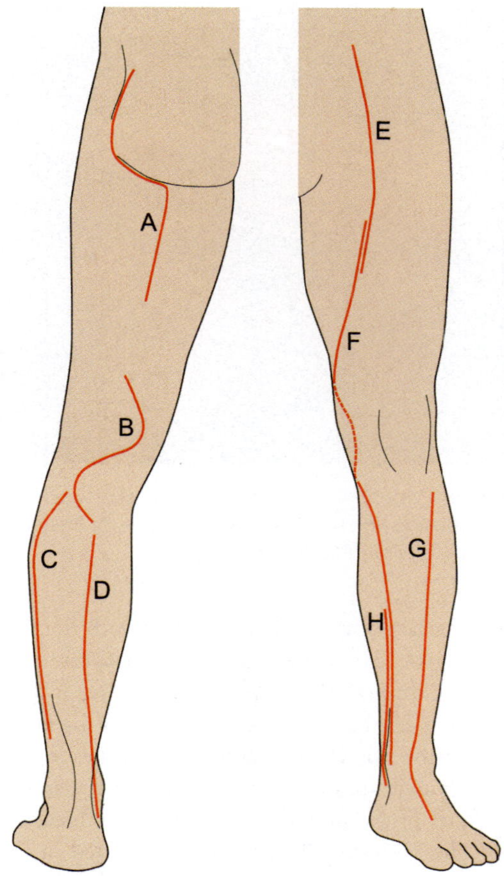

FIGURE 4-14 Incisions for lower extremity vessels and nerves. (**A**) Sciatic nerve. (**B**) Popliteal fossa, including popliteal artery and vein, sciatic nerve, proximal anterior and posterior tibial arteries and veins, proximal tibial and common peroneal nerves, and proximal lesser saphenous vein. (**C**) Common, superficial, and deep peroneal nerves. (**D**) Sural nerve, lesser saphenous vein, posterior tibial artery and vein, and tibial nerve. (**E**) Common femoral artery and vein and femoral nerve. (**F**) Greater saphenous vein. (**G**) Anterior tibial artery and vein and dorsalis pedis artery and vein. (**H**) Posterior tibial artery and vein and tibial nerve.

The popliteal artery can be palpated within the popliteal fossa with the knee in flexion. It enters the popliteal fossa superomedially and courses inferolaterally. A transverse or a "lazy S" incision is made in the popliteal fossa to prevent scar contracture. The popliteal fossa is most easily exposed in the prone position; it can, however be exposed from the supine position with the legs flexed at the hip and knee and externally rotated ("frog-leg position") and the contralateral hip elevated by a cushion. The tibial nerve lies most superficial followed by the vein and then the artery. The tibial nerve crosses the vessels from lateral to medial following the tendon of the biceps femoris muscle. The popliteal artery is medial to the popliteal vein.

The posterior tibial artery and vein lie along a line 1 to 2 cm medial to the midline at the level of the fibular neck and the midpoint between the medial malleolus and bony calcaneus,

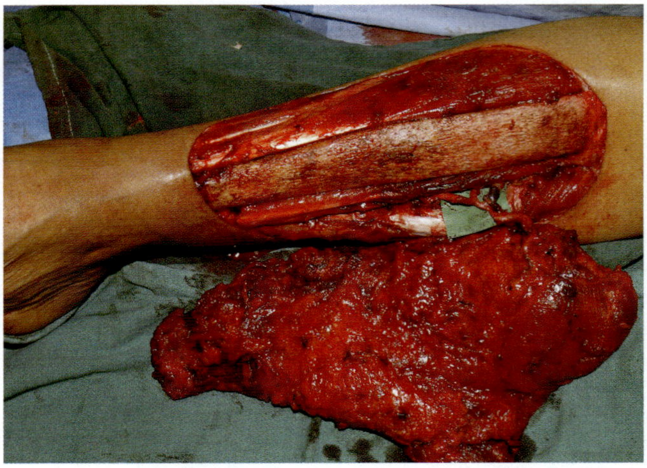

FIGURE 4-15 Posterior tibial artery and vein as recipient blood vessels using an end-to-side anastomosis for free flap reconstruction of a pretibial wound.

where the arterial pulse can be palpated beneath the skin at the level of the ankle. For a lower leg reconstruction, an incision along this line through the deep fascia of the leg is made (35). This dissection can be performed prone or in the lateral position lying on the side of the defect. The two heads of the gastrocnemius muscle are split in the midline, and then the soleus is also divided in the midline far enough to achieve adequate exposure. The posterior tibial vessels are located in the plane between the soleus (posterior) and the flexor digitorum longus (anterior) muscles, which may also be approached medially for more distal wounds (Figure 4-15). In the region of the ankle, the posterior tibial vessels lie beneath the flexor retinaculum. The posterior tibial and flexor digitorum longus tendons lie anterior to the vessels, and the tibial nerve and flexor hallucis longus tendon lie posterior. The distal approach to the posterior tibial vessels can be limited to an incision behind the medial malleolus, along the palpable pulse of the posterior tibial artery, for reconstructions of the foot and ankle.

The anterior tibial artery and vein lie beneath an imaginary line joining a point 2.5 cm distal to the medial side of the fibular head and a point midway between the malleoli anteriorly. The dorsalis pedis artery can then be palpated lateral to the tendon of the extensor hallucis longus muscle on the dorsum of the foot. The anterior tibial vessels can be exposed by making an incision 1 to 2 cm lateral to the lateral edge of the tibial bone (36). The vessels lie between the tibialis anterior muscle medially and the extensor hallucis longus and extensor digitorum longus tendons laterally. The deep peroneal nerve runs beside the anterior tibial vessels.

The two main superficial veins of the lower extremity, the greater and lesser saphenous veins, run superficial to the fascia lata of the thigh and the fascia cruris. Exposure is along their course described earlier. The greater saphenous vein will be encountered when approaching the anterior tibial vessels in the lower leg. As mentioned, it courses behind the medial femoral epicondyle and then moves to a more anterior position, ending at the femoral vein in the inguinal region. The lesser saphenous vein will be encountered when dissecting the posterior tibial vessels through a posterior midline leg approach. It then moves to the posterior midline and ends near or in the popliteal fossa.

Nerve Exposure

The femoral nerve is exposed in the same way as the femoral artery and vein, beginning with an incision 2 to 3 cm below and parallel to the inguinal ligament curving downward along the medial border of the sartorius muscle. The deep fascia of the thigh is incised parallel to the medial border of the sartorius, and the femoral nerve, artery, and vein are exposed.

To achieve exposure of the sciatic nerve at the level of the sciatic notch, the patient is placed in a prone position. A line from the posterior iliac spine toward the greater trochanter is imagined. An incision is made along the distal aspect of this line and curved underneath the crease of the gluteus maximus muscle (37). The incision is carried through the soft tissue to the muscle, which may be partly transected close to its insertion on to the femur, iliotibial band, and fascia lata. The gluteus maximus is then retracted superiorly to expose the sciatic nerve as it exits beneath the piriformis muscle. Care is taken to protect the inferior gluteal artery because it provides some of the blood supply to the nerve. In the posterior thigh, the sciatic nerve is exposed with a vertical incision. It is located by retracting the biceps femoris muscle medially in the upper thigh and laterally in the lower thigh. In the lower thigh, a curved or zigzag incision over the popliteal fossa is made, and the nerve is seen to divide into common peroneal and tibial branches between the biceps femoris muscle laterally and the semitendinosus and semimembranosus muscles medially. The femur is palpable directly beneath the nerve.

The proximal common peroneal and tibial nerves are exposed in the popliteal fossa just as the popliteal artery and vein are, with an incision that does not cross the fossa vertically, to prevent scar contracture. They often bifurcate from the sciatic nerve superior to the fossa. The common peroneal nerve hugs the border of the biceps femoris muscle and then passes around the lateral aspect of the proximal fibula, where it is palpable just below the prominence of the fibular head. It is in this region that the nerve is most vulnerable to injury. To expose the common peroneal nerve, a transverse popliteal incision is again made and then curved inferiorly over the lateral aspect of the leg. The deep peroneal nerve can be accessed by extending the incision over the anterior aspect of the leg, lateral to the border of the tibia, as in exposure for the anterior tibial artery. The nerve and artery are located between the tibialis anterior and extensor hallucis longus muscles.

The tibial nerve descends through the middle of the popliteal fossa between the heads of the gastrocnemius muscle where it lies next to the posterior tibial artery. Proximally, the tibial nerve gives off many branches, including two branches to the gastrocnemius, branches to the popliteus muscle, and branches to the plantar flexors of the foot. More distally, it gives branches to the flexor digitorum longus and hallucis longus. Proximal exposure is via a popliteal fossa approach, with division of the medial and lateral heads of the gastrocnemius and proximal soleus. Distal exposure can be achieved through an incision made along the medial border of the gastrocnemius muscle extending inferiorly behind the medial malleolus. It is usually easier to locate the nerve inferiorly, medial to the Achilles tendon and trace it superiorly. At the level of the calf, the medial head of the gastrocnemius is retracted, and the soleus muscle is visualized. It is necessary to detach the medial soleus muscle from the tibia to visualize the midportion of the nerve along the medial aspect of the transverse intermuscular septum. After this fascial layer is opened vertically, the tibial nerve and posterior tibial vessels are exposed behind the tibia.

The sural nerve, which is made up of the medial sural cutaneous nerve and branches of the lateral sural cutaneous nerve, runs along the midline of the calf and then courses laterally, posterior to the lateral calcaneus within the flexor retinaculum to end in the fifth digit. It lies in close proximity to the lesser saphenous vein, which is posterior and medial. It is often easiest to locate it at the ankle and then trace it distally or proximally as needed.

POSTOPERATIVE CARE

In addition to vigilant monitoring of the flap, the recipient vessel site must be carefully checked to avoid potential complications. Drains as well as dressings, splints, and tracheostomy ties must be placed in such a way as to not put pressure on the flap pedicle or the recipient vessels proximal to the anastomosis. The incision line as well as the native skin flaps, whether cervical, mastectomy, or extremity skin, must be carefully observed for wound dehiscence or necrosis, particularly in the setting of prior surgery, radiation, or trauma. Although wounds occurring over noncritical structures can often be treated conservatively, those that occur over recipient and free flap vessels need to be addressed aggressively to prevent infection, exposure, thrombosis, or rupture. In cases of poor-quality skin flaps overlying the recipient vessel site, prophylactic replacement by the free flap or a second pedicled or free flap should be considered at the time of the initial surgery.

REFERENCES

1. Takamatsu A, Harashina T, Inoue T. Selection of appropriate recipient vessels in difficult microsurgical head and neck reconstruction. *J Reconstr Microsurg* 1996;12:499.
2. Nahabedian MY, Sing N, Deune, EG, et al. Recipient vessel analysis for microvascular reconstruction of the head and neck. *Ann Plast Surg* 2004;52:148.
3. Harunobu S, von Luedinghausen M, Ohno K, et al. Anatomy of microvascular anastomosis in the neck. *Plast Reconstr Surg* 1998;101:33–41.
4. Yagi S, Nakayama B, Kamei Y, et al. Posterolateral cervical vein as a recipient vein in reconstructive microvascular surgery of the head and neck. *J Reconstr Microsurg* 2007;23:19.
5. Graham BB, Varvares MA. End-to-side venous anastomosis with the internal jugular vein stump: a preliminary report. *Head Neck* 2004; 26:537.
6. Shimizu F, Lin MP, Ellabban M, et al. Superficial temporal vessels as a reserve recipient site for microvascular head and neck reconstruction in vessel-depleted neck. *Ann Plast Surg* 2009;62:134.
7. Hanasono MM, Barnea Y, Skoracki RJ. Microvascular surgery in the previously operated and irradiated neck. *Microsurgery* 2009;29:1.
8. Mulholland S, Boyd JB, McCabe S, et al. Recipient vessels in head and neck microsurgery: radiation effect and vessel access. *Plast Reconstr Surg* 1993;92:628.
9. Jacobson AS, Eloy JA, Park E, et al. Vessel-depleted neck: techniques for achieving microvascular reconstruction. *Head Neck* 2008;30:201.
10. Head C, Sercarz JA, Abemayor E, et al. Microvascular reconstruction after previous neck dissection. *Arch. Otolaryngol Head Neck Surg* 2002; 128:328.
11. Yu P. The transverse cervical vessels as recipient vessels for previously treated head and neck cancer patients. *Plast Reconstr Surg* 2005;115:1253.
12. Horng SY, Chen MT. Reversed cephalic vein: a lifeboat in head and neck free-flap reconstruction. *Plast Reconstr Surg* 1993;92:752.
13. Kim KA, Chandrasekhar BS. Cephalic vein in salvage microsurgical reconstruction in the head and neck. *Br J Plast Surg* 1998;51:2.
14. Urken ML, Higgins KM, Lee B, et al. Internal mammary artery and vein: recipient vessels for free tissue transfer to the head and neck vessel-depleted neck. *Head Neck* 2006;28:797.
15. Clark CP 3rd, Rohrich RJ, Copit S, et al. An anatomic study of the internal mammary veins: clinical implications for free-tissue-transfer breast reconstruction. *Plast Reconstr Surg* 1997;99:400.
16. Harris JR, Lueg E, Genden E, et al. The thoracoacromial/cephalic vascular system for microvascular anastomoses in the vessel-depleted neck. *Arch Otolaryngol Head Neck Surg* 2002;128:319.
17. Aycock JK, Senson KM, Gottlieb LJ. The thoracoacromial trunk: alternative recipient vessels in reoperative head and neck microsurgery. *Plast Reconstr Surg* 2008;121:88.
18. De Gier HH, Balm AJ, Bruning PF, et al. Systematic approach to the treatment of chylous leakage after neck dissection. *Head Neck* 1996;18:347.
19. Babin RW, Panje WR. The incidence of vasovagal reflex activity during radical neck dissection. *Laryngoscope* 1980;90:1321.
20. Ninkovic MM, Schwaegger AH, Anderl H. Internal mammary vessels as a recipient site. *Clin Plast Surg* 1998;25:213.
21. Moran SL, Nava G, Benham AH, et al. An outcome analysis comparing the thoracodorsal and internal mammary vessels as recipient sites for microvascular breast reconstruction: a prospective study of 100 patients. *Plast Reconstr Surg* 2003;111:1876.
22. Yap LH, Whiten SC, Forster A, et al. Sensory recovery in the sensate free transverse rectus abdominis myocutaneous flap. *Plast Reconstr Surg* 2005; 115:1280.
23. Temple CL, Tse R, Bettger-Hahn M, et al. Sensibility following innervated free TRAM flap for breast reconstruction. *Plast Reconstr Surg* 2006;117:2119.
24. Sacks JM, Chang DW. Rib-sparing internal mammary vessel harvest for microvascular breast reconstruction in 100 consecutive cases. *Plast Reconstr Surg* 2009;123:1403.
25. Saint-Cyr M, Chang DW, Robb GL, et al. Internal mammary perforator recipient vessels for breast reconstruction using free TRAM, DIEP, and SIEA flaps. *Plast Reconstr Surg* 2007;120:1769.
26. Fisher J, Bostwick J 3rd, Powell RW. Latissimus dorsi blood supply after thoracodorsal vessel division: the serratus collateral. *Plast Reconstr Surg* 1983;72:502.
27. Kerr-Valentic MA, Gottlieb LJ, et al. The retrograde limb of the internal mammary vein: an additional outflow option in DIEP flap breast reconstruction. *Plast Reconstr Surg* 2009;124:717.
28. Johnson RK, Spinner M, Shrewsbury MM. Median nerve entrapment syndromes in the proximal forearm. *J Hand Surg*4(suppl A):48,1979.
29. Miller TT, Reinus WR. Nerve entrapment syndromes of the elbow, forearm, and wrist. *AJR Am J Roentgenol* 2010;195:585.
30. Palmer BA, Hughes TB. Cubital tunnel syndrome. *J Hand Surg Am* 2010;35:153.
31. Cobb TK, Carmichael SW, Cooney WP. Guyon's canal revisited: an anatomic study of the carpal ulnar neurovascular space. *J Hand Surg* 1996;21(suppl A):861.
32. Abrams RA, Ziets RJ, Lieber RL, et al. Anatomy of the radial nerve motor branches in the forearm. *J Hand Surg* 1997;22(suppl A):232.
33. Abrams RA, Brown RA, Botte MJ. The superficial branch of the radial nerve: an anatomic study with surgical implications. *J Hand Surg* 1992; 17(suppl A):1–37.
34. Kim D, Orron DE, Skillman JJ. Surgical significance of popliteal artery variants: a unified angiographic classification. *Ann Surg* 1989;210:776.
35. Park S, Han SH, Lee TJ. Algorithm for recipient vessel selection in free tissue transfer to the lower extremity. *Plast Reconstr Surg* 1999;103:1937.
36. Godina M, Arnez ZM, Lister GD. Preferential use of the posterior approach to blood vessels of the lower leg in microvascular surgery. *Plast Reconstr Surg* 1991;88:287.
37. Patil PG, Friedman AH. Surgical exposure of the sciatic nerve in the gluteal region: anatomic and historical comparison of two approaches. *Neurosurgery* 2005;56;165.

CHAPTER 5

Monitoring Microsurgical Flaps and Replanted Tissues

William Lineaweaver

Most clinicians monitor revascularized tissue after microsurgical flap and replant procedures (1). The objectives of postoperative tissue monitoring have become increasingly sharply defined, but their achievement can remain elusive.

Simply stated, tissue monitoring should detect significant circulatory complications in revascularized tissue. Detected complications should be of a magnitude associated with failure of the flap or replant. The principal outcome of effective postoperative monitoring is a demonstrated improvement in salvage of compromised flaps and replants after intervention triggered by the monitor (2). Secondary outcomes can include specificity (e.g., minimal false alarms leading to unnecessary interventions) and cost savings related to salvaged flaps (based on estimates of secondary procedures and morbidities associated with flap failures), as well as facility savings related to effective monitoring outside of intensive care units (ICUs) (3–5).

Postoperative monitoring can range from clinical examinations to sophisticated devices that measure tissue blood flow, directly assess pedicle vessel patency, or detect metabolic changes associated with tissue ischemia (6). A great number of monitoring techniques have been described over the past 4 decades, testifying to the failure of any one technique to convincingly deliver definitive results. Few monitoring techniques have been rigorously evaluated by outcome analyses (7,8).

This chapter reviews current monitoring techniques, a format followed since the early days of microsurgery (6,9). Each technique will be defined and its applications summarized. This review will attempt to extend beyond simple cataloging with a concluding discussion of monitoring outcome studies.

CLINICAL MONITORING

Monitoring revascularized flaps and replants by repeated clinical examination is the most commonly used technique of postoperative microsurgical tissue assessment (1,7,10). Applied to flaps and replants, clinical monitoring requires visible tissue components and regular examinations by experienced observers. As summarized by McKee, the parameters of clinical monitoring include tissue color, capillary refill, tissue turgor, and temperature (11). A well-perfused unit of revascularized tissue is pink with brisk, equilibrating capillary refill; grossly normal turgor; and a warm temperature. Arterial insufficiency is characterized by pale or cyanotic tissue, decreased or absent capillary refill, deflated turgor, and a relatively cool temperature. Venous obstruction results in progressive cyanosis, increased rates of capillary refill, congested turgor, and decreased temperature.

These examinations can be impaired by the lack of a skin component in the revascularized tissue or precluded entirely with buried flaps. Some surgeons have advocated maintaining a skin island on muscle flaps and externalized components (island skin flaps or exposed segments jejunal tissue) for clinical assessment of buried flaps (12,13). Pigmented skin, ambient temperature, and subtotal flap ischemia remain as problems that can confound clinical monitoring.

Reports of the efficacy of clinical monitoring serve as a standard by which other techniques can be measured. A recent analysis of a large flap series managed with clinical postoperative monitoring reported a 63% salvage rate in complicated flaps and a 0.4% incidence of false positive examinations leading to unnecessary reexplorations (14).

TEMPERATURE MONITORING

Evaluation of the temperature of revascularized tissue has been intermittently used as a monitor throughout the history of clinical microsurgery. The technology of temperature measurement has included surface temperature probes, implantable thermocouple probes, needle electrodes, and "sticker type" skin surface indicators (15–18).

Generally, the temperature of the monitored tissue should decrease with compromise of the vascular pedicle. The values and rates of such decreases must be interpreted within empirically derived guidelines to establish clear definitions of critical values.

Temperature monitoring as a technique is confounded by great variabilities in patient temperatures in postoperative periods. These problems have led different investigators to use different types of temperature detectors as noted. Data interpretation must be based on trends and derived comparison values rather than immediate readings (19).

Such difficulties have resulted in infrequent use of temperature as a monitoring parameter. Some authors, however, have reported salvages of complicated replants monitored with temperature detectors, while Khouri and Shaw achieved a salvage rate of 87% in complicated flaps monitored by comparative readings from surface temperature digital thermometers applied to flaps and control sites (15,17,19).

SURFACE DOPPLER

Ultrasound Doppler devices convert sound waves reflected by columns of moving blood cells into audible signals or wave form tracings (6). The most commonly used device includes a pencil-shaped probe connected by a wire to a transmission-receiver box that contains an amplifier and speaker. Loss of signals from pedicle vessels indicate compression or occlusion of the vessels.

These portable, handheld devices have long been used to examine the patencies of flap pedicle vessels (20). The signals can be misleading if the pedicle vessel sites are poorly marked and if the Doppler picks up signals from deep or adjacent vessels. Therefore, it is important to clearly mark the site of the vessels that are to be examined and determine at flap inset that the pedicle signals are distinct from other vessels in the region (21).

Pencil Doppler probes may also be used to monitor the signals obtained from perforating vessels reaching the skin as terminal branches of the vascular pedicle. These points are identified intraoperatively and marked with a fine suture so that the ICU staff can locate them for monitoring purposes.

Surface Doppler examinations are rarely reported as an independent technique. Rather, the Doppler is used in a context of regular physical examinations. Disa and coworkers reported a salvage rate of 77% in complicated flaps with surface components monitored with clinical examination and Doppler signals. No complicated buried flaps were salvaged, indicating that Doppler monitoring requires a visible flap component for successful interpretation (22).

IMPLANTABLE DOPPLER

Several strategies have been used to increase the efficacy of Doppler monitoring by implanting small Doppler probes so that they are in direct contact with pedicle vessels and produce a continuous signal generated by pedicle blood flow. Different probe placements have included arterial probes and probes placed on both the artery and vein of a flap pedicle (23,24). Most investigators now recommend placing a probe on the pedicle vein because such a probe can most readily detect either arterial or venous thrombosis (25).

The reported utility of implantable Doppler probe monitoring has been inconsistent. Kind and coworkers reported 100% salvage of 16 complicated flaps monitored with Doppler probes implanted on pedicle veins (26). de la Torre and coworkers reported salvage of seven of eight flaps (83%) monitored with probes placed on the artery and vein of each pedicle (24). Paydar and coworkers reported salvage of three of four (75%) complicated buried flaps monitored with Doppler probes placed on pedicle veins (25). Two other large series, however, found no significant differences in salvage rates between flaps monitored with implantable Doppler probes and flaps monitored clinically (27,28).

LASER DOPPLER

Laser Doppler technology uses shifts in light reflection (rather than sound) to detect the density and velocity of moving particles. A laser Doppler probe placed on the surface of a flap detects changes in the wave length of laser light reflected off moving red blood cells in capillaries near the surface of the flap.

Arterial and venous obstructions become detectable to the laser Doppler as capillary blood flow diminishes, and the monitor registers such decrease as changes in perfusion units (6,29).

Clinton and coworkers reported that their salvage rate for complicated flaps monitored with the laser Doppler was 82%, a significant improvement from their 50% salvage rate achieved with clinical examination (30). Problems associated with laser Doppler monitoring include false positives, the need for interpretation of the monitor's readings, fracturing of fiberoptic cables with use, and the expense of the probes (6,8,29).

PULSE OXIMETER

Pulse oximeter probes transmit two distinct wave lengths of light, one of which is absorbed by oxygenated hemoglobin; the other is absorbed by deoxygenated hemoglobin. The device can then calculate arterial oxygen saturation while also displaying underlying pulsations in the monitored tissue. Pedicle thromboses generally result in decreasing oxygen saturation and diminished or absent pulses (31).

Pulse oximetry has been associated with an 80% salvage rate in complicated replanted fingers (31). Use of pulse oximetry for flap monitoring is anecdotal, and application of pulse oximetry to flaps is limited by the configuration of available probes that do not readily fix to flap surfaces (32).

TISSUE OXIMETRY

This technology measures tissue oxygen saturation by the measurement of scattering and absorption of near-infrared and visible red light projected onto a tissue surface by a surface probe. Changes in these light patterns reflect changes in

TABLE 5-1 Salvage Rates Associated with Microsurgical Monitoring Technique

Technique	Salvage Rates (%)	Applications	References
Clinical examination	50–66	Flaps with visible components	2,27,30
Temperature	87	Flaps with visible components	19
Surface Doppler	77	Flaps with visible components	(2
Implantable Doppler	69–100	Surface flaps and buried flaps	24,26–28
Laser Doppler	82	Flaps with visible components	30
Pulse oximeter	80	Replanted digits	31
Tissue oximetry	100	Flaps with visible skin components	33

oxygenation of tissue hemoglobin, and an attached computer console translates these data into a tissue oxygen saturation percentage. Criteria for tissue oxygenation changes over time must be established to determine thresholds for monitor alarms (33).

Keller reported salvage of 100% of 5 complicated flaps monitored with this device (33).

OTHER MONITORING TECHNIQUES

Other techniques of microsurgical monitoring have been sporadically reported over the past 4 decades of clinical microsurgery. Pratt and coauthors recently summarized such techniques, which include tissue pH, photoplethysmography, fluorometry, microdialysis, color duplex ultrasonography, impedance plethysmography, and confocal microscopy. These monitoring techniques are supported by clinical reports that usually contain anecdotal, uncontrolled evidence. Quantitative fluorometry has been shown to improve salvage rates in cutaneous flaps and transplanted toes compared with clinical examinations, but performance of these studies is complicated enough to have resulted in limited use of this technology (2). Further details of these techniques can be obtained through the bibliography of Pratt's thorough review (7).

OUTCOME ANALYSES AND MICROSURGICAL MONITORING

This review has summarized the most common monitoring systems and strategies currently described in clinical reports. Each of these monitors appears to work for some clinicians in some scenarios a set of circumstances that probably reveals that microsurgical monitoring is a mixture of technique and personnel. None of these techniques (except for clinical examinations) has achieved truly widespread use, an indication that no single type of monitoring has sufficiently obvious utility and sufficient ease of application to become a standard.

How should reports of monitoring techniques be evaluated?

The setting for microsurgical monitoring evaluation can be illustrated by a hypothetical case series of 100 microsurgical flaps. Typically, such a series today will have 95 successful flaps and five failures (2,7). How can a monitoring technique be useful in such a series?

A basic mistake is to equate monitor function with the detection of successful, uncomplicated flaps. In the above series, a monitor that was unplugged and inert could be interpreted as detecting 95 successful flaps while missing any signs of problems in the five failed flaps, thereby achieving a 95% rate of "successful monitoring" (23). Such a measure of monitor function does not demonstrate any real utility of a monitoring technique. Although this principle is increasingly recognized (3), reports of clinical monitoring with no evidence of active monitor function continue to appear (34,35).

Monitors should be evaluated in terms of their active performance. The active performance of a monitor includes false positives leading to unnecessary interventions; true positives whereby the monitor correctly indicates significant flap complications; and most importantly, flap salvage, indicating that the monitor led to improved outcomes in the management of complicated flaps (35,36). In the hypothetical case series, a monitor must show a significant effect in salvaging some or all of the 5% of failed flaps. No other measure of monitor function is clinically meaningful.

Table 5-1 summarizes the performance of the reviewed monitoring techniques within these parameters. No technique shows a clear and consistent improvement over clinical monitoring. Innovative monitoring techniques and strategies should demonstrate advantages over clinical monitoring to claim real utility, and future innovations must submit to these analyses to establish a convincing basis for clinical use.

Do I have a prediction for the future of microsurgical monitoring? I believe that reduction in costs and size of color duplex ultrasonography will allow a small, inexpensive iteration of this device to become a bedside microsurgical monitor that can clearly and directly visualize flow in pedicle vessels with interval examinations (37).

REFERENCES

1. Jallali N, Ridha H, Butler P. Postoperative monitoring of free flaps in UK plastic surgery units. *Microsurgery* 2005;25:469.
2. Whitney T, Lineaweaver W, Billy JB, et al. Improved salvage of complicated microvascular transplants monitored with quantitative fluorometry. *Plast Reconstr Surg* 1992;90:105.

3. Iglher N, Eisenhardt SU, Penna V, et al. A new evaluation tool for monitoring devices and its application to evaluate the implantable Doppler probe. *J Reconstr Microsurg* 2010;26:265.
4. Haddock NT, Gobble RM, Levine JP. More consistent postoperative care and monitoring can reduce costs following microvascular free flap reconstruction. *J Reconstr Microsurg* 2010;26:435.
5. Rozen WM, Enajat M, Whitaker I, et al. Postoperative monitoring of lower limb free flaps with the Cook-Swartz implantable Doppler probe. *Microsurgery* 2010;30:354.
6. Buncke HJ, Lineaweaver W, Valauri F, Buncke GH. Monitoring. In Buncke HJ (ed). *Microsurgery.* Philadelphia: Lea & Febiger, 1991, pp. 715–721.
7. Pratt GF, Rozen WM, Chubb D, et al. Modern adjuncts and technologies in microsurgery. *Microsurgery* 2010;30:657.
8. Whitaker I, Olver DW. Monitoring: The Evidence for Plastic Surgery. Stone C (ed).Shrewsbury, UK: tfm Publishing, 2008, pp. 225–234.
9. Harrison DH, Girling M, Mott G. Methods of assessing the viability of free flap transfer during the postoperative period. *Clin Plast Surg* 1983;10:21.
10. Whitaker I, Cantab AB, Rozen WM, et al. Postoperative monitoring of free flaps in autologous breast reconstruction. *J Reconstr Microsurg* 2010;26:409.
11. McKee N. Operative complications and the management of intraoperative flow failure. *Microsurgery* 1993;14:158.
12. Hammer H, Bugyi I, Zellner P. Soft tissue reconstruction of the anterior surface of the lower leg. Scand. J. *Plast Reconstr Surg* 1986;20:137.
13. Cho BC, Shin DP, Byun JS, et al. Monitoring flap for buried free tissue transfer. *Plast Reconstr Surg* 2002;110:1249.
14. Chubb D, Rozen W, Whitaker I, et al. The efficacy of clinical assessment in the postoperative monitoring of free flaps: a review of 1140 consecutive cases. *Plast Reconstr Surg* 2010;125:1157.
15. Stirrat CR, Seaber A, Urbaniak J, et al. Temperature monitoring in digital replantation. *J Hand Surg* 1978;3:342.
16. May JW, Lukash F, Gallico G, et al. Removable thermocouple probe microvascular patency monitor. *Plast Reconstr Surg* 1983;72:366.
17. Reagan D, Grundberg A, George MJ. Clinical evaluation and temperature monitoring in predicting viability in replantations. *J Reconstr Microsurg* 1983;10:1.
18. Aihara M, Tane N, Matsuzaki K, et al. The sticker-type temperature indicator in replantation. *J Reconstr Microsurg* 1993;9:191.
19. Khouri R, Shaw WW. Monitoring of free flaps with surface temperature recordings. *Plast Reconstr Surg* 1992;89:495.
20. Solomon GA, Yaremchuk M, Manson PN. Doppler ultrasound surface monitoring of both arterial and venous flow in clinical free tissue transfers. *J Reconstr Microsurg* 1986;3:39.
21. Tsuzuki K, Yanai A, Bandoh Y. A contrivance for monitoring skin flaps with a Doppler flow meter. *J Reconstr Microsurg* 1990;6:363.
22. Disa JJ, Cordeiro P, Hidalgo D. Efficacy of conventional monitoring techniques in free tissue transfer. *Plast Reconstr Surg* 1999;104:97.
23. Swartz WM, Jones NF, Cherup L, et al. Direct monitoring of microvascular anastomoses with the 20-MHz ultrasonic Doppler probe. *Plast Reconstr Surg* 1988;81:149.
24. de la Torre J, Hedden W, Grant JW, et al. Retrospective review of the internal Doppler probe for intra- and postoperative microvascular surveillance. *J Reconstr Microsurg* 2003;19:287.
25. Paydar K, Hansen SL, Chang DS, et al. Implantable venous Doppler monitoring in head and neck free flap reconstruction increases the salvage rate. *Plast Reconstr Surg* 2010;125:1129.
26. Kind G, Buntic RF, Buncke GM, et al. The effect of an implantable Doppler probe on the salvage of microvascular tissue transplants. *Plast Reconstr Surg* 1998;101:1268.
27. Rozen WM, Chubb D, Whitaker J, et al. The efficacy of postoperative monitoring. *Microsurgery* 2010;30:105.
28. Smit JM, Werker PMN, Liss AG, et al. Introduction of the implantable Doppler system did not lead to an increased salvage rate of compromised flaps. *Plast Reconstr Surg* 2010;125:1710.
29. Hovius SER, van Andrichem LNA, Mulder HA, et al. The predictive value of the laser Doppler flow meter for postoperative microvascular monitoring. *Ann Plast Surg* 1993;31:307.
30. Clinton MS, Sepka RS, Bristol D, et al. Establishment of normal ranges of laser Doppler blood flow in autologous tissue transplants. *Plast Reconstr Surg* 1991;87:299.
31. Graham B, Paulus D, Caffee HH. Pulse oximetry for vascular monitoring in upper extremity replantation surgery. *J Hand Surg* 1986;11(suppl A):687.
32. Menick FJ. The pulse oximeter in free muscle flap surgery. *J Reconstr Microsurg* 1988;4:331.
33. Keller A. A new diagnostic algorithm for early prediction of vascular compromise in 208 microsurgical flaps using tissue oxygen saturation measurements. *Ann Plast Surg* 2009;62:538.
34. Ferguson RH, Yu P. Techniques of monitoring buried fasciocutaneous flaps. *Plast Reconstr Surg* 2009;123:525.
35. Lineaweaver W. Techniques of monitoring buried fasciocutaneous flaps [letter]. *Plast Reconstr Surg* 2009;124:1729.
36. Lineaweaver W. The implantable Doppler probe [letter]. *Plast Reconstr Surg* 1988;82:1099.
37. Rosenberg JJ, Fornage BD, Chevray PM. Monitoring buried free flaps: limitations of the implantable Doppler and use of color duplex sonography as a confirmatory test. *Plast Reconstr Surg* 2006;118:109.

CHAPTER 6

Microvascular Failure: Avoidance, Rescue, and Salvage

Chih-Hung Lin and Steven Lo

The management of the failing and the failed microvascular free flap remains one of the most challenging and controversial areas in microsurgery from both a technical and pharmacologic standpoint. With failure rates decreasing to less than 5% in most major centers, experience in flap salvage is conversely decreasing, and conversely studies require increasing statistical power to demonstrate any benefit from therapeutic interventions. Nonetheless, flap thrombosis or pedicle compromise still occurs in 10% of cases, with a subsequent salvage rate of 69% to 85% (1,2). The dilemmas in flap salvage center around three main questions. First, what is the proven role of pharmacologic agents such as dextran in reducing the risk of postoperative flap failure? Second, when all surgical options have been exhausted in reexploration of the failing flap, what is the role of thrombolytic agents? Third, in flaps that eventually result in total failure, what is the next step in the reconstructive algorithm? The answers to these questions are controversial, and despite numerous studies published in the literature, few are of sufficient quality to merit strong recommendations.

PHARMACOLOGIC ADJUNCTS TO POSTOPERATIVE FLAP CARE

Pharmacologic Agents: Lack of Benefit or Lack of Statistical Power?

Postoperative pharmacologic agents remain controversial, with clinicians using a variety of their own preferred agents or none at all, reflecting the lack of consensus on their use. In assessing the benefits of such therapies, it must be remembered that virtually none of the studies published on the subject have sufficient statistical power to show any difference. Given a flap success rate of 95%, investigation of a therapeutic agent for a 3% increase in success would require 1000 cases to have a 90% power of detecting a difference at a significance level of 0.05. Likewise, a 2% increase in success would require 4000 cases (3). Furthermore, thrombotic tendencies in free flap models in animals do not necessarily reflect those seen in humans and should be interpreted with caution. Animal models provide only level V evidence and should not be used as the basis of clinical practice, particularly if higher levels of evidence such as human trials are available.

Aspirin

Although the antiplatelet agent aspirin has been shown in animal models to reduce venous thrombosis (4), no clear benefit has been demonstrated in humans (5,6). Some studies suggest it has a preferential effect in preventing arterial rather than venous thrombosis (7).

Dextran

Likewise, dextran, a polysaccharide available in 40,000- and 70,000-kD molecular lengths, has not been demonstrated to have beneficial effects in clinical trials. Theoretically, it has been used as a volume expander to reduce viscosity and improve the rheological characteristics of blood flow and by decreasing platelet aggregation by conferring an increased electronegative charge (8). However, the complication profile of dextran is a source of major concern. One prospective study comparing dextran 40 with aspirin did not come to any firm conclusions regarding flap failures in 100 head and neck cases because no flap failures occurred. However, systemic complications associated with volume expansion such as heart failure, myocardial infarction, pleural effusion, and pulmonary edema were significantly higher with dextran 40 than with aspirin, between 3.9 to 7.2 times greater (9).

Heparin

Heparin, a cofactor of antithrombin III that exerts its downstream effects via inhibition of the common pathway of fibrinogen to fibrin conversion, has been used in a variety of forms. Most commonly, it is used as an intraoperative irrigation solution but also as a postoperative infusion or as subcutaneous thromboembolic prophylaxis. Notably, animal models suggest an effective intraoperative concentration of 100 units/mL, but in clinical practice, some centers continue to use lower concentrations of 5000 units/L of normal saline (5 units/mL) (10,11). Khouri et al.'s multicenter prospective study involving 493 patients from 23 centers assessed the use of heparin irrigation and infusion and subcutaneous heparin. Heparin irrigation did not influence flap failure (3.9% with and 4.1% without) (12). Postoperative heparin infusion was confounded by its use "off protocol" when a flap was deemed to be in trouble, and therefore appropriate analysis of its efficacy was not possible. Only subcutaneous heparin was associated with a reduced risk of postoperative thrombosis (odds ratio [OR], 0.27; $P = 0.038$). The rationale for the efficacy of heparin over aspirin may come from animal models that suggest that the fibrin pathway (heparin) is more important in microvascular thrombosis than the thromboxane pathway (aspirin) (12). Furthermore, it has been implicated as having greater importance in venous rather than arterial occlusion (7).

Comparative Trials of Pharmacologic Agents

Strong recommendations cannot be made for the use of any particular pharmacologic agent. A retrospective study comparing low-molecular-weight heparin (5000 units subcutaneous) and aspirin (325 mg) in 505 patients found no difference in major outcomes regarding flap failure or bleeding-related complications (6). In contrast, Khouri et al.'s study found that only subcutaneous heparin had any beneficial effect in reducing thrombosis (2). Although this trial concluded that most antithrombotic agents are a "useless crutch" to aid microvascular surgery, these conclusions are only partially valid. Lack of statistical power may render this and other studies prone to type II errors (false negatives), and they should be interpreted as such. Therefore, clinical studies on pharmacologic agents do not demonstrate conclusively that aspirin, dextran, or heparin has no benefit in preventing thrombosis, simply that the power of the trials is likely to be insufficient. However, the risk-to-benefit profile of certain agents, such as dextran, strongly suggests that its use should be discontinued in clinical practice.

DECISION TO REEXPLORE

Detection of Flap Compromise and Bedside Maneuvers

The detection of flap compromise may be on a clinical basis alone or aided by a variety of invasive and noninvasive monitoring techniques. These are covered separately in another chapter. After compromise has been detected, a number of bedside maneuvers must be performed to exclude any readily reversible factors before returning the patient to the operating room. Nonetheless, while these maneuvers are being performed, it is prudent to alert and prepare the operating room for possible flap reexploration.

Bedside maneuvers may be divided into local or systemic maneuvers. Local factors that should be addressed include the removal of all dressings, selective removal of tensioning sutures, and assessment of adequate drain functioning. A hematoma should not simply be removed at the bedside because it may serve as an indicator of venous hypertension or occlusion rather than inadequate hemostasis and mandates return to the operating room. Furthermore, we have encountered clinical cases of pedicle avulsion when local evacuation of hematoma has been performed. Systemic maneuvers include altering the positioning of the patient, elevation of the blood pressure, reversal of hypovolemia, and assessment of and correction of hemoglobin and hematocrit parameters. Drug charts should also be reviewed to ensure that vasoconstrictive agents have not been given.

Timing of Surgical Reexploration

The decision to reexplore should be made as early as possible, once appropriate bedside maneuvers have been performed. Early reexploration has been demonstrated in numerous studies to be the key determinant of successful flap salvage (13,14). Nonetheless, the exact time limits at which a flap should be reexplored remain undefined. One study found that successful flap salvage occurred in flaps that were reexplored on average 4 hours after detection of flap compromise, but unsuccessful salvage attempts were performed at 9 hours (15). Furthermore, we have previously shown that the majority of problems with flap compromise occur within the first 72 hours (95% cases) and that greater care and monitoring are required within this time period (1). Certain caveats exist that mandate a lower threshold for return to operating room; these include double free flaps, chronic wounds and cases in which vein grafts have been used. In double free flaps, a compromise in one free flap may result in loss of the second flap, especially if sequential linking of pedicles is performed. We have also previously shown a higher risk of free flap venous pedicle compression (21%) when a second flap (pedicled pectoralis major) is used in combination for extensive head and neck defects (16). Chronic wounds and the use of vein grafts are both independent factors for an increase in flap failure, with ORs of 2.9 and 2.5, respectively (2). Given these data, a lower threshold for reexploration of free flaps with these characteristics should be considered.

SURGICAL MANAGEMENT OF THE FAILING FLAP

Primary Revision of Anastomosis

In Khouri et al.'s study, identification of intraoperative thrombus during the primary surgery occurred in 41 out of 493 free flaps (12). Primary revision of the anastomosis resulted in failures rates no higher than for flaps without primary intraoperative thrombosis (failure rates of 4.9% vs. 4.1%). An emphasis on meticulous surgical technique is therefore critical to overall success even in cases with "on-table" thrombosis (2).

Secondary Revision of Anastomosis

Assessment

The most critical aspect in flap salvage is assessment. This should be performed in a careful and systematic manner and should not be immediately directed at the anastomosis. Errors in flap planning or inset may be as likely to contribute as inadequate technical execution of the anastomosis, and revision of the anastomosis alone will not solve these problems. Drain placement, tensioning sutures, and pedicle of excessive redundancy or kinking should be assessed for potential compressive effects on the pedicle. Position of the flap in relation to the pedicle must be checked for potential shearing, tensions, kinking, or twisting, particularly at vulnerable points such as the pedicle–fascial interface in single perforator flaps. Furthermore, any significant changes in pedicle position with patient positioning should be assessed, such as the effects of rotation of the head on neck pedicles and inclination of the patient with breast reconstruction flaps.

Arterial versus Venous Insufficiency

In a study from our institution, venous thrombosis was commoner than arterial thrombosis (57% vs. 42%), but flap salvage rates were higher in cases with venous thrombosis (1). Success rates in venous thrombosis were 91% compared with arterial at 75% ($P = 0.024$). This may be partially attributable to distal collection of thrombus from arterial occlusion, which may occlude the small caliber perforating vessels. In venous insufficiency it must also be remembered that mottling discoloration of supposed venous stasis may be due to impaired arterial inflow. It is essential therefore that the artery is assessed even in cases of apparent isolated venous thrombosis and that a low threshold for revision of arterial anastomosis maintained. Furthermore, although Doppler assessment combined with Acland's test may be deemed adequate, the simple maneuver of opening a side branch in the arterial pedicle can give a more cogent confirmation of the adequacy of arterial inflow. During revision of the venous anastomosis, it is essential that a side branch or secondary vein is kept open during the entire revision to prevent rethrombosis caused by intraflap flow stasis.

Embolectomy

Embolectomy with Fogarty catheters must be done with great caution because there is a risk of secondary intimal damage at the level of the smaller caliber perforating vessels. An alternative approach is to remove thrombus via side branches at the level of the distal perforator. Furthermore, resection of an entire thrombosed vascular segment can be performed and reconstituted with vein graft. Gentle manual pressure on the flap can also occasionally dislodge venous thrombosis present in small-caliber perforating vessels.

Accessory Pedicles and Vein Grafts

In the head and neck, numerous options exist, particularly in the contralateral neck. Other sites, such as the extremities and breast, have fewer recipient pedicles, with some requiring preservation in case of secondary pedicled flap salvage. Numerous accessory venous pedicles are available in breast reconstruction, such as cephalic vein turndown, distal branch of internal mammary vein, external jugular vein, and the thoracodorsal vessels. However, although an ipsilateral pedicled latissimus dorsi can still be used based on reverse flow from the serratus branch, sacrificing the thoracodorsal vessels should still be performed judiciously. The lower extremity poses a greater challenge and often requires vein grafting to a more proximal vessel out with the zone of injury and thrombosis. In accordance with the hemodynamics of blood flow, Poiseuille's law ($Q = \Delta P \pi r^4/8\eta\, l$ where Q is blood flow, P is perfusion pressure, r is the diameter of the vessel, η is viscosity, and l is the length of the vessel) tells us that blood flow is related to higher inflow pressure and lower resistance. Thus, it is better to have high-pressure inflow such as the external carotid artery or the superficial temporal artery using end-to-side anastomosis and a larger diameter vein graft such as the great saphenous whose length is kept as short as possible.

However, the effect of vascular diameter is to the fourth power, making its contribution to flow greater than of all the other variables. Thus a sizable greater or lesser saphenous vein graft plays an important role in maximizing any increment in blood flow (17). To overcome muscle spasm within the wall of a constricted vascular conduit, heparin solution can be infused to the lumen under pressure to expand the vein graft and produce less resistance to flow. When vein grafting is not feasible, cross-leg flaps—random or axial or a contralateral recipient pedicle for the free flap—can be used as a salvage maneuver.

OUTCOMES

Microsurgical salvage rates vary in the literature but are something of a moot point. The single greatest factor influencing salvage rates has been shown repeatedly to be early timing of reexploration, and this must be borne in mind rather than overall flap salvage rates per se. Nonetheless, in our series of 113 flap reexplorations in 1142 free flaps, we noted an overall complete salvage rate of 63.7% and a further 20.4% partially salvaged (1).

PHARMACOLOGIC AGENTS IN THE FAILING FLAP

Thrombolytic Agents: Mode of Action

Thrombolytic agents act, as their names suggest (e.g., tissue plasminogen activator [TPA]), by activating plasminogen to form the fibrinolytic enzyme plasmin. One of the earliest and most widely available agents is streptokinase, with a half-life of 20 minutes. Its risk profile is higher than other drugs, with an allergic response in 6% (8). Urokinase has superseded streptokinase in the treatment of other thrombotic conditions such as myocardial infarction and pulmonary embolism because of its hypoallergenicity and because it has an equivalent efficacy and half-life to streptokinase. TPA has a shorter half-life than either uro- or streptokinase and has specificity for fibrin rather than its precursor substrate fibrinogen.

Technique of Use

There is no consensus as to when or how to use thrombolytic therapies. Generally, when all surgical maneuvers have failed, it can be considered but will be ineffective if the no-reflow phenomenon has occurred at a molecular level. However, distinguishing intravascular thrombus caused by mechanical flow stasis and thrombus secondary to the endothelial dysfunction seen in the no-reflow phenomenon is not yet possible. One must adopt local hospital policies regarding the off-label use of thrombolysis and in particular pay attention to medical contraindications to its use. Doses that have been used in previous studies include streptokinase or urokinase at between 100,000 and 250,000 units and TPA at 15 mg infused over half an hour. These can be infused via an arterial side branch without disrupting the arterial anastomosis. The venous pedicle should be taken down completely during the infusion to minimize systemic side effects and the flap allowed to freely elute for 30 minutes. The anesthetist must be aware of the timing of the infusion to assess potential allergic reactions and loss of blood volume during flap elution.

Outcomes

Because there is no consensus as to when thrombolytic therapy is required, studies on its use are unsurprisingly confounded by numerous variables such as the use of thrombolytics in flaps with already restored venous outflow. Furthermore, the majority of clinical evidence comes from case reports and small series, making the actual efficacy of thrombolytics debatable. Two larger retrospective series include those of Yii et al. (13) and Panchapakesan et al. (14), neither of which conclusively demonstrates a statistical benefit with the use of flap thrombolysis. Yii et al. studied 1733 free flaps, with 41 flaps presenting with pedicle thrombosis (13). Of these, 68% were salvaged, and 32% ultimately failed. A comparison between these two groups was made concerning the use of thrombolytics, with urokinase used in seven flaps (100,000 units) and TPA in one case (15 mg). No significant benefit was demonstrated in the use of thrombolytics between flaps that were salvaged and flaps that ultimately failed. And there was no benefit demonstrated in the use of Fogarty catheters. The main and only significant factor in determining flap salvage appeared to be the time to reexploration (salvage group = 1.5 days; failure group = 4.2 days; $P = 0.007$). Likewise, Panchapakesan et al. retrospectively analyzed 590 flaps, of which 44 flaps suffered from pedicle thrombosis (14). Of these 44 patients, 20 received thrombolytics of which six patients (30%) eventually survived (25). Streptokinase or urokinase was used at a dose of 250,000 units in 50 cc of saline infused into the flap over 30 minutes. Again, time was demonstrated to be of great importance. In flaps receiving thrombolysis, the time to reexploration was demonstrated to be the major factor in flap salvage (salvaged, 32.8 hr vs. failure, 63.8 hr; $P = 0.05$). This study did not, however, separately analyze the statistical efficacy of thrombolysis between flap failure and salvage groups. Simple contingency analysis (salvaged flaps thrombolysis, 6; not thrombolyzed, 13; failed flaps thrombolysis, 14; not thrombolyzed, 11; Fisher's exact test $P = 0.15$) of the data presented in this study does not suggest that thrombolysis has a significant association with flap salvage.

NO-REFLOW PHENOMENON

Ames et al. described the no-reflow phenomenon in 1968 in a rabbit cerebral ischemia model after noting that cerebral vascularization after tissue reperfusion was nonhomogeneous (18). The no-reflow phenomenon is defined as the failure of microvascular perfusion despite adequate arterial inflow (18). There are two continuing problems in this field. First, it still remains only partially elucidated. Second, its relevance to clinical practice is limited by the failure of translation of laboratory interventions into successful clinical therapies. On a histological level, the no-reflow phenomenon is characterized by swelling of the vascular endothelium and loss of its normal integrity, ultimately resulting in exposure of subendothelial collagen and consequent platelet aggregation. This leads to flow stasis and irreversible microvascular thrombosis. Although these changes are postulated in animal models to be reversible up to 12 hours after ischemic onset, it is not possible to correlate this time limit with clinical studies unless intraoperative biopsies are performed (19).

Modern theories regarding changes at the molecular level are more complex, with two main stages involved. During the first stage of tissue ischemia, adenosine triphosphate is used as an energy substrate with formation of hypoxanthine. The protease xanthine oxidase is also formed during this time because of increased intracellular calcium levels. The second stage occurs during reperfusion, with xanthine oxidase converting hypoxanthine to xanthine and in doing so releasing reactive oxygen species (ROS) such as superoxide free radicals (20). These free radicals are thought to be ultimately responsible for loss of endothelial cell integrity, disrupting cell membrane lipids and cell death. The xanthine oxidase system is thought to be the predominate mechanism in endothelial cells, but a contribution is also made from the nicotinamide adenine dinucleotide phosphate (NADPH) oxidase system in neutrophils (21). Thus, although the process is initiated by ischemia, the actual damage occurs during reperfusion. With the activation of cytokine by the reactive oxygen metabolite, several adhesion molecules are presented on the surface of endothelium and neutrophil, such as P-selectin, E-selectin, L-selectin, intercellular adhesion molecule 1 (ICAM-1), and integrin. Because of the ligands between the adhesion molecules, the neutrophil–endothelial interaction will result in extravasation of neutrophil and subsequent parenchymal tissue damage,

Therapeutic Agents Targeted Against Reperfusion Injury

Numerous laboratory studies have investigated the mechanism responsible for reperfusion injury and the no-reflow phenomenon. Despite this, no clinically effective therapies have yet been developed. It should be noted that thrombolytic therapies are sometimes erroneously said to target the no-reflow phenomenon. This is incorrect because they only aid in dissolution of thrombus but cannot reverse the loss of endothelial integrity nor prevent the production of superoxide free radicals that characterize true no-reflow. Actual therapies that target certain steps during the reperfusion stage include xanthine oxidase inhibitors, free radical scavengers, and neutrophil inhibitors. Rodent flap models have shown benefits from the xanthine oxidase inhibitor allopurinol (22), the free radical scavenger superoxide dismutase (22), the antioxidant ascorbic acid (23), and immunosuppressants that reduce neutrophil influx (24). Nonetheless, none of these therapies have found a significant application in clinical studies, and attempting to salvage a flap that has reached the critical no-reflow stage is currently futile.

SURGICAL MANAGEMENT OF THE FAILED FLAP

Three General Approaches to the Failed Primary Free Flap

Our approach to the patient with primary free flap failure was described in a group of 3361 free flaps (25). In this large series, there were 1235 free flaps for head and neck reconstruction and 2126 for extremities over a 7-year period. Primary failures occurred in 42 head and neck patients and 52 extremity cases. The general approach thereafter was second free flap, regional flap, or conservative management. In the head and neck cases, 40% underwent a second free flap, 36% a regional flap, and 24% conservative management. For the extremities, the respective figures were 29%, 5%, and 63%. Additionally, 3% of extremity cases underwent secondary limb amputation.

Indications for a Second Free Flap

Critical defects in the head and neck may be life threatening, such as those that may result in carotid blowout or intracranial infection, such as skull base resections. The Crane principle and use of conservative measures do not apply in such instances and mandate the use of second flap. Although the proportion of cases in which a secondary free flap and secondary pedicled flap was similar (40% vs. 36%), the pedicled flaps had a very high complication rate, requiring revision with a second free flap in one third of cases (25). Thus, we advocate a second free flap as the primary choice of reconstruction in critical head and neck defects.

Regarding the extremities, the philosophy differs. First, critical means limb rather than life threatening, with primary free flap failure resulting in a secondary amputation rate of 3.4%. Second, the Crane principle and use of conservative measures can be applied successfully in many cases because the lower limb rarely has exposure of critical structures such as the great vessels. Salvage was possible in 63% of cases of failed primary free flaps with conservative treatment alone. Other groups suggest reasonable salvage rates after free flap failure of 36.5% (26). The lower limb is not amenable to many ipsilateral regional flaps, particularly when a free flap has been considered as appropriate for the primary defect, largely because of zone of injury issues. The standard cross-leg flap, however, remains a possibility. In our series, only 5% proceeded to regional flap reconstruction (25).

Technical Points in Secondary Free Flaps

The same flap should be performed when possible, and bone should be replaced with bone when possible because the functional results and secondary revision rates are still significantly better. Points to note in the design of a second free flap include the need for a larger flap dimension caused by debridement at the recipient site, longer length of pedicle to allow access to vessels outside the zone of trauma, or in a differing anatomical region. If possible, the original vessels should not be used because of the presence of vasculitis and the potential for occult intimal changes. In head and neck free flaps, the contralateral neck was used in 35% of cases, and in the lower limb, if necessary, the contralateral leg may be used for vascularization of the second free flap (16). An illustrative case of a failed free flap in an extensive oromandibulofacial defect is given in Figures 6-1 to 6-7, in which a second free flap was chosen in preference to a regional flap in view of the poor outcomes of salvage with regional flaps.

Outcomes of Secondary Free Flaps

The philosophy of our unit, therefore, is that a second free flap should be attempted in most cases with few contraindications, particularly given the high complication rate of "rescue" pedicled flaps. Contraindications are relative and may include deteriorating health of the patient or local uncontrolled infection.

The success rates of second free flaps in head and neck cases do not differ significantly to primary free flaps at 94%, perhaps reflecting the availability of vessels in nontrauma zones and without previous surgery. Some caution is advocated in

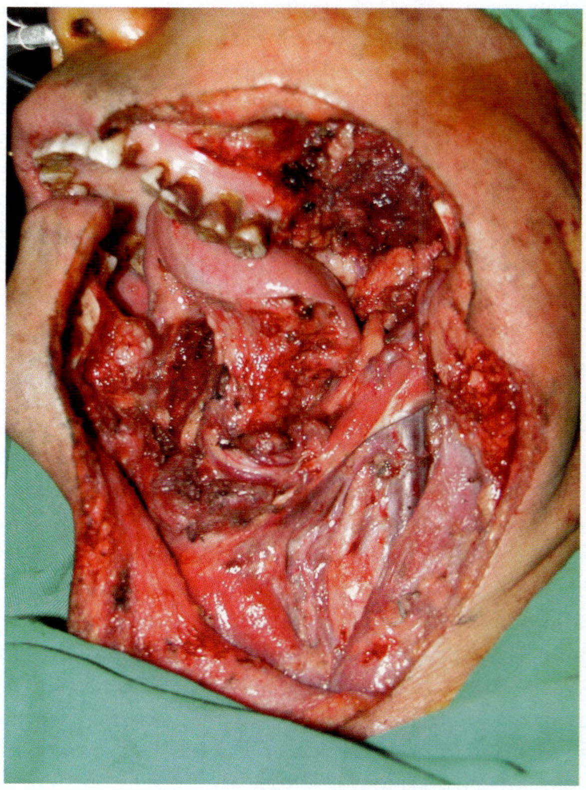

FIGURE 6-1 Extensive composite oromandibulofacial defect after resection of a primary buccal SCC (stage IV).

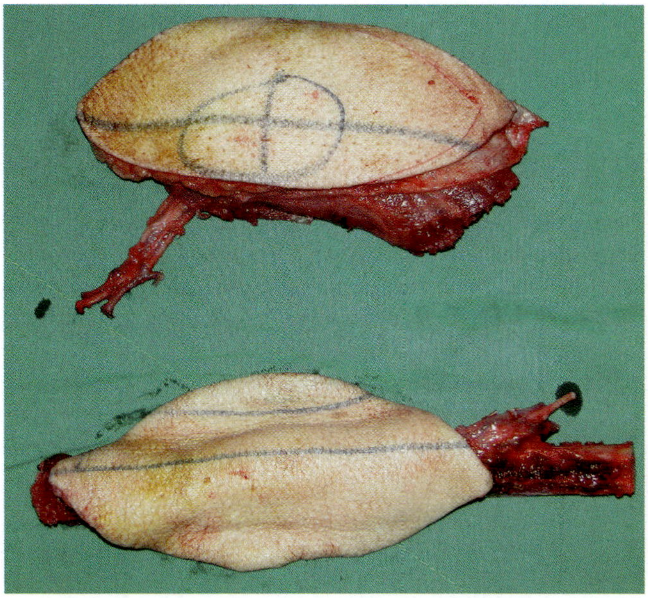

FIGURE 6-2 Two free flaps raised for reconstruction of the defect: fibula osteoseptocutaneous flap and antero-lateral thigh flap (ALT) with vastus lateralis. The arterial anastomoses were facial artery for the fibula and superior thyroid for the antero-lateral thigh flap with vastus lateralis (ALT-VL). The venous anastomoses for both flaps were to the branches of the internal jugular vein.

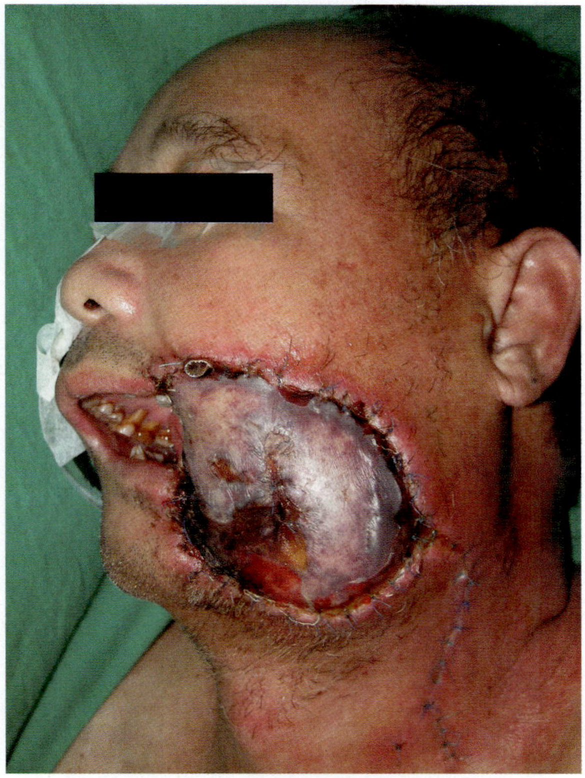

FIGURE 6-3 The external ALT-VL flap was reexplored on postoperative day 1 for venous congestion. No obvious problem was noted regarding compression or kinking of the pedicle, and thrombectomy and revision of anastomosis to a separate branch of the internal jugular vein. Despite attempts at revision, the flap suffered complete necrosis after 1 week. This photograph was taken 1 week later.

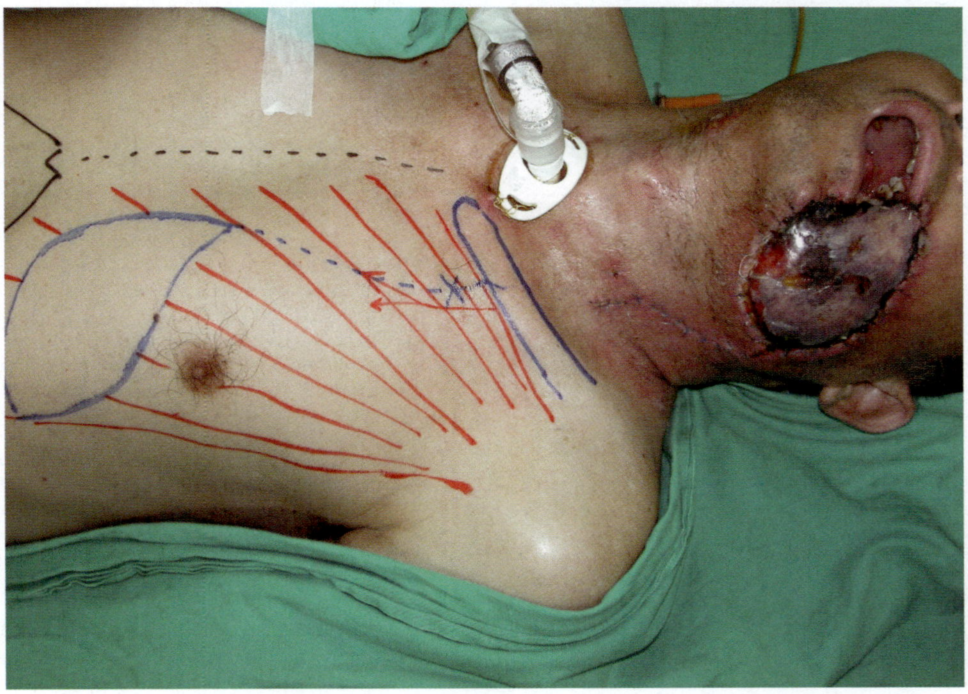

FIGURE 6-4 Although a design for a pedicled pectoralis major flap was made for this defect, it was not used for the secondary reconstruction.

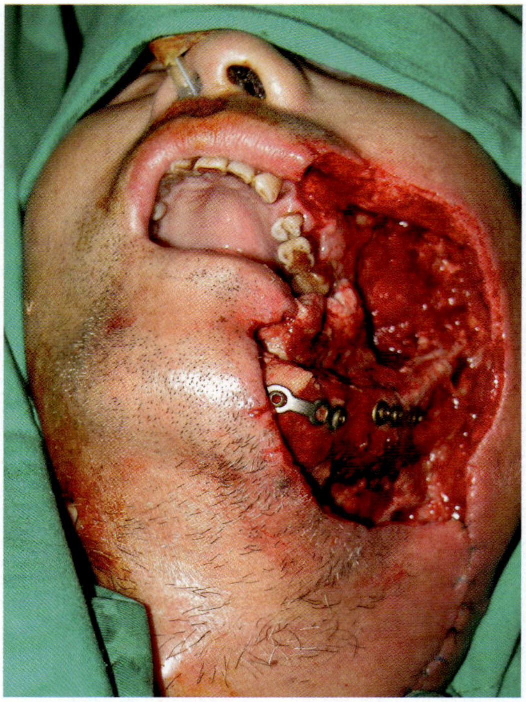

FIGURE 6-5 Defect after removal of the failed external flap. Erythema is noted around the ipsilateral neck, therefore, the superficial temporal vessels were used in the second procedure.

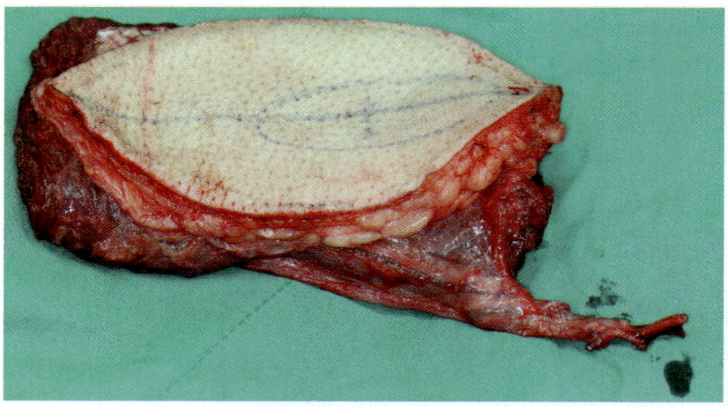

FIGURE 6-6 A second free ALT-VL was raised as our first choice, according to our protocol after free flap failure in head and neck cases.

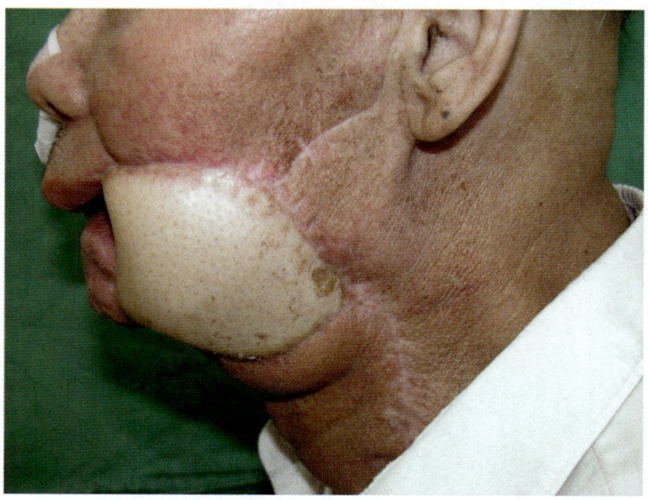

FIGURE 6-7 The replacement free flap survived without postoperative complications.

attempting a second free flap in the extremities given a lower success rate of 82%. Despite this, the majority of cases in our series were salvageable with conservative measures alone (25).

CONCLUSIONS

The technical aspects of flap salvage are not particularly controversial and are similar in most microsurgical units. However, three questions were posed earlier in this chapter. First, what is the proven role of pharmacologic agents such as dextran in reducing the risk of postoperative flap failure?

The role of most agents has not been proven, and dextran, in particular, has been demonstrated to have significant adverse effects. Only subcutaneous heparin has been shown to have any beneficial effect. However, given the low rates of flap failure, the power required to reach appropriate conclusions and avoid type II errors has not been reached in any single trial.

Second, when all surgical options have been exhausted in reexploration of the failing flap, what is the role of thrombolytic agents? Again, studies do not suggest a clear clinical benefit, with analyses suggesting that timing of reexploration is the single most important factor in determining success of flap salvage. Thrombolysis has not been shown to be a statistically significant factor in flap rescue.

Third, in flaps that eventually go on to complete failure, what is the next step in the reconstructive algorithm? In most cases, if a free flap was deemed to be the correct primary indication, then it remains the correct secondary indication. This is particularly the case in head and neck reconstruction but may be less applicable in reconstruction of the breast and extremities.

REFERENCES

1. Chen KT, Mardini S, Chuang DCC, et al. Timing of presentation of the first signs of vascular compromise dictates the salvage outcome of free flap transfers. *Plast Reconstr Surg* 2007;120:187–195.
2. Khouri RK, Cooley BC, Kunselman AR, et al. A prospective study of microvascular free-flap surgery and outcome. *Plast Reconstr Surg* 1998;102:711–721.
3. Lerman J. Study design in clinical research: sample size estimation and power analysis. *Can J Anesth* 1996;43(2):184–191.
4. Peter FW, Franken RJPM, Wang WZ, et al. Effect of low dose aspirin on thrombus formation at arterial and venous microanastomoses and on the tissue microcirculation. *Plast Reconstr Surg* 1997;99:1112–1121.
5. Chien W, Varvares MA, Hadlock T, et al. Effects of aspirin and low-dose heparin in head and neck reconstruction using microvascular free flaps. *Laryngoscope* 2005;115:973–976.
6. Ashjian P, Chen CM, Pusic A, et al. The effect of postoperative anticoagulation on microvascular thrombosis. *Ann Plast Surg* 2007;59:36–40.
7. Li X, Cooley BC. Effect of anticoagulation and inhibition of platelet aggregation on arterial versus venous microvascular thrombosis. *Ann Plast Surg* 1995;35:165–169.
8. Hanasono MM, Butler CE. Prevention and treatment of thrombosis in microvascular surgery. *J Reconstr Microsurg* 2008;24(5):305-314. doi: 10.1055/s-2008-1080530. Epub 2008 Jul 9. Review.
9. Disa JJ, Polvora VP, Pusic AL, et al. Dextran-related complications in head and neck micro- surgery: do the benefits outweigh the risks? A prospective randomized analysis. *Plast Reconstr Surg* 2003;112:1534–1539.
10. Cox GW, Runnels S, Hsu HSH, Das SK. A comparison of heparinized saline irrigation solutions in a model of microvascular thrombosis. *Br J Plast Surg* 1992;45:345–347.
11. Andresen DM, Barker JH, Hjortdal VE. Local heparin is superior to systemic heparin in preventing arterial thrombosis. *Microsurgery* 2002;22:265–272.

12. Khouri RK, Cooley BC, Kunselman AR, Landis JR, Yeramian P, Ingram D, Natarajan N, Benes CO, Wallemark C. A prospective study of microvascular free-flap surgery and outcome. *Plast Reconstr Surg* 1998;102(3): 711-721.
13. Yii NW, Evans GR, Miller MJ, et al. Thrombolytic therapy: what is its role in free flap salvage? *Ann Plast Surg* 2001;46(6):601–604.
14. Panchapakesan V, Addison P, Beausang E, et al. Role of thrombolysis in free-flap salvage. *J Reconstr Microsurg* 2003;19(8):523–530.
15. Bui DT, Cordeiro PG, Hu QY, et al. Free flap reexploration: indications treatment and outcomes in 1193 free flaps. *Plast Reconstr Surg* 2007;119:2092–2100.
16. Chen HC, Demirkan F, Wei FC, Cheng SL, Cheng MH, Chen IH. Free fibula osteoseptocutaneous-pedicled pectoralis major myocutaneous flap combination in reconstruction of extensive composite mandibular defects. *Plast Reconstr Surg* 1999;103(3):839-845.
17. Lin CH, Mardini S, Lin YT, Yeh JT, Wei FC, Chen HC. Sixty-five clinical cases of free tissue transfer using long arteriovenous fistulas or vein grafts. *J Trauma* 2004;56(5):1107-1117.
18. Ames A III,Wright L, Kowada M, et al. Cerebral ischemia, 11: the no-reflow phenomenon. *Am J Pathol* 1968;52:437–447.
19. May JW Jr,Chait LA, O'Brien BM, Hurley JV. The no-reflow phenomenon in experimental free flaps. *Plast Reconstr Surg* 1978;61(2):256–267.
20. Calhoun KH, Tan L, Seikaly H. An integrated theory of the no-reflow phenomenon and the beneficial effect of vascular washout on no-reflow. *Laryngoscope* 1999;109(4):528–535.
21. van den Heuvel MG, Buurman WA, Bast A, et al. Review: ischaemia-reperfusion injury in flap surgery. *J Plast Reconstr Aesthet Surg* 2009;62(6):721–726.
22. Im MJ, Manson PN, Bulkley GB, et al. Effects of superoxide dismutase and allopurinol on the survival of acute island skin flaps. *Ann Surg* 1985;201:357–359.
23. Zaccaria A, Weinzweig N, Yoshitake M, et al. Vitamin C reduces ischemia-reperfusion injury in a rat epigastric island skin flap model. *Ann Plast Surg* 1994;33:620–623.
24. Cetinkale O, Bilgic L, Bolayirli M, et al. Involvement of neutrophils in ischemia-reperfusion injury of inguinal island skin flaps in rats. *Plast Reconstr Surg* 1998;102:153–160.
25. Wei FC, Demirkan F, Chen HC, Chuang DC, Chen SH, Lin CH, Cheng SL, Cheng MH, Lin YT. The outcome of failed free flaps in head and neck and extremity reconstruction: what is next in the reconstructive ladder? *Plast Reconstr Surg* 2001;108(5):1154-1160; discussion 1161-1162.
26. Benacquista T, Kasabian AK, Karp NS. The fate of lower extremities with failed free flaps. *Plast Reconstr Surg* 1996;98(5):834-840; discussion 841-842.

CHAPTER 7

Microsurgery and Brain Plasticity

Anders Björkman and Göran Lundborg

With the introduction of microsurgical techniques several decades ago, a new dimension was introduced in reconstructive surgery. Stereoscopic magnification combined with atraumatic surgical techniques and new surgical materials created new possibilities in the revascularization of injured body parts, the reconstruction of damaged nerve structures, the replantation of severed digits, and the introduction of many other micro-level reconstructive procedures. Microsurgery has indeed revolutionized our possibilities to restore structure and function after trauma, tumor ablation, and severe congenital defects.

However, what is not so well known is the fact that all reconstructive procedures, whether we are dealing with finger replantation, hand transplantation, nerve reconstruction, or nerve transfer, introduce profound changes in the central nervous system (CNS). More than 80 years ago, it was discovered that all body parts have their own representation in the brain, constituting a "cortical body map" known as the sensory and motor homunculi. During open brain surgery in conscious patients, Penfield and Boldrey (1) demonstrated that tactile stimulation of various areas on the brain surface triggered the perception of sensory stimuli in various anatomical regions and could also produce muscle contractions in various parts of the body. It was found that stimulation of specific brain areas produced perception of tactile stimuli or muscle contraction primarily in the opposite side of the body. In this way, Penfield and Boldrey were able to map the body on the brain surface (Figure 7-1). They were able to identify a sensory area posterior to the central sulcus where direct cortical stimulation produced sensory perceptions from different bodyparts and another area anterior to the central sulcus where cortical stimulation produced muscle contractions. These observations have later been verified by direct cortical recording techniques in primates and by the use of various brain imaging techniques in humans (2–6). The hand and the face have disproportionately large representational areas in the motor as well as sensory cortex, reflecting the extremely well-developed sensory and motor functions in these areas. The hand representational area in the sensory cortex presents a size of about 10 to 15 mm with the individual digital representations well separated (Figure 7-2), the thumb showing a larger representation than the fingers (see Figure 7-1).

Activation of the hand's motor area is reflected in movements of the contralateral hand. Although simple tasks involving gross grip are associated with activation primarily of the contralateral motor area, fine precision movements induce recruitment of other cortical motor areas in the parietal and frontal lobes, also including the ipsilateral hemisphere (7). Planning and initiation of motor tasks are associated with activation of the premotor areas situated in the frontal lobe (7). From studies in animals and healthy humans, it is known that it is the *pattern of movement* rather than separate anatomical body parts or muscles that are represented in the primary motor cortex (8). Furthermore, the motor areas are well integrated with the somatosensory system in the parietal lobe and with the cerebellum (9). In 1952, Sharrington showed that sensory afferent information is needed to execute well-coordinated movement (10). Thus, in most voluntary-controlled motor functions, a cortical sensorimotor network is required to produce the required movement.

Stimulation of cutaneous mechanoreceptors in the hand generates impulses that pass through the dorsal root ganglia and spinal cord to the somatosensory brain cortex after traversing intermediate relay stations in the cuneate nucleus in the brain stem and the ventroposterior lateral (VPL) nucleus in the thalamus. Such signals activate primarily the contralateral hemisphere but information is also sent to the ipsilateral hemisphere (11,12). The primary somatosensory cortex (S1) contains four cytoarchitecturally different areas: area 3a, 3b, 1, and 2 (2,13). Area 3b and 1 receive most of their information from receptors in the skin (2,14), and area 3a and 2 receive most of their information from the muscles and joints. Furthermore, it has been shown (15) that different areas are activated by different forms of stimuli so that whereas area 3b and 1 are activated by all types of stimuli, area 3a is stimulated

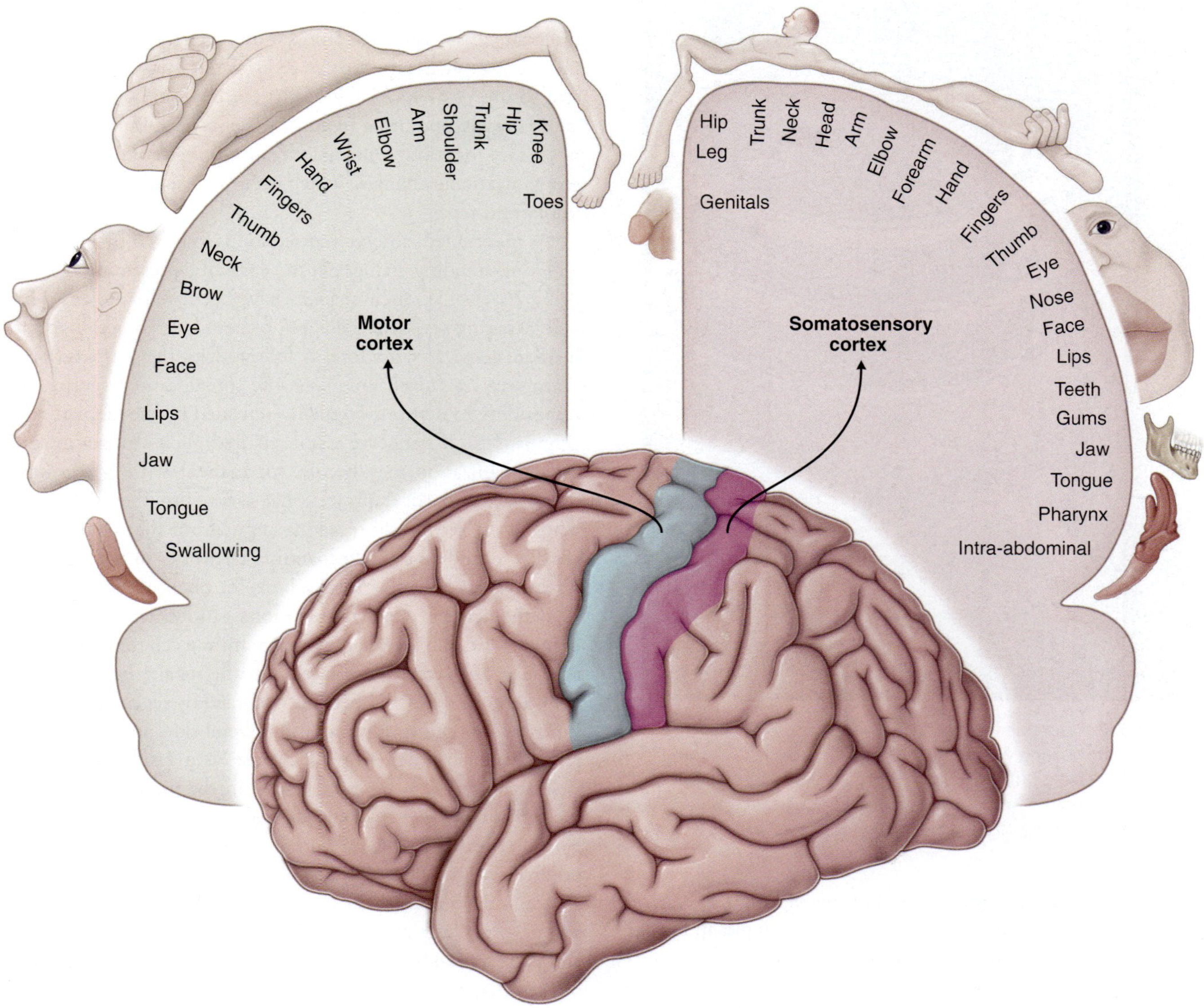

FIGURE 7-1 Schematic illustration of human primary sensory and motor cortex. Body parts are projected over the brain surface in specific order, the face and hand localized laterally and inferiorly. Sensory cortex is posterior to the central sulcus, and the motor cortex is anterior to the sulcus.

only when also motor activation occurs. Area 2 is activated by all mechanical stimuli but has been shown to be activated mainly by the detection of surface curvature differences and the recognition of shape. Each area in S1 contains a complete map of the body. However all four areas in S1 are extensively interconnected.

BRAIN PLASTICITY

One of the most interesting questions in neuroscience concerns the manner in which the nervous system can modify its organization and ultimately its function throughout an individual's lifetime based on sensory input, experience, learning, and injury (16,17), a phenomenon often referred to as *brain plasticity* (18,19).

Classical teaching held that the cortical body map is already firmly established at birth and cannot be changed thereafter; however, concepts evolving over the past few decades indicate that the brain is very adaptive and can change its functional organization in response to changes in activity and sensory inflow from the periphery (2,4,20–26). Both the motor and the somatosensory cortices can rapidly reorganize their synaptic networks as a response to changes in sensory inflow and peripheral motor activity. For instance, professional violin players may increase the cortical projections of their string hand as a response to intense training (27,28), and it is also known that extensive use of fingers, as in Braille reading, results in enlargement of the corresponding cortical projectional areas in the primary somatosensory cortex (29). On the other hand, decreased sensory inflow and motor activity, as well as immobilization of a limb, is associated with synaptic depression and shrinkage of the corresponding cortical areas (30). Rapid reorganizations of the somatosensory cortex are seen after local anesthesia of a finger, and this is associated with expansion of the adjacent cortical finger projections (31,32). Such rapid reorganizational changes illustrate constant ongoing "cortical competition" among various body parts—deafferentation of

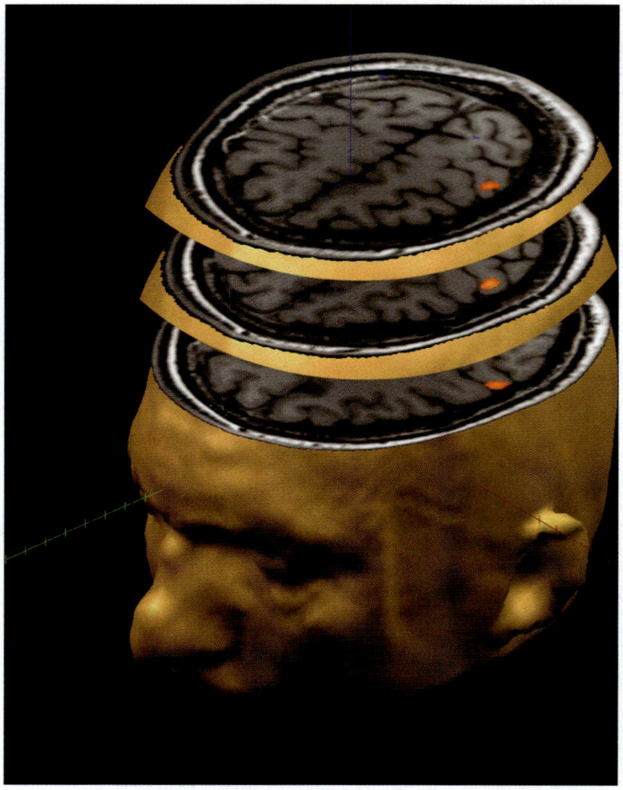

FIGURE 7-2 Magnetic resonance imaging investigation of a normal brain showing well-separated projectional sites for the thumb (lower position), index finger (intermediate layer), and little finger (upper layer). (Courtesy by Andreas Weibull, Medical Radiation Physics, Malmö, Skåne University Hospital, Malmö, Sweden.)

one part is rapidly followed by expansion of adjacent cortical body representations. Such changes can be very rapid and occur within minutes, illustrating a rapid shift in balance between excitation and inhibition of synapses in the brain. An example is the unmasking of present but normally inhibited synapses (25,26).

More long-standing functional reorganizations in the cerebral cortex, as well as at subcortical level, can be seen after chronic denervation, such as in amputation, and over time such changes can become established and permanent (33–35). Dramatic cortical reorganizations have been seen after arm amputation when the "empty" cortical arm representation is rapidly occupied by the nearby face representation. This may lead to very striking phenomena as soon as 24 hours afterward: the amputated hand can remain partially mapped in the new expanded facial area so that touch to various areas of the face can give rise to tactile sensations in the missing hand (36–38). The cortical reorganizational changes that occur after amputation is the basis for phantom sensation and phantom pain, which often occur as a complication to such an injury (39–41).

THE CORTICAL RESPONSE TO MICROSURGICAL PROCEDURES

Injuries to peripheral nerves represent a major microsurgical challenge. Although the severed nerve ends can be meticulously repaired using microsurgical techniques, there is no real way to control the outgrowth of axonal sprouts, which as a result are often largely misdirected. For example, in hand axons originally ment to supply the thumb can re-grow out into the index finger and so on. (22,24,42). Clinically, the outcome of nerve repair is usually disappointing in adult patients with limited recovery of sensory function. One major reason is the prominent cortical reorganizational changes, which occur in association with nerve injury and repair.

As mentioned, a nerve transection is followed by immediate and long-standing changes in the cortical representational areas (4,25,26,43–45). Such changes have been well studied in animal experiments, especially on primates. Transection of the median nerve at wrist level is followed by the formation of a silent area—a "black hole"—in the somatosensory cortex corresponding to neurons originally activated by the median nerve (Figure 7-3). If the nerve is not repaired, such changes in cortical reorganization may become permanent with expansion of the adjacent cortical projectional areas into that silent area. Thus, areas previously receiving input from the median nerve are now occupied by the expanding territories of the radial and ulnar nerves. This may form a basis for phantom sensations.

If the nerve is repaired new axonal sprouts traverse the zone of injury and reinnervate the distal Schwann cell tubes. However, as a result of axonal misdirection at the repair site (46), many Schwann cell tubes will become occupied by regenerating axons from heterotopic regions, and peripheral skin areas will not be reinnervated by their original axons. As a result, the original well-organized hand representations in the motor and somatosensory cortices will be changed into a dysorganized, mosaic-like pattern, preventing the median nerve from recapturing all of its original territory (4,21,22,24). The boundaries between separate anatomical skin areas and individual finger representations disappear, and the hand representation is changed into dispersed and discontinuous islands (see Figure 7-3). Due to misdirection of the outgrowing axons the hand now "speaks a new language to the brain," and this new language cannot easily be understood in an adult. Studies in monkeys have shown that after the repair of a nerve transection, such representational changes occur at subcortical as well as cortical levels (45,47). Sensory reeducational programs after nerve repair may substantially help to compensate for the changes in the cortical hand representation (48–50). The effects of such sensory reeducation can be enhanced by training programs, especially those addressing the plasticity of the brain. To use the CNS's adaptive ability for therapeutic purposes, guided plasticity (51) is an attractive concept with promising results. For example, this potential for cerebral plasticity can be used clinically to strengthen and promote CNS functions that are lost or weakened.

Nerve Transfer

When tension-free direct coaptation of distal and proximal nerve stumps not are possible because of a large nerve gap, an autologous nerve graft is the option of choice (24).

Nerve transfers, which involve the use of a proximal expendable sensory or motor nerve as the donor of regenerating axons to reinnervate the distal target organ, are alternatives to autologous nerve grafts when the nerve gap is substantial or when

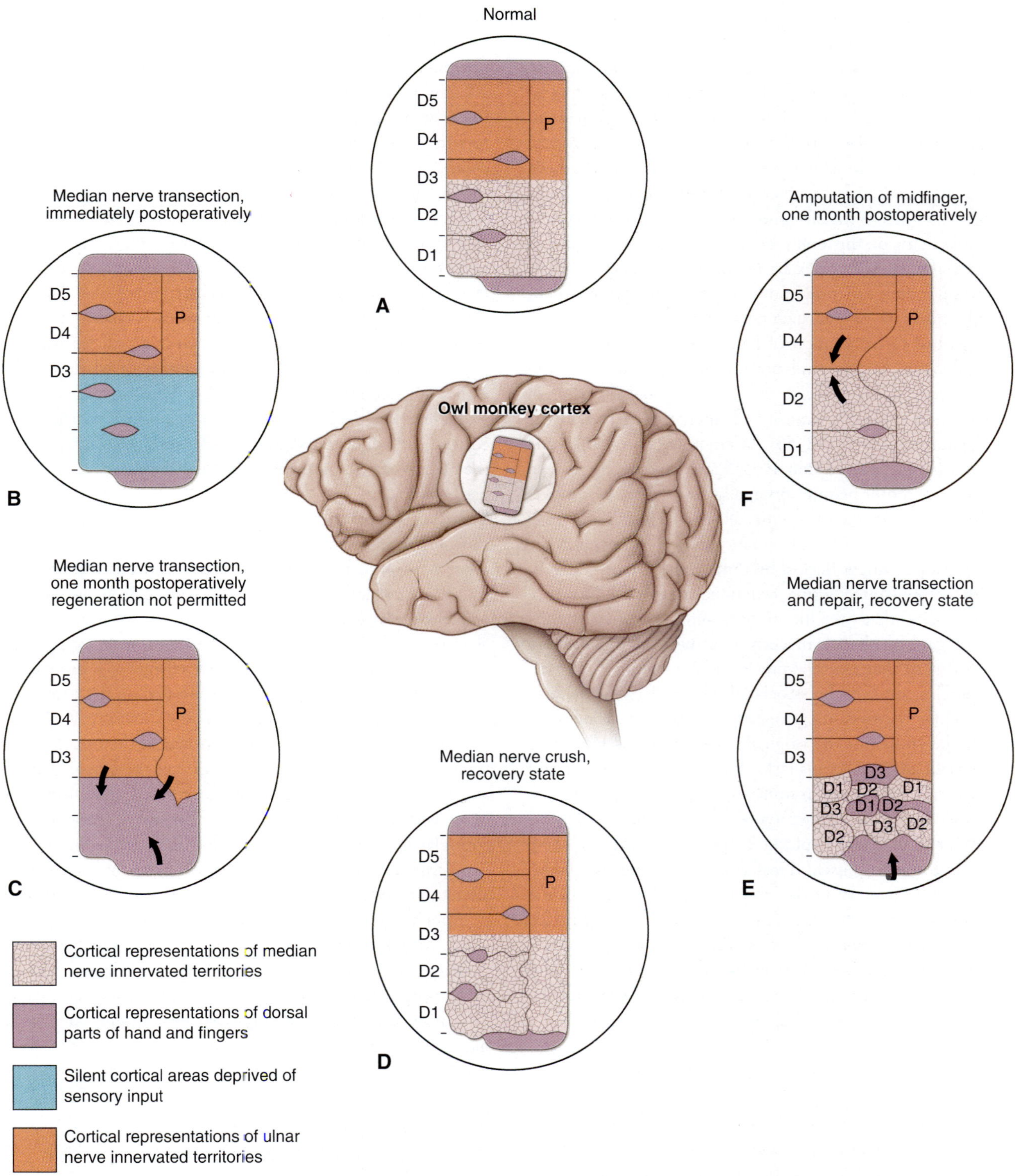

FIGURE 7-3 Changes in cortical mapping (area 3b of an owl monkey) as a result of deafferentation such as amputation and nerve injury followed by axonal outgrowth. (**A**) Normal cortical representation of the fingers. (**B**) Transection of the median nerve immediately after surgery. The cortical area corresponding to the median nerve becomes silent because of acute deprivation of afferent inflow. (**C**) One month after median nerve transection, regeneration is not permitted. The cortical area, previously receiving input from the median nerve, is now occupied by expanding cortical representations of dorsal radial-innervated skin and ulnar-innervated skin of the hand. (**D**) The median nerve in the recovery phase after a crush injury. The mapping of fingers and palm has returned to practically normal because of intact Schwann cell tubes guiding the regenerating fibers to the correct peripheral targets. (**E**) Transection of the median nerve, repair and axonal regeneration. Recovery phase. The cortical median nerve representation is now totally remodeled and characterized by small discontinuous patches, some of them overlapping, responding to inputs in a somatotopic disorganized pattern. (**F**) Amputation of the midfinger. Representations of the second and fourth digits have expanded, now occupying the area previously receiving input from the midfinger.

there is no proximal nerve end to be found. Nerve transfers offer a promising surgical alternative for restoration of function by providing motor axons close to the end organ, thus minimizing the time needed for reinnervation. Because the denervated target is reinnervated by a foreign motor neuron pool, relearning based on CNS plasticity is needed to achieve a functional outcome (24,52). Various nerve transfer procedures have been described for restoration of function in the arm as well as the face (53). Such nerve transfer procedures are highly dependent on the plasticity of the brain because populations of motor neurons in the cerebral cortex are required to reinnervate "new" muscles and induce function in muscle groups that they did not originally innervate. Several such nerve transfer procedures have been described for restoration of hand and arm function after peripheral nerve damage and brachial plexus injuries. A frequently used procedure for restoration of elbow function in brachial plexus injuries is transfer of intercostal nerves to the musculocutaneous nerve (52–55). After reinnervation following such a transfer, elbow flexion is facilitated by taking a deep breath because motor neurons originally devoted to chest movements now are redirected to induce elbow flexion. With time, breathing is not needed to facilitate elbow flexion, and the motor control of elbow flexion becomes more independent. It has been demonstrated, using functional magnetic resonance imaging studies, that over the months and years after surgery, there is a gradual change in cortical activity in the primary motor cortex so that neurons previously controlling the intercostal muscles comes to be associated with activity in the arm (52,55). Thus, the dynamic properties of the brain allow it to adapt to the situation, the original motor neurons becoming active in their original motor tasks despite a nerve transfer and a different cerebral input. Presumably, cortical reorganizational changes occur in many other types of motor nerve transfers routinely used in brachial plexus surgery. Not only in nerve transfers but also in muscle transferring procedures is restoration of function dependent on reorganizational changes in the motor cortex. For instance, a finger extensor muscle may be used to restore lost opposition of the thumb, and a wrist flexor can be used to restore finger extension. Both procedures require substantial reorganizational changes in the motor cortex for the desired movements to become spontaneous.

Flaps

Noninnervated flaps used for simple coverage of tissue defects can acquire some degree of sensibility through peripheral reinnervation. A neurosensory flap, or "innervated flap," may restore sensation immediately if pedicled on its neurovascular axis or in a delayed fashion if it is transferred and the nerve anastomosed to a suitable recipient. Not only does the inclusion of a peripheral nerve in flap provide the possibility for immediate sensory innervation, but it may also improve flap circulation because the vascularity of the flap depends on vasoregulatory nerves in the vessel walls. Sensate flaps have particular application in areas where protective sensibility is desirable such as the hands. When a pedicled neurosensory flap is used, the afferent nerve supply from the skin is intact, resulting in a normal sensory afferent flow to the brain. However, because the flap is moved to a new location, the sensory information is initially misinterpreted, resulting in an anatomic misdirection of sensory stimulation. As a result of these changes in afferent signal pattern, a cortical reorganization takes place. Over time, the cortical projection of information from receptors in the transferred skin area may be transferred in sensory cortex to the location that normally innervates the area, resulting in a more normal sensory perception.

Free neurosensory flaps are similar to pedicled flaps with the exception that the recipient nerve has to reinnervate the distal nerve territory. This reinnervation process occurs over an extended time period and is prone to misdirection of the outgrowing nerves. Therefore, the clinical result when it comes to return of sensory function often is inferior to that in a pedicled flap.

When it comes to muscle flaps, much of what was stated earlier for pedicled and free sensory flaps is true. A cortical reorganization occurs, resulting in a gradual transfer of the cortical control of transferred muscle from the original place to the place where the control of the function that is reconstructed has been located.

In both experimental animals and in humans, it has been shown that transfer of C7 nerve from one side of the body to the other to restore function in a brachial plexus injury induces significant cortical reorganizational changes. Initially, the ipsilateral cortex controls the function, but this is followed by gradual changes in which both hemispheres assume a form of joint control. Finally, there is a progressive change to a more contralateral control of the function. This is based on the strong interhemisperic plasticity that is seen in many situations. A change in one hemisphere is immediately mirrored in the opposite hemisphere (25). However, both in the case of the cross-C7 transfer and in nerve injuries in general, the cortical activation pattern never returns to normal when the majority of the activation is contralateral to the stimulation. This likely represents a cortical compensation; the brain tries to compensate for the changes in afferent and efferent nerve signaling by using both hemispheres.

After surgical reconstruction of nerves and muscles, there is always a relearning process. The afferent signal pattern is changed, and this results in both cortical and subcortical reorganization. It is well known from several studies that this reorganization process can be improved by training—sensory and motor relearning. This relearning process aims at preserving the cortical organization as much as possible (48–50).

HAND REPLANTATION AND TRANSPLANTATION

Amputation of a hand is followed by rapid cortical organizational changes. The projectional site of the amputated body part disappears (silent area, black hole), and the adjacent cortical areas expand into the deafferented area and use of the neurons usually supplying the amputated hand. However, after replantation, the hand recaptures its original projectional site in the somatosensory cortex, a phenomenon that parallels function in the replanted hand (56). Interestingly, the hand projection appears not only in the contralateral hemisphere but also to a larger extent in the ipsilateral hemisphere, an expression of interaction between the two hemispheres to optimize function. Also, after transplantation of a hand, an autologous phenomenon occurs: the transplanted donor's hand, replanted onto the recipients forearm, becomes projected in the recipient's brain in the "correct" hand position (56–58).

REFERENCES

1. Penfield W, Boldrey E. Somatic motor and sensory representations in the cerebral cortex of man as studied by electrical stimulation. *Brain* 1937;60:389–443.
2. Merzenich MM, Kaas JH, Sur M, et al. Double representation of the body surface within cytoarchitectonic areas 3b and 1 in S1" in the owl monkey (*Aotus trivirgatus*). *J Comp Neurol* 1978;181:41–74.
3. Kaas JH, Florence SL. Mechanisms of reorganization in sensory systems of primates after peripheral nerve injury. *Adv Neurol* 1997;73:147–158.
4. Merzenich MM, Jenkins WM. Reorganization of cortical representations of the hand following alterations of skin inputs induced by nerve injury, skin island transfers, and experience. *J Hand Ther* 1993;6:89–104.
5. Blankenburg F, Ruben J, Meyer R, et al. Evidence for a rostral-to-caudal somatotopic organization in human primary somatosensory cortex with mirror-reversal in areas 3b and 1. *Cereb Cortex* 2003;13:987–993.
6. van Westen D, Fransson P, Olsrud J, et al. Fingersomatotopy in area 3b: an fMRI-study. *BMC Neurosci* 2004;5:28.
7. Ehrsson HH, Fagergren A, Jonsson T, et al. Cortical activity in precision-versus power-grip tasks: an fMRI study. *J Neurophysiol* 2000;83:528–536.
8. Schieber MH, Constraints on somatotopic organization in the primary motor cortex. *J Neurophysiol* 2001;86:2125–2143.
9. Roland PE, Zilles K. Functions and structures of the motor cortices in humans. *Curr Opin Neurobiol* 1996;6:773–781.
10. Sharrington CS. *The Interactive Action of the Nervous System.* Cambridge, 1952.
11. Hansson T, Brismar T. Tactile stimulation of the hand causes bilateral cortical activation: a functional magnetic resonance study in humans. *Neurosci Lett* 1999;271:29–32.
12. Bodegård A, Geyer S, Naito E, et al. Somatosensory areas in man activated by moving stimuli. *Neuroreport* 2000;11:187–191.
13. Geyer S, Schleicher A, Zilles K. Areas 3a, 3b, and 1 of human primary somatosensory cortex. *Neuroimage* 1999;10:63–83.
14. Jones EG, Friedman DP. Projection pattern of functional components of thalamic ventrobasal complex on monkey somatosensory cortex. *J Neurophysiol* 1982;48:521–544.
15. Bodegård A. F*unctional mapping of somatosensory cortices in the human brain.* Thesis. Stockholm: Division of Human Brain Research, Department of Neuroscience, Karolinska Institute, 2001.
16. Kaas J. Plasticity of sensory and motor maps in adult mammals. *Ann Rev Neurosci* 1991;14:137–168.
17. Donoghue JP, Hess G, Sanes JN. Motor cortical substrates and mechanisms for learning, InJR Bloedel, TJ Ebner, SP Wise (eds). *Acquisition of Motor Behaviour in Vertebrates.* Cambridge, MA: MIT, 1996, pp. 363–386.
18. Purves D, Augustine GJ, Fitzpatrick D, et al. *Neuroscience.* Sunderland, MA: Sinauer Associates, 2004.
19. Kandel ER, Schwartz JH, Jessel TM. *Principles of Neural Science.* New York: McGraw-Hill, 2000.
20. Bach-y-Rita P. The brain beyond the synapse: a review. *Neuroreport* 1994;5:1553–1557.
21. Lundborg G. Brain plasticity and hand surgery: an overview. *J Hand Surg Br* 2000;25:242–252.
22. Lundborg G: Richard P. Bunge memorial lecture Nerve injury and repair—a challenge to the plastic brain. *J Peripher Nerv Syst* 2003;8:209–226.
23. Allard T, Clark SA, Jenkins M, et al. Reorganization of somatosensory area 3b representations in adult owl monkeys after a digital syndactyly. *J Neurophysiol* 1991;66:1048–1058.
24. Lundborg G. *Nerve Injury and Repair. Regeneration, Reconstruction and Cortical Remodelling.* Philadelphia: Elsevier, 2004.
25. Chen R, Cohen LG, Hallett M. Nervous system reorganization following injury. *Neuroscience* 2002;111:761–773.
26. Wall JT, Xu J, Wang X. Human brain plasticity: an emerging view of the multiple substrates and mechanisms that cause cortical changes and related sensory dysfunctions after injuries of sensory inputs from the body. *Brain Res Brain Res Rev* 2002;39:181–215.
27. Pascual-Leone A, Hamilton R. The metamodal organization of the brain. *Prog Brain Res* 2001;134:427–445.
28. Elbert T, Pantev C, Wienbruch C, et al. Increased cortical representation of the left hand in string players. *Science* 1995;270:305–307.
29. Pascual-Leone A, Wassermann EM, Sadato N, et al. The role of reading activity on the modulation of motor cortical outputs to the reading hand in Braille readers. *Ann Neurol* 1995;38:910–915.
30. Huber R, Ghilardi MF, Massimini M, et al. Arm immobilization causes cortical plastic changes and locally decreases sleep slow wave activity. *Nat Neurosci* 2006;9:1169–1176.
31. Calford MB, Tweedale R. Acute changes in cutaneous receptive fields in primary somatosensory cortex after digit denervation in adult flying fox. *J Neurophysiol* 1991;65:178–187.
32. Rossini PM, Martino G, Narici L, et al. Short-term brain plasticity in humans: transient finger representation changes in sensory cortex somatotopy following ischemic anesthesia. *Brain Res* 1994;642:169–177.
33. Code RA, Eslin DE, Juliano SL. Expansion of stimulus-evoked metabolic activity in monkey somatosensory cortex after peripheral denervation. *Exp Brain Res* 1992;88:341–344.
34. Manger PR, Woods TM, Jones EG. Plasticity of the somatosensory cortical map in macaque monkeys after chronic partial amputation of a digit. *Proc R. Soc Lond B Biol Sci* 1996;263:933–939.
35. Pons T, Preston E, Garraghty K. Massive cortical reorganization after sensory deafferentiation in adult macaques. *Science* 1991;252:1857–1860.
36. Elbert T, Flor H, Birbaumer N, et al. Extensive reorganization of the somatosensory cortex in adult humans after nervous system injury. *Neuroreport* 1994;5:2593–2597.
37. Flor H, Elbert T, Wienbruch C, et al. Phantom-limb pain as a perceptual correlate of cortical organization following arm amputation. *Nature* 1995;375:482–484.
38. Borsook D, Becerra L, Fishman S, et al. Acute plasticity in the human somatosensory cortex following amputation. *Neuroreport* 1998;9: 1013–1017.
39. Flor H, Nikolajsen L, Staehelin J ensen T. Phantom limb pain: a case of maladaptive CNS plasticity? *Nat Rev Neurosci* 2006;7:873–881.
40. Wilkins KL, McGrath PJ, Finley GA, et al. Phantom limb sensations and phantom limb pain in child and adolescent amputees. *Pain* 1998;78: 7–12.
41. Saadah ES, Melzack R. Phantom limb experiences in congenital limb-deficient adults. *Cortex* 1994;30:479–485.
42. Lundborg G. Enhancing posttraumatic nerve regeneration. *J Peripher Nerv Syst* 2002;7:139–140.
43. Lundborg G, Rosen B. Hand function after nerve repair. *Acta Physiol (Oxf)* 2007;189:207–217.
44. Silva AC, Rasey SK, Wu X, et al. Initial cortical reactions to injury of the median and radial nerves to the hands of adult primates. *J Comp Neurol* 1996;366:700–716.
45. Taylor KS, Anastakis DJ, Davis KD. Cutting your nerve changes your brain. *Brain* 2009;132:3122–3133.
46. Witzel C, Brushart T. Morphology of peripheral axon regeneration. *J Periph Nerv Syst* 2003;8:75–76.
47. Hansson T, Brismar T. Loss of sensory discrimination after median nerve injury and activation in the primary somatosensory cortex on functional magnetic resonance imaging. *J Neurosurg* 2003;99:100–105.
48. Dellon AL. Sensibility and Re-education of Sensation in the Hand. Baltimore: Williams & Wilkins, 1981.
49. Rosén B, Balkenius C, Lundborg G. Sensory re-education today and tomorrow. Review of evolving concepts. *Br J Hand Ther* 2003;8:48–56.
50. Wynn-Parry CB, Salter M. Sensory re-education after median nerve lesions. *Hand* 1976;8:250–257.
51. Duffau H. Brain plasticity: from pathophysiological mechanisms to therapeutic applications. *J Clin Neurosci* 2006;13:885–897.
52. Malessy MJ, Bakker D, Dekker AJ, et al. Functional magnetic resonance imaging and control over the biceps muscle after intercostal-musculocutaneous nerve transfer. *J Neurosurg* 2003;98:261–268.
53. Mackinnon SE, Novak CB. Nerve transfers. New options for reconstruction following nerve injury. *Hand Clin* 1999;15:643–666, ix.
54. Chuang DC, Yeh MC, Wei FC. Intercostal nerve transfer of the musculocutaneous nerve in avulsed brachial plexus injuries: evaluation of 66 patients. *J. Hand Surg* 1992;17(suppl A):822–828.
55. Mano Y, Nakamuro T, Tamura R, et al. Central motor reorganization after anastomosis of the musculocutaneous and intercostal nerves following cervical root avulsion. *Ann Neurol* 1995;38:15–20.
56. Bjorkman A, Waites A, Rosen B, et al. Cortical sensory and motor response in a patient whose hand has been replanted: one-year follow up with functional magnetic resonance imaging. *Scand J Plast Reconstr Surg Hand Surg* 2007;41:70–76.
57. Roricht S, Machetanz J, Irlbacher K, et al. Reorganization of human motor cortex after hand replantation. *Ann Neurol* 2001;50:240–249.
58. Lanzetta M, Perani D, Anchisi D, et al. Early use of artificial sensibility in hand transplantation. *Scand J Plast Reconstr Surg* 2004;38:106–111.

CHAPTER 8

Rectus Abdominis Flaps

David W. Chang

HISTORY

Brown et al. (1) are credited with being the first to use abdominal cutaneous flaps based on the perforators of the rectus abdominis muscle. Drever's (2) report of the epigastric "island flap" also recognized the potential for transferring an "island" of skin supplied by a segment of the underlying rectus abdominis muscle. Drever (2) described a vertically oriented musculocutaneous flap based on the deep superior epigastric vascular supply that was transferred to a chest wall defect.

Pennington and Pelly (3) published the first report of transferring a free rectus abdominis musculocutaneous flap based on the deep inferior epigastric artery (DIEA) and vein (DIEV). This flap was used to repair an infraclavicular defect (3). Since then, free rectus abdominis muscle and musculocutaneous flaps have been widely used in reconstruction for defects in the head and neck, breast, and upper and lower extremities.

Since it was first described in 1979, the free transverse rectus abdominis myocutaneous (TRAM) flap has become one of the most popular and reliable methods of microsurgical breast reconstruction. Over time, the free TRAM flap has evolved to include the muscle-sparing (MS)-TRAM flap and the deep inferior epigastric perforator (DIEP) flap, both of which minimize disease at the donor site by harvesting less muscle and less anterior rectus fascia.

ANATOMY

Rectus Abdominis Muscle

The rectus abdominis muscles are a pair of muscles that flex the spine and tighten the intraabdominal wall (Figure 8-1). They arise from the symphysis pubis and the pubic crest and insert on the linea alba and at the fifth, sixth, and seventh costal cartilages, interdigitating with the pectoralis major muscles. The rectus abdominis muscles are long, straight muscles enclosed by a thick sheath except for the posterior part below the arcuate line, which is usually located midway between the umbilicus and symphysis pubis. Although the rectus abdominis muscle in situ measures approximately 30 cm × 10 cm, postharvest contraction limits the useful size to approximately 20 cm × 8 cm.

The rectus abdominis muscle is subdivided by two to five tendinous inscriptions. Moon and Taylor (4) reported that 93.5% of a series that included more than 108 rectus abdominis muscles had three tendinous inscriptions, with the most caudal one at the level of the umbilicus. The inscriptions are adherent to the overlying anterior sheath but not to the posterior sheath. They do not usually extend completely through the muscle and may pass only halfway across it (5).

Rectus Sheath

A rectus sheath encloses each rectus abdominis muscle. This unique fascial isolation of the muscle facilitates the dissection of the flap. The rectus sheath is attached to the anterior aspect of the muscle by fusion to its inscriptions. The aponeurotic extensions of the muscles of the intraabdominal wall merge to form the anterior portion of the rectus sheath fascia. The composition of the rectus sheath varies at different locations between the symphysis pubis and xiphoid process. Above the costal margin, the anterior sheath is formed by an extension of the external oblique aponeurosis. In the upper two thirds of the rectus abdominis muscle, the anterior sheath is formed by the external oblique aponeurosis and a contribution from the internal oblique aponeurosis (5).

An important transition is in the posterior sheath at the arcuate line, which is a semicircular line also called the arc of Douglas or Douglas line. The arcuate line is generally located halfway between the umbilicus and pubic crest, although its location is variable. The arcuate line marks the transition point where the internal oblique aponeurosis ceases to split and the aponeuroses of all three muscles pass ventral to the rectus abdominis muscle. The transversalis fascia is the only layer present below the arcuate

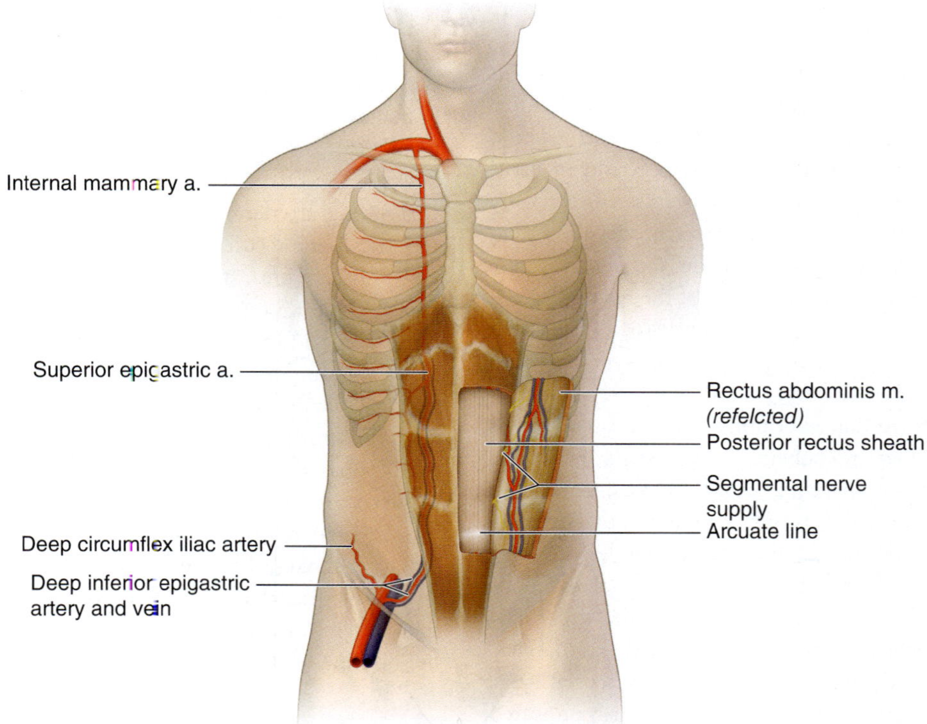

FIGURE 8-1 Anatomy of the rectus abdominis muscle. a, artery; DCIA, deep circumflex iliac artery; m, muscle.

line, and this region between the umbilicus and pubic crest is a region of weakness and potential herniation after flap dissection.

The linea alba represents the decussation of the fused aponeuroses in the midline. The linea alba is wider in the region of the xiphoid process and narrows to a fine line below the umbilicus. The lateral border of the rectus sheath is often discernable externally and is referred to as the linea semilunaris.

Blood Supply

According to the classification system of Mathes and Nahai (6), the rectus abdominis muscle is a type III muscle with two dominant vascular pedicles—one composed of the deep superior epigastric artery (DSEA) and vein (DSEV) and the other composed of the DIEA and DIEV. The DSEA and DSEV and DIEA and DIEV pedicles arborize as they approach each other longitudinally under the surface of the rectus abdominis muscle. These two vascular systems connect above the umbilicus through a system of small-caliber vessels that Taylor and Palmer (7) referred to as "choke" vessels.

The DSEA arises from the internal mammary artery at the level of the sixth intercostal space. The length of the DSEA from its origin to its entrance into the rectus abdominis muscle ranges from 3 to 6 cm. The diameter at its origin ranges from 1 to 4 mm; the diameter at its entrance into the rectus abdominis muscle ranges from 1 to 3 mm. The vessel generally has two venae comitantes, of which the diameter at the origin ranges from 1.5 to 4.0 mm and the diameter at the muscular entrance ranges from 1 to 3 mm.

The DIEA usually originates 1 cm above the inguinal ligament from the medial aspect of the external iliac artery directly opposite the deep circumflex iliac artery. Rarely, the DIEA originates from the internal iliac artery as a branch of the obturator artery. In 20% of cases, the DIEA may itself give off an anomalous obturator artery. The main DIEA pierces the transversalis fascia and enters the rectus sheath just below the arcuate line, approximately midway between the umbilicus and pubic crest. The DIEA then ascends obliquely and medially between the rectus abdominis muscle and the posterior wall of the sheath. Generally, the DIEA divides into two or three large branches below the level of the umbilicus. These vessels pass upward into the rectus abdominis muscle to communicate with the superior epigastric system above the level of the umbilicus.

The length of the DIEA from its origin to its entrance into the rectus abdominis muscle ranges from 6 to 15 cm. In a series of 25 cadaver dissections reported by Boyd et al. (8), the mean diameter of the DIEA was 3.4 mm. The artery has two venae comitantes, which usually join to form a single vein before their junction with the external iliac vein. In the study by Boyd et al. (8), the DIEV entered the external iliac vein as a single trunk in 68% of cases and as a double trunk in 32% of cases. The mean diameter of the DIEV was approximately 3.5 mm (8).

The DIEA communicates with the terminal intercostal artery branches that course between the transversalis abdominis and internal oblique muscles to enter the rectus sheath. The DIEA then divides into multiple branches that course within the muscle to anastomose with branches of the DSEA. The DIEA has peritoneal branches and an umbilical branch in addition to muscular branches. The vessels between the watershed areas of the upper and lower vascular systems are difficult to demonstrate grossly, although there is ample physiological proof that they exist. There is a small branch of the DSEA that courses along the costal margin to join the intercostal artery lateral to the rectus sheath (8).

The DIEA is the dominant vessel of the rectus abdominis muscle. Dye injected into this vessel will stain the abdominal wall as high as midway between the umbilicus and xiphoid process, but dye injected into the DSEA rarely results in staining below the umbilicus. Cadaveric studies were used to classify the degrees of arborization of the DIEA into three types. In the type 1 pattern, the DIEA does not divide and remains as a single vessel as it courses under the surface of the rectus abdominis muscle (29%). The type 2 pattern refers to a DIEA that divides into two dominant branches (57%). The type 3 pattern is a trifurcation of the DIEA (14%) (9,10).

The blood supply to the abdominal wall is a two-tiered arrangement of muscular and subcutaneous vascular networks. The superior and inferior epigastric artery systems form a deep longitudinal blood supply. This supply is linked to the lower six intercostal vessels and the ascending branch of the deep circumflex iliac artery within the muscles of the abdominal wall. The subcutaneous network consists of branches of the superficial epigastric artery, superficial circumflex iliac artery, external iliac artery, superficial superior epigastric artery, and intercostal arteries. The subcutaneous and deep vascular systems are connected by perforators that traverse the rectus abdominis muscles.

Extensive studies of the venous circulation of the TRAM flap have revealed superficial and deep vascular systems (11). The veins of the superficial system are above Scarpa's fascia and communicate extensively across the midline. The superficial veins drain into the deep venous system by way of the veins accompanying the musculocutaneous arterial perforators. The valves located in the connecting veins regulate the direction of blood flow from the superficial toward the deep system.

Perforators

The deep arteries supply the overlying abdominal skin by a system of perforators (Figure 8-2). These vessels are terminal branches of the DIEA and DIEV. Cadaveric studies performed by Taylor and Palmer (7) demonstrated a rich connection between the DIEA system and the abdominal wall skin. Many perforating arteries emerge through the anterior rectus sheath, but the highest concentration of major perforators is in the periumbilical area; the largest of these major perforators is greater than 0.5 mm in diameter. The fewest number of perforators is found in the suprapubic area.

The perforators communicate with the other regional superficial vessels through a system of "choke" vessels that link these territories with one another and allow the design of large skin islands based on the DIEA. The dominant connections between these systems occur within the subdermal plexus.

The branches of the periumbilical perforators look like the radiating spokes of a wheel with the hub located at the umbilicus. Thus, incorporation of the periumbilical perforators permits harvest of a skin flap with virtually any orientation from the midline (12).

Innervation

The rectus abdominis muscles are innervated in a segmental fashion from the lower six intercostal nerves, derived from T7 to T12, that traverse the plane between the transversus abdominis and internal oblique muscles. These nerves are mixed motor and sensory nerves, providing innervation to the rectus muscle and sensory supply to the overlying skin. The intercostal nerves enter the mid portion of the muscle at its posterior surface (13).

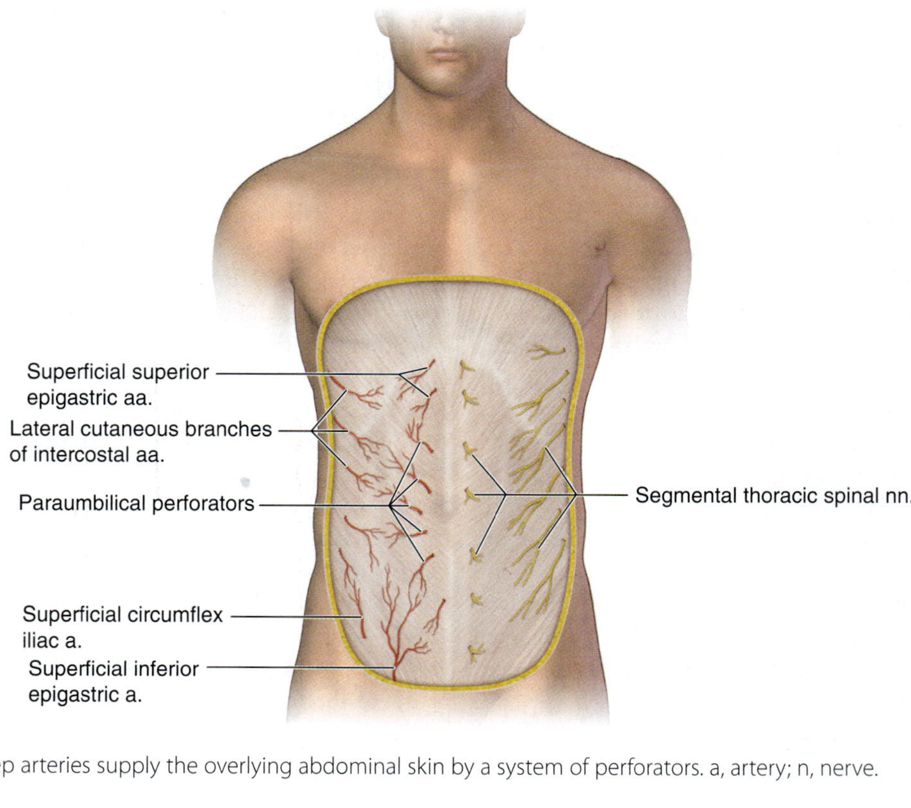

FIGURE 8-2 The deep arteries supply the overlying abdominal skin by a system of perforators. a, artery; n, nerve.

Anatomic Variations

In a series of 115 cadaver dissections, Milloy et al. (14) reported no cases of an absent DIEA or DIEV and only three cases in which the DSEA and DSEV could not be identified. In the vast majority of cases, the DIEA courses along the deep surface of the rectus abdominis muscle. Occasionally, the DIEA–DIEV pedicle can be tracked for an unusual distance along the lateral aspect of the muscle before it takes a medial intramuscular route. Another anomalous course has been described in which the DIEA–DIEV pedicle winds around the medial aspect of the muscle without providing feeders to the muscle and ends as a perforator. In this anomaly, the perforator to the skin runs directly through the anterior rectus sheath without traversing the muscle (15).

VARIANTS OF THE FLAP

The rectus abdominis muscle may be transferred alone as a muscle flap or with the fascia, skin, and subcutaneous tissue as a musculocutaneous flap. Many factors influence the flap design, including the defect's size and volume as well as the defect's proximity to the appropriate recipient vessels.

The choice of skin incision for a pure muscle flap depends on the amount of muscle required and the patient's preference regarding scar placement. A vertical paramedian incision is quick and efficient but leaves a noticeable scar. A transverse suprapubic incision with abdominal wall undermining provides sufficient access to the lower muscle and the vascular pedicle. A variable length of muscle can be included depending on the recipient site requirements.

There is great flexibility in the design of the skin island in terms of size, shape, orientation of its axis relative to that of the muscle, and location over the muscle. The skin of a significant portion of the abdomen may be reliably transferred because of a network of subcutaneous vessels emanating from the musculocutaneous perforators in the periumbilical region. The nature of the abdominal blood supply allows large skin islands to be oriented along almost any axis relative to the muscle, although some orientations are preferable to others. The skin island may be oriented transversely, vertically, or more obliquely. It is also safe to design a skin island across the midline. In general, at least part of the skin island should be located near the umbilical system where the number of perforators is greatest.

A vertical rectus abdominis musculocutaneous (VRAM) flap is commonly used when a reliable, bulky flap is desired (Figure 8-3). With a VRAM flap, a vertically oriented skin paddle that overlies the entire length of the rectus abdominis muscle may be harvested from the region of the symphysis pubis to the xiphoid process. The blood supply to the skin paddle of a VRAM flap is robust, and the entire skin flap can be used reliably.

Another commonly used flap design is the TRAM flap (Figure 8-4) (16). Popularized for use in breast reconstruction, a TRAM flap incorporates skin from the entire lower abdomen. Four different skin zones have been identified that can be included in a TRAM flap. Zone 1 refers to the skin overlying each lateral rectus abdominis muscle. Zone 2 denotes the skin

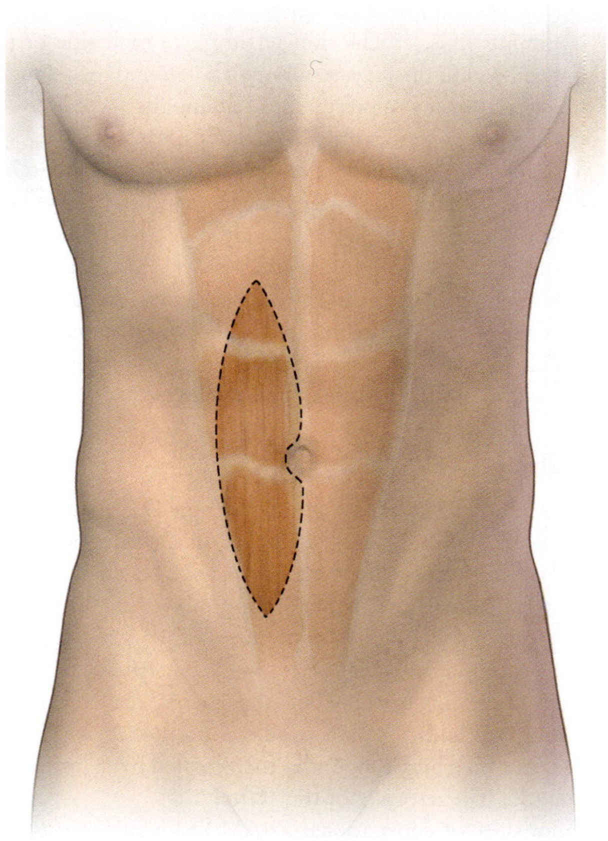

FIGURE 8-3 A vertical rectus abdominis musculocutaneous flap.

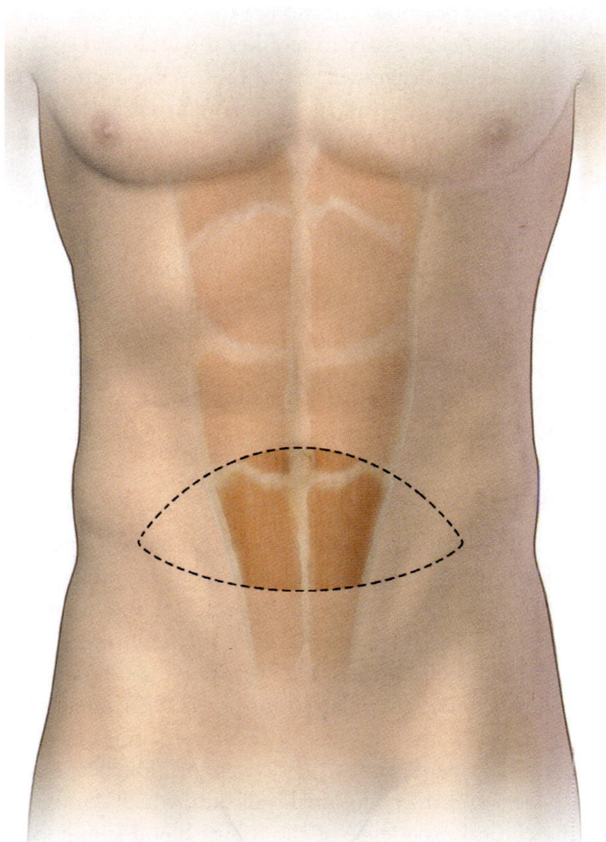

FIGURE 8-4 A transverse rectus abdominis musculocutaneous flap.

of the contralateral lower abdomen overlying the opposite rectus abdominis muscle. The skin territory on each side of the abdomen lateral to the linea semilunaris is referred to as zone 3; the skin lateral to the opposite linea semilunaris is zone 4. The blood supply to zone 4 is the most tenuous.

There are few disadvantages to the use of a rectus abdominis flap. Obese patients are usually poor candidates for rectus abdominis flaps because they frequently have a very thick panniculus supported by a thin atrophic muscle. The presence of previous abdominal scars can interfere with flap design or preclude the use of a rectus abdominis flap altogether. Some patients may object to the location of the donor site scar. However, scarring can be minimized by using a low transverse incision.

Pedicled TRAM Flap

The conventional TRAM flap is based on the DSEA and necessitates sacrifice of all or most of the rectus abdominis muscle. An ipsilateral or contralateral pedicle may be selected, depending on the planned inset configuration; however, the surgeon must ensure that the blood supply or outflow is not compromised by kinking, twisting, or compression. After being tunneled through an opening in the medial aspect of the inframammary fold, the skin paddle is positioned within the breast defect. The breast mound is then created by tailoring and insetting the flap vertically or transversely.

Donor sites for conventional TRAM flap breast reconstruction usually leave a fascial defect that necessitates repair with a synthetic mesh. The repair should provide adequate anterior abdominal wall integrity without displacing the umbilical stalk from its midline position. Plication of the contralateral abdominal fascia may be necessary to recenter the umbilical stalk and to provide contour symmetry. Closure of the rectus sheath should end 1 to 2 cm below the pedicle to avoid vascular compromise of the skin paddle. Undermining of the remaining abdominal skin may be necessary to facilitate a tension-free closure; however, it is usually not necessary to release the tissues past the border of the costal margin. Draping of the abdominal skin is simulated to mark the umbilical window. Creation of the window can be performed before or after the abdominal closure as long as the surgeon's technique allows for the nontraumatic retrieval of the umbilical stalk. The superficial fascial system, Scarpa fascia, is reapproximated before closure of the dermis and final closure of the skin.

Free TRAM Flap

The free TRAM flap has several features that make it well suited for breast reconstruction in the appropriate candidate. The DIEA is the dominant vessel of the rectus abdominis muscle and the TRAM flap. Dye injected into this vessel will stain the abdominal wall as high as midway between the umbilicus and xiphoid process, but dye injected into the DSEA rarely results in staining below the umbilicus. Cadaveric studies by Taylor and Palmer (7) demonstrated a rich connection between the DIEA system and the abdominal wall skin, which corresponds with the clinical experience of the robust blood supply of the free TRAM flap.

Muscle-Sparing TRAM Flap

In the traditional TRAM flap, the rectus abdominis muscle is taken with the skin and subcutaneous tissue paddle, not necessarily to provide extra volume to the reconstructed breast but rather because it is the structure through which branches of the DIEA travel. These perforating branches carry blood to and from the abdominal skin that is essential for recreating a breast mound. Because the muscle itself is only necessary to the free flap because of the vascular vessels passing through it in route to the desired skin and subcutaneous tissues, surgeons have decreased the amount of muscle harvested with the free flap. This has come to be termed a MS-TRAM (muscle-sparing TRAM) flap. There are three types of free MS-TRAM flap procedures: (1) the medial portion of the rectus abdominis muscle can be preserved and a lateral portion of the rectus muscle harvested with the flap (MS-1M); (2) a lateral portion of the muscle can be preserved and the medial portion of the rectus muscle harvested with the flap (MS-1L); or (3) a small cuff of muscle around the perforators can be harvested with the flap, leaving the majority of the muscle intact (MS-2) (Figure 8-5).

The type of free MS-TRAM flap harvested is, for the most part, dependent on the location and orientation of the perforators. If the perforators are located very medially, then the MS-1L flap is usually used. If the perforators are located in the middle of the muscle, usually the MS-2 flap is used. If the perforators are located laterally, then the MS-1M flap can be harvested. Also, the orientation of the perforators within the rectus muscle is a determining factor in how much of the rectus abdominis muscle will be taken with the perforators. If the perforators are coming directly up through the muscle, then only a small amount of muscle needs to be sacrificed. However, if the perforators are coursing obliquely through the muscle, then more muscle will need to be sacrificed.

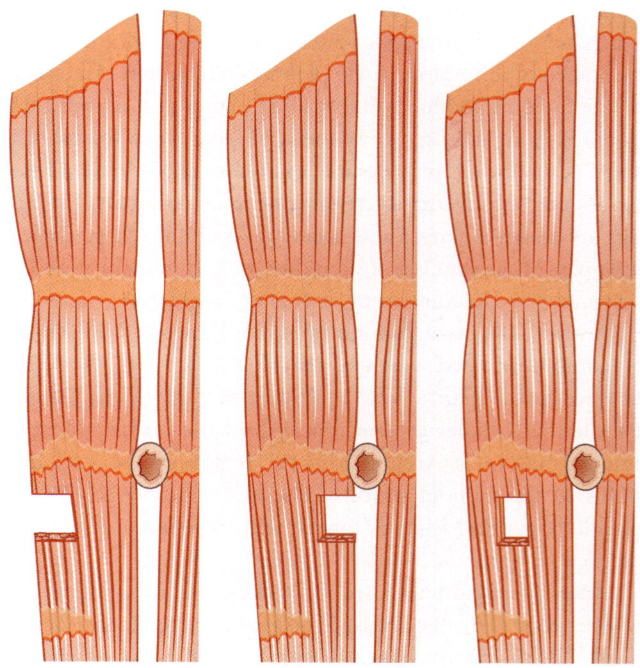

FIGURE 8-5 Muscle-sparing transverse rectus abdominis myocutaneous flaps.

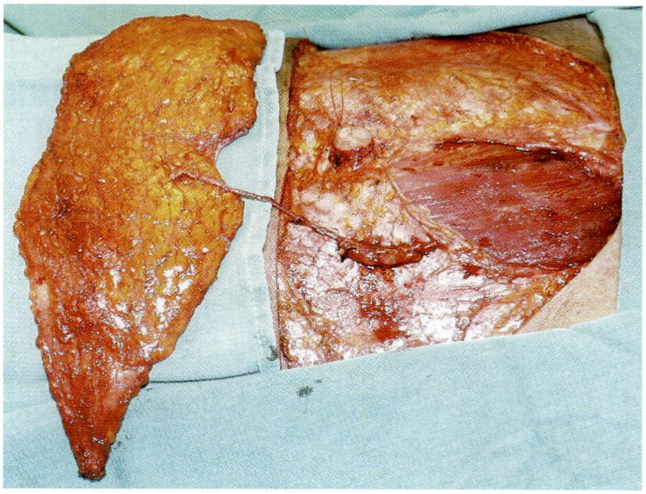

FIGURE 8-6 A deep inferior epigastric perforator flap.

DIEP Flap

A DIEP flap refers to sparing of the rectus abdominis muscle and harvesting only the perforating vessels (Figure 8-6). The greatest benefit of sparing the muscle entirely is the reduction of morbidity at the donor site. However, studies have shown that there is no statistically significant clinical difference between a DIEP donor site and a donor site in which a major portion of the rectus abdominis is spared (MS-2) (17).

A major concern regarding the use of a DIEP flap, which may have fewer perforators than a free MS-TRAM flap, is that complications of the reconstructed breast mound can arise secondary to an insufficient blood supply. A suboptimal blood supply to the transferred tissue will result in fat necrosis in the breast mound. Patient selection and intraoperative decision making are crucial to maximizing the potential benefit of DIEP flap breast reconstruction.

Innervated Flap

The rectus abdominis muscles are innervated in a segmental fashion from the lower six intercostal nerves, derived from T7 to T12. These nerves are mixed motor and sensory nerves, providing innervation to the rectus muscle and sensory supply to the overlying skin. By stimulating one of the segmental nerves, it is possible to select a portion of the rectus abdominis muscle for use in functional muscle transplantation.

Innervated TRAM flaps have been used to facilitate sensory return to the reconstructed breast. The TRAM flap is innervated by the T6 to T12 spinal nerves, which have been shown to carry a significant number of sensory fibers. Anatomical dissections have demonstrated that these nerves pierce the anterior rectus fascia and enter the overlying subcutaneous tissues after giving off motor branches through their intramuscular course. Neurophysiologic studies have confirmed sensory distributions of 8 × 8 cm areas of skin supplied by a single perforating neurovascular bundle. Although spontaneous recovery of sensation has been reported in the reconstructed breast, the results have been inconsistent and variable.

GUIDELINES FOR DISSECTION AND HARVEST

Rectus Abdominis Muscle Flap

The rectus abdominis muscle and musculocutaneous flaps are ideal for repair of anterior defects when the patient can be placed in a supine position so that the ablative and reconstructive surgical teams can work simultaneously. Surface markings include a midline, lateral muscle extent, and iliofemoral axis. The level of the DIEA is marked approximately 1 cm above the inguinal ligament, where the artery enters the deep lateral side of the muscle midway between the umbilicus and pelvic crest.

After a skin incision is made, the anterior rectus sheath is exposed and incised in the middle to expose the anterior surface of the rectus abdominis muscle. The rectus sheath attachments are divided to the medial and lateral borders of the muscle. Care must be taken when separating the inscriptions to the anterior rectus sheath because the inscriptions are densely adherent. The intercostal branches are isolated and ligated. The inferior epigastric vascular pedicle is identified at the lateral border of the lower part of the muscle above the pubic tubercle. The segmental nerves accompanying the vessels may be preserved for functional transfers. The rectus abdominis muscle is separated from the posterior sheath (Figure 8-7).

The rectus abdominis muscle is then gently retracted to expose the inferior epigastric vessels that course beneath it. After the vascular pedicle has been identified and isolated, the inferior muscle attachment at the symphysis pubis and pubic crest is detached to facilitate exposure of the deep inferior epigastric pedicle and its dissection. The deep inferior epigastric

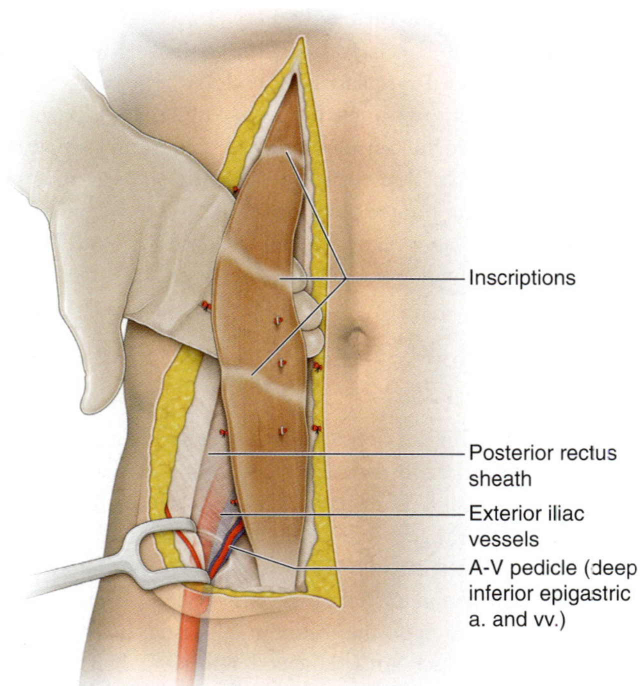

FIGURE 8-7 A rectus abdominis muscle flap showing the deep inferior epigastric arteriovenous pedicle. Ex, exterior.

pedicle is traced toward its origin from the external iliac vessels to maximize vascular pedicle length.

Rectus Abdominis Musculocutaneous Flap

If a skin island is planned, an ellipse is drawn in a vertical, transverse, or oblique orientation depending on the donor scar, previous abdominal incisions, and recipient site requirements. Irrespective of flap design, care should be taken to include the large periumbilical perforators in the flap.

The border of the skin island is incised down to the rectus sheath fascia. The skin and subcutaneous tissues are elevated off the anterior rectus sheath from lateral to medial until the lateral perforators are seen. The cutaneous flap is then elevated from the contralateral side to expose the medial row of perforators. The cutaneous flap is carefully dissected off the rectus sheath, preserving all perforators. After all the major perforators are identified, a decision can be made as to which perforators will be included with the rectus abdominis flap.

A fascia-sparing technique is used to open the rectus sheath fascia, incorporating only a small cuff of fascia around the perforators and then connecting these islands of fascia to each other. When the fascia is opened in this manner, only a minimal amount of fascia is sacrificed, facilitating primary closure of the fascia without undue tension or use of synthetic mesh. The rectus sheath incision is extended inferiorly and laterally to expose the underlying rectus abdominis muscle. The lateral border of the muscle is identified and dissected inferiorly where the DIEA–DIEV pedicle is found. The anterior rectus sheath fascia is dissected off the underlying rectus abdominis muscle and its inscriptions. Several intercostal nerves and vessels will be seen on the surface of the posterior rectus sheath.

As much or as little muscle can be taken as needed. If muscle preservation is desired, then only a small cuff of the muscle around the perforators is harvested with the flap. However, if a large amount of well-vascularized muscle is desired, then the entire rectus abdominis muscle from the costal margin down to its inferior attachment can be harvested. The muscle may be divided just past the skin island or the entire muscle may be used, depending on the recipient site. After the recipient site is prepared and the flap is ready for transfer, the DIEA and DIEV are divided, and the flap is transferred to the recipient site.

Free TRAM, MS-TRAM, and DIEP Flaps

Free TRAM Flap

For patients with high-risk factors such as smoking and obesity, optimizing perfusion to the flap by including as many major perforators as possible is a priority (18,19). In these instances, a full-muscle TRAM flap may be the best choice.

The TRAM flap is carefully dissected off the rectus sheath, preserving all major perforators on the preferred side. A fascia-sparing technique is used to open the rectus sheath fascia, incorporating only a small cuff of fascia around the perforators and then connecting these islands of fascia to each other (Figure 8-8). When the fascia is opened in this manner, only a minimal amount of fascia is sacrificed, facilitating primary closure of the fascia without tension or use of synthetic mesh. The rectus sheath incision is extended inferiorly and laterally to expose the underlying rectus abdominis muscle.

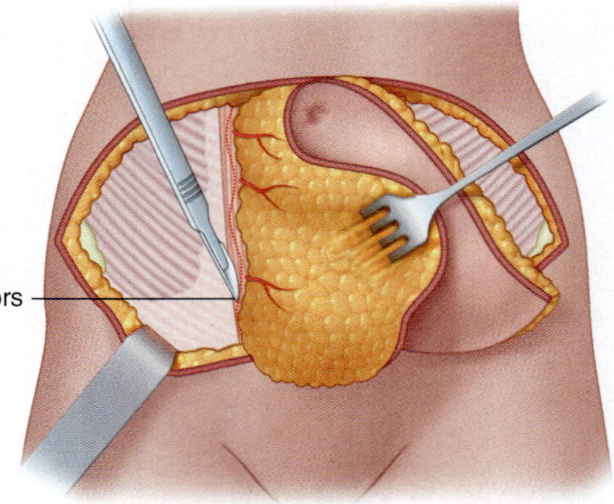

FIGURE 8-8 A fascia-sparing technique.

The anterior rectus sheath fascia is dissected off the underlying rectus abdominis muscle and its tendinous inscriptions. The rectus sheath attachments are divided to the medial and lateral borders of the muscle. Care must be taken when separating the inscriptions to the anterior rectus sheath, where they are densely adherent. Several intercostal nerves and vessels will be seen on the surface of the posterior rectus sheath. The intercostal branches are isolated and ligated. The lateral border of the muscle is identified and dissected inferiorly, where the DIEA pedicle is found at the lateral border of the lower part of the muscle above the pubic tubercle. The rectus abdominis muscle is separated from the posterior sheath.

The rectus abdominis muscle is then gently retracted to expose the deep inferior epigastric vessels that course beneath it. After the vascular pedicle has been identified and isolated, the inferior muscle attachment at the symphysis pubis and pubic crest is detached to facilitate exposure and dissection of the deep inferior epigastric pedicle. The deep inferior epigastric pedicle is traced toward its origin at the external iliac vessels to obtain optimal vascular pedicle length. The upper muscle attachment is divided, and the DSEA and DSEV are ligated. Superiorly, the muscle can be divided at any level above the perforators to the flap, even at its insertion at the costal margin if necessary. The deep inferior epigastric pedicle is left intact until the recipient site is prepared.

After the recipient vessels are dissected and the mastectomy pocket is prepared, the TRAM flap harvesting is completed by individually ligating the DIEA and DIEV using either hemoclips or suture ligatures. After the flap is harvested, the muscle is secured to the overlying flap with several sutures to minimize any undue tension on or twisting of the perforators.

MS-TRAM Flap

With the MS-TRAM flap, the skin and subcutaneous tissues are elevated off the anterior rectus sheath from lateral to medial until the lateral perforators are seen (Figure 8-9). At this time, lateral perforators from both the right and left sides are evaluated, and the decision is made regarding which perforators will be included with the flap. The size, number, and orientation of the perforators should be considered when making this evaluation.

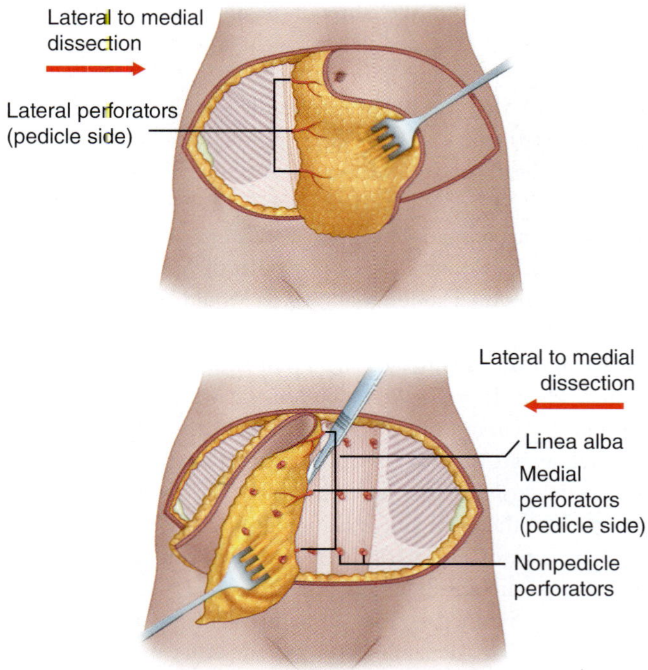

FIGURE 8-9 The skin and subcutaneous tissues are elevated off the anterior rectus sheath from lateral to medial.

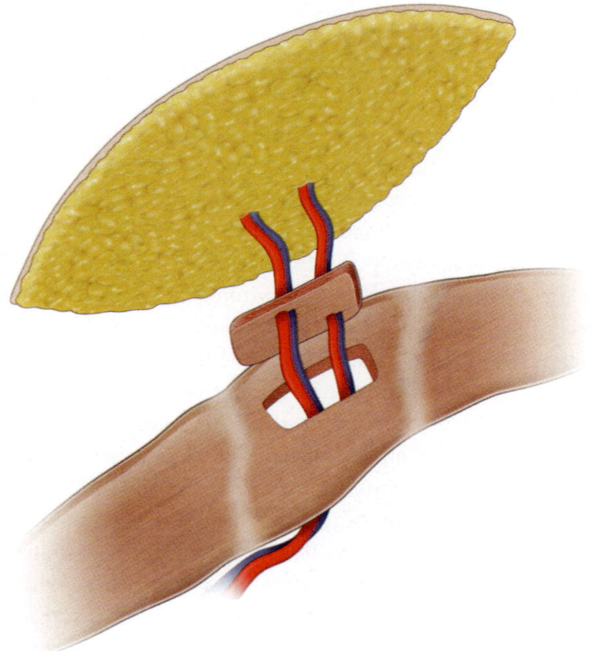

FIGURE 8-10 A free muscle-sparing transverse rectus abdominis myocutaneous flap.

The lateral row of perforators on the side that will not be used are hemoclipped and divided, and then the flap is elevated to expose the medial row of perforators. Again, perforators on both sides are evaluated, the preferred perforators are kept, and the others are hemoclipped and divided. This maneuver is continued until two or more of the best perforators remain and have been selected for inclusion in the flap. All things being equal, the author prefers medially located perforators contralateral to the breast defect. Medial perforators provide longer pedicles, and their harvest results in less functional damage to the remaining rectus muscle because the muscle is innervated from lateral to medial. Also, compared with the laterally located perforators, medially located perforators may provide better perfusion to the tissues across the midline of the flap. Generally, two or three moderate to large perforators will provide sufficient circulation to the MS-TRAM flap in most cases.

The anterior rectus sheath fascia is dissected off the underlying rectus abdominis muscle and its inscriptions, and the orientation and course of the perforators within the rectus muscle are evaluated. The decision to perform an MS-TRAM or a DIEP flap procedure is made based on the number, caliber, and location of perforators as well as the orientation and course of the perforators within the rectus muscle. If the perforators are located in different intramuscular layers, the muscle fibers between the perforators would need to be divided for a DIEP flap; under these circumstances, a small cuff of muscle fibers between and around the perforators is incorporated, and a free MS-TRAM flap is performed (Figure 8-10).

After the extent of muscle that needs to be taken with the flap is decided, the muscle is split in the direction of the muscle fibers within the intramuscular septum medially and laterally down to the posterior rectus sheath. Under the rectus abdominis muscle, the main branch to the perforators can usually be visualized at this time. Inferior to the most inferior perforator, the muscle fibers between the lateral and medial dissected plane are then divided. A bipolar device is preferred for dividing the muscles to minimize bleeding. All vascular branches should be either hemoclipped or cauterized with the bipolar device. It is important to maintain a hemostatic, clean operative field to optimize visualization and exposure. After the inferior portion of the muscle is divided, the main pedicle should be exposed. The rectus muscle fibers are then split inferiorly to further expose and dissect out the main pedicle. With a free MS-TRAM or DIEP flap, usually the pedicle does not need to be dissected all the way down to the origin because the pedicle is already fairly long. Finally, the muscle fibers at the superior aspect of the perforators are divided between the medially and laterally dissected plane of the rectus muscle. At this time, the superior blood supply to the rectus muscle is seen and ligated.

After the recipient vessels are dissected and the recipient site is prepared, the flap harvesting is completed by individually ligating the DIEA and DIEV using either hemoclips or suture ligatures. After the flap is harvested, the muscle is secured to the overlying flap with several sutures to minimize any shearing forces on the perforators.

DIEP Flap

If the perforating vessels are skeletonized, sparing the entire rectus abdominis muscle, the resulting flap is referred to as a DIEP flap. Sparing the entire muscle potentially reduces donor site morbidity, including abdominal bulge and weakness. However, whether use of DIEP flaps reduces these complications significantly more than does use of free MS-TRAM flaps has not been clearly established.

The flap is elevated as described for the free MS-TRAM flap. A DIEP flap is selected when there is a single large perforator or when two or more perforators are located within the same intramuscular septum. The optimal situation for a DIEP flap is when it can be harvested without significant damage to the rectus abdominis muscle.

After the perforators are identified, each perforator is followed down into the intramuscular septum. The muscle is then split bluntly and sharply, and the perforators are dissected to the main branch. The main branch is then followed until the deep inferior epigastric pedicle is visualized. In an ideal condition for a DIEP flap, there is a minimal need for cutting or resecting the rectus muscle. The remainder of the flap dissection is as described for free MS-TRAM flap procedure.

Because a DIEP flap may have fewer perforators than a free TRAM flap, there is concern that the reconstructed breast mound might have an insufficient blood supply, causing fat necrosis in the breast mound. Patient selection and intraoperative decision making are crucial to maximizing the potential benefit of DIEP flap breast reconstruction. The surgeon's goal should be to perform a reconstruction that will leave the patient with the least donor site morbidity possible while at the same time providing her with the greatest chance at a successful reconstruction.

TRICKS AND TIPS FROM THE AUTHOR

All flap and recipient site dissection is performed under loupe magnification, and the author recommends the use of a headlight for optimal visualization of the operative field. The first step of the flap harvest procedure is to dissect out the umbilicus. It helps to make four small stab incisions with a #11 blade at the 12, 3, 6, and 9 o'clock positions. Skin hooks are then placed into the stab incisions to provide retraction while incisions are made to connect the stab incisions. Using tenotomy scissors, the umbilical stalk is dissected down to its base. There is no need to make the umbilical stalk overly thin or thick. A marking stitch is placed at the 12 o'clock position of the umbilicus for use as a guide during the insetting of the umbilicus and to prevent twisting of the umbilical stalk.

The border of the skin island is incised down to the abdominal wall. The superficial inferior epigastric vein (SIEV) and the superficial inferior epigastric artery (SIEA) are identified and preserved. If the SIEA is significant in size and the patient is a good candidate, a SIEA flap can be used for breast reconstruction (discussed in Chapter 46). Even if a SIEA flap is not planned, it is important to preserve and dissect out the SIEV for about 4 to 5 cm. With the increasing use of DIEP and free MS-TRAM flaps with fewer and smaller perforators being included with the flap, occasionally the SIEV needs to be used as a secondary means of venous drainage if deep venous drainage alone is not adequate.

MANAGEMENT OF THE DONOR SITE

Meticulous closure of the donor defect is required to prevent a weakening or herniation of the anterior abdominal wall. There is tremendous controversy regarding the optimum method for closing the abdominal wall defect after the rectus abdominis flap harvest. There are two major camps of thought on the issue, and they are divided over the necessity of introducing a synthetic mesh for closure of the anterior rectus sheath. Drever and Hodson-Walker (20) described a technique of placing a synthetic mesh of the exact dimensions to the area of the anterior rectus sheath that was removed with the flap. Lejour and Dome (21) reported using a double-layer synthetic mesh between the posterior sheath and the direct closure of the anterior sheath. Hartrampf (22) argued for direct approximation of the residual anterior fascial margins to achieve a centralization of the remaining muscles; by doing so, he believed that the mechanical advantage of the residual abdominal muscles would be restored.

If the fascia is harvested using a fascia-sparing technique, the medial and lateral cuffs of the anterior sheath can be closed primarily where it was split longitudinally without creating any tension, even in most cases of bilateral flap harvest (Figure 8-11). The rectus fascia sheath is closed primarily with a nonabsorbable suture using either an interrupted or running technique. However, if the overlying fascia integrity is poor or if a significant amount of fascia has been harvested and a tension-free primary closure is difficult, a synthetic mesh is used to reinforce the closure. Synthetic mesh can be placed using an inlay or an onlay technique, depending on the surgeon's preference. The anterior sheath should be carefully repaired below the level of the arcuate line where herniation is more likely to occur because the posterior rectus sheath is deficient in this area. Closed-suction drains are placed above the fascia closure in the subcutaneous tissue.

Removal of rectus abdominis along with the portion of overlying fascia creates a potential weakness in the intraabdominal wall that may predispose the patient to ventral herniation or a midline bulge. Fortunately, there have not been significant problems with muscle weakness postoperatively, and donor site morbidity because of a loss of fascial support has been very low (23,24). Although patients who participate in active sports or engage in other physical activities may experience an impact on their lifestyles, few reports quantify the actual effects of removing the rectus abdominis (25).

DONOR-SITE COMPLICATIONS

The driving force behind the development of variations of the free TRAM flap, such as the MS-TRAM and DIEP flaps, has been the desire to reduce abdominal donor site morbidity. One way to minimize abdominal donor site morbidity, particularly hernia or bulge, is to ensure an optimal tension-free fascial closure. The author prefers to use a fascia-sparing technique in the harvesting of most free TRAM flaps regardless of how much rectus abdominis muscle is sacrificed. Thus, even in bilateral cases, the rectus fascia sheath can be closed primarily with minimal tension. However, if the overlying fascia integrity is poor or if a tension-free primary closure is difficult, synthetic mesh can be used to reinforce the closure.

RECONSTRUCTIVE INDICATIONS

As a superiorly based pedicle flap, the rectus abdominis flap has been used extensively in breast reconstruction (26–28). It has also been used for cases of sternal dehiscence and other chest wall defects. As an inferiorly based pedicle flap, it has

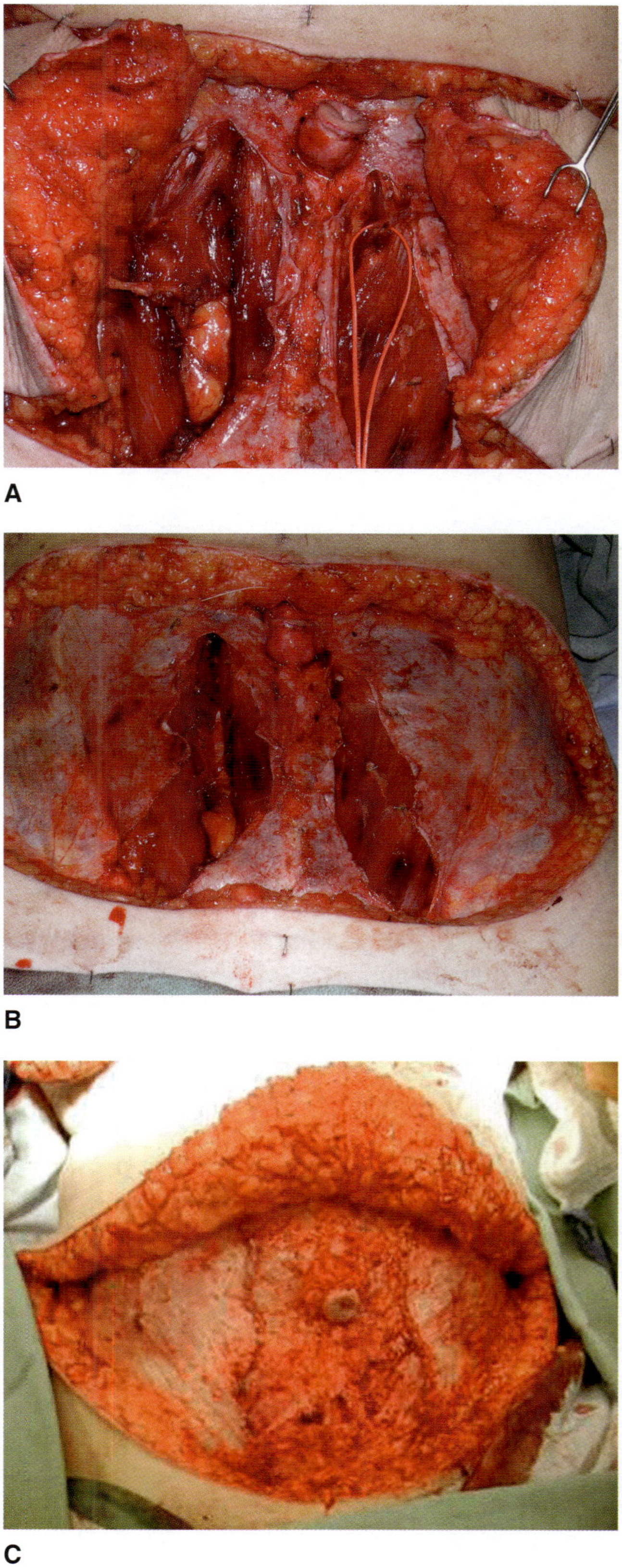

FIGURE 8-11 (**A**) A bilateral flap harvest; right muscle-sparing transverse rectus abdominis myocutaneous flap and left deep inferior epigastric perforator flap. (**B**) The donor site defect. (**C**) The rectus fascia sheath is closed primarily with minimal tension.

been used for coverage of lower abdominal wall and groin defects and thigh defects (29). As a free flap based on the inferior epigastric vessels, this flap has been used for head and neck defects, upper and lower extremity defects, and breast reconstruction (30).

The rectus abdominis muscle and musculocutaneous flaps have assumed important roles in head and neck reconstruction because they are easy to harvest, have long vascular pedicles, and are tremendously reliable. The rectus abdominis musculocutaneous flap can serve as a source of skin for external coverage when regional flaps are not available or are unsuitable because of the defect's size or distance from the donor site. For example, a VRAM flap is useful for reconstruction after a total glossectomy because the VRAM flap can supply sufficient soft tissue bulk and height for approximation of the new tongue to the palate without the use of a palatal augmentation prosthesis.

The rectus abdominis flap has also become the flap of choice for many skull-base defects that require free tissue transfer. The versatility of the rectus abdominis flap design is extremely useful when trying to achieve a water tight closure of a defect that involves the nasal, oral, or intracranial cavities, and multiple epithelial surfaces are required for a successful outcome. The epithelialized portions of the flap can be used to enhance the contour of regions such as the infratemporal fossa or the orbit after ablation. Finally, the extremely reliable nature of this flap is a critical factor in ensuring protective coverage to exposed portions of the brain or dura.

Another use for the rectus muscle flap has been in upper and lower extremity reconstruction. The muscle is long and thin and thus is well suited for extremity defects. The rectus flap, when transferred as a muscle-only flap with a skin graft, often atrophies and conforms to the defect, thus providing a good contour.

Perhaps one of the greatest uses for this flap has been in breast reconstruction. The development of the TRAM flap has revolutionized postmastectomy breast reconstruction. Particularly, the free TRAM flap has become the gold standard for autologous tissue breast reconstruction, and since first described in 1979, it has spawned numerous variations, including the free MS-TRAM flap, the free DIEP flap, and the free SIEA flap. These flaps have many features that make them well suited for breast reconstruction. Most patients have adequate lower abdominal skin and subcutaneous tissue available for incorporation into the flap to reconstruct a breast. The rectus abdominis muscle's vascular pedicle is large, long, constant, and reliable. The robust blood supply of the free TRAM flap reduces the risk of fat necrosis and enables aggressive folding, trimming, and shaping of the flap to optimize the aesthetic outcome in breast reconstruction. In addition, the free TRAM flap requires minimal donor site sacrifice in most cases. And finally, the free TRAM flap can be harvested with the patient in a supine position while a mastectomy is being performed. With proper patient selection and safe surgical technique, each of these flaps can transfer the lower abdominal skin and subcutaneous tissue to provide an aesthetically pleasing breast reconstruction with minimal donor site morbidity (Figure 8-12).

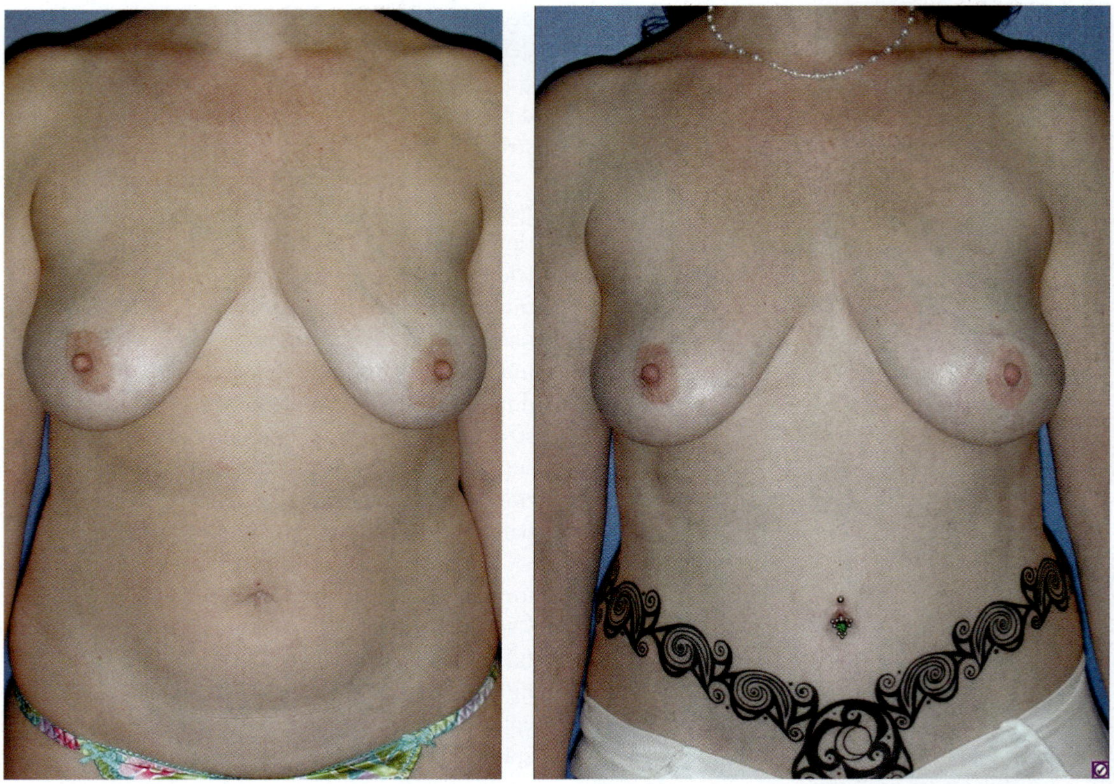

A B

FIGURE 8-12 (**A**). A young woman with left breast cancer. (**B**) After immediate reconstruction with a free deep inferior epigastric perforator flap, a staged nipple–areolar reconstruction was done.

COMPARE FLAP WITH SIMILAR FREE TISSUE TRANSFERS

The rectus abdominis muscle and musculocutaneous flaps have been widely used for reconstructing various moderate to large defects requiring well-vascularized tissue. The rectus abdominis muscle has many features that make it well suited for microvascular transfer. Its vascular pedicle contains large vessels and is constant, reliable, and long. The rectus abdominis muscle is versatile—it can be used alone or with the overlying skin as a musculocutaneous flap. In most patients, abundant subcutaneous tissue is available for incorporation into the flap, and various sizes, shapes, and orientations of the skin island are possible. Furthermore, rectus abdominis flaps are relatively easy to dissect and can be harvested with the patient in a supine position.

The latissimus dorsi flap is the most similar tissue transfer to the rectus flap. It too is an expendable muscle and musculocutaneous unit with a large dominant vessel and reasonable pedicle length. However, the patient needs to be turned for harvesting, and the flap cannot generally carry sufficient tissue for autologous breast reconstruction. Merits of the donor scars may be debated, but only that of the rectus has the potential for resembling that of a cosmetic operation. The latissimus muscle does the advantage of having a large surface area, an asset when large wounds need cover. Another comparable free tissue transfer is the anterior lateral thigh flap with or without the vastus lateralis muscle. The donor defect here is very much dependent on the size of flap taken and the need for skin grafting. Nevertheless, it rarely carries sufficient tissue for breast reconstruction, and its donor site can be disfiguring when the skin component is extensive.

There are a number of alternative flaps for breast reconstruction, but most are considered to be backup options for when rectus based flaps are unavailable. These are discussed elsewhere.

REFERENCES

1. Brown R, Vasconez L, Jurkiewicz M. Transverse abdominal flaps and the deep epigastric arcade. *Plast Reconstr Surg* 1975;55:416.
2. Drever J. The epigastric island flap. *Plast Reconstr Surg* 1977;59:343.
3. Pennington DG, Pelly AD. The rectus abdominis myocutaneous free flap. *Br J Plast Surg* 1980;33:277.
4. Moon H, Taylor GI. The vascular anatomy of the rectus abdominis musculocutaneous flaps based on the deep superior epigastric system. *Plast Reconstr Surg* 1988;82:815.
5. Gray H. Anatomy of the Human Body, 29th American edition. Goss C (ed). Philadelphia: Lea and Febiger, 1973, p. 424.
6. Mathes S, Nahai F. *Clinical Applications for Muscle and Musculocutaneous Flaps.* St. Louis: CV Mosby, 1982, p. 44.
7. Taylor G, Palmer J. The vascular territories (angiosomes) of the body: experimental and clinical applications. *Br J Plast Surg* 1987;40:113.
8. Boyd JB, Taylor GI, Corlett R. The vascular territories of the superior and deep inferior epigastric systems. *Plast Reconstr Surg* 1984;73:1.
9. Miyamoto Y, Harada K, Kodama Y, et al. Cranial coverage involving scalp, bone and dura using free inferior epigastric flap. *Br J Plast Surg* 1986;39:483.
10. Sadove R, Merrell J. The split rectus abdominis free muscle transfer. *Ann Plast Surg* 1987;18:179.
11. Carramenha E, Costa M, Carriquiry C, et al. An anatomic study of the venous drainage of the transverse rectus abdominis musculocutaneous flap. *Plast Reconstr Surg* 1987;79:208.
12. Taylor GI, Corlett R, Boyd JB. The extended deep inferior epigastric flap: a clinical technique. *Plast Reconstr Surg* 1983;72:751.

13. Duchateau J, Declety A, Lejour M. Innervation of the rectus abdominis muscle: implications for rectus flaps. *Plast Reconstr Surg* 1988;82:223.
14. Milloy F, Anson B, McAfee D. The rectus abdominis muscle and the epigastric arteries. *Surg Gynecol Obstet* 1960;110:293.
15. Godfrey P, Godfrey N, Romita M. The "circummuscular" free TRAM pedicle: a trap. *Plast Reconstr Surg* 1994;93:178.
16. Sheflan M, Dinner MI. The transverse abdominal island flap: part I. Indications, contraindications, results, and complications *Ann Plast Surg* 1983;10:24.
17. Bajaj AK, Chevray PM, Chang DW. Comparison of donor-site complications and functional outcomes in free muscle-sparing TRAM flap and free DIEP flap breast reconstruction. *Plast Reconstr Surg* 2006;117:737–746;discussion 747–750.
18. Chang D, Wang B, Robb G, et al. The effect of obesity on flap and donor site complications in free TRAM flap breast reconstruction. *Reconstr Surg* 2000;105(5):1640–1648.
19. Chang D, Reece G, Wang B, et al. Effect of smoking on complications in patients undergoing free TRAM flap breast reconstruction. *Plast Reconstr Surg* 2000;105(7):2374–2380.
20. Drever J, Hodson-Walker N. Closure of the donor defect for breast reconstruction with rectus abdominis myocutaneous flaps. *Plast Reconstr Surg* 1985;76:558.
21. Lejour M, Dome M. Abdominal wall function after rectus abdominis transfer. *Plast Reconstr Surg* 1991;87:1054.
22. Hartrampf CR. Discussion of article by Drever JM, Hodson Walker N: closure of the donor defect for breast reconstruction with rectus abdominis myocutaneous flaps. *Plast Reconstr Surg* 1985;76:563.
23. Hartrampf CR. Abdominal wall competence in transverse abdominal island flap operations. *Ann Plast Surg* 1984;12:139.
24. Scheflan M, Dinner M. The transverse abdominal island flap. Part II. Surgical technique. *Ann Plast Surg* 1983;10:120.
25. Bunkis J, Walton RL, Mathes SJ, et al. Experience with the transverse lower rectus abdominis operation for breast reconstruction. *Plast Reconstr Surg* 1983;72:819.
26. Dinner MI, Labandter HP, Dowden RV. The role of the rectus abdominis myocutaneous flap in breast reconstruction. *Plast Reconstr Surg* 1982;69:209.
27. Drever JM. The lower abdominal transverse rectus abdominis myocutaneous flap for breast reconstruction. *Ann Plast Surg* 1983;10:179.
28. Gandolfo EA. Breast reconstruction with a lower abdominal myocutaneous flap. *Br J Plast Surg* 1982;25:452.
29. Rees R, Shack B, Hulsey T, et al. A new technique for reconstruction of an open above knee amputation. *Plast Reconstr Surg* 1983;72:882.
30. Urken ML, Turk J, Weinberg H, et al. The rectus abdominis free flap in head and neck reconstruction. *Arch Otolaryngol Head Neck Surg* 1991;117:857.

CHAPTER 9

Anatomy and Elevation of the Posterior Thigh Perforator Flap for Breast Reconstruction

Neil Tanna, Steven M. Levine, and Robert J. Allen, Sr.

NOTE

None of the authors has a financial interest in any of the products, devices, or drugs mentioned in this manuscript.

The posterior thigh has long served as a source of autologous tissue for reconstructive surgery. Hurwitz described the use of a posterior thigh musculocutaneous flap based on the inferior gluteal artery (1). Angrigiani et al. described the transfer of posterior and medial thigh skin based on profunda femoris perforators (2). Song et al. discussed the use of the posterior thigh perforator free flap (3). Flaps based on this circulation have also been routinely used for pressure sores (4).

The posterior thigh region is bordered by the inferior gluteal fold superiorly, the iliotibial tract laterally, the adductor muscles medially, and the popliteal fossa inferiorly. Flaps from the posterior thigh have been based on either the profunda femoris artery or descending branch of the inferior gluteal artery. Cadaver studies have shown that the dominant blood supply to the posterior thigh is from the profunda femoris artery perforators (5).

The profunda femoris artery arises from the lateral aspect of the femoral artery and passes into the posterior compartment of the thigh, dividing into medial and lateral branches. The lateral branches are perforating arteries, piercing the adductor magnus muscle insertion. Between four and six perforators continue as musculocutaneous (35%) or septocutaneous (65%) vessels, most often extending into a line from the ischium to the lateral femoral condyle. These vessels range from 2 to 4 mm for proximal branches and 1 to 2 mm for distal branches.

The posterior femoral cutaneous nerve (S1–S3) is found in the subfascial plane in the posterior midthigh, which provides the possibility of transferring a sensitized flap with branches from this nerve.

Flap names in the posterior thigh region have been based on anatomical location, muscle origin, or arterial pedicle flap type (5). Recently, the senior author described the posterior thigh as a new option for women with inadequate abdominal tissue (Figure 9-1) (6). The posterior thigh soft tissue supplies the profunda artery perforator (PAP) flap or thigh gluteal artery perforator (TGAP) flap.

In the majority of patients, the posterior thigh contains a dominant perforator from the profunda femoris artery. This allows the harvest of a PAP flap. Less often, inadequate PAPs will be present. Instead, the dominant perforator to the posterior thigh tissue arises from the descending branch of the inferior gluteal artery. In distinction to the PAP flap, a flap from similar posterior thigh distribution based on this will be deemed a TGAP flap. The latter deserves mention as distinct from GAP flaps. Although both share a similar source vessel, the GAP flaps are harvested from the gluteal region, but the TGAP from the posterior thigh.

PREOPERATIVE IMAGING

Magnetic resonance angiography or computed tomography angiography of the pelvis and thigh with contrast assists with preoperative planning (Figures 9-1 to 9-4). It is performed in the planned operative position. Planning may be augmented with a handheld Doppler to identify the dominant skin perforator(s). Typically, there are both medial and lateral perforators. However, pursuing a medial perforator will allow ease of

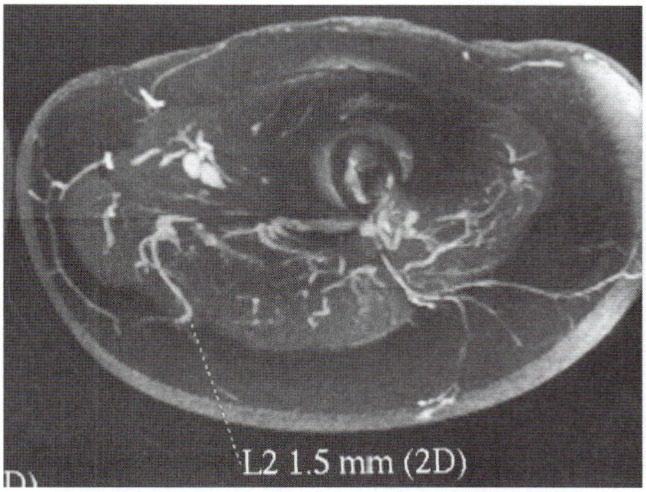

FIGURE 9-1 Computed tomography angiogram shows a dominant perforator (labeled L2) located in the posteromedial left thigh and measuring approximately 1.5 mm in diameter.

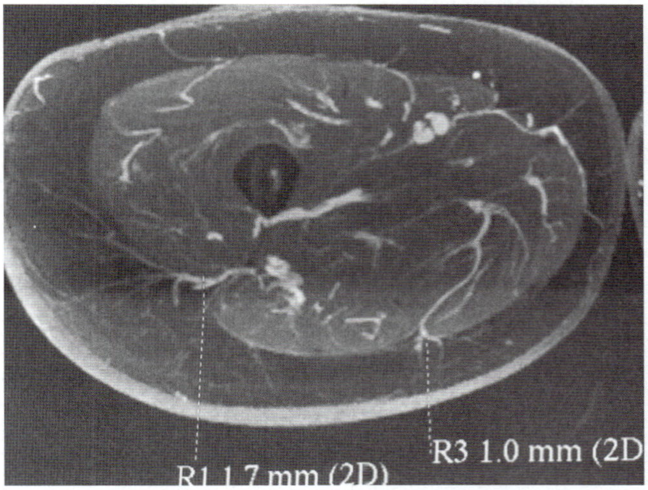

FIGURE 9-2 Computed tomography angiogram shows one of two perforators (labeled R3) located in the posteromedial right thigh that measures approximately 1.0 mm in diameter. Choosing medial perforators allows for ease of harvest in the supine position.

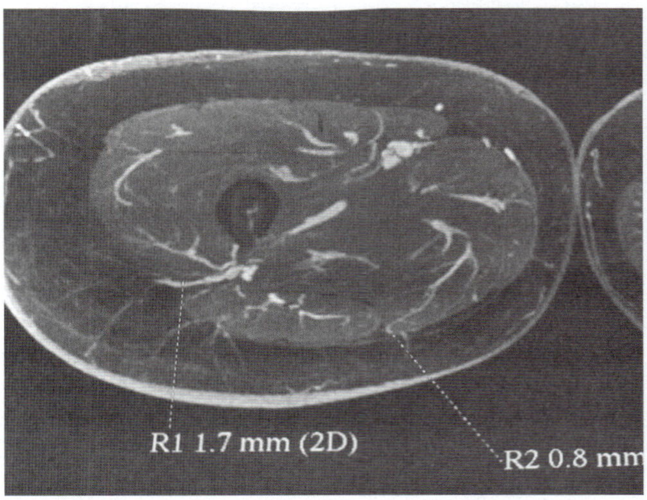

FIGURE 9-3 Computed tomography angiogram also shows another posteromedial right thigh perforator (labeled R2) located in the postero-medial right thigh that measures approximately 0.8 mm in diameter.

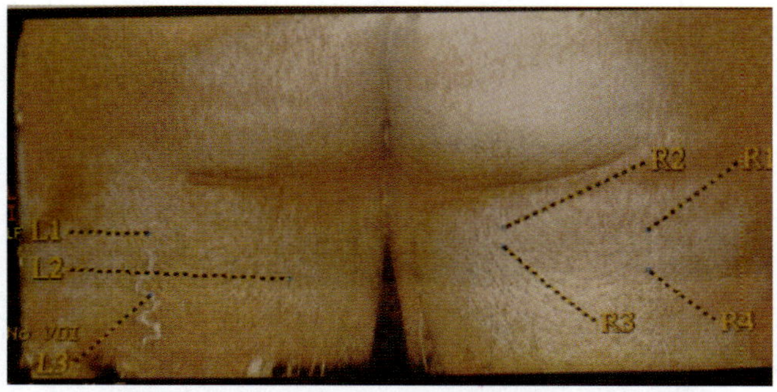

FIGURE 9-4 Reconstructed images of Figures 9-1 to 9-3 allow for preoperative identification of L2, R2, and R3 as ideal perforators for bilateral profunda artery perforator flap harvest.

harvest in the supine position. Additionally, this medial perforator tends to be larger and enter posterior to the gracilis muscle.

MARKINGS

If possible, the patient is marked in the office the day before surgery (Figures 9-5 and 9-6). The chest is marked, including the inframammary fold and breast footprint. The dimensions and volume needed for reconstruction are estimated.

An elliptical skin paddle measuring approximately 27 cm × 7 cm is drawn approximately 1 cm inferior to the gluteal fold.

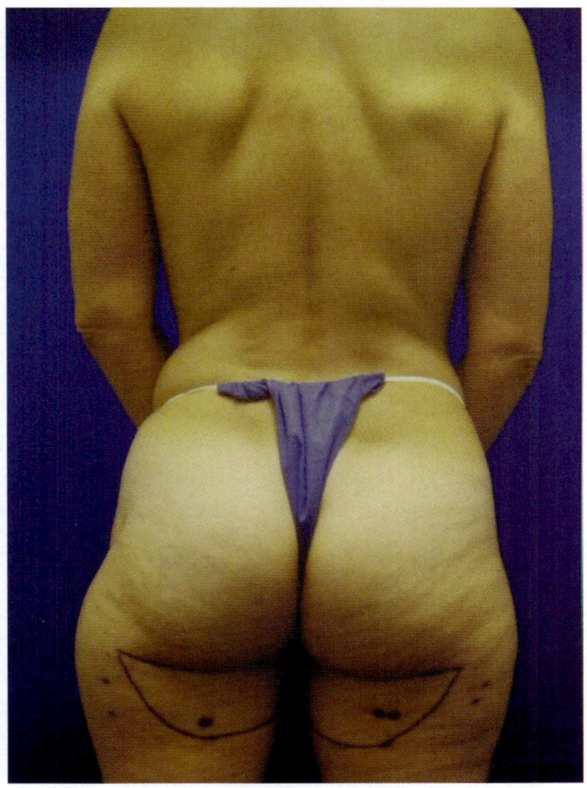

FIGURE 9-5 Using preoperative imaging (Figures 9-1 to 9-4) and a Doppler, the profunda artery perforator flaps and corresponding perforators are marked out bilaterally. The patient is not a candidate for abdominally based autologous reconstruction.

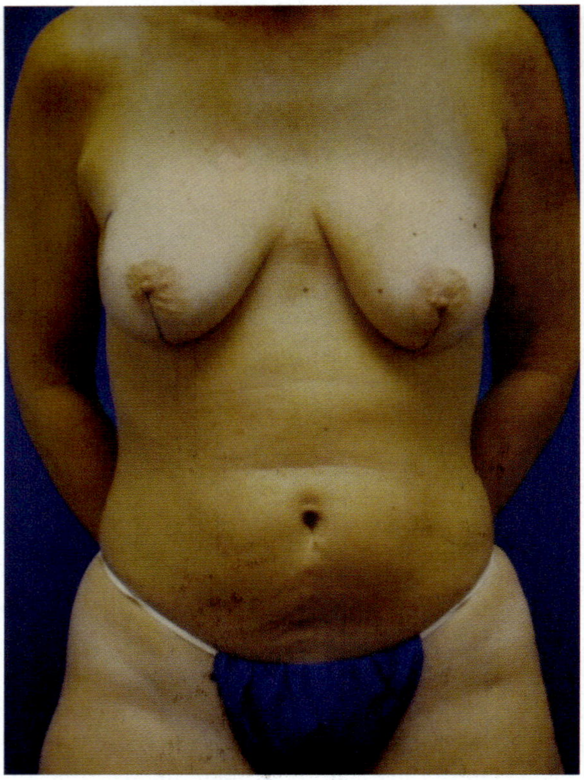

FIGURE 9-6 The patient in Figure 9-5 will undergo bilateral nipple-sparing mastectomies with immediate reconstruction.

The flap is designed as an ellipse so the scar does not extend onto the visible lateral or medial thigh outside of the gluteal fold. The transverse length is usually 27 cm. The planned amount of outward beveling is also estimated and marked. Beveling in the lateral thigh helps to increase flap volume but should be limited superiorly to avoid disturbing the contour of the inferior buttock and gluteal fold.

INTRAOPERATIVE POSITIONING

The PAP or TGAP flaps can be harvested in the supine or prone position. The supine position, assisted by a frog-legged posture, is the preferred harvest approach of the senior author, and this will be described. It offers the advantage of decreased operative time by eliminating the need for repositioning. Harvest can proceed concomitantly with mastectomy or recipient vessel exposure. Additionally, it allows for rapid dissection from a medial approach.

TECHNIQUE

All skin incisions are injected with local anesthesia with epinephrine (Figure 9-7). The patient is then prepped and draped in sterile fashion. The elliptical incision is made, and dissection proceeds through the subcutaneous tissue. Harvest of the medial portion of the flap is easily performed in the supine, frog-legged position noted earlier (Figure 9-8). Internally rotating the hip permits easy dissection of the lateral portion of the flap. Beveling in the lateral thigh can increase flap volume and

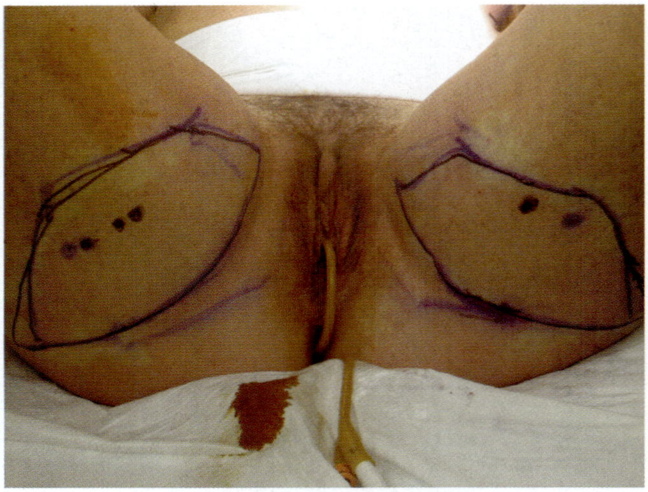

FIGURE 9-7 The incisions have been infiltrated with local anesthesia before sterile prepping and draping.

potentially help with postoperative donor site contour. Beveling should be limited superiorly to avoid disturbing the contour of the inferior buttock and gluteal fold.

After an island of skin and subcutaneous tissue are created in the posterior thigh (Figure 9-9), attention is paid to the superior incision. Suprafascial dissection, from anterior to posterior, proceeds over the gracilis muscle. Halfway through the width of the gracilis muscle, the fascia is incised. Subfascial dissection continues to the posterior border of the gracilis muscle (Figure 9-10). The muscle is retracted anteriorly to identify the adductor magnus. Subfascial dissection continues over the adductor magnus. The vascular pedicle is precisely identified according to the preoperative angiography. After the key perforator is identified, standard perforator dissection proceeds to harvest the desired pedicle length and vessel diameter (Figures 9-11 to 9-13). The donor site is closed in a multilayer fashion over a drain.

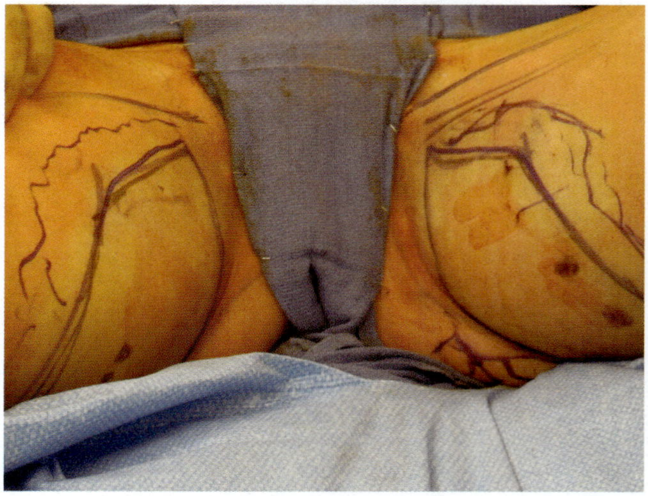

FIGURE 9-8 Harvest of the flap is completed in the supine position. Harvest of the medial flap is best done in the frog-legged position, with the hips externally rotated. Internal rotation of the hip allows for lateral harvest.

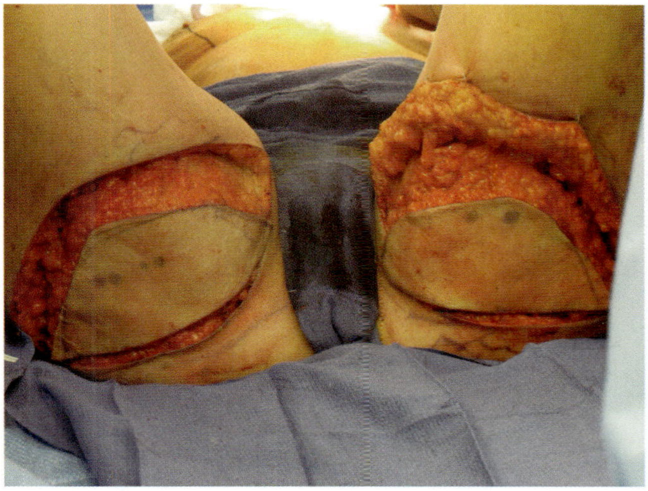

FIGURE 9-9 With the lower extremities elevated, bilateral islands of posterior thigh skin and subcutaneous tissue can be seen.

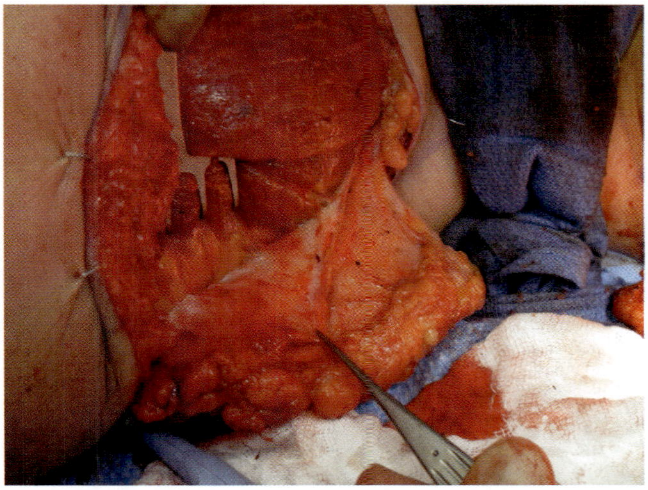

FIGURE 9-10 During harvest of the right profunda artery perforator flap, subfascial dissection is performed. The gracilis muscle is retracted anteriorly while the fascia (within the surgical forceps) is elevated with the flap.

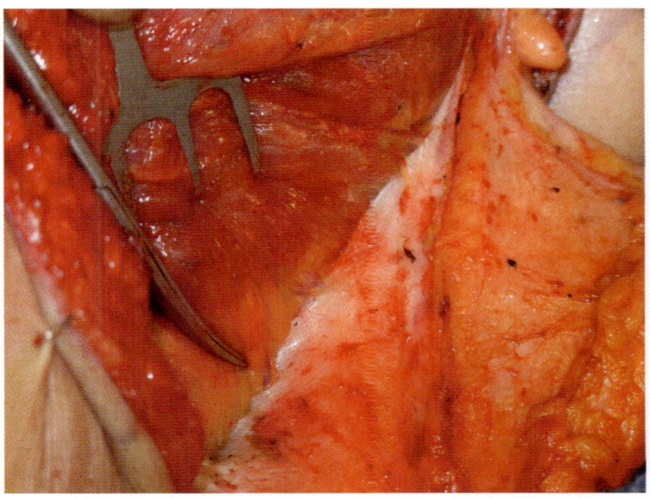

FIGURE 9-11 With the gracilis muscle retracted anteriorly, the surgical scissors point to the identified perforator of the right profunda artery perforator flap.

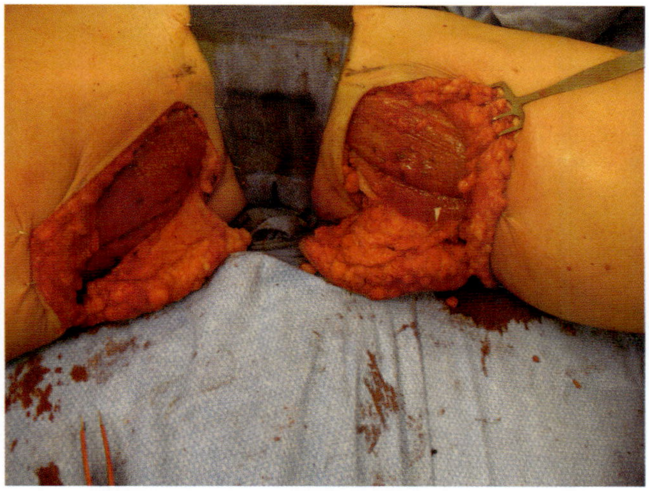

FIGURE 9-12 During harvest of the left profunda artery perforator flap, a perforator is visualized posterior to the gracilis muscle. The white arrowhead rests on the adductor magnus and points to the perforator.

The internal mammary vessels are the preferred recipient site. These vessels are accessed between the second and third or third and fourth costal cartilages. Partial rib resection may be needed for adequate exposure (Figures 9-14 and 9-15).

After recipient site preparation, the anastomosis is performed (Figure 9-16). This long narrow flap can be coned and inset with absorbable suture rather like the transverse upper gracilis (TUG) flap described elsewhere. For reconstruction of nipple-sparing mastectomies, the flap is deepithialized and buried under the breast skin for a one-stage reconstruction (Figure 9-17).

In the supine or prone position, a PAP flap can be raised in approximately 80 minutes.

POSTOPERATIVE CARE

Standard postoperative free flap care and monitoring is performed. The patient is monitored in the postanesthesia care unit for 1 to 2 hours before transfer to her room. She can ambulate on postoperative day 1 but should avoid any strenuous exercise for 4 weeks. The length of hospital stay is two to four days.

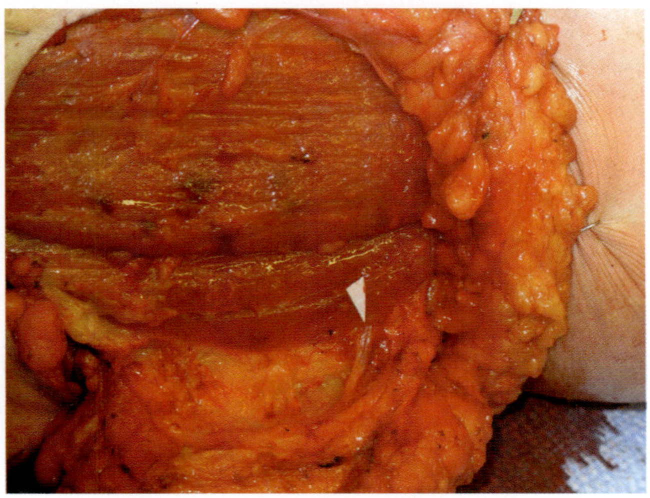

FIGURE 9-13 Close-up view of Figure 9-12.

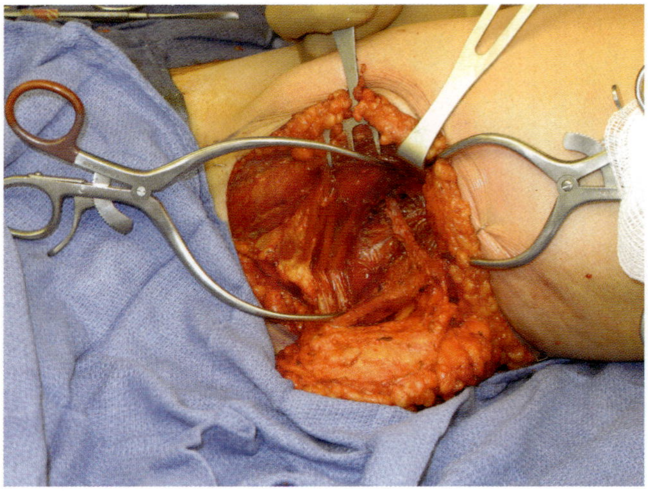

FIGURE 9-14 Standard perforator dissection proceeds to harvest the desired pedicle length and vessel diameter.

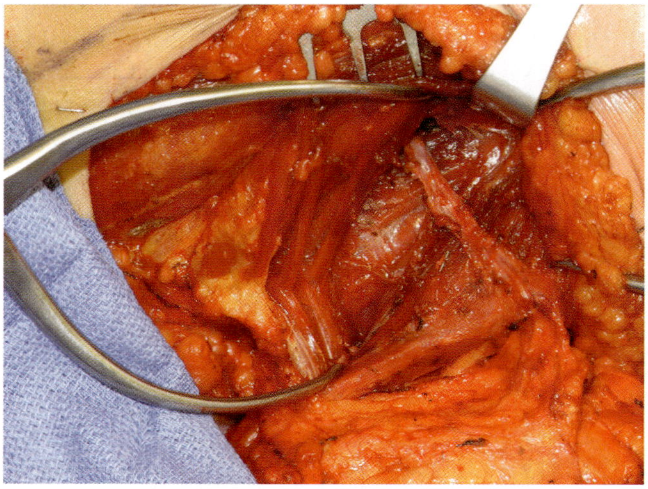

FIGURE 9-15 Close-up view of Figure 9-14.

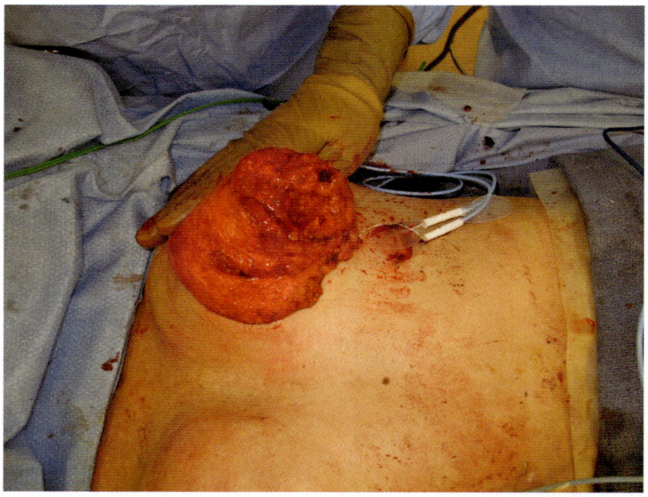

FIGURE 9-16 After microvascular anastomosis, the long elliptical design provides an ideal shape for coning to create natural breast.

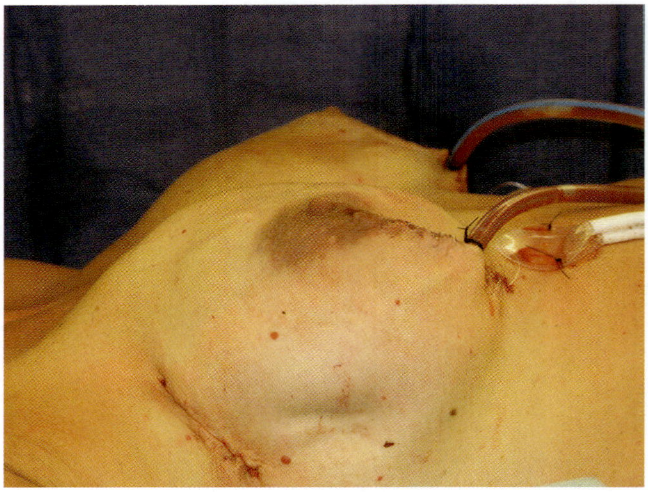

FIGURE 9-17 For reconstruction of nipple-sparing mastectomies, the flap is deepithialized and buried under the breast skin for a one-stage reconstruction. The flap is monitored postoperatively with implantable Doppler.

REFERENCES

1. Hurwitz DJ. Closure of a large defect of the pelvic cavity by an extended compound myocutaneous flap based on the inferior gluteal artery. *Br J Plast Surg* 1980;33:256–261.
2. Angrigiani C, Grilli D, Thorne CH. The adductor flap: a new method for transferring posterior and medial thigh skin. *Plast Reconstr Surg* 2001;107:1725–1731.
3. Song YG, Chen GZ, Song YL. The free thigh flap: a new free flap concept based on the septocutaneous artery. *Br J Plast Surg* 1984;37:149–159.
4. Paletta C, Bartell T, Shehadi S. Applications of the posterior thigh flap. *Ann Plast Surg* 1993;30:41–47.
5. Ahmadzadeh R, Bergeron L, Tang M, et al. The posterior thigh perforator flap or profunda femoris artery perforator flap. *Plast Reconstr Surg* 2007;119:194–200; discussion 201–192.
6. Allen RJ, Haddock NT, Ahn CY, Sadeghi A. Breast reconstruction with the profunda artery perforator (PAP) flap. *Plast Reconstr Surg* 2012;129(1):16e–23e.

CHAPTER 10

Free-Style Free Flaps and Supermicrosurgery

Isao Koshima and Naoya Sawamoto

The introduction of "supermicrosurgery," which implies the anastomosis and dissection of small-caliber vessels ranging from 0.3 to 0.8 mm in diameter, has led to the development of new reconstructive techniques. Applications of supermicrosurgery include crushed fingertip replantations using venule grafts, toetip transfers for fingertip loss, partial auricular transfers for total tracheal and eyelid defects, and lymphaticovenular anastomoses for lymphedema. Other forms of supermicrosurgery involve perforator-to-perforator anastomosis ("free-style free flaps") and include deep inferior epigastric perforator (DIEP) and paraumbilical perforator (PUP), gluteal artery perforator (GAP), thoracodorsal artery perforator (TAP), anterolateral thigh (ALT) perforator, superficial circumflex iliac perforator (SCIP), tensor fascia lata (TFL) perforator, and medial plantar artery perforator (MPAP) flaps. Such short-pedicled flaps have now been used for extremity and facial defects, and their success rate is almost the same as that for conventional free flap transfers with large-diameter vessels and long pedicles. The advantages of these "pure" perforator flaps are the simplicity of surgery; short elevation time, and concealable donor sites. Disadvantages include the need for supermicrosurgical expertise and an intrinsic anatomical variation in the anatomy of the perforators.

WHAT IS SUPERMICROSURGERY?

"Supermicrosurgery" is a technique of microneurovascular anastomosis for smaller vessels and single nerve fascicles and includes the microneurovascular dissection of these small structures whose diameters are less than 0.8 to 0.3 mm. It requires ultra-delicate microsurgical instruments (EMI Factory Company Ltd., Japan) and fine suture materials (Crown Jun Company Ltd., Japan) with needles less than 80 to 30 microns in size. This technique has spawned new forms of reconstructive microsurgery using "pure" perforator flaps (in which the anastomoses are at the perforator level) as well as nerve and fascicular flaps.

HISTORY OF SUPERMICROSURGERY

Supermicrosurgical techniques were established in the early 1980s during research on an experimental model for vascularized nerve grafting using the rat's sciatic nerve. Fine dissection of the nerve's vascular pedicle—a muscle perforator originating from the femoral artery—necessitated a special supermicrosurgical technique (1,2). Later, this technique was applied clinically for the dissection of human muscle perforator-to-perforator flaps; subsequently, many such perforator flaps were established. From 1989 onward, a new era of perforator flaps for reconstructive microsurgery was established.

Meanwhile, supermicrosurgery techniques were enjoying high success rates in the following scenarios:

1. Finger replantation distal to the distal interphalangeal (DIP) joint (3,4).
2. Vascularized toenail/nailbed transfers for finger nail losses (5).
3. Vascularized DIP joints transfers.
4. Toetip transfers for fingertip reconstruction (6).
5. Recently, successful arteriole graft for fingertip replantation has been reported (7).

Using supermicrosurgery, new "short T-pedicled" in addition to "pure" perforator flaps were proposed (8) (Figure 10-1). Both have the advantages of rapid elevation and transfer to practically anywhere in the body.

Free perforator-to-perforator flaps are now frequently performed. These are "pure" perforator flaps in which small

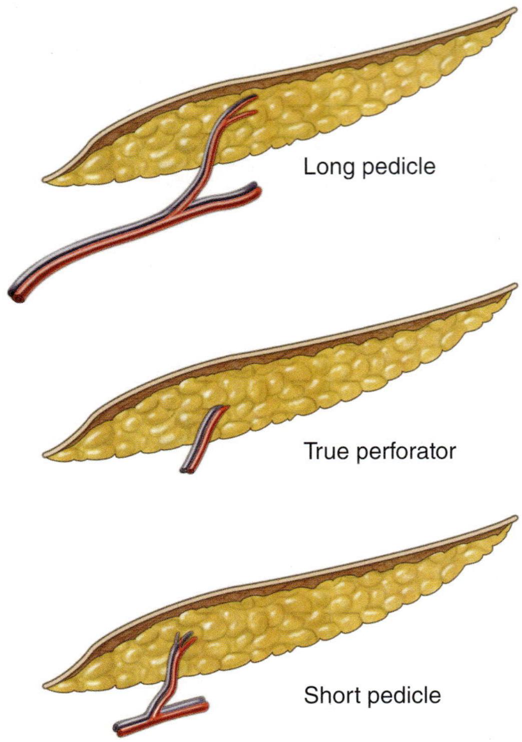

FIGURE 10-1 Classification of free perforator flaps.

perforators of less than 0.8 mm diameter from the flap are anastomosed to similarly sized vessels at the recipient site. Reports of such flaps include the PUP adiposal flap or DIEP flap for breast reconstruction and soft tissue facial augmentation (9–12). Other "pure" perforator flaps include the TAP flap (for the extremities) (13), the ALT flap (extremities) (8,14), the TFL perforator flap (hand) (15), the medial thigh perforator flap (foot) (16), the GAP flap (facial augmentation) (17), the posterior tibial flap (hand) (18), and the medial plantar perforator flap for finger pulp coverage (19–22). In addition, the free SCIP flap (23), the digital artery perforator (DAP) flap (24), the TAP and capillary perforator (TAPcp) flap (13) have further extended the scope of supermicrosurgery.

Clinical application of these techniques led to a concept that was first proposed at the Japanese Society of Reconstructive Microsurgery in the early 1990s. In 1996, it was presented internationally at the Morning Lecture at the Brigham Women's Hospital in Boston and in the following year at the First International Course on Perforator Flaps at Gent in Belgium (25). In addition, many new free tissue transfers involving supermicrosurgery have been developed, including appendix transfer for urethral loss (26), partial auricular transfer for upper eyelid reconstruction (27–32) as well as for defects of the trachea (33), toe-web transfers for oral commissure replacement (34), vascularized nerve flaps with perforator vessel anastomosis (35,36), and fascicular turnover flaps for nerve gaps (37). Additionally, vascularized adiposal flaps elevated on their perforators are now used in facial and breast augmentation (38). Current lymphaticovenular anastomotic techniques used in the treatment of lymphedema may also be considered to be supermicrosurgery (39,40).

IMPORTANCE OF MICROANATOMY

An expanding knowledge of microanatomy coupled with increasing microsurgical skills has facilitated the vascularized transfer of tissues of small volume containing nerves, lymph ducts, and so on. For example, microanatomy contributed the development of vascularized lymphatic transfer from the first web space of the foot. Knowledge of the communication between the dorsalis pedis artery and the medial planter artery facilitated the fabrication of the reversed medial malleolar (or *medialis pedis*) flap. Supermicrosurgical technique is also essential for the elevation of these flaps.

HAND SURGERY

Supermicrosurgery has a vital part to play in hand surgery; especially in the replantation of amputated digits. Supermicrosurgery has improved the clinical outcomes in many aspects of hand surgery. For example, the success rate of replantation of fingertip amputations was dramatically improved as a result of this technique. Even crushed fingertips can be restored with a success rate of 88% by anastomosing subdermal venules. Distal phalangeal replantation in children has also now become possible with supermicrosurgery.

TECHNIQUE OF SUPERMICROSURGERY

For the anastomosis of vessels 0.5 mm in diameter, 50- or 30-μm sized needles are used (Crown Jun Company, Japan). Usually six to eight sutures are needed. A special needle holder has been invented by another Japanese company, in which the author is the creative supervisor (Emi Company, Japan). This device has an ultra-fine tip, which makes it easier to hold and suture with small needles.

In supermicrosurgery, especially during vessel anastomosis, a one-handed suture technique is required. With conventional microsurgery, a counterforce is applied by opening the vessel with jeweler's forceps and passing the needle with a driver held in the other hand. But in supermicrosurgery, the vessel is too tiny for the tip of the forceps to be inserted into the lumen. This makes conventional suture technique difficult. Thus, a one-handed suture technique is used. The surgeon must accelerate the needle through the external wall of the vessel into the lumen using only the dominant hand. After the needle is pulled through with the needle driver, the needle tip is inserted into the lumen of the opposite vessel and again accelerated through the wall using the dominant hand. This time, however, counterforce may be gently applied on the external wall using the closed tips of the jeweler's forceps as necessary.

NEUROANASTOMOSIS

Peripheral nerves consist of many nerve fascicles. Each fascicle is covered with perineurium, the diameter of which is around 0.3 mm. Supermicrosurgery has enabled the anastomosis of small individual fascicles or terminal fibers. This is used in fascicular grafting and in the fascicular turnover flap method for nerve gaps (37).

THE FUTURE OF SUPERMICROSURGERY

In the near future, anastomosis of structures less than 100 µm in diameter will be possible. With the use of supermicrosurgical techniques, many new flaps and existing flaps elevated on their true perforators rather than on their major feeding vessels will become available.

APPLICATIONS OF SUPERMICROSURGERY

Case 1: Distal Phalangeal Replantation

Case Report

A 47-year-old man amputated the distal phalanx of the left middle finger (Figure 10-2A). Under a digital block, the proximal arteriole of the radial digital artery was anastomosed to the distal radial volar cutaneous venule, and the distal ulnar venule was anastomosed to the proximal cutaneous vein using an arteriolar graft to complete the drainage system. A distal subdermal venule (0.3 mm) was joined to a proximal subdermal venule after surgery (Figure 10-2B). The finger survived completely without congestion (Figure 10-2C).

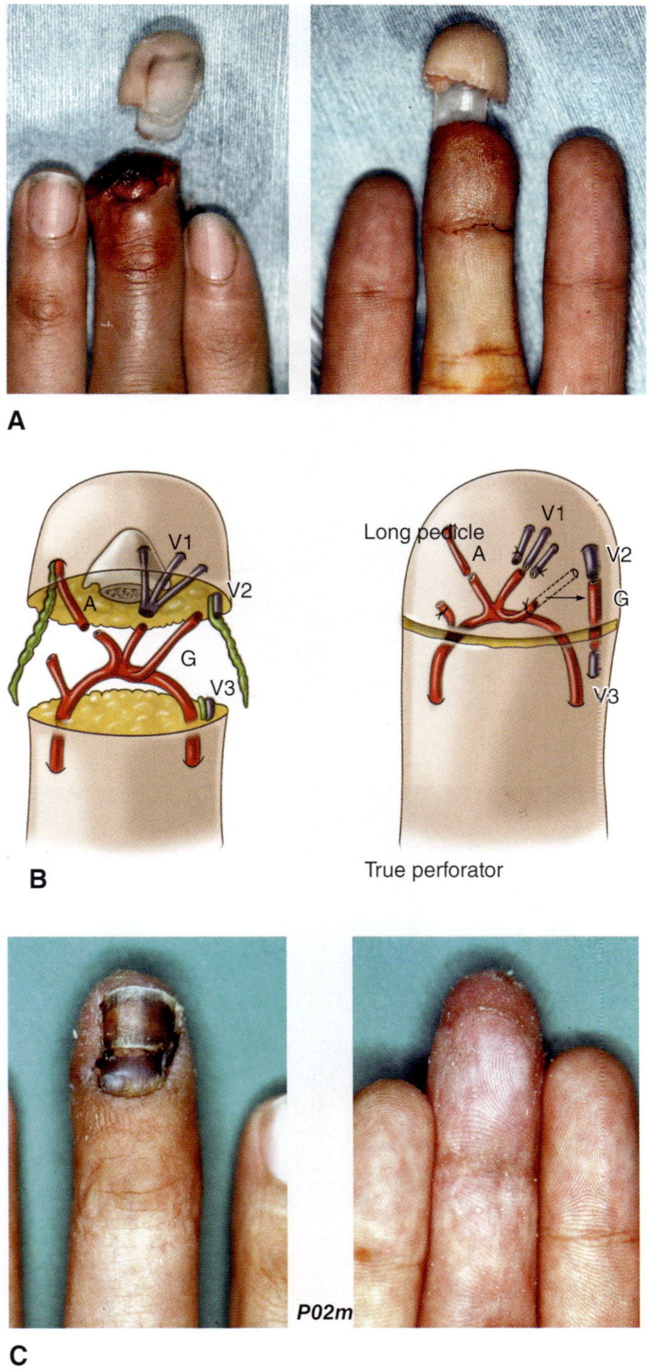

FIGURE 10-2 Atypical fingertip replantation distal to the terminal arch of the digital artery. (**A**) Amputation at the level of the nai . (**B**) An arteriole (G) was used for venous drainage (V2–V3). (**C**) Two months after surgery.

Trimmed Second Toe Tip Transfer

A trimmed second toe tip transfer is a good indication for claw nail deformity of any digit except the thumb. The medial neurovascular bundle is used as a pedicle with minimal tissue taken from the toe tip. This has been reported using a corticocancellous bone graft, but the nonvascularized bone tends to be absorbed. However, a beautiful fingertip can be made with a combination vascularized nail bed and underlying bone transfer.

Vascularized Nerve Flap

Vascularized Peroneal Nerve Flap The deep peroneal nerve is located lateral to the tibia along with anterior tibial artery and vein. The distal part of the nerve is used as a vascularized nerve graft with the anterior tibial artery and vein as pedicles. This flap can be elevated with skin paddle, which can be used as a monitoring flap. The pedicle length can be as long as 20 cm.

Case 2: Vascularized Lateral Femoral Cutaneous Nerve Flap

The vascular pedicle of this flap consists of perforators of the lateral circumflex femoral artery. Donor site morbidity is extremely low.

Case Report

A 28-year-old woman had rhabdomyosarcoma arising in the biceps muscle. Radical tumor excision included the brachial artery and median nerve. An ALT flap was harvested from the right thigh. The median nerve was reconstructed with a vascularized lateral femoral cutaneous nerve graft based on the descending branch of lateral circumflex femoral artery. The nerve gap was 15 cm long. A saphenous vein graft was used to reconstruct the brachial artery. The biceps muscle was reconstructed with a fascia lata graft. Seven months after surgery, the Tinel sign had reached the wrist, and the sensory recovery yielded a two-point discrimination of 25 mm (Figure 10-3).

Lymphaticovenous Anastomosis

The effectiveness of lymphaticovenous anastomosis (LVA) for lymphedema has already been reported. Recently, early stage or "prophylactic LVA" has also been described. The authors have performed LVA for 22 years in more than 600 cases. LVA is minimally invasive and can even be performed under local anesthesia. In reviewing our data, compression therapy was unnecessary in 75% of cases after LVA.

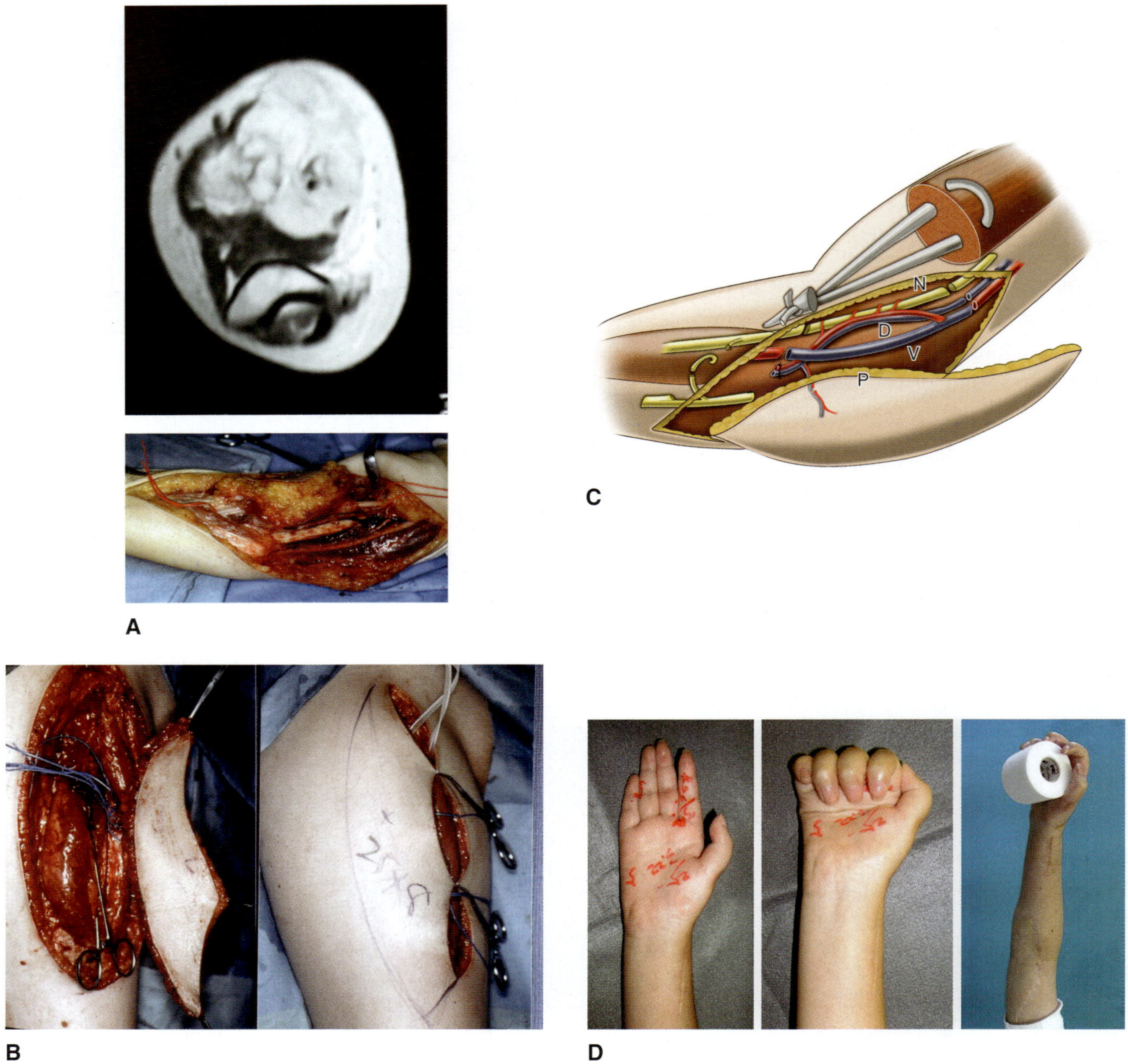

FIGURE 10-3 An anterolateral thigh (ALT) "true" perforator flap and nerve flap for a massive elbow defect. (**A**) The wide defect after resection of rhabdomyosarcoma together with brachial artery and median nerve. (**B**) The free ALT "true" perforator flap from the right thigh was transferred. (**C**) The donor vessel was the perforator (P) of the descending branch (D) of lateral circumflex femoral system. The defect in the brachial artery was bridged with saphenous vein graft (V), which also served as the recipient artery; and the median nerve gap was repaired with a vascularized lateral femoral cutaneous nerve flap (N). The recipient vein was a brachial vena comitans. (**D**) Five years after surgery. Semmes-Weinstein and moving 2PD values were 3.22 and 25 mm on the palm. (Reproduced with permission from Koshima I, Nanba Y, Tsutsui T, et al. Vascularized femoral nerve graft with anterolateral thigh "true" perforator flap for massive defects after cancer ablation in the upper arm. *J Reconstr Microsurg* 2003;19:299–302.)

Case 3: Lymphaticovenular Anastomosis for Obstructive Lymphedema

Case Report

A 64-year-old woman had secondary lymphedema and complete brachial nerve palsy of the left upper arm for 11 years. Five years earlier, she had received a mastectomy and radiation. Two lymphaticovenular anastomoses were performed in the forearm. There was remarkable clinical improvement of the affected arm after surgery, and the patient needed neither postoperative compression nor physiotherapy. The authors believe that the smooth muscle cells within the anastomosed lymphatics regenerated secondary to the surgical bypass effect, allowing the arm to regain active lymphatic function (Figure 10-4).

Pure Perforator Flaps

With the development of supermicrosurgery, perforators can be dissected directly and anastomosed to small recipient vessels smaller than 1 mm in diameter. The diameter of perforator is often

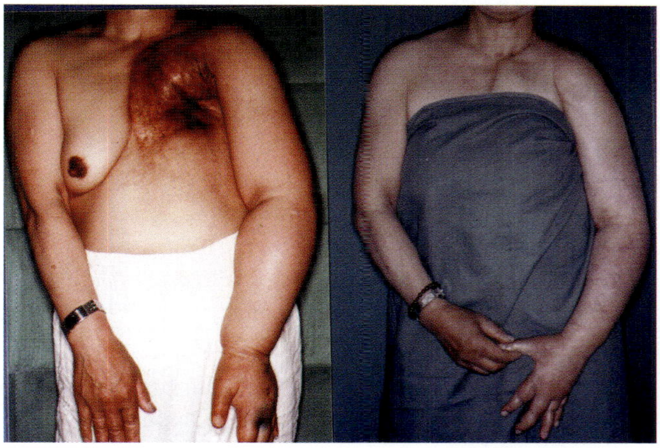

A

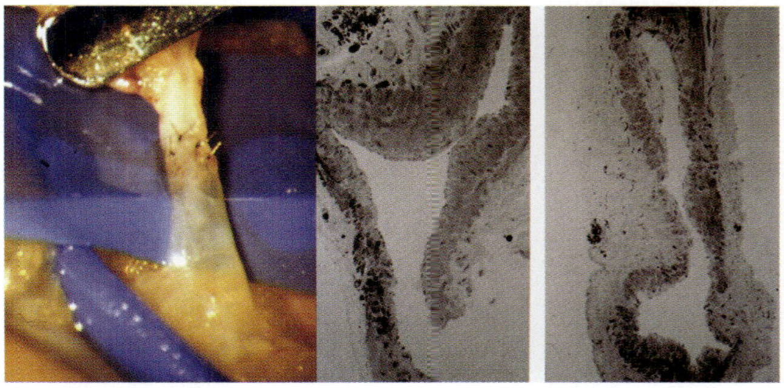

B

FIGURE 10-4 Long-standing lymphedema of the upper arm. (**A**) *Right,* preoperative view. Only two lymphaticovenular anastomoses were performed. *Left,* postoperative view at 8 years without any postoperative compression therapy. (**B**) *Right,* lymphaticovenous anastomosis was established. *Left,* biopsied lymphatic channel from the elbow shows degeneration and regeneration of smooth muscle cells. (Reproduced with permission from Koshima I, Kawada S, Morigichi T, Kajiwara Y. Ultrastructural observation of lymphatic vessels in lymphedema in human extremities. *Plast Reconstr Surg* 1996;97(2):397–405.)

about 0.8 mm. Such a flap reduces donor site morbidity compared with equivalent muscle or musculocutaneous flaps. Furthermore, flaps can often be raised from concealed areas. Operation time is also reduced because of the simplicity of the procedure. Success rates are the same as with conventional free flaps.

However, the technique of flap positioning and anastomosis is comparatively difficult. A flap elevated with a perforator forming the pedicle, is termed a "pure" perforator flap.

TECHNICAL PEARLS

Recipient Vessel Selection

Smaller branches of the main vessels such as the temporal, facial, and frontal arteries can and should be used as recipient vessels to match the vessel diameters of the flap perforators and minimize donor site morbidity.

Perforator-to-Perforator Anastomosis

Both short T-pedicled and "pure" perforator flaps have been developed (see Figure 10-1). Free perforator-to-perforator flaps are becoming increasingly popular. As mentioned earlier, these "pure" perforator flaps involve the anastomosis of small flap perforators with those at the recipient site and have diameters smaller than 0.8 mm. Tiny vein grafts are sometimes required.

T-Shaped Pedicle or Flow-Through Vascular Anastomosis

The authors now frequently use "flow-through" vascular anastomosis using a T-shaped pedicle vessel (see Figure 10-1). This can help preserve blood flow at the recipient site. Multiple flap transfers may then be performed in a limb without losing distal perfusion.

Vein Grafting

Tiny vein grafts from the volar aspect of the wrist and the dorsum of the foot are frequently used in the performance of supermicrosurgery.

Preoperative Management

A thorough knowledge of the vascular anatomy of both the donor and recipient site is important. Doppler ultrasonography and computed tomography angiography may be used for preoperative evaluation. But if the surgeon is well accustomed to the specific microvascular dissection, these examinations may not be needed. In other words, the surgeon should be able to elevate flaps without preoperative study. Unanticipated absence or loss of perforators during surgery may require the surgeon to switch to another perforator flap.

Dominance of Perforators, Combined Flaps, and Multiple Anastomoses

Adjacent perforators often have a reciprocal relationship to each other: if one is large and dominant, the other is often hypoplastic. This phenomenon is frequently seen with the ascending branch of the superficial circumflex iliac artery (SCIA) and with the superficial inferior epigastric artery (SIEA). In such cases, the surgeon should choose the largest perforator or use both perforators for pedicles. With perforator flaps in the inguinal area, where flap elevation typically begins with an incision near the inguinal ligament, multiple perforators from the SCIA, SIEA, superficial inferior epigastric vein (SIEV), or DIEP can be found. The surgeon can choose the dominant one or select a number of perforators, including the dominant one; this is then called a *combined flap.* Multiple vascular anastomoses contribute to a higher success rate.

Vascular Anomalies

The anatomy of the vascular system varies from person to person, especially with regards to the distribution of tiny perforating vessels. The surgeon should therefore anticipate vascular anomalies during perforator supermicrosurgery. When the surgeon cannot find the anticipated perforator, an adjacent usable perforator will always exist. Sometimes such vessels may appear extremely small. However, this may be due to spasm. The application of topical vasodilators such as papaverine hydrochloride or Xylocaine may allow better appreciation of their true size.

"Sparking" Dissection

Meticulous hemostasis using bipolar cautery is essential because any blood staining of the tissues makes the dissection of the tiny vessels difficult. The authors like to use a Bovie with a straight blade for flap elevation. This technique is called "sparking dissection." The blade can be used as a blunt dissector by moving it perpendicular to its flat surface as well as for electrical cutting and coagulation. With care, dissection of the perforator is greatly facilitated using the Bovie in this manner.

Vascular Spasm During Surgery

Perforators and other small vessels can go into spasm very easily, and this may prove to be problematic during flap elevation. The surgeon should therefore apply topical vasodilators frequently during the operation.

DONOR SITE CLOSURE

Vascularization from the flap bed is very important for long-term flap integration and survival. Multiple drains are placed under the flap and retained for few days after surgery to prevent the collection of blood or serum, which would serve to impede this phenomenon.

Plastic surgery is often a battle between aesthetics and blood flow. Perforator flaps decrease donor site morbidity by avoiding the sacrifice of blood flow at the donor site. Thus, "true" perforator flaps—transferred by supermicrosurgery—are potentially revolutionary in overcoming this historic antagonism.

The surgeon should pay particular attention for donor site closure. Completion of an anastomosis with a demonstrable blood flow is not the end of the operation. Skin closure should be comfortable without undue tightness. The suture lines should be coated with antibiotic ointment, and a light gauze dressing should be applied generously windowed to facilitate monitoring. The surgeon should always be mindful of aesthetics at both the donor and recipient sites. Donor site closure is not just subcontract work for the most junior house staff.

POSTOPERATIVE CARE

The authors generally use divided intravenous infusions of prostaglandin E_1 (PGE_1) as antithrombotic therapy for 5 to 7 days after surgery.

The tiny vessels involved in supermicrosurgery are very susceptible to compression. Compressive dressings or bandages should therefore be avoided. Rather than closing the wound under tension, a split-thickness skin graft is used, or the wound is temporarily left open and covered with a synthetic skin substitute to avoid pressure on the pedicle(s).

FREE-STYLE FREE PERFORATOR FLAPS

By using meticulous microsurgical technique, the perforator can be dissected in a retrograde fashion until adequate length or size of vessel is obtained. This permits free flaps to be elevated from virtually any part of body. This concept has led to the term *free-style free (perforator) flaps*. Great versatility in donor site selection is the hallmark of free-style free flaps. However, in seeking increasingly smaller vessels, random perforators, or individualized free-style free flaps, anatomic variation is frequently encountered. Surgeons performing supermicrovascular procedures must be comfortable not only with microdissection and small vessel microanastomosis but also with the possibility of encountering unfamiliar anatomy (41).

APPLICATIONS

Digital Artery Perforator Flap

Digital arteries have many branches and also perforators. This perforator facilitate the DAP flap, which is useful for resurfacing fingertip. Subdermal venulae are used for venous drainage.

Case Report

A 48-year-old woman presented with a chronic ulcer on the left thumb secondary to a burn injury. A digital artery perforator was identified as the pivot point of the flap, which was elevated for ulcer coverage. The donor site was closed using a split skin graft (Figure 10-5).

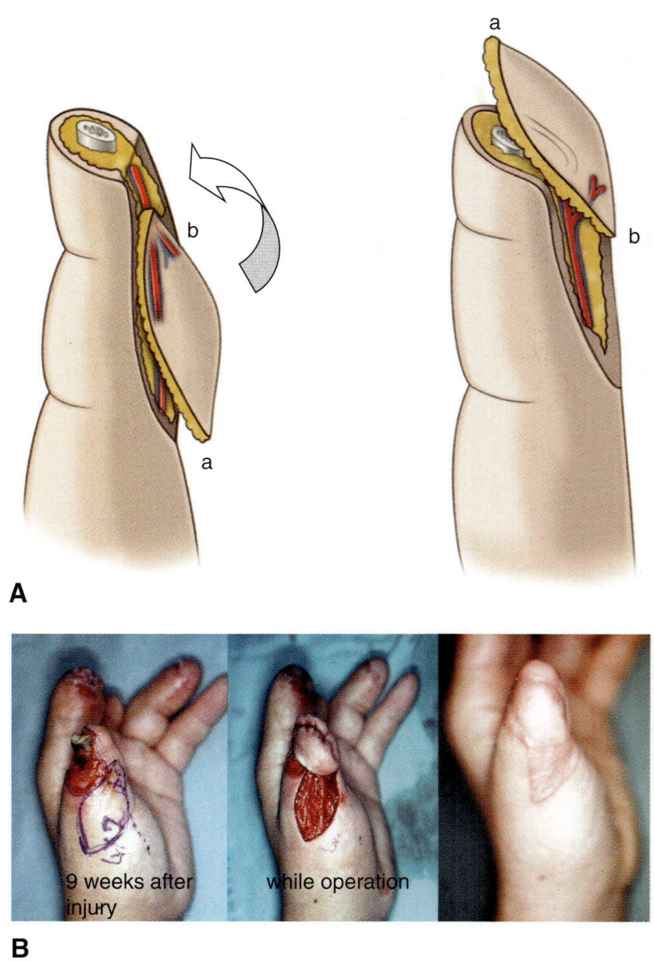

FIGURE 10-5 Digital artery perforator (DAP) flap. (**A**) Diagram of a DAP flap showing 180 degree rotation of the flap. (**B**) Case repaired with an island DAP flap. (Reproduced with permission from Koshima I, Urushibara K, Fukuda N, et al. Digital artery perforator flaps for fingertip reconstructions. *Plast Reconstr Surg* 2006;118(7):1579–1584.)

Superficial Circumflex Iliac Artery Perforator Flap

This flap is based on a perforator of the SCIA. Its characteristics include a long pedicle; low donor site morbidity; thin, supple consistency; and rapid elevation. The SCIP flap can be used with vascularized iliac bone, which is a good option for mandibular, cranial, limb, and phalangeal replacement. When raised with adipose tissue alone, it is also good for the restoration of facial contour. Its long pedicle facilitates urethral, penile, and vaginal reconstruction. As a thin cutaneous flap; it is good for resurfacing hands; and when elevated with the lateral femoral cutaneous nerve, it can be used as vascularized nerve graft.

Case Report

A 53-year-old woman presented with a severe contracture of right buccal mucosa together with a right maxillary defect after resection of an adenoid cystic carcinoma (Figure 10-6B). A vascularized free adiposal flap was transferred with a short pedicle consisting of the SCIA, SIEA, and SIEV (Figures 10-6A and 10-6C). The recipient vessels were the preauricular branch

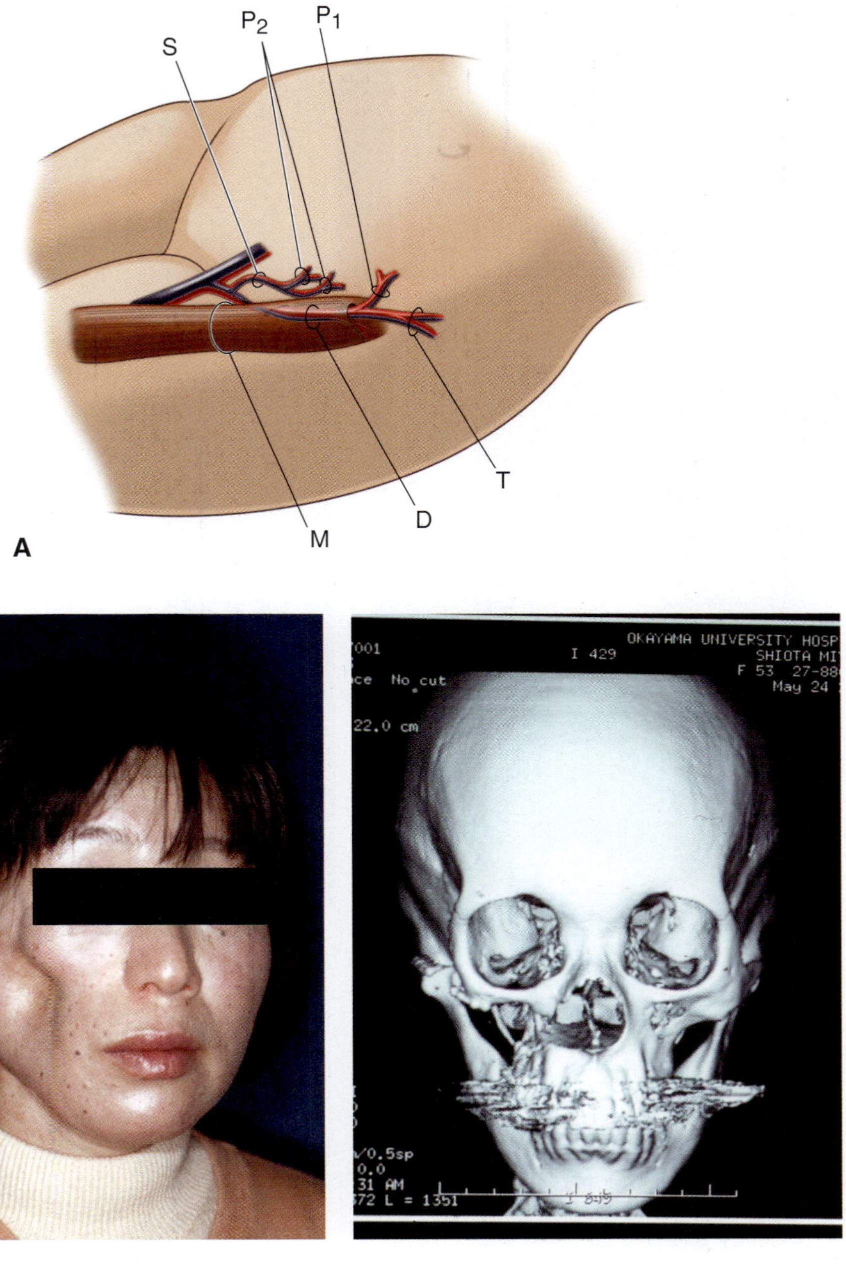

FIGURE 10-6 Superficial circumflex iliac artery perforator (SCIP) flap. (**A**) Anatomical schematic of the SCIP flap. D, deep branch; M, sartorius muscle; P1, skin perforator; P2, skin perforators; S, superficial branch; T, transverse branch. (From Koshima I, Nanba Y, Tsutsui T, et al. Superficial circumflex iliac artery perforator flap for reconstruction of limb defects. *Plast Reconstr Surg* 2004;113(1):233–240.) (**B**) Case with facial deformity after the excision of an acinic cell carcinoma. (**C**) A combined SCIP and superficial inferior epigastric (SIEA) adiposal flap was transferred from the right abdominal region. (**D**) Ten months after surgery. (Reproduced with permission from Koshima I. Short pedicle superficial inferior epigastric artery adiposal flap: new anatomical findings and the use of this flap for reconstruction of facial contour. *Plast Reconstr Surg* 2005;116(4):1091–1097.)

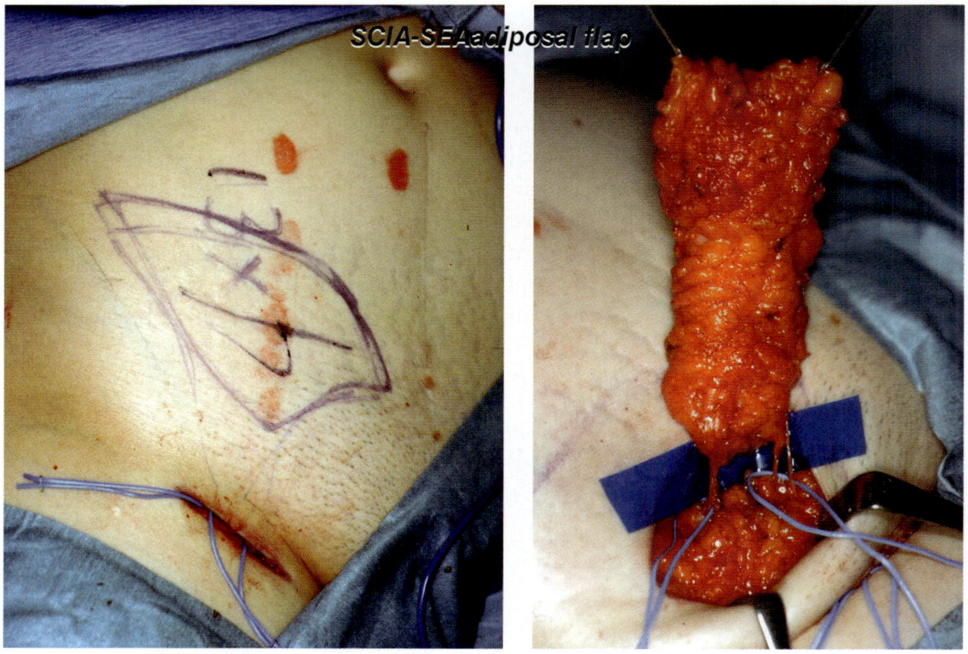

C

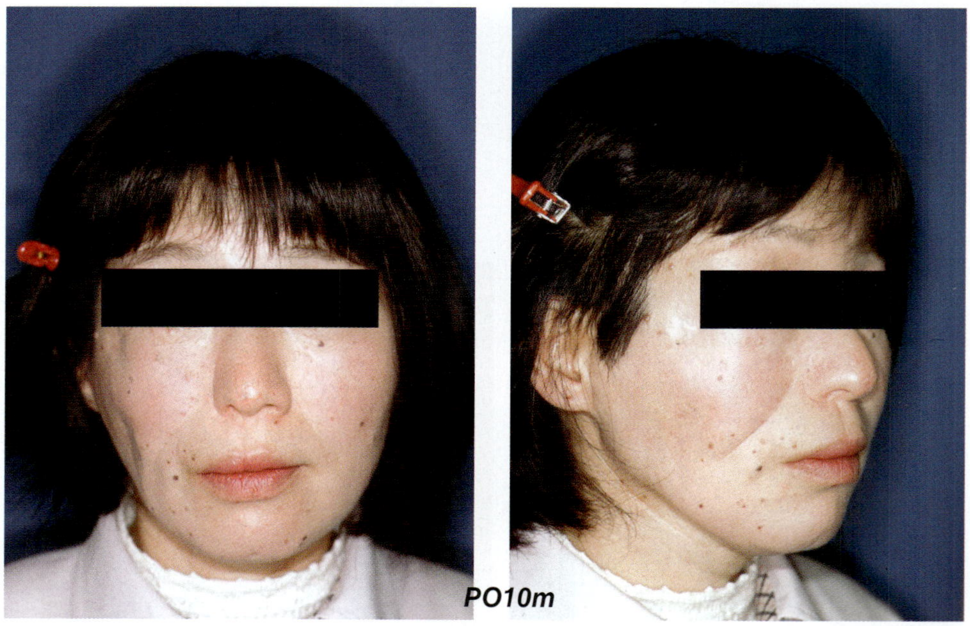

D

FIGURE 10-6 *(Continued)*

and frontal branch of the superficial temporal artery (STA) (0.8 mm each) and the superficial temporal vein (STV). Ten months after surgery, there was no flap atrophy or necrosis (Figure 10-6D).

Thoracodorsal Artery Perforator Flap

The pedicle is a perforator of the thoracodorsal (TD) artery. This flap does not include muscle. The characteristics are low donor site morbidity with preservation of latissimus function and a less conspicuous scar. A serious complication of latissimus dorsi flaps in children is scoliosis. The TAP flap, by preserving the muscular branch of the TD nerve, helps prevents scoliosis.

Case Report

A 51-year-old man presented with a severe scar contracture in his left hand caused by a burn injury (Figure 10-7A). Release of the contracture was performed, and a TAP flap was harvested from his left chest wall (Figure 10-7B). The effects of the contracture were abolished and an acceptable contour restored (Figure 10-7C).

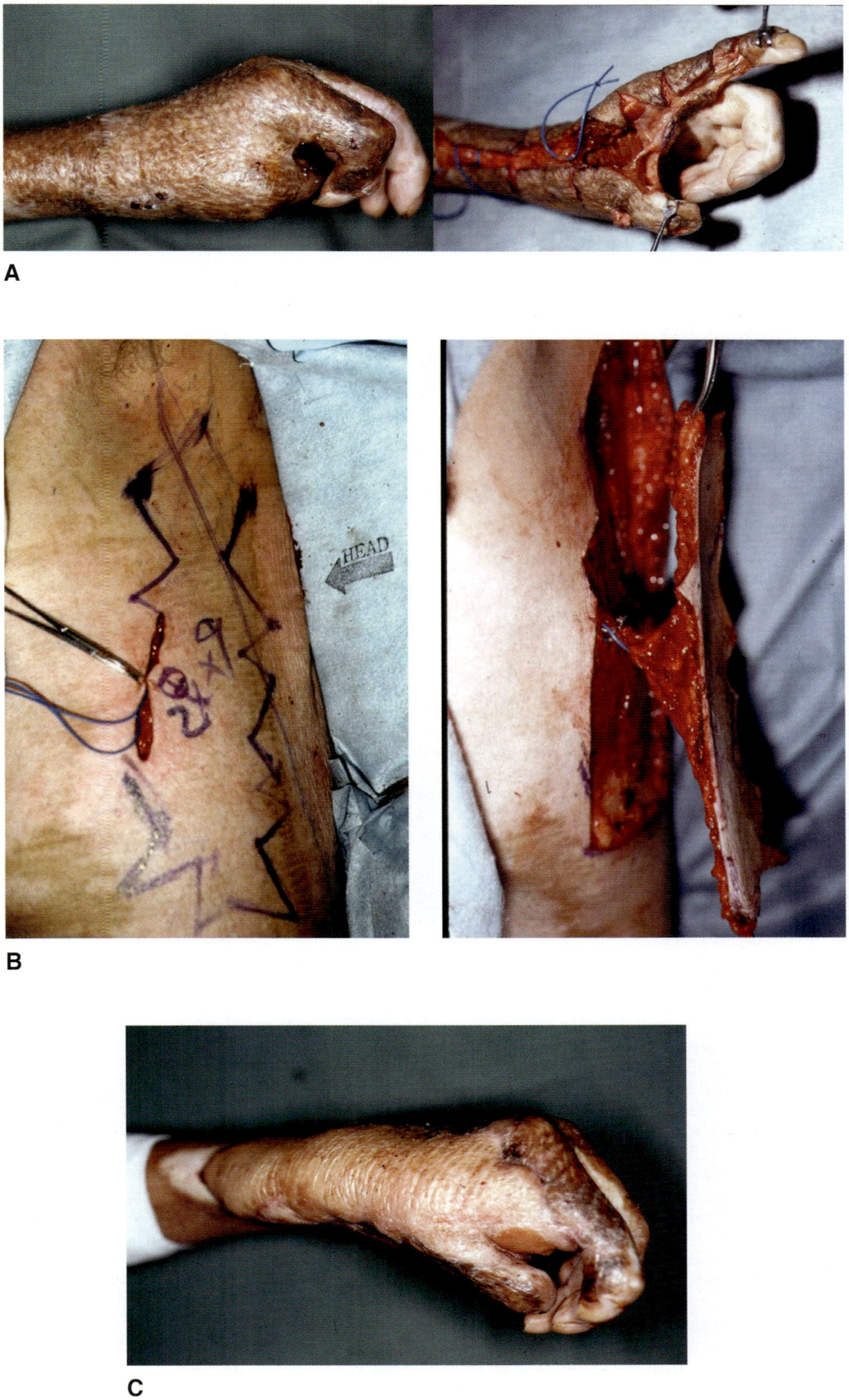

FIGURE 10-7 Thoracodorsal artery perforator (TAP) flap. (**A**) A severe burn contracture was released. (**B**) A TAP flap was elevated from the left midaxillary region with the patient in the supine position. (**C**) Postoperative view. (Reproduced with permission from Koshima I, Narushima M, Mihara M, et al. New thoracodorsal artery perforator (TAPcp) flap with capillary perforators for reconstruction of upper limb. *J Plast Reconstr Aesthet Surg* 2010;63(1):140–145).

ACKNOWLEDGMENT

A part of this work was reported at the First International Course on Perforator Flaps in Gent in June 13, 1997, at the First and 2nd Congresses of World Society of Reconstructive Microsurgery in Taipei and Heiderberg in October and November 2001 and June 2003, respectively, and the Twelfth Congress of the International Plastic Reconstructive and Aesthetic Surgery in Sydney in October 2001 and August 14, 2003.

I would like to thank Dr Katsuyuki Urushibara, my esteemed coworker from the Kawasaki Medical School, for his vital contributions to the development of supermicrosurgery and perforator flaps. Tragically, he died in a traffic accident at 44 years of age on August 22, 2009.

REFERENCES

1. Koshima I. Harii K. Experimental study of vascularized nerve grafts: Multifactorial analyses of axonal regeneration of nerves transplanted into an acute burn wound. *J Hand Surg* 1985;10(suppl A):64–72.
2. Koshima I, Harii K. Experimental study of vascularized nerve grafts: Morphometric study of axonal regeneration of nerves transplanted into silicone tubes. *Ann Plast Surg* 1985;14:235–243.
3. Yamano Y. Replantation of the amputated distal part of the fingers. *J Hand Surg Am* 1985;10:211–218.
4. Koshima I, Soeda S, Moriguchi T, et al. The use of arteriovenous anastomosis for replantation of the distal phalanx of the fingers. *Plast Reconstr Surg* 1992;89(4):710–714.
5. Koshima I, Soeda S, Takase T, Yamasaki M. Free vascularized nail grafts. *J Hand Surg* 1987;13(suppl A):29–32.
6. Koshima I, Inagawa K, Urushibara K, et al. Fingertip reconstructions using partial-toe transfers. *Plast Reconstr Surg* 2000;105:1666–1674.
7. Koshima I. Atypical arteriole anastomoses for fingertip replantations under digital block. *J Plast Reconstr Aesthet Surg* 2008;61:84–87.
8. Koshima I, Fujitsu M, Ushio S, et al. Flow-through anterior thigh flaps with a short pedicle for reconstruction of lower leg and foot defects. *Plast Reconstr Surg* 2005;115(1):155–162.
9. Koshima I, Inagawa K, Jitsuiki Y, et al. Scarpa's adipofascial flap for repair of wide scalp defects. *Ann Plast Surg* 1998;102:88–92.
10. Koshima I, Inagawa K, Urushibara K, et al. Paraumbilical perforator flap without deep inferior epigastric vessels. *Plast Reconstr Surg* 1998;102: 1052–1057.
11. Koshima I, Inagawa K, Yamamoto M, et al. New microsurgical breast reconstruction using free PUP (paraumbilical perforator) adiposal flaps. *Plast Reconstr Surg* 2000;106:61–65.
12. Koshima I, Inagawa K, Urushibara K, et al. Onestage facial contour augmentation with intraoral transfer of a paraumbilical perforator adiposal flap. *Plast Reconstr Surg* 2001;108:988–994.
13. Koshima I, Narushima M, Mihara M, et al. New thoracodorsal artery perforator (TAPcp) flap with capillary perforators for reconstruction of upper limb. *J Plast Reconstr Aesthet Surg* 2010;63(1):140–145.
14. Koshima I, Nanba Y, Tsutsui T, Takahashi Y. New anterolateral thigh perforator flap with a short pedicle for reconstruction of defects in the upper extremities. *Ann Plast Surg* 2003;51:30–36.
15. Koshima I, Urushibara K, Inagawa K, Moriguchi T. Free tensor fasciae latae perforator flap for the reconstruction of defects in the extremities. *Plast Reconstr Surg* 2001;107:1759–1765.
16. Koshima I, Hosoda M, Inagawa K, et al. Free medial thigh perforator-based flaps: new definition of the pedicle vessels and versatile application. *Ann Plast Surg* 1996;37:507–515.
17. Koshima I, Tsutsui T, Takahashi Y, Nanba Y. Free gluteal artery perforator flap with a short, small perforator. *Ann Plast Surg* 2003;51:200–204.
18. Koshima I, Soeda S. Free posterior tibial perforator-based flaps. *Ann Plast Surg* 1991;26:284–288.
19. Inoue T, Kobayashi M, Harashina T. Finger pulp reconstruction with a free sensory medial plantar flap. *Br J Plast Surg* 1988;41:657.
20. Ishikura N, Heshiki T, Tsukada S. The use of a free medialis pedis flap for resurfacing skin defects of the hand and digits: results in five cases. *Plast Reconstr Surg* 1995;95:100.
21. Lee HB, Tark KC, Rah DK, et al. Pulp reconstruction of fingers with very small sensate medial plantar free flap. *Plast Reconstr Surg* 1998;101:999.
22. Koshima I, Urushibara K, Inagawa K, et al. Free medial plantar perforator flaps for the resurfacing of finger and foot defects. *Plast Reconstr Surg* 2001;107:1753–1757.
23. Koshima I, Nanba Y, Tsutsui T, et al. Superficial circumflex iliac artery perforator flap for reconstruction of limb defects. *Plast Reconstr Surg* 2004;113(1):233–240.
24. Koshima I, Urushibara K, Fukuda N, et al. Digital artery perforator flaps for fingertip reconstructions. *Plast Reconstr Surg* 2006;118(7):1579–1584.
25. Koshima I. *Microsurgery in the Future: Introduction to Supra-microsurgery and Perforator Flaps.* Presented at the First International Course on Perforator Flap and Arterialized Skin Flaps. Special invited lecture. Gent, Belgium,June 13,1997.
26. Koshima I, Inagawa K, Okuyama N, et al. Free vascularized appendix transfer for reconstruction of penile urethra with severe fibrosis. *Plast Reconstr Surg* 1999;103:964–969.
27. Fujino T, Harashina T, Nakajima T. Free skin flap from the retroauricular region to the nose. *Plast Reconstr Surg* 1976;57:338.
28. Parkhause N, Evance D. Reconstruction of the ala of the nose using a composite free flap from the pinna. *Br J Plast Surg* 1985;38:306–313.
29. Shenaq SM, Dinh TA, Spira M. Nasal ala reconstruction with an ear helix free flap. *J Reconstr Microsurg* 1989;5:63–67.
30. Pribaz JJ, Falco N. Nasal reconstruction with auricular microvascular transplant. *Ann Plast Surg* 1993;31:289–297.
31. Tanaka Y, Tajima S, Tsujiguchi K, et al. Microvascular reconstruction of nose and ear defects using composite auricular free flaps. *Ann Plast Surg* 1996;36:298–302.
32. Koshima I, Urushibara K, Okuyama H, et al. Ear helix flap for reconstruction of total loss of the upper eyelid. *Br J Plast Surg* 1999;52:314–316.
33. Koshima I, Umeda N, Moriguchi T, et al. A full-thickness chondrocutaneous flap from the auricular concha for repair of tracheal defects. *Plast Reconstr Surg* 1997;99:1887–1893.
34. Koshima I, Inagawa K, Urushibara K, Moriguchi T. Combined submental flap with toe web for reconstruction of the lip with oral commissure. *Br J Plast Surg* 2000;53:616–619.
35. Koshima I, Okumoto K, Umeda N, et al. Free vascularized deep peroneal nerve grafts. *J Reconstr Microsurg* 1996;12:131–141.
36. Koshima I, Nanba Y, Tsutsui T, et al. Vascularized femoral nerve graft with anterolateral thigh "true" perforator flap for massive defects after cancer ablation in the upper arm. *J Reconstr Microsurg* 2003;19:299–302.
37. Koshima I, Narushima M, Mihara M, et al. Fascicular turnover flap for nerve gaps. *J Plast Reconstr Aesthet Surg* 2010;63:1008–1014.
38. Koshima I. Short pedicle superficial inferior epigastric artery adiposal flap: new anatomical findings and the use of this flap for reconstruction of facial contour. *Plast Reconstr Surg* 2005;15:(116):1091–1097.
39. Koshima I, Kawada S, Moriguchi T, Kajiwara Y. Ultrastructural observations of lymphatic vessels in lymphedema in human extremities. *Plast Reconstr Surg* 1996;97(2):397–405.
40. Koshima I, Inagawa K, Urushibara K, et al. Supermicrosurgical lymphaticovenular anastomosis for the treatment of lymphedema in the upper extremities. *J Reconstr Microsurg* 2000;16:437–442.
41. Mardini S, Tsai FC, Wei FC. The thigh as a model for free style free flaps. *Clin Plast Surg* 2003;30(3):473–480.

CHAPTER 11

Prefabricated Flaps

Jacques Baudet, Vincent Casoli, Philippe Pelissier, and Vincent Pinsolle

For many years, conventional plastic surgery procedures (grafts of various tissues; local, regional, or distant flaps) have been the only solution to problems of simple or composite defects. In most cases, whenever these techniques were appropriately applied, the end results were highly satisfactory.

But it is obvious that they would not guarantee a satisfactory result for extensive and compound defects, especially in the head and neck. Free flap transfers have opened up a new field and have constituted a significant progress in reconstructive surgery.

In the early 1980s, new ideas were born of the need to achieve better functional and cosmetic results while minimizing adverse donor site sequelae. New concepts led to the description and utilization of the so-called "prefabricated flaps" described in 1982 (1), 1987, and 1992 (2) by multiple authors. In 1994 (3), an article on "prelaminated flaps," a different technical entity, was first published.

Prefabricated or prelaminated flaps may be either a choice or a necessity. Experienced surgeons may *choose* them when they are convinced that these flaps offer the best solution to fulfill the functional and cosmetic requirements of the area to be reconstructed. They can be a necessity, in some rare situations, when there is no adequate donor site available for a simpler alternative.

What, then, is the concept of the "prefabricated flap?" A prefabricated flap is constructed in familiar donor sites for pedicled or free tissue transfers (e.g., Chinese forearm flap, scapular or parascapular flap, lateral arm flap [LAF], scalp flap, fibula flap, supraclavicular flap, anterolateral thigh flap) based on axial vessels and often a sensory nerve supply. The idea is to achieve—in one or several stages—complete preparation of a composite flap before its transfer. Different tissue components, either free or vascularized, are incorporated within the donor site (e.g., skin, mucosa, bone, cartilage, nerve), and transfer is achieved when the prefabricated flap seems capable of fulfilling the expected reconstructive goal. This technique is most applicable for head and neck reconstruction such as trachea, larynx, and esophagus, but there are various indications for its use in other parts of the body. We will discuss them later.

A variety of adjunct techniques expand the indications and reconstructive potential of prefabricated flaps. These include delay of the flap, flap preexpansion, induced neovascularization, and induced neovascularization. However, in the future, tissue engineering holds the potential for even greater application of this technique.

TECHNIQUES OF FLAP PREFABRICATION

Apart from the basic technique, the following technical modalities are currently used.

Delay

The delay procedure has been successfully used for a long time to improve the viability of random flaps such as cross-leg and extended latissimus dorsi flaps (the latter down to the iliac crest) (4). In a first stage, two parallel incisions are made, and the resulting bipedicle flap is raised. (The opportunity should be taken at this first stage to skin graft the donor site.) Two weeks later, if necessary, additional incisions can be made partially dividing the flap's tip from the donor site. This itself may be staged. This delay procedure is highly reliable and can be applied to most types of prefabricated flap.

Expansion

There are a number of reasons to consider skin expansion. One is to obtain the greatest surface area of flap that still permits primary closure of the donor site. Another is to obtain an extremely thin flap so as to meet the requirements of a specific recipient area. An important benefit is that the capsule formed under the flap and around the expander participates in increasing its vascularity and viability. Expansion can be performed under an island flap or, as some authors have shown both experimentally and clinically, under a "neovascularized skin territory" (5).

Vascular Induction

In this modality, an arteriovenous pedicle (e.g., the radial artery and its venae comitantes) is placed under the prospective flap; it can be based proximal to the donor site or distal (6–8). The implanted arteriovenous pedicle with a surrounding segment of fascia or muscle can be harvested from the area surrounding the prefabricated flap or transferred there by microvascular surgery from another part of the body. The selection of the donor site depends on the ability of this "neoflap" to incorporate and carry the required tissue components (after being implanted); the texture, thickness, and color match of the skin; and the anticipated donor deficit after transfer is complete. If the final transposition of the flap is to be pedicled rather than free, then its location is also a major consideration.

Prefabricated Induced Expanded Flap

Here a tissue expander is placed under the arteriovenous pedicle of an induced flap (9,10). The advantages of induction and expansion mentioned earlier are thus combined. Some authors have suggested wrapping the base of the pedicle with a short segment of Gore-Tex (polytetrafluoroethylene) or a thin silicone sheet to prevent adhesion to the surrounding tissues and facilitate later elevation of the flap. The expander should be inflated for 8 weeks (11).

THE MAIN DONOR SITES FOR PREFABRICATED FLAPS

The detailed anatomy of these donor sites is detailed in other chapters. However, a brief overview of the anatomy for each donor site is given here. Their main clinical applications as prefabricated flaps as well as results and postoperative complications are discussed.

Scalp Flap

The scalp and adjacent underlying structures consists of four layers: hair-bearing skin, subcutaneous tissue, superficial temporal fascia (STF), and deep temporal fascia (DTF) (12). It is well vascularized supplied by the temporal artery (TA), which divides into the superficial temporal artery (STA) and the middle temporal artery (MTA). The venous drainage is provided by accompanying veins. A secondary blood supply is provided by the occipital artery and vein and the posterior auricular artery and its comitant vein.

A temporoparietal fascial flap (TPFF) is a thin layer, which can be pedicled for local use or transferred as a free flap to cover defects up to a 15-cm diameter.

Sensation of the temporal scalp is mainly by the auriculotemporal nerve, which runs close to the superficial temporal artery. Harvesting the hair-bearing scalp has a limited coverage potential when unipedicled (~4-cm width × 13-cm length) but up to 36-cm length if pedicled on *both* superficial temporal arteries. A composite regional flap can include part of the temporal muscle and even an osteoperiosteal bone segment. The scalp flap is used most the time as a regional flap for post traumatic or burn alopecia and eyebrow, cheek, and lip reconstruction. But the temporoparietal fascia may be used as a free flap in many other head and neck scenarios, as well as in the upper and lower extremity.

Prefabricated Scalp Flap

Various modalities of prefabrication have enlarged the indications of this donor site.

Pretransfer Expansion

Extensive alopecia is a strong indication for the use of one or more tissue expanders for pretransfer expansion. For many years, the preexpanded forehead flap has been pedicled down to cover defects of the nose, leaving a minimal donor defect. A prefabricated expanded flap with a skin graft for lining can be transferred as a bipedicled "visor flap" for mustache and beard reconstruction (13). Furthermore, the temporoparietal fascia covered by a skin graft provides a thin, viable lining for oral or nasal cavity reconstruction (14), and a composite transfer with an island scalp flap (based on the anterior branch of the superficial temporal artery) can be used to reconstruct eyelids, eyelashes, and an exenterated orbital cavity (15).

Prefabricated Induced Expanded Scalp Flap

This flap has been used to resurface the mustache and beard areas in a patient with extensive head and neck burns for whom it was the only suitable solution (11). In the first stage, the occipital area was selected as the donor site, and a fascial forearm flap based on the radial pedicle was inserted subcutaneously with a skin expander positioned beneath it. The facial vessels were selected as recipients. To facilitate dissection of the pedicle at the time of transfer, the authors recommended wrapping the pedicle with a Gore-Tex sheet. After 8 weeks' expansion, the prefabricated flap was transferred on its pedicle to the right cheek and upper lip and a satisfactory result achieved with the expectation of normal hair growth.

Disadvantages

Apart from the classical complications related to the use of tissue expanders, the scalp has a tendency for hair loss whenever the donor site is closed under excessive tension. It can be corrected if needed by a secondary expansion of the surrounding scalp area. Finally, distortion of the eyebrow or ear, although unusual, may need some correction.

Submental Flap

The submental flap, which was described initially in 1993 (16), is supplied by the submental artery, a horizontal terminal branch of the facial artery. It runs under the platysma muscle as far as the midline of the neck and is accompanied by small venae comitantes.

Its main indications are reconstruction of the corner of mouth, the cheek, and the lips. Defects may be posttraumatic, the result of tumor resection, or a consequence of noma disease. Here the submental flap has contributed to vastly improved results.

Less frequently, it has been used to reconstruct the tip of the nose, and because the submental artery supplies the inferior border of the mandible, an osteocutaneous flap can be harvested for remodeling a composite ipsilateral maxillary defect as a pedicled flap. In more distant locations, it can be used as a free flap. The donor site can be closed easily with minimal scarring hidden under the chin (17).

Prefabricated Submental Flap

A skin expander with a full-thickness skin graft inserted under the platysma muscle enlarges the coverage potential and vascularization of a bipedicled submental flap and thins it out to match the thickness of the lips and cheek while allowing easy closure of the donor site (11).

For reconstruction of the columella, some authors have used a reverse-flow prefabricated submental flap with a cartilage implant (18).

Disadvantages

A careful dissection of this donor site prevents injury to the facial nerve, and the cosmetic sequelae are almost nonexistent.

Supraclavicular Flap

After key anatomical studies performed by a number of authors (19), further research and clinical application have led to the description of a "supraclavicular neurovascular free flap" (20).

A triangular skin territory measuring 20 × 12 cm is supplied by the cutaneous branch of the transverse cervical artery, which originates from the thyrocervical trunk or directly from the subclavian artery.

The venous drainage is dependent on numerous small veins that drain via the transverse cervical and supraclavicular veins into the external jugular vein and ultimately into the subclavian vein. But this anatomy is somewhat inconsistent.

The sensory nerves are derived from the lateral supraclavicular branches of the superficial cervical plexus. One branch is associated with the artery and can therefore be included in the flap to restore sensation.

If necessary, a tangential segment of the clavicle can be harvested with the flap for an osteocutaneous reconstruction.

Prefabricated Supraclavicular Flap

The supraclavicular area fulfills many of the requirements for a rather satisfactory donor site for head and neck reconstruction, but two parameters can be improved by prefabricating and inducing a preexpanded flap: (1) the bulkiness of the skin may be thinned by the expansion procedure, and (2) the length of the pedicle may be increased by inserting a temporoparietal fascia flap vascularized by superficial temporal vascular pedicle immediately beneath it. The blood supply of the flap is also thereby improved (21). Central facial reconstruction including the nose is well handled by this technique (22).

Disadvantages

Apart the visible scar at the donor site, which is quite acceptable, regional functional disability is unlikely.

Scapular and Parascapular Flaps

The subscapular branch of the axillary artery divides into the thoracodorsal and circumflex scapular arteries. The scapular flap (23,24) and the parascapular flap (25) are supplied by two main branches of the circumflex scapular artery: the transverse and the descending, respectively. The descending branch supplies the parascapular flap and the lateral border of the scapula, which can be harvested as an independent vascular unit. Because the subscapular artery gives origin to the thoracodorsal vessels, it is possible to harvest a "chimeric flap" including both scapular and parascapular flaps with the lateral border of the scapula, the latissimus dorsi muscle with the ninth rib, and the serratus anterior muscle with the sixth rib. This donor site clearly has the largest reconstructive potential of any in the body, and it is not surprising therefore that there are a few instances of prefabricated flaps designed in this area.

Prefabricated Scapular and Parascapular Flaps

A prefabricated composite pedicled scapular flap bearing endosteal implants has been used to fit a maxillary defect (26). After a careful preoperative planning based on three-dimensional modeling, endosteal implants are inserted into the bone, and the flap is covered by a split-thickness skin graft and by a Gore-Tex sheet. After 3 to 4 weeks, the transfer is achieved by anastomosis with the facial vessels. In a final stage, a dental prosthesis is fitted on the implants.

Preexpansion is indicated when a large skin surface has to be harvested with primary closure of the donor site. Furthermore, a preexpanded free tissue transfer is the ideal solution to restore a satisfactory contour to several facial aesthetic units. In some rare situations, when the subscapular pedicle has been previously ligated, a preexpanded neovascularized flap using an arteriovenous radial pedicle has been successfully resorted to.

Disadvantages

The donor site has no functional impairment, and the cosmetic result is acceptable unless numerous aesthetic units require reconstruction.

Latissimus Dorsi Myocutaneous Flap

Initially described as a pedicled flap for breast reconstruction (27,28), the era of microsurgical surgery opened the way for more extensive anatomical research and use of the latissimus dorsi flap for free tissue transfers (29,30). This flap is mainly supplied by the thoracodorsal artery, a branch of the subscapular artery. The secondary blood supply is by the perforating branches of the posterior intercostal arteries. Venae comitantes accompany the artery, and the thoracodorsal nerve innervates the muscle. It can be used for restoration of the muscle function. This flap is one of the most commonly used free flaps; its constant anatomy is responsible of its extreme reliability; and apart from the large surface it can provide, as mentioned earlier, it can be harvested on a single pedicle as a chimeric flap with mainly components.

Prefabricated Latissimus Dorsi Myocutaneous Flap

There are few indications for prefabrication in this donor site, except when a large skin surface is needed with primary closure of the donor site. However, a flap providing thin skin coverage is often a better choice (31,32).

Disadvantages

Functional impairment of the regional area is uncommon.

Lateral Arm Flap

Initially described in 1982 (33), a further anatomical study was published in 1987 dealing with the sensory nerve supply of this donor site (34).

The LAF is a septocutaneous flap supplied by a branch of the profunda brachii artery (PBA), the posterior radial collateral artery (PRCA). That branch enters the intermuscular septum between the triceps posteriorly and the brachialis and brachioradialis muscles anteriorly and supplies the flap by several septocutaneous perforators.

The venous drainage is provided by a superficial network, which drains into the cephalic vein and deep venae comitantes of the PRCA. Both are anastomosed whenever possible.

The LAF has a dual nerve supply: the first is the posterior cutaneous nerve of the forearm (PCNF), which runs in the septum alongside the artery. It innervates the proximal part of the forearm and provides sensation to the extended lateral arm flap (ELAF), a variation of the flap that is harvested more distally than the basic LAF increasing its coverage potential. The PCNF can also be used as a vascularized nerve to bridge a defect at the recipient site. The second nerve is the posterior cutaneous nerve of the arm (PCNA), which actually supplies the skin of the LAF enabling its use as a neurosensate flap.

The LAF is a reliable fasciocutaneous flap that may be pedicled or used as a free tissue transfer. The skin is rather thin, and the local anatomy of the region permits the harvest of a composite flap with bone (a segment of distal humerus), tendons (lateral head of the triceps, brachialis, and brachioradialis muscles), and nerves (PCNF, PCNA; see earlier).

The main indications are reconstructive procedures in the head and neck, the upper extremity, and less frequently the lower extremity and trunk.

In the head and neck, almost any external local defect in need of a three-dimensional reconstruction (the LAF is thicker than the ELAF) can be dealt with using this flap or a variant thereof, but the best indications are for intraoral defects and partial upper esophageal or pharyngeal defects. In the upper extremity, including composite defects of the hand and fingers (skin, bone, tendon, and nerves), the LAF is highly effective. Apart from contour and scarring sequelae at the donor site, flap harvesting leaves a sensory deficit proximally in the posterior forearm.

Prefabricated Lateral Arm Flap

Most techniques of prefabrication can be applied to this donor site (35).

Disadvantages

Hypoesthesia or dysesthesia in the proximal portion of the posterior forearm can be encountered without significant disability.

Radial Forearm Flap

Described in 1981 (36) and 1982 (37), the forearm flap is supplied by both the radial and ulnar arteries, the terminal branches of the brachial artery. Apart from supplying the whole anterior compartment of the forearm, they give off the anterior and posterior interosseous arteries, which vascularize the posterior aspect of the forearm. The radial forearm flap (RFF) is harvested on the radial system and the ulnar forearm flap (UFF) on the ulnar.

The venous drainage of the RFF is provided by the two venae comitantes of the radial artery, which join the median cubital vein and by a superficial network constituted by the cephalic and basilic veins.

The sensory nerve supply is twofold: the median cutaneous nerve of the forearm (MCNF) with an anterior branch adjacent to the basilic vein, the lateral cutaneous nerve of the forearm (LCNF) parallel to the cephalic vein.

The RFF is a septocutaneous flap with the arterial pedicle located in the septum between the brachioradialis and the flexor carpi radialis, providing perforating branches for the overlying fascia and skin. Deep branches supply tendons, muscles, nerves, bone.

It follows that a composite prefabricated flap can include nerves, tendons (palmaris longus, brachioradialis, and flexor carpi radialis), or the radius (an osteoperiosteal tangential segment) (38–40).

Prefabricated Forearm Flap

The flap is usually outlined over the distal third of the forearm, but its design, length, and width depend on the requirements of the surface to be reconstructed, the components to be included within it, and the length of pedicle required for adequate vessel access (the venous pedicle may be lengthened by dissecting the cephalic or basilic vein proximally).

The design and elevation of the fasciocutaneous and osteofasciocutaneous RFF is described elsewhere in this text and will not be repeated here.

The forearm is the best choice for many prefabrications.

Anterolateral Thigh Flap

This flap was first described in 1984 (48). It is based on septocutaneous or musculocutaneous perforators of the descending branch of the lateral circumflex femoral artery. Venous drainage is provided by venae comitantes accompanying the arterial network. It can be a composite flap incorporating different muscles of the thigh, fascia, and skin. If necessary, a reinnervated part of the vastus lateralis can be included in the flap to restore motor function.

The lateral femoral cutaneous nerve, which innervates its cutaneous territory, may be taken with the flap and anastomosed to a recipient sensory nerve to restore sensory innervation.

Since the original description, this flap has acquired a large spectrum of indications as a pedicled but mainly as a free flap in the head and neck, trunk, and upper and lower extremity. The donor site has to be skin grafted if a wide flap is harvested, but techniques of prefabrication can facilitate primary closure.

Prefabricated Anterolateral and Medial Thigh Flap

Any technique of prefabrication can be applied to this donor site. If a wide surface has to be harvested, flap delay in several steps can improve its blood supply and prevent partial skin necrosis.

Preexpansion Transfer

To adapt the thickness of the skin to the requirements of the recipient site for resurfacing a burn scar contracture or to facilitate primary closure of the donor site, preliminary tissue expansion is the ideal solution for this flap (49).

Vascularized Induced Flap

The anterolateral thigh can be the donor site of the descending lateral circumflex pedicle to be dissected out and transferred under the medial thigh area for neovascularization. The first such successful case was reported for the treatment of an extensive scar contracture of the neck (11). Transfer was achieved 6 weeks after implantation of the pedicle (the descending lateral circumflex artery and the great saphenous vein), which was ultimately anastomosed to the facial vessels. Complete success was achieved. This technique is one solution to common anatomic anomalies (e.g., the lack of perforators) encountered during the dissection of a anterolateral thigh flap.

Preexpanded Induced Median Thigh Flap (11)

Several authors have reported the successful use of this technique for the same indications as for other preexpanded and induced flaps. An excellent aesthetic result was obtained after two thinning procedures.

Disadvantages

The considerable length of the donor site scar does not constitute a significant cosmetic detriment.

Fibula Flap

The fibula is the most commonly used osseous free tissue transfer for extensive defects because of its considerable length, constant blood supply, and capacity to be harvested as a composite transfer with a skin paddle (based on septocutaneous perforators), muscles (lateral half of the soleus, the whole soleus or the flexor hallucis longus), or as an osteomusculocutaneous flap.

Initially described in 1975 (50) and later in 1983 (51) and followed by extensive clinical appraisal it was in 1982 and 2000 that the same authors reported the successful transfer of the so called "composite fibula and soleus" flap for compound extensive defects of the lower extremity (52,53).

The arterial blood supply is derived from the peroneal artery. The popliteal artery bifurcates into the anterior tibial artery and the common peroneotibial trunk, the latter dividing into the posterior tibial artery and the peroneal artery. The peroneal artery gives off a nutrient medullary branch—which enters the fibula in its middle third—periosteal and muscular branches and about six cutaneous perforators.

The venous drainage of the flap is via the venae comitantes of the peroneal artery.

The flap's sensory innervation is provided for the lateral side of the leg by the lateral sural cutaneous nerve, and the motor branches to the soleus can be theoretically anastomosed to a recipient nerve to restore function.

The fibula donor site thus offers a reliable potential to supply various anatomical modalities for reconstruction in the tibia, femur, radius, mandible, and trunk.

There are therefore few indications for prefabrication because highly sophisticated reconstruction can usually be achieved in one stage without it.

Disadvantages

Mild transitory ambulatory difficulty or visible scarring at the donor site when it has been skin grafted are minor issues compared with the exceptional reconstructive potential of this donor site.

Prefabricated Fibula Flap

A great number of maxillary and mandible reconstructions have been reported (54) using a prefabricated fibula by the insertion of dental implants positioned with a drilling template in a preplanned position and covered by a split-thickness skin graft. Six weeks later, the flap is transferred and a bar construction with overdentures attached to the implants. Apart from some failures related to flap necrosis or implant loss, a 95% success rate was observed, and the authors described this procedure as a "powerful tool." The forearm is the best donor site for a prefabricated phalloplasty, but some authors have reported prefabrication on the lateral aspect of the leg to minimize the cosmetic sequelae.

Because the "tube within a tube" principle for the prefabrication of a neourethra would be responsible for an excessively wide transverse skin defect on the leg, some surgeons have suggested the initial creation of a neourethra by wrapping a full-thickness skin graft around a N° 30 catheter inserted subcutaneously along the longitudinal lateral aspect of the leg (55). In a second stage, a bifoliate *longitudinal* skin flap is raised to include the neourethra and a segment of fibula harvested proximally to obtain some rigidity. Phalloplasty is completed by suturing together the distal and proximal leaves of the skin flap. Similar prefabricated phallus procedures have been reported by other authors (56).

To restore some sensibility, the lateral sural cutaneous nerve (LSCN) is anastomosed to the two dorsal or clitoral recipient nerves.

The authors report restoration of a satisfactory sensibility and penile rigidity using this technique.

DISADVANTAGES

Some impairment of the motion of the ankle and some discomfort in the distal segment of the leg have been reported.

UTILIZATION OF PREFABRICATED FLAPS

Nasal Reconstruction

The flap is usually outlined over the distal third of the forearm, but its length and width depend on the requirements of the surface to be reconstructed and the potential extension of the defect to the surrounding areas (eyelids, cheek, and lips). In the skin markings, the tip of the nose (nostrils and columella) is designed as a trefoil flap, the lateral lobes longer than the middle, so each can be rolled in to form a nostril and maintained in that position by an intranasal bolus.

In terms of prefabrication, a full-thickness skin graft is inserted under the flap at the subcutaneous level to provide lining to the reconstructed nasal cavity. To rebuild a total framework, the bony component is harvested at the time of the transfer and split in two parts (nasal dorsum and anterior septum) while carefully maintaining the periosteal lining to preserve a satisfactory blood supply (2,41). Alternatives include a carved costal cartilage graft inserted under the forearm fascia or the use of an alloplastic support, taking into account the known problems of infection and extrusion related to this last material. To provide a better contour to the nostrils, carved cartilage grafts from the ear concha can be added to the rims.

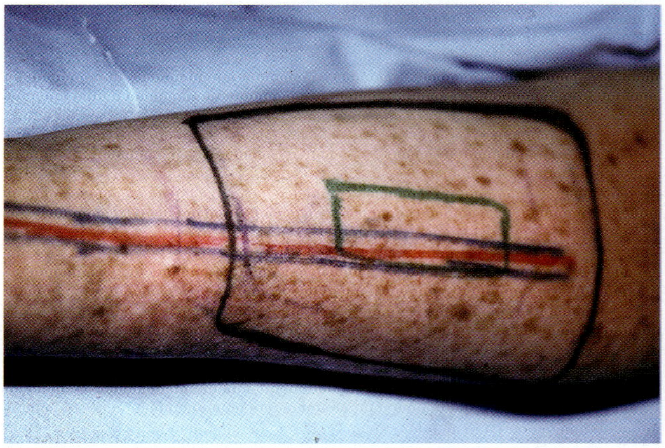

FIGURE 11-2 Design on the left forearm of the skin territory anticipated for nasal reconstruction. At the center of the flap, a rectangle is outlined corresponding to the vascularized segment of the radius to be included to provide reconstruction of the nasal framework.

The donor site is covered primarily by a split-thickness skin graft, and the prefabricated flap is transferred 1 month later, the facial vessels acting as the recipient pedicle (Figures 11-1 to 11-7).

There are two main advantages, (1) avoid visible scarring at the most usual donor site for nasal reconstruction: the forehead,

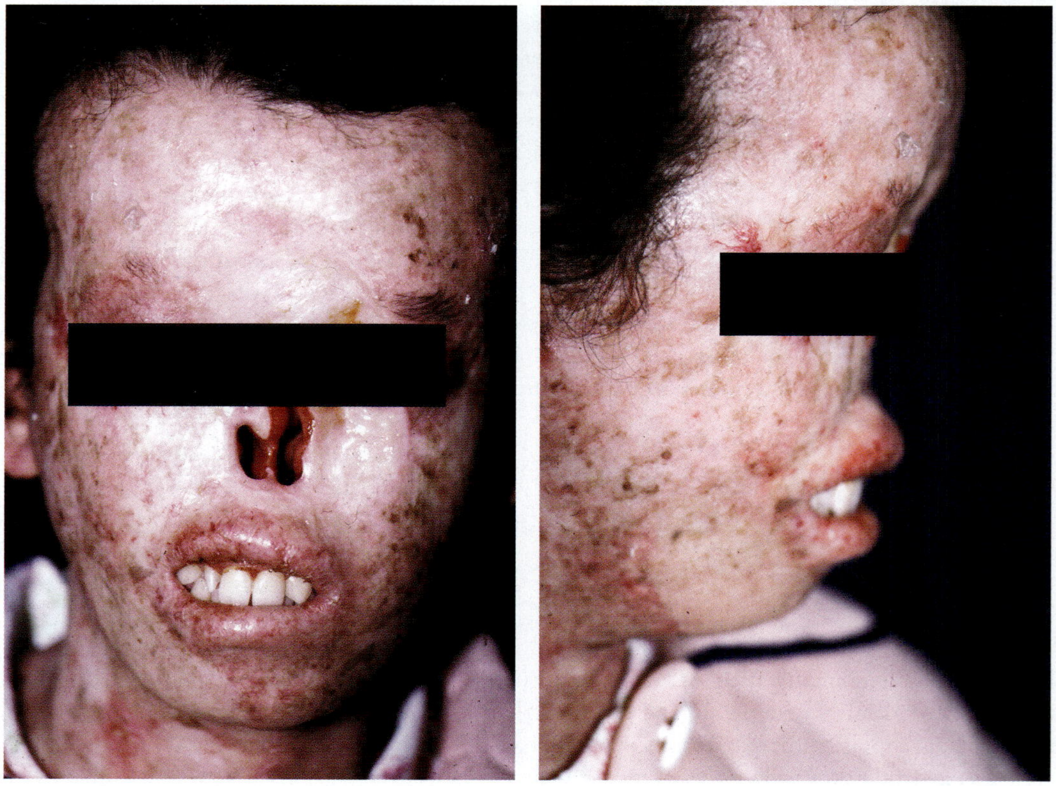

A B

FIGURE 11-1 (**A**) and (**B**) Xeroderma pigmentosum in a young woman with a history of numerous destructive basal cell carcinomas and superficial malignant melanomas. Her nose, upper and lower eyelids, and both eyebrows require reconstruction.

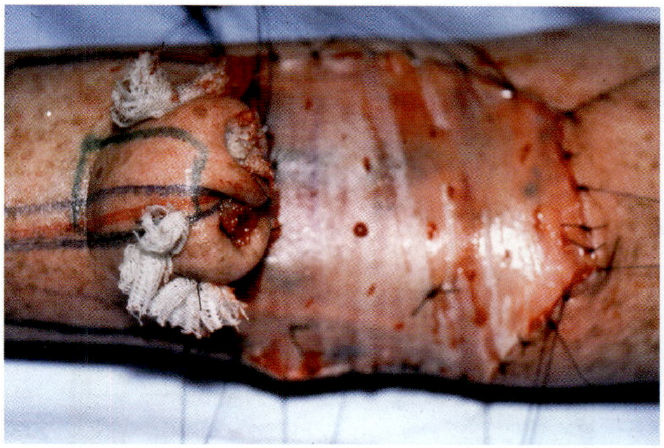

FIGURE 11-3 View of the prefabricated nose and skin grafting of the donor site.

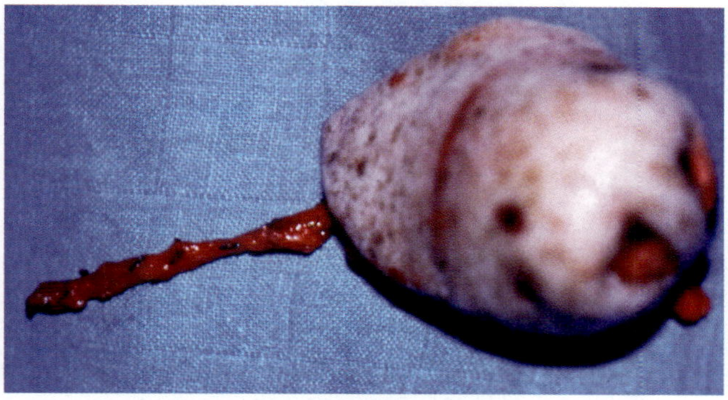

FIGURE 11-5 The prefabricated nose is ready to be revascularized. The facial artery and vein are selected as recipient vessels.

and (2) transfer a composite reconstruction only after satisfactory results have been obtained at the donor site.

Ear Reconstruction

Whenever a patient has damaged or abnormal skin around the injured ear (after burns, traumatic scalp avulsion, tumor resection, or failure of a previous attempt at classical reconstruction using a temporoparietal fascia flap), a prefabricated forearm flap is indicated (42).

A carved autogenous costal cartilage is inserted under the donor site, with forearm fascia being a better choice than forearm skin because the latter is not thin enough to reveal the surface contours of the carved graft. A skin graft is then used to resurface the anterior or posterior aspects of the fascia. Another possibility for obtaining a thin covering skin layer is to perform an initial expansion of the donor site. A silicone framework is always an alternative to an autogenous cartilage graft, but the risks of infection and extrusion are higher.

There is no real advantage of a prefabricated flap for routine microtia reconstruction because the traditional reconstructive procedures do not leave any significant adverse sequela in the scalp area.

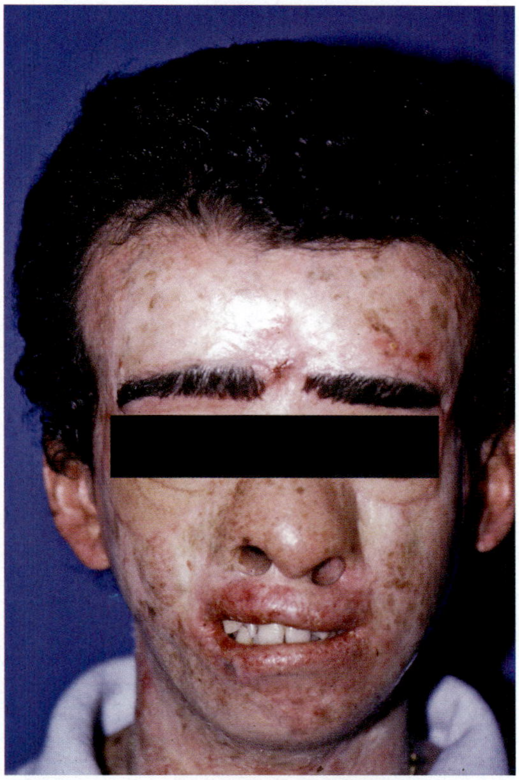

FIGURE 11-6 Final result with satisfactory shape and nose projection. The eyebrows and upper and lower eyelids have been reconstructed by a unipedicled galea and scalp flap and skin graft.

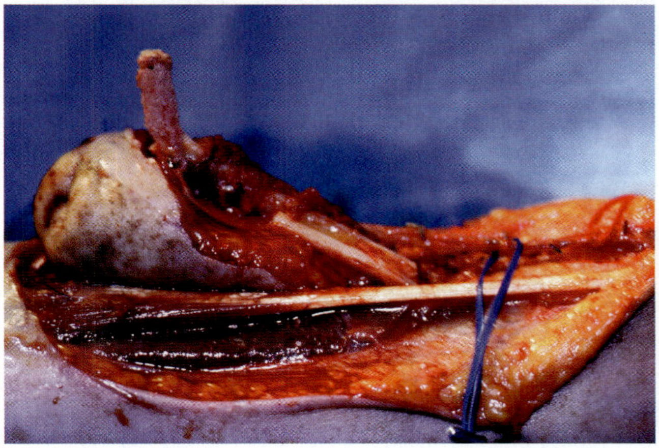

FIGURE 11-4 One month later, the prefabricated nose is harvested with part of the radius divided in a horizontal segment for the dorsum of the nose and a vertical one for the columella.

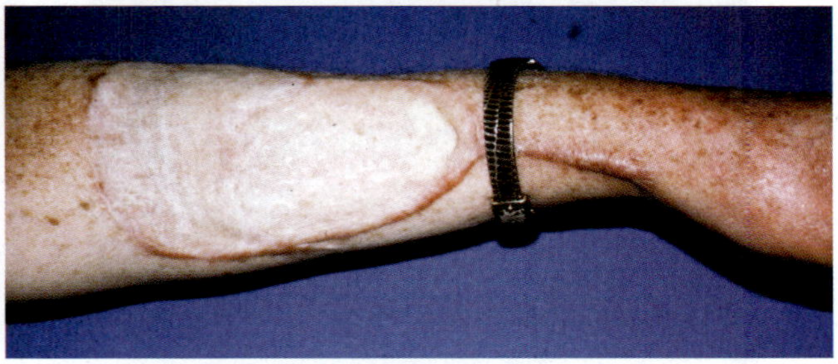

FIGURE 11-7 View of the donor site.

Prefabricated ear reconstruction is therefore only considered when conventional techniques are impossible or have failed.

Eyebrow, Eyelids, Cheek, and Lips Reconstruction

Attempts to reconstruct several facial anatomical units using a single-stage free tissue transfer followed by numerous revisions is often associated with unforeseen complications and an imperfect outcome.

Prefabrication along the lines described earlier presents a viable alternative (41). Any branch of the external carotid can be selected as the recipient artery and the external jugular system sourced for the vein.

Thanks to the generous diameter of the radial artery and the forearm veins, additional free tissue components such as a scalp flap for eyebrow reconstruction can be transferred with satisfactory results (Figures 11-8 to 11-13).

The prefabricated forearm flap has been used for through-and-through defects localized to the cheek using different approaches: a prefabricated forearm with a skin expander under a subfascial skin graft or a subfascial mucosal graft above silicone sheeting.

Mandible Reconstruction

There are several donor sites for reconstruction of the mandible as conventional bone graft or free tissue transfer. The radius can be used for midsize defects and transferred in one stage as single revascularized unit or as composite osteocutaneous flap (39).

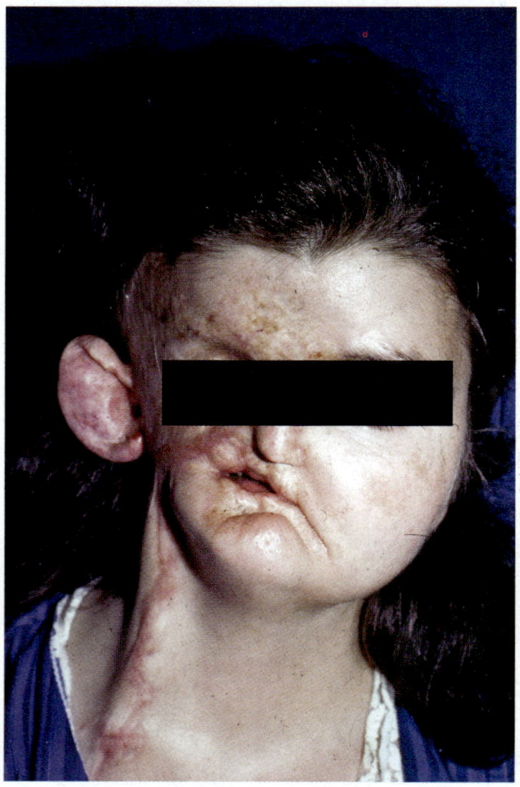

FIGURE 11-8 Patient with sequelae of radiotherapy in childhood for an immature hemangioma.

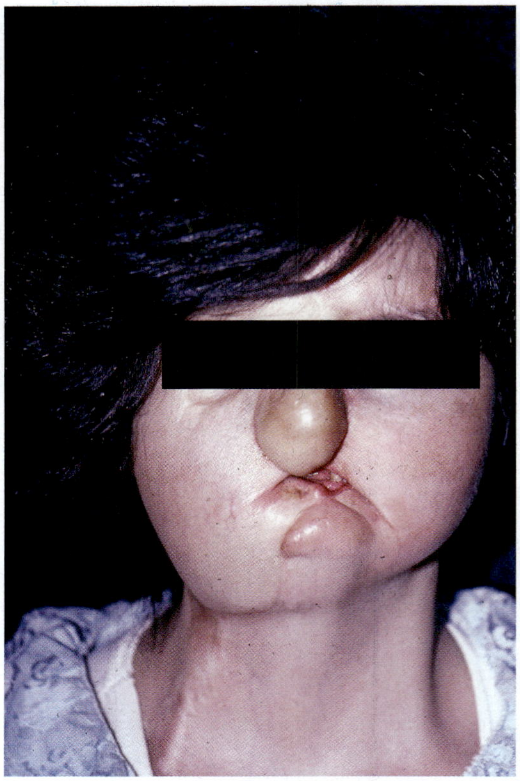

FIGURE 11-9 Appearance after two microsurgical operations: A groin flap to the cheek and a composite flap consisting of the dorsum of the foot and second metatarsal for nasal reconstruction.

Prefabrication is indicated whenever a through-and-through defect has to be reconstructed and dental implants can be inserted with satisfactory results (43).

Neck Reconstruction

Severe neck contractures after burn injury are very common, and after their release, a medium-thickness skin graft is the simplest reconstructive procedure. However, in addition to contracting less, a flap provides a better color match and elasticity.

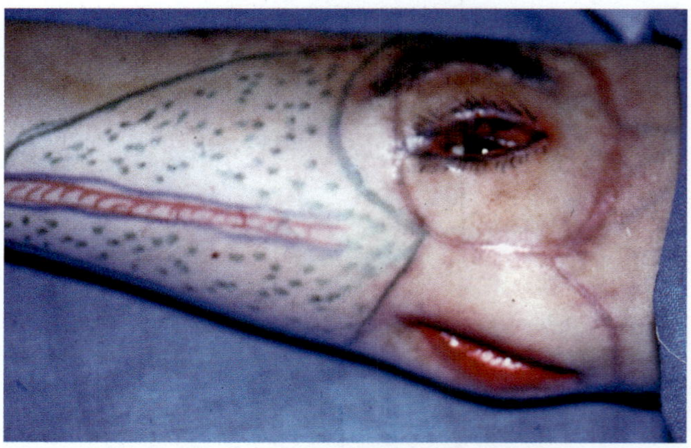

FIGURE 11-10 View of the prefabricated multiple anatomical units on the forearm. The inner lining of the orbital cavity and both lips have been achieved by a full-thickness skin graft. The eyebrow has been reconstructed by a free scalp flap revascularized by an end-to-side anastomosis with the radial pedicle.

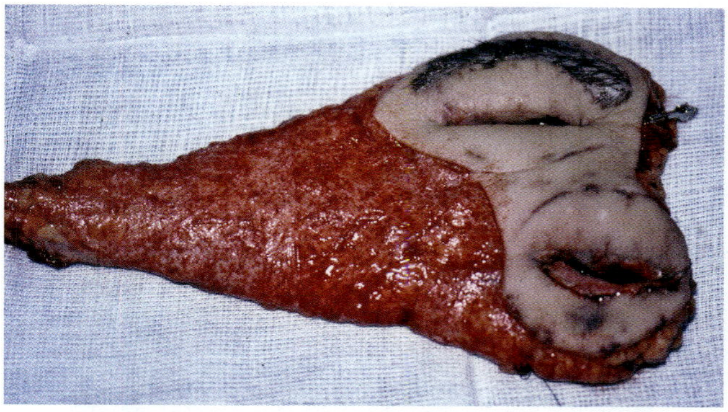

FIGURE 11-11 The radial pedicle has been divided, and the flap will be transferred with inset under the groin flap after deepithelialization of its proximal part.

A preexpanded forearm flap can provide the adequate amount of tissue for midsize defects whenever there is no healthy local tissue available. But for large defects, the thigh and upper chest are preferred as donor sites for prefabricated induced expanded flaps (11).

Trachea and Larynx Reconstruction

Tracheal reconstruction is a real challenge because it is mandatory to restore an adequate hollow stability for satisfactory airway patency. A prefabricated bilaminar radial forearm free flap has been transferred to successfully close a tracheoesophageal fistula (44). For a total tracheal reconstruction, a prefabricated radial free flap including a trimmed costal cartilage has provided both internal and external resurfacing (45). Many other

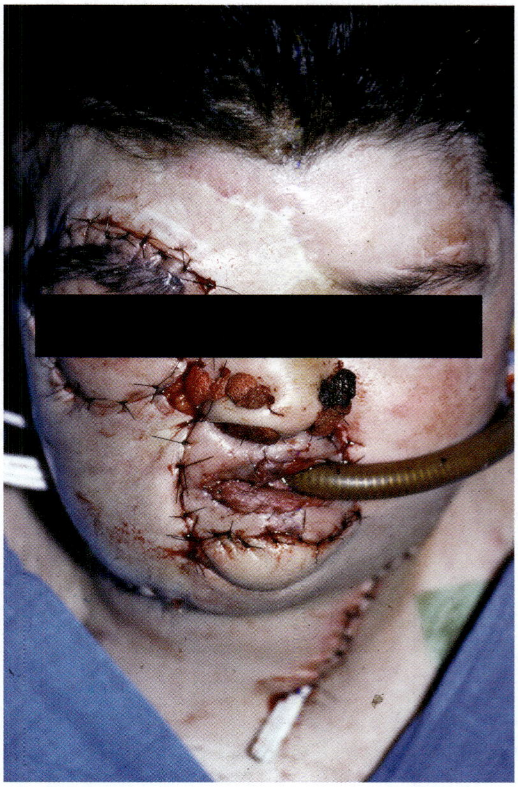

FIGURE 11-12 Immediate postoperative appearance.

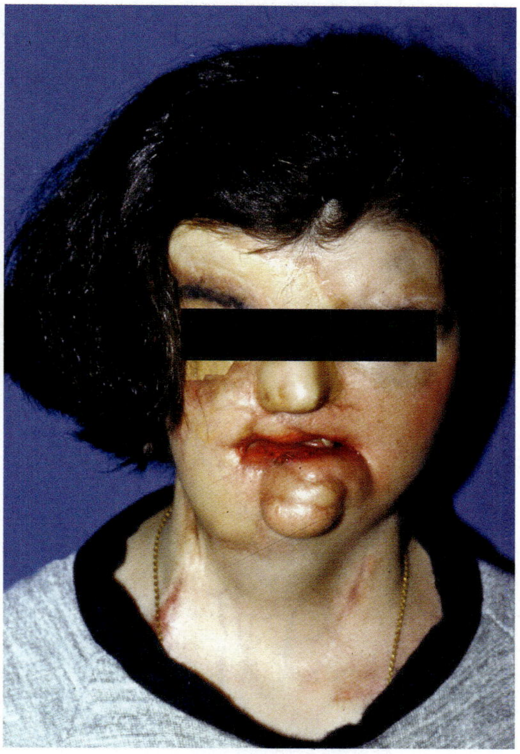

FIGURE 11-13 Final result of this complex reconstruction after two free transfers of a prefabricated flap used to reconstruct multiple facial units.

donor sites have undergone prefabrication to attain a similar goal, but the appropriate choice depends on a careful evaluation of local anatomical requirements. A significant advance would be to incorporate a reliable synthetic prosthesis, but they are currently unpredictable in terms of integration.

Esophageal Reconstruction

For pharyngeal or cervical esophageal fistulae or strictures after resection of malignant tumors, the ideal solution is a free microvascular transfer of a segment of the gastrointestinal tract (46). But when this is contraindicated or a previous attempt has failed, a prefabricated skin tube may be considered. The forearm is selected for midsized defects. The tubed skin flap is sutured in two layers and transferred 2 weeks later after the absence of leakage is established. The recipient artery can be the transverse cervical or the facial artery, and the external jugular vein serves well as the recipient vein. For more extensive defects, a prefabricated tensor fascia lata musculocutaneous flap has been suggested, supplied by the transverse branch of the lateral circumflex femoral artery. These prefabricated flaps can be inserted subcutaneously or under the sternum depending on recipient requirements.

Phalloplasty

There are many indications for phalloplasty, including congenital malformations, posttraumatic amputation, self-mutilation, surgical resection for tumor, and female-to-male transsexualism. The first single-stage phallus reconstruction was achieved in 1984 using a free forearm flap (40). Phalloplasty is certainly one

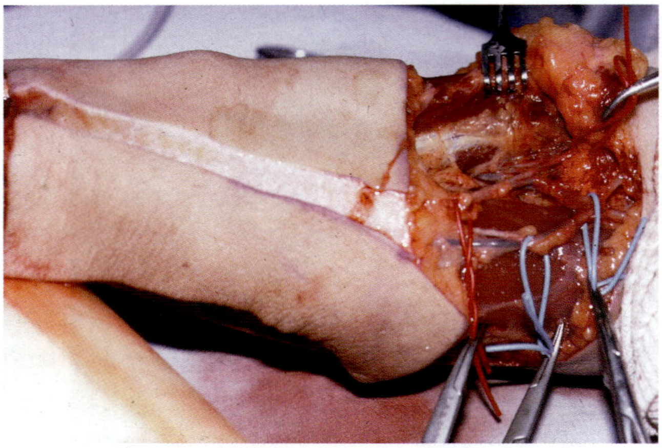

FIGURE 11-14 Operative view at the time of prefabrication.

of the most challenging surgeries because it is here that the reconstruction is expected to resemble as closely as possible the normal anatomy. After the risk of early postoperative microsurgical complications such as partial or total necrosis has passed, mid- and long-term follow-up is required to rule out of the latent development of urethral fistula or stricture, which might necessitate surgical revision. For patients who demand a sexually functional phalloplasty or when the surgeon has suggested that this may be achieved, insertion of a costal cartilage or alloplastic penile prosthesis at the time of the one-stage transfer increases the rate of these complications. To prevent these problems or at least diminish their incidence, we recommend a prefabricated phalloplasty on the forearm (Figures 11-14 to 11-16).

The neophallus is outlined on the forearm approximately 17 cm in length and 18 cm in width. On the central axis of the flap in the midline, a 3-cm-wide strip is outlined for the neourethra. On either side of this, a 1-cm-wide longitudinal strip is deepithelialized. Using absorbable sutures, the edges of this central skin band are sutured together over a Foley catheter to form a tube that will form the neourethra. The glans penis is modeled according the surgeon's own technique and preference. The donor site is skin grafted. This prefabricated phalloplasty is transferred about 1 month later after satisfactory healing of all structures has been affirmed. Sensory function can be obtained by anastomosing the cutaneous nerves (the lateral and medial antebrachial cutaneous nerves) to the dorsal or clitoral nerves (41). Some authors have harvested part of the

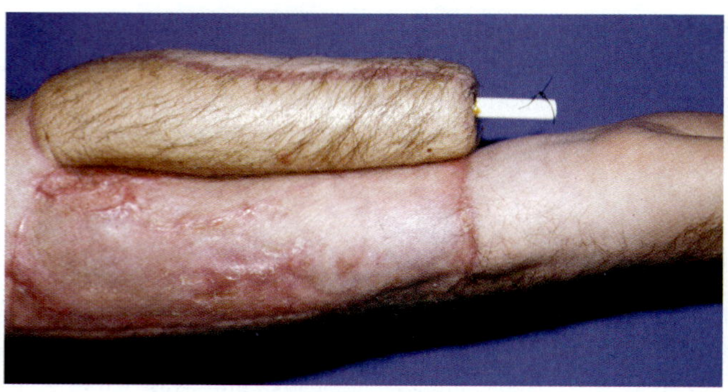

FIGURE 11-15 Prefabricated phallus before its transfer 1 month later.

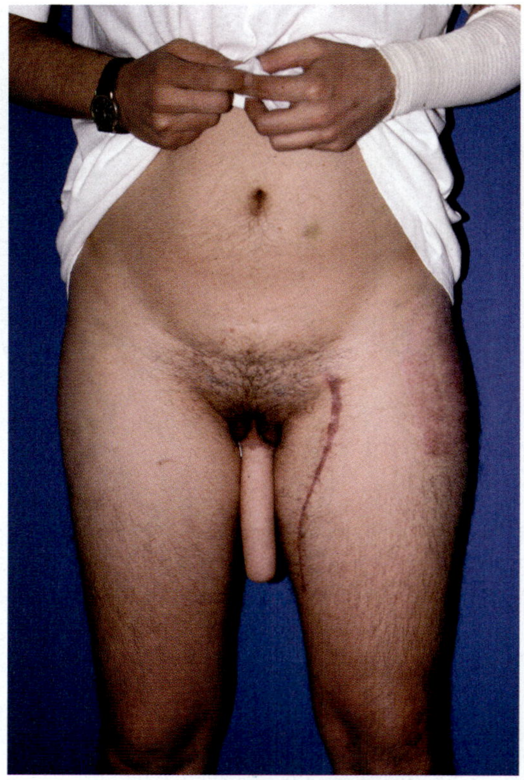

FIGURE 11-16 Satisfactory cosmetic result and voiding.

radius in the prefabricated penis to provide some structural support (47).

Disadvantages

There is a massive cosmetic defect as the result of skin grafting to most of the anterior forearm. However, this can be mitigated by a delayed skin expansion on the dorsal aspect of the forearm to cover the anterior excised surface. Localized dysesthesia or anesthesia in the cutaneous territory of the radial nerve is commonly encountered usually without significant discomfort.

THE FUTURE OF THE PRINCIPLE OF PREFABRICATED FLAPS

The potential of prefabricated flaps will be expanded as the result of basic science and clinical research as well as by the wider use of the successful clinical applications already reported.

Prefabricated Flaps with Bioengineering

Prefabricated Tissue Engineered INTEGRA Free Flap

In 2007, a case of a prefabricated flap using INTEGRA as the outer layer was reported (57). An unsuccessful attempt to raise an anterolateral thigh flap led the authors to save the descending branch of the lateral circumflex vessels with a distal segment of muscle and to place them over the vastus lateralis muscle. An INTEGRA sheet was then used to cover the pedicle. Two weeks later, a split-thickness skin graft was applied over the INTEGRA, and finally this prefabricated flap was successfully transferred.

Prefabricated Engineered Bone Flaps

Bone formation using biotechnological methods has led many authors to seek to create a substitute to autologous bone grafts. In an athymic mouse, human bone marrow stromal cells have been injected into the latissimus dorsi muscle, which contained a porous hydroxyapatite ceramic scaffold (58). Eight weeks later, well-shaped bony formation was obtained. This research opens the way for the clinical application of tissue engineering to avoid donor site morbidity and to accurately configure the shape and size of the desired bone graft. Similar research into bone formation within an interconnected porous hydroxyapatite implant has been performed. The implant was inserted in the groin area of a rat, the superficial inferior epigastric vessels being included in the mold, and 10 mg of bone morphogenic protein was added to it. At 3 weeks, satisfactory bone formation was obtained.

Angiogenesis Factors

Vascular Endothelial Growth Factors

Vascular endothelial growth factor (VEGF) has the potential of angiogenesis. Its effect on flap viability was demonstrated experimentally in a rat model. An autologous tail artery loop was implanted under the lower abdomen after anastomosis to the femoral artery and vein. Under this prefabricated flap, VEGF in topical polyvinyl alcohol was injected. Compared with a control group, greater maturation in the vascular development was demonstrated in the VEGF-treated flaps (59).

Basic Fibroblast Growth Factor

The effect of basic fibroblast growth factor on induced flaps was investigated in pigs by inserting a Gelfoam sponge carrier of the growth factor at the musculosubcutaneous tissue interface of a latissimus dorsi musculocutaneous flap (60).

The skin survival rate was higher in the growth factor treated animals than in the control group in relation to the induced angiogenesis.

Adipose Derived Stem Cells

Adipose-derived stem cells (ASCs) have been injected under a prefabricated abdominal flap in rats (constructed by the implantation of a femoral loop) (61). Capillary genesis and flap survival proved to be more reliable in the stem cell group than in other control groups.

ASCs contain the same angiogenesis cytokine as VEGF. ASCs, which are more readily available, therefore have a great potential for clinical use in multiple fields. They have opened up a new and promising era of research and potential therapy.

Apart from these bioengineered tissue products, human cell cultures (e.g., chondrocytes, bone, muscle cells, peripheral nerves, medullary stem cells) are obviously a very promising avenue of research with respect to prefabricated flaps.

CONCLUSION

Prefabricated and prelaminated flaps can be credited with a significant advance in the reconstruction of extensive and composite defects, mainly in the head and neck area. But, more recently, composite tissue allotransplantation, especially for the face and upper limb, have opened a new and promising era. In some patients with posttraumatic injuries of the face such as a dog bite or a congenital malformation such as a neurofibromatosis, excellent results have been obtained after facial allotransplantation. Other patients with total single or double hand amputations have regained highly useful function and an excellent cosmetic appearance.

But the lifetime administration of immunosuppressive drugs to lessen the risk of rejection and their side effects should be taken into account when considering allotransplantation. The informed consent of the patient together with the agreement of the internal review board and the medical ethics committee is mandatory before undertaking such surgery, even if it seems fully justified and is urged by the patient.

It is not inappropriate to contemplate a rosy future for the various modalities of tissue reconstruction, some of which remain experimental, but others have already been successfully used in clinical applications. But in our field of reconstructive microsurgery, until we can achieve simpler and safer solutions to solve extensive and compound defects by auto or allotransplantations, tissue manufacture by prefabrication seems, at the moment, to be a reasonable solution.

REFERENCES

1. Shen TY. Vascular implantation into skin flap. Experimental study and clinical applications. A preliminary report. *Plast Reconstr Surg* 1981;68:404.
2. Baudet J, Pelissier P, Martin D, et al. Prefabricated free flap transfer. Presented at the 3rd Annual meeting of the American Society for Reconstructive Microsurgery September 12 to 13, San Antonio, 1987. InSwartz WM, Banis JC Jr (eds). *Head and Neck Microsurgery* Baltimore: Williams Wilkins 1992.
3. Pribaz JJ, Fine NA. Prelamination defining the prefabricated flap: a new case report and review. *Microsurgery* 1994;15:618.
4. Taylor GI, Corlett RG, Caddy CM, et al. An anatomic review of the delay phenomenon II: Clinical applications. *Plast Reconstr Surg* 1992;89:408.
5. Maitz PKM, Pribaz JJ. Hergrueter CA. Impact of tissue expansion on flap prefabrication: an experimental study in rabbits. *Microsurgery* 1996;1:35.
6. Orticochea M. A new method for total reconstruction of the nose. The ears as donor area. *Br J Plast Surg* 1991;24:225.
7. Shen TY. Microvascular transplantation of prefabricated thigh flap (letter). *Plast Reconstr Surg* 1982;69:568.
8. Hirase Y, Valauri FA, Buncke HJ. Customized prefabricated neovascularized free flaps. *Microsurgery* 1987;8:218.
9. Khoury RK, Ozbek MR, Hruza GJ, et al. Facial reconstruction with prefabricated induced expanded (PIE) supraclavicular flap. *Plast Reconstr Surg* 1995;95:1007.
10 Pribaz JJ, Fine N, Orgill DP. Flap prefabrication in the head and neck surgery. A ten years experience. *Plast Reconstr Surg* 1999;103:808–820.
11. Guo L, Pribaz JJ. Prefabrication and prelamination. InWei FC, Mardini S (eds). *Plastic and Reconstructive Surgery.* St. Louis: Saunders Elsevier, 2009, p. 103.
12. Moran SL. Temporoparietal fascia flap, in Plastic and reconstructive surgery. InWei FC, Mardini S (eds). *Plastic and Reconstructive Surgery.* St. Louis: Saunders Elsevier, 2009, p. 159.
13. Tsoutos D, Gravvanis A, Ioannovich J. Prefabricated hair bearing temporal flap for two different facial aesthetic subunits reconstruction. Case report. *Eur J Plast Surg* 2005;27:394.
14. Upton S, Ferraro N, Healy G, Khoury RK. The use of prefabricated fascia flap for lining of the oral and nasal cavity. *Plast Reconstr Surg* 1994; 94:573.
15. Altindas M, Yucel A, Ozturk G, et al. The prefabricated temporal island flap for eyelid and eye socket reconstruction in total orbital exenteration patients: a new method. *Ann Plast Surg* 2010;65:177.
16. Martin D, Pascal JF, Baudet J, et al. The submental island flap: a new donor site. Anatomy and clinical applications as a free or pedicled flap. *Plast Reconstr Surg* 1993;92:867.
17. Pistre V, Pelissier P, Martin D, et al. Ten years of experience with the submental flap. *Plast Reconstr Surg* 2001;108:1576.

18. Tan O, Kiroglu FA, Bekir A. Reconstruction of the columella using the prefabricated reverse flow submental flap. *Head Neck* 2006;28:653.
19. Lamberty BGH. The subclavian axial patterned flap. *Br J Plast Surg* 1979;32:207.
20. Baudet J, Martin D, Ferreira R, et al. The supraclavicular neurovascular free flap. Anatomy and clinical applications. In Brunelli G (ed). *Textbook of Microsurgery.* G . Milan: Masson, 1988, p. 169.
21. Khouri RK, Ozbek MR, Hruza GJ, et al. Facial reconstruction with prefabricated induced expanded (PIE) Supraclavicular skin flaps. *Plast Reconstr Surg* 1995;95:1007.
22. Guo L, Pribaz JJ. Pre-expanded ultra thin supraclavicular flap for (full face) reconstruction with reduced donor site morbidity and without the need for microsurgery. *Plast Reconstr Surg* 2005;11:1845.
23. Dos Santos LF. [The scapular flap: a new microsurgical free flap]. *Rev Bras Cir* 1980;70:133.
24. Gilbert A, Teot L. The free scapular flap. *Plast Reconstr Surg* 1982; 69:601.
25. Nassif TM, Vidal L, Bovet JL, et al. The parascapular flap: a new cutaneous microsurgical free flap. *Plast Reconstr Surg* 1982;69:591.
26. Vinzenz KG, Holle J, Wuringer E, et al. Revascularized composite grafts with inserted implants for reconstructing the maxilla-improved flap design and flap prefabrication. *Br J Oral Maxillofac Surg* 1998;36:346.
27. Tansini I. Nuovo processo per l'amputation della mammaella per cancre. *Reform Med* 1986;12:3.
28. Olivari N. The latissimus flap. *Br J Plast Surg* 1976;29:126.
29. Baudet J, Guimberteau JC, Nascimento E. Successful clinical transfer of two free thoracodorsal axillary flaps. *Plast Reconstr Surg* 1976;58:680.
30. Maxwell GP, Manson PM, Hoopes JE. Experience with thirteen latissimus dorsi myocutaneous flaps. *Plast Reconstr Surg* 1979;64:1.
31. Vergote T, Revol M, Servant JM, et al. Lambeaux musculocutanés de grand dorsal expansés microanastomosés. *Ann Chir Plast Esthet* 1993; 38:323.
32. Hirase Y, Valauri FA, Buncke HJ. Prefabricated sensate myocutaneous and osteomyocutaneous free flap. An experimental model. Preliminary report. *Plast Reconstr Surg* 1988;82:440.
33. Song R, Song Y, Yu Y, Song Y. The upperarm free flap. *Clin Plast Surg* 1982;9:27.
34. Rivet D, Buffet M, Martin D, et al. The lateral arm flap: an anatomic study. *J Reconstr Microsurg* 1987;3:121.
35. Shenaq JM. Pretransfer expansion of a sensate lateral arm free flap. *Ann Plast Surg* 1987;19:558.
36. Yang G, Chen B, Gao Y, et al. Forearm free skin flap transplantation. *Natl Med J China* 1981;61:139.
37. Song R, Gao Y, Song Y, et al. The forearm flap. *Clin Plast Surg* 1982; 9:21.
38. Biemer E, Stock W. Total thumb reconstruction. A one stage reconstruction using an osteocutaneous forearm flap. *Br J Plast Surg* 1983;36:52.
39. Soutar DS, Schecker LR, Tanner NSB, et al. The radial forearm flap: a versatile method for intraoral reconstruction. *Br J Plast Surg* 1983;36:1.
40. Chang TS, Hwang WY. Forearm flap in one stage reconstruction of the penis. *Plast Reconstr Surg* 1984;74:251.
41. Baudet J, Martin D. Principles of prefabricated flaps. In Strauch B, Vasconez LO, Hall-Findlay E (eds). *Grabb's Encyclopedia of Flaps,* 2nd ed. Philadelphia: Lippincott-Raven, 1998.
42. Akin S. Burn ear reconstruction using a prefabricated free radial forearm flap. *J Reconstr Microsurg* 2001;17:233.
43. Orringer JS, Shaw WW, Borud LJ, et al. Total mandibular and lip reconstruction with a prefabricated osteocutaneous free lower flap. *Plast Reconstr Surg* 1999;104:793.
44. Wreesmann VB, Smeele LE, Hilgers FJM, et al. Closure of tracheoesophageal fistula with prefabricated revascularized bilaminar radial forearm free flap. *Head Neck* 2009;31:838.
45. Fujiwara T, Nishino K, Numajiri T. Tracheal reconstruction with a prefabricated and double folded radial forearm free flap. *J Plast Reconstr Aesthet Surg* 2009;62:790.
46. Chen HC, Kuo YR, Huang TB, et al. Microvascular prefabricated free skin flap for oesophageal reconstruction. *Ann Thorac Surg* 1999;67:911.
47. Ramesh S, Serjius A, Wong TB, et al. Two stage penile reconstruction with free sensate radial forearm osteocutaneous flap. *Med J Malaysia* 2008;63:343.
48. Song YG, Chen GZ, Song YL The free thigh flap: a new free flap concept based on the septocutaneous artery. *Br J Plast Surg* 1984;37:149.
49. Hallock GG. The pre-expanded anterolateral thigh flap. *Ann Plast Surg* 2004;53:170.
50. Taylor GI, Miller GD, Ham FJ. The free vascularized bone graft. A clinical extension of microvascular techniques *last. *Reconstr Surg* 1975;55:533.
51. Chen ZW, Yan W. The study and clinical applications of osteocutaneous flap of fibula. *Microsurgery* 1983;4:11.
52. Baudet J, Panconi B, Caix P, et al. The composite fibula and soleus free transfer. *Int J Microsurg* 1982;4:10.
53. Pelissier P, Casoli V, Demiri E, et al. Fibula free transfer in the lower extremity. *Plast Reconstr Surg* 2000;105:567.
54. Rohner D, Jaquiery C, Kunz C, et al. Maxillofacial reconstruction with prefabricated osseous free flaps: a 3-year experience with 24 patients. *Plast Reconstr Surg* 2003;112:748.
55. Hage JJ, Wintres HAH, Lieshout JV. Fibula free flap phalloplasty: modification and recommendations. *Microsurgery* 1996;17:358.
56. Capelouto CC, Orgill DP, Louglin KR. Complete phalloplasty with a prelaminated osteocutaneous fibula flap. *J Urol* 1997;158:2238.
57. Houle JM, Neumeister MW. A prefabricated tissue engineered INTEGRA free Flap. *Plast Reconstr Surg* 2007;120:1322.
58. Akita S, Tamai N, Myoui A, et al. Capillary vessel network by inserting a vascular pedicle enhances bone formation in tissue engineered bone using interconnected porous hydroxyapatite ceramics. *Tissue Eng* 2004;10(5-6): 789–795.
59. Li QF, Reis ED, Zhang WX, et al. Accelerated flap prefabrication with vascular endothelial growth factor. *J Reconstr Microsurg* 2000;16:45.
60. Haws MJ, Erdman D, Bayati S, et al. Basic fibroblast growth factor induced angiogenesis and prefabricated flap survival. *J Reconstr Microsurg* 2001;17:39.
61. Li H, Zan T, Li Y, et al. Transplantation of adipose-derived stem cells promotes formation of prefabricated flap in a rat model. *J Exp Med* 2010;22:131.

CHAPTER 12

Latissimus Dorsi Flaps

Claudio Angrigiani

The latissimus dorsi flap is one of the most versatile and reliable options available for reconstructive surgery. It can be used as a musculocutaneous unit, as a muscle flap, or as a skin island based on the cutaneous branches of the vascular pedicle of the muscle.

HISTORY

The latissimus dorsi musculocutaneous flap was originally defined and performed by Tansini (1) as refinement of his original back flap for breast reconstruction based on the superficial circumflex scapular vessels (2) (Figure 12-1). He incorporated the latissimus dorsi muscle because he observed the contribution of the thoracodorsal vascular pedicle to the blood supply of the back skin. Tansini's method was mentioned in the literature by D'Este and Purpura (3,4); however it fell in disfavor mainly because of Halsted's policy of radical mastectomy without reconstruction (5). Gillies's base-to-length ratio philosophy for flap design also contributed to the delayed enthusiasm for musculocutaneous flaps (6).

The latissimus dorsi musculocutaneous flap was reinvented for reconstructive surgery in the 1970s by Olivari, who used it to cover a large radiation ulcer of the chest wall (7). Quillen el al. published on its use in head and neck reconstruction, and Muhlbauer proposed its use for breast reconstruction (8,9). Bostwick was the first to describe the latissimus dorsi musculocutaneous flap for breast reconstruction in English medical literature (10). Maxwell described the use of the latissimus dorsi as a free flap (11).

The literature is replete with many different uses of the latissimus dorsi musculocutaneous flap both as an island and free with microvascular anastomosis (12–14). The bulkiness of the flap was considered a major drawback for certain clinical problems. This problem was solved by diminishing the muscle volume (tailoring the distal end with a fasciocutaneous extension) or by dividing the muscle along its intramuscular pedicle (15–16).

Identification and isolation of the skin perforators derived from muscular branches of the pedicle permitted the elevation of the so-called latissimus dorsi musculocutaneous flap "without the muscle" (17). This technique is known as the thoracodorsal artery perforator [TDAP] flap (Figure 12-2). Although it is time consuming and demands a more delicate surgical technique, it is possible to completely spare the muscle and its innervation and to considerably reduce the volume of the flap. Further reports showed helpful modifications and increasing applicability of this technique (18,19). Koshima initiated the perforator flap era with his publication on rectus abdominis perforator flaps (20). A classification of perforator flaps was proposed by Geddes et al. The source of the flap vessel is considered as well as the anatomical structures pierced. In this case, the thoracodorsal perforator is denominated as TDAP/LT if the cutaneous branch pierces the muscle or TDAP/S if it is a direct septal branch (21).

A rib bone segment may also be incorporated in the flap as an osteomyocutaneous unit (22). A 12-cm segment of the ninth and tenth ribs may be harvested in combination with the flap based on the communication between the thoracodorsal and the periosteal vessels of the ribs. This mixed osteocutaneous flap is now considered unreliable and is not frequently used. The tip of the scapula may be incorporated in the flap as a vascularized bone, supplied by the osseous branch of the thoracodorsal artery.

A "reverse musculocutaneous flap" can be harvested using the posterior intercostal branches as the source of muscle vascularization. This flap is used for repair of midline cutaneous defects (23).

ANATOMY OF VESSELS, NERVES, AND SKIN TERRITORY

The latissimus dorsi is a large subcutaneous muscle, the back counterpart of the pectoralis major. It has a broad origin from an aponeurosis, which arises from spinous processes of the 7th to 12th thoracic vertebrae, the lumbar and sacral spinous

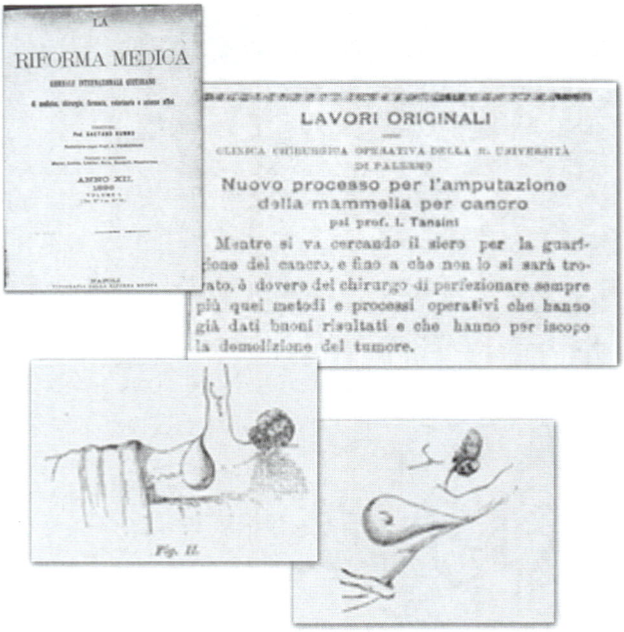

FIGURE 12-1 Front page of Tansini's paper and diagrams.

processes, and the posterior and middle outer rim of the iliac crest via the thoracodorsal fascia. The trapezius muscle covers the superomedial part of the latissimus dorsi muscle. The remaining part of the muscle is subcutaneous. It covers a portion of the paraspinal muscles and the majority of the serratus anterior. In its middle portion, there is a slight attachment to the 10th, 11th, and 12th ribs and interdigitations with serratus anterior fibers.

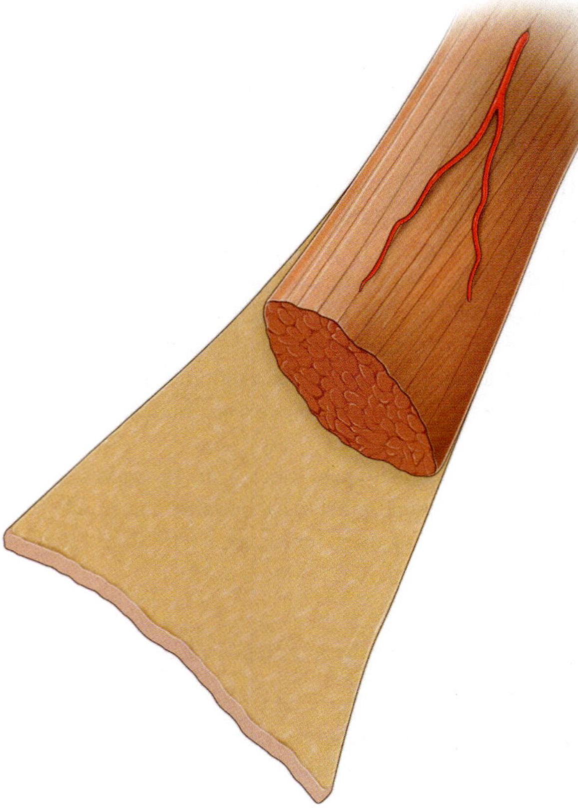

FIGURE 12-2 Muscle sectioning for decreasing flap volume.

Laterally, it inserts into the lesser tubercle of the humerus and the medial lip of the intertubercular groove. The muscle functions as an extender, adductor, and medial rotator of the humerus. It holds the inferior angle of the scapula against the chest wall and stabilizes and elevates the pelvis when bringing the lower extremity forward.

The latissimus dorsi muscle has a dominant vascular pedicle (thoracodorsal artery and vein) and secondary blood supply from the posterior intercostal perforators as mentioned.

The thoracodorsal artery arises from the subscapular artery, which originates from the axillary artery. It divides into the thoracodorsal and the circumflex scapular arteries 3 to 4 cm from its origin (Figure 12-3). The subscapular artery may share a common trunk at its origin with the posterior circumflex humeral artery in one third of cases. The thoracodorsal artery gives off an important branch (which might be considered a division of this artery) to the serratus anterior muscle. The branch to the serratus gives off itself a branch to the latissimus muscle. Therefore, there are several arterial connections between the serratus and the latissimus dorsi arterial systems that allow harvesting of the latissimus dorsi muscle even when the thoracodorsal artery is sectioned at its origin.

The thoracodorsal artery ranges from 6 to 12 cm in length and 3 mm in diameter in a normal man. It enters the muscle from underneath at site located at approximately 4 cm distal to the inferior scapular border and 2.5 cm lateral to the medial border of the latissimus dorsi muscle (24). The muscle's vascular pedicle divides into two main branches inside the muscle, the horizontal (medial or transverse) and descending oblique (lateral or vertical). They parallel the superior and the lateral border of the muscle approximately. The lateral branch is usually a little larger than the horizontal one; it runs parallel to the lateral border of the muscle approximately 2.5 cm from its edge. These branches anastomose with each other within the muscle and with the intercostal perforators (the secondary blood supply of the muscle). These anastomoses are profuse and large in diameter.

The two main intramuscular divisions of the thoracodorsal artery give off four to seven cutaneous branches through the muscle (perforators) within an 8- to 10-cm radius of the muscle hilus. The diameter of the cutaneous perforators ranges between 0.5 and 1.1 mm. Generally, the most proximal one is the largest. In the author's experience, there are three perforators coming from the vertical muscle branch and two from the horizontal one in most cases.

The thoracodorsal artery generally gives off a cutaneous branch just before entering the muscle (70% of the cases). This branch (which is referred to as "septocutaneous") was first noticed by Tansini. De Connick mentioned it, and it was clinically used by Baudet for his thoracodorsal free flap (25,26). It is curious that it neither courses through nor pierces any septum or fascia. Although it is frequently present, it is not always adequate to perfuse a free flap. When it is small, there is a compensatory muscle perforator of larger diameter.

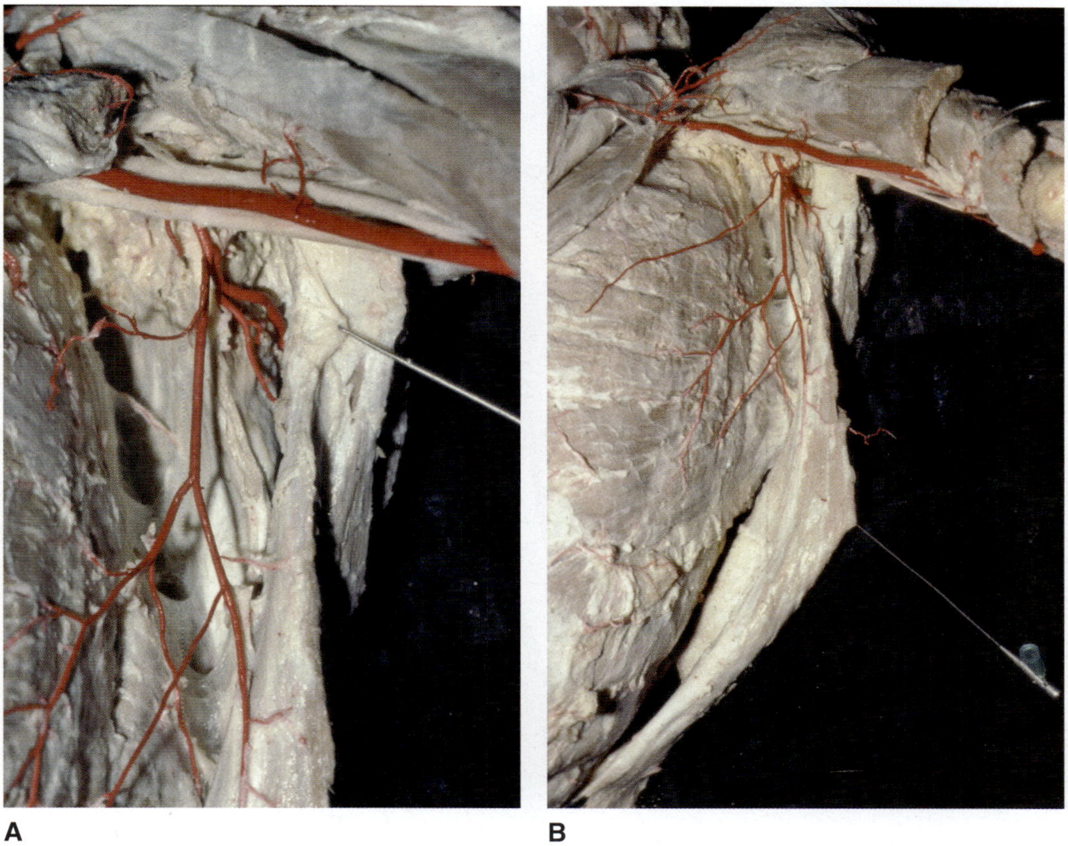

FIGURE 12-3 Anatomical specimen injected with colored latex. Axillary, subscapular, thoracodorsal, and their branches are clearly observed. (**A**) The anterior border of the latissimus dorsi muscle is retracted by the hook). (**B**) The close-up view shows the origin and the proximal part of the circumflex scapular).

The 9th, 10th, and 11th posterior intercostal vessels are the three largest of the medial dorsal branches to the latissimus dorsi muscle (secondary pedicles). These are the major vascular pedicles on which the reverse latissimus dorsi musculocutaneous flap is based.

Veins

The two venae comitantes of the thoracodorsal artery drain into a large subscapular vein (7–9 mm).

Nerves

The thoracodorsal nerve accompanies the vascular pedicle inferiorly and divides into a lateral and a medial branch. Although intimately related to the vascular pedicle, it can be spared during flap harvesting; and this is of utmost importance when a TDAP is performed to maintain full muscle function.

Cutaneous Territory Angiosome

Carl Manchot initiated "the cutaneous territories era" when he published his famous work *Die Hautarterien des Menschliches Körpers* in 1889 (27). As a result of his magnificent anatomical investigation of the arteries of the skin, he described the anatomical cutaneous territories summarized in the final illustration of his book. Michel Salmon investigated the vascular anatomy of the muscles and skin through radiopaque intraarterial injections. The use of radiology revealed the cutaneous territories in greater anatomical detail (28) Nakajima studied some of the anatomical cutaneous territories in vivo by selective angiography with prostaglandin E. (29). Cormack and Lamberty developed the concept of dynamic and potential territories in addition of the classical anatomical territories (30). Behan and Wilson proposed the term *angiotome* for "any area of skin than can be cut as a flap, which is supplied by an axial vessel but may be extended by its communications with branches of an adjacent vessel" (31).

The primary anatomical territory of the cutaneous branches of the thoracodorsal artery is an area of 255 cm^2 in the upper part of the muscle (Figure 12-4).The dynamic clinical cutaneous territory of the thoracodorsal artery through its cutaneous branches is an area of approximately 30 × 20 cm (600 cm^2). This has been proven by clinical experience (Figure 12-5). This area might even be enlarged further by delay procedures that would extend the potential uses of this flap. According to the original description of an "angiosome" by Taylor et al. (32)—a composite block of tissue supplied by a source artery—the thoracodorsal angiosome would be the upper part of the latissimus dorsi muscle, the serratus anterior muscle, the attached deep fascia, the overlying skin, subcutaneous tissue, and the tip of the scapula. Nowadays, the angiosome concept is frequently

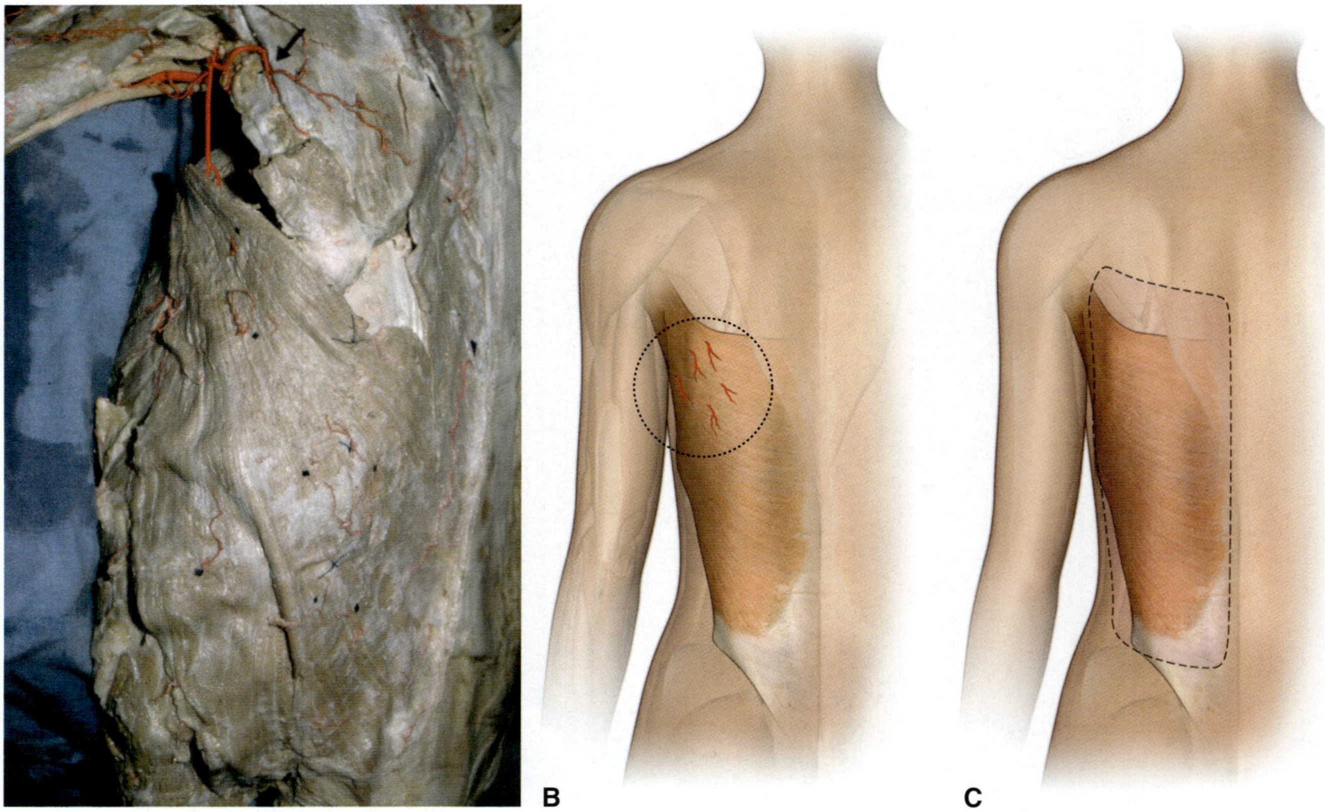

A B C

FIGURE 12-4 (**A**) Anatomical specimen injected with colored latex (above left). The skin and subcutaneous tissue have been resected. The muscle perforators are observed at the superficial surface of the latissimus dorsi muscle. (**B**) Diagram of the muscle perforators originated from the thoracodorsal artery (above right). The anatomical area of distribution is marked. (**C**) Dynamic territory; possible flap based on the thoracodorsal pedicle approximately.

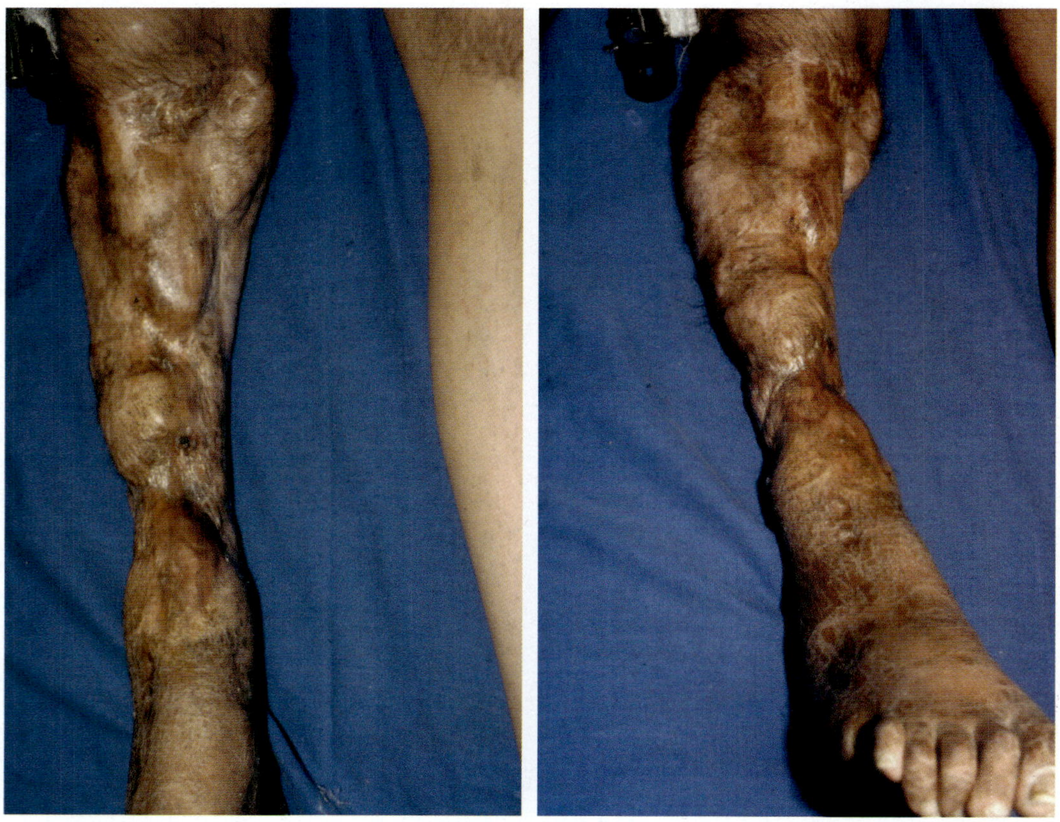

A B

FIGURE 12-5 (**A** to **I**) Unstable skin coverage of a posttraumatic lower limb treated with a large musculocutaneous latissimus dorsi flap.

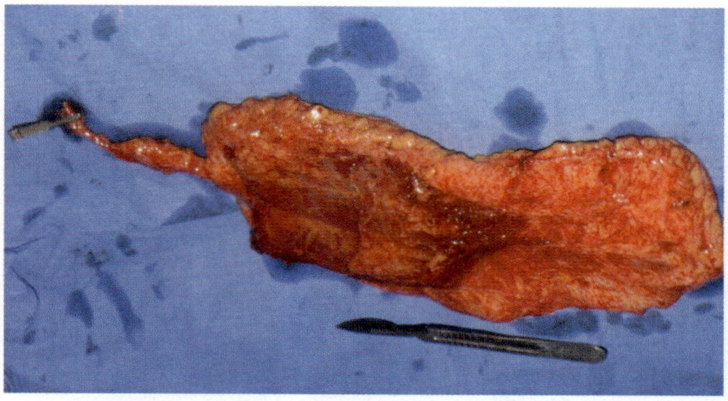

C

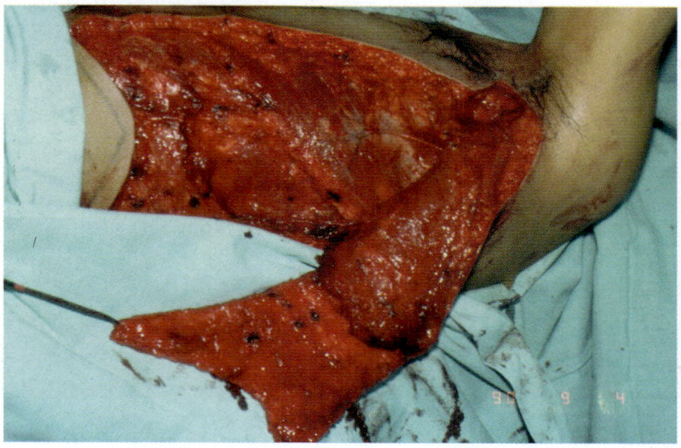

D

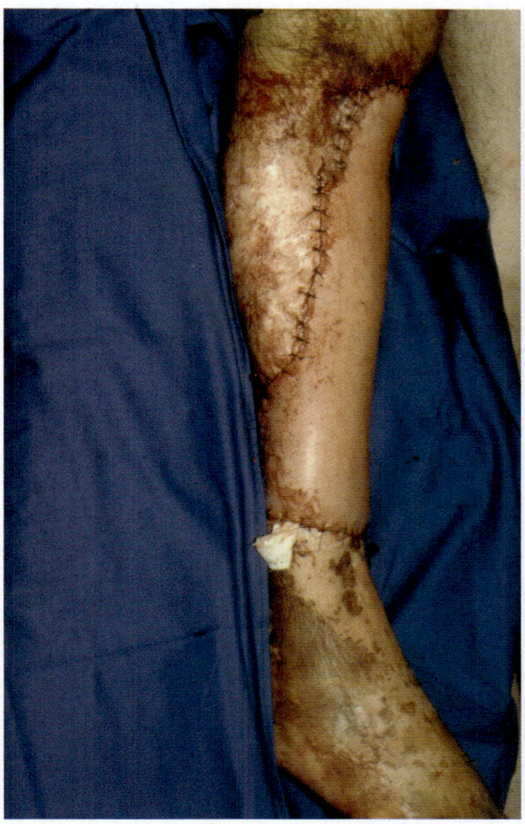

E

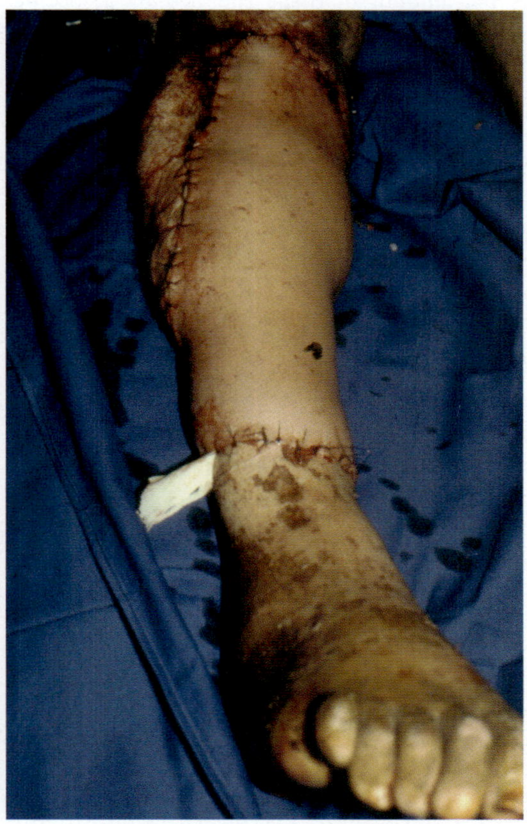

F

FIGURE 12-5 *(Continued)*

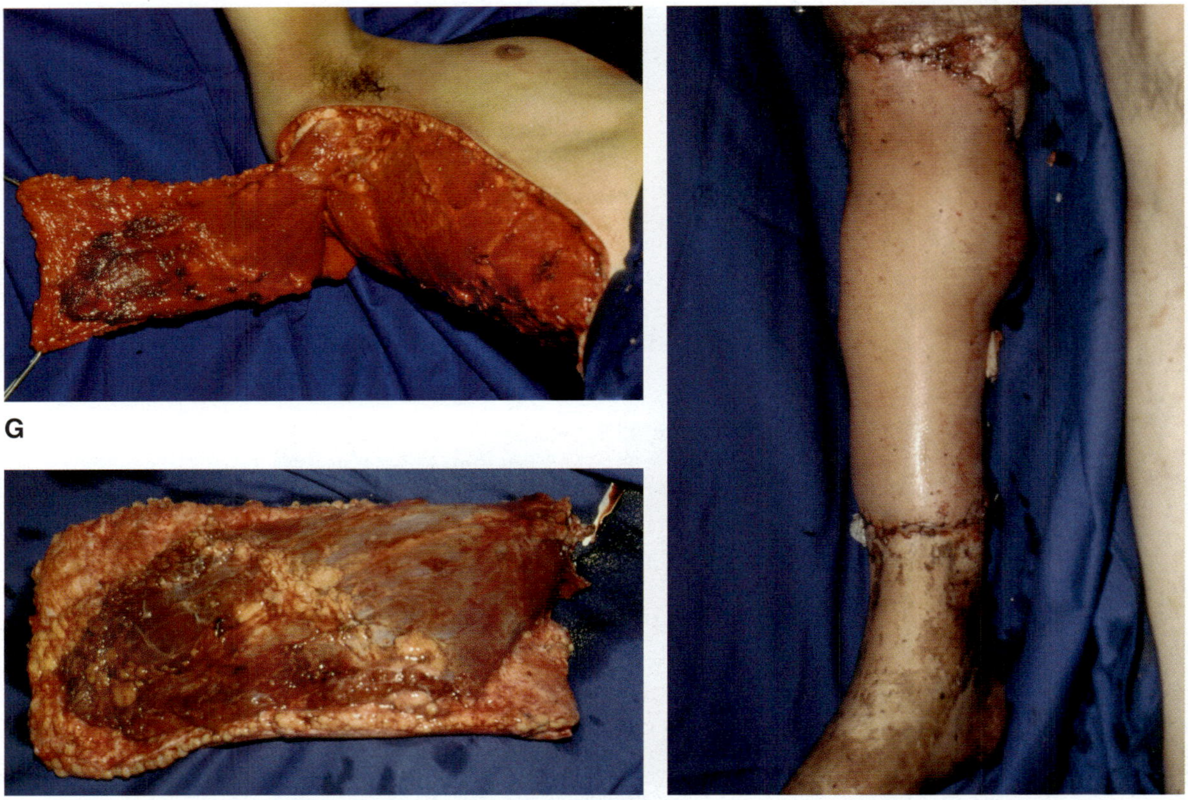

G I H

FIGURE 12-5 *(Continued)*

used to name the amount of tissue supplied by a specific artery and is more generally applied to the skin. The thoracodorsal angiosome would thus be the area of skin and subcutaneous tissue perfused by the cutaneous branches of the thoracodorsal artery and might be considered synonymous with its dynamic territory.

DETAILED SURGICAL TECHNIQUE

Muscle Flap

The latissimus dorsi muscle may be easily exposed through a horizontal straight or lazy curved 8- to 10-cm incision 6 to 8 cm inferior to the axillary fold. This approach permits wide exposure of the thoracodorsal pedicle up to its origin from the subscapular trunk and direct visualization of the skin branches through or around the anterior border of the muscle (Figure 12-6).

Blunt dissection is performed on the superficial face of the muscle. The skin arteries (perforators) appearing at the muscle surface are ligated (or coagulated) and divided. After the superficial surface is exposed, the dissection continues on the deep surface of the muscle. Coagulation of the intercostal perforators must be done carefully. The fascial muscle origin from the iliac crest is incised as well as that from the thoracic spine. The muscle is elevated, and the deep surface is exposed. The vascular pedicle is identified under 4x loupe magnification. Collateral branches are ligated and divided. The branch to the serratus anterior is sectioned last of all. It is preserved to the last moment because it protects the pedicle from involuntary traction.

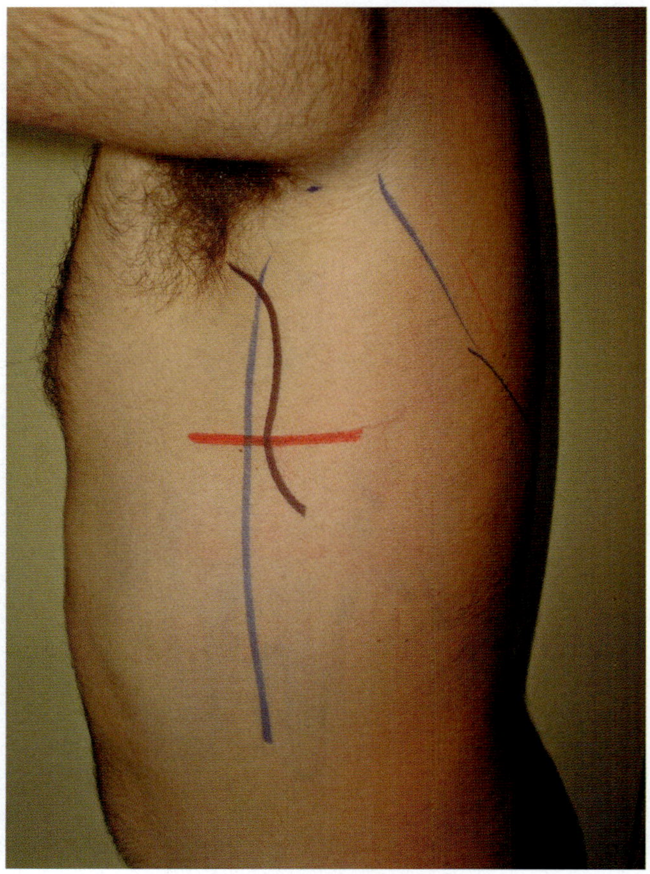

FIGURE 12-6 Diagram of possible approaches for muscle flap elevation.

The vascular pedicle is then liberated from the proximal part of the muscle. The humeral muscle insertion is exposed as its tendon swings around that of the teres major. After it is separated from the teres major, it may be sectioned.

It is possible to reach all points of the latissimus dorsi from the initial skin incision. Shorter incisions may be performed if an endoscopic technique is used to reach distal portions of the muscle. The muscle may then be transposed locally or completely liberated by sectioning the vascular pedicle.

Musculocutaneous Flap

Flap Design

The skin island may be designed over the muscle depending on recipient site requirements as well as preferences for the position of the donor site scar. It is preferable to design the skin island overlying direct musculocutaneous perforators derived from the thoracodorsal vessels. With such perforators incorporated in the flap, it is possible to orientate the skin island in any direction without considering the direction of muscle fibers. Usually a better esthetic result is obtained when the flap is designed perpendicular to the direction of the muscle fibers, thereby placing its axis in the relaxed skin tension lines. In cases of severe burn scarring, it is reasonable to place the skin island in an uninvolved area if one is present. A 30-cm-long flap can be safely harvested (Figure 12-7).

It is possible to design the skin island over any part of the muscle, but here one must rely on intramuscular anastomoses as well as the presence of a muscle perforator within the designated area. The chances of complete survival are less when the skin island is small because with a randomly designed flap, there would be less chance of incorporating a perforator. Thus, small skin islands designed in the distal part of the muscle (near the iliac crest) tend to be unreliable.

Flap Elevation

The skin of the inferior border of the flap is incised down to the muscle fascia. The superficial surface of the muscle beyond the skin island is dissected free. After the anterior border of the muscle is exposed, dissection is carried beneath it, and any attachments to the rib cage are released. Direct muscle branches from the intercostal arteries are ligated and divided.

The muscle is elevated, and the vascular pedicle is exposed. The vascular hilum is identified, and the direction of the thoracodorsal muscular branches is observed on the deep muscle surface. The main direct cutaneous muscle perforators from the thoracodorsal artery are located within 6 to 8 cm of the hilum. After the vascular pedicle is identified and isolated, the desired amount of muscle to be harvested distally is marked and divided.

The superior border of the skin island is then incised. The latissimus dorsi tendon is exposed under the teres major. The vascular pedicle is gently retracted and protected as the tendon is divided proximally. Then the vascular pedicled is defined by ligation and section of the various branches. The branch to the serratus anterior is sectioned last. Local transposition of the flap is then carried out or the pedicle is sectioned for free transfer.

Thoracodorsal Artery Perforator Flap

The TDAP flap was originally described as a method that, by excluding muscle, minimized bulk—an inconvenience in some cases. The perforator flap technique allows identification of specific cutaneous arteries and elevation of a skin flap without the underlying muscle The TDAP flap is indicated when the surgeon needs a thin cutaneous flap with the advantages of the thoracodorsal pedicle (e.g., length, reliability, arc of rotation).

The perforator flap concept also allows independent movement of the skin island from the underlying muscle when a "traditional" musculocutaneous flap is harvested. This technique occasionally facilitates flap inset.

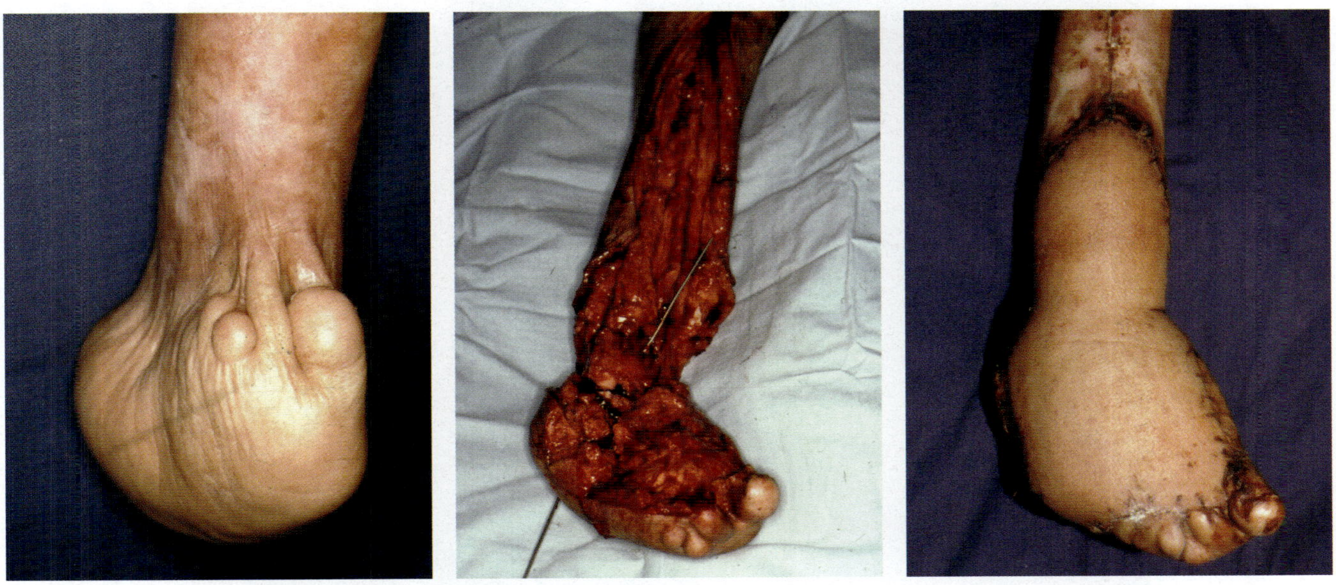

A B C

FIGURE 12-7 (**A** to **C**) Severe burn sequelae of the anterior ankle and foot that prevents plantar flexion and normal gait. Retraction release produces a large defect that was resurfaced with a "tailored" latissimus dorsi musculocutaneous flap to diminish flap volumen.

Flap Design

A point is marked at the lateral border of the latissimus dorsi muscle 8 cm inferior to the axillary fold. A 6-cm-diameter circle is designed centered in this point. The point represents the emergence of the vascular pedicle into the subcutaneous tissue, with the circle enclosing the likely location of the largest perforators of the thoracodorsal artery (Figure 12-8). As long as this area is included in the flap design, its axis may be placed in any direction.

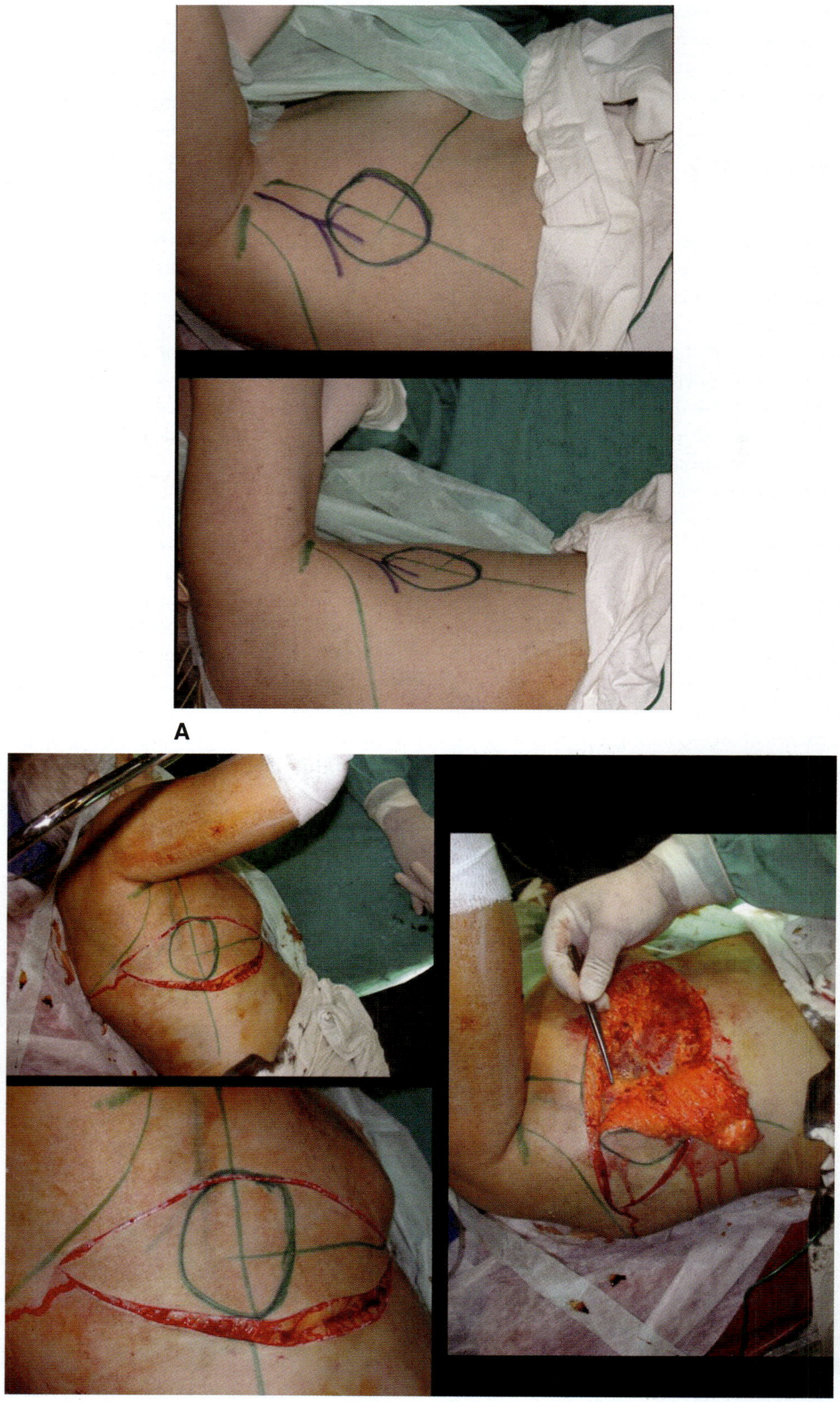

A

B

FIGURE 12-8 (**A** to **H**) Thoracodorsal artery perforator flap design and elevation.

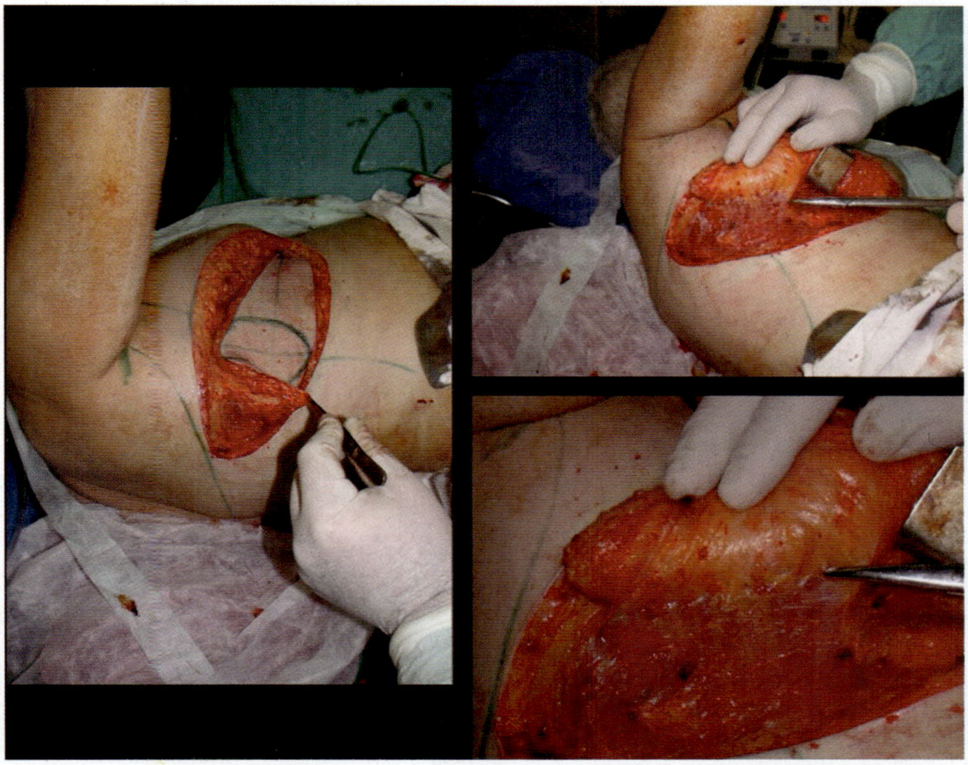

C

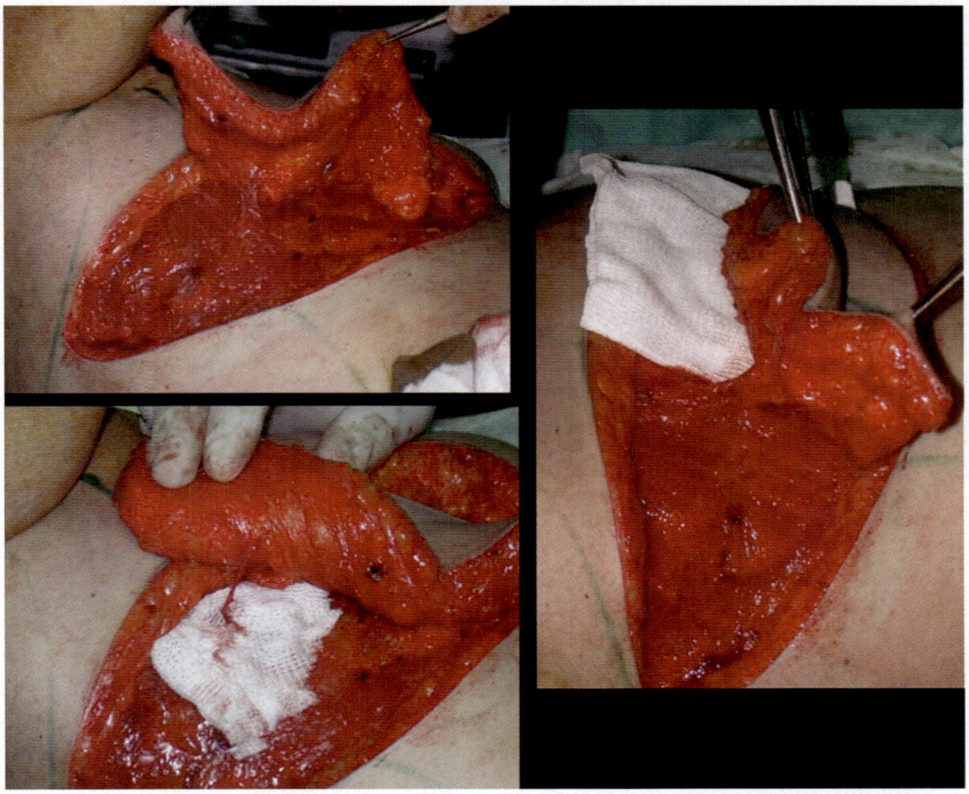

D

FIGURE 12-8 *(Continued)*

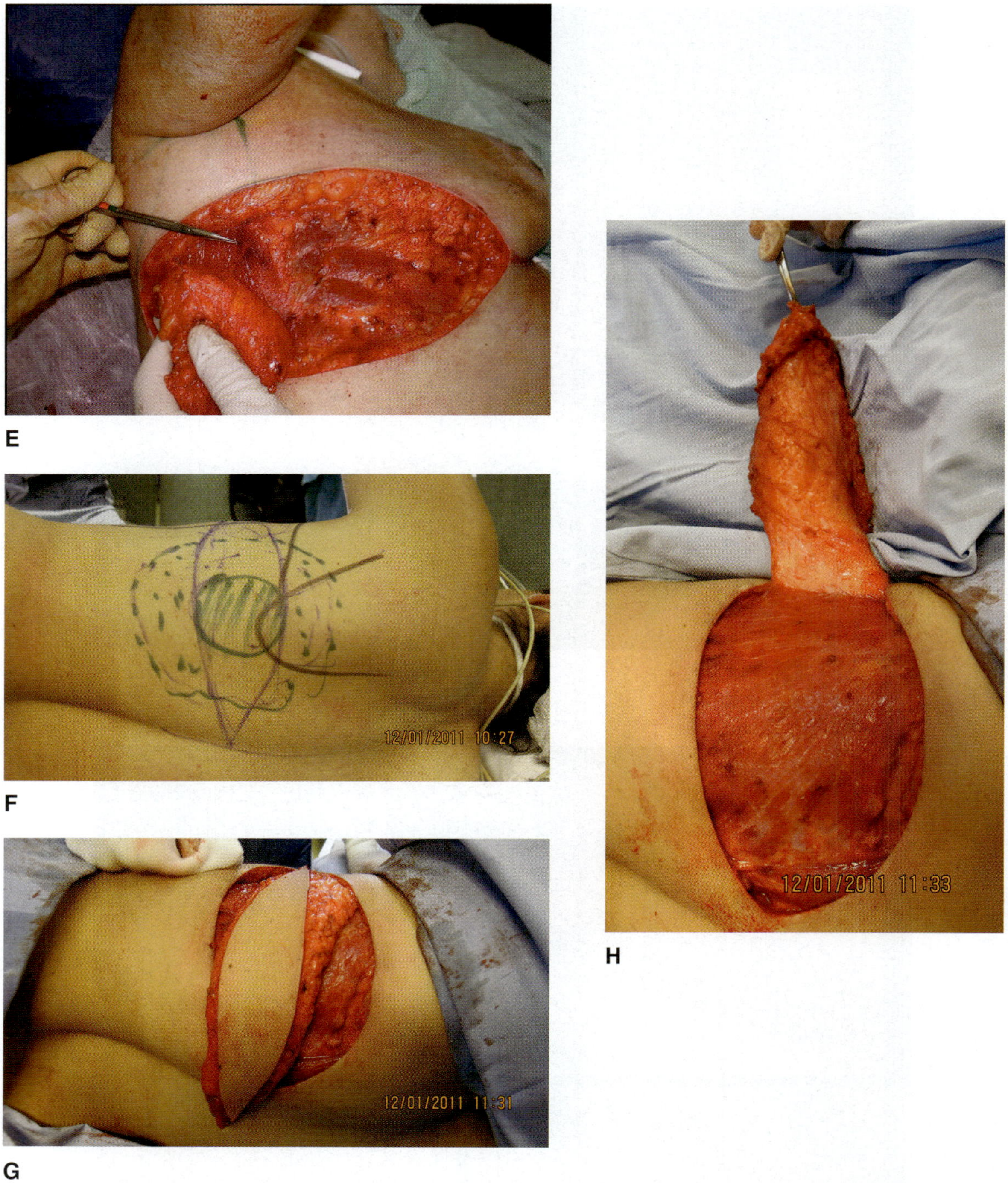

FIGURE 12-8 *(Continued)*

Flap Elevation

The skin is incised at the inferior border of the flap. The lateral border of the muscle is exposed. Careful dissection under 4x magnification is carried proximally over the lateral border of the muscle few centimeters anterior and posterior.

The dissection is performed superficial to the deep fascia. Cutaneous branches of the thoracodorsal artery passing through the muscle (perforators) are exposed as well as direct cutaneous branches given off before it enters the muscle. The latter are frequently, but not always, present. Accordingly, the largest cutaneous artery is selected and either dissected through the muscle or around its border to the parent vessel. In the author's experience, the largest cutaneous branch of the thoracodorsal artery is usually a direct branch, located at the lateral border of the muscle or a perforator positioned a few millimeters medial to the lateral border of the muscle. The author has observed that the compensatory law of Dubreuil Chambardell (33) is applicable in this area: when the muscular perforator is large, the direct cutaneous branch is small and vice versa.

The presence of a direct cutaneous branch renders the operative procedure easier and faster.

The skin island is completely isolated on the cutaneous artery and venae comitantes. The vascular pedicle is dissected up to its origin at the subscapular trunk as with a conventional musculocutaneous flap (Figure 12-9).

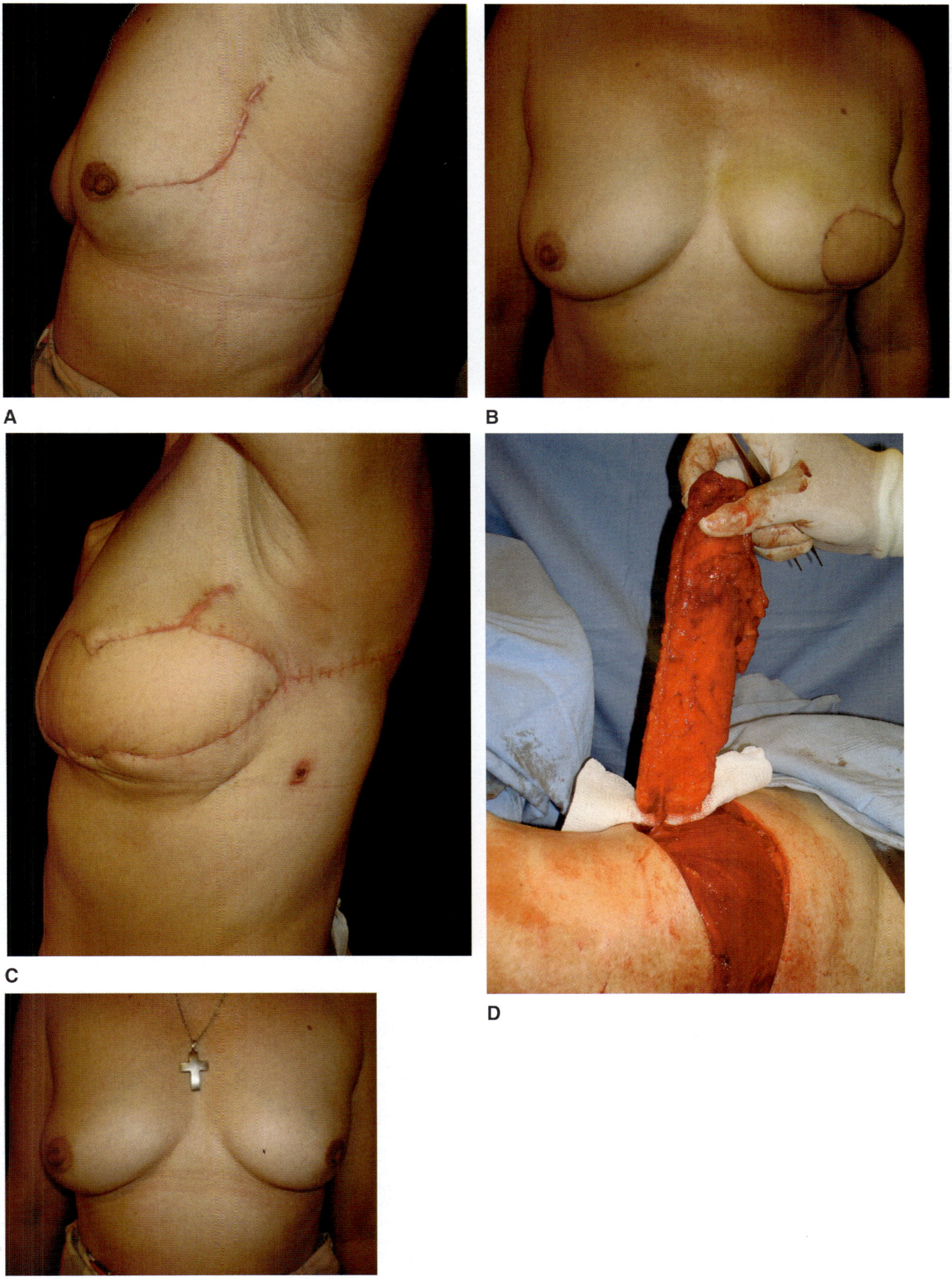

FIGURE 12-9 (**A** to **E**) A thoracodorsal perforator island flap is used for immediate breast reconstruction in a 44-year-old patient who will undergo a complete mastectomy. Muscle preservation produced better donor site morbidity and esthetic appearance. Volume was completely replaced by the flap without a prosthesis.

Closure of the Donor Site

Direct closure of donor site is usually possible with flaps up to about 8 cm wide. Larger flaps may necessitate skin grafting the donor site. The orientation of the skin island makes a difference: when perpendicular to the muscle fibers (orientated favorably with regards to the relaxed skin tension lines), a 12- to 14-cm-wide flap donor site can be easily closed directly (depending on skin laxity and age).

Potential Donor Defect

There is no noticeable function deficit in normal individuals when latissimus dorsi muscle is absent. It is advisable to preserve latissimus dorsi muscle in patients with paraplegia for pelvic stability. Patients who require the use of crutches may also have a functional loss when the latissimus dorsi is taken (34). There is no functional deficit with the TDAP flap. Spread or hypertrophic scars are frequently observed at the donor site, but keloids are rare.

DONOR SITE COMPLICATIONS

Seroma formation is a common complication when the muscle is harvested even with adequate and prolonged suction drainage. It may be troublesome to eradicate and may result in a bursa formation that eventually may need surgical excision. Wound dehiscence and widened scars may occur, especially at the anterior border when the flap is designed horizontally. Patient complaints about scar appearance are extremely common.

There may be a volume deficit compared with the contralateral side, and the tip of the scapula may be more prominent. This may be avoided by suturing the remaining inferior part of the muscle to the infraspinatus fascia. Irregular contour compared with the contralateral site may be ameliorated by fat injection.

LIST OF INDICATIONS

Pedicled Transfer

- Local pedicled muscle flap: elbow flexion: biceps replacement; anterior axillary fold reconstruction in Poland's syndrome
- Local musculocutaneous or TDAP: anterior and posterior chest wall defect repair, breast reconstruction, tegument reconstruction of anterior and posterior arm down to the elbow
- Local reverse flap: coverage of medial lower thoracic and lumbar defects

Distant Transfer (As a Free Flap)

- Head and neck: coverage of intraoral defects, including mandibular, maxillary, and orbital reconstruction combined with scapula and rib
- Lower extremity: major coverage problems, pseudoarthrosis
- Upper extremity: coverage defects distal to the elbow
- Abdomen: abdominal wall reconstruction

The pedicled latissimus dorsi flap (musculocutaneous or TDAP) has regained popularity for breast reconstruction. It is widely used, especially in immediate breast reconstruction after periareolar skin-sparing mastectomy. It allows immediate closure of the defect and provides considerable volume (~400 cc), which may be sufficient to match the contralateral side in small- to medium-sized breasts. Although its use as a free flap is still extremely valuable for lower limb reconstruction, it has lost some popularity because of the use of more convenient regional flaps as anterolateral thigh flap or local perforator flaps, which do not require patient repositioning.

REFERENCES

1. Tansini I. Sopra il nuovo mio processo di amputazione della mammilla. *La Gazzetta Medica* 1906;12:757.
2. Tansini I. Nuovo processo per l'amputazione della mammella per cancro. *La Riforma Medica Napoli* 1896.
3. d'Este S. La technique de l'amputation de la mammelle pour carcinome mammaire. *Rev Chir* 1912;45:164.
4. Purpura F. Tansini method for cure of cancer of the breast. *Lancet* 1908; 1:634.
5. Halstead WS. The results of radical operations for the cure of cancer of the breast Tr. *Am Surg A* 1907;25:61.
6. Gillies H. *Plastic Surgery of the Face.* London: Hodder and Stoughton, 1920.
7. Olivari N. The latissimus dorsi flap. *Br J Plast Surg* 1976;29:126.
8. Quillen CG, Serafin JC, Georgiade NG. Use of latissimus dorsi musculocutaneous island flap for reconstruction of the head and neck area. *Plast Reconstr Surg* 1976;62:113.
9. Muhlbauer W, Olbrisch R. The latissimus dorsi musculo cutaneous flap for breast reconstruction. *Chir Plast* 1977;4:27.
10. Bostwick J, Vasconez L, Jurkiewicz MJ. Breast reconstruction after radical mastectomy *Plast Reconstr Surg* 1978;61:682.
11. Maxwell GP, Stueber K, Hoopes JE. A free latissimus dorsi musculocutaneous flap. *Plast Reconstr Surg* 1978;62:462.
12. Schneider WJ, Hill HL, Brown RG. Latissimus dorsi myocutaneous flap for breast reconstruction. *Br J Plast Surg* 1977;30:277–281.
13. Hokin JA. Mastectomy reconstruction without prosthetic implant. *Plast Reconstr Surg* 1983;72:810.
14. Marshall DR, Anstee EJ, Stapleton MJ. Soft tissue reconstruction of the breast using the extended composite latissimus dorsi myocutaneous flap. *Br J Plast Surg* 1984;37:361.
15. Hayashi A, Maruyama Y. The "reduced" latissimus dorsi musculocutaneous flap. *Plast Reconstr Surg* 1989;84(2):290.
16. Godina M. The tailored latissimus dorsi free flap. *Plast Reconstr Surg* 1987;80:304.
17. Angrigiani C, Grilli D, Siebert J. Latissimus dorsi flap without muscle. *Plast Reconstr Surg* 1995;96(7):1608.
18. Kim JT, Koo BS, Kim SK. The thin latissimus dorsi perforator-based free flap for resurfacing. *Plast Reconstr Surg* 2001;107:374.
19. Cavadas PC, Teran-Saavedra PP. Combined latissimus dorsi-thoracodorsal artery perforator free flap: the "razor flap." *J Reconstr Microsurg* 2002;18:29.
20. Koshima I, Soeda S. Inferior epigastric artery skin flaps without rectus abdominis muscle. *Br J Plast Surg* 1989;42:645.
21. Geddes CR, Morris SF, Neligan PC. Perforator flaps: evolution, classification, and applications. *Ann Plast Surg* 2003;50:90.
22. Maruyama Y, Onishi K, Iwahira Y, et al. Free compound rib-latissimus dorsi osteomusculocutaneous flap in reconstruction of the leg. *J Reconstr Microsurg* 1986;3:13.
23. Bostwick J III, Scheflan M, Nahai F, Jurkiewicz MJ. The "reverse" latissimus dorsi muscle and musculocutaneous flap: anatomical and clinical considerations *Plast Reconstr Surg* 1980;65(4):395.
24. Thomas BP, Geddes CR, Tang M, et al. The vascular basis of the thoracodorsal artery perforator flap. *Plast Reconstr Surg* 2005;116:819–822.
25. De Coninck A, Boeckx W, Vanderlinden E, Claessen G. Autotransplants avec microsutures vasculaires. Anatomiedes zones donneuses. *Ann Chir Plast* 1975;20:163–170.
26. Baudet J, Guimberteau JC, Nascimento E. Successful clinical transfer of two free thoracodorsal axillary flaps. *Plast Reconstr Surg* 1976;58:680.
27. Manchot C. *Die Hautarterien des Menschliches Körpers.* Leipzig: FCW Vogel, 1889.
28. Salmon M. *Artères de la Peau.* Paris: Masson, 1936.

29. Nakajima H, Maruyama Y, Koda E. The definition of vascular skin territories with prostaglandin E: the anterior chest, abdomen and thigh-inguinal region. *Br J Plast Surg* 1981 34:258–263.
30. Cormack GC, Lamberty BGH. *The Arterial Anatomy of Skin Flaps.* Edinburgh: Churchill Livingstone, 1986.
31. Behan FC, Wilson JSP. *The Vascular Basis of Laterally Based Forehead Island Flaps and Their Clinical Applications.* II Congress of the European Section of the International Confederation of Plastic and Reconstructive Surgery, Madrid,1973.
32. Taylor GI, Palmer JH. The vascular territories (angiosomes) of the body: experimental study and clinical applications. *Br J Plast Surg* 1987;40:113.
33. Dubreuil-Chambardel L. *Traité des variations du système artériel.* Paris: Masson, 1925.
34. Russell RC. Pribaz J, Zook EG, et al. Functional evaluation of latissimus dorsi donor site. *Plast Reconstr Surg* 1986;78:336.

CHAPTER 13

Scapular and Parascapular Flaps

Summer E. Hanson and John W. Siebert

HISTORICAL PERSPECTIVE

The scapular and parascapular flaps are variations of skin, fascia, muscle, or bone based on the subscapular artery and its branches located in the posterior trunk between the axilla and midline and are used to address a variety of soft tissue defects. Primarily a fasciocutaneous flap with a type B pattern of circulation, there are several modifications that make this flap both reliable and versatile. The first description of the scapular fasciocutaneous flap based on the circumflex scapular artery (CSA) was done more than 3 decades ago, and further modifications have been made based on extensive study of the vascular supply (1,2). The CSA gives off several periosteal branches, making the lateral border of the scapula a reliable source of vascularized bone (3). Batchelor and Sully first described incorporation of the latissimus dorsi muscle with the parascapular or scapular flap for additional tissue in a scalp defect (4). The CSA system offers a reliable pedicle with a robust, branching vascular pattern, which has become a workhorse free tissue transfer in facial reconstruction.

ANATOMY

The subscapular artery and vein are branches from the third portion of the axillary vessels (Figure 13-1). There are two major branches of the subscapular artery: (1) the thoracodorsal artery (TDA), which predominantly supplies the latissimus dorsi and serratus anterior muscles as well as the tip of the scapular bone for use in osteocutaneous flaps, and (2) the CSA, which runs through the triangular space formed by the teres major, teres minor and long head of the triceps, and branches to the transverse and descending cutaneous branches associated with the scapular and parascapular fasciocutaneous flaps (Figure 13-2). The CSA pedicle is approximately 2.5 mm in diameter and has a length of 5 to 6 cm. Two venae comitantes run with the CSA and drain to the thoracodorsal vein. Sensory innervation of the skin paddle is through the lateral and posterior cutaneous nerves of the third, fourth, and fifth intercostal nerves, although these are divided in flap elevation.

Whereas the periosteal branches of the CSA supply the lateral aspect of the scapula, the tip is more commonly supplied by the TDA. Up to 10 cm of bone can be harvested in adult women and closer to 14 cm in men (5). The distinct blood supply to the lateral border of the scapula and the scapular tip allows for two separate vascularized bone segments to be included in the flap if needed. Conventionally, the parascapular skin paddle is positioned longitudinally along the lateral border of the scapula, and a scapular flap to include bone is positioned transversely along the scapula. These are designed to orient the skin paddle over the descending branch of the CSA in the parascapular flap or the transverse branch supplying the scapula bone, with an average length or 10 to 15 cm and a width of 5 to 7 cm. These dimensions may be increased depending on posterior skin laxity and soft tissue defect.

VARIATIONS OF THE FLAP

A number of combinations of tissues can be harvested based on a single vascular pedicle, and thus flaps can be tailored to the defect being addressed, including the scapular or parascapular fasciocutaneous flap, scapular or parascapular osteocutaneous flap, or dorsal thoracic fascia flap. Two separate segments of bone from the scapula can be harvested based on the lateral aspect supplied by the periosteal branches of the CSA as well as the tip of the scapula supplied by the angular artery from the TDA or as a branch from the serratus collaterals (6). The medial border of the scapula has been included with the standard scapular harvest based on the distal branches of the CSA.

Tissue expansion of the flap or adjacent skin may be performed in advance of harvest to increase the flap dimensions while maintaining direct closure of the donor site. The parascapular flap can be used in a vertical, horizontal, or oblique

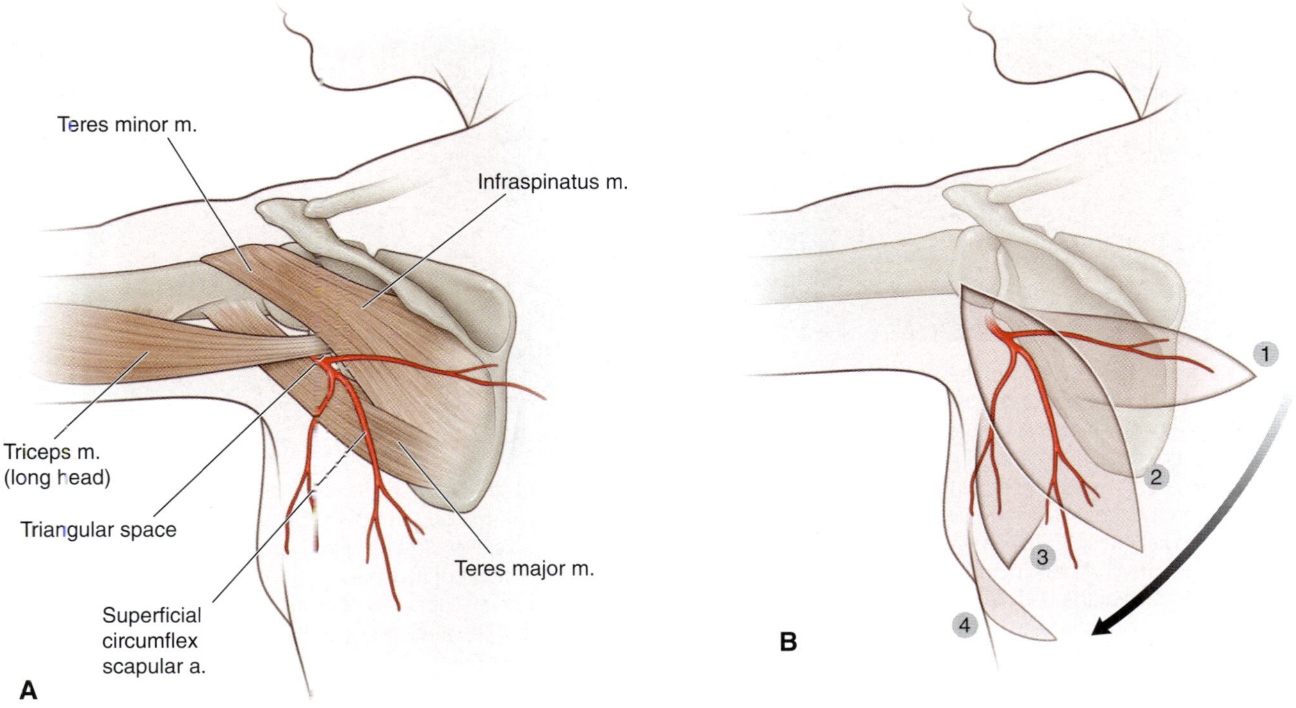

FIGURE 13-1 Illustration of the anatomic relationship in the circumflex scapular and parascapular flaps. (**A**) Artistic representation of the left triangular anatomic space and the origin of the circumflex scapular artery. The anterior arterial branch is noted along with the descending and transverse branches. (**B**) The flap design can be rotated progressively in an anterior direction to fall within the inframammary fold. A, artery; M, muscle.

fashion depending on tissue distensibility or position of the scar as long as the CSA pedicle is captured in the flap design (see Figure 13-1). For example, the skin paddle may be positioned more laterally in the female patient, positioning the incision in the ipsilateral inframammary fold, the so-called inframammary extended circumflex scapular flap (7). Alternatively, the fascia and subcutaneous tissues can be harvested without the overlying skin, reducing the donor site morbidity.

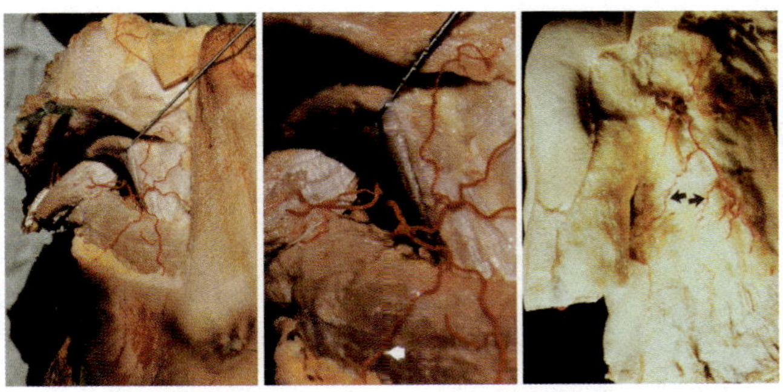

FIGURE 13-2 Anatomic dissections illustrating branching patterns of the circumflex scapular artery (CSA) system. (**A**) Posterior view of cadaver dissection showing the left CSA and its numerous cutaneous branches exiting in a radial pattern from the triangular space. (**B**) Close-up view of the same cadaver specimen, demonstrating the anterior cutaneous branch (arrow) originating from the proximal descending branch of the left CSA. (**C**) Posterior view of the left upper back in a different cadaver dissection, demonstrating the anterior course of the anterior arterial branches (arrows). (Reproduced with permission from Siebert JW, Longaker MT, Angrigiani C. The inframammary extended circumflex scapular flap: an aesthetic improvement of the parascapular flap. *Plast Reconstr Surg* 1997;99(1):70–77.)

Pedicle length for microvascular transplantation can be extended by carrying the dissection of the CSA until it joins the TDA to form the subscapular artery. If further length is required, the TDA can be divided, increasing the pedicle to include the subscapular vessels. Here, the incision is carried out toward the axilla for proximal exposure. Pedicle length in standard rotational flap transposition can only be carried out to the level of the triangular space unless the teres minor muscle is divided. Although the scapular and parascapular flaps are commonly used in microvascular transplantation, direct flap transposition can be achieved to the adjacent posterior trunk or axilla or less commonly tunneled as an island flap.

DETAILED TECHNIQUE OF THE DISSECTION AND HARVEST

The flap is usually harvested from the same side as the recipient site, although consideration could be given to use the nondominant arm. Traditionally, the patient is positioned in the lateral decubitus position and secured with a vacuum bean bag and safety straps to maintain positioning. An axillary roll should be used to avoid traction on the contralateral brachial plexus. The authors prefer to have the patient in the supine position with a bump under the ipsilateral shoulder. The flap

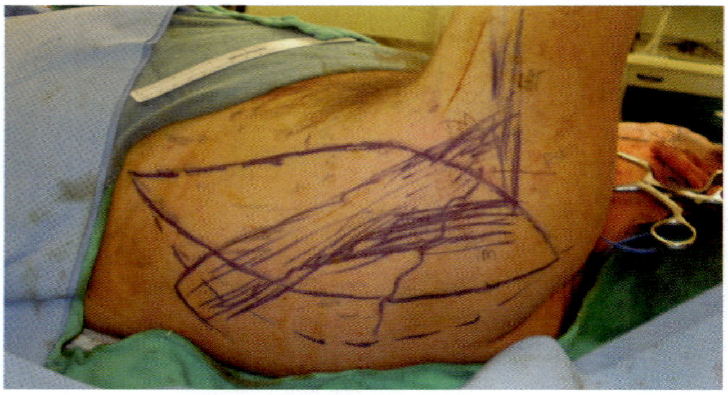

FIGURE 13-3 Preoperative set up. The patient is placed in the supine position with a bump under the ipsilateral shoulder. The ipsilateral arm is positioned at 90 degrees with tension on the teres muscles. The tip of the scapula is palpated. The triangular space is made up by the long head of the triceps (LHT), the teres minor (Tm), and the teres major (TM) illustrated in the figure. The circumflex scapular artery (CSA) exits through the triangular space and gives off a transverse branch and a descending branch. The anticipated positions of the pedicle and two branches are marked in the photograph. Doppler may be used to confirm positioning of the CSA. The skin paddle is position to maximize capture of these branches based on the size of the defect (solid line). Additionally, the subcutaneous dissection can be extended to incorporate dorsal thoracic fascia as needed for contouring the flap as in facial reconstruction. This is indicated by the dashed line. The arm is prepped and kept in the sterile field for manipulation during flap elevation.

may be harvested simultaneously with recipient site preparation, and thus the arm and back can be prepped out at the beginning of the case. The arm should be positioned keeping the humerus abducted, placing some tension on the teres major and minor.

Begin by palpating the triangular space (teres major, teres minor, and long head of the triceps) and tip of the scapula (Figure 13-3). The pedicle is located in the subfascial plane. Doppler may be used to confirm the position of the CSA in the triangular space. The skin paddle is drawn in an ellipse based on the anticipated defect. The scapular flap traditionally begins with a horizontal skin paddle centered over the triangular space approximately 2 cm above the posterior axillary crease extending from the axillary border of the scapula to the midline. The parascapular flap skin island is oriented obliquely centered over the triangular space extending toward the posterior iliac spine, although many variations of the skin paddle are illustrated in Figure 13-1. Capturing the CSA in the flap design is the only requirement, and many variations of the skin paddle have been described to suit the defect.

Scapular and parascapular free flap elevation has been described via a lateral approach with direct pedicle identification or through a retrograde dissection approach. In the lateral approach, the incision overlying the triangular space medial to the axillary border of the scapula is carried out through the skin and subcutaneous tissues. The triceps, teres major, and teres minor are identified and retracted to expose the CSA and venae comitantes in the triangular space. After the pedicle is identified and the flap design confirmed, the remaining incision is carried out through the dorsal thoracic fascia. The distal flap is

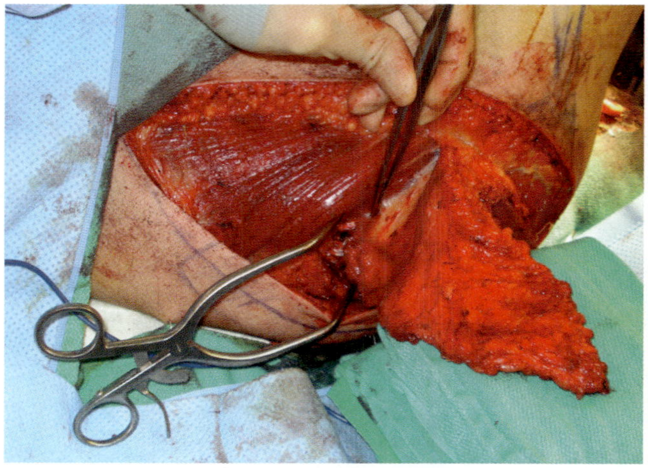

FIGURE 13-4 Retrograde flap elevation. The skin incisions are made and dissection carried down to the level of the dorsal thoracic fascia. The distal or surrounding subcutaneous tissue is elevated to incorporate the additional fascial extensions. The flap is elevated in the subfascial plane from the distal end retrograde to the level of the teres major and minor muscles at the distal triangular space.

elevated from the underlying subscapularis, trapezius, and teres minor and major muscles. The transverse and descending branches of the CSA are visualized as they join the CSA.

The authors typically favor a retrograde approach (Figure 13-4). The distal flap incisions are made through the skin and subcutaneous tissues to the dorsal thoracic fascia. The flap is elevated in the subfascial plane until the teres minor and major muscles are visualized at the triangular space and the CSA identified. The lateral and medial flap incisions are carried out in the subfascial plane to isolate the flap on its vascular pedicle. Proximal dissection of the pedicle will increase length. The teres minor and triceps muscles are retracted and the CSA and paired venae comitantes identified (Figure 13-5).

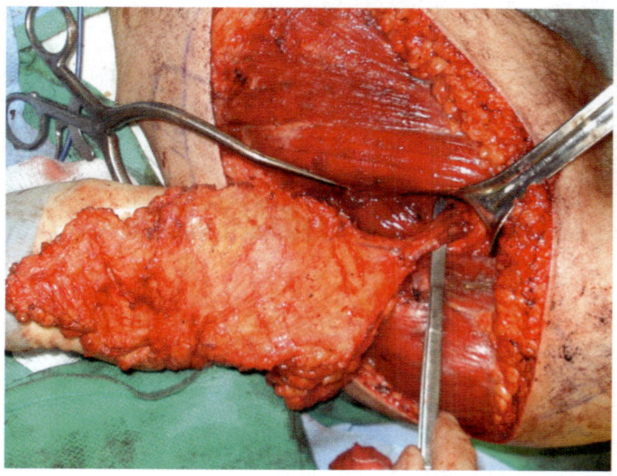

FIGURE 13-5 Proximal dissection of the pedicle is carried out with sequential Gelpy retractors. Careful attention is paid when dividing the branches to the periosteum of the scapula in a purely soft tissue flap. Proximal dissection of the pedicle is carried to the junction of the thoracodorsal artery to attain length while preserving continuity with the subscapular artery.

The muscular branches to the teres major and minor muscles are divided as well as the infrascapular branches. Proximal pedicle dissection is generally carried to the junction with the TDA to preserve continuity with the subscapular artery. The TDA can be divided, leaving the CSA in continuity with the subscapular system for maximal pedicle length. The authors prefer to maintain continuity between the TDA and subscapular artery for latissimus and serratus perfusion.

If vascularized bone is to be included, the dissection is carried out to identify the descending muscular branch off of the CSA along the axillary border of the scapula. The fibers of the teres major are divided at their origin to leave a small cuff of muscle enveloping the artery. The appropriate sized segment of bone is harvested with an osteotome or sagittal saw, preserving continuity of the periosteal perforators with the CSA and venae comitantes. The inferior third of the axillary border of the scapula receives periosteal vascular supply directly from the TDA; thus, if continuity is maintained between the TDA and the CSA in dissecting the pedicle, two separate vascularized segments may be included in the flap design.

TRICKS AND TIPS FROM THE AUTHOR

The authors prefer the patient be in a supine position on the operating table, with a bump under the left shoulder. A sterile ether screen is suspended and draped with a Mayo stand drape, two Kerlex, and a Coban. The arm is included in the prep, draped with a stockinet, and wrapped with two sterile Kerlix wraps and suspended from the sterile screen with Cochers at the elbow and wrist. The table can then be rotated away from the operator as needed.

The flap is designed with the patient positioned with a bump under the ipsilateral shoulder and the arm abducted at 90 degrees to put tension on the teres major. The tip of the scapula is palpated as well as the border of the latissimus muscle, the teres major, and the lateral border of the scapula. The width of the teres muscle is approximately two fingers breadth, or 4 cm, and parallel to the lateral border of the scapula. The triangular space is located at the edge of the scapula at a height of two finger breadths above an axis formed by the lateral border of the scapula. The widest portion of the skin paddle is positioned over the triangular space where the pedicle is expected.

CLOSURE OF THE DONOR SITE

This particular donor site is commonly closed primarily in a multilayered fashion over a 19-Fr Blake drain. A skin paddle width greater than 8 to 10 cm may make direct closure of the donor site challenging. The use of a skin graft is associated with contour deformity, posterior unfavorable scarring, and decreased graft take because of mobility of the scapula. If a vascularized bone flap from the axillary border of the scapula is included, reattachment of the teres major may be necessary. If a larger donor site skin paddle is anticipated, tissue expansion may be included to achieve primary closure of the donor site. Alternatively, Liu and colleagues described their use of a free-style pedicled TDA perforator flap for donor site closure of a large parascapular free flap (8), essentially extending the back scar but avoiding tension on the closure or skin grafting.

DONOR SITE COMPLICATIONS

The parascapular flap is a versatile tool in reconstruction because it may be harvested as a fasciocutaneous or osteocutaneous flap with or without dorsal thoracic fascial extensions to tailor to a variety of complex defects. With this in mind, a number of possible complications and adverse effects have been described. The most common of these is an unfavorable scar. The donor site is most often closed primarily, and with tension or the mobility of the shoulder, there can be widening of the scar or, rarely, delayed healing. Additionally, seroma, hematoma, and infection are rare complications. Scapular dyskinesis, weakness of internal and external shoulder rotation, and limited range of motion have all been discussed with division of the teres muscles and harvest of scapular bone with this flap. Roll and colleagues reported specifically on their experience with parascapular flap donor site complications in a series of 20 patients and found three patients to have limited shoulder function, two patients with delayed wound healing, and one patient with a brachial plexus neuropathy related to prolonged shoulder abduction (9). The most common complication seen in our practice is unfavorable posterior scar, although this is not been a complaint of most patients.

RECONSTRUCTIVE INDICATIONS

Given the variability of tissue that can be incorporated into the parascapular and scapular flaps, these are the flaps of choice for a variety of complex, multidimensional defects, including orbital, skull base, midfacial, and mandibular bony reconstruction, as well as soft tissue reconstruction as in cases of hemifacial microsomia or atrophy (Figure 13-6). Additionally, parascapular and scapular flaps have been used in reconstruction of upper and lower extremity defects, both with or without bone, and in limb salvage (10,11). In particular, scapular and parascapular flaps have been described as a workhorse for facial soft tissue reconstruction in patients with Parry-Romberg syndrome, Treacher Collins syndrome, and other conditions causing facial asymmetry or deficiency (12–15) (Figures 13-7 to 13-9). This flap system has been described for use in oromaxillofacial and oromandibular defects requiring an intraoral lining, bone, and an external skin paddle for coverage, including sinus obliteration, alveolar reconstruction, or periorbital or skull base support (4,16–19). Particularly useful for head and neck reconstruction, the scapular flap has been described with up to 14 cm of bone harvest from the lateral border with bone stock dense enough

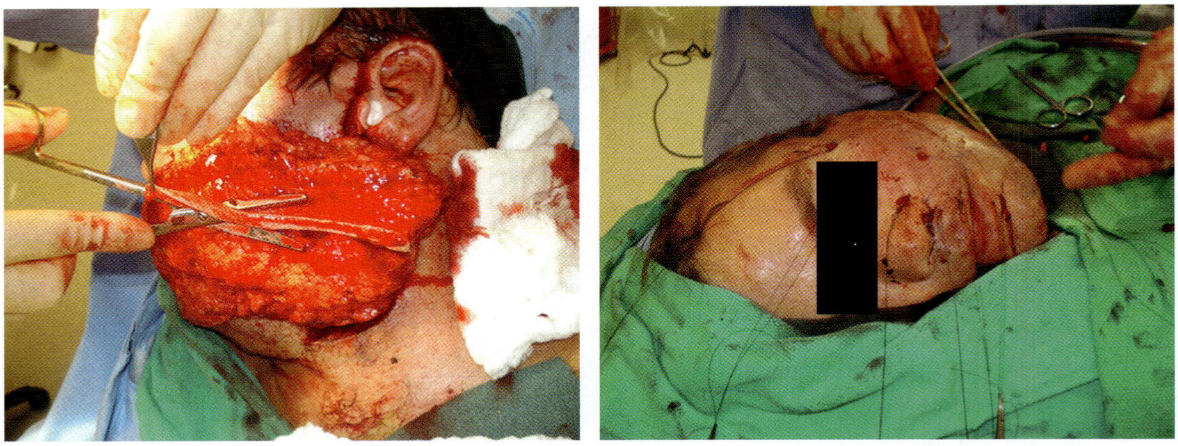

A B

FIGURE 13-6 (**A**) The parascapular and scapular flap has become a workhorse in facial reconstruction. The authors recommend deepithelializing the flap and tailoring the distal margins. (**B**) The flap is inset with tie-over bolsters. See Chapter 34 for more detailed description of facial reconstruction.

to take osseointegrated implants or dental implants (20,21), although it is not as reliable as the fibula for use with dental implants or if osteotomies of the bone are required for shaping. It is particularly useful with bone for reconstructive cases of the mandibular ramus requiring soft tissue. Depending on the patient body habitus, this flap offers a reliable volume of tissue for larger soft tissue reconstruction.

Evaluation of the patient also includes eliminating any associated shoulder pathology, restricted motion, or vascular insufficiency. A previous history of axillary node dissection or mastectomy may call into question the viability of the vascular supply to the flap.

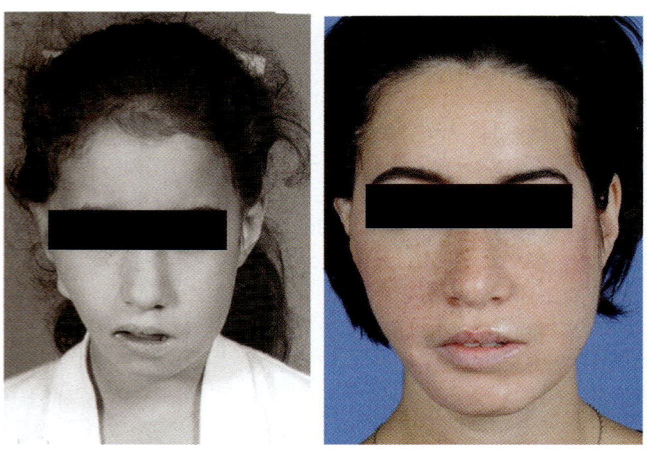

A B

FIGURE 13-7 (**A**) Preoperative frontal view of a 6-year-old girl with right-sided hemifacial microsomia. She underwent facial reconstruction with a scapular flap, including a portion of bone to reconstruct the mandibular ramus. She went on to have distraction osteogenesis of the right mandible, including the portion of transferred scapula and overlying soft tissue fascia. (**B**) Postoperative frontal view 20 years after reconstruction.

COMPARISON OF FLAP WITH SIMILAR FREE TISSUE TRANSFER

Similar flaps may be designed to correct the variety of tissue defects addressed by the parascapular flap, including the anterolateral thigh, superficial inferior epigastric artery, superficial circumflex iliac artery, and deep circumflex iliac artery, among others. The parascapular flap, with its dorsal thoracic fascial extensions, offers customizable tissue thickness with the ability to correct severe soft tissue defects separated within the same flap. It allows fascia, subcutaneous fat, and skin based on distinct, robust branching patterns that are unmatched elsewhere in the body. The scapular flap should be considered when a straight bone segment is needed but a

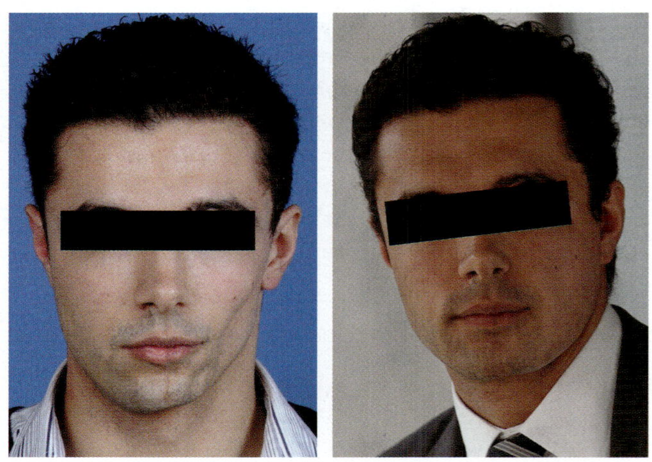

A B

FIGURE 13-8 (**A**) Preoperative frontal view of a 24-year-old man with left-sided hemifacial atrophy. He underwent free tissue transfer with an ipsilateral parascapular flap. (**B**) Postoperative frontal view 2 years after reconstruction.

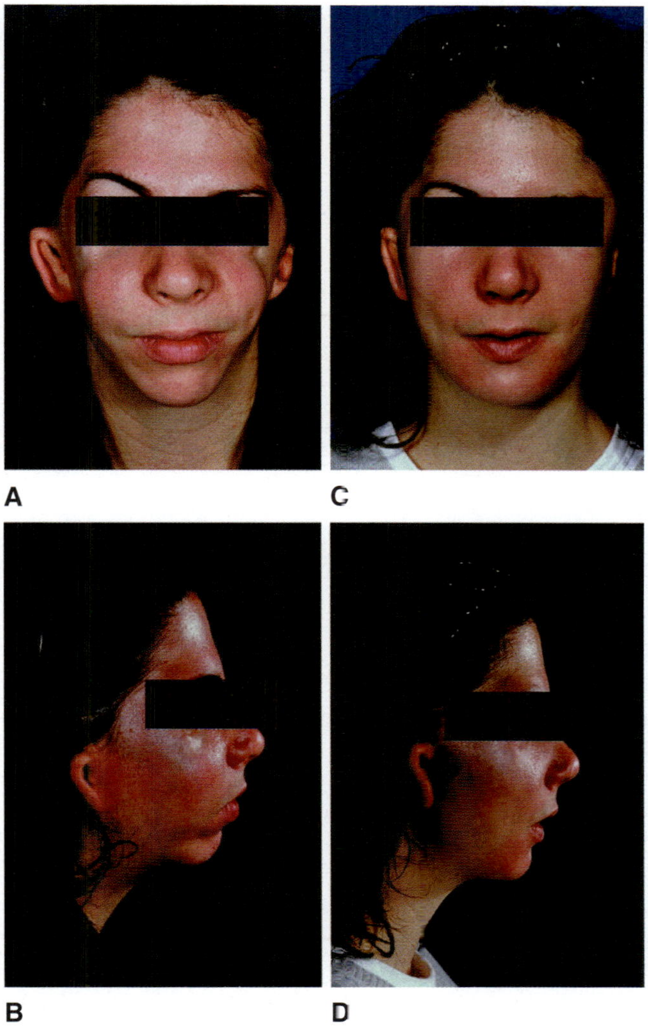

FIGURE 13-9 A 19-year-old woman with Treacher Collins syndrome who had previously undergone multiple nonvascularized reconstructive procedures. (**A**) Preoperative frontal view. Note the severe bilateral maxillary deficiency, which is worse on the left. (**B**) Preoperative lateral view. (**C**) Postoperative frontal view 7 years after staged bilateral parascapular flap reconstruction. Secondary procedures included flap debulking and genioplasty. (**D**) Postoperative lateral view. (Reproduced with permission from Saadeh PB, Chang CC, Warren SM, et al. Microsurgical correction of facial contour deformities in patients with congenital malformations: a 15-year experience. *Plast Reconstruct Surg* 2008;121(6):368e–378e.)

fibula is not available because of vascular insufficiency or inadequate collateral circulation in the lower extremity or if there is a concern for donor site morbidity associated with the iliac crest.

REFERENCES

1. Saijo M. The vascular territories of the dorsal trunk: a reappraisal for potential flap donor sites. *Br J Plast Surg* 1978;31(3):200–204.
2. dos Santos LF. The vascular anatomy and dissection of the free scapular flap. *Plast Reconstr Surg* 1984;73(4):599–604.
3. Gilbert A, Teot L. The free scapular flap. *Plast Reconstr Surg* 1982;69(4):601–604.
4. Batchelor AG, Sully L. A multiple territory free tissue transfer for reconstruction of a large scalp defect. *Br J Plast Surg* 1984;37(1):76–79.
5. Swartz WM, Banis JC, Newton ED, et al. The osteocutaneous scapular flap for mandibular and maxillary reconstruction. *Plast Reconstr Surg* 1986;77(4):530–545.
6. Coleman JJ III,Sultan MR. The bipedicled osteocutaneous scapula flap: a new subscapular system free flap. *Plast Reconstr Surg* 1991;87(4):682–692.
7. Siebert JW, Longaker MT, Angrigiani C. The inframammary extended circumflex scapular flap: an aesthetic improvement of the parascapular flap. *Plast Reconstr Surg* 1997;99(1):70–77.
8. Liu Y, Song B, Jin J, et al. A freestyle pedicled thoracodorsal artery perforator flap aiding the donor-site closure of a parascapular flap. *J Plast Reconstr Aesthet Surg* 2010;63(3):e280–e282.
9. Roll C, Prantl L, Feser D, et al. Functional donor-site morbidity following (osteo-) fasciocutaneous parascapular flap transfer. *Ann Plast Surg* 2007;59(4):410–414.
10. Cerkes N, Erer M, Sirin F. The combined scapular/parascapular flap for the treatment of extensive electrical burns of the upper extremity. *Br J Plast Surg* 1997;50(7):501–506.
11. Chen D, Jupiter JB, Lipton HA, Li SQ. The parascapular flap for treatment of lower extremity disorders. *Plast Reconstr Surg* 1989;84(1): 108–116.
12. Longaker MT, Siebert JW. Microvascular free-flap correction of severe hemifacial atrophy. *Plast Reconstr Surg* 1995;96(4):800–809.
13. Longaker MT, Siebert JW. Microsurgical correction of facial contour in congenital craniofacial malformations: the marriage of hard and soft tissue. *Plast Reconstr Surg* 1996;98(6):942–950.
14. Saadeh P, Reavey PL, Siebert JW. A soft-tissue approach to midfacial hypoplasia associated with Treacher Collins syndrome. *Ann Plast Surg* 2006;56(5):522–525.
15. Saadeh PB, Chang CC, Warren SM, et al. Microsurgical correction of facial contour deformities in patients with craniofacial malformations: a 15-year experience. *Plast Reconstr Surg* 2008;121(6):368e–378e.
16. Chiu ES, Sharma S, Siebert JW. Salvage of silicone-treated facial deformities using autogenous free tissue transfer. *Plast Reconstr Surg* 2005;116(5):1195–1203; discussion 1204–1205.
17. Upton J, Albin RE, Mulliken JB, Murray JE. The use of scapular and parascapular flaps for cheek reconstruction. *Plast Reconstr Surg* 1992;90(6):959–971.
18. Urken ML, Weinberg H, Buchbinder D, et al. Microvascular free flaps in head and neck reconstruction. Report of 200 cases and review of complications. *Arch Otolaryngol Head Neck Surg* 1994;120(6):633–640.
19. Urken ML, Bridger AG, Zur KB, Genden EM. The scapular osteofasciocutaneous flap: a 12-year experience. *Arch Otolaryngol Head Neck Surg* 2001;127(7):862–869.
20. Frodel JL Jr, Funk GF, Capper DT, et al. Osseointegrated implants: a comparative study of bone thickness in four vascularized bone flaps. *Plast Reconstr Surg* 1993;92(3):449–455; discussion 456–458.
21. Moscoso JF, Keller J, Genden E, et al. Vascularized bone flaps in oromandibular reconstruction. A comparative anatomic study of bone stock from various donor sites to assess suitability for endosseous dental implants. *Arch Otolaryngol Head Neck Surg* 1994;120(1):36–43.

CHAPTER 14

The Free Groin Flap

Robert I.S. Winterton, Waseem Bhat, and Simon P.J. Kay

The use of an axial pattern flap based on the superficial circumflex iliac artery (SCIA) and the superficial venous network of the groin was first reported by McGregor and Jackson in 1972 (1). Their seminal paper provided the first anatomical description of this flap.

During the early 1970s, the groin flap was initially used as a pedicled flap. The axial pattern flaps described by McGregor and Morgan in 1973 (2) stimulated the development of free tissue transfer using microvascular techniques, and the first use of the groin for microsurgical reconstruction was reported by Daniel and Taylor (3), who transferred a flap based on the superficial inferior epigastric artery (SIEA). In the same year, O'Brien described a free groin flap based on the SCIA (4). The groin flap is of particular historical interest because it was the first fasciocutaneous free flap performed successfully in a human subject (3). The groin flap is thin, especially if harvested in the flexural crease, and the donor scar is well disposed compared with other flaps. The advantageous donor site is the reason this flap has been particularly popular in women and children, with the flap having been successfully transferred in children as young as 3 months old (5). The reconstructive potential of the flap increased when it was discovered that it could safely be raised as an osseofasciocutaneous flap by including the iliac bone (6). The flap can be lateralized to make it less bulky and used successfully as a mega-flap to cover very large defects. Additionally, it has been used solely as a cutaneous flap by leaving the fascia behind, which also allows for optimization of the donor site. The free groin flap is most useful for skin and fat transfer and is not generally combined with other tissues as a composite or chimera flap.

Its use has gradually declined over the past decade, in part because of technical difficulties such as a variable vascular origin and narrow-caliber vessels but also because of the development of other donor sites and the recent advances in the potential of perforator-based flaps. However, this flap remains a safe reconstructive modality, providing a large area of soft, pliable, generally hairless skin, with the advantage of an excellent donor site.

Despite passing through a phase of varying popularity, it will certainly remain part in the essential repertoire of microsurgeons because of its availability and uniquely satisfactory donor site.

ANATOMY

The free groin flap is centered over the axis of the superficial circumflex iliac vessels. Both cadaveric and clinical studies investigating this vasculature have demonstrated considerable anatomical variation (7–9).

The work of Taylor and Daniel (7) on 100 cadaveric dissections provides the most descriptive account of the vascular anatomy in this region. They showed that in 14%, there was a common origin of the SCIA and SIEA, and in 17%, there was a separate origin of the SIEA and SCIA. In 35%, the SIEA was absent, and there was a large SCIA, and in 17% cases, the artery arose from vessels other than the femoral. Figure 14-1 shows common variations in the origin of the SCIA and SIEA vessels. In only one third of dissections was the anatomy symmetrical on either side. With regards to the size of the vessel: in 87%, the artery diameter was larger than 1 mm; it was exactly 1 mm 11% of the time; and it was smaller than 1 mm in 2% cases. The vascular variations in this region have become notorious and have been the subject of much scrutiny. It is, however, the authors' opinion and experience that it is not necessary to know this anatomy before raising the flap in individual cases but that the surgeon may rely upon there being an SCIA present, and by raising the flap from lateral to medial, the surgeon will discover the anatomy in the fullness of time without compromising his or her dissection.

As the SCIA leaves the femoral triangle, it passes for a short length from deep to superficial before turning laterally and crossing parallel to the inguinal ligament, approximately one patient's thumb breadth caudal, before reaching the medial

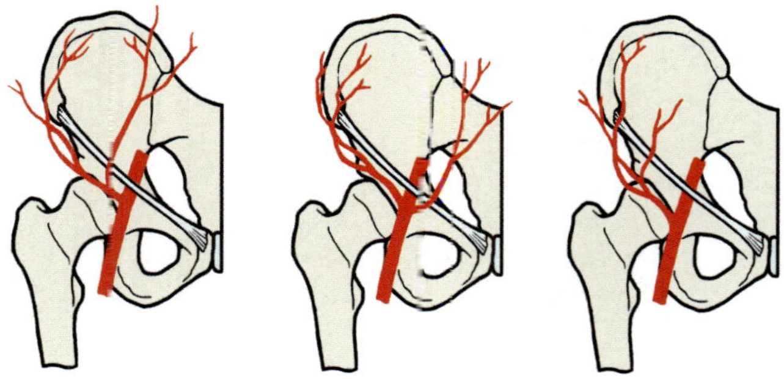

FIGURE 14-1 The three most common variations in the vascular anatomy of the origin of the superficial circumflex iliac artery (SCIA) and superficial inferior epigastric artery systems.

border of the sartorius. It continues its course laterally, but before it does so, it gives a constant branch that pierces the fascia investing sartorius. This branch supplies the muscle but in addition sends its greater contribution along the same axis as the SCIA but deep to the sartorius fascia. This vessel that runs deep to the sartorius fascia terminates in a perforator lateral to the lateral cutaneous nerve of thigh (Figure 14-2), and this perforator must be included in larger flaps that extend lateral to a line passing vertically through the anterior superior iliac spine (ASIS) or include the fat pad that lies immediately caudal to be lateral iliac crest. Because this perforator arises lateral to the lateral cutaneous nerve of the thigh, this nerve must inevitably be divided and repaired to allow inclusion of this perforator in the flap. Inclusion of this lateral perforator is not required in smaller flaps limited in lateral extent to a line passing through the ASIS.

Particular care should be taken to understand the venous anatomy of this flap. The superficial circumflex iliac vein (SCIV) and the superficial inferior epigastric vein (SIEV) are usually located superficial to Scarpa's fascia. The SCIV in most cases drains into the long saphenous vein adjacent to the saphenofemoral junction (10), but the SCIV and SIEV may alternatively join to form one large vein that joins the femoral vein directly (11). The vein draining the flap is most definitely not the long saphenous vein itself, which may be found in the medial extent of the flap and may tempt the surgeon by its easy availability and large size. This vein only drains the most medial third of the flap, and reliance on it will result in venous infarction distally (laterally).

The SCIA venae comitantes are small and can seem daunting at first to the microsurgeon. However, careful preparation of the vessels will allow this vein to be dissected cephalad toward the inguinal ligament, and it will then be appreciated that there is a substantial length of vein of acceptable caliber if required.

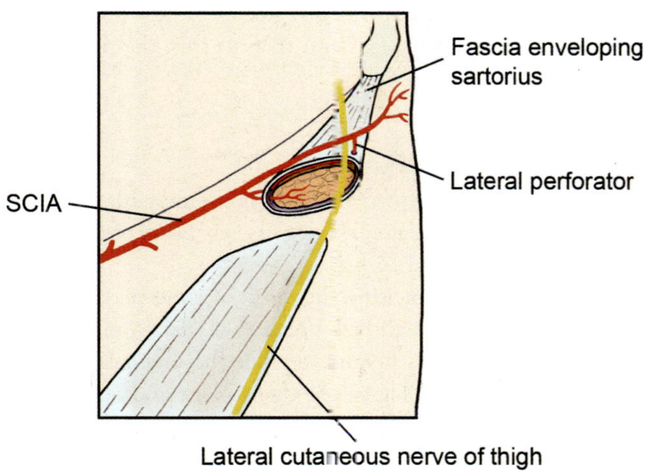

FIGURE 14-2 The relationship of the lateral cutaneous nerve of the thigh, sartorius fascia, and superficial circumflex iliac artery (SCIA) perforator that passes lateral to the nerve before piercing the fascia and entering the flap.

Superficial Circumflex Iliac Artery

The SCIA is 1.5 to 3.0 cm in length and has a diameter of 0.8 to 2.0 mm (7). Although the groin skin can be supplied by multiple systems, the main supply for the flap is by the SCIA. The SCIA arises from the anterolateral aspect of the femoral artery within the femoral triangle 2 to 3 cm below the inguinal ligament in close proximity to the origin of the superficial epigastric, circumflex femoral, and profunda femoris arteries. The SCIA runs lateral, inferior, and parallel to the inguinal ligament, initially running superior the iliacus fascia toward the medial border of the sartorius muscle, where it divides into the deep and superficial branches.

The superficial branch runs superficial to the sartorius fascia, continuing laterally to supply the skin beyond the ASIS, and then heads cranially toward the midaxial line. The deep branch perforates the sartorius fascia at the medial border and runs superolaterally until it reaches the lateral border of the sartorius, where it becomes suprafascial, giving off several perforators in the anterolateral part of the groin.

The groin flap based on the direct cutaneous perforators from the SCIA has been a workhorse in reconstructive surgery since it was first described in 1972 (1,12). This flap has the advantage of being easy to dissect in experienced hands, given the superficial nature of the source artery, but the flap is subject to having a variable length and caliber artery. The SCIVs are of a large caliber and can be incorporated into the flap to augment venous drainage (13).

Superficial Inferior Epigastric Artery

The SIEA has a length of 4 to 7 cm and a diameter of 0.75 to 3.5 mm (7). THE SIEA is a direct cutaneous perforator artery from the anterior aspect of the common femoral artery. The vessels are found 1 to 3 cm below the inguinal ligament as either an independent trunk or together with the SCIA (7). The artery perforates the deep fascia of the femoral triangle and passes superiorly and laterally in the subcutaneous tissue superficial to the linea semilunaris.

When a dominant SIEA is present, it can reach an external diameter of 2 mm, and its course may run approximately 10 cm into the integument before arborizing into terminal lateral and medial branches. These terminal branches form anastomoses with perforators of the deep epigastric artery and lateral branches of the posterior intercostal arteries.

Recent work has shown that the SIEA can be identified in 72% of specimens, and the arterial diameter is 1.6 mm (0.75–3.5 mm) at the level of the inguinal ligament. In 58% of cases, the artery is present bilaterally. The length of the pedicle ranges from 4 to 7 cm (14).

Venous Drainage (Superficial Circumflex Iliac Vein)

The SCIV has a length of 2 to 4 cm and a diameter of 1.5 to 2 mm (7). The groin is drained by two systems, the SCIV and the SIEV. Both of these are located superficial to Scarpa's fascia. The main drainage of the region is the SCIV, which runs into the femoral triangle superficial to the artery. The SCIV and SIEV in many cases join to form a common trunk with a diameter of 2.5 mm (10). Rarely does the SCIV drain directly into the femoral vein, with most instances draining into the saphenous system (10).

The vena comitantes are generally small vessels. If only one vein is present, the average size is 0.5 to 1.8 mm, and if two are present, than the size ranges from 0.2 to 1.8 mm. If the two veins join to form a common trunk, the size of the vessels can range from 0.4 to 2.8 mm (10).

Anatomy of the Regional Nerves

The groin is supplied by the segmental branches of T12 and L1. These cross the iliac crest 5 cm posterior to the ASIS. The lateral femoral cutaneous nerve of the thigh emerges medial to the ASIS and passes deep to the flap. Care must be taken to preserve this. Generally, no sensory nerves are included in the flap, but the lateral cutaneous branch of intercostal nerve T12 can be included if required.

Doppler Mapping

The anatomy of the region can be variable, and preoperative Doppler ultrasonography or duplex color investigation may be useful in detecting the exact location of the SIEA and SCIA vascular systems and determining which one is dominant. Several authors advocate its use (8,15), and they suggest that the presence of a weak signal would contraindicate the use of the flap. It is not the authors' normal practice to map the SCIA or its perforators, having found that in clinical practice in more than 100 cases, the vessel is constant and the perforator is reliable. However, where a very narrow flap is to be raised or for a surgeon undertaking their first few flaps of this sort, Doppler mapping is very simple and can reliably indicate the SCIA and the perforator lateral to the lateral cutaneous nerve of the thigh. It also serves to emphasize that the course of the artery is not transverse from medial to lateral but that it passes obliquely in a proximal and lateral course to run parallel to the inguinal ligament.

TECHNIQUE FOR FLAP HARVEST

Flap Design

The flap should be designed after the key anatomical landmarks have been marked. These include the inguinal ligament identified as passing between the palpable pubic tubercle and the ASIS. The axis of the artery is one thumb's breadth caudal to the inguinal ligament, and the flap is centered on this line. A standard flap can be extended up to 10 cm beyond the ASIS, especially if bone is to be harvested with the flap. Wide flaps of 10 cm or more may still allow their donor sites to be closed primarily (Figure 14-3).

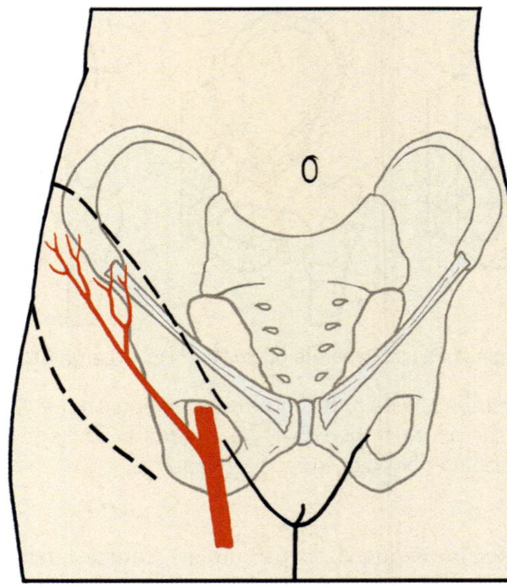

FIGURE 14-3 The design of a standard groin flap.

The pedicle's origin overlies the femoral artery, and some of the flap may extend medially to this if required (although adult hair patterns should be anticipated). Equally, the skin paddle of the flap need not overlie the origin of the pedicle provided it includes at least one perforator from the region of the lateral thigh or lateral sartorius muscle, which may allow a longer pedicle to be dissected. Usually, however, the flap will be centered over the axis of the vessel and will overlie the origin of the pedicle.

Where a narrow flap is to be chosen (most often when selecting a small flap to resurface the first web space of the hand), it is prudent either to use Doppler to confirm the exact location of the pedicle and vascular axis or to raise a wider flap to be sure to include the axis and then to trim the flap before transfer.

Raising the Flap

The preferred position of the patient is supine with a padded sand bag under the ipsilateral hip to ease exposure of the lateral aspect of the flap (Figure 14-4).

Surgery begins by incising the entire perimeter of the skin flap (Figure 14-5). The authors prefer to dissect from lateral to medial, and meticulous hemostasis must be maintained at all times. Any bleeding will stain the tissue plane and obscure the distinctions necessary for a successful elevation of the flap. The senior author raises the flap with a monopolar diathermy until the femoral triangle is reached when he reverts to scissor dissection aided by bipolar diathermy. By this means, it is possible to keep a virtually bloodless field and identify every structure (Figure 14-6).

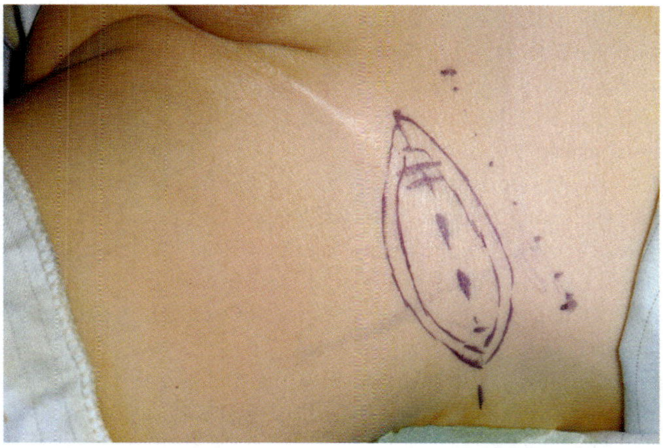

FIGURE 14-4 The preoperative markings of the flap before dissection. The axis of the flap is one patient's thumb breadth below the inguinal ligament, passing obliquely cephalad and lateral, parallel to the inguinal ligament, and need not overlie the vascular origin.

In flaps that include significant tissue overlying the lateral hip, as one moves from lateral to medial, a decision must be made whether to harvest just superficial fat or that fat pad (of different appearance and consistency) that fills the hollow below the iliac crest. For most instances, elevation of the flap at the level of the superficial fascia suffices, and this plane leads one directly onto the fascia investing the lateral thigh and sartorius. As the lateral border of sartorius is approached, a vessel will be seen coursing on the fascial undersurface of the flap and arising from a large perforator lateral to the lateral cutaneous nerve of the thigh. Depending on the amount of tissue lateral to this point, a decision must be made whether to include this perforator in the flap. Doing so necessitates division of the lateral cutaneous nerve of the thigh.

We will first consider the case in which this perforator is not included in the flap. In these circumstances, the perforator is divided, and the flap elevation continues in the plane immediately superficial to the fascia investing sartorius muscle. Through this fascia may be seen the corresponding deep vessel described as the deep branch of the SCIA above. When the dissection

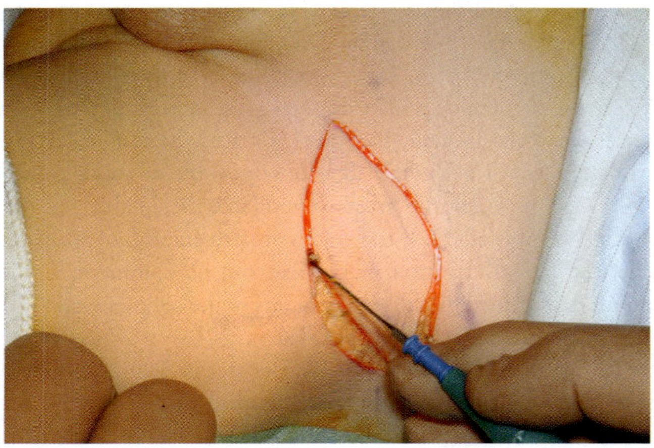

FIGURE 14-5 The entire flap incised, and dissection proceeds with monopolar diathermy, thus maintaining meticulous hemostasis to preserve anatomical detail.

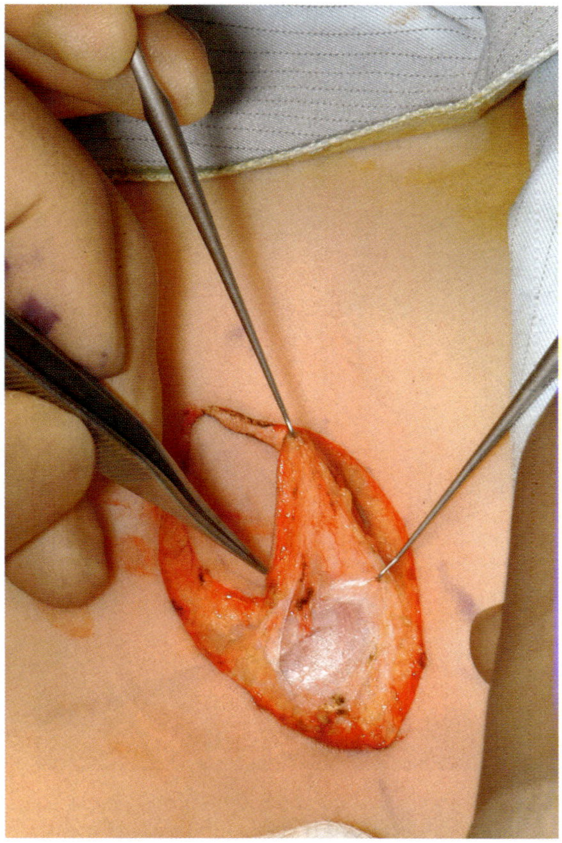

FIGURE 14-6 The flap is raised from lateral to medial in an almost bloodless field. The perforator arising lateral to the lateral cutaneous nerve of thigh has been sharp divided in this case and will be repaired.

reaches the medial border of sartorius, this deep branch of the SCIA that pierces the muscle must be carefully divided. At this point, dissection switches to blunt gentle separation of the tissues and bipolar cautery as the pedicle passes superficial to the femoral nerve and the source of the pedicle is approached.

The superior, inferior, and medial borders of the flap are also dissected toward the same point. After being identified at the lateral border of sartorius, the SCIA is visible and can now confidently be traced down to the femoral artery (Figure 14-7). This vessel is always found arising from the femoral artery, so advanced knowledge of the anatomy is not required. At the same time, one preserves the accompanying vein but divides the superior and inferior branches, including the SIEA if it arises from the same pedicle. The vessels are skeletonized at this point, and the vein will be found to have a variable course of running toward the femoral vein but often first coursing parallel to the femoral artery over some distance. When the vessels are the only attachments remaining, the vascularity of all territories of the flap is confirmed before final division of the pedicle (Figure 14-8). At the point of pedicle division, it is the senior author's practice to clip and divide the vein, ensuring there is greater length on the vein than the artery, to protect it from tension after anastomosis at the recipient site. This allows the vein to fill and become turgid before division of the artery, which may prove helpful in selecting the diameter of the recipient vein where a choice exists.

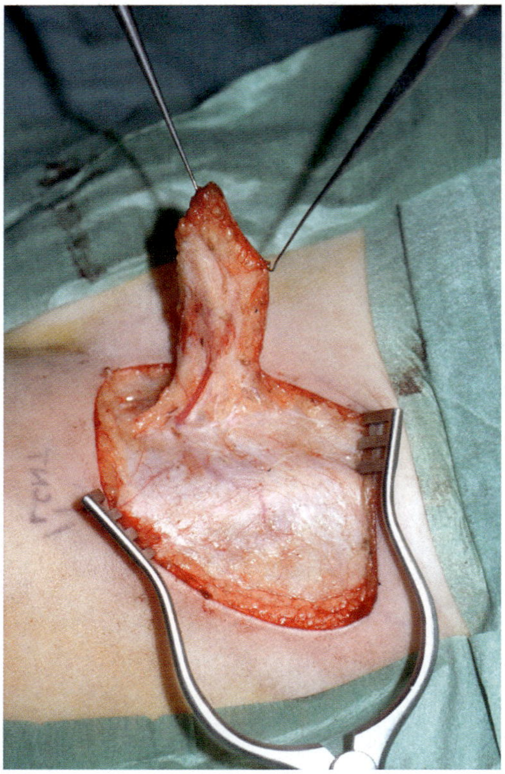

FIGURE 14-7 The flap raised above the sartorius fascia. The vascular pedicle is clearly visible on the underside of the flap.

Although when first approached, the SCIA at its junction with the femoral artery may seem surprisingly large and robust to an inexperienced surgeon, by the time of division, it may seem less so. The authors' practice is to place a Satinsky aneurysm clamp on the femoral artery to completely isolate this vascular junction and then to harvest the flap by incising with microsurgical scissors a diamond-shaped cuff of femoral vessel. Before removal of the artery clamp, the small defect can be closed directly with a fine monofilament vascular suture. This cuff offers greater choice at the time of vascular repair at the recipient site.

Returning to the situation in which the lateral perforator is included with the flap, the lateral cutaneous nerve of the thigh must be divided and repaired. The authors' preference is to divide this away from the axis of the flap and therefore position the subsequent neurosynthesis in a position not directly beneath the donor site scar. The perforator and the deep branch of the SCIA, which runs deep to the sartorius fascia, are elevated until the medial border of sartorius is approached. Here the branch directly into muscle is divided and the connection between the SCIA and the subfascial vessel preserved, whence the dissection proceeds as described earlier.

In 2004, Koshima et al. (13) described a superficial circumflex iliac perforator flap (SCIP flap) based on this vessel alone. Their paper describes using the flap for reconstruction of limb defects, and it has subsequently been used as a sensate flap in head and neck reconstruction (16). The dissection of a fasciocutaneous paddle laterally allows for a predictably hairless flap to be raised and allows a longer vascular pedicle to be dissected for cases in which a short vascular pedicle would not suffice.

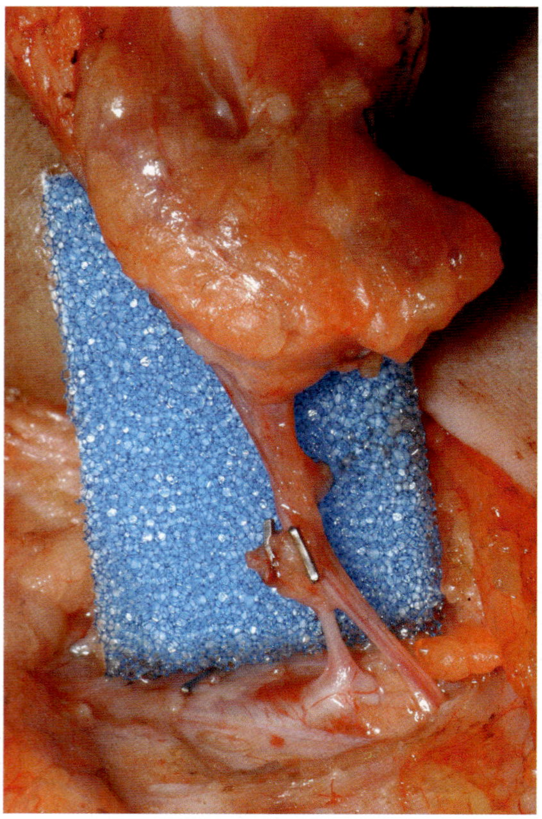

FIGURE 14-8 The flap raised on the vascular pedicle alone.

Alternative Technique

Some authorities hold that dissection of the groin flap from medial to lateral allows the surgeon to quickly ensure the vascular supply for the flap is adequate (9,12). In this technique, the initial incision passes over the femoral vessels, and the incision is extended inferiorly to define the long saphenous vein. This is then traced superiorly to just before its termination in to the femoral vein, where it receives the SCIV emerging in the superficial subcutaneous plane. The SCIV is traced into the flap to allow access to the arterial system, which is situated laterally and in a deeper plane. The femoral artery is progressively cleared until the origin of the SCIA is located, usually 1 cm below the inguinal ligament on the lateral side. After the SCIA origin has been located, the vessel is traced laterally to clear a workable length of pedicle. It is now possible to make a decision as to whether the arteriovenous axis is suitable for free groin flap transfer (9). If the vessels are present and of adequate size, the lateral elevation of the flap can be commenced, the extent determined by the requirements of the recipient site. The flap is thinned laterally to the ASIS.

Although it is tempting for the novice raising this flap to start medially and confirm the anatomy of the vessels, the authors urge the lateral to medial approach. The problem with medial exploration first is that it is very easy to mistake the vessels and come upon them abruptly or unexpectedly and so injure them. If the dissection proceeds from lateral to medial, the course of the vessels is progressively revealed, and their origin can be reached rapidly and safely.

Closure of the Donor Site

The limitation of the groin flap size is generally that which can be closed directly because the main attraction of this flap is the hidden donor site. When closed, this usually leaves the linear scar just caudal to the inguinal skin crease, which may pass laterally around the flank. If a flap of any size has been harvested, then it is usual to close the wound over a suction drain in three layers. For donor sites where large flaps have been raised, slight hip flexion can be helpful to reduce the tension while closing the wound. The hip can then be extended over the course of a few days, with the decision regarding walking delayed until the wound seems stable (1).

POSTOPERATIVE CARE

The recipient site is managed as for any flap, with monitoring of the flap viability according to local protocols (17). Any indication of flap compromise should warrant immediate reexploration, following the dictum "things are a lot worse than they look" (15).

No specific care is required for the donor site, but seromas may be managed by aspiration if they become painful for the patient or develop any signs of infection. The postoperative outcome of the donor site is generally regarded as excellent because the scar is hidden or concealed with clothing.

Patients should generally expect to remain in the hospital for up to 1 week, which depends on the indication for the procedure.

ADVANTAGES AND DISADVANTAGES OF THE FREE GROIN FLAP

Advantages

One of the main advantages of the groin flap remains the minimal donor defect left after it is raised (Figure 14-9). The scar is easily concealed with clothing, and although it may stretch over time, this can be easily revised if the patient so desires.

Just as with the pedicled groin flap, the size of the free groin flap can be remarkable. A very large area of groin skin is supplied by the SCIA vessels, and free flaps larger than 30 × 15 cm can be transferred. The limitation is most commonly that which can be closed primarily rather than the vascular territory itself. Where a very large flap is required, the skin territory may be extended by including the SIEA flap territory, or alternatively, it may be extended on the lateral flank in continuity with a latissimus dorsi musculocutaneous flap, furnishing a very long wide flap that can resurface a very major part of one limb.

The time taken to raise the flap is relatively short, and may usually be undertaken without recourse to turning the patient if the recipient site can be reached in the supine position. The flap is also hairless, excepting the most medial part of the flap.

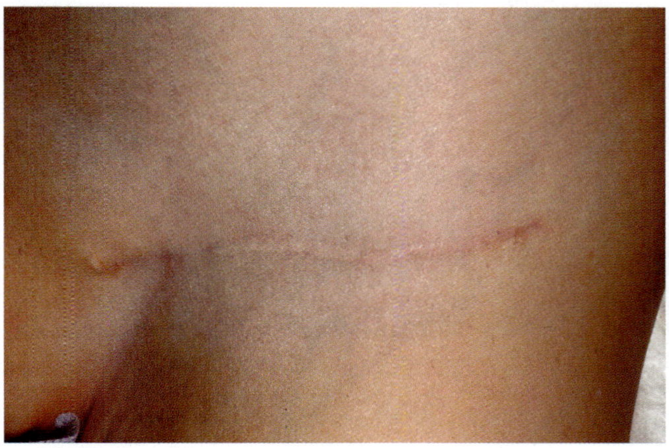

FIGURE 14-9 The healed donor site in a child.

Disadvantages

There can be technical difficulties such as a variable vascular origin, narrow-caliber vessels, and short pedicle length; however, when designed properly and raised judiciously, the resultant flap is expected to do well.

The reconstruction may on occasion be too bulky, thus requiring secondary procedures for optimal esthetic outcome. The color of the groin flap is also paler than many other skin areas, leading to a potential color mismatch.

Subcutaneous seroma is a common complication of the donor site, and patients can develop meralgia paresthetica (18), a sensory neurologic disorder presenting as dysesthesia over the anterolateral aspect of thigh caused by neuritis of the lateral femoral cutaneous nerve of the thigh. Entrapment of the nerve in scar tissue is another cause of meralgia paresthesia. In most cases, this will improve in time and does not present a significant postoperative problem provided the patient is pre-warned of the event.

RECONSTRUCTIVE INDICATIONS FOR THE GROIN FLAP

The groin flap based on the SCIA or SIEA can be applied for many reconstructive purposes, some examples of which are:

- Epithelial defect closure of all types (Figures 14-10 and 14-11)
- Deepithelialized flaps may be used to reconstruct subcutaneous volume defects such as in Poland's syndrome and hemifacial atrophy.
- Osteofasciocutaneous flaps may be used to reconstruct defects of the wrist and forearm (6) or large mandibular defects (19).
- The groin flap may form part of a "mega-flap" to cover large defects where one flap is not sufficient. For instance, the flap may be used in continuity with a latissimus dorsi free flap (20,21) or the tensor fascia lata myocutaneous flap (22).
- Unusually, this flap may be used to transfer vascularized lymph nodes for upper or lower extremity edema treatment.

GROIN FLAPS IN CHILDREN

Harii and Ohmori (23) published the first report of free groin flap use in children in 1975, using it to cover defects after lower limb trauma. Two years later, Ohmori et al. (5) reported

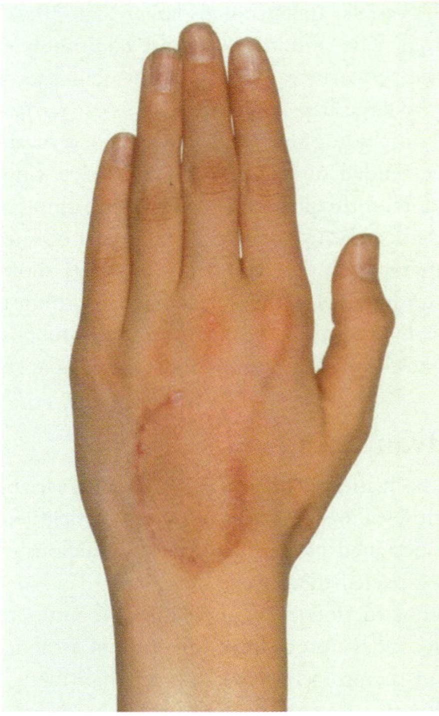

FIGURE 14-10 Closure of an extravasation injury defect on the dorsum of the hand.

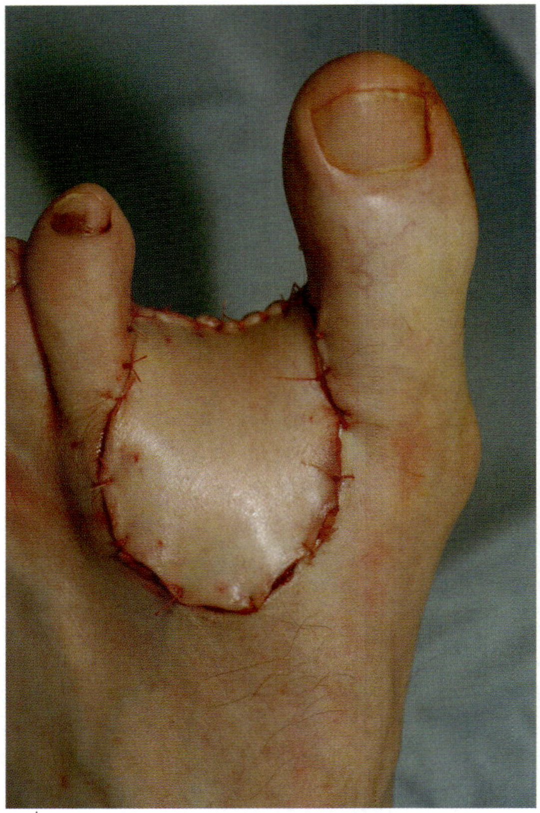

FIGURE 14-11 Closure of a defect after resection of the second toe for malignancy.

successful use of a free groin flap after a burn injury to the upper limb in a 3-month-old baby. Since then, free groin flaps have been widely used for the reconstruction of congenital hand anomalies (Figure 14-12), reconstruction of trauma wounds including exposed metalwork after fracture fixation (Figure 14-13), reconstruction of skin after burn scar contracture release, and soft tissue coverage after excision of osteomyelitis.

All types of microvascular procedure have been undertaken in children, including premature babies, and neither vessel size nor patient age is a contraindication to surgery. In a series of 22 microvascular transfers in children, Parry et al. (24) found that vessel size in children (0.8–1.5 mm compared with

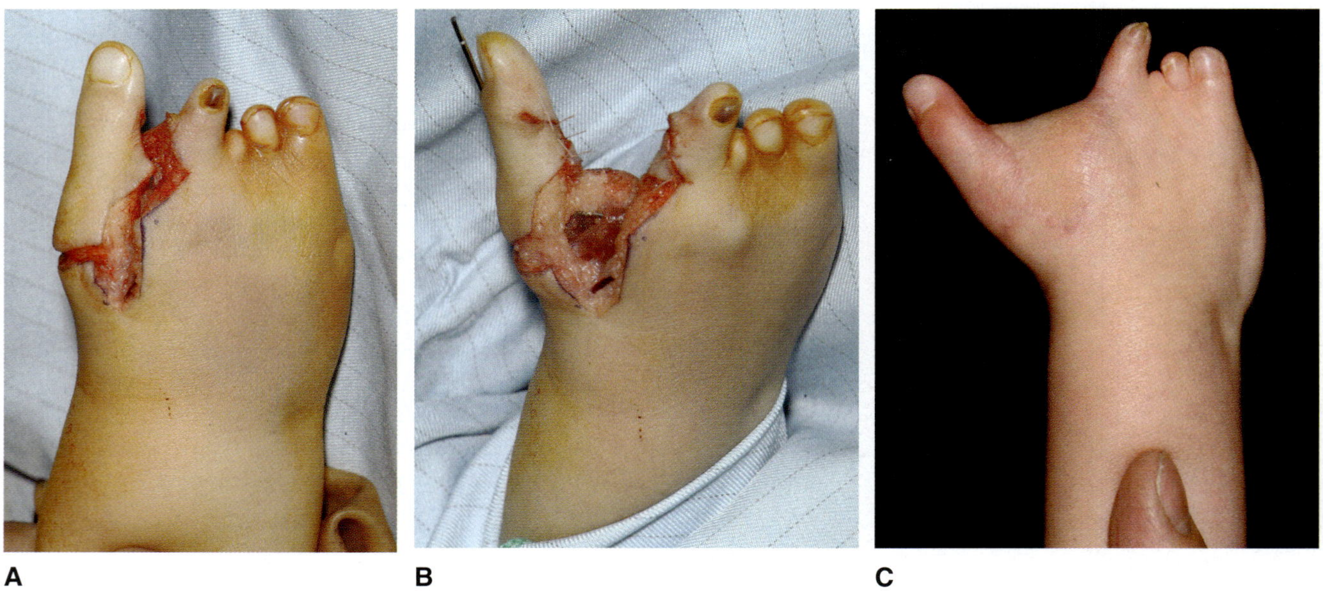

FIGURE 14-12 A child's hand with the digits approximated too closely for a useful pincer grip (**A**). After separation of the digits and a rotation osteotomy (**B**), a groin flap is used to reconstruct the defect to good effect (**C**). This case in which the recipient vessels lie within the wound is ideal for the groin flap because pedicle length is not an issue.

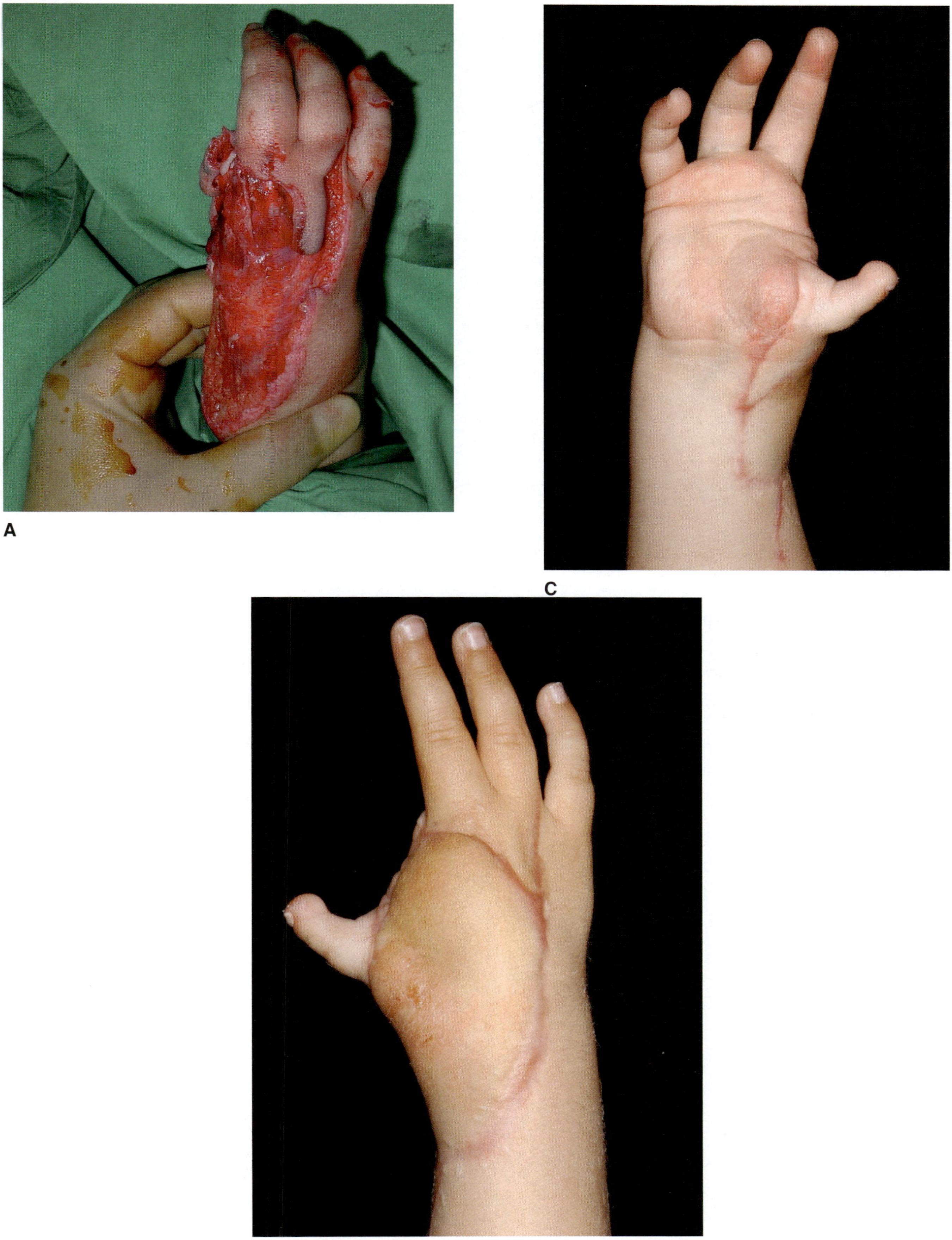

FIGURE 14-13 A child's hand after an injury that has obliterated the index finger and thumb along with dorsal soft tissue (**A**). Reconstruction with free groin flap and the free second toe results in a functional and well-balanced hand (**B** and **C**).

1.0–3.0 mm in adults) posed no technical problems. Similarly, vessel size was not a limiting factor in a series of 43 microvascular procedures performed at the authors' institution (25) with the smallest anastomoses being 0.4 mm.

The groin flap can be a very good option for reconstruction in children with excellent success rates, and furthermore, it need not be associated with any more risk than seen in adults (26,27).

CONCLUSION

The free groin flap is a classic workhorse flap and should form part of the repertoire for most microsurgical practitioners. The flap may initially seem daunting to raise given that the vasculature can be variable and of narrow caliber, but careful planning allows this flap to be raised safely and experience allows it to be raised relatively quickly. The donor site is excellent, and the free groin flap is a potentially large and versatile flap suitable for a wide variety of reconstructive indications.

REFERENCES

1. McGregor IA, Jackson IT. The groin flap. *Br J Plast Surg* 1972;25:3–16.
2. McGregor IA, Morgan G. Axial and random pattern flaps. *Br J Plast Surg* 1973;26:202–213.
3. Daniel RK, Taylor GI. Distant transfer of an island flap by microvascular anastomoses. A clinical technique. *Plast Reconstr Surg* 1973;52:111–117.
4. O'Brien BM, MacLeod AM, Hayhurst JW, Morrison WA. Successful transfer of a large island flap from the groin to the foot by microvascular anastomoses. *Plast Reconstr Surg* 1973;52:271–278.
5. Ohmori K, Harii K, Sekiguchi J, Torii S. The youngest free groin flap yet? *Br J Plast Surg* 1977;30:273–276.
6. Acarturk S, Ozmen E. Composite osteo-cutaneous groin flap for the reconstruction of wrist and forearm defects. *Br J Plast Surg* 1984;37:388–393.
7. Taylor GI, Daniel RK. The anatomy of several free flap donor sites. *Plast Reconstr Surg* 1975;56:243–253.
8. Baudet J, LeMaire JM, Guimberteau JC. Ten free groin flaps. *Plast Reconstr Surg* 1976;57:577–595.
9. Omori K, Harii K. Free groin flaps: their vascular basis. *Br J Plast Surg* 1975;28:238–246.
10. Penteado CV. Venous drainage of the groin flap. *Plast Reconstr Surg* 1983;71:678–684.
11. Goodstein WA, Buncke HJ Jr.Patterns of vascular anastomoses vs. success of free groin flap transfers. *Plast Reconstr Surg* 1979;64:37–40.
12. O'Brien B MW. *Microvascular Reconstructive Surgery.* Edinburgh: Churchill Livingstone, 1977.
13. Koshima I, Nanba Y, Tsutsui T, et al. Superficial circumflex iliac artery perforator flap for reconstruction of limb defects. *Plast Reconstr Surg* 2004;113:233–240.
14. Ninkovic M. *Superficial Inferior Epigastric Artery Perforator Flap.* St Louis: Quality Medical Publishing, 2006.
15. Karkowski J, Buncke HJ. A simplified technique for free transfer of groin flaps, by use of a Doppler Probe. *Plast Reconstr Surg* 1975;55:682–686.
16. Iida T, Mihara M, Narushima M, Koshima I. A sensate superficial circumflex iliac perforator flap based on lateral cutaneous branches of the intercostal nerves. *J Plast Reconstr Aesthet Surg* 2012;65:538–540.
17. Winterton RI, Pinder RM, Morritt AN, et al. Long term study into surgical re-exploration of the "free flap in difficulty." *J Plast Reconstr Aesthet Surg* 2010;63:1080–1086.
18. Moscona AR, Hirshowitz B. Meralgia paresthetica as a complication of the groin flap. *Ann Plast Surg* 1980;4:161–163.
19. Harrison TJ, Quillen CG. Free osteocutaneous groin flap in the reconstruction of large mandibular defects. A case study. *Arch Otolaryngol* 1983;109:485–488.
20. Harii K, Iwaya T, Kawaguchi N. Combination myocutaneous flap and microvascular free flap. *Plast Reconstr Surg* 1981;68:700–711.
21. Dzwierzynski WW, Sanger JR, Matloub HS, Yousif NJ. Combination latissimus dorsi and groin free flap with double microvascular transfer. *Ann Plast Surg* 1995;34:631–634.
22. Watson AC, McGregor JC. The simultaneous use of a groin flap and a tensor fasciae latae myocutaneous flap to provide tissue cover for a completely degloved hand. *Br J Plast Surg* 1981;34:349–352.
23. Harii K, Ohmori K. Free groin flaps in children. *Plast Reconstr Surg* 1975;55:588–592.
24. Parry SW, Toth BA, Elliott LF. Microvascular free-tissue transfer in children. *Plast Reconstr Surg* 1988;81:838–840.
25. Devaraj VS, Kay SP, Batchelor AG, Yates A. Microvascular surgery in children. *Br J Plast Surg* 1991;44:276–280.
26. Hough M, Fenn C, Kay SP. The use of free groin flaps in children. *Plast Reconstr Surg* 2004;113:1161–1166.
27. Pinder RM, Hart A, Winterton RI, et al. Free tissue transfers in the first 2 years of life—a successful cost effective and humane option. *J Plast Reconstr Aesthet Surg* 2010;63:616–622.

CHAPTER 15

Anterolateral Thigh and Tensor Fascia Lata Flaps

Peirong Yu

ANTEROLATERAL THIGH FLAPS

The anatomy of the anterolateral thigh (ALT) flap was first described in Chinese literature in 1983 by Zhou et al. (1). The same group of investigators provided more detail on the anatomy and clinical applications of the flap in the following year (2–4). The first report in the English literature appeared in the *British Journal of Plastic Surgery* in 1984 (5). This flap did not gain popularity for more than a decade, although several case reports were published from China and Japan in the late 1980s and early 1990s (6–10). The main reason for the delayed adaption of this flap was thought to be the rather confusing and inconsistent anatomy of the vascular pedicle. In the early 1990s, however, Japanese authors reported larger series of the ALT flap, and the perforator flap concept was introduced (10–12). Since then, this flap gradually gained attention among reconstructive surgeons (13–22). However, the ALT flap did not reach the same enthusiasm in Western countries because of the variations of vascular anatomy, tedious perforator dissection, and a difficult and steep learning curve. In 2004, a simple perforator classification system was introduced by the author (23,24), making it much easier to learn for beginners. Because of obesity in Western countries, this flap can be too thick, and flap thinning is sometimes required. The concept of flap thinning was first introduced by Koshima et al. in 1993 (11) and Kimura et al. in 2001 (19). Because of the unique vascular anatomy, several components including skin and muscle can be included in the same flap; thus, the Chimeric flap concept was introduced by Koshima in 1993 (11,12). In the past several years, the ALT flap has become one of the most popular soft tissue flaps for various applications. It is particularly useful for head and neck reconstruction.

Anatomy of the Anterolateral Thigh Flap

Arterial Anatomy

The lateral circumflex femoris artery from the profundus femoris artery gives rise to three branches: the ascending branch to the gluteus minimus muscle, the transverse branch to the tensor fascia lata (TFL) muscle, and the descending branch to the vastus lateralis muscle. In most (96%) cases, the main pedicle artery of the ALT flap is the descending branch of the lateral circumflex femoris artery (Figure 15-1). The descending branch sends out one to three cutaneous perforators to supply the ALT flap skin (type I) (Figures 15-2 and 15-3). The descending branch usually travels in the intermuscular space between the rectus femoris and the vastus lateralis and intermedius muscles. Soon after its take-off from the lateral circumflex femoris artery, it sends out a rectus femoris branch supplying the rectus femoris muscle and another branch supplying the vastus intermedius muscle (Figure 15-4). The main descending branch continues to descend along the medial edge of the vastus lateralis muscle and sends out numerous branches to supply this muscle. The diameter of the descending branch is usually between 2 and 2.5 mm immediately below the rectus femoris branch and 2.5 to 3.5 mm above the rectus femoris branch.

In 2% of cases, the cutaneous perforator derives from the transverse branch of the lateral circumflex femoris artery (type II) (Figures 15-2 and 15-5). The perforator travels longitudinally within the vastus lateralis muscle for its entire length before it enters the fasciocutaneous flap and requires tedious intramuscular dissection for a long distance. To obtain a larger pedicle vessel, the transverse branch needs to be included.

In the remaining 2% of cases, the cutaneous perforators pierce the rectus femoris muscle and derive from the rectus femoris branch of the descending branch (type III)

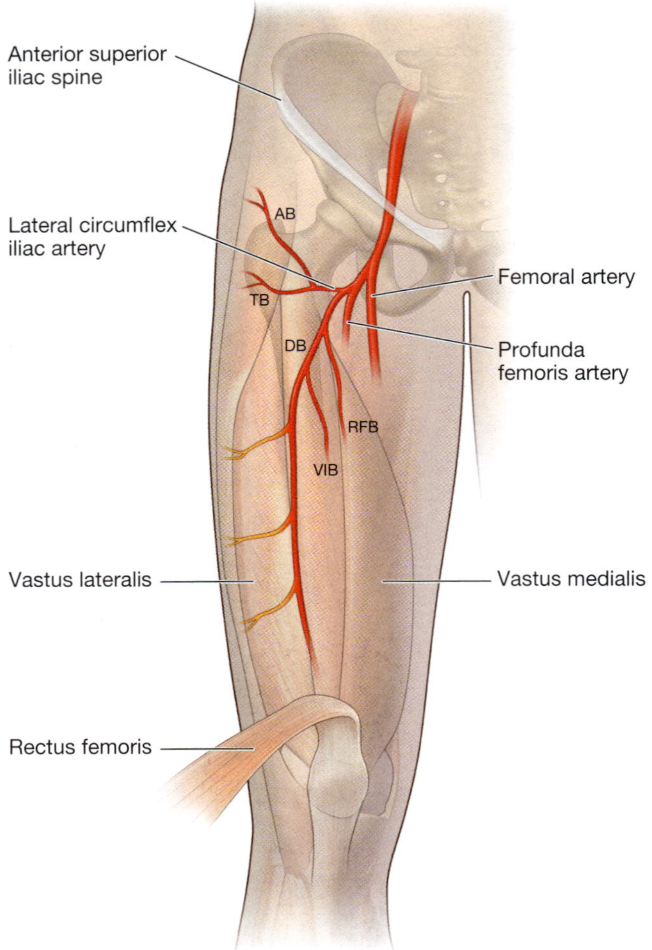

FIGURE 15-1 Anatomy of the lateral circumflex femoris artery and its branches. AB, ascending branch; ASIS, anterior superior iliac spine; DB, descending branch; LCF, lateral circumflex femoris artery; PFA, profundus femoris artery; RF, rectus femoris muscle; RFB, rectus femoris branch; SFA, superficial femoral artery; TB, transverse branch; VIB, vastus intermedius branch.

(Figure 15-6). The perforator can be traced back through intramuscular dissection to the main vessel.

Venous Anatomy

Two venae comitantes accompany the perforator artery and then travel alongside the descending branch artery throughout its course. There are numerous H connections between the two venae comitantes; therefore, using either one of them should provide adequate venous drainage. The two venae comitantes usually converge above the rectus femoris branch of the descending branch artery. Immediately below their convergence, the medial venae comitante is usually slightly larger than the lateral one with a diameter from 2 to 3.5 mm. After the two venae comitantes converge, the vein is significantly larger, with a diameter from 3 to 5 mm.

Sensory Nerve Anatomy

The lateral femoral cutaneous nerve (L2–L3) can be included with the flap for sensory reinnervation. This nerve enters the thigh through the lateral end of the inguinal ligament and travels in the plane immediately above the deep fascia (Figure 15-7). At approximately 10 cm below the inguinal ligament, the nerve branches into a lateral branch and a medial branch. The former continues to travel along or lateral to the line connecting the anterior superior iliac spine (ASIS) and the supralateral corner of the patella (AP line), and the latter turns medially and descends approximately 2 to 3 cm medial to the AP line. The lateral branch is within the ALT flap and can be taken for sensory reinnervation while the medial one can be left intact. The diameter of the femoral cutaneous nerve in the proximal thigh before the bifurcation is usually between 1.5 and 2 mm.

Motor Nerve Anatomy

Various amounts or even the entire vastus lateralis muscle can be included in the ALT flap when indicated. Several motor nerves derive from the femoral nerve innervate the vastus lateralis muscle. One of the main motor nerve branches travels closely with the vascular pedicle, the descending branch. Proximal in the thigh, the motor nerve travels lateral to the descending branch vessels (see Figure 15-4). Before the descending branch vessels enter the vastus lateralis muscle, the motor nerve takes a turn underneath the descending branch and travels medially alongside the descending branch vessels. The nerve then sends out numerous small branches that accompany the vascular branches to innervate the vastus lateralis muscle. The main nerve branch continues to travel alongside the descending branch vessels and eventually terminates in the vastus lateralis muscle. During flap dissection, the motor nerve should be separated from the vessels and preserved if the corresponding muscle is not taken with the flap. The vastus lateralis muscle, however, can be harvested as a functional muscle flap by including the motor nerve.

Perforator Anatomy: The Surface Location of Cutaneous Perforators—The "ABC System"

The surface location of the cutaneous perforators appears to follow a pattern. The perforator that is most consistently present is located near the midpoint of the AP line. Approximately 5 cm more proximal and distal to that, a second and third perforator may be found. Based on this pattern, the location of the cutaneous perforators may be classified as perforator A (most proximal), perforator B (middle), and perforator C (most distal), thus the "ABC system" (Figure 15-8). The average distances (longitudinally, the y-axis) measured from the ASIS to perforators A, B, and C are 18.4 ± 2.2 cm, 23.5 ± 2.0 cm, and 28.6 ± 2.3 cm, respectively, in a Western population (data from 244 ALT free flaps). Therefore, these three perforators are separated from each other by approximately 5 cm (see Figure 15-8).

The measured distance between the ASIS and the cutaneous perforators obviously depends on the height of the patient. The relative location of each perforator between the ASIS and superolateral patella can be determined, with the ASIS being point 0, the superolateral patella being point 1.0 and the midpoint being point 0.5. The location, number, size, and types of perforators are summarized in Table 15-1 and Figure 15-8.

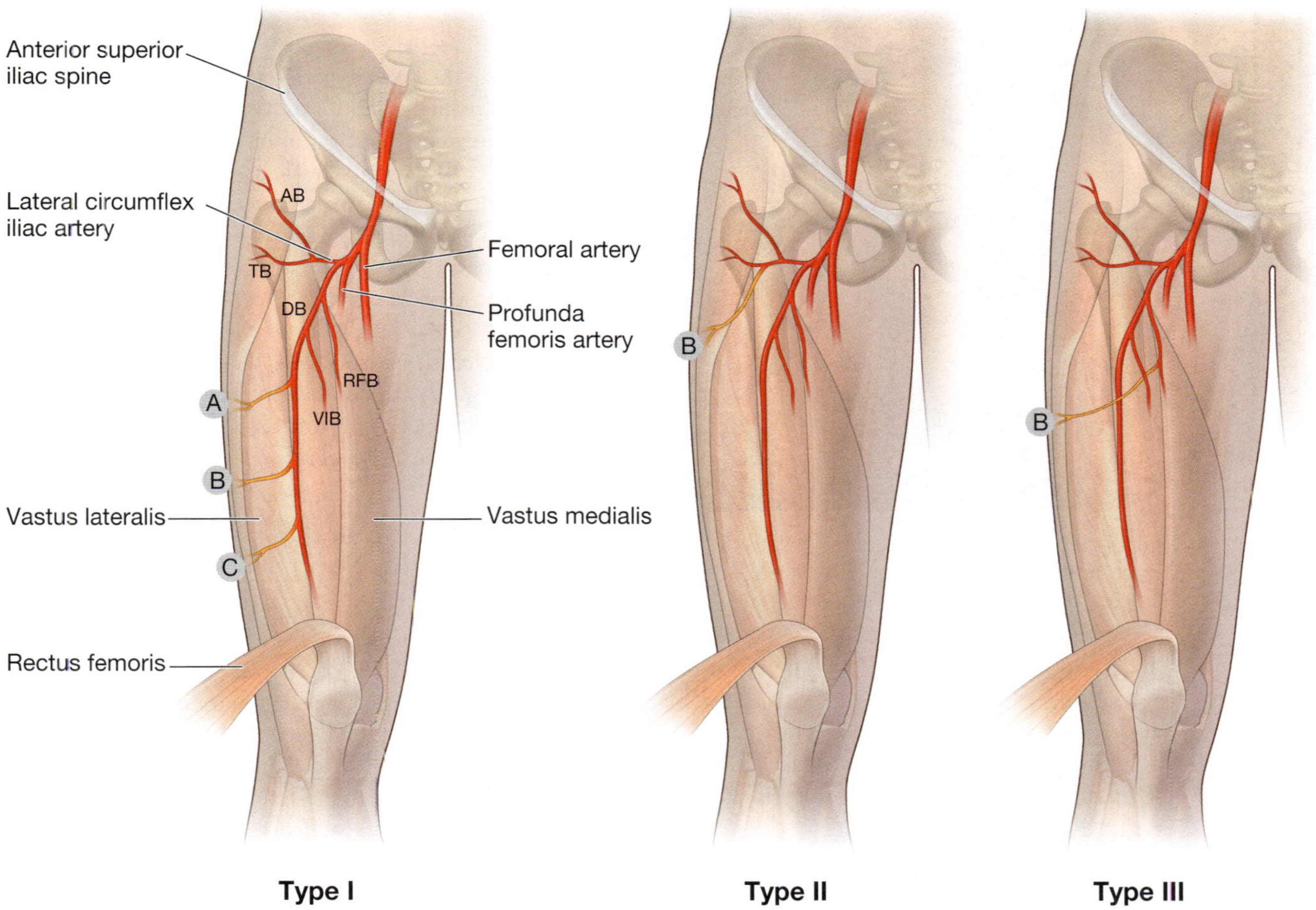

FIGURE 15-2 Types of vascular supply to the anterolateral thigh flap. In type I, perforators originate from the descending branch. In type II, perforators originate from the transverse branch via the vastus lateralis muscle. In type III, perforators originate from the rectus femoris branch via the rectus femoris muscle. AB, ascending branch; ASIS, anterior superior iliac spine; DB, descending branch; LCF, lateral circumflex femoris artery; PFA, profundus femoris artery; RF, rectus femoris muscle; RFB, rectus femoris branch; SFA, superficial femoral artery; TB, transverse branch; VIB, vastus intermedius branch; VL, vastus lateralis muscle; VM, vastus medialis muscle.

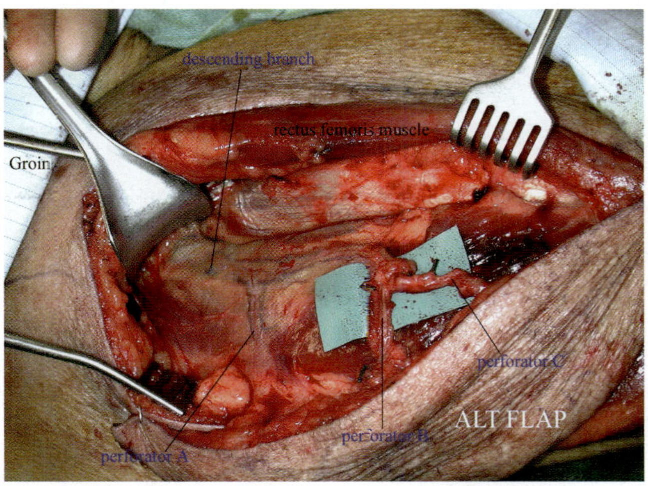

FIGURE 15-3 A type I blood supply to the anterolateral thigh (ALT) flap in which the perforators originate from the descending branch.

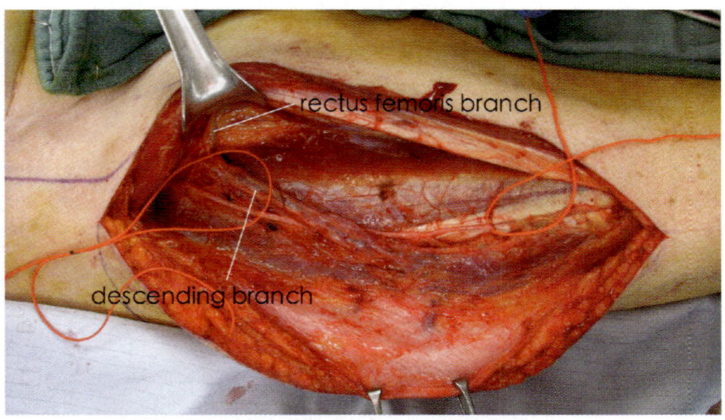

FIGURE 15-4 The descending branch gives rise to the rectus femoris branch that supplies the rectus femoris muscle and travels within the muscle. The motor nerve travels closely with the descending branch.

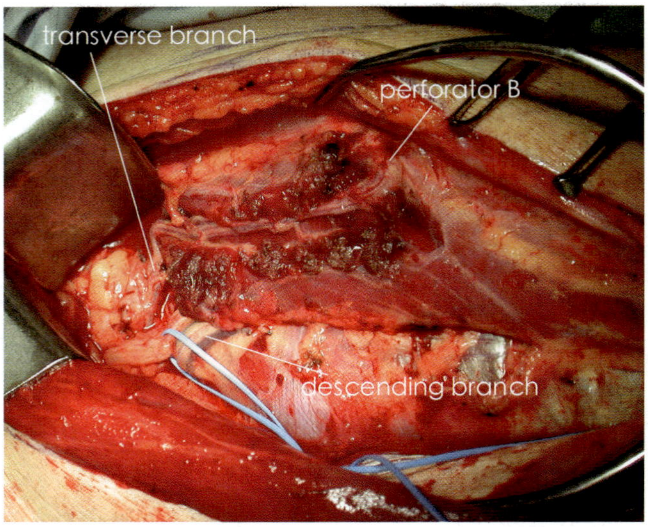

FIGURE 15-5 The cutaneous perforator originates from the transverse branch (type II) and travels within the vastus lateralis muscle for the entire path, making perforator dissection more difficult.

Horizontally (the x-axis), the cutaneous perforators are located, on average, 1.5 cm lateral to the AP line. Twenty-six percent of flaps had a single perforator, most commonly perforator B; 49% had two perforators; and 25% had three perforators (Table 15-2).

Occasionally (12% in our series), although perforators B and C originate from the descending branch, perforator A may originate from the bifurcation of the descending branch and transverse branch (Figure 15-9). This branch is also called the "oblique branch" (25).

Flap Thickness

The ALT flap is consistently thicker proximally, becoming progressively thinner distally (Figure 15-10); the exceptions are very thin flaps (6 mm or less), the thickness of which does not change significantly. The flap thicknesses are 18.3 ± 8.8 mm, 15 ± 7 mm, and 12.5 ± 6.4 mm at the level of perforator A, B, and C, respectively. Compared with the thickness at the level of perforator B, the flap is 20 ± 14% thicker at perforator A and 18.4 ± 11.5% thinner at perforator C.

The mean flap thickness at perforator B in female patients is 19.9 ± 6.9 mm, which is significantly greater (P = 0.004) than that in male patients (12.9 ± 6.0 mm). In contrast, the mean body mass index (BMI) in female patients (24.7 ± 4.3) is slightly lower than that in male patients (26.0 ± 4.4). As a result, the difference in flap thickness per BMI between male and female patients (0.48 ± 0.17 and 0.80 ± 0.20, respectively) is even greater. Overall, flap thickness correlates with BMI fairly well (R = 0.6; P = 0.00001). The correlation is greater in male patients than in female patients. The ALT flap in Asian population is generally much thinner than in the Western population. For instance, the average flap thickness is 6 mm in Japanese man and 10 mm in Japanese women (10,26).

Accuracy of Preoperative Handheld Doppler Examination

As observed by many surgeons, handheld Doppler can be inaccurate. Therefore, a study was conducted to examine the accuracy of two commonly used handheld Doppler devices, the Huntleigh Mini Dopplex D-900 used in the clinic and the Koven ES-100X MiniDoppler with sterile probes used in the operating room, in 100 ALT flaps (24). For perforator B, the Huntleigh had a sensitivity of 100% but a specificity of 0%. The Koven had a sensitivity of 91% and a specificity of 55%. The Doppler signal was within 1 cm of the actual perforator B in approximately 70% of flaps for both Doppler devices. Overall, the Huntleigh was thought to be too sensitive, giving a false-positive signal in all flaps without a perforator, but the Koven is less sensitive and slightly more specific but requires longer time to locate a perforator. After the first 100 ALT flaps, the author no longer uses preoperative Doppler examination for the ALT flap design. The "ABC system" is reproducible and more reliable than the Doppler examination. In thin patients, however, Doppler examination may be more accurate than in obese patients, and the beginners may find it useful in flap design. Because of its low specificity, Doppler examination should be verified with the "ABC system."

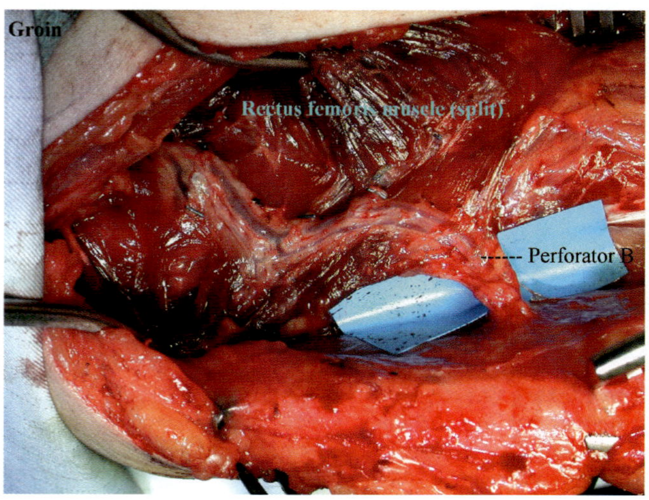

FIGURE 15-6 The perforator originates from the rectus femoris branch and travels within the rectus femoris muscle (type III).

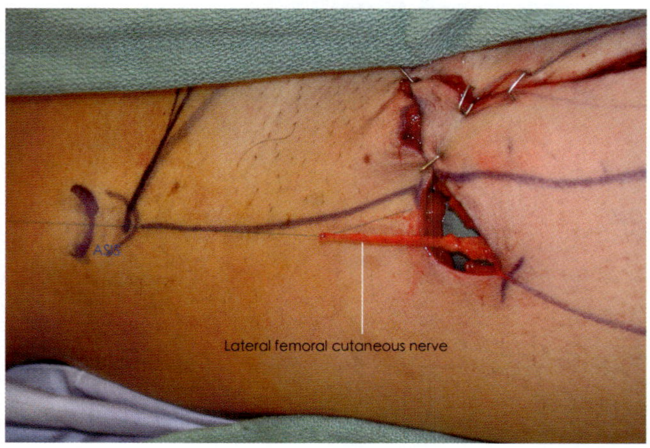

FIGURE 15-7 The lateral femoral cutaneous nerve, a sensory nerve to the anterolateral thigh flap, can be included for sensory innervation.

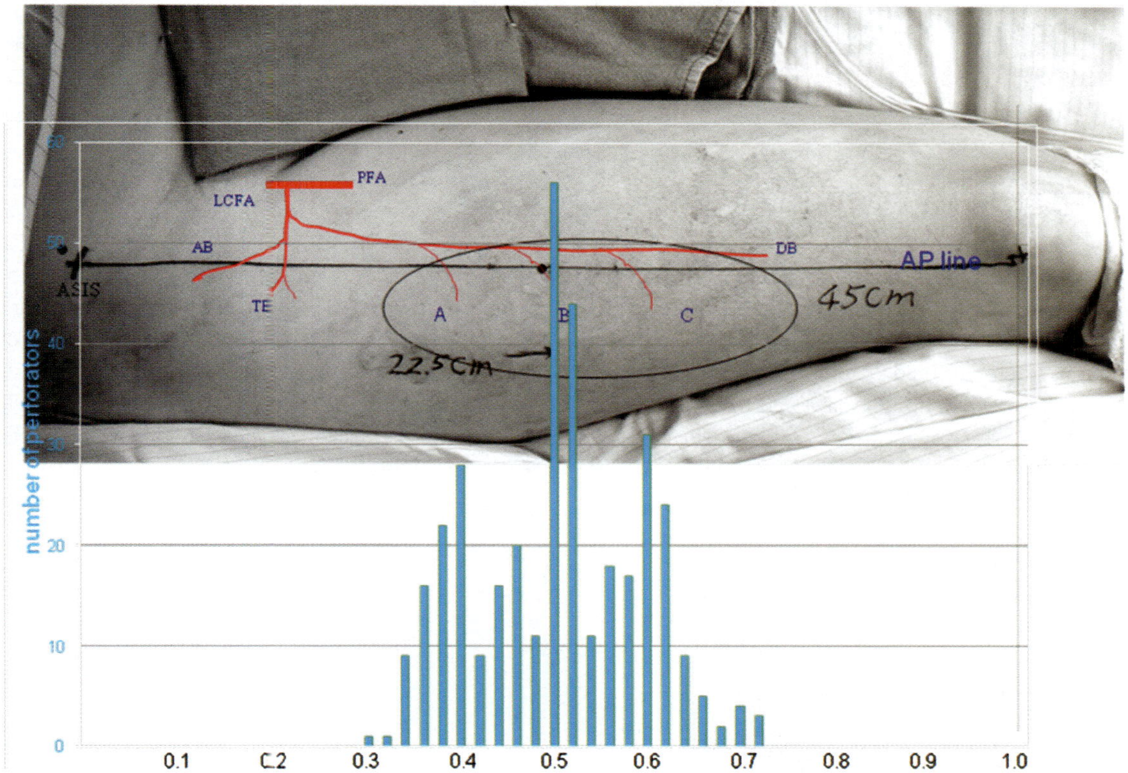

FIGURE 15-8 Surface locations of the cutaneous perforators of the anterolateral thigh flap. Based on the locations, the cutaneous perforators are classified as perforator A, B, and C. AB, ascending branch; ASIS, anterior superior iliac spine; DB, descending branch; LCFA, lateral circumflex femoris artery; PFA, profundus femoris artery; TB, transverse branch.

Surgical Techniques

Patient Positioning

The patient is placed in a supine position on the operating table. With the patient under general anesthesia, the lower extremities tend to rotate outward (supination), making the identification of landmarks and perforators inaccurate and potentially leading to failure of flap harvesting. This is particularly true in obese patients with thick subcutaneous tissue. Therefore, it is critical to place the lower extremity in a neutral position with the knee and foot pointing to the ceiling. To keep the leg in a neutral position, it may be necessary to wrap a towel around the foot and clip the towel to the table or to the towel around the other foot (Figure 15-11). Skin is prepared from the level of the ASIS down to below the patella. It is not necessary to prepare the thigh circumferentially; "table-to-table" preparation of the thigh is adequate.

Flap Design

With the leg in a neutral position, the most prominent point of the ASIS and the supralateral corner of the patella are marked with a marking pen. A straight line is drawn to connect these two landmarks. As mentioned, this is called the AP line. The length of the line is measured and its midpoint is identified. The presumed location of perforator B is then marked 1.5 cm lateral to the AP line and slightly distal (3–5 mm) to the

TABLE 15-1 Perforator Locations and Characteristics Based on 244 Anterolateral Thigh Flaps

Perforators	A	B	C
Presence (%)	53	87	59
Septocutaneous (%)	46	19	12
y-axis	18.4 ± 2.2 cm Point 0.4*	23.5 ± 2.0 cm Point 0.5*	28.6 ± 2.3 cm Point 0.6*
x-axis	1.4 ± 0.6 cm	1.4 ± 0.7 cm	1.5 ± 0.6 cm
Size†: small (%)	18	17	72
Size: medium (%)	27	37	19
Size: large (%)	55	46	9

*Relative location between the anterior superior iliac spine and superolateral patella.
†Small, <0.5 mm; medium, 0.5 to 1 mm; large, >1 mm.

TABLE 15-2 Presence of Perforators

Single: 26%			Double: 49%			Triple: 25%
A	B	C	A + B	B + C	A + C	ABC
3%	20%	3%	18%	24%	7%	25%

midpoint (Figure 15-12). Next, the presumed locations of perforators A and C are marked 5 cm proximal and distal to the presumed perforator B, respectively, in adults. The estimated flap dimension is then outlined, centering on perforator B, bearing in mind that the flap design may need to be recentered based on the actual perforator locations. A handheld Doppler device can be used to help detect perforator B, which may be helpful for beginners and teaching. After perforator B signal is identified, perforators A and C are marked as described earlier. However, handheld Doppler examination can be inaccurate and misleading, also as outlined earlier.

Flap Dissection as a Perforator Flap

An anterior incision approximately 15 cm long spanning across all three presumed perforators is made first down to the fascia over the rectus femoris muscle (Figure 15-13). For a flap width of 7 to 10 cm, the anterior incision is usually 1.5 to 2.0 cm medial to the AP line. The fascia is incised, and subfascial dissection proceeds laterally. Although suprafascial dissection is preferred by some surgeons, subfascial dissection is easier for beginners because the "septum" between the vastus lateralis and rectus femoris muscles can be easily identified in the subfascial plane. In addition, the fascia can be a useful layer of tissue in reconstruction. The fascia is retracted laterally with three Allis

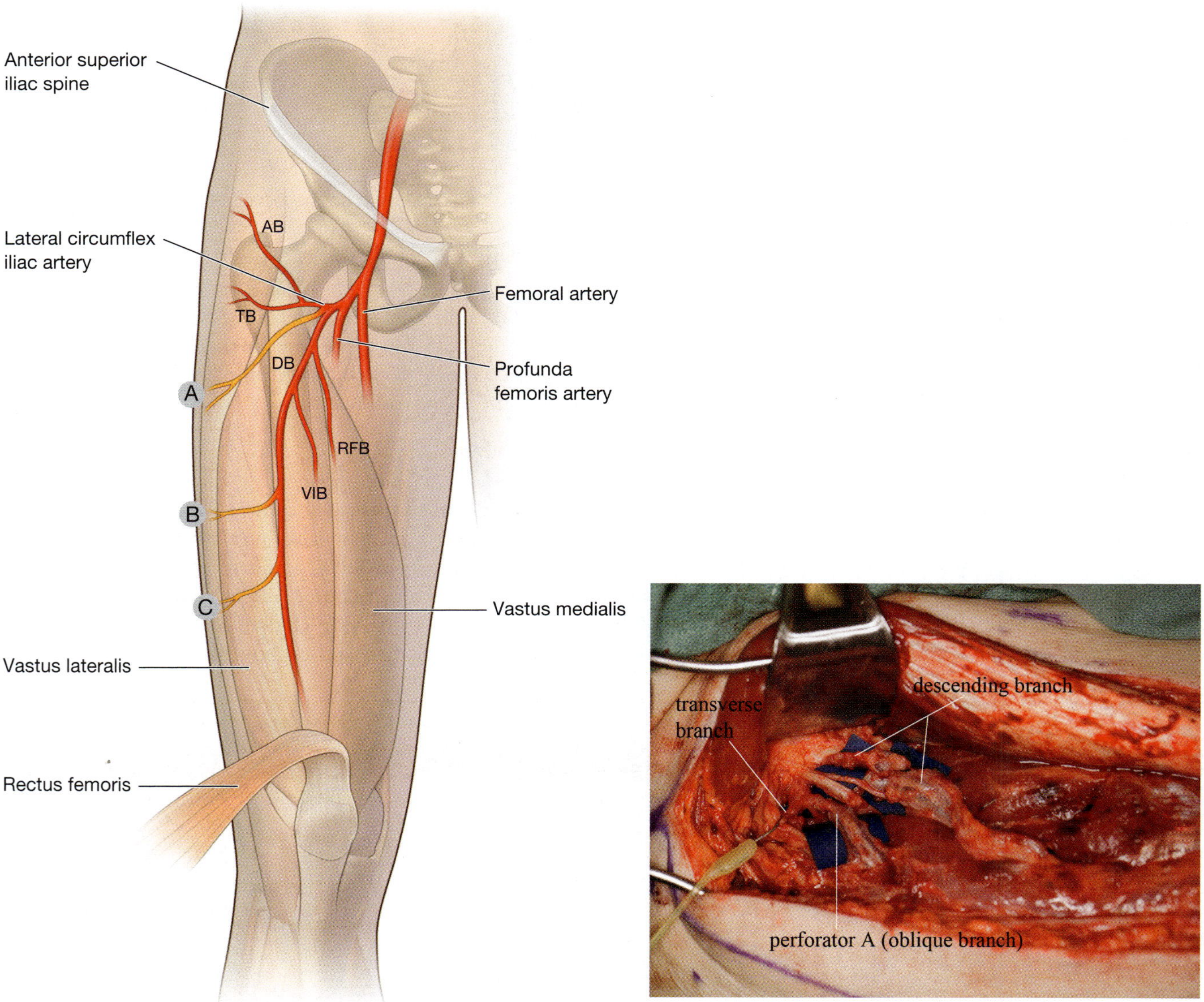

A B

FIGURE 15-9 (A) and (B) Perforator A originates from the bifurcation of the transverse and descending branch, and perforators B and C originate from the descending branch. AB, ascending branch; ASIS, anterior superior iliac spine; DB, descending branch; LCF, lateral circumflex femoris artery; PFA, profundus femoris artery; RF, rectus femoris muscle; RFB, rectus femoris branch; SFA, superficial femoral artery; TB, transverse branch; VIB, vastus intermedius branch; VL, vastus lateralis muscle; VM, vastus medialis muscle

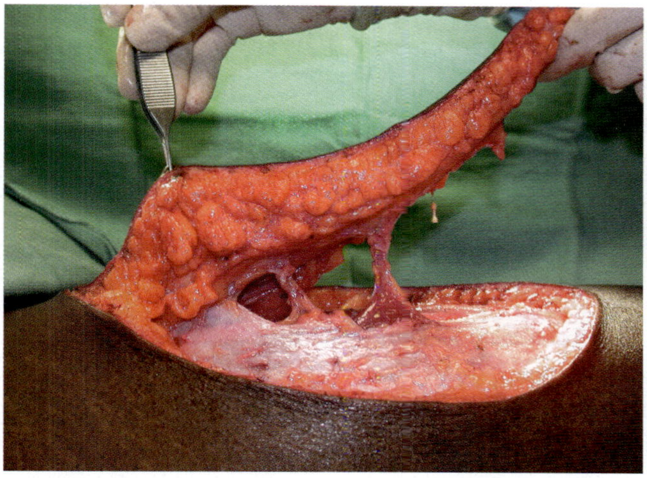

FIGURE 15-10 The anterolateral thigh flap is thicker proximally and thinner distally.

clamps, each one positioned at a perforator location. The septum appears as a strip of light brown fatty tissue through which the intermuscular space can be entered by blunt dissection (Figure 15-14). The rectus femoris muscle is retracted medially, exposing the descending branch (Figure 15-15). Septocutaneous perforators can be seen running in this intermuscular space and traced back to the descending branch. Otherwise, dissection is continued laterally over the vastus lateralis muscle until musculocutaneous perforators piecing this muscle are seen. The surface locations of the visualized perforators are marked with a 5-0 suture on the skin surface, and the flap is recentered as needed.

Next, the descending branch of the lateral circumflex femoris artery is identified in the intermuscular space, running along the medial edge of the vastus lateralis muscle above the vastus intermedius muscle. With both the perforators and the descending branch in the view, the perforators are dissected out toward the descending branch.

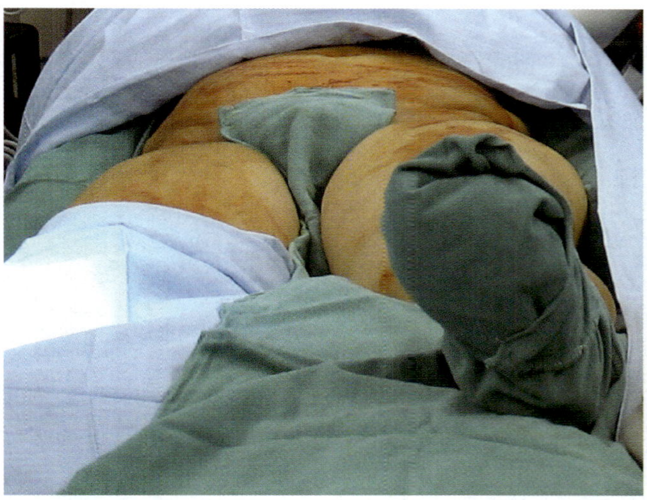

FIGURE 15-11 The leg position should be neutral with the toes straight up pointing to the ceiling. To prevent leg rotation, the foot is wrapped with a towel and clipped to the drape or to the towel on the other foot.

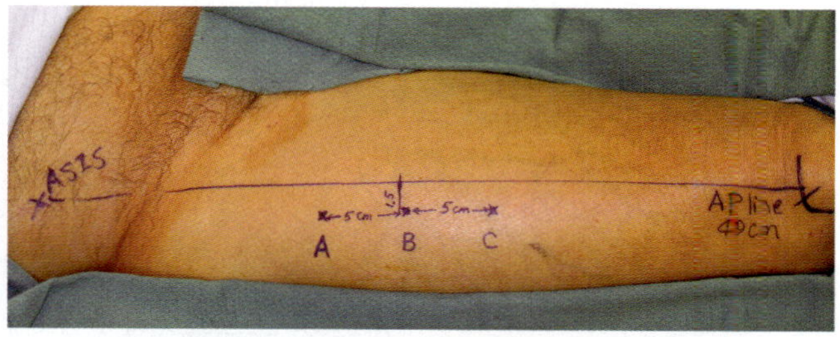

FIGURE 15-12 Marking the locations of the three cutaneous perforators based on the "ABC" system. ASIS, anterior superior iliac spine.

For septocutaneous perforators, the dissection is straightforward. There are usually two venae comitantes accompanying each perforator artery. There may be numerous small branches off the perforators supplying the vastus lateralis. These branches are ligated and divided to completely free the perforators. Small motor nerves may also be seen accompanying the perforators. If possible, these nerves should be separated and preserved (Figure 15-16). All perforators are then traced back to the descending branch. The descending branch vessels distal to the last perforator are ligated and divided. Care should be taken to identify and separate the motor nerve that travels closely with the descending branch before its division. The motor nerve should be traced back to its main trunk in the proximal thigh so that its entire length can be separated from the vessels and preserved (see Figure 15-4). Occasionally, a motor nerve may travel between two perforators (Figure 15-17). If both perforators need to be included, the nerve is then divided to release the perforators and reanastomosed. All of the flap dissections can be performed through the anterior incision only. It is important not to island the flap before identifying and dissecting out the perforators. In the event no suitable cutaneous perforators are found, the anterior incision may simply be closed.

For musculocutaneous perforators, intramuscular dissection begins at the fascial level where the perforators exit the muscle. With loupe magnification, the muscle fibers are carefully separated for a few centimeters long along the fiber direction with a pair of tenotomy scissors. Such dissection continues following the direction of the perforators toward the main vessel (Figure 15-18). Tiny muscular branches off the perforators should be cauterized using fine bipolar tips. Larger branches are

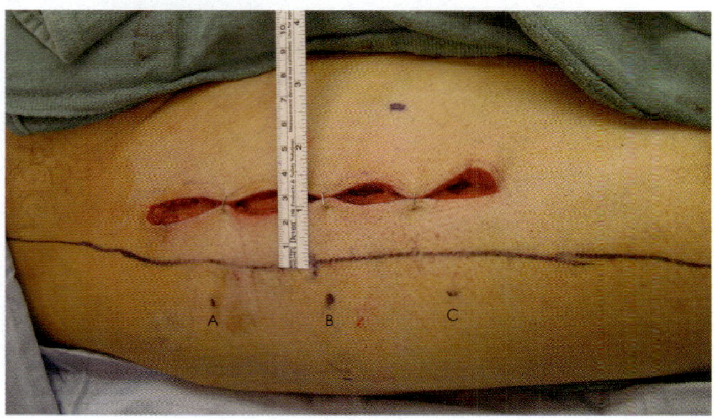

FIGURE 15-13 Only the anterior incision is made initially over the rectus femoris muscle long enough to cover all three perforators.

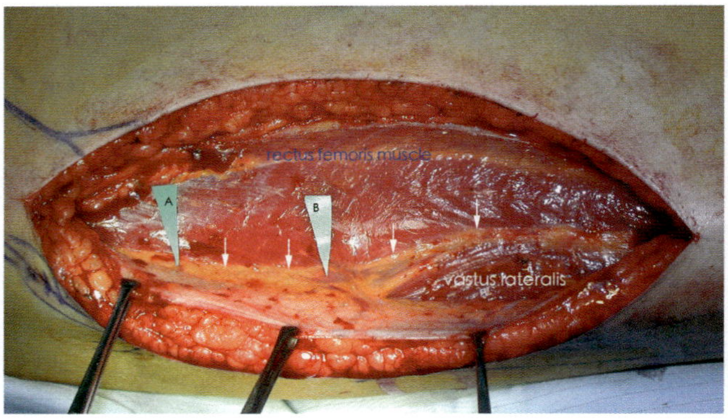

FIGURE 15-14 Three Allis clamps are placed on the fascia to retract it laterally during subfascial dissection. The intermuscular space (septum) between the rectus femoris and vastus lateralis muscles is identified as a yellow fat line (arrows). Two perforators are seen lateral to the septum.

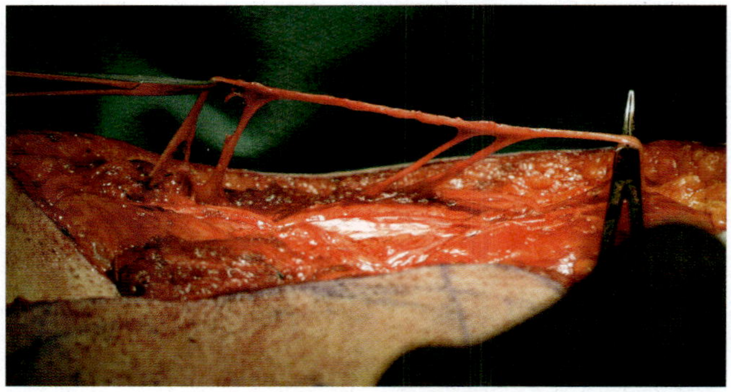

FIGURE 15-16 The motor nerves that supply the vastus lateralis muscle should be separated from the vascular pedicle and preserved if possible.

clipped with microsurgical clips or ligated with very fine sutures to avoid avulsion of the perforators. The perforators should gradually become larger toward the main vessel, and dissection becomes easier. In most cases, there is only a thin layer of muscle (2–3 cm wide and less than 1 cm thick) covering the perforator. The muscle can be divided to free the perforator. If the perforator is deep in the muscle, it is best not to divide the muscle to minimize functional deficit.

Flap design is finalized according to the dimensions of the final defect and exact locations of the perforators. The flap may be recentered if necessary. The distal and posterior borders of the flap are incised and the flap raised off the vastus lateralis muscle relatively quickly, with the surgeon's fingers protecting the perforators. The proximal border of the flap is incised last. When a sensate flap is needed, the lateral femoral cutaneous nerve is identified through the proximal incision (27). An additional 5 cm of nerve is harvested via proximal subcutaneous dissection (see Figure 15-7). After the recipient vessels are prepared, the vascular pedicle is divided either below or above the rectus femoris branch depending on the needs and sizes of the vessels. A 19-Fr Blake drain is placed in the thigh wound. The majority of the donor sites (85%) can be closed primarily. The lower extremity is wrapped with an ACE wrap from the foot all the way to the groin for 1 week. Ambulation is resumed as soon as the patient is able to. If skin grafting is required to cover the donor site, a knee immobilizer is placed, and the patient can ambulate with the knee immobilizer on and with a walker or cane.

Relationship of the Anterolateral Thigh Flap to Other Local Thigh Flaps

A combination of flaps based on the same vascular system (i.e., "chimeric" flaps) can be raised from the anterior and lateral aspects of the thigh.

1. The most common combination is probably the ALT fasciocutaneous flap with the vastus lateralis muscle flap. Both flaps are based on the descending branch. Depending on the size of the defect, various amounts of muscle can be harvested based on either a muscular branch or the entire descending branch. The vastus lateralis muscle is a large

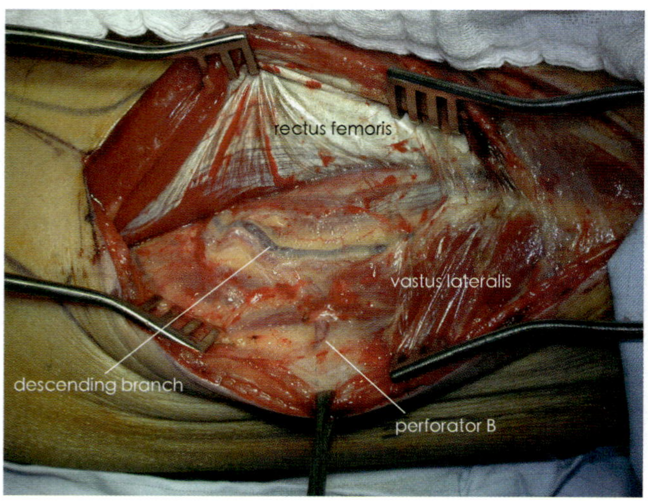

FIGURE 15-15 The rectus femoris muscle is retracted medially to expose the descending branch.

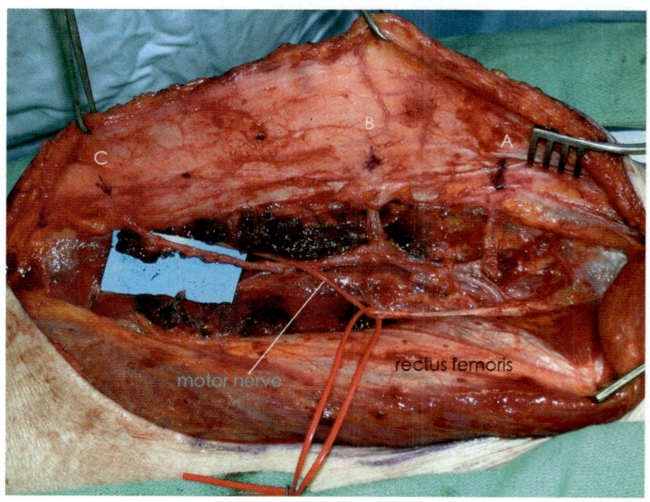

FIGURE 15-17 If the motor nerve travels between two perforators, the nerve is divided to release the perforators and reanastomosed.

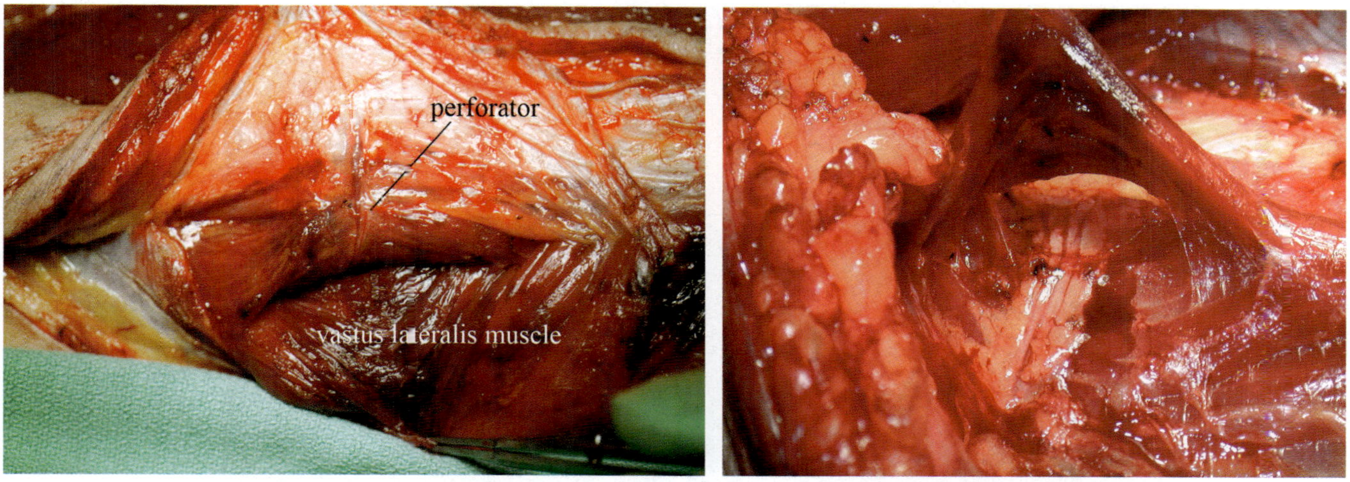

A B

FIGURE 15-18 (A) and (B) Intramuscular dissection of perforators.

muscle, and in most cases, only a portion of the muscle is needed. The superficial half of the muscle is usually taken to avoid exposure of the femur and minimize donor site morbidity. Dissection is carried out below (deeper to) the descending branch so that the descending branch is included in the muscle flap. The remaining vastus lateralis muscle also receives blood supply from direct branches of the profundus femoris artery that supply the posterior thigh muscle groups. Necrosis of the whole or remaining vastus lateralis muscle after taking out the descending branch has not been observed in the author's experience.

2. Combination of the TFL flap and the ALT flap: This is a useful combination of flaps for extensive abdominal wall reconstruction as pedicled flaps. To increase the arc of rotation, both the transverse and descending branch may need to be dissected out as island flaps.
3. Combination of ALT and anteromedial thigh (AMT) flaps: The blood supply to the AMT flap is a perforator from the rectus femoris branch that descends medially along the medial border of the rectus femoris muscle. The cutaneous perforator travels between the sartorius and rectus femoris muscles to enter the AMT skin. Sometimes the rectus femoris branch travels within the muscle and gives rise to a musculocutaneous perforator to the skin. The combination of ALT and AMT flaps can provide large amount of skin coverage and several independent skin islands (Figure 15-19). However, the vascular anatomy of the AMT flap is variable. In the author's experience in exploring 100 AMT flaps, a cutaneous perforator from the rectus femoris branch was present only in 50% of the cases. Because the rectus femoris branch arises from the descending branch, the rectus femoris muscle can be harvested with the ALT flap based on the same vascular pedicle.
4. Including the iliac crest bone: The ascending branch of the lateral circumflex femoris artery also provides blood supply to the outer cortex of the iliac crest bone (11,28). Therefore, a segment of the outer cortex of the iliac crest can be included in the ALT flap by including the ascending branch, although dissection can be tedious.

Donor Site Morbidity of the Anterolateral Thigh Flap

1. Surgical scar: With primary close of the donor site, a surgical scar can be inconspicuous (Figure 15-20A), although closure under tension may result in a widened scar. Skin grafting on the donor site heals well with minimal deformity (Figure 15-20B). The author routinely takes some fascia with the ALT flap, and the fascial defect

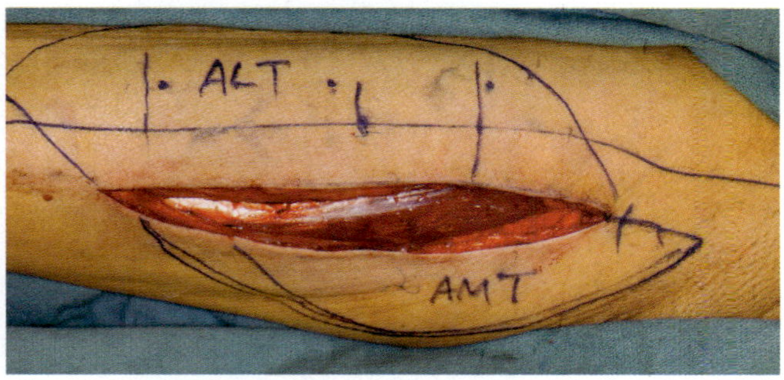

A

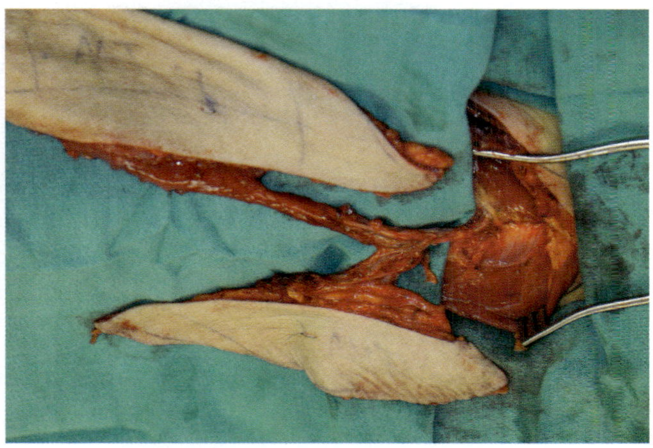

B

FIGURE 15-19 (A) and (B) Chimeric flap with both the anterolateral thigh (ALT) and anteromedial thigh (AMT) flaps based on the same vascular pedicle, the descending branch.

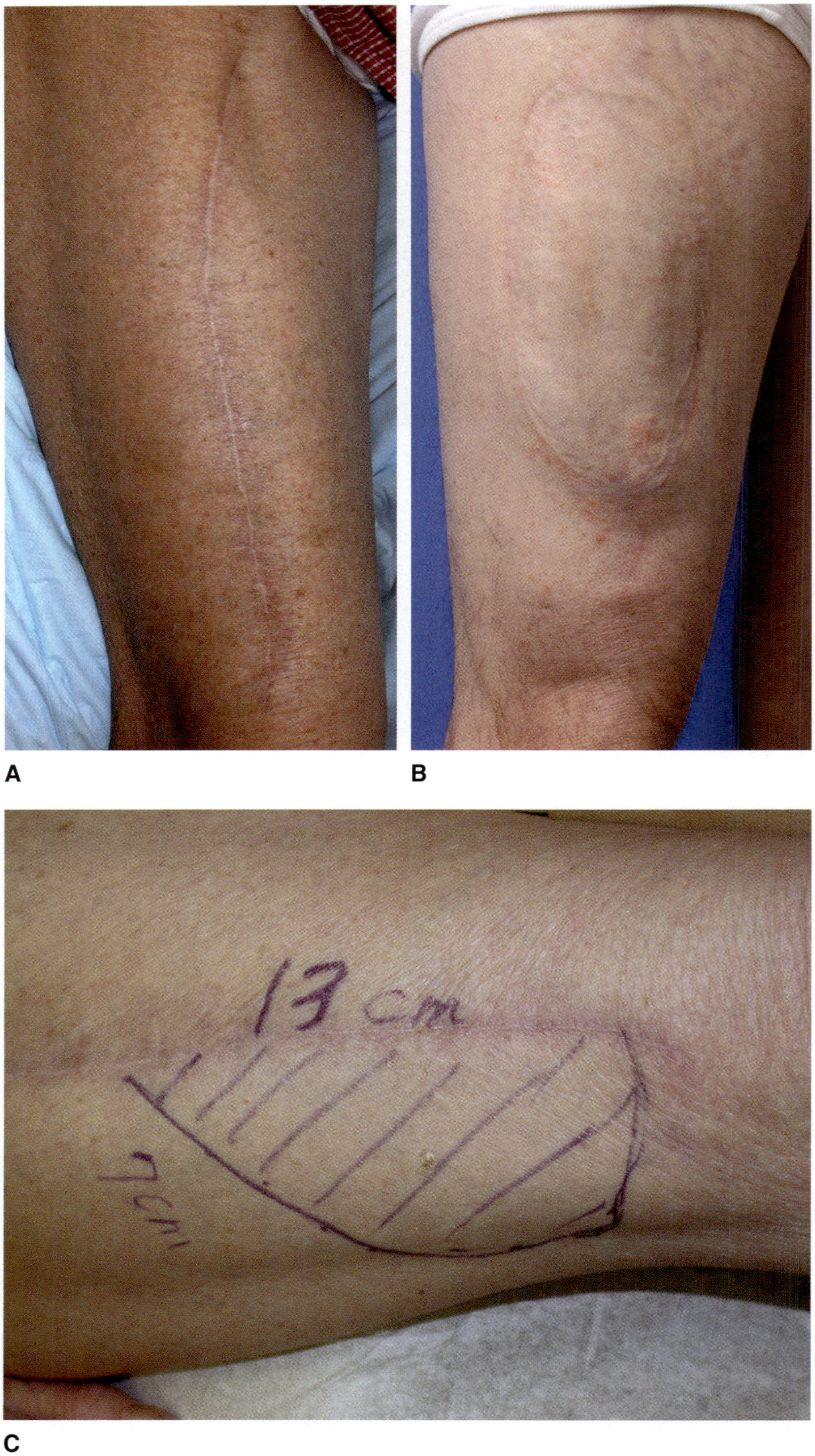

FIGURE 15-20 Donor site scar after primary closure (**A**) and skin grafting (**B**). There is an area of numbness in the inferolateral thigh above the knee (**C**).

is not closed. Bulging of the muscle through the fascial defect actually results in an even surface after skin grafting (flush with the surrounding skin). Skin grafting over a closed fascia may form a concavity, especially in obese patients. The author has not seen any functional consequences of muscle bulging.

2. Numbness: Because the lateral femoral cutaneous nerve travels within the ALT flap, harvesting the flap results in permanent numbness in the inferior lateral thigh (Figure 15-20C). With time, however, the area of numbness may decrease, and patients become less aware of it.
3. Functional deficits: Kuo et al. (20) reported no differences in isometric power testing between the donor and normal thighs in 20 patients who had a cuff of vastus lateralis muscle harvested. Isokinetic peak torque including concentric and eccentric contraction test also showed no differences except a mild weakness of the donor thigh on the concentric contraction test of the quadriceps muscle. Kimata et al. (18) reported that all patients could perform daily activities normally; however, damaging the vastus lateralis muscle or skin grafting to the donor site could cause some weakness and slightly decreased range of motion of the hip and knee. Our recent prospective study of more than 200 patients (29) has shown that all patients regained their preoperative level of activity after harvesting the ALT flap. Overall, 7% of patients complained temporary leg weakness, which usually revolves within 1 to 6 months. When the entire vastus lateralis muscle was taken, 25% of the patients complained of weakness. Taking a cuff to half of the vastus lateralis muscle did not increase the rate of leg weakness. Skin grafting the donor site and dividing one or more of the motor nerve branches also did not show an increase of weakness.
4. Neuroma formation: Two patients (1%) complained of tingling and pain at the donor scar with a positive Tinel sign consistent with neuroma. They were explored, and a small neuroma was found at the proximal and distal cutting end of the lateral femoral cutaneous nerve, respectively (Figure 15-21). Symptoms disappeared after the removal of the neuroma. The cutting end of the nerve should be buried deep when closing the donor site.
5. Other complications: In the author's experience, seroma occurred in 10% of patients, hematoma in 3%, and wound dehiscence in 1%.

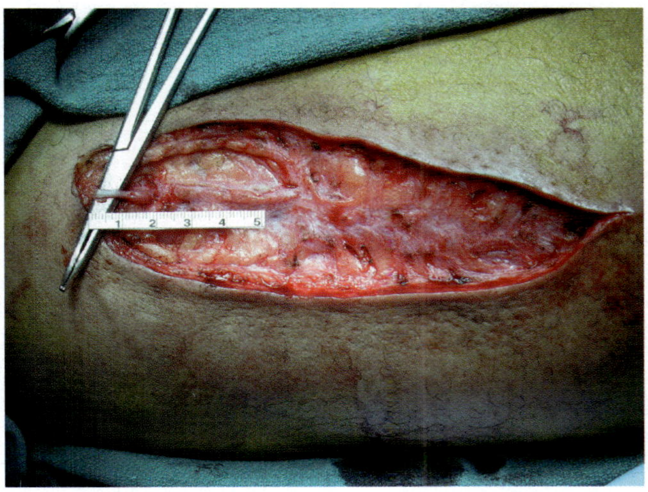

FIGURE 15-21 An unusual donor site morbidity, neuroma formation at the proximal cutting end of the lateral femoral cutaneous nerve.

Clinical Applications

Although, as a free flap, the ALT flap can be used virtually anywhere in the body, it may be too bulky to cover hand defects unless aggressive thinning is performed. This flap is particularly useful for the following reconstructions.

1. Head and neck reconstruction as a free flap (30–32)

   The ALT flap is the author's flap of choice for a variety of head and neck defects (Table 15-3). It has the following advantages in addition to its minimal donor site morbidity and quick postoperative recovery:

   a) The flap thickness is usually appropriate to provide enough bulk, which is retained much better than a muscle flap.
   b) Various amounts of vastus lateralis muscle depending on the needs can be included in the flap to seal the cranial base, fill a deep defect, and cover the carotid artery.
   c) A long vascular pedicle can easily reach the neck when the flap is used for orbital and maxillary reconstruction or reach the transverse cervical vessels in the lower neck to avoid jeopardizing the carotid artery system in patients who have undergone previous surgeries, radiotherapy, and chemotherapy.
   d) Simultaneous two-team approach and no need to change positions.
   e) Can be used as a sensate flap (27).
   f) When two cutaneous perforators are present, the flap can be split into two separate skin islands. One skin island is used for tongue, pharyngeal, and esophageal reconstruction, and the other skin island can be used to resurface

TABLE 15-3 Clinical Applications of the Anterolateral Thigh Flap

Clinical Application	Number of flaps
Pharyngoesophageal	89
Craniofacial	54
Floor of mouth and tongue	45
Posterior mandible and oropharynx	25
Double free flap with a fibula	17
Other head neck soft tissue	5
Scalp	2
Trachea	1
Trunk and extremity	6
Total	244

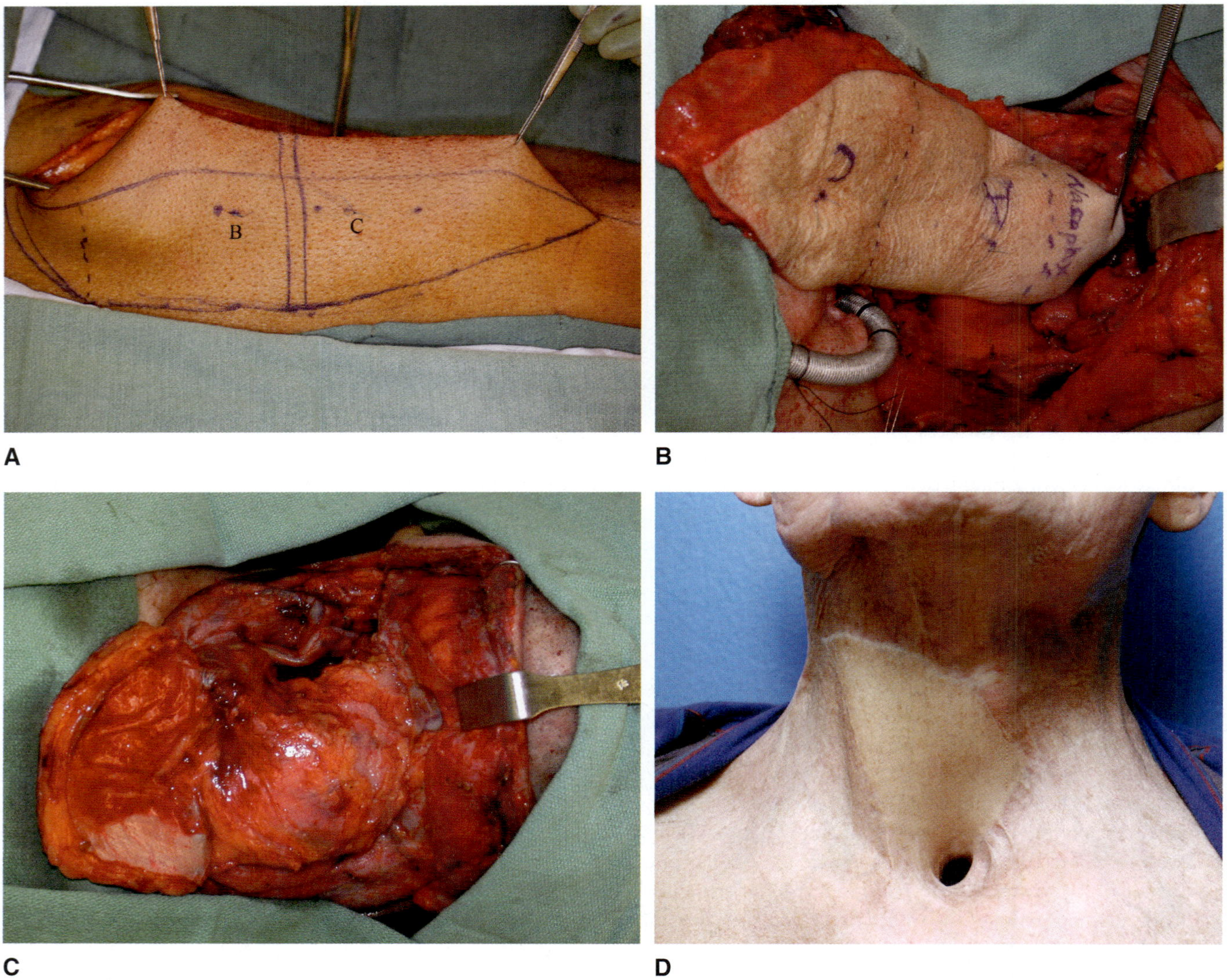

FIGURE 15-22 A two-skin island anterolateral thigh flap can be designed based on two separate perforators (**A**). One skin paddle is used for pharyngoesophageal reconstruction (**B** and **C**) and the other for neck resurfacing (**D**).

the neck in patients with skin involvement of the tumor or radiation damage (Figure 15-22). The multi-island ALT flap can also be used to reconstruct three-dimensional craniofacial defects (Figure 15-23).

2. Lower abdominal, groin, scrotal, vaginal, perineal, and ischial reconstruction as an island flap

As a pedicled island flap with a long vascular pedicle, the flap can reach the lower abdomen even above the umbilicus in some patients for abdominal wall or hernia reconstruction. It certainly reaches the groin easily even the contralateral groin (33) (Figure 15-24). A small amount of muscle can be included to cover the femoral vessels. This flap can be used to reconstruct a total scrotal defect with excellent contour and protection of the testes (21) (Figure 15-25). We have also successfully used this flap for ischial pressure ulcer reconstruction when other options have been exhausted (21). In patients with recurrent rectal cancer when the rectus abdominis muscle is unavailable because of bilateral ostomies or compromised abdominal wall integrity, the ALT can be used as a pedicled island flap for vaginal reconstruction (Figure 15-26) or reconstruction of total pelvic exenteration defects (34) (Figure 15-27).

Conclusions

The ALT flap is a useful and versatile tool in reconstructive surgery. The anatomic variations and difficulties of flap elevation have probably been exaggerated. Recognizing the patterns of perforator anatomy may simplify flap dissection and increase the success rate of flap harvesting.

TENSOR FASCIA LATA FLAPS

The TFL muscle originates from the iliac crest from the ASIS posteriorly. The muscle is approximately 3 to 4 cm wide and 10 to 12 cm long. It continues distally with the iliotibial tract. The clinical application of the TFL flap was first described by

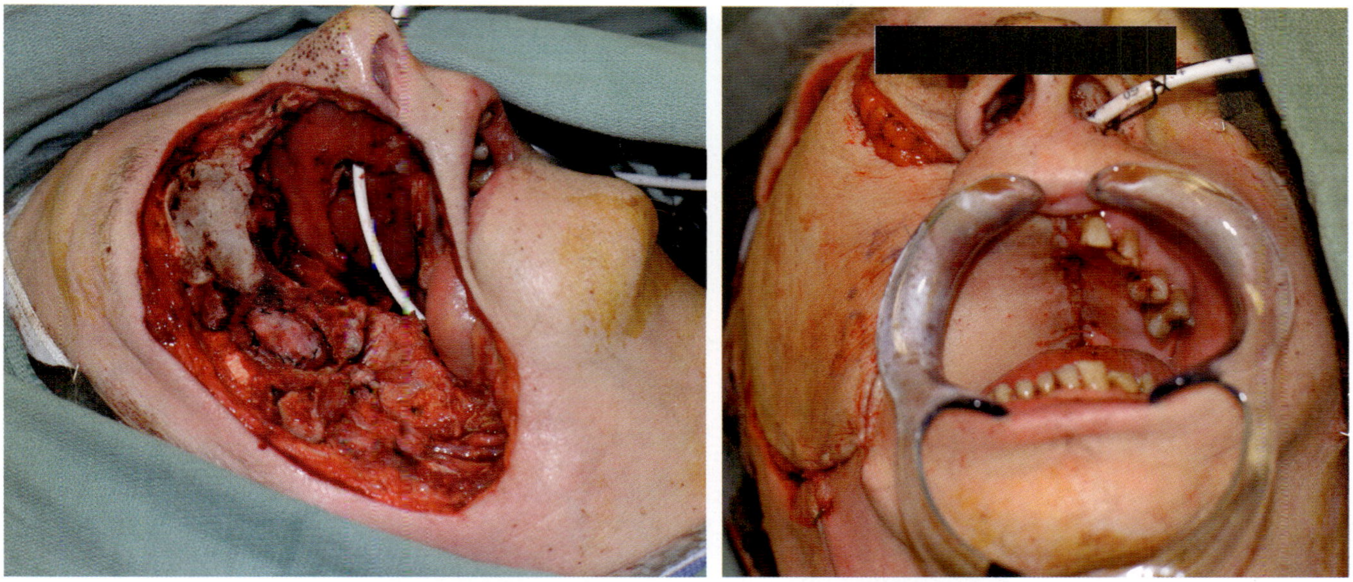

A B

FIGURE 15-23 (A) and (B) The multi-island anterolateral thigh flap is also an excellent option for three-dimensional reconstruction of craniofacial defects.

Nahai et al. in 1978 (35,36) and has been commonly used as a pedicled flap for lower abdominal wall and pressure ulcer reconstruction (35–39). The TFL flap can be raised as a fasciocutaneous flap or myocutaneous flap including the TFL muscle. It is rarely used as a free flap in modern-day practice because many other flaps may be more advantageous.

Anatomy of the Tensor Fascia Lata Flap

Vascular Anatomy

The description of the vascular anatomy of the TFL flap has been controversial. Since Nahai et al.'s original report, the transverse branch of the lateral circumflex femoris artery has been widely accepted as the main blood supply to this flap (35–37,40). However, other reports seem to suggest that the ascending branch is the vascular pedicle of the TFL flap (41–43). In a recent cadaver dissection study, the ascending branch was found to be the blood supply of the TFL muscle in all 45 specimens, and all cutaneous perforators were branches of the ascending branch (44). However, clinical experiences seem to suggest that the transverse branch also contributes to the blood supply to the TFL in some cases (Figure 15-28). Nevertheless, the vascular pedicle enters the TFL muscle at 6 to 8 cm below the ASIS and branches out into the muscle and

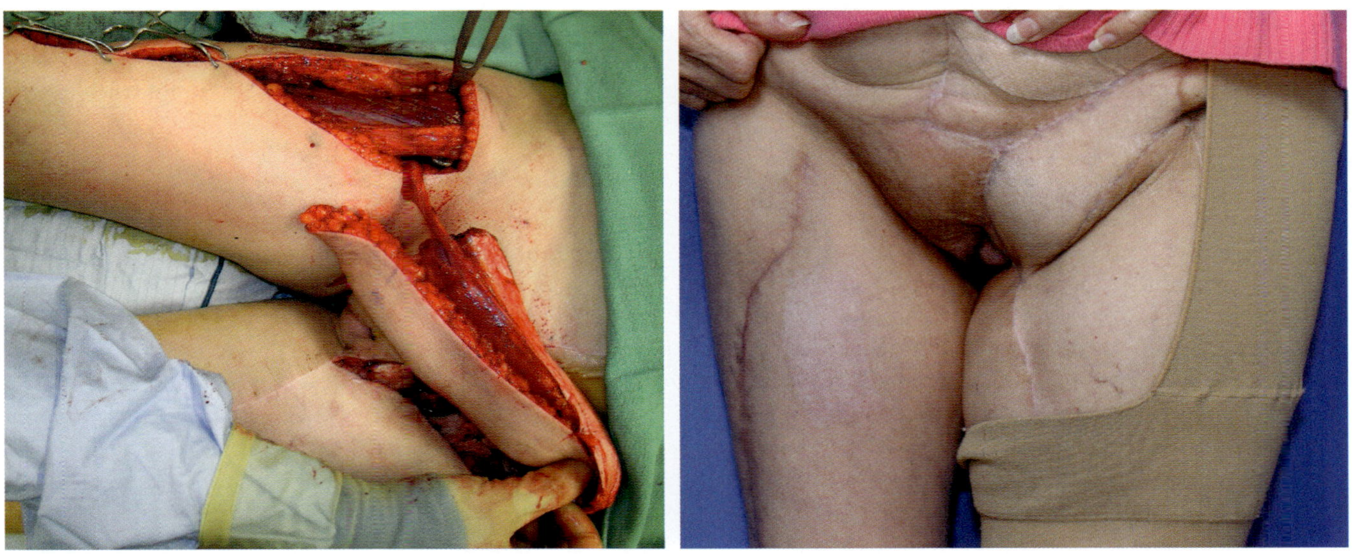

A B

FIGURE 15-24 A pedicled anterolateral thigh (ALT) island flap can reach the contralateral groin (A). It was used to cover a groin defect with exposed radiated femoral vessels in a patient with a previous ipsilateral ALT flap reconstruction (B).

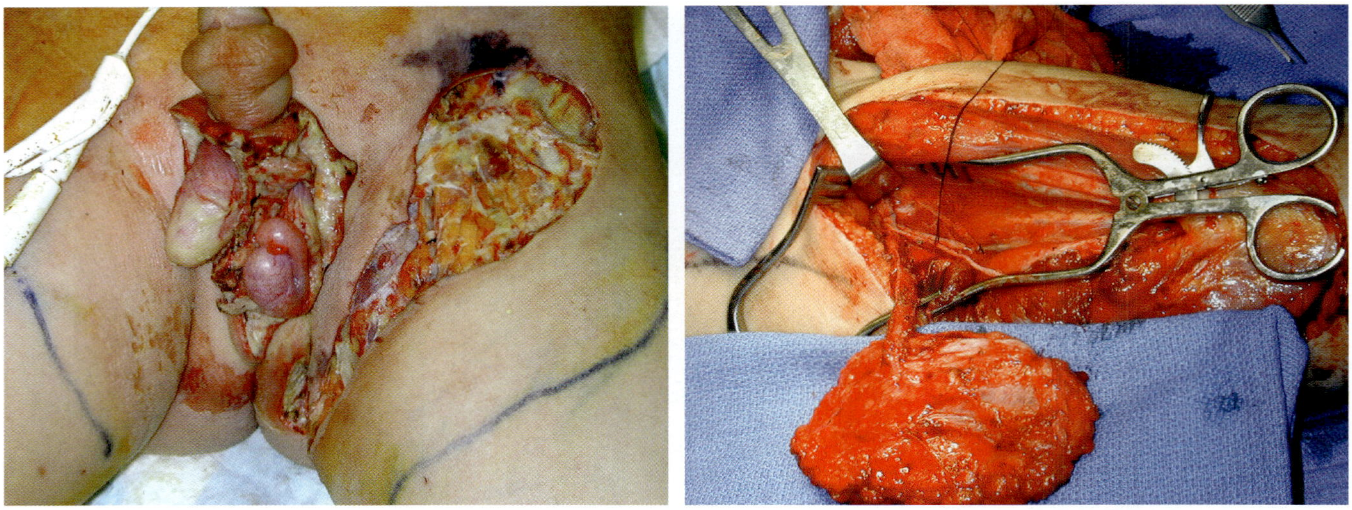

A B

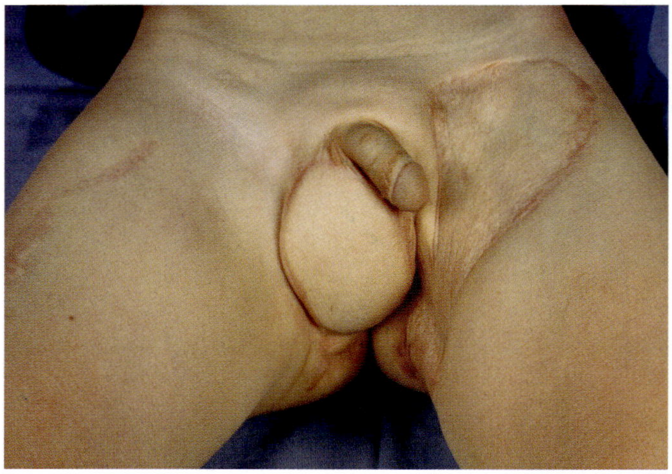

C

FIGURE 15-25 Fournier's gangrene in a 9-year-old boy with exposed testes (**A**). The groin defect was skin grafted, and the scrotal defect was reconstructed with a pedicled anterolateral thigh flap (**B** and **C**).

the overlying skin. The upper branch supplies the proximal portion of the TFL muscle and the outer cortex of the iliac crest in some cases. The lower branches supply the rest of the TFL muscle and the TFL fascia below the muscle. The skin territory of the TFL flap can be divided into three zones: the proximal zone, middle zone, and the distal zone (45). Based on their injections studies, Gosain et al. found that injection into the lateral circumflex femoris artery only stained the proximal zone over the TFL muscle while injection into the superior lateral genicular artery stained the distal zone, leaving the middle zone unstained (45). Injection into the ascending branch also only stained the skin overlying the TFL muscle in a separate study (44). With recent advances in the perforator anatomy of the ALT flap, we now understand that the middle zone of the TFL flap territory is primarily supplied by musculocutaneous perforators from the descending branch (same as the ALT flap) (46,47), and the posterior (lateral) thigh flap skin is supplied by the third perforator of the profundus femoris artery. This anatomy explains why the distal portion (8–10 cm above the knee) of the TFL flap is not reliable when based on its proximal pedicle.

Nerve Supply

The skin territory of the TFL flap is innervated by the lateral cutaneous branch of the twelfth thoracic nerve and the lateral femoral cutaneous nerve (L2–L3) (same as the ALT flap). The former pierces the internal and external oblique muscles and descends below the iliac crest about 6 cm posterior to the ASIS. It provides skin sensation over the iliac crest and the upper half of the TFL muscle. This nerve is usually smaller than 1 mm in diameter. The lateral femoral cutaneous nerve enters the thigh below the inguinal ligament immediately anterior to the ASIS. It travels above the deep fascia and divides into two branches 6 to 8 cm below the inguinal ligament. At this point, the nerve has a diameter of approximately 2 mm. The lateral branch travels along the line connecting the ASIS to the lateral patella

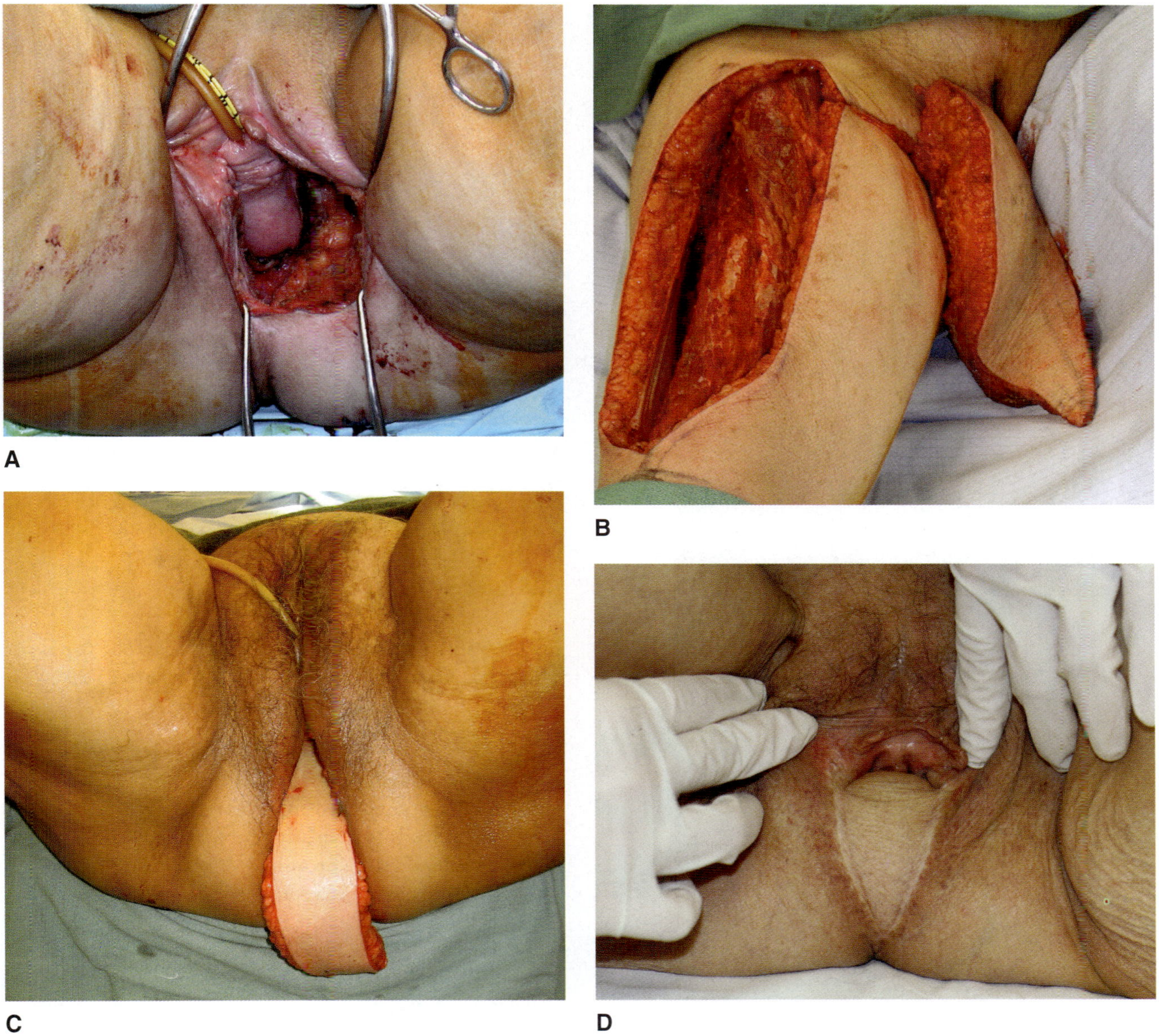

FIGURE 15-26 (A) to (D) Reconstruction of a vaginal defect with an anterolateral thigh flap with the vastus lateralis muscle in a patient with recurrent rectal cancer involving the vagina undergoing a posterior pelvic exenteration. The flap was brought to the perineal defect via a subcutaneous tunnel in the medial thigh (perineal route).

and can be harvested with the TFL flap. The medial branch travels along the anterior midline of the thigh.

Surgical Techniques

A line is drawn from the ASIS to the lateral tibial condyle in a supine or standing position (Figure 15-28A). This line serves as the central axis of the TFL flap. A flap with a width of 10 cm can be designed centering on this line. However, primary closure of the donor site can be difficult with a flap width beyond 8 cm. The flap should not be designed beyond a point 8 to 10 cm above the patella because the distal portion is unreliable. Surgical delay has been suggested for the "extended TFL flap," but it is rarely used in modern-day practice because of the availability of other flaps. The posterior border of the flap is incised, and flap dissection usually starts distally in the subfascial plane to include the skin and fascia. The skin is sutured to the fascia to prevent shearing. Proximally, the TFL muscle may be included in the flap if muscle is needed. At 6 to 8 cm below the ASIS, the vascular pedicle enters the muscle. The flap above the vascular pedicle can be divided and the vascular pedicle dissected out to serve as an island flap or free flap. The TFL flap can also be raised as a perforator flap by identifying the musculocutaneous perforators in the suprafascial plane. Over the TFL muscle, the fascia is densely adherent to the muscle and not easily separated. Above the fascia, however, there is a clear and loose tissue plane within which the perforators can be easily identified. Handheld Doppler examination may help identify the perforators. As a local rotational flap, the musculocutaneous perforators are

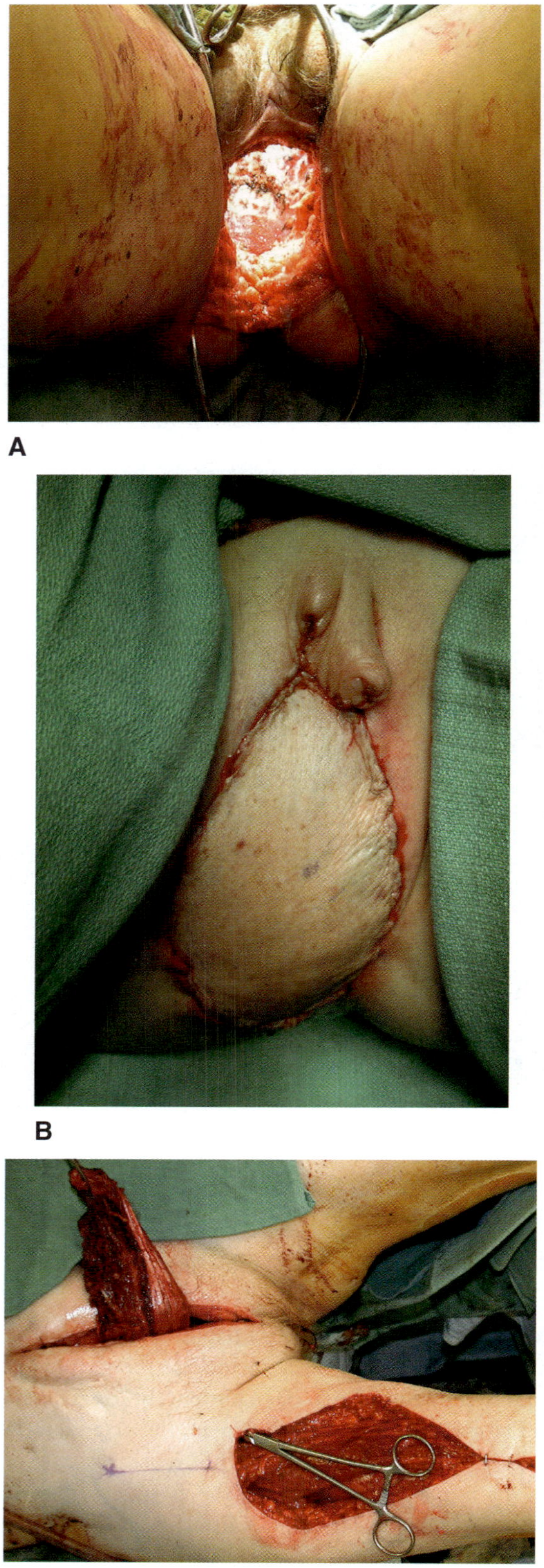

A

B

C

FIGURE 15-27 A total pelvic exenteration defect (**A**) was reconstructed with an anterolateral thigh flap with the vastus lateralis muscle (ALT-VL) from one thigh and a second vastus lateralis muscle flap from the contralateral thigh. The ALT-VL flap was brought to the perineal defect through the perineal route (**B**). The contralateral vastus lateralis muscle was turned over the inguinal ligament to the pelvis (**C**).

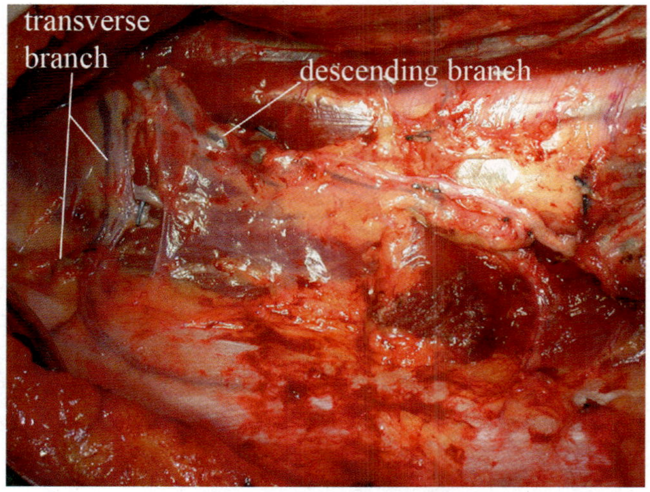

FIGURE 15-28 Vascular anatomy. The transverse branch of the lateral circumflex femoris artery travels laterally and enters the tensor fasciae latae muscle. It also sends a small branch to the fascia. The descending branch travels inferiorly to supply the vastus lateralis muscle.

usually not dissected out through the muscle. The flap is simply rotated based on the perforators (see Figure 15-29).

Donor Site Morbidity

Donor site morbidity from harvesting the TFL flap is usually minor. Contour deformity may be the most common complaint. This is particularly problematic when skin grafting of the donor site is required, when the TFL muscle is taken, and when used as a rotational flap with a bulky pivot point. Sensory deficit in the lateral thigh is also present but with minimal consequences. Severe functional deficit has not been reported. However, because the most common indication of this flap is pressure ulcers in patients with paraplegia, functional deficits and contour deformity are negligible.

The most common flap-related complication is necrosis of the distal portion of the flap when used as a pedicled flap. This can be frustrating because this is usually the part most needed. Therefore, it is important to realize the limitations of this flap during flap design.

Indications

When this flap was first described, it became a very versatile flap for various reconstructive indications. It is most commonly used as a pedicled flap for pressure ulcer, groin defect, and lower abdominal wall reconstruction (35–39). It is also used as a free flap with or without the iliac crest bone for head and neck and extremity reconstruction (37,40,41). However, it has been less commonly used as a free myocutaneous flap in the past 1 to 2 decades because of the availability of other well-known myocutaneous flaps such the rectus abdominis and latissimus dorsi flaps (48). It is also rarely used as a free fasciocutaneous flap in recent years because of the popularity of the ALT flap and other fasciocutaneous flaps.

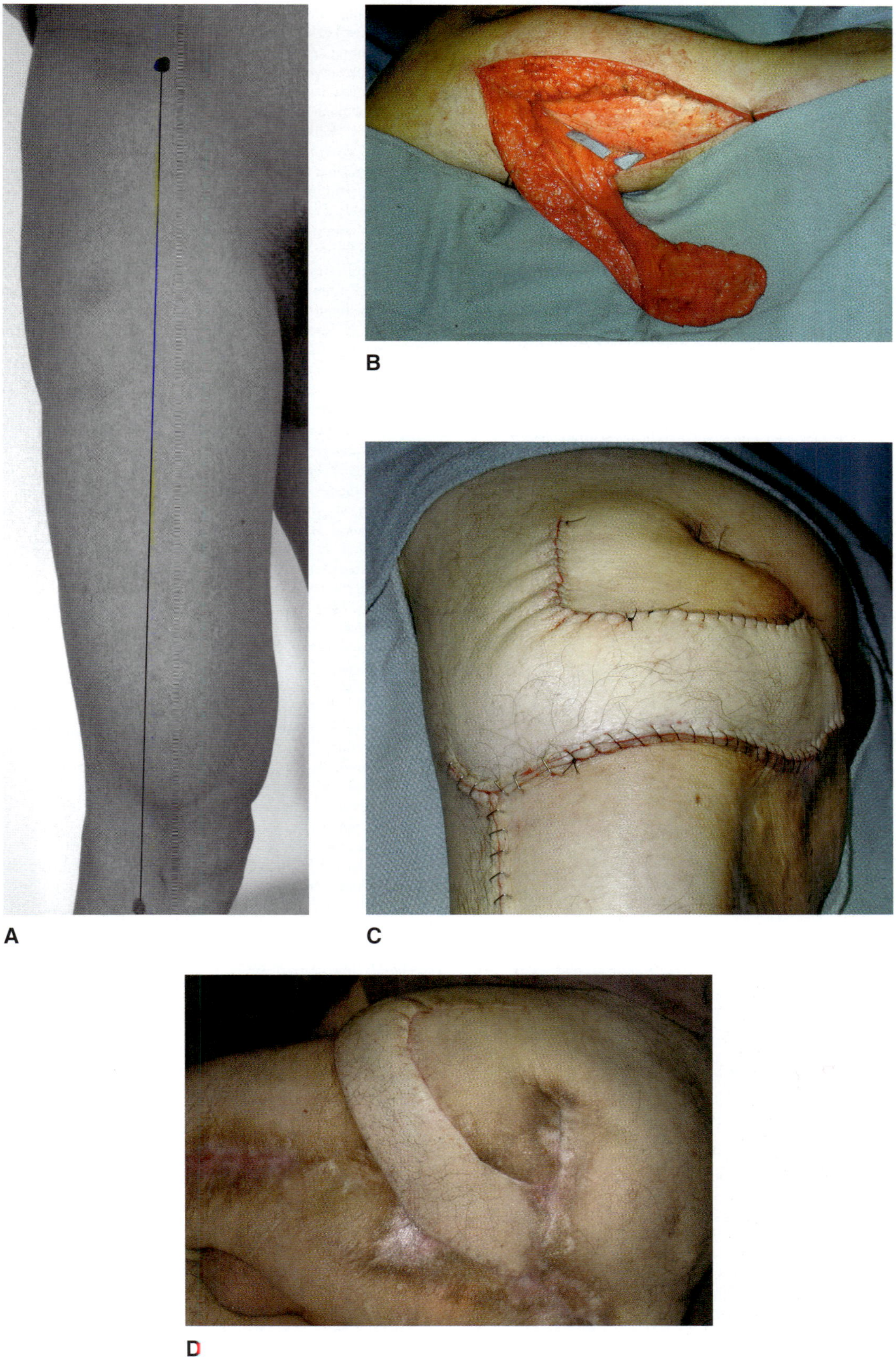

FIGURE 15-29 A line is drawn to connect the anterior superior iliac spine (ASIS) and the tibial condyle (**A**). This line serves as the central axis of the tensor fasciae latae (TFL) flap. The TFL flap can be raised as a perforator flap based on a musculocutaneous perforator (**B**). The flap is rotated posteriorly to reconstruct a recurrent ischial ulcer (**C** and **D**).

REFERENCES

1. Zhou CM, Zhong SZ, Liu MZ. Anatomy of the anterolateral leg flap. *Chin J Appl Anat* 1983;1:97.
2. Xu DC, Zhong SZ, Kong JM, et al. Anatomy of the anterolateral thigh flap. *Chin J Appl Anat* 1984;2:158–160.
3. Gao JH, Luo LS, Chen LF, Li YN. Surface location of main cutaneous vessels in the anterolateral thigh skin flap. *Chin J Appl Anat* 1984;2:161–163.
4. Luo LS, Gao JH, Chen LF, Li YN. A new free skin flap-anterolateral thigh skin flap: its anatomy and clinical application. *Chin J Plast Surg Burns* 1985;1:50–52.
5. Song YG, Chen, GZ, Song YL. The free thigh flap: a new free flap concept based on the septocutaneous artery. *Br J Plast Surg* 1984;37:149.
6. Xu DC, Zhong SZ, Kong JM, et al. Applied anatomy of the anterolateral thigh flap. *Plast Reconstr Surg* 1988;82:305–310.
7. Zhang GL. Clinical application and improvement of an anterolateral thigh flap. *Chin J Plast Surg Burns* 1989;5:269–270.
8. Koshima I, Fukuda H, Utunomiya R, Soeda S. The anterolateral thigh flap: variations in its vascular pedicle. *Br J Plast Surg* 1989;42:260–262.
9. Zhou G, Qiao Q, Chen GY, et al. Clinical experience and surgical anatomy of 32 free anterolateral thigh flap transplantations. *Br J Plast Surg* 1991;44:91–96.
10. Koshima I, Fukuda H, Yamamoto H, et al. Free anterolateral thigh flaps for reconstruction of head and neck defects. *Plast Reconstr Surg* 1993;92:421.
11. Koshima I, Hosoda M, Moriguchi T, et al. A combined anterolateral thigh flap, anteromedial thigh flap, and vascularized iliac bone graft for a full-thickness defect of the mental region. *Ann Plast Surg* 1993;31:175.
12. Koshima I, Yamamoto H, Hosoda M, et al. Free combined composite flaps using the lateral circumflex femoral system for repair of massive defects of the head and neck regions: an introduction to the chimeric flap principle. *Plast Reconstr Surg* 1993;92:411.
13. Pribaz JJ, Orgill DP, Epstein MD, et al. Anterolateral thigh free flap. *Ann Plast Surg* 1995;34:585–592.
14. Kimata Y, Uchiyarna K, Ebihara S, et al. Versatility of the free anterolateral thigh flap for reconstruction of head and neck defects. *Arch Otolaryngol Head Neck Surg* 1997;123:1325.
15. Kimata Y, Uchiyarna K, Ebihara S, et al. Anatomic variations and technical problems of the anterolateral thigh flap: a report of 74 cases. *Plast Reconstr Surg* 1998;102:1517–1523.
16. Luo S, Raffoul W, Luo J, et al. Anterolateral thigh flap: a review of 168 cases. *Microsurgery* 1999;19:232–238.
17. Shieh SJ, Chiu HY, Yu JC, et al. Free anterolateral thigh flap for reconstruction of head and neck defects following cancer ablation. *Plast Reconstr Surg* 2000;105:2349.
18. Kimata Y, Uchiyama K, Ebihara S, et al. Anterolateral thigh flap donor site complications and morbidity. *Plast Reconstr Surg* 2000;106:584.
19. Kimura N, Satoh K, Hasumi T, Ostuka T. Clinical application of the free thin anterolateral thigh flap in 31 consecutive patients. *Plast Reconstr Surg* 2001;108:1197.
20. Kuo YR, Jeng SF, Kuo MH, et al. Free anterolateral thigh flap for extremity reconstruction: clinical experience and functional assessment of donor site. *Plast Reconstr Surg* 2001;107:1766.
21. Yu, P, Sanger JR, Matloub HS, et al. Anterolateral thigh fasciocutaneous island flaps in perineoscrotal reconstruction. *Plast Reconstr Surg* 2002;109:610.
22. Wei FC, Celik N, Chen HC, et al. Have we found an ideal soft-tissue flap? An experience with 672 anterolateral thigh flaps. *Plast Reconstr Surg* 2002;109:2219.
23. Yu P. Characteristics of the anterolateral thigh flap in a Western population and its application in head and neck reconstruction. *Head Neck* 2004;26:759–769.
24. Yu P, Youssef A. Efficacy of the handheld Doppler in preoperative identification of the cutaneous perforators in the anterolateral thigh flap. *Plast Reconstr Surg* 2006;118:928–933.
25. Wong CH, Wei FC, Fu B, et al. Alternative vascular pedicle of the anterolateral thigh flap: the oblique branch of the lateral circumflex femoral artery. *Plast Reconstr Surg* 2009;123:571–577.
26. Nakayama B, Hyodo I, Hasegawa Y, et al. Role of the anterolateral thigh flap in head and neck reconstruction: advantages of moderate skin and subcutaneous thickness. *J Reconstr Microsurg* 2002;18:141–146.
27. Yu P. Reinnervated anterolateral thigh flap for tongue reconstruction. *Head Neck* 2004;26:1038–1044.
28. Dorafshar AH, Seitz IA, DeWolfe M, et al. Split lateral iliac crest chimera flap: utility of the ascending branch of the lateral femoral circumflex vessels. *Plast Reconstr Surg* 2010;125:574.
29. Hanasono MM, Skoracki RJ, Yu P. A prospective study of donor site morbidity after anterolateral thigh fasciocutaneous and myocutaneous free flap harvest in 220 patients. *Plast Reconstr Surg* 2010;125:209–214.
30. Yu P. One-stage reconstruction of complex pharyngoesophageal, tracheal, and anterior neck defects. *Plast Reconstr Surg* 2005;116:949–956.
31. Yu P, Robb GL. Reconstruction for total and near-total glossectomy defects. *Clin Plast Surg* 2005;32:411–419.
32. Yu P, Hanasono MM, Skoracki RJ, et al. Pharyngoesophageal reconstruction with the anterolateral thigh flap following total laryngopharyngectomy. *Cancer* 2010;116:1718–1724.
33. Ver Halen J, Yu P. Reconstruction of extensive groin defects with contralateral anterolateral thigh-vastus lateralis muscle flaps. *Plast Reconstr Surg* 2010;125:130e.
34. Wong S, Garvey P, Skibber JM, Yu P. Reconstruction of pelvic exenteration defects with the anterolateral thigh-vastus lateralis muscle flaps. *Plast Reconstr Surg* 2009;124:1177–1185.
35. Nahai F, Silverton J, Hill H, Vasconez L. The tensor fascia lata musculocutaneous flap. *Ann Plast Surg* 1978;1:372.
36. Hill H, Nahai F, Vasconez L. The tensor fascia lata musculocutaneous free flap. *Plast Reconstr Surg* 1978;61:517.
37. Nahai F, Hill H, Hester TR. Experiences with the tensor fascia lata flap. *Plast Reconstr Surg* 1979;63:788.
38. Williams JK, Carlson GW, deChalain T, et al. Role of tensor fasciae latae in abdominal wall reconstruction. *Plast Reconstr Surg* 1998;101:713.
39. Foster RD, Anthony JP, Mathes SJ, Hoffman WY. Ischial pressure sore coverage: a rationale for flap selection. *Br J Plast Surg* 1998;51:260.
40. Lin CH, Wei FC, Lin YT, et al. Lateral circumflex femoral artery system: Warehouse for functional composite free-tissue reconstruction of the lower leg. *J Trauma* 2006;60:1032–1036.
41. Bulstrode NW, Kotronakis I, Baldwin MAR. Free tensor fasciae latae musculofasciocutaneous flap in reconstructive surgery: a series of 85 cases. *J Plast Reconstr Aesthet Surg* 2006;59:130–136.
42. Dabernig J, Shilov B, Schumacher O, et al. Functional reconstruction of Achilles tendon defects combined with overlying skin defects using a free tensor fasciae latae flap. *J Plast Reconstr Aesthet Surg* 2006;59:142.
43. Siddharth P, Smith NL, Mason RA, Giron F. Variational anatomy of the deep femoral artery. *Anat Rec* 1985;212:206–209.
44. Hubmer MG, Schwaiger N, Windisch G, et al. The vascular anatomy of the tensor fasciae latae perforator flap. *Plast Reconstr Surg* 2009;124:181.
45. Gosain AK, Yan JG, Aydin MA, et al. The vascular supply of the extended tensor fasciae latae flap: how far can the skin paddle extend? *Plast Reconstr Surg* 2002;110:1655.
46. Wei FC, Celik N, Chen HC, et al. Have we found an ideal soft-tissue flap? An experience with 672 anterolateral thigh flaps. *Plast Reconstr Surg* 2002;109:2219.
47. Yu P. Characteristics of the anterolateral thigh flap in a Western population and its application in head and neck reconstruction. *Head Neck* 2004;26:759–769.
48. Nahai F. Discussion: the vascular supply of the extended tensor fasciae latae flap: how far can the skin paddle extend? *Plast Reconstr Surg* 2002;110:1662.

CHAPTER 16

The Gracilis Muscle Free and Pedicled Flap

Jennifer L. Giuffre and Alexander Y. Shin

HISTORY OF THE GRACILIS MUSCLE FLAP

Reconstructive surgery has been revolutionized by the discovery of muscle and musculocutaneous flaps. One of the first flaps to be recognized and used was the gracilis muscle. In 1952, Pickerell et al. (1) described transposing the gracilis to correct anal incontinence and later (1956) urinary incontinence (2). Orticochea reported, in 1970, that he had indirectly transferred a compound flap including the gracilis muscle to the sole of a foot (3). He described that the flap was being supplied by blood flow from the muscle. Later in 1972, Orticochea (4) described how to reconstruct a penis with the gracilis muscle and its overlying skin. Pers and Medgyesi (5) reported a number of uses of the gracilis including repair of a vesicovaginal fistula. Other uses for the gracilis muscle flap were described by Bartholdson and Hulten (6) in which the gracilis muscle was transposed into large perineal sinuses after proctocolectomy.

The first large "island" musculocutaneous flap experience using the gracilis muscle was reported by McCraw et al. (7) for vaginal reconstruction. The segmental vascular territories of the gracilis muscle and the overlying skin were detailed and studied by injecting a thin latex suspension into the major muscular arteries of 12 live mongrel dogs (8). Subsequent latex injection studies in human specimens illustrated a discrete and independent musculocutaneous vascular territory (8). In 1976, Harii et al. used the direct transfer of a free gracilis musculocutaneous flap by microvascular anastomosis for the reconstruction of three different defects: a facial defect, an unstable scar over the tibia, and a scalp defect (9).

The evolution of the use of the gracilis muscle led to a free, innervated functioning muscle to replace finger flexor musculature destroyed by Volkmann's ischemic contracture in 1975 (10). Harii et al. (11) similarly described using the gracilis muscle as a free functional flap; however, in this case, it was used to replace muscles of facial expression in long-standing Bell's palsy. The first noted application of using the gracilis muscle flap in the reconstruction of chronic nonobstetrical brachial plexus injuries was by Ikuta et al. in 1979, when a free-functioning gracilis muscle was transferred to restore elbow flexion in a boy with a 10-year-old brachial plexus injury (12). Since then, the use of the free innervated musculocutaneous gracilis flaps in brachial plexus reconstruction has become an invaluable tool to restore elbow flexion, prehension, and rudimentary grasp. Doi et al. (13) reported the transfer of two free innervated gracilis muscles within 6 weeks of each other to obtain such results (13).

GRACILIS MUSCLE ANATOMY

The gracilis muscle is situated in the medial thigh and is the most superficial of the adductor muscle group (Figure 16-1). It originates from the lower half of the symphysis pubis and the medial portion of the inferior pubic ramus by a thin aponeurosis. This muscle is flat proximally and courses distally and longitudinally, ending in a round tendon that passes posterior to the medial condyle of the femur and inserts into the medial surface of the upper portion of the tibia at the pes anserinus. The gracilis is one of three adductors of the thigh that flexes and medially rotates the leg. It is the smallest of the three adductors, which also includes the adductor magnus and adductor longus muscles.

GRACILIS MUSCLE VASCULAR ANATOMY

The gracilis muscle is a type 2 muscle (one dominant pedicle and minor pedicle or pedicles) per the Mathes and Nahai's classification of the vascular anatomy of muscles (14). The larger dominant vascular pedicle is capable of sustaining the circulation to the muscle after elevation of the flap and division of the distal and minor pedicles (Figure 16-2).

The proximal dominant vascular pedicle is the medial femoral circumflex artery and venae comitantes originating from the

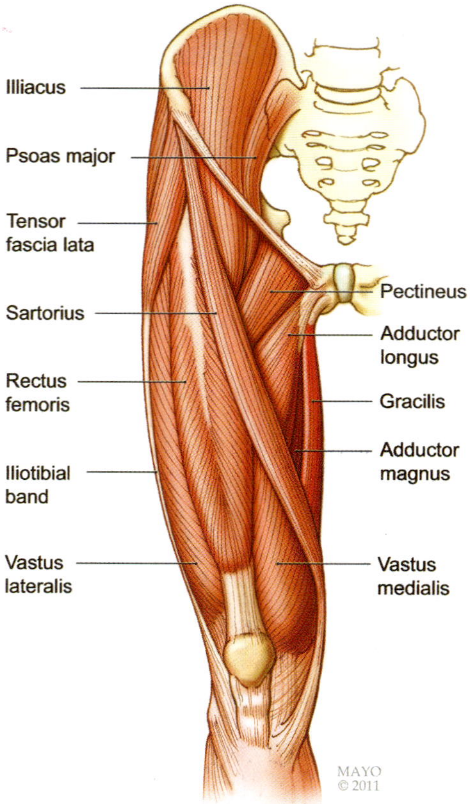

FIGURE 16-1 The gracilis muscle is situated in the medial thigh and is the most superficial of the adductor muscle group. (Used with permission of Mayo Foundation for Medical Education and Research, all rights reserved.)

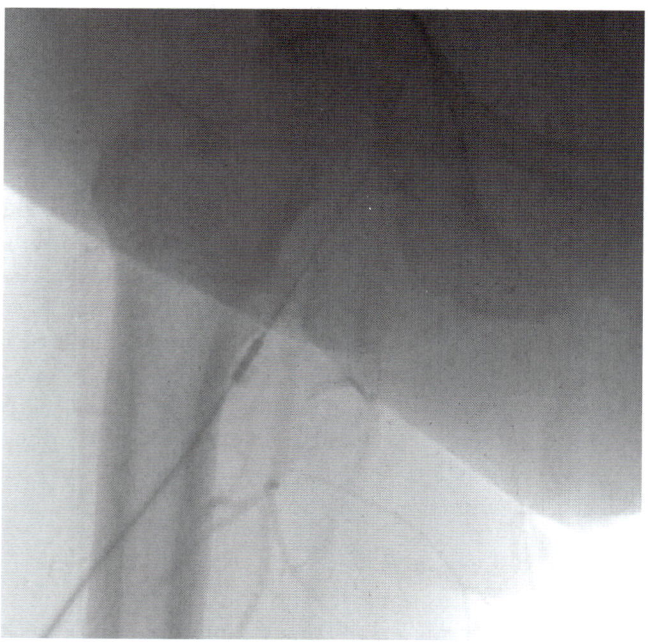

FIGURE 16-2 The medial circumflex artery is the dominant vascular pedicle to the gracilis that courses beneath the adductor longus muscle and superficial to the adductor magnus muscle, entering the medial, deep aspect of the gracilis muscle, approximately 10 cm inferior to the pubic tubercle. The angiogram depicts the dominant artery arising directly from the profunda femoris artery. (Reproduced with permission from Drs. T.E. Hayakawa and E.W. Buchel, University of Manitoba, Canada.)

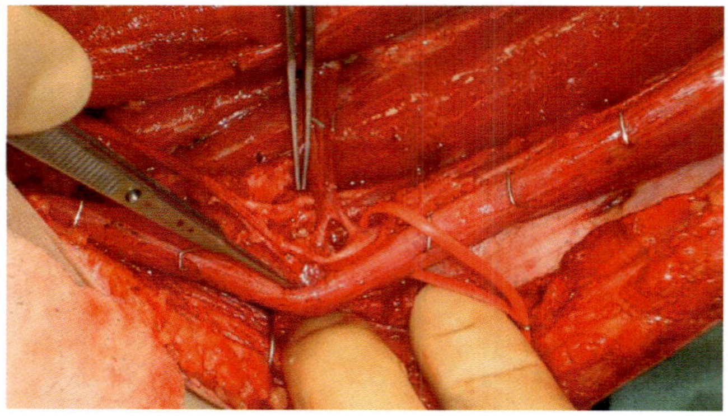

FIGURE 16-3 The pedicle terminates as two or three branches entering the medial, deep aspect of the gracilis muscle, approximately 10 cm inferior to the pubic tubercle. (Reproduced with permission from Drs. T.E. Hayakawa and E.W. Buchel, University of Manitoba, Canada.)

profunda femoris artery and vein. Typically, the vascular pedicle to the gracilis is located approximately 7 to 12 cm from the groin crease but can be highly variable. There are many vascular variations in the origin of the nutrient vessels to the gracilis muscle. They may branch directly from either the profunda femoris vessels or the medial circumflex femoral vessels (9). However, without exception, the pedicle courses beneath the adductor longus muscle and superficial to the adductor magnus muscle, providing vascular branches to each of these muscles. The pedicle terminates as two or three branches entering the medial, deep aspect of the gracilis muscle, approximately 10 cm inferior to the pubic tubercle (Figure 16-3). The length of the pedicle is 6 to 8 cm from the profunda femoris vessels and has a vessel diameter of approximately 1.6 to 1.8 mm.

The veins of the gracilis muscle are located with the arterial pedicle as paired venae comitantes. The entire muscle and proximal half of the cutaneous territory are adequately drained by the paired venae comitantes associated with the medial femoral circumflex artery. The venae eventually drain into the deep veins associated with profunda femoris artery. The proximal veins of the dominant pedicle have an external lumen diameter of 1.5 to 2.5 mm and a pedicle length of 6 to 8 cm.

The minor vascular pedicle(s) include one or two branches of the superficial femoral artery and venae comitantes. These pedicles are approximately 2 cm in length and 0.5 mm in diameter. They are located within the inferior half of the muscle.

GRACILIS MUSCLE NEURAL ANATOMY

The motor nerve of the gracilis muscle is the anterior branch of the obturator nerve (L2, L3, L4). The nerve enters the muscle approximately 2 to 3 cm superior to the point of entrance of the major vascular pedicle and nearly constantly at a 45-degree angle to the muscle (Figure 16-4). The motor nerve may be dissected proximally between the adductor longus and adductor magnus muscles to increase donor nerve length. This motor nerve also gives branches to the adductor longus and magnus muscles. To further increase the length of the nerve harvested with the gracilis muscle, when a long nerve pedicle is required, the nerve branches to the adductor muscles can be carefully dissected off of the gracilis motor branch in an interfascicular fashion.

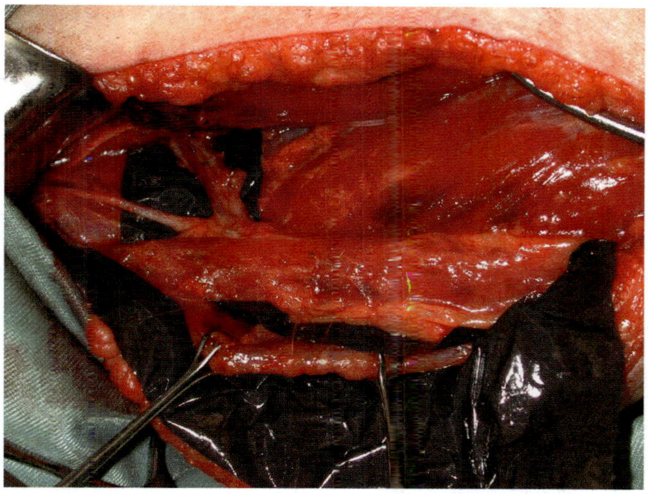

FIGURE 16-4 The nerve enters the muscle approximately 2 to 3 cm superior to the point of entrance of the major vascular pedicle and nearly constantly at a 45-degree angle to the muscle. (Reproduced with permission from Drs. T.E. Hayakawa and E.W. Buchel, University of Manitoba, Canada.)

The motor nerve runs with the sensory nerve along the medial surface of the adductor longus muscle. Small sensory branches from the obturator nerve enter the medial thigh skin, although no specific sensory branch can be located consistently. The skin territory of the gracilis is innervated by branches of the anterior femoral cutaneous nerve of the thigh (L2 and L3).

GRACILIS MUSCLE FLAP AND MUSCULOCUTANEOUS FLAP

Gracilis Muscle Flap Dimensions

The gracilis muscle measures approximately 5 to 6 cm in width, 24 to 30 cm in length and has an additional 10 to 12 cm of tendon (Figure 16-5). If the gracilis muscle is harvested with a cutaneous portion, the musculocutaneous flap reliably measures 6 to 8 cm in width and 24 cm in length. The muscle is thin and flat proximally (measuring 2–5 cm in thickness, depending on the size of the individual), becomes round in the midportion, and tapers to the size of the gracilis tendon distally.

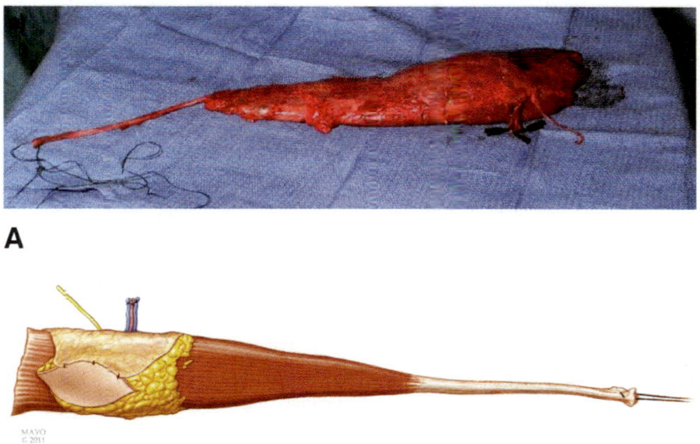

A

B

FIGURE 16-5 (**A**) The gracilis muscle measures approximately 5 to 6 cm in width and 24 to 30 cm in length and has an additional 10 to 12cm of tendon. (**B**) The vascular pedicle and the nerve are illustrated entering the deep surface of the muscle. (Used with permission of Mayo Foundation for Medical Education and Research, all rights reserved.)

Pedicled Gracilis Muscle Flap: Arc of Rotation

The entire muscle may be elevated reliably on its dominant vascular pedicle and transposed locally around the perineal and pelvis region (Figure 16-6). A proximally based flap is reliable. Although distally based flaps have been described to reach the knee (15), this flap is unreliable and rarely indicated. The distally based gracilis muscle flap is based on the distal minor pedicle; therefore, a delay is recommended 2 weeks before flap transposition to improve the likelihood of flap viability (15). If the minor pedicle is not located within the distal third of the muscle, the flap will not have adequate arc of rotation for knee coverage. Additionally, because the minor pedicle is not visualized during the delay procedure, the status and location of the minor pedicle are unknown until the second procedure. For this reason, this flap is rarely indicated for knee coverage and is unreliable.

Gracilis Muscle Flap Skin Territory

The medial thigh skin is not entirely vascularized by musculocutaneous perforating vessels from the gracilis. The clinically reliable island of skin based on the gracilis measures 8 × 24 cm

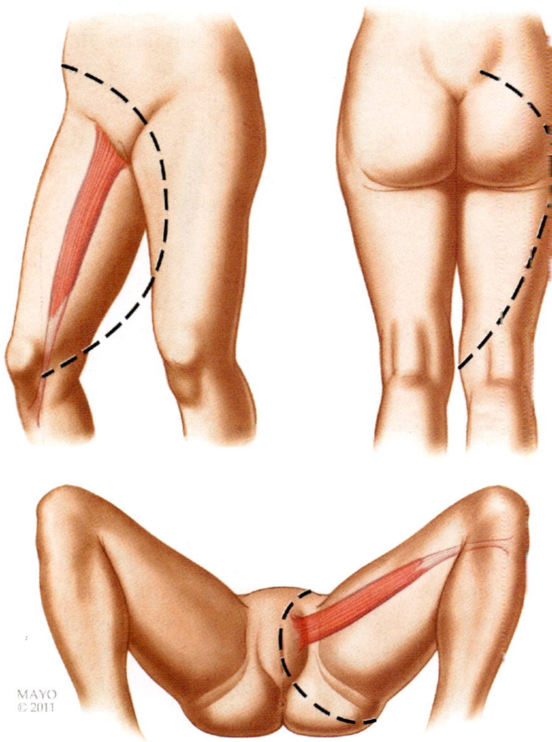

FIGURE 16-6 The entire muscle may be elevated reliably on its dominant vascular pedicle and transposed locally around the perineal and pelvis region. (Used with permission of Mayo Foundation for Medical Education and Research, all rights reserved.)

and is usually designed over the proximal two thirds of the muscle (8,15). Survival of the proximal cutaneous territory requires adequate localization of the skin territory over the muscle and careful preservation of the musculocutaneous perforating vessels. Perforating musculocutaneous arteries are small (<0.5 mm in diameter) and are distributed mostly over the proximal portion of the muscle (15). The skin over the distal third of the muscle is not reliable with division of the minor pedicles(s). Local transposition or free transfer of the gracilis with the proximal two thirds skin island is a reliable flap.

McCraw and Dibbell (8) described the relationship of cutaneous blood supply to subadjacent muscle vascular territories by injecting a thin latex suspension into human specimens. They demonstrated hundreds of minute vessels passing to the skin through the deep fascia. At the level of the deep fascia (not the investing muscular fascia), there is a dense lateral arborization of vessels on either side of the fascia. These minute vessels form a plexus on the superficial surface of the deep fascia. From this location, the vessels pass perpendicularly outward to the skin. To help improve the survival of the skin flap, it is best to include the fascia within the flap (8).

Innervated Free Functional Gracilis Flap

The strength of a muscle is directly proportional to the physiological cross-sectional area of the muscle fibers. It has been suggested that after transplantation, the muscle will atrophy to 25% to 50% of the pretransfer size (11,16).

It can be estimated that with maximum contraction, a muscle can shorten between 40% and 57% of its fully stretched length (17,18). This allows for a rough calculation of a muscle's contractile range by measuring the muscle fiber length. In a strap muscle, such as the gracilis, the muscle fibers are arranged parallel to the line of pull of the muscle, and the bundles of muscle fibers run the full length of the muscle. Therefore, the degree of shortening of the gracilis, with a 30-cm-long muscle belly, would be at least 12 cm in its normal state (30 cm × 40%) (10).

Manktelow and McKee (10) explained that a muscle develops its greatest contractile force at its physiological stretched resting length and has less amount of contractile force as the muscle shortens. As such, they recommended that if the gracilis is to be used as a functional muscle for finger flexion, it is desirable to insert the muscle into the forearm so that it is stretched maximally when the fingers and wrist are extended. This will give the desired contractile force when the wrist and fingers are in the neutral position. They also noted that if the full range of contraction is used, the last portion of the range of contraction usually cannot be carried out against significant resistance; therefore, the last few centimeters of contraction should not be expected to be useful in finger flexion where the requirement is for good strength at full finger flexion. A muscle should then be selected that normally has an amplitude of motion greater than the desired range of motion in its transplanted site.

Technique of Gracilis Muscle Flap Harvest

The gracilis flap may be designed with or without a cutaneous portion for local or distant coverage of defects or as a functional muscle. The gracilis musculocutaneous flap requires careful planning because the muscle is narrow, and the overlying skin is not adherent to the muscle.

Although there are many different methods of harvest, a majority, if not all, harvest methods begin proximally. The indication of the gracilis flap will determine the technique of harvest. If a small innervated gracilis is needed for facial reanimation, a proximal incision is used. However, if a complete length gracilis muscle and tendon with or without a skin paddle is required for restoration of elbow flexion or prehension in patients with brachial plexus injuries, it has been the experience of the authors to commence with a distal dissection either at the distal insertion of the gracilis at the pes anserinus or at the distal medial thigh at the musculotendinous junction. This method of harvest allows reliable identification of the overlying skin paddle, particularly in patients who have redundant or obese medial thighs. The following section will describe the proximal-incision-first technique followed by the distal-incision-first technique.

In the standing position, the gracilis muscle can be topographically identified by drawing a line between the proximal pubic tubercle and the distal gracilis muscle tendinous insertion at the pes anserinus (Figure 16-7). The topographic guideline drawn onto the patient should be drawn before the patient is placed in lithotomy or any other position involving flexion of the knee and hip because the landmarks may migrate and become inaccurate with posture changes. If a cutaneous portion of the flap is to be included, it is outlined slightly posterior to the line drawn from the pubic tubercle to the pes anserinus of the knee. The anterior border of the skin paddle should lie on this topographic line and may be extended posterior 6 to 9 cm, centered over the gracilis muscle. Alternatively, the skin paddle can be determined after the distal gracilis tendon has been identified as described later in the chapter. The location of the dominant vascular pedicle into the medial muscle belly,

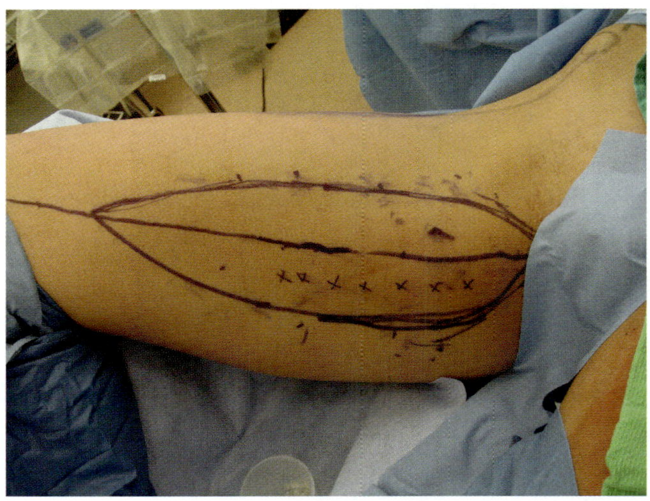

FIGURE 16-7 The gracilis muscle can be topographically identified by drawing a line between the proximal pubic tubercle and the distal gracilis muscle tendinous insertion at the pes anserine. (Used with permission of Mayo Foundation for Medical Education and Research, all rights reserved.)

approximately 10 cm from the pubic tubercle, must be considered in the design of the skin island on the muscle belly. In the operating room, the patient is positioned supine with the legs externally rotated and abducted.

Proximal Dissection First (Small Gracilis Muscle Flap, Facial Reconstruction) Technique

An incision is made just posterior to the drawn topographic line if a gracilis-only muscle flap is required or along the anterior border of the proposed cutaneous skin paddle in a musculocutaneous flap. The dissection is carried though the superficial fascia toward the muscle bellies. The gracilis muscle is identified by the progression of muscles from the adductor longus anteriorly to the gracilis muscle medially, and the semimembranosus muscle posteriorly. The gracilis can also be recognized by its flat muscle and rounded tendon configuration. Skin and subcutaneous tissue are elevated from the muscle to identify the anterior and posterior borders of the gracilis muscle. If a musculocutaneous flap is designed, temporary sutures approximating the skin edge to the underlying gracilis are placed to avoid shear and traction on the musculocutaneous perforating vessels.

The adductor longus muscle is retracted anteriorly 10 cm inferior to the pubic tubercle to expose the medial circumflex artery and paired venae comitantes coursing between the adductor longus and adductor magnus and entering the deep surface of the gracilis muscle. After the pedicle is visualized, it is mobilized proximally by dividing muscular branches to the adductor longus and adductor magnus muscles until the profunda femoris artery and vein are reached. The motor nerve is identified entering the deep surface of the gracilis and dissected as far proximal as possible if the gracilis flap will be used as an innervated flap. The nerve is harvested to the appropriate length. The anterior border of the gracilis muscle is then elevated with the adjacent deep muscle fascia of the adductor longus and adductor magnus muscles. Posteriorly, the semimembranosus and magnus fascia are elevated with the flap. The gracilis is dissected completely from its surrounding tissue proximally and distally. Distally, secondary minor pedicles are identified and ligated. The gracilis flap, although ready for transfer, is maintained in position until the recipient site has been prepared. After the recipient site is prepared, the gracilis is transferred either locally or distantly. The gracilis muscle may be passed through a subcutaneous or submuscular tunnel to the desired recipient site or the distal and proximal extends of the gracilis can be transected followed by division of the neurovascular pedicle for free muscle transfer.

The donor site is closed primarily over drains. The donor deficit is minimal and the donor scar is an acceptable longitudinal medial thigh scar. The loss of this muscle is not clinically detected because it is compensated by the stronger adductor longus and adductor magnus muscles.

Distal Dissection First (Full-Length Musculocutaneous Innervated Flap for Brachial Plexus Elbow or Forearm Flexor Reconstruction) Technique

If a full length gracilis is needed, the gracilis tendon at the pes anserinus can be identified via a 3-cm longitudinal incision over the pes anserinus and a 4-cm longitudinal incision in the distal medial thigh (Figure 16-8). At the pes anserinus, the gracilis tendon can be easily palpated as the most superior tendinous insertion. The inferior tendon at the pes anserinus is the semitendinosus tendon. The gracilis and semitendinosus tendons are covered by sartorius fascia (Figure 16-9). A longitudinal incision is made over the tendons, and the sartorius fascia is elevated. Dissection is carried between the tendons until the

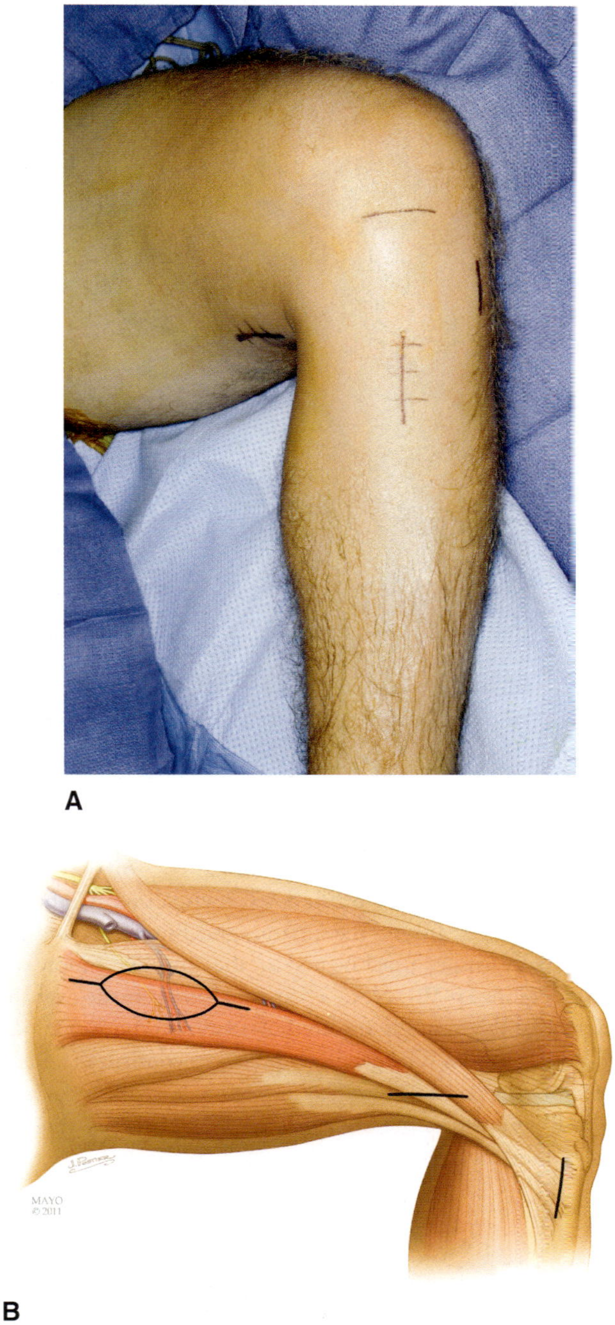

FIGURE 16-8 When a full-length gracilis is needed, the harvest begins distally where the gracilis tendon at the pes anserine can be identified via 3-cm longitudinal incision over the pes anserine (**A**) and a 4-cm longitudinal incision in the distal medial thigh (**B**) and a proximal thigh incision or skin paddle. (Used with permission of Mayo Foundation for Medical Education and Research, all rights reserved.)

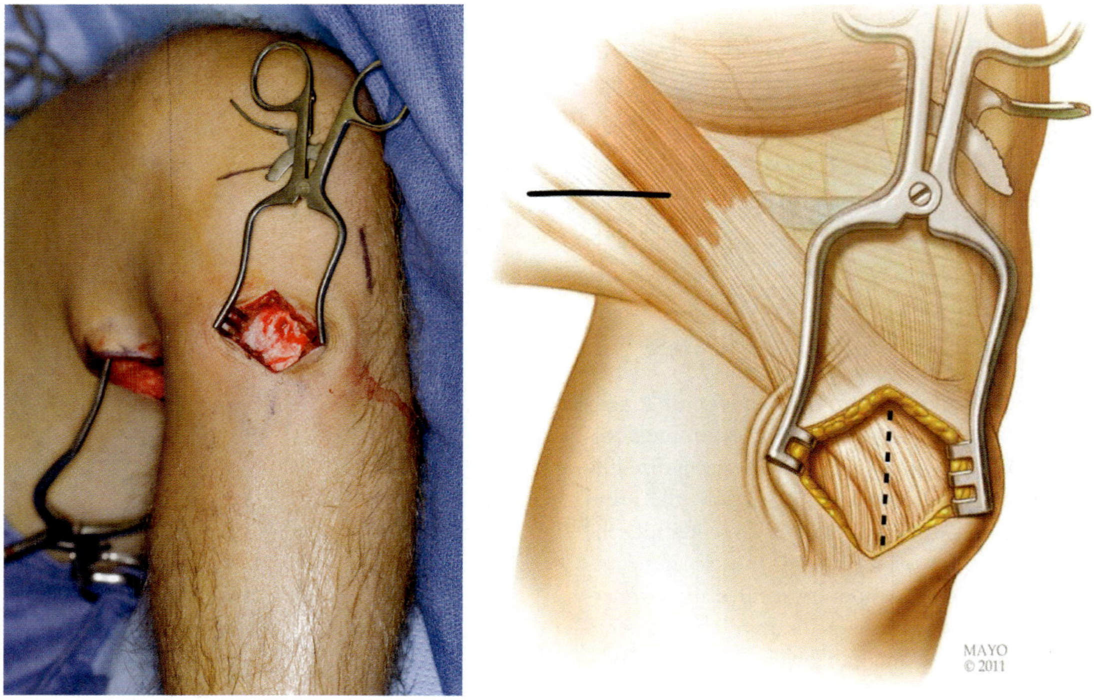

A B

FIGURE 16-9 The gracilis and semitendinosus tendons are covered by sartorius fascia, which is demonstrated in an intraoperative photograph (**A**) as well as a line drawing (**B**). (Used with permission of Mayo Foundation for Medical Education and Research, all rights reserved.)

medial collateral ligament of the knee is visualized. Umbilical tape is then placed around the superior gracilis tendon, and the multiple soft tissue attachments to the gracilis tendon are divided (Figure 16-10). Next, a 4-cm incision is made over the distal medial thigh, where the musculotendinous portion of the gracilis is identified. The gracilis is pulled to confirm the gracilis tendon previously identified inserting into the proximal tibia. All soft tissues attachments to the gracilis are divided between these two incisions (Figure 16-11).

After the gracilis muscle and tendon has been identified, traction can be applied to the muscle and tendon proximally, causing the entire muscle to "bowstring," thus outlining the specific area of cutaneous territory overlying the muscle that

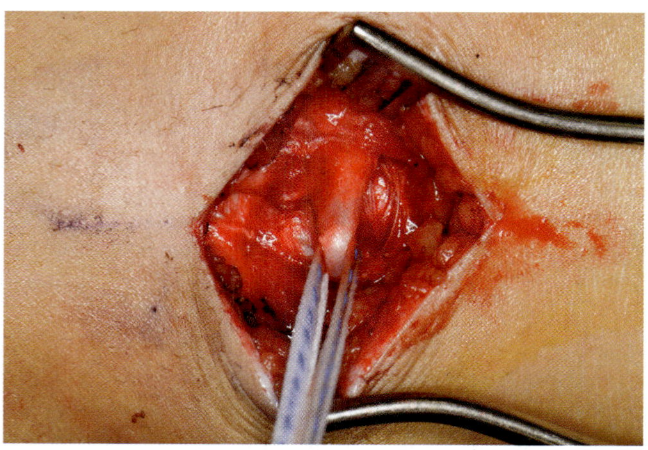

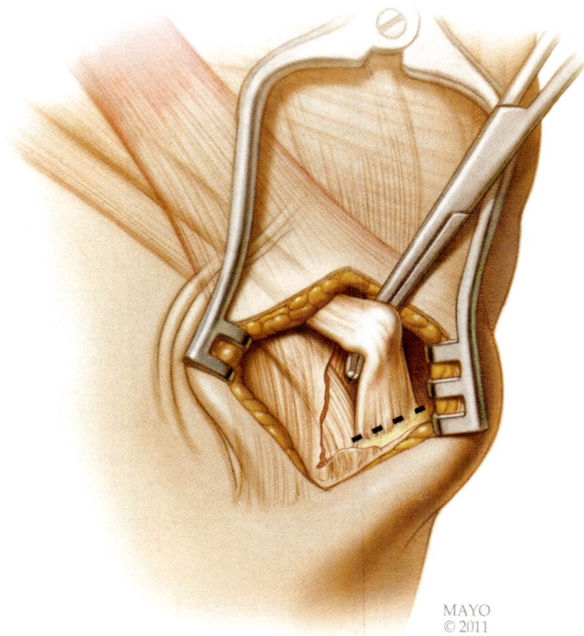

A B

FIGURE 16-10 (**A**) After the overlying sartorius fascia is divided, umbilical tape is placed around the superior gracilis tendon, and the multiple soft tissue attachments to the gracilis tendon are divided. (**B**) At the pes anserine, the gracilis tendon is the most superior tendinous insertion; the inferior tendon is the semitendinosus tendon. (Used with permission of Mayo Foundation for Medical Education and Research, all rights reserved.)

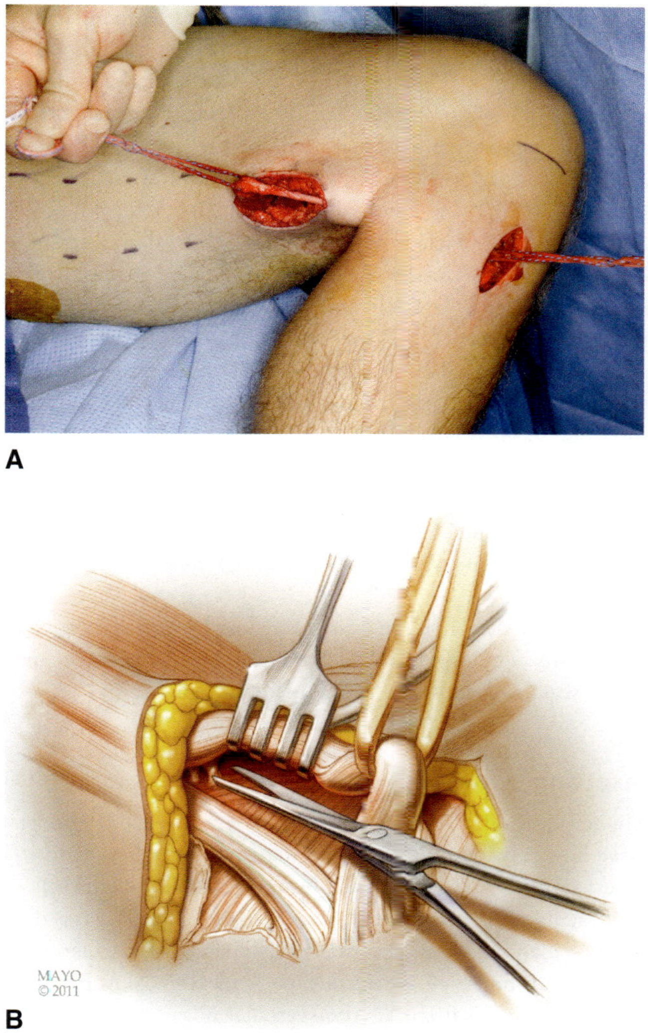

FIGURE 16-11 All soft tissues attachments to the gracilis are divided between the two incisions at the pes anserine and the distal medial thigh as seen in an intraoperative photograph (**A**) as well as a line drawing (**B**). (Used with permission of Mayo Foundation for Medical Education and Research, all rights reserved.)

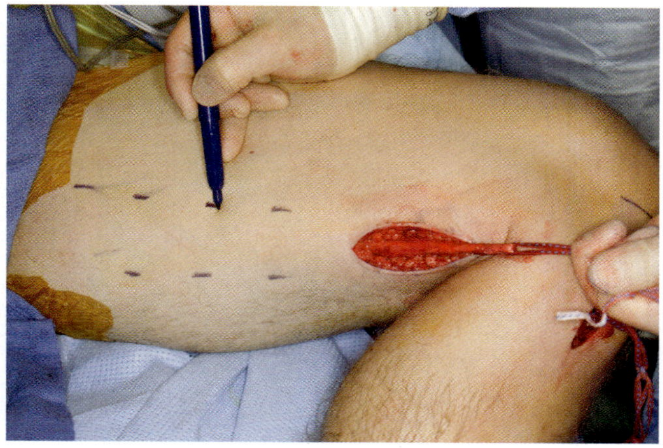

FIGURE 16-12 After the gracilis muscle or tendon has been identified, traction can be applied to the muscle or tendon proximally, causing the entire muscle to "bowstring," thus outlining the specific area of cutaneous territory overlying the muscle that may be incorporated into the musculocutaneous flap if required. (Used with permission of Mayo Foundation for Medical Education and Research, all rights reserved.)

may be incorporated into the musculocutaneous flap if required (Figure 16-12). When the skin island is placed directly over the muscle, the skin dimensions may include the proximal two thirds of the medial thigh skin with a maximum width of 8 cm. The location of the dominant vascular pedicle into the medial muscle belly, approximately 10 cm from the pubic tubercle, must be considered in the design of the skin island on the muscle belly. A handheld, sterile Doppler device can be used to identify and mark skin perforators overlying the proximal gracilis muscle (Figure 16-13). An elliptical shaped incision is drawn slightly anterior to the anterior border of the gracilis muscle, centered about the identified skin perforators.

Next, the proximal thigh incision is made along the anterior border of the skin paddle, and dissection is carried toward the adductor longus (Figure 16-14). The fascia of the adductor longus is incised longitudinally, and the fascial edge is sewn to the skin paddle edge to avoid shear and traction on musculocutaneous perforating vessels. In the interval between the adductor longus and gracilis muscles, the fascia of the adductor longus is gently retracted to expose the obturator nerve and the dominant proximal artery and venae comitantes (Figure 16-15). The adductor longus is retracted medially and superiorly while the vascular perforators to the adductor longus are carefully dissected and ligated. Caution to aggressive dissection should be made as the medial femoral circumflex vessels are tented up against the adductor longus and can be iatrogenically injured. After the perforators to the adductor longus are ligated, the vessels are dissected to the profunda femoral artery and vein. The artery and vein are isolated proximally, and vessel loops are placed around each vessel. If an innervated flap is to be used, the obturator nerve is identified entering the deep surface of the gracilis obliquely to the vascular pedicle and stimulated with a disposable nerve stimulator to verify contraction. A vessel loop is placed around the

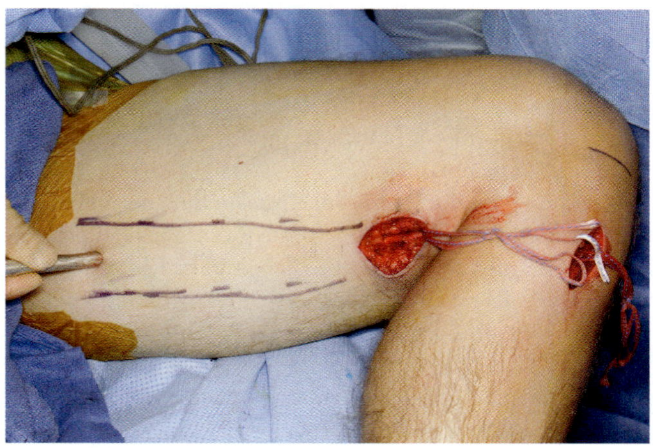

FIGURE 16-13 A handheld, sterile Doppler device can be used to identify and mark the skin perforators overlying the proximal gracilis muscle. (Used with permission of Mayo Foundation for Medical Education and Research, all rights reserved.)

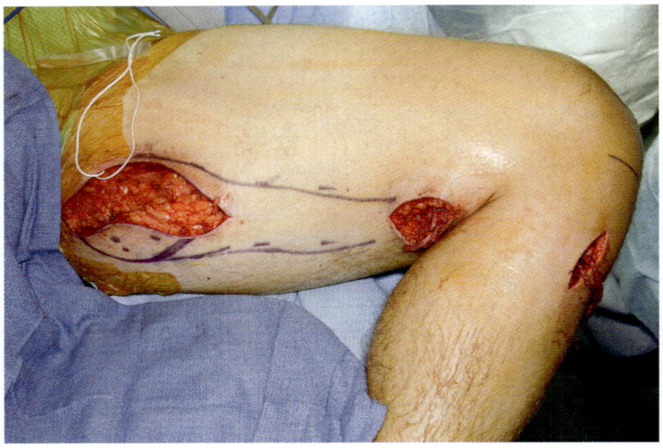

A

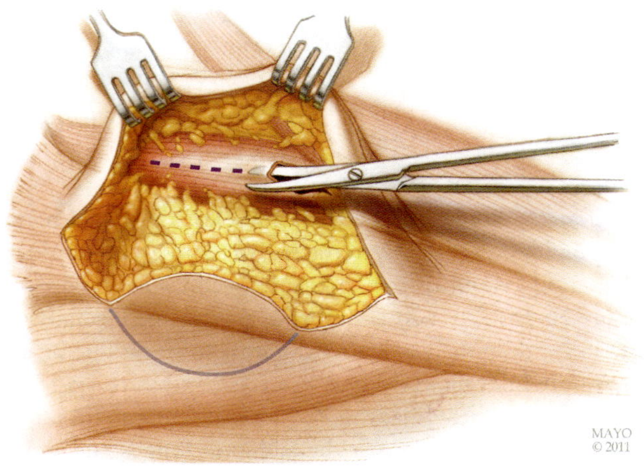

B

FIGURE 16-14 (**A**) An elliptical-shaped incision is drawn slightly anterior to the anterior border of the gracilis muscle, centered about the identified skin perforators. The proximal thigh incision is made along the anterior border of the skin paddle, and dissection is carried toward the adductor longus. (**B**) Fascia of the adductor longus is incised longitudinally. (Used with permission of Mayo Foundation for Medical Education and Research, all rights reserved.)

nerve, and the dissection progresses as far proximal as possible. To gain nerve length, the nerve branches to the adductor muscles are carefully dissected in an interfascicular fashion from the gracilis motor branch. Typically, a nerve pedicle of 8 to 12 cm can be obtained.

Next, the posterior skin paddle incision is made, and dissection is carried to the level of the adductor magnus muscle. The adductor magnus fascia is incised longitudinally and reflected with the gracilis muscle (Figure 16-16). Care should be made not to expose the gracilis or perforate the gracilis fascia. Ultimately, a fascial sleeve around the proximal gracilis (the adductor longus, adductor magnus, and semitendinosus fascia) and its skin paddle remain.

Between the two thigh incisions, blunt-finger dissection is performed in a subfascial plane. The secondary pedicle can often be felt or seen and is ligated. The distal tendon of the gracilis is then detached from the pes anserinus and passed first into the distal thigh incision and then passed to the proximal thigh incision. The gracilis muscle is gently delivered out of the proximal incision (Figure 16-17). The fascia of the adductor magnus is transversely divided at the distal edge of the gracilis. At this point, the only attachments of the gracilis are to the tendinous origin at the pubic tubercle and the vascular pedicle (Figure 16-18).

The gracilis muscle is replaced back into its native bed, and the proximal attachment is addressed. The proximal attachment is tendinous laterally and more muscular medially. The tendon is dissected off the adductor longus tendon and adductor magnus muscles, and using an angled electrocautery tip (bent by the surgeon), the gracilis tendon is detached from the pubic rami (Figure 16-19). The flap harvest is now complete, and the gracilis is perfusing only from its dominant pedicle. A papaverine-soaked sponge is placed over the vessels until the recipient site has been prepared. After the recipient site is ready for the transfer, the pedicle of the gracilis is ligated and divided.

The three donor site incisions are closed primarily over suction drains. The donor deficit is minimal, and the three small donor scars are acceptable in the medial thigh.

Insetting of the Free Innervated Gracilis Flap

The application of the free innervated gracilis flap will determine how it is inset, what vessels are used, and what nerve will innervate the flap. Secure and strong proximal attachments of the gracilis at the recipient site are first performed followed by the vascular anastomosis. Reestablishment of vascular flow within 60 minutes of ischemia time is ideal and has been the goal of our surgical team. After vascular anastomosis, coaptation of the donor motor nerve to the obturator branch of the gracilis is performed under an operating microscope. Finally, tensioning of the gracilis is performed. Placement of sutures every 5 cm into the muscle to obtain ideal resting length of the muscle has been recommended by Manktelow and McKee (10). In brachial plexus reconstructions, however, the authors have found that tensioning the gracilis flap such that the elbow is maintained in 30 degrees of flexion at rest is a reliable way of tensioning the muscle.

ADVANTAGES OF THE GRACILIS FLAP

The gracilis muscle harvested as a flap is reliable, and the anatomy is consistent with few anatomic variants. The muscle is pliable, with minimal bulk, and can be tailored to fill the dimensions of a small defect. A cutaneous skin paddle may be incorporated into the flap to supplement the reconstruction or monitor the flap. Alternatively, the gracilis muscle can be harvested without a cutaneous component and covered by a skin graft. During harvest of the gracilis muscle flap, a simultaneous recipient site may be prepared. The gracilis muscle flap may be innervated for functional use in facial reanimation or upper extremity movement restoration. The muscle is usually split in facial muscle replacement. About 30% to 40% of the muscle is ideal. Selection of the appropriate segment is aided by splitting

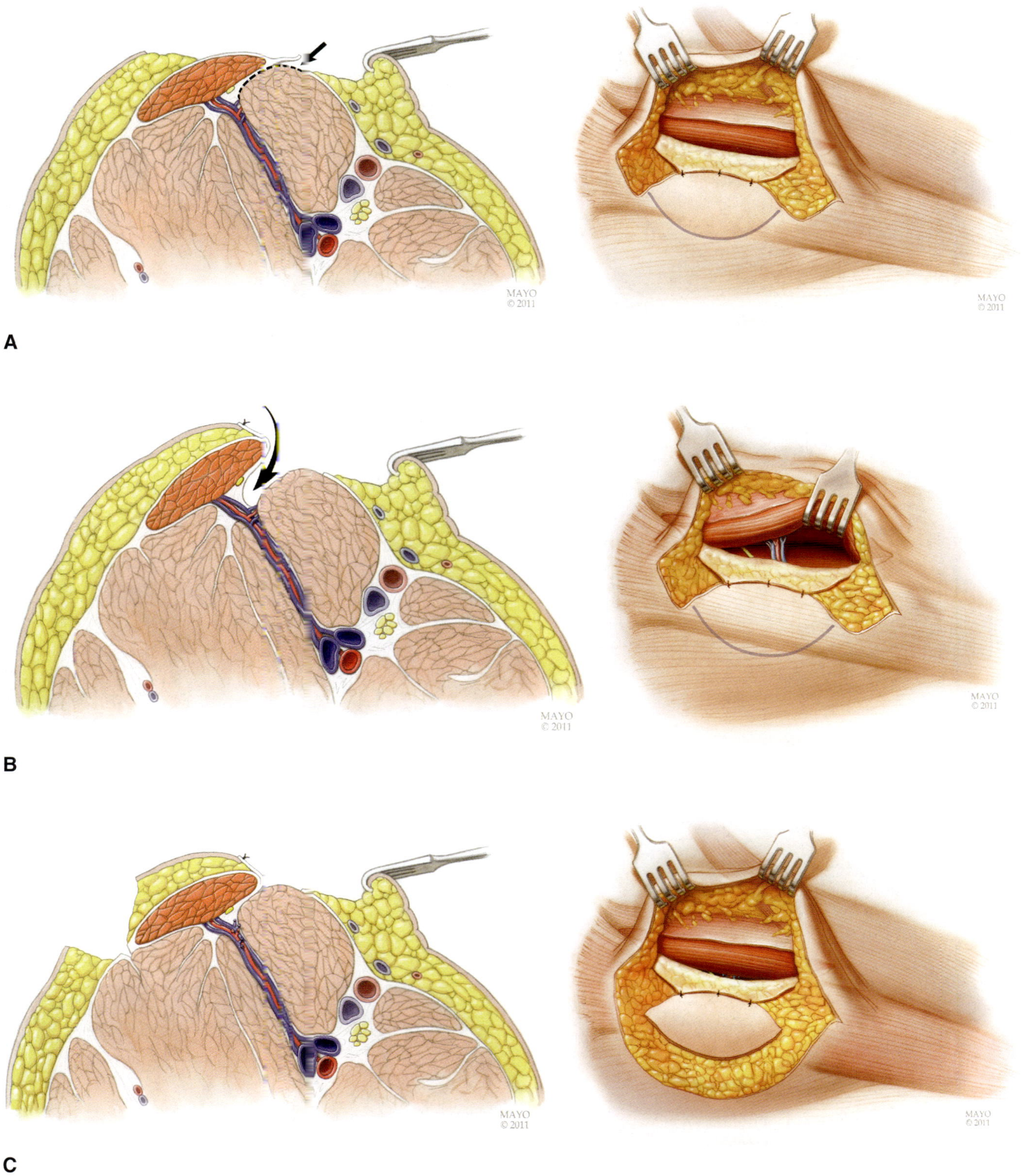

FIGURE 16-15 The fascia of the adductor longus is incised longitudinally (**A**), and the fascial edge is sewn to the skin paddle edge to avoid shear and traction on musculocutaneous perforating vessels (**B**). In the interval between the adductor longus and gracilis muscles, the fascia of the adductor longus is gently retracted to expose the obturator nerve and the dominant proximal artery and venae comitantes (**C**). (Used with permission of Mayo Foundation for Medical Education and Research, all rights reserved.)

the nerve into its two to three fascicles and then using a nerve stimulator to select the corresponding one. The donor site is closed with an acceptable medial thigh scar and without a donor site functional deficit.

Prerequisites for using a free, functional, innervated flap in the upper extremity include an intact antagonist muscle group; appropriately located recipient vessels; an undamaged synergistic recipient motor nerve and an expendable donor muscle

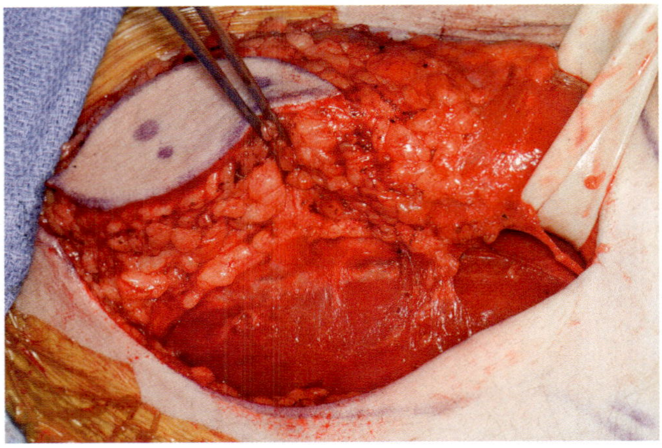

A

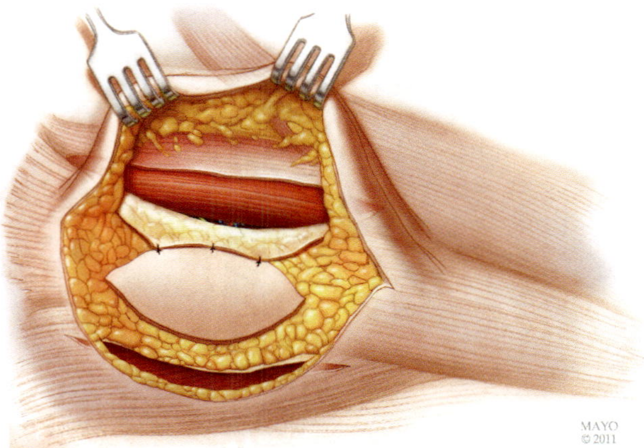

B

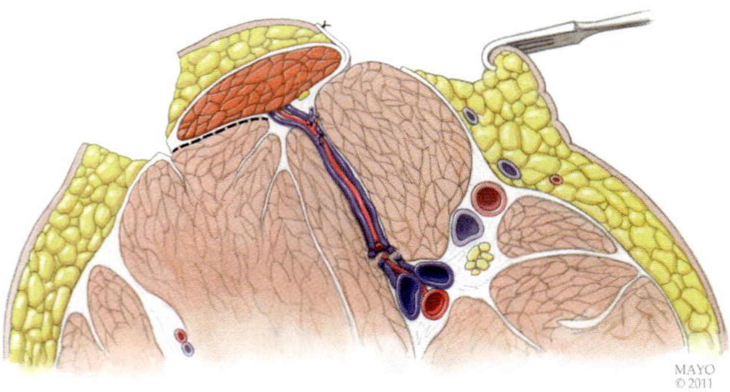

C

FIGURE 16-16 The adductor magnus fascia is incised longitudinally and reflected with the gracilis muscle as seen in an intraoperative photograph (**A**) and a line drawing (**B**). (**C**) Cross-section view. (Used with permission of Mayo Foundation for Medical Education and Research, all rights reserved.)

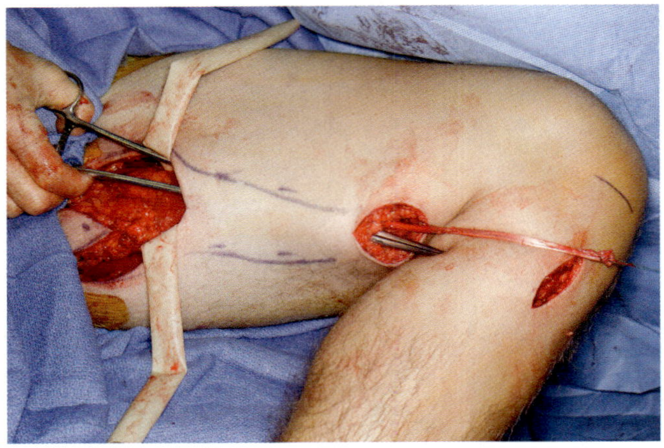

A

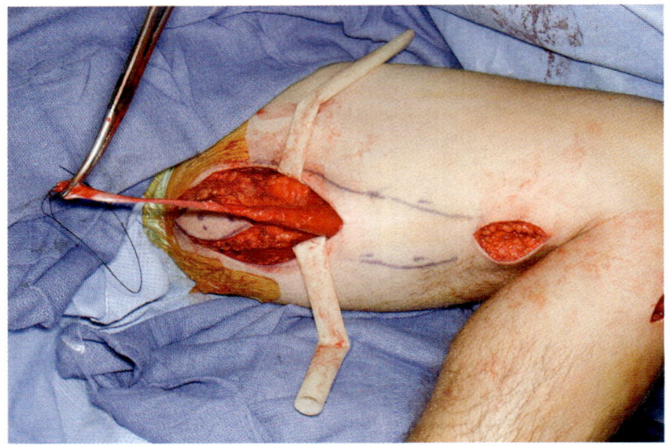

B

FIGURE 16-17 (**A**) The distal tendon of the gracilis is then detached from the pes anserine and passed first into the distal thigh incision and then passed to the proximal thigh incision. (**B**) The gracilis muscle is gently delivered out of the proximal incision. (Used with permission of Mayo Foundation for Medical Education and Research, all rights reserved.)

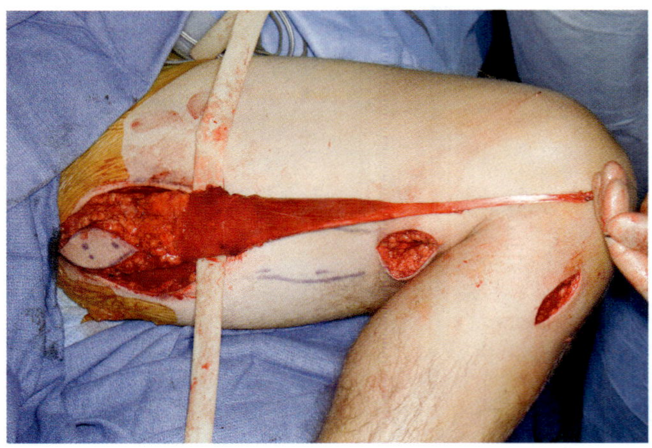

FIGURE 16-18 The only attachments of the gracilis are to the tendinous origin at the pubic tubercle and the vascular pedicle. (Used with permission of Mayo Foundation for Medical Education and Research, all rights reserved.)

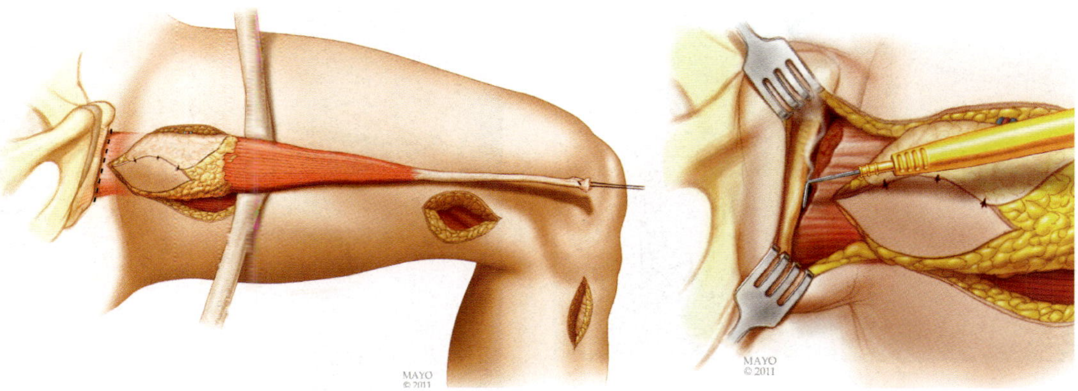

FIGURE 16-19 (**A**) The proximal attachment is tendinous laterally and more muscular medially. (**B**) The tendon is dissected off the adductor longus tendon and adductor magnus muscles, and using an angled electrocautery tip (bent by the surgeon), the gracilis tendon is detached from the pubic rami. (Used with permission of Mayo Foundation for Medical Education and Research, all rights reserved.)

supplied by a single major neurovascular pedicle with adequate excursion, strength, and contractility. Additional factors potentially affecting the speed and extent of muscle recovery after transfer appear to be related to ischemia time, the distance from the neurorrhaphy to the muscle flap motor end plates, and the technical adequacy of the neurorrhaphy. The maximum ischemia time of a muscle at room temperature is unknown. Kuzon et al. (19) examined the isometric contractile function after recovery of free, vascularized gracilis muscle transfers in 15 dogs subjected to graded periods of intraoperative ischemia. They reported that, on average, the replanted gracilis muscles had significantly less twitch and tetanic tension than in the control dogs; however, there were several individual reports of dogs regaining 100% of the control's maximal tetanic tension. The study did not find a correlation between intraoperative ischemia time of up to 4 hours and functional return (19). Despite this, the authors' preference is to restore blood flow within 60 minutes.

DISADVANTAGES OF THE GRACILIS FLAP

Without the cutaneous component of the gracilis flap, the muscle is covered with a skin graft. The muscle power and bulk may be excessive in facial reconstruction but not adequate enough in upper extremity reconstruction. An occasional complaint of patients has been hyperesthesia, particularly in the distal thigh, presumably caused by iatrogenic injury to the cutaneous branch of the obturator nerve, which courses near the vascular pedicle. Patients may also complain of the scarring to the medial aspect of the thigh.

INDICATIONS FOR THE GRACILIS FLAP

A functional gracilis flap has been described for facial reanimation, elbow flexion, and finger and wrist flexion and extension in brachial plexus injury patients. Recently, transverse upper gracilis (TUG) flaps have been described for breast reconstruction after a skin-sparing mastectomy. The gracilis muscle has also been used to restore quadriceps function (Figure 16-20) and anterior tibialis function (Figure 16-21). Other reconstructive indications for this flap include coverage of any small defects, vaginal and penile reconstruction, coverage of pressure sores in the groin and perineum, rectal sphincter reconstruction, reconstruction of urethrocutaneous and vesicocutaneous fistulas as well as vesicovaginal and rectovaginal fistulas, and correction of intractable vaginal prolapse (Table 16-1).

Facial Reanimation

In cases of irreversible facial paralysis, the free gracilis muscle can be used to reanimate the face, specifically concentrating on reconstructing the smile (Figure 16-22). If the facial paralysis is a consequence of a tumor resection including sacrifice of the facial nerve, the transected facial nerve stump will be available as a motor source for innervating the free gracilis in the recipient paralyzed face. The gracilis muscle flap is harvested in the described manner. The recipient site is approached through a preauricular incision. A cheek flap is raised, and the facial nerve and vessels (either the facial vessels or the superficial temporal vessels) are identified and prepared for the anastomosis and neurorrhaphy. After revascularization and neurorrhaphy of the gracilis muscle, the two ends of the gracilis are fixed to the zygoma and the upper and lower lips and modiolus region under proper tension (20,21).

In cases of long-standing facial paralysis when the ipsilateral facial nerve stump is not available as the motor source, a cross-facial nerve graft from an intact contralateral facial nerve branch has the potential to innervate the transferred gracilis using a sural nerve graft.

Innervation to the muscle will usually occur 8 to10 months after surgery. The muscle's contractile power will increase over the subsequent 2 years after surgery (20).

Zuker (21) describes using a portion of the gracilis muscle in facial reanimation to avoid excess bulk. He states that the volume of the gracilis muscle is assessed in the thigh and usually about 40% to 50% of the circumference of the muscle is sufficient for use in reconstructing the smile (Figure 16-23). Because of the parallel orientation of the muscle fibers and the

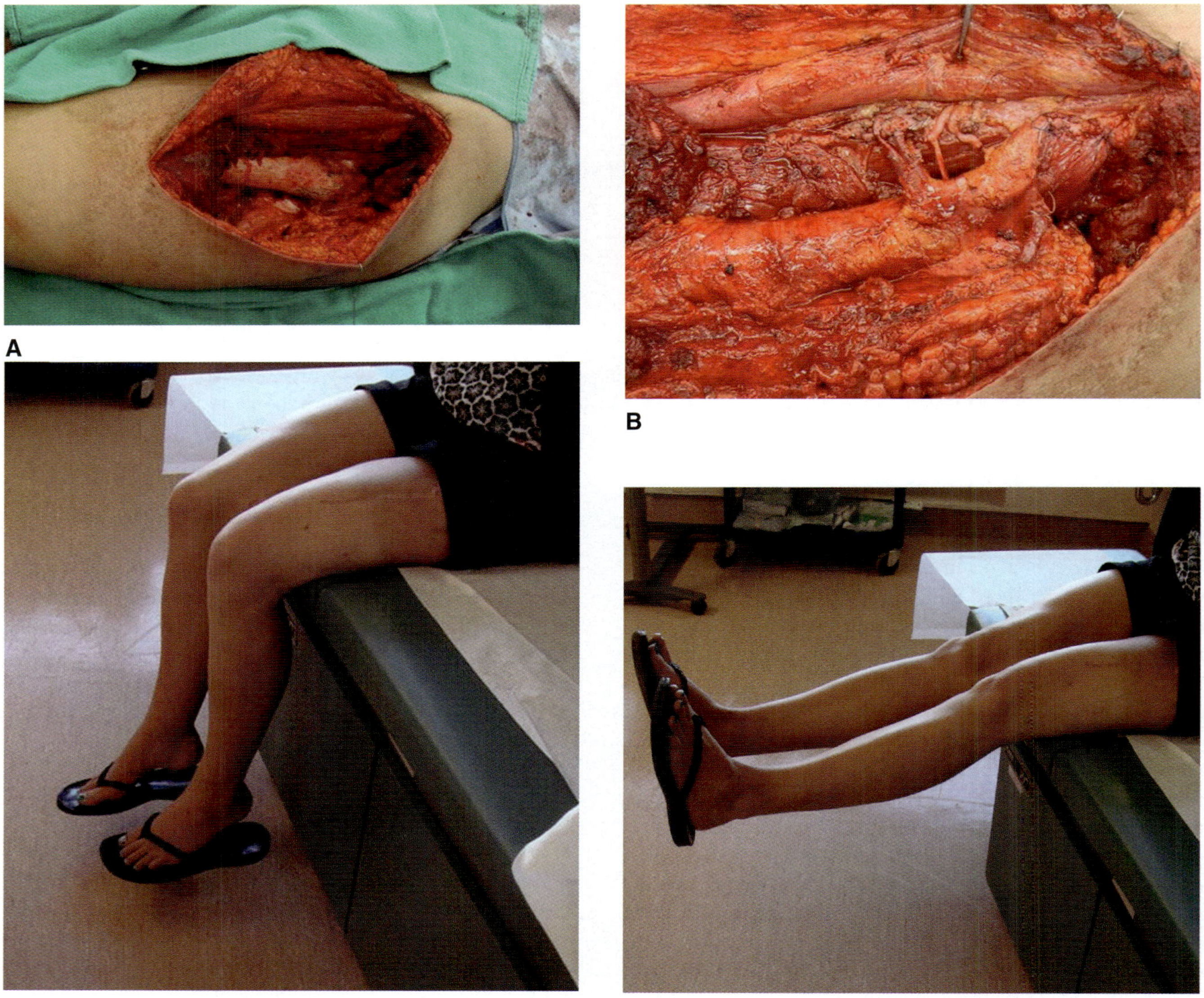

FIGURE 16-20 Reconstruction of a quadriceps muscle using a free-functioning innervated gracilis muscle from the contralateral leg. (**A**) The debrided quadriceps muscle is seen in the top left. (**B**) The free-functioning innervated gracilis attached proximally into the origin of the rectus femoris muscle and distally into the remnant of the quadriceps tendon. Postoperative flexion (**C**) and extension (**D**) photographs taken at 18 months. (Reproduced with permission from Drs. T.E. Hayakawa and E.W. Buchel, University of Manitoba, Canada.)

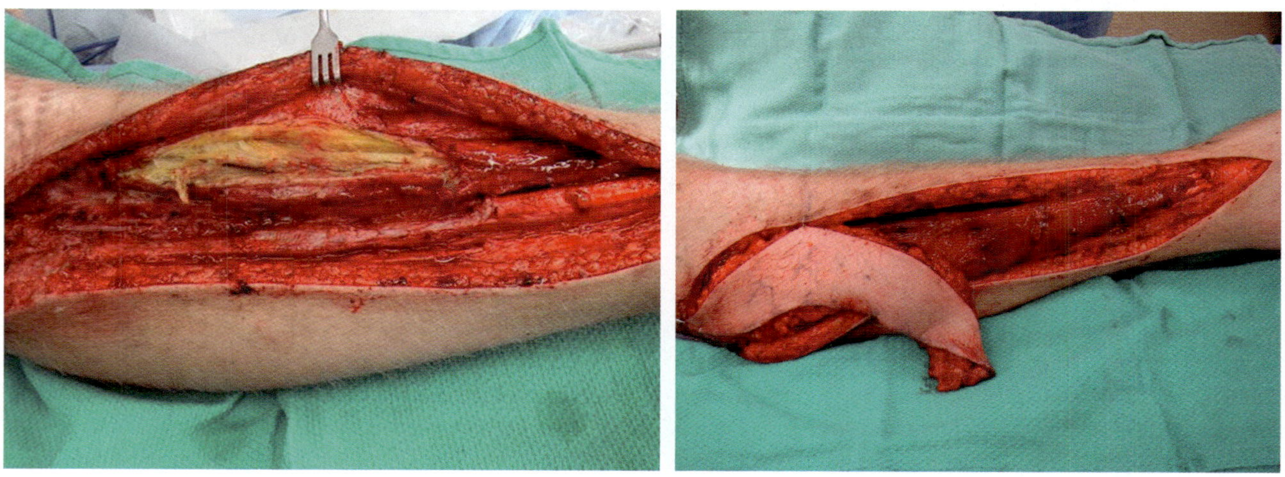

FIGURE 16-21 (**A**) Complete necrosis of the anterior tibialis muscle secondary to anterior compartment syndrome. (**B**) Reconstruction of anterior tibialis muscle using an innervated free-functioning gracilis muscle. (Reproduced with permission from Drs. T.E. Hayakawa and E.W. Buchel, University of Manitoba, Canada.)

TABLE 16-1. Indications for the Gracilis Flap

	References	Advantages	Disadvantages
Genitourinary reconstruction • Vaginal reconstruction • Penile reconstruction • Anal sphincter reconstruction	McCraw et al (7) Cronje and Van Zyl (30) Soper et al. (31) Nahai (32) Mathes and Nahai (15) Orticochea (4) Hester et al. (33) Song et al. (34)	Brings vascularity and bulk to fill the soft tissue deficit Pliable Epithelial surface in musculocutaneous flaps for lining Hastens recovery after radical ablative surgery for tumor resection, especially in cases with adjunctive radiotherapy	Location and bulk of the vascular pedicle may hinder flap mobility Upper thigh bulge of tissue secondary to rotated gracilis flap Atrophy Aesthetics Possible prolapse
Small wound defect coverage • Perineal and pelvis • Extremity • Facial defects (orbital exenteration, maxillectomy • Contour defects (hemifacial atrophy)	Mathes and Nahai (15) Conway and Griffith (35) Foster et al. (36)	Promotes healing by introducing vascular supply Has greater bulk for obliterating dead space	Muscle is more susceptible to ischemic necrosis than skin or subcutaneous tissue
Facial reanimation	Frey (22) Harii et al. (11) Harii and Asato (20) Zuker (21)	Muscle fibers are parallel and show a long amplitude of contraction Thin muscle with minimal bulk A portion of the muscle can be used	Muscle power and bulk may be excessive for facial reanimation
Upper extremity movement restoration	Ikuta et al. (12) Mankelow and McKee (10) Doi et al. (13) Shin et al. (24) Bishop (23)	Long tendon length Able to achieve M4 muscle strength Adequate excursion and contractility	Not all patients achieve M4 muscle strength
Breast reconstruction	Yousif et al (25) Furnas (26) Wechselberger and Schoeller (27)	Can be an option in thin women without adequate abdominal, buttock or back subcutaneous tissue used in other flaps Discrete donor site scarring Allows esthetic shaping, contouring and projection of the reconstructed breast	For reconstruction of small to medium sized breasts Possible complications of wound dehiscence and lymphedema Upper thigh contour defect

long amplitude of contraction, contraction of the gracilis muscle within the recipient bed can give a natural-appearing smile (22).

Elbow Flexion in Brachial Plexus Patients

When the time from brachial plexus injury to presentation is more than 9 to 12 months, a free-functioning muscle transfer in conjunction with an extraplexal motor nerve transfer to restore elbow function is recommended. Free-functioning muscles transferred for a specific purpose should have the strength and excursion comparable to the paralyzed muscles they are replacing (23). A variety of free-functioning muscles can be transferred, including the latissimus dorsi (thoracodorsal nerve), the rectus femoris (femoral nerve), and the gracilis (anterior division of the obturator nerve). The gracilis has become a commonly transferred muscle because of its reliable, proximally based neurovascular pedicle (allows earlier reinnervation), and its long tendon length (which has the potential to restore elbow flexion, wrist extension, or finger flexion) (24). The free-functioning muscle transfers may be powered by either two intercostal motor nerves or the spinal accessory

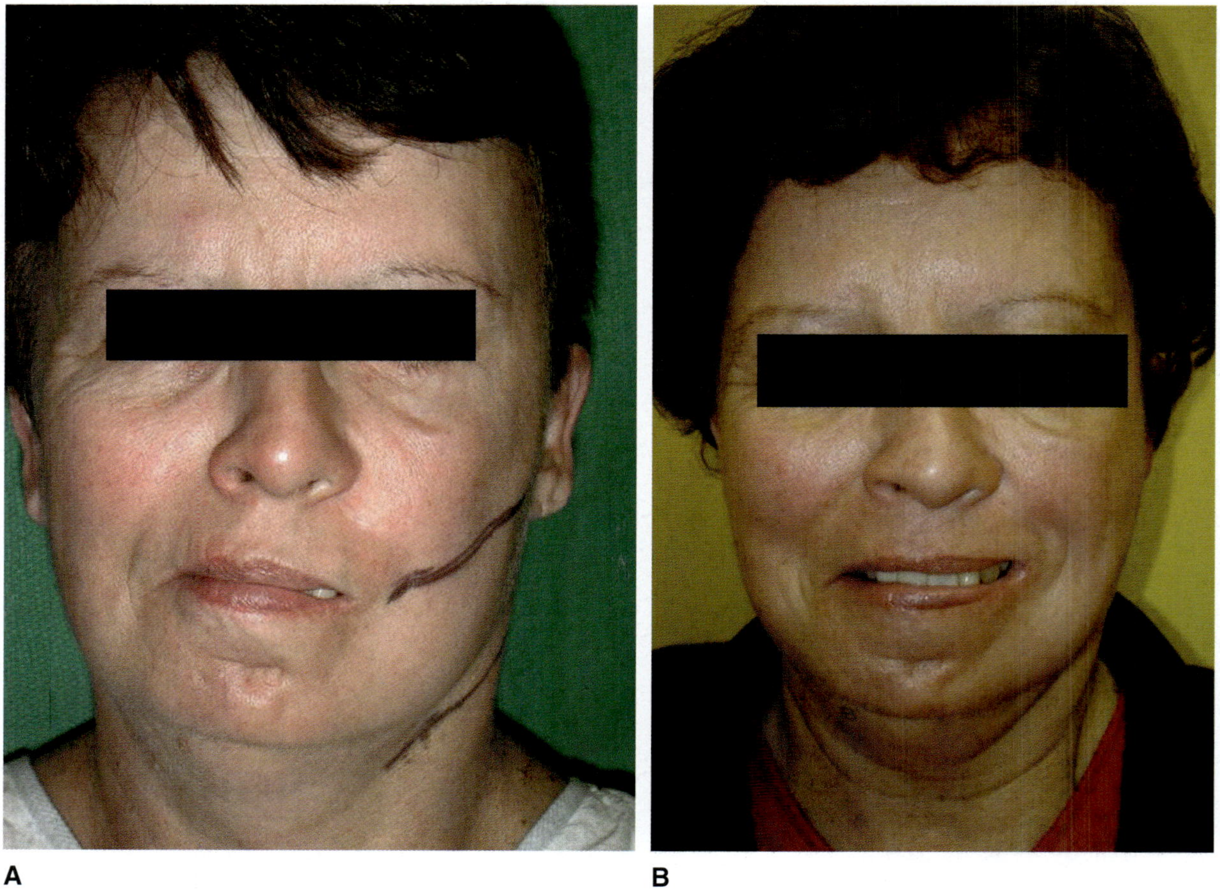

FIGURE 16-22 In cases of irreversible facial paralysis, the free gracilis muscle can be used to reanimate the face, specifically concentrating on reconstructing the smile. Pre- (**A**) and postoperative (**B**) photographs. (Reproduced with permission from Drs. T.E. Hayakawa and E.W. Buchel, University of Manitoba, Canada.)

nerve. Proximally, the gracilis is secured to the clavicle while distally the gracilis tendon is woven into the biceps tendon (Figure 16-24). Seventy-nine percent of the gracilis free-functioning muscle transfers for elbow flexion alone achieved at least M4 strength (23).

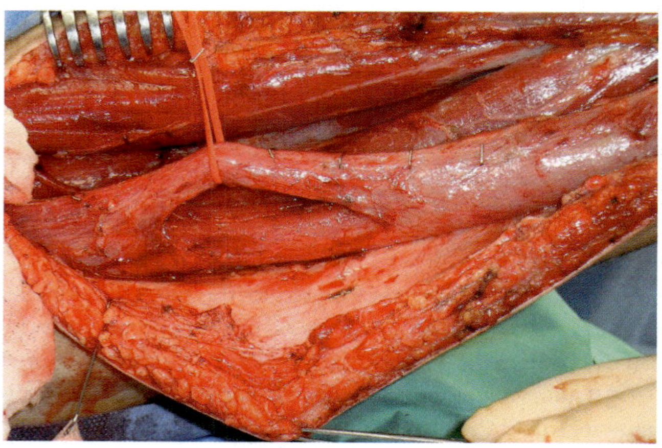

FIGURE 16-23 Zuker (21) states that the volume of the gracilis muscle is assessed in the thigh and usually about 40% to 50% of the circumference of the muscle is sufficient for use in reconstructing the smile. (Reproduced with permission from Drs. T.E. Hayakawa and E.W. Buchel, University of Manitoba, Canada.)

Hand Function Restoration in Brachial Plexus Patients

Despite favorable results for early nerve grafting and transfer techniques for shoulder and elbow function, reported results of grafting or nerve transfers for hand function have been less favorable (23). Hand function requires restoration of both grasp and release in addition to the adequate positioning of the hand in space. Intrinsic muscle function and wrist or digital movement cannot readily be restored by nerve transfers; therefore, either a single or double gracilis free-functioning muscle transfer has been proposed.

Doi et al. (13) described a double gracilis transfer to provide shoulder stability and function combined with flexion and extension of the elbow, hand sensibility, and rudimentary hand grasp and release. In the first muscle transfer, the gracilis muscle is neurotized by the spinal accessory nerve and anastomosed to the thoracoacromial trunk to produce elbow flexion and finger or wrist extension. Proximally, the gracilis is attached to the clavicle and routed distally under the brachioradialis to the radial wrist and finger extensors (Figure 16-25). In the second transfer, the gracilis is neurotized to motor intercostal nerves and anastomosed to the thoracodorsal artery to create finger flexion (Figure 16-26). The sensory intercostal nerves are neurotized to the lateral cord contribution to the median nerve for

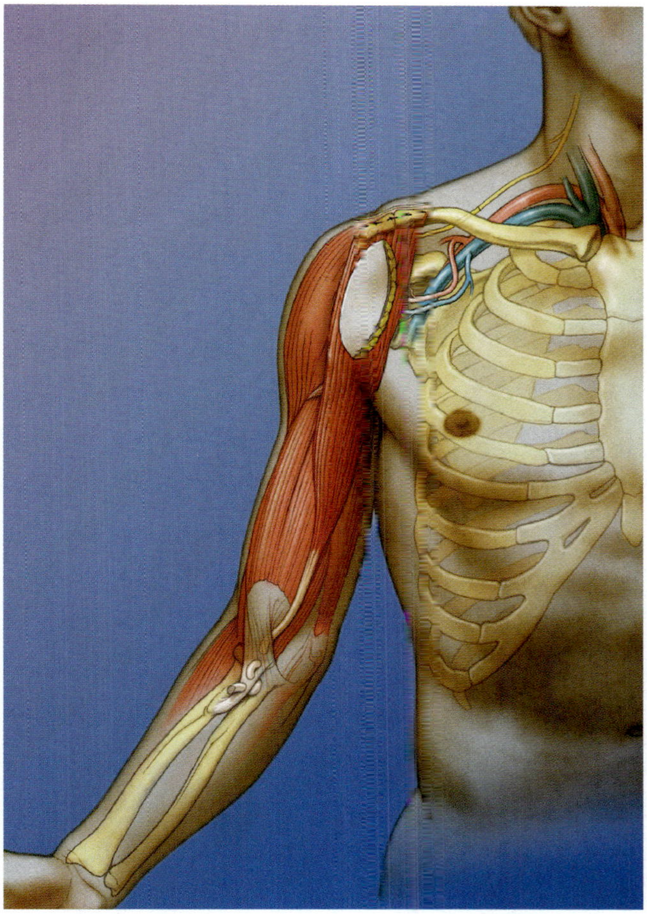

FIGURE 16-24 Proximally, the gracilis is secured to the clavicle while distally the gracilis tendon is woven into the biceps tendon. (Used with permission of Mayo Foundation for Medical Education and Research, all rights reserved.)

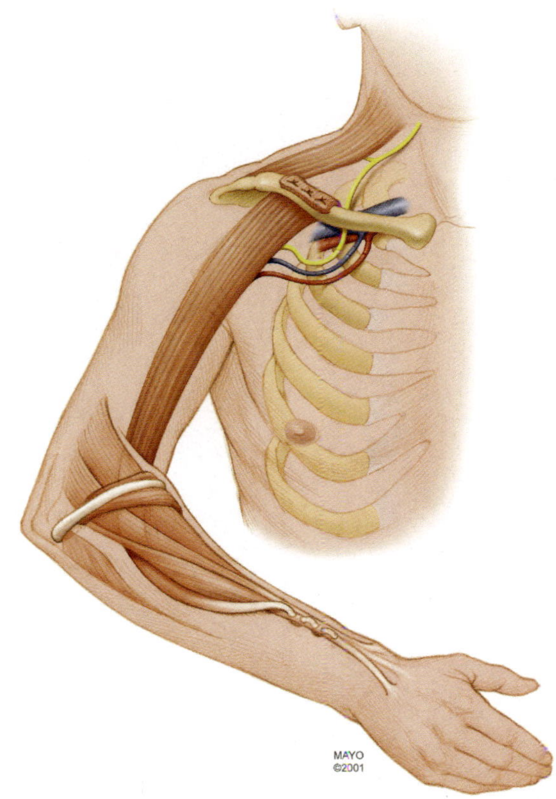

E1014709-002-0

FIGURE 16-25 In Doi et al.'s (13) first muscle transfer, the gracilis is attached to the clavicle proximally and routed distally under the brachioradialis to the radial wrist and finger extensors. (Used with permission of Mayo Foundation for Medical Education and Research, all rights reserved.)

hand sensation. Proximally, the gracilis is attached to the second rib, routed subcutaneously along the medial aspect of the arm, and attached to the finger flexor tendons.

The senior author (AYS) and his colleague (Dr. A.T. Bishop) have made modifications to the gracilis free muscle transfer originally described by Doi et al. (13). A single gracilis muscle transfer is performed to restore elbow flexion and finger flexion. The gracilis is secured proximally to the clavicle with several suture anchors. The muscle is tunneled into the forearm beneath the pronator teres to create a pulley effect and is provisionally placed in its final position. The vascular anastomosis is preferentially performed end to end to the thoracoacromial trunk. The neurorrhaphy is completed with two motor intercostal nerves, or alternatively, the spinal accessory or phrenic nerves. Distally, the flexor digitorum profundus and flexor pollicis longus tendons are identified and sutured together in a position that creates key pinch and grasp with traction. The gracilis tendon is then woven into the prepared flexor digitorum profundus and flexor pollicis longus tendons using a Pulvertaft weave. The graft is tensioned to allow the fingers to extend with elbow flexion and allow the fingers and thumb to close with elbow extension (Figure 16-27).

Breast Reconstruction After Skin-Sparing Mastectomy

The TUG flap was initially described by Yousif et al. (25) and further popularized by Furnas (26) and Wechselberger and Schoeller (27). The TUG flap is designed with a semilunar skin paddle transverse to the longitudinal axis of the gracilis muscle in the proximal inner thigh. The superior aspect of the flap is marked one or two fingerbreadths below the groin crease anteriorly and centrally and continues posteriorly in the gluteal fold. The anteroposterior dimensions of the flap can measure up to 28 cm. The width of the flap harvested is judged by pinching the skin together to allow an easy tension-free closure (Figure 16-28). The flap width has been designed as wide as 8 to 10 cm. A handheld, sterile Doppler device is used to identify skin perforators over the gracilis muscle. These perforators are incorporated into the skin paddle design. The anterior thigh incision is made first. The flap is elevated superficial to the muscular fascia until the adductor longus muscle is reached (Figure 16-29). When the adductor longus muscle is reached, an incision is made through the adductor longus fascia. The adductor longus is then retracted to expose the neurovascular pedicle entering the gracilis on the deep aspect of the muscle. The pedicle is isolated and dissected proximally.

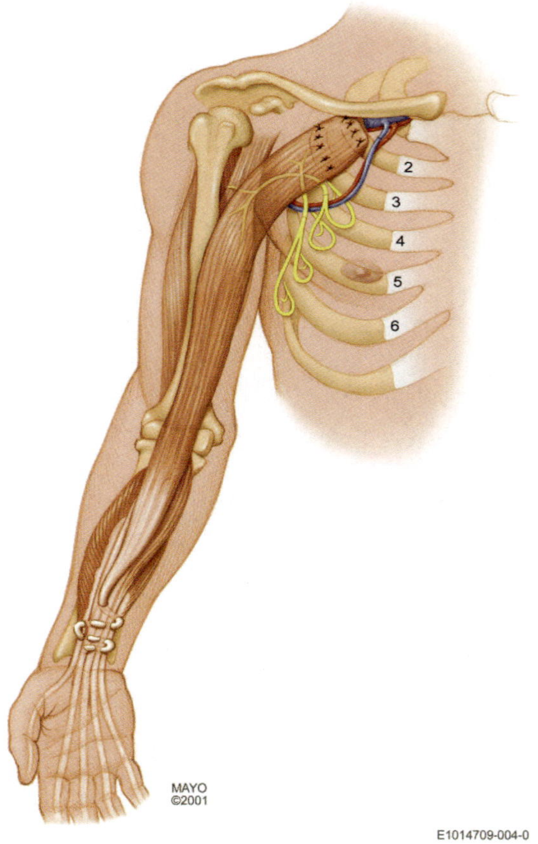

FIGURE 16-26 In Doi et al.'s (13) second transfer, the gracilis is neurotized to motor intercostal nerves and anastomosed to the thoracodorsal artery to create finger flexion. (Used with permission of Mayo Foundation for Medical Education and Research, all rights reserved.)

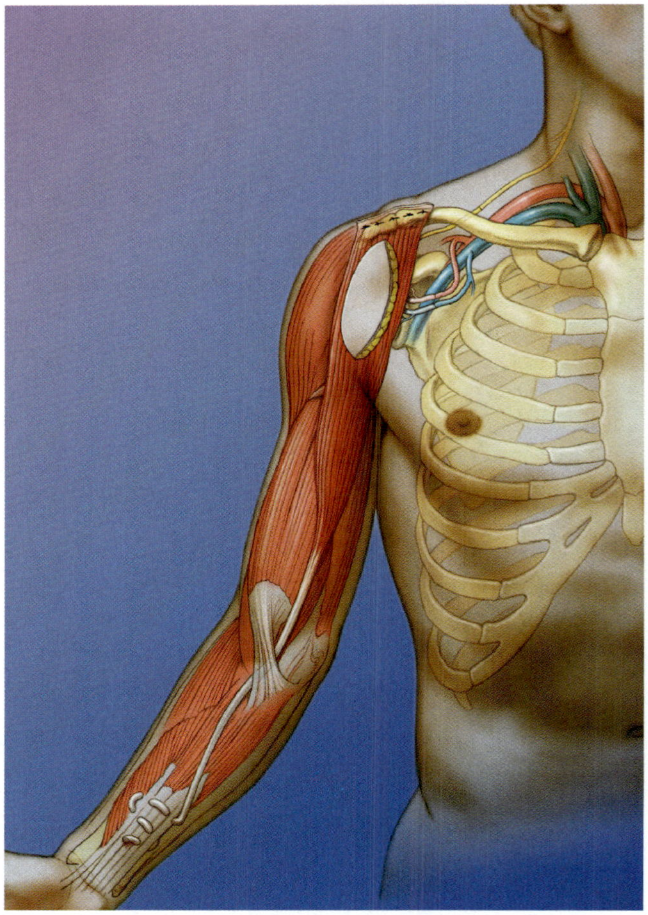

FIGURE 16-27 The graft is tensioned to allow the fingers to extend with elbow flexion and allow the fingers and thumb to close with elbow extension. (Used with permission of Mayo Foundation for Medical Education and Research, all rights reserved.)

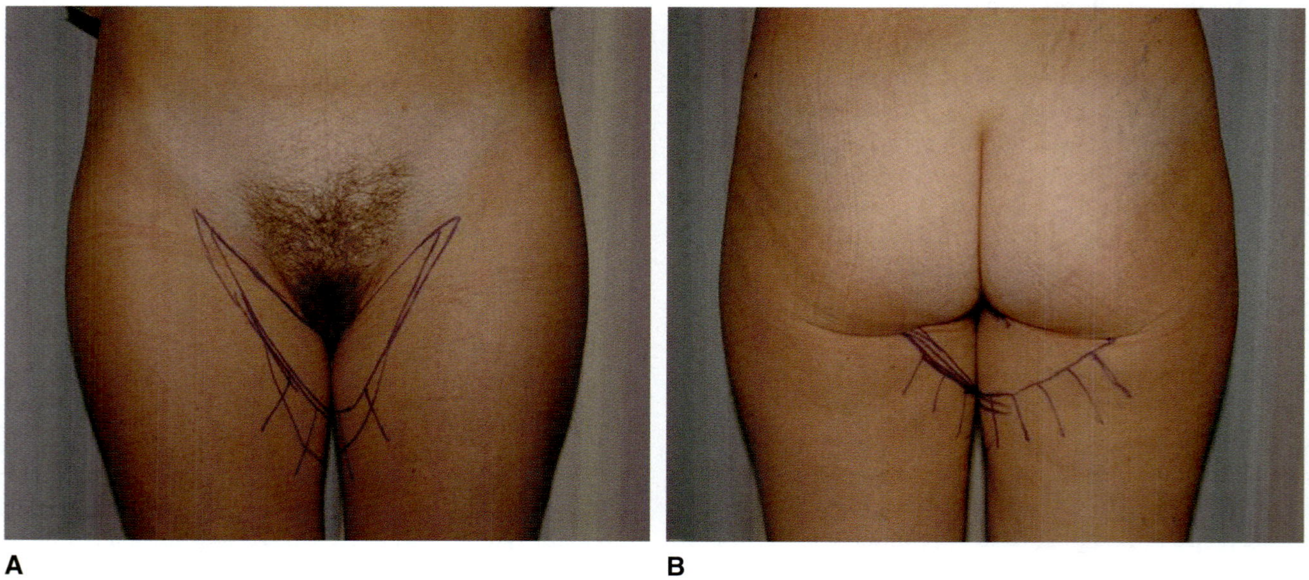

FIGURE 16-28 The transverse upper gracilis flap is designed with a semilunar skin paddle transverse to the longitudinal axis of the gracilis muscle in the proximal inner thigh an anterior view (**A**) of the markings and a posterior view (**B**) of the markings. (Reproduced with permission from Drs. T.E. Hayakawa and E.W. Buchel, University of Manitoba, Canada.)

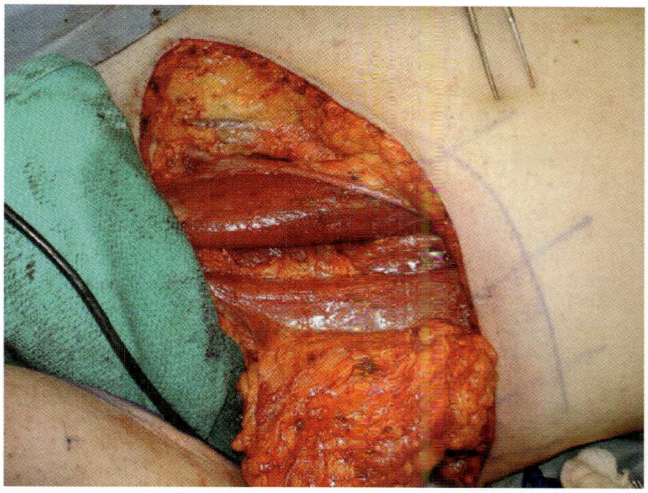

FIGURE 16-29 The flap is elevated superficial to the muscular fascia until the adductor longus muscle is reached. (Reproduced with permission from Drs. T.E. Hayakawa and E.W. Buchel, University of Manitoba, Canada.)

The obturator nerve is divided. Next the posterior skin paddle incision is made, and the dissection continues in a plane superficial to the muscular fascia. An incision through the muscular fascia occurs at the posterior aspect of the gracilis muscle. Without disrupting the skin paddle overlying the gracilis, the gracilis is freed of surrounding tissue proximally and distally. The gracilis muscle is transected superior and inferior, taking only the muscle directly below the skin paddle (Figure 16-30). After the recipient site is prepared, the vascular pedicle to the TUG flap is divided as proximal as possible to obtain length of the pedicle. The flap consisting of skin, subcutaneous tissue, and muscle is then coned (Figure 16-31) into the shape of a breast and placed into the skin-sparing mastectomy pocket for microvascular anastomosis to the internal mammary vessels and inset. The donor site is closed primarily over drains. This is a viable option for small to medium-breasted women who do not have excess abdominal tissue, buttock tissue, or back tissue for a transverse rectus abdominis myocutaneous, deep inferior epigastric perforator, superficial inferior epigastric artery, inferior gluteal artery perforator, superior gluteal artery perforator, or latissimus dorsi flap (Figure 16-32).

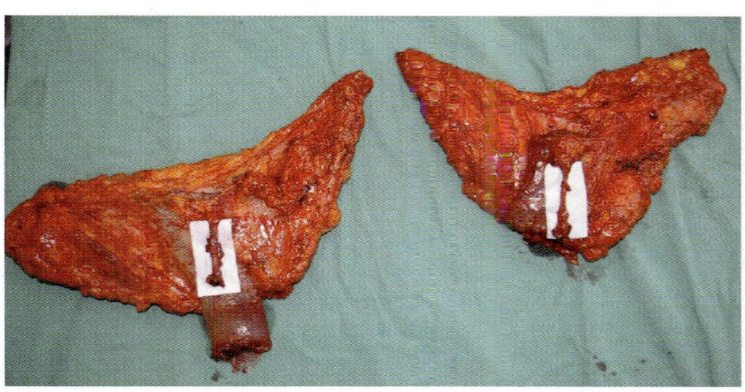

FIGURE 16-30 The gracilis muscle is transected superior and inferior, taking only the muscle directly below the skin paddle. (Reproduced with permission from Drs. T.E. Hayakawa and E.W. Buchel, University of Manitoba, Canada.)

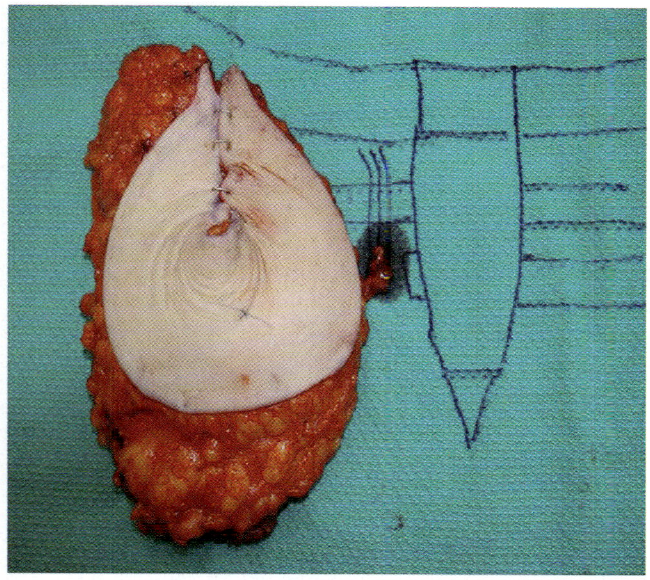

FIGURE 16-31 The flap consisting of skin, subcutaneous tissue, and muscle is then coned to give the shape of a breast. (Reproduced with permission from Drs. T.E. Hayakawa and E.W. Buchel, University of Manitoba, Canada.)

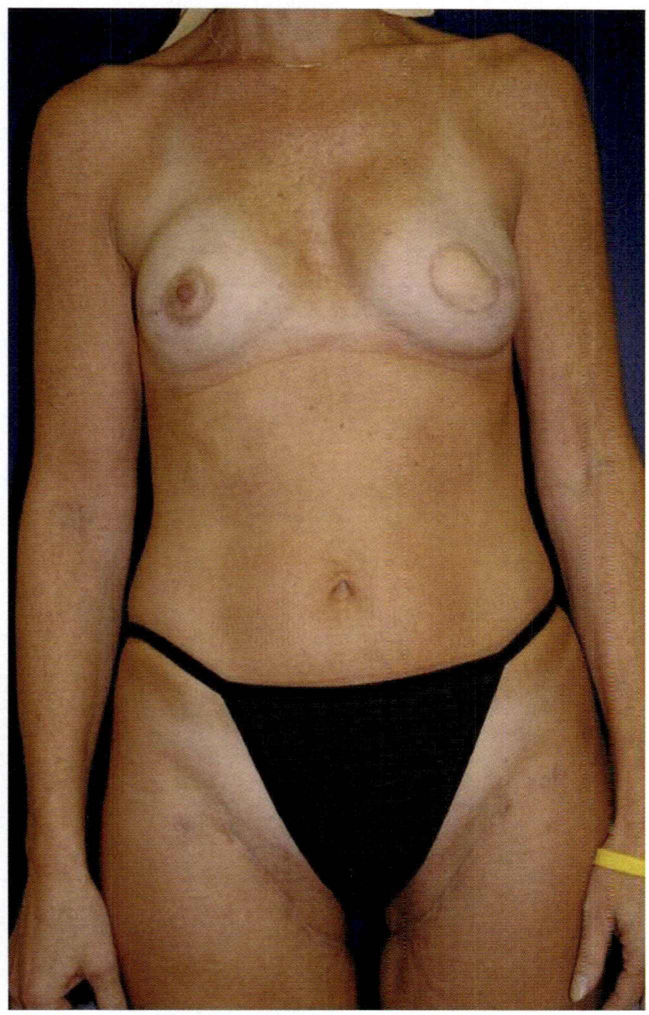

FIGURE 16-32 Postoperative picture of a transverse upper gracilis breast reconstruction. (Reproduced with permission from Drs. T.E. Hayakawa and E.W. Buchel, University of Manitoba, Canada.)

CONCLUSION

Recent advances in the harvest of the gracilis flap have concentrated on reducing the length of the scars to the medial thigh for an aesthetic improvement.

Various minimally invasive techniques have been proposed, all of which aim to reduce scar formation. An endoscopic free gracilis muscle harvest has been described. Lin et al. (28) compared the conventional gracilis harvest with that of an endoscopic harvest. They found the endoscopic technique to be safe, relatively simple, and cost effective and to have a shorter scar length (6.5 cm compared with 15 cm in the conventional technique) and reduced donor site morbidity. They state, however, that the endoscopic technique requires training and an extensive learning period. Because of the drawbacks of endoscopic techniques, including the steep learning curve as well as the need for special equipment, Bannasch (29) described a semi-open approach to the gracilis muscle flap without endoscopic assistance. This approach involves a short inconspicuous transverse incision in the groin area with a counterincision distally. The mean incision length was 8.8 cm. The authors prefer to harvest the gracilis muscle with three small incisions: a 2- to 3-cm longitudinal incision at the pes anserinus, a 2- to 3-cm transverse incision in the medial-posterior aspect of the distal thigh, and an incision approximately 7 cm in length to remove the muscle and skin paddle in the medial thigh.

Regardless of the technique in harvesting the flap, the gracilis muscle flap is a reliable, versatile, expendable muscle that can be used for static coverage of wounds and as a dynamic muscle transfer.

REFERENCES

1. Pickerell K, Broadbent TR, Masters FW, Metzger JT. Construction of a rectal sphincter and restoration of anal continence by transplanting the gracilis muscle. *Ann Surg* 1952;135:853.
2. Pickerell K, Georgiade N, Crawford H, et al. Gracilis muscle transplant for correction of urinary incontinence in male children. *Ann Surg* 1956;143:239.
3. Orticochea M. The musculocutaneous flap method: an immediate and heroic substitute for the method of delay. *Br J Plast Surg* 1972;25:106.
4. Orticochea M. A method of total reconstruction of the penis. *Br J Plast Surg* 1972;25:347.
5. Pers M, Medgyesi S. Pedicle muscle flaps and their application in the surgery of repair. *Br J Plast Surg* 1973;26:313.
6. Bartholdson L, Hulten L. Repair of persistent perineal sinuses by means of a pedicle flap of musculus gracilis. *Scand J Plast Reconstr Surg* 1975;9:74.
7. McCraw JB, Massey FM, Shanklin KD, Horton CE. Vaginal reconstruction with gracilis musculocutaneous flaps. *Plast Reconstr Surg* 1976;58:176–183.
8. McCraw JB, Dibbell DG. Experimental definition of independent musculocutaneous vascular territories. *Plast Reconstr Surg* 1977;60(2):212–220.
9. Harii K, Ohmori K, Sekigughi J. The free musculocutaneous flap. *Plast Reconstr Surg* 1976;57(3):294–303.
10. Manktelow R, McKee N. Free muscle transplantation to provide active finger flexion. *J Hand Surg* 1978;3(5):416–426.
11. Harii K, Ohmori K, Torii S. Free gracilis muscle transplantation with microneurovascular anastomoses for the treatment of facial paralysis. *Plast Reconstr Surg* 1976;57:133.
12. Ikuta Y, Yoshioka K, Tsuge K. Free muscle graft as applied to brachial plexus injury-case report and experimental study. *Ann Acad Med Singapore* 1979;8(4):454–458.
13. Doi K, Muramatsu K, Hattori Y, et al. Restoration of prehension with the double free muscle technique following compete avulsion of the brachial plexus. Indications and long-term results. *J Bone Joint Surg* 2000;82(suppl A):652–666.
14. Mathes SJ, Nahai F: Classification of the vascular anatomy of muscles: experimental and clinical correlation. *Plast Reconstr Surg* 1981;67(2):177.
15. Mathes SJ, Nahai F. *Clinical Applications for Muscle and Musculocutaneous Flaps*. St. Louis: C.V. Mosby, 1982.
16. Terzis JK, Dykes RW, Williams HB. Recovery of function in free muscle transplants using microneurovascular anastomoses. *J Hand Surg* 1978;3:37–59.
17. Haines R. The laws of muscle and tendon growth. *J Anat* 1932;66:578.
18. Pfuhl W. *Anatomy for Surgeons: Back and Limbs*. New York: Harper & Row, 1969,p. 23.
19. Kuzon WM Jr,McKee NH, Fish JS, et al. The effect of intraoperative ischemia on the recovery of contractile function after free muscle transfer. *J Hand Surg Am* 1988;13(2):263–273.
20. Harii K, Asato H. Microneurovascular free gracilis muscle transfer for facial reanimation. In *Grabb's Encyclopedia of Flaps*,vol. I. 2008.
21. Zuker R. Microneurovascular free transfer of a partial gracilis muscle to the face. In *Grabb's Encyclopedia of Flaps*, vol. I. 2008.
22. Frey M. Smile reconstruction using the gracilis muscle. *Operat Tech Plast Reconstr Surg* 1999;6(3):180–189.
23. Bishop AT. Functioning free-muscle transfer for brachial plexus injury. *Hand Clin* 2005;21(1):91–102.
24. Shin AY, Spinner RJ, Steinmann SP, Bishop AT. Adult traumatic brachial plexus injuries. *J Am Acad Orthop Surg* 2005;13:382–396.
25. Yousif NJ, Matloub HS, Kolachalam R, et al. The transverse gracilis musculocutaneous flap. *Ann Plast Surg* 1992;29(6):482–490.
26. Furnas HJ. The transverse gracilis musculocutaneous flap. *Ann Plast Surg* 1993;30(5):480.
27. Wechselberger G, Schoeller T. The transverse musculocutaneous gracilis flap: a valuable tissue source in autologous breast reconstruction. *Plast Reconstr Surg* 2004;114(1):69–73.
28. Lin CH, Wei FC, Lin YT. Conventional versus endoscopic free gracilis muscle harvest. *Plast Reconstr Surg* 2000;105:89–93.
29. Bannasch MA. The semi-open approach to the gracilis muscle flap: aesthetic refinements in gracilis muscle harvest. *J Reconstr Microsurg* 2009;25(1):63–67.
30. Cronje HS, Van Zyl JS. Resurfacing the vulva and vagina. *Int J Gynecol Obstet* 1988;27:113.
31. Soper JT, Larson D, Hunter VJ, et al. Short gracilis musculocutaneous flaps for vulvovaginal reconstruction after radical pelvic surgery. *Obstet Gynecol* 1989;74(5):823.
32. Nahai F. Muscle and musculocutaneous flaps in gynecologic surgery. *Clin Obstet Gynecol* 1981;24:1277.
33. Hester TR, Hill HL, Jurkiewicz MJ. One stage reconstruction of the penis. *Br J Plast Surg* 1978;31:279.
34. Song R, Song Y, Yu Y. Anal reconstruction by a modified Pickerell procedure. *Clin Plast Surg* 1982;9:109.
35. Conway H, Griffith BH. Plastic surgery for closure of decubitus ulcers in patients with paraplegia: based on experience of 1000 cases. *Am J Surg* 1956;91:946.
36. Foster RD, Anthony JP, Lathes SJ, et al. Flap selection as a determinant of success in pressure sore coverage. *Arch Surg* 1997;132(8):868.

CHAPTER 17

The Deep Circumflex Iliac Flap

G. Ian Taylor, Russel J. Corlett, and Andrew Ives

BACKGROUND

The iliac crest was one of three bones dissected by us in 1973 as a potential donor site for vascularized transfer to be used to repair a 12.5-cm defect of the tibia in a young man after trauma. In a cadaver, the bone was raised on the deep circumflex iliac artery (DCIA) vessels but the idea was abandoned because only a 6- to 8-cm straight segment of bone was available. Ultimately, the fibula was chosen and transferred successfully (1).

Then in 1976, the iliac crest was evaluated again in the search for a composite skin and bone free flap, needed to repair compound leg injuries in two patients with bone defects of up to 9 cm. Again, the DCIA pedicle was examined in a fresh cadaver. It was dissected but not injected with ink, and the blood supply to the skin seemed to be tenuous from small vessels. So the superficial circumflex iliac artery (SCIA) vessels were chosen instead, especially because a large skin flap was needed (2).

Finally, in 1978, challenged by a patient with a massive defect of the hemipelvis after tumor ablation, the DCIA supply to the iliac crest was reevaluated and compared with that of the SCIA. In a large series of fresh cadavers, this time using injections of the vessels with different colored inks, the blood supply to the skin and the bone was evaluated (3). This revealed not only the blood supply to the soft tissues and the bone from each vessel, but also, to our delight, that there was a significant supply to the skin from the DCIA (Figure 17-1).

Histology showed ink-stained branches from the DCIA supplying the iliac crest from the anterior superior iliac spine (ASIS) back to and beyond the tuberosity of the crest, the ilium between the ASIS and the anterior inferior iliac spine (AIIS), and the attached musculature. The pathway of the DCIA, its branches, and its connections were displayed by dissection and by radiology using injections with radiopaque lead oxide (Figures 17-2 and 17-3). In 50 subjects, the variations in the anatomy of the DCIA and its accompanying veins were assessed (3) (Figure 17-4).

After successful reconstruction of the hemipelvis in 1978 with the DCIA skin and bone flap (Figure 17-5), this composite unit was used successfully the same year to reconstruct the lower jaw in a young man after an extended hemimandibulectomy to ablate an osteosarcoma. Not only was the shape of the jaw restored, but a functional reconstruction was also achieved by incorporating various soft tissues to reconstruct the temporomandibular joint and floor of the mouth (4) (Figures 17-6 and 17-7).

Although an excellent functional and aesthetic result was achieved, the jaw was a bit bulky, and removal of the full thickness of the iliac crest left a dent in the hip. To improve on the result in 1980, the rim of the iliac crest was split along its length (5), taking the inner cortex in the flap and leaving the outer cortex for hip contour and a more robust closure of the donor site (6,7) (Figure 17-8). Additional modifications include opening or closing osteotomies to straighten or adjust the curvature of the bone; different bone flap designs from either the ipsilateral or contralateral hips for jaw reconstruction (Figures 17-9 and 17-10), with the inclusion of nerve grafts and osseointegrated titanium implants into the bone to provide a functional result (8); limb reconstruction (9–12); and deleting the bone as a musculocutaneous flap for breast and leg reconstruction (4).

ANATOMY

The DCIA, measuring between 1 and 3 mm in diameter, arises from the terminal portion of the external iliac artery (EIA), adjacent to the origin of the deep inferior epigastric artery (DIEA), lying deep to the inguinal ligament. It courses characteristically in a straight line upward and laterally toward the ASIS in a shallow V-shaped tunnel. Its roof is formed by the

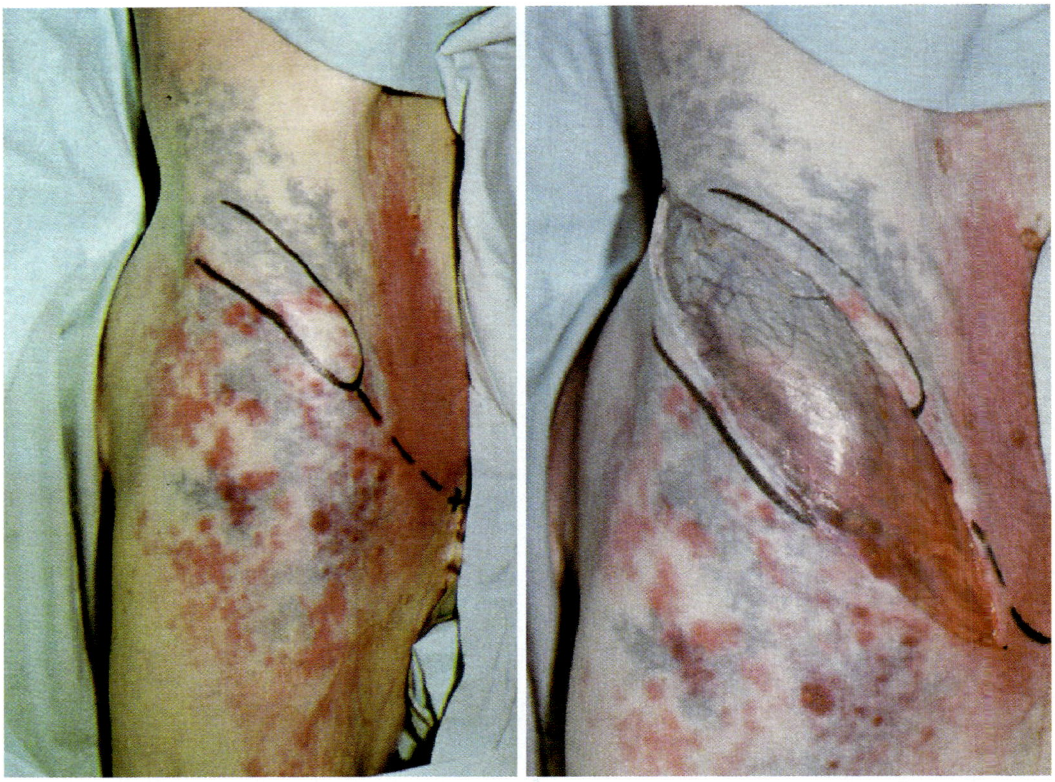

FIGURE 17-1 The deep circumflex iliac artery (black ink) and the superficial circumflex iliac artery (red ink) injected in a fresh cadaver with dissection showing anastomosis between these two vessels in the loose areolar layer over the external oblique muscle and fascia and their supply to the deep tissues.

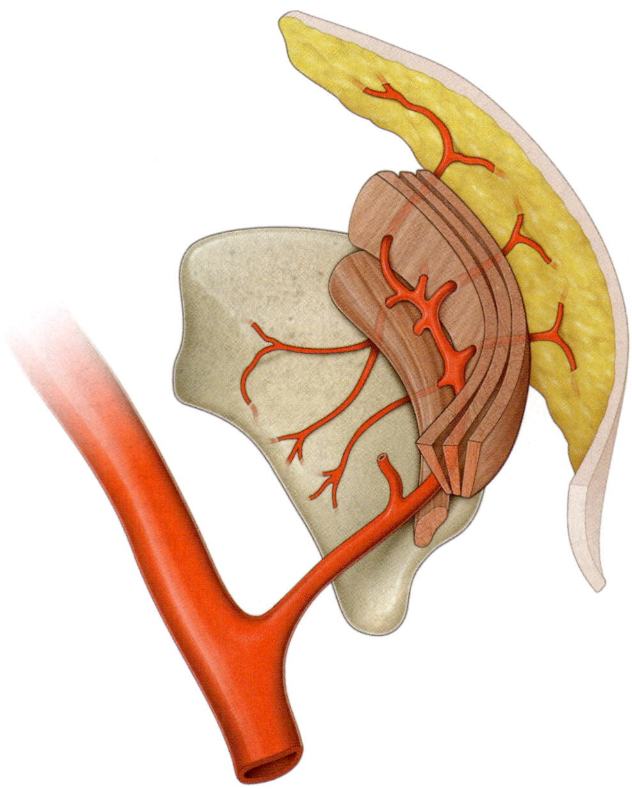

FIGURE 17-2 Diagram of the deep circumflex iliac artery with the ascending branch (divided), musculocutaneous perforators piercing the three muscles of the abdominal wall, and the supply to iliacus and the bone.

transversalis fascia and its walls by the iliacus muscle medially and the transversus abdominis laterally (Figure 17-11).

Approaching the ASIS, the DCIA usually provides a large ascending branch (see Figure 17-4). This artery pierces the transversus muscle to lie between it and the internal oblique muscle. The DCIA also provides branches that pierce the iliacus, supply it, and contribute to the anastomosis around the ASIS. *One of these is often large and short before piercing iliacus and is easily torn if the pedicle is retracted too vigorously.*

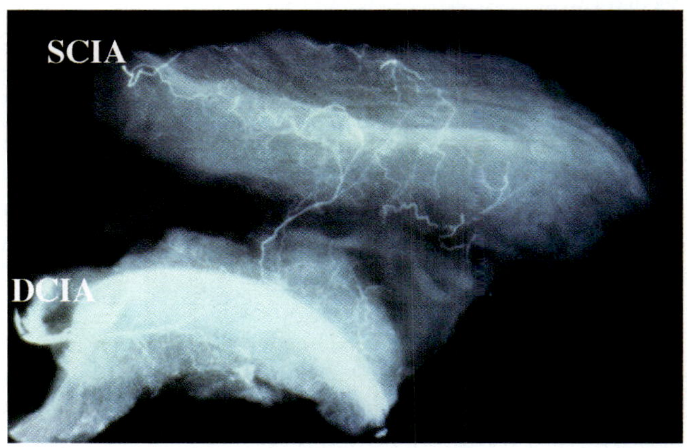

FIGURE 17-3 The deep circumflex iliac artery (DCIA) injected with lead oxide; its supply to the iliac crest; and in this case, its continuation as a large perforator to anastomose with branches of the superficial circumflex iliac artery (SCIA) (arrow) to supply the skin.

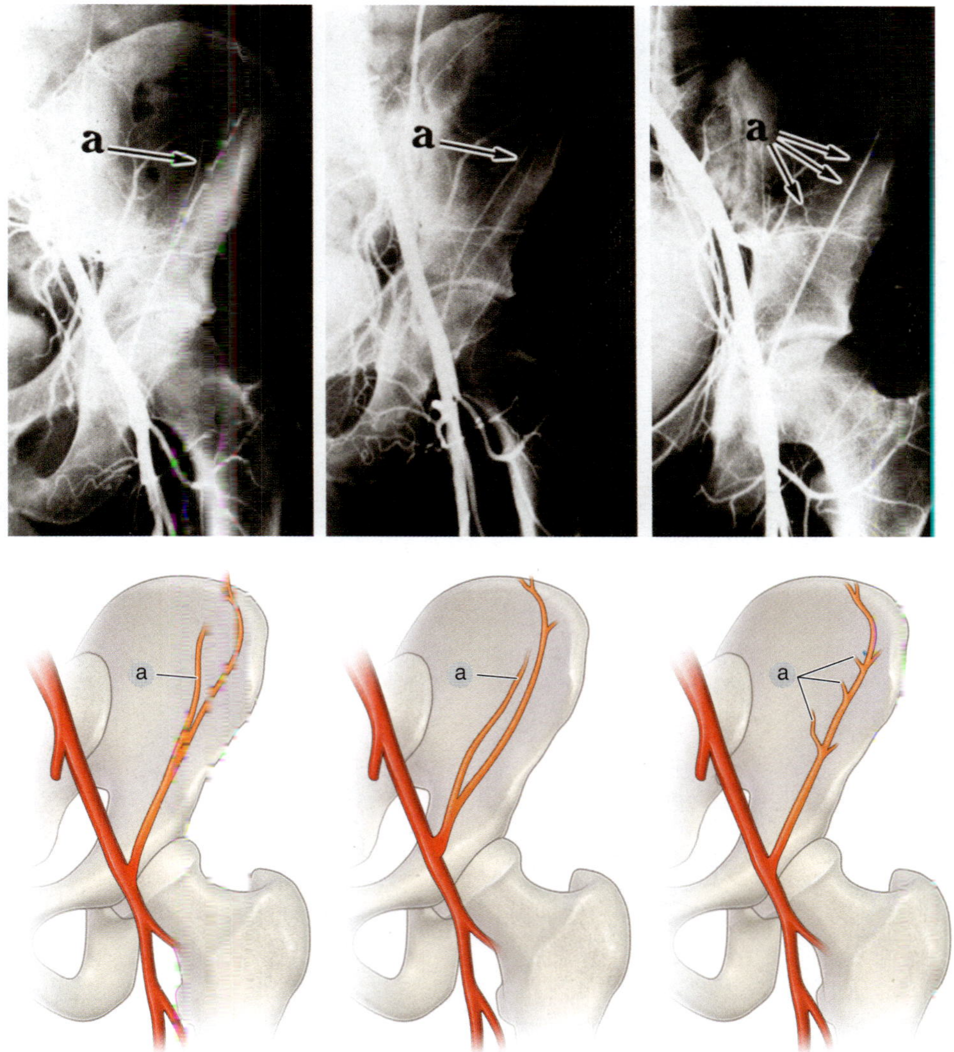

FIGURE 17-4 The variations in the origin of the ascending branch (a) as seen in angiographic studies of the deep circumflex iliac artery. The schematic below also illustrates these variations, which occurred in 62% *(left)*, 16% *(center)*, and 22% *(right)* of the cadaver dissections.

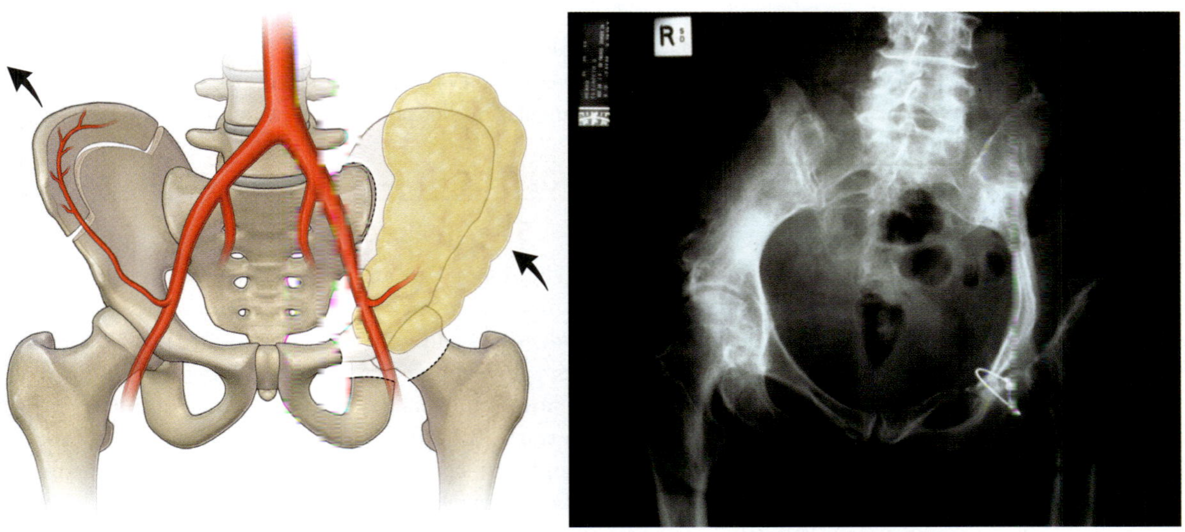

A B

FIGURE 17-5 Diagram (**A**) and result (**B**) at 6 months showing reconstruction of the pelvic ring on the left side with a right deep circumflex iliac artery free bone flap.

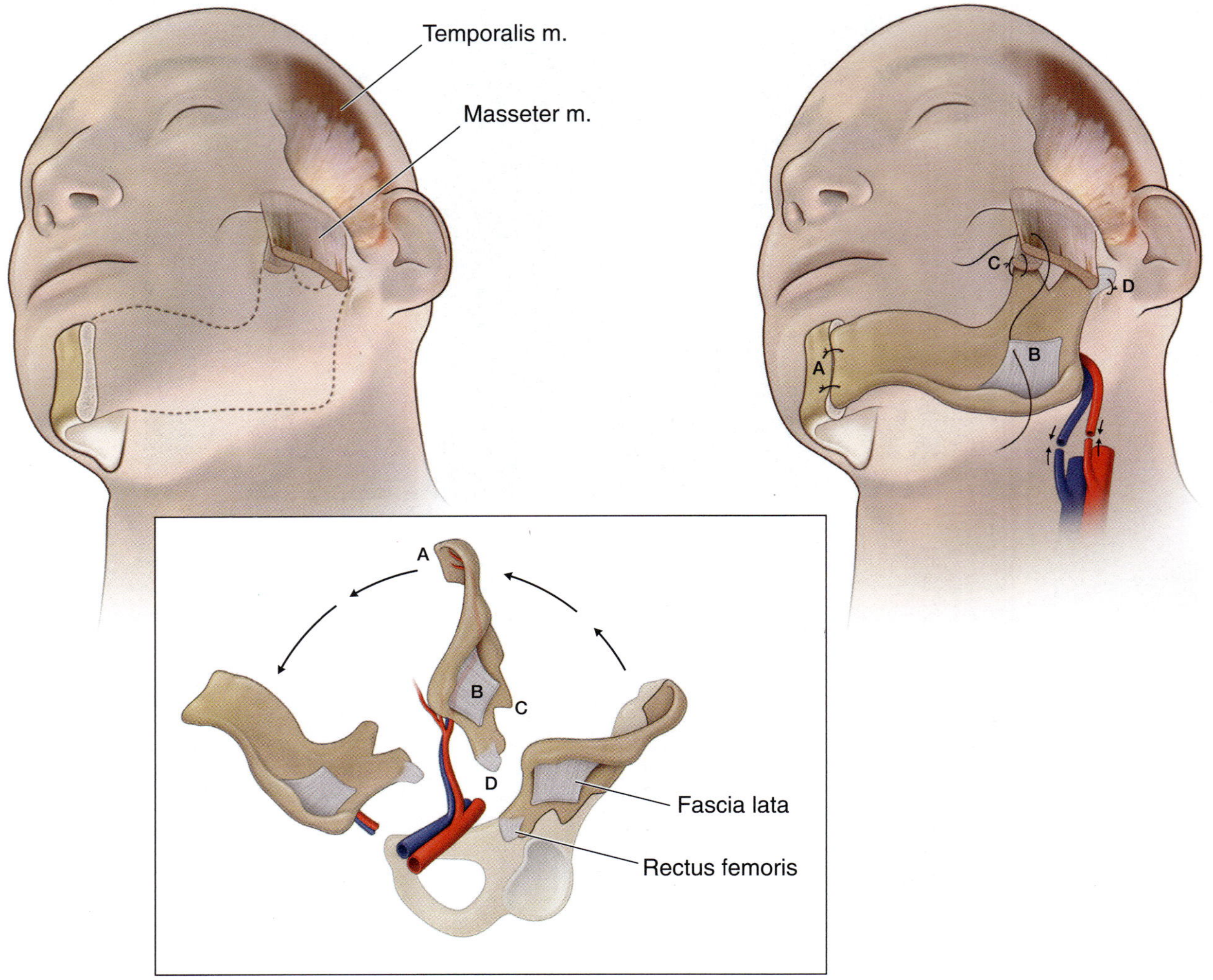

FIGURE 17-6 The operative procedure. *(Left)* The defect after an extended hemimandibulectomy and resection of soft tissue (dotted line). *(Center)* The design of the compound flap nourished by the deep circumflex iliac vessels. *(Right)* The free living bone flap is fixed in position, with anastomoses of its vessels to the facial vessels. The anterior margin of the bone is wired to the stump of the mandible in the region of the right first premolar (**A**). The retained masseter muscle is reattached to a flap of fascia lata in the compound flap (**B**). The temporalis tendon is fixed to the newly fashioned coronoid process (**C**). The capsule of the temporomandibular joint is reconstructed from a portion of the tendinous origin of the rectus femoris muscle in the free flap (**D**).

Thereafter, the DCIA follows the curved inner surface of the iliac crest, 1 to 2 cm from the rim, supplies the bone, and continues in the groove between iliacus and transversus abdominis, being overlapped often by a down-hanging fold of the latter muscle (see Figure 17-11). Usually 8 to 10 cm beyond, the ASIS the DCIA pierces obliquely the three muscles of the abdominal wall—transversus, internal, and external oblique—anastomoses with the iliolumbar artery coming from behind, and emerges often as a large cutaneous perforator (see Figures 17-2 and 17-3). During its course beyond the ASIS, the DCIA provides a number of small branches that also pierce the abdominal wall musculature, forming a fine mobile anastomotic lattice on the surface of external oblique that joins with twigs from the SIEA (see Figures 17-1 and 17-3).

The DCIA is accompanied by two venae comitantes that join to form a single vein averaging 5 mm. This vein characteristically diverges upwards and medially to cross either in front (usually) or behind the EIA to reach the external iliac vein (EIV) (see Figure 17-11). As it diverges from the artery there is always a small tributary that "anchors" the deep circumflex iliac vein (DCIV) at this point and passes deep to the inguinal ligament, another point to be aware of when tracing the pedicle.

DISSECTION

Step 1: Preoperative

The donor flap and the recipient site are marked out *before* surgery. The area is shaved and the ASIS and pubic tubercle identified and joined with a marking pen. The femoral artery is palpated and marked, and an incision line is drawn 2 cm above and parallel to the inguinal ligament to expose the pedicle. If a skin flap is required, it is designed beyond the ASIS and parallel to the iliac crest, two thirds above and one thirds below (Figure 17-12).

The recipient vessels are identified and marked to alert the ablative or reconstructing surgeons so that care can be taken to avoid and preserve them. The other important preoperative step is to ensure that the bowel is empty.

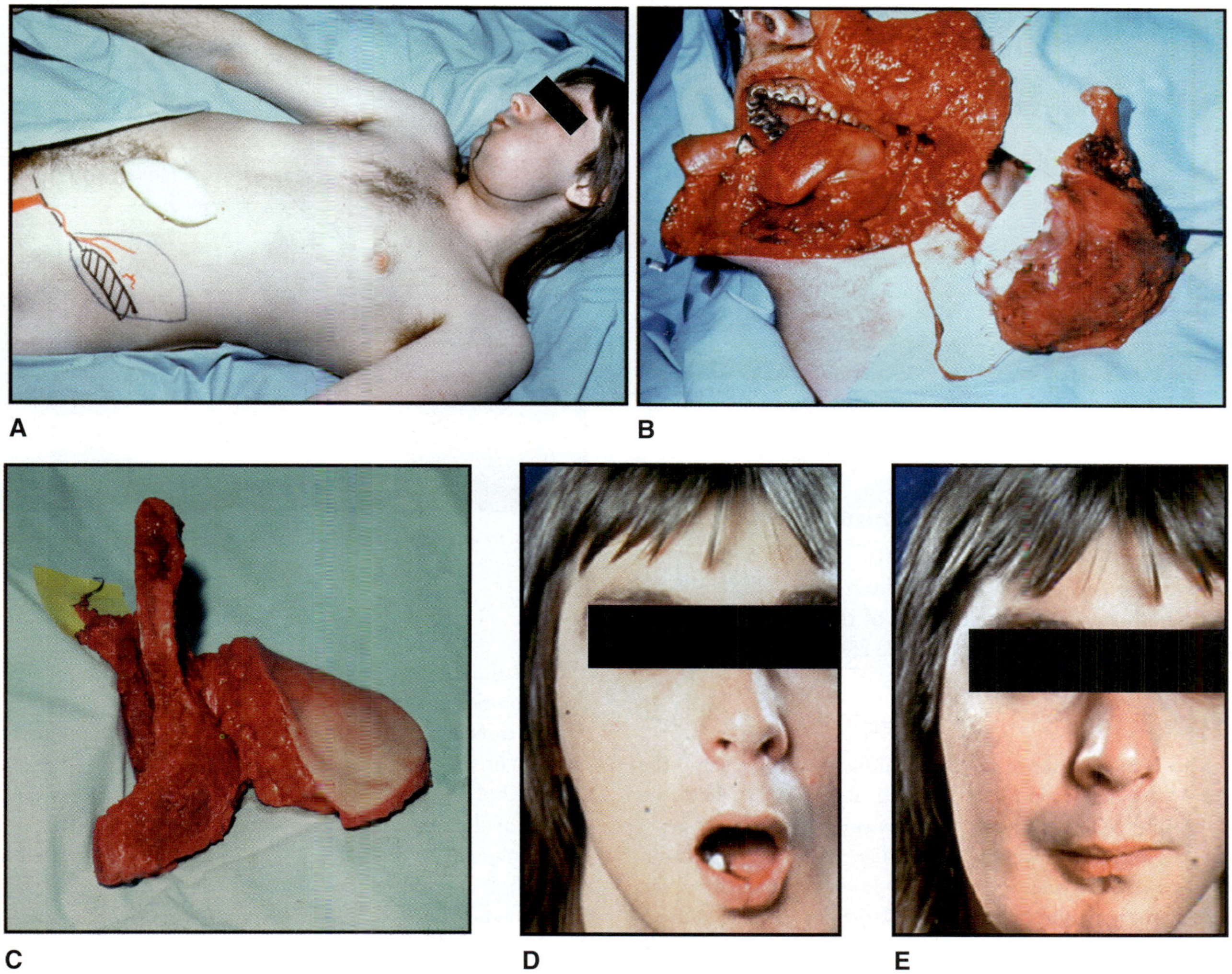

FIGURE 17-7 The incisions marked preoperatively on the groin and the jaw (**A**), the osteosarcoma resected (**B**), the composite skin muscle and bone flap (**C**), and the result (**D** and **E**) at 8 months in our first jaw reconstruction. (Reproduced with permission from Taylor G, The Angiosome Concept and Tissue Transfer. Taylor and Francis Group LLC Books.)

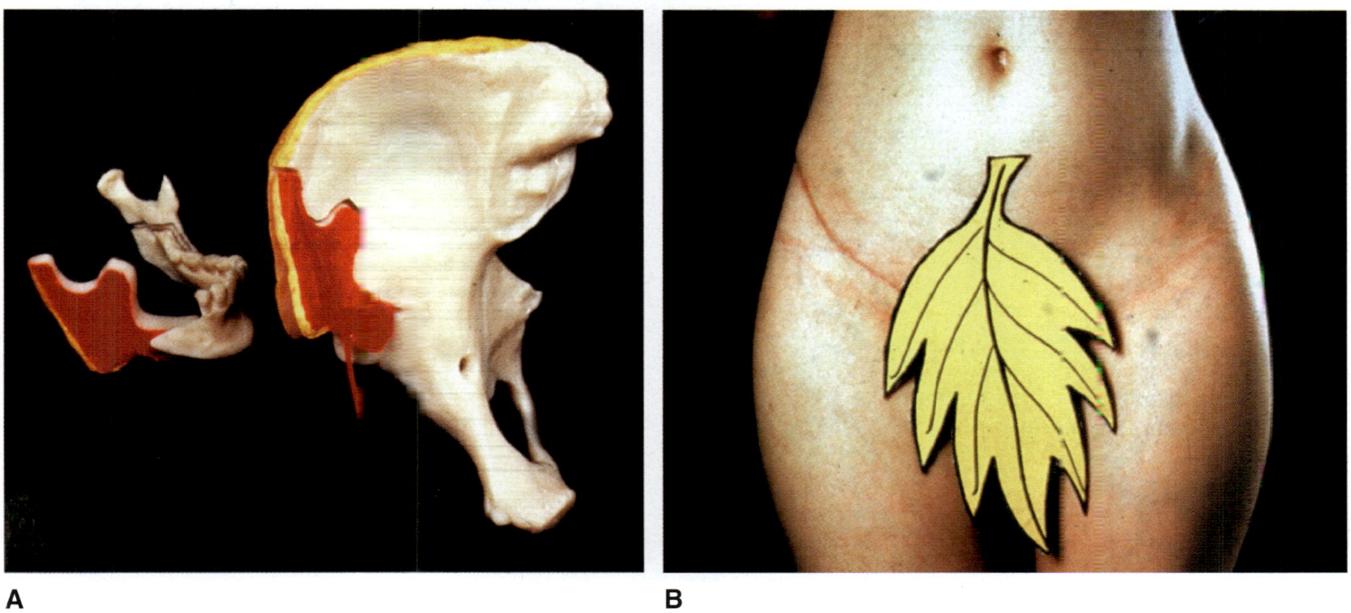

FIGURE 17-8 The refined procedure showing splitting of the iliac crest (**A**) to take the inner cortex as the bone flap in one of our deep circumflex iliac artery flap designs and (**B**) the superior aesthetic and functional result in this patient in whom previously a full-thickness bone graft had been harvested from her left hip.

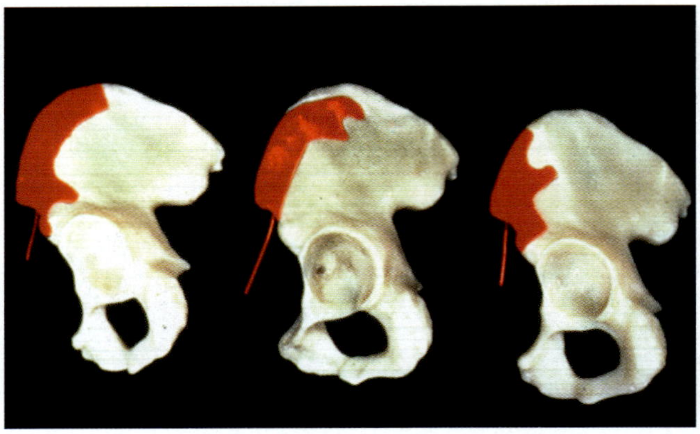

FIGURE 17-9 Various bone flap designs taken from the ipsilateral (*left* and *right*) or contralateral (*center*) hip.

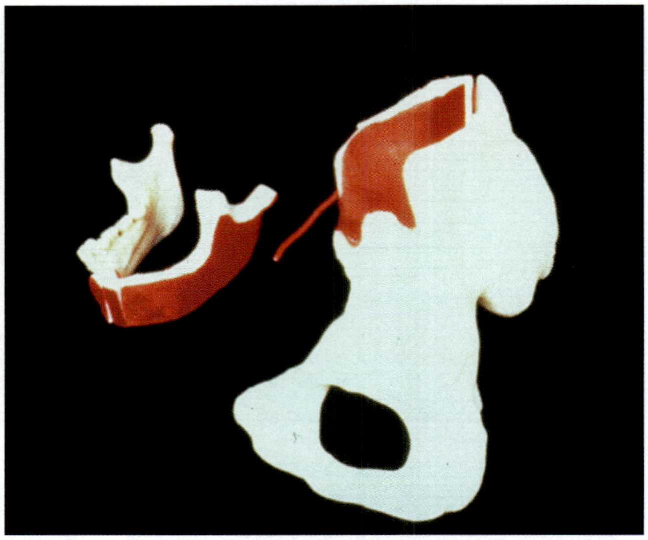

FIGURE 17-10 Model to show refined trimming of the iliac crest for better jaw shape and osteotomy to cross the midline of the new jaw.

Step 2: Positioning the Patient

In the operating room, the patient is placed supine with a sandbag under the *opposite* hip. This facilitates easier dissection of the pedicle because of the curvature of the pelvis and can be removed subsequently if necessary (see Figure 17-3).

Step 3: Identifying the Pedicle

The skin is incised above the inguinal ligament and along the upper border of the skin flap. The skin flap, together with the loose areolar layer of anastomotic arterioles over the external oblique, is reflected down toward the iliac crest, stopping within 2 to 3 cm of the bone where usually small branches from the DCIA can be seen and preserved. If a large skin flap is required, the continuation of the DCIA as a cutaneous perforator can be often identified 8 to 10 cm beyond the ASIS in the vicinity of the tuberosity of the crest.

The three muscles of the abdominal wall and the transversalis fascia are incised to produce a "keyhole" usually 2 cm above and behind the ASIS. During this procedure, the ascending branch of the DCIA is usually encountered and can be traced back to the DCIA if necessary. The index finger is inserted into the keyhole and passed medially above and parallel to the inguinal ligament where, unless the patient is obese, the pulsation of the DCIA can be felt.

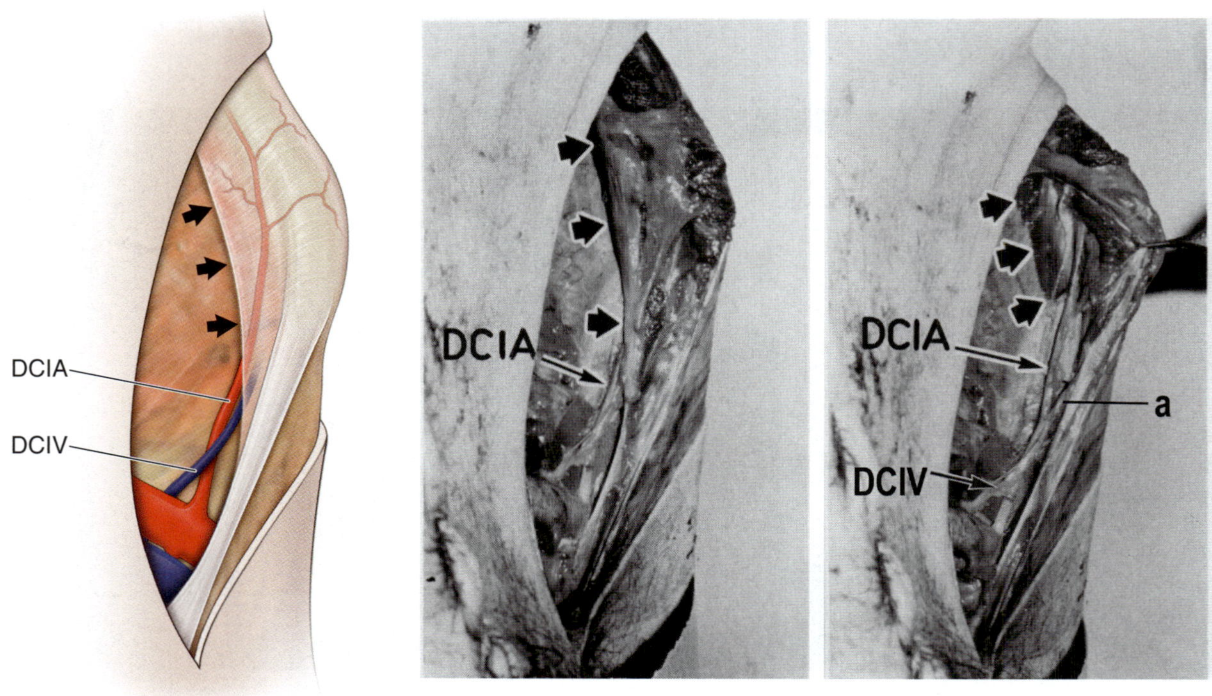

FIGURE 17-11 Progressive cadaver dissection showing the fusion of the transversalis fascia to the iliacus fascia (arrows). The deep circumflex iliac vessels (DCIVs) lie between this groove and the inner lip of the iliac crest. Note the deep circumflex iliac vein DCIV diverging from its artery to pass behind the external iliac artery in this dissection. The ascending branch (a) is seen in the right picture.

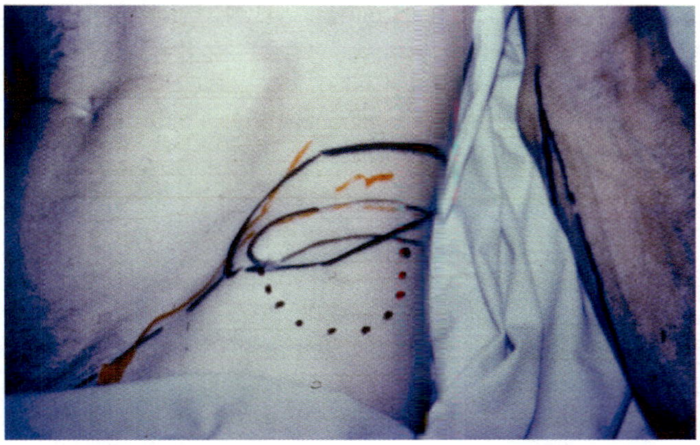

FIGURE 17-12 Skin flap designed beyond the anterior superior iliac spine. If needed, an additional flap of subcutaneous tissue and fascia lata (dotted) can be included.

With the finger protecting the DCIA, the external oblique and the conjoined tendons of the internal oblique and transversus abdominis are incised above and parallel to the inguinal ligament, preserving the ilioinguinal nerve and the spermatic cord in male patients. The DCIA and its venae comitantes lie in an areolar tunnel. Its roof, the fascia transversalis, and its continuation over the iliacus muscle is formally incised to identify the pedicle (see Figure 17-11).

The pedicle is traced medially ligating branches, often small but usually large near the ASIS. Within 2 to 3 cm from the EIA, the venae comitantes join, and the deep circumflex iliac vein (DCIN) diverges upward, away from the DCIA, crossing usually in front of the EIA to reach the EIV (see Figure 17-11).

During its course, the DCIV receives a small tributary as it diverges from the artery, accompanied usually by a branch of the DCIA that must be identified carefully with magnification and ligated. To add to this tedious part of the dissection, there is often a lymph node, sometimes quite large, in this vascular triangle. The DCIV, as it approaches the EIV, is joined by other tributaries, often the DIEV, and may be 1 cm in diameter or larger as it reaches its destination.

The ascending branch of the DCIA is usually large and pierces the transversus muscle at a variable point medial to the ASIS (see Figures 17-4 and 17-11). It must not be confused with the main trunk as the DCIA may be smaller beyond the origin of its ascending branch. Even more confusing can be an early origin of the ascending branch that may be as far medial as to appear to be a duplication of the DCIA and may not pierce the transversus abdominis until close to the ASIS (see Figure 17-4, center).

Finally, mention should be made of the relationship of the DCIA to the lateral cutaneous nerve of the thigh. The nerve lies medial to the ASIS and passes in front of the artery from which it receives many short branches, as well as from the accompanying veins. Although it is possible to preserve the nerve or use it as a vascularized nerve flap, it is often divided because (1) the unbranched *intrapelvic* portion of the nerve can always be harvested as a nerve graft to restore continuity, for example, between the inferior dental and mental nerves, and (2) the area of anesthesia on the lateral side of the thigh is rarely troublesome and usually recovers within 12 to 18 months.

Step 4: The Superolateral Dissection

When a skin flap is required, the skin perforators are identified beyond the ASIS and preserved, retaining a 2-cm cuff of abdominal muscles attached to the iliac crest. Because the DCIA pierces the three abdominal wall muscles and then crosses the iliac crest about 10 cm posterior to the ASIS, there is no point in keeping muscle attached to the flap beyond that point because it only increases the bulk of the flap unnecessarily, damages the abdominal wall, and makes wound closure difficult (Figure 17-13). At this point in the dissection, the iliac crest curves directly backward and inferiorly, and it is a common mistake to continue too far superiorly. The pedicle passes obliquely across the inside of the pelvis in its fascial tunnel, lying on the iliacus muscle near its lateral attachment. This muscle is incised medial to the pedicle and swept medially from the bone by blunt dissection to preserve the periosteal vessels on the surface of the ilium.

Step 5: The Inferolateral Dissection

If for any reason there have been problems dissecting the pedicle or flap at this stage, the procedure can be aborted with minimal morbidity. Otherwise, the lower border of the skin flap is incised and elevated up to the *outer* lip of the iliac crest. The incision is deepened along this line, down to bone, and the attached muscles detached by sharp dissection from the outer half of the bone.

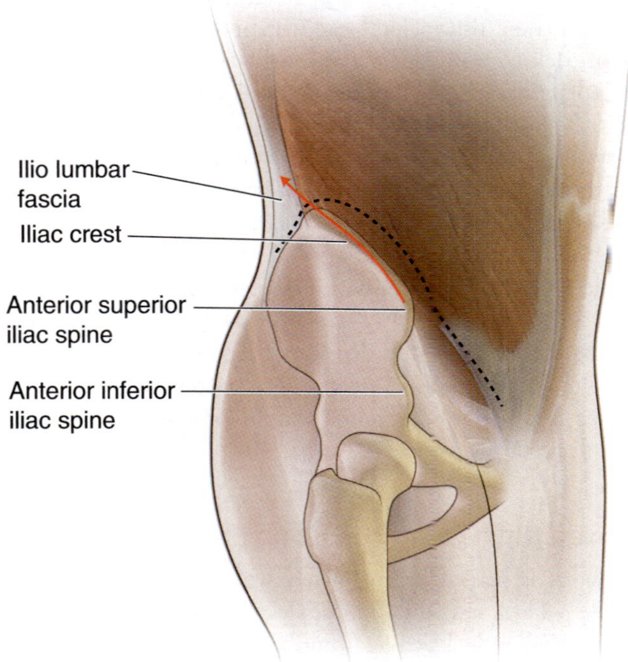

FIGURE 17-13 Incision (dotted) is shown on the external oblique muscle (brown), its aponeurosis, and the underlying muscles above the iliac crest. Beyond the posterior border of the muscle in the vicinity of the tuberosity, the incision follows the curvature of the bone. The axis of the skin flap (arrow) is indicated, which diverges upward from the iliac crest at the tuberosity (A). The ASIS (B) and the AIIS (C) are labeled as well as the iliolumbar fascia (D).

Unless the full thickness of the iliac crest is required, the iliac crest is split along its length from the ASIS to the tuberosity, beyond which the crest is thinner and the full thickness is included. To ensure in depth that an adequate thickness of the inner surface of the iliac crest and wing of the ilium is obtained, especially for jaw reconstruction, one hand is placed inside the pelvis to guide the direction of the osteotome. Usually the osteotome exits through the outer cortex 2 to 3 cm below the iliac crest, leaving a crescent of bone, not unlike the segment of an orange, with the gluteal muscles attached.

The remaining gluteal muscles are detached from the outer surface of the bone. This is quite bloody, particularly in the posterior part, where good hemostasis with either cutting diathermy or a good firm pack may be required.

Step 6: The Inferomedial Dissection

The medial dissection between the ASIS and the AIIS requires some care so as to avoid inadvertent damage to the pedicle. The inguinal ligament is detached from the ASIS; the iliacus muscle is divided; and the rectus femoris tendon attached to the AIIS identified and incised, leaving a cuff of tendon attached to the AIIS. This cuff of tendon is important because it represents the future ligaments of the temporomandibular joint and is used to secure the new head of the mandible (AIIS) in place after transfer. It is prudent to leave a small amount of iliacus muscle around the pedicle for protection while the bone flap is mobilized.

Step 7: Dividing the Bone

The bone flap is divided using a reciprocating saw. For jaw reconstruction, this includes the AIIS and most of the crest. A useful trick is to drill a hole at the angle between the vertical and horizontal segments of the ilium to allow the point of the saw to be inserted and to cut in each direction; otherwise, it can be awkward to "turn the corner." It is important to remember that the crest turns inferiorly as it passes posteriorly; otherwise, the saw may cut through the iliac crest prematurely. To avoid this mistake and remembering that the male (android) and female (gynecoid) pelvises have different shapes, the iliac crest is cut across at right angles *posteriorly* to the required depth and the saw cuts joined. After division of the bone, the flap is left for 15 to 20 minutes to overcome any spasm in the vessels, and the flap is sutured to the wound margin to prevent any kinking or avulsion of the pedicle.

Step 8: Shaping the Bone Flap

The bone is shaped approximately while still attached by its pedicle with a saw and "pineapple" burr and its circulation assessed. Often the bleeding from the bone is so brisk that bone wax is required for hemostasis. Where full-thickness bone is present in the flap, multiple holes are drilled in the outer cortex to assist in revascularization should the anastomoses fail. On two occasions when this occurred and was detected early, the soft tissue were removed, and the bone survived as a graft, probably because the iliac crest is composed of 90% cancellous bone in contrast to the fibula, which is 90% cortical bone.

A plastic model, taken from a range of shapes and sizes, is used to match the shape and size of the bone flap to that of the removed mandible (Figure 17-14). The pedicle is divided, and any final shaping of the bone is done on a side table before transferring the flap.

Step 9: Flap Transfer and Inset

The DCIA flap is the ideal reconstruction for defects of the body and ramus of the mandible because the shape of the ipsilateral iliac bone closely matches the mandible (see Figure 17-10), and the DCIA pedicle sits comfortably over the branches of the external carotid vessels in the neck and is long enough to reach these without the need for vein grafts. The tendon of rectus femoris is used to suspend the head of the neo mandible from the meniscus of the TM joint (see Figure 17-6). The other bone end—and the osteotomy if required—is fixed with interosseous wires and crossed Kirschner wires. This method of fixation is preferred because:

1. Screws do not hold well in cancellous bone and may become loose before bone union.
2. The crossed K-wires provide rigid fixation, especially at the osteotomy site, and they allow for easy adjustment to achieve the desired new jaw contour. The figure-of-8 interosseous wires compress the bone ends, and these are tightened *after* the vascular anastomoses.
3. At a later date, these wires can be removed easily through one or two small incisions, especially if osteointegrated implants are planned (Figures 17-14 and 17-15).

After completing the vascular anastomoses *the arterial clamp is removed first* to ensure bright bleeding from all tissues as they fill up "like a bucket." The bone and muscle bleed first, and it may be a minute or two before the circulation reaches the skin and the venous anastomosis. If the vein clamp is removed first, and especially if joined end to side to the internal jugular vein, backbleeding into the flap and especially the bone may give a false-positive result.

Step 10: Closure of the Donor Site

A second team, well conversant with the anatomy of the region, repairs the donor site. It is vital to reconstruct the abdominal wall to prevent herniation, and this requires careful identification of tissue layers, especially the cut end of the inguinal ligament that has been tagged usually with a stout suture.

Because the iliacus muscle has little fascial connective tissue at its pelvic attachment, sutures do not hold well. Therefore drill holes are made along the cut edge of the ilium to receive heavy interrupted monofilament nylon sutures. A good trick is to insert temporarily 23-gauge needles into each hole as they are drilled because these holes are easily lost as the wound is closed. Bone wax is often required at the cut edge of the bone for hemostasis.

The transversus abdominis and the internal oblique muscles are sutured to these drill holes, commencing posteriorly, until the previous site of the ASIS is reached. The repair is then continued along the conjoined tendon.

A drain tube is inserted. The external oblique is sutured to the glutei muscles and their attached split bone "crescent" to

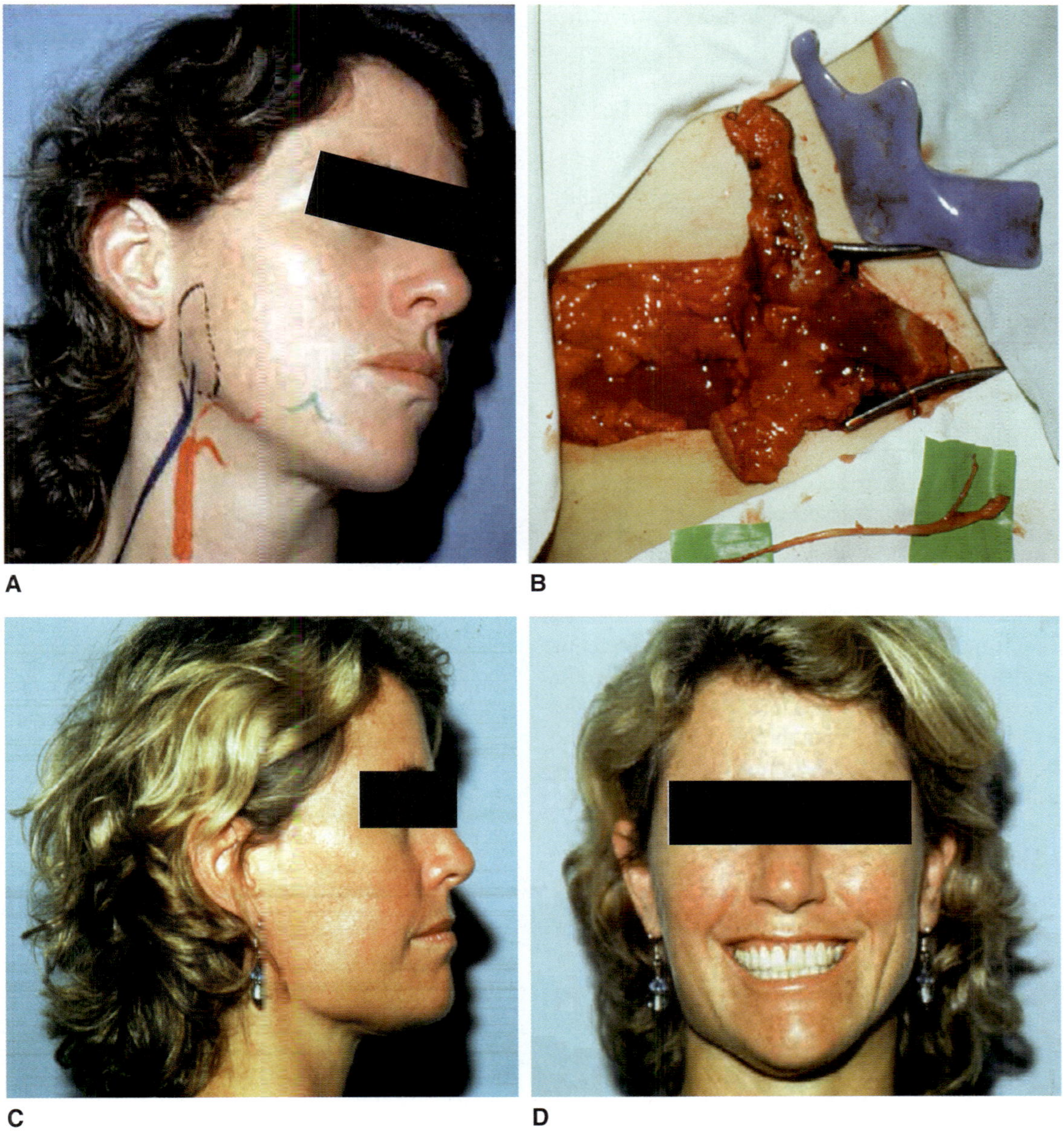

FIGURE 17-14 Preoperative marking of recipient vessels and bulge (dotted) of the ameloblastoma (**A**). Shaping of the bone flap to match the acrylic model with an intrapelvic graft of the lateral cutaneous nerve of the thigh ready for insertion (**B**). Note the burr holes in the outer cortex of the new ramus and the bleeding from the cancellous bone of the split iliac crest, which forms the new body of the mandible. The final result at 12 months is shown in (**C** and **D**) after osseointegrated implants on the patient's right side. (Reproduced with permission from Taylor G. The Angiosome Concept and Tissue Transfer. Taylor and Francis Group LLC Books.)

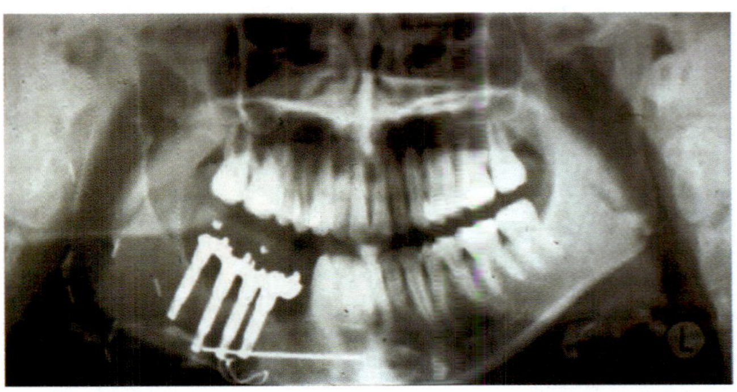

FIGURE 17-15 Union and osseointegrated implants in the same patient. Note that one of the Kirschner and one of the interosseous wires still remain at the chin point.

restore hip contour, the inguinal ligament is reattached to this bone, and the repair is continued along the anterior wall of the inguinal canal. The skin is closed by direct approximation.

COMPLICATIONS

Abdominal Hernia

Early in our series, two cases of hernia occurred laterally. This complication has been eliminated by:

1. Suture of the transversus and internal oblique muscle to drill holes in the remaining wing of the ileum.

2. Avoiding unnecessary muscle bulk by incising down to the iliac crest, 8 to 10 cm beyond the ASIS and near the tuberosity, leaving only a thin shaving of muscle and periosteum attached to the bone beyond this point (see Figure 17-13).
3. Making sure the bowel is empty before surgery
4. Making sure the surgeon repairing the donor site is familiar with the anatomy and should have been involved in dissecting the flap

Nerve Injury

Anesthesia or hypothesia of the lateral thigh is common and recovers spontaneously after 12 to 18 months. It is due to division of the lateral cutaneous nerve of the thigh, which can be preserved, and branches of the subcostal nerve that flow across the iliac crest from above. There have been no cases of injury to the femoral nerve or major vessels in our series of more than 160 cases.

Blood Loss

The procedure is quite vascular, especially (1) at the posterior region of the dissection where a large compression pack left for some time solved the problem and (2) from the cut ends of the bone where bone wax provided the solution. Blood should be typed and cross-matched, especially if doing the procedure for the first time.

Bulky Skin Flap

Although the subcutaneous component can be thinned at a later date if the skin flap is placed externally, either in the head and neck or elsewhere (9,10). However, if placed intraorally, it is often too bulky if the patient is "well padded" and the blood supply to the skin is often kinked or twisted. In these situations, we combine the procedure with a radial forearm free flap, especially because the size of the deep circumflex vessels matches almost exactly the distal end of the radial vessels and the cephalic vein, and sensation can be included in the radial flap (Figure 17-16).

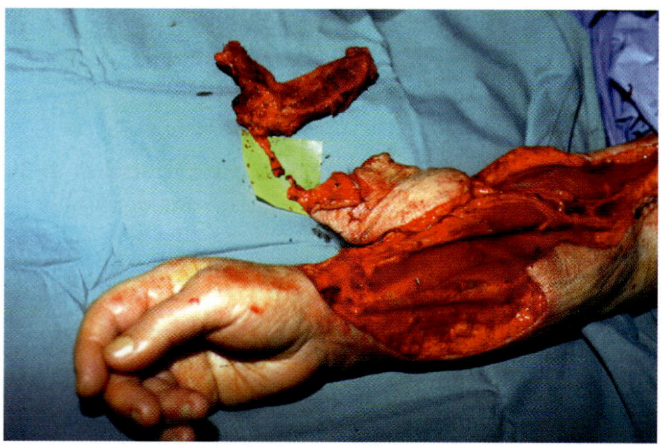

FIGURE 17-16 Deep circumflex iliac artery bone flap about to be anastomosed to the distal end of a radial forearm flap on the side table. The circulation to both flaps is established before transferring these combined flaps.

Bone Flap Exposure

This sometimes occurs intraorally if the closure is a bit tight or the bone flap is too large. Because the iliac crest is so vascular, it granulates, and free mucosal cell "seeding" will heal the area between 1 and 2 weeks. We have observed this on seven occasions, and no surgical intervention was required except in one case when excessive bone was trimmed and a successful secondary suture was performed at 1 week when the complication was discovered.

INDICATIONS

The DCIA flap can be used:

1. As a composite skin, muscle, and bone flap
2. As a bone only flap
3. As a musculocutaneous flap
4. As a perforator flap

We have not attempted a perforator flap because most of the vessels supplying the skin are very small except for the continuation posteriorly of the DCIA as a skin perforator, and this is not a large vessel in a significant number of cases. Computed tomography angiography may help in this situation because it has been successful in assessing perforators in other donor sites for free flap transfer.

Although the authors have used the musculocutaneous flap for breast and limb reconstruction (4), the main use has been to provide vascularized bone. Our other mainstay bone flap is the fibula (1), and the choice is usually between these two, although radial osteocutaneous and free rib flaps have been used as well (8,13).

Ideally, the DCIA is used for *curved* bone defects and the fibula for *straight* long bones. However, osteotomies can be performed in either bone to straighten the former or curve the latter.

Mandible Reconstruction

The curvature of the iliac crest matches closely that of the mandible to the chin point. Therefore, the authors believe this is ideal, especially in a young patient, for reconstruction of the ramus and body of the mandible where there is sufficient bone to reach the opposite angle of the jaw with an opening osteotomy if required. The height of the reconstructed body of the mandible can be matched to the normal side and is ideal for osseointegrated implants (see Figure 17-15).

Alternatively, the fibula is preferred for reconstruction of the body of the mandible from angle to angle, especially in edentulous patients, with usually two closing osteotomies at the chin and with a thin reinnervated skin flap for lining. (8,13)

Maxillary Reconstruction

We have found the fibula to be ideal for the arch of the upper jaw and the DCIA, although not ideal, has been used to reconstruct the body of the maxilla.

Long Bones

The DCIA has been used to reconstruct bone defects of the tibia of up to 8 cm taken from where the anterior portion of the iliac crest is straight. In one patient, a step osteotomy of the bone was used to straighten the bone and used successfully to repair a 12-cm defect (10).

Otherwise, the authors believe that the fibula is the best choice because it matches exactly the radius and ulna and fits snugly into the medullary cavity of the femur, tibia, and distal humerus (9–11).

Bone Union

A most interesting observation has been the rate of bone union of the fibula and lilac crest, which seems to be related to the status of the recipient bone. Although the iliac rest appears to unite more rapidly, the union time of the bone flap is approximately the same as that of a fracture of the recipient bone.

In other words, unless complicated by radiotherapy or infection union usually occurs in the jaw within 6 to 8 weeks, in the upper extremity by 8 to 10 weeks, and in the lower limb between 3 and 4 months.

REFERENCES

1. Taylor GI, Miller G, Ham FJ. The free vascularised bone graft. *Plast Reconstr Surg* 1975;55:533.
2. Taylor GI, Watson N. One stage repair of compound leg defects with revascularised flaps of groin skin and iliac bone. *Plast Reconstr Surg* 1978;61:494.
3. Taylor GI, Townsend PL, Corlett RJ. Superiority of the deep circumflex iliac vessels as the supply for free groin flaps: experimental work. *Plast Reconstr Surg* 1979;64:595.
4. Taylor GI, Townsend PL, Corlett RJ. Superiority of the deep circumflex iliac vessels as the supply for free groin flaps: clinical work. *Plast Reconstr Surg* 1979;64:745.
5. Taylor GI, Corlett RJ. Refinements of the free iliac osteocutaneous flap designed on the deep circumflex iliac vessels. *Plast Surg Forum* 1980;97:185.
6. Taylor GI. Reconstruction of the mandible with free composite iliac bone grafts. *Ann Plast Surg* 1982;9:361.
7. Taylor GI. microsurgical repair of hemifacial microsomia: osteocutaneous free tissue transfer. In Brent B (ed). *The Artistry of Plastic Surgery.* St. Louis: CV Mosby, 1987.
8. Taylor GI. Keeping a head. 23rd Gillies Memorial Lecture. *Br J Plast Surg* 2002;55:543.
9. Taylor GI. The current status of free vascularized bone grafts. *Clin Plast Surg* 1983;10:185.
10. Taylor GI. Composite tissue transfer to the lower limb. *Recent Adv Plastic Surg* 1985;3:83.
11. Taylor GI. Free composite bone flaps. In *Operative Surgery,* 4th ed. Butterworths, 1986, p. 159–181.
12. Taylor GI, Corlett RJ. Microvascular free transfer of a compound deep circumflex groin and iliac crest transfer to the upper extremity. In Strauch B, Vasconez L, Hall-Findlay B (eds). *Grabb's Encyclopedia of Flaps.* Little Brown, 1990, p. 1197.
13. Taylor GI. Discussion of Hidalgo D and Rekow A. A review of 60 consecutive fibula free flaps. *Plast Reconstr Surg* 1995;96(3):597–602.

CHAPTER 18

Vascularized Fibular Bone Graft and Free Fibular Osteocutaneous Flap

Neil F. Jones

HISTORY

The free vascularized fibular bone graft was first described by Ueba and Fujikawa (1) in 1974 and by Taylor et al. (2) in 1975. Harvesting of the fibular bone alone evolved to harvesting a small overlying "buoy" skin flap for postoperative monitoring described by Yoshimura et al. (3) and subsequently to the fibular osteocutaneous flap described by Chen and Yan (4). Transfer of a vascularized segment of fibular bone with or without a skin component has become the preferred technique for reconstruction of segmental defects of the long bones of the upper and lower extremities (5) and for mandibular reconstruction (6,7).

ANATOMY

The adult fibula provides 25 to 30 cm of bone vascularized by the peroneal artery and its two accompanying vena comitantes. The peroneal artery provides a dual blood supply: an endosteal supply through a nutrient artery that enters the fibula at the junction of the proximal and middle thirds and a periosteal supply through multiple segmental perforators (Figure 18-1A). The nutrient artery divides into a short ascending and a long descending artery (3). The epiphysis is supplied by branches from the anterior tibial artery and the medial genicular artery. The anatomy of the vascularized fibular epiphyseal transfer is described separately in Chapter 86. At their origin from the posterior tibial artery and vein, the peroneal artery and vena comitantes are quite large at 2 to 3 mm in diameter (see Figure 18-3D), and the pedicle of the peroneal vessels is approximately 4 to 6 cm in length.

A skin paddle over the lateral aspect of the middle and distal thirds of the lower leg can be incorporated as an osteocutaneous flap (Figure 18-1B) based on one or more septal perforators (4,5,8–12), which traverse laterally in the thin posterolateral crural septum separating the soleus and peroneus longus and brevis muscles in the middle third of the leg and the flexor hallucis longus and peroneal muscles in the distal third of the leg (Figure 18-2). Multiple cadaveric dissections have investigated the blood supply to the lateral aspect of the lower leg (3–5, 8–12). Yoshimura et al. (3) described three types of perforators. Type A includes musculocutaneous perforators, which are usually located in the proximal third of the leg and primarily pass through the peroneus longus muscle and less frequently through the soleus muscle. Type B septocutaneous perforators are found throughout the entire lower leg and pass between the soleus and peroneal muscles but give off branches to these adjacent muscles. Type C septocutaneous perforators are found in the middle and distal thirds of the lower leg and pass between the soleus and peroneal muscles but without providing any branches to these muscles. Beppu et al. (8) confirmed that perforators in the proximal third of the lower leg always traveled an intramuscular course, but perforators in the distal two thirds of the lower leg usually traveled in the posterolateral septum. Although Chen and Yan (4) had recommended preserving an additional cuff of soleus muscle to preserve the type B musculocutaneous perforators described by Yoshimura et al. (3), Wei et al. (5) concluded that the septocutaneous perforators in the posterolateral crural septum were sufficient to provide perfusion to a fibular osteocutaneous flap and therefore advocated that it was not necessary to harvest the fibula with a portion of the soleus muscle. However, Schusterman et al. (9) found that several perforators passed through the soleus muscle before reaching the skin and therefore recommended that a cuff of soleus be harvested to improve the reliability of the skin island of a fibular osteocutaneous flap. Jones et al. (10) demonstrated that the septocutaneous perforators were concentrated around

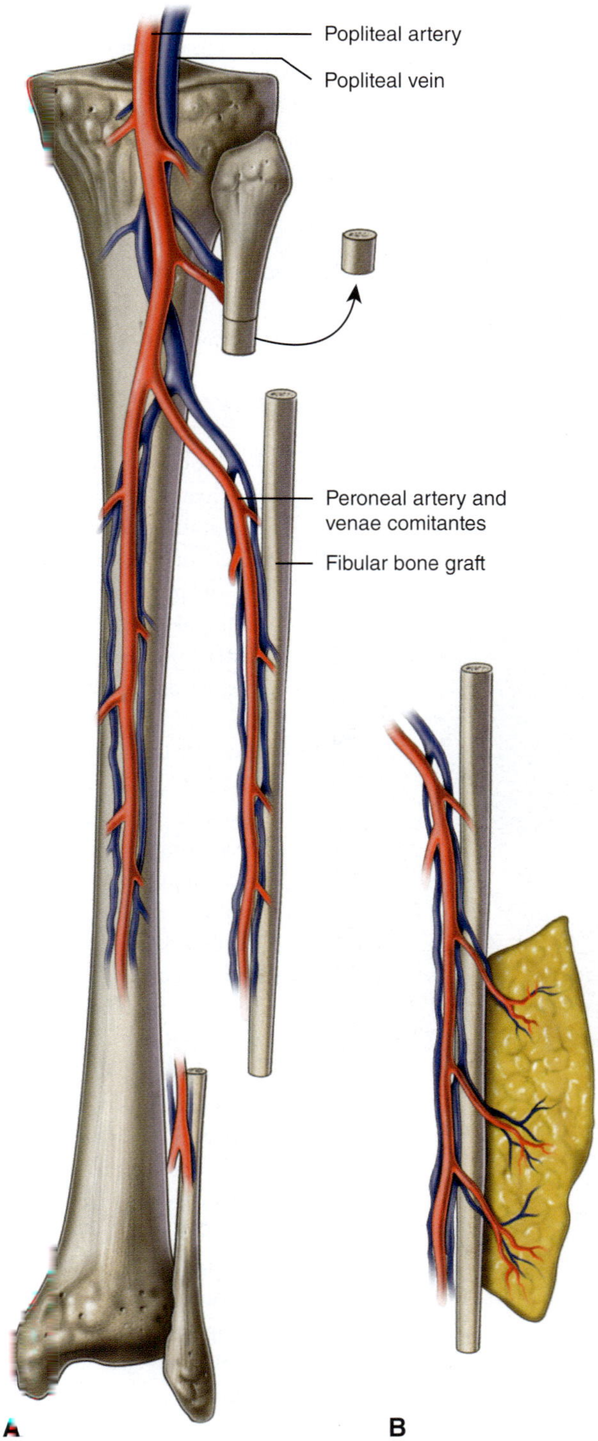

FIGURE 18-1 Anatomy of the vascularized fibular bone graft (**A**) and the fibular osteocutaneous flap (**B**).

the junction of the middle and distal thirds of the lower leg and the largest septocutaneous perforator was usually approximately 8 to 10 cm above the lateral malleolus. One hundred percent viability of the skin paddle of fibular osteocutaneous flaps was achieved in flaps that were based solely on septocutaneous perforators without incorporating any cuff of the soleus or flexor hallucis longus muscles. Therefore, Jones et al. (10) also confirmed that it was not necessary to incorporate any portion of the soleus muscle as long as the skin flap was designed over the junction of the middle and distal thirds of the lower leg. From a prospective study of perforators in 24 fibular osteocutaneous flaps, Cho et al. (11) concluded that if a fibular osteocutaneous flap is designed 10 to 20 cm from the fibular head, a cuff of soleus and flexor hallucis longus muscle should be included to incorporate intramuscular perforators; however, if a fibular osteocutaneous flap is designed 20 to 30 cm from the fibular head, it is possible to elevate the flap without incorporating a cuff of the soleus or flexor hallucis longus muscles.

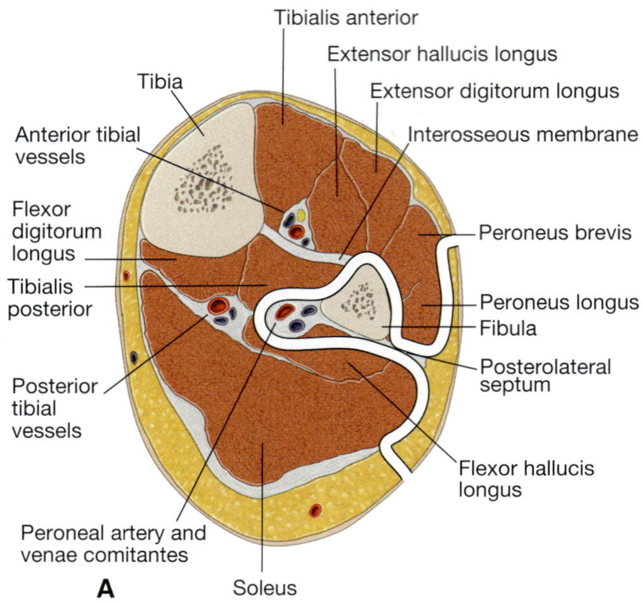

A

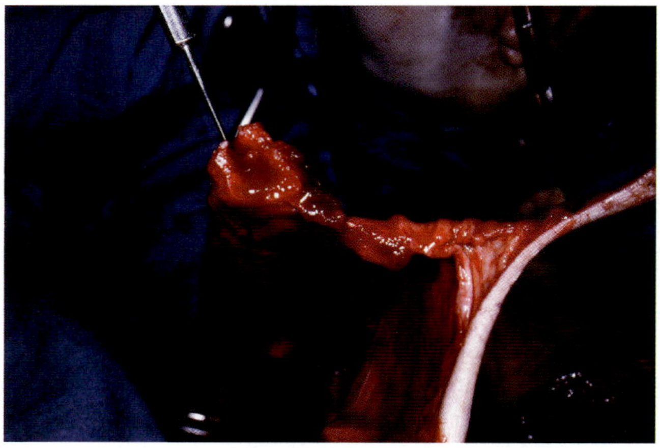

B

FIGURE 18-2 (**A**) Cross-sectional anatomy at the junction of the middle and distal thirds of the lower leg showing the septocutaneous perforators in the posterolateral septum. (**B**) The posterolateral septum itself in a fibular osteocutaneous flap. EDL, extensor digitorum longus; EHL, extensor hallucis longus; FDL, flexor digitorum longus; FHL, flexor hallucis longus; PB, peroneus brevis; PL, peroneus longus; TA, tibialis anterior; TP, tibialis posterior.

Thirty-four percent of the cutaneous perforators from the peroneal artery were found to be musculocutaneous and 66% septocutaneous (12). Musculocutaneous perforators were found predominantly in the upper two thirds, and septocutaneous perforators were located in the lower two thirds of the lower leg.

Despite multiple anatomical studies, the reliability of the skin island of a fibular osteocutaneous flap has been questioned by several authors (7,9). This is directly attributable to the fragile nature of the lateral intermuscular septum itself, the location and identification of septocutaneous perforators, and the surgeon's technical ability to dissect the septum without injuring it or while performing osteotomies. However, if the surgeon understands the anatomy, the fibular osteocutaneous flap is extremely reliable (10).

The lateral portion of the soleus muscle or the flexor hallucis longus muscle can be harvested together with the fibula for obliteration of any associated dead space. Very rarely, intramuscular dissection of a perforator through the soleus muscle (see Figure 18-5B) may be required if a single septocutaneous perforator supplying the skin paddle is judged to be of insufficient caliber or if no septocutaneous perforators are visible during flap harvest (13). The lateral portion of the soleus muscle based on a separate muscle perforator can also be harvested as one of the components of a chimeric osteomyocutaneous peroneal artery perforator flap (14,15). The skin paddle of a fibular osteocutaneous flap can potentially be innervated using the lateral sural cutaneous nerve (16).

PREOPERATIVE INVESTIGATIONS

The popliteal, posterior tibial, and dorsalis pedis pulses should be palpated preoperatively. Harvest of a vascularized fibular bone graft or fibular osteocutaneous flap is probably contraindicated in patients with symptomatic peripheral vascular disease or previous trauma to the lower leg (17) or absent peripheral pulses. The value of preoperative angiography or vascular imaging still remains controversial (18–32). Many surgeons do not routinely perform preoperative angiography, but it should be considered if the foot pulses are abnormal or if the donor leg has been affected by significant previous trauma (18–23). Some surgeons prefer to perform a conventional angiogram preoperatively (18,20,22); others prefer computed tomography angiography (CTA) (26–28) or magnetic resonance angiography (MRA) (29–32) to exclude the very rare likelihood of a vascular anomaly.

Young et al. (18) reported that preoperative angiography of the leg altered the operative plan in 25% of patients. Angiography revealed an 11% incidence of abnormal peroneal artery anatomy. The decision of which leg to be harvested was changed in 12.5%. Seres et al. (19) reported a 15.6% incidence of vascular anomalies in 39 patients undergoing preoperative angiography before a fibular flap harvest and therefore recommended preoperative vascular imaging to be essential. However, from a retrospective review of more than 400 free fibular flaps, Jones (20) concluded that there was no need for preoperative angiography of the donor leg. Lutz et al. (21) also confirmed that routine angiography of the donor leg was not necessary in a prospective study of 120 free fibular flaps. Color Doppler flow imaging has also been recommended as a cost-effective, noninvasive technique for preoperative assessment prior to a fibular flap (24,25). More sophisticated noninvasive imaging has evolved using CTA, (26–28) and MRA (29–32). The fibula was excluded as a donor site in 9% of 32 patients evaluated by MRA (30).

The most feared complication after harvest of a vascularized fibular bone graft or fibular osteocutaneous flap is devascularization of the foot caused by the unrecognized vascular anomaly peroneal arteria magna. According to Lippert and Pabst (33), the peroneal artery becomes the major nutrient artery to the foot in 7% to 12% of the population, either because of a congenital anomaly or because of occlusive disease of the anterior and posterior tibial arteries. The peroneal artery can be congenitally absent in fewer than 0.1%, but the incidence of an abnormal peroneal artery (peroneal arteria magna) has been estimated at 0.2% to 3.5%. Rosson and Singh (34) performed a cost-effective analysis of preoperative vascular imaging before fibular harvest using MRA and traditional angiography, which demonstrated a prevalence of peronea arteria magna of 5.3%. They concluded that MRA of the donor limb before free fibular transfer is cost effective. Even though there are several large series of vascularized fibular bone graft and fibular osteocutaneous flap harvests without any preoperative vascular imaging and no adverse devascularizing sequelae (20,21), there is one report of acute ischemia of the lower leg caused by peronea arteria magna (35). Mureau et al. (36) also described total occlusion of the peroneal artery, but this was only discovered after the fibular flap had been harvested. Otherwise, these authors had never encountered any peroneal artery abnormalities leading to complications in the donor leg, if normal ankle pulses were palpable, in a series of 95 consecutive fibular flaps over a 14-year period.

SURGICAL TECHNIQUE OF FLAP HARVEST

Taylor et al. (2) initially described a posterior approach to harvest the fibula, but the lateral approach described by Gilbert (37–39) is much simpler and faster (Figures 18-3 and 18-4A). The patient is positioned supine with a sandbag under the ipsilateral hip to internally rotate the leg and a second sandbag to stabilize the foot and hold the knee fully flexed. The entire fibula bone is outlined over the lateral aspect of the lower leg by palpating the fibular head at the knee and the lateral malleolus at the ankle and the anterior and posterior borders of the fibula (see Figure 18-3A). The length of the fibula can then be divided into thirds, and the junction of the proximal third and middle third can be marked as a rough guide to the entrance of the nutrient artery from the peroneal artery. Using an 8-mHz Doppler pencil probe, septal perforators can be identified and marked (Figure 18-5A). These septal perforators usually arise approximately 1 cm posterior to the fibula, and the largest is usually around the junction of the middle and distal thirds of the fibula (10) (Figure 18-5C).

Dissection of a vascularized fibular bone graft or a fibular osteocutaneous flap is performed under a thigh tourniquet inflated to 350 mm Hg after exsanguination of the leg with an Esmarch bandage. If only bone is to be harvested, a longitudinal incision is made at the posterior margin of the fibula starting approximately 5 cm below the head of the fibula and ending 5 cm above the lateral malleolus. During the proximal subcutaneous dissection just below the fibular head, great care

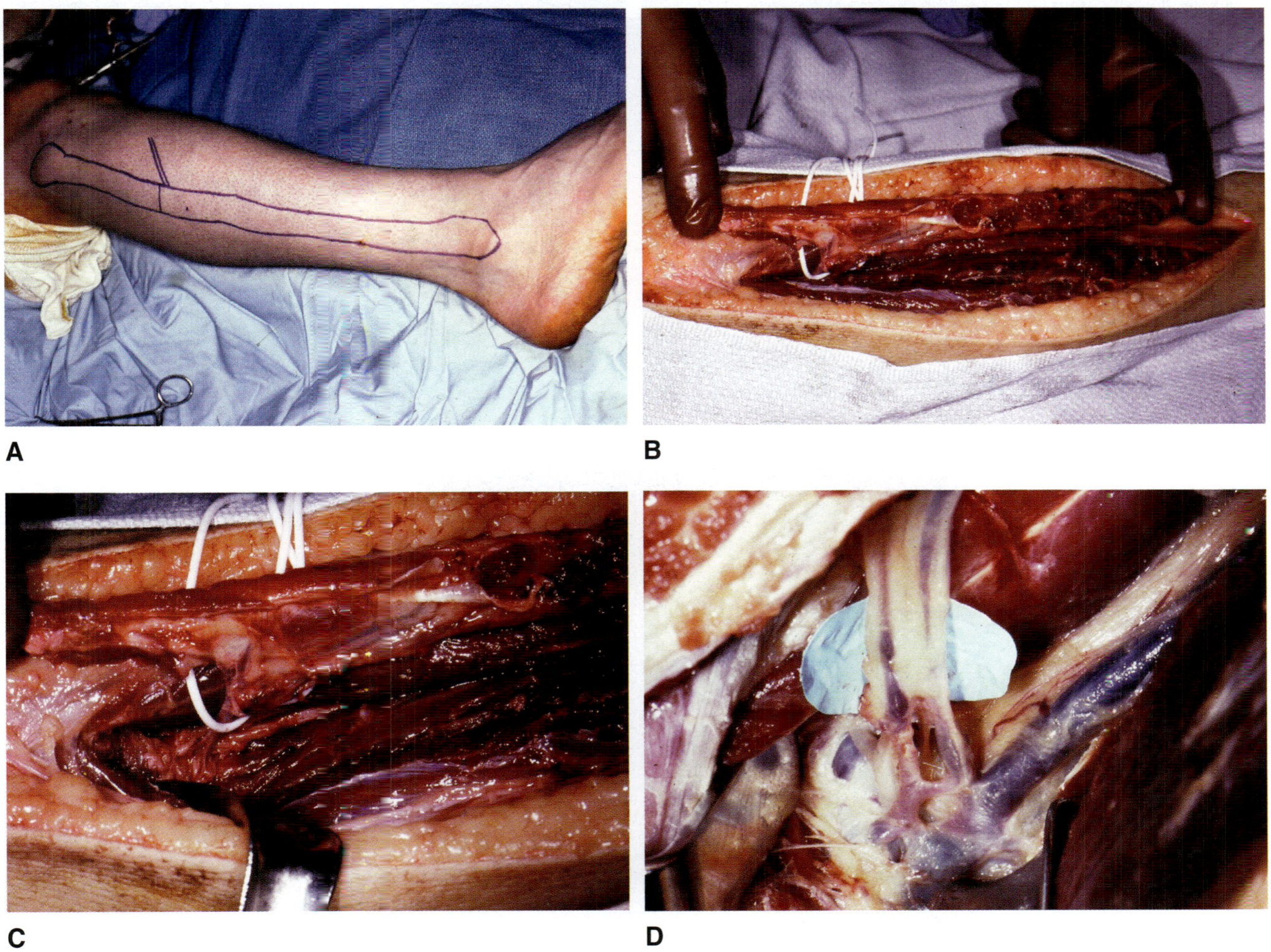

FIGURE 18-3 Lateral approach to harvest a vascularized fibular bone graft (**A** and **B**) showing the entry of the nutrient branch into the fibula bone (**C**) and a close-up view of the origin of the peroneal artery and two venae comitantes from the posterior tibial vessels (**D**).

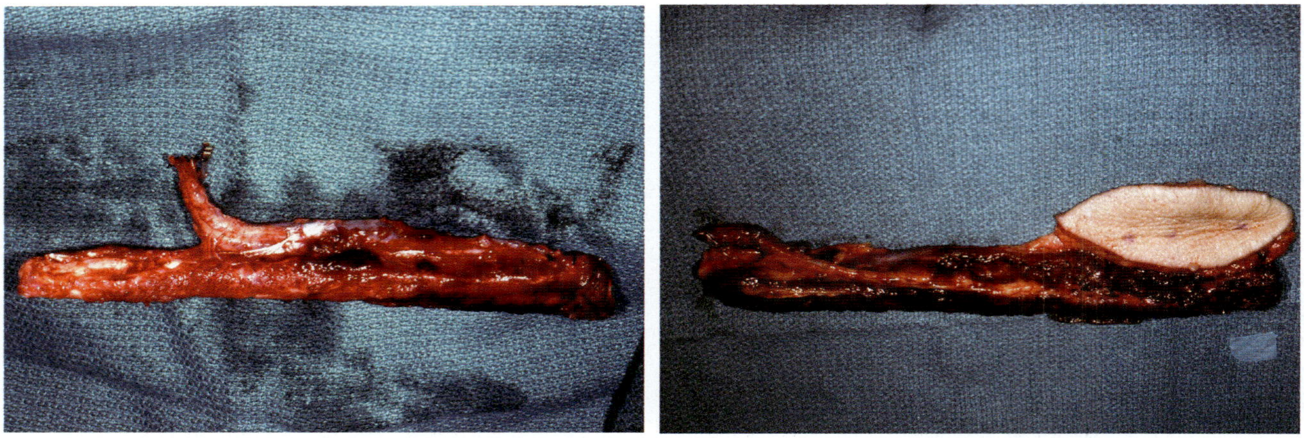

A B

FIGURE 18-4 (**A**) Vascularized fibular bone graft. (**B**) Small "buoy" flap for postoperative monitoring.

must be maintained to prevent any injury to the common peroneal nerve. The incision is carried down through the subcutaneous tissues to identify the fascia separating the soleus and peroneus muscles in the middle third of the leg and the flexor hallucis longus and peroneal muscles in the distal third of the leg. Dissection is then exactly similar to that described for the now more usual dissection of a fibular osteocutaneous flap (see later discussion; see Figures 18-3 and 18-4A).

A template of the soft tissue defect is made using a piece of Esmarch bandage or surgical glove wrapper and transferred

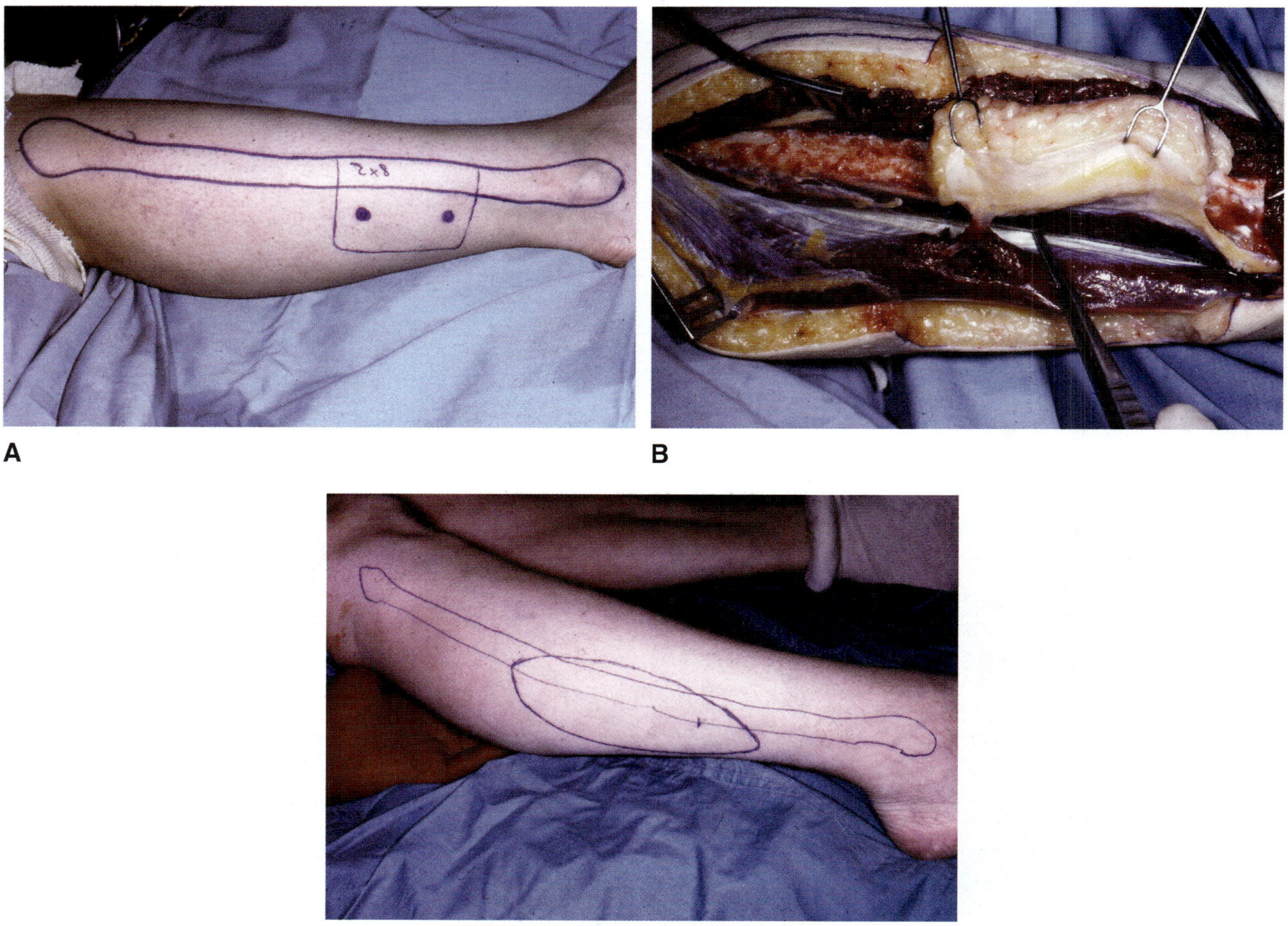

A B

C

FIGURE 18-5 (**A**) Design of a fibular osteocutaneous flap with preoperative mapping of the cutaneous perforators using a handheld 8 mHz Doppler probe. (**B**) One of these identified perforators is a musculocutaneous perforator passing through the soleus muscle. (**C**) Design of a fibular osteocutaneous flap over the junction of the middle and distal thirds of the lower leg.

onto the lateral aspect of the lower leg centered over the most dominant perforator (see Figure 18-5A). Alternatively, the template can be incorporated into an elliptical-shaped skin island centered over the dominant perforator (Figure 18-5C). The outlined skin island is then extended superiorly and inferiorly with a longitudinal incision to just below the fibular head and to just above the lateral malleolus. The inferior portion of the longitudinal incision should be incised first before the margins of the skin island are incised to identify the interval between the soleus and the peroneus longus muscles in the distal third of the lower leg. Developing this interval distally between these two muscles allows the surgeon to understand the location and plane of the lateral intermuscular septum before beginning the anterior or posterior dissection of the skin island itself.

Anterior Dissection of the Posterolateral Septum

The anterior margin of the skin island is incised first and extended down through the subcutaneous tissues and through the fascia overlying the peroneal muscles. Dissection beneath the fascia proceeds in a posterior direction until the anterior surface of the posterolateral septum is reached (Figure 18-6A). Small perforators may be seen in the septum corresponding to previous Doppler identification.

Dissection of the Lateral and Anterior Muscle Compartments

Starting inferiorly, the peroneus longus and peroneus brevis muscles are elevated upward off the lateral surface of the fibula,

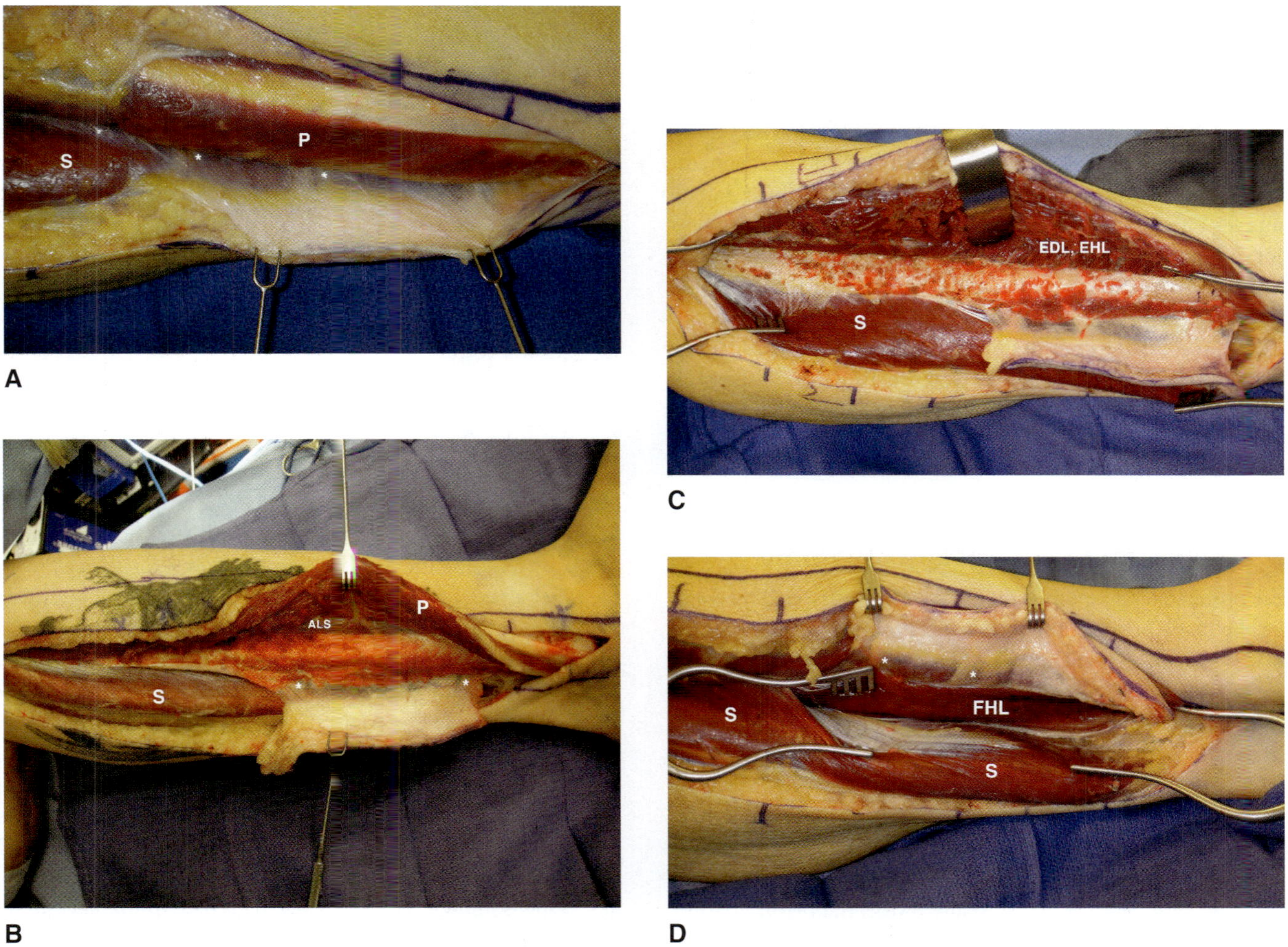

FIGURE 18-6 The right fibula viewed from laterally; the knee is to the left and the ankle to the right. (**A**) The anterior margin of the skin island has been incised with dissection beneath the fascia overlying the peroneus longus and brevis muscles (P) to the anterior surface of the posterolateral septum. Two septocutaneous perforators (marked with an asterisk) are visible in the septum. (**B**) The peroneus longus and brevis muscles (P) are elevated off the lateral surface of the fibula. The anterolateral septum (ALS) separating the peroneus longus and brevis muscles in the lateral compartment from the extensor digitorum longus and extensor hallucis longus muscles in the anterior compartment can be seen. (**C**) The anterolateral septum has been incised, and the extensor digitorum longus (EDL) and extensor hallucis longus (EHL) muscles are being swept away from the tibial surface of the fibula toward the tibia, with great care taken to protect the anterior tibial artery and deep peroneal nerve. The soleus muscle (S) is seen superiorly still attached to the posterior aspect of the fibula. (**D**) The posterior margin of the skin island has been incised with dissection beneath the fascia overlying the soleus (S) and flexor hallucis longus muscles to the posterior surface of the posterolateral septum. The plane between the soleus and flexor hallucis longus (FHL) muscles is shown. Two septocutaneous perforators (marked with an asterisk) are visible in the septum.

leaving a 1-mm or smaller cuff of muscle attached to the lateral surface of the fibula (Figure 18-6B). Superiorly, the peroneal muscles are separated from the soleus muscle and elevated up to the superior crest of the fibula, where the thinner anterolateral septum separating the anterior and lateral compartments of the leg is incised. The muscles of the anterior compartment, the extensor digitorum longus and extensor hallucis longus, are now elevated downward and medially off the medial or tibial surface of the fibula toward the tibia (Figure 18-6C). The anterior tibial artery and deep peroneal nerve may be seen superiorly during this dissection and must be protected by mobilization of these muscles in a medial or tibial direction away from the fibula. Eventually, at the completion of the anterior compartment dissection, the entire length of the interosseous membrane can be visualized, and the distal 5 cm of interosseous membrane is incised in a distal-to-proximal direction to facilitate the distal osteotomy (see Figure 18-6C).

Posterior Dissection of the Posterolateral Septum

The posterior margin of the skin island is now incised down through the skin and subcutaneous tissues and through the fascia overlying the soleus muscle and flexor hallucis longus muscle. The sural nerve may be encountered during this posterior dissection and must be identified and protected. Dissection then proceeds beneath the fascia in an anterior direction until the posterior surface of the posterolateral septum is reached (Figure 18-6D). The perforators in the septum are usually more obvious on the posterior surface (Figure 18-7A). The posterolateral septum is incredibly thin and fragile and slightly more posterior than expected.

Dissection of the Posterior Muscle Compartment and Distal Osteotomy

The posterolateral aspect of the fibula is now dissected by entering the plane between the soleus and the flexor hallucis longus muscle distally (see Figures 18-6D and 18-7A) and then by releasing the soleus muscle from the proximal half of the fibula. The site of the distal osteotomy is selected leaving 6 to 8 cm of fibula above or proximal to the lateral malleolus to preserve the stability of the ankle joint. The periosteum is sharply incised on the lateral, tibial, and posterior surfaces, and the distal osteotomy is performed using either an oscillating saw or a Gigli saw. Lateral traction can then be applied to the distal end of the fibula with a large bone hook. This usually reveals the peroneal artery and two vena comitantes approximately 5 mm posterior and slightly medial or tibial to the fibula lying between the tibialis posterior and flexor hallucis longus muscles. The distal peroneal artery and vena comitantes are clamped, ligated, and divided.

The distal end of the osteotomized fibular segment is grasped with a Dingman bone holder and strongly retracted outward to allow division of the interosseous membrane 1 mm away from the tibial surface of the fibula in a distal-to-proximal direction, all the way up to the anticipated site of the proximal osteotomy. This reveals the anterior aspect of the tibialis posterior muscle, which has the appearance of a V-shaped decussation (Figure 18-7B). The muscle is dissected in this V to expose the location of the peroneal vessels, and the tibialis posterior muscle fibers are then carefully separated away from the vascular pedicle in a tibial direction but preserving a cuff of tibialis posterior muscle between the peroneal vessels and the tibial surface of the fibula, which maintains the periosteal blood supply to the fibula. This dissection can be continued in a distal-to-proximal direction for approximately 5 cm. More proximal dissection can only be facilitated after performing the proximal osteotomy of the fibula.

Proximal Osteotomy

This should be performed approximately 6 cm distal to the fibular head; otherwise, it becomes exceedingly difficult to dissect the peroneal artery and vena comitantes back to their origin from the posterior tibial vessels. The proximal osteotomy has to be performed very carefully because the peroneal vessels are immediately posterior to the fibula and can be injured by inadvertent blunt dissection. The osteotomy is performed using an oscillating saw or a Gigli saw after careful protection of the vessels posteriorly with a retractor. After the proximal osteotomy has been completed, lateral traction can then be applied to both the proximal and distal ends of the fibula bone using two strong bone hooks or Dingman bone holders to further define the V-shaped decussation of the tibialis posterior muscle fibres (see Figure 18-7B).

Dissection of the Tibialis Posterior and Flexor Hallucis Longus Muscles

The peroneal vessels can be visualized from both the anterior surface of the tibialis posterior muscle and the posterior surface of the flexor hallucis muscle by flipping the fibula bone segment upward and downward using the two bone holders (Figures 18-7C and 18-7D). Anteriorly, the dissection is completed by releasing the tibialis posterior muscle fibers away from the tibial aspect of the peroneal vessels all the way superiorly in a distal-to-proximal direction but maintaining a cuff of muscle between the peroneal vessels and the tibial surface of the fibula, which contains the periosteal branches of the peroneal artery (see Figure 18-7C). Posteriorly, the flexor hallucis longus muscle fibers are separated laterally away from the lateral aspect of the peroneal vessels but carefully maintaining a cuff of muscle between the peroneal vessels and the posterior surface of the fibula, which contains the periosteal branches of the peroneal artery (see Figure 18-7D). The proximal origin of the flexor hallucis longus muscle is completely detached from the middle third of the fibula, revealing the posterior aspect of the peroneal vessels (see Figure 18-7D), but the motor nerve branch to flexor hallucis longus from the posterior tibial nerve must be preserved.

Dissection of the Pedicle of the Peroneal Vessels

As the dissection proceeds more proximally, large muscular branches from the peroneal vessels passing into the soleus muscle may be encountered and need to be ligated and divided. The peroneal artery and two vena comitantes pass toward the tibia to

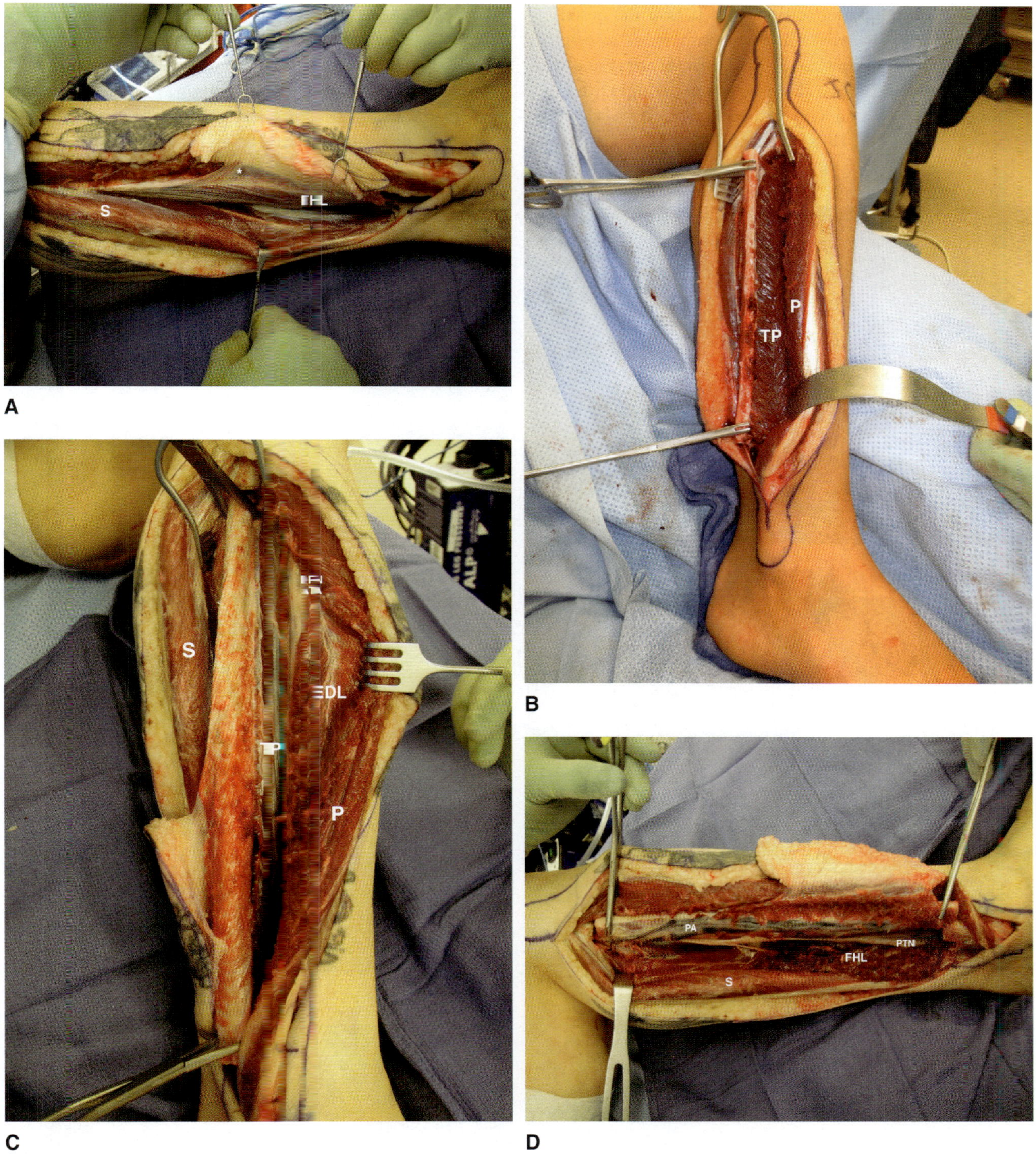

FIGURE 13-7 (**A**) The posterior surface of the posterolateral septum containing two septocutaneous perforators (one marked with an asterisk). The plane between the soleus (S) and flexor hallucis longus (FHL) muscles has been developed. Superiorly, the soleus is being detached from the inferior border of the fibula. (**B**) After incising the interosseous membrane, the V-shaped decussation of the tibialis posterior (TP) muscle is clearly seen. (**C**) Starting inferiorly, the TP muscle fibers are dissected away from the underlying peroneal vessels in a tibial direction. The deep peroneal nerve (DPN) and anterior tibial artery (ATA) are seen superiorly beneath the extensor digitorum longus (EDL) muscle. (**D**) The FHL muscle fibers are separated away from the peroneal vessels (PA) in a lateral direction. The fibular bone graft held in two Dingman bone holders can be flipped from anterior to posterior so that the peroneal vessels can always be visualized with respect to the flexor hallucis longus FHL and tibialis posterior muscles as well as the posterior tibial nerve and artery (PTN).

their origin from the posterior tibial vessels, and the posterior tibial nerve will become visible and obviously needs to be protected. Under loupe magnification, the peroneal artery and two vena comitantes are dissected all the way to their origin from the posterior tibial artery and vein and separated on vessel loops (Figures 18-3B, 18-3D, 18-8A, and 18-8B). The tourniquet is deflated, and punctate bleeding from the proximal and distal ends of the fibula should be seen. Perfusion to the skin paddle of a fibular osteocutaneous flap is confirmed by capillary refill or by documenting an audible pulse in one of the septocutaneous perforators using the pencil Doppler probe, and this can be marked with a suture (Figure 18-8C and 18-8D).

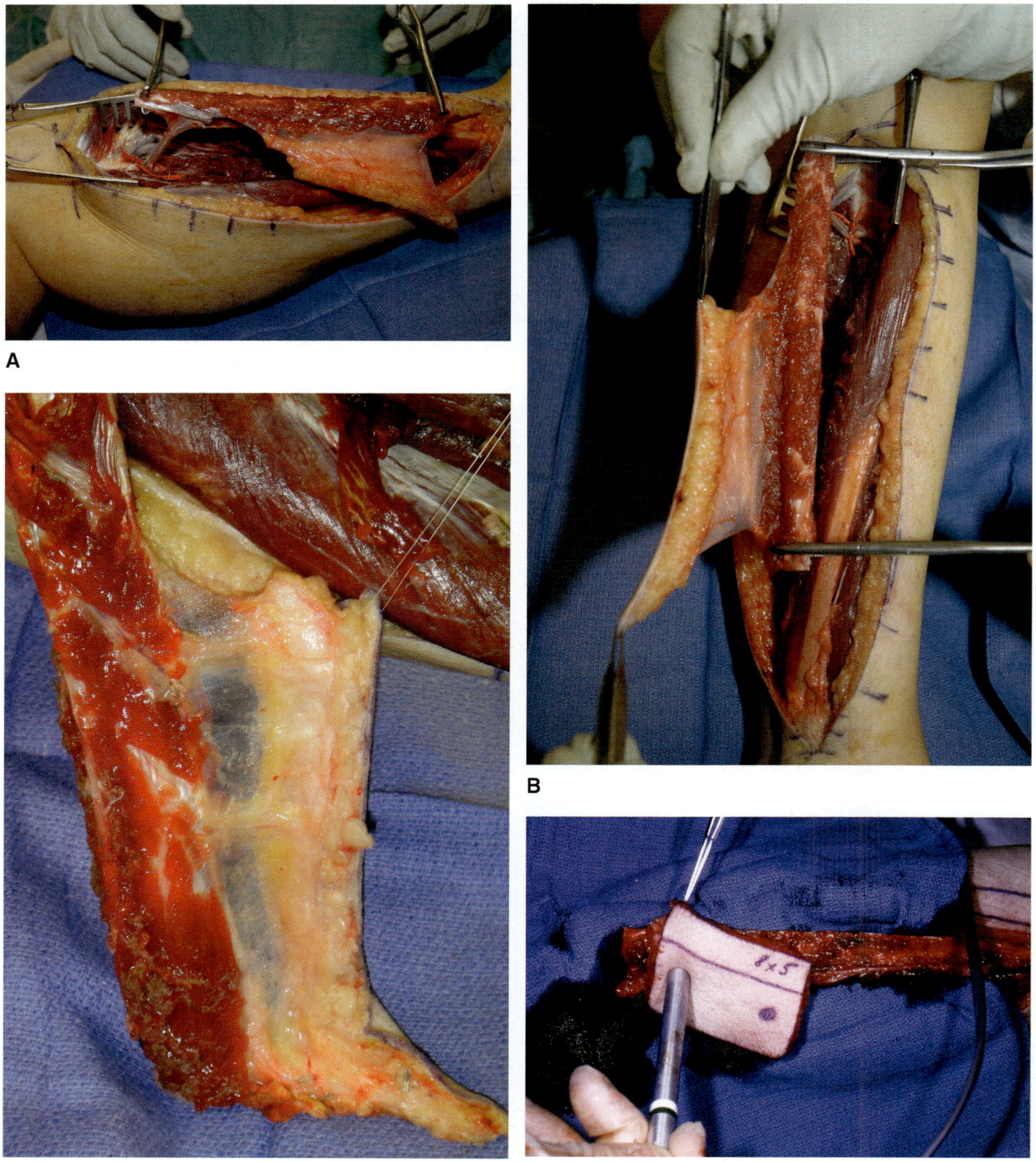

A B C D

FIGURE 18-8 (**A**) The peroneal artery and two venae comitantes are dissected to their origin from the posterior tibial vessels. (**B**) Posterolateral septum of the skin island demonstrating the extreme thinness of the septum (**C**). (**D**) After deflation of the tourniquet, the 8-mHz pencil Doppler can be used to confirm flow in a septocutaneous perforator.

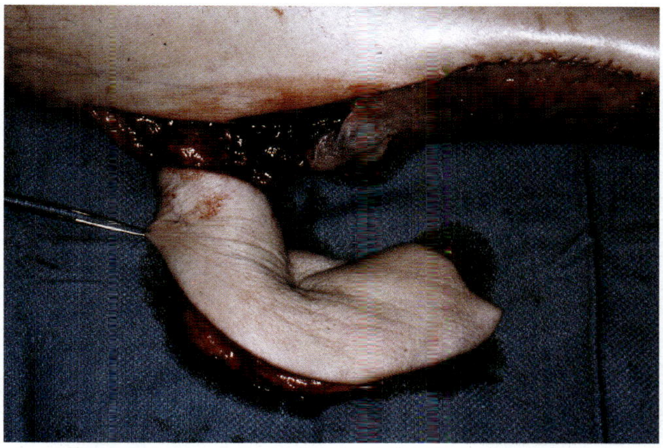

FIGURE 18-9 Fibular osteocutaneous flap for mandibular reconstruction, with the osteotomies and fixation to a reconstruction plate being performed while the flap is still perfused in-situ in the leg before ligation of the peroneal vessels.

After reperfusion of the fibula osteocutaneous flap for 15 minutes, the leg can be reexsanguinated and the tourniquet reinflated to allow precise ligation of the peroneal artery and two vena comitantes to allow transfer of the flap to the recipient site. For mandibular reconstruction, some surgeons prefer to fabricate the new mandible in situ by performing osteotomies on the fibula and fixating the fibular segments to a reconstruction plate with the peroneal vessels still perfusing in continuity in the leg (Figure 18-9) rather than performing the osteotomies and plate fixation on a back table after ligation and division of the vascular pedicle (Figure 18-10). This is described in the chapter on mandibular reconstruction (Chapter 32).

The normal 4- to 6-cm length of the peroneal vascular pedicle can be elongated by elevating the periosteal cuff from the proximal fibula down to the estimated length of fibular bone that will be required for reconstruction of the segmental bone defect; the proximal fibula bone is then excised (Figure 18-11A). Alternatively, if the distance between the segmental bone defect to be reconstructed and the recipient vessels is much greater than the length of the normal peroneal vascular pedicle, an interposition vein graft can be anastomosed between the peroneal artery and one of the vena comitantes under the operating microscope on a back table to create an AV loop (Figure 18-11B).

Closure of the Donor Site

The tourniquet is deflated and hemostasis achieved in the donor site. One or two suction drains are placed into the depths of the defect beneath the muscles. The proximal fascial envelope of the flexor hallucis longus muscle is sutured to the remnant of the interosseous membrane still attached to the tibia to restore the resting tension of this muscle. Its motor nerve branch from the posterior tibial nerve should have been preserved during harvesting of the fibula. The fascia overlying the soleus and peroneal muscles is approximated in the proximal half of the incision, and the fascia overlying the soleus, flexor hallucis longus, and peroneal muscles is approximated in the distal half of the incision. If only fibula bone has been harvested or if only a narrow skin paddle has been harvested, primary skin closure can be achieved. For osteocutaneous flaps with a width greater than 2 cm, the donor defect should be skin grafted. The skin margins are tacked down to the underlying muscles so that a smooth shallow bed is created, and a fenestrated 17/1000-inch split-thickness skin graft applied. The donor site in the lower leg is similar to the donor site of a radial forearm flap. The graft is covered with a sheet of Xeroform or Adaptic gauze and a stent of 1 inch foam rubber applied or a vacuum-assisted closure (VAC) device is applied. The lower leg is then immobilized in a plaster of Paris posterior splint with the ankle in neutral position. The split-thickness skin graft is inspected 5 to 7 days after surgery, and if there has been complete "take" of the skin graft, the patient can start gentle mobilization with a pressure dressing over the skin graft. If there is less than perfect "take" of the split-thickness skin graft over the peroneus longus and brevis tendons, this should be treated with dressing changes and will gradually granulate, contract, and reepithelialize.

A valgus deformity of the ankle may occur after harvest of a vascularized fibular bone graft in children; therefore, some surgeons recommend performing a distal tibiofibular syndesmosis prophylactically with iliac crest bone graft and screw fixation (see Chapter 62).

COMPLICATIONS RELATED TO THE DONOR SITE

Youdas et al. (40) reported no gait abnormalities or significant loss of knee or ankle motion in patients more than 10 months after surgery, although there was some loss of muscle strength in foot inversion and eversion. Anthony et al. (41) reported an immediate postoperative morbidity of 17% caused by infection, wound separation, or partial skin graft loss, but patients had pain-free ambulation and were able to engage in all recreational activities an average of 7 months after surgery. Seventy-two percent were free of any pain in the donor leg, and 28% had only occasional mild discomfort. A total of 41% of patients reported ankle stiffness and 10% ankle instability. Seven percent exhibited peroneal nerve palsy and sensory loss, but these resolved in all patients. Vail and Urbaniak (42) reviewed 247 lower limbs in 198 patients between 24 and 144 months after harvesting of a vascularized fibular bone graft. Five percent of the limbs had sensory deficits at 3 months, which increased to 12% at 5 years after surgery. Ankle pain increased over time from 1.6% at 3 months to 11.5% at 5 years. Pain in other sites in the lower limb other than the ankle also increased over time from 3.6% at 3 months to 9% at 5 years. Shpitzer et al. (43) evaluated the donor site in 38 fibular osteocutaneous flaps and nine vascularized fibular bone grafts. A total of 27% of patients had late donor site morbidity with weakness of the great toe, ankle instability and stiffness, pain, and edema. Tang et al. (44) analyzed the subjective complaints and objective findings of 39 patients who underwent vascularized fibular bone grafting for avascular necrosis of the femoral head. Forty-two percent of patients had a sense of instability and 37% a sense of weakness, but no objective instability could be documented, and only great toe flexion (29%) and extension (43%) were found to be

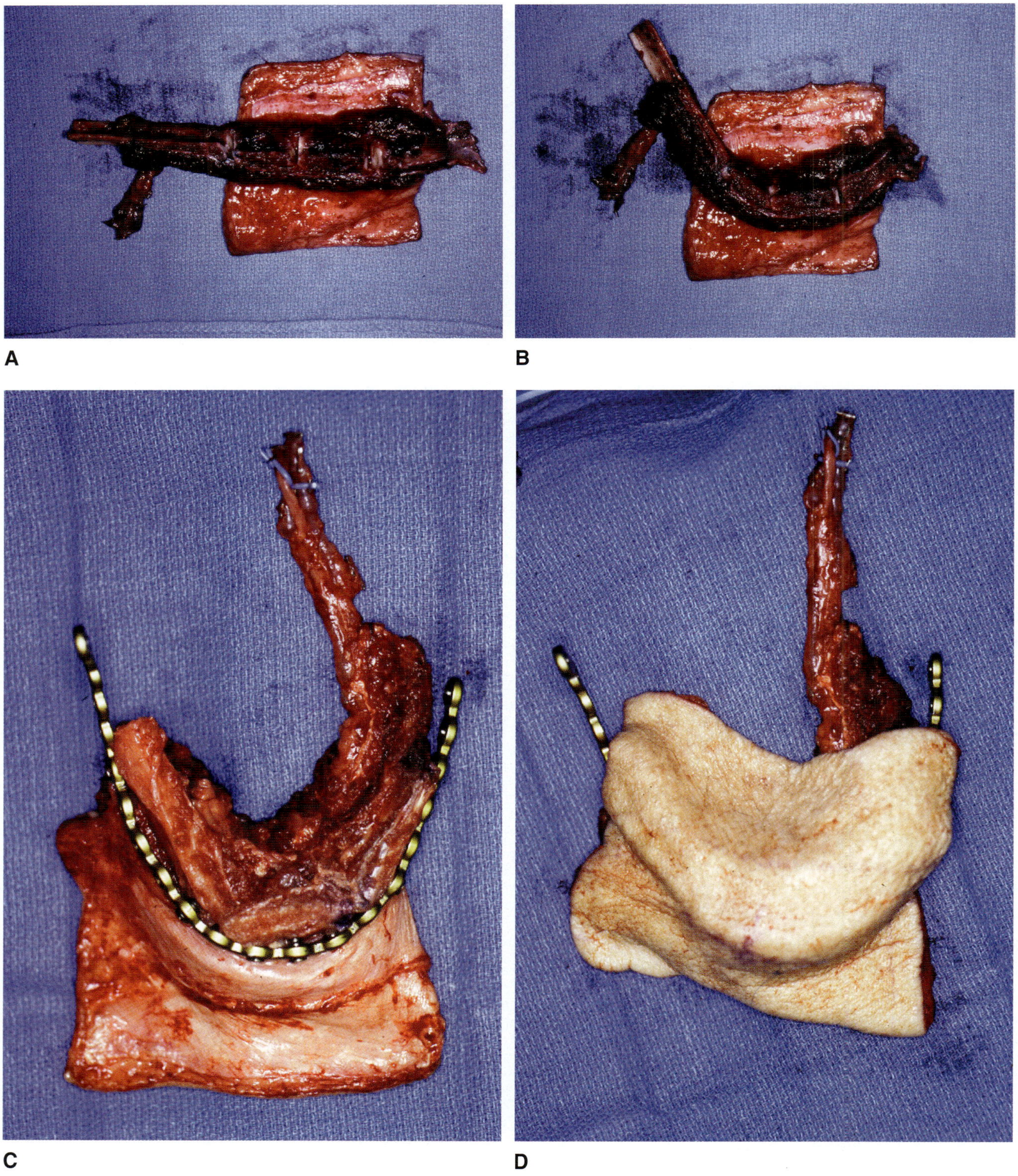

FIGURE 18-10 Fibular osteocutaneous flap for mandibular reconstruction with the osteotomies (**A** and **B**) and fixation to a reconstruction plate (**C** and **D**) being performed on a back table after removal of the flap from the leg.

mildly weak. Eighty-nine percent of patients were pain free, and all patients had similar range of motion of the knee and ankle compared with the nonoperated leg. Babovic et al. (45) reviewed 72 vascularized fibular bone grafts and 28 fibular osteocutaneous flaps at an average follow-up of 17 months. There was a 30% complication rate. Fifteen percent had limited maximum walking distance, 10% had numbness in the foot, 8% had loss of the split-thickness skin graft, 7% had wound dehiscence, 5% had exposure of the peroneal tendons, and 6% had hammer toe deformity. Lee et al. (46) performed gait analysis before surgery and at 1 and 3 months after surgery after fibular flap harvest. Initially, there was significant loss of plantar

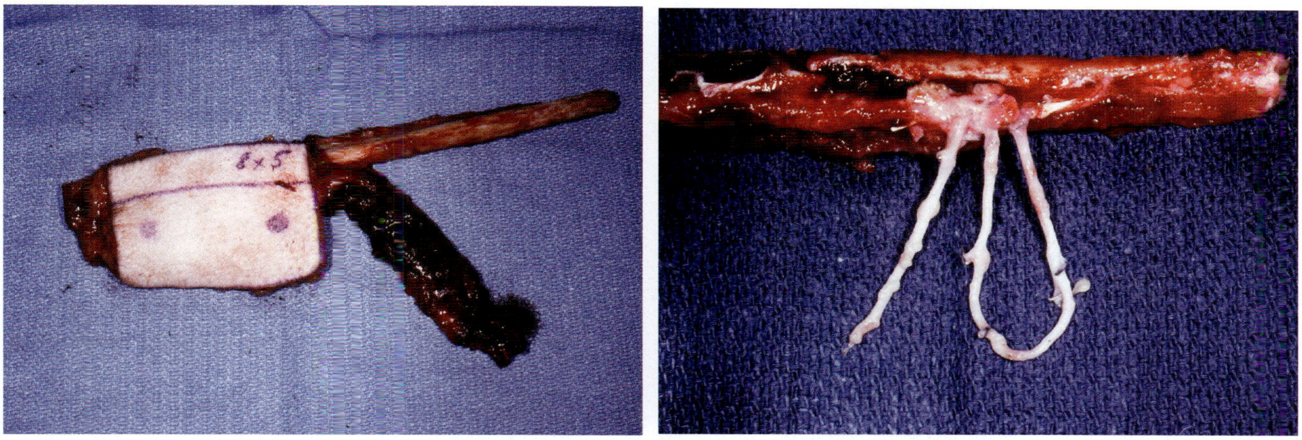

FIGURE 18-11 (**A**) Stripping the periosteum and vascular pedicle away from the proximal fibula will lengthen the vascular pedicle. (**B**) Anastomosis of an interposition vein graft to create an AV loop between the peroneal artery and one vena comitans.

flexion, but this returned to normal within 3 months after surgery. Momoh et al. (47) reported a complication rate of 31% after fibular flap harvest, including cellulitis (10%), wound dehiscence (8%), skin graft loss (15%), and abscess (1%). There was no difference in complication rates between primary skin closure and skin grafting of the donor defect. Long-term morbidity occurred in 17% of patients, including weakness (8%), ankle instability (4%), contracture of the great toe (9%), and decreased ankle motion (12%), but 96% of patients returned to their preoperative level of ambulation.

In summary, the overall donor site morbidity after harvest of a vascularized fibular bone graft or fibular osteocutaneous flap is reported to be up to 30%. Early complications include cellulitis; infection; wound dehiscence; skin graft loss; subjective sensory deficits in the foot; and much more rarely, compartment syndrome, peroneal nerve palsy, and stress fracture of the ipsilateral tibia. Late complications include weakness or contracture of the great toe, decreased range of motion of the ankle, ankle instability, and discomfort or pain with vigorous activity.

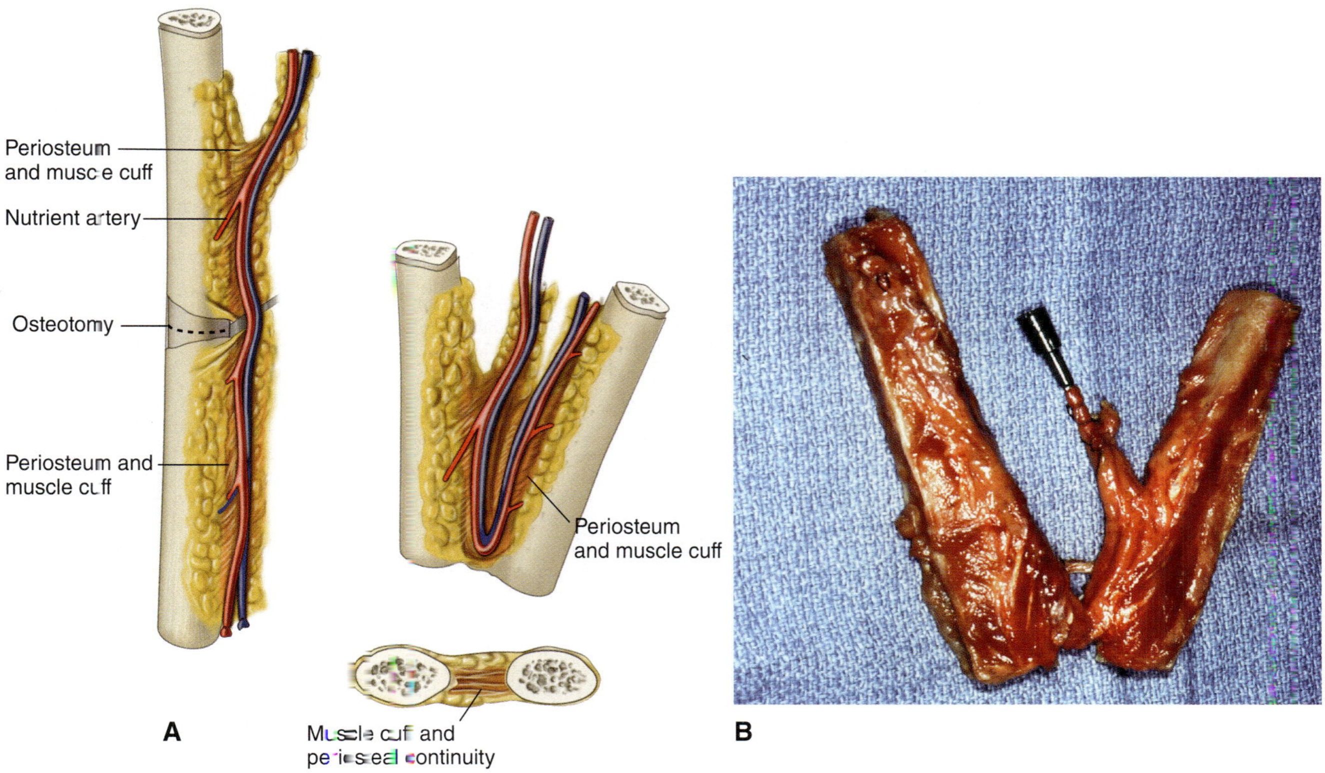

FIGURE 18-12 Diagrammatic representation (**A**) and photograph (**B**) of a "double-barrel" vascularized fibular bone graft. An osteotomy divides the fibula into two parallel segments. Whereas the superior segment is vascularized by both an endosteal supply from the nutrient artery and by periosteal branches from the peroneal artery, the distal segment is only vascularized by periosteal branches from the peroneal artery.

VARIATIONS OF VASCULARIZED FIBULAR BONE GRAFTS AND FIBULAR OSTEOCUTANEOUS FLAPS

1. Fibular bone alone (1,2) (see Figure 18-4A)
2. "Double-barrel" fibula (48–54) (Figure 18-12)

   Jones et al. (48) and O'Brien et al. (49) established the principle of osteotomizing a vascularized fibular bone graft into two or more bony segments but maintaining vascularity to these bony segments. Whereas the proximal segment is vascularized by both an endosteal and a periosteal blood supply, the distal segment or segments are vascularized by a periosteal blood supply alone. These experimental studies provided the basis for performing two or three osteotomies in the fibula to create the shape for mandibular reconstruction (6,7) but also the concept of a "double-barrel" fibular bone graft in which two fibular bone segments are folded back on each other (see Figure 18-12) to produce twice the cross-sectional area of a single fibular bone graft (48,49). This technique has been applied for reconstruction of segmental bone defects of the femur and pelvis (48–52) and even to increase the vertical height of the fibula in mandibular and maxillary reconstruction (53,54). This "double-barrel" technique will also allow simultaneous reconstruction of bony defects of the radius and ulna (48).
3. Multiple osteotomies (6,7) (see Figure 18-10)
4. Fibular osteocutaneous flap (4,5) (see Figures 18-2, 18-4B, and 18-9)
5. "Double skin paddles": deepithelialized or two separate perforators (55,56)

   A single large skin island of a fibular osteocutaneous flap can be separated into two skin paddles either by deepithelializing the intervening segment of skin to create a "double-paddle" fibular osteocutaneous flap (55), or a single skin island can be divided into two totally separate skin flaps based on two separate individual septocutaneous perforators (56). Both of these techniques can be used to reconstruct both the mucosal defect and the external skin defect of composite "through-and-through" mandibular defects.
6. With soleus muscle to obliterate dead space (13)
7. Chimeric osteomyocutaneous peroneal artery perforator flap with separate perforators to the skin and soleus muscle (14,15)
8. With flexor hallucis longus muscle to obliterate dead space
9. Sensate flap including the lateral sural cutaneous nerve (16)

RECONSTRUCTIVE INDICATIONS FOR VASCULARIZED FIBULAR BONE GRAFTS AND FIBULAR OSTEOCUTANEOUS FLAPS

1. Segmental bone defects greater than 6 cm of the humerus, radius, and ulna caused by trauma, tumor resection, and infection; occasionally for reconstruction of complex bony defects of the metacarpals (Chapter 60)
2. Segmental bone defects greater than 6 cm of the femur (using a "double-barrel" fibular bone graft) and tibia caused by trauma, tumor resection, or infection; occasionally for reconstruction of complex bony defects of the foot (Chapter 81)
3. Composite bone and soft tissue defects of the upper and lower extremities. (Chapters 60 and 81)
4. Complex arthrodeses of the shoulder, elbow, wrist, and knee and ankle after failed conventional treatment (Chapters 60 and 81)
5. Complex fusion of the cervical and lumbar spine
6. Complex pelvic reconstruction after tumor resection (Chapter 81)
7. Avascular necrosis of the femoral head (Chapter 85)
8. Transfer of the vascularized proximal fibular epiphysis to maintain growth in the upper or lower extremities of children (Chapter 86)
9. Mandibular reconstruction after resection of tumors of the floor of the mouth, primary bone tumors of the mandible, or osteoradionecrosis of the mandible and for posttraumatic reconstruction (Chapter 32)
10. Reconstruction of the maxilla after tumor resection and trauma (Chapter 31)

REFERENCES

1. Ueba Y, Fujikawa S. Nine years follow-up of a vascularized fibular graft in neurofibromatosis; a case report and literature review. *Orthop Trauma Surg* 1983;26:595.
2. Taylor GI, Miller GD, Ham FJ. The free vascularized bone graft: A clinical extension of microvascular techniques. *Plast Reconstr Surg* 1975;55:533–544.
3. Yoshimura M, Shimamura K, Iwai Y, et al. Free vascularized fibular transplant. A new method for monitoring circulation of the grafted fibula. *J Bone Joint Surg* 1983;65(suppl A):1295–1301.
4. Chen ZW, Yan W. The study and clinical application of the osteocutaneous flap of fibula. *Microsurgery* 1983;4:11–16.
5. Wei FC, Chen HC, Chuang CC, Noordhoff MS. Fibular osteoseptocutaneous flap: anatomic study and clinical application. *Plast Reconstr Surg* 1986;78:191–200.
6. Hidalgo DA. Fibula free flap: a new method of mandible reconstruction. *Plast Reconstr Surg* 1989;84:71–79.
7. Hidalgo DA, Rekow A. A review of 60 consecutive fibula free flap mandible reconstructions. *Plast Reconstr Surg* 1995;96:585–596; discussion 597–602.
8. Beppu M, Hanel DP, Johnston GHF, et al. The osteocutaneous fibula flap: an anatomic study. *J Reconstr Microsurg* 1992;8:215–223.
9. Schusterman MA, Reece GP, Miller MJ, Harris S. The osteocutaneous free fibula flap: Is the skin paddle reliable? *Plast Reconstr Surg* 1992;90:787–793; discussion 794–798.
10. Jones NF, Monstrey S, Gambier BA. Reliability of the fibular osteocutaneous flap for mandibular reconstruction: anatomical and surgical confirmation. *Plast Reconstr Surg* 1996;97:707–716; discussion 717–718.
11. Cho BC, Kim SY, Park JW, Baek BS. Blood supply to osteocutaneous free fibula flap and peroneus longus muscle: prospective anatomis study and clinical applications. *Plast Reconstr Surg* 2001;108:1963–1971.
12. Heitmann C, Khan F, Levin LS. Vasculature of the peroneal artery: an anatomic study focused on the perforator vessels. *J Reconstr Microsurg* 2003;19:157–162.
13. Wong CH, Tan BK, Wei FC, Song C. Use of the soleus musculocutaneous perforator for skin paddle salvage of the fibula osteoseptocutaneous flap: anatomical study and clinical confirmation. *Plast Reconstr Surg* 2007;120:1576–1584.
14. Yazar S, Cheng MH, Wei FC, et al. Osteomyocutaneous peroneal artery perforator flap for reconstruction of composite maxillary defects. *Head Neck* 2006;28:297–304.
15. Cheng MH, Saint-Cyr M, Ali RS, et al. Osteomyocutaneous peroneal artery-based combined flap for reconstruction of composite enbloc mandibular defects. *Head Neck* 2009;31:361–370.
16. Wei FC, Chuang SS, Yim KK. The sensate fibula osteoseptocutaneous flap: a preliminary report. *Br J Plast Surg* 1994;47:544–547.
17. Grewal R, Otsuka NY, Jones NF. Successful transfer of a vascularized fibular osteocutaneous bone graft harvested distal to a previously fractured fibula. *Plast Reconstr Surg* 2007;120:2127.

18. Young DM, Trabulsy PP, Anthony JP. The need for preoperative leg angiography in fibula free flaps. *J Reconstr Microsurg* 1994;10:283–287.
19. Seres L, Csaszar J, Voros E, Borbely L. Donor site angiography before mandibular reconstruction with fibula free flap. *J Craniofac Surg* 2001;12:608–613.
20. Jones NF. The need for preoperative leg angiography in fibular free flaps. *J Reconstr Microsurg* 1994;10:287–289.
21. Lutz BS, Wei FC, Ng SH, et al. Routine donor leg angiography before vascularized free fibula transplantation is not necessary: a prospective study in 120 clinical cases. *Plast Reconstr Surg* 1999;103:121–127.
22. Carroll WR, Esclamado R. Preoperative vascular imaging for the fibular osteocutaneous flap. *Arch Otolaryngol Head Neck Surg* 1996;122:708–712.
23. Whitley SP, Sandhu S, Cardozo A. Preoperative vascular assessment of the lower limb for harvest of a fibular flap: the views of vascular surgeons in the United Kingdom. *Br J Oral Maxillofac Surg* 2004;42:307–310.
24. Futran ND, Stack BC Jr, Zaccardi MJ. Preoperative color flow Doppler imaging for free fibula tissue transfer. *Ann Vasc Surg* 1998;12:445–450.
25. Smith RB, Thomas RD, Funk GF. Fibular free flaps: The role of angiography in patients with abnormal results on preoperative color flow Doppler studies. *Arch Otolaryngol Head Neck Surg* 2003;129:712–715.
26. Karanas YL, Antony A, Rubin G, Chang J. Preoperative CT angiography for free fibula transfer. *Microsurgery* 2004;24:125–127.
27. Chow LC, Napoli A, Klein MB, et al. Vascular mapping of the leg with multi-detector row CT angiography prior to free-flap transplantation. *Radiology* 2005;237:353–360.
28. Ribuffo D, Atzeni M, Saba L, et al. Clinical study of peroneal artery perforators with computed tomographic angiography: implications for fibular flap harvest. *Surg Radiol Anat* 2010;32:329–334.
29. Bretzman PA, Manaster BJ, Davis WL, Coleman DA. MR angiography for preoperative evaluation of vascularized fibular grafts. *J Vasc Interv Radiol* 1994;5:603–610.
30. Lorenz RR, Esclamado R. Preoperative magnetic resonance angiography in fibular-free flap reconstruction of head and neck defects. *Head Neck* 2001;23:844–850.
31. Kelly AM, Cronin P, Hussain HK, et al. Preoperative MR angiography in free fibula flap transfer for head and neck cancer: clinical application and influence on surgical decision making. *Am J Roentgenol* 2007;188:268–274.
32. Fukaya E, Saloner D, Leon P, et al. Magnetic resonance angiography to evaluate septocutaneous perforators in free fibula flap transfer. *J Plast Reconstr Aesthet Surg* 2010;63:1099–1104.
33. Lippert H, Pabst R. Arteries of the lower leg. In H. Lippert and R. Pabst (eds). *Arterial Variations in Man: Classification and Frequency.* Munich: Bergmann Verlag, 1985, pp. 63–64.
34. Rosson GD, Singh NK. Devascularizing complications of free fibula harvest: peronea arteria magna. *J Reconstr Microsurg* 2005;21:533–538.
35. Astarci P, Siciliano S, Verhelst R, et al. Intra-operative acute leg ischemia after free fibular flap harvest for mandible reconstruction. *Acta Chir Belg* 2006;106:423–426.
36. Mureau MA, Flood SJ, Hofer SO. Total peroneal artery occlusion during fibula free flap harvesting: salvage using the venous flow-through principle. *Plast Reconstr Surg* 2006;117:101e–106e.
37. Gilbert A. Vascularized transfer of the fibular shaft. *Int J Microsurg* 1979;1:100–102.
38. Gilbert A. Free vascularized bone graft. *Int Surg* 1981;66:27–31.
39. Collin T, Sugden P, Ahmed O, Ragbir M. Technical consideration of fibular osteocutaneous flap dissection. *J Plast Reconstr Aesthet Surg* 2008;61:1503–1506.
40. Youdas JW, Wood MB, Cahalan TD, Chao EY. A quantitative analysis of donor site morbidity after vascularized fibula transfer. *J Orthop Res* 1988;621–629.
41. Anthony JP, Rawnsley JD, Benhaim P, et al. Donor leg morbidity and function after fibula free flap mandible reconstruction. *Plast Reconstr Surg* 1995;96:146–152.
42. Vail TP, Urbaniak JR. Donor-site morbidity with use of vascularized autogenous fibular grafts. *J Bone Joint Surg* 1996;78(suppl A):204–211.
43. Shpitzer T, Neligan P, Boyd B, et al. Leg morbidity and function following fibular free flap harvest. *Ann Plast Surg* 1997;38:460–464.
44. Tang CL, Mahoney JL, McKee MD, et al. Donor site morbidity following vascularized fibular grafting. *Microsurgery* 1998;18:383–386.
45. Babovic S, Johnson CH, Finical SJ. Free fibula donor-site morbidity: the Mayo experience with 100 consecutive harvests. *J Reconstr Microsurg* 2000;16:107–110.
46. Lee JH, Chung CY, Myoung H, et al. Gait analysis of donor leg after free fibular flap transfer. *Int J Oral Maxillofac Surg* 2008;37:625–629.
47. Momoh AO, Yu P, Skoracki RJ, et al. A prospective cohort study of fibular free flap donor-site morbidity in 157 consecutive patients. *Plast Reconstr Surg* 2011;128:714–720.
48. Jones NF, Swartz WM, Mears DC, et al. The "double barrel" free vascularized fibular bone graft. *Plast Reconstr Surg* 1988;81:378–385.
49. O'Brien BM, Gumley GJ, Dooley BJ, Pribaz JJ. Folded free vascularized fibula transfer. *Plast Reconstr Surg* 1988;82:311–318.
50. Yajima H, Tamai S. Twin-barrelled vascularized fibular grafting to the pelvis and lower extremity. *Clin Orthop Relat Res* 1994;303:178–184.
51. Sakuraba M, Kimata Y, Iida H, et al. Pelvic ring reconstruction with the double-barreled vascularized fibular free flap. *Plast Reconstr Surg* 2005;116:1340–1345.
52. Coulet B, Pflieger JF, Arnaud S, et al. Double-barrel fibular graft for metaphyseal areas reconstruction around the knee. *Orthop Traumatol Surg Res* 2010;96:868–875.
53. Guyot L, Richard O, Cheynet F, et al. "Axial split osteotomy" of free fibular flaps for mandible reconstruction: preliminary results. *Plast Reconstr Surg* 2001;108:332–335.
54. Chang YM, Tsai CY, Wei FC. One-stage, double barrel fibula osteoseptocutaneous flap and immediate dental implants for functional and aesthetic reconstruction of segmental mandibular defects. *Plast Reconstr Surg* 2008;122:143–145.
55. Jones NF, Vögelin E, Markowitz BL, Watson JP. Reconstruction of composite through-and-through mandibular defects with a double-skin paddle fibular osteocutaneous flap. *Plast Reconstr Surg* 2003;112:758–765.
56. Yang KC, Leung JKW, Chen JS. Double paddle peroneal tissue transfer for oromandibular reconstruction. *Plast Reconstr Surg* 2000;106:47–55.

CHAPTER 19

Radial Forearm Flaps

J. Brian Boyd

BRIEF HISTORY

Originally termed the "Chinese" flap, the radial forearm flap (RFF) was first described by Song et al. in the early 1980s (1). As its popularity caught on in the West, it was subsequently used as a reverse pedicled flap in hand reconstruction (2) and an osteocutaneous flap for reconstruction of oromandibular defects (3). Although numerous other fasciocutaneous, osteocutaneous, and perhaps perforator flaps have lately encroached on its clinical turf, particularly because of the prominent donor scar of the RFF and the skeletal weakening when bone is harvested, the RFF remains unique in the soft, thin supple nature of its cutaneous constituents, its ability to be reinnervated at the recipient site, and its capacity to be folded upon itself for the reconstruction of complex structures such as the penis, nose, lip, and oral cavity. Although the indications for this flap have declined, it still has an important role to play in reconstructive surgery.

ANATOMY

The RFF is based on the fasciocutaneous perforators from the radial artery that pass between the tendons and muscle bellies of the flexor carpi radialis and those of the brachioradialis (Figure 19-1). Tiny veins accompany these perforators, permitting the flap to be raised on the radial artery and its venae comitantes. Alternatively, the venous drainage may be supplied by any of the subcutaneous veins passing through the flap itself. These are often traced proximally to larger veins such as the cephalic or basilic where larger diameters simplify anastomosis. The size of flap that may safely be elevated has not been precisely defined, but it includes most of the anterior and lateral forearm skin.

Accompanying the cephalic and basilic veins in the antecubital fossa are the lateral (LABC) and medial antebrachial cutaneous (MABC) nerves, respectively (see Figure 19-1). At this level, the nerves are large structures and are easily identified lying on either side of the biceps tendon just superficial to the deep fascia. The LABC is usually found just medial to the cephalic vein (4). However, as these nerves pass distally, they branch repeatedly and become smaller, more superficial, and harder to find. For these reason, when elevating innervated RFFs, the nerves are first located proximally and then traced distally until they or their branches are seen to enter the flap.

The osseous component of the RFF comprises the anterolateral aspect of the distal radius between the pronator tubercle and a point just proximal to the radial styloid (see Figure 19-1). For mechanical reasons, harvest is limited to no more than one third of the cross-sectional area of the intact bone. As the radial artery passes into the distal forearm, it lies on the anterior surface of the flexor pollicis longus muscle. It is through this muscle that branches from the radial artery pass to supply the underlying radius. Thus, when an osteocutaneous flap is taken, some of the muscle must be included to guarantee vascularity of the bone. This comprises the radial half of the muscle clothing the flat anterior surface of the radius in its distal third. The osteotomy passes from the anterior midline of the radius posterolaterally to its bare area to harvest 33% of the cross-section of the radius and incorporate the radial half of the flexor pollicis longus muscle belly to preserve blood supply to the graft. In an average man, the length of bone that may be harvested is no more than 12 to 14 cm.

It is possible to raise the RFF as a fasciocutaneous flap and leave the skin behind (5). In this case, medial and lateral skin flaps are elevated off the deep fascia, which is then raised with the radial vessels. The wound is closed without the need for a skin graft.

VARIANTS

Standard Radial Forearm Flap

The RFF is most commonly raised from the forearm as a distal skin paddle lying over the wrist and centered on the axis

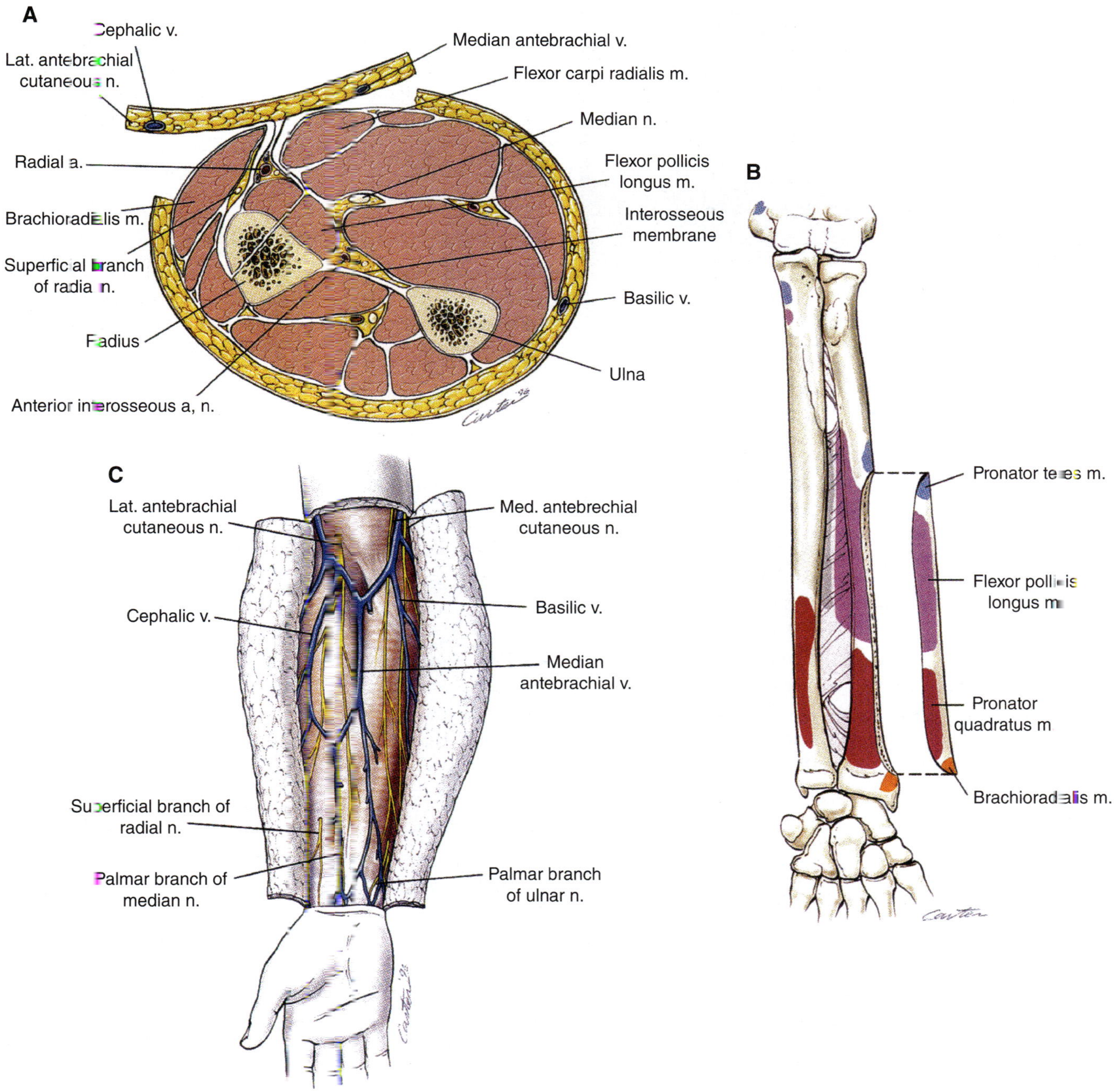

FIGURE 19-1 Diagrams illustrating the anatomy of the radial forearm flap. (**A**) Section of the distal forearm showing the relationship of the radial artery to the vascular septum, the flexor pollicis longus, and the radial osteotomy. About one third of the cross-sectional area is taken and it passes from the midpoint of the anterior surface dorsolaterally to the "bare area" of the radius. The cephalic vein is included in the skin paddle. (**B**) Muscular attachments to the left anterior radius and ulna. The bone graft extends between the insertions of the brachioradialis and pronator teres tendons, and the osteotomy is "boat shaped" (see text). (**C**) Disposition of the nerves and subcutaneous veins in the forearm. For most purposes, the lateral antebrachial cutaneous nerve is all that is needed to innervate the entire anterior and lateral forearm. However, when an "extended" flap is taken, the medial antebrachial cutaneous nerve should be taken as well. The nerves are found in close association with the cephalic and basilic veins, respectively, in the proximal forearm. a, artery; lat, lateral; m, muscle; med, median; n, nerve; v, vein. (Reprinted from Operative Techniques in Plastic and Reconstructive Surgery, Vol. 3, J. Brian Boyd, Mandible reconstruction with the radial forearm flap, 241-247, Copyright 1996, with permission from Elsevier.)

of the radial artery. Many surgeons position the skin paddle so that it also overlies the cephalic vein on the radial side of the wrist (Figure 19-2). This vein is very robust and an easy match for large recipient veins such as the external jugular or the saphenous. However, the surgeon should ascertain whether or not the cephalic vein has been recently canalized because thrombosis would preclude its use. The radial artery is dissected to its origin. Either of the venae comitantes or the cephalic vein can provide adequate venous drainage alone. The advantage of the cephalic vein, apart from its size, is that

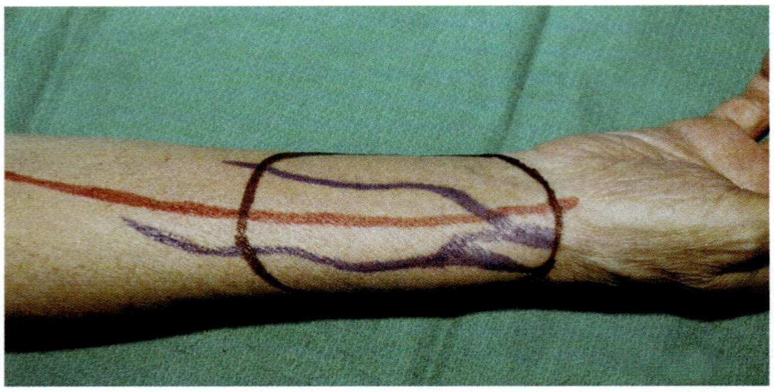

FIGURE 19-2 Preoperative marking of a typical skin paddle: It overlies the cephalic vein as well as the septum between the brachioradialis and the flexor carpi radialis. Although the resulting scar is more conspicuous than a more anterior positioning, the large vein facilitates vessel access in the head and neck.

being completely separate from the arterial pedicle, it is freer to access recipient vessels at a distance from the arterial anastomosis.

Reverse Pedicled Radial Forearm Flap

Although technically not a microsurgical flap, the reverse pedicled RFF should be considered here. The flap was described by Stock et al. (2) for thumb reconstruction and consisted of radial bone pedicled distally on the radial artery and its venae comitantes. However, larger skin flaps have been safely raised consisting of most of the anterior forearm skin. There has been extensive debate about how the flap develops an adequate venous drainage in view of the presence of valves restricting retrograde flow. Although the possibility that extreme dilatation causing the valves to become incompetent cannot be dismissed, it would seem more probable that the venous blood finds its way around the valves by means of ladderlike cross-connections between the tiny vaso vasorum (6).

Innervated Radial Forearm Flap

The skin of the anterior forearm derives its nerve supply from the LABC and the MABC nerves. The watershed between the two lies down the midline of the forearm, but there is considerable overlap, so much so that a flap consisting of the full width of the anterior wrist retains normal sensation if elevated on the LABC nerve alone (7,8).

However, when *extended* RFFs are taken, such as in penile reconstruction, it is probably wise to dissect out both the LABC and the MABC nerves and connect each to a recipient nerve at the site of reconstruction (9).

Innervated flaps are typically used in intraoral (10), lower lip (11), penile (12), and sole of foot reconstruction (13).

Osteocutaneous Radial Forearm Flap

As mentioned earlier, the osteocutaneous RFF can provide thin, supple, potentially innervated skin together with a 12- to 14-cm segment of vascularized bone (Figures 19-1 and 19-3). The bone, although dense and strong, is thin and unicortical. Moreover, its harvesting weakens the donor radius by about 76% (14). It is very useful in reconstructing short, straight segmental defects of the mandible, its skin paddle providing the associated oral lining. Although it may be osteotomized (Figure 19-4), it cannot be recommenced for extensive anterior bony defects because of its insubstantial nature and lack of bone height. It is best used laterally (15). The elevation of this flap and the handling of the donor site are discussed below.

Radial Forearm Fascial Flap

The use of a fascial RFF is somewhat limited, but it certainly spares the donor site the necessity of a skin graft (4). Here the deep fascia is elevated rather than a skin paddle. The operation starts with the elevation of medial and lateral skin flaps to expose the deep fascia of the forearm. This deep fascia is then elevated with the radial artery and its venae comitantes in the same way as one would elevate a standard RFF. Such a flap with the addition of a skin graft may be used for the closure of small wounds requiring thin cover (e.g., the foot, hand, and ear).

Prefabricated Radial Forearm Flaps

The RFF has been modified in a staged procedure to better handle complex defects. The simplest form of prefabrication is a tissue expansion performed on the flap after elevation but before transfer at a later date. Other forms of prefabrication include the addition of cartilage and skin grafts for complex facial and tracheal reconstruction. Prefabricated flaps are dealt with elsewhere.

TECHNIQUE OF DISSECTION AND HARVEST

Before raising a RFF, the surgeon should perform an Allen test to ensure that the ulnar artery is intact and capable of perfusing the forearm and hand after the radial artery is taken. That said, it is preferable to take the flap from the patient's nondominant arm for obvious reasons. After the patient has been seen for the first time, the operation should be explained and great emphasis placed on not permitting venepuncture in the affected side. While in the office, the venous pattern should be noted and thrombosis of the superficial veins excluded. Scars should be sought and damage to the radial artery ruled out.

The operation is performed under tourniquet control. Although some degree of exsanguination is desirable, complete exsanguination should be avoided because the radial artery and smaller superficial veins may become difficult to identify. Rather than using an Esmarch bandage, an Ace bandage may be used. Alternatively, the Esmarch bandage can be wrapped gently. Total exsanguination may lead to serious problems when a superficial ulnar artery is present. The bloodless vessel may be mistaken for a vein and ligated, rendering the hand completely ischemic (16).

The operation is best planned in reverse, taking a template of the defect and superimposing it on the distal forearm. Often, however, this is not possible because of the need for simultaneous dissection, so an estimate will have to be made. In any case, the flap is designed on the distal forearm proximal to the wrist crease. Typically, the flap overlies both the radial artery and the

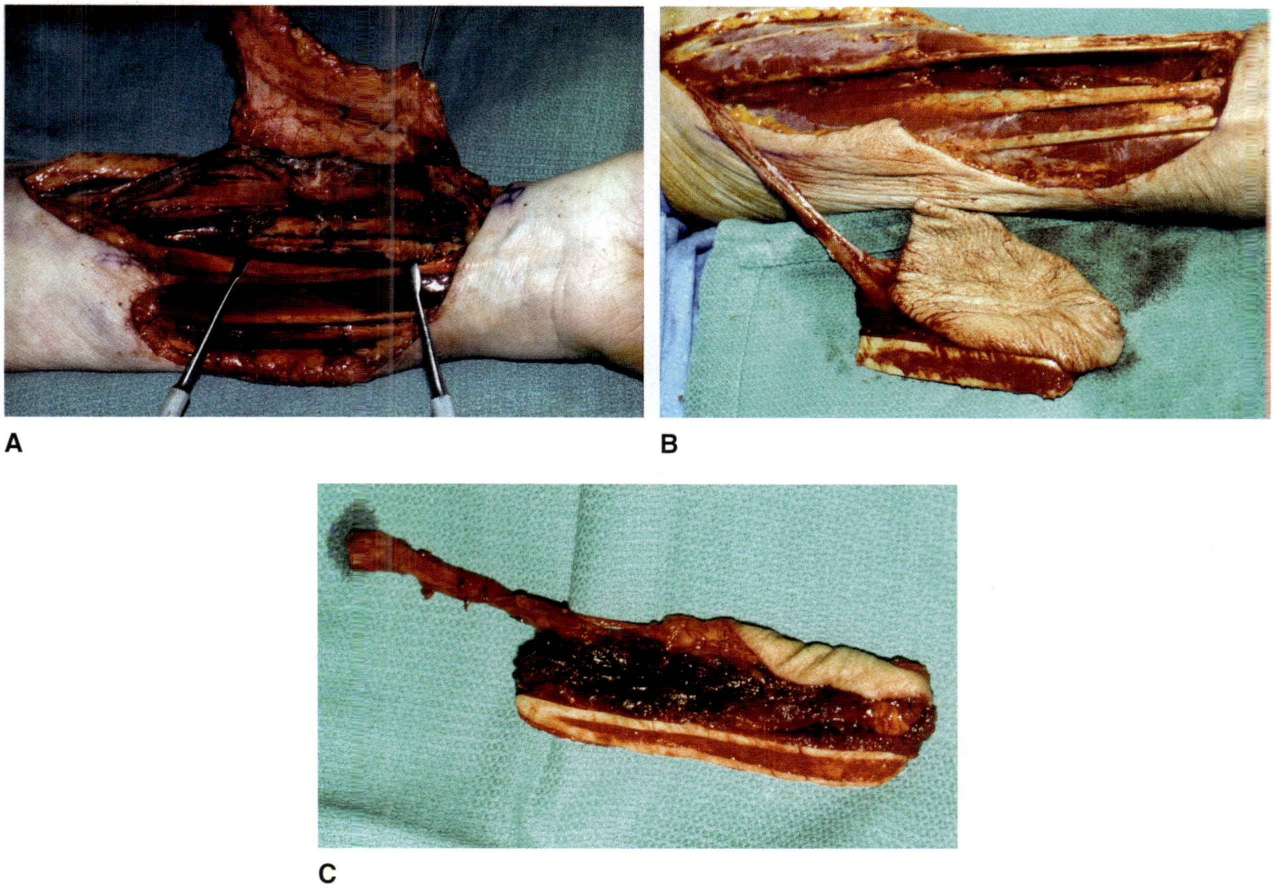

FIGURE 19-3 (**A**) The hand is on the right. Elevation of an osteocutaneous flap showing the radial artery giving small perforating branches to the skin paddle as well as to the underlying flexor pollicis longus and pronator quadratus. It is through these muscles that the bone graft derives its circulation. (**B**) and (**C**) The flap is separated using the boat-shaped cut described in the text.

cephalic vein (see Figure 19-2). If the flap needs to be larger, it can extend proximally up the forearm to its full length and ulnarward to the medial border of the forearm. It does not need to overlie the cephalic vein if it has been decided to use the venae comitantes, but it does need to overlie the septum between the brachioradialis and the flexor carpi radialis (see Figure 19-1), which transmits the perforators from the radial artery.

The arm is then gently exsanguinated and the tourniquet inflated to 100 mm Hg above systolic blood pressure. Generally, dissection begins distally, but in the case of innervated flaps, the

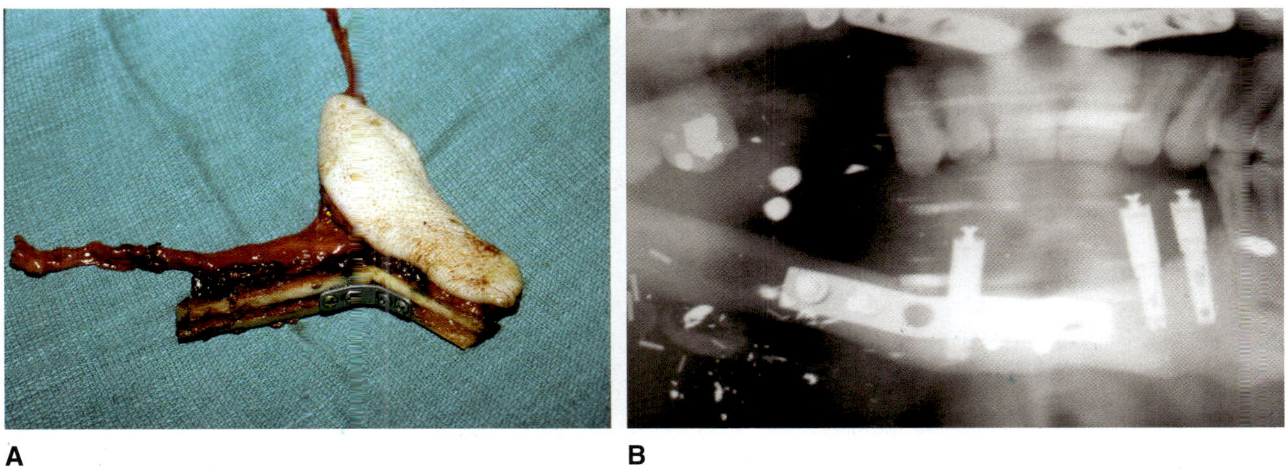

FIGURE 19-4 (**A**) and (**B**) An osteotomy performed on a small radial bone graft to deal with the curvature of a short mandibular parasymphyseal defect. The bone graft does not do well in extensive anterior defects. (**B**) A panoramic radiograph showing solid bony union and an osteointegrated implant in the radial bone graft.

nerves are located at the start of the operation. Through a midline axial incision, the LABC and MABC nerves may be located on either side of the biceps tendon in the proximal forearm, where they lie deep and are associated with the cephalic and basilic veins, respectively (see Figure 19-1). Together with the vein(s), they are traced distally as far as the proximal margin of the flap. After this has been done, the RFF is elevated conventionally.

The distal border of the flap in incised, and dissection is carried down to the deep fascia. Superficial veins are tied off, and the radial artery sought between the tendons of the brachioradialis (BR) and the flexor carpi radialis (FCR). Laterally the superficial radial nerve is preserved. The artery is divided between ligatures. This distal dissection confirms the position of the radial artery, the BR and FCR tendons, and the fascial septum between them.

On the ulnar side of the flap, the skin incision continues down to but not through the deep fascia. Dissection then passes radially at this level until the midpoint of the FCR tendon. Here, the deep fascia is incised, and dissection proceeds below it but superficial to the paratenon. At the radial border of the FCR tendon, the tendon is hugged as dissection proceeds around its radial border. The radial artery is now visible, and the septum carrying perforating vessels to the overlying skin is apparent (see Figure 19-3).

A similar approach is taken as the radial aspect of the flap is raised. Here, though, there are two structures to identify and preserve. One is the cephalic vein, and the other is the terminal branch of the radial nerve. The former must be taken with the flap, but the latter must be carefully dissected out and left behind. Sometimes a small branch of the nerve may have to be sacrificed because of its location within the flap, but the main trunk can always be preserved. As the tendon of the brachioradialis is encountered, the dissection passes over its radial border, and then, at about its center, the deep fascia is incised, and dissection proceeds on the surface of the paratenon toward the tendon's ulnar margin. Passing closely around this structure, the radial artery becomes evident with a thin mesentery of tissue—the septum—conducting perforators to the overlying skin (see Figure 19-3). This delicate structure, now isolated from both sides, is carefully preserved along the full length of its connection with the overlying skin flap.

The radial artery, with its venae comitantes, is now elevated from its bed (the flexor pollicis longus). Deep branches are clipped or coagulated. Proceeding distal to proximal, the vascular pedicle is dissected from between the muscle bellies of the FCR and the BR, again dividing small branches to the surrounding tissues. Dissection of the artery stops at its origin from the brachial artery in the proximal forearm. At this point, the venous connections can be complex. Often there is a communicating vein between the deep and superficial systems. Some advocate preserving this connection to maximize venous drainage (17), but it is probably unnecessary; the flap survives well on either system alone.

When ready for transfer, the vessels are ligated and divided to maximal length. If the flaps are innervated, the nerves are taken also and the flap passed to the recipient site.

Harvesting of an osteocutaneous RFF flap entails some modifications to the above. The dissection is the same distally, medially, and laterally until the point where the radial artery itself is about to be elevated from its bed. As mentioned, the arterial pedicle lies on the muscle belly of the flexor pollicis longus (see Figures 19-1 and 19-3). The origin of this muscle clothes the flat anterior surface of the distal radius, and it is through this muscle that branches from the radial artery reach the underlying bone. Therefore, the muscle must not be excessively stripped from the bone to facilitate the required osteotomy. Because the muscle is attached intimately to the bone, the bone itself is not visible. It can be palpated, however, between index finger and thumb. Grasping the bone thus as a guide, an incision is made down through the muscle and the periosteum at the midline of its flat anterior surface. This incision is on the ulnar side of the radial artery. Periosteum is stripped on either side of the incision for a short distance medially and laterally. Stripping is obviously safer in an ulnar direction because the intended bone harvest lies radial. The incision curves laterally just proximal to the insertion of the BR insertion on the radial styloid and passes under that tendon toward the bare area of the radius. Proximally, it passes laterally just distal to the insertion of the pronator teres (PT) tendon. To "steal" an extra couple of centimeters, the PT insertion can be divided and the proximal limit of bone resection and thereby extended. Before performing the osteotomy, it is important to visualize the complete pathway of the bony cut. This lies along the mid anterior surface of the anterior radius and curves laterally between the insertions of the PT and BR onto the bare area.

Cutting the bone is intimidating at first. It helps to have a couple of assistants with retractors and saline irrigation. The plane of the osteotomy is dorsoradial, taking about one third of the cortex. It may be performed with an oscillating saw, but with experience, a reciprocating saw with a narrow blade is smoother and faster. A straight osteotomy with a right-angled cut at each end is acceptable, but it has been shown that a continuous "boat-shaped" cut (using the narrow blade) avoids stress risers and does not weaken the residual radius to the same degree (18). Nevertheless, the radius is weakened considerably (by 76%) and is susceptible to fracture after relatively minor trauma, particularly in the first 3 months. For this reason, it is advocated that the forearm and wrist be immobilized in an above-elbow cast for 12 weeks. Others have suggested prophylactic plating (19,20), but this may not be cost effective (21). Splinting is still required.

At the final release of the tourniquet, the vascularity of the hand must be inspected, and if it is found to be deficient, the radial artery must be immediately reconstructed with a vein graft. With a favorable—and even sometimes with an *un*favorable—preoperative Allen test result, this should not be required. However, there should be no hesitation in carrying it out if necessary. Unexpected ischemia in the face of a normal preoperative Allen test result usually means damage to the ulnar artery (16).

TRICKS AND TIPS

Many tricks and tips have been included in the description of flap elevation, and by way of emphasis, they are listed here together with some others:

1. Work distal to proximal except when elevating an innervated flap.
2. First find the sensory nerves in the proximal forearm when elevating an innervated flap.
3. Shift the skin paddle in an ulnar direction to avoid hair in individuals who are hirsute. This generally precludes use of the cephalic vein.
4. Always check if the cephalic vein has been previously cannulated and palpate for thromboses before deciding to use it.
5. Dissection does not need to be subfascial until the septum between the BR and FCR is about to be entered unless one is elevating a fascial flap.
6. Always preserve the option of using either the deep or the superficial venous systems (or both).
7. The LABC nerve alone is sufficient to innervate the anterior and radial aspects of the wrist.
8. In some individuals, it is possible to raise a small flap, up to 6 cm wide and 4 cm long, positioned just proximal to the wrist crease and close the defect without a skin graft. A long rotation flap based on the ulnar artery and incised along the radial border of the forearm is rotated distally and a proximal defect closed as a V to Y (Figure 19-5).

CLOSURE OF THE DONOR SITE

The only area presenting a problem is the distal forearm from which the skin paddle itself was harvested. Preservation of deep fascia and paratenon is vital in producing a vascularized bed that will receive a skin graft. The paratenons of the FCR and BR are approximated with 4.0 chromic catgut. The palmaris longus tendon may be removed if necessary and the wound edges advanced to decrease the size of the defect. An unmeshed skin graft is usually applied with either a traditional tie-over or a Vac dressing, and the wrist splinted. Some have advocated delayed skin grafting and the initial use of Integra with the Vac. One week later, the silicone sheet may be removed and a thin split-thickness skin graft applied. This seems like an expensive and unnecessary step, but there is no substitute for meticulous technique and appropriate care of tissues. In time, the donor site scar settles to a lesser or greater extent (Figure 19-6).

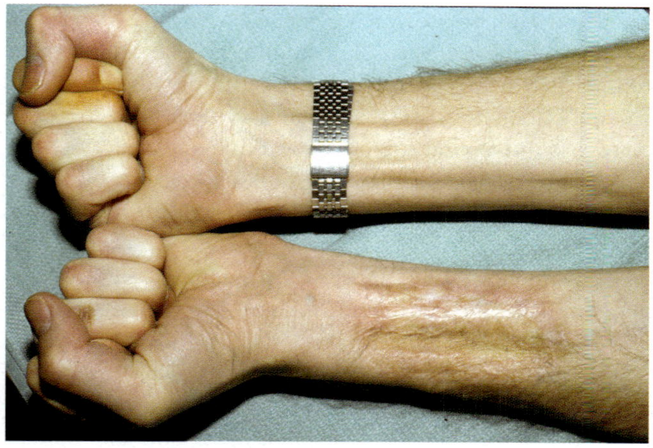

FIGURE 19-6 A typical donor site appearance at 1 year.

DONOR SITE COMPLICATIONS

If the operation is performed in the absence of a favorable Allen test result, there is a possibility of devascularizing the hand (although, surprisingly, this is still uncommon). For this reason, the capillary refill is carefully assessed after the flap has been removed and after the tourniquet has been released. There are also reports of damage to an aberrant ulnar artery lying in a superficial position (16). If necessary, the radial artery must be reconstructed using a reverse vein graft. Another method of reconstructing the radial artery while at the same time closing the skin defect has been described using a simultaneous anterolateral thigh flow-through flap (22), but this may seem excessive to some.

A more frequent complication is delayed healing or breakdown in the skin-grafted area. This is caused by infection, seroma, hematoma, or excessive wrist movement or because the

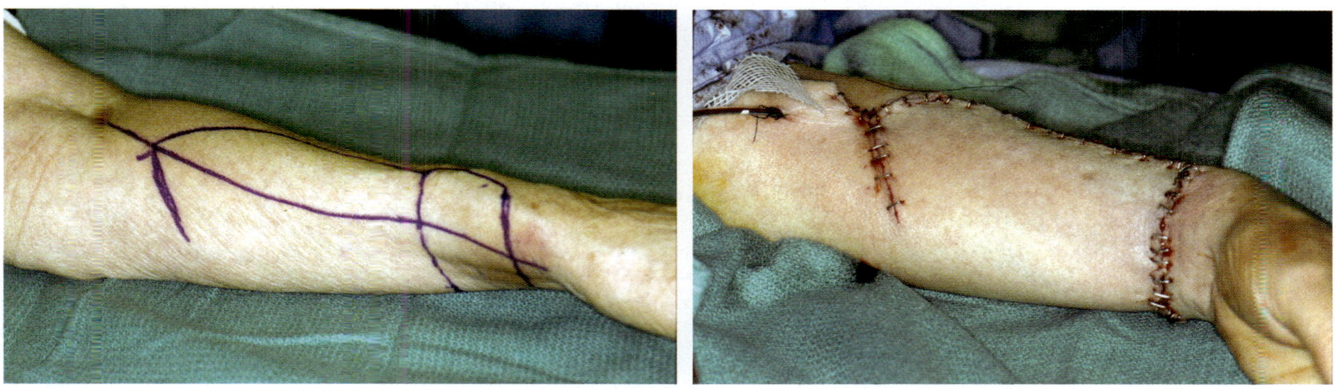

A B

FIGURE 19-5 (**A**) and (**B**) To improve the donor site appearance, it is possible to plan a primary closure after harvest of a small radial forearm flap (up to 6 x 4 cm). An ulnar-based flap is designed, and the elevation of the flap is performed through its radial border. The flap is rotated distally, closing the proximal forearm in a V-Y manner. It is vital to preserve the perforators from the ulnar artery, making this a sort of pedicled ulnar artery forearm flap.

paratenon was not adequately preserved over the BR and FCR tendons. The result is usually tendon exposure. Treatment by conservative means; debridement, wet-to-dry dressings, and immobilization are usually adequate. However, in severe cases, other forms of wound closure may be contemplated.

Radial nerve neuroma pain might be expected following the necessary damage to some of its distal branches. Oddly, this is extremely uncommon, if it occurs at all.

As mentioned earlier, fracture of the radius is a serious complication when the radial bone has been harvested. The operation weakens the radius in the order of 76%, rendering it susceptible to relatively minor trauma. To avoid this, some surgeons have advocated the application of a plate to the donor radial defect (21). Prolonged splinting is still appropriate, however.

Other nonspecific complications may occur but are not discussed here (23).

INDICATIONS FOR THE RADIAL FOREARM FLAP

1. Intraoral reconstruction
2. Nasal reconstruction
3. Sensate reconstruction (general)
4. Perioral reconstruction
5. Hand or upper limb reconstruction (reverse pedicled or free)
6. Penile reconstruction
7. Burn scar release
8. Mandibular reconstruction (small bone defects)
9. Lower limb coverage
10. Ear reconstruction (fascial flap)

COMPARISON WITH SIMILAR FREE TISSUE TRANSFERS

It is reasonable to compare the RFF with other fasciocutaneous flaps as well as with rival osteocutaneous transfers. The RFFs most important qualities are its soft, supple, and delicate nature; its lack of bulk; its long pedicle; its large vessels; and its capacity to be innervated. The ability of the flap to carry bone is a plus, but the bone itself is suboptimal for many clinical scenarios. Furthermore, the donor site is very conspicuous when a skin graft has been used to close it and very weak when bone has been harvested.

The ulnar forearm flap (UFF) (24) shares many of the qualities of the RFF except its ability to carry bone. The scar resulting from an UFF is somewhat less conspicuous because it lies on the less visible ulnar side of the forearm. It, too, may be innervated, and its skin paddle is generally less hairy. Dissection involves the ulnar nerve in the UFF, but no comparable nerve is at risk when elevating the RFF.

In some centers, the anterolateral thigh (ALT) flap has replaced the RFF for many clinical problems (25). However, it remains significantly more bulky, particularly in the West, where obesity is more prevalent. Nevertheless, it can be thinned (26), and donor site healing has been shown to be superior with the ALT (27). The RFF retains a more consistent anatomy (and ease of elevation) and a greater potential for reinnervation.

When comparing the osteocutaneous RFF with other osteocutaneous transfers for mandibular reconstruction, the only advantages it has are the thinness of its skin paddle and its suitability for reinnervation. For certain lateral mandibular defects, it works extremely well, but lack of bony height and the difficulty in performing osteotomies make it unsuitable for anterior or use with extensive bony defects.

Yet the RFF remains one of the most common free tissue transfers performed today. Its anatomy is constant, and it is easy to elevate; its blood vessels are large and its pedicle is long; the elevation is rendered bloodless by tourniquet; and the donor site generally permits a two-team approach. Special advantages of the flap include thinness, reinnervation potential, and the capacity to carry small yet strong pieces of vascularized bone. Although use of the osteocutaneous flap has declined, use of the innervated flap has increased. The RFF remains one of the essential flaps in reconstructive microsurgery.

REFERENCES

1. Song R, Gao Y, Yu Y, et al. The forearm flap. *Clin Plast Surg* 1982;9:21–26.
2. Stock W, Biemer E, Mühlbauer W. Forearm flap with its various possibilities of application. *Handchir Mikrochir Plast Chir* 1984;16:201–203.
3. Soutar DS, Scheker LR, Tanner NS, et al. The radial forearm flap: a versatile method for intra-oral reconstruction. *Br J Plast Surg* 1983;36:1–8.
4. Wongkerdsook W, Agthong S, Amarase C, et al. Anatomy of the lateral antebrachial cutaneous nerve in relation to the lateral epicondyle and cephalic vein. *Clin Anat* 2011;24:56–61.
5. Schoofs M, Bienfait B, Calteux N, et al. The forearm fascia flap. *Ann Chir Main* 1983;2:197–201.
6. Lin SD, Lai CS, Chiu CC. Venous drainage in the reverse forearm flap. *Plast Reconstr Surg* 1984;74:508–512.
7. Boyd B, Mulholland S, Gullane P, et al. Reinnervated lateral antebrachial cutaneous neurosome flaps in oral reconstruction: are we making sense? *Plast Reconstr Surg* 1994;93:1350–1359;discussion 1360–1362.
8. Boyd JB, Kim SS, Granzow J, et al. Documenting the density of innervation in a sensate radial forearm flap based on the lateral antebrachial cutaneous nerve. *Plast Reconstr Surg* 2009;123:216e–217e.
9. Boutros S, Yuksel E, Weinfeld AB, et al. Neural anatomy of the radial forearm flap. *Ann Plast Surg* 2000;44:375–380.
10. Matthews RN, Hodge RA, Eyre J, et al. Radial forearm flap for floor of mouth reconstruction. *Br J Surg* 1985;72:561–564.
11. Sadove RC, Luce EA, McGrath PC. Reconstruction of the lower lip and chin with the composite radial forearm-palmaris longus free flap. *Plast Reconstr Surg* 1991;88:209–214.
12. Semple JL, Boyd JB, Farrow GA, et al. The "cricket bat" flap: a one-stage free forearm flap phalloplasty. *Plast Reconstr Surg* 1991;88:514–519.
13. Chicarilli ZN, Price GJ. Complete plantar foot coverage with the free neurosensory radial forearm flap. *Plast Reconstr Surg* 1986;78:94–101.
14. Swanson E, Boyd JB, Mulholland RS. The radial forearm flap: a biomechanical study of the osteotomized radius. *Plast Reconstr Surg* 1990;85:267–272.
15. Zenn MR, Hidalgo DA, Cordeiro PG, et al. Current role of the radial forearm free flap in mandibular reconstruction. *Plast Reconstr Surg* 1997;99:1012–1017.
16. Fatah MF, Nancarrow JD, Murray DS. Raising the radial artery forearm flap: the superficial ulnar artery "trap." *Br J Plast Surg* 1985;38:394–395.
17. Gottlieb LJ, Tachmes L, Pielet RW. Improved venous drainage of the radial artery forearm free flap: use of the profundus cubitalis vein. *J Reconstr Microsurg* 1993;9:281–284;discussion 284–285.
18. Bardsley AF, Soutar DS, Elliot D, et al. Reducing morbidity in the radial forearm flap donor site. *Plast Reconstr Surg* 1990;86:287–292; discussion 293–294.

19. Nuñez VA, Pike J, Avery C, et al. Prophylactic plating of the donor site of osteocutaneous radial forearm flaps. *Br J Oral Maxillofac Surg* 1999;37:210–212.
20. Waits CA, Toby EB, Girod DA, et al. Osteocutaneous radial forearm free flap: long-term radiographic evaluation of donor site morbidity after prophylactic plating of radius. *J Reconstr Microsurg* 2007;23:367–372.
21. Rockwell GM, Thoma A. Should the donor radius be plated prophylactically after harvest of a radial osteocutaneous flap? A cost-effectiveness analysis. *J Reconstr Microsurg* 2004;20:297–306.
22. Chang KP, Lai CH, Liang WL, et al. Alternative reconstruction of donor defect of free radial forearm flap in head and neck cancer. *Scand J Plast Reconstr Surg Hand Surg* 2010;44:31–36.
23. Smith A, Bowen VA, Boyd JB. Donor site deficit of the osteocutaneous radial forearm flap. *Ann Plast Surg* 1994;32:372–376.
24. Lovie MJ, Duncan GM, Glasson DW. The ulnar artery forearm free flap. *Br J Plast Surg* 1984;37:486–492.
25. Wei FC, Jain V, Celik N, et al. Have we found an ideal soft-tissue flap? An experience with 672 anterolateral thigh flaps. *Plast Reconstr Surg* 2002;109:2219–2226; discussion 2227–2230.
26. Kimura N, Satoh K. Consideration of a thin flap as an entity and clinical applications of the thin anterolateral thigh flap. *Plast Reconstr Surg* 1996;97:985–992.
27. Kesting MR, Hölzle F, Wales C, et al. Microsurgical reconstruction of the oral cavity with free flaps from the anterolateral thigh and the radial forearm: a comparison of perioperative data from 161 cases. *Ann Surg Oncol* 2011;18(7):1988–1994.

CHAPTER 19

CHAPTER 20

Ulnar Forearm Flap

Ming-Huei Cheng and Jung-Ju Huang

BRIEF HISTORY: ORIGINAL DESCRIPTION AND SUBSEQUENT EVOLUTION

The forearm region is now one of the most commonly selected donor sites for free flap transfer for reconstructive microsurgery. The radial and ulnar arteries can independently perfuse the forearm and hand. A free forearm flap can therefore be harvested based on either one of the vessels. Leaving the other vessel as the dominant blood supply for the donor site is generally safe and widely accepted.

Harvesting one of the two major vessels of the forearm for a free flap was first introduced in 1982. Song et al. designed a forearm flap based on the radial artery and later popularized it because of the ease of flap harvest and its reliability (1). Two years later, the ulnar artery forearm flap was introduced by Lovie et al. in 1984 with similar clinical applications (2). The ulnar artery forearm flap can be designed as a free or reverse pedicle flap. It is used frequently in intraoral reconstructions as well as the lower extremity reconstructions (2).

Basically, the ulnar forearm flap (UFFs) has the same advantages of the radial forearm flap. The flap is thin and pliable and is therefore versatile for three-dimensional flap design and flap inset, especially in head and neck reconstruction. The pedicle is lengthy and sizable for microvascular anastomosis. However, because of the historical reason and the long-term belief that the ulnar artery is the dominant vessel in the forearm and hand, the radial artery forearm flap is much more widely used than the ulnar artery forearm flap.

There are some disadvantages of the radial forearm flap that makes this flap less preferred by some surgeons. Although suprafascial dissection in radial forearm flap harvest to minimize the donor site morbidity has been recommended, this surgical technique is still considered difficult by some surgeons. Additionally, the radial donor site is hairy, and the scar is more conspicuous than that in the ulnar forearm region. The UFF is therefore often preferable. The ulnar forearm donor site also contains more muscle and therefore has better take of skin grafts.

In the beginning, the UFF was designed as a free fasciocutaneous flap for reconstruction of head and neck cancer (2). Two years after its introduction, the same group successfully used the UFF for penile reconstruction (3). In 1988, Glasson and Lovie further described their experience of using the UFF as a proximally based or distally based island flap for hand reconstruction (4). The usage of UFF may be further expanded with the inclusion of the medial antebrachial nerve as a sensate flap.

Many surgeons now use the UFF for head and neck reconstruction, extremity reconstruction, and penis reconstruction (5–10). With better understanding of its anatomy, the flap design is further advanced with the inclusion of the dorsal ulnar artery (11) for distal forearm or hand reconstruction. Because several perforators are available, the ulnar forearm can be designed as a chimeric flap to reconstruct two adjacent defects such as an intraoral and an external cheek defect. The UFF can be further split into two separate flaps for two different defects such as for bilateral buccal defects (26).

ANATOMY OF THE VESSELS, NERVES, AND SKIN TERRITORY

The UFF is based on the ulnar artery, which originates from the brachial artery. Distal to the bicipital aponeurosis, the brachial artery divides into two main branches, the radial and ulnar arteries, to supply the forearm and hand. The radial artery runs between the pronator teres muscle and brachioradialis muscle, and the ulnar artery passes under and across the pronator teres muscle, flexor carpi radialis muscle, and flexor digitorum superficialis muscle. The ulnar artery gives off the common interosseous artery shortly after the bifurcation of the brachial artery. In a rare variation, the ulnar artery branches off the brachial artery, 5 to 7 cm distal to the elbow joint. In this situation, the common interosseous artery may originate either from the radial

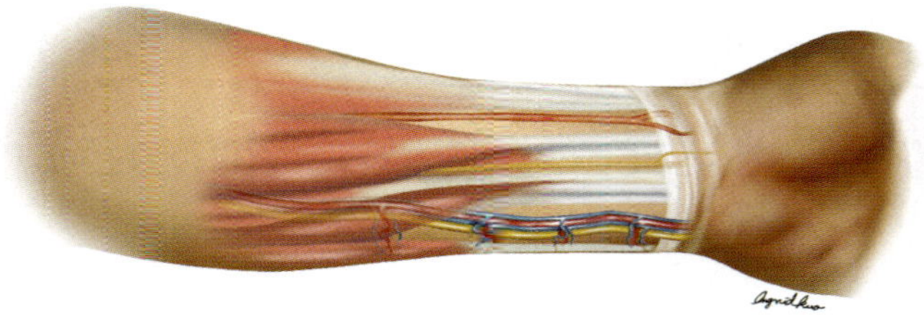

FIGURE 20-1 The anatomy of the ulnar forearm flap. The ulnar vessels are located under the tendinous part of the flexor carpi ulnaris and are in close proximity to the ulnar nerve. Distally, the ulnar pedicle gives off septocutaneous perforators to the skin paddle. (Reproduced with permission from Ingrid Kuo.)

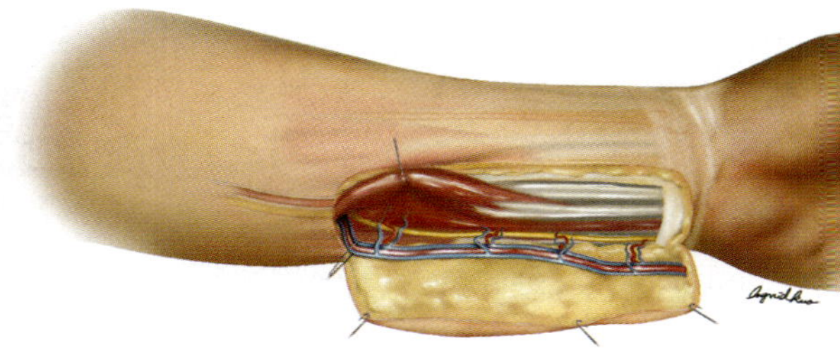

FIGURE 20-3 After an incision is made from the radial side of the flap and suprafascial dissection is performed, multiple septocutaneous perforators can be identified. By inclusion of at least one of the perforators, the ulnar forearm flap can be raised safely. (Reproduced with permission from Ingrid Kuo.)

artery or directly from the brachial artery. The distal ulnar artery then runs medially and distally and reaches the medial aspect of the forearm at the level about half the way between the elbow and wrist. During its course, the ulnar nerve runs close to the ulnar vessels and therefore requires careful separation from the ulnar vessels during flap dissection (Figure 20-1). The ulnar artery runs distally under the tendon of the flexor carpi ulnaris (FCU) until it joins the superficial palmar arch. In most of the cases, an ulnar dorsal artery branch can be found approximately 5.3 cm proximal to the pisiform bone. A retrograde ulnar dorsal flap can also be designed based on this small branch.

Although in most cases, the ulnar artery runs deep between the flexor carpi ulnaris and flexor digitorum superficialis, it can be found running superficially to these structures in 0.7% to 9.38% of patients (12–14). In these situations, the radial artery usually takes a high origin from the brachial artery, proximal to the take-off of this superficial ulnar artery. In very rare cases, the superficial ulnar artery originates directly from the axillary artery. In its course over the forearm, the superficial ulnar artery runs superficial to the pronator teres and flexor muscles and may be either superficial or deep to the fascia of these muscles. In this kind of anomaly, the palmaris longus tendon is often absent.

Distal to the origin of the common interosseous artery, the ulnar artery gives off three to seven septocutaneous perforators on its way to the superficial palmar arch (Figure 20-2). Usually the most distal septocutaneous perforator lies within 5 cm of the proximal palmar crease. This allows a flap designed over the distal forearm to obtain a long pedicle. The distance between the most distal, and the most proximal septocutaneous perforator ranges from 3 to 16.5 cm. The large separation of these

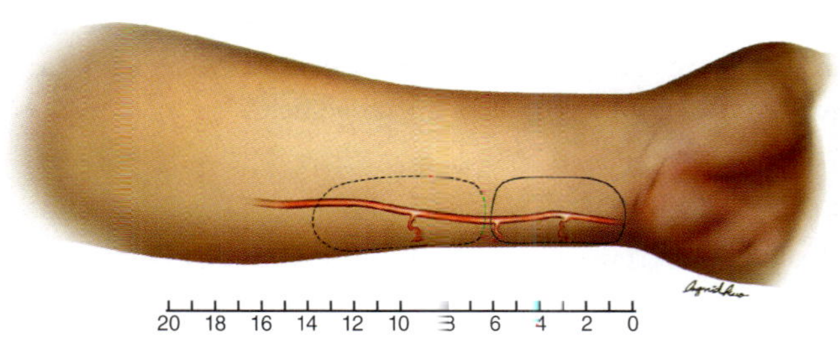

FIGURE 20-2 Flap design is based on the septocutaneous perforators. The ulnar forearm flap (UFF) can be designed as a pedicled flap, a single free flap, a chimeric flap, or separate individual flaps. A single UFF may be split into two separate free flaps based on individual septocutaneous perforators. By dividing the pedicle of the distal flap close to the perforator of the proximal flap, a lengthier pedicle can be obtained for the distal flap. (Reproduced with permission from Ingrid Kuo.)

septocutaneous perforators allows great freedom in flap design, including a chimeric flap or the possibility of harvesting two independent skin flaps based on separate perforators from the same main pedicle (Figure 20-3) (26).

The ulnar artery and vein are quite sizable for microvascular anastomosis. The average arterial diameter is 2.3 mm and venous diameter is 1.7 mm (26). For head and neck reconstruction, the arterial diameter is compatible in size to commonly used recipient arteries such as the facial and superior thyroid. However, size discrepancy is commonly encountered with the vein. Although some surgeons like to include the basilic vein for the venous anastomosis, the author has found the small ulnar concomitant vein to be quite adequate in nearly all cases. However, sometimes a vein graft is required when the pedicle length is insufficient (26).

SURGICAL TECHNIQUE

Indications for the Ulnar Forearm Flap

The UFF is one of the commonly applied soft tissue flaps in head and neck reconstruction. Table 20-1 lists the commonly used fasciocutaneous flaps in head and neck reconstruction and the characteristics of each flap. Among them, the ulnar and radial forearm flaps are considered the thinnest flaps with good surface area, pedicle length, and vessel caliber for anastomosis.

Because of its thin characteristics, the UFF is the flap of choice in buccal mucosa reconstruction and for palatal reconstruction. It is also a good choice in tongue reconstruction when the tongue defect is less than 50%.

Aside from head and neck reconstruction, the UFF is also indicated in urethral and penile reconstruction in which a thin flap with a lengthy pedicle is required.

Preoperative Evaluation: Allen Test

The Allen test is the easiest and most commonly performed examination before the harvest of a free flap from the forearm region. Before performing the Allen test, the hand and forearm are squeezed to push the blood out of the extremity. Then the patient is asked to make a tight fist. Both the radial and arteries are then compressed by the examiner. The radial artery is then released to check the perfusion status of the ulnar artery. The same procedure is then performed while releasing the compression over the ulnar artery to examine the perfusion of the radial artery. The Allen test result is considered negative if both arteries can perfuse the hand well. A positive Allen test result indicates

TABLE 20-1. Comparisons of Different Flaps and Ulnar Forearm Flap

Flap Character Flap Type	Flap Dimension	Flap Thickness	Pedicle Size	Pedicle Length	Dissection Difficulty
Radial forearm flap	Excellent	Thin	Good	Excellent	Excellent
Ulnar forearm flap	Excellent	Thin	Good	Excellent	Excellent
Lateral arm flap	Fair	Moderate	Fair	Poor	Good
RAM flap	Good	Thick	Excellent	Good	Excellent
ALT—FC flap	Excellent	Moderate	Excellent	Excellent	Fair
TAP flap	Good	Moderate	Good	Good	Fair
MSAP	Good	Thin	Good	Excellent	Fair

ALT-FC, anterolateral thigh fascio-cutaneous flap; MSAP, medial sural artery perforator flap; RAM, rectus abdominis musculocutaneous flap; TAP, thoracodorsal artery perforator flap.

a deficiency of perfusion from either the radial or ulnar artery and is therefore a contraindication for taking a forearm flap.

The authors performed the Allen test in 50 healthy volunteers on bilateral forearms. All patients had a negative Allen test result bilaterally. The refilling time of both radial and ulnar artery was recorded. The results showed that 54% of the forearms had faster refilling time on the radial artery, but 30% of the forearms had faster refilling time on the ulnar artery. The others had equal refilling times for both radial and ulnar arteries. The authors suggest using the Allen test and refilling time on the radial and ulnar artery for preoperative screening and decision making when choosing the radial or UFF.

Severe vascular compromise resulting from ulnar artery harvesting is rare. Preoperative patient selection is very important to eliminate such kind of problems. Patients with positive Allen test result should not receive ulnar or radial artery forearm flaps to prevent any severe vascular compromise after flap harvest.

Preoperative Doppler scan over the radial or the ulnar artery is also a quick and easy way to examine the status of the radial and ulnar arteries. It also helps to locate the septocutaneous perforators of the ulnar artery for a more accurate flap design.

When the Allen test result is equivocal and reconstruction with a free UFF is recommended or in patients with a history of forearm trauma, preoperative computed tomography angiography or magnetic resonance angiography can be considered. However, this is unnecessary in patients with negative Allen test results.

SELECTION BETWEEN THE RADIAL AND ULNAR FOREARM FLAP

Because the forearm is perfused by two vessels, the harvest of one of the two major vessels as a donor vessel raises the concern about the residual perfusion of the hand. The change of blood flow in the remaining artery after one vessel is ligated for free tissue transfer has been studied in an animal model (15). Although ligation of one major vessel results in increased blood flow in the remaining artery, the total blood flow to the distal limb is decreased (15). Therefore, it is recommended to harvest the nondominant vessel for flap transfer. In the forearm region, the radial and ulnar artery both contribute equally to its perfusion; thus, the issue of which of the vessels is the dominant one is controversial. The ulnar artery was considered dominant in the past. However, in a recent study performed by Haerle and colleagues using color Doppler sonography and plethysmography, the ulnar artery was found to be dominant proximal to the common interosseous artery, but the radial artery was dominant distal to the common interosseous artery (16). They suggest using the UFF rather than a radial forearm flap for reconstruction because the ulnar artery is nondominant distal to the common interosseous artery. Smoking reduces blood flow in large and small vessels. Ali and Srivastava showed in a clinical study (17) that although the Allen test result is usually normal, 44% and 55% of the ulnar arteries in the dominant and nondominant hands, respectively, could not be palpated in smokers. The flow of the ulnar artery is also reduced in smokers. The radial artery is considered less susceptible to damage by smoking in this patient group (Table 20-2).

Flap Design

The ulnar artery, which is located underneath the flexor carpi ulnar is tendon, is marked by palpation (see Figure 20-1). A straight line between the pisiform bone and the medial epicondyle is drawn. This line marks the course of the ulnar artery from the midpoint of the forearm to the wrist. A pencil Doppler can be used to identify locations of the septocutaneous perforators. This is particularly important when harvesting a chimeric flap or two or more separate flaps from a single donor pedicle. The skin paddle is designed centered over the ulnar artery. The entire procedure can be performed under tourniquet control with a bloodless operative field.

Flap Harvest

Flap harvest is started by incising along the radial border of the flap with the forearm in supination. A suprafascial dissection is then carried out with a blade. An incision is made along the fascia to reach the subfascial plane when the flexor digitorum superficialis muscle is reached. The dissection proceeds in the subfascial plane until the ulnar pedicle and ulnar nerve are encountered. The flexor digitorum superficialis is retracted laterally and the flexor carpi ulnaris medially to expose the intermuscular space. This allows exposure of the ulnar pedicle and ulnar nerve. After the pedicle is identified, the skin incision can

TABLE 20-2. Comparisons of Radial and Ulnar Forearm Flaps

	Radial Forearm Flap	Ulnar Forearm Flap
Nondominant artery (%)	30	54
Artery diameter (mm)	2–4	2–4
Vein diameter (mm)	1–2	1–2
Sensory nerve	Lateral antebrachial cutaneous	Medial antebrachial cutaneous
Perforators numbers	All tiny perforators	Three to seven
Perforators size	Smaller	Bigger
Skin territory, thickness	Thin	Thinner
Hair	Hair bearing in whites	Hairless
Ease for dissection	Easy (30–40 min)	Easier (20–30 min)
Donor site scar	Conspicuous	Inconspicuous

be extended proximally to expose the entire vascular pedicle (see Figure 20-2). The distal part of the pedicle close to the wrist is then divided. The pedicle is dissected out while the ulnar nerve is preserved in situ. The flap is elevated in the subfascial plane with the vascular pedicle. Occasionally a few ulnar nerve branches wrap around the pedicle. These nerve branches can be preserved by careful dissection. The incision on the ulnar site of the skin flap is then made. During the dissection, the medial antebrachial cutaneous nerve can be explored and included for a sensate flap if necessary. The flap harvest time is around 30 minutes for an experienced surgeon and 60 to 90 minutes for residents and fellows.

TRICKS AND TIPS FROM THE AUTHORS

Although it is rare, the ulnar pedicle is more vulnerable to injury when it is located superficially. It is recommended to use tenotomy scissors or blade dissection rather than cauterization when starting the flap dissection from the incision over the radial side of the flap to prevent any possible injury to the superficial ulnar artery. In addition, it is easier to expose the ulnar artery in rare cases when it is located superficially.

It is important during UFF harvest to avoid injury to the ulnar nerve. Sometimes the ulnar nerve has separate branches going across the ulnar pedicle that require careful dissection under loupe magnification. To not to damage the ulnar nerve, it is recommended to dissect the ulnar nerve off the ulnar pedicle before the incision and dissection from the ulnar side of the flap. This allows easier, faster flap dissection without accidental injury to the ulnar nerve.

The UFF can be elevated as a perforator flap. However, when the perforators are very tiny, to avoid detachment of the pedicle from the skin flap, the pedicle can be sutured to the skin flap on its distal end after it has been divided. The suture helps to keep the pedicle attached to the skin flap to ensure the tiny branches between the pedicle and the skin flap remain intact.

Donor site morbidity from wound closure is a concern after harvesting a forearm flap. A suprafascial dissection is recommended to preserve the paratenons to allow better skin graft take.

CLOSURE OF THE DONOR SITE

After elevation of the UFF, most of the donor site has to be closed with a skin graft. If the flap's width is less than 2.5 cm, primary closure may be possible. To enhance skin graft viability, a suprafascial dissection of the flap is recommended to preserve the fascia. During closure of the donor site, the ulnar nerve should be positioned between the flexor digitorum superficialis and the flexor carpi ulnaris with several simple perineurial sutures to avoid nerve exposure.

Before the wound is grafted, a running purse-string suture between the dermis and the fascia is performed along the wound edge to help reduce the donor site defect and to keep the skin margins in place. This helps to avoid tethering of the skin graft when the patients move their forearms or hands. Furthermore, the dermis-to-fascia sutures smooth the gap between skin graft and forearm skin, avoiding a step-off and producing a better cosmetic result.

The donor site can be closed with a split- or full-thickness skin graft. A full-thickness skin graft is recommended for better cosmesis, less scar contracture, and better donor site function. A tie-over bolster should be placed for 5 days to enhance skin graft take, and a short-arm split is used for 2 weeks.

Although some surgeons advocate the usage of a sliding radial based forearm flap to close the donor site, most surgeons prefer a skin graft to reduce the risk of donor site morbidities (18)

A vacuum-assisted closure system may be used for the donor site closure to decrease tendon exposure if the fascia is not well preserved (19).

COMPLICATIONS OF THE DONOR SITE

The donor site complications from an UFF harvest can be divided into acute and chronic.

Acute complications include total or partial skin graft loss, vascular insufficiency, and transient or permanent ulnar nerve palsy. To prevent skin graft loss, a suprafascial dissection had been recommended to leave the forearm fascia intact to facilitate better skin graft take. Furthermore, a tie-over bolster on the skin graft for 5 days and volar short-arm splint to prevent hand flexion are also recommended for better immobilization of the skin graft. Concerns about limitation of volar flexion in the forearm and hand distal to the donor site caused by skin graft contracture involving underlying flexor tendons are theoretical rather than real.

A few patients may experience transient numbness over the ulnar nerve territories, especially the ring finger and little finger, for variable time periods after surgery. Most of these symptoms will recover within 3 months.

Although acute severe vascular compromise is rare, a minor vascular insufficiency can happen after sacrificing the ulnar artery (20).

Rodriguez and colleagues evaluated the donor site morbidities after UFF harvest by performing postoperative high-resolution color duplex ultrasonography of bilateral forearms and arms and photoplethysmography of the distal digits (20). Grip strength over hand and two-point discrimination over the digits were also evaluated. The grip strength and sensation were not statistically significant between donor and nondonor hands. None of their patients presented with cold intolerance or symptoms of hand claudication 2 months after surgery. Radial artery flow velocity "increased" 17.5% as compensation for loss of the ulnar artery in the donor forearm compared with the normal contralateral forearm. However, the perfusion to the distal digits of the donor hand was quite comparable to that over the nondonor hand.

In well-selected patients and with careful and delicate flap dissection to preserve the ulnar nerve and intact fascia to minimize the donor site morbidities, the UFF can prove to be a reliable and versatile flap for reconstruction.

CLINICAL APPLICATIONS

Head and Neck Reconstructions (Buccal, Tongue, Palate, Nose, Prefabricated)

The forearm skin is thin and pliable. According to Sieg's report, the skin over the ulnar region is thinner than that on the radial region, making the UFF an even better choice in reconstructions when a thin flap is required (6). The outcome is comparable to that of the radial forearm flap, but it has better donor site cosmesis. In head and neck reconstruction, the UFF is a good choice for buccal mucosa (Figure 20-4) and hemitongue reconstruction (21) (Figure 20-5).

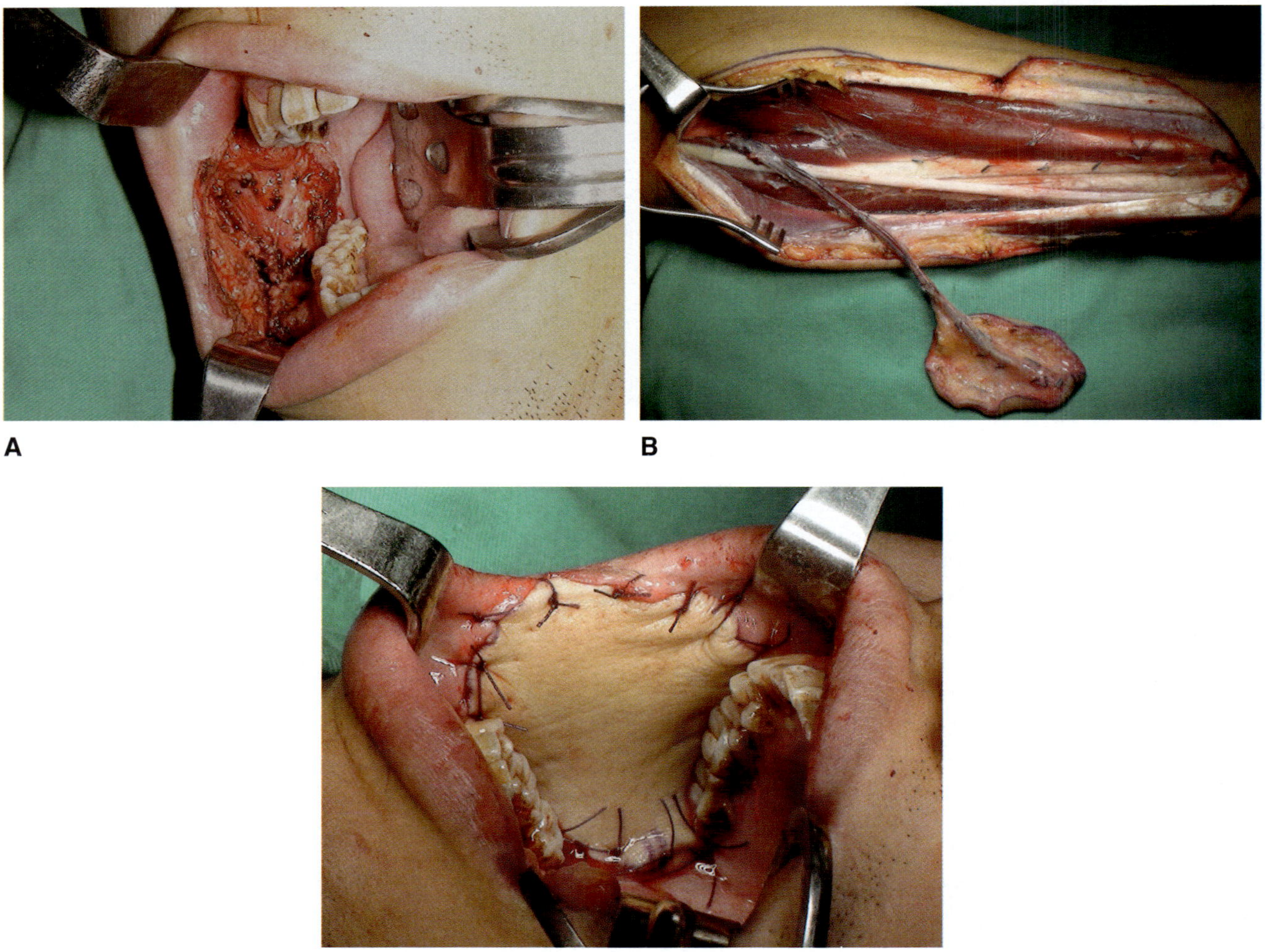

FIGURE 20-4 A 32-year-old male patient presented with right buccal cancer, staged T2N0M0. After wide excision of the cancer lesion, a free ulnar forearm flap (UFF) was designed for reconstruction. (**A**) The buccal mucosa lesion after cancer ablation. (**B**) A free UFF measuring 4 x 7 cm was harvested from his left forearm. (**C**) The immediate postoperative appearance after reconstruction.

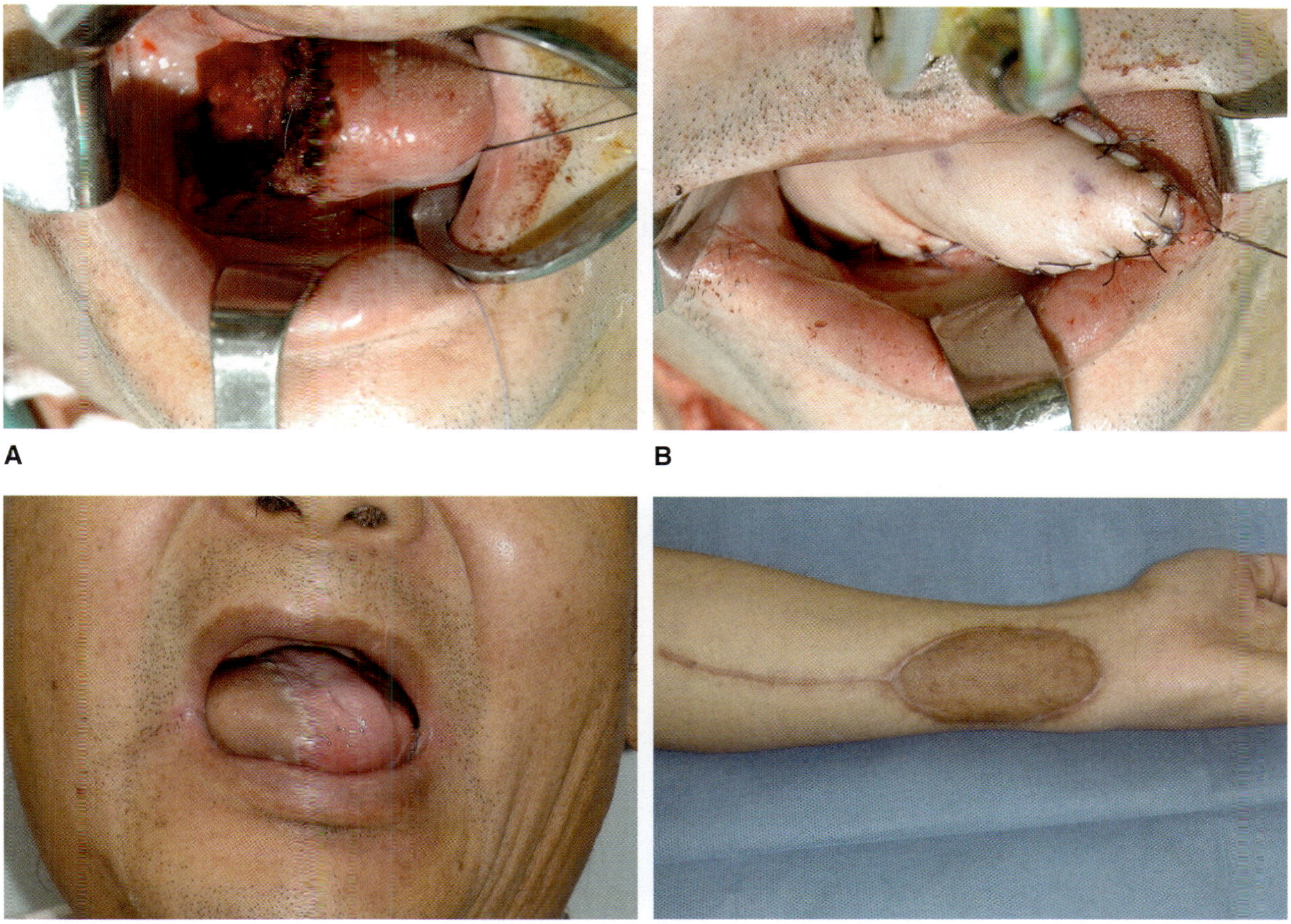

A B C D

FIGURE 20-5 A 59-year-old male patient presented with an exophytic tongue tumor over his right tongue. Biopsy revealed squamous cell carcinoma. After hemiglossectomy, a free ulnar forearm flap was elevated from his left forearm for hemitongue reconstruction. (**A**) Hemiglossectomy performed by the surgical oncologist. (**B**) The immediate postoperative result of a free ulnar forearm flap measured 9 x 5 cm for right tongue reconstruction. (**C**) At a follow-up of 8 months, the patient was satisfied with both functional and cosmetic outcomes. (**D**) The donor site appearance after flap elevation and full-thickness skin graft.

The pliability allows a free three-dimensional flap inset, resulting in better postoperative function. This is particular relevant in hemitongue reconstruction to where it permits better tongue mobility for swallowing as well as speech function (8,9). The inclusion of the palmaris longus tendon as a sling allows for simultaneous lip reconstruction.

As mentioned in the anatomy section, there are usually three to five sizable septocutaneous perforators emerging from the ulnar pedicle distal to the common interosseous artery. Thus, two or more skin paddles can be harvested as a chimeric flap or as two (or more) separate skin flaps each based on different perforators but each having a separate segment of the ulnar artery as its pedicle. This is particular useful for trismus reconstruction or with oral cancer reconstruction in patients who present with bilateral malignant or premalignant lesions (Figures 20-3 and 20-6). The lengthy vascular pedicle can reach the commonly used recipient vessels in the head and neck region without the requirement of vein grafts.

Although a small piece of ulna bone can be transferred as part of an osteocutaneous flap for bony reconstruction, it is not recommended for the mandible because even 40% of the thin distal ulna has insufficient stock for a functional reconstruction. There is also a high incidence of donor site ulna fractures.

Extremity Reconstruction

The UFF has been applied in upper extremity reconstruction with satisfactory results (4). Glasson and Lovie introduced the proximally and distally based UFFs in hand and forearm reconstruction (4). Furthermore, Jawad and Harrison applied the sensate UFF with the inclusion of the medial antebrachial nerve for coverage of an elbow joint prosthesis (22). The sensate UFF preserved sensation over the joint and prosthesis and therefore lessened the risk of pressure ulcer. A reverse UFF can be designed with proximally or distally based pedicle to cover wrist or elbow defects with satisfactory results. With the inclusion of the ulnar dorsal artery, wrist and hand defects can be covered with a pedicled ulnar dorsal artery flap if the defect is close to the donor site (11).

Although many reconstructive surgeons have used the UFF in upper extremity reconstruction, it is not commonly used in lower extremity reconstruction.

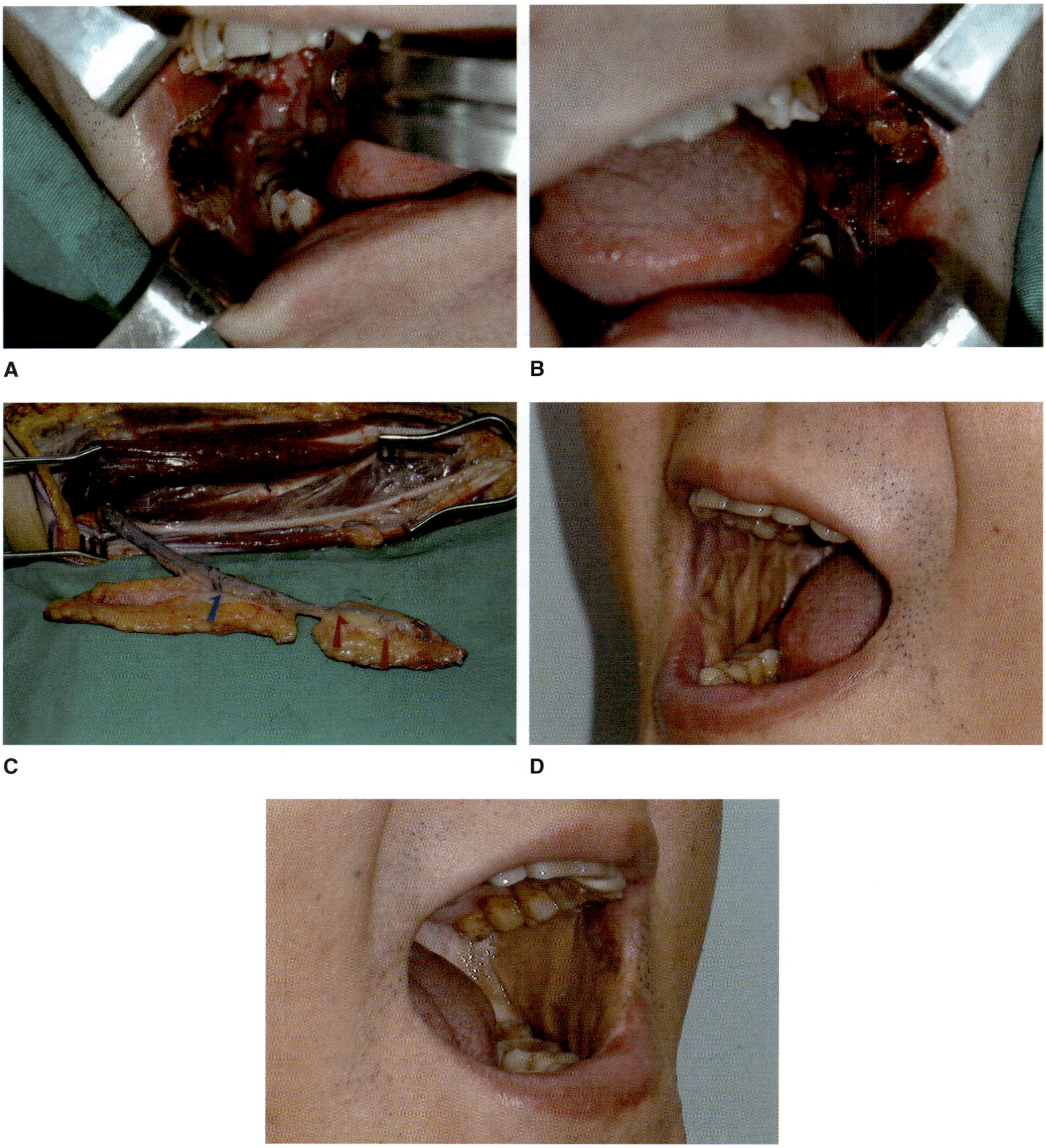

FIGURE 20-6 A 37-year-old male patient with history of betel nut chewing for more than 10 years presented with trismus (preoperative interincisor distance of 1 cm). After release of the submucosal fibrosis, two separate free ulnar forearm flaps (UFFs) were harvested from the left forearm for reconstruction of bilateral buccal mucosa defects. (**A**) Defect over the right buccal mucosa after release of the fibrosis. (**B**) Left buccal mucosa defect. (**C**) Two free UFFs were harvested from the left forearm. (**D**) and (**E**) At a follow-up of 15 months, the patient was satisfied with the swallowing and speech functions with an interincisor distance of 5 cm.

Penis and Urogenital Reconstruction

Urethral reconstruction using free tissue transfer requires a donor tissue that is thin, durable, sufficiently large enough, hairless if possible, and with a long and large neurovascular pedicle for safe flap transfer (23). The radial forearm flap has been used for urethral and penile reconstruction with good results (23). However, the radial side of the forearm is a hair-bearing region. The ulnar forearm, on the other hand, is usually hairless. Elimination of hair over the reconstruction flap is important for urethral reconstruction to reduce recurrent infections from the hair follicles. Common indications for penile and urethral reconstructions using free flap include recurrent urethral strictures and failed hypospadias reconstruction. Several flap designs have been introduced using the radial forearm flap (23–25) for urethra and penis reconstruction and can be applied to the UFF as well. A "cricket bat" design for urethral reconstruction has been introduced for urethral and penile reconstruction to prevent scar contracture (25). Furthermore, Biemer modified the flap for a subtotal penis reconstruction to include urethra and glands reconstruction (24). The UFF can be folded or separated into two skin paddles for urethral and penis reconstruction. Recipient vessels may include the groin vessels or the external pudendal vessels.

Nasal Reconstruction

The free radial forearm flap has been applied in nasal reconstruction for years. In reconstruction of the nasal inner lining, a free flap is often required because of the tissue insufficiency from the surrounding regions in patients with severe trauma or burn or in cancer surgeries. A thin free flap is required to provide three-dimensional reconstruction of the nasal inner lining. Although the forehead flap is usually the first choice in reconstruction of the nose, in patients who have failed surgery or who have a severe scar over the forehead region, a free flap is still required. Because the UFF is even thinner than the radial forearm flap with a more concealed donor scar, the authors recommend the UFF as a reliable option for nasal reconstruction.

CONCLUSION

The UFF has the advantages of being a soft, thin, and pliable flap with a long vascular pedicle containing vessels of good diameter for safe microvascular anastomoses. A rich supply of septocutaneous perforators also allows versatile flap design. It is therefore a good donor site for head and neck, upper extremity, and peno-urethral reconstruction. The donor site morbidity is minimal and the donor site cosmesis is acceptable.

REFERENCES

1. Song R, Gao Y, Song Y, et al. The forearm flap. *Clin Plast Surg* 1982;9(1):21–26.
2. Lovie MJ, Duncan GM, Glasson DW. The ulnar artery forearm free flap. *Br J Plast Surg* 1984;37(4):486–492.
3. Glasson DW, Lovie MJ, Duncan GM. The ulnar forearm free flap in penile reconstruction. *Aust N Z J Surg* 1986;56(6):477–479.
4. Glasson DW, Lovie MJ. The ulnar island flap in hand and forearm reconstruction. *Br J Plast Surg* 1988;41(4):349–353.
5. Gilbert DA, Schlossberg SM, Jordan JH. Ulnar forearm phallic construction and penile reconstruction. *Microsurgery* 1995;16(5):314–321.
6. Sieg P [Ulnar versus radial forearm flap in orofacial reconstruction]. *Mund Kiefer Gesichtschir* 2000;4(1):35–38.
7. Gabr EM, Kobayashi MR, Salibian AH, et al. Role of ulnar forearm free flap in oromandibular reconstruction. *Microsurgery* 2004;24(4):253–258.
8. Salibian AH, Allison GR, Armstrong WB, et al. Functional hemitongue reconstruction with the microvascular ulnar forearm flap. *Plast Reconstr Surg* 1999;104(3):654–660.
9. Salibian AH, Allison GR, Krugman ME, et al. Reconstruction of the base of the tongue with the microvascular ulnar forearm flap: a functional assessment. *Plast Reconstr Surg* 1995;96(5):1081–1089; discussion 1090–1091.
10. Li KK, Salibian AH, Allison GR, et al. Pharyngoesophageal reconstruction with the ulnar forearm flap. *Arch Otolaryngol Head Neck Surg* 1998;124(10):1146–1151.
11. Vergara-Amador E. Anatomical study of the ulnar dorsal artery and design of a new retrograde ulnar dorsal flap. *Plast Reconstr Surg* 2008;121(5):1716–1724.
12. Devansh. Superficial ulnar artery flap. *Plast Reconstr Surg* 1996;97(2):420–426.
13. Fadel RA, Amonoo-Kuofi HS. The superficial ulnar artery: development and surgical significance. *Clin Anat* 1996;9(2):128–132.
14. Sieg P, Jacobsen HC, Hakim SG, Hermes D. Superficial ulnar artery: curse or blessing in harvesting fasciocutaneous forearm flaps. *Head Neck* 2006;28(5):447–452.
15. Olazabal AE, Morrison WA, O'Brien BM. Immediate and short-term effect on arterial flow of clamping or stripping one vessel of a two vessel limb in a dog model. *Microsurgery* 1994;15(10):722–725.
16. Haerle M, Häfner HM, Dietz K, et al., Vascular dominance in the forearm. *Plast Reconstr Surg* 2003;111(6):1891–1898.
17. Ali SN, Srivastava S. Study of ulnar and radial arteries at wrist level in smokers. *Scand J Plast Reconstr Surg Hand Surg* 2008;42(6):320–324.
18. Hallock GG. Closure of the ulnar forearm free flap donor site using a local radial forearm flap. *Br J Plast Surg* 1992;45(2):94–96.
19. Andrews BT, Smith RB, Chang KE, et al., Management of the radial forearm free flap donor site with the vacuum-assisted closure (VAC) system. *Laryngoscope* 2006;116(10):1918–1922.
20. Rodriguez ED, Mithani SK, Bluebond-Langner R, Manson PN. Hand evaluation following ulnar forearm perforator flap harvest: a prospective study. *Plast Reconstr Surg* 2007;120(6):1598–1601.
21. Engel H, Huang JJ, Lin CY, et al. A strategic approach for tongue reconstruction to achieve predictable and improved functional and aesthetic outcomes. *Plast Reconstr Surg* 2010;126(6):1967–1977.
22. Jawad AS. Harrison DH. The island sensate ulnar artery flap for reconstruction around the elbow. *Br J Plast Surg* 1990;43(6):695–698.
23. Harashina T, Inoue T, Tanaka I, et al. Reconstruction of penis with free deltoid flap. *Br J Plast Surg* 1990;43(2):217–222.
24. Biemer E. Penile construction by the radial arm flap. *Clin Plast Surg* 1988;15(3):425–430.
25. Semple JL, Boyd JB, Farrow GA, Robinette MA. The "cricket bat" flap: a one-stage free forearm flap phalloplasty. *Plast Reconstr Surg Plast Reconstr Surg* 1991;88(3):514–519.
26. Huang JJ, Wu CW, Lam WL, Nguyen DH, Kao HK, Lin CY, Cheng MH. Anatomical basis and clinical application of the ulnar forearm free flap for head and neck reconstruction. *Laryngoscope* 2012;122(12):2670–2676. doi: 10.1002/lary.23565. Epub 2012 Oct 15.

CHAPTER 21

Lateral Arm Flap

Jason H. Ko and Douglas P. Hanel

BRIEF HISTORY

In the early 1980s, numerous authors described a novel fasciocutaneous flap from the lateral aspect of the proximal arm—the lateral arm flap (LAF)—beginning with Song et al. in 1982 (1), Cormack and Lamberty in 1983 (2), and Katsaros et al. in 1984 (3). The traditional LAF, extending from the insertion of the deltoid muscle to the lateral epicondyle, quickly gained popularity because of its anatomic consistency, straightforward dissection, and versatility as a pedicled or free fasciocutaneous flap (4–7). As indications for use of the LAF expanded, surgeons began designing composite LAFs that included vascularized bone from the humerus, vascularized tendon from the triceps, or vascularized sensory nerve (4,8,9). In 1991 both Katsaros et al. and Kuek and Chuan reported the use of an "extended" LAF (ELAF) that included skin distal to the lateral epicondyle as a modification of the LAF (9,10), representing a thin, pliable flap that was a viable alternative to the radial forearm flap (Figure 21-1). Although the initial popularity of the LAF has diminished over time, the LAF continues to be an excellent option for various reconstructive challenges throughout the body. In addition, some surgeons have recently moved away from the radial forearm flap because of concerns about the vascular sequelae of harvesting the radial artery (11), thereby creating a mild resurgence for the LAF and ELAF in reconstructive microsurgery.

ANATOMY

The profunda brachii artery (PBA) arises from the posterolateral aspect of the brachial artery just distal to the lower border of teres major. Passing along the spiral groove with the radial nerve, it lies in the deep intermuscular septum and divides into the middle collateral artery and the radial collateral artery (RCA). The RCA accompanies the radial nerve distally, branching into the anterior radial collateral artery (ARCA) and posterior radial collateral artery (PRCA). The traditional LAF is based on four or five septocutaneous perforators from the PRCA, which courses distally through the lateral intermuscular septum between the triceps posteriorly and the brachialis and brachioradialis anteriorly (Figure 21-2). The length of the RCA pedicle is 6 cm (range, 4–8 cm), with a vessel caliber of 1.5 to 3 mm. There are usually two (75%)—and less often one (25%)—accompanying venae comitantes with diameters of 2.5 to 3 mm that drain into the profunda brachii veins. If dissection proceeds proximally to the level of the PBA, the caliber of the artery increases to 3 to 5 mm in diameter, as described by Moffett et al. (6). When performing the ELAF, the most distal septocutaneous perforator, located approximately 4 cm proximal to the lateral epicondyle, should be included with the flap, effectively increasing the pedicle length to 9 to 16 cm. The ARCA, which travels through the lateral intermuscular septum between the brachialis and lateral head of the triceps muscle, is a minor pedicle of the traditional LAF, with a length of 2 to 6 cm and diameter of 0.5 to 1.2 mm. Another minor pedicle of the LAF is the radial recurrent artery (RRA), which is a branch of the radial artery that courses laterally and superiorly along the medial surface of the brachioradialis, anastomosing proximally with the ARCA. The RRA is the major blood supply for the distally based pedicled LAF and has a length of 8 cm and a diameter of 0.8 to 2 mm (7,12).

The radial nerve travels with the PBA between the medial and lateral heads of the triceps before traveling between the brachioradialis and brachialis muscles distally. The lower lateral brachial cutaneous nerve (LBCN) is a proximal branch of the radial nerve that arises superior to the origin of the PBA and pierces the brachial fascia posterior to the deltoid insertion. The LBCN provides sensory innervation to the skin of the posterolateral upper arm to the level of the olecranon, which is the skin territory for the standard LAF. The posterior antebrachial cutaneous nerve (PACN) is a branch of the radial nerve that arises at the level where the RCA divides into the ARCA and PRCA.

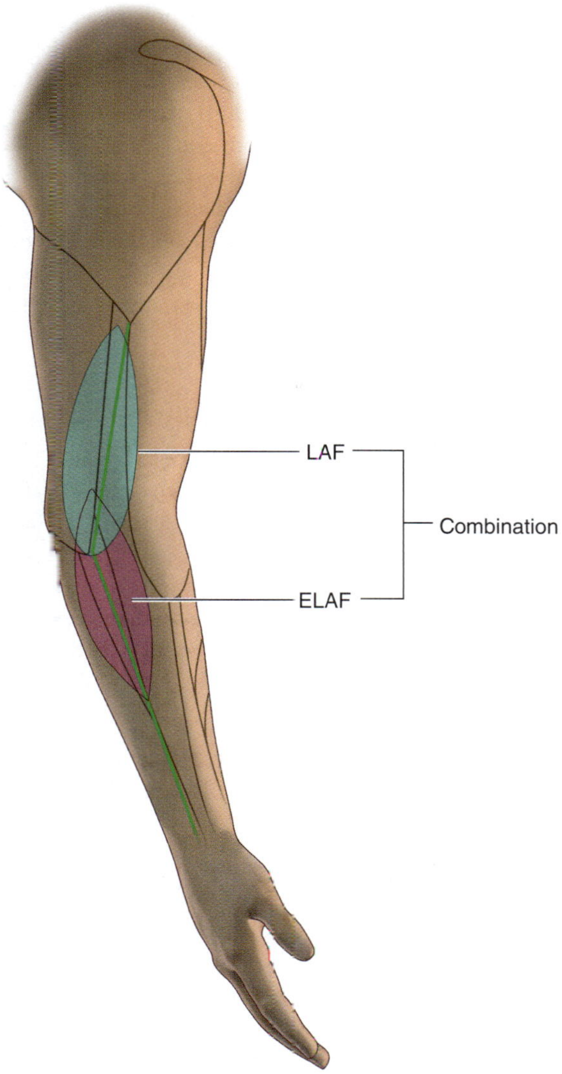

FIGURE 21-1 Flap markings of the standard lateral arm flap (LAF) and the extended lateral arm flap (ELAF).

The PACN travels with the PRCA, perforating the lateral head of the triceps at its attachment to the humerus. In the distal upper arm, the PACN divides into an upper branch that supplies the posterior-inferior upper arm and a lower branch that supplies the lateral side of the arm and elbow, which is the skin territory for the ELAF. By including the LBCN or PACN with the traditional LAF or ELAF, respectively, the flap can be raised as a neurosensory flap.

The LAF can be harvested as an osteofasciocutaneous flap because of a rich supply of vascular connections from the PRCA to the posterolateral humerus, extending from the supracondylar ridge to the lateral epicondyle (3,13). The majority of vascular connections are between 2 and 7 cm proximal to the lateral epicondyle. Therefore, the LAF and ELAF can be harvested with a portion of vascularized bone from the humerus. The width of the harvested bone should be no more than one third of the diameter of the humerus (1–1.5 cm in width), with a length up to 15 cm. To maximize vascular connections within the intermuscular septum, a cuff of the brachioradialis and medial head of the triceps should be included with the osseous flap. Because of the vascular connections between the PRCA and lateral head of the triceps muscle, the LAF can be harvested with a portion of triceps muscle to increase bulk (8). In addition, a strip of vascularized triceps tendon, measuring up to 2 × 10 cm in dimensions, can also be included with the flap.

The LAF and ELAF can also be harvested as a fascia-only or adipofascial flap, providing thin and pliable tissue that works well for hand reconstruction and creates a smooth gliding surface for tendons (3,5,9). In addition, a fascia-only or adipofascial LAF can be split based on perforators to reconstruct individual fingers, and because no skin is harvested with the flap, the donor site can be closed primarily.

VARIANTS

Traditional Lateral Arm Flap

The LAF is a fasciocutaneous flap with a skin paddle centered over a line between the insertion of the deltoid and the lateral

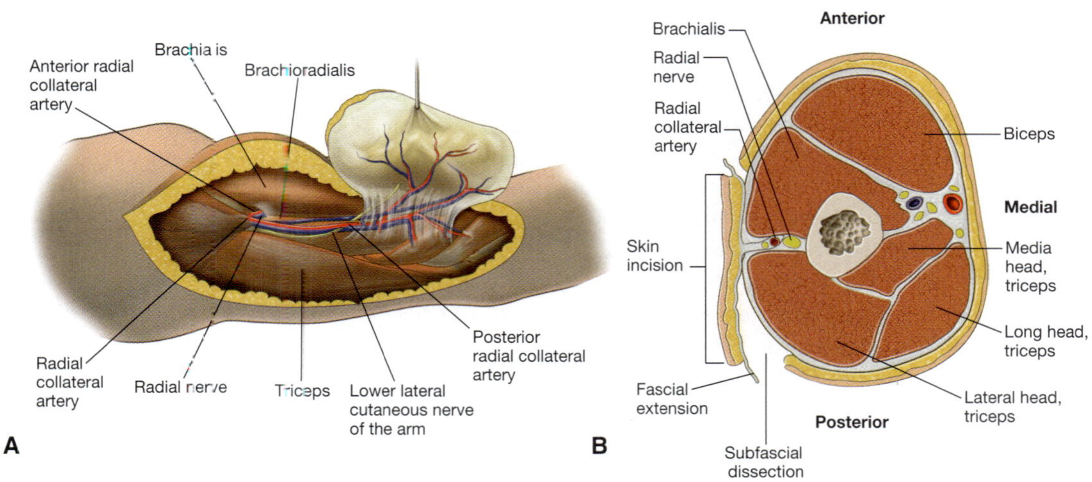

FIGURE 21-2 (**A**) The standard lateral arm flap (LAF) is based on septocutaneous perforators from the posterior radial collateral artery. The lower lateral brachial cutaneous nerve can be included as a neurosensory flap. (**B**) A cross-sectional view of the proximal arm demonstrates the subfascial plane of dissection for the LAF with inclusion of the vascular pedicle within the lateral intermuscular septum. This illustration demonstrates the importance of identifying and protecting the radial nerve early in the flap dissection. a, artery; Ant, anterior; m, muscle.

epicondyle. The standard LAF is based on septocutaneous perforators from the PRCA, with its major blood supply from the RCA. If a longer pedicle or vessels of larger caliber are required, more proximal dissection of the pedicle to the level of the PBA can also be performed (6).

Extended Lateral Arm Flap

The ELAF is a fasciocutaneous flap with a skin paddle designed distal to the lateral epicondyle (10,14). The ELAF is based on the most distal perforator of the PRCA, which is typically located 4 cm proximal to the lateral epicondyle. Using the ELAF enables lengthening of the pedicle up to 9 to 16 cm while providing thin, pliable skin even in obese patients. For this reason, the ELAF is a viable alternative to the radial forearm free flap.

Pedicled Lateral Arm Flap and Extended Lateral Arm Flap

The LAF can be raised either as a proximally or distally based pedicled flap. The proximally based pedicled LAF or ELAF, based on the RCA, can be used to reconstruct the posterior shoulder; because of the course of the PRCA, it is more difficult to reconstruct anterior shoulder defects with the standard LAF. However, by dissecting proximally to the level of the PBA, the pedicled LAF can reach the anterior shoulder or axilla in a tension-free manner (6).

The distally based, or reverse, pedicled LAF is based on retrograde flow through the RRA and used to reconstruct elbow defects (7,12). Prior injury to the radial artery proximally may compromise flow through the reverse LAF. In addition, rotating the reverse LAF 180 degrees may lead to venous insufficiency of the flap, so the surgeon should consider performing a microvascular venous anastomosis of a cephalic vein branch within the flap to a nearby recipient vein if venous congestion is noted during flap inset.

Innervated Lateral Arm Flap and Extended Lateral Arm Flap

The LBCN provides sensation to the skin paddle of the LAF, whereas the PACN supplies the skin territory of the ELAF. The aforementioned cutaneous nerves can be included with the LAF and ELAF, respectively, when designing a neurosensory flap. The LBCN and PACN are relatively large at this level in the upper extremity, so nerve dissection is straightforward. When elevating a neurosensory flap, the sensory nerve to be included in the flap should be dissected proximally at the beginning of the procedure to not only protect the nerve but to also obtain sufficient length for nerve coaptation before harvesting the LAF or ELAF.

Osteofasciocutaneous Lateral Arm Flap and Extended Lateral Arm Flap

The LAF and ELAF can be harvested with a segment of vascularized bone from the posterolateral humerus based on consistent vascular connections from the PRCA to the periosteum of the humerus located between 2 and 7 cm proximal to the lateral epicondyle (3,13). Vascularized bone can be harvested along the length of the skin paddle (10–15 cm), but only bone with a width up to 1 or 1.5 cm (one third of the diameter of the humerus) should be removed to prevent iatrogenic fracture of the humerus. The vascularized bone is unicortical in nature—although dense and strong—and should be obtained between 3 and 6 cm above the lateral epicondyle to maximize blood supply. The inclusion of a cuff of brachioradialis and medial head of the triceps helps to capture vascular connections to the bone within the intermuscular septum.

Musculotendinous Lateral Arm Flap and Extended Lateral Arm Flap

If increased bulk is required, a segment of the lateral head of the triceps muscle can be included with the LAF or ELAF based on vascular connections from the PRCA (3,8,9). These vascular connections travel through the lateral triceps into the triceps tendon, allowing for inclusion of a vascularized tendon graft (2 × 10 cm) with the LAF or ELAF without affecting elbow extension (8).

Fascia-Only or Adipofascial Lateral Arm Flap and Extended Lateral Arm Flap

To achieve an even thinner, more pliable flap, the LAF and ELAF can be harvested as a fascia-only or adipofascial flap (3,5,9). Generally, the fascial flap should be harvested with at least a thin layer of fat and can measure up to 15 × 9 cm in area (5). These flaps conform well to the contour of the fingers and can be split based on individual perforators. In addition, both the deep and superficial surfaces of the adipofascial flap provide excellent platforms for tendon gliding in hand and foot reconstruction. An added benefit of the fascial LAF and ELAF is that the donor site can be closed primarily without requiring a skin graft.

Prefabricated Lateral Arm Flap and Extended Lateral Arm Flap

Pretransfer tissue expansion of the LAF can be performed for staged reconstructions of complex defects. Such tissue expansion can increase the size of the flap to 11 × 18 cm while promoting primary closure of the donor site (15). Other forms of prefabrication include placement of skin grafts before definitive transfer in complex penile reconstruction (16).

TECHNIQUE OF DISSECTION AND HARVEST

Markings

The landmarks for a standard LAF are the insertion of the deltoid proximally and the lateral epicondyle distally, and the skin paddle should be centered over this axis (Figure 21-3). A pinch test can be performed to determine the maximum width of the skin paddle that will allow for primary closure (Figure 21-4); however, direct closure can typically be obtained with a width of 6 cm. In elderly patients, flap widths up to 8 cm can be

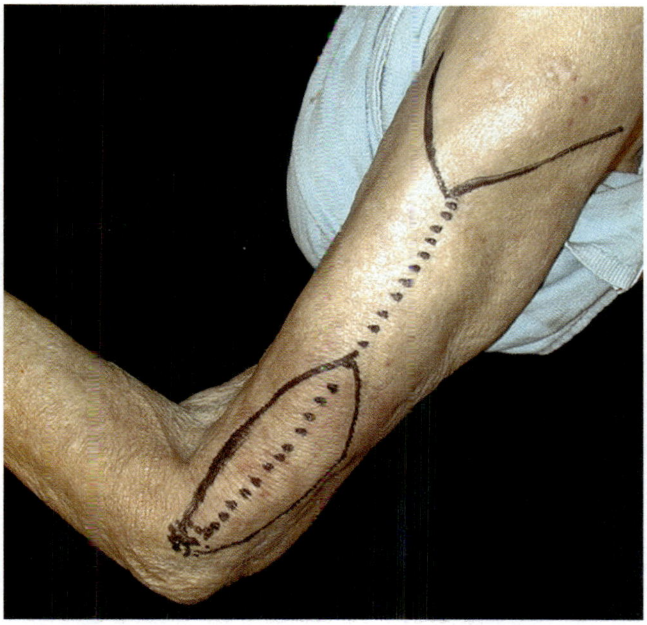

FIGURE 21-3 Preoperative marking of a typical skin paddle for the lateral arm flap. The landmarks are the insertion of the deltoid muscle and the lateral epicondyle, and the skin paddle should be designed along the axis between those two points.

closed primarily. Flap lengths of 5 to 20 cm can be achieved, but extension of the flap proximally over the deltoid makes primary closure more difficult. Although not necessary for the standard LAF, a handheld Doppler can be used to locate the septocutaneous perforators before incision. When designing the ELAF, the surgeon should locate the distalmost perforator (~4 cm proximal to the lateral epicondyle) with a handheld Doppler to aid with flap design. The ELAF can extend 12 to 15 cm beyond the lateral epicondyle and is typically designed over the epicondylar region or the proximal radial forearm. The width of the ELAF depends on the defect to be reconstructed, and the pinch test can help determine whether the donor site can be closed primarily.

Standard Lateral Arm Flap Technique

Although some surgeons do not advocate the use of the tourniquet for a standard LAF, many surgeons use a sterile tourniquet placed as proximally as possible for at least the distal aspects of flap elevation. If a tourniquet is used, it will have to be removed during proximal dissection of the pedicle regardless. After the LAF is designed, flap elevation is started posteriorly because this dissection is more straightforward than the anterior dissection, and similar to the septocutaneous perforators of a free fibula flap, the perforators of the LAF skin paddle travel slightly posteriorly. Therefore, the incision is

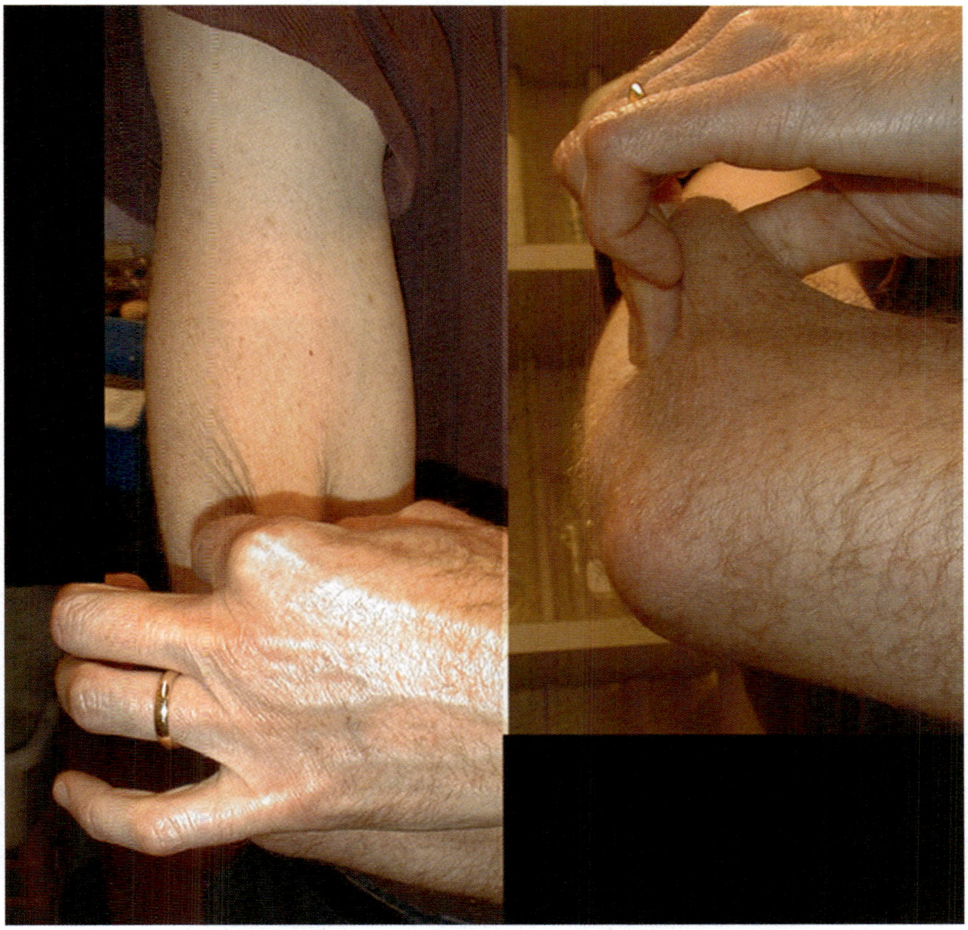

FIGURE 21-4 The width of the skin paddle can be determined by performing a "pinch test." Typically, a skin paddle 6 cm wide can be closed primary, and in older patients, the width can be increased to 8 cm and still allow for primary closure.

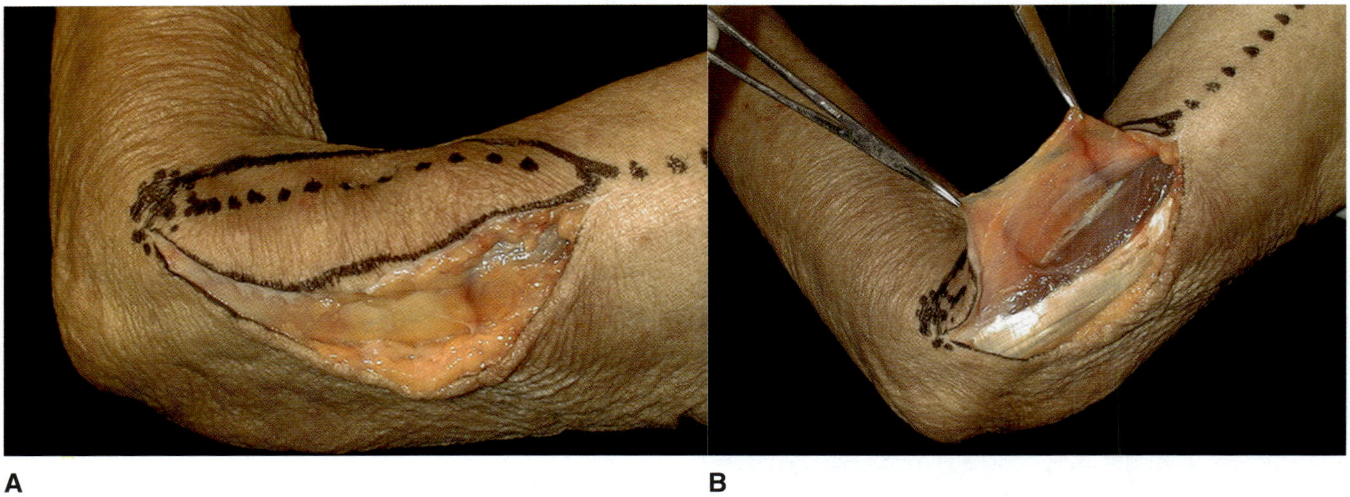

FIGURE 21-5 (**A**) Dissection of the lateral arm flap begins posteriorly in the subfascial plane. (**B**) The septocutaneous perforators are identified posteriorly as they emerge from the lateral intermuscular septum.

made along the posterior edge of the flap, continuing down through the posterior fascia to expose the lateral head of the triceps (Figure 21-5). At this stage, it is helpful to suture the fascia to the overlying skin and subcutaneous fat layer to prevent shearing of the perforators during flap elevation. Dissection proceeds anteriorly in the subfascial plane until the lateral intermuscular septum is reached. The septocutaneous perforators are visualized superficial to the deep fascia as they travel from the intermuscular septum through the fascia. After the perforators are identified, the anterior incision can be made (Figure 21-6). As mentioned previously, the anterior dissection is slightly more difficult because tissue planes are less clear, and the fascia is more adherent to the underlying muscle. The anterior fascia is incised over the brachioradialis and brachialis muscles, and dissection proceeds posteriorly in the subfascial plane to the level of the intermuscular septum. When both anterior and posterior dissections have reached the intermuscular septum, the distal fascia is incised down through the periosteum of the humerus, and the intermuscular septum—along with the overlying flap—is dissected subperiosteally in a proximal direction to the level of the deltoid insertion (Figure 21-7). After the PRCA and associated venae comitantes are located as they enter the intermuscular septum, the surgeon should dissect out the PRCA proximally until the ARCA and radial nerve are encountered. The radial nerve is located anterior to the PRCA and protected throughout the remainder of the procedure. The ARCA is then ligated, allowing for proximal dissection of the PRCA as it joins the RCA. As mentioned previously, further dissection can be performed to the level of the profunda brachii vessels to obtain increased pedicle length and caliber (6).

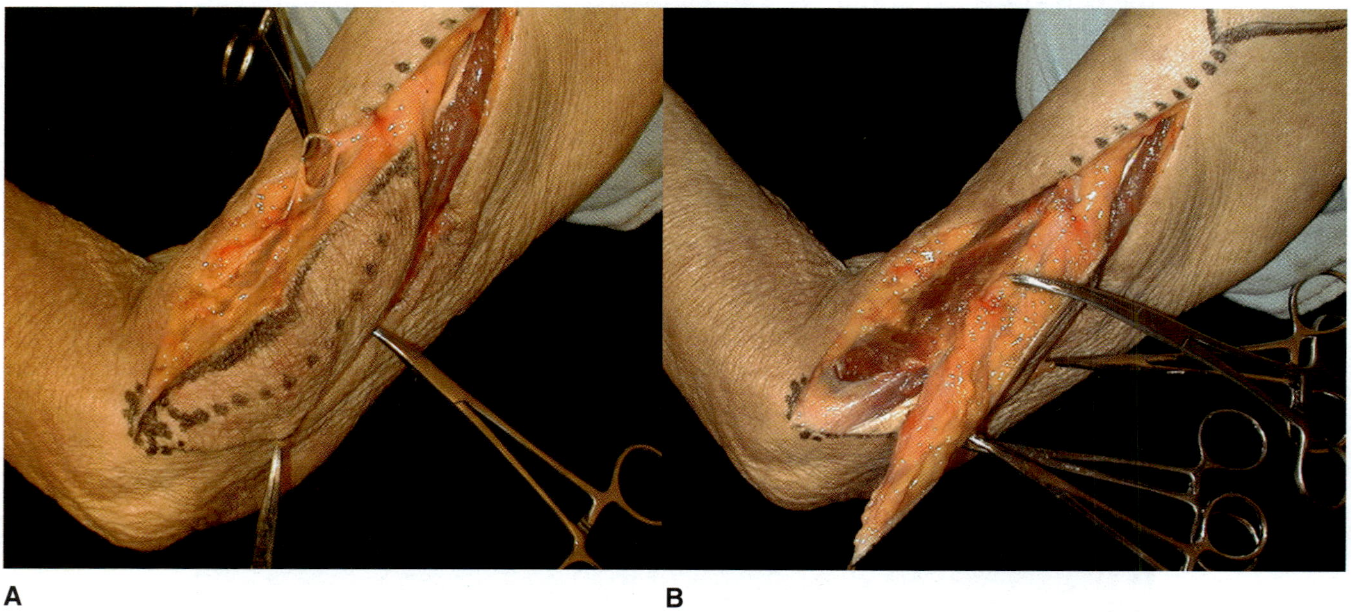

FIGURE 21-6 (**A**) The anterior dissection is begun subfascially over the brachialis and brachioradialis, and the lateral brachial cutaneous nerve is identified. (**B**) The anterior dissection proceeds to the level of the intermuscular septum.

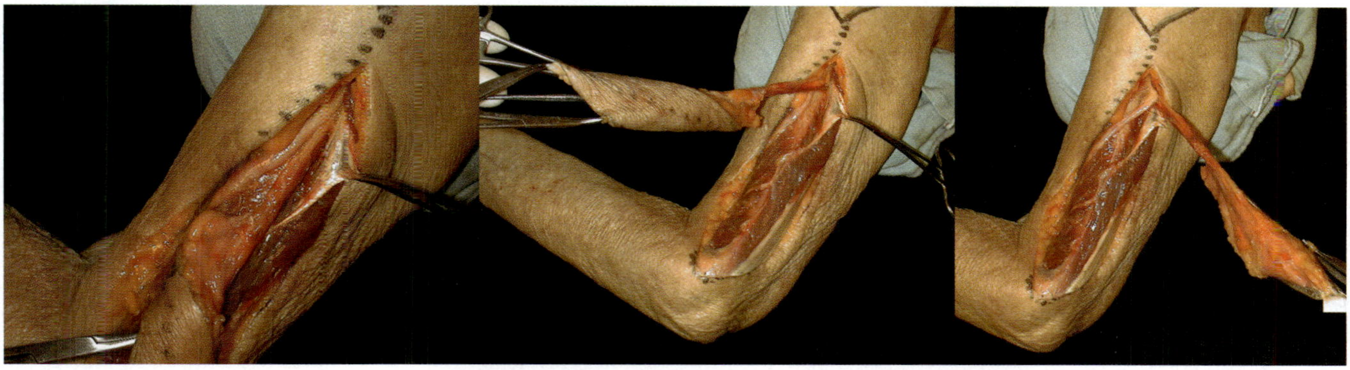

A B C

FIGURE 21-7 After dissecting the flap both posteriorly and anteriorly, the intermuscular septum—along with the overlying flap—is dissected subperiosteally in a proximal direction to the level of the deltoid insertion. The posterior radial collateral artery (PRCA) should be dissected proximally until the anterior radial collateral artery and radial nerve are encountered. (**A**) The radial nerve is located anterior to the PRCA and protected throughout the remainder of the procedure. (**B**) and (**C**) Dissection of the flap should continue proximally to the level of the RCA.

At the level of the deltoid insertion, the radial nerve is susceptible to injury; therefore, identifying and gently retracting the radial nerve is essential during proximal dissection of the vascular pedicle. Distally, the PACN is encountered and divided at the distal end of the flap, resulting in numbness or hypesthesia in the proximal lateral forearm. Although some authors recommend sparing the PACN (17), this dissection is tedious, and preservation of the PACN distally is typically unnecessary in our experience. Proximally, the LBCN enters the cutaneous territory of the LAF at the level of the deltoid insertion. If a neurosensory flap is planned, proximal dissection of the LBCN should be performed at the beginning of the procedure to prevent injury to the nerve. Otherwise, the LBCN can be sacrificed, and the surgeon should consider directing the transected LBCN stump into a nearby muscle in an effort to prevent neuroma pain.

Extended Lateral Arm Flap Technique

When harvesting the ELAF, a sterile tourniquet is generally recommended, and as mentioned previously, the most distal perforator should be located with a handheld Doppler to aid with flap design. After marking out the flap over the epicondylar and proximal forearm regions, dissection begins distally in the forearm and posteriorly over the triceps in a subfascial plane toward the lateral epicondyle. The PACN is elevated with the flap in the forearm, allowing for a neurosensory flap, if the surgeon desires. When the lateral epicondyle is reached, the intermuscular septum is visible posteriorly, and flap elevation should include the terminal portion of the PRCA with septocutaneous perforators from the lateral epicondyle. By including the deep fascia of the forearm region, it is easier to capture the distal PRCA perforators at the epicondylar level, making the dissection more straightforward. At least 3 cm of the intermuscular septum proximal to the lateral epicondyle should be harvested to include the distalmost septocutaneous perforators in the flap. After reaching the intermuscular septum, the remainder of the ELAF pedicle dissection is the same as that for the LAF. It may be helpful to identify the radial nerve between the brachioradialis and brachialis early in the dissection to prevent injury during vascular pedicle dissection.

Pedicled Lateral Arm Flap and Extended Lateral Arm Flap

Elevation of a proximally based pedicled LAF or ELAF is similar to that of the corresponding free flap. However, to reach the axilla or anterior shoulder in a tension-free manner, pedicle dissection should proceed proximally to the level of the profunda brachii vessels. For the distally based, or reverse, pedicled LAF, the distal perforators should be identified with a handheld Doppler before flap harvest. Similar to dissection of the standard LAF, the flap is elevated posteriorly and then anteriorly. The intermuscular septum is then exposed proximally, and the PRCA is dissected at the level of the deltoid insertion and ligated. The flap, along with the intermuscular septum, is then raised subperiosteally in a proximal-to-distal direction to the level of the lateral epicondyle. Although stopping the dissection approximately 2 cm proximal to the lateral epicondyle is safer, continuing the dissection to the lateral epicondyle, or 1 to 2 cm beyond the epicondyle, will provide increased mobility of the reverse LAF. The distally based LAF, based on blood supply from the RRA, can then be rotated into the elbow region or antecubital fossa without tension. However, rotation of 180 degrees may increase the risk of venous congestion of the flap, so the surgeon should consider performing a microvascular venous anastomosis to a nearby vein to improve flap survival.

Innervated Lateral Arm Flap and Extended Lateral Arm Flap

The LAF can be elevated as a neurosensory flap by including the LBCN, which enters the cutaneous territory of the flap at the level of the deltoid insertion. When harvesting an innervated LAF, the LBCN should be identified at the proximal edge of the flap early in the procedure, and sufficient length of the

LBCN should be dissected to achieve tension-free nerve coaptation after transfer. To harvest a neurosensory ELAF, the PACN should be included with the flap, providing up to 12 to 16 cm of vascularized nerve. The PACN is found early in the ELAF dissection lying superficial to the brachioradialis. The nerve can be traced proximally as it enters the deep fascia anterior to the intermuscular septum in the distal third of the upper arm. The nerve can be followed, running parallel to the vascular pedicle, to the level of the deltoid insertion, where it joins the radial nerve at the bifurcation of the PBA.

Osteofasciocutaneous Lateral Arm Flap and Extended Lateral Arm Flap

The LAF and ELAF can include a segment of vascularized bone from the distal posterolateral humerus because of consistent branches from the PRCA located 2 to 7 cm proximal to the lateral epicondyle (13). Flap dissection is similar, except the intermuscular septum is left intact over the bone to be harvested. As mentioned previously, the width of the bone should not exceed 1 to 1.5 cm—which corresponds to one-third of the diameter of the humerus—to decrease the risk of iatrogenic fracture of the humerus, and lengths up to 15 cm can be achieved. The bone should be harvested with the intermuscular septum en bloc, and capturing the bone between 3 and 6 cm proximal to the lateral epicondyle will ensure a more reliable vascular supply. In addition, incorporating a cuff of brachioradialis and medial head of the triceps helps to maintain vascular connections to the bone.

Musculotendinous Lateral Arm Flap and Extended Lateral Arm Flap

The LAF and ELAF can be elevated with a segment of the lateral head of the triceps muscle for increased bulk. Dissection is similar to standard flap harvest, but muscle fibers are left attached to the intermuscular septum as the rest of the muscle is separated from the humerus. Vascularized tendon (up to 2 × 10 cm) can also be included with the flap based on vascular connections from the PRCA that traverse the lateral triceps to reach the tendon (8).

Fascia-Only or Adipofascial Lateral Arm Flap and Extended Lateral Arm Flap

A fascial LAF or ELAF can measure up to 15 × 9 cm in area (5). Dissection is the same as for a standard flap except without the skin paddle. At least a thin layer of fat should be harvested with the fascial flap, and the amount of fat will depend on the recipient site. The main benefit of the fascial flap, in addition to providing a thinner, more pliable flap than the fasciocutaneous LAF and ELAF, is that it allows for primary closure of the donor site without the need for skin grafts. When reconstructing soft tissue defects on the fingers, for example, the fascial flap can be split based on individual perforators within the flap. In addition, tendon grafts can be placed either deep to the fascial flap or through the superficial fat layer of the flap, which promotes excellent tendon gliding in hand and foot reconstruction.

TRICKS AND TIPS

Although many tricks and tips have already been included in the description of flap elevation, the following represents a summary of recommendations from the authors:

1. When harvesting the LAF or ELAF flap, start by elevating the posterior aspect of the flap to visualize the septocutaneous perforators as they arise from the intermuscular septum before raising the anterior portion of the flap.
2. At the level of the deltoid insertion, the radial nerve is susceptible to injury. It is helpful to identify and protect the radial nerve early in the pedicle dissection for both the LAF and ELAF. When harvesting the ELAF, it is also wise to identify the radial nerve between the brachialis and brachioradialis proximally early in the flap dissection.
3. The caliber of the flap's vessels is relatively small, so dissection should proceed proximally beyond the bifurcation of the ARCA and PRCA to obtain vessels of appropriate diameter. More proximal dissection to the level of the PBA will result in larger vessels and a longer pedicle.
4. When performing a neurosensory LAF or ELAF, find the sensory nerves (LACN or PACN) proximal to the flap before elevating the skin paddle.
5. Limit the width of vascularized bone to 1 to 1.5 cm, which corresponds to one-third of the diameter of the distal humerus, to decrease the risk of late fracture with an osteofasciocutaneous LAF or ELAF.
6. By limiting the width of vascularized triceps tendon to 2 cm, there should be no appreciable effect on elbow extension.
7. Raising an ELAF flap will allow lengthening of the vascular pedicle to 9 to 16 cm compared with a pedicle length of 6 cm for the standard LAF.
8. Typically, a skin paddle 6 cm wide can be closed primarily, and in elderly patients, the width can increase to 8 cm without requiring a skin graft.
9. Although the standard LAF is generally a thin, pliable fasciocutaneous flap, it can be quite thick in overweight individuals, potentially limiting its use for certain indications. However, even in obese patients, the skin over the lateral epicondyle is relatively thin, so the ELAF is a thin flap in almost all patients. For this reason, the ELAF represents a viable alternative to the radial forearm free flap in most patients.

CLOSURE OF THE DONOR SITE

Performing a pinch test before surgery will help determine the maximum width of skin paddle that can be closed primarily. A general rule of thumb is 6 cm wide in most patients and 8 cm in elderly patients. Anything larger will require a skin graft; however, the skin graft can potentially be excised in a serial fashion. Typically, a split-thickness sheet graft is used to close larger donor sites, and this is covered with either a compression bolster or negative-pressure dressing. One advantage of the fascial LAF and ELAF is that the donor site can be closed primarily without requiring a skin graft. After harvesting a fascial LAF or ELAF, a subcutaneous drain can be used to close down

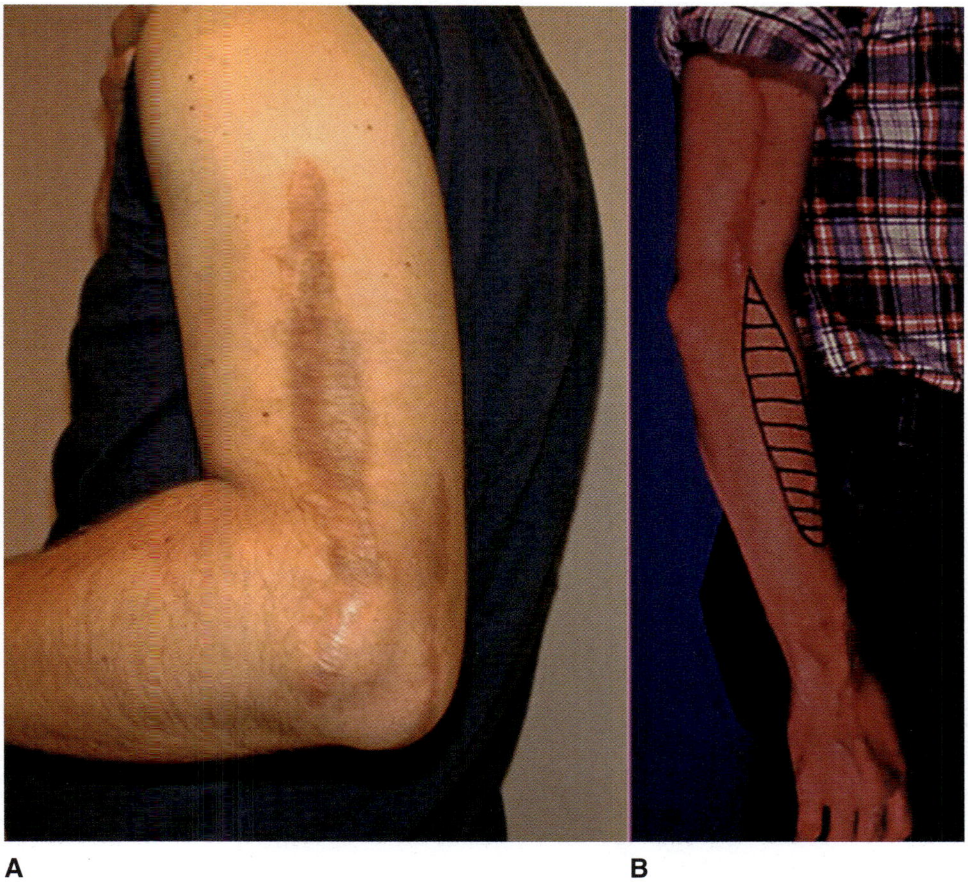

FIGURE 21-8 Donor site complications. (A) Widening of the lateral arm flap donor site scar. (B) Area of hypesthesia in the anterolateral forearm after transection of the posterior antebrachial cutaneous nerve.

any dead space. However, when primary closure is obtained with a standard LAF or ELAF, a drain is usually unnecessary.

DONOR SITE COMPLICATIONS

The main concern with the LAF and ELAF is donor site scar. When the donor site is closed primarily, the closure is usually performed under some tension, which can result in scar widening or hypertrophy (Figure 21-8). Although male patients can tolerate these scars well, female patients may be unhappy with a widened scar in the proximal arm and even more unhappy with a scar in the proximal forearm. When skin grafts are used to close the donor site, these complaints are amplified. In these cases, scar revision (or serial skin graft excision) is an option as a secondary procedure. Concerns regarding donor site scarring have led to the LAF and ELAF falling out of favor despite their initial popularity, although recently there seems to be a renewed interest in the ELAF as an alternative to the radial forearm flap (11).

Fifty-nine percent of patients experience hypesthesia of the proximal lateral forearm skin caused by transection of the PACN during harvest (see Figure 21-8) (17); however, this is less of a concern with the ELAF because most of the affected skin is included in the flap. Another major concern is heavy hair growth on the flap in male patients, which is more prevalent with the ELAF than the LAF because most patients do not have significant hair growth in the proximal arm. Hair growth on the flap is only a significant concern when the flap is placed intraorally in head and neck reconstruction, and other flaps should be considered in these circumstances. Patients may also experience pain in the region of the lateral epicondyle, which may be related to dissection of the mobile wad. In addition, tight closure of the donor site of an ELAF may contribute to this elbow pain, although patients do not develop any functional deficits in the elbow.

INDICATIONS FOR THIS FLAP

1. Hand and upper extremity reconstruction (distally based reverse pedicled or free flap) (Figures 21-9 and 21-10)
2. Reconstruction of the shoulder and axilla (proximally based pedicled flap)
3. Lower extremity reconstruction (Figure 21-11)
4. Head and neck (intraoral) reconstruction
5. Penile reconstruction
6. Burn scar reconstruction
7. Neurosensory reconstruction

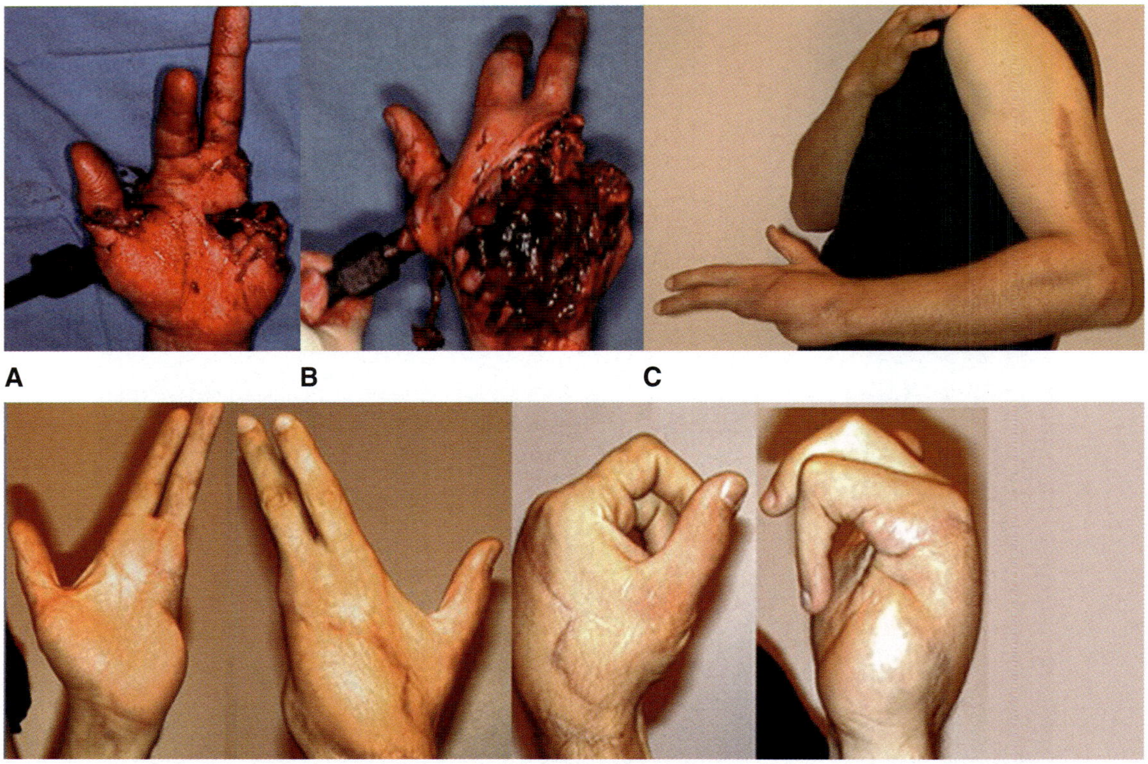

A B C

D E F G

FIGURE 21-9 An ipsilateral lateral arm flap is used to reconstruct a significant soft tissue injury along the dorso-ulnar aspect of the left hand, demonstrating excellent contour and good functional result.

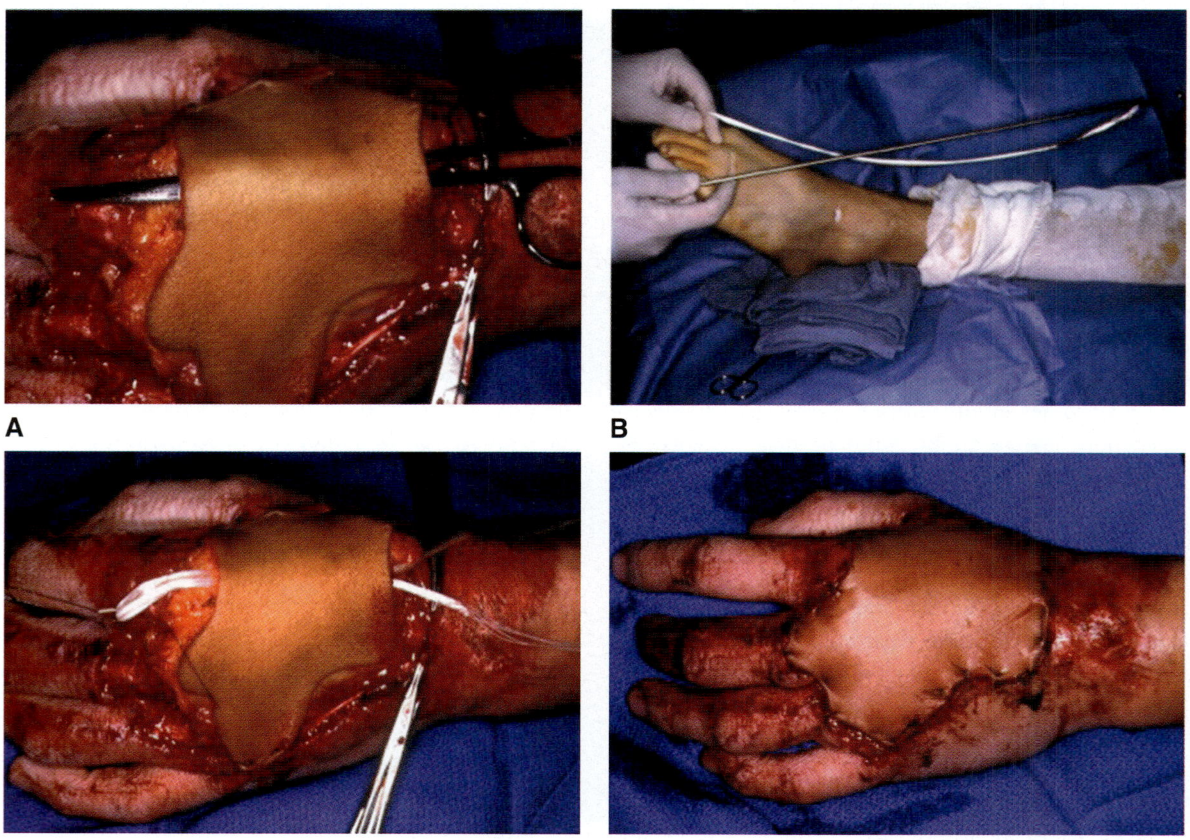

A B

C D

FIGURE 21-10 Reconstruction of the dorsum of the hand using tendon grafts placed in the subcutaneous plane—between the fascia and the skin—of the lateral arm flap, resulting in smooth contour, tendon gliding, and excellent function.

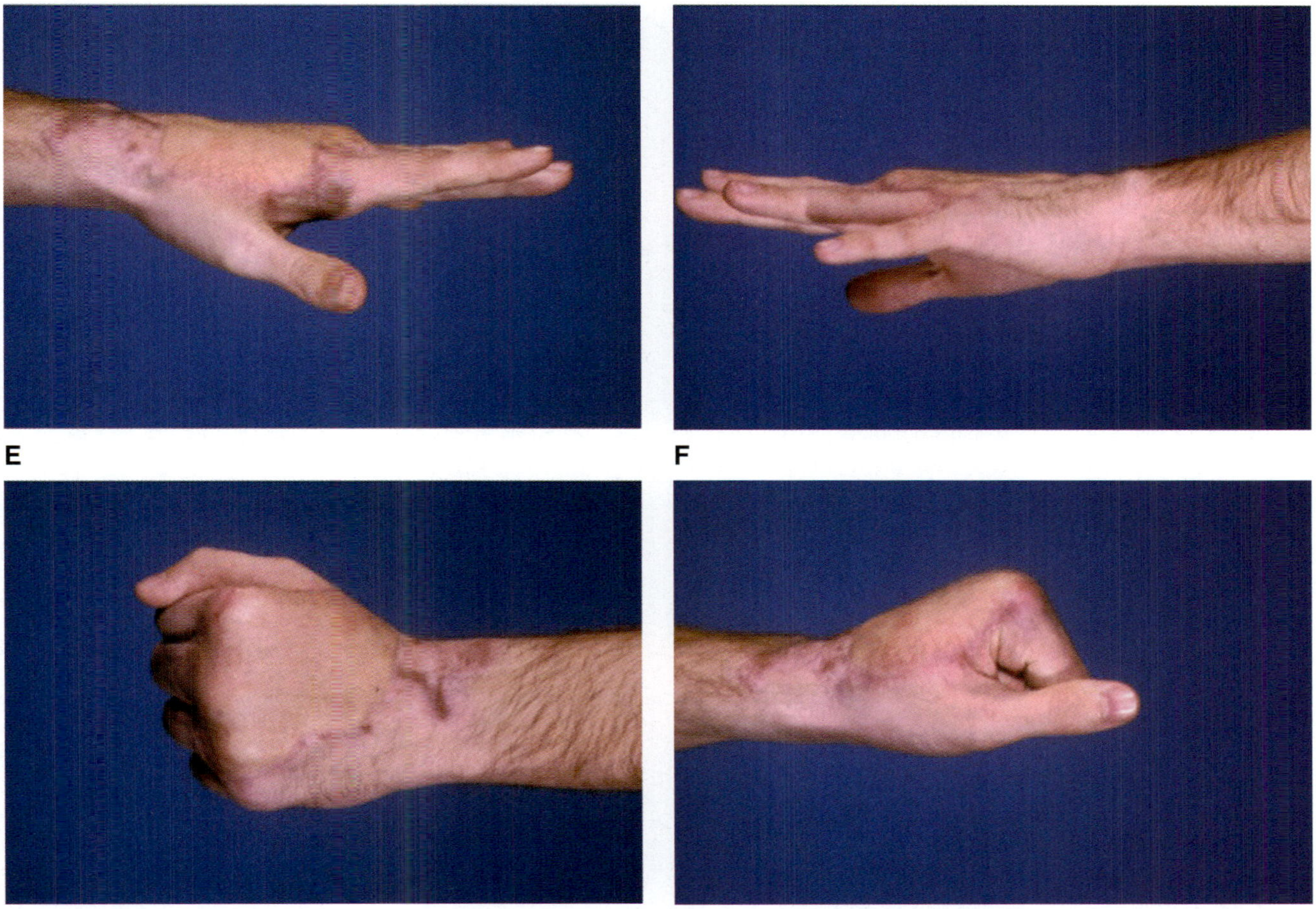

E F

G H

FIGURE 21-10 *(Continued)*

COMPARISON WITH SIMILAR FREE TISSUE TRANSFERS

Although the standard LAF was widely performed after its initial description, its use has declined over the years because of concerns regarding the donor site. In addition, newer fasciocutaneous flaps, namely the anterolateral thigh (ALT) flap, have surpassed the LAF and radial forearm flap in popularity. However, the ELAF is currently experiencing a resurgence as a potential alternative to the radial forearm flap.

The radial forearm flap is a thin, pliable flap that possesses a longer and larger pedicle than the LAF, making it a better

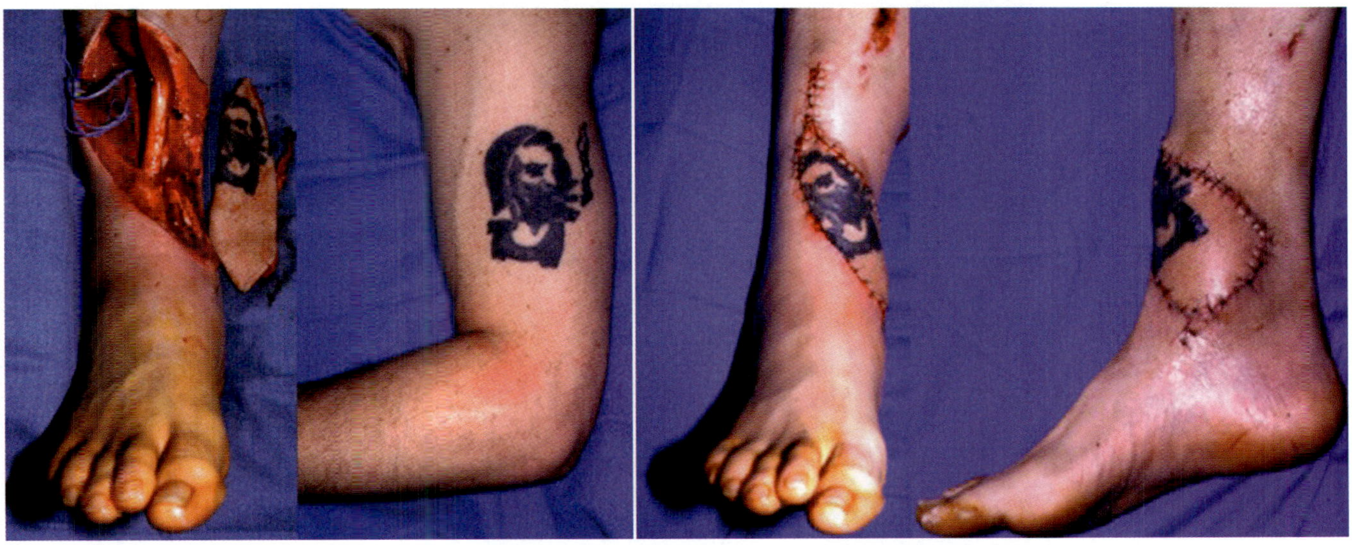

A B C D

FIGURE 21-11 Lower extremity reconstruction using a lateral arm flap from the contralateral arm.

option for many head and neck and lower extremity reconstructive surgeries. However, there is a growing concern that harvesting the radial artery with the radial forearm flap may result in cold intolerance and long-term digital ischemia (11), so some surgeons are turning to the ELAF as their flap of choice when they need a thin, pliable free flap. Even in obese patients, the skin overlying the lateral epicondyle is relatively thin, which is one of the major advantages of the ELAF compared with other fasciocutaneous flaps.

Another alternative is the ulnar forearm flap, which undoubtedly possesses some of the vascular concerns that the radial forearm flap does, if not more. One additional concern with the ulnar forearm flap is potential injury to the ulnar nerve during harvest. A flap that continues to gain popularity worldwide is the ALT flap, which is now the workhorse free flap for most reconstructive surgeons because of its fasciocutaneous nature, long pedicle, relatively low donor site morbidity, and ability to be thinned primarily. However, in Western countries especially, the ALT flap can be quite bulky in heavy patients, making it less ideal in certain situations.

Although the popularity of the LAF has declined over the years, the LAF and ELAF are still commonly performed. The anatomy of these flaps is constant, and the dissection is straightforward. Although the caliber of the vascular pedicle is relatively small, the pedicle is long, and pedicle size and length can be increased with more proximal dissection. Whereas the LAF is relatively thin in many patients, the ELAF is thin in almost all patients. In addition, the ability to harvest vascularized bone, tendon, or nerve with the flap makes the LAF and ELAF useful in various reconstructive scenarios. For these reasons, the LAF and ELAF continue to be two of the essential flaps in reconstructive microsurgery.

REFERENCES

1. Song R, Song Y, Yu Y, Song Y. The upper arm free flap. *Clin Plast Surg* 1982;9(1):27–35.
2. Cormack GC, Lamberty BG. Fasciocutaneous vessels in the upper arm: application to the design of new fasciocutaneous flaps. *Plast Reconstr Surg* 1984;74(2):244–250.
3. Katsaros J, Schusterman M, Beppu M, et al. The lateral upper arm flap: anatomy and clinical applications. *Ann Plast Surg* 1984;12(6):489–500.
4. Scheker LR, Kleinert HE, Hanel DP. Lateral arm composite tissue transfer to ipsilateral hand defects. *J Hand Surg Am* 1987;12(5 Pt 1):665–672.
5. Housif NJ, Warren R, Matloub HS, Sanger JR. The lateral arm fascial free flap: its anatomy and use in reconstruction. *Plast Reconstr Surg* 1990;86(6):1138–1145; discussion 1146–1147.
6. Moffett TR, Madison SA, Derr JW Jr, Acland RD. An extended approach for the vascular pedicle of the lateral arm free flap. *Plast Reconstr Surg* 1992;89(2):259–267.
7. Maruyama Y, Takeuchi S. The radial recurrent fasciocutaneous flap: reverse upper arm flap. *Br J Plast Surg* 1986;39(4):458–461.
8. Gosain AK, Matloub HS, Yousif NJ, Sanger JR. The composite lateral arm free flap: vascular relationship to triceps tendon and muscle. *Ann Plast Surg* 1992;29(6):496–507.
9. Katsaros J, Tan E, Zoltie N, et al. Further experience with the lateral arm free flap. *Plast Reconstr Surg* 1991;87(5):902–910.
10. Kuek LB, Chuan TL. The extended lateral arm flap: a new modification. *J Reconstr Microsurg* 1991;7(3):167–173.
11. Higgins JP. A reassessment of the role of the radial forearm flap in upper extremity reconstruction. *J Hand Surg Am* 2011;36(7):1237–1240.
12. Culbertson JH, Mutimer K. The reverse lateral upper arm flap for elbow coverage. *Ann Plast Surg* 1987;18(1):62–68.
13. Haas F, Rappl T, Koch H, et al. Free osteocutaneous lateral arm flap: anatomy and clinical applications. *Microsurgery* 2003;23(2):87–95.
14. Kuek LB. The extended lateral arm flap: a detailed anatomical study. *Ann Acad Med Singapore* 1992;21(2):169–175.
15. Shenaq SM. Pretransfer expansion of a sensate lateral arm free flap. *Ann Plast Surg* 1987;19(6):558–562.
16. Khouri RK, Young VL, Casoli VM. Long-term results of total penile reconstruction with a prefabricated lateral arm free flap. *J Urol* 1998;160(2):383–388.
17. Fogdestam I, Tarnow P, Kalaaji A. Extended free lateral arm flap with preservation of the posterior cutaneous nerve of the forearm. *Scand J Plast Reconstr Surg Hand Surg* 1996;30(1):49–55.

CHAPTER 22

The Temporoparietal Fascia Flap

William Swartz

The temporoparietal fascia (TPF) flap was first described by Monks (1), who used it for eyelid reconstruction in 1898, and has since been used extensively as a pedicled flap for the eyelid, coverage of ear cartilage, temporomandibular joint, and palate reconstruction.

It was first described as a free flap by R.A. Smith, who used it for lower extremity coverage (2). Its main attribute is that it is thin and pliable and easily supports skin grafts and tendon gliding. As a free flap, it has been used mostly for upper extremity coverage, particularly on the back of the hand and digits (3). Using it as a two-layered flap, tendons can be passed between the layers, thus allowing tendon gliding in the aponeurotic layer between the superficial and deep layers (4). Because it is thin and durable, it has been used for coverage of the Achilles tendon and malleoli of the foot and ankle. Another unique application is for provision of nasal lining in complex maxillofacial wounds. In each of these applications, thicker skin flaps would not be applicable.

ANATOMY

The TPF flap consists of two layers of fascia overlying the temporal region. The superficial fascia (TPF, epicranial aponeurosis) lies immediately deep to the hair follicles. It is a continuation of the subcutaneous musculoaponeurotic system (SMAS), which includes the orbicularis and frontalis muscles anteriorly. It continues as the galea above and SMAS layers of the face below the zygomatic arch. Yano et al. (5) consider this flap a thin muscle flap because of these relationships. Beneath the TPF, a loose areolar plane separates it from the deep temporal fascia, which invests the temporalis muscle and attaches to bone above and around the muscle. Inferiorly it attaches to the periosteum of the zygomatic arch (Figure 22-1).

The blood supply to both the superficial and deep layers is derived from the superficial temporal artery and vein, the terminal branches of the external carotid system. The vessels themselves are always found above the TPF. Above the zygomatic arch, the artery has a variable branching pattern. The most common is an anterior and posterior branches of roughly equal size, with minor variation (Figure 22-2).

The blood supply of the deep fascia is supplied by the middle temporal artery, a branch of the temporal artery, which consistently branches 1 to 3 cm below the arch and superficial to it. This vessel is best seen after reflecting the superficial fascia as it originates on the underside of the temporal artery. It enters the deep temporal fascia immediately above the fascia's attachment to the arch. This vascular arrangement gives opportunity for developing the flap in two layers.

The superficial temporal artery and vein lie just in front of the ear and may be dissected through the tail of the parotid gland. The diameter of the superficial temporal artery ranges from 0.8 to 2.1 mm, and the vein is consistently greater than 2.0 mm. The pedicle length can be up to 8 cm; however, 3 to 5 cm is more common. The flap size may be up to 14 by 12 cm or 8 by 10 cm for the deep fascia.

The temporal branch of the facial nerve lies in the anterior most extent of the TPF flap dissection. Its course is deep to the TPF and is at risk in this area (Figure 22-3).

TECHNIQUE OF ELEVATION

The dissection is started through a preauricular incision extended superiorly as a T or Y within the hair-bearing scalp. The level of dissection is just below the hair follicles. The course of the superficial temporal artery is mapped with the Doppler to identify its course in the scalp and its major branches. Lidocaine with epinephrine is injected to facilitate dissection and minimize bleeding. Use of the needle-tipped electrocautery permits near bloodless surgery and minimizes damage to hair follicles. Numerous small blood vessels to the scalp are cauterized using the bipolar device, making the dissection somewhat tedious. After the hair-bearing scalp is elevated, the superficial

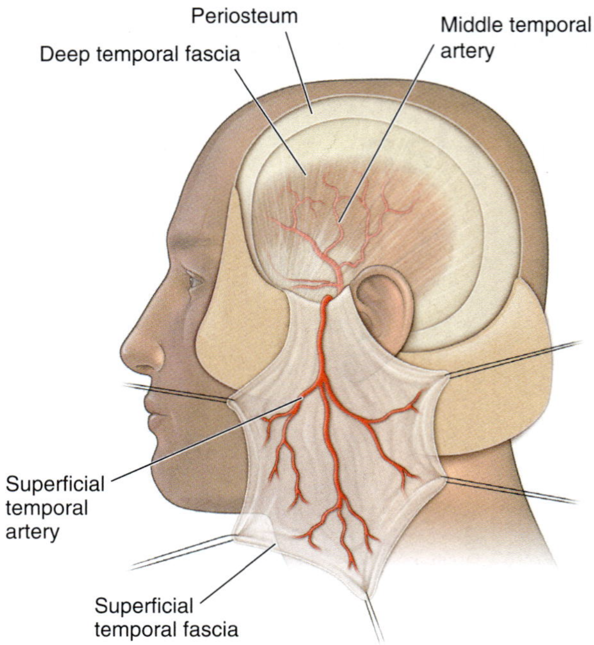

FIGURE 22-1 Temporoparietal fascia and its related anatomy. The fascia is composed of both a superficial and a deep layer supplied by the superficial temporal artery and vein.

fascia is incised around the periphery based on required flap dimensions and then elevated in a retrograde fashion toward the flap base at the zygoma. This is readily accomplished because an avascular plane exists between the TPF and the deep temporal fascia. The dissection then proceeds to isolate the superficial temporal artery and vein below the zygomatic arch. If a second layer of tissue is desired, the deep temporal fascia is then dissected from the underlying temporal muscle. This fascia attaches directly to the pericranium around its periphery and is also dissected from peripheral to central. The deep temporal artery must not be divided during the proximal dissection. Finally, the superficial and deep fascias are detached from the zygomatic arch, and the vessels are dissected proximally until they are of sufficient size for microsurgical anastomosis. Proximal branches of the superficial temporal artery maybe ligated to extend the pedicle length.

Endoscopic dissection of this flap has been described whereby a preauricular incision is used for access of the endoscope permitting dissection of the flap from beneath the hair follicles. A second incision at the distal extension of the flap permits access to the peripheral dissection. The superficial temporal fascia is readily elevated endoscopically in the areolar plane. The authors advocate this technique to reduce donor scar morbidity and increase patient acceptance of this flap. They report no alopecia and one temporary frontal branch palsy in

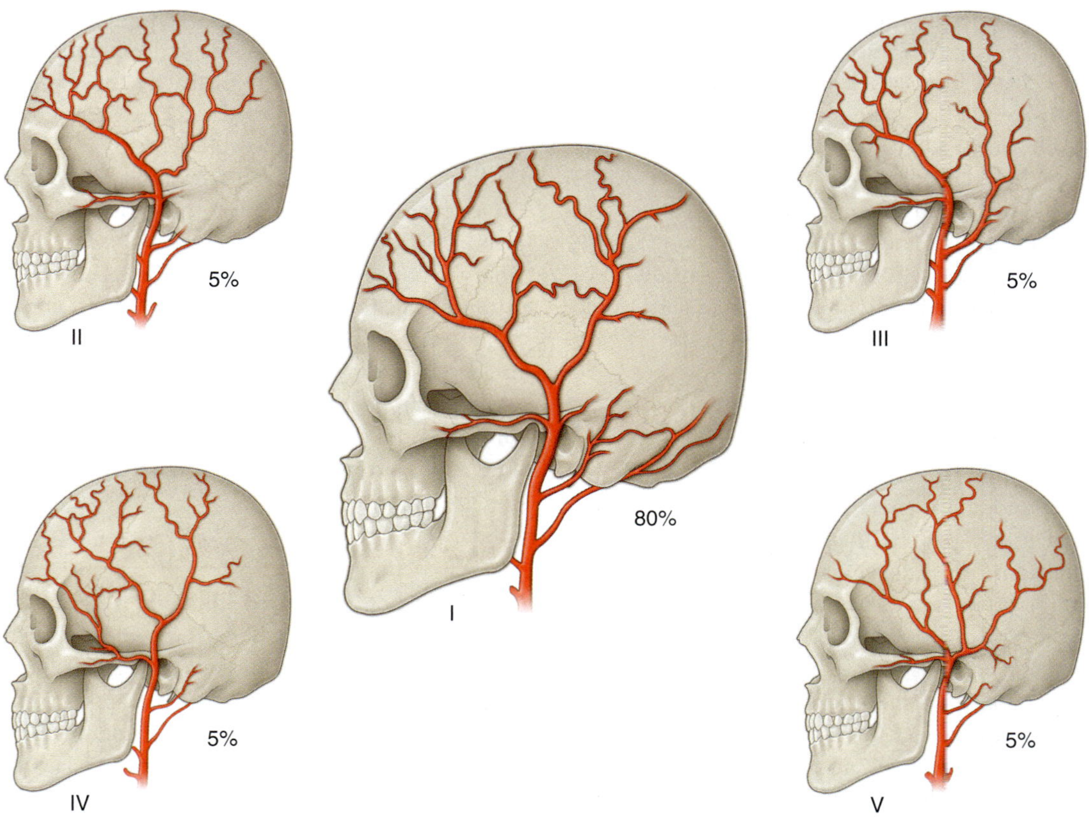

FIGURE 22-2 Vascular anatomy of the temporoparietal fascia flap. The superficial temporal artery arborizes into anterior, central, and posterior branches distal to the zygomatic arch. A deep branch at the arch supplies the deep fascia layer.

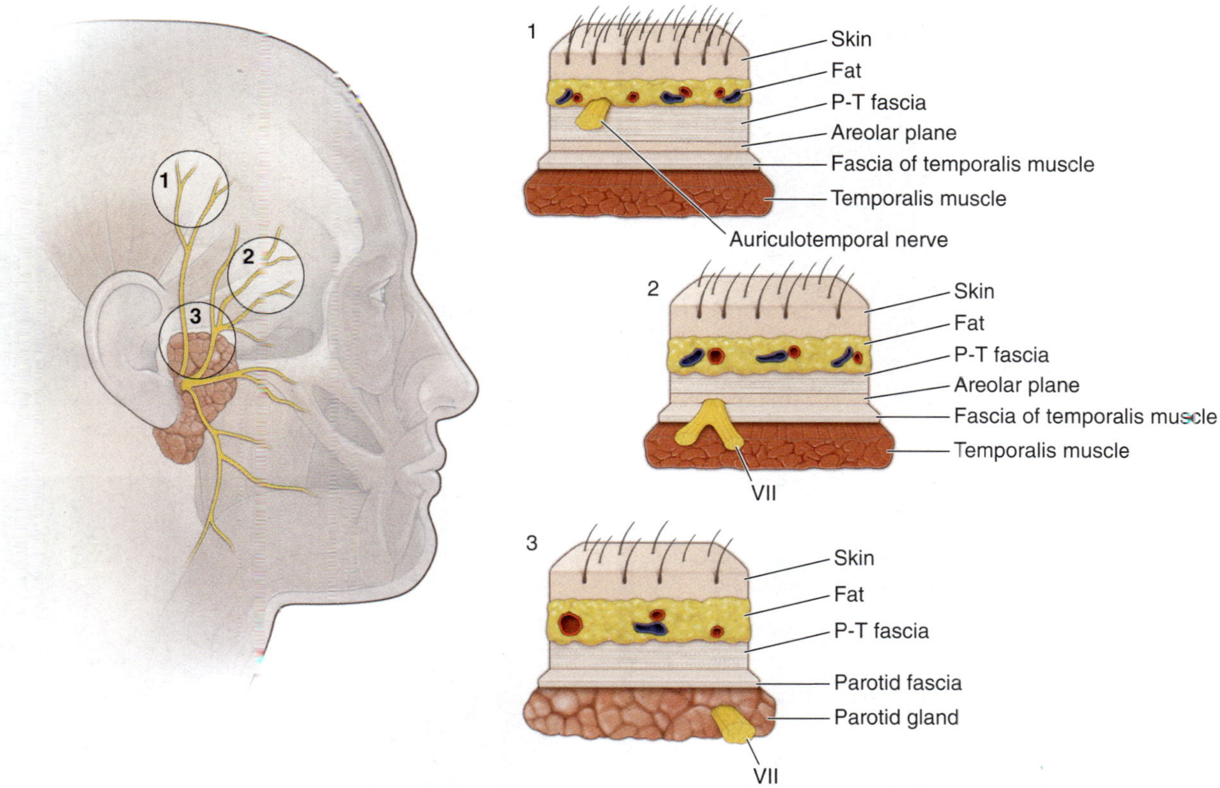

FIGURE 22-3 Anatomy of the facial nerve. The facial nerve emerges from deep to parotid gland at the stylomastoid foramen to a plane of areolar tissue between the fascia of the temporalis muscle and the more superficial temporoparietal fascia above the zygomatic arch.

five patients reported (6). Chung et al. reported endoscopic harvest of the flap without placing the second scar in the hair-bearing scalp through a limited incision in the preauricular area only. In their technique, they used scissors connected to electrocautery to minimize bleeding in the layer between the fascia and hair-bearing scalp. Endoscopic harvest took less than 1 hour in the latter cases of their series. No patients experienced alopecia or frontal branch injury (7). This technique would be most appropriate in patients whose hair pattern would make a scalp scar otherwise unacceptable.

CLOSURE OF THE DONOR SITE

The donor site incisions are closed over a suction drain using interrupted sutures or staples. Buried sutures tend to place hair follicles at risk for alopecia and should be avoided.

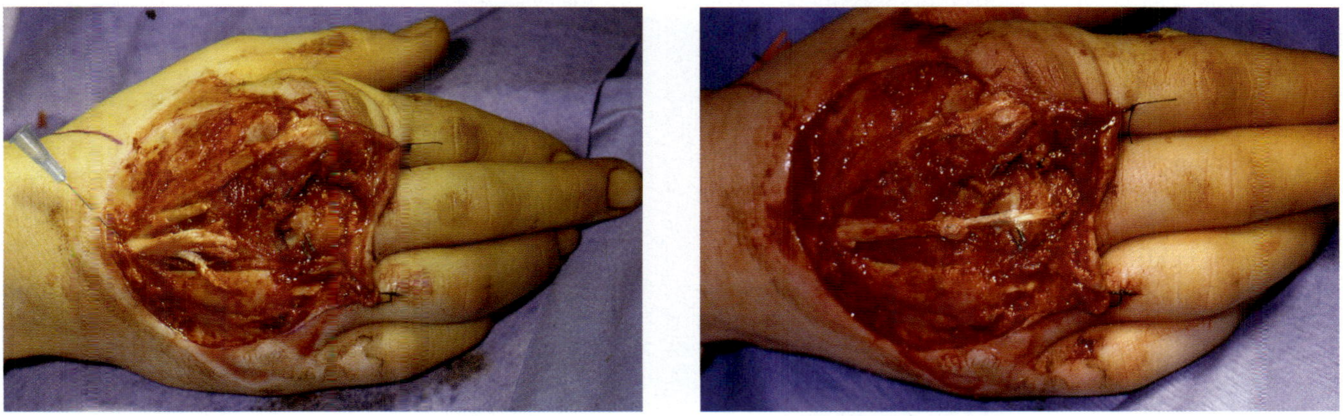

A B

FIGURE 22-4 A 23-year-old woman with a crush injury of the hand involving loss of the dorsal skin, tendon avulsions, and metacarpal fracture. (**A**) Debrided wound. The third metacarpal fracture is pinned with K-wires. (**B**) Extensor tendons repaired and grafted. (**C**) The temporoparietal flap elevated. The temporal artery and vein are isolated at the level of the tragus. (**D**) The skin graft placed on the temporoparietal fascia; the fascia was split to isolate the tendon graft from the fracture. (**E**) and (**F**) Early active range of motion.

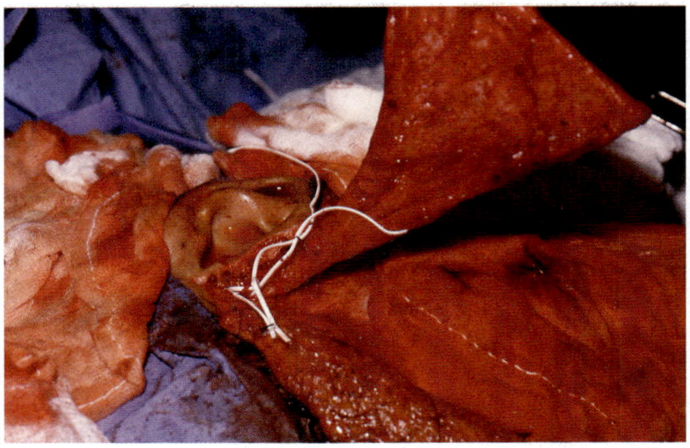

C

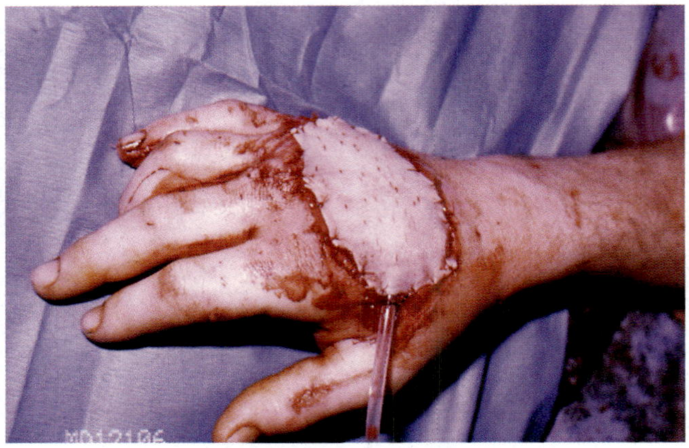

D

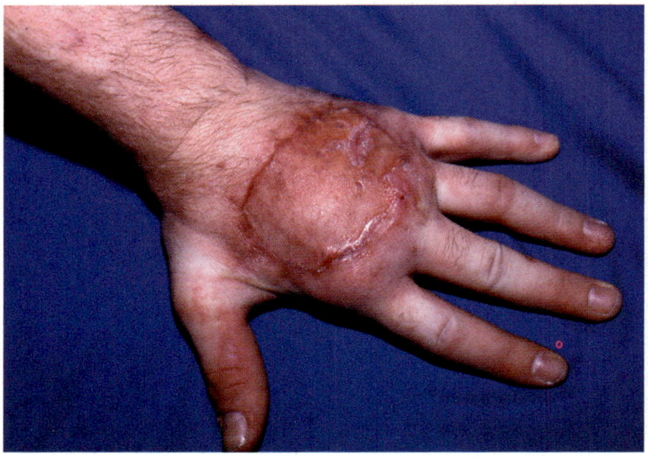

E

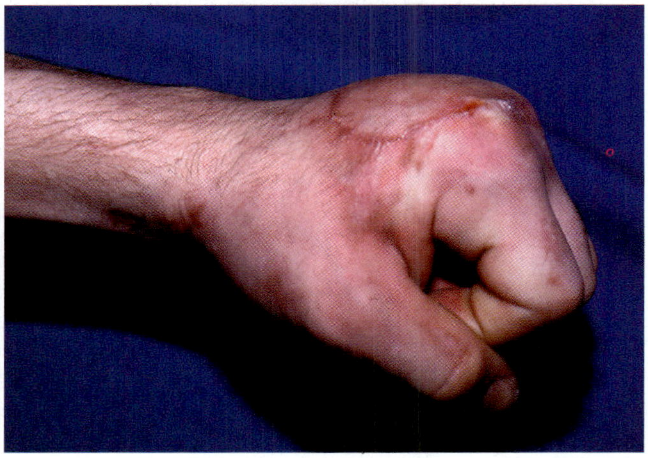

F

FIGURE 22-4 *(Continued)*

DONOR SITE COMPLICATION

The most common complication of TPF harvest is alopecia. This can be avoided by judicious use of electrocautery. This author prefers a needle-tipped cautery for dissection and bipolar coagulation for larger vessels. In long-haired individuals, the scar can be hidden, but in persons with short hair, the scar can be objectionable. Endoscopic harvest should be considered in special cases.

A second complication is injury to the frontal branch of the facial nerve. Care should be taken to end the anterior dissection well behind the known course of this structure. A nerve stimulator is useful in identifying the nerve at the level of the zygomatic arch and lateral orbital rim. Where larger flaps are desired, the incorporation of fascia posteriorly is preferable and safer than extending the flap anteriorly.

REFERENCES

1. Monks G. Restoration of a lower eyelid by a new method. *Boston Med J* 1898;139:385–387.
2. Smith RA. The free fascia scalp flap. *Plast Reconstr Surg* 1980;66:204.
3. Upton J, Rogers C, Durham-Smith G, Swartz W. Clinical applications of free temporoparietal flaps in hand reconstruction. *J Hand Surg* 1986;11(suppl A):475–483.
4. Biswas G, Dip NB, Ishwar L, Padmanabha S. The sandwich temporoparietal fascia free flap for tendon gliding. *Plast Reconstr Surg* 2001;108(6):1639–1645.
5. Yano H, Nishimura G, Kaji S, Murakami R, and Fujii A Clinical and histological comparison between free temporoparietal and scapular fascial flaps. Plast Reconstr Surg 1995;95:452-462.
6. Yano H, Fukui M, Yamada K, Nishimura G. Endoscopic harvest of a free temporoparietal fascia free flap to improve donor site morbidity. *Plast Reconstr Surg* 2001;107:1003–1008.
7. Chung K, Cederna P. Endoscopic harvest of temporoparietal fascia free flaps for coverage of hand wounds. *J Hand Surgery* 2002;27(suppl A): 525–533.

CHAPTER 23

Enteric and Omental Flaps

Albert H. Chao, Michael J. Miller, and Peirong Yu

The abdominal cavity is an abundant source of tissue for reconstructive surgery. Portions of the stomach, small intestine, colon, and omentum may be used for a variety of soft tissue restorations. In fact, the first clinical free tissue transfer involved the small bowel and was reported by Seidenberg et al. in 1959 (1). Intraabdominal tissue harvest offers advantages in certain circumstances and with minimal functional morbidity or deforming scars. Currently, the greater omentum and small bowel are the most useful intraabdominal flaps. This chapter focuses on these two donor tissues with particular focus on indications, patient preparation, anatomy, technique of flap harvest, method of inset, postoperative patient care, and how to manage possible complications.

THE OMENTAL FLAP

History

The greater omentum was first used in surgery in the 19th century to reinforce intestinal repairs (2) and to treat portal hypertension. O'Shaughnessy (3) first reported extraperitoneal reconstruction in 1937 using pedicle omental flaps to revascularize ischemic myocardium. Thompson and Pollock (4) later reported using it to treat bronchopleural fistula. Over the years, it has proven useful as a pedicled flap for a variety of soft tissue problems of the chest and abdominal wall. The first microsurgical transfer of the omentum was reported by McLean and Buncke in 1972 (5). They used an omental free flap in a 29-year-old man to cover a large scalp defect after tumor resection. Microvascular surgery extended the application of the omentum to reconstruction on the head and neck and extremities. The omentum has many favorable characteristics that support its continued use: large surface area and volume, malleability, rich blood supply, immunologic and angiogenic properties, long pedicle length, large-diameter vessels, predictable anatomy, and low donor site morbidity. The primary disadvantages are the need for a laparotomy and the requirement for skin grafting on exposed surfaces, which can result in an irregular contour and poor color match depending on the location. With the development of other flap options, the omentum is most often considered a secondary tissue source today, especially as a free flap. Nevertheless, it remains an important option, and reconstructive microsurgeons should be comfortable using it.

Anatomy

The omentum is composed of two distinct parts, the greater and lesser omentum. The lesser omentum extends from the liver to the lesser curvature of the stomach and first part of the duodenum. It is not used in reconstructive surgery; only the greater omentum has relevance as a flap donor tissue.

The greater omentum is a large sheetlike structure composed primarily of adipose tissue on a supporting fibrovascular framework. It stores fat and provides mechanical protection to the viscera. It also contains a rich network of lymphatic tissue with characteristic "milky spots" composed of numerous macrophage and lymphocyte aggregations that act as a first line of immune defense for the peritoneal cavity. Topologically, the greater omentum is a double sheet of peritoneum. The anterior leaf attaches to the greater curvature of the stomach, proximal duodenum, and gastrosplenic ligament. It drapes a variable distance anterior to the small and large intestines and then folds onto the posterior leaf, which ascends to join the antimesenteric border of the transverse colon and gastrocolic ligament.

The greater omentum has a well-characterized vascular anatomy with a type III blood supply, according to the Mathes and Nahai classification (6). The right and left gastroepiploic arteries provide two dominant pedicles and either may be used to transfer the flap (Figure 23-1). These vessels course within the anterior leaf of the omentum approximately 1.5 cm inferior to the greater curvature of the stomach. The right gastroepiploic

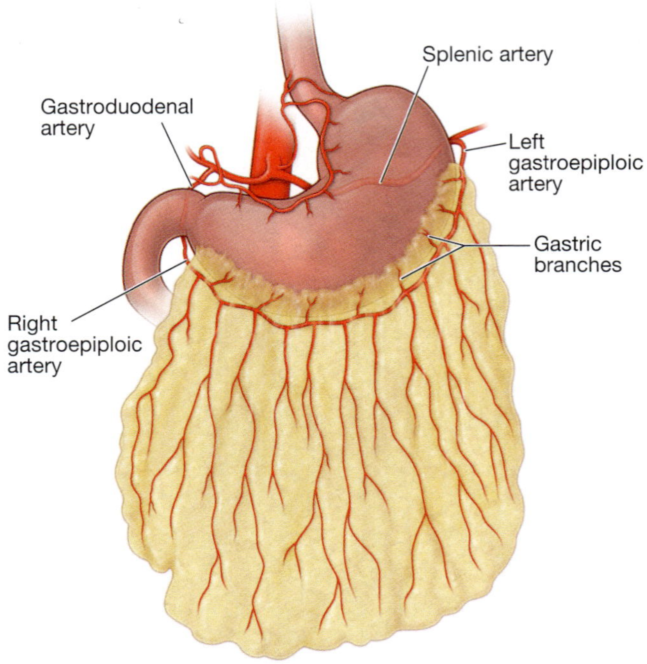

FIGURE 23-1 Anatomy of the greater omentum. The vascular pedicle of the flap is the right or left gastroepiploic artery.

artery originates from the gastroduodenal artery and travels from right to left along the greater curvature of the stomach. The left gastroepiploic artery originates from the splenic artery and runs from left to right along the greater curvature. They join together to form one large, continuous vessel. At its origin, the right gastroepiploic artery generally has a slightly larger diameter (~2–3 mm) compared with the left (~2 mm). Venous anatomy mirrors the arterial except that the right gastroepiploic vein is a branch of the superior mesenteric vein. These are large vessels that are well suited to microvascular tissue transfer.

Within the omentum, there are three major arteries that arise from the gastroepiploic vessels and course inferiorly. These are the right, left, and middle omental arteries. The middle artery terminally bifurcates and joins the other two, forming a distal arcade. This arrangement allows the omentum to be lengthened and folded to accommodate various defects and facilitate pedicled transfer to more distant locations.

Variations

There are few natural variations in the basic anatomy, but different patterns can occur in the vascular arcades depending on the level of terminal bifurcation of the middle omental artery (7). In some patients, the middle artery can be absent altogether. If plans include lengthening of the flap or harvesting a portion of the omentum only, the specific anatomy of the individual patient must be confirmed. Acquired variations can be encountered secondary to previous surgery or bouts of intraabdominal inflammation, which cause scaring, contraction, adherence, and loss of volume. By carefully dividing adhesions, the omentum can usually be unfolded and separated from the peritoneal linings of the abdominal wall, viscera, mesenteries, and itself. The amount of tissue available can vary greatly based on the patient's body habitus and history. Because of its dual blood supply and the vascular pattern within the omentum, the flap may also be harvested segmentally using only the right or left half. Furthermore, because the right and left gastroepiploic arteries form essentially a single large vessel, a flow-through flap can be designed. Finally, a portion of the greater curvature of the stomach can be harvested with the omentum, the gastro-omental flap, for pharyngoesophageal reconstruction.

Flap Dissection

Harvesting the greater omentum may be performed through either an endoscopic or open approach. In each case, a nasogastric tube and urinary catheter are placed first. Although recommended by some, a bowel preparation is generally not necessary. The endoscopic approach is based on conventional minimally invasive techniques (8,9). For patients in whom a strictly endoscopic approach might be unfavorable (e.g., previous abdominal surgery), an endoscopic-assisted approach can be considered. This combines a limited laparotomy with minimally invasive techniques.

Open harvest of the greater omentum is most common and begins with an upper midline laparotomy incision. The omentum is usually encountered immediately upon entering the abdomen. If the patient has had previous abdominal surgery, it will likely be adherent to the anterior abdominal wall or viscera or even incarcerated in small ventral hernias. This does not render the omentum unusable, but adhesions must be carefully taken down to preserve the integrity of the blood supply to the omentum. After being identified and freed, it is first reflected cranially to expose the attachments of the posterior leaf to the transverse colon. These are taken down to isolate the omentum on the anterior attachments to the greater curvature of the stomach, the first portion of the duodenum, and gastrosplenic ligament (Figure 23-2).

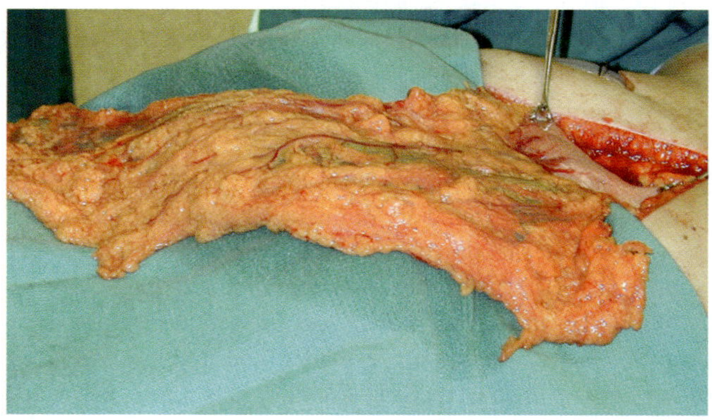

FIGURE 23-2 The posterior leaf of the omentum is detached from the transverse colon. The greater omentum is now isolated on the anterior attachments to the greater curvature of the stomach. The flap is more commonly based on the right gastroepiploic vessels. The omentum is then taken down from the stomach starting from the left side.

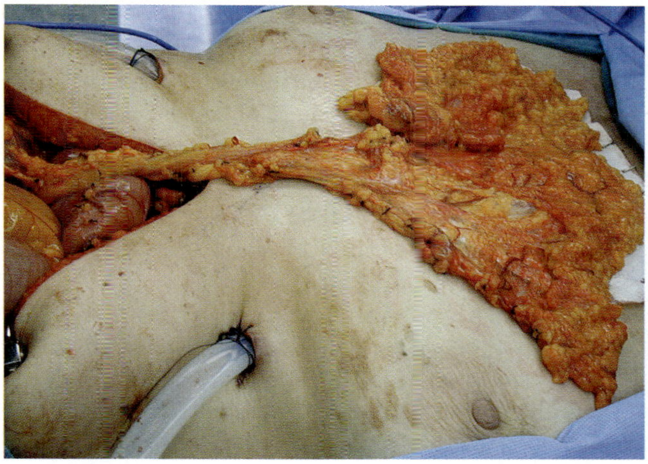

FIGURE 23-3 The omental flap is now completely islanded based on the right gastroepiploic vessels and pulled up to the chest.

When used as a pedicled flap, the omentum can be raised on either the right or left gastroepiploic vessels. The flap is more commonly based on the right gastroepiploic vessels (Figure 23-3). The left gastroepiploic artery and vein are ligated and divided immediately distal to their takeoff from the splenic vessels. The dissection proceeds along the greater curve of the stomach, ligating each short gastric branch between the stomach and the gastroepiploic arcade (Figure 23-4). If it is preferable to base the flap on the left side, then the right gastroepiploic vessels are ligated just proximal to the pylorus, and the dissection proceeds from right to left. All of these vessels are high flow, and it is essential to meticulously control them to avoid serious intraabdominal bleeding complications after surgery. After complete isolation of the flap and preparation of the recipient site, the flap pedicle is ligated, and the tissue is transferred to the defect for reconstruction.

For thoracic defects, a pedicled omental flap may be transferred either via a transdiaphragmatic route or through a subcutaneous tunnel. A transdiaphragmatic approach can reduce the chance of developing an epigastric hernia, but diaphragmatic hernias may also occur. The xyphoid is usually resected, and a small portion of the anterior diaphragm immediately below the xyphoid is opened to allow the omental flap to be pulled through. The diaphragmatic defect is closed with heavy Prolene sutures to minimize the risk of diaphragmatic hernia but not to strangulate the vascular pedicle. Except when buried, split-thickness skin grafting of the omentum is usually required (Figure 23-5).

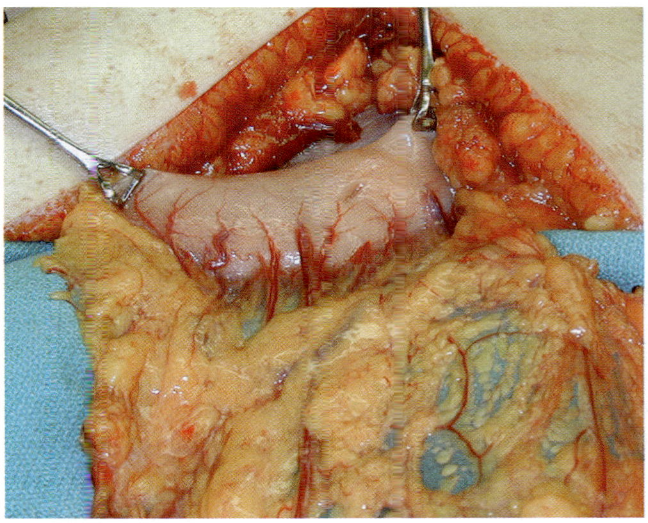

FIGURE 23-4 The short gastric branches between the stomach and the gastroepiploic vessels are ligated and divided. Great care should be taken to secure these vessels to prevent intraabdominal hemorrhage after surgery.

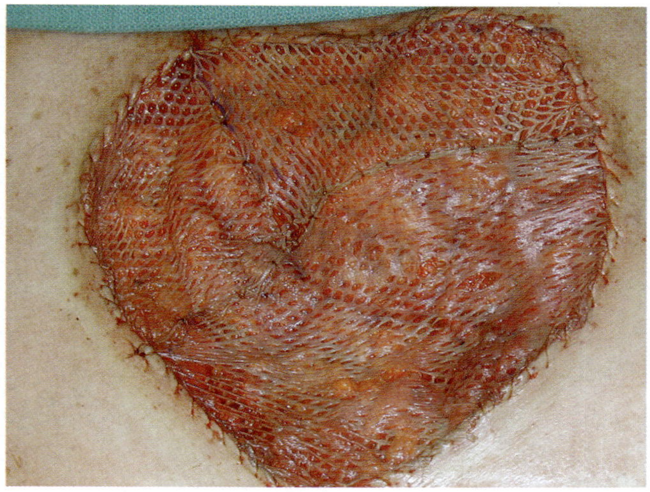

FIGURE 23-5 Unless the omental flap is buried, skin grafting is usually required.

Tricks and Tips

Successful reconstruction using the omentum requires thoughtful patient selection, matching the reconstructive requirements to the anticipated amount and type of tissue available. If possible, avoid using it in a setting of previous abdominal surgery or history of significant episodes of inflammation (e.g., diverticulitis, perforated viscus). Anticipate anatomic variations when planning to lengthen the flap. Use a fiberoptic light source to transilluminate the tissue, identifying the location of the omental arteries and arcades before fashioning the flap. For microvascular transfer, harvest the flap based on the right gastroepiploic vessels. They are usually larger in caliber and less hazardous to dissect because they are not in proximity to the spleen. When the omental flap is used for posterior trunk defects, mobilization of the colon from its retroperitoneal position is usually necessary to deliver the flap to the recipient site. Work with a general abdominal surgeon to harvest the flap unless you have a good background and experience working in the abdominal cavity, especially if there has been previous abdominal surgery. For sternal wound reconstruction, care should be taken to ensure that the bony edges of the lower sternum are smoothened out with a burr to prevent injury to the vascular pedicle (Figure 23-6).

Donor Site

The laparotomy incision is closed in standard fashion. Ventral hernia is a recognized morbidity after omental flap harvest that

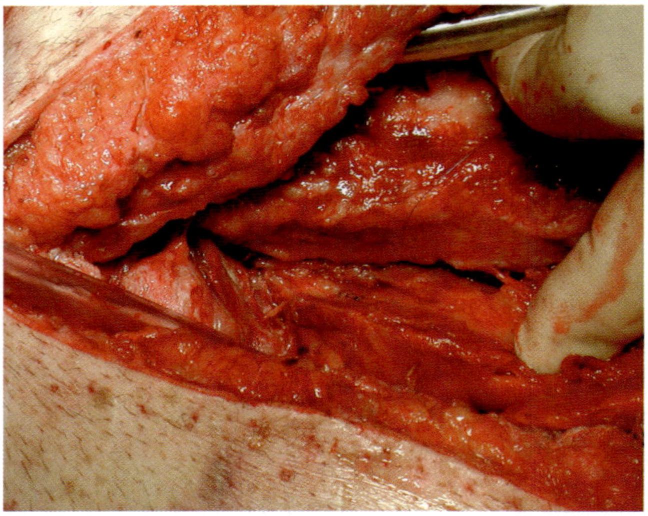

FIGURE 23-6 In this case, the omental flap was used for sternal wound reconstruction. The sharp deep edge of the sternum caused laceration of the pedicle artery and postoperative hemorrhage. Therefore, the sharp edges of the sternum should be buried down to prevent such vascular injury.

can occur at a rate as high as 21%, especially when the flap is transferred subcutaneously. Laparoscopic harvest may help to reduce this risk. Abdominal wall infections occur not infrequently, and standard sequelae of intraabdominal surgery such as ileus or obstruction may occur. Given the important role of the omentum as a peritoneal defense organ, potential physiologic morbidity has also been investigated and thought not to be significant, although only limited studies in small animal models have been performed.

Indications

Careful patient selection is essential. The type and amount of tissue expected from the omentum should be anticipated and matched to the reconstructive needs.

Pedicled Omental Flap

The single most common indication for a pedicled omental flap is sternal wound reconstruction. These wounds are usually complications from heart surgery but have become less common in recent years. After several surgical debridements, the wound is reconstructed with well-vascularized tissue. The upper middle sternal wound can also be reconstructed with pedicled pectoralis major muscle flaps. The lower sternal wound can be reconstructed with a pedicled rectus abdominis muscle flap. For a sternal wound that involves the entire sternum, however, the omental flap can be a good option to cover the entire wound (Figure 23-7). In addition, the omentum is more malleable than a muscle flap and can be used to fill small dead spaces.

Other indications for a pedicled omental flap include pelvic, abdominal, and back defects (10,11). For abdominal wall defects, the omental flap is typically combined with mesh and can be positioned either on the underside or the superficial surface by tunneling it through a separate opening. In the pelvis, the omentum may be used to fill the pelvic dead space after a pelvic exenteration, to reconstruct the pelvic floor or vagina, as an interposition for the treatment of fistulas, and in the management of perineal wounds. Although it can extend to the posterior trunk and proximal lower extremity, this is most often done in salvage situations because other more suitable local options usually exist for those sites.

Free Omental Flap

As a free tissue transfer, the omental flap is most often used for defects of the scalp and upper extremity, where its properties as a thin and malleable flap are particularly valuable (12–14). It can also be used to cover radiation-induced brachial plexus injury (Figure 23-8) after breast cancer treatment. It has been shown that microvascular omental transfer after neurolysis is most effective in treating these lesions (15). By including part of the greater curvature of the stomach, the gastro-omental flap has been used to reconstruct defects of the upper aerodigestive tract, such as pharyngoesophageal defects, especially when concurrent intraoral or cervical skin resurfacing is necessary (16).

THE JEJUNAL FLAPS

History

Clinical reconstructive microvascular surgery began with the use of enteric flaps in the head and neck. This era was foreshadowed in 1947 when Longmire (17) modified the Roux technique of pedicled bowel transfer for esophageal reconstruction. He augmented the blood supply of the distal bowel by anastomosing a mesenteric vessel to the internal mammary artery. The concept was extended to complete revascularization of the transferred tissue with pioneering work conducted on free intestinal transfers in animals. Finally, in 1959, Seidenberg et al. (1) reported the first clinical case of a free jejunal transfer performed for esophageal reconstruction. This was actually the first free tissue transfer performed in humans. Several more successful jejunal flap reconstructions were reported in the 1960s (18–20). Although these early reports demonstrated a possibility of this technique, the lack of proper magnification, microsurgical instruments, and sutures severely limited its use until the 1980s. The free jejunal flap enjoyed its popularity since early 1980s and became the workhorse flap for pharyngoesophageal reconstruction in many centers (21–29).

Segments of jejunum may be transferred in two ways. Individual isolated units based on a single mesenteric arcade are referred to as free jejunal transfers. Free jejunal flaps, which are often used in cases of hypopharyngeal and cervical esophageal carcinoma, are limited to partial esophageal defects because of the segmental blood supply. When the esophageal defect is greater than 20 cm, another reconstructive option must be used because each mesenteric vessel only supplies up to 20 cm of jejunum (30–32). The jejunal flap must therefore be based on multiple arcades with some vessels pedicled from the superior mesenteric artery (SMA) and vein and some revascularized using microsurgery.

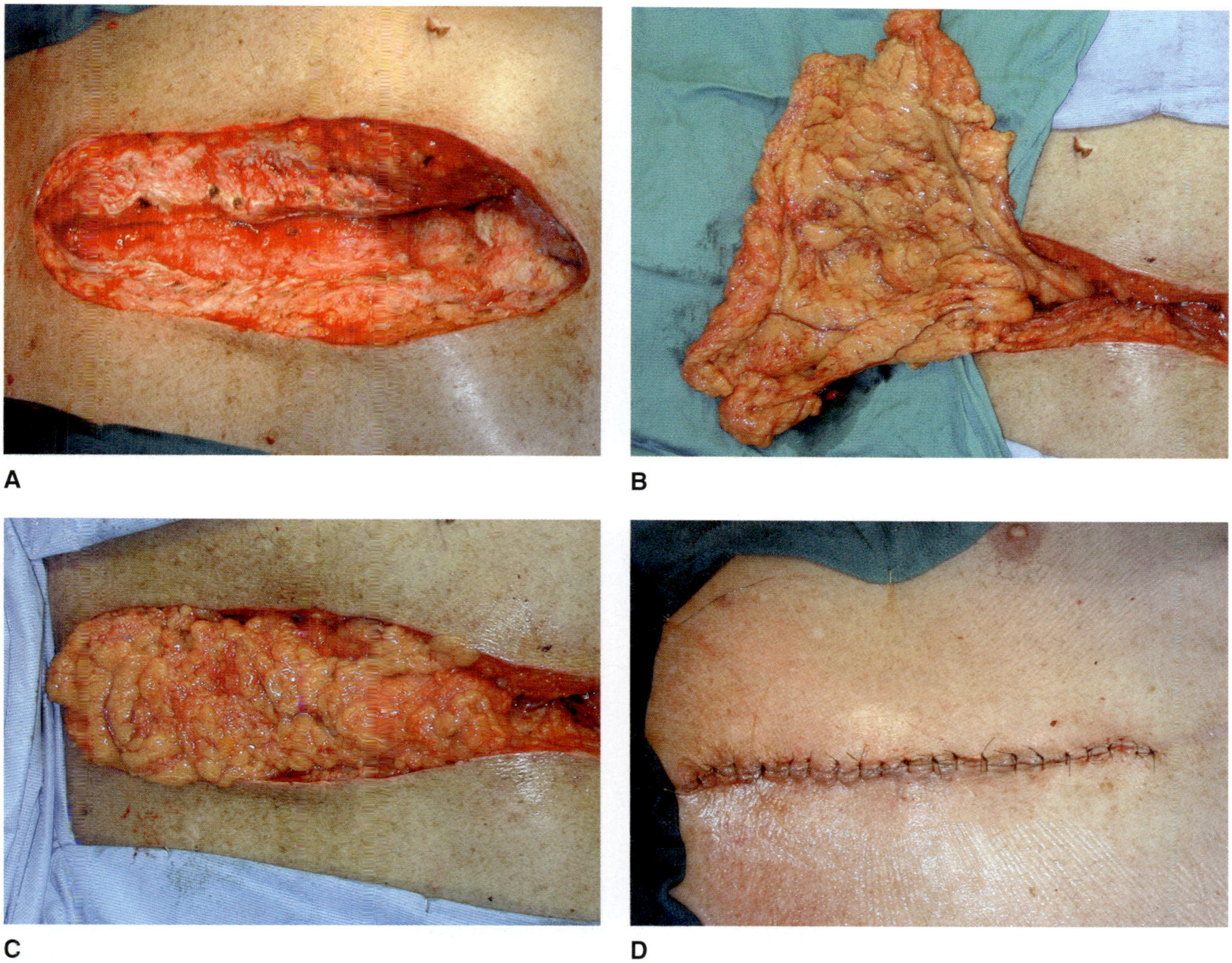

FIGURE 23-7 The most common indication for a pedicled omental flap is a full-length sternal wound after heart surgery. Serial debridement is performed before definitive reconstruction (**A**). The omental flap is elevated based on the right gastroepiploic vessels and pulled up to the chest wound through a small incision in the anterior diaphragm below the xyphoid (**B**). The flap covers the entire sternal wound completely (**C**). The flap is buried and the incision closed primarily (**D**).

The addition of microsurgical techniques has allowed for the replacement of the entire esophagus using longer conduits through "supercharging." Longmire described the first supercharged jejunal flap for esophageal reconstruction in 1947 (17). Since then, the field of microsurgery has advanced significantly, and the use of these techniques has become more widespread, making the supercharged jejunal flap a viable option for total esophageal reconstruction when the stomach is unavailable (33–37).

Anatomy

The small intestine consists of the duodenum, jejunum, and ileum. In adults, it measures approximately 22 to 23 feet in length and functions primarily in digestion and absorption of enteric contents. The duodenum is the first and shortest segment, which directly follows the stomach and transitions into the jejunum at the ligament of Treitz. No distinct line of demarcation distinguishes the jejunum from the ileum, although the ileum tends to contain more mesenteric fat and have a smaller caliber than the jejunum. The jejunum and ileum are suspended from the posterior wall of the abdomen by mesentery, which allows them to move freely within the abdominopelvic cavity.

The small intestine receives its blood supply from the SMA, with the exception of the duodenum, whose proximal portion is supplied by the gastroduodenal artery. The SMA originates from the abdominal aorta, anterior to L1 and approximately 1 cm inferior to the takeoff of the celiac artery. From there, it proceeds inferiorly, passing behind the neck of the pancreas and the splenic vein, before giving rise to several jejunal and ileal arteries (also termed mesenteric branches), which run in parallel to each other within the layers of the mesentery (Figure 23-9). As they travel toward the small intestine, the jejunal and ileal arteries divide into branches, which possess anastomoses with adjacent branches to form a series of arterial arcades. The collateral flow conferred by these anastomoses is the basis for the ability to divide select mesenteric branches without causing ischemia. The venous drainage of the small intestine occurs through the superior mesenteric vein, which

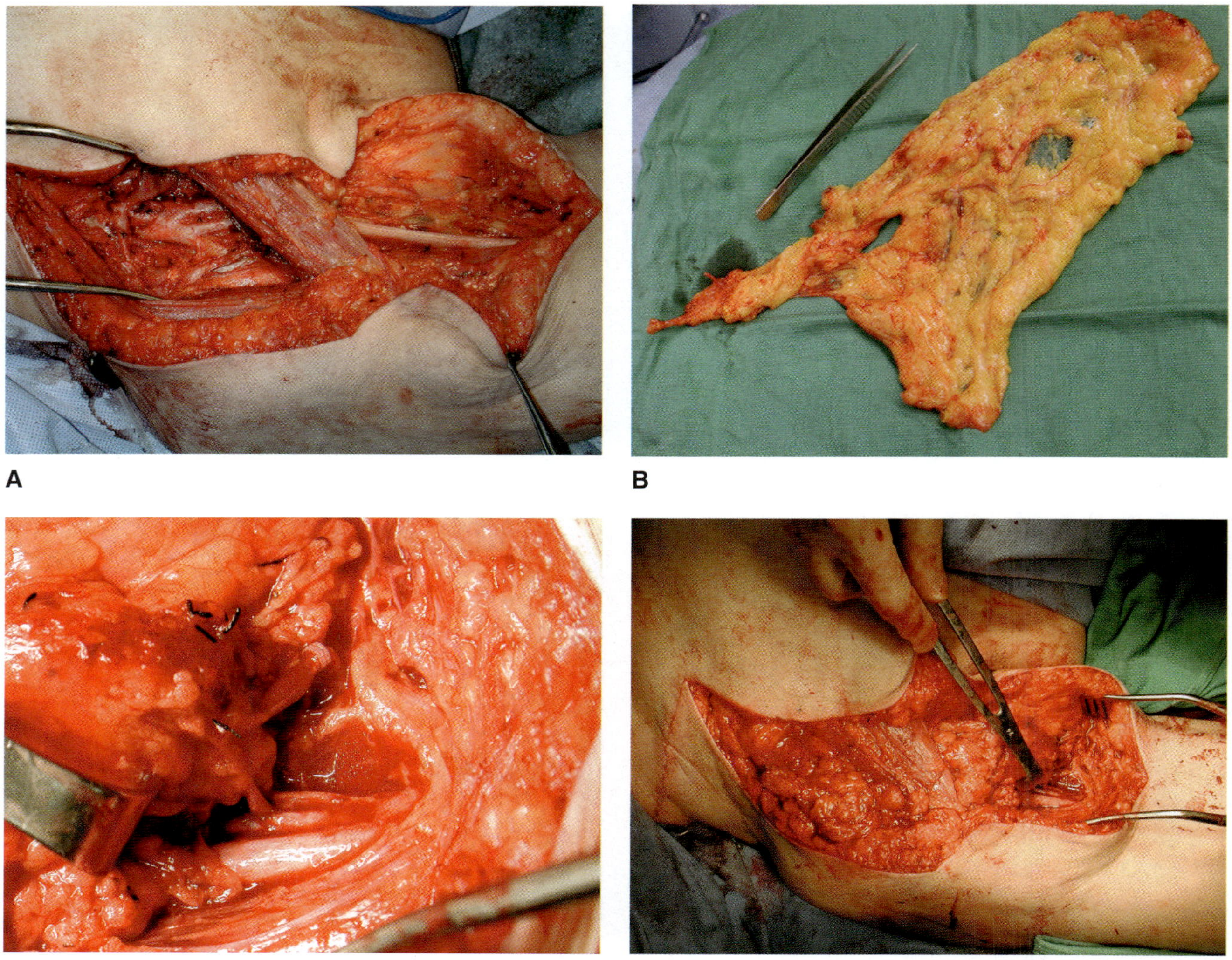

A B C D

FIGURE 23-8 Radiation injury to the brachial plexus after breast cancer treatment (**A**). A small segment of the omentum was harvested (**B**). The omental flap was transferred to the axilla as free flap (**C**) and covers the brachial plexus nicely (**D**).

ultimately joins the splenic vein to empty into the portal system.

Patient Preparation

Informed consent involves some special considerations. Jejunal flaps are used to reestablish alimentary tract continuity. Leaks and strictures might occur as well as functional swallowing difficulties. The possible donor site complications are essentially the same as with any intraabdominal surgery involving a small bowel resection with gastrostomy and jejunostomy feeding tube placements.

Preoperative assessment includes evaluation of the patient's cardiopulmonary, renal, and nutritional status. The age of many cancer patients is often in the sixth and seventh decades, an age group with a high incidence of concomitant cardiovascular disease and renal disease. In addition to common preoperative screening tests such as a complete blood count and chemistry profile, chest radiograph, and electrocardiogram, it is often advisable to obtain pulmonary function tests, cardiac stress test, and a nutritional assessment (including total serum protein, albumin, and transferrin). If the patient is malnourished, preoperative nutritional therapy is indicated. Each of these areas should be optimized if possible before surgery. A multidisciplinary team approach is preferred with each area addressed. In addition, the patient is seen preoperatively by the speech therapist in anticipation of future rehabilitation if a laryngectomy is to be performed.

Surgical Preparation

On the day before surgery, the patient is asked to consume only liquids. A mechanical bowel preparation is ordered, which may consist of magnesium citrate or other mild oral agent followed in the evening by a gentle cleansing enema. The patient is admitted to the hospital on the morning of surgery.

Close communication with anesthesia staff is important before and during the procedure. Nasotracheal intubation is preferred using a reinforced tube that directs the ventilator tubing away from the surgical field. An arterial line is placed to

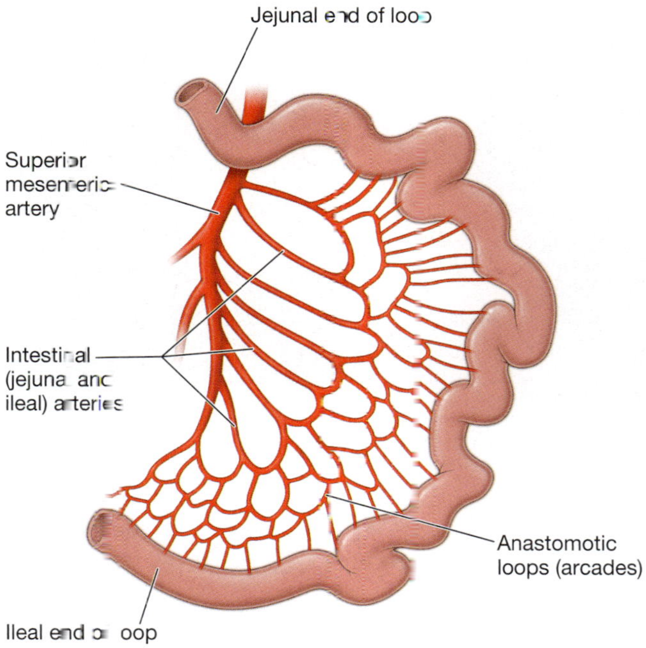

FIGURE 23-9 Vascular anatomy of the small intestine. The small bowel receives segmental blood supply from several mesenteric branches of the superior mesentery artery.

provide monitoring of blood pressure and arterial blood oxygenation and a ready access for intraoperative blood drawing during the prolonged surgical procedure. Central venous access is planned to avoid interference with the surgical field at the neck and upper chest. The patient is positioned on the table with a roll behind the shoulders to extend the neck and facilitate access to the neck. Surgical skin preparation is carried out from the margin of the mandible to the pubic bone. If a saphenous vein graft is anticipated, then one lower extremity might also be prepared. Prophylaxis for deep vein thrombosis is provided. Perioperative antibiotics are administered before the surgical incision is made.

The Free Jejunal Flap

An approach using three surgical teams is most expedient in cases of immediate reconstruction after tumor resection. The extirpative team begins the resection and confirms the need for pharyngoesophageal reconstruction. Approximately 1 hour before the completion of the tumor ablation, the reconstructive surgeons may start the abdominal portion of the procedure. In most patients, the two teams can work simultaneously without interfering with each other's progress. It is important to maintain separate sets of instrumentation and for personnel to avoid moving from the head and neck field to the abdomen to prevent contamination of the abdominal wound with oral flora or exfoliated tumor cells. When the ablative surgeons are finished, the reconstructive team may transfer the flap to the head and neck and begin the inset. At this time the third team, consisting of general surgeons, may join in the procedure and reestablish continuity of the small intestine, place gastrointestinal (GI) tubes, and complete the abdominal wound closure. Three teams working together allow overlap of each portion of the procedure and reduce operative time.

Flap Harvest

The abdomen is entered through an upper midline incision. A thorough intraabdominal exploration is carried out. It is important to identify the presence of gallstones, liver disease, synchronous GI malignancies, or other processes that may affect the patient's prognosis or postoperative course. The entire small bowel is examined before final attention is focused on the proximal jejunum and its vascular arcades.

A portion of bowel is selected beginning as proximally as possible where well-formed arcades begin to occur, usually approximately 40 cm from the ligament of Treitz. A segment measuring 15 to 20 cm in length is designed based on one of the mesenteric branches, usually the second. The vascular anatomy is best assessed by transilluminating the outstretched mesentery and directly palpating the vessels (Figure 23-10). A sterile fiberoptic light source works very nicely for this purpose.

Isolating the vascular pedicle begins the dissection. The assistant holds up the bowel segment with the mesentery expanded. The surgeon creates a window through the mesentery between the terminal vessels immediately adjacent to the bowel at each proposed line of resection. A fan-shaped portion of mesentery is dissected with the apex located at the point of the mesenteric vessel on which the flap is based (Figure 23-11). The peritoneum is incised, and significant vessels crossing to adjacent portions of the mesentery are individually ligated with silk ties. Ties are preferred because hemoclips can be dislodged with manipulation of the flap. Meticulous control of crossing vessels is important because even small vessels can form a significant mesenteric hematoma and threaten the safety of the flap. The vessels of the pedicle are cleaned of peritoneal lining, lymphatics, and fat for about 2 cm. This facilitates ligation and division of the vessel and later identification when they are divided and tend to retract into the mesentery. A final inspection of the vascular anatomy is done to ensure that it will be possible to harvest the flap without injury to the SMA or other vessels supplying the remainder of the bowel.

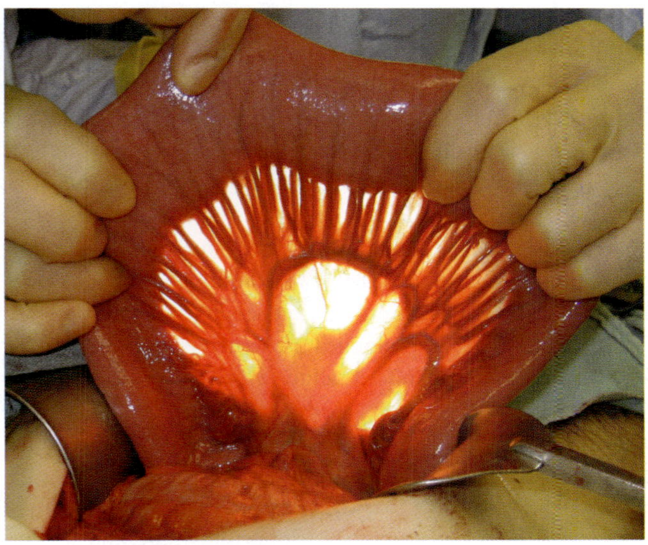

FIGURE 23-10 The anatomy of the mesenteric vessels can be nicely visualized with a fiberoptic light as backlighting.

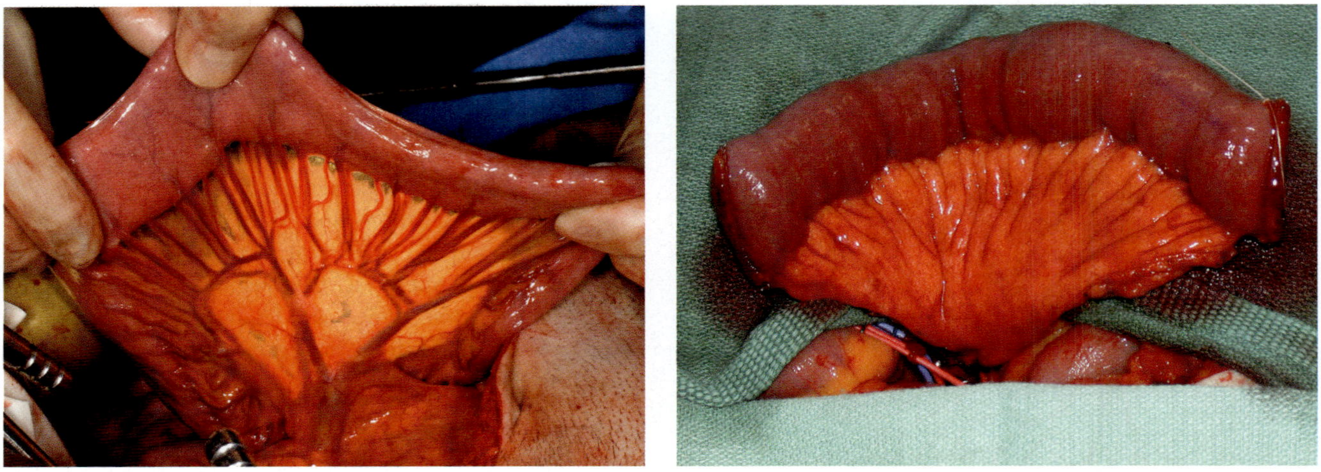

A B

FIGURE 23-11 The second mesenteric branch is chosen as the vascular pedicle for the jejunal flap (**A**). The mesentery on both sides of the vascular pedicle is divided followed by the division of the small bowel using a gastrointestinal stapler (**B**).

After isolation of the vascular pedicle, the bowel is ready to be divided. A GI stapling device may be used for this purpose. The bowel is divided perpendicular to the longitudinal axis (Figure 23-11B). A marking suture is placed at the proximal resection line to ensure orientation of the loop in an isoperistaltic direction at the time of inset in the neck. With the jejunal loop completely isolated, adequate perfusion is demonstrated by a healthy pink color in the serosa of all portions of bowel, particularly on the antimesenteric side adjacent to the staple line. Other evidence of satisfactory vascularity includes palpable and visible pulsations in the arcades, filling of small vessels on the serosal surface, and continued peristalsis of the loop. With these signs confirmed, the flap is ready for transfer (Figure 23-11B). It is covered with warm, moist laparotomy pads while final preparations are made in the recipient site.

After completing preparations in the neck, it is time to divide the pedicle and transfer the flap from the abdomen. The artery is usually taken first. It is cross-clamped, and the stump is double ligated with 2-0 silk. A record of ischemia time is begun. The vein is then ligated and divided in a fashion similar to the artery. The flap is removed from the abdominal field, and the area is inspected to ensure perfect vascular control. The lumen of the bowel segment is irrigated with normal saline to remove mucus or other intestinal contents. Various techniques have been described for protecting the bowel from ischemic injury during the transfer. Some authors believe that cooling is an essential part of graft preservation during the ischemic period. Our conclusion is that 1 to 2 hours of ischemia is well tolerated, and reperfusion can generally be accomplished within that time. If prolonged ischemia is anticipated, the bowel may be bathed in iced saline.

Donor Site Closure

At this time, an abdominal surgery team, if available, may begin bowel anastomosis, placement of jejunostomy tube, and abdominal closure while the reconstructive team continues work in the neck. Small bowel continuity may be restored with stapling devices or by sutured anastomosis. A feeding jejunostomy tube is placed distal to the bowel anastomosis, and a layered abdominal closure completes this portion of the procedure. A gastrostomy tube may also be placed, or, alternatively, a nasogastric tube can be passed through the reconstructed esophagus into the stomach. If the latter option is chosen, the tube must be securely fixed to prevent premature removal after surgery.

Inset and Revascularization

Proper planning during this part of the procedure is vital to smoothly complete a successful reconstruction. The sequence of steps is to (1) complete the proximal inset by performing pharyngojejunal anastomosis, (2) tailor the flap to the proper length and perform a portion of the distal inset at the esophageal resection line, (3) revascularize the flap, and (4) complete the distal inset. Details of reconstruction are discussed in other chapters.

After completing the vascular anastomoses and flap insetting, a portion of vascularized jejunum, approximately 3 cm long, is used as a postoperative monitor to assess flap perfusion. This segment of jejunum is isolated on a terminal arcade vessel and brought outside the neck through the neck incision (Figure 23-12). It may be covered with a petroleum gauze dressing. A 2-0 silk tie is placed around the terminal arcade vessel so that the vessel can be ligated by simply tying the suture when it is ready to remove the monitoring segment. It is usually removed 7 days after surgery at bedside before the patient is discharged from the hospital.

Indications

The standard indication for the free jejunal flap is for reconstruction of circumferential defects of the hypopharynx and cervical esophagus. This circumstance is usually associated with:

1. Cancer of the hypopharynx, piriform sinus, or larynx
2. Recurrent cancer at the tracheal stoma after laryngectomy
3. Thyroid cancer involving the esophagus

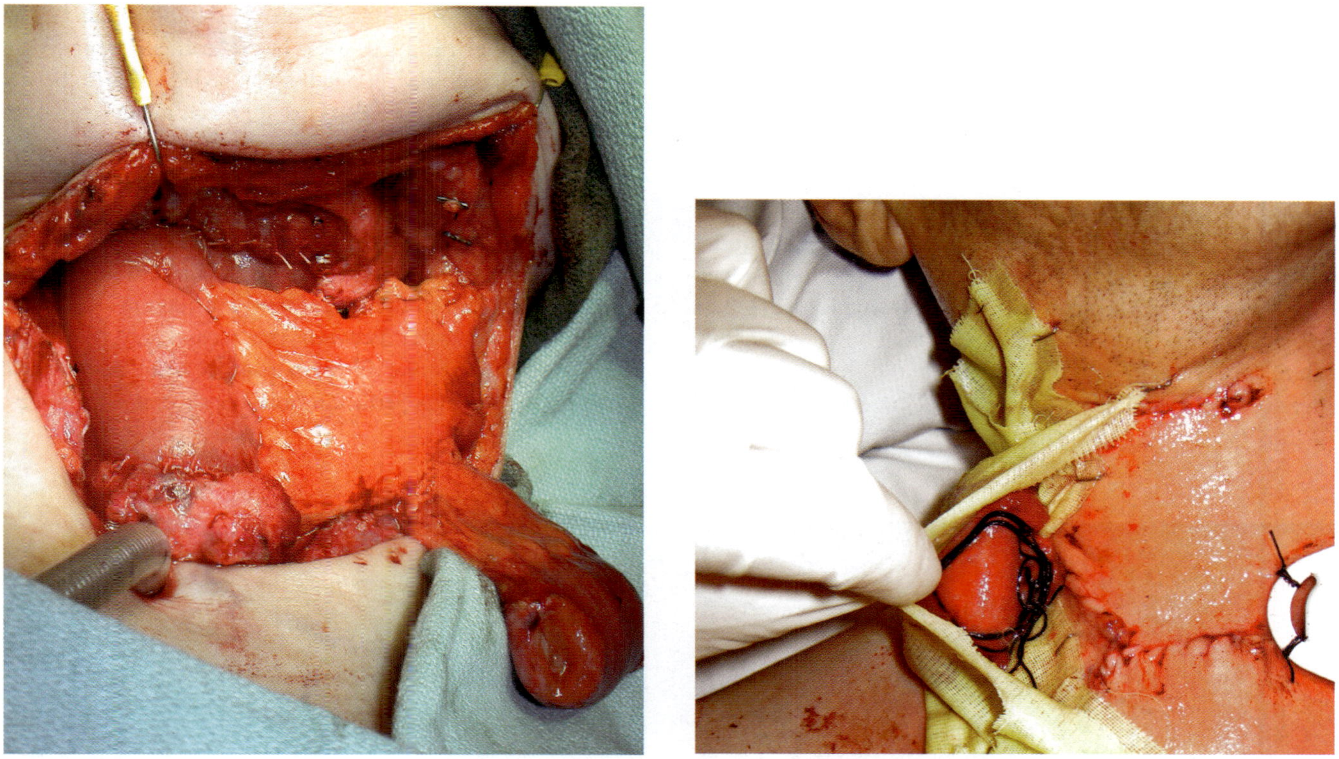

A **B**

FIGURE 23-12 The main jejunal flap is used for pharyngoesophageal reconstruction while a small segment of bowel based on one or two terminal arcade vessels is externalized for monitoring purpose (**A** and **B**). 2-0 silk ties were placed around the terminal arcade vessel for easy removal of the monitoring segment at the bedside before the patient is discharged from the hospital, usually 7 to 10 days after surgery.

4. Benign strictures refractory to dilation, such as radiation induced strictures or ingestion of lye
5. Nonhealing pharyngocutaneous fistula after prior reconstruction or radiotherapy

Compared with fasciocutaneous flaps for pharyngoesophageal reconstruction such as the anterolateral thigh flap, the jejunal flap heals well with low fistula rates and no delayed fistulas. Therefore, patients may start an oral diet sooner, usually 1 to 2 weeks after surgery, but delayed fistulas have been seen after fasciocutaneous flap reconstruction; thus, an oral diet is usually delayed for 2 to 6 weeks depending on whether patients have received prior radiotherapy (38,39). The disadvantages of the jejunal flap compared to fasciocutaneous flaps include (1) added abdominal and bowel surgery and thus higher surgical risks and longer postoperative recovery and (2) lower success rate for speech rehabilitation and poor tracheoesophageal speech quality (40).

The Supercharged Jejunal Flap

Meticulous operative planning and intraoperative execution are essential. The authors use a three-team approach in most cases. The thoracic or general surgeons (or both) perform the esophagectomy and gastrectomy when necessary. The surgical approach is either through two incisions (abdominal and cervical) as in a transhiatal esophagectomy or three incisions with the addition of a right thoracotomy. To minimize the operating time, it is important to establish a coordinated flow among the various teams. If a thoracotomy is required, the patient is first placed in lateral decubitus position and then switched to supine. While the ablative surgical team is operating in the abdomen, the reconstructive surgeons can start to prepare recipient vessels in the neck. The teams then change positions. The reconstructive surgeons now prepare the jejunal flap while the ablative surgeons expose the proximal esophagus through the neck incision and remove the manubrium and clavicular head if a substernal approach is desired. The jejunal conduit is then passed through the chest and into the neck, and the teams switch positions again. The reconstructive surgeons revascularize the proximal jejunum, complete the esophagojejunal anastomosis in the neck, and fashion the monitoring segment while the other surgical team restores GI continuity in the abdomen. When properly organized, no time is wasted for all teams involved. Clear communication among surgical teams and anesthesia regarding fluid resuscitation and avoidance of vasopressor medications is imperative because different disciplines may manage these issues differently.

Flap Harvesting

When resection is complete, the length of the esophageal defect is measured to estimate the length of the conduit needed (33). The mesentery of the proximal and midjejunum is closely examined using a fiberoptic light to transilluminate the tissues and elucidate the vascular anatomy. The first mesenteric branch beyond the ligament of Trietz is identified and preserved to maintain blood supply to the distal duodenum and most proximal portion of jejunum, which is used to reestablish enteric continuity.

Typically, the second mesenteric branch is dissected down to the level of the SMA and vein and ultimately divided to serve as the vascular pedicle for supercharging the proximal flap. In the simplest cases, the mesentery between the second and third branches is divided up to the serosal border, allowing the jejunal segment to unfurl (Figure 23-13). This step helps straighten the natural sinusoidal properties of the small bowel and reduce redundancy. If more length is required, the third mesenteric branch is ligated and divided (Figure 23-14). Secondary arcade vessels between the third and fourth mesenteric branches are preserved so that the segment of bowel normally supplied by the third branch is now supplied by the pedicled fourth branch through intact arcade vessels. This approach is the most common setup.

If still greater length is required, such as in patients with very long torsos or a concomitant total laryngopharyngectomy, the fourth mesenteric branch can also be ligated and divided. In these cases, only the mesentery between the third and fourth branches is divided to the serosal border while the arcade connections are preserved between the second and third and between the fourth and fifth branches (Figure 23-15). The third segment receives perfusion from the supercharged second

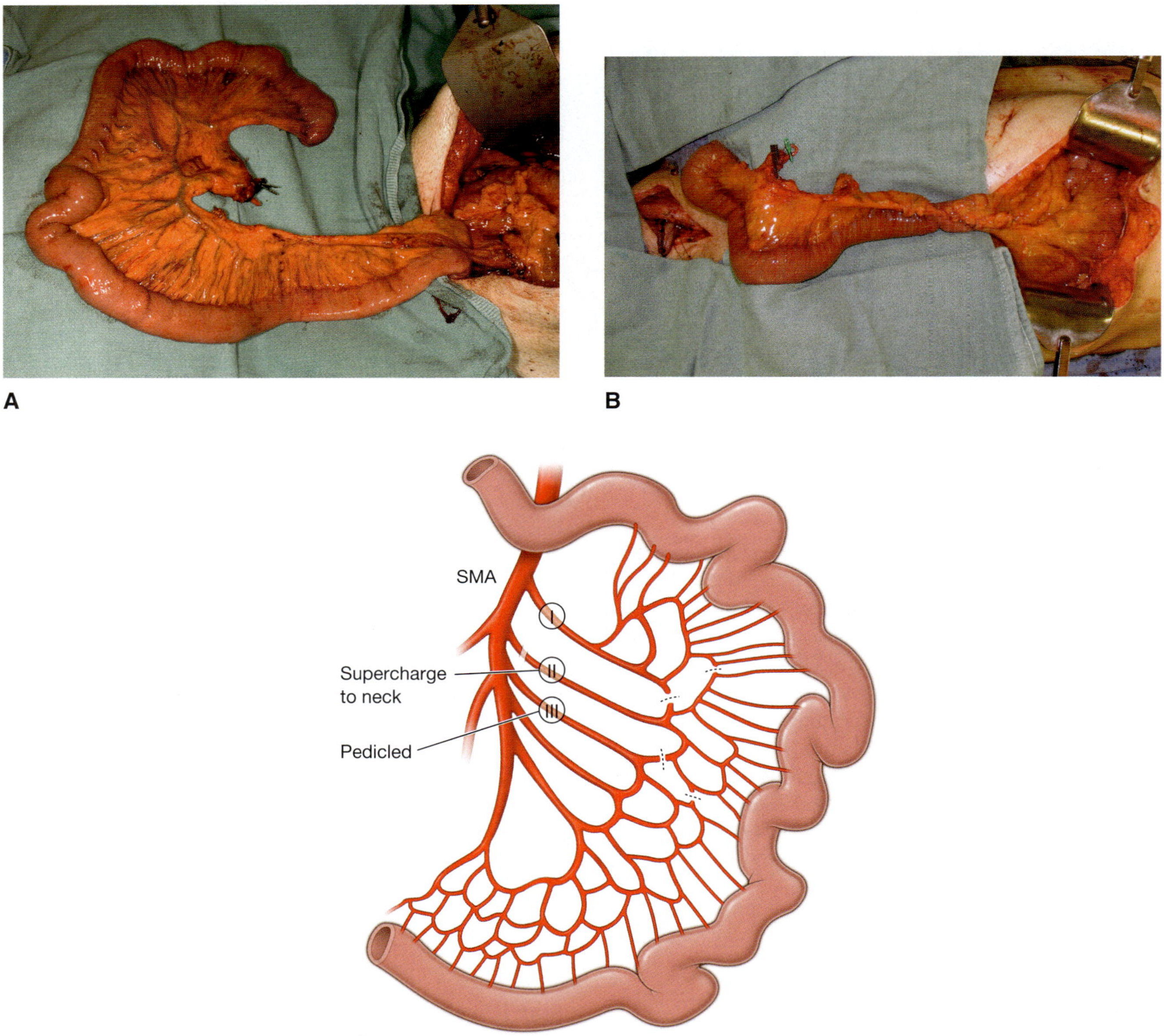

FIGURE 23-13 (A) to (C) In preparation of the supercharged jejunal flap, the mesentery between the second and third mesenteric branch vessels is divided up to the serosal border, allowing the jejunal segment to unfurl. The second mesenteric vessels are "supercharged" to the vessels in the neck or the internal mammary vessels. The third mesenteric vessels are left intact to serve as the vascular pedicle for pedicled portion of the jejunal flap. SMA, superior mesenteric artery.

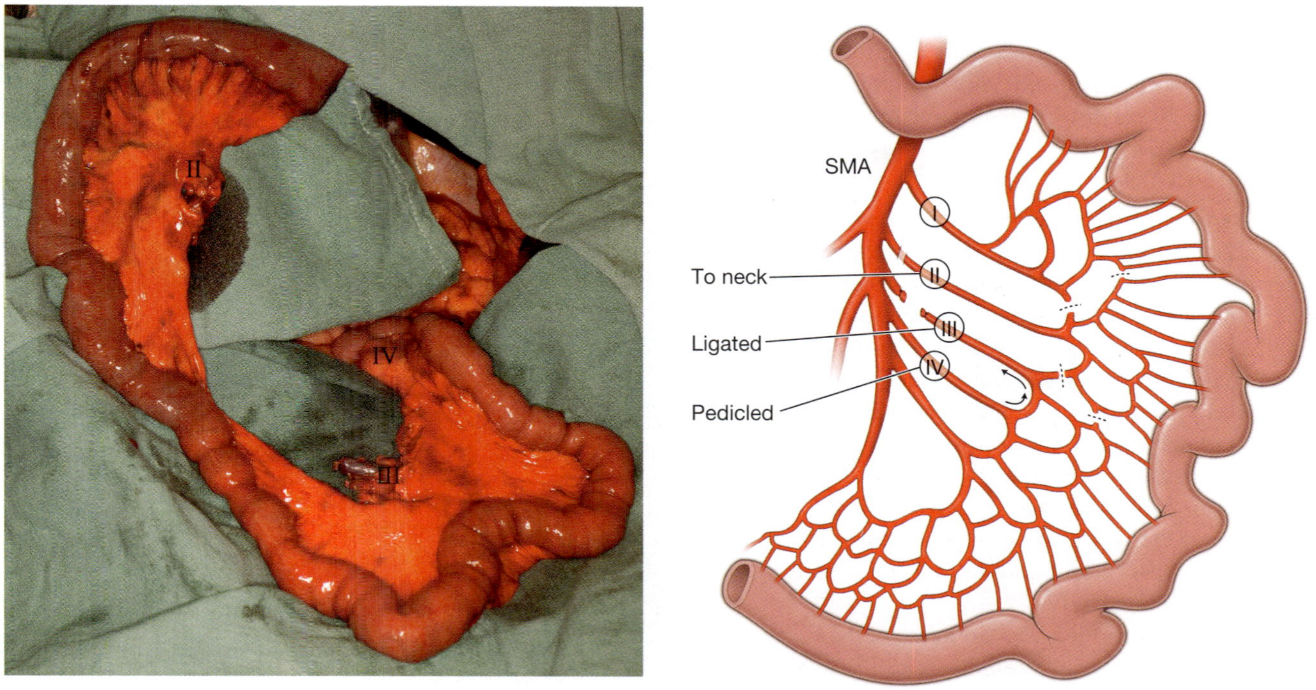

A B

FIGURE 23-14 (A) and (B) When more length is needed, the third mesenteric branch is ligated and divided. The mesentery between the second and third mesenteric vessels is divided to the serosal border of the jejunum while the arcade vessels between the third and fourth mesenteric vessels are kept intact so that the small bowel normally perfused by the third branch can be perfused by the pedicled fourth branch via these arcade connections.

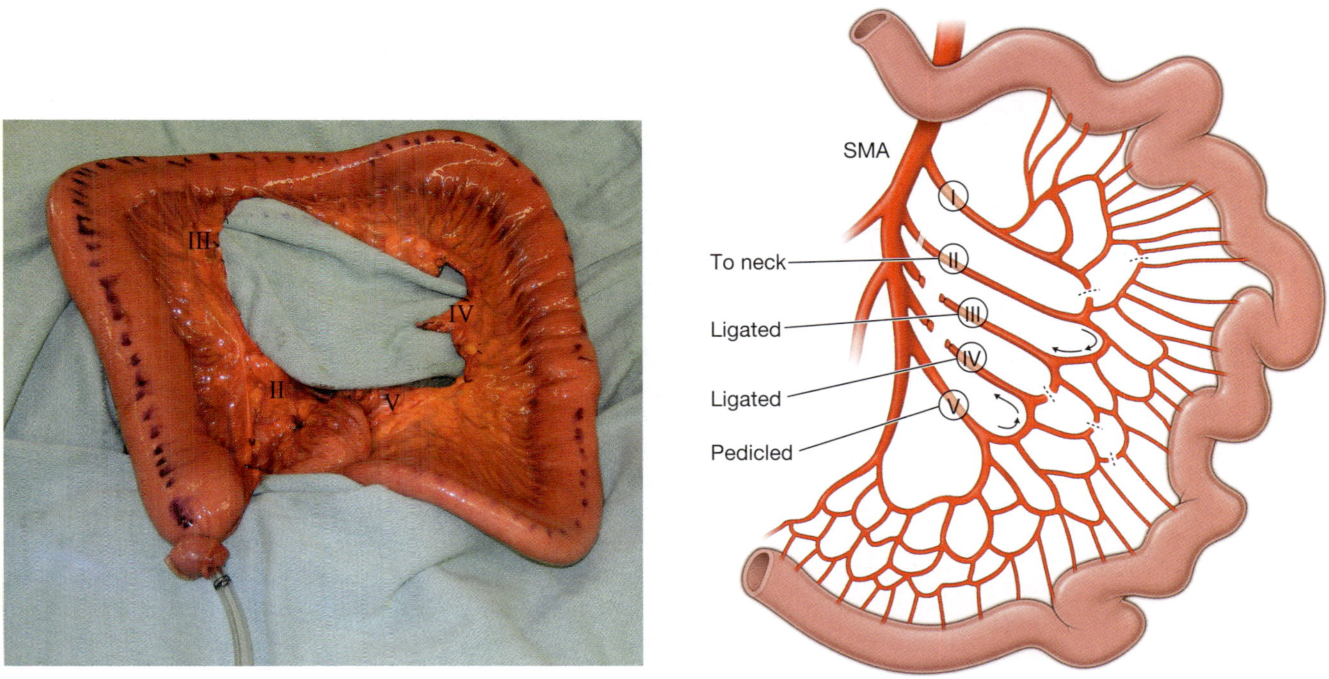

A B

FIGURE 23-15 (A) and (B) If still greater length is required, the fourth mesenteric branch can also be ligated. In these cases, only the mesentery between the third and fourth branches is divided to the serosal border while arcade connections are preserved between the second and third and between the fourth and fifth branches.

segment, and the fourth segment receives perfusion from the pedicled fifth branch. When adequate length is achieved, the jejunum is divided proximally with a linear cutting stapler, typically 30 to 40 cm distal to the ligament of Treitz.

Flap Transfer

There are two potential routes for transferring the jejunal flap to the neck, retrocardiac, which is the orthotopic route, or substernal, which is the heterotopic route (Figure 23-16). The former is used in patients undergoing immediate reconstruction. The latter is usually reserved for patients undergoing a delayed reconstruction after previous failed esophageal reconstruction. In these cases, a portion of the manubrium, clavicular head, and first rib are removed to enlarge the thoracic inlet and avoid constriction on the jejunal conduit. Whether the retrocardiac or substernal route is selected, transfer is accomplished using a sterile laparoscopic camera bag to protect the conduit and prevent traction and shearing forces on the delicate arcade vessels (Figure 23-17).

After the jejunal flap is pulled up to the neck, vascular anastomoses are performed, most commonly to the internal mammary vessels or the transverse cervical vessels. After the proximal jejunum is revascularized, any excess length of jejunal conduit is removed to minimize redundancy in the neck. The proximal 3 to 5 cm of jejunum based on one or two terminal arcade vessels is exteriorized as a postoperative monitoring segment as with free jejunal flap reconstruction (Figure 23-12B). The esophagojejunal anastomosis is then performed in the neck using a single layer of 3-0 Vicryl or polydioxanone (PDS) suture in an end-to-end fashion. In patients with a total laryngopharyngectomy, the proximal pharynx or base of tongue is larger than the jejunal diameter, so an end-to-side anastomosis is performed to accommodate the size discrepancy.

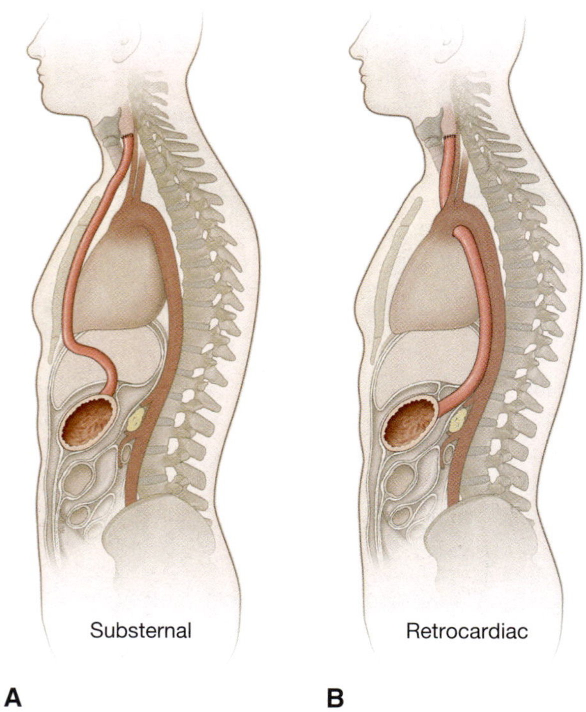

FIGURE 23-16 Schematic showing the substernal *(left)* and retrocardiac *(right)* pathways to pull the jejunal conduit to the neck.

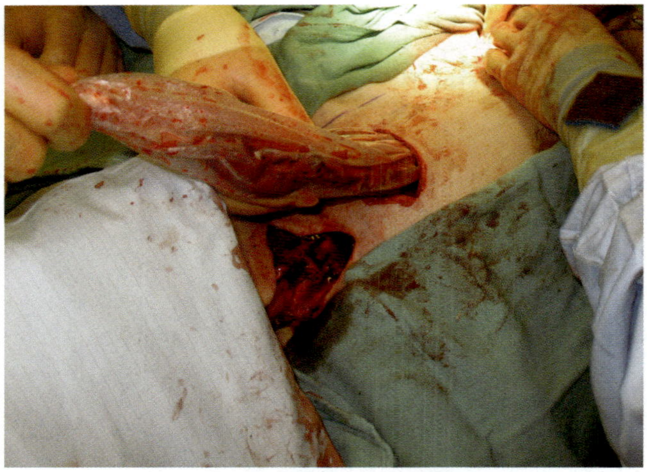

FIGURE 23-17 The small bowel and its mesentery are placed in a plastic bag and pulled to the neck through the chest. The bag protects the mesentery vessels from avulsion injury.

Tricks and Tips

Technically, three key steps are required in such a complex reconstruction: selecting the appropriate jejunal segment, choosing the optimal recipient vessels for microsurgical anastomosis, and creating a suitable conduit passageway.

Careful consideration of the mesenteric anatomy is the most critical component in surgical planning. If possible, the most proximal jejunum beyond the first mesenteric branch should be included to avoid wasting of the proximal bowel. Thus, the second mesenteric branch is often selected for supercharging. However, this selection also depends on the anatomy of the mesentery since it is the arc length of the mesentery between branches, not the bowel itself, which determines the reach of the flap. Therefore, the segment of bowel with longer mesenteric vessels and wider mesenteric intervals between the vessels should be selected so the conduit can be adequately unfurled and lengthened.

The choice of recipient vessels is another critical factor in the decision-making algorithm. In general, recipient vessels lower in the neck (transverse cervical vessels) or in the chest (internal mammary vessels) are preferred to facilitate reach of the mesenteric pedicle. The choice of recipient vessels also depends on conduit pathway, which is dictated by the clinical scenario of each individual patient (e.g., immediate vs. delayed reconstruction). A reconstructive algorithm is created to assist with surgical planning (Figure 21-18).

For delayed reconstruction, the substernal pathway is chosen because the retrocardiac route is scarred from previous surgery or infection. The left manubrium and clavicular head are resected, and the internal mammary vessels are easily exposed, making them the recipient vessel of choice. The vascular anastomosis is then completed in the upper chest in the space where

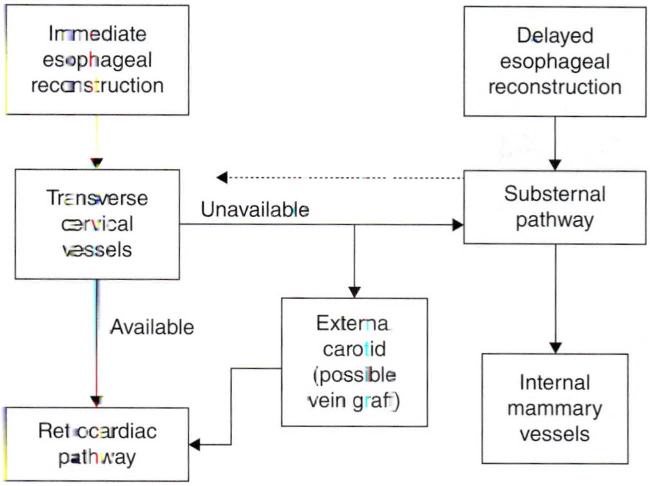

FIGURE 23-18 Algorithm for choosing recipient vessels and transthoracic pathways for total esophageal reconstruction with the supercharged jejunal flap.

the manubrium and clavicular head were removed. The left transverse cervical vessels are an alternate option.

For immediate reconstruction, the native retrocardiac pathway is available and preferred to avoid unnecessary resection of the manubrium and clavicular head. This pathway is also slightly shorter than the substernal pathway. The internal mammary vessels, which are located anteriorly, are not a good option with this pathway. The transverse cervical vessels lower in the neck are preferred to avoid vein grafting to the external carotid system. The substernal pathway, however, should be considered during an immediate reconstruction in the following clinical circumstances: (1) the transverse cervical vessels are unavailable, which may occur in 23% of the unilateral necks (41), or (2) the patient has severe kyphosis. One contraindication for choosing the substernal pathway is in patients with previous coronary artery bypass surgery where the internal mammary artery was used as the bypass graft. Therefore, for immediate reconstruction, the authors now prefer exploring the left transverse cervical vessels first. If they are adequate, the retrocardiac pathway is chosen. If not, then the authors opt for the substernal pathway and the use of the internal mammary vessels. The second option is to proceed with the retrocardiac pathway and use the external carotid system, such as the superior thyroid artery and internal jugular vein as recipient vessels. This option is less desirable because a vein graft is often necessary, making an already complex reconstruction even more so.

Donor Site Closure

Intestinal continuity is reestablished in the abdomen by the thoracic or general surgical team through a gastrojejunal anastomosis using the posterior wall of the stomach or through a Roux-en-Y jejunojejunal anastomosis if a gastrectomy was performed. A feeding jejunostomy tube is routinely placed. The midline abdominal incision is closed with heavy Prolene sutures.

Indications

The primary indication for a supercharged jejunal flap is total esophageal reconstruction. Total esophageal reconstruction is a demanding procedure for both the patient and surgeon alike. A gastric conduit is the first choice for reconstruction because of its robust blood supply and need for only a single bowel anastomosis to reestablish continuity with good results (42,43). However, in certain situations, the stomach may be unavailable. Colon interposition has been used for several decades as an alternative to the gastric conduit (44–48). However, patients with atherosclerosis; inappropriate vascular anatomy; previous colon resection; or intrinsic colon disease such as inflammatory bowel disease, cancer, or diverticulosis are not candidates. The jejunum closely approximates the size of the native esophagus, possesses peristaltic activity, and is typically free of intrinsic diseases.

Indications for the supercharged jejunal flap for total esophageal reconstruction include:

1. Previous gastric surgery: stomach unavailable or inadequate
2. Radiated stomach: high risk for gastric necrosis if pulled up
3. Total esophagectomy plus total laryngectomy: stomach would not reach the base of the tongue
4. Failed gastric pull-up reconstruction: these are life-threatening complications with mediastinal infection and sepsis. A diversion procedure is usually performed first after thorough debridement of the necrotic stomach with a spit fistula and G-tube and J-tube placement (Figure 23-19). Definitive esophageal reconstruction with a supercharged jejunal flap is performed several months later when the patient is fully recovered from the complication (see Figure 23-19).

Relative contraindications for jejunal flaps include inflammatory small bowel disease, atherosclerotic vascular disease with severe mesenteric involvement, and portal hypertension. Advanced patient age or concurrent medical illnesses should not necessarily be considered contraindications to microvascular reconstruction unless they are judged severe enough to preclude the extirpative surgery.

Postoperative Care

Requirements for postoperative care are similar to those for any patient after major head and neck or thoracic surgery with some special considerations. The gastrostomy tube is maintained on intermittent suction until return of active bowel sounds. Jejunostomy feeding may be initiated on the second postoperative day. A modified barium swallow study is performed to confirm healing and to assess swallowing function 7 to 14 days after surgery depending on whether previous radiotherapy was given. If satisfactory healing and function are confirmed, the patient may be started on a liquid diet, which may be advanced to a regular diet usually within the next several days. The feeding tube may be removed when the patient reliably demonstrates an ability to take adequate nutrition by mouth.

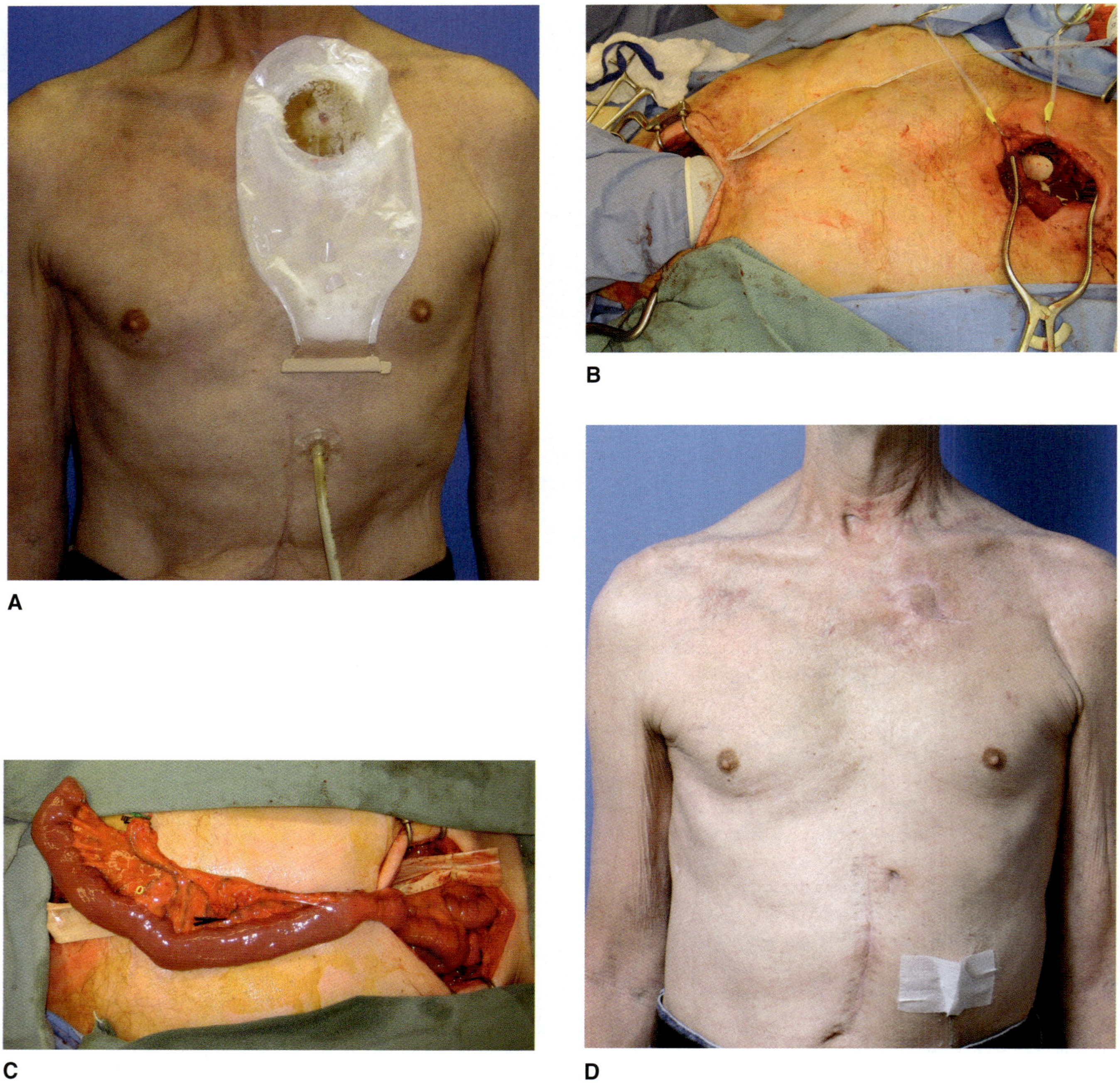

FIGURE 23-19 A patient with a life-threatening tracheoesophageal fistula was initially managed with a diversion procedure (**A**) and a latissimus dorsi muscle flap to repair the tracheal defect. Six months later, total esophageal reconstruction was performed with a supercharged jejunal flap via the substernal pathway (**B** and **C**). He was able to tolerate a regular diet after reconstruction without the need for tube feeding (**D**).

REFERENCES

1. Seidenberg B, Rosenak SS, Hurwitt ES, Som ML. Immediate reconstruction of the cervical esophagus by a revascularized isolated jejunal segment. *Ann Surg* 1959;149:162–171.
2. Bloomhardt SL, Andrews CF, Hetherington RR. Surgical research of the great omentum. *Surg Gynecol Obstet* 1917;24:474–479.
3. O'Shaughnessy L. Surgical treatment of cardiac ischaemia. *Lancet* 1937;1:185.
4. Thompson SA, Pollock B. The use free omental grafts in the thorax: An experimental study. *Am J Surg* 1945;70:227.
5. McLean DH, Buncke HJ. Jr. Autotransplant of omentum to a large scalp defect, with microsurgical revascularization. *Plast Reconstr Surg* 1972;49:268–274.
6. Mathes SJ, Nahai F. *Reconstructive Surgery: Principles, Anatomy & Technique.* New York: Churchill Livingstone, 1997.
7. Alday ES, Goldsmith HS. Surgical technique for omental lengthening based on arterial anatomy. *Surg Gynecol Obstet* 1972;135:103–107.
8. Salameh JR, Chock DA, Gonzalez JJ, et al. Laparoscopic harvest of omental flaps for reconstruction of complex mediastinal wounds. *JSLS* 2003;7:317–322.
9. Saltz R. Endoscopic harvest of the omental and jejunal free flaps. *Clin Plast Surg* 1995;22:747–754.
10. Hultman CS, Carlson GW, Losken A, et al. Utility of the omentum in the reconstruction of complex extraperitoneal wounds and defects: donor-site complications in 135 patients from 1975 to 2000. *Ann Surg* 2002;235:782–795.
11. Mathes DW, Thornton JF, Rohrich RJ. Management of posterior trunk defects. *Plast Reconstr Surg* 2006;118:73e–83e.
12. Losken A, Carlson GW, Culbertson JH, et al. Omental free flap reconstruction in complex head and neck deformities. *Head Neck* 2002;24:326–331.

13. Seitz IA, Williams CS, Wiedrich TA, et al. Omental free-tissue transfer for coverage of complex upper extremity and hand defects—the forgotten flap. *Hand (N Y)* 2009;4:397–405.
14. Maloney CT Jr, Wages D, Upton J, Lee WP. Free omental tissue transfer for extremity coverage and revascularization. *Plast Reconstr Surg* 2003;111:1899–1904.
15. Brunelli G, Brunelli F. Surgical treatment of actinic brachial plexus lesions: free microvascular transfer of the greater omentum. *J Reconstr Microsurg* 1985;1:197–200.
16. Patel RS, Gilbert RW. Utility of the gastro-omental free flap in head and neck reconstruction. *Curr Opin Otolaryngol Head Neck Surg* 2009;17: 258–262.
17. Longmire WP. A modification of the Roux technique for antethoracic esophageal reconstruction. *Surgery* 1947;22:94–1008.
18. Roberts RE, Douglas FM. Replacement of the cervical esophagus and hypopharynx by a revascularized free jejunal segment. *N Engl J Med* 1961;264:342–344.
19. Nakayama K, Yamamoto K, Tamiya T, et al. Experience with free autografts of the bowel with a new venous anastomosis apparatus. *Surgery* 1964;55:796–802.
20. Jurkiewicz MJ. Vascularized intestinal graft for reconstruction of the cervical esophagus and pharynx. *Plast Reconstr Surg* 1965;36:507–509.
21. Hester TR, McConnell FMS, Nahai F, et al. Reconstruction of cervical esophagus hypopharynx, and oral cavity using free jejunal transfer. *Am J Surg* 1980;140:487–491.
22. Gluckman JL, McCafferty GJ, Black RJ, et al. Complications associated with free jejunal graft reconstruction of the pharyngoesophagus: a multiinstitutional experience with 52 cases. *Head Neck Surg* 1984;7: 200–205.
23. Coleman JJ, Searles JM, Hester TR, et al. Ten years experience with the free jejunal autograft. *Am J Surg* 1987;154:389–393.
24. Coleman JJ, Tan KC, Searles JM, et al. Jejunal free autograft: analysis of complications and their resolution *Plast Reconstr Surg* 1989;84: 589–595.
25. Schusterman MA, Shestak K, de Vries EJ, et al. Reconstruction of the cervical esophagus: free jejunal transfer versus gastric pull-up. *Plast Reconstr Surg* 1990;85:16–21.
26. Reece GP, Schusterman MA, Miller MJ, et al. Morbidity and functional outcome of free jejunal transfer reconstruction for circumferential defects of the pharynx and cervical esophagus. *Plast Reconstr Surg* 1995;96:1307.
27. Cordeiro PG, Shah K, Santamaria E, et al. Barium swallows after free jejunal transfer: Should they be performed routinely? *Plast Reconstr Surg* 1999;103:1167.
28. Chang DW, Hussussian C, Lewin JS, et al. Analysis of pharyngocutaneous fistula following free jejunal transfer for total laryngopharyngectomy. *Plast Reconstr Surg* 2002;109:1522.
29. Disa JJ, Pusic AL, Hidalgo DA, Cordeiro PG, et al. Microvascular reconstruction of the hypopharynx: defect classification, treatment algorithm, and functional outcome based on 165 consecutive cases. *Plast Reconstr Surg* 2003;111:652.
30. Okazaki M, Asato H, Takushima A, et al. Secondary reconstruction of failed esophageal reconstruction *Ann Plast Surg* 2005;54:530–537.
31. Dowson HMP, Strauss D, Ng R, Mason R. The acute management and surgical reconstruction following failed esophagectomy in malignant disease of the esophagus. *Dis Esophagus* 2007;20:135–140.
32. Chana JS, Chen HC, Sharma R, et al. Microsurgical reconstruction of the esophagus using supercharged pedicled jejunum flaps: special indications and pitfalls. *Plast Reconstr Surg* 2002;110:742–748.
33. Poh M, Selber JC, Skoracki R, et al. Technical challenges of total esophageal reconstruction using a supercharged jejunal flap. *Ann Surg* 2011;253:1122–1129.
34. Heitmiller RF, Gruber PJ, Swier P, Singh N. Long-segment substernal jejunal esophageal replacement with internal mammary vascular augmentation. *Dis Esophagus* 2000;13:240–242.
35. Sekido M, Yamamoto Y, Minakawa H, et al. Use of the "supercharge" technique in esophageal and pharyngeal reconstruction to augment microvascular blood flow. *Surgery* 2003;134:420–424.
36. Sakuraba M, Kimata Y, Hishinuma S, et al. Importance of additional microvascular anastomosis in esophageal reconstruction after salvage esophagectomy. *Plast Reconstr Surg* 2004;113:1934–1939.
37. Hirabayashi S, Miyata M, Shoji M, et al. Reconstruction of the thoracic esophagus with extended jejunum used as a substitute with the aid of microvascular anastomosis. *Surgery* 1993;113:515–519.
38. Yu P, Robb GL. Pharyngoesophageal reconstruction with the anterolateral thigh flap: a clinical and functional outcomes study. *Plast Reconstr Surg* 2005;116:1845–1855.
39. Yu P, Hanasono MM, Skoracki RJ, et al. Pharyngoesophageal reconstruction with the anterolateral thigh flap after total laryngopharyngectomy. *Cancer* 2010;116:1718–1724.
40. Yu P, Lewin JS, Reece GP, Robb GL. Comparison of clinical and functional outcomes and hospital costs following pharyngoesophageal reconstruction with the anterolateral thigh free flap versus the jejunal flap. *Plast Reconstr Surg* 2006;117:968–974.
41. Yu P. The transverse cervical vessels as recipient vessels for previously treated head and neck cancer patients. *Plast Reconstr Surg* 2005;115:1253–1258.
42. Orringer MB, Marshall B, Chang AC, et al. Two thousand transhiatal esophagectomies—changing trends, lessons learned. *Ann Surg* 2007;246:363–372.
43. Young MM, Deschamps C, Trastek VF, et al. Esophageal reconstruction for benign disease: early morbidity, mortality and functional results. *Ann Thorac Surg* 2000;70:1651–1655.
44. DeMeester TR, Johansson KE, Franze I, et al. Indications, surgical technique, and long-term functional results of colon interposition or bypass. *Ann Surg* 1988;208:460–474.
45. DeMeester SR. Colon interposition following esophagectomy. *Dis Esophagus* 2001;14:169–172.
46. Mansour KA, Bryan FC, Carlson GW. Bowel-interposition for esophageal replacement: twenty-five year experience. *Ann Thorac Surg* 1997;64:752–756.
47. Cense HA, Visser MR, Van Sandick JW, et al. Quality of life after colon interposition by necessity for esophageal cancer replacement. *J Surg Oncol* 2004;88:32–38.
48. Klink CD, Binnebosel M, Schneider M, et al. Operative outcome of colon interposition in the treatment of esophageal cancer: a 20-year experience. *Surgery* 2010;147:491–496.

CHAPTER 24

Medial Condylar Flap

Allen T. Bishop

HISTORY

Vascularized bone grafts have great utility in reconstructing bony defects and promoting fracture union. In contrast to conventional (nonvascularized) grafting, transfer of vascularized bone has the potential to revascularize necrotic bone in the setting of avascular necrosis and has superior structural properties (1). Small vascularized grafts with a reliable endosteal blood supply and acceptable donor site morbidity are of use for a variety of indications and in many anatomic sites.

Periosteal grafts are less commonly used clinically but have been demonstrated experimentally to produce predictable new bone formation provided they have adequate vascularity (2). A variety of donor sites have been identified, including clavicle, fibula, ilium, humerus, tibia. An ideal periosteal flap should provide thin corticoperiosteal tissue including the cambium layer to reliably generate new bone at the recipient site. It should be sufficiently flexible to allow it to conform to small tubular bones or cover larger surfaces like a "patch."

MEDIAL FEMORAL CONDYLE FLAP

The medial femoral condylar flap was described initially as a potential pedicled periosteal flap based on branches of the descending genicular artery by Hertel and Masquelet in 1989 (3). It was proposed to be of use for bone healing problems of the mid and distal third of the femur as well as the proximal tibia. The ability to include periosteum, bone, and muscle on the vascular pedicle provided potential usefulness for treatment of nonunions, segmental tibial defects, and revascularization of aseptic necrosis about the knee joint. Its use as a free corticoperiosteal transfer was subsequently developed by Sakai and Doi and applied for treatment of persistent nonunions of the humerus, ulna, and metacarpals (4–6).

Its potential as a vascularized bone flap was more recently recognized. It is at present an increasingly used flap providing vascularized periosteum, bone, or both for a variety of increasing indications, including nonunions or defects in the mandible, orbit, clavicle, distal tibia, small finger joints, scaphoid, radius, and ulna (6). It has proved particularly valuable in treating radiation- and trauma-induced avascular necrosis in the talus, clavicle, humerus, and carpal bones (7–14).

ANATOMY

The anatomy of the medial femoral condylar flap is based on a reliable extraosseous blood supply from two potential sources, enabling elevation of a corticoperiosteal flap, a vascularized bone, or an osteocartilaginous flap with or without an associated fasciocutaneous monitoring paddle (Bouy flap) (15).

Extraosseous Blood Supply (Figure 24-1)

Two arteries and their accompanying pair of venae comitantes provide direct circulation to the medial aspect of the distal femur. They are the *descending genicular artery*, arising from the superficial femoral vessels just proximal to the hiatus in the adductor magnus muscle, and the *medial superior genicular artery*, which is identified at the proximal aspect of the medial femoral condyle and easily traced toward the posterior midline, where it arises from the popliteal artery.

This blood supply has been recognized by anatomists for decades based on studies of bone vascular foramina. The dual circulation described above was published by Scapinelli in 1968, with considerable detail (16).

Although a bone or periosteal flap may be transferred on either pedicle in most cases, an understanding of the variations commonly seen clinically is important before undertaking elevation of this flap.

The descending genicular vessel arises from the superficial femoral artery a mean 13.7 cm proximal to the medial aspect of the knee joint (17) (Figure 24-2). It divides commonly into

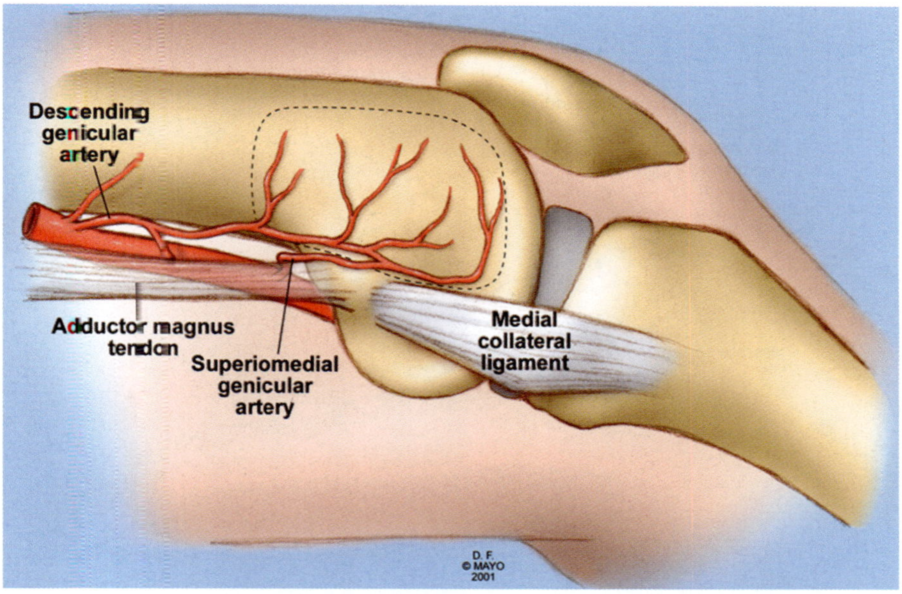

FIGURE 24-1 Both the descending genicular and medial superior genicular vessels potentially supply the medial femoral condyle flap. They supply the broad surface of the distal medial femoral metaphysis with a robust blood supply, including both periosteum and multiple nutrient arteries. (By permission of Mayo Foundation for Medical Education and Research. All rights reserved.)

two or three of the branches, which include an osteoarticular branch, one or more muscular branches, and a saphenous branch that supplies adjacent skin innervated by the saphenous nerve (Figure 24-3). The descending genicular vessels travel along the saphenous nerve within the adductor canal deep to the sartorius muscle. A recent anatomic study investigated both the extra- and intraosseous blood supply to the medial aspect of the distal femur (17). The descending genicular artery was found to have an average diameter of 1.5 mm (range, 1–2 mm) proximally. The osteoarticular, muscular and saphenous components generally branch from the descending genicular artery proper but at times may arise directly from the superficial femoral artery.

The osteoarticular branch of the descending genicular artery, of interest for bone flap elevation, is not invariably present. It was found in 89% of knee specimens, arising 11.3 cm (range, 5.5–15 cm) from the knee joint with an internal diameter of 1.1 mm (range, 0.63–1.5 mm) (see Figures 24-2

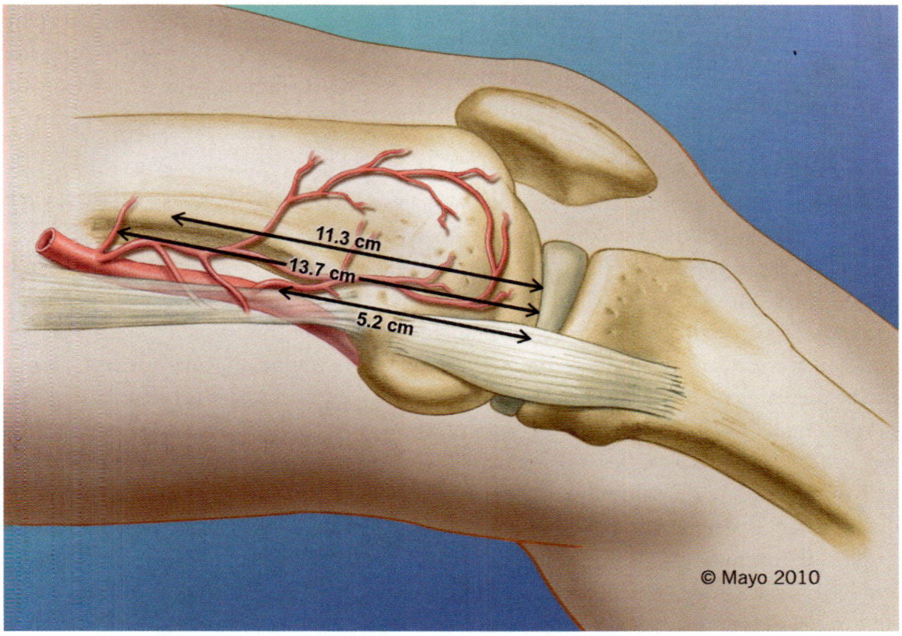

FIGURE 24-2 Mean distance of vessel origin as measured from the knee joint line. The descending genicular vessels are typically longer, are easily identified, and are the preferred pedicle for periosteal bone grafting. (By permission of Mayo Foundation for Medical Education and Research. All rights reserved.)

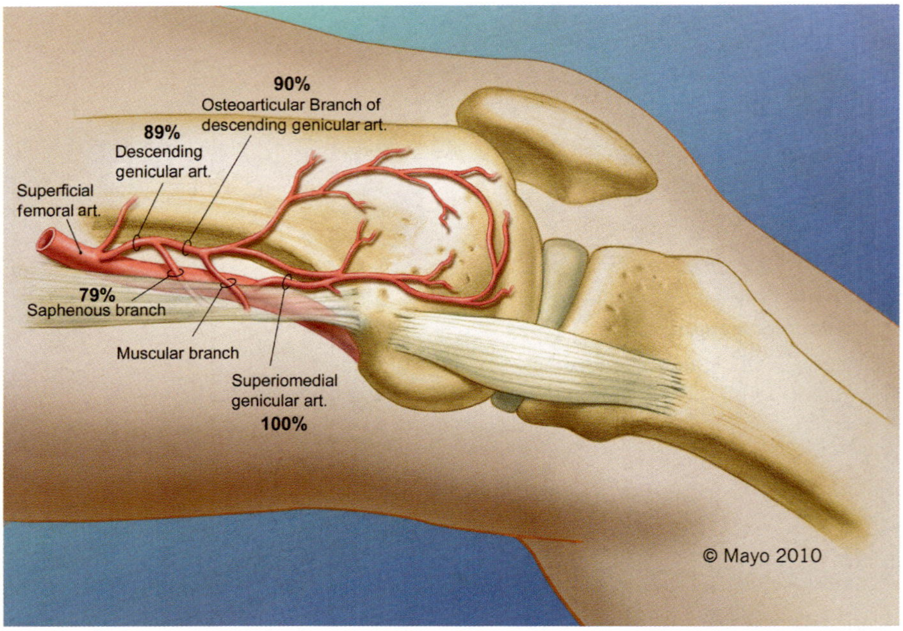

FIGURE 24-3 The superomedial genicular artery and descending genicular artery and its major branches are shown. Percentages refer to the frequency with which the vessels were found in the author's anatomic study (17). (By permission of Mayo Foundation for Medical Education and Research. All rights reserved.)

and 24-3). It lies just deep or lateral to the adductor magnus tendon along the posterior aspect of the medial intermuscular septum. As it reaches the metaphysis of the femur, it divides into an anteriorly and another posteriorly directed branch with contributions from the medial superior genicular artery. These vessels form a circularly arranged network of branches covering the face of the medial femoral condyle extraarticularly and providing multiple nutrient vessels that penetrate the thin cortical surface of the femur.

The saphenous branch was present in 79% of the specimens, branching off the descending genicular vessel an average of 11.7 cm (range, 9.5–18 cm) from the knee joint with an average internal diameter of 0.97 mm (range, 0.75–1.25 mm) (see Figures 23-2 and 23-3). It travels with the saphenous nerve deep to the sartorius to supply skin and subcutaneous tissues.

The superior medial genicular artery was present in all the specimens and originated from the popliteal artery an average of 5.2 cm (range, 3.5–6.5 cm) above the knee joint, with an internal diameter of 0.78 mm (range, 0.38–1.4 mm) (see Figures 23-2 and 23-3). It crosses from behind the adductor magnus tendon to anastomose with the osteoarticular branch of the descending genicular artery, contributing to the perforating vessels. The superior medial genicular artery was the dominant vessel supplying the medial femoral condyle in two of the specimens (11%).

It can be seen from these data that although the descending genicular vessels are often larger and longer than the medial superior vessels, they are not invariably so. In a recent series of 12 medial femoral condylar grafts, the descending genicular was used in 10 cases and the medial superior genicular in two (8). Both vessels should be inspected and an intraoperative decision made regarding the pedicle of choice based on availability, pedicle length, and vessel diameter.

Intraosseous Blood Supply

Yamamoto et al. found an average of 30 nutrient perforators supplying the medial femoral metaphysis based on the osteoperiosteal system of vessels (17). These nutrient vessels arise from the two major anterior and posterior branches that together cover the face of the medial femoral metaphysis. They are visible by direct inspection and may be seen to enter the surface of the bone through the thin outer cortex. The authors examined the intraosseous vessels within the bone after microangiography with Batson's compound and Spalteholz clearing. They found most nutrient vessels to be directed roughly perpendicular to the cortex, extending to an average depth of 13 mm (range, 9.4–18.3 mm). Importantly, the greatest number of perforators was detected in the posterior-distal quadrant of the medial distal femoral metaphysis (Figure 24-4).

VARIANTS OF THE FLAP

Corticoperiosteal Flap

Vascularized periosteal flaps have been known to have some osteogenic capability for many years, although the extent of new bone formation has been inconsistent and occasionally unsatisfactory (4). It is likely that the manner in which the flap is raised is of critical importance. In particular, the cambium layer must be included, requiring inclusion of a thin, fragmented layer of cortical bone with the periosteum. The inclusion of this bone does not hamper the flexibility of the flap because the medial femoral condylar cortex is exceedingly thin. It may be included without risk of mechanical compromise of the femur, making this location ideal as a periosteal flap donor. Given that bone is routinely included in the flap, it is more properly termed as "corticoperiosteal" rather than a periosteal flap.

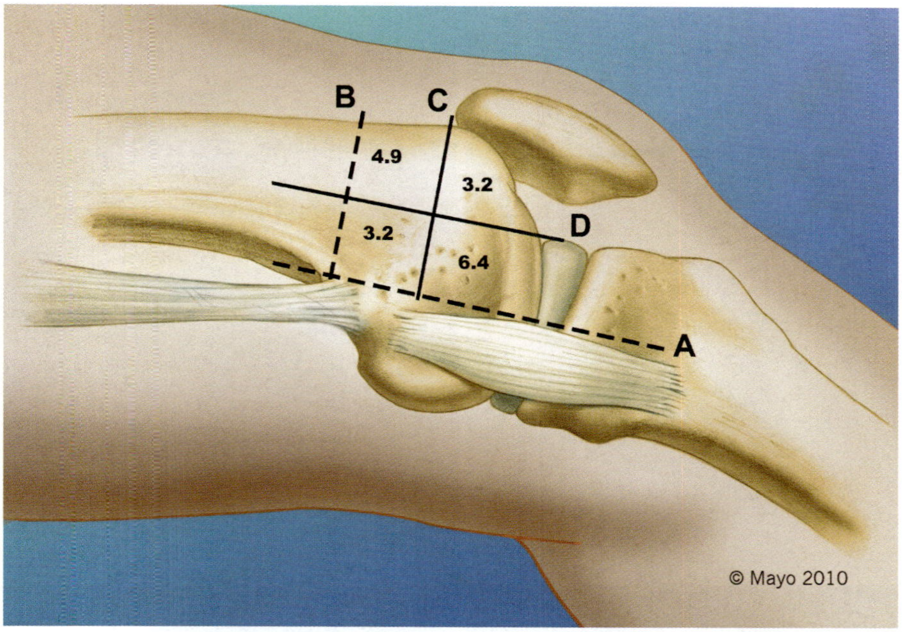

FIGURE 24-4 The average number of perforating vessels per quadrant of the medial femoral condyle. The quadrants are formed by drawing lines along the insertions of the hamstring and medial collateral ligament (**A**), from the insertion of the adductor magnus (**B**), and then from the proximal pole of the patella (**C**) and the anterior margin of the medial meniscus (**D**). (By permission of Mayo Foundation for Medical Education and Research. All rights reserved.)

Vascularized Bone Flap

The medial femoral condyle graft offers several advantages in the setting of combined avascular necrosis and scaphoid foreshortening. Because it is dissected free from all connections, the graft may be reshaped and manipulated to fit the defect with less risk of possible torsion or damage to the vascular pedicle. Cancellous bone quality is excellent: it is similar if not higher in density to the scaphoid and noticeably more robust than the distal radius. These small grafts are easily obtained from the medial femoral condyle, although the dissection of the proximal vasculature requires meticulous technique. Bone grafts are limited in dimension because of the anatomic constraints of the region. Care must be taken not to raise the flap proximally into the femoral diaphysis, resulting in mechanical compromise and possible later fracture of the bone. Grafts as long as 3 cm may be raised. An anteroposterior width and depth of 1 to 2 cm is easily obtained. No fractures have been reported to date in the literature from this donor site.

Osteocartilaginous Flap

A small portion of the medial patellar facet cartilage can be included with vascularized bone, described recently to resurface the proximal aspect of the scaphoid destroyed by avascular necrosis with a successful outcome (15).

DETAILED TECHNIQUE

General

Although either femur may be used as a donor, for upper extremity indications, the ipsilateral side is generally chosen to enable use of a crutch or cane in the opposite hand if needed after surgery. The patient is positioned supine on the operating table with the hip and knee flexed and externally rotated. A pneumatic tourniquet is used during elevation.

Exposure

A medial incision is made centered over the distal portion of the vastus medialis extending from the joint line of the knee proximally 20 cm (Figure 24-5).

The vastus medialis muscle is identified at its medial border and elevated from its fascial compartment. The descending genicular and medial superior genicular vessels are then identified.

The investing fascia of the vastus medialis is incised and the muscle retracted anteriorly. The descending genicular vessels are then easily visualized on the floor of the muscle compartment proximally, as are the periosteal vessels on the surface of the medial femoral condyle distally (Figure 24-6). The superomedial genicular vessels also contribute to the condylar blood supply and are identified at the metaphyseal level (Figure 24-7). The smaller vessels are generally ligated and the larger selected and dissected for microvascular connections. Generally, the descending genicular artery is larger and is mobilized proximally to its superficial femoral origin. In the illustrated example, the medial superior genicular artery is larger and has been followed to its popliteal artery origin, with the surgeon identifying and ligating small articular branches that would limit pedicle length as encountered.

Harvest of the Corticoperiosteal Flap

After exposure of the medial femoral surface and dissection of the vascular pedicles, the corticoperiosteal flap is raised. With

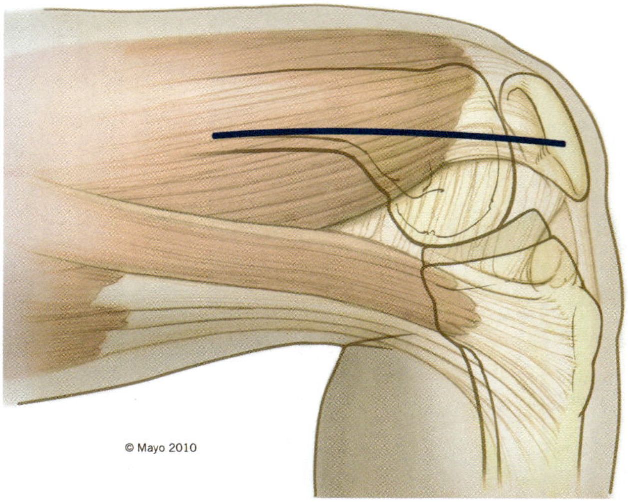

A

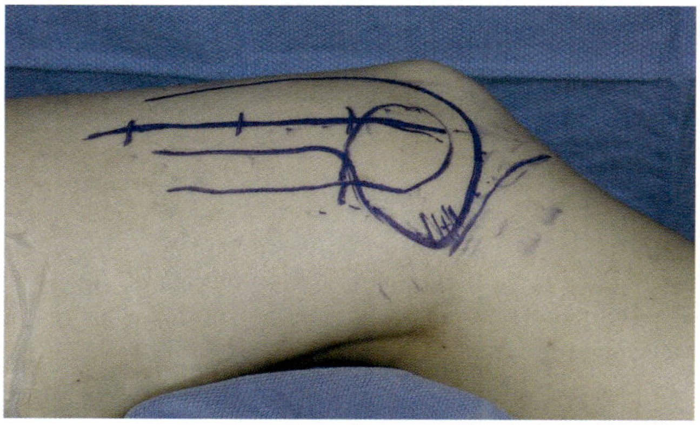

B

FIGURE 24-5 (A) and (B) Exposure of the medial femoral condyle. To harvest the vascularized periosteal bone graft, the incision is positioned over the medial femur at the posterior border of the vastus medialis. The incision begins at the articular edge of the distal femur, extending some 18 to 20 cm proximally. (By permission of Mayo Foundation for Medical Education and Research. All rights reserved.)

the vastus musculature reflected anteriorly, a large and easily visible network of anastomotic vessels derived from the system is seen to cover the medial surface of the distal femoral metaphysis (see Figure 24-6). The vessels supplying the face of the medial femoral distal metaphysis are next inspected and compared. Although in most cases the descending genicular vessels are larger, at times the medial superior vessels provide most of the blood flow (see Figure 24-7). After this distribution of genicular vessels is evaluated, the graft is outlined on the supracondylar periosteum to include the blood supply. It extends approximately 8 cm in length from the metaphyseal–diaphyseal junction proximally to the distal joint capsular reflection distally. Its width (typically measuring 6 cm) is limited by the posterior border of the femur and medial collateral ligament posteriorly and the medial patellar facet anteriorly. Flap elevation is performed without violating the joint capsule.

With the graft margins identified, the periosteum is progressively elevated with a curved, sharp osteotome. Elevation of the

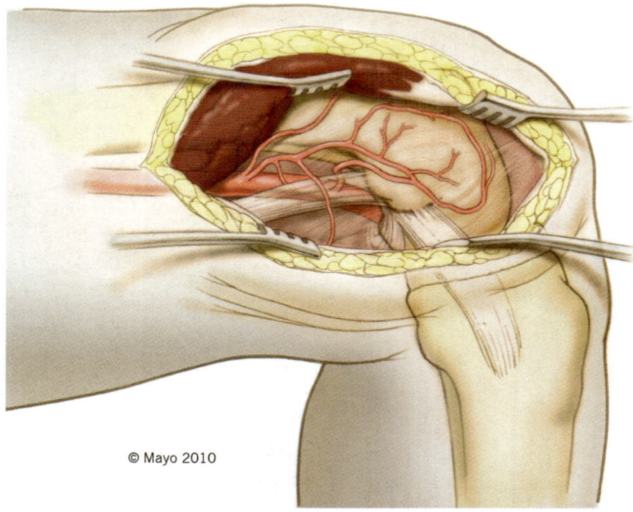

A

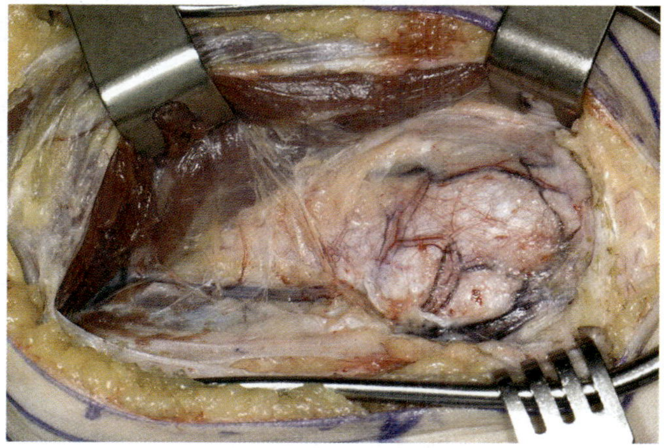

B

FIGURE 24-6 (A) The fascia is incised. (B) The vastus lateralis is elevated, and the medial femoral condyle is identified. The descending genicular vessels are visible running horizontally at left. (By permission of Mayo Foundation for Medical Education and Research. All rights reserved.)

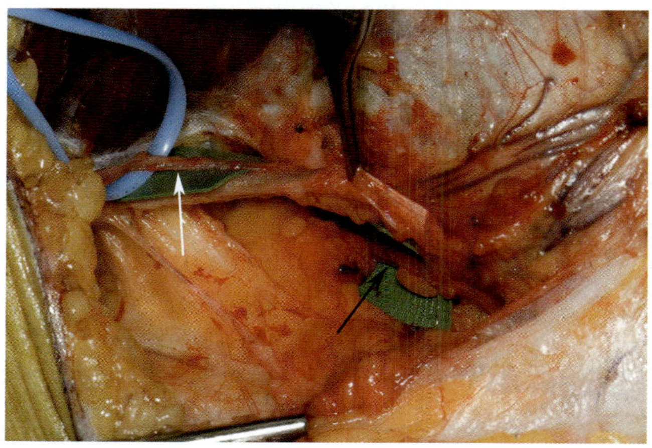

FIGURE 24-7 The descending genicular and medial superior genicular vessels are dissected, visible lying on the background material. (By permission of Mayo Foundation for Medical Education and Research. All rights reserved.)

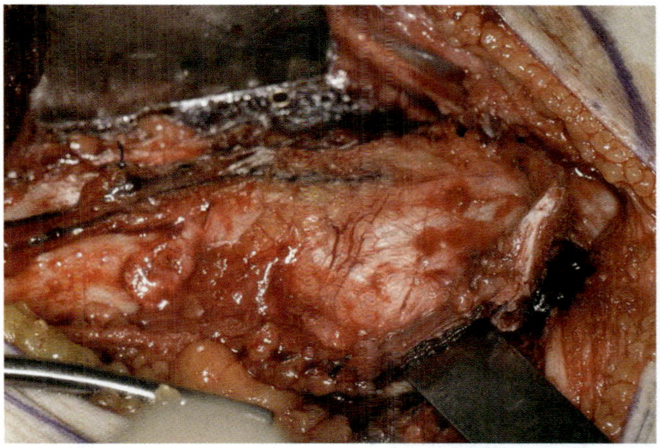

FIGURE 24-8 The corticoperiosteal graft is elevated carefully with a curved osteotome. (By permission of Mayo Foundation for Medical Education and Research. All rights reserved.)

graft proceeds from the margins toward the center by gentle advancement of the osteotome a few millimeters at a time using a combination of shallow cuts with the mallet and (most importantly) prying of the graft from underlying cancellous bone (Figure 24-8). Dissection in this fashion preserves the cambium layer and results in a thin flap that includes the periosteum and connected fragments of cortical bone.

Next, the vascular pedicle of the graft is dissected proximally to its origin from the superficial femoral vessels in Hunter's canal (Figure 24-9). Because the harvested graft is thin and pliable (Figure 24-10), it may be wrapped around small tubular bones such as the clavicle, radius, or ulna and secured with heavy nonabsorbable sutures or bone anchors. When used to promote healing in larger bones, it may be applied to cross the nonunion site as a "patch," generally held in place with suture anchors or transosseous sutures. Once positioned and secured, microvascular anastomoses are completed to prepared recipient vessels, and this is easily done given the 1 to 2 mm diameter of the proximal descending genicular vessels.

Vessel patency and a bleeding flap surface confirm a successful transfer. The flap circulation may be continuously monitored postoperatively with a cutaneous Bouy flap raised with the saphenous branch of the descending genicular, an implanted laser, or ultrasound probe or confirmed later with a bone scan performed in the first week after surgery.

Harvest of Vascularized Bone Segment

A vascularized segment of bone may be taken for reconstruction of small bone defects. The most common indication has been for scaphoid waist nonunion, when a wedge or structural graft is required to both restore scaphoid length and revascularize the proximal portion of the bone. It may be used for a variety of purposes, however, including for talus revascularization, craniofacial reconstruction, or metacarpal defects.

The graft is limited in length by the proximal transition from thin expendable metaphyseal bone to the thick cortical bone of the femoral diaphysis. Fractures of the femur have not been reported from harvest of this graft but could conceivably

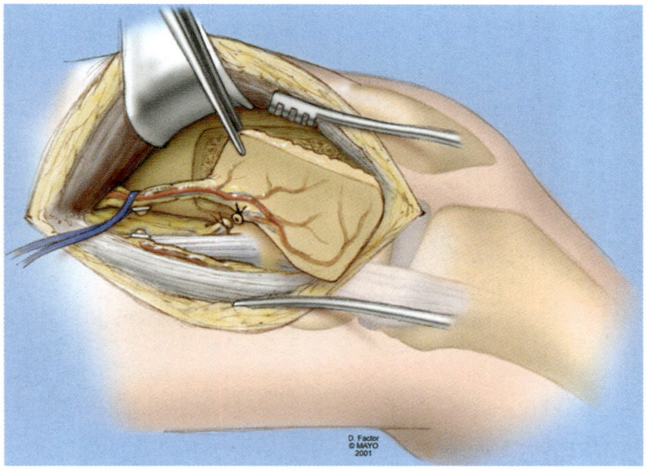

A

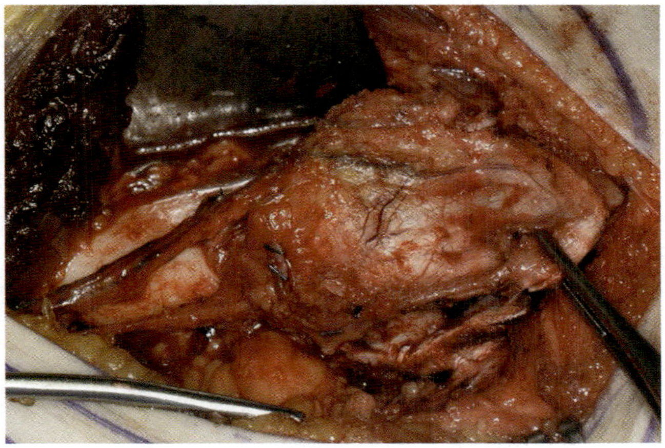

B

FIGURE 24-9 (A) and (B) The flap elevation completed. (By permission of Mayo Foundation for Medical Education and Research. All rights reserved.)

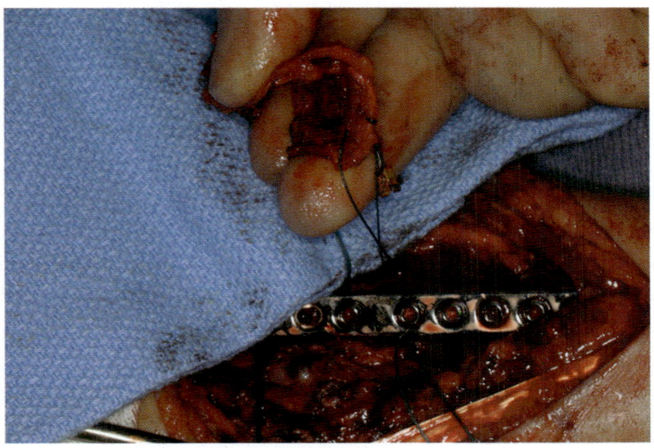

FIGURE 24-10 The pliability of the flap enables it to be "tubed," in this case to wrap around a forearm nonunion site. It may be held in position with sutures or bone anchors. (By permission of Mayo Foundation for Medical Education and Research. All rights reserved.)

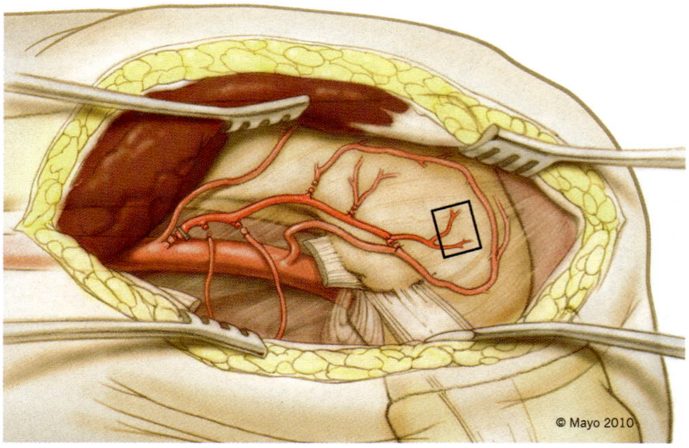

FIGURE 24-11 A site for bone graft elevation is outlined, to be of appropriate size and include the maximal number of nutrient vessels. In general, the distal and posterior quadrant of the metaphyseal surface is selected for this purpose. (By permission of Mayo Foundation for Medical Education and Research. All rights reserved.)

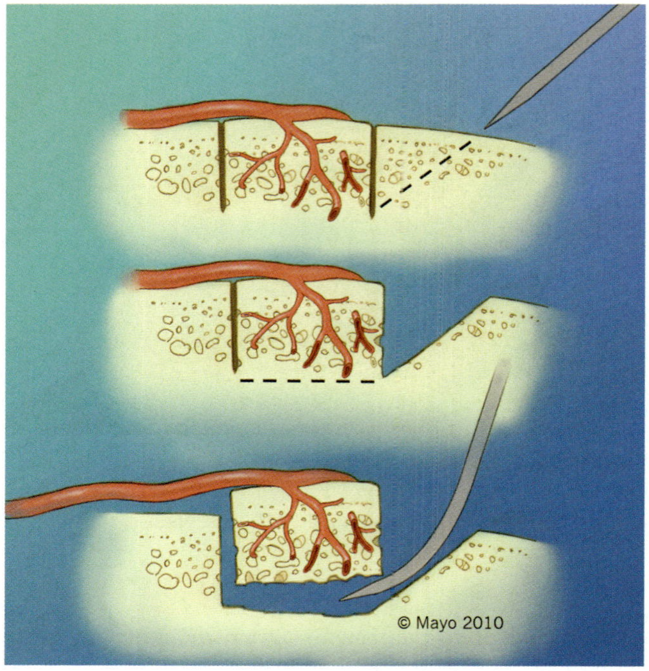

FIGURE 24-12 Care must be taken to avoid separation of the cortical and underlying compact cancellous bone during harvest. We make an additional oblique cut distal to the bone graft and removing an additional wedge of bone. This allows the graft to be mobilized on its deep surface without a prying motion. (By permission of Mayo Foundation for Medical Education and Research. All rights reserved.)

occur with an overzealous harvest, including diaphyseal cortex. Up to 3 cm in length is generally possible.

When possible, a site containing a number of visible nutrient foramina is used, most generally in the distal posterior quadrant. Other locations may be more favorable upon inspection based on individual variations in surface vessels as well as the size and shape of the bone or need to include articular cartilage. Generally, either the posterior or anterior branch of the osteoarticular vessel is used. The other branches are ligated or cauterized with a bipolar cautery.

The area to be included is outlined with surgical marker and its borders incised using bipolar cautery as needed for small crossing vessels distally, posteriorly, and anteriorly (Figure 24-11). The medial collateral ligament and the joint capsule should not be disturbed. With a small osteotome or a microsagittal saw, the outer cortex is then cut vertically in continuity with the periosteum. When making the osteotomy on the side of the vascular pedicle, the vascular pedicle is lifted gently out of the way with a vessel loupe followed by use of an osteotome to make the cut.

As the graft is mobilized, care must be taken to avoid separation of the cortex and periosteum from the cancellous portion of the graft during elevation. This can be prevented by making an additional cut distal to the graft at a 45-degree angle, allowing the graft to be elevated from its deep surface (Figure 24-12).

Next, it is necessary to carefully elevate the vessels proximal to the area of graft elevation from the surface of the bone to which they are adherent. This is done with great care under magnification, including venae comitantes and a small "tongue" of surrounding periosteum as needed to avoid injury to the blood supply. Small nutrient or articular branches may be ligated or cauterized with a fine-tipped bipolar cautery. Proximally, the smaller of the two genicular vessel pedicles is ligated and the dissection completed, following the other to its origin.

The tourniquet may be released at this time, allowing the bone flap to perfuse, permitting an immediate assessment of bone blood flow, which is generally excellent with visible pulsation in the pedicle and bleeding from the margins of the flap.

TRICKS AND TIPS

The most difficult part of the flap elevation is the mobilization of the osteoarticular vessels proximal to the bone or periosteal flap. These vessels are adherent to the bone surface and contain other nutrient branches. This is best accomplished by gently separating the vessels and a surrounding cuff of periosteum from the underlying bone using sharp dissection. Provided one does not elevate cortical bone with the pedicle, this does not result in heterotopic ossification of the pedicle.

We strive to prevent peripheral vasospasm during the flap elevation by maintaining the patient's core temperature with ambient temperature control and use of a Bair-Hugger warm air blanket, as well as topical vasodilators during pedicle dissection. Confirmation of adequate circulation may then be immediately obtained by release of the thigh tourniquet, allowing the bone or corticoperiosteal flap to briefly perfuse in situ. Two teams are used to simultaneous prepare the recipient site and elevate the flap, greatly shortening the surgical procedure. Flap elevation is accomplished in less than 1 hour because of the ease of exposure of the medial femoral condyle.

DONOR SITE CLOSURE AND AFTERCARE

After periosteal flap elevation, we loosely approximate the vastus fascia and close the skin and subcutaneous tissues in layers. When vascularized bone is removed, the defect may be filled with a bone substitute if desired. A compressive dressing is applied. A knee immobilizer is worn for the first few days and thereafter used occasionally as needed for comfort.

DONOR SITE MORBIDITY AND COMPLICATIONS

To date, the morbidity and complications from the donor site have been minimal and rare. A review of the literature demonstrates one case of a "stitch abscess" and two cases of saphenous nerve dysesthesia (9). No fracture, deep infection, or knee internal derangement has been reported.

There is some morbidity at the donor site, however. Harvest of either periosteum or bone results in a visible scar on the anteromedial distal thigh. This is certainly more visible than the iliac crest donor site but no more problematic than other commonly used flaps such as the fibula or scapula. All patients experience some medial distal thigh pain with knee flexion and extension for a period of days to weeks after surgery. A few will desire the use of a cane or crutch for a few days, and intermittent use of a knee immobilizer improves comfort during the immediate postoperative period.

INDICATIONS

Vascularized Bone Graft

Numerous pedicled and free vascularized bone grafts have been described for the treatment of scaphoid nonunions. A pedicled vascularized graft from the dorsal radius has been among the most popular such grafts, originally described by Zaidemberg and anatomically defined by Sheetz et al. based on the 1,2 intercompartmental supraretinacular artery (ICSRA) (18,19). However, the 1,2 ICSRA graft has been shown to fail in the special circumstance of scaphoid waist nonunions with a humpback deformity, associated carpal collapse, and an avascular proximal pole (20). In this circumstance, improved results have recently been reported with a vascularized wedge from the medial femoral condyle, with 100% union in the initial series of patients (8). Virtually any area requiring enhanced bone healing or reconstruction of small defects in cases with recalcitrant nonunion, radionecrosis, avascular necrosis, or other situations with poorly vascularized soft tissue beds are potential indications for this flap.

Corticoperiosteal Flap

The ability of a periosteal flap to enhance bone healing in a site without a large defect makes it an attractive, less bulky alternative to vascularized bone grafting when conditions are not favorable for conventional graft treatment. It has been used after failed conventional treatment of fractures, particularly when infection and scarring limit conventional cancellous graft efficacy. Pathologic fracture after radiotherapy is effectively treated with this method (11) as are allograft–host junction nonunions after tumor reconstruction (7).

REFERENCES

1. Jones DB Jr, Burger H, Bishop AT, Shin AY. Treatment of scaphoid waist nonunions with an avascular proximal pole and carpal collapse. Surgical technique. *J Bone Joint Surg Am* 2009;2:169.
2. King KF. Periosteal pedicle grafting in dogs. *J Bone Joint Surg* 1976;58 (suppl B):117.
3. Hertel R, Masquelet AC. The reverse flow medial knee osteoperiosteal flap for skeletal reconstruction of the leg. Description and anatomical basis. *Surg Radiol Anat* 1989;11:257.
4. Sakai K, Doi K, Kawai S. Free vascularized thin corticoperiosteal graft. *Plast Reconstr Surg* 1991;87:290.
5. Doi K, Sakai K. Vascularized periosteal bone graft from the supracondylar region of the femur. *Microsurgery* 1994;15:305.
6. Sammer DM, Bishop AT, Shin AY. Vascularized medial femoral condyle graft for thumb metacarpal reconstruction: case report. *J Hand Surg Am* 2009;34:715.
7. Choudry UH, Bakri K, Moran SL, et al. The vascularized medial femoral condyle periosteal bone flap for the treatment of recalcitrant bony nonunions. *Ann Plast Surg* 2008;60:174.
8. Jones DB Jr, Burger H, Bishop AT, Shin AY. Treatment of scaphoid waist nonunions with an avascular proximal pole and carpal collapse. A comparison of two vascularized bone grafts. *J Bone Joint Surg Am* 2008;90:2616.
9. Jones DB Jr, Moran SL, Bishop AT, Shin AY. Free-vascularized medial femoral condyle bone transfer in the treatment of scaphoid nonunions. *Plast Reconstr Surg* 2010;125:1176.
10. Pelzer M, Reichenberger M, Germann G. Osteo-periosteal-cutaneous flaps of the medial femoral condyle: a valuable modification for selected clinical situations. *J Reconstr Microsurg* 2010;26:291.
11. Fuchs B, Steinmann SP, Bishop AT. Free vascularized corticoperiosteal bone graft for the treatment of persistent nonunion of the clavicle. *J Shoulder Elbow Surg* 2005;14:264.
12. Benlidayi ME, Gaggl A, Buerger H, et al. Comparison of vascularized osteoperiosteal femur flaps and nonvascularized femur grafts for reconstruction of mandibular defects: an experimental study. *J Oral Maxillofac Surg* 2009;67:1174.
13. Bakri K, Moran SL. Initial assessment and management of complex forearm defects. [review]. *Hand Clin* 2007;23:255.
14. Henry M. Genicular corticoperiosteal flap salvage of resistant atrophic non-union of the distal radius metaphysis. *Hand Surg* 2007;12:211.
15. Kaelicke T, Buerger H, Mueller EJ. [A new vascularized cartilage-bone-graft for scaphoid nonunion with avascular necrosis of the proximal pole. Description of a new type of surgical procedure]. [German]. *Unfallchirurg* 2008;111:201.
16. Scapinelli R. Studies on the vasculature of the human knee joint. *Acta Anat* 1968;70:305.
17. Yamamoto H, Jones DB Jr, Moran SL, et al. The arterial anatomy of the medial femoral condyle and its clinical implications. *J Hand Surg Eur* 2010;35:569.
18. Sheetz KK, Bishop AT, Berger RA. The arterial blood supply of the distal radius and ulna and its potential use in vascularized pedicled bone grafts. *J Hand Surg Am* 1995;20:902.
19. Zaidenberg C, Siebert JW, Angrigiani C. A new vascularized bone graft for scaphoid nonunion. *J Hand Surg Am* 1991;16:474.
20. Chang MA, Bishop AT, Moran SL, Shin AY. The outcomes and complications of 1,2-intercompartmental supraretinacular artery pedicled vascularized bone grafting of scaphoid nonunions. *J Hand Surg Am* 2006;31:387.

CHAPTER 25

Venous Flaps

Sang-Hyun Woo

BRIEF HISTORY AND SUBSEQUENT EVOLUTION

The survival of a conventional free flap depends heavily on the dynamic flow between the arterial inflow and venous outflow much like in the normal circulation. However, there are some limitations in elevating a conventional flap such as the sacrifice of significant peripheral arteries and the time-consuming meticulous technique for dissection. Furthermore, when a very thin skin flap is needed, especially in head and neck and hand reconstruction, conventional flaps frequently prove too bulky.

In an effort to overcome these disadvantages, many experimental studies are underway using a thin skin flap based on the subcutaneous venous network. A venous flap is defined here as a skin flap with the inclusion of veins only. In 1985, Baek et al. (1) first described this concept. A venous flap, having only venous channels, survived by a "to-and-fro" flow in capillaries and venules without any arterial inflow. The oxygen content in the venous blood pulsating in the venous flap was hoped to be sufficient to meet the basic requirements for flap survival. However, this flap remained prone to ischemia irrespective of the number of venous pedicles connected because of the low pO_2 on the venous side of the circulation. A small surviving area and the uncertainty of flap survival at all limited the clinical application of Baek's venous flap (2–4).

To ensure flap survival, arterial inflow would seem to be the first prerequisite. The "arterialized venous flap" is a skin flap that has arterial inflow through one vein (the "afferent" vein) and venous outflow through one or more "efferent" veins. Arterialization of the venous system results in high-pressure blood flow with abundant oxygen and nutrients delivered through the venous system. This concept was first introduced by Nakayama et al. (5) in 1981 and was followed up by several reports of animal studies (6–10) and clinical trials (11–15).

Since then, arterialized venous flaps have been used in a wide variety of reconstructions, including the upper and lower extremities (16–18), face, and neck (19–21). "Flow-through venous flaps," they have been used for simultaneous reconstruction of arteries and overlying soft tissue (22–24). Interestingly, two separate defects on the foot or digit have been covered with bilobed arterialized venous flaps (25,26). Furthermore, composite defects have been reconstructed with tendocutaneous venous flaps (16,18,27–29), osteocutaneous venous flaps (13), and even neurocutaneous flaps (18,30,31). Initially, the size of venous flaps was as small as 2 × 2 cm (Figure 25-1). Later relatively large defects were covered with arterialized venous flaps ranging from 14 × 9 cm to 14 × 16 cm (17,32). However, severe postoperative swelling, discoloration, and bullae formation and unpredictable partial necrosis persist as major problems associated with arterialized venous flaps. Many experimental studies have focused on finding out both the basic physiology of the flap and techniques to improve flap survival (33–37).

GENERAL CONSIDERATIONS

Anatomy of Vein, the Venosome, and Associated Tissues

The peripheral venous system is subdivided into a superficial or epifascial and a deep or subfascial system by the superficial fascia (38). The two systems are interconnected by the transfascial system consisting of perforating veins. Deep veins accompany the arteries. Venous flaps always include a superficial venous channel above the underlying muscle fascia.

Various characteristics of venous territories have been described in the anatomic study of the veins of the human body by Taylor et al. in 1990 (39). The venous architecture is arranged as a continuous network of vascular arcades. This arrangement exists within all tissues and between adjacent tissues. The venous

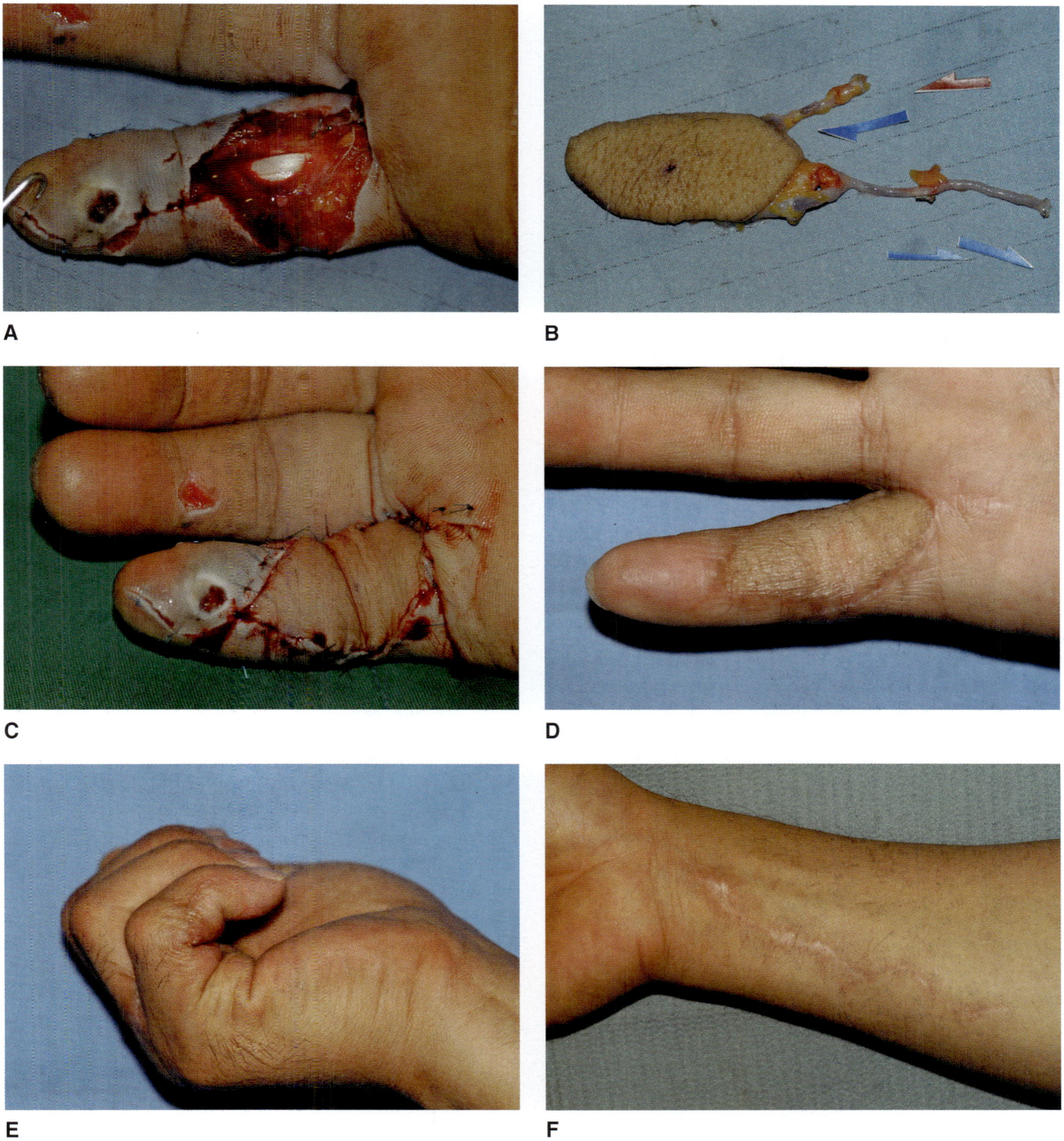

FIGURE 25-1 One of the most common indications of the arterialized venous flap is resurfacing of the volar defect of the small finger. (**A**) On the small finger, a soft tissue defect exposes the flexor tendon. (**B**) Harvested venous flap with two veins. (**C**) Immediate postoperative view. One afferent vein was anastomosed to the ulnar digital artery, and the efferent vein was passed through a subcutaneous tunnel and anastomosed to a dorsal vein of the small finger. (**D**) and (**E**) Postoperative views 10 months later. (**F**) Donor site, volar aspect of the forearm.

network consists of linked valvular and avalvular channels that allow equilibration of flow and pressure. Avalvular segments of the venous network, called oscillating veins, connect and allow free flow between valved channels of adjacent venous territories. Veins hitchhike with nerves, making it possible to design innervated venous flaps. This pattern can be found in the medial forearm and lower leg involving the medial antebrachial cutaneous nerve with the basilic vein in the former case and the long and short saphenous veins with the saphenous and sural nerves in the latter.

Suggested Survival Mechanism

Survival of a conventional flap depends heavily on the dynamic interchange between arterial inflow and venous outflow much like in normal circulation. In the pure venous flap, venous blood is less oxygenated, has a slower flow rate, and is therefore prone to thrombosis (40). In the arterialized venous flap, high-pressure arterial blood with its high pO_2 as well as contained nutrients is essential for the survival of the flap. Because at least 50% of the blood oxygen is extracted even before it reaches the capillaries (41), an arterialized venous flap is able to survive with just a precapillary and postcapillary venous system while in an ischemic state.

The sudden rise in venous pressure of an arterialized venous flap right after the anastomosis causes active congestion (42). If the efferent venous drainage is not efficient, deoxygenated hemoglobin accumulates in the flap, causing ischemia. If this condition persists, it produces swelling, discoloration, and bullae formation and finally results in partial necrosis in the region where oxygen and nutrient extraction is minimal. Unlike a conventional flap with normal circulation, if the arterialized flap has only one draining vein, the interstitial fluid in the tissues stagnates and blood flow is only effective near that single vascular channel. This eventually causes partial necrosis in the flap. However, as the number of draining veins increase, the venous channels become more extensive within the flap, and this facilitates more efficient exchange of oxygen and nutrients enhancing flap survival. Sasa et al. (7) also reported that if the efferent vein is well maintained, the rearterialization process of the flap could be accelerated. Also, if the arterialized venous flap has a healthy recipient vascular bed, this hastens neovascularization from underneath the flap, which can also improve the chance of flap survival (35).

The principal outcome of neovascularization is to decrease the high pressure in the afferent venous system. Neovascularization may be partially replaced by an adaptation of the vascular network in the flap. A delay procedure consisting of an arteriovenous fistula 3 weeks before raising the flap might help avoid the consequences of high pressure in the venous system. Neovascularization of the arterialized venous flaps can be explained in two possible ways (18). The first is horizontal neovascularization between the flap margins and the edges of the recipient site, which plays a more important role from 3 to 5 days after surgery. The second is formation of neovessels vertically between the recipient bed and the flap. This, according to the author, plays a critical role in ameliorating postoperative venous congestion approximately 1 week after surgery. If the recipient bed is totally avascular, this postoperative congestion resolves very slowly. This is one of the main causes of flap necrosis in venous flaps. Although there is a report of survival of arterialized venous flaps performed to achieve coverage of exposed bone without periosteum (13), there is no doubt that flap survival rate is much greater in recipient sites that have at least some degree of vascularity than in sites totally devoid of vessels.

In arterialized venous flaps, severe edema and discoloration, not usually seen with conventional flaps, are frequently noted after surgery and last several weeks. The swelling is most pronounced in the first week and gradually starts to subside thereafter. It is thought that the venous valves are subject to high arterial pressures, causing dilation and stagnation of the interstitial fluid within the tissues. Sufficient oxygen and nutrients can be absorbed from the blood flowing through the veins and from the stagnant interstitial fluid, but accumulation of toxic metabolites and deoxygenated hemoglobin results in flap necrosis (Figure 25-2).

Direction of the Intravenous Valve

Direction of flow is considered important in vein grafts because of the presence of valves. In some situations, the direction of flow in venous flaps is not reversed to avoid size discrepancy during the anastomosis of the vessels. Both animal (36,41,43,44) and human trials (18,32,45) have verified that the direction of the valves is irrelevant to the survival of the flap. In arterialized venous flaps, good blood circulation to the periphery is imperative for flap survival and may take place even in the presence of competent venous valves (9,35,46). In the studies, surgical denervation during flap elevation caused vasoparalysis, which induced arteriovenous shunts to open up. In addition, high-pressure arterial blood flow rendered minor valves within the veins nonfunctional. However, it is recommended that the direction of flow in the efferent vessels be aligned with the valves of the recipient draining vessels whenever possible to ease drainage.

Clinically, arterialized venous flaps usually look pale immediately after vessel anastomosis between the artery and afferent vein of the flap. After several hours, opening of the arteriovenous shunts appears to be triggered by ischemia in the overlying skin. This results in capillary refill being restored. In the through-valve type of venous flap, the flap assumes a pinkish tint along the course of the afferent vein. However, in the case of arterial inflow through afferent vein against valves, the flap assumes a color change similar to that of "parading troops" advancing from the anastomotic site toward the distal part of the flap (Figure 25-3). Over the next few days, congestion, ecchymoses, bullae formation, and discoloration obscure the evaluation of capillary refill. After the congestion is resolved approximately 10 days after surgery, the flap assumes a normal color. In cases of superficial epidermolysis on the flap, it is removed, uncovering healthy tissue.

Causes of Unpredictable Flap Necrosis

The occurrence of postoperative necrosis along with unstable changes in the venous flap was more common in the early period of the author's experience. It occurred in cases in which the procedure was performed despite inappropriate indications. In patients with diabetes, flap failure or partial necrosis resulted when flaps were used to achieve coverage of chronic open wounds with ongoing infection or with a totally avascular beds. On sites devoid of any ongoing infection and with at least a partially vascularized recipient bed, it is more appropriate to use venous flaps.

Problems related to flap size were also encountered. Arterialized venous flaps proved best at reconstructing small to medium-sized defects but not large defects. Currently, when there is an extensive soft tissue defect of the hand or forearm, a perforator flap is the first choice. Failures also resulted because

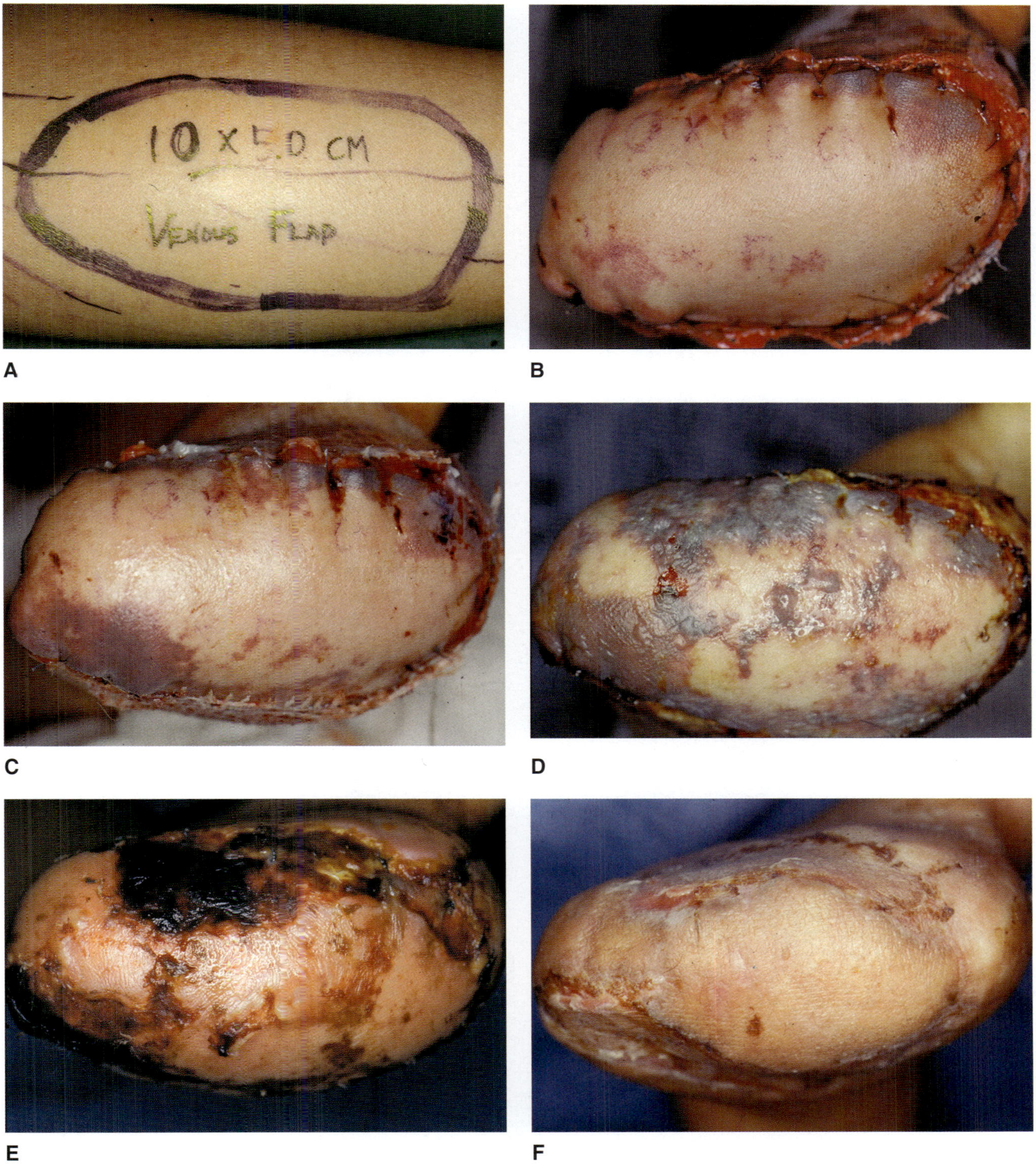

FIGURE 25-2 Typical postoperative sequence of an arterialized venous flap. (**A**) A soft tissue defect over the metacarpal area was covered with an arterialized venous flap 5 × 10 cm. The flap, which included four veins, was harvested from the volar aspect of the forearm. The second common digital artery was anastomosed to one afferent vein against its valves (antidromic). Three efferent veins were anastomosed to superficial veins on the dorsum of the hand. (**B**) Marginal discoloration appeared 30 hours after surgery. (**C**) Purplish discoloration expanded from the margin to the center of the flap on the fourth day after surgery. (**D**) Multiple bullae and mottled discoloration were noticed on the entire surface of the flap on postoperative day 8. (**E**) and (**F**) On day 16, there was a necrotic area at the margin of the flap (~25%), which was debrided and resurfaced with a split-thickness skin graft.

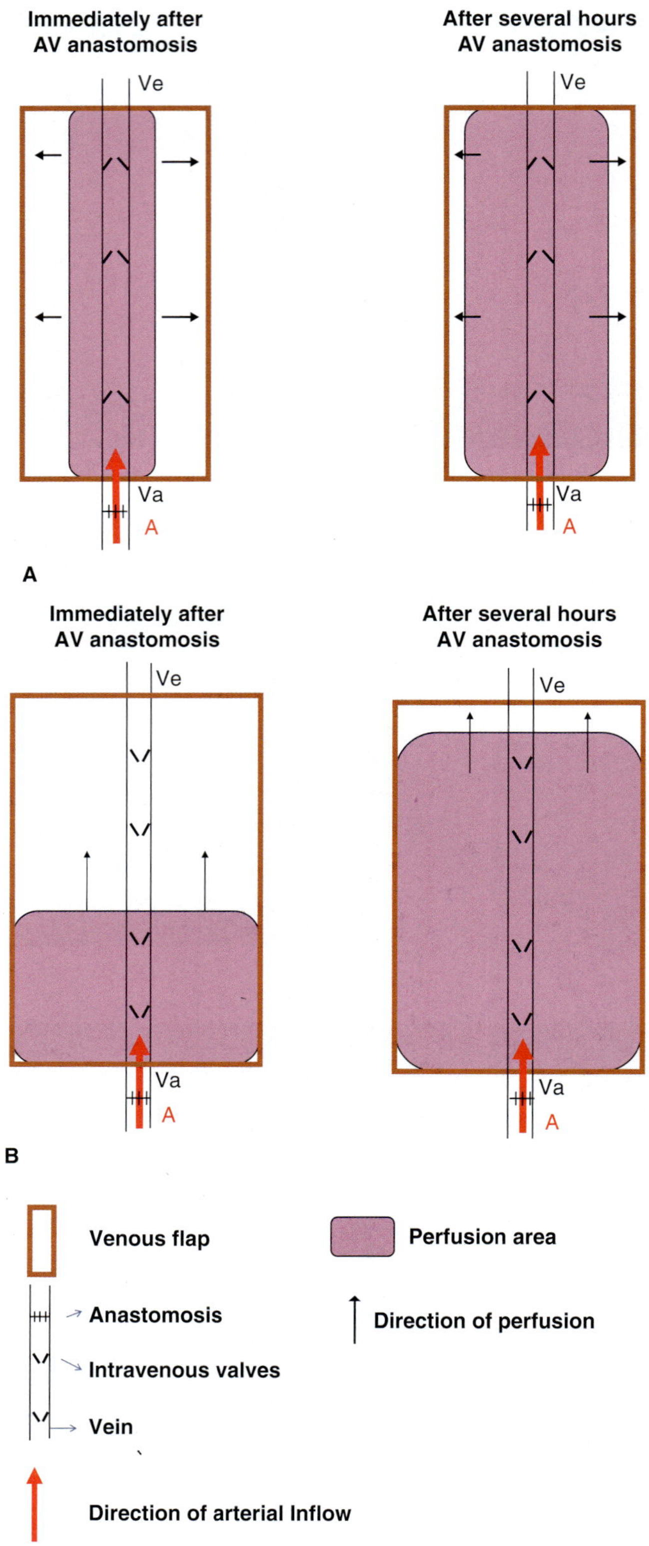

FIGURE 25-3 Suggested perfusion pattern of the arterialized venous flap. (**A**) In the orthodromic type of venous flap, the flap assumes a pinkish tint along the course of the afferent vein (Va). However, in the case of arterial inflow through afferent vein against valves (antidromic), the flap assumes a color change similar to the so-called "parading troops" pattern, which appears to "march" from the anastomotic site to the distal part of the flap. In type I, venous flap of the "through-valve" or orthodromic type, immediately after operation, perfusion is possible around the venous pedicle. Several hours after the microanastomosis, perfusion of the flap progresses from the axis of venous pedicle to the both lateral margins of the flap. (**B**) In the "against-valve" (antidromic), venous flap, perfusion produces a gradual color change similar to troops parading from the anastomotic site to the distal part of the flap. Immediately after the operation, perfusion is possible to the first intravenous valve. Several hours after arteriovenous (AV) anastomosis, perfusion of the flap progresses to the distal part of the flap. A, artery; Va, afferent vein; Ve, efferent vein.

of difficulties in postoperative monitoring. In the early period of our clinical experience, it was not easy to differentiate typical venous congestion of the flap from anastomotic thrombosis of the afferent or efferent vein. When monitoring a venous flap, observation of capillary refill or surface temperature are unreliable modalities. If the flap's condition is suspicious, puncturing it with a needle or blade and observing bright red bleeding is more reliable.

VARIANTS OF THE FLAP

Flap Classifications According to Size

Based on the characteristics of the venous flap, flaps smaller than 10 cm^2 were classified as small, and those larger than 25 cm^2 were classified as large. Those in between were classified as medium-sized flaps.

Flap Compositions

Although typical venous flaps only consist of skin and subcutaneous tissue, compound venous flaps may include two structures, such as tendon, nerve, or blood vessels along with the skin flap. Innervated venous flaps contain sensory nerves, tendocutaneous flaps, extensor tendons, and conduit venous flaps, and integrated vein grafts. Composite flaps including three different types of tissue (vessel, nerve, and tendon, as well as skin) have been used for the reconstruction of composite defects of the hand.

Suggested Flap Types

On the basis of my basic research and clinical experience, I would like to suggest three types of arterialized venous flap (18). This classification takes into consideration the presence of the valves, the venous network of the donor site, and the location, as well as the number of veins at the recipient site (Figure 25-4).

Type I is an "orthodromic flow-through venous flap," which mimics the blood flow in a standard vein graft. It may be a straight or Y-shaped pattern. The width-to-length ratio of the flap is 1:3 or 1:4. This is good for small flaps or long and narrow flaps. One efferent vein may be anastomosed to the distal part of the recipient artery instead of a recipient vein. Clinically, it may be applied as a conduit venous flap for reconstruction of an arterial defect with an associated soft tissue deficiency as in finger replantation. However, in this type, there would be a long scar at the donor site because of the linear incision resulting from the harvest of both flap and pedicles.

Type II is an antidromic venous flap in which the arterial inflow is against the valve through the afferent vein. A reversed Y- or H-shaped venous network is good for medium-sized flaps.

In Type III venous flaps, venous flow drains through efferent veins against valves in the recipient vessels. This is appropriate for large flaps. The presence of multiple veins at the recipient site is mandatory. In the event that the third or fourth draining vein in the recipient bed is unavailable, the third or fourth efferent vein may be ligated.

In both type II and type III venous flaps, one of the efferent veins is also anastomosed to a recipient artery for the reconstruction of arterial defects.

Flap Donor Sites

Certain characteristics of venous flaps, such as the absence of valves in the veins, extensive networking, and intimate association and support of the overlying skin, play an important role in the selection of donor site. As a result, there are some preferable donor sites for venous flaps. These are the volar aspect of the forearm, the volar aspect of the distal wrist including the thenar area, the dorsum of the foot, and the medial aspect of the calf. In cases of hand reconstruction, the most common donor site is the volar aspect of the ipsilateral forearm. The forearm is the most common donor site for large flaps. The volar aspect of the distal wrist and thenar area are appropriate for small- to medium-sized flaps. These may be used for reconstruction of defects of the pulp and the volar aspects of the fingers.

The dorsum of the foot is also one of the most favored donor sites for innervated venous flaps. It has a rich venous network and branches of the superficial peroneal nerve beneath skin much thinner than that of the forearm. Ideally, the volar side of the finger should be reconstructed with glabrous skin such as the palm or instep. The innervated arterialized venous flap can provide excellent functional and cosmetic coverage of severe avulsion injuries of the finger (47). Small arterialized venous flaps that use medial plantar skin are useful for finger pulp reconstruction (48). However, it is difficult to harvest a thin, pliable, and sufficiently arterialized venous flap to cover a completely denuded finger from the medial plantar skin. It is also not easy to elevate enough long cutaneous veins and cutaneous branches of medial plantar nerve in the instep venous flap.

Both lateral sides of the thenar and hypothenar region contain a branch of the dorsal cutaneous vein. The durable glabrous skin from these areas makes them appropriate donor sites for venous flaps in finger pulp reconstruction (49). When elevating the flap, a segment of the branch of the dorsal cutaneous vein, the subcutaneous tissue, and deep fascia of the thenar or hypothenar muscles are included. At the recipient site, a proper digital artery and dorsal vein are prepared at the interphalangeal joint level.

An anatomical study has shown that the scalp has few or no valves and is potentially one of the best donor sites of arterialized venous free flaps (39).

Flap Variants

Tendocutaneous Compound Venous Flap

To reconstruct a compound defect involving soft tissue and tendons, a venous flap that includes the palmaris longus tendon from the distal wrist has been harvested in a number of clinical cases (18,27–29). Most flaps incorporated two veins. The tendons were repaired first using multiple figure-of-8 or modified Becker's sutures under appropriate tension, and then the vessels were anastomosed. Rehabilitation was started on postoperative

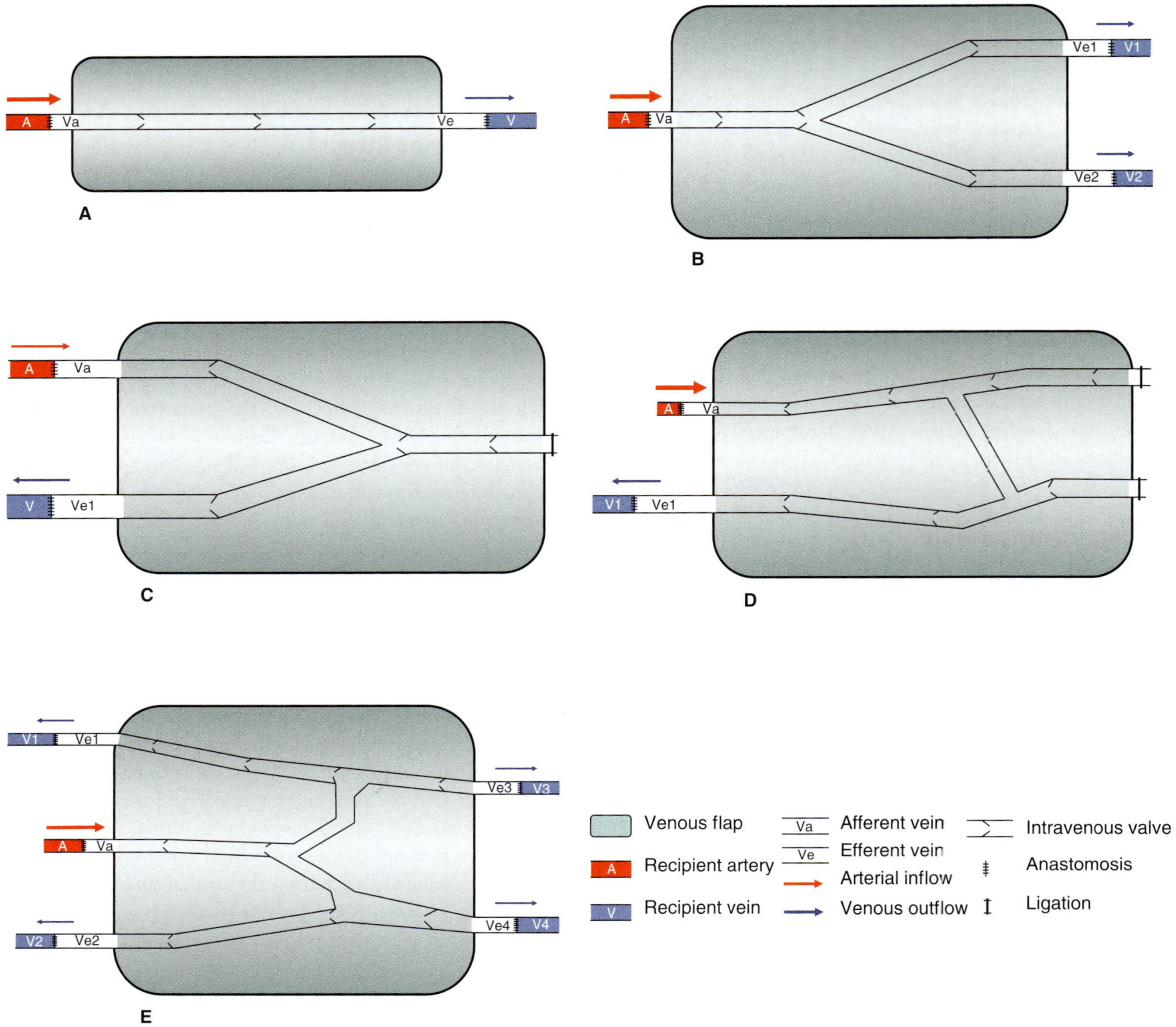

FIGURE 25-4 Classification of arterialized venous flaps. This classification is based on the presence and direction of the intravenous valves, the venous network of the donor site, and the location and number of veins in the recipient site. (**A**) Type I, through-valve type with a flow-through pattern. (**B**) Type I, through-value type with a Y-shaped pattern. (**C**) Type II, against-valve type with a reversed Y-shaped pattern. (**D**) Type II, against-valve type with an H-shaped pattern. (**E**) Type III, mixed pattern through and against the valves. A, artery; V, vein; Va, afferent vein; Ve, efferent vein.

day 10—when the circulation within the flap was stable—using a dynamic splint with a volar block to restrict finger flexion.

Illustrative Case: Tendocutaneous Compound Venous Flap A 38-year-old woman sustained a crushing injury to the right index finger resulting in a compound tissue defect. There was a transverse fracture at the shaft of the middle phalanx, a 2-cm defect of the extensor tendon in zones I and II, and an overlying soft tissue defect. After debridement, a 2 × 2 cm venous flap with 2.5 cm of the palmaris longus tendon and containing two veins was harvested from the ipsilateral wrist. It was designed as a reversed Y-shaped venous network. The afferent vein was anastomosed to the ulnar digital artery of the index finger, and the efferent vein was anastomosed to the dorsal vein of the finger against the direction of its valves. The donor site was resurfaced with a full-thickness skin graft from the inner upper arm. The transferred tendon was sutured with multiple figure-of-8 sutures to the remnant of the extensor tendon. The flap survived without any complications. Ten months after the operation, the range of motion was 0 to 90 degrees at the metacarpophalangeal joint, 10 to 90 degrees at the proximal interphalangeal joint, and 25 to 55 degrees at the distal interphalangeal joint. Total active range of motion was 200 degrees (Figure 25-5).

Innervated Venous Flap

In forearm cases, using the cephalic vein as a guide, the anterior branch of the medial or lateral antebrachial cutaneous nerve of

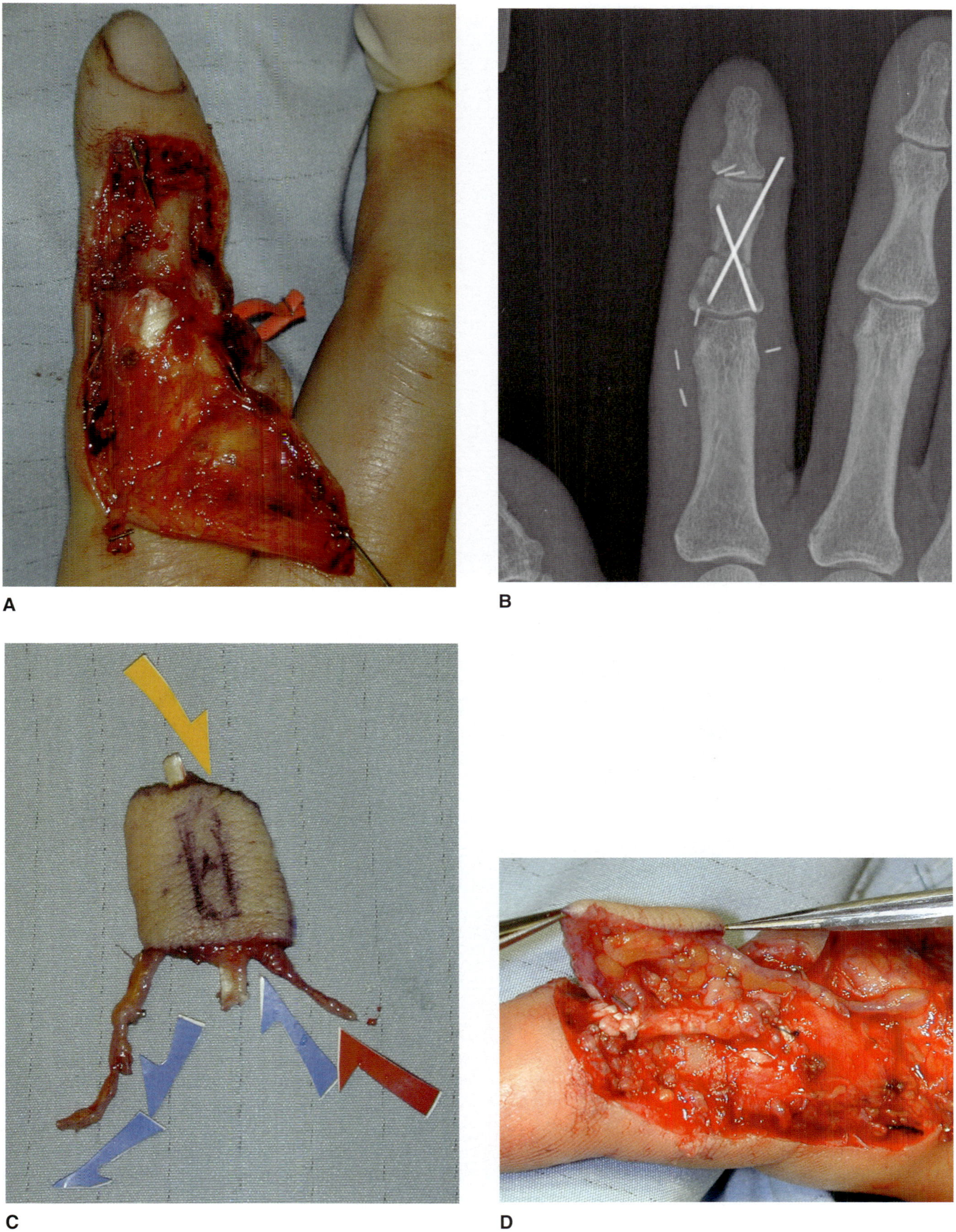

FIGURE 25-5 Tendocutaneous arterialized venous flap. (**A**) Preoperative view of a compound defect on the dorsal aspect of the right index finger. (**B**) A middle phalangeal bone fracture was reduced and fixed with two Kirschner wires. (**C**) Dissected 2 × 2 cm compound venous flap, including the palmaris longus tendon and two veins. (**D**) Repaired extensor tendon using tendon graft in zone I and II using a multiple "figure-of-8" technique.

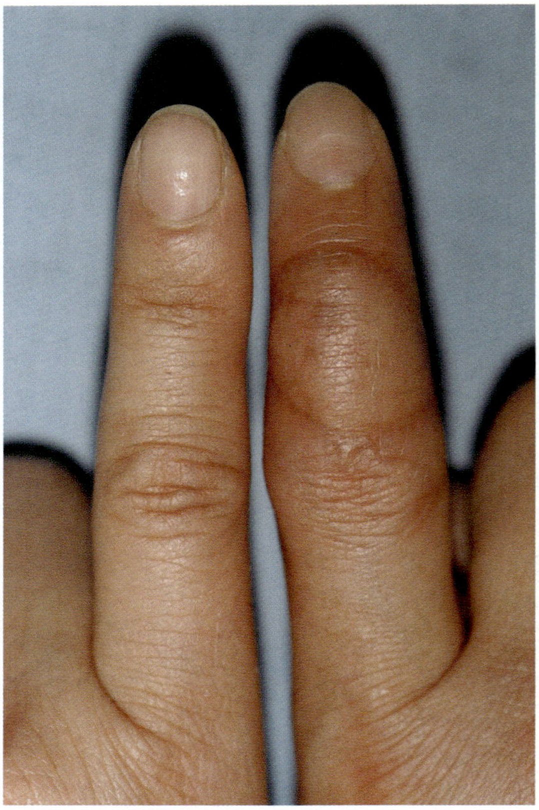

E

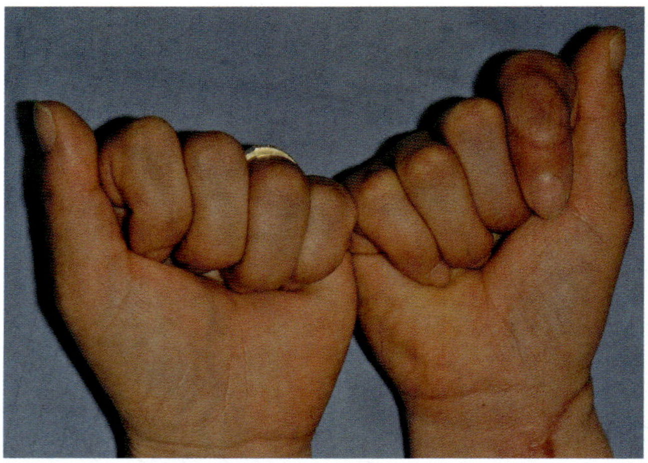

F

FIGURE 25-5 (*Continued*) (**E**) and (**F**) Postoperative appearance 10 months later. The active ranges of motion of the proximal interphalangeal joint and the distal interphalangeal joint are about 80 (10/90) degrees and 30 (25/55) degrees, respectively.

the forearm may be included in the design of an innervated venous flap. From the dorsum of the foot the dorsal lateral cutaneous nerves can also be harvested together with the lateral veins to craft an innervated flap. The distribution of nerves and vessels must first be checked through an incision proximal to the flap, which is then harvested as described earlier. Innervated venous flaps have been used to reconstruct soft tissue defects of the palmar side of the digits or hand with a segmental defect of the nerve.

Illustrative Case: Innervated Conduit Venous Flap A 38-year-old woman was referred after primary treatment following a crush injury to the forearm by a press machine. Reduction of distal radius fracture, K-wire transfixation of radius and ulna, and debridement of devitalized soft tissue was performed initially. A soft-tissue defect approximately 3 × 7 cm in size as well as a 5.5-cm ulnar bone defect and a 10-cm defect of both the ulnar artery and the ulnar nerve were evident. A 4 × 7 cm venous flap that included the sural nerve and lesser saphenous vein was harvested to reconstruct the ulnar artery and nerve. Another 10 cm of the sural nerve was also harvested as a cable nerve graft. The conduit venous flap was designed with a Y-shaped venous pattern. Two of the veins were anastomosed to the proximal and distal ulnar artery, and one vein was attached to a subcutaneous vein in the wrist as the draining vein. The donor site was resurfaced with a split-thickness skin graft. The flap developed some discoloration and bulla formation at the edges but eventually healed without any signs of necrosis. Twenty months after surgery, static two-point discrimination was 9 and 13 mm for the ring and small fingers, respectively. Pinch and grasp was 7 and 17 lb, which was 44% and 38% that of the intact contralateral hand, respectively. Claw hand deformity was not observed, but atrophy of the first interdigital web space and external rotational deviation on extension of the small finger was evident (Figure 25-6).

Illustrative Case: Large Venous Flap A 44-year-old man sustained a belt injury from a roller machine to the index, long, and ring fingers. After debridement of nonviable tissues, there was a soft tissue defect on the dorsal aspect around the middle phalanx. The extensor tendons were partially devitalized, and the middle phalangeal bone was exposed. A 12 × 3 cm venous flap, which contained three veins, was harvested from the ipsilateral forearm. The blood supply was provided by anastomosis between one afferent vein of the flap and the ulnar digital artery of the ring finger. Two draining veins were sutured to the dorsal veins on the dorsum of the hand. The flap survived completely. After 10 days, gentle motion of each finger joint was commenced. The flap was divided and defatted 4 weeks after the first operation. Eight months after the operation, total active range of motion of the index, long, and ring fingers was 160, 175, and 180 degrees, respectively (Figure 25-7).

Preexpanded Venous Flap

Prefabrication of conventional free flaps with tissue expansion has many advantages, including increasing flap size, decreasing donor site morbidity, and thinning of the flap. The experimental research of Leighton et al. (50) concluded that expansion induced an increase in capillary density within the flap, increased vascularity of the expander capsule, and produced thinning of the overlying soft tissue by the increased intraluminal pressure.

Using rabbits, the author has shown that expansion of arterialized venous flaps resulted in a more than three times greater survival area than in nonexpanded control group (51). After 3 weeks' expansion, a venogram demonstrated dilated veins to

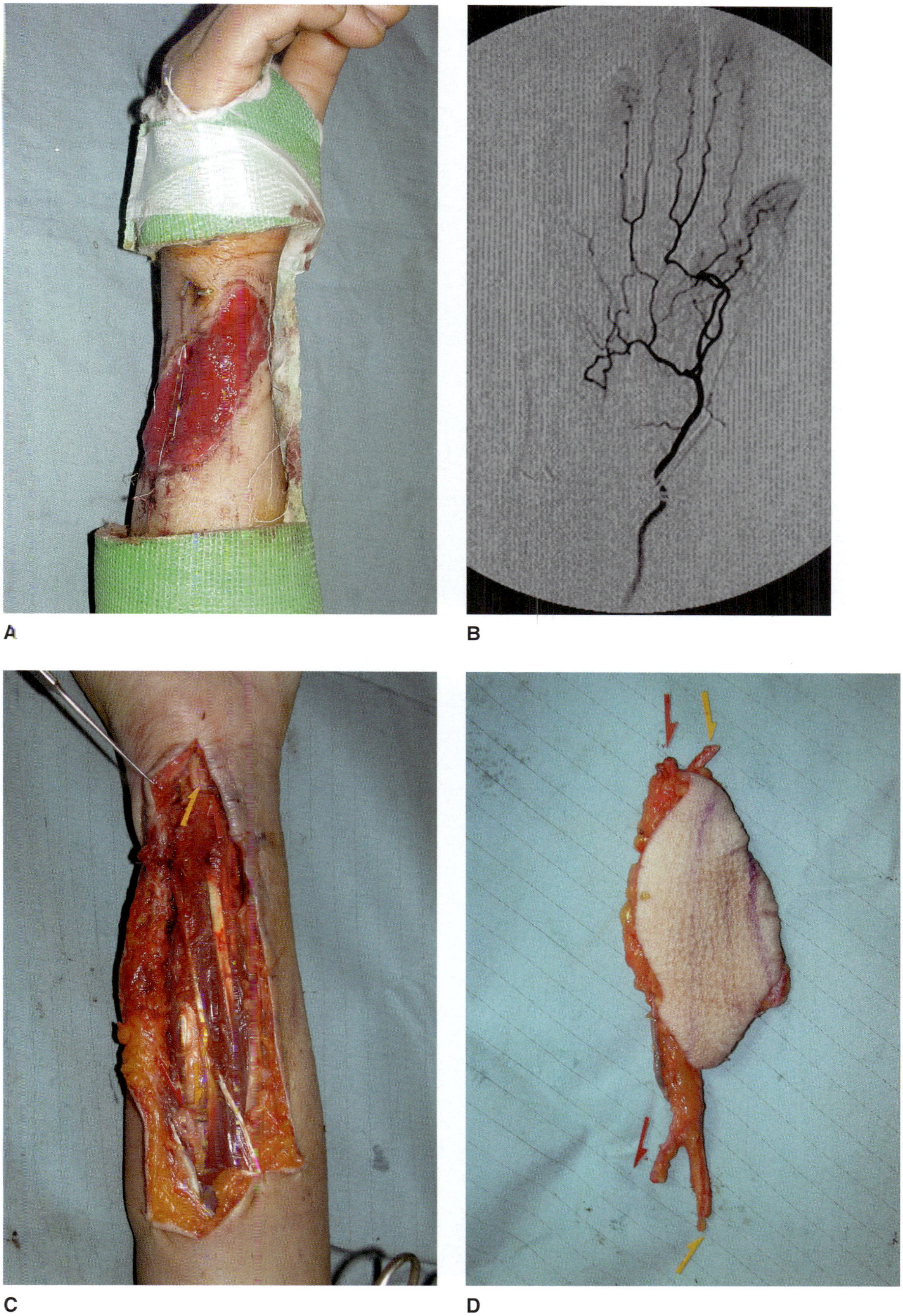

FIGURE 25-6 Innervated conduit venous flap. (**A**) Composite defect of the distal ulnar area of the right forearm. (**B**) Preoperative angiogram shows a defect of the ulnar artery in the distal forearm. (**C**) Intraoperative view shows the defect of the ulnar artery and ulnar nerve, each about 10 cm in length with an overlying soft tissue defect about 4 × 7 cm in size. (**D**) An innervated conduit venous flap was harvested from the left lower leg based on the small saphenous vein and the sural nerve.

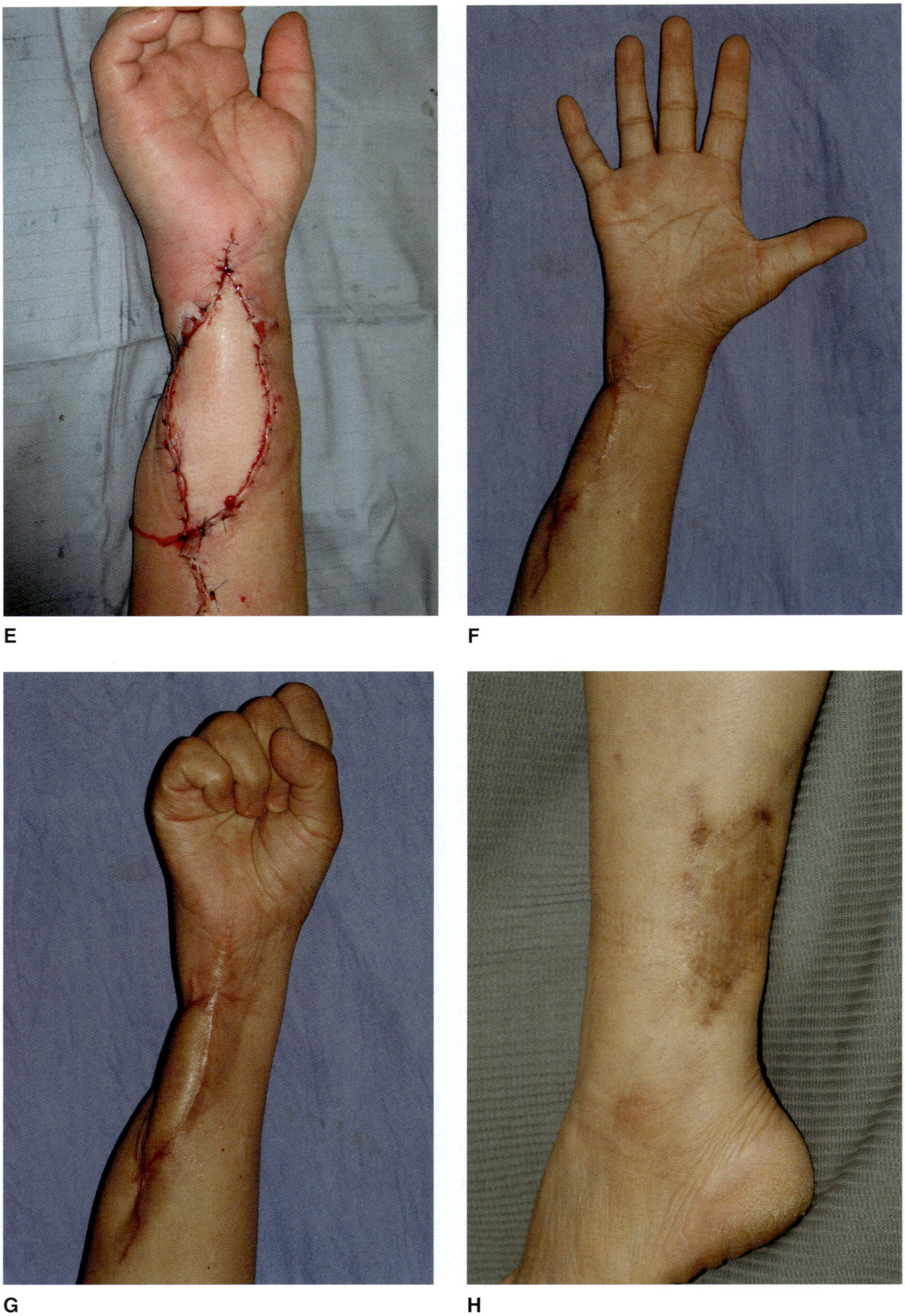

FIGURE 25-6 (*Continued*) (**E**) Immediate postoperative view. (**F**) and (**G**) Postoperative view 14 months later. Note there is no claw hand deformity. (**H**) Postoperative view of the donor site, which was covered with split-thickness skin graft.

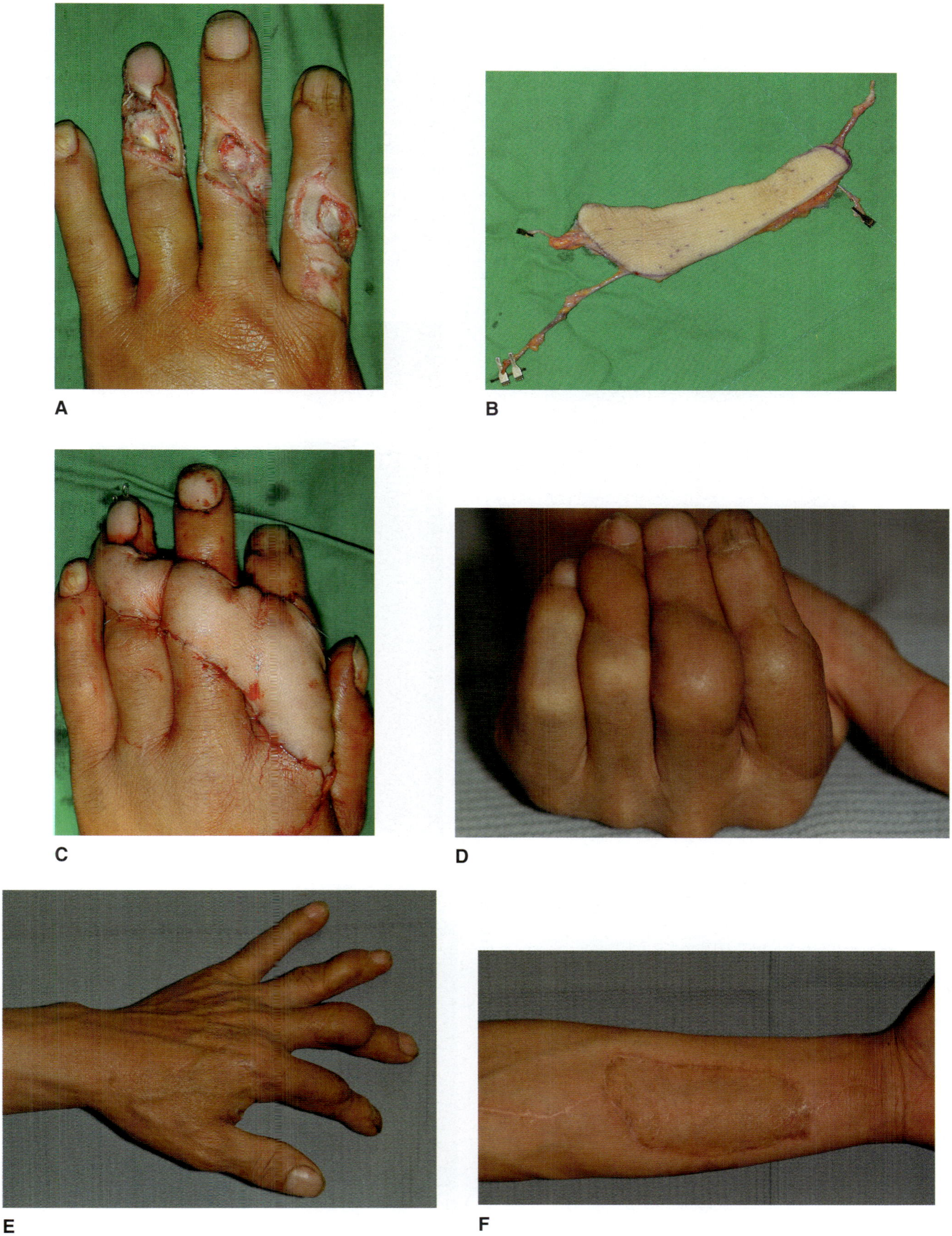

FIGURE 25-7 Large venous flap. (**A**) Preoperative view of multiple soft tissue defects of the dorsal aspect of the left index, long, and ring finger. (**B**) A venous skin flap about 12 × 3 cm including four veins from the anterior aspect of the ipsilateral forearm. (**C**) Immediate postoperative view of surgical syndactyly state. (**D**) to (**F**) Postoperative view of the donor and recipient site 8 months later.

the flap tip and a newly formed venous network throughout the entire flap. Mutaf et al. (52) showed that expansion of a venous flap increases the area of flap survival. Expansion induces rapid revascularization, and the very rich, dilated venous plexus between the recipient bed and the venous flap facilitates plasmatic imbibition. They concluded that the improved survival of the venous flap resulted from the better drainage of harmful metabolites.

Preexpansion is required to transfer larger arterialized venous flaps to the cervicofacial region (20) because it is not easy to find additional veins that will drain the arterialized venous flap in this region (Figure 25-8). Some authors have applied various delay procedures to arterialized venous flaps to increase their vascularity (53). Although it may increase the surviving area of the flap, surgical delay itself limits flap size. Furthermore, the pharmacologic effects of some drugs, which have been used in chemical delay (54), may cause unwanted systemic side effects.

Preexpanded arterialized venous flaps require a two-stage operation, prolonging the treatment period. Expander insertion also introduces its own potential complication. However, preexpansion confers many advantages over conventional arterialized venous flaps. These include no sacrifice of major arteries; easier, less time-consuming dissection; long vascular pedicles;

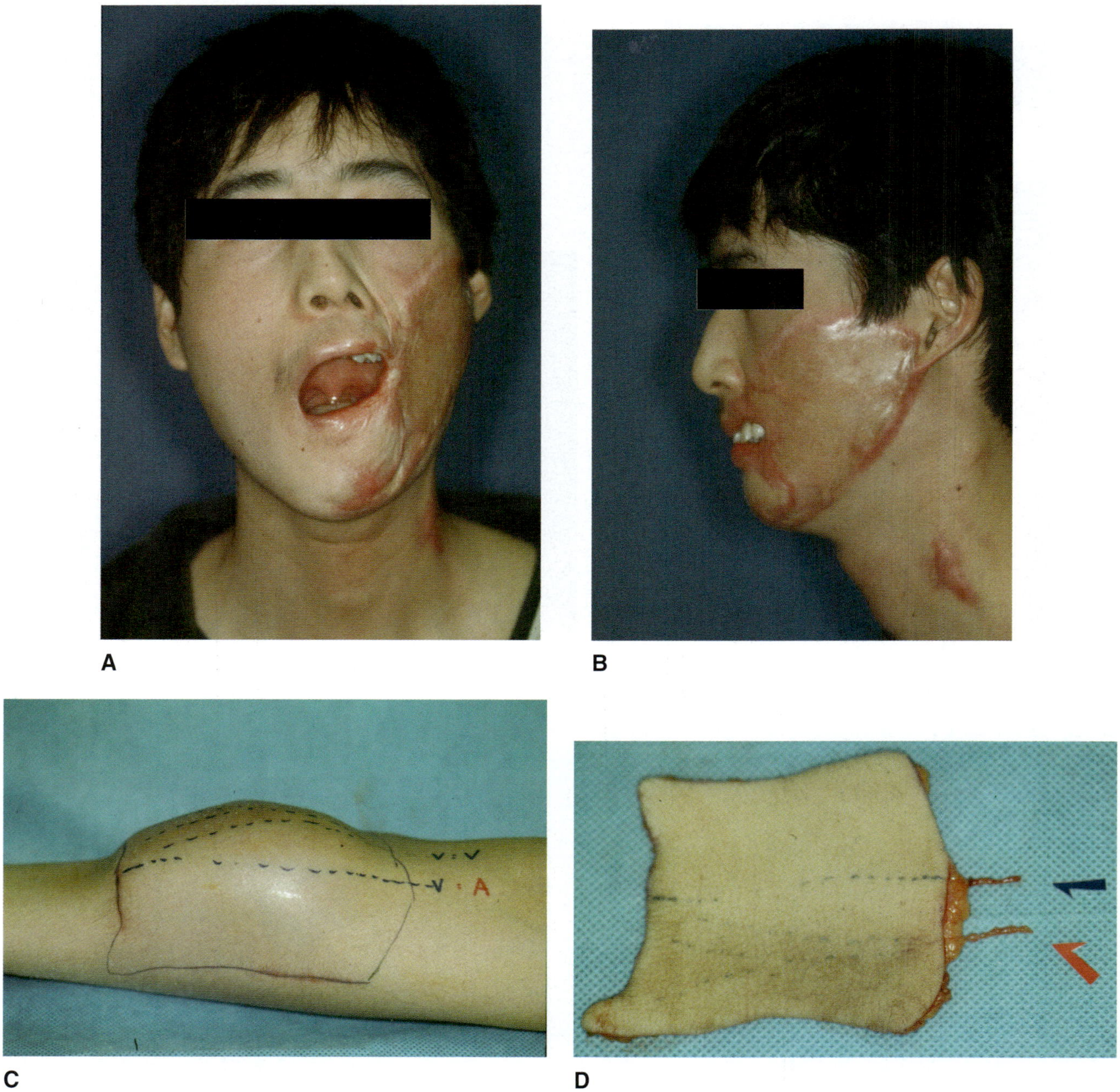

FIGURE 25-8 Preexpanded venous flap. (**A**) and (**B**) Preoperative views of a contact burn on the left cheek showing severe postburn scar contracture. (**C**) A rectangular tissue expander of 250 cm^3 was placed under the subcutaneous tissue, preserving venous networks on the flexor aspect of the forearm. The expander was inflated to a volume of 310 cm^3 over a period of 40 days. (**D**) The harvested expanded venous flap, which was about 10 × 12 cm in size, and which included two veins. The afferent vein was connected to the facial artery and the other sutured to the facial vein.

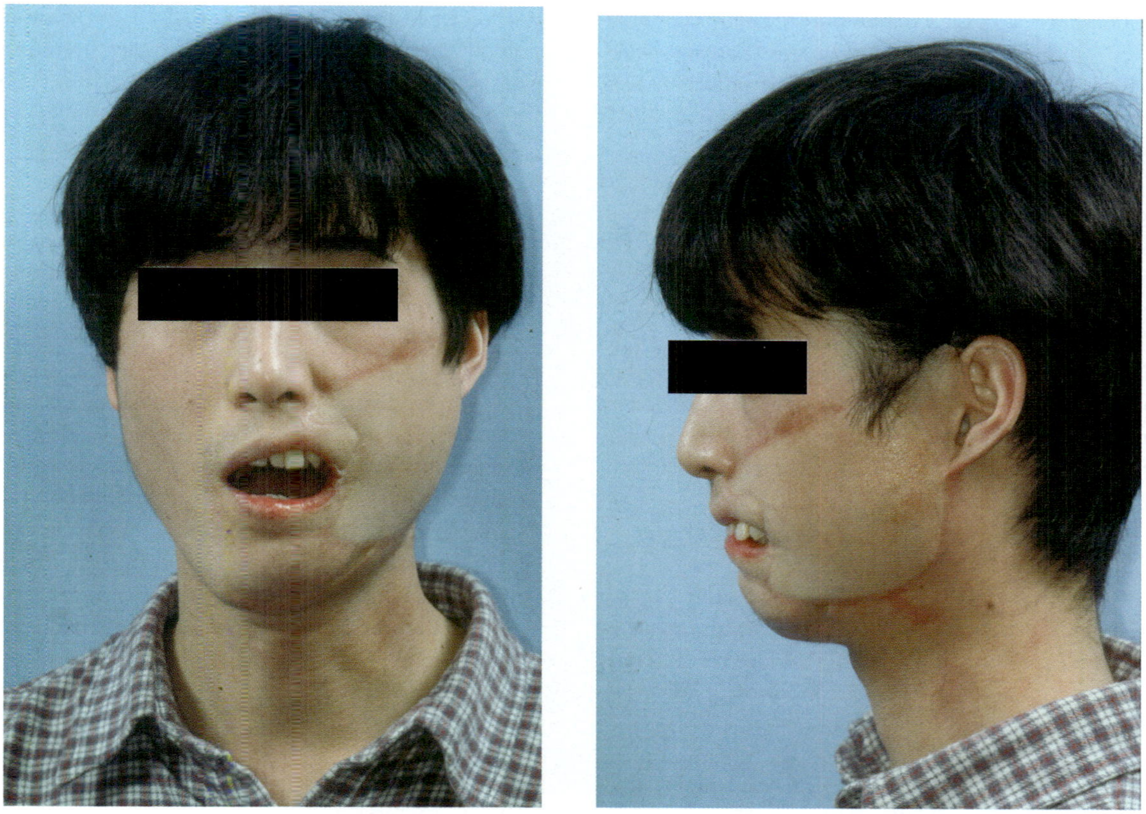

E F

FIGURE 25-8 (*Continued*) (**E**) and (**F**) Ten months after surgery, the arterialized venous flap is well matched in both texture and thickness to the facial skin. But a vermilion contracture of the left oral commissure still needs secondary correction.

abundant donor sites (any skin area with a venous network); custom design of the flap; and a thin, well-textured skin. Furthermore, preexpansion decreases donor site morbidity, eliminates postoperative instability, and results in total flap survival.

Delayed Venous Flap

Excellent experimental studies (53,54) have demonstrated the effects of surgical delay procedures on the survival of large arterialized venous flaps in the rabbit ear model. Surgical delay procedures significantly increased the survival of arterialized venous flaps in this model. Chemical and surgical-chemical delays have also been carried out. Doxazocin mesylate and nitroglycerine patches have been applied in the same animal model. By combining surgical and chemical delays, the extent of the delay could be reduced. Based on these experimental results, acute soft tissue and tendon defects in the hand were treated by dorsalis pedis tendocutaneous delayed arterialized venous flaps (16). The advantage of the tendocutaneous delayed arterialized venous flap is that a larger flap can be obtained than when using undelayed venous or arterialized venous flaps. The survival rate of the arterialized venous flap also increases, permitting the use of a composite flap. Unlike with a dorsalis pedis free flap, the main artery of the donor site is preserved; thin, pliable tissue is used; and elevation is easy, without the need for a deep dissection. The disadvantages are the two-stage operation, donor-site scarring, and weakening of toe extension.

Operation Technique

Flap Design and Dissection

A tourniquet is applied proximal to the donor site using a pressure of 100 mm Hg, which allows the veins to become engorged. The distribution of the veins is traced on the skin with a marking pen. The flap is centered on the area where the vein distribution is most abundant. To allow for postoperative swelling and edema, the flap should be larger than the recipient defect. Flaps are elevated superficial to the muscle fascia and include only skin, subcutaneous tissues, and veins. The recipient vessels are dissected out away from the "zone of injury" through separate incisions. Additional vein length proximal and distal to the cutaneous portion of the flap is harvested and the vessels passed through a subcutaneous tunnel to reach these recipients. This strategy also allows the surgeon to perform arterial and venous anastomoses proximal to the injury site, where the vessel size match is better. For reconstruction of the dorsal aspect of the hand or the wrist, the superficial radial artery and vein may be used as recipient vessels.

Generally, small- and medium-sized flaps, or those smaller than 25 cm^2, should include two veins suitable for anastomosis. When the venous pedicle of one afferent and one efferent vein is located on the same side of the flap, arterial blood is supplied through the afferent vein against the venous valves (antidromically) and drained through the efferent vein in the normal direction of flow. The relatively smaller vein is used as the afferent vein and the larger vein as the efferent vein. The length of the venous pedicle of the afferent vein should be as short as possible to minimize the number of intravenous valves, which create resistance to inflowing arterial blood. Even though the recipient artery is anastomosed to the afferent vein, there is often no venous drainage through the efferent vein. In this situation, one can often see venous engorgement around the first valve distal to the anastomosis. To facilitate the passage of arterial inflow through the obstructing valves, catheterization with heparin solution is required through a branch distal to anastomosis but proximal to the first valve. The tip of the catheter is pressed against the valve leaflets, mechanically destroying or disabling each valve in succession. If successful, one should see blood draining through the efferent veins. The length of the efferent vein is tailored according to the requirement at the recipient site. If possible, two efferent veins are anastomosed in medium-sized flaps. In large flaps, as many veins are included as possible. One or two veins are used as afferent and two or more as efferent veins.

Postoperative Management

The flaps were monitored intensely for 7 days after surgery. During this period, patients should be at rest as with other free flap surgery. After surgery, capillary refill, surface temperature, color, and bulla formation of the flap are monitored. When the flap is congested and capillary refill obscured, palpation of pulse, Doppler evaluation, and surface temperature monitoring are helpful for evaluating flap viability. However, the bleeding pattern from stab wounds in the flap is the most useful tool for differentiating the typical congestion of venous flaps from true anastomotic thrombosis. Routine anticoagulation therapy with 60 mg of prostaglandin E1 and 5000 units of heparin are administered for approximately 1 week, and 100 mg of baby aspirin is prescribed orally for 1 month.

As mentioned, postoperative monitoring of arterialized venous flaps is not easy because signs of vascular insufficiency and characteristic edema and congestion of venous flaps are difficult to differentiate. In standard free flaps, the perfusion of the flap can easily be monitored by means of the color and surface temperature of the flap as well as by physical examination. However, with venous flaps, the color is light purple tinged with red for the first 2 to 3 days, becoming darker thereafter. It is easy to confuse the normal postoperative course with venous insufficiency of the flap. Setting aside color changes, if the capillary refill is good and brisk and if there is bright red bleeding from the edge of the flap or from a stab wound, normal circulation exists. Occasionally, suboptimal flap survival manifests itself as flap edge maceration or epidermolysis over the whole flap surface. These conditions often improve after flap edema subsides and neovascularization from the recipient bed occurs. Difficulty in postoperative monitoring of the flap is a disadvantage for the inexperienced. In cases of venous congestion, flap viability can be monitored only by palpating the pulse or by laser Doppler probe analysis.

TRICKS AND TIPS FROM THE AUTHOR

In an arterialized venous flap, the actual dissection is easy and relatively quick, so it can be used as free flap on an emergency basis. But there are some important considerations in the first operation. Below are a few tips from the author on the basis of clinical experience.

- Try a small flap first. In small flaps, if the anastomoses are good, survival of the flap is predictable.
- Use venous flaps for the coverage of acute, fresh, partially avascular recipient wounds and avoid using them to resurface chronic, infected, and totally avascular beds.
- Design the venous flap to be larger than the conventional flap to allow for postoperative swelling. The venous channel should be located along the center of the flap.
- In a large venous flap, it is better to anastomose as many efferent veins as possible.
- If a very large and thin skin flap is required in elective cases, consider preexpansion or a surgical delay procedure first or select a perforator flap.
- When anastomosing afferent veins with the flow directed against the valves, the afferent vein should be as short as possible and the vein diameter as small as possible. For efferent veins, the length and the diameter of the vein can vary depending on the recipient vein network.
- When monitoring the flap, one must distinguish between usual postoperative congestion of the venous flap and true vascular insufficiency.

DONOR SITES: CLOSURE AND COMPLICATIONS

One of the most common donor sites of the venous flap is the flexor surface of the forearm. The donor sites of small flaps were usually closed primarily if less than 3 cm wide. When it is not possible for the donor site to be closed primarily, a full-thickness skin graft is recommended.

Regarding donor-site morbidity, it is better to avoid the forearm as a donor site for large flaps or in young women because of the cosmetic disfigurement. After elevation of the radial forearm flap, there is delayed wound healing associated with split-thickness skin graft in 19% to 53% of cases (55,56). Partial necrosis of the grafted skin may be caused by deep dissection of the forearm, resulting in exposure of the flexor tendons. Dissection of the donor site for a venous flap is not as deep as that for a radial forearm flap. This is analogous to suprafascial dissection of the radial forearm flap. According to Lutz et al. (57), the aesthetic outcome was rated as good or fair in 98% of cases. This was attributed to complete skin graft take on a smooth recipient bed. Full-thickness skin grafts, when securely anchored and properly splinted, achieved the same success rate but with a superior appearance.

In elevation of innervated flaps, dysesthesia distal to the donor site usually consists of mild numbness. Distal sensory loss is often inevitable, but with a typical venous flap, only small branches of the important sensory nerves are dissected and harvested. In the forearm, extensive cross-innervation by the superficial radial nerve, the medial, and the lateral antebrachial cutaneous nerves ensures that the sensory loss is minimal or absent. Nevertheless, accidental injury or unnecessary division of superficial radial nerve should be avoided.

In cases of harvesting from the posterior part of the lower leg or dorsum of the foot, postoperative scarring may be improved with a split-thickness skin graft.

RECONSTRUCTIVE INDICATIONS

The main advantage of an arterialized venous flap is the ease of harvesting a thin flap without the need to sacrifice a major artery at the donor site. The length of vascular pedicle to be harvested can be as long as desired. Compared with other free flaps, flap elevation is very rapid, and under the one tourniquet, the donor site and recipient bed are in a single operative field. The design of venous flaps is very easy because of direct visualization of the venous plexus through the thin overlying skin. There is no limitation in donor site selection because it is possible to find a venous network in almost any anatomical site.

There are advantages to using arterialized venous flaps over standard flaps in resurfacing multiple digit injuries. First, these thin venous flaps more closely resemble the skin over the fingers or dorsum of the hand, and second, they can easily be harvested because subcutaneous fat can be minimized in places other than around the venous pedicle (as opposed to standard flaps, which are thick because of the inclusion of a deep-seated and more difficult to dissect vascular pedicle). Third, to repair multiple injuries with one flap, diverse flap shapes must be harvested; however, it is not easy to obtain such a variety of shapes with standard flaps. With venous flaps, the venous distribution can be seen clearly under the tourniquet, and various flap designs are possible. Although a state of surgical syndactyly exists after resurfacing multiple digits with one flap, it is possible to perform active and passive movement of the joints 1 week after surgery, and a considerable range of motion can be attained before separation is carried out.

In addition to an unstable postoperative course, there are some pitfalls to using arterialized venous flaps. When the venous network is not evident because of opaque or thick skin, it is difficult to design the flap. Also, when a glabrous skin flap is needed, non–hair-bearing donor sites are very limited.

Skin coverage for soft tissue defects after elective burn contracture release in the hand and immediate reconstruction for resurfacing exposed tendon or joint in acute hand trauma provide other reasonable indications for use of venous flaps.

Despite their numerous advantages, arterialized venous flaps are not commonly selected as the first choice for microsurgical reconstruction because of the unstable postoperative recovery sequence that involves severe postoperative swelling, discoloration, and bullae formation. In addition, unpredictable necrosis of the flap causes many surgeons to hesitate in selecting it. Postoperative monitoring of the flap is not easy. Purple discoloration or bullae formation in the flap is easily confused with anastomotic problems.

As outlined earlier, venous flap transfer along with nerve, tendon, or vessel is clinically and theoretically possible. There has been only one report of an osteocutaneous venous flap (13). Here the tibia was carried on a venous flap based on the long saphenous vein. We have not attempted to transfer the osteocutaneous venous flap because it is not easy to dissect the venous flap and retain the vascularity of the bone within it. Furthermore, in the event of partial necrosis of the venous flap, the exposed bone would require coverage with another flap.

Blood flow through a persistent arteriovenous shunt can lead to high-output cardiac failure, especially in patients with preexisting heart disease. However, in our experience, there were no heart problems after venous flap surgery because the flow in the arteriovenous shunts was generally minimal. One may need to check postoperative electrocardiography regularly in high-risk patient cases. If problems occur, simple ligation of vessels is the solution.

In our experience, the success rate of arterialized venous flaps in reconstructing soft tissue compound injuries is similar to that of conventional flaps. We propose specific indications for their use in the reconstruction of hand defects (Table 25-1).

FLAP COMPARISON

The arterialized venous flap has a big advantage over conventional flaps because any skin and subcutaneous region with a venous network may be used as a flap, solving the problem of donor site selection. There is also no need to sacrifice major arteries. Virtually any venous system with enough length can be

TABLE 25-1 Reconstructive indications of arterialized venous flaps for the hand according to the tissue defects

Tissue defects	Reconstructive options
• Soft tissue defect, only	Venous skin flap
small or medium size defect (<25 cm^2)	small venous flap with 2 veins (1A & 1V)*
large size defect (> 25 cm^2)	
defect on the multiple digits	long & narrow venous flap with 3 veins (1A & 2V)*
defect on the hand or forearm	large venous skin flap with 4 or 5 veins (1A or 2A & 2V or 3V)*
• Compound tissue defects	Compound venous flap
tendon + soft tissue defects	tendocutaneous venous flap
nerve + soft tissue defects	innervated venous flap
vessel + soft tissue defects	conduit venous flap
• Composite tissue defects	Composite venous flap
tendon + nerve + soft tissue defects	innervated tendocutaneous venous flap
nerve + vessel + soft tissue defects	Innervated conduit venous flap

*1A or 2A: One or two arteries anastomosis with one or two afferent veins of the flap
1V or 2V: One or two veins anastomosis with one or two efferent veins of the flap

used to base a thin, customized, shaped flap in a relatively short time. If the survival of the arterialized venous flap can be accurately predicted without using the delay procedure or prefabrication, it can be expected to gain popularity in many scenarios, especially for resurfacing of the hand or the head and neck area. To optimize the survival rate of the flap, careful preoperative design is needed to site the venous network over the entire area of the flap. After the arterialization of the flap is completed, an effort must be made create as many efferent veins as possible to maximize flap survival. When an arterialized venous flap is centered on the main venous network and is drained by two or more efferent veins, the survival pattern and rate are as good as with conventional flaps (36).

The dorsal hand and wrist are not only of great functional importance but are also aesthetically conspicuous. When tendons and bone are exposed after degloving and crush injuries, there are many options for reconstruction such as fasciocutaneous, muscle, fascial, and venous flow-through flaps. Parrett et al. (58), found a significant difference between these options: venous flaps had the best overall aesthetic outcome. Venous flaps required no debulking in this study and had the best color, contour, and texture match compared with the other types of flaps. The only limiting factor in the use of arterialized venous flaps is defect size. In cases of small to moderate-sized defects, the venous flap could be the first choice. Larger wounds require larger conventional flap reconstruction, resulting—inevitably—in more sizable donor site defects.

Various fasciocutaneous flaps such as the radial forearm flap, groin flap, and scapular flap have been described to cover postburn defects of the cervicofacial region. These flaps should be considered as primary options for reconstruction. For more demanding reconstruction with thinner and larger flaps, technical modification is needed. Preexpanded flaps from the radial forearm and anterolateral thigh can provide good postoperative results. However, pedicle dissection is tedious because the pedicle is located under the fascia or the capsule of the expander. Moreover, the first operation and the subsequent serial expansions produce dense scarring around the pedicle. This may increase the risk of flap failure.

Perforator flaps minimize the donor defect by preserving muscle. They can be thinned during elevation and may be of large area. Nevertheless, there are technical difficulties involved in harvesting flaps, particularly if they have been preexpanded. "Supramicrosurgical" techniques (59) are often required to dissect and anastomose the small-caliber vessels, and there may be potential problems with circulatory compromise to the distal regions of the flap.

REFERENCES

1. Baek SM, Weinberg H, Song Y, et al. Experimental studies in the survival of venous island flap without arterial inflow. *Plast Reconstr Surg* 1985;75:88.
2. Honda T, Nomura S, Tamauchi S, et al. The possible applications of composition skin and subcutaneous vein graft in the replantation of amputated digits. *Br J Plast Surg* 1984;37:607.
3. Yoshimura M, Shimada T, Imura S, et al. The venous skin graft method for repairing skin defects of the fingers. *Plast Reconstr Surg* 1987;79:243.
4. Chia SL, Cheng HH, Mao L. Free transplantation of venous network pattern skin flap. *Plast Reconstr Surg* 1988;82:892.
5. Nakayama Y, Soeda S, Kasai Y. Flaps nourished by arterial inflow through the venous system: an experimental investigation. *Plast Reconstr Surg* 1981;67:328.
6. John CM, William RP. Creation of free flaps by arterialization of venous system. *Arch Otolaryngol* 1984;110:221.
7. Sasa M, Xian W, Breidenbach W, et al. Survival and blood flow evaluation of canine venous flaps. *Plast Reconstr Surg* 1988;82:319.
8. Germann, GK, Eriksson E, Russel RC. Effects of arteriovenous flow reversal on blood flow and metabolism in a skin flap. *Plast Reconstr Surg* 1987;79:375.
9. Thatte MR, Kumta SM, Purohit SK, et al. Cephalic venous flap: a series of 8 cases and a preliminary report on the use of 99mTc labeled RBCs to study the saphenous venous flap in dogs. *Br J Plast Surg* 1989;42:193.
10. Matsushita K, Firrell JC, Ogden L, et al. Blood flow and tissue survival in the rabbit venous flap. *Plast Reconstr Surg* 1993;91:127.
11. Tsai TM, Matiko JD, Breidenbach W, et al. Venous flaps in digital revascularization and replantation. *J Reconstr Microsurg* 1987;3:113.
12. Inoue G, Maeda N, Suzuki K. Resurfacing of skin defect of the hand using the arterialised venous flap. *Br J Plast Surg* 1990;43:135.
13. Koshima I, Soeda Y, Nakayama Y. An arterialized venous flap using the long saphenous vein. *Br J Plast Surg* 1991;44:23.
14. Hisashi O, Kazuma O. A free arterialized venous loop flap. *Plast Reconstr Surg* 1992;89:965.
15. Inada Y, Fukui S, Tamai S, et al. The arterialised venous flap: experimental studies and clinical case. *Br J Plast Surg* 1993;46:61.
16. Cho BC, Lee JH, Byun JS, et al. Clinical applications of the delayed arterialized venous flap. *Ann Plast Surg* 1997;39:145.
17. De Lorenzi F, van der Hulst RR, den Dunnen WF, et al. Arterialized venous free flaps for soft-tissue reconstruction of digits: a 40-case series. *J Reconstr Microsurg* 2002;18:569.
18. Woo SH, Kim KC, Lee GJ, et al. A retrospective analysis of 154 arterialized venous flaps for hand reconstruction: an 11-year experience. *Plast Reconstr Surg* 2007;119:1823.
19. Kovacs AF. Comparison of two types of arterialized venous forearm flaps for oral reconstruction and proposal of a reliable procedure. *J Craniomaxillofac Surg* 1998;26:249.
20. Woo SH, Seul JH. Pre-expanded arterialised venous free flaps for burn contracture of the cervicofacial region. *Br J Plast Surg* 2001;54:390.
21. Safak T, Akyurek M. Cephalic vein-pedicled arterialized anteromedial arm venous flap for head and neck reconstruction. *Ann Plast Surg* 2001;47:446.
22. Nishi G, Shibata Y, Kumabe Y, et al. Arterialized venous skin flaps for the injured finger. *J Reconstr Microsurg* 1989;5:357.
23. Titley OG, Chester DL, Park AJ. A-a type, arterialized, venous, flow-through, free flap for simultaneous digital revascularization and soft tissue reconstruction, revisited. *Ann Plast Surg* 2004;53:185.
24. Deune EG, Rodriguez E, Hatef D, et al. Arterialized venous flow-through flap for simultaneous reconstruction of a radial artery defect and palmar forearm soft-tissue loss from sarcoma resection. *J Reconstr Microsurg* 2005;21:85.
25. Cheng TJ, Chen YS, Tang YB. Use of a sequential two-in-one free arterialised venous flap for the simultaneous reconstruction of two separate defects on the foot. *Br J Plast Surg* 2004;57:685.
26. Hyza P, Vesely J, Stupka I, et al. The bilobed arterialized venous free flap for simultaneous coverage of 2 separate defects of a digit. *Ann Plast Surg* 2005;55:679.
27. Chen CL, Chiu HY, Lee JW, et al. Arterialized tendocutaneous venous flap for dorsal finger reconstruction. *Microsurgery* 1994;15:886.
28. Inoue G, Tamura Y, Suzuki K. One-stage repair of skin and tendon digital defects using the arterialized venous flap with palmaris longus tendon: an additional four cases. *J Reconstr Microsurg* 1996;12:93.
29. Kim JS, Woo SH, Yoon JH, et al. Arterialized venous free flap with palmaris longus tendon for the one-stage reconstruction of defect of skin and extensor tendon. *J Korean Orthop Assoc* 2004;39:278.
30. Takeuchi M, Sakurai H, Sasaki K, et al. Treatment of finger avulsion injuries with innervated arterialized venous flaps. *Plast Reconstr Surg* 2000;106:881.
31. Kayikcioglu A, Akyurek M, Safak T, et al. Arterialized venous dorsal digital island flap for fingertip reconstruction. *Plast Reconstr Surg* 1998;102:2368.
32. Woo SH, Jeong JH, Seul JH. Resurfacing relatively large skin defects of the hand using arterialized venous flaps. *J Hand Surg* 1996;21 (suppl B):222.
33. Kim SE, Woo SH, Seul JH. The comparison of survival rate of the arterialized venous flaps utilizing delay procedure and number of draining veins. *J Korean Soc Reconstr Hand Surg* 1995;1:62.
34. Woo SH, Kim SE, Seul JH. The comparison of survival rate of the arterialized venous flaps dependant on the number of draining vein used. *J Korean Soc Plast Reconstr Surg* 1996;23:371.

35. Pittet B, Chang P, Cederna P, et al. The role of neovascularization in the survival of an arterialized venous flap. *Plast Reconstr Surg* 1996;97:621.
36. Woo SH, Kim SE, Lee TH, et al. Effects of blood flow and venous network on the survival of the arterialized venous flap. *Plast Reconstr Surg* 1998;101:1280.
37. Pittet B, Quinodoz P, Alizadeh N, et al. Optimizing the arterialized venous flap. *Plast Reconstr Surg* 2008;122:1681.
38. Hochauf S, Sternitzky R, Schellong SM. Structure and function of the peripheral venous system. *Herz* 2007;32:3.
39. Taylor GI, Caddy CM, Watterson PA, et al. The venous territories (venosomes) of the human body: experimental study and clinical implications. *Plast Reconstr Surg* 1990;86:185.
40. Hume M. Venous thrombosis: mechanisms and treatment. *Adv Exp Med Biol* 1978;102:215.
41. Nichter LS, Jazayeri MA. The physiologic basis for nonconventional vascular perfusion. *Plast Reconstr Surg* 1995;95:406.
42. Cotran RS, Kumar V, Robbins SL. Fluid and hemodynamics derangement. In *Robbin's Pathologic Basis of Disease*, 4th ed. Philadelphia: Saunders, 1989,p. 87.
43. Yuen QM, Leung PC. Some factors affecting the survival of venous flaps: an experimental study. *Microsurgery* 1991 12:60.
44. Choi BC. *Effects of Intravenous Valves on the Survival of the Arterialized Venous Flap* [thesis]. Department of Plastic Surgery, Graduate School of Yeungnam University, Degree of Master of Medicine, 1998,p. 1.
45. Inoue G, Tamura Y. The use of afferent arteriovenous fistula in digit replantation surgery: A report of two cases. *Br J Plast Surg* 1991;44:230.
46. Ozek C, Zhang F, Lineaweaver WC, et al. Arterialization of the venous system in a rat lower limb model. *Br J Plast Surg* 1997;50:402.
47. Takeuchi M, Sakurai H, Sasaki K, et al. Treatment of finger avulsion Injuries with innervated arterialized venous flaps. *Plast Reconstr Surg* 2000;4:881.
48. Lee HB, Tark KC, Rah DK, et al. Pulp reconstruction of fingers with very small sensate medial plantar free flap. *Plast Reconstr Surg* 1998;101:999.
49. Iwasawa M, Ohtsuka Y, Kushima H, et al. Arterialized venous flaps from the thenar and hypothenar regions for repairing finger pulp tissue losses. *Plast Reconstr Surg* 1997;99:1765.
50. Leighton WD, Russell RC, Marcus DE, et al. Experimental pre-transfer expansion of free flap donor sites: I. Flap viability and expansion characteristics. *Plast Reconstr Surg* 1988;82:69.
51. Shin HJ, Woo SH, Jeong JH, et al. Survival pattern of previously expanded arterialized venous flaps. *J Korean Soc Plast Reconstr Surg* 1997;24:459.
52. Mutaf M, Tasaki Y, Fujii T. Expansion of venous flaps: an experimental study in rats. *Br J Plast Surg* 1998;51:393.
53. Byun JS, Constantinescu MA, Lee WPA, et al. Effects of delay procedures on vasculature and survival of arterialized venous flaps: an experimental study in rabbits. *Plast Reconstr Surg* 1995;96:1650.
54. Cho BC, Lee MS, Lee JH, et al. The effects of surgical and chemical delay procedures on the survival of arterialized venous flaps in rabbits. *Plast Reconstr Surg* 1998;102:1134.
55. Bardsley AF, Soutar DS, Elliot D, et al. Reducing morbidity in the radial forearm flap donor site. *Plast Reconstr Surg* 1990;86:287.
56. Richardson D, Fisher SE, Vaughan ED, et al. Radial forearm flap donor-site complications and morbidity: a prospective study. *Plast Reconstr Surg* 1997;99:109.
57. Lutz BS, Wei FC, Chang SC, et al. Donor site morbidity after suprafascial elevation of the radial forearm flap: a prospective study in 95 consecutive cases. *Plast Reconstr Surg* 1999;103:132.
58. Parrett BM, Bou-Merhi JS, Buntic RF. Refining outcomes in dorsal hand coverage: consideration of aesthetics and donor-site morbidity. *Plast Reconstr Surg* 2010;126:1630.
59. Koshima I, Yamamoto T, Narushima M, et al. Perforator flaps and supermicrosurgery. *Clin Plast Surg* 2010;37:683.

CHAPTER 26

Toe and Joint Transfers to Include Dorsalis Pedis Flaps

Mauricio Kuri, Bauback Safa, Rudolf Buntic, and Gregory M. Buncke

BRIEF HISTORY: ORIGINAL DESCRIPTION AND SUBSEQUENT EVOLUTION

Thumb reconstruction and attempts to improve function date back to French author Huguier in 1874, when he deepened the first web space to improve grasp (1). In 1887, Guermoprez performed the first digit transfers from mutilated mangled hands to the thumb (2). In 1897, Nicoladoni introduced the concept of thumb reconstruction in stages with the combination of bone grafting and a thoracic skin flap prepared into the shape of a glove (3). In addition, in 1900 he developed the first toe-to-thumb reconstructions using a pedicle of the second toe as a cross-pedicle second toe-to-thumb flap and dividing the pedicle in a second-stage procedure. However, because of the inconvenience of attaching the foot to the hand and the advent of microsurgery, this technique fell out of favor. In 1918, Noesske performed the first pollicization of the index finger (4). The technique was further modified and has since gained general acceptance, particularly in the pediatric population.

The first successful replantation of an amputated thumb came in 1965 in Japan by Komatsu and Tamai (5). With the development of new microsurgical instruments and the advent of microsurgical techniques in the 1960s and 1970s, one-stage thumb reconstruction became possible. In 1966, Buncke reported a successful toe-to-thumb transplant in rhesus monkeys (6) and in 1967 a vascularized island metacarpophalangeal (MCP) joint transfer in a traumatized finger (7). With these innovations, vascularized joint transfers using microsurgical techniques began to emerge (8–11). Cobbett performed a human great-toe-thumb transfer in 1969, and Dongyue followed with transfer of the second toe (12,13).

Other techniques were developed to reconstruct damaged thumbs in single-stage procedures while trying to minimize the donor site morbidity of the great toe transfer, such as the "wrap-around" flap. Described originally by Morrison and colleagues in 1980 (14) and later by Urbaniak (15), the "wrap-around" flap provides soft tissue coverage consisting of innervated glabrous skin and an esthetic appearance and minimizes donor site morbidity. In the late 1980s, Wei et al. introduced the "trimmed" great toe and Upton and Mutimer "a modification of the great toe transfer," essentially the same concepts, both primarily addressing the aesthetic concerns of sculpting a toe to look like a thumb by reducing the bony and soft tissue elements (16,17).

As the revolution of microsurgery evolved to repair and restore function of mangled hands, it also incorporated more complex flaps that addressed multilevel upper extremity injuries, such as the use of composite flaps. The dorsalis pedis flap, originally described by McCraw and Furlow (18) as a pedicled flap and later by Ohmori and Harii (19) as a free flap, was used not only for its pliability, sensory potential, and long pedicle but also because of its utility to incorporate surrounding structures such as the extensor tendons, great toe, or joints that provide different options for composite reconstruction (20–23). Unfortunately, the dorsalis pedis flap has fallen out of favor because of its donor site morbidity; on the other hand, some authors have reported minimal complications with its use (21,22,24).

Reconstructive options for mangled hands have evolved dramatically in the past 50 years. The advent of microsurgical centers with multidisciplinary teams has revolutionized upper and lower extremity reconstruction and limb salvage, providing not only improvements in limb function but also appearance. This chapter addresses the anatomy and surgical dissection of the various toe transfers, as well as vascularized joint transfers and the dorsalis pedis flap.

SURGICAL ANATOMY OF TOE TRANSFERS

Venous Network

The venous drainage of the foot consists of deep and superficial systems and a dorsal and plantar system. The deep system consists essentially of the vena comitantes of the dorsalis

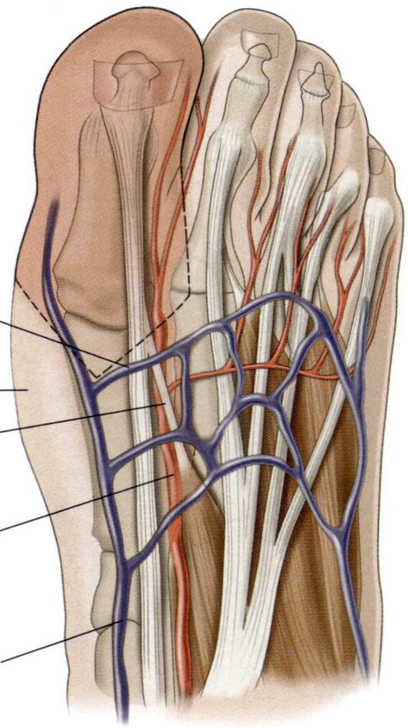

FIGURE 26-1 The superficial venous system. The dorsal digital veins coalesce to form the dorsal metatarsal veins, which drain into the dorsal venous arch. The dorsalis pedis artery crosses above the tarsus and lies between the extensor hallucis longus and the extensor digitorum longus, passing deep beneath the superior and inferior extensor retinaculum. a, artery.

pedis artery. The superficial system is formed from the dorsal digital veins. At the web space, they coalesce to form the dorsal metatarsal veins, which drain into the dorsal venous arch (Figure 26-1). In turn, the dorsal venous arch forms the greater and lesser saphenous veins. The former passes over the anterior aspect of the medial malleolus, and the latter is posterior to the lateral malleolus.

The plantar venous system is composed of a superficial plantar and a deep plantar venous network. The superficial plantar network is formed by thin intradermal and subcutaneous veins, which drain into the dorsal arcade. The midplantar veins drain into the venous arcade at the base of the toes. The deep plantar venous network accompanies the medial and lateral plantar arteries. For venous drainage, the venae comitantes of the dorsalis pedis may be used; however, the superficial venous network provides veins of larger caliber and the option of more length.

Arterial Anatomy

The arteries supplying toe transfers, vascularized joint transfers, and the dorsalis pedis flap are based on the terminal branches of the dorsalis pedis artery. However, for the great toe or second toe with a plantar-dominant system, the plantar metatarsal arteries provide the inflow. The first branch of the tibioperoneal trunk, the anterior tibial artery, continues to become the dorsalis pedis artery. The dorsalis pedis artery lies between the extensor hallucis longus and the extensor digitorum longus, passing deep beneath the superior and inferior extensor retinaculum. It travels intimately with the deep peroneal nerve, located laterally to the artery. The dorsalis pedis artery courses above the tarsus and crosses the extensor hallucis brevis accompanied by two venae comitantes. The artery gives off five branches: lateral and medial tarsal, arcuate, first dorsal metatarsal artery (FDMA), and deep plantar arteries. The arcuate artery provides the second, third, and fourth dorsal metatarsal arteries. Before diving plantar, the dorsalis pedis artery gives off the FDMA, passing dorsal to the intermetatarsal ligament, giving off terminal branches, the dorsal digital arteries, supplying the lateral side of the great toe, the medial side of the second toe, and the communicating branch to the first plantar metatarsal artery (FPMA) (25). In relationship to the interosseous muscle, the course of the FDMA is variable; it may lay superficial, within, or deep to the muscle (Figure 26-2). In 50% to 70% of patients, the FDMA is larger in caliber than the FPMA, and in 20% to 40% of patients, the FPMA is larger than the FDMA (26).

The plantar arterial system originates from the posterior tibial artery, which branches into the medial and lateral plantar arteries. The lateral plantar artery continues obliquely to the base of the fifth metatarsal bone and completes the deep plantar arch. The deep plantar arch gives rise to the plantar metatarsal arteries, which travel between the metatarsal bones, dividing into the plantar digital arteries. The plantar digital arteries to the great toe originate from the FPMA.

Nerves

The superficial and deep peroneal nerves and the sural nerve supply the sensory innervation of the foot. The superficial peroneal nerve pierces the fascia in the distal third of the leg and divides into medial dorsal and intermediate dorsal cutaneous nerves, passing superficial to the extensor retinaculum and innervating the peroneus longus and brevis muscles. The terminal branches of the nerve provide sensory innervation to the dorsum of the foot, with the exception of the first web space. The deep peroneal nerve begins at the bifurcation of the peroneal nerve and travels

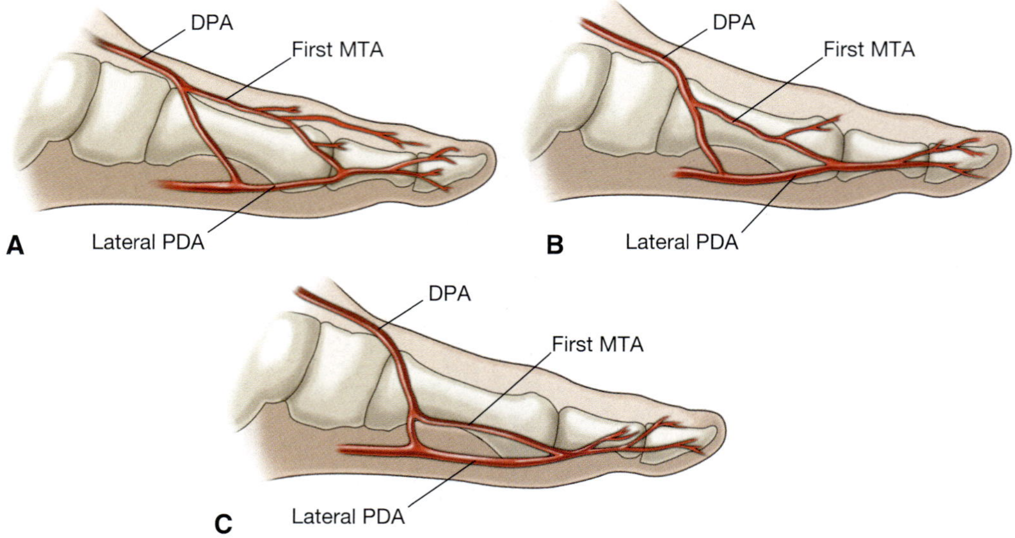

FIGURE 26-2 The dorsalis pedis artery gives off the first dorsal metatarsal artery (FDMA). The takeoff of the FDMA is variable and clinically has been observed dorsally, midway through the muscle, or plantar.

deep to the extensor digitorum longus on the interosseus membrane with the anterior tibial artery. Proximally, the deep peroneal nerve innervates the muscles of the anterior compartment of the leg. Distally, it lies just medial to the dorsalis pedis artery and divides into the medial and lateral branches. The medial branch provides cutaneous innervation to the first web space of the foot. The lateral branch innervates the extensor digitorum brevis and extensor hallucis brevis.

Tendons and Joints

The extensor tendons on the dorsum of the foot include the extensor digitorum longus and brevis and the extensor hallucis longus and brevis. The extensor digitorum longus divides on the anterior surface of the ankle and inserts into the lateral four toes. The extensor hallucis longus, whose function is to extend the great toe and assist in foot eversion and inversion, inserts on the dorsal aspect of the distal phalanx of the great toe. The extensor hallucis brevis, closely involved with the dorsalis pedis artery in its course, inserts on the proximal phalanx of the great toe.

The metatarsophalangeal (MTP) joint of the great toe has a strong capsule and volar plate. It has a wide range of motion and can hyperextend up to 70 degrees and flex up to 45 degrees, unlike the MCP joint, which can hyperextend an average of 35 degrees and flex an average of 75 degrees (27). Therefore, because the great toe has a greater range of motion, especially in extension, pinning of the new MTP joint on the hand is done in neutral position.

DETAILED SURGICAL TECHNIQUE OF DISSECTION AND HARVEST

Great Toe Transfer

The ideal toe-to-thumb reconstructions are for amputations at the level of the proximal phalanx of the thumb, sparing the MCP joint. The great toe provides excellent functional results of pinch and grasp and provides pulp, nail, and "like-with-like" tissue replacement. The main disadvantage of the great toe is the donor site morbidity. The most common complication is wound breakdown or delayed healing at the donor site (28). However, although rare, unsteady gaits and impairment in walking and running have been reported (29). Overall, foot function after great toe transfer is well preserved, and daily activities are not impaired (28). Despite the functional advantages that the great toe provides, the cosmetic appearance with increased diameter of the toe and increased width of the nail can make the aesthetic result less pleasing.

A key consideration before toe-to-thumb transfer is to evaluate the recipient blood supply in the injured hand. Arteriograms are an important part of the preoperative workup, as well as a two-team approach that involves two surgeons, two scrubs, multiple overhead lights, tourniquet control, and loupe magnification. Recipient venous vessels such as the venous arch or the cephalic vein can be used for outflow. If these are destroyed, the vena comitans of the radial artery can be used. Recipient nerves can usually be found at the level of the amputation. If destroyed, nerve transfers from other digital nerves can be performed but will affect adjacent fingers. Branches of the superficial radial nerve can be used if the thumb palmar digital nerves are not available.

Great toe dissection begins with the marking the superficial venous system. The surgeon should plan to have a tension-free closure of the donor foot and avoid taking more skin than necessary to allow primary closure of the donor site. Split-thickness skin grafting of the recipient site is preferred over the donor site to minimize donor site morbidity. A V-shaped incision is made at the base of the great toe distal to the MTP joint medially and into the first web space laterally. The plantar incision passes from the medial aspect of the great toe obliquely connecting to the lateral incision

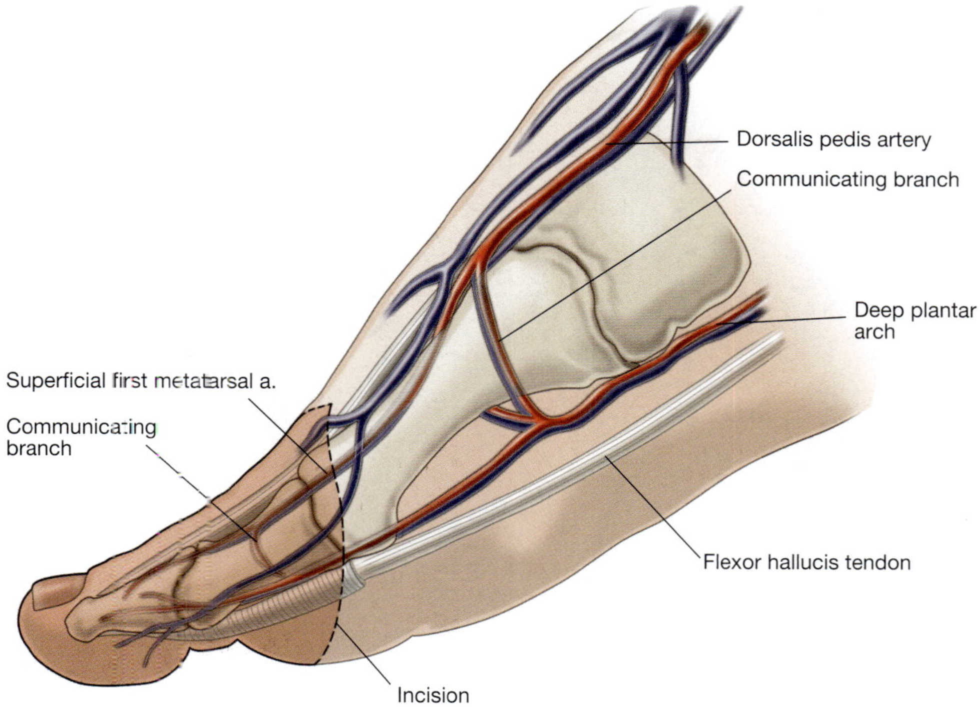

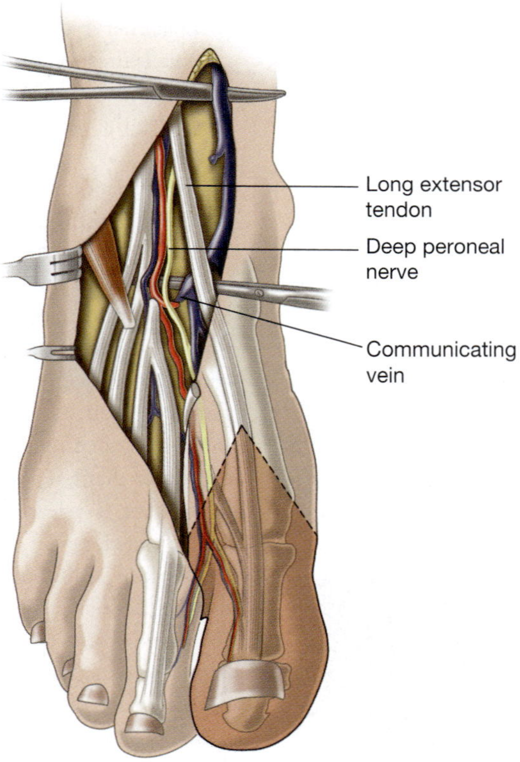

FIGURE 26-3 (A) Planned medial incision for the great toe dissection. (B) Lateral dissection identifies the dorsalis pedis artery, deep peroneal nerve, and a draining vein. Note how the extensor hallucis brevis has been released. a, artery; n, nerve; v, vein.

(Figure 26-3A). The saphenous vein medial to the malleolus fans out over the dorsum. Dissection is performed through the skin, identifying the venous tributaries and following them to the outflow vein. The structures to identify next are the FDMA, extensor tendon, and deep peroneal nerve (Figure 26-3B). The FDMA continues as a dominant branch of the DP in approximately 60% (28). The artery can be identified and dissected distally toward the first web space and proximally to the dorsalis pedis (Figure 26-4). The deep peroneal nerve will be located lateral to the FDMA and should be preserved and coapted to the dorsal sensory branch of the radial nerve.

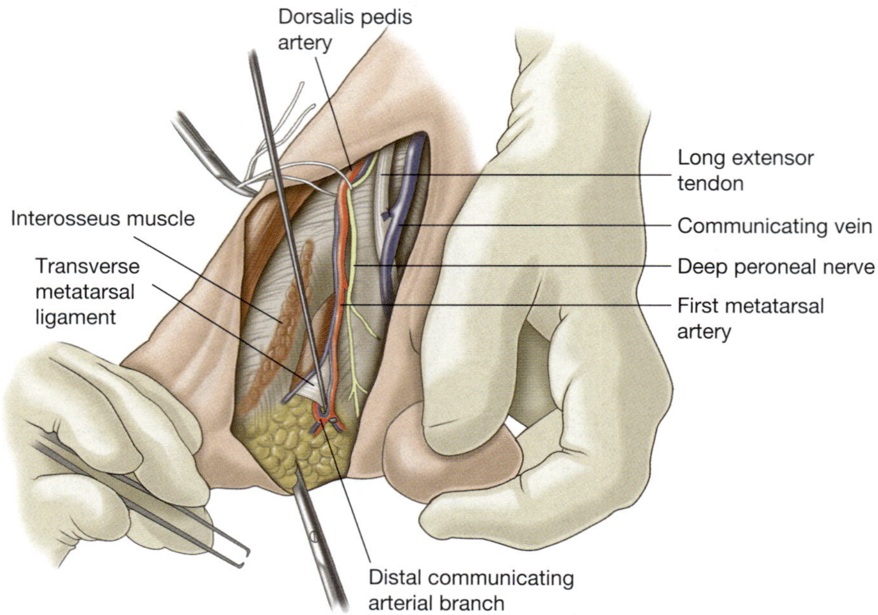

FIGURE 26-4 The dissection is carried distally, identifying the distal communicating artery, the intermetatarsal ligament (which should be released to improve plantar exposure), and the digital vessels. m, muscle

If the patient does not have a suitably large FDMA, dissection proceeds deep to the intermetatarsal ligament, which is divided to facilitate exposure. A corresponding V-shaped incision is made plantarly through the skin, subcutaneous tissue, and plantar fascia to identify the lateral plantar digital artery and nerve (Figure 26-5). The artery can be traced proximally to the bifurcation of the FPMA into the medial digital artery to the second toe and the lateral digital artery to the great toe. At this point, there may be multiple interconnections between the dorsal and plantar systems, and there is great variability of the vascular anatomy in this region.

Protecting and mobilizing the venous pedicle on the medial side of the flap, the long flexor tendon is dissected proximally. On the dorsum of the foot, the long extensor is transected at the appropriate length, and the dorsalis pedis artery and deep peroneal nerve are protected in a vascular loop. The MTP joint capsule is incised and the toe disarticulated, protecting the long flexor tendon. At this point, the surgical team on the hand measures the length required for the artery, vein, nerves, and tendons.

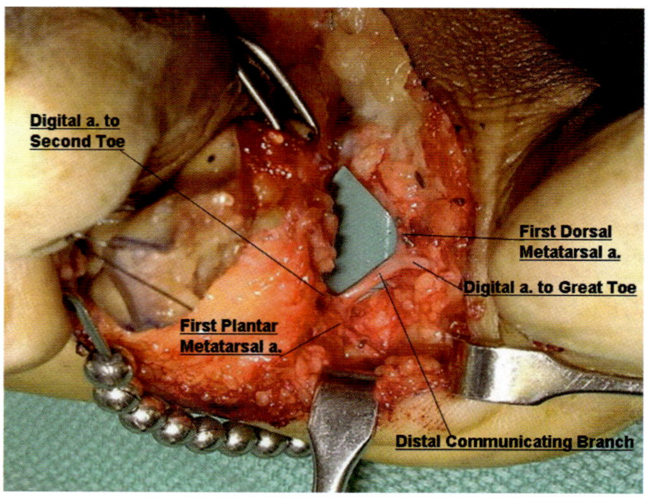

FIGURE 26-5 Dissection of the first web space.

After the joint has been disarticulated and while the vascular pedicle is still attached, the tourniquet is deflated, and any vascular bleeders are clamped and ligated. The flexor tendon is left attached to prevent avulsion of the pedicle (Figure 26-6). When the tourniquet is released, papaverine and warm irrigation are used to relieve spasm. A Serafin Clamp can be used to clinically evaluate the dominant perfusion of the toe. Selective clamping and a pencil Doppler can be used to determine the dominance of the dorsal and plantar systems. Generally, the larger diameter vessels are the dominant system. After the tourniquet is released, the toe is reperfused for 20 minutes before transfer.

Working simultaneously, the second surgical team prepares the recipient site. The incisions should provide access to both volar and dorsal structures and should incorporate the skin flaps from the donor toe. A volar incision exposes the carpal tunnel structures, including the median nerve and the flexor pollicis longus (Figure 26-7). Depending on the injury, the flexor pollicis longus have retracted into the carpal tunnel. The extensor pollicis longus and brevis tendons are easily identified and can be located through a dorsal incision extending into the snuffbox. The dorsal branch of the radial artery is identified and dissected. Similarly, a dorsal vein such as the cephalic vein is identified in the snuffbox.

The ideal osteosynthesis situation is when there is a remnant of the proximal phalanx of the thumb, which can be used as a peg to fit inside the proximal phalanx of the great toe (27,28). An oscillating saw is used to trim the articular cartilage from the base of the proximal phalanx of the great toe. A high-speed burr

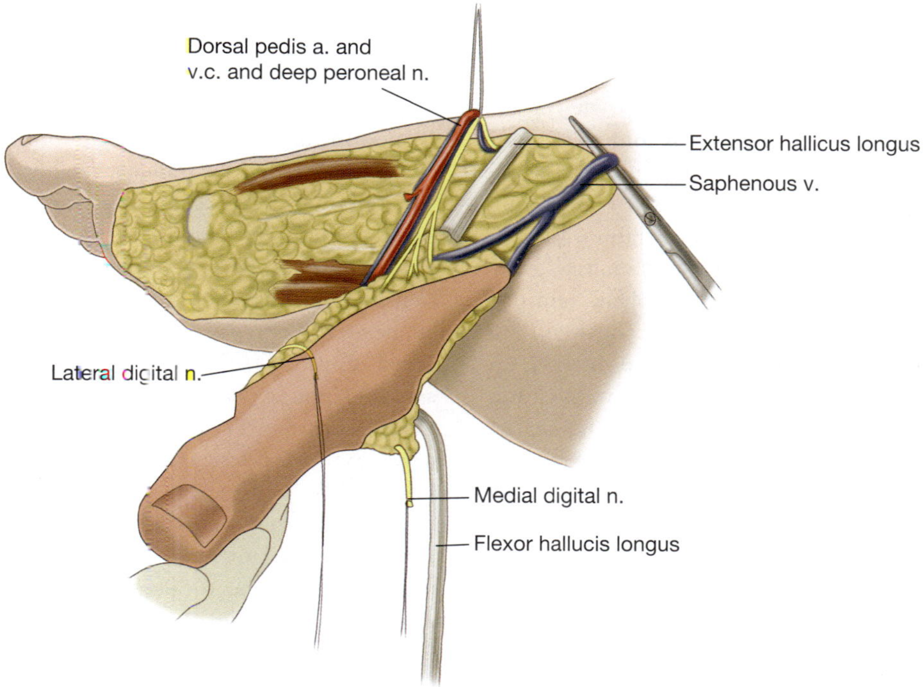

FIGURE 26-6 After the toe is disarticulated, the tourniquet is released and perfusion to the toe confirmed. a, artery; n, nerve; v, vein; vc, vena contaminates.

is used to increase the diameter of the intramedullary canal of the proximal phalanx of the great toe to accommodate the proximal phalanx of the thumb. There should be an overlap of at least 4 mm (30). The construct is secured with one or two self-tapping cortical screws that cross all four cortices or interosseous wires. After osteosynthesis is achieved, fluoroscopy is used to confirm appropriate alignment of the great toe (Figure 26-8).

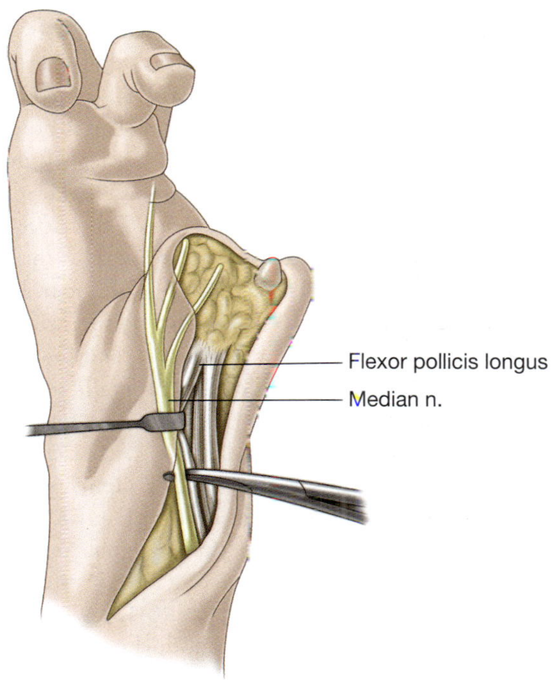

FIGURE 26-7 Palmar incision exposing the nerve stumps of the median nerve, radial artery, and flexor pollicis longus. n, nerve.

In the situation of a thumb amputation sparing the metacarpal articular surface, a composite MCP joint can be fabricated by harvesting the toe MTP joint capsule.

After osteosynthesis is completed, the extensor tendon is repaired first. Often the hand is reexsanguinated and a second tourniquet time is used to perform the bone, tendon, and nerve repairs and even the anastomoses. A Pulvertaft weave or simple figure-of-8 sutures are used to repair the extensor tendon. The flexor tendon repair is performed preferably proximal to the A1 pulley, with a four-strand technique plus an epitendinous suture. The authors favor release of the A1 pulley. The microscope is brought into the field for the arterial anastomosis. The arteries are prepared by removing excess adventitial tissue and trimming just enough to allow a tension-free anastomosis but

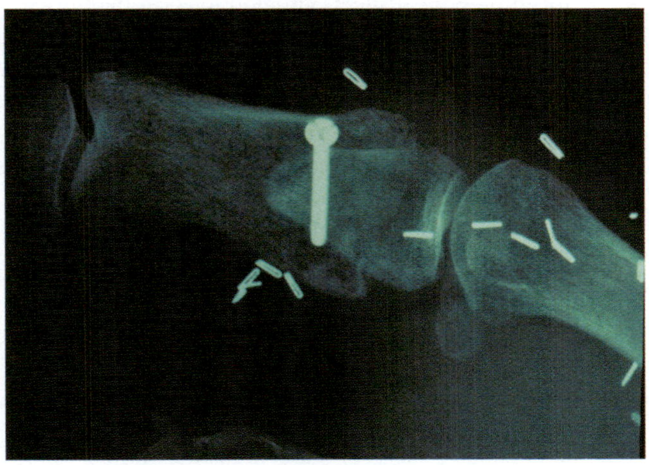

FIGURE 26-8 Osteosynthesis showing the peg fitting inside the proximal phalanx of the great toe, secured by a cortical screw.

also allow for expansion and prevention of kinking after perfusion is established. End-to-side or end-to-end anastomoses are performed between the FDMA and a dorsal branch of the radial artery. If the plantar system is dominant, the medial plantar artery of the great toe or the FPMA is connected to the ulnar digital artery of the thumb or to a dorsal branch of the radial artery using an interposition vein graft. Even under tourniquet, the authors recommend the use of Serafin Clamp to stabilize the vessels when performing the anastomoses. Next, the vein is anastomosed end to end to the cephalic vein or a dorsal vein that matches the caliber of the saphenous vein. The digital nerves are coapted. Warm irrigation and papaverine are used routinely to prevent spasm and reestablish flow. In closure of the recipient site, the skin flaps are loosely approximated, and skin grafts are used if the skin closure is tight. Skin grafts have been placed over vascular anastomoses without any problems. A well-padded dressing is placed with a protective thumb spica splint.

The great toe donor site is closed primarily with a tension-free closure (Figure 26-9). In the pediatric population, absorbable sutures are used. The authors avoid using skin grafts on the donor site and remove the minimal amount of skin necessary when harvesting the toe to minimize donor site morbidity. Before closure, meticulous hemostasis should be ensured, and a closed suction drain is also used. The authors often remove the dorsal two thirds of the metatarsal head, leaving the sesamoids intact. The sesamoids are then advanced over the weight-bearing area of the metatarsal head and held in place with through-and-through sutures through the metatarsal head and the sesamoids to provide appropriate padding on the plantar surface of the foot (27). Others have advanced the flexor hallucis brevis into the metatarsal head for extra padding (30). The foot is immobilized in a posterior well-padded splint with the ankle at 90 degrees for 1 week. Heel weight bearing with a boot is allowed at 4 weeks. Full weight bearing on the plantar surface is allowed at 6 weeks.

Immediately after the anastomoses are performed, an infusion of dextran 40 at 25 cc/hr is started and continued until postoperative day 5. Aspirin is given before surgery and continued for 30 days after surgery. Heparin is not used routinely except in circumstances of take-backs or intraoperative susceptibility for thrombosis. Patients are monitored in the intensive care unit for 48 hours and then transferred to a lower level of care. Toe transfers are monitored clinically, checking skin color, temperature, and capillary refill every 2 hours for the first 48 hours after surgery. The average hospital stay is 6 days. The patients are discharged with a custom-made protective orthoplastic splint.

"WRAP-AROUND" FLAP

Morrison et al. first described the "wrap-around" flap in 1980, prompted mainly because of the size discrepancy between the great toe and the thumb in an attempt at partial preservation of the great toe (14). The diameter of the proximal phalanx of the great toe is about 30% (16) wider than the thumb. In the "wrap-around" flap, most of the soft tissues of the thumb, including the nail, are transferred to the thumb. The bony framework for the thumb is either the native thumb itself in an avulsion injury where there is an intact bony framework or an ICBG.

The advantages of this flap are the preservation of the framework of the great toe, an improved appearance to the reconstructed thumb, stability, length, and a sensate reconstruction (14,15). However, disadvantages of this flap include bone resorption of the skeletal framework (30), its limited use to amputations proximal to the MCP joint, and contraindication in children because of a lack of epiphyses. In children a whole great toe transfer or pollicization provides a better functional result (31). The ideal indications for this flap include avulsion injuries in which the bony framework and tendon mechanisms are still intact, and all that is needed is soft tissue coverage that can resemble the appearance of the contralateral thumb (32).

The Morrison "wrap-around" flap uses the ipsilateral great toe because the lateral side of the toe is used leaving behind a medial flap on the toe, and when transposed, the FDMA aligns better with the dorsal radial artery. The flap incorporates the nail and the lateral and plantar aspects of the great toe but leaves a proximal-based flap of medial skin, approximately 1 cm in width, that tapers around the tip of the toe. The width of this flap is equivalent to the difference between the circumference of the great toe and the contralateral normal thumb (Figure 26-10). The dissection around the nail should be at the subperiosteal level to prevent injury to the nail matrix. If the plantar arterial system is dominant, the dissection proceeds in a similar fashion as the great toe transfer following the lateral digital artery proximally to the first plantar metacarpal artery.

For amputations through the metacarpal head, the iliac crest bone graft (ICBG) is angulated in approximately 20 degrees of flexion or contoured with a slightly flexed shape. If an ICBG is used, the proximal phalanx or metacarpal is reamed out to accommodate the ICBG, which is fixed with Kirschner wires or screws (as described in the great toe-to-thumb transfer). After the bony framework is secured and the recipient vessels exposed, the "wrap-around" flap is brought to the hand and the medial (now radial) border of the flap sutured from distal to proximal. The nail bed is transfixed to the bony framework with a Kirschner wire. The vascular pedicle is either tunneled to the snuffbox, or a lazy S-incision is extended to reach the radial artery and cephalic vein. In most cases, a subcutaneous tunnel is sufficient; however, if there is any indication of tension on the skin, we extend the incision. In addition, we do not hesitate to use skin grafts to keep the closure as tension free as possible. The dominant artery of the "wrap-around" flap is anastomosed end to end or end to side to the radial artery. The draining vein or saphenous vein is anastomosed end to end to a dorsal vein. The lateral digital nerve of the toe is coapted to the ulnar digital nerve of the thumb and the deep peroneal nerve to a branch of the superficial branch of the radial nerve (Figure 26-11).

The donor defect is closed with full-thickness skin grafting and a local flap. The distal half of the distal phalanx of the toe is resected, and the proximal-based medial flap is advanced. The dorsal defect with exposed bone is usually covered with a

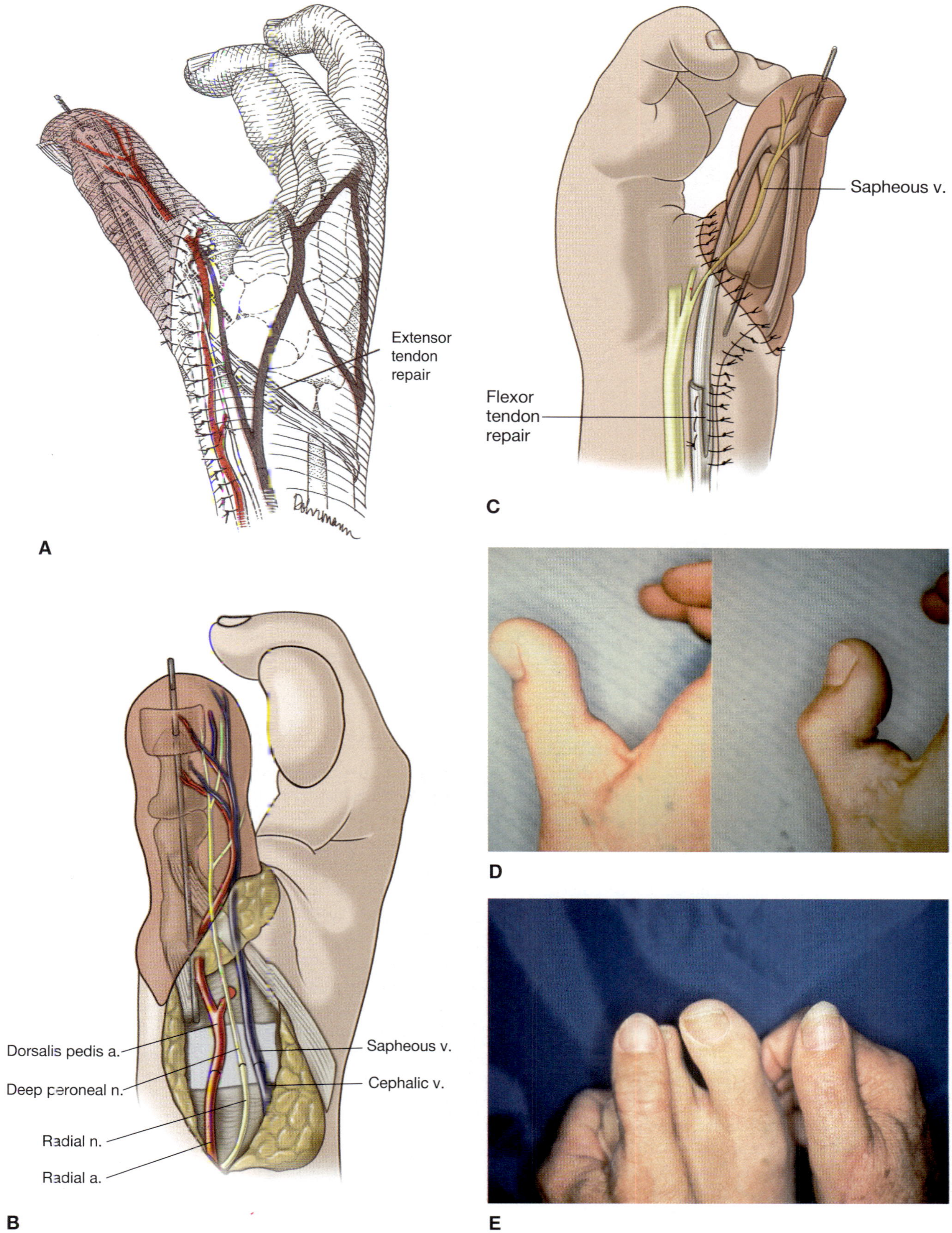

FIGURE 26-9 Great toe after transfer. The osteosynthesis is usually performed with K-wires, and the skin is loosely closed. The dorsalis pedis artery is anastomosed end to end to the dorsal branch of the radial artery, and the saphenous vein is anastomosed end to end to the cephalic vein. The deep peroneal nerve is coapted to a branch of the superficial radial nerve. (D) Interphalangeal joint flexion of a great toe transfer. (E) Great toes atrophy over time so that their size resembles the opposite normal thumb. a, artery; n, nerve; v, vein.

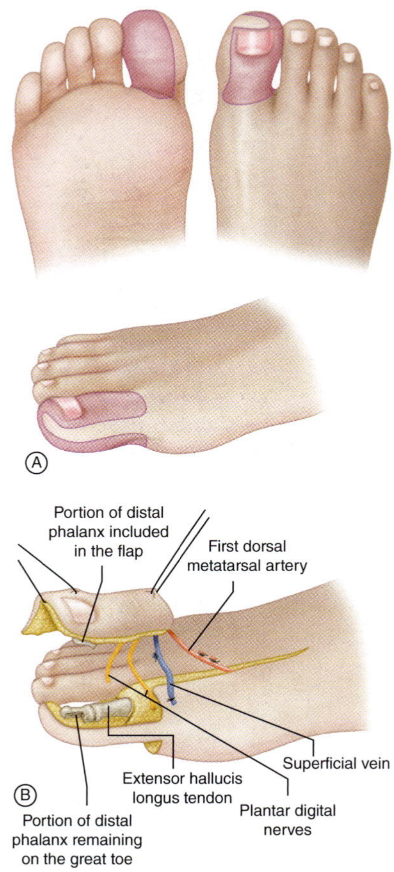

FIGURE 26-10 Design of the wrap-around flap. Note the medial strip of skin that is used to cover the residual stump of the great toe.

plantar cross toe flap from the second toe, which is divided around postoperative day 10 to 14. The plantar defect is covered with a full-thickness skin graft. Alternatively, the distal phalanx and a portion of the proximal phalanx of the great toe can be excised, and the proximal-based medial flap is used to cover the defect.

The most common complications of the donor site include wound dehiscence and ulceration. Some series report callous formation, but these resolved without any significant morbidity (32). In the recipient site, the most common complications include partial skin loss and bone resorption, although flap failure, malunion, fracture (especially in heavy laborers) bulging of the pulp, skin atrophy, and nail deformity have also been reported (33,34).

TRIMMED GREAT TOE TRANSFER

The "trimmed" great toe transfer described by Wei et al. is a technique that involves reduction of both bone and soft tissue components of the great toe (16). It is used for thumb reconstruction at or distal to the MCP joint and is indicated when there is a significant size discrepancy between the great toe and the thumb. It provides a similar size match to the normal thumb while preserving flexion and extension at the interphalangeal (IP) joint of the new thumb. In addition, because the epiphyses are preserved, growth is expected, unlike with the "wrap-around" flap.

The design and dissection are similar to the "wrap-around" technique. The width of the normal thumbnail is measured, and this measurement is transposed to the great toe nail so the excess nail plate is excised medially (Figure 26-12). The circumference of the normal thumb is measured at the base of the nail, the IP joint, and the midproximal phalanx, and these measurements are transposed to the great toe, leaving the excess skin medially. This medial skin flap, which is based proximally, tapers at its tip and is used to close the donor site in a similar fashion as the "wrap-around" flap. The dissection proceeds by elevating the medial proximally based flap but protecting the medial neurovascular bundle. The medial collateral ligament and joint capsule are incised longitudinally along the midaxial medial surface of the proximal and distal phalanges and elevated subperiosteally to create superior and inferior flaps. Longitudinal osteotomies are made, trimming about 2 to 4 mm from the medial aspect of both the distal and proximal phalanges. The medial collateral ligament and joint capsule are repaired. The toe harvest proceeds in a similar fashion to the whole great toe technique, with either a transverse osteotomy at the base of the proximal phalanx or disarticulation through the MTP joint.

The donor site is closed primarily with the medial proximal-based flap used to assist in a tension free closure. If the amputation is at the IP joint, the remaining stump can be closed in a similar technique as the "wrap-around" flap. In the original series, patients were satisfied with size, sensory two-point discrimination was 6 to 30 mm (mean, 20 mm), IP joint motion averaged 18 degrees, and all patients had normal gait on gross observation (16).

DORSALIS PEDIS FLAP

Originally described by McCraw and Furlow in 1975 as a local transposition flap (18), the dorsalis pedis free flap was first described by Ohmori and Harii in 1976 (19). It has been used for a wide variety of defects, including the head and neck, upper extremity, and lower extremity. Some of its advantages include thinness and pliability, sensibility, reliable vascularity, long vascular pedicle, and the ability to incorporate other structures such as the extensor tendons, the MTP joint, or the whole great toe or second toe (21–23,35). In addition, by including the superficial or deep peroneal nerves in the flap, sensation can be restored to the recipient hand (21,22,35). The main disadvantage of the dorsalis pedis flap is the donor site morbidity, including wound breakdown, chronic pain, paresthesias, hypersensitivity, and in rare cases ischemia of the foot (19,36–38).

The dorsalis pedis flap is supplied by the dorsalis pedis artery, a terminal branch of the anterior tibial artery, which lies between the extensor hallucis longus and the extensor digitorum communis deep to the extensor retinaculum (Figure 26-13A). The branches of the dorsalis pedis artery include the lateral and medial tarsal arteries and the arcuate artery terminating in the FDMA (39). Because the FDMA may be rudimentary (28), if a great toe is to be incorporated with a dorsalis pedis flap, the FPMA must be preserved and included in the flap dissection.

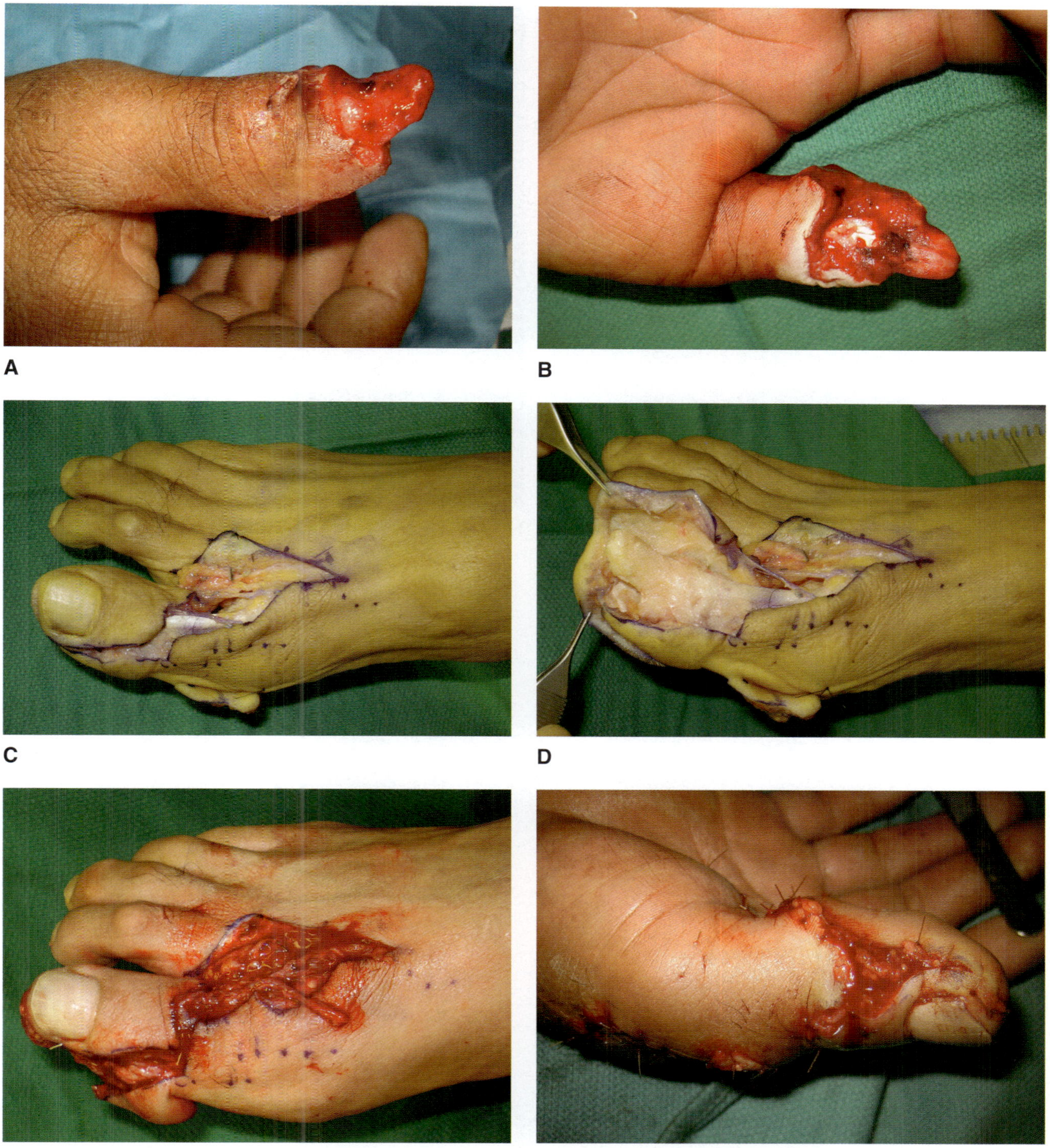

A B C D E F

FIGURE 26-11 (A) and (B) This patient sustained an avulsion injury to the distal soft tissues of the thumb, but the extensor and flexor tendons remained intact. (C) Markings and identification of key structures. (D) The flap has been elevated off the periosteum with preservation of the nail bed. (E) Perfusion of the flap after the tourniquet was deflated. (F) After skin closure.

Before harvest, the vascular supply of the DP is traced with a Doppler. The venous network is marked and incorporated into the flap design. Dissection is done under tourniquet control. An incision is made along the medial margin of the flap, incorporating the draining vein (Figure 26-13B). The arterial pedicle is located either at the proximal or distal end of the flap design (Figure 26-13C). After the artery is located, the septocutaneous perforators between the artery and the skin must be preserved. If the dissection is begun distally, the FDMA is ligated and traced back proximally unless the flap incorporates the first web space or the great toe (Figure 26-14D). The flap is then elevated deep to the fascia, leaving the paratenon intact.

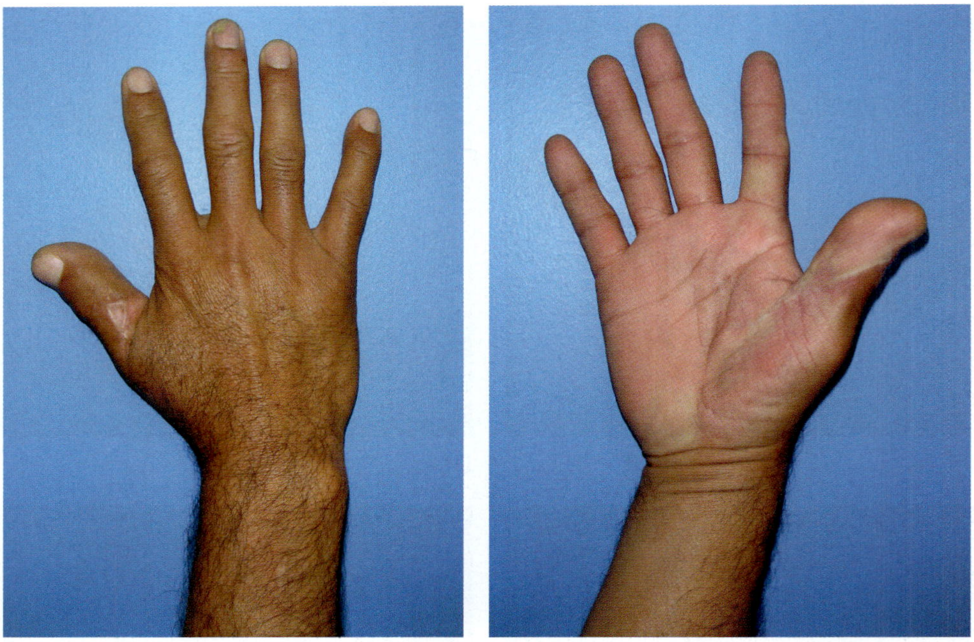

G H

FIGURE 26-11 (*Continued*) (**G**) and (**H**) Six months after surgery.

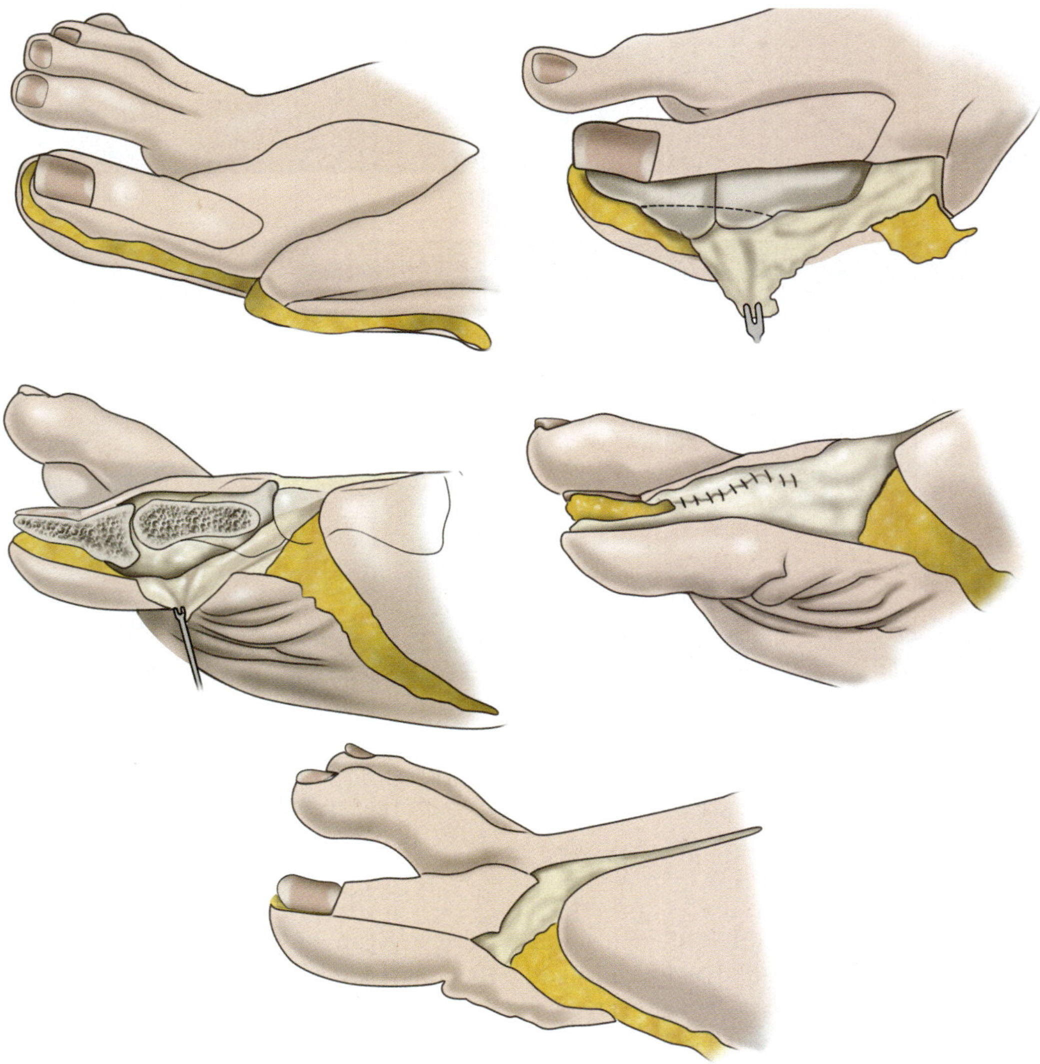

FIGURE 26-12 Design of a trimmed toe transfer.

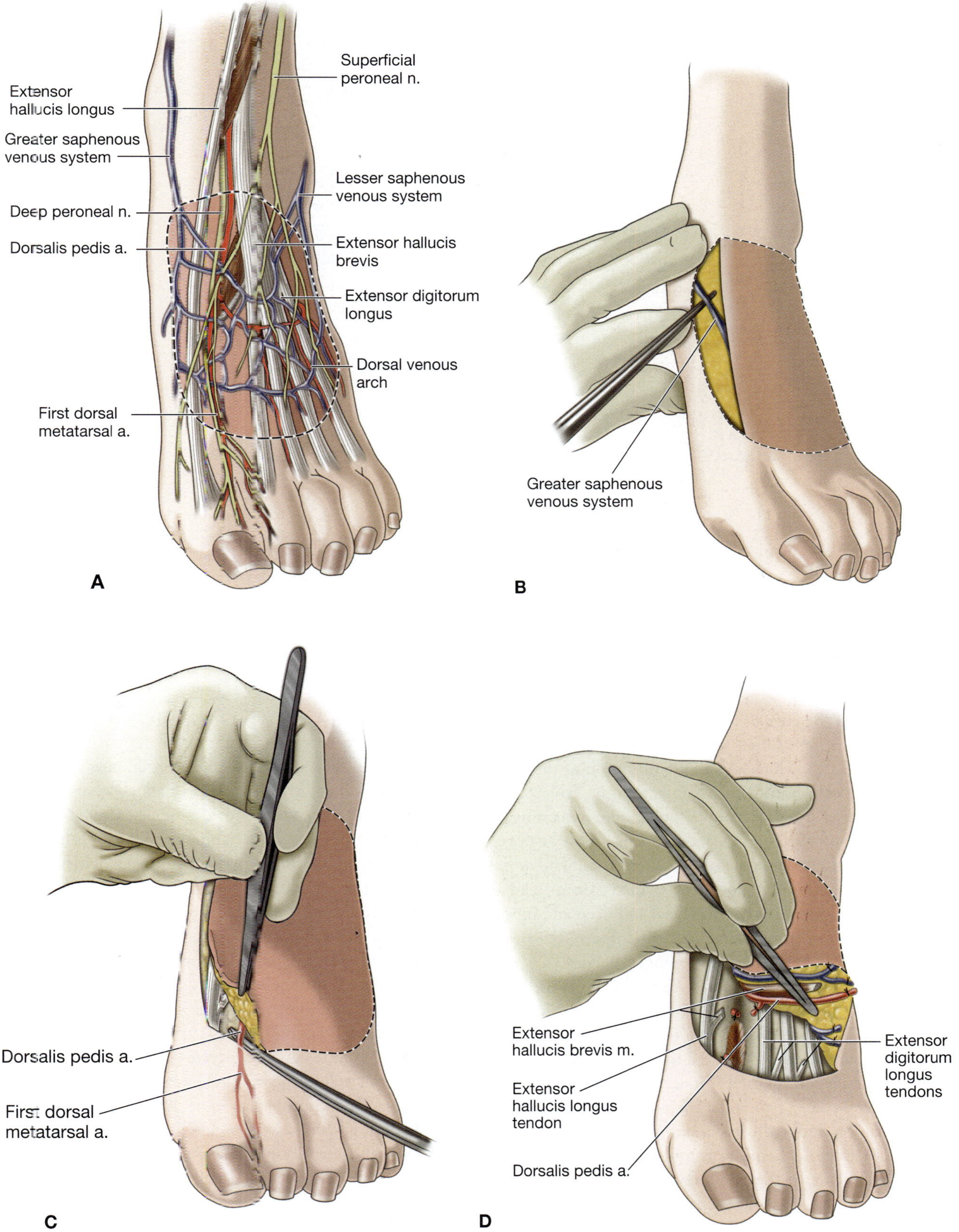

FIGURE 26-13 Dorsalis pedis flap: (A) The anterior tibial artery lies between the extensor hallucis longus and the extensor digitorum communis deep to the extensor retinaculum. The dorsalis pedis flap is marked centered over the septocutaneous perforators. (B) Dissection is started medially, incorporating the draining vein. (C) to (F) Identification of the first dorsal metatarsal artery distally. a, artery; n, nerve; vc, vena contaminates.

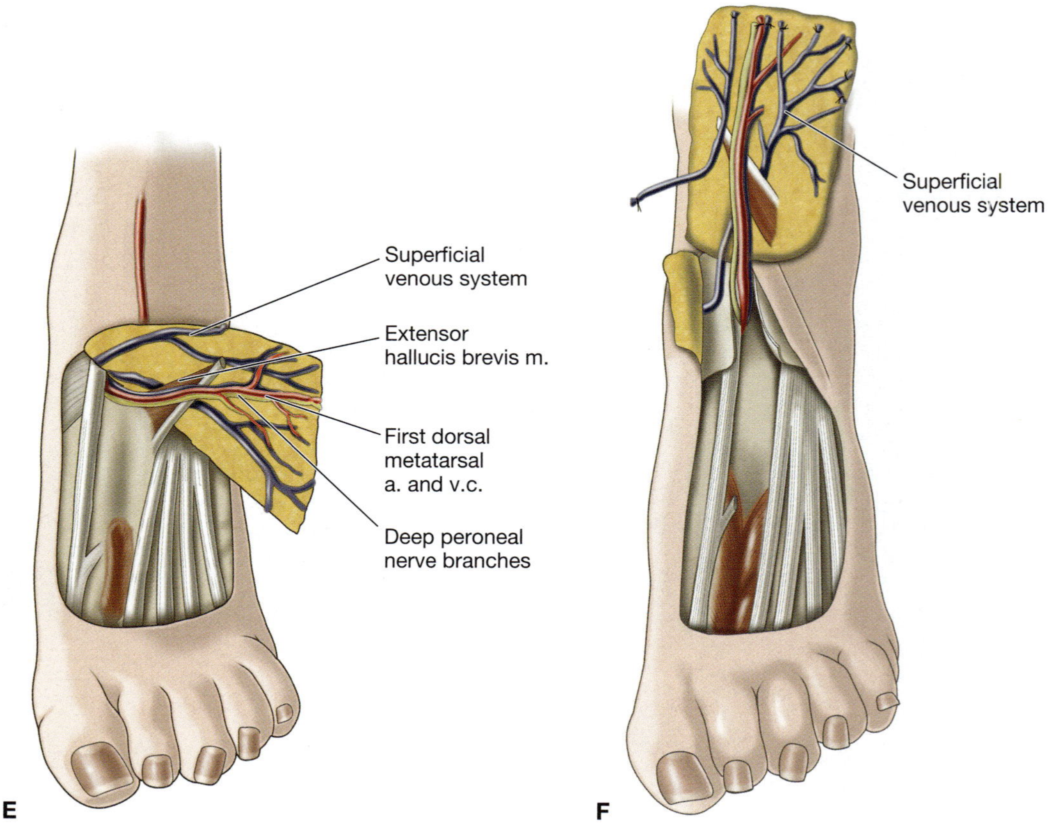

FIGURE 26-13 *(Continued)*

Sutures between the edge of the flap and the fascia can be used to prevent shearing. Often the extensor hallucis brevis is included in the flap, which aids in identification of the correct plane (38). Paratenon must be left intact on the extensor digitorum communis, extensor hallucis longus, and remaining part of the extensor brevis. The FDMA originates from the dorsalis pedis artery at the base of the second metatarsal. The dorsalis pedis then dives deeply to form the plantar system, and the takeoff of the FDMA may be superficial and deep and in some cases originate from the plantar surface (Figure 26-14). The deep peroneal and superficial peroneal nerves can easily be harvested with the flap. After the flap is elevated with arteries, veins, nerves, and the extensor hallucis brevis, the pedicle is traced proximally until the appropriate length is achieved. The tourniquet is released to confirm adequate blood flow of the flap before transfer (Figure 26-15).

As a general rule, a flap wider than 3 cm on the dorsum of the foot requires a split-thickness skin graft to close the donor site (38). Meticulous hemostasis and careful inspection and repair of any rents in the paratenon are critical for healing. The most common complications are "nontake" of the skin graft, wound breakdown, and delayed healing (36). However, infections, scarring, contracture, hyperesthesias, and ischemia have been reported (36). This flap should not be used in patients with a history of peripheral vascular disease or problems with wound healing (36,40). However, when the flap is harvested as a fascial flap, donor site complications have been lower (39).

COMBINED DORSALIS PEDIS TRANSFERS

The dorsalis pedis flap can be converted into a composite flap or chimeric flap (as described by Hallock) that includes bone, tendon, and toes, which provides single-stage reconstruction in complex upper extremity trauma (21,22,41). It has the advantage of incorporating replacement tissues with similar functional and structural functions while addressing the reconstruction in a single stage. While providing soft tissue coverage, the composite dorsalis pedis flap can minimize the number of operative procedures and provide several tissue components based on one reliable vascular pedicle with the ability to incorporate a joint and extensor tendons that can maximally restore hand function (21–23).

Design of the flap incorporates the designated toe, toe pulp, or joint as well as the proximal extension of the fasciocutaneous flap. Dissection begins in a similar fashion as the dorsalis pedis flap (Figure 26-16). However, the key is to locate the FDMA and identify its takeoff from the dorsalis pedis artery proximally and its course distally dorsal to the intermetatarsal ligament. Injury to the dorsalis pedis artery or FDMA will lead to flap necrosis. If the toe or toe pulp is to be included, the dissection proceeds as previously described for the whole great toe.

Closure of the donor site requires split-thickness skin grafting of the dorsum of the foot, but the donor site of the toe or toe pulp is closed primarily as for the whole great toe. The foot is splinted in dorsiflexion and immobilized for 1 week. Weight

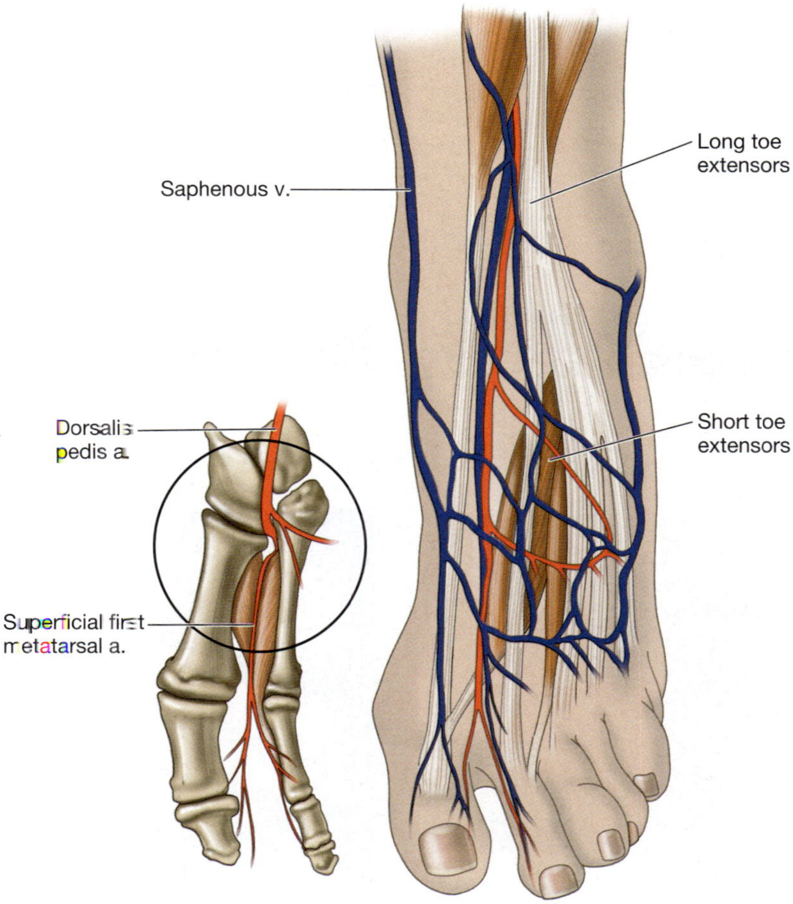

FIGURE 26-14 The first dorsal metatarsal artery (FDMA) originates from the dorsalis pedis artery at the base of the second metatarsal. The dorsalis pedis dives down to form the plantar system, and the takeoff of the FDMA may be superficial and deep and in some cases originates on the plantar surface. a, artery; v, vein.

bearing on the heel is allowed after 2 weeks. Complications from this composite flap are similar to those from the dorsalis pedis flap—delayed healing, wound edge necrosis, and occasionally pain with ambulation (21–24).

VASCULARIZED JOINT TRANSFERS

Reconstruction of single joints with vascularized joint transfers has been well documented (9,42–44). Previously, nonvascularized joint transfers have had disappointing results (45,46). Animal studies have shown that nonvascularized bone and joint undergoes morphologic changes of joint space narrowing, growth arrest, and fibrous invasion (8). Vascularized bone grafts have been shown to preserve hyaline cartilage and maintain subchondral bone and structural integrity (10). Moreover, by preservation of the epiphysis, children have demonstrated longitudinal growth compared with the toe on the contralateral foot (43).

The first vascularized finger joint island transfer was done by Buncke et al. in 1967 (7). Foucher and Merle performed the first whole vascularized toe joint transfer in 1976 (47). Vascularized joint transfers allow the incorporation of soft tissues, flexor, and extensor tendons and produce stable long-term joints with growth potential, lateral stability, and minimal degenerative changes (35,44,48).

Vascularized joint transfers can be classified as partial or complete (9). Partial joint transfers enter the capsule and disrupt the synovium and congruency of joint surfaces (35). Total joint transfers are a single unit respecting the synovium and articular congruency of the joint. In addition, transferring a joint with an overlying skin paddle allows monitoring of vascular perfusion and protection of tendon gliding and enables a tension-free closure.

Vascularized joint transfers are indicated in young, active, motivated patients who have sustained trauma with extensive bony loss or a failed arthroplasty or arthrodesis (9,35,44). In children, the indications include congenital anomalies and traumatic defects with bony loss in which vascularized joints with intact epiphyses provide the potential for longitudinal growth (35,43).

The second toe is most commonly chosen for vascularized bone grafts or joint transfers (9). Before harvest, an elliptical skin island is designed over the joint and preserved (Figure 26-17). After identifying the dorsalis pedis and FDMAs, the FDMA is followed distally preserving the medial digital artery to the second toe and ligating the lateral digital artery to the great toe. As the dissection approaches the intermetatarsal ligament, the communication between the FDMA and FPMA systems is identified and the most dominant system selected, preserving the medial digital artery to the second toe. Perforators to the

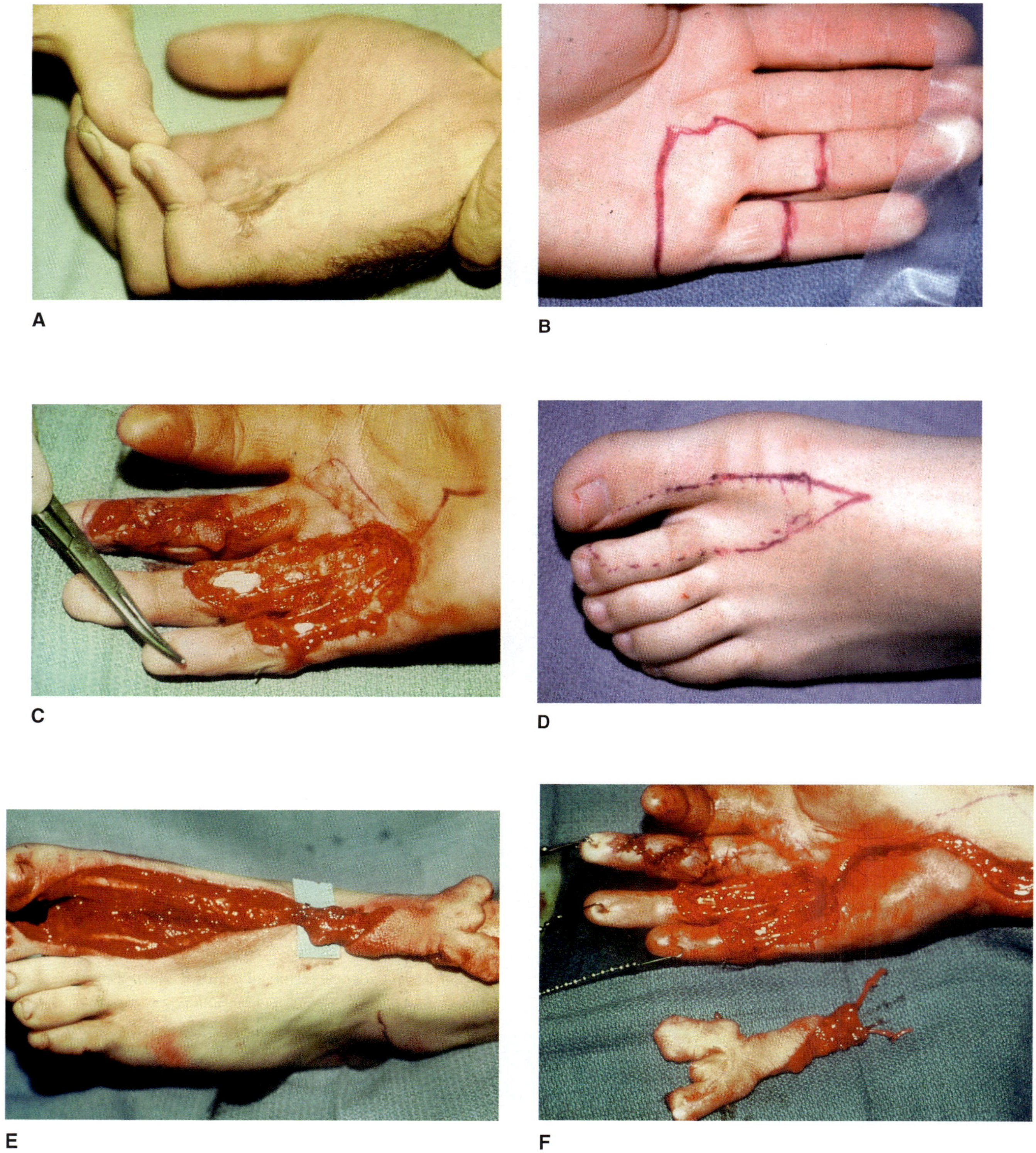

FIGURE 26-15 (A) This patient sustained a deep electrical burn to the distal palm of the small, ring, and long fingers. Previous attempts to release the scar with full-thickness skin grafting failed, resulting in this deformity. (B) Template obtained from the opposite hand. (C) Fingers after contracture release. The long finger was released with multiple Z-plasties. Note the exposed tendon and neurovascular structures. (D) The template is superimposed on the first and second toes. The flap is based on an extension of the dorsalis pedis artery and the first dorsal metatarsal artery. (E) The flap is elevated and the tourniquet released to verify perfusion. (F) The flap is placed next to the recipient defect. Microvascular anastomoses are performed.

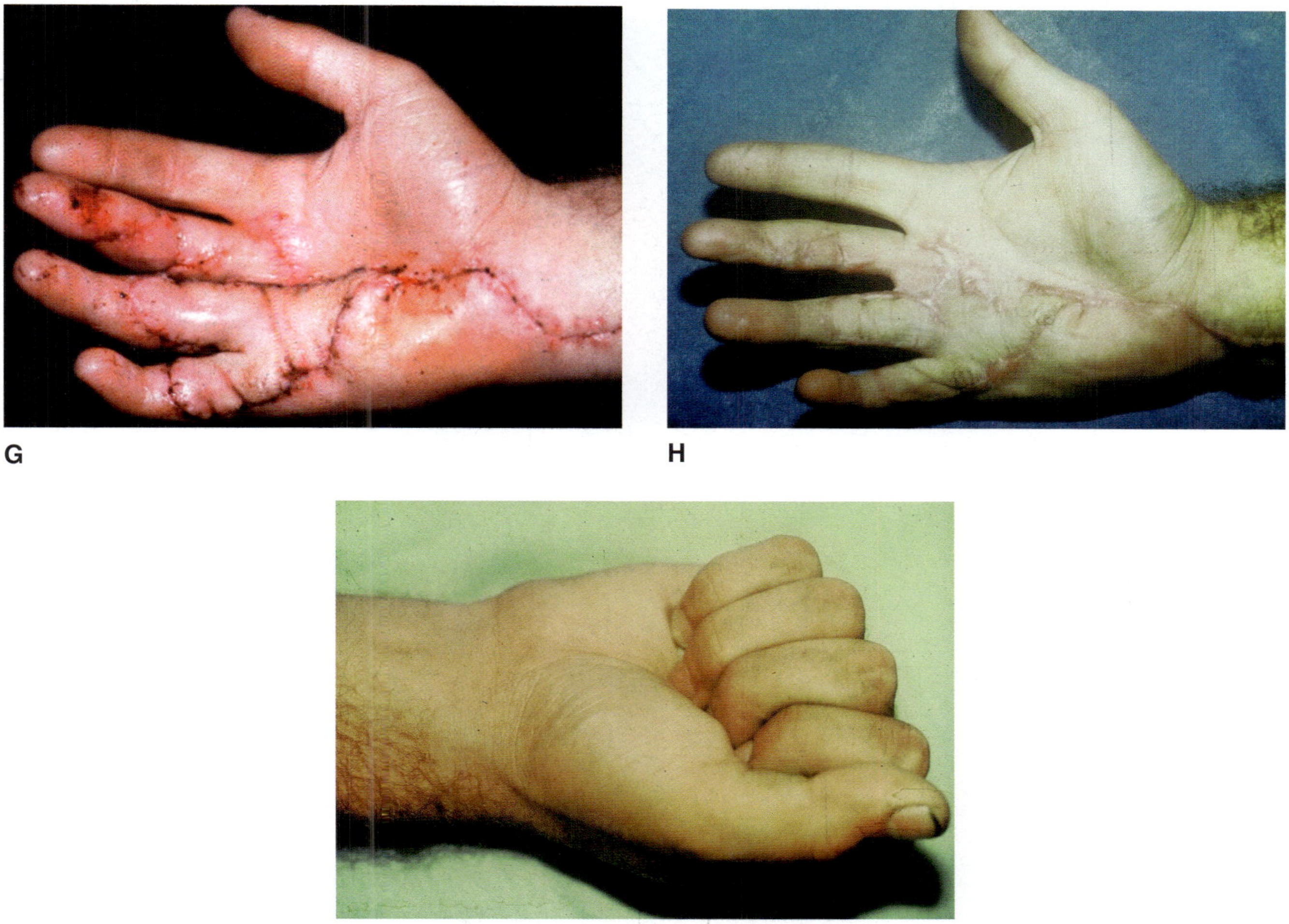

G H I

FIGURE 26-15 (*Continued*) (**G**) The wound is loosely closed, and the proximal interphalangeal joint is pinned in extension. Five months after surgery, extension (**H**) and flexion (**I**).

dorsal skin flap of the second toe are carefully preserved throughout the dissection. If the extensor and flexor tendons also need to be reconstructed, these tendons are harvested at the appropriate length en bloc with the toe proximal interphalangeal joint (PIP) joint by disarticulating the distal interphalangeal joint (DIP) joint and an osteotomy proximally through the proximal phalanx or disarticulation through the MTP joint. At this point, the joint is only tethered by the pedicle, the tourniquet is released, and the vascularity of the monitoring skin flap is evaluated.

In the recipient site, bony fixation of the proximal and middle phalanges is achieved by step-cut osteotomies or a peg and dowel technique (9) and skeletal stability secured with K-wires or interosseous wires or by mini-plate fixation if there is adequate bone stock. The proximal and distal extensor tendon repairs are made as far distally from the transferred joint to reduce tendon scarring. Early postoperative movement is encouraged.

To achieve closure of the donor site defect, the toe remnants are excised, and the donor site is closed primarily over a small Penrose drain. Alternatively, the PIP joint can be bone grafted with Kirschner wire fixation if there is enough skin to close the donor defect. Finally, the second toe can be shortened with osteosynthesis of the middle phalanx to the proximal phalanx and closure of the residual wound with a full-thickness skin graft (49). Postoperative care of the donor site is similar to a great toe transfer (Figure 26-18).

Common complications of vascularized joint transfers, including infection, tendon adhesions, stiffness, skeletal malalignment, bowstringing, and total failure of the vascularized joint, have all been reported (9,35,42,49). Range of motion depends on multiple factors that include the patient's age, etiology, donor site, recipient site, and comorbidities.

Children regain better range of motion than adults (11,35,44). Tsai et al. reported that the transferred epiphyses remained open and growth was proportional or increased compared with the contralateral toe (43). The improved range of motion in children might be related to the ability of the transferred joint to adapt during growth.

COMPLICATIONS

The most common intraoperative and immediate postoperative complication is vasospasm (29). Many of these cases can be resolved with adventitial stripping; use of papaverine,

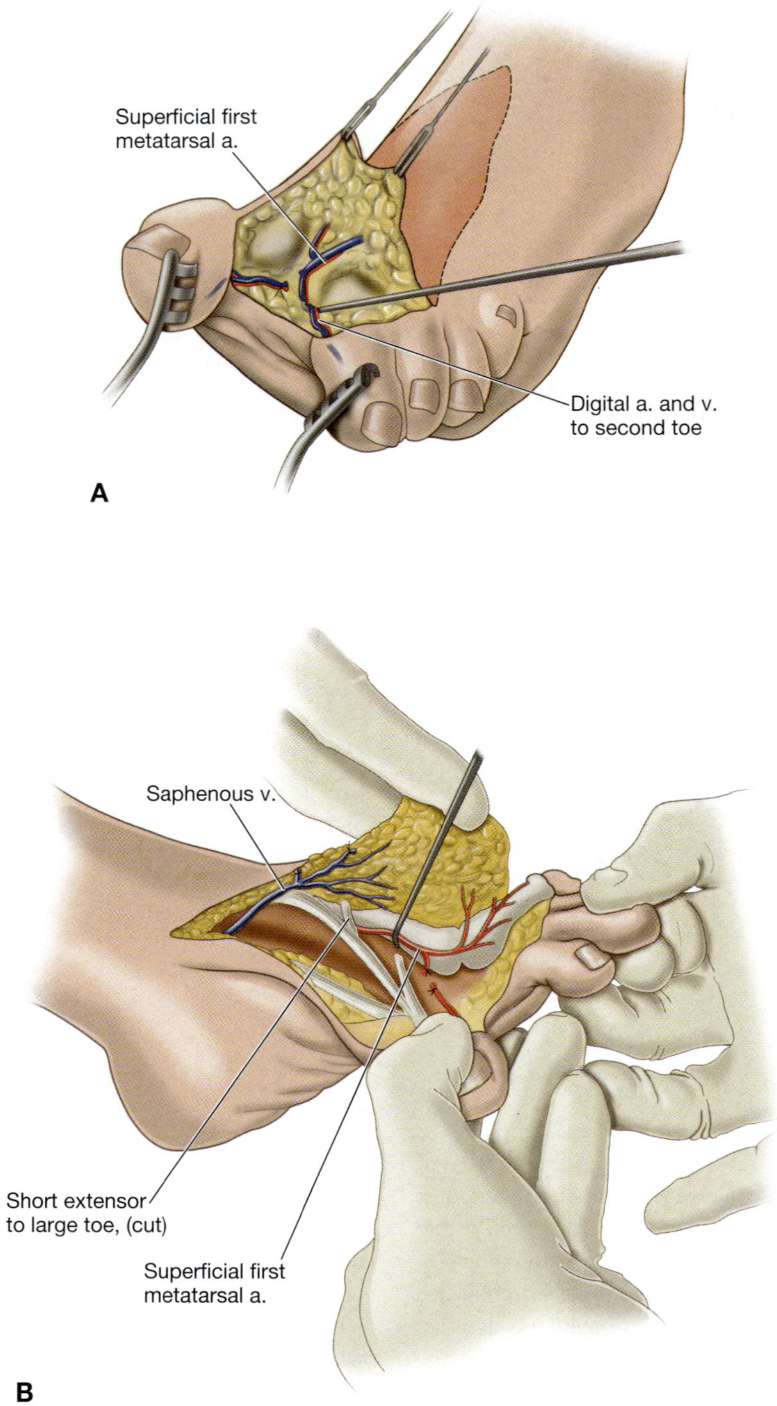

FIGURE 26-16 Combined dorsalis pedis flap with vascularized metatarsal bone graft and metatarsophalangeal (MTP) joint. (**A**) After marking the flap, dissection begins distally to identify the digital vessels and more proximally the first dorsal metatarsal artery (FDMA). (**B**) After visualization of the FDMA, transection of the intermetatarsal ligament allows exposure of the vessels and proximal dissection of the flap. If the MTP joint is to be incorporated, a cuff of intrinsic muscle is included to preserve the blood supply to the bone. As the dissection proceeds proximally, the draining vein is identified and preserved. It is important to preserve the septocutaneous perforators to maintain viability of the skin flap.

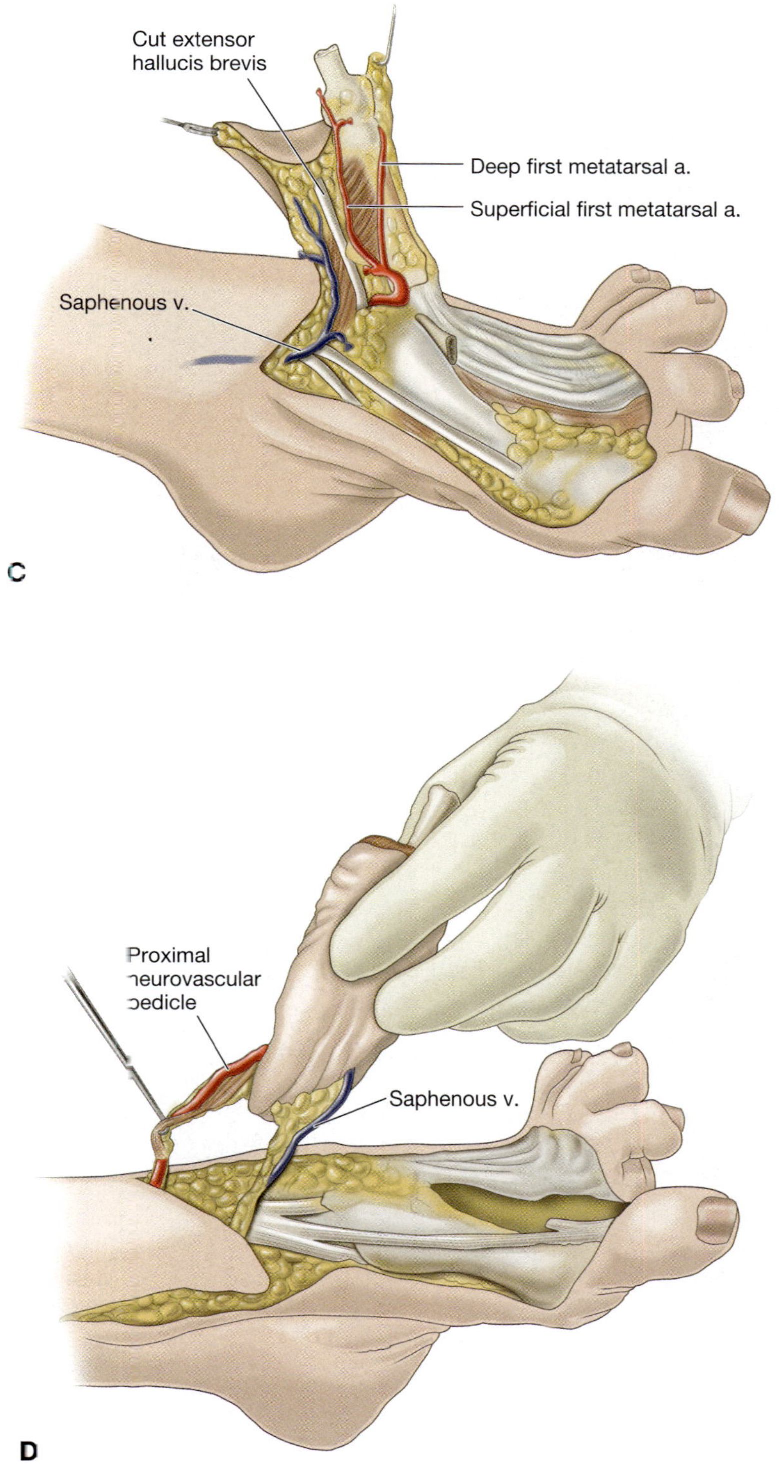

FIGURE 26-16 (*Continued*) (C) The second toe is sacrificed, and the osteocutaneous flap is elevated. It is important to preserve the paratenon on the extensor hallucis longus to support skin grafting if necessary. (D) Flap elevated on its pedicle. a, artery; v, vein.

lidocaine, and mechanical expansion; or inspecting for small side branches that have not been clipped. The use of vein grafts is recommended if there is tension on the anastomosis. However, usually the dorsalis pedis artery and cephalic vein provide enough length to preclude their use. After surgery, chlorpromazine will help prevent vasospasm, especially in children (50). Failure of toe-to-hand transfers is rare and is reported at 5% (9,26,51).

The most common secondary procedures for toe-to-hand transfers are for tendon adhesions and include tenolyses, tendon transfers, and tenorrhaphies (52). Other reported complications include extension lag, joint stiffness, neuroma formation, tendon rupture, and nonunions (52,53). Donor site complications include delayed wound healing, hyperkeratosis, and weakness in pushoff; however, claw toe, varus/valgus deformities, cold intolerance, and pain have also been reported (54).

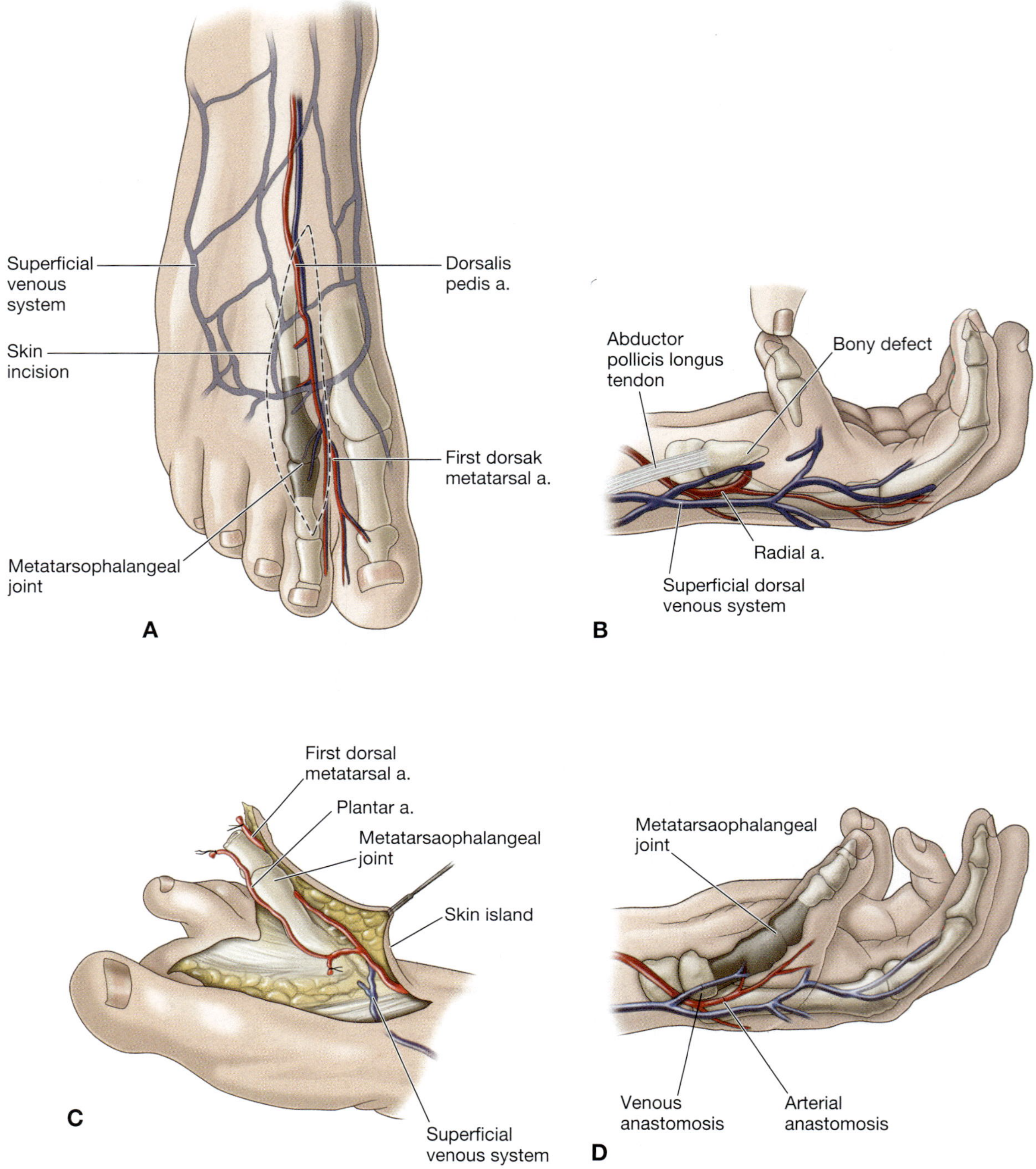

FIGURE 26-17 (A) Anatomy of the vascularized metatarsophalangeal (MTP) joint of the second toe, dorsalis pedis artery, first dorsal metatarsal artery (FDMA), and digital arteries to the first and second toes. Any of the three joints of the second toe may be used—MTP, proximal interphalangeal joint (PIP), or distal interphalangeal joint (DIP)—depending on the recipient area. (B) Example of a potential segmental defect of the MTP joint of the thumb. (C) The vascularized MTP joint transfer has been harvested with an overlying skin island for postoperative monitoring. (D) Insetting of the vascularized joint transfer. Osteosynthesis is usually done with K-wires and anastomoses to the cephalic vein and dorsal branch of the radial artery. If a skin paddle is used, the deep peroneal nerve can be coapted to the dorsal sensory branch of a digital nerve. a, artery.

REHABILITATION

Therapy is highly individualized for each patient. However, most therapy addresses tendon gliding, recovery of sensibility, bony stability, and soft tissue edema control. Rehabilitation of a toe transfer usually starts on postoperative day 5 after the surgeon performs the first dressing change. The hand therapist fabricates a dorsal protective thumb spica splint with the wrist in a neutral position (28). Therapy is started with gentle passive range of motion of the carpometacarpal joint. Passive and active range of motion is started on uninvolved digits. On days 10 to 14, gentle passive MCP and IP (if free) range of motion is performed. On days 18 to 21, active range of motion of the MCP and IP joints is started. At 3 to 4 weeks, the Kirschner wire is removed, and MCP joint active and passive motion are started. Care is taken to avoid lateral motion if the collateral ligaments were reconstructed. During the fourth and

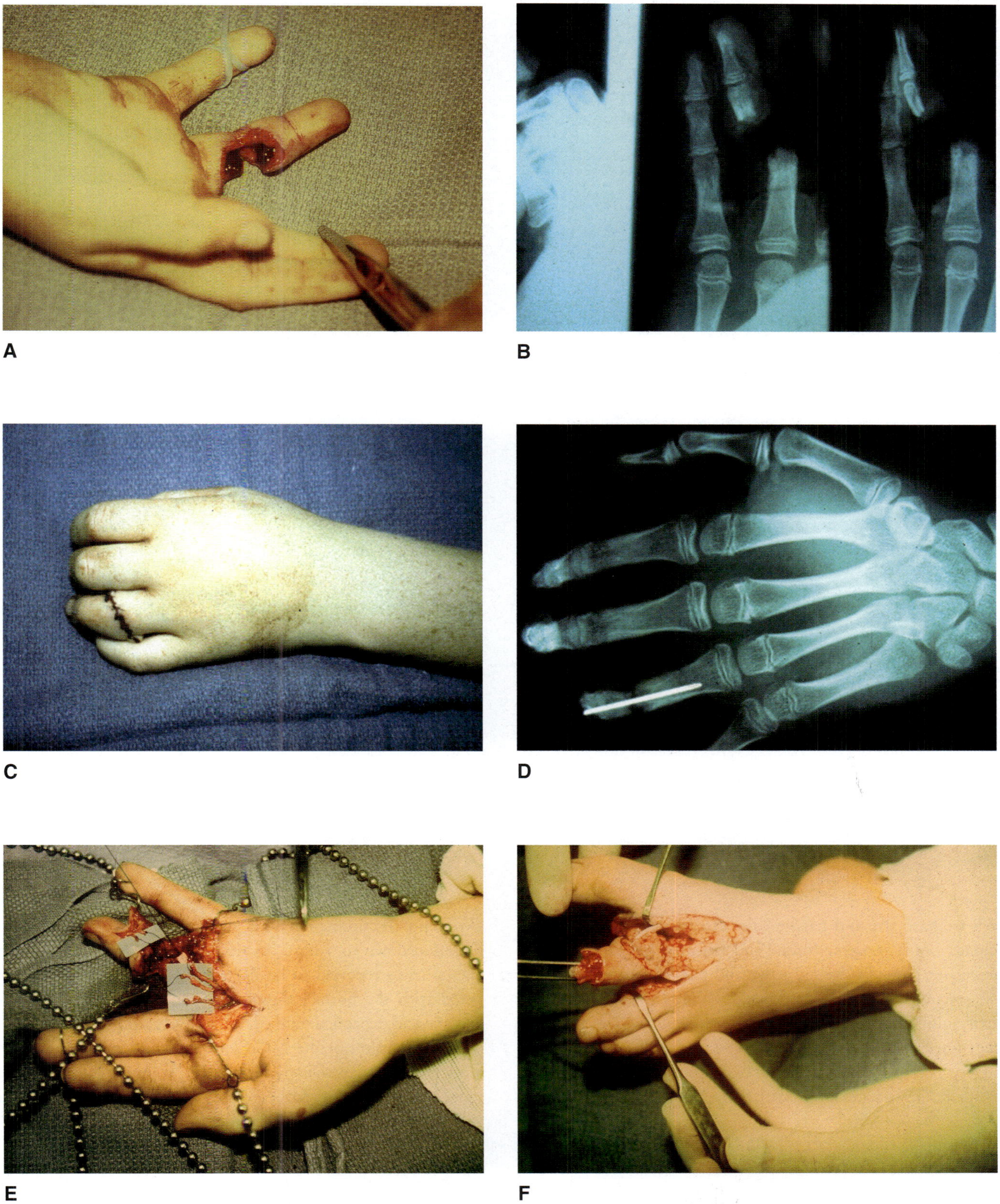

FIGURE 26-18 A 14-year-old boy sustained segmental loss of the proximal interphalangeal joint (PIP) joint of his left ring finger after a bicycle spoke wheel accident. (A) The ulnar neurovascular bundle was intact, and the distal tip was perfused. (B) Segmental loss of the PIP joint. (C) The wound was closed primarily after irrigation. (D) Bony stabilization was achieved with a K-wire, and he subsequently underwent an elective vascularized joint transfer. (E) The proximal and distal neurovascular bundles were dissected. (F) Simultaneously, a second team harvested the ipsilateral second toe, preserving the medial neurovascular bundle.

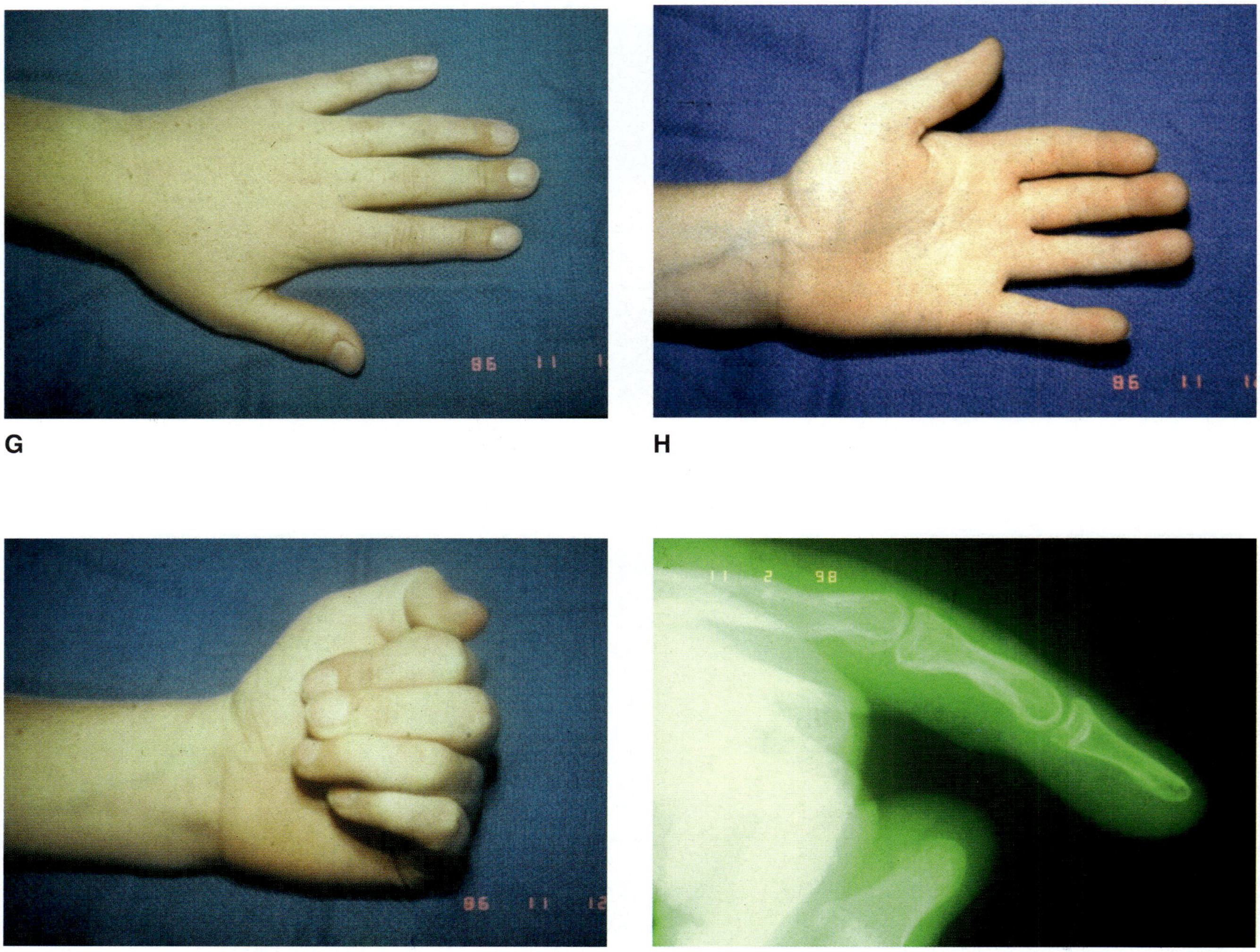

G H I J

FIGURE 26-19 (*Continued*) (**G**) Five months after surgery. (**H**) Extension. (**I**) Flexion. (**J**) Radiograph showing that congruency of the PIP joint space has been maintained.

fifth weeks, active and passive wrist extension beyond neutral is started, as well as edema control and scar massage reduction techniques. At around 6 weeks, active and passive composite thumb movements are begun, and a blocking splint is made to allow isolated joint motion. Light functional activities are initiated. Functional electrical stimulation can begin as early as 5 weeks after surgery. At 6 to 8 weeks, the splint is discontinued, and by the eighth week, strengthening exercises are initiated (28).

SENSORY REHABILITATION AND FUNCTIONAL RESULTS

Sensory rehabilitation is started as soon as the patient can perceive a 30-cps tuning fork in the proximal portion of the repaired nerve (55). Sensory rehabilitation progresses by differentiating static from dynamic stimuli and different shapes and textures (28). Patients can continue the therapy as an outpatient home program (56). Two-point discrimination has been reported as low as 8 mm (53,57). Buncke et al. reported a total of 161 great toe transfers between 1972 and 2004 (27) with an average two-point discrimination of 8 mm and a range of protective sensation down to 5 mm. In addition, grip strength and pinch strength was reported to be 77% and 67%, respectively, compared with the normal thumb. Thumb range of motion was variable and depended on the level, type of reconstruction, inclusion or exclusion of the MCP joint, scarring, and compliance with postoperative therapy. Buncke et al. reported an average range of motion at the MCP joint of 44 degrees (63% of normal side) and 40 degrees at the IP joint (59% of the normal side).

REFERENCES

1. Huguier PC. Du remplacement du pouce par son metacarpien, par l'agrandissement du premier espace interosseux. *Arch Gen Med* 1874;1:78.
2. Guermonprez F. *Notes sur quelques r{233}sections et restaurations dii pouce.* Paris: P. Asselin, 1887.
3. Nicoladoni C. Daumenplastik und organischer Ersatz der Fingerspitze (Anticheiroplastik und Daktyloplstik). *Arch Klin Chir* 1900;61:606.
4. Noesske H.Ueber Ersatz des samt Metakarpus verlorenen Daumens durch operative Umstellung des Zeigefingers. *Munchener Medizinische Wochenschrift* 1920;67:465.
5. Komatsu S, Tamai S. Successful replantation of a completely cut-off thumb: case report. *Plast Reconstr Surg* 1968;42:374–377.

6. Buncke HJ Jr, Buncke CM, Schulz WP. Immediate Nicoladoni procedure in the Rhesus monkey, or hallux-to-hand transplantation, utilising microminiature vascular anastomoses. *Br J Plast Surg* 1966;19(4):332–337.
7. Buncke HJ Jr, Daniller AI, Schulz WP, et al. The fate of autogenous whole joints transplanted by microvascular anastomoses. *Plast Reconstr Surg* 1967;39(4):333–341.
8. Entin MA, Alger JR, Baird RM. Experimental and clinical transplantation of autogenous whole joints. *J Bone Joint Surg* 1962;44A(8):1518–1536.
9. Buncke HJ, Valauri F. Vascularized joint transplantation. InBuncke HJ (ed). *Microsurgery: Transplantation-Replantation*. Philadelphia: Lea & Febiger, 1991.
10. Tsai TM, Ogden L, Jaeger SH, et al. Experimental vascularized total joint autografts—a primate study. *J Hand Surg* 1982;7(suppl A):140–146.
11. Singer DI, O'Brien BM, McLeod AM, et al. Long-term follow-up of free vascularized joint transfers to the hand in children. *J Hand Surg Am* 1988;13(5):776–783.
12. Cobbett JR. Free digital transfer. Report of a case of transfer of a great toe to replace an amputated thumb. *J Bone Joint Surg Br* 1969;51(4):677–679.
13. Dongyue Y, Yudong G. Thumb reconstruction utilizing second toe transplantation by microvascular anastomosis: report of 78 cases. *Chin Med J (Engl)* 1979;92(5):295–309.
14. Morrison WA, O'Brien BM, MacLeod AM. Thumb reconstruction with a free neurovascular wrap-around flap from the big toe. *J Hand Surg (Am)* 1980;5:575–583.
15. Urbaniak JR. Wrap-around procedure for thumb reconstruction. *Hand Clin* 1985;1(2):259–269.
16. Wei FC, Chen HC, Chuang CC, et al. Reconstruction of the thumb with a trimmed-toe transfer technique. *Plast Reconstr Surg* 1988;82(3):506–515.
17. Upton J, Mutimer K. A modification of the great-toe transfer for thumb reconstruction. *Plast Reconstr Surg* 1988;82(3):535–538.
18. McCraw JB, Furlow LT Jr. The dorsalis pedis arterialized flap. A clinical study. *Plast Reconstr Surg* 1975;55(2):177–185.
19. Ohmori K, Harii K. Free dorsalis pedis sensory flap to the hand, with microneurovascular anastomoses. *Plast Reconstr Surg* 1976;58(5):546–554.
20. Chang TS, Wang W, Wu JB. Free transfer of the second toe combined with dorsalis pedis flap using microvascular technique for reconstruction of the thumb and other fingers. *Ann Acad Med Singapore* 1979;8(4):404–412.
21. Zhang YX, Wang D, Zhang Y, et al. Triple chimeric flap based on anterior tibial vessels for reconstruction of severe traumatic injuries of the hand with thumb loss. *Plast Reconstr Surg* 2009;123(1):268–275.
22. Eo S, Kim Y, Kim JY, Oh S. The versatility of the dorsalis pedis compound free flap in hand reconstruction. *Ann Plast Surg* 2008;61(2):157–163.
23. Caroli A, Adani R, Castagnetti C, et al. Dorsalis pedis flap with vascularized extensor tendons for dorsal hand reconstruction. *Plast Reconstr Surg* 1993;92(7):1326–1330.
24. Del Piñal F, García-Bernal FJ, Delgado J, et al. Overcoming soft-tissue deficiency in toe-to-hand transfer using a dorsalis pedis fasciosubcutaneous toe free flap: surgical technique. *J Hand Surg Am* 2005;30(1):111–119.
25. Greenberg BM, May JW Jr. Great toe-to-hand transfer: role of the preoperative lateral arteriogram of the foot. *J Hand Surg Am* 1988;13:411–414.
26. Wei FC, Santamaria E. Toe to finger reconstruction. InGreen DP, Hotchkiss RN, Pederson WC (eds). *Green's Operative Hand Surgery*. Philadelphia: Churchill Livingstone, 1993.
27. Buncke GM, Buncke HJ, Lee CK. Great toe-to-thumb microvascular transplantation after traumatic amputation [review]. *Hand Clin* 2007;23(1):105–115.
28. Buncke HJ. Great toe transplantation. In Buncke HJ (ed). *Microsurgery: Transplantation-Replantation*. Philadelphia: Lea & Febiger, 1991.
29. Gu YD, Cheng DS, Zhang GM, et al. Long-term results of toe transfer: retrospective analysis. *J Reconstr Microsurg* 1997;13:405–408.
30. Vedder NB, Maser BM. Thumb reconstruction: microvascular methods. In Mathes SJ (ed). *Plastic surgery*, vol. 7. Philadelphia: Elsevier, 2006, p. 253.
31. Taghinia AH, Littler JW, Upton J. Refinements in pollicization: a 30-year experience. *Plast Reconstr Surg* 2012;130(3):423e–433e.
32. Doi K, Hattori Y, Dhawan V. The wrap-around flap in thumb reconstruction. *Tech Hand Up Extrem Surg* 2002;6(3):124–132.
33. Lee KS, Che IJ, Hahn SB. Thumb reconstruction with a free neurovascular wrap-around flap from the big toe: long-term follow up of thirty cases. Microsurgery 1995;16:692–697.
34. Doi K, Kuwata N, Kawai S. Reconstruction of the thumb with a free wrap-around flap from the big toe and an iliac bone graft. *J Bone Joint Surg Am* 1985;67:439–445.
35. Hierner R, Berger AK. Long-term results after vascularized joint transfer for finger joint reconstruction. In Eisenmann-Klein M, Neuhann-Lorenz C. *Innovations in Plastic and Aesthetic Surgery*. New York: Springer, 2008, pp. 95–103.
36. Samson MC, Morris SF, Tweed AE. Dorsalis pedis flap donor site: acceptable or not? *Plast Reconstr Surg* 1998;102:1549–1554.
37. Zuker RM, Manktelow RT. The dorsalis pedis free flap: technique of elevation, foot closure, and flap application. *Plast Reconst Surg* 1986;77:93.
38. Buncke GM, Buncke HJ. The dorsalis pedis flap. In Buncke HJ (ed). *Microsurgery: Transplantation-Replantation*. Philadelphia: Lea & Febiger, 1991.
39. Ritz M, Mahendru S, Somia N, Pacifico MD. The dorsalis pedis fascial flap. *J Reconstr Microsurg* 2009;25(5):313–317.
40. Furlow LT. The dorsalis pedis flap. In Strauch B, Vasconez LD, Hall-Findlay EJ (eds). *Grabb's Encyclopedia of Flaps*. Boston: Little Brown and Company, 1990, pp. 1654–1660.
41. Hallock GG. Further clarification of the nomenclature for compound flaps. *Plast Reconstr Surg* 2006;117:151e–160e.
42. Foucher G. Vascularized joint transfer. In Green DP (ed). *Operative Hand Surgery*, 3rd ed, vol 2. New York: Churchill Livingstone, 1993, pp. 1201–1221.
43. Ishida O, Tsai TM. Free vascularized whole joint transfer in children. *Microsurgery* 12:196–206,1991.
44. Tsai TM, Wang WZ. Vascularized joint transfers: Indications and results [review]. *Hand Clin* 1992;8(3):525–536.
45. Barsky AJ. *Congenital Anomalies of the Hands and Their Surgical Treatment*. Springfield, IL: Thomas, 1958.
46. Peacock EE. Reconstructive surgery of hands with injured central metacarpophalangeal joints. *J Bone Joint Surgery* 1956;38(suppl A):291–302.
47. Foucher G, Merle M. Transfert articulaire au niveau d'un doigt en microchirurgie. *G. A. M. lettre d'information du GAM* 1976;7:15.
48. Foucher G, Lenoble E, Smith D. Free and island vascularized joint transfer for proximal interphalangeal reconstruction: a series of 27 cases. *J Hand Surg Am* 1994;19(1):8–16.
49. Chen SH, Wei FC, Chen HC, et al. Vascularized toe joint transfer to the hand [review]. *Plast Reconstr Surg* 1996;98(7):1275–1284.
50. Urbaniak JR. Replantation in children. InSerafin D, Georgiade N (eds). *Pediatric Plastic Surgery*. St. Louis: CV Mosby, 1984, pp. 1168–1185.
51. Poppen NK, Norris TR, Buncke HJ Jr. Evaluation of sensibility and function with microsurgical free tissue transfer of the great toe to the hand for thumb reconstruction. *J Hand Surg Am* 1983;8(5 Pt 1):516–531.
52. Yim KK, Wei FC. Secondary procedures to improve function after toe-to-hand transfers. *Br J Plast Surg* 1995;48(7):487–491.
53. Rosson GD, Buncke GM, Buncke HJ. Great toe transplant versus thumb replant for isolated thumb amputation: critical analysis of functional outcome. *Microsurgery* 2008;28(8):598–605.
54. Lin PY, Sebastin SJ, Ono S, et al. A systematic review of outcomes of toe-to-thumb transfers for isolated traumatic thumb amputation. *Hand (N Y)* 2011;6(3):235–243.
55. Mackinnon SE, Dellon AL. Surgery of the *Peripheral Nerve*. New York: Thieme, 1988.
56. Wei FC, Ma HS. Delayed sensory reeducation after toe-to-hand transfer. *Microsurgery* 1995;16:583–585.
57. Woo SH, Kim JS, Seul JH. Immediate toe-to-hand transfer in acute hand injuries: overall results, compared with results for elective cases. *Plast Reconstr Surg* 2004;113:882–892.

CHAPTER 27

Surgical Exposure of the Brachial Plexus

Robert J. Spinner

COMMON EXPOSURES OF THE BRACHIAL PLEXUS

Exposure of the brachial plexus is necessary for treatment of injuries, entrapments, and tumors. Exposure to all levels from spinal nerves to terminal branches can be achieved through standard approaches. These approaches can be performed individually or in combination as determined by the pathology. Posterior approaches allow full exposure of posterior terminal branches. Roots themselves are intradural. Surgical approaches can only be performed and appreciated with a good knowledge of normal anatomy and common variations (1).

Anterior Exposures

Supraclavicular

The supraclavicular exposure is facilitated by positioning of the patient with a bump between the shoulders. The head of the bed is elevated. The neck is turned away from the side being operated. The field is prepped widely, including the neck, chest, complete upper limb, and both legs. In some cases, exposure posteriorly to the scapula may be deemed necessary. In this case, the ipsilateral shoulder is elevated with a bump. A bump is also placed under the buttock to externally rotate the leg if exposure to the ipsilateral leg for sural nerve harvesting is needed.

The brachial plexus is commonly exposed through a standard zig-zag type incision, especially when combined with an infraclavicular approach (Figure 27-1). This provides the most generous exposure of neural (and vascular) elements. An incision is made paralleling the posterior aspect of the sternocleidomastoid muscle from the midneck to the clavicle. This is combined with a transverse limb across the clavicle. This incision is then extended with an incision in the deltopectoral interval to expose the infraclavicular brachial plexus.

I prefer a transverse incision in the supraclavicular region which can be undermined sufficiently to allow generous exposure. The incision is planned using one of Langer's lines, several finger breadths above the clavicle. The incision runs from the middle of the sternocleidomastoid laterally toward the trapezius (Figure 27-2). Exposure to the upper elements of the brachial plexus is easier when the incision is made higher; exposure to the lower elements is easier with a lower incision.

The incision is deepened with sharp dissection through the platysma. Care is taken to develop the avascular subplatysmal plane cranially and caudad because this is necessary to gain ample exposure to the plexus. The external jugular vein and supraclavicular nerves are seen and preserved (Figure 27-3). A longitudinal dissection is now performed through the fatty tissues from the lateral border of the midsternocleidomastoid to the clavicle, keeping the external jugular vein medially. The external jugular vein is typically preserved, but it can be sacrificed. The transverse cervical artery is ligated. The clavicular insertion of the sternocleidomastoid can be released. The omohyoid is identified and serves as an important landmark. It is mobilized in a vasoloop. The dissection on the omohyoid stays on its superficial surface initially. The lateral dissection opens up the plane toward the scapula; it is usually not scarred here. Dissection of the medial portion of the omohyoid opens up the space beneath the sternocleidomastoid. Medial dissection is done until the internal jugular vein or undulations from it are appreciated. The internal jugular vein and carotid artery are medial to the brachial plexus. The omohyoid is divided at the bowtie and tagged on tension medially and laterally (Figure 27-4). This step improves visualization and frees up an assistant retracting medially.

Key neural structures lie beneath the omohyoid. The fat pad is dissected longitudinally using bipolar cautery and is retracted laterally. The scalene anterior muscle is seen and the phrenic nerve (C3–C5) is identified first on its surface and confirmed with a nerve stimulator and protected. The phrenic nerve is traced cephalad. It and the small nerve to the subclavius are the only nerves of the brachial plexus that run from superolaterally to inferomedially. The phrenic nerve is traced to its C5 contribution and mobilized carefully. The phrenic nerve continues

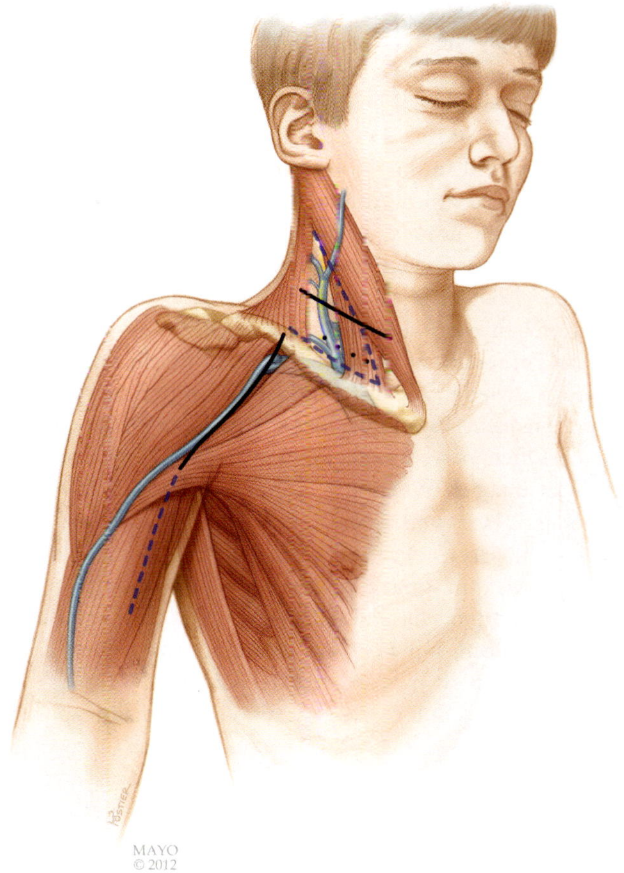

FIGURE 27-1 Planned incisions for brachial plexus exposures: solid lines, preferred. (By permission of Mayo Foundation for Medical Education and Research. All rights reserved.)

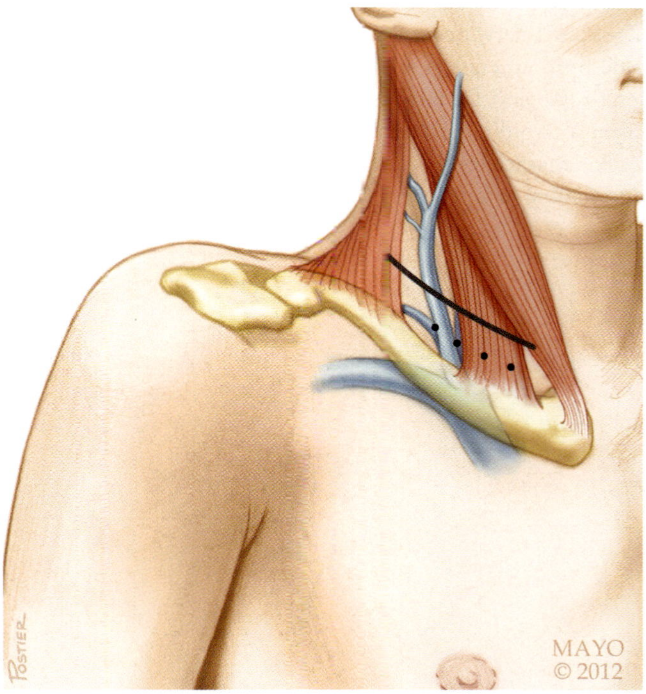

FIGURE 27-2 Planned supraclavicular incisions. Dashed line for thoracic outlet surgery. (By permission of Mayo Foundation for Medical Education and Research. All rights reserved.)

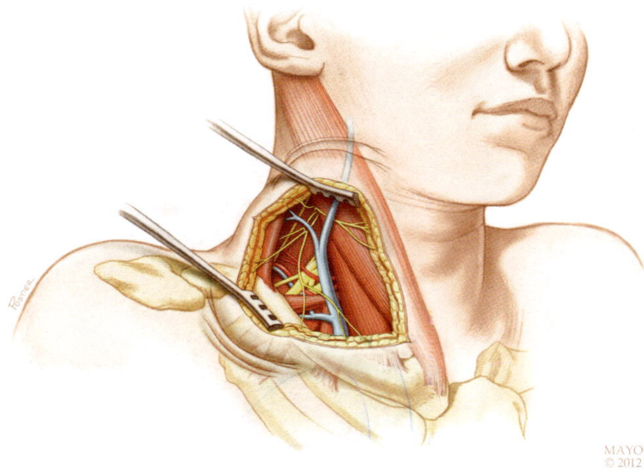

FIGURE 27-3 Superficial exposure, external jugular vein. (By permission of Mayo Foundation for Medical Education and Research. All rights reserved.)

just lateral to the scalene anterior above its C5 contribution. Care is taken to avoid injury to an accessory phrenic nerve which should be protected when present.

Alternatively, dissection can be done initially laterally to the anterior scalene (and phrenic nerve). The upper trunk or its divisions can be identified or palpated even through scar. Dissection then proceeds proximally and distally.

In many cases of brachial plexus trauma, the upper trunk is scarred. Dissection then proceeds toward the clavicle, where injury is less prominent. The suprascapular nerve is first identified on the lateral border. It heads obliquely, running beneath but along the same path as the omohyoid to the scapular notch. Next the anterior and posterior divisions of the upper trunk are identified; the anterior division is more medially located. The anterior division supplies the biceps brachii; the posterior division supplies the deltoid. Sometimes this dissection can be facilitated by mobilizing the clavicle subperiostally and retracting on it. In some cases of preganglionic injury, the suprascapular nerve can be found below the clavicle. Dissecting in the retroclavicular space is facilitated by ligating the suprascapular vessels early in the procedure and widely as well as dividing the subclavius muscle.

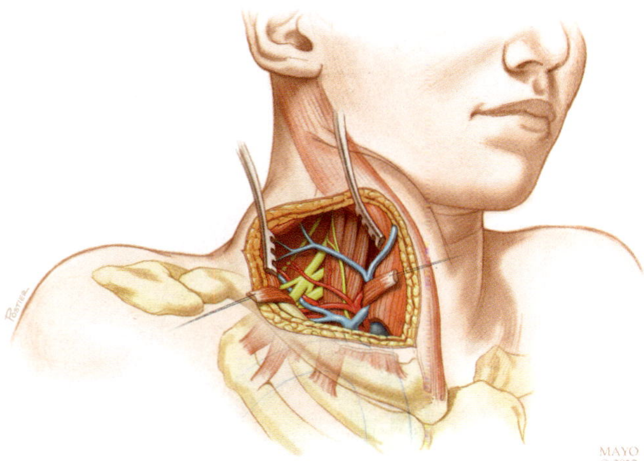

FIGURE 27-4 Division and retraction of omohyoid muscle. (By permission of Mayo Foundation for Medical Education and Research. All rights reserved.)

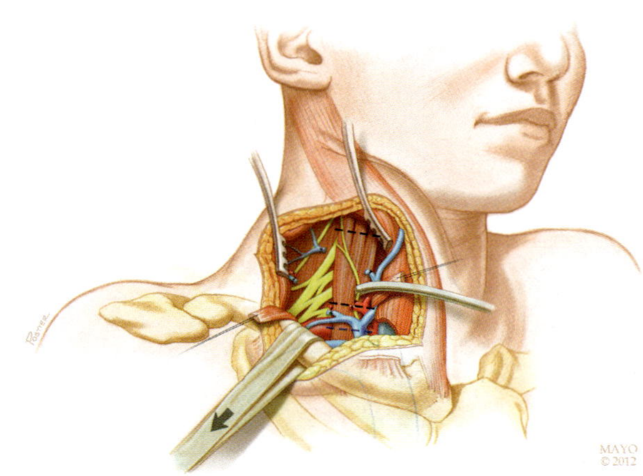

FIGURE 27-5 Identification of phrenic nerve. Planned resection of scalene anterior (black dash is for routine BP exposure; blue dash indicates the caudal extent of routine muscle resection). (By permission of Mayo Foundation for Medical Education and Research. All rights reserved.)

For proximal exposure, the phrenic nerve must be mobilized. Division of the anterior scalene is then done proximally at the level of the C5 nerve (Figure 27-5). A portion of the muscle is divided or, preferably, resected. The upper trunk can be traced to C6, which is then followed. The C7 nerve and middle trunk are next identified in the interscalene triangle. The dorsal scapular artery is ligated. Exposure to the level of the foramina is obtained at these levels (Figure 27-6).

Two nerves deserve specific comment because of their proximal innervation. Intraoperative stimulation of these branches may produce muscle contractions and help identify normal proximal nerve. The dorsal scapular nerve is the most proximal nerve, derived from C5 (and C4) near the intervertebral foramen. It pierces the scalene medius and supplies the rhomboids and the levator scapulae. The long thoracic nerve receives separate contributions from C5, C6, and C7 and penetrates the scalene medius. Its contribution from the undersurface of C6 consistently provides another way besides the phrenic to identify the proximal neural elements in cases of severe fibrosis. The long thoracic nerve can also be identified deep to the omohyoid and the suprascapular nerve and continues on to supply the serratus anterior on the chest wall.

More proximal exposure of these neural elements is often necessary to identify healthy nerve in cases of severe injury. This entails dissecting proximal to the C5 contribution of the phrenic nerve or proximal to the C6 contribution of the long thoracic nerve. Additional scalene anterior fibers can be removed. Bony dissection, when deemed necessary, should be done carefully using Kerrison or Leksell rongeurs. Venous bleeding can be controlled with hemostatic agents. The location (and proximity) of the vertebral artery should be considered.

In cases of trauma or tumor involving the brachial plexus, the anatomy is altered by the pathology, and dissection may be quite tedious. Frequent use of the nerve stimulator helps confirm anatomy. Often, nerve stimulation does not produce visible contraction of muscles. When scar is apparent, the lack of muscle contraction is easily understandable. When there is little scarring involving the nerve or the scalene muscles and no muscle contraction is seen with stimulation, there usually has been a preganglionic injury. After supraclavicular exposure of the spinal nerves has been obtained, intraoperative recordings can be performed using somatosensory- or motor-evoked potentials.

For the typical adult brachial plexus post-traumatic exposure, C5 to C7 are exposed. C8 and T1 are not exposed. In my opinion, identification of these lower nerves does not change management. In panplexal lesions, the lower elements are often avulsed. Furthermore, even if postganglionic injuries are present, these proximal nerves would not be used as donors for nerve grafting due to the distance from distal targets.

If desired, the lower trunk can be exposed next. It lies more medial and posterior than the upper and middle trunks. The subclavian artery is usually identified and mobilized before identification of the lower trunk. The subclavian artery is posterior and the subclavian vein is anterior to the scalene anterior. The spinal nerves comprising the brachial plexus run in a cascade from anterior and lateral for C5 to posterior and medial for T1. C8 and T1 can be exposed (Figure 27-7). Care must be taken to avoid pleural tear or chyle leak.

For thoracic outlet syndrome exposures, a lower skin incision is used (Figure 27-8). Dissection is performed medial to

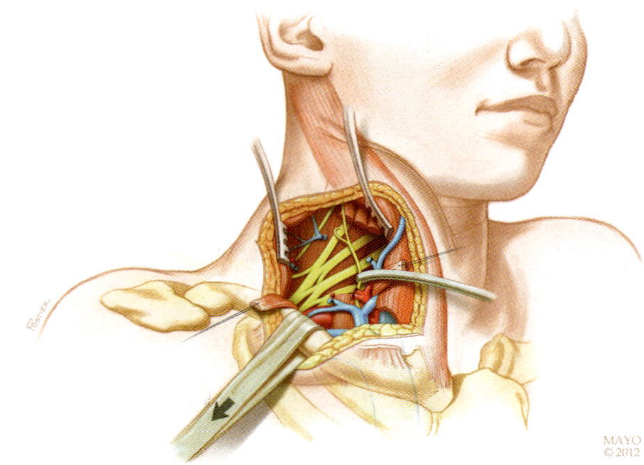

FIGURE 27-6 Exposure of C5 to C7 for typical supraclavicular exploration. (By permission of Mayo Foundation for Medical Education and Research. All rights reserved.)

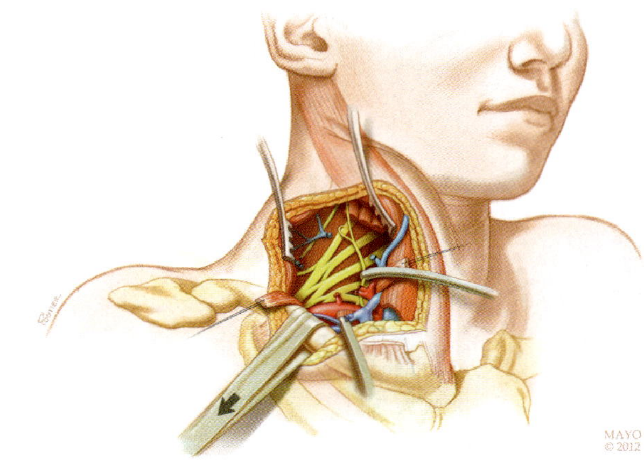

FIGURE 27-7 Exposure of C5 to T1 for thoracic outlet surgery exploration. (By permission of Mayo Foundation for Medical Education and Research. All rights reserved.)

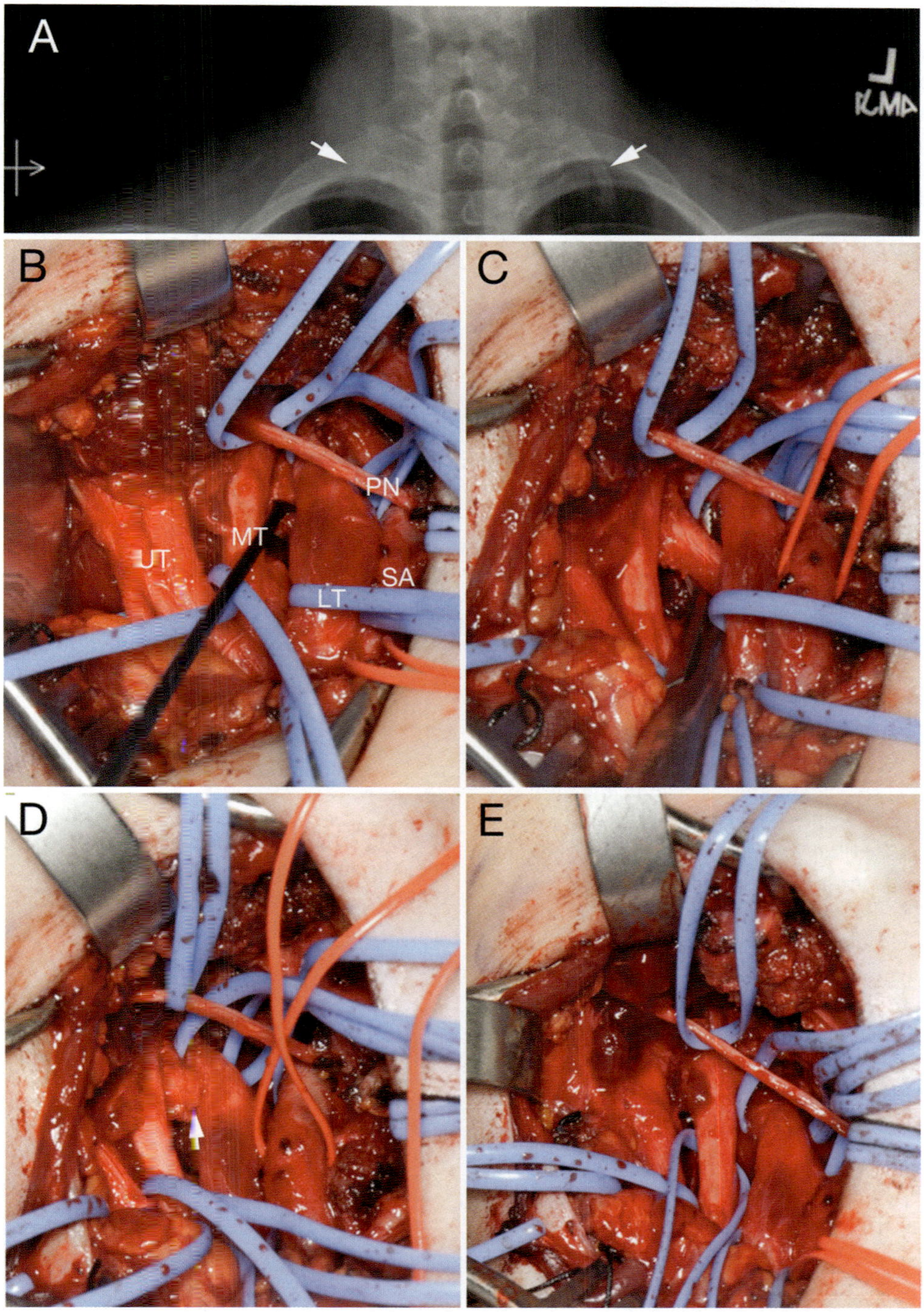

FIGURE 27-8 Supraclavicular exposure for neurogenic thoracic outlet syndrome. This 15-year-old girl presented with a several year history of progressive overhead-related symptoms of dysesthesias radiating into the ulnar side of her right dominant hand. She had weakness in finger extensors, finger flexors, thenar muscles, and interossei. She had a Tinel's sign in the supraclavicular fossa and positive thoracic outlet maneuvers and noninvasive vascular studies. Electrophysiologic testing confirmed a lower trunk plexopathy with active denervation. Cervical magnetic resonance imaging (MRI) did not show any abnormalities. Brachial plexus MRI showed T2 hyperintensity of the lower trunk. One year after surgery, her pain had resolved. Her neurologic examination improved to a moderate extent. She started developing mild positional symptoms without neurologic findings in the opposite limb. (**A**) Chest X-ray shows bilateral cervical ribs (arrows). The left side is larger than the right one. (**B**) The right brachial plexus has been exposed. Scalene anterior muscle has been largely resected. The cervical rib is seen (probe). Discoloration of the lower trunk (LT) and subclavian artery (SA) is seen. MT, middle trunk; PN, phrenic nerve; UT, upper trunk. (**C**) The tip of the tonsil clamp is beneath the scalene medius fibers, which are tenting up the lower trunk. (**D**) The scalene medius fibers have been divided at the inferior aspect of the cervical rib (arrow). The distortion of the lower trunk has been corrected. (**E**) The cervical rib has been resected.

the external jugular vein. A similar dissection is carried out. The pathology is close to the foramina. The scalene anterior is removed widely off the first rib, and the scalene medius is divided. Bony prominences, such as a cervical rib or an elongated C7 transverse process, are removed. The subclavian artery is mobilized beyond the thyrocervical trunk, sometimes to the vertebral artery take-off.

Spinal Accessory Nerve

The spinal accessory nerve can easily be identified in the lateral portion of the zig-zag or transverse incision just described. The spinal accessory nerve is frequently used as a nerve transfer (such as to the suprascapular nerve or to a free-functioning muscle transfer). It is easier to identify it more distally. The medial border of the trapezial fascia is identified. The dissection is deepened. The supraclavicular nerve or its branches may be seen more superficially. The spinal accessory nerve is then identified. When stimulated, it causes strong contraction of the trapezius. The spinal accessory nerve is traced more deeply. This is critical for direct nerve transfer and is necessary when additional length is required, such as in the cases of scarred or retracted target nerves or for free muscle transfers anchored to the clavicle and supplied by the thoracoacromial artery. During the distal dissection, a connection to the cervical plexus is appreciated medially. The spinal accessory nerve runs along with a neighboring vessel. Below the clavicle, in the deep dissection, several branches are given off. At this level, the nerve is transected and prepared for neurotization, but a proximal branch to the trapezius must be preserved.

More proximally, the spinal accessory nerve may also be identified at the cephalad portion of the exposure. It runs along with the accessory lymph nodes obliquely in the posterior triangle. Other cervical plexus elements also course obliquely in this region (some of which may have motor fibers and produce some weaker contraction). The easiest way for me to locate the nerve more proximally is by dissecting about 1.5 cm above the great auricular nerve coursing around the sternocleidomastoid. Stimulation of the nerve is performed. In addition, the branch to the sternocleidomastoid may also be stimulated in a retrograde manner or be specifically identified several centimeters proximally.

Infraclavicular

The infraclavicular approach to the brachial plexus is usually fairly straightforward in unoperated circumstances. In contrast, in cases of previous surgery, such as for arterial reconstruction, dissection can be quite difficult.

An incision is made either by itself or incorporated into the previously described zig-zag incision. The incision extends from the clavicle diagonally toward the proximal arm region (Figure 27-9). Distally, the incision is kept away from the axilla and is extended into the arm as necessary. The dissection is deepened. The deltopectoral groove is identified (Figure 27-10). The cephalic vein is mobilized laterally. The interval between the deltoid and pectoralis major is developed (Figure 27-11). The pectoralis minor is identified (Figure 27-12) with its origin from the ribs and its tendinous insertion into the coracoid.

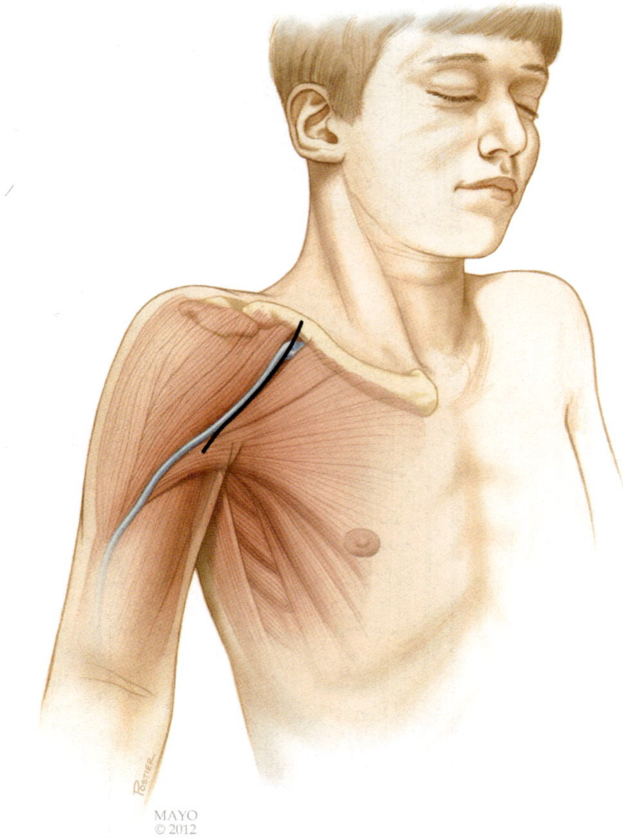

FIGURE 27-9 Infraclavicular exposure. Skin incision. (By permission of Mayo Foundation for Medical Education and Research. All rights reserved.)

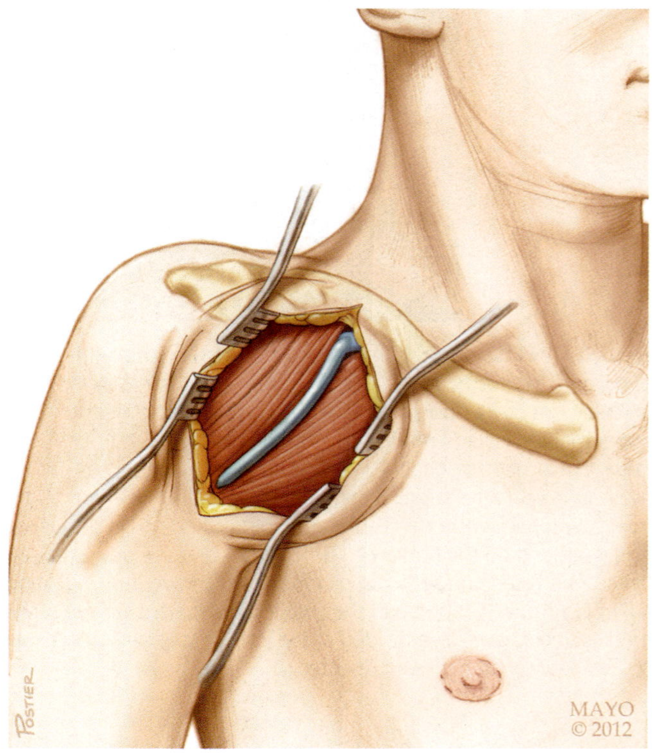

FIGURE 27-10 Deltopectoral interval. (By permission of Mayo Foundation for Medical Education and Research. All rights reserved.)

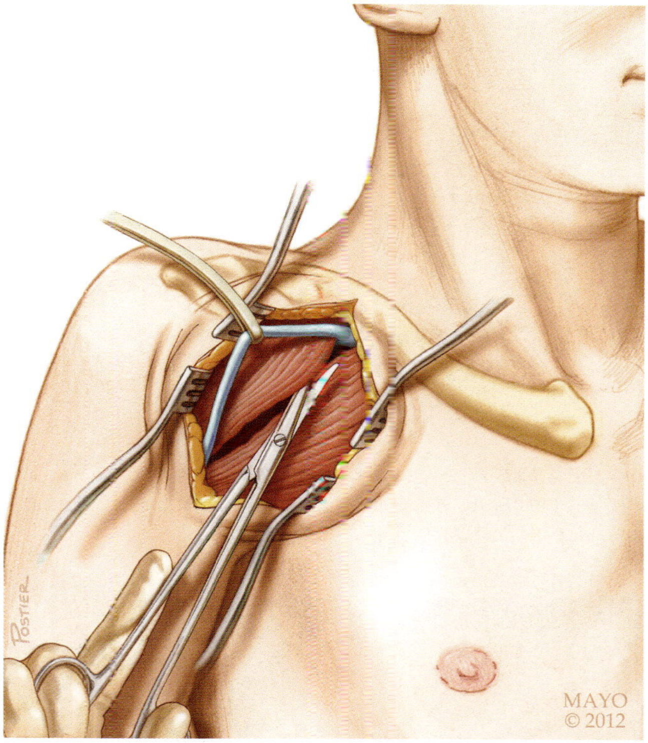

FIGURE 27-11 Deepening the deltopectoral interval. (By permission of Mayo Foundation for Medical Education and Research. All rights reserved.)

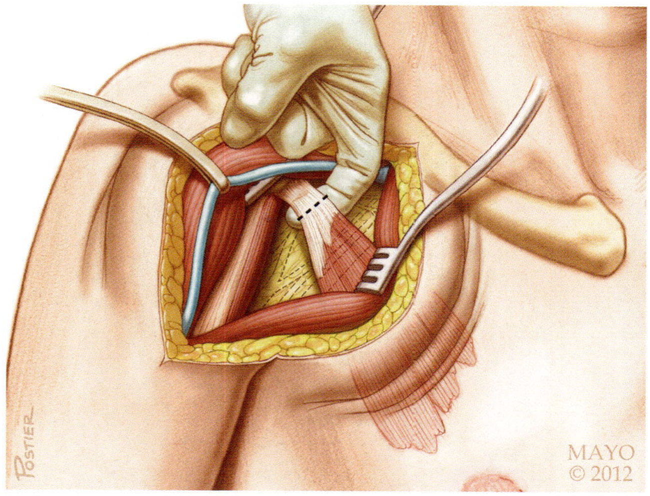

FIGURE 27-13 Mobilization of the pectoralis minor. (By permission of Mayo Foundation for Medical Education and Research. All rights reserved.)

The surgeon's index finger is used to mobilize the muscle (Figure 27-13), which is divided at its tendinous attachment near the coracoid for planned reattachment during closure. The tagged pectoralis minor muscle is reflected with its suture kept on tension to aid in its retraction (Figure 27-14). The fat pad is swept away. Curved self-retainers are placed with care to maintain the teeth superficial to the level of the coracoid. The lateral cord comes into view first and is mobilized. It is traced distally to identify the musculocutaneous nerve and the lateral cord contribution to the median nerve. The axillary artery is next identified more medially and protected. The branch to the coracobrachialis is seen arising from the musculocutaneous nerve. Brachial plexus surgeons must be aware that the musculocutaneous nerve may not be identified in the infraclavicular region because of a low take-off in approximately 10% of cases. The median nerve is next identified and traced back to its medial cord contribution. It is traced to the medial cord and the ulnar nerve as necessary. More proximally, pectoral branches and the ansa connecting them can be seen. The thoracoacromial branch can be identified more proximally near the medial pectoral nerve. This anatomic orientation facilitates quick and easy identification of the "M" of the superficial terminal branches of the brachial plexus (Figure 27-15). The use of appropriately colored vasoloops also helps to facilitate rapid differentiation of nerves and vessels.

The plane of dissection for the dissection of the posterior neural elements is then developed lateral to the lateral cord and the musculocutaneous nerve (Figure 27-16). These nerves are retracted gently with the axillary artery. More proximally, the posterior cord is identified. Subscapular branches, including

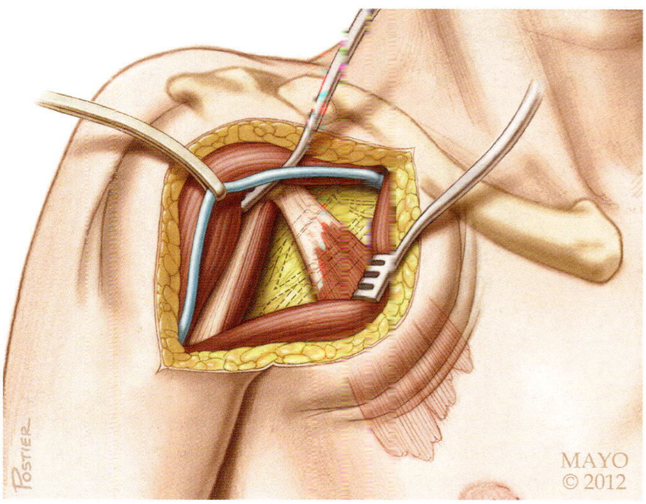

FIGURE 27-12 Identification of the pectoralis minor. (By permission of Mayo Foundation for Medical Education and Research. All rights reserved.)

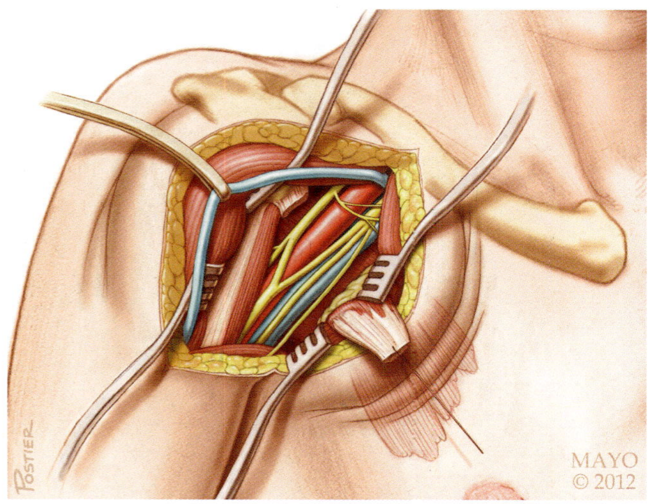

FIGURE 27-14 Release of the tendinous insertion of the pectoralis minor. (By permission of Mayo Foundation for Medical Education and Research. All rights reserved.)

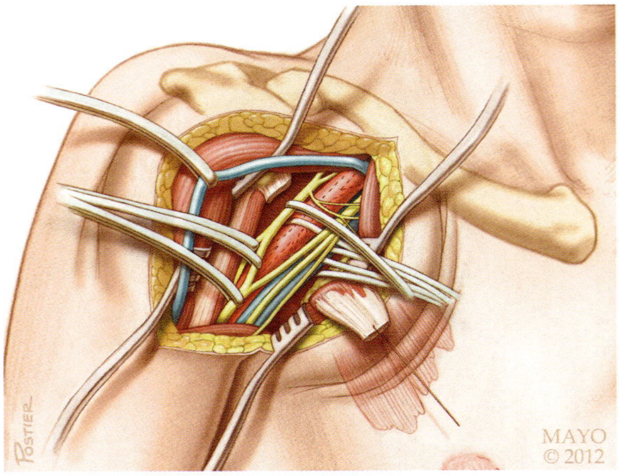

FIGURE 27-15 Exposure of the "M" of the brachial plexus. (By permission of Mayo Foundation for Medical Education and Research. All rights reserved.)

the thoracodorsal nerve, from the posterior cord are preserved. The axillary and radial nerves are seen and mobilized (Figure 27-17). The axillary nerve is smaller and runs obliquely to the quadrangular space. The radial nerve is larger. Branches of the triceps brachii can be identified.

In cases of scar, dissection is slow. Use of a portable Doppler may help map the artery or a bypass graft. Additional exposure can be obtained by releasing part of the origin of the pectoralis major from the clavicle, or by taking down part of or the entire pectoralis major insertion from the humerus. Alternatively, the origin of the conjoined tendon can be taken down to help identify or dissect the axillary nerve more distally. If either of these tendinous structures is completely released, it should be marked and repaired at the end of the case. A period of immobilization is necessary to protect these repairs.

After exposure of the pathology, nerve action potentials can be performed across the lesions.

Retroclavicular

Occasionally, a retroclavicular exposure is necessary by itself. This may be deemed necessary, especially when the clavicle has been fractured or fixated (Figure 27-18) or with tumors lying

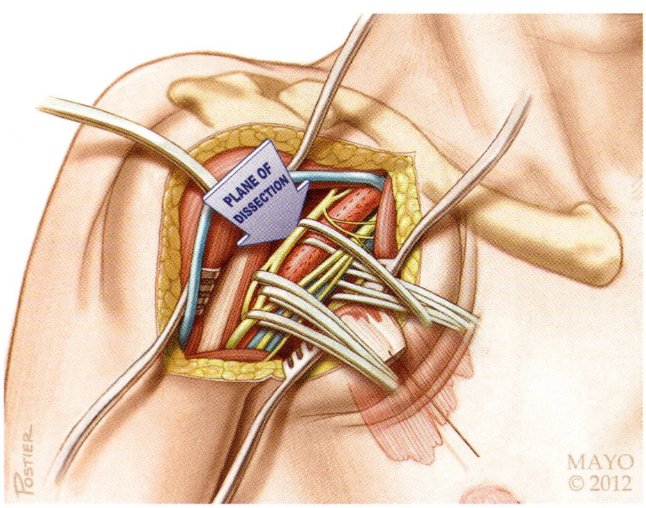

FIGURE 27-16 Plane of dissection to the posterior cord, axillary nerve, and radial nerve. (By permission of Mayo Foundation for Medical Education and Research. All rights reserved.)

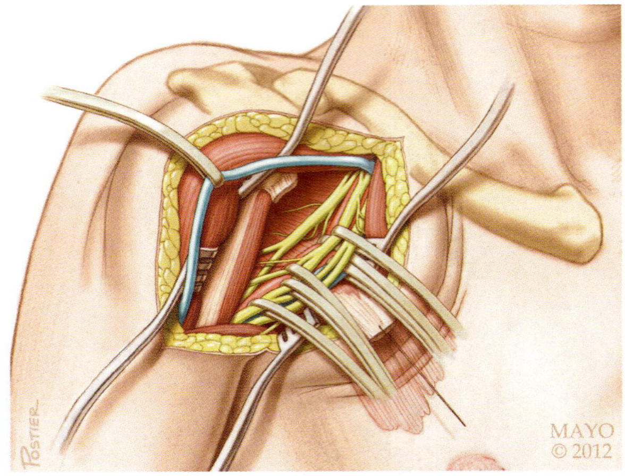

FIGURE 27-17 Exposure of the posterior cord, axillary nerve, and radial nerve. (By permission of Mayo Foundation for Medical Education and Research. All rights reserved.)

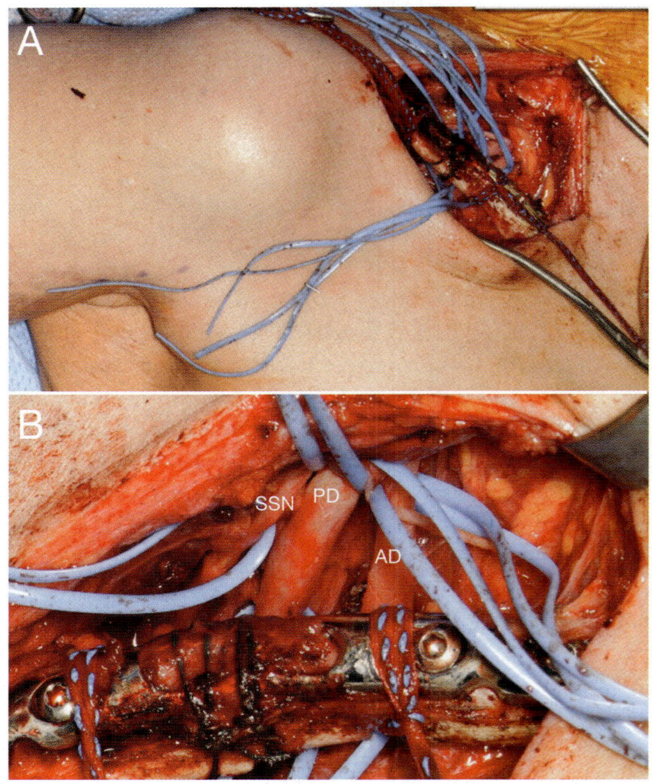

FIGURE 27-18 Retroclavicular exposure. This 43-year old woman sustained a communited clavicle fracture from a fall. She underwent open reduction and internal fixation of this fracture 5 days after injury. She was found to have weak shoulder abduction several months after surgery. Electrophysiologic testing at first suggested an axillary nerve palsy. Several months later, a repeat study showed no activation and denervation in the brachioradialis as well as the deltoid, suggestive of an injury to the posterior division of the upper trunk. She developed a nonunion of the clavicle. At operation 7 months after injury, nerve action potentials were obtained across the lesion, and neurolysis was performed. She underwent autogenous bone grafting. She made good clinical and electrophysiological recovery over the next year, and her clavicle united. **(A)** The retroclavicular approach was used. The clavicle has been mobilized. Proximal and distal control of neural elements has been obtained above and below the clavicle. **(B)** A neuroma in continuity involving the posterior division (PD) of the upper trunk can be seen. AD, anterior division of upper trunk; SSN, suprascapular nerve.

beneath the clavicle, particularly involving the divisions. A transverse incision is used. Dissection is performed down onto the clavicle, which is mobilized superiorly. Soft tissue flaps are raised. From the supraclavicular vantage point, the omohyoid is identified and retracted superiorly on tension. The upper trunk, its divisions, and the suprascapular nerve are identified above the clavicle. Note how close these neural elements are to the clavicle. Depending on the injury or extent of the dissection, these may be the only structures that need to be identified. The suprascapular vessels are ligated. From the infraclavicular vantage point, distal control of nerves should be obtained. A window can be developed above the transverse course of the cephalic vein, which can be maintained in a vasoloop. The clavicle is retracted either cephalad or caudad, and dissection is continued beneath the clavicle. The subclavius muscle and fascia are divided. The divisions lie beneath the clavicle. Dissection is difficult beneath the clavicle, and good lighting is necessary. The remainder of the retroclavicular dissection can be done at this time. The suprascapular nerve can be dissected distally to the notch through this approach (2). If necessary, the retroclavicular approach can be incorporated into a more formal supraclavicular or infraclavicular exposure.

Osteotomy of the clavicle has not been deemed necessary even in cases of retroclavicular injuries or benign tumors. By working above and below the clavicle patiently, I have been able to obtain good exposure in this location. If absolutely necessary, a preplating technique with a low contour reconstruction plate is performed before the osteotomy.

Arm

The deltopectoral incision can be extended distally, or a separate approach can be done extending from the level of the axillary crease distally to the midarm. The arm is abducted and externally rotated on an arm board. Through a relatively short incision, all of the major nerves in the arm can be identified (Figures 27-19 and 27-20). The fascia is incised, and the musculocutaneous nerve is identified superficial to the humerus beneath the biceps brachii and coracobrachialis muscles. The musculocutaneous nerve is traced distally, first to the branch to the biceps brachii and second to the branch to the brachialis and then to the lateral antebrachial cutaneous nerve. The medial antebrachial cutaneous nerve is identified just beneath the fascia and mobilized. The brachial artery is seen with the

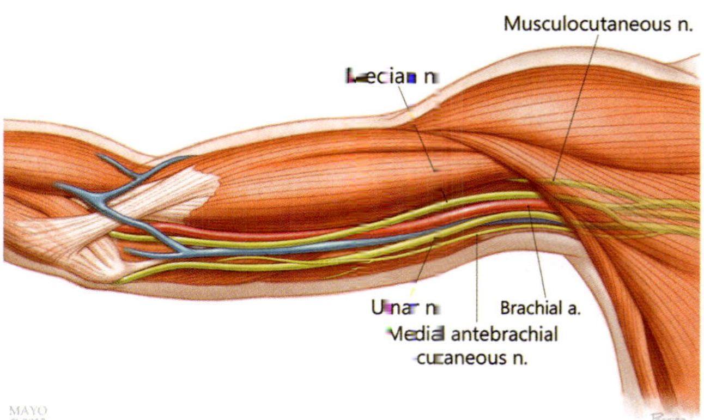

FIGURE 27-19 Medial arm anatomy showing the course of the major nerves. (By permission of Mayo Foundation for Medical Education and Research. All rights reserved.)

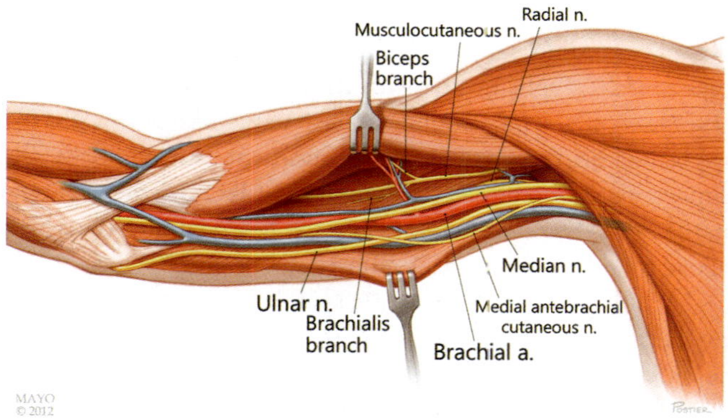

FIGURE 27-20 Medial arm anatomy showing branches of the musculocutaneous nerve and their relationship to the median and ulnar nerves. a, artery; n, nerve. (By permission of Mayo Foundation for Medical Education and Research. All rights reserved.)

brachial veins. The median nerve can be identified just deep to these vessels. Posteriorly and medially, the ulnar nerve can be identified and mobilized. The radial nerve can be identified in two locations, either posterior to the humerus in the proximal third of the arm or more proximally, deep to the brachial artery. If desired, the approach can be extended proximally to allow identification of the axillary nerve. A nerve stimulator can be used to confirm the anatomy. Knowledge of this anatomy is important when performing common distal nerve transfers (3,4).

Posterior Exposures

Occasionally during brachial plexus surgery, posterior approaches are necessary for additional exposure. These may be performed together with other procedures or in isolation. These approaches can be done either with the patient in a lateral position (because the ipsilateral sural nerve may also have to be prepped). Alternatively some prefer to perform the anterior and posterior procedures separately (by repositioning the patient), such as for nerve transfers, thereby offering more anatomic perspectives for the surgeon.

For example, the suprascapular nerve may be separately compressed or injured at the suprascapular notch beneath the transverse scapular ligament. Release of this ligament may also help mobilize the nerve if trying to gain extra length during a repair (2). Similarly, the axillary nerve can be identified posteriorly in normal anatomy to facilitate a pull-through interposition nerve graft from the site of injury to just distal to the bifurcation of the axillary nerve from the posterior cord. In addition, common nerve transfers, such as transfer of a triceps branch to the anterior branch of the axillary nerve (5) or transfer of the spinal accessory nerve to the suprascapular nerve, can be performed posteriorly (6) closer to the target muscle end organ. Finally, a posterior subscapular approach to the brachial plexus has been described by Kline et al. (7), especially for proximal dissections or revision operations for lower neural elements, such as tumors or thoracic outlet surgery.

Suprascapular and Spinal Accessory Nerves

A transverse incision is made just above the scapular spine. The incision is centered on the coracoid which is palpated anteriorly.

The suprascapular nerve is approximately halfway between the acromion and the superior border of the scapula (6). The trapezius muscle is split in line with its fibers or elevated from the scapular spine. The atrophic supraspinatus muscle is reflected exposing the transverse scapular ligament. Alternatively, the supraspinatus can be elevated subperiosteally from the supraspinatus fossa. The nerve runs below the ligament and the artery above it and the ligament is released.

For a distal nerve transfer, the spinal accessory nerve may be exposed either through the same (longer) incision used for the suprascapular nerve or a separate more medial incision near the medial portion of the scapula. The trapezius is split. The spinal accessory nerve is identified just medial to the medial border of the scapula. It can be found at a point approximately 40% between the midline of the spinous processes and the acromion along the superior aspect of the scapula (6).

Axillary and Radial Nerves

A longitudinal incision is made from the posterior acromion to the midposterior arm. The deltoid is reflected anteriorly. Care should be taken during the superficial dissection. If the superior lateral cutaneous nerve is identified, it can be traced to the posterior branch of the axillary nerve. The quadrangular space is bounded by the teres minor superiorly, the teres major inferiorly, the long head of the triceps brachii medially, and the surgical neck of the humerus laterally. Within the quadrangular space, the main trunk of the axillary nerve or the anterior or posterior branches can be identified near the posterior humeral circumflex vessels.

The interval between the long and lateral heads of the triceps brachii is defined and deepened. The triangular interval is bounded by the teres major superiorly, the long head of the triceps brachii medially, and the lateral head of the triceps brachii (and the lateral border of the humerus) laterally. The radial nerve is identified in the triangular interval and radial nerve branches to the triceps can be identified, tested, and used for nerve transfers.

REFERENCES

1. Shin AY, Spinner RJ. Clinically relevant surgical anatomy and exposures of the brachial plexus. In Bishop AT, Spinner RJ, Shin AY (eds). In *Brachial Plexus Injuries in Adults. Hand Clinics* 2005, pp. 21:1–11.
2. Bodily KD, Spinner RJ, Shin AY, Bishop AT. Clinical significance of suprascapular nerve mobilization. *Clin Anat* 2005;18:573–579.
3. Liverneaux PA, Diaz LC, Beaulieu JY, et al. Preliminary results of double nerve transfer to restore elbow flexion in upper type brachial plexus palsies. *Plast Reconstr Surg* 2006;117:915–919.
4. Oberlin C, Béal D, Leechavengvongs S, et al. Nerve transfer to biceps muscle using a part of ulnar nerve for C5-C6 avulsion of the brachial plexus: anatomical study and report of four cases. *J Hand Surg* 1994;19(suppl A):232–237.
5. Witoonchart K, Leechavengvongs S, Uerpairojkit C, et al. Nerve transfer to deltoid muscle using the nerve to the long head of the triceps, part I: an atomic feasibility study. *J Hand Surg* 2003;28(suppl A):628–632.
6. Colbert SH, Mackinnon S. Posterior approach for double nerve transfer for restoration of shoulder function in upper brachial plexus palsy. *Hand* 2006;1:71–77.
7. Kline DG, Hudson AR, Kim DH. *Atlas of Peripheral Nerve Surgery.* Philadelphia: WB Saunders, 2001.

SECTION 2

HEAD AND NECK

CHAPTER 28

Scalp Replantation

Kaixiang Cheng, Yixin Zhang, and Fuguo Chen

SCALP ANATOMY

Skin

Scalp skin is deep, compact, and rich in blood vessels, sweat glands, and hair follicles. Its dermis is very thick, through which hair follicles enter the subcutaneous tissue. Because of this, split-thickness skin graft can be harvested repeatedly without any adverse effects on scalp healing.

Subcutaneous Tissue

The subcutaneous tissue is resilient and compact, with many blood vessels, nerves, many adnexal structures, and abundant collateral anastomoses. Because there is a fibrous scaffold in the subcutaneous tissue, blood vessels do not readily contract after division or avulsion; as a result, bleeding is prolonged. On the other hand, infection does not spread easily after trauma or surgery.

Galea

The galea aponeurotica is a tough and resilient layer of fibrous tissue that covers the skull and forehead and is continuous with the frontalis and the superficial musculoaponeurotic system (SMAS). It attaches to the crest and periosteum of the superciliary arch in the forehead and to the external occipital protuberance and superior nuchal lines of the occipital bone.

Subgaleal Loose Connective Tissue

The small arteries and veins in the loose connective tissue between the galea and periosteum supply the periosteum, and the emissary veins here are valveless normally draining the external veins of the skull and superficial veins in the scalp into the dural venous sinuses. Because of this arrangement, a hematoma is likely to form here upon vessel injury, and the emissary veins may conduct infection intracranially. Furthermore, because of the loose subgaleal connective tissue, the scalp is often avulsed at the subgaleal level.

Pericranium

The pericranium is a layer of compact fibrous tissue closely adherent to the skull and is supplied by blood vessels from the diploe. It is analogous to the periosteum of other bones. In the event of serious injury, scalp avulsion sometimes includes the pericranium. The skull cannot produce new bone after the loss of its pericranium. Skull fractures, in addition to the openings for the diploic vessels are possible channels for the spread of infection (Figure 28-1).

Blood Vessels and Nerves in the Scalp

Arteries accompany veins and nerves in the scalp, and they can be divided into three groups: the anterior group, the middle group, and the posterior group. In front are the supratrochlear and supraorbital arteries, in the middle are the superficial temporal and posterior auricular arteries, and behind are the occipital arteries along with the greater occipital and lesser occipital nerves (Figure 28-2). The supratrochlear and supraorbital arteries mainly supply forehead skin and scalp, and the superficial temporal artery supplies the scalp in the occipital, occipitonuchal, and postauricular areas. The three vessel groups join with each other via abundant anastomoses.

The blood supply of the scalp is so rich that scalp necrosis is rare after avulsion injury as long as a narrow pedicle containing at least one of these vessels remains connected. The occipital artery originates from external carotid artery and travels posteriorly and superiorly beneath posterior belly of digastric muscle. It winds backward along the medial side of mastoid process and enters the occipital area between trapezius and the insertion of the sternocleidomastoid muscle. The artery mainly supplies the occipital and posterior parietal areas and anastomoses with the superficial temporal artery.

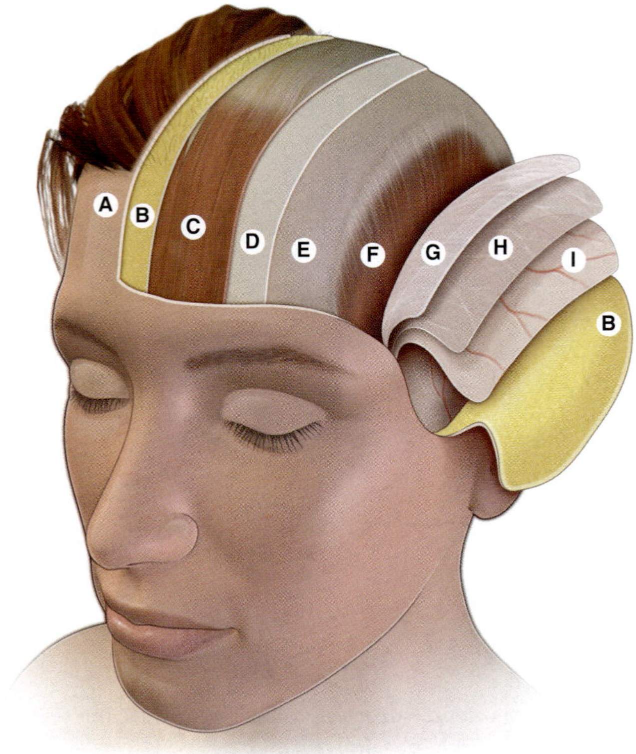

FIGURE 28-1 Anatomy of the skull and scalp: A, skin; B, subcutaneous tissue; C, frontalis muscle and galea aponeurotica; D, pericranium; E, cranium; F, temporalis muscle; G, deep temporalis fascia; H, loose areolar tissue; I, temporoparietal fascia with superficial temporal vessels.

BRIEF HISTORY OF SCALP RECONSTRUCTION

Conventional Options

Total scalp avulsion follows severe trauma, often caused by a shearing force applied obliquely to the long hair-bearing scalp by a rapidly rotating gear or belt. In the early stages of industrialization, scalp avulsion was very common because of improper safety management. Young women were often the victims.

Scalp avulsion injury was often complicated by massive hemorrhage and other severe injuries. The volume of blood loss can be 800 to 2000 mL after total scalp avulsion. The patient may develop shock after rapidly losing 1000 mL of blood. Associated injuries include partial skin avulsion of the face, laceration of the pinna or eyelid, skull bone fracture, skull and brain injury, fracture of cervical vertebra, bone fracture of the upper limb, and thoracic injury.

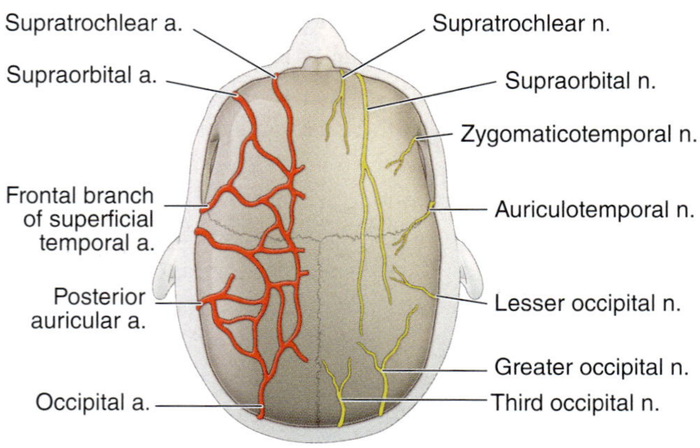

FIGURE 28-2 Blood vessels and nerves within the scalp.

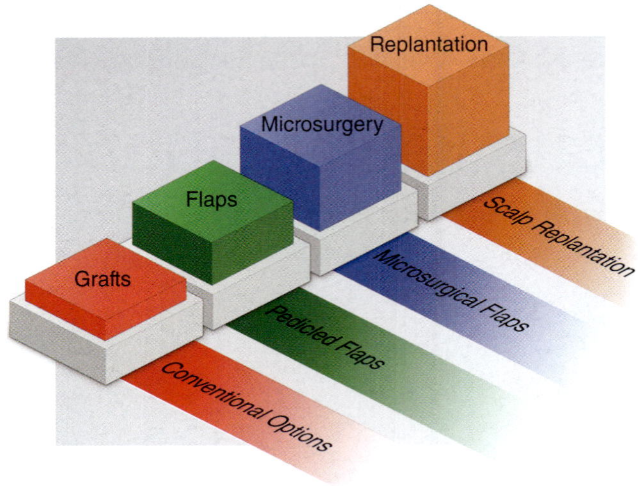

FIGURE 28-3 Four main stages of scalp reconstruction after avulsion.

Treatment of total scalp avulsion has gone through four stages. Initially, it was treated by decortication of the skull and split-thickness skin grafting; later local flaps were used. With the onset of microsurgery, free tissue transfer was used to provide well-vascularized cover. However, nowadays every effort is made to carry out replantation in the acute stage (Figure 28-3).

In 1939, Farmer (1) reported repair of a scalp wound using an intermediate split-thickness skin graft. He drilled the skull's outer cortex and skin grafted several days later after granulation tissue had spread out over the bone. In 1967, Orticochea (2) reported repair of scalp avulsion by pedicled flaps. These approaches were used to treat scalp avulsion until the late 1970s, and even now they are still used when replantation is impossible or fails.

Microsurgical Free Flaps

Microsurgical transfer of flaps is an available method for reconstruction of moderate-sized scalp defects. A number of microsurgical free flaps, such as the latissimus dorsi myocutaneous flap, the rectus abdominis flap, the radial forearm flap, and the anterolateral thigh fasciocutaneous flap, may be used for the scalp reconstruction (3–7). Anastomosis to the superficial temporal vessels is reliable and simplifies reconstruction. Neck vessels are also commonly used as recipients (e.g., the external jugular vein, the facial artery and vein, the internal jugular vein, and the superior thyroid vessels). Occasionally, vein grafts are required.

The omentum flap, combined with a split-thickness skin graft, has also been well described for the repair of scalp defects (8–12). Providing effective coverage and restoration of contour, this flap may be used for total or near total defects. In addition, the inherent capability of the omentum to combat infection and form an ideal bed for the establishment of skin or bone grafts provides further indications for its use.

Replantation of the Avulsed Scalp

In 1976, Miller et al. (13) announced the first successful scalp replantation. In 1970s, there were a large number of single case reports on successful scalp replantation (14–18). Since then, emergency replantation has become the first option after scalp avulsion (19–29). Zhou et al. (30), Chen and Wan (31), and Yin et al. (32) reported series with multiple cases of successful scalp replantations. In the 1990s, Cheng et al. (33) replanted 18 entire scalp avulsions and two partial scalp avulsions successfully and summarized their experience using anastomoses with simultaneous vein grafts to both recipient and donor vessels, as well as their preference for not using vasodilators or anticoagulants either intraoperatively or postoperatively, so as to lessen the risk of hemorrhagic complications (see later discussion).

EMERGENCY MANAGEMENT OF SCALP AVULSION INJURY

In the emergency scenario, hemostasis and the application of a wound dressing are the first steps in patient management. After the patient is stabilized, the avulsed scalp should be cleaned, wrapped by normal saline gauze, and placed in a sterile container. Blood pressure and other vital signs are closely monitored, and biochemical analysis, radiographs, or computed tomography (CT) scanning is performed as indicated.

Resuscitation with intravenous fluids, including blood, is begun immediately. At the same time, associated life-threatening injuries, such as pneumothorax, cervical fracture or dislocation, skull fracture, intracranial bleeding, and limb and major abdominal trauma should be assessed and treated. Scalp replantation may only proceed after shock and other complications are under control and the vital signs are stable (Figure 28-4).

If the replantation cannot be performed at the initial hospitalization, then the patient should be stabilized as discussed, and the avulsed scalp prepared for transport. It should be cleaned, wrapped in normal saline gauze, sealed in a plastic bag, and then placed in ice water to reduce warm ischemia time. The warm ischemia time may exceed 6 hours in winter but must be somewhat less in summer for an equivalent outcome (33).

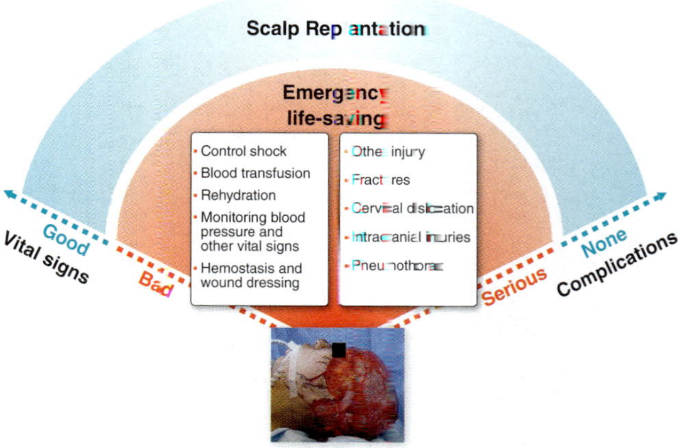

FIGURE 28-4 The scalp should be microsurgically replanted after shock and complications are under control and the vital signs are stable.

However, the avulsed scalp may be safely stored for up to 15 to 21 hours in its sealed plastic bag covered with ice water.

In some severe cases, the avulsed scalp may be badly contused or crushed, and the avulsion can involve significant adjacent areas, including scalp, face, forehead, eyebrow, ears, and even the mouth (Figure 28-5).

In the operating room, the surgeon explores the recipient and donor vessels, assesses the overall condition of the avulsed scalp, and decides whether to carry out a replantation or to cover the wound with a split-thickness skin graft. *However, every attempt should be made to replant or revascularize major scalp avulsions.* It's helpful even if only part of the scalp survives. Partial replantation, although not ideal, is often useful in the coverage of exposed bone, thereby simplifying the remaining wound closure.

SCALP REPLANTATION

Scalp replantation, then, is always the first choice. Even the scalp is crushed, partially missing, or torn into several major pieces, a microsurgical replantation is still recommended as long as a recipient blood supply is available.

Scalp replantation is routinely performed under general anesthesia by three teams: one for scalp debridement, one for skull debridement, and one for harvesting a vein graft from a limb (Figure 28-6). This arrangement improves working efficiency, shortens warm ischemia time, and increases the probability of success.

The first team of surgeons explores the avulsed scalp for donor blood vessels and carries out any further debridement. The vessels will be later checked under the microscope for damage to their walls or lining and will be trimmed back to where they have a healthy appearance. The lead surgeon will decide whether the final recipient vessels have a normal structure and record relevant details such as the diameter of the vessels and their distance from the verge of the lacerated scalp. These data are important when it comes to harvesting the donor vein.

Exploration of the superficial temporal and occipital vessels is always done first because of their size and predictability (Figure 28-7). Next in line come the supratrochlear vessels. Although these three vessels are all easy to locate and have a decent diameter for microvascular anastomosis, they do have a tendency to be damaged by the initial injury. In reviewing the reported cases, most authors seem to have chosen to use bilateral superficial temporal vessels, but others have selected unilateral superficial temporal vessels and contralateral supratrochlear vessels. Nahai et al. (16) and Wilhelmi et al. (28) reported scalp replantation with the anastomosis of a single temporal artery and vein. There are even some reports of survival of part of a scalp reattached as a composite graft in children *without* microvascular anastomoses. Such successes as these must be considered fortuitous, and the treatment is not recommended by the present authors.

If the scalp is found to be severely injured during the debridement, such as having lacerations in the temporal and occipital galea, the corresponding vessels will likely have been severely damaged, too. These vessels should be strictly avoided for anastomotic purposes. The anastomosis is only as reliable as

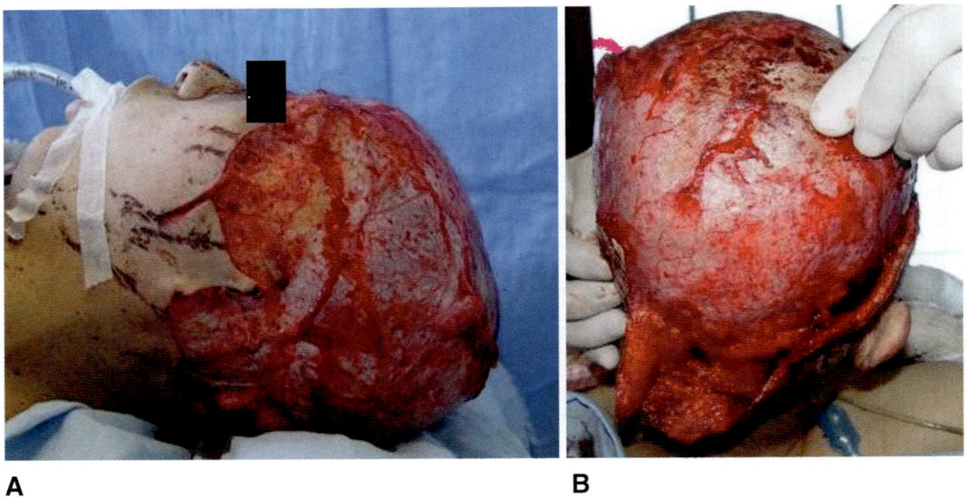

FIGURE 28-5 (**A**) and (**B**) Severe scalp avulsion involved part of the face, forehead, left eyebrow, left ear, and left temporoparietal-occipital region.

the condition of the vessels selected. Vessels subject to extensive trauma should therefore be avoided.

The key vessels are all tagged and labeled by the first team. Those badly damaged are simply ligated. The supraorbital and supratrochlear vessels should be routinely dissected out and tagged. They may become vital if, because of vessel injury, anastomosis of the superficial temporal or occipital arteries were to fail.

The second team of surgeons debrides the skull and prepares the recipient vessels. After debridement, the surgeons will assess whether there is skull fracture so as to avoid misdiagnosis and delayed treatment. Then the surgeons will secure hemostasis, remove devitalized tissue, and partially suture the lacerated scalp.

As for the recipient vessels, the first choice is the superficial temporal vessels. Next come the occipital, the supratrochlear, and the supraorbital vessels. The superficial temporal vessels are located beneath the deep fascia in front of the ear. The vessels are seldom affected by trauma, rarely lacerated, and easy to expose. However, if the scalp *is* lacerated in the region of the superficial temporal fascia near the superficial temporal vessels, careful judgment under the microscope will be needed to see whether the vessels are usable. *Assessment with the naked eye is not reliable in this situation*. If other vessels will obviously require vein grafting, it is recommended to abandon these recipient vessels and choose the superficial temporal vessels in front of the ear preferentially. All of the arteries to be used in the scalp replantation should be perfused with 0.1% heparin in normal saline flushes until exudate emerges at the wound borders. The intra-arterial perfusion helps prevent thrombosis after anastomosis.

If the facial skin, lateral scalp, ear, or part of the parotid are lacerated, the superficial temporal vessels are likely to have been traumatized. In this case, the surgeon should select bilateral occipital vessels or occipital vessels in combination with the contralateral supratrochlear or supraorbital vessels. In rare cases of extensive trauma to both superficial temporal and occipital vessels, the anterior vessels may be used together. In summary, the surgeon must find a pair of vessels from the above vessel groups as recipients. The usual pairs are as follows: bilateral superficial temporal vessels, bilateral occipital vessels, superficial temporal vessels with contralateral occipital vessels, occipital vessels with contralateral supratrochlear or supraorbital vessels.

The artery-to-vein ratio is ideally 1:2 in scalp replantation. In severe trauma, because of lack of undamaged veins, it might be as low as 1:1, when the risks of subcutaneous hematoma and partial scalp necrosis are greatly increased. After a decision is

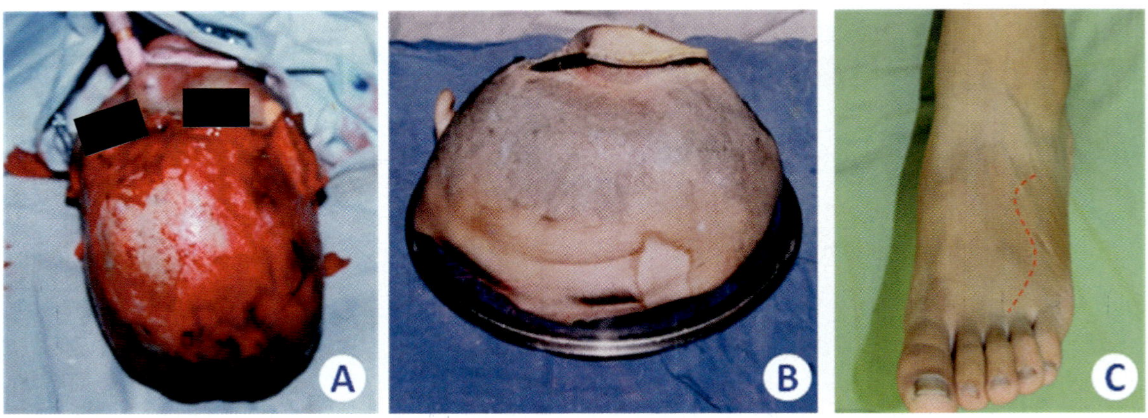

FIGURE 28-6 Scalp replantation is routinely performed under general anesthesia by three teams: skull debridement (**A**), scalp debridement (**B**), and harvesting of the vein graft (**C**).

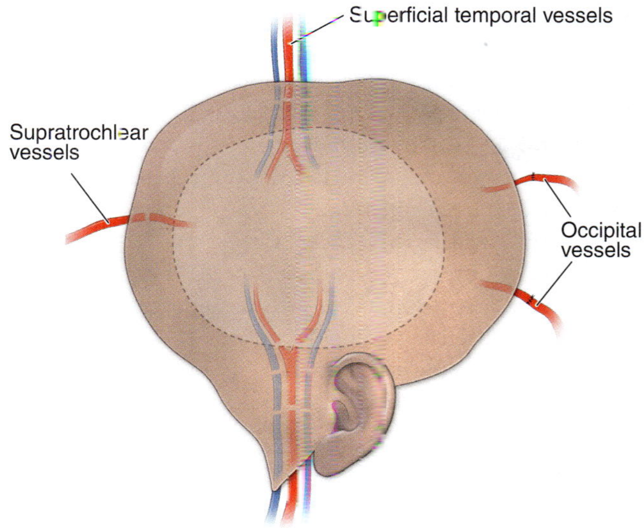

FIGURE 28-7 Schematic diagram of vessels in scalp replantation.

made on recipient vessel selection in the recipient site, the distance of each vessel to the wound edge as well as its diameter should be determined. The diameter and length of vein grafts are calculated by combining this data with that from the scalp.

The third surgical team then harvests vein grafts of appropriate length and diameter from the dorsum of foot or the medial side of forearm. If the measurements are taken from the donor and recipient vessels at an early stage, simultaneous dissection is facilitated (see Figure 28-8).

The great saphenous, cephalic, and basilic veins are absolutely excluded because of their excessively large diameters (>2.5 mm), thick walls, and lots of valves, making them a poor match for those in the scalp. These large vein grafts would slow the blood velocity and produce turbulence at the anastomoses. This can lead to bleeding or thrombosis and account for scalp replantation failure. Conversely, their secondary branches are good sources of grafts because they match well those in the scalp, being smaller and having thinner walls with fewer valves. We feel strongly that the more accurate the vessel match, the fewer the anastomotic problems. Each individual vein graft is generally 4 to 5 cm in length and 6 to 7 cm in very rare cases. Anastomoses of, say, six vessels needs a total vein harvest of 25 to 30 cm. For more than this, the surgeon may have to harvest from a second limb.

ANASTOMOSES OF BLOOD VESSELS AND CUTANEOUS NERVE

After preparations are complete, the donor and recipient vessels will be anastomosed. In 1996, Cheng et al. (33) reported simultaneous grafting of donor and recipient vessels, which greatly increases operation efficiency. With this method, a vein graft is connected to the artery in the recipient (skull) area, while another is connected to the equivalent vein in the avulsed scalp. The two groups of surgeons perform vein grafting in different donor and recipient sites at the same time, which reduces the anastomotic time, facilitates multiple repairs, and increases the patency rate. The avulsed scalp is repositioned on the skull, where it is trimmed to eliminate redundancy and restore normal scalp tension. The anastomoses are then completed (see Figure 28-9).

The order of repair depends on scalp ischemia time. With an ischemia time exceeding 6 to 8 hours, the artery should be anastomosed first. After arterial anastomosis, the vein should be left open to reduce backpressure and allow arterial perfusion to reverse long-term scalp ischemia. Meanwhile, subcutaneous bleeding points will be easily detected and controlled, which is helpful in reducing exudation and oozing under the scalp after surgery. After bilateral anastomoses have been performed, however, the central underside of the scalp becomes inaccessible for hemostasis because it can no longer be turned over. Further

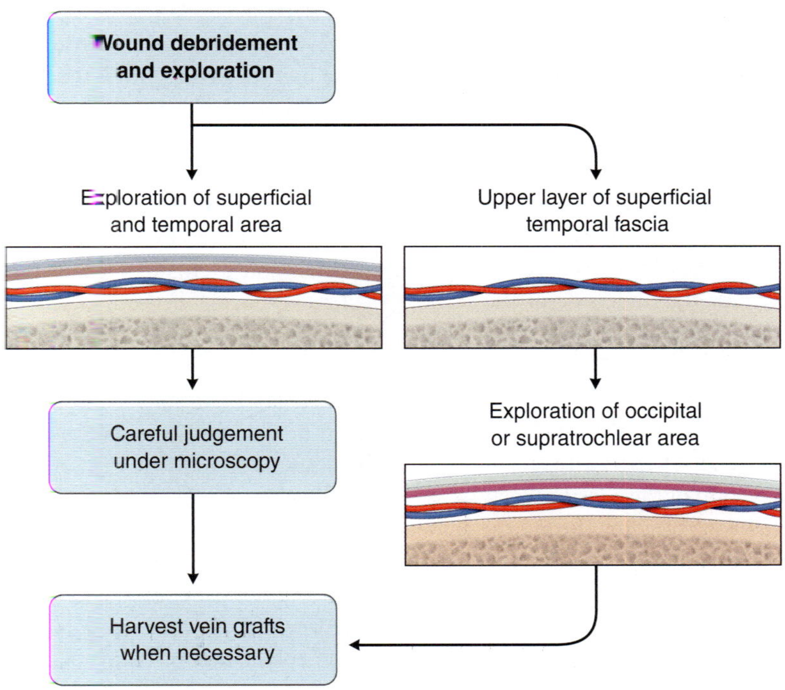

FIGURE 28-8 Schematic diagram regarding the exploration of avulsed scalp before.

SECTION 2

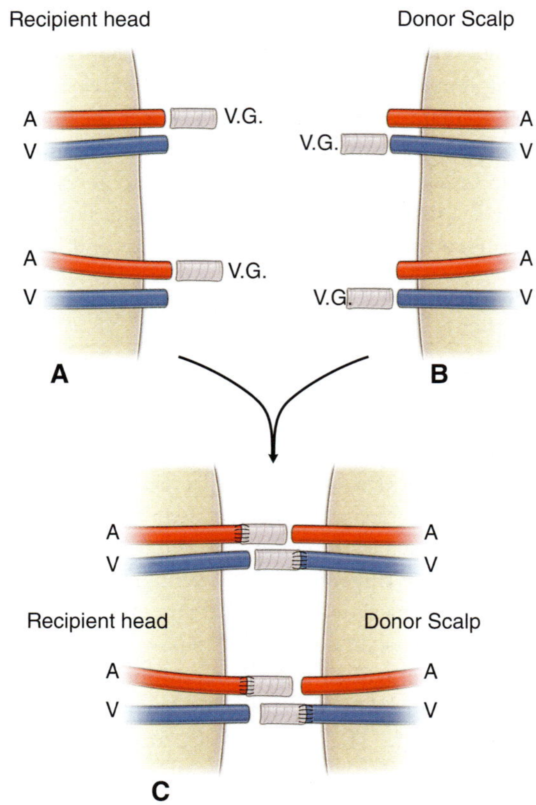

FIGURE 28-9 Diagram of simultaneous vein grafting to donor and recipient pedicles. (1). Vein grafts to the arteries on the recipient head by one operating team. (2). Simultaneously, vein grafts to the veins on the donor scalp by another operating team. (3) During the final anastomoses, only half the number of vascular anastomoses have to be done, thus shortening the operative time significantly. A, artery; V, vein; VG, vein graft.

hemostasis relies on the restoration of normal physiological scalp tension as described earlier. After the arteries are repaired, the veins expand with blood and are easily anastomosed themselves. In the time taken for veins to be clamped and joined on the first side, ongoing venous and arterial bleeding on the second may produce excessive blood loss. The need for reperfusion after a prolonged ischemia time versus the importance of minimizing blood loss may be reconciled by intermittent clamping of the artery proximal to its anastomosis during the venous repairs.

If warm ischemia time is kept within 4 to 5 hours, we recommend that the veins be done first. This results in minimal bleeding from the wound edge or the underside of the scalp, leaving the operative field clear for uncomplicated microvascular anastomoses.

However, because many of our patients reach us late, the microsurgical procedure generally starts with anastomosis of one artery followed by repair of all of the veins on the same side. It is concluded by reconnection of the contralateral vessels. In the case of massive subcutaneous bleeding during the anastomosis of a vein, the surgeon should obtain hemostasis under direct vision if possible, judiciously clamping the already anastomosed artery to reduce bleeding. If the arterial perfusion seems inadequate after anastomosis of the arteries on one side, the surgeon should immediately check the arterial anastomoses as well as the position and direction of the vein grafts. If good flow is identified, the surgeon may proceed to anastomose the contralateral arteries and finally the veins.

In our experience, the longer the scalp ischemia time, the longer the time interval between arterial anastomosis and perfusion. Extensive loss of blood and serum is commonly observed after the onset of arterial perfusion. Large hematomas may develop under a replanted scalp after surgery because after bilateral vessel repairs have been carried out, it cannot be turned over to inspect the undersurface for bleeding points. Suction drains may help prevent such accumulations but are of little help with arterial bleeding. When arterial perfusion is seen to decrease, the scalp will be less likely to survive. This may be related to endothelial injuries of the vessels caused by long-term ischemia and anoxia of the tissues within the scalp.

During dissection of the donor and recipient vessels, exploration of the sensory nerves of the scalp is worthwhile so that sensation may be restored to the replanted scalp. We repair the supraorbital and greater occipital nerves if possible because these are responsible for sensation of forehead skin and most of the scalp. The sensory function of the replanted scalp will gradually recover within 6 to 8 months after the surgery if these nerves have been repaired (Figure 28-10).

POSTOPERATIVE MANAGEMENT

After replantation, bilateral suction drains are placed under the scalp, and the wound is given a light pressure dressing to reduce the risk of hematoma or seroma.

After surgery, the patient should be kept supine, with a head ring in the occipital area. The head should be turned every 2 hours to avoid necrosis of the flap secondary to pressure. The patient will be brought into a semi-sitting position 48 hours after surgery if stable. He or she should be given oxygen via nasal prongs and receive routine observations. The room temperature should be kept at 25°C. The complete blood count and electrolytes should be checked daily for three days after surgery and abnormalities treated appropriately.

Broad-spectrum antibiotics and vasodilators may be given, but anticoagulants should be used cautiously or avoided. At 48 hours after surgery, anticoagulants *may* be used provided the hemoglobin is within normal limits. The use of anticoagulants within 48 hours is contraindicated because long-term scalp ischemia followed by reperfusion will have resulted in overexpansion and overcongestion of the replanted scalp, leading to extensive oozing beneath it. In addition, large quantities of crystalloid given in the perioperative phase will dilute the blood and prolong coagulation time. Because the replanted scalp is secured in the recipient area before the complete reestablishment of a blood supply and the scalp cannot be turned over for hemostasis, the only way to control the bleeding is by restoring proper physiological tension as the scalp is positioned, trimmed, and sutured into the recipient site. Under these circumstances, anticoagulants would be extremely risky to both the replanted scalp and the patient in general.

After 2 to 4 weeks of good perfusion, the partial or total scalp replantation will likely survive assuming appropriate postoperative management. Normal hair growth in replanted area should occur 6 months after surgery (Figure 28-11).

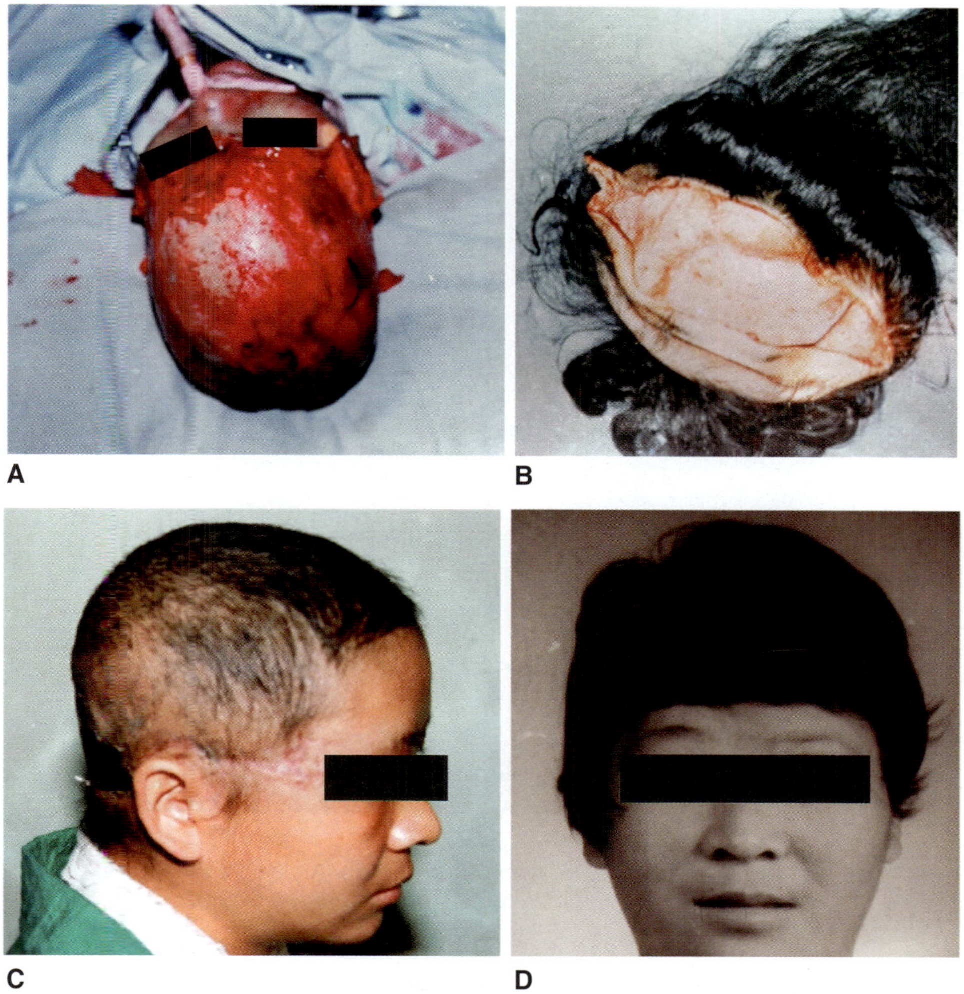

FIGURE 28-10 A 35-year-old woman who sustained a total avulsion of the entire scalp. View of the patient's head (**A**) and amputated scalp (**B**). (**C**) and (**D**) Nearly 2 years after surgery, the final result with luxuriant regrowth of hair. The patient has latterly regained full sensation of the replanted scalp.

MANAGEMENT OF VASCULAR PROBLEMS

Volume of negative pressure drainage, capillary response, and scalp temperature and color are the major indicators for survival of the replanted scalp. The normal scalp is grayish white, which is much different from skin in other areas. Therefore, it is very difficult to judge the scalp on the basis of color change. To make a sound and precise judgments, the surgeons should take all the indicators into account.

After surgery, the scalp may present with signs of insufficient blood supply such as a grayish white color, cool temperature (less than 28°C), slow capillary response, and low volume of suction drainage, indicating thrombosis or spasm at the arterial anastomotic site or the associated vein graft. Arterial perfusion is at risk, and prompt intervention required. This is often seen when large-diameter graft veins are used to bridge the vascular defect and their length exceeds 6 cm. Persistent vascular spasm is a major reason for disturbed arterial perfusion.

Too rapid a capillary response, a drop in skin temperature, hemorrhage under the scalp, over 200 to 300 mL/hr of negative pressure drainage, and progressive cyanosis suggest thrombosis at the venous anastomotic site or spasm of the vein graft on the venous side. With other factors excluded, arterial spasm improves with warming, hydration, and the passage of time, but thrombosis has no remission. For thrombosis, exploration is mandatory.

Negative pressure drainage of over 200 mL/hr within 6 hours of surgery, along with blood accumulation under the scalp, indicates extensive exudation, blood leakage at the anastomotic site, failure to ligate bleeders, venous thrombosis, or too much resistance in the draining veins. At this time, surgical exploration is urgent. If artery-to-vein ratio is 1:1, more draining veins should be connected—with vein grafts as necessary—to reduce backpressure and decrease the exudation of blood. Thrombosed anastomoses may need to be revised, perhaps with longer vein grafts.

Leech therapy is an option to improve venous hemodynamics if venous inadequacy cannot be remedied by surgery and if such circumstances become sustained or occur repeatedly. This is often caused by persistent spasm after reestablishing blood circulation, a result of prolonged warm ischemia time and severe microvascular injury within the avulsed scalp.

With close monitoring in the postoperative period, a vascular crisis should be detected early and explored immediately. Large hematomas should also be eliminated as early as possible after being detected. If all goes well, the replanted scalp should then survive successfully with a luxuriant regrowth of hair (Figure 28-12).

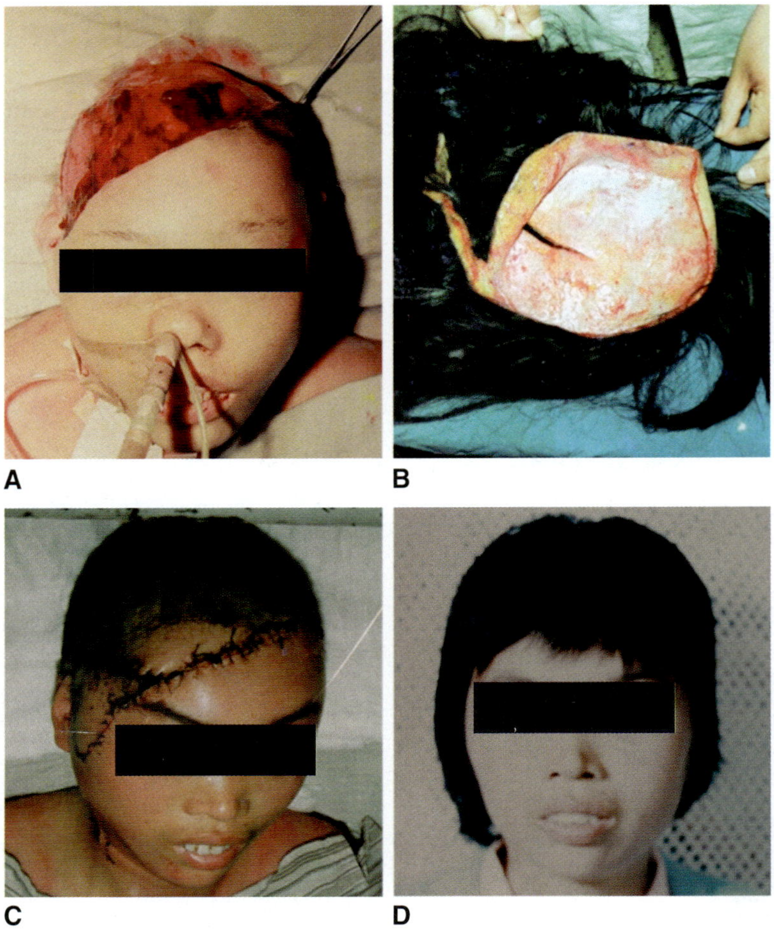

FIGURE 28-11 A 34-year-old woman who sustained nearly total avulsion of the scalp. (**A**) View of the head following scalp avulsion. (**B**) View of the avulsed scalp. (**C**) Appearance a few days after surgery. (**D**) Postoperative view showing normal hair growth in the replanted scalp 6 months after surgery.

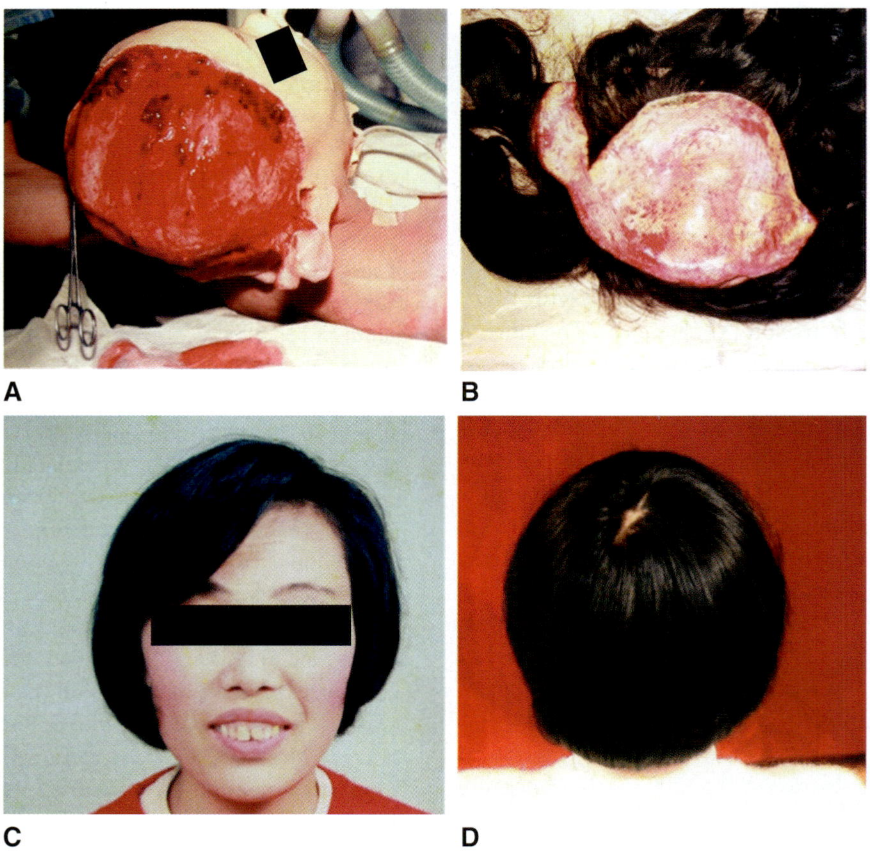

FIGURE 28-12 A 31-year-old woman who sustained a complete avulsion of the scalp. (**A**) and (**B**) View of patient's head and amputated scalp. (**C**) and (**D**) Result nearly 2 years after surgery.

REFERENCES

1. Farmer AW. Treatment of avulsed skin flaps. *Ann Surg* 1939;110(5):951.
2. Orticochea M. Four flap scalp reconstruction technique. *Br J Plast Surg* 1967;20(2):159.
3. Chang TS. Experiences in microsurgery in the People's Republic of China. *J Microsurg* 1979;1(2):154.
4. Furnas H, Lineaweaver WC, Alpert BS, et al. Scalp reconstruction by microvascular free tissue transfer. *Ann Plast Surg* 1990;24(5):431.
5. Lee B, Bickel K, Levin S, et al. Microsurgical reconstruction of extensive scalp defects. *J Reconstr Microsurg* 1999;15:255.
6. Mccombe D, Donato R, Hofer S, et al. Free flaps in the treatment of locally advanced malignancy of the scalp and forehead. *Ann Plast Surg* 2002;48:600.
7. Newman M, Hanasono M, Disa J, et al. Scalp reconstruction: a 15-year experience. *Ann Plast Surg* 2004;52:501.
8. McLean DH, Buncke HJ Jr. Autotransplant of omentum to a large scalp defect, with microsurgical revascularization. *Plast Reconstr Surg* 1972;49(3):268.
9. Browning FS, Eastwood DS, Price DJ, et al. Scalp and cranial substitution with autotransplanted greater omentum using microvascular anastomosis. *Br J Surg* 1979;66(3):152.
10. Sanger J, Maiman D, Matloub H, et al. Management of chronic osteomyelitis of the skull using vascularized omental transfer. *Surg Neurol* 1982;18(4):267.
11. Irons GB, Witzke DJ, Arnold PG, et al. Use of the omental free flap for soft-tissue reconstruction. *Ann Plast Surg* 1983;11(6):501.
12. Shen YM, Shen ZY. Greater omentum in reconstruction of refractory wounds. *Chin J Traumatol* 2003;6(2):81.
13. Miller GD, Austee EJ, Shell JA. Successful replantation of an Avulsed scalp by microvascular anastomoses. *Plast Reconstr Surg* 1976;58(2):133.
14. Buncke HJ, Rose EH, Brownstein MJ, et al. Successful replantation of two avulsed scalps by microvascular anastomosis. *Plast Reconstr Surg* 1978;61(5):666.
15. Biemer E, Stock W, Wolfensberger C, et al. Successful replantation of a totally avulsed scalp. *Br J Plast Surg* 1978;32(1):19.
16. Nahai F, Aurteau J, Vasconez LO. Replantation of an entire scalp and ear by microvascular anastomoses of only 1 artery and 1 vein. *Br J Plast Surg* 1978;31(4):339.
17. Spira M, Daniel RK, Agris J. Successful replantation of totally avulsed scalp, with profuse regrowth of hair: case report. *Plast Reconstr Surg* 1978;62(3):447.
18. Chater NL, Buncke HJ, Brownstein M. Revascularization of the scalp by microsurgical techniques after complete avulsion. *Neurosurgery* 1978;2(3):269.
19. Gatti JE, La Rossa D. Scalp avulsions and review of successful replantation. *Ann Plast Surg* 1981;6(2):127.
20. Hentz VR, Palma CR, Elliott E, et al. Successful replantation of a totally avulsed scalp following prolonged ischemia. *Ann Plast Surg* 1981;7(2):145.
21. Fogdestam I, Lilja J. Microsurgical replantation of a total scalp avulsion. Case report. Scand. J. *Plast Reconstr Surg* 1986;20(3):319.
22. Sakai S, Soeda S, Ishii Y. Avulsion of the scalp: which one is the best artery for anastomoses? *Ann Plast Surg* 1990;24(4):350.
23. Eren S, Hess J, Larkin GC. Total scalp replantation based on one artery and one vein. *Microsurgery* 1993;14:266.
24. McCann J, O'Donoghue J, Ghazal SK, et al. Microvascular replantation of a completely avulsed scalp. *Microsurgery* 1994;15:639.
25. Arashiro K, Ohtsuka H, Ohtani K, et al. Entire scalp replantation: case report and review of the literature. *J Reconstr Microsurg* 1995;11:245.
26. Barisoni D, Lorenzini M, Governa M, et al. Two cases of scalp reimplantation based on one artery and one vein with interposed vein grafts. *Eur J Plast Surg* 1997;20:51.
27. Lee B, Bickel K, Levin S. Microsurgical reconstruction of extensive scalp defects. *J Reconstr Microsurg* 1999;15(4):255;discussion 263.
28. Wilhelmi BJ, Kang RH, Kiumars M, et al. First successful replantation of face and scalp with single-artery repair: model for face and scalp transplantation. *Ann Plast Surg* 2003;50:53.
29. Liu T, Dong J, Wang J, et al. Microsurgical replantation for child total scalp avulsion. *J Craniofac Surg* 2009;220(1):81.
30. Zhou S, Chang T, Guan W, et al. Microsurgical replantation of the avulsed scalp: report of six cases. *J Reconstr Microsurg* 1993;9(2):121.
31. Chen IC, Wan HL. Microsurgical replantation of avulsed scalps. *J Reconstr Microsurg* 1996;12(2):105.
32. Yin JW, Matsuo JM, Hsieh CH, et al. Replantation of total avulsed scalp with microsurgery: experience of eight cases and literature review. *J Trauma* 2008;64(3):796.
33. Cheng K, Zhou S, Jiang K, et al. Microsurgical replantation of the avulsed scalp: report of 20 cases. *Plast Reconstr Surg* 1996;97:(6).

CHAPTER 29

Ear and Lip Replantation

Johnny T. Chang, Bauback Safa, Mauricio Kuri, and Gregory M. Buncke

Traumatic amputations of facial structures carry unique significance because of the magnitude of their functional, aesthetic, and psychosocial impact. In addition, such injuries are not uncommon, given their prominent positions on the face. Unfortunately, replantation of these amputated parts is challenging, and reports of success are rare in the literature. However, without efforts at replantation, reconstruction poses some of the greatest challenges to surgeons in terms of recovering critical functions, matching and maintaining local anatomy and symmetry, and preempting adverse changes over time such as scarring and contracture.

In this chapter, amputations of the ear, lips, and tongue are grouped together because of similarities in the techniques necessary for successful replantation. Amputation of these parts is generally by avulsion, most often resulting from either traumatic shearing in motor vehicle collisions or ripping and tearing from human or dog bites. Replantation is made significantly more difficult by the broad zones of injury and loss of intact vessel length. Vessels for suitable venous anastomoses are difficult to find and even when found cannot adequately drain the entire part. Because of this, successful replantation of these parts requires intensive postoperative care directed at providing adequate venous outflow during the period of neovascularization through strategies such as anticoagulation, bleeding, and leeching.

Although replantation of these parts is technically and clinically challenging, success can provide results that cannot be matched by existing reconstructive techniques (1). Moreover, attempts at replantation typically do not preclude future reconstructive efforts in case of failure, and partial salvage of amputated parts can provide additional native tissue to facilitate later reconstructive efforts. Therefore, every attempt should be made at replantation as a first course of action if at all possible, including expedient transfer to a specialized microsurgical center if such expertise is not immediately available.

EAR

The external ear sits in a prominent and relatively unprotected position on the face. Avulsion frequently occurs because of motor vehicle collisions as well as human and dog bites. Although the functional impacts of ear amputations are less significant and debilitating than loss of other facial parts, the aesthetic impact is significant, especially in patients with short or thin hair who cannot mask their loss with changes in hairstyle.

Reconstruction of the ear has remained one of the most challenging problems in plastic surgery because of its complex shape and unique component tissues. The combination of delicate cantilevered cartilage covered by relatively thin skin presents a challenge in terms of finding, shaping, and sculpting donor tissue to match the natural contours of the ear while preventing the inevitable scarring and contracture from distorting the final result. Although successful outcomes are possible, reconstruction typically requires multiple stages, results are generally far from ideal, and the final appearance of the reconstructed ear is unpredictable.

Attempts at replantation of the amputated ear are therefore particularly compelling. Although difficult, the challenge of ear replantation is somewhat ameliorated by the relatively low metabolic demands of cartilage and thin skin (1). The significant vascularity of the face also provides multiple options for inflow through the superficial temporal artery, the posterior auricular artery, and their multiple branches.

TONGUE

Amputation of the tongue, conversely, imparts a much larger functional than aesthetic loss. Furthermore, the psychosocial sequelae can be tremendous because the tongue is critical not only for speech and articulation—the basis for human communication and social interaction—but also for taste and thus gustatory enjoyment of food. The tongue also contributes to mastication in the form of food bolus control, deglutition, and airway protection (2). Its loss clearly produces a considerable functional impairment.

Anatomically, the tongue is unique in that it is composed almost entirely of muscle. Although muscle has relatively high metabolic demands, making it much more sensitive to ischemic insults, successful replantation has been reported after significant periods of ischemia. Reconstruction of the amputated tongue generally requires complex microvascular tissue transfer (2). In terms of replantation, the difficulties that the microsurgeon faces revolve around access and exposure, both intraoperatively and postoperatively. Attention to intraoperative setup and preparation is critical for success. Most important, consideration must be given to obtaining and securing adequate airway control, starting with the patient's initial presentation to the trauma bay, continuing intraoperatively with the decision of whether to perform a formal tracheostomy, and extending into postoperative recovery with proper sedation and edema management.

LIPS

Amputation of the lips results in significant functional, aesthetic, and psychosocial sequelae. Functionally, the lips are critical for oral competence and speech and contribute a minor role in deglutition. In addition, they have a significant role in nonverbal communication in the form of facial expression. Loss or deformity of the lips is consequently severely debilitating.

The lips are structurally complex and difficult to reconstruct, with subtle features such as the gradual but distinct vermilion border, the curves of the Cupid's bow and tubercle, and the unsupported soft tissue philtral columns. These structures are challenging to reproduce with non-native tissue. Furthermore, the dry mucosa of the lip is unique and cannot satisfactorily be replaced by other mucosal tissue such as intraoral wet mucosa.

Nevertheless, compared with replantation of the ear and tongue, replantation of the lips poses certain advantages. Access and exposure are relatively simple, and arterial anatomy is straightforward. Although alignment of anatomic features is critical and not always easy in the presence of complex avulsion injuries, small postoperative revisions can ultimately provide significant benefits. Numerous secondary techniques are also available, ranging from simple scar revisions to more complex local and regional flaps that can provide significant improvement. Regardless, replantation of the lips requires very similar intraoperative and postoperative techniques to ear and tongue replantation because of frequently inadequate venous outflow.

HISTORY AND LITERATURE REVIEW

Ear

Although Buncke first reported the successful replantation of a total ear in a rabbit using microvascular techniques in 1966, the first report of successful ear replantation in humans did not appear until 1980 with publication of Pennington's successful reattachment of an avulsed ear using vein grafts to the superficial temporal artery and vein (1,3–5). In all, a total of 31 cases of successful ear replantation have been reported in the literature, after ischemia times of up to 33 hours. Twelve resulted from motor vehicle collisions, eight from human or dog bites, and only five from sharp trauma (1,4,6–20).

Arterial repairs were performed in all cases, although in two cases, inflow was established via arterialization of the venous system in the amputated part through arteriovenous anastomoses. Twelve cases were performed in artery-only fashion, relying on postoperative outflow augmentation measures to combat congestion. Reported intraoperative techniques for establishing inflow and outflow included direct repair to superficial temporal or posterior auricular branches, vein grafting, and use of the pedicled superficial temporal vascular leash. In addition, Wong et al. (21) reported one case in which the ear was temporarily perfused on the forearm using a perforator from the radial artery and a superficial forearm vein. The construct consisting of amputated part, radial artery, and vein graft was then transferred to the superior thyroid artery and external jugular vein, respectively, resulting in essentially full take without postoperative congestion (21).

Postoperatively, some form of chemical or mechanical leeching was required in 20 of the 31 cases. In seven cases, no additional postoperative outflow measures were instituted, although iatrogenic hemodilution was used in one patient, and prolonged systemic anticoagulation of 18 days was required in another. Three reports did not specify whether postoperative congestion was encountered. Nineteen of 31 patients required blood transfusions ranging from 2 to 13 units; only four required none. Eight reports did not specify whether transfusions were given.

Lip

Lip replantation has a similar history, with the first report of partially successful replantation published in 1976 (22). Since that time, 29 cases of successful lip replantation have been reported, after ischemia times of up to 17 hours (22–38). Twenty-five of those cases resulted from human or dog bites. Arterial repairs were performed in all cases, although one case required arterialization of venous channels in the amputated part through an arteriovenous anastomosis (29). Vein grafting was required in only one case. Venous repairs were performed in nine of the 29 cases, retrograde arteriovenous anastomoses were used in three cases for outflow, and the remaining 17 cases were artery-only replants. Local vessels used included labial, angular, and facial vessels depending on the location of the amputation.

After surgery, leeches were required in 21 of the 29 cases, and mechanical or chemical leeching was used in five additional cases to treat venous congestion. Taylor and Andrews reported a case of staged inset to ameliorate postoperative congestion, a technique subsequently replicated by Hendrick with success, although in both cases leeches and blood transfusions were still necessary (25,29). Twenty-five of the 29 cases required blood transfusions ranging from two to 16 units, one did not require transfusions, and three reports did not comment on transfusions.

Tongue

As rare as successful lip and ear replantations may be, reports of successful tongue replantation are even fewer in number with only three cases in the English literature. Buntic reported the first such case in 1998, in a patient involved in a motor vehicle collision (2). The 5 × 4 cm amputated segment was replanted using a single left lingual artery and a vein graft from the ipsilateral left lingual vena comitantes through the floor of the mouth to the left facial vein. Airway control was secured with a tracheostomy. No leeching was necessary.

Subsequently in 2001, Davis and Armstrong reported an initially successful case in which a 5 × 3.5 cm tongue segment amputated by human bite was reattached using a left lingual artery and contralateral ventral vein (39). The patient did well and was discharged on postoperative day 4, only to return on day 6 with complete necrosis after resuming cigarette smoking. Egozi et al. then reported a successful case in 2006 of a large near-total amputation of the anterior two thirds of the mobile tongue in a motorcycle collision (40). Revascularization was achieved through the left lingual artery and a contralateral right-sided vein, and the majority of the part survived with only 1 cm of distal necrosis.

In 2007, Kim et al. (41) reported a third successful case of tongue replantation using an artery-only approach with postoperative leeching for outflow. The authors expressed ambivalence regarding the benefits of tongue replantation but noted that their amputated part was significantly smaller than previously reported cases. In their case, the part measured 2.5 cm wide by only 0.8 to 1.7 cm long; the authors commented that in cases of such small amputations, direct closure of the tongue might suffice or even prove more effective.

ANATOMY

Ear

The external ear consists of multiple convoluted and complex features that present both challenges and landmarks in terms of proper alignment in replantation and repair (Figure 29-1). Care should be taken to examine the contralateral ear for symmetry during inset of the amputated part, although this may be difficult depending on the degree of trauma as well as associated injuries such as to the cervical spine. The auricle is composed of a thin cartilaginous framework, its overlying perichondrium, minimal subcutaneous tissue, and intermediate thickness skin. Auricular cartilage is similar to nasal cartilage in terms of its flexibility and tendency to warp in the presence of external forces such as soft tissue and perichondrial scarring.

Vascular supply to the ear consists of a branch of the superficial temporal artery anteriorly that enters at the root of the helix and the posterior auricular artery that enters at the inferior aspect of the concha (Figures 29-2 and 29-3) (1,42–44). In 7% of patients, the occipital artery rather than the posterior auricular artery provides the dominant blood supply to the posterior surface of the ear (44). The posterior auricular artery gives off multiple branches as it courses superiorly that can be

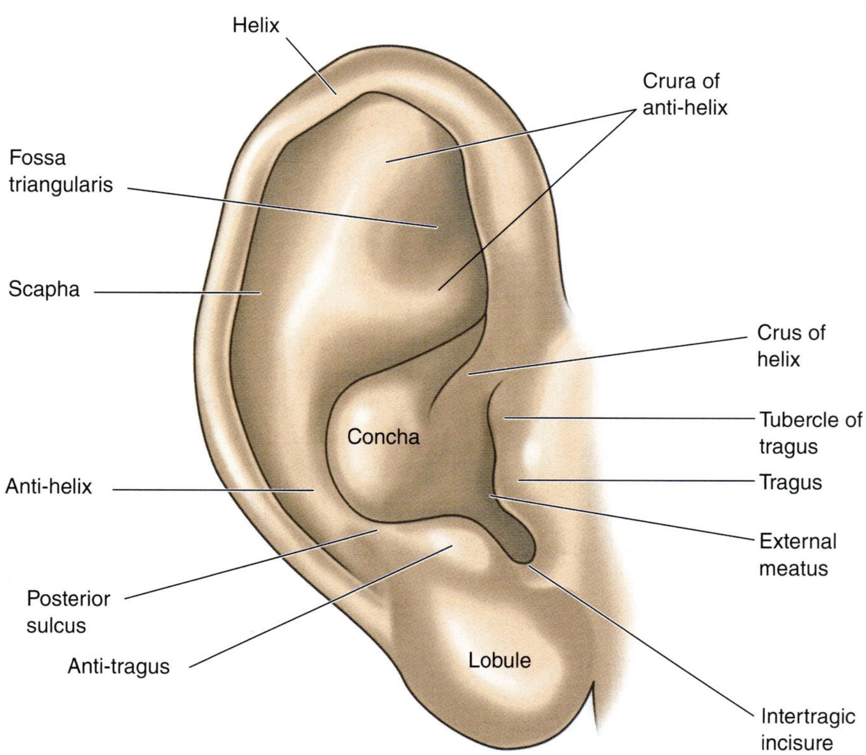

FIGURE 29-1 Features and landmarks of the external ear, or auricle.

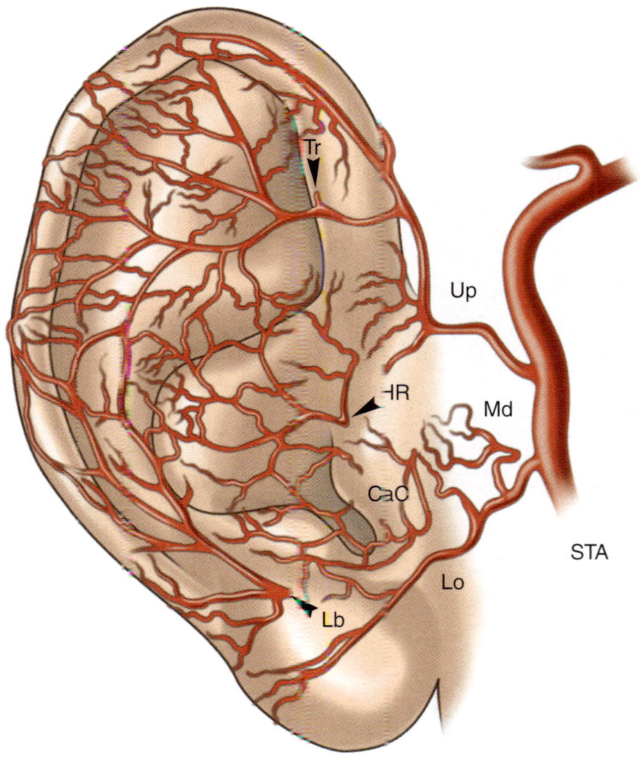

FIGURE 29-2 Arterial supply to the anterior ear. The superficial temporal artery (STA) provides upper, middle, and lower branches (Up, Md, Lo) to the anterior ear. Branches of the posterior auricular artery come through the triangular fossa (Tr), the concha (HR and CaC), and the earlobe (Lb).

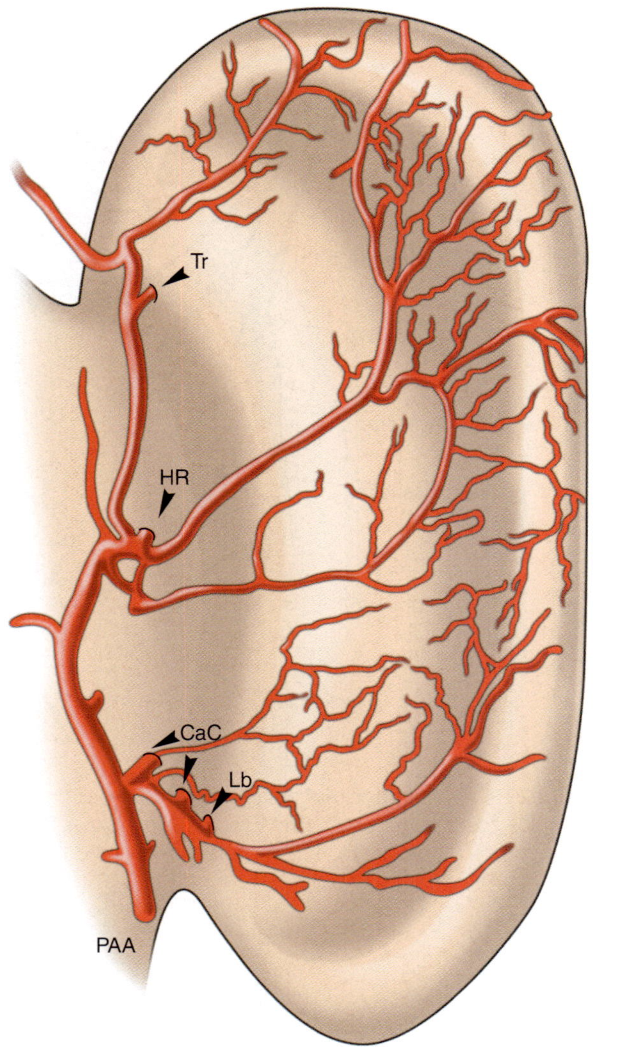

FIGURE 29-3 Arterial supply to the posterior ear. The posterior auricular artery (PAA) sends branches to throughout the posterior ear and perforators to the anterior ear at the triangular fossa (Tr), cymba conchae (CyC), helical root (HR), cavum conchae (CaC), and earlobe (Lb).

used for inflow in replantation, as well as branches that supply a portion of the anterior surface of the ear. Veins typically follow these arteries but are usually avulsed and retracted, making it impossible to find specific targets for venous anastomoses. Furthermore, venous outflow from the ear, as with the lips and tongue, depends significantly on diffuse and segmental subdermal networks that are not amenable to microvascular repair.

Nerves adequate for repair are typically not found, but in time patients generally recover adequate sensibility anyway. The auriculotemporal and lesser occipital nerves supply the superior portions of the anterior and posterior ear, respectively. The great auricular nerve supplies the inferior portion of the ear. Arnold's nerve supplies the concha and part of the external auditory canal (1,42–44).

Tongue

The tongue is composed of eight muscles, four of which are attached directly to bone and are termed *extrinsic*, and four, attached only to other muscles, called *intrinsic* (Figures 29-4). The extrinsic muscles affect tongue position and consist of the genioglossus, hyoglossus, styloglossus, and palatoglossus. The intrinsics affect tongue shape and consist of the superior longitudinal, inferior longitudinal, verticalis, and transversus muscles. This distinction between intrinsic muscles is largely academic, however, because identifying them is neither clinically practical nor necessary. Because of the intraoral and intrapharyngeal location of the tongue, amputations tend to affect only the distal tongue with preservation of its base. Thus, both in reconstruction and replantation, replacing distal bulk rather than functional muscle is the primary goal.

Vascular supply to the tongue is provided by the paired left and right lingual arteries, which course through the ventral or inferior substance of the tongue as the deep lingual arteries (Figure 29-5) (42,45). They are separated by a median fibrous septum, which allows few interconnecting channels between the two vessels; nonetheless, reports of successful replantation have all described single arterial anastomoses without significant contralateral tissue loss (2,39,41). Because their course is, by definition, intramuscular, the vascular structures tend to retract

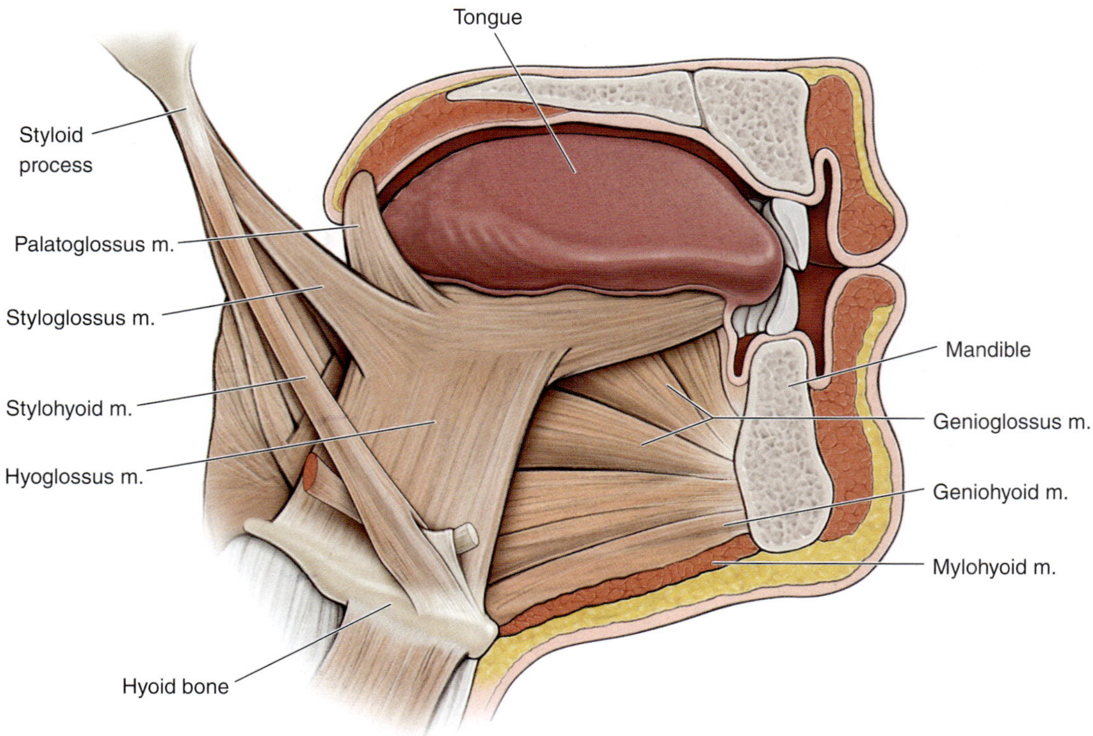

FIGURE 29-4 The extrinsic muscles of the tongue consist of the genioglossus, hyoglossus, styloglossus, and palatoglossus muscles. (Reproduced with permission from Morton, D., Foreman, K.B., Albertine, K. Gross Anatomy: The Big Picture, 1st Edition. Available at http://accessmedicine.mhmedical.com.)

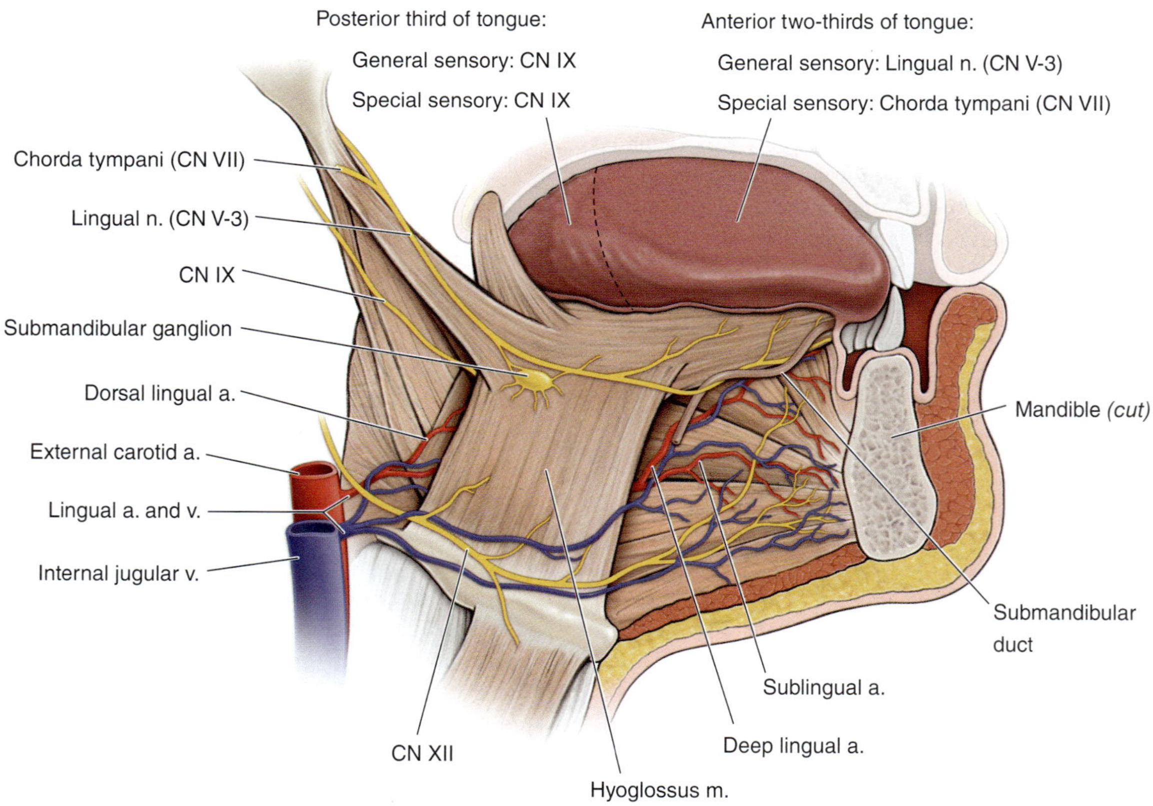

FIGURE 29-5 The paired lingual arteries and veins run through the ventral substance of the tongue on either side of the median septum of the tongue. (Reproduced with permission from Morton, D., Foreman, K.B., Albertine, K. Gross Anatomy: The Big Picture, 1st Edition. Available at http://accessmedicine.mhmedical.com.)

within the substance of the tongue and present great difficulties in dissection. Veins are rarely accessible for anastomosis.

The nerve supply to the tongue consists of motor branches from the hypoglossal and vagus nerves deep within the head and neck and outside the zone of amputation, general somatic sensory nerves, and gustatory sensory nerves for taste. The glossopharyngeal nerve provides both general sensory and taste fibers for the posterior third of the tongue. The lingual nerve and the chorda tympani provide general sensory and taste fibers, respectively, for the anterior two thirds.

Lips

The lips consist of several complex but subtle features, the upper lip more so than the lower lip, making reconstruction and repair of the upper lip more challenging and critical (Figure 29-6). In addition, the dry mucosa of the lip, which comprises the majority of the visible vermilion, is unique and to some extent irreplaceable. Common vermilion replacement strategies use intraoral mucosa, but this wet mucosa is prone to painful chapping when exposed to ambient air.

Intrinsic muscular control of the lips is provided by the orbicularis oris and allows pursing of the lips and maintenance of oral competence (Figure 29-7). The fibers of the orbicularis oris muscle circumscribe the oral aperture and originate from multiple locations: the mandible, the maxilla, and the deep dermis. At the commissures, the superior and inferior fibers originate from a chiasma called the modiolus. The superior fibers travel parallel to the upper lip to insert into the contralateral philtral columns (26,42).

Extrinsic muscular control, which provides mouth opening and expressions such as smiling and frowning, is provided by the perioral muscles of facial expression. The upper lip is activated by levator labii superioris, levator anguli oris, and zygomaticus major. The lower lip is activated by the mentalis, depressor labii inferioris, depressor anguli oris, and platysma.

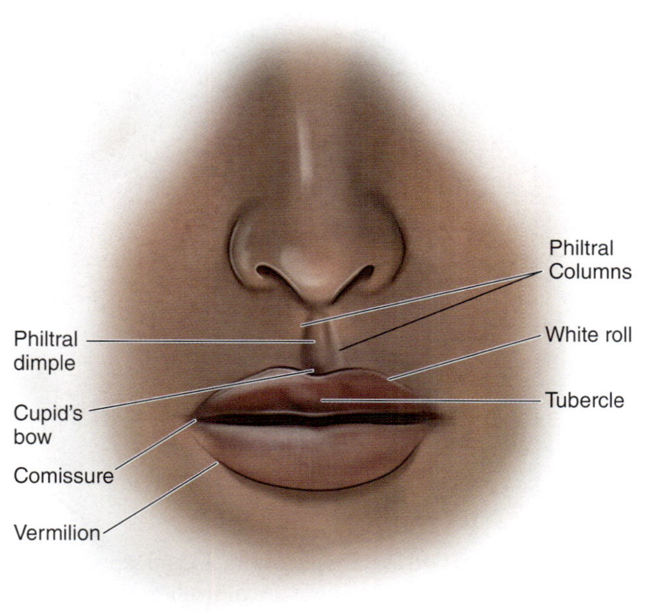

FIGURE 29-6 Features of the lips.

Vascular supply to the lips is provided by the left and right superior and inferior labial arteries (Figure 29-8). The arteries originate from the respective facial arteries lateral to the commissures and course medially just deep to the vermilion border or mucocutaneous junction, superficial to the orbicularis oris muscle. The superior labial artery gives off several branches to supply

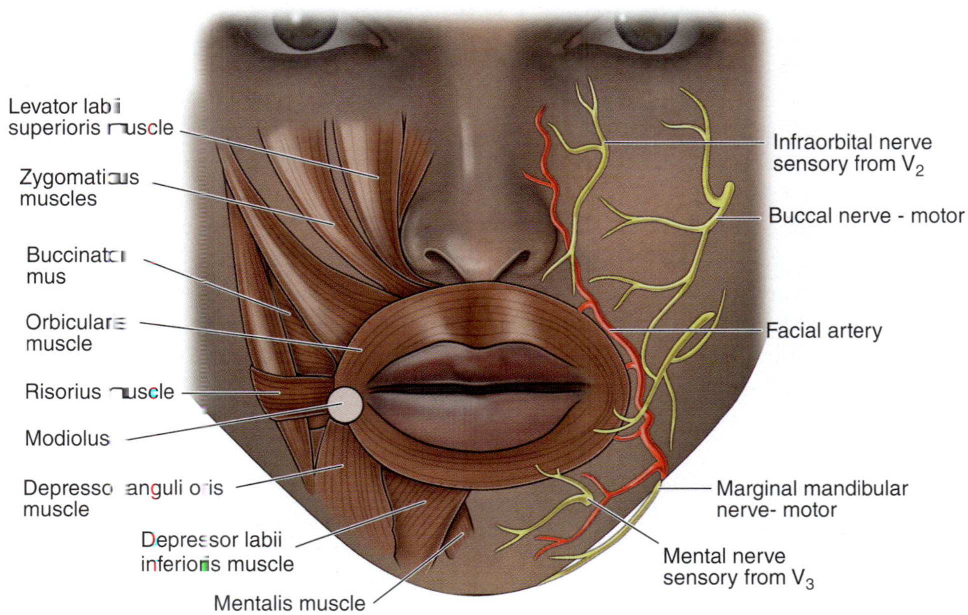

FIGURE 29-7 Perioral musculature.

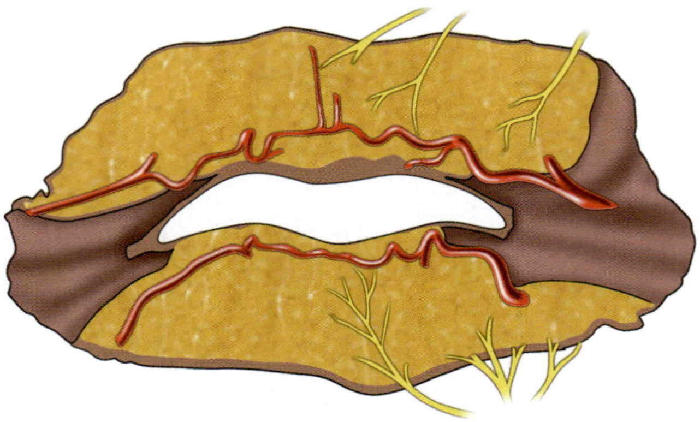

FIGURE 29-8 Superior and inferior labial arteries after takeoff from the facial artery.

the cutaneous lip as well as the nasal columella and septum. Small veins do travel with the arteries but are difficult to find, difficult to repair, and contribute only partly to the venous drainage of the lips with significant dependence on subdermal venous networks.

PREOPERATIVE CONSIDERATIONS

As with amputations of any body part, there are no absolute indications or contraindications for replantation. All indications and contraindications are relative, and each situation should be considered individually in light of the patient, the history, and concomitant injuries. The pros and cons should be weighed carefully, and a frank discussion with the patient is mandatory, covering the risk of failure, the lengthy and taxing postoperative course with the likely need for transfusions, the potential need for further revisionary surgeries, and the possibility of suboptimal aesthetic and functional outcomes despite survival of the replanted part (4,11,46–51).

Indications and Contraindications

First and foremost, the basic tenets of trauma care should be considered and addressed before any consideration of replantation. In all situations, but particularly in the case of lip and tongue amputations, the patient's airway should be secured, with intubation or tracheostomy if necessary. After an adequate airway has been confirmed, the patient's cardiovascular status and concomitant injuries should be evaluated. Hypotension and other severe cardiopulmonary disturbances are likely to preclude attempts at replantation, especially if vasopressor support is required. Neurosurgical and neurologic disabilities may not be absolute contraindications but should be considered carefully: in cases of cervical spine injury, the need for significant manipulation of the head and neck in replantation of facial parts should be discussed with the neurosurgery service (1).

Comorbidities should also be considered in deciding whether to replant. Advanced age, decreased mental status, and diminished mental capacity are relative contraindications. Atherosclerosis and peripheral vascular disease may not be contraindications but do portend potential technical difficulties with microvascular anastomoses resulting from vessel delamination and intimal damage. The patient's psychiatric status, especially in cases of self-inflicted injuries, is important to consider as well. However, it is often difficult or impossible to determine acutely whether the patient has an untenable baseline condition that precludes replantation or simply a psychiatric aberration that can be managed postoperatively with adequate psychiatric care. Replantation can frequently be beneficial in these cases, especially in light of the significant psychosocial impact of facial amputations.

Social history can also play a significant role in the decision to replant. Smoking is not necessarily a contraindication but does contribute to a higher risk of failure, partial loss, and healing complications (52,53). Anecdotally, vessels tend to be smaller in caliber. Furthermore, the patient's ability to abstain completely from smoking in the postoperative period needs to be assessed honestly because any intermittent vasoconstriction will certainly doom the replanted part to failure. The patient's religious and personal convictions may preclude postoperative transfusions, which in the case of ear, lip, and tongue replants is nearly inevitable. Finally, the patient's social support resources should be assessed to best plan for the extensive postdischarge care and recovery that will be necessary.

Next, the condition of the part and the amputation stump should be assessed. Severe multilevel injuries, severe contamination, and severe crush and avulsion injuries are relative but significant contraindications. Multilevel and mutilating injuries can result in parts that cannot be entirely perfused despite reconstitution of vascular inflow, leaving distal parts ischemic. Contaminated parts and wounds can often be adequately debrided, cleaned, and addressed with intravenous (IV) antibiotics, but contamination with chemical substances such as grease is often untenable. Although severe crush and avulsion injuries are classic contraindications to replantation, as noted earlier, this is nearly always the case with ear, lip, and tongue amputations. Successful replantation in these cases requires recognition of the expanded zones of injury. Prolonged ischemia, especially warm ischemia, is often noted as a contraindication, but successful digital replantations have been reported after warm ischemia of up to 33 hours and cold ischemia of up to 94 hours (50). The ear has low metabolic demands similar to the digits, but the tongue and lips, because of their muscular component, are more sensitive to ischemia.

Nevertheless, when the patient's condition can tolerate it, when the amputation is total or near total, when the part is a single intact piece of tissue, and when an inflow vessel can be found upon dissection, it is generally worthwhile to attempt replantation. Most pediatric amputations, although technically more difficult, warrant replantation because of the tremendous healing potential of young children and because of the potentially higher psychosocial cost of amputation.

Alternatives to Replantation

Alternatives to replantation should always be considered and discussed with the patient. Although there is no evidence-based size cutoff for replantation, composite nonvascularized grafting is a reasonable option in amputations of the ear when the maximum distance from a vascularized bed is less than 1 to

1.5 cm. This does not hold true for the tongue or the lips because muscular tissue has significantly higher metabolic demands than cartilage and cannot tolerate the temporary ischemia inherent in composite grafting. On the other hand, the tongue and lips can tolerate greater tissue loss without significant residual deformity or functional impact. Defects of up to a quarter of the upper lip or a third of the lower lip can often be closed directly. Even larger defects may be reconstructed with relative ease and with excellent results using various lip-sharing and lip-switch procedures (25). However, these procedures become more challenging and less effective when the subtle and complex features of the lips are involved, including Cupid's bow and the tubercle, the philtral columns, and the commissures. In these situations, replantation of smaller defects may be worthwhile as a first attempt at reconstruction without precluding other reconstructive attempts in the long term if loss or partial loss occurs.

For ear amputations that are larger, numerous alternatives have been described for preserving tissue without replantation. Removal of skin and banking of the cartilage in abdominal or retroauricular pockets for delayed reconstruction has frequently been described but almost always results in significant warping or resorption. Some authors have reported greater success after covering the banked part with fascial flaps such as the temporoparietal fascial flap, but such strategies expend tissue that is often needed for later reconstruction. Ultimately, such banked cartilage generally results in distorted shapes and poor definition (1,10,44).

For partial amputations with devascularized segments, Elsahy and Mladick et al. described techniques for augmenting perfusion to the ischemic tissues with local flaps. In Elsahy's technique, a local skin flap is elevated and inset into a denuded portion of the amputated cartilage, and then the skin flap is divided at a later time (10). Mladick et al., on the other hand, proposed deepithelializing the entire partially amputated segment, burying it in a retroauricular pocket until perfusion is reestablished, and then removing it from the pocket and allowing the denuded ear to reepithelialize secondarily without additional coverage (10,47,54). It is critical in this technique to maintain as much dermis as possible to maximize viability and minimize subsequent warping; some authors have reported success using dermabrasion for this purpose.

SURGICAL TECHNIQUE

Anesthesia

In the case of tongue and lip replantation, preoperative planning and discussion with the anesthesia staff is particularly important. Oral intubation may be adequate for certain lip replantations if the endotracheal tube can be kept out of the way, but in general, nasal Rae tubes are preferred. In certain situations, especially in cases of tongue amputation when significant airway obstruction may be present or expected, tracheostomy is the safest option (2,39). In addition, patients may need to remain intubated postoperatively while edema and bleeding resolve. Perioperative airway control is the first and most important issue to consider in all cases, and it is easy to underestimate the potential for rapidly developing obstruction from bleeding, edema, or a retracted and shortened tongue.

Preparation of the Part

Frequently in cases of complete amputation, a period of time is available after the surgeon finishes evaluating the patient but before the patient arrives in the operating room (OR), during which the amputated part can be prepared. A separate table is set up in the OR where exploration and tagging of structures is performed under loupe or microscope magnification. A target artery is requisite for replantation; however, adequate target veins are difficult or impossible to identify; and, when found, are usually avulsed and badly damaged. As many vessels as possible are identified and tagged at this stage. Cavadas reported a case of ear replantation in which four submillimeter vessels were repaired (two arterial, one venous, and one arteriovenous), resulting in essentially full take without postoperative congestion (7). When nerves are encountered during dissection, they should also be tagged for possible repair.

The part is washed gently with bacteriocidal solution or soap. The amputated edge is inspected for any visible vascular lumens. On the tongue and lips, the anatomy is relatively constant with single dominant vessels in consistent locations; this is less true with the ear, which has not only two separate vascular supplies but also branches from those major vessels that may be the best options for inflow. The part is tacked to a sterile towel with a suture to help hold it in place. Short skin incisions should be made directly over any visualized lumen(s) or in the approximate anatomic locations of known vessels if no lumen is seen. Careful dissection is performed to expose any vessels and to release them from the surrounding soft tissue to minimize tension on the eventual repair. The ends of the vessels are then tagged with microclips, and the part is placed back on ice in a sterile container.

Preparation of the Amputation Site

Because the feasibility of replantation is limited by the availability of adequate target vessels on the amputated part, any target vessels identified on it will guide the search for vessels at the amputation site. First, the amputation site is irrigated with copious amounts of warm saline. This not only serves to dilute any tissue contamination but is also invaluable in clarifying anatomic structures. The amputation stump is inspected for exposed vascular lumens, guided by both anatomy as well as the locations of target vessels identified on the amputated part. Access incisions are then made directly over these locations, either to chase visualized lumens or to identify vessels if no lumens are seen. Any vessels that are identified are then carefully freed from surrounding tissue to reduce tension on the anastomoses, as well as to allow some latitude in trimming to healthy vessel outside the zone of injury. The vessel ends are then tagged with microclips.

If no vessels are found on the amputation site near the target vessels, alternate sources of inflow must be considered. Vein grafts can be quickly and easily harvested from the volar forearm or the foot and anastomosed in reverse manner to nearby vessels for inflow (46). For ear replantation, the use of the pedicled superficial temporal artery leash has been reported by multiple authors (1,55). Other authors caution that sacrifice of the superficial temporal artery precludes use of the temporoparietal fascia flap for future reconstruction. Alternative vascular pedicles for the ear have been described as well, although in isolated case reports. Wong et al. reported the use of a radial artery perforator and a superficial forearm vein, performed in situ in the forearm, and then transferred to the superior thyroid artery and external jugular vein (21). They reported no postoperative congestion requiring mechanical or chemical leeching and a small area of lobule necrosis that healed without intervention or residual deformity. Last, in cases of ear or lip amputation when a suitable arterial stump cannot be identified on the part, retrograde arterialization of venous channels with an arteriovenous anastomosis has been used with success (1,7,15,20,29).

Vascular Anastomosis and Inset

After target vessels have been identified, the part should be inset as much as possible without restricting access for microvascular repairs. Key anatomic features should be aligned at this point; the vermilion border is particularly sensitive to misalignment. For ear replantation, the cartilage should be secured with as few sutures as possible to facilitate orientation of the part and compared with the contralateral ear for symmetry. In some situations, for example, anastomoses in the posterior auricular sulcus, inset may be postponed, and the part may be temporarily positioned to maximize exposure for microsurgery (1,15).

Based on a series of three cases, Cavadas reported success and improved ease of access via an anterior approach to the ear made possible by excising the conchal cartilage (7). He described insetting the posterior skin first and then excising the conchal cartilage to allow excellent anterior exposure for microvascular anastomoses. When this is possible, it can facilitate microsurgery greatly and obviate the potential for vascular kinking that exists when the ear has to be retracted anteriorly for posterior access.

The artery is generally repaired first, mainly because the absence of inflow results in collapse of the outflow veins, making them difficult to visualize and repair. Many different techniques are used by different surgeons for microvascular repair, with good outcomes. However, our preference is the backwall technique. First, the vessels are trimmed to length, conservatively in case intimal damage necessitates further trimming. In general, it is better to place the vessels on slight tension rather than have redundant vessel length that promotes kinking. The vessels are secured with Serafin clamps, which are atraumatic and narrow in profile, which is ideal when there is limited vessel length. The clamps position the vessels, relieve tension during repair, and prevent intraluminal blood from collecting and obscuring the lumen and intima. The vessels are gently dilated with dilating forceps and irrigated with a small amount of heparin solution using a microcatheter to clear intraluminal blood and clots. The intima is inspected at this point for damage and delamination.

The repair is then performed in simple interrupted fashion, typically with 9-0, 10-0, or 11-0 nylon. The first suture is placed at the center of the back wall and subsequent sutures successively from back to front on either side of it. This allows the most difficult suturing to be done when the lumen is still open and visible and the easiest when preceding sutures largely obscure the lumen. Each stitch should be carefully inserted under direct vision of the lumen and intima, taking care to avoid backwalling or partial depth bites.

After the repair is complete, the Serafin clamps are released, and the anastomosis is inspected for patency and leakage. The vessel is bathed with a topical vasodilator, such as papaverine or high-concentration lidocaine, and copious amounts of warm saline. Small leaks will generally seal on their own, but pulsatile leaks should be repaired with interrupted sutures. The part is then inspected for reperfusion with particular attention paid to skin color, bleeding from distal skin edges, and pinprick if necessary. Frequently, part reperfusion is delayed by as much as 15 to 30 minutes, likely because of vessel spasm at the anastomosis as well as within the part itself. If the anastomosis was technically sound and flow is seen through the anastomosis, it is reasonable to proceed with inset despite the lack of visible reperfusion in the part. Ultimately, lack of initial perfusion or inflow before final inset is caused by one of the following factors: technical problems with the anastomosis, vasospasm, inadequate inflow from the proximal vessel, or unrecognized distal injury in the target vessel or part (50).

Inset is then completed, with care taken to avoid kinking or compressing the vascular pedicle. The primary aim should be to stabilize the part and protect the pedicle rather than obtain an optimally aesthetic inset at this point. There are few aesthetic sequelae from a loose inset, and those sequelae can more easily be addressed at a later stage. Alternatively, staged inset in the acute period over the first 2 weeks has been reported with good success (25).

Interrupted sutures should be used to allow individual stitches to be removed as needed to relieve compression on the vessels. If inset results in kinking that cannot be resolved, it is best to take the time to resect additional vessel length and repeat the anastomosis (1). If soft tissue coverage over the anastomosis cannot be obtained without undue tension, a small split-thickness skin graft can be laid directly over the vessels (1). The graft can easily be shaved from either the part itself or nearby using a #10 blade and secured with one or two absorbable stitches.

If venous congestion is expected, which is the case in nearly all ear, lip, and tongue replants, a small ellipse of skin can be excised to allow for outflow and monitoring. Deepithelialization of the posterior surface of the ear has been reported as well for this purpose, although some congestion can still be expected despite these maneuvers (55).

POSTOPERATIVE MANAGEMENT

The overall goal of our postoperative protocol is to support and maintain adequate inflow and outflow during the period of time when damaged vessels are undergoing intimal repair and prone to thrombosis and spasm and when new venous channels are being regenerated. In our experience, for straightforward cases with adequate arterial and venous anastomoses, this is a period of approximately 5 days; when venous outflow is inadequate, the period of venous neovascularization is closer to 7 to 12 days. Our strategy includes the following key components:

- Strategies to minimize vessel spasm, including pharmaceutical interventions, avoidance of mechanical disturbances, dietary restrictions, temperature control, and abstinence from nicotine
- Anticoagulation to prevent intraluminal thrombosis caused by intimal damage
- Anticoagulation and mechanical strategies to maintain external bleeding in cases when there is inadequate venous outflow

Patients are kept in bed until postoperative day 5 to minimize the risk of vasospasm. Although a designated "warm room" is not used, patients are kept away from cold drafts and excessive temperature drops. When there is significant concern for vasospasm, for example, with significant avulsive mechanisms and submillimeter vessels, chlorpromazine is sometimes prescribed as both an antispasmodic (α-blocker) and an anxiolytic. It is particularly helpful in pediatric patients in whom both spasm and anxiety seem to be more prevalent.

Monitoring of replanted parts is based primarily on clinical examination of color, turgor, capillary refill, and temperature. However, in our institution, we also obtain valuable information from quantitative fluorimetry, which provides objective data about inflow and outflow dynamics. By measuring the increase and subsequent decrease in cutaneous fluorescence after IV injection of fluorescein, we can supplement our clinical findings with quantitative indicators of inflow and outflow, respectively.

There are many differing views and studies regarding the use of anticoagulation in replantation surgery. It is our belief that in the case of traumatic amputations with concomitant intimal damage, some form of anticoagulation is beneficial with minimal risk of morbidity. When a venous anastomosis is not performed, the case for anticoagulation is even more compelling because outflow must be maintained in the form of external bleeding.

When there is an adequate venous anastomosis, which is rare in such replantations, our protocol is to start dextran-40 at a rate of 25 mL/h at the time of anastomosis. In addition, aspirin is started immediately after surgery. The dextran-40 is discontinued on postoperative day 5 if the part is doing well, and aspirin is continued for 1 month. If there is significant vessel damage, which is almost always the case, a heparin infusion titrated to bleeding or clinical examination is strongly considered.

In general, however, ear, lip, and tongue replants do not have adequate venous outflow even when venous anastomoses are performed. Although numerous different protocols have been reported by various authors in case reports and short case series, we apply a protocol for artery-only digital replantation, which we previously published based on a series of 19 cases (Figure 29-9) (56). In addition to aspirin and dextran, a heparin infusion is started immediately. The heparin is titrated to a controlled bleed and relief of venous congestion rather than laboratory values, although blood work does need

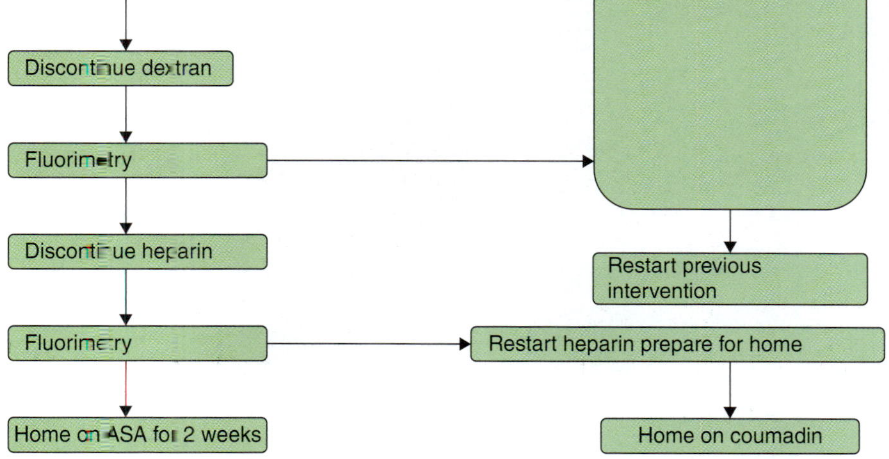

FIGURE 29-9 Artery-only pharmacologic protocol for digital replantation. We use subvisual quantitative fluorimetry as a complementary modality to clinical examination; however decisions may be based on clinical examination alone if fluorimetry is not available.

to be performed to avoid excessive anticoagulation. Mechanical scrubbing with heparin-soaked gauze can be performed on any exposed wounds or denuded skin. Leeches are used both to relieve venous congestion and for a local anticoagulation effect from the hirudin found in their saliva. Because *Aeromonas* spp. have been cultured from leech saliva, targeted prophylactic antibiotics such as a fluoroquinolone should be administered if they are used (57). Various other mechanical and chemical leeching maneuvers have been reported in literature, including deepithelialization, punctures and small incisions, and local injection of anticoagulants such as subcutaneous heparin.

About postoperative day 6, if the part is doing well, leeches and scrubs are discontinued. If the part continues to do well, this is followed by discontinuation of the dextran and then the heparin infusion. If the part does well initially but becomes congested after discontinuation of the heparin infusion, transition to postdischarge oral Coumadin for a period of several weeks is considered.

OUTCOMES, CASES, AND PHOTOS

Case 1: Ear Replantation

A 21-year-old male driver was involved in a motor vehicle rollover, sustaining an avulsion amputation of his entire right ear, as well as a cervical spine compression fracture (Figure 29-10A). While the patient was being evaluated and stabilized, the amputated part was brought to a tagging table in the OR, where a 0.5-mm artery was identified at the junction of the middle and upper thirds of the ear (Figure 29-10B). A nearby vein was also identified. An artery was found on the patient in the postauricular area but was deemed too damaged for use as inflow. Therefore, the superficial temporal vessels were elevated and divided in the temporoparietal area and then transposed for anastomosis to the artery and vein on the part using 11-0 nylon. The ear perfused immediately, and IV dextran-40 was started at 25 mL/h. The ear was then loosely inset with 4-0 and 5-0 nylons (Figure 29-10C). Aspirin was administered perioperatively.

After surgery, the ear became congested within several hours, so a heparin drip was started and titrated to congestion and bleeding. Intermittent leech therapy was used as well (Figure 29-10D). The congestion resolved except for an area isolated to the lobule. The heparin was discontinued on postoperative day 5, the dextran-40 was discontinued on postoperative day 10, and the patient was discharged home on postoperative day 13 with a viable ear except for a small area of necrosis on the distal lobule. In total, the patient received 8 units of packed red blood cells. The necrotic portion of the lobule was excised and closed primarily 4 weeks after surgery and ultimately healed well (Figure 29-10E).

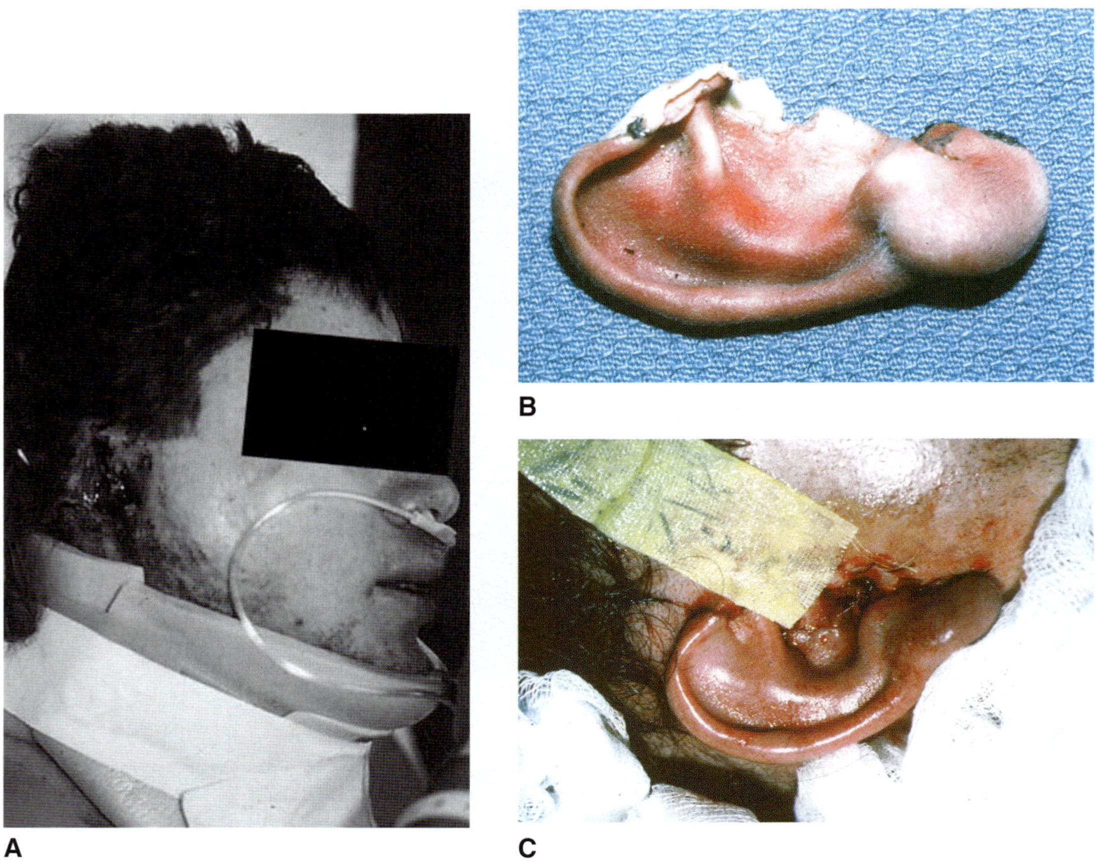

FIGURE 29-10 Case 1. (**A**) A 21-year-old male involved in a motor vehicle rollover, sustaining an avulsion amputation of his right ear, as well as a cervical spine compression fracture. (**B**) The amputated ear, a 0.5-mm artery, and a nearby vein were identified at the junction of the middle and upper thirds of the ear. (**C**) The amputated ear loosely inset after arterial and venous anastomoses.

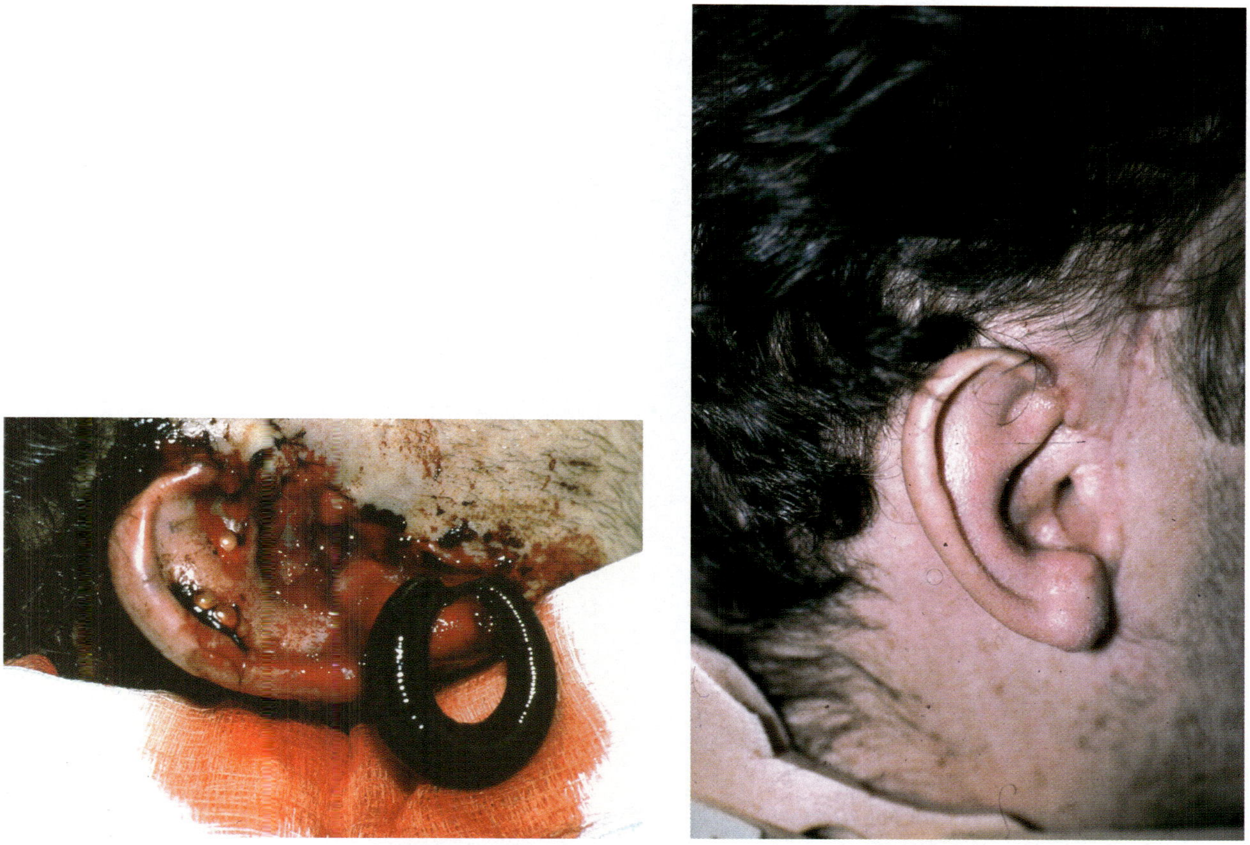

D E

FIGURE 29-10 (*Continued*) (**D**) The congested ear treated with a heparin drip and intermittent leech therapy in addition to dextran-40 and aspirin. (**E**) Follow-up several months after replantation demonstrated an aesthetic outcome.

Case 2: Lip Replantation

A 35-year-old male patient was involved in an altercation, resulting in a human bite amputation of his central lower lip (Figure 29-11A). Before the patient's arrival in the OR, the part was brought to a tagging table where a single 0.5-mm right labial artery was identified (Figure 29-11B). No adequate veins could be found. Intubation was performed via a nasal Rae tube.

After surgery, the patient was managed using an artery-only replant protocol. Leeches were used for the first few days as needed to treat congestion (Figure 29-11C). Aspirin and dextran-40 were administered for 5 days. A heparin drip, titrated to bleeding, was discontinued on postoperative day 7. A total of 2 units of packed red blood cells was transfused. The patient was discharged on postoperative day 7 with the replanted lip fully viable (Figure 29-11D). Subsequent follow-up demonstrated full survival of the replanted segment with good oral competence (Figure 29-11E).

Case 3: Tongue Replantation

An unrestrained 15-year-old male patient was involved in a motor vehicle collision and bit down on his tongue on impact, amputating 4 cm from the distal tip. Upon presentation to the emergency department, the patient had significant intraoral bleeding, which was managed by lateral decubitus positioning for airway protection and clipping of the lingual arteries. While a tracheostomy was being performed under ketamine sedation and local anesthetic, the part was brought to a tagging table in the OR (Figure 29-12A). Both lingual arteries along with accompanying veins were identified on the part. The left lingual artery measured 1.5 mm in diameter and was significantly larger than the diminutive right lingual artery.

Intraoperatively, the patient's alveolar fractures were treated first to avoid any significant manipulation within the oral cavity after replantation. The proximal stump of the tongue was retracted forward to the level of the incisors using heavy silk sutures (Figure 29-12B). The left lingual artery was repaired without excessive tension. However, the accompanying vein was retracted into the stump and too friable to use for venous outflow. A dorsal foot vein was harvested and anastomosed from the distal part to the ipsilateral facial vein through the floor of the mouth. A bite block was left in place. Total ischemia time was 8 hours, and operative time was 6 hours.

After surgery, as expected, the tongue became extremely edematous. Clinical assessment supplemented with quantitative fluorimetry was used for monitoring. Aspirin and dextran-40 were administered for 5 days. A total of 5 units of packed red blood cells was transfused. The tracheostomy was decannulated on postoperative day 12, and the patient progressed from a liquid diet to a solid diet over the next 2 months. Sensory return was noted 1 cm past the amputation site at that point despite the lack of a nerve repair. Functional mobility of the tongue was essentially normal, as were speech and articulation (Figures 29-12C to 29-12E).

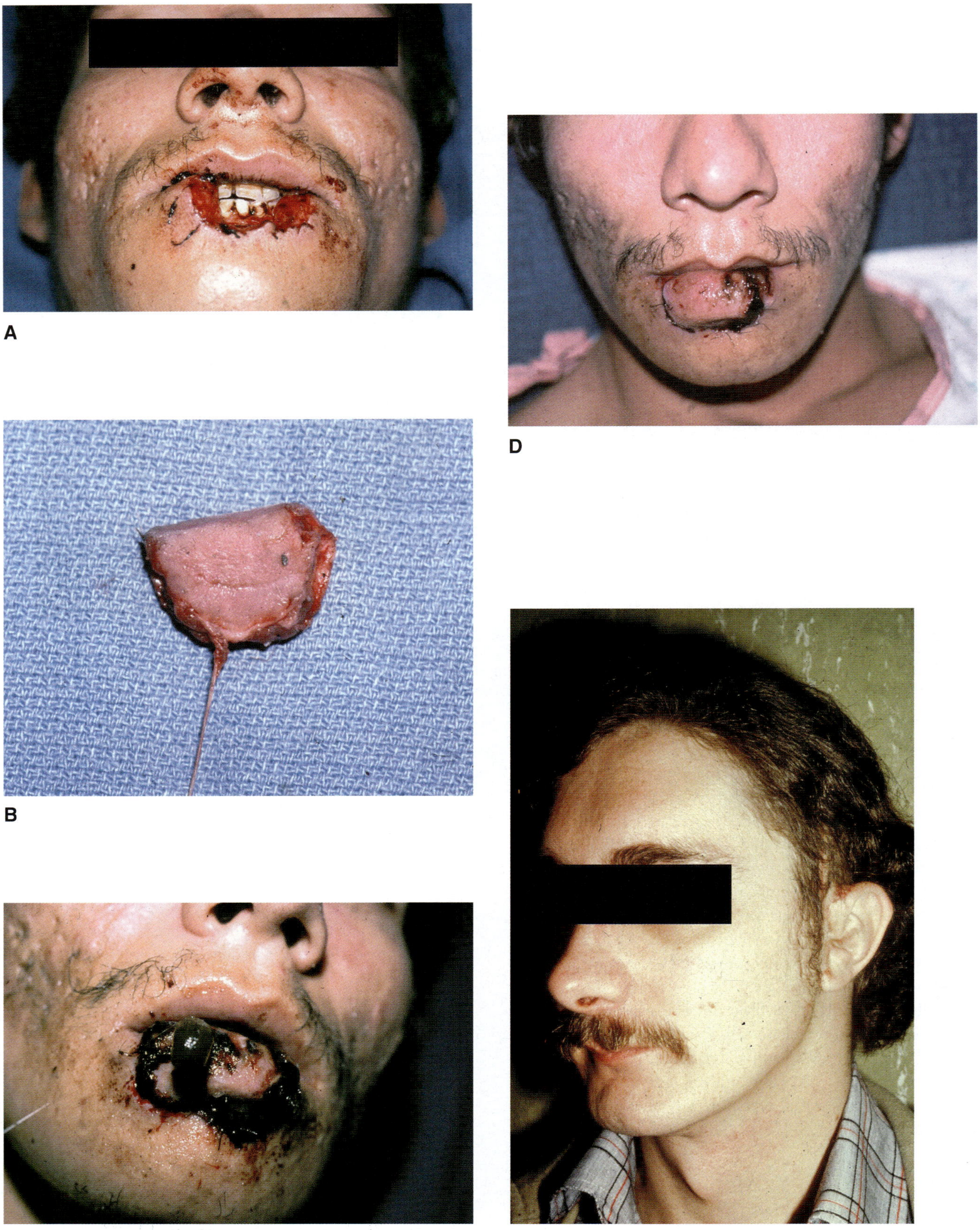

FIGURE 29-11 Case 2. (**A**) A 35-year-old male patient involved in an altercation, resulting in a human bite amputation of his central lower lip. (**B**) The amputated lower lip segment; a 0.5-mm right labial artery was identified, but no adequate vein could be found. (**C**) Leeches were used for the first few days as needed to treat congestion in addition to a heparin drip, dextran-40, and aspirin. (**D**) The fully viable replanted lip upon discharge on postoperative day 7. (**E**) Subsequent follow-up demonstrated full survival of the replanted segment with good oral competence.

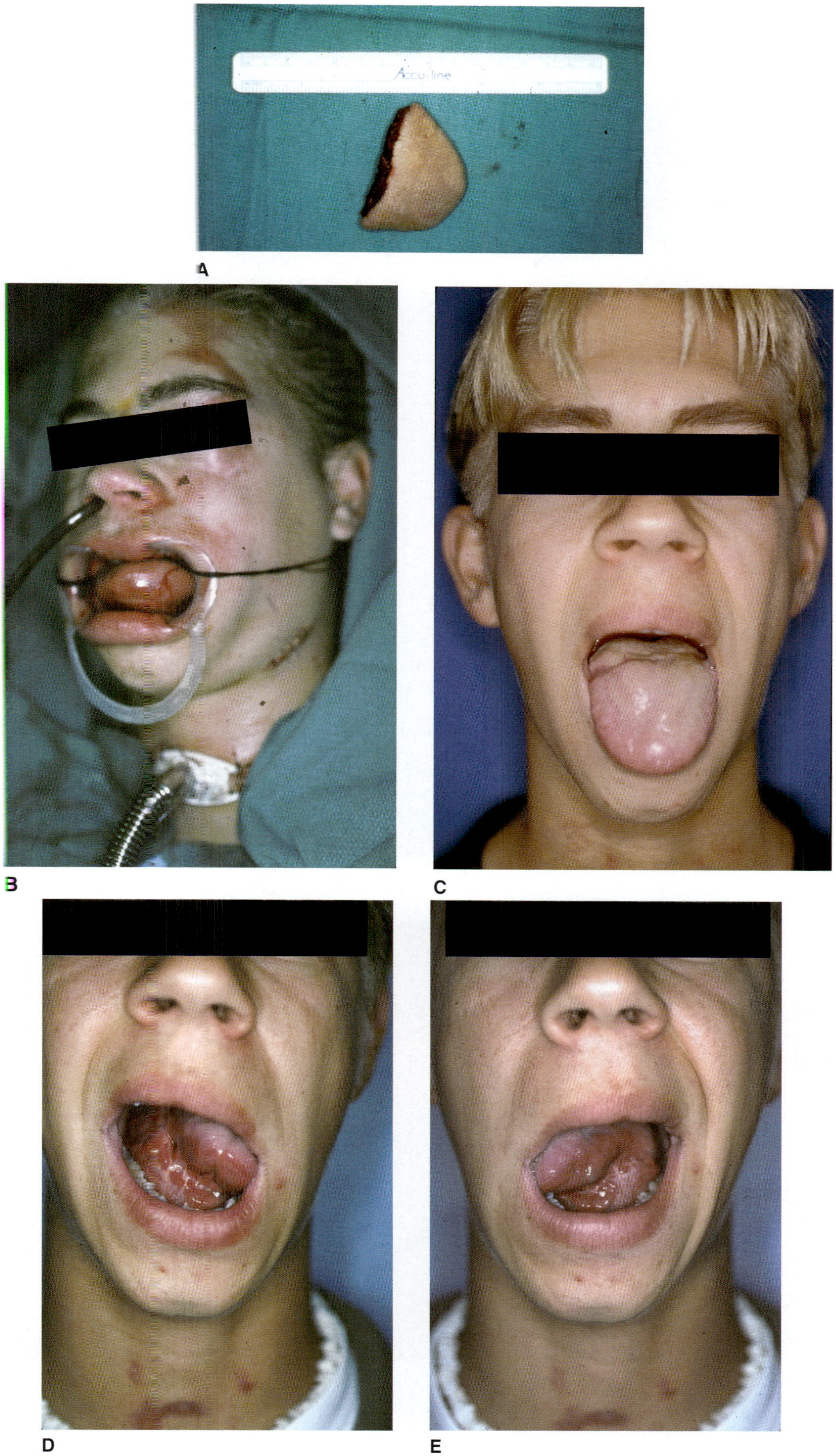

FIGURE 29-12 Case 3. (**A**) The amputated tongue measuring 4 cm long by 5 cm wide. (**B**) The proximal stump of the tongue retracted forward to the level of the incisors using heavy silk sutures. (**C**) to (**E**) Essentially normal functional mobility of the tongue, as well as normal speech and articulation on follow-up.

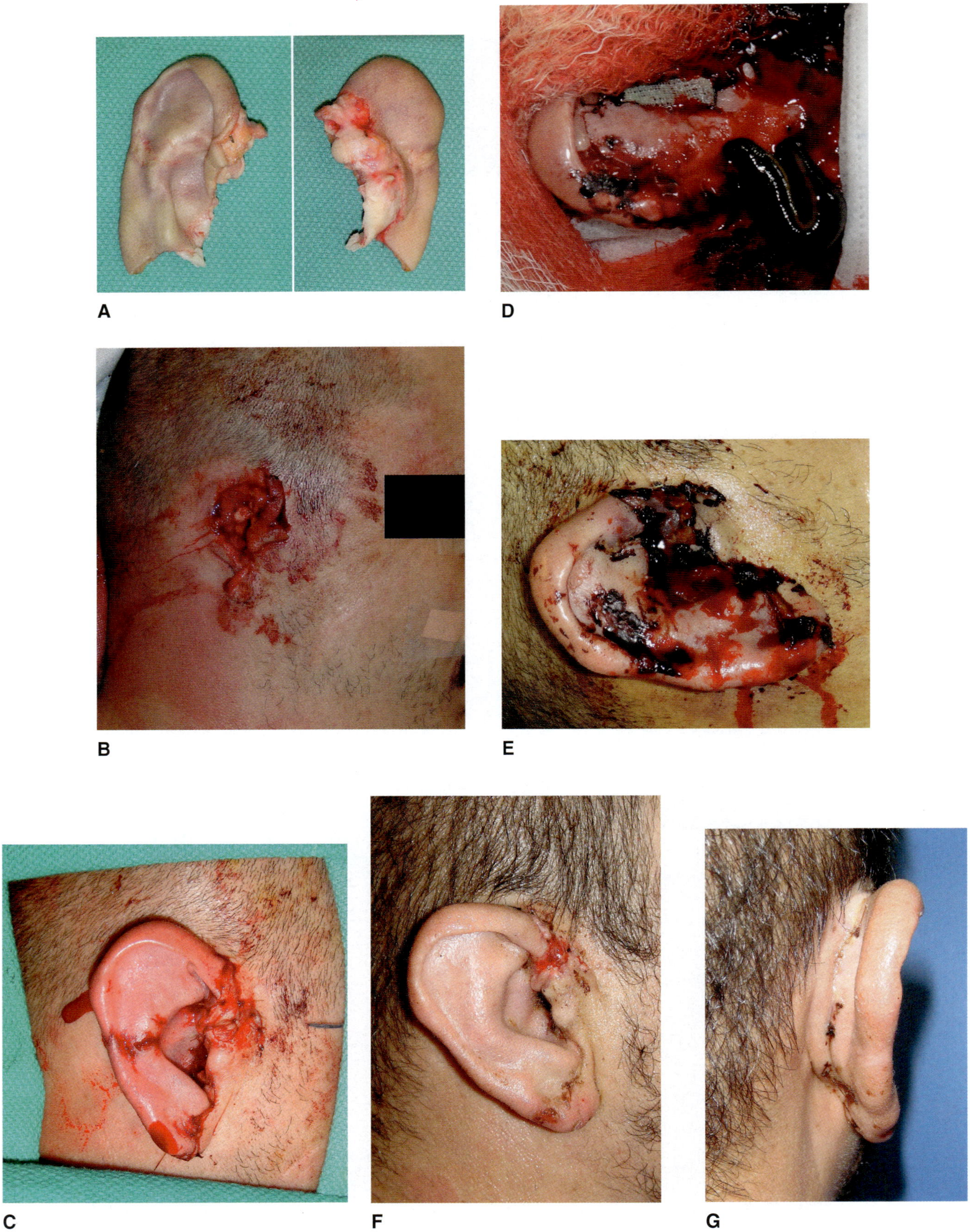

FIGURE 29-13 Case 4. (**A**) A 20-year-old prisoner with a human bite amputation of 90% of his right ear. (**B**) A small inferior portion of the lobule remained intact. (**C**) After arterial anastomosis and loose inset, the ear immediately became pink and perfused. (**D**) A small ellipse of skin near the lobule was excised for postoperative bleeding and monitoring. Medicinal leeches were placed on this wound as needed to treat congestion. (**E**) On postoperative 7, after discontinuation of dextran-40, heparin, and medicinal leeches, the ear remained viable without evidence of congestion. (**F**) and (**G**) Full survival of the replanted ear at 3-week follow-up.

Case 4: Partial Ear Replantation

A 20-year-old male prisoner was involved in an altercation in which he sustained a human bite amputation of 90% of his ear, leaving only part of the lobule intact (Figures 29-13A and 29-13B). On the tagging table, an artery and vein were found at the level of the lobule, and two additional arteries measuring less than 0.5 mm in diameter were found posteriorly at the mid-ear level. A branch of the posterior auricular artery was also found at that level. The ear was first inset anteriorly using absorbable sutures and then retracted forward with skin staples to provide access for microvascular anastomosis. Under the microscope, it was clear that the lobular vessels were inadequate because of multilevel injury. An anastomosis was performed between one of the postauricular vessels and the posterior auricular artery branch using simple interrupted 11-0 nylon sutures. The ear turned pink immediately upon release of the clamps. The staples were then released, and the posterior inset was performed with loose interrupted absorbable sutures (Figure 29-13C). A small ellipse of skin was excised for postoperative bleeding and monitoring.

After surgery, we placed the patient on our artery-only digital replantation protocol with a dextran-40 infusion, a heparin infusion titrated to bleeding and congestion, aspirin, and medicinal leeches (Figure 29-13D). On postoperative 6, the leeches and dextran-40 infusion were discontinued. The ear remained viable without evidence of ischemia or congestion, so the heparin drip was discontinued on postoperative day 7 (Figure 29-13E). On postoperative day 9, the patient was discharged to prison. He received a total of 8 units of packed red blood cells. Follow-ups at 3 and 8 weeks demonstrated full survival of the replanted part (Figures 29-13F and 29-13G).

REFERENCES

1. Kind GM. Microvascular ear replantation. *Clin Plast Surg* 2002;29(2):233–248.
2. Buntic RF, Buncke HJ. Successful replantation of an amputated tongue. *Plast Reconstr Surg* 1998;101(6):1604–1607.
3. Buncke HJ, Schulz WP. Total ear reimplantation in the rabbit utilising microminiature vascular anastomoses. *Br J Plast Surg* 1966;19(1):15–22.
4. Steffen A, Katzbach R, Klaiber S. A comparison of ear reattachment methods: a review of 25 years since Pennington. *Plast Reconstr Surg* 2006;118(6):1358–1364.
5. Pennington DG, Lai MF, Pelly AD. Successful replantation of a completely avulsed ear by microvascular anastomosis. *Plast Reconstr Surg* 1980;65(6):820–823.
6. Akyürek M, Safak T, Kecik A. Microsurgical ear replantation without venous repair. *Ann Plast Surg* 2001;46(4):439–442.
7. Cavadas PC. Supramicrosurgical ear replantation: case report. *J Reconstr Microsurg* 2002;18(5):393–395.
8. Cho BH, Ahn HB. Microsurgical replantation of a partial ear, with leech therapy. *Ann Plast Surg* 1999;43(4):427–429.
9. Concannon MJ, Puckett CL. Microsurgical replantation of an ear in a child without venous repair. *Plast Reconstr Surg* 1998;102(6):2088–2093.
10. Elsahy N. Ear replantation. *Clin Plast Surg* 2002;29(2):221–231.
11. Finical SJ, Keller KM, Lovett JE. Postoperative ramifications of total ear replantation. *Ann Plast Surg* 1998;41(6):657–670.
12. Horta R, Costa-Ferreira A, Costa J, et al. Ear replantation after human bite avulsion injury. *J Craniofac Surg* 2011;22(4):1457–1459.
13. Jung S-N, Yoon S, Kwon H, Yim Y-M. Successful replantation of an amputated earlobe by microvascular anastomosis. *J Craniofac Surg* 2009;20(3):822–824.
14. Kim KS, Kim ES, Hwang JH, Lee SY. Microsurgical replantation of a partial helix of the ear. *Microsurgery* 2009;29(7):548–551.
15. Kind G, Buncke G. Total ear replantation. *Plast Reconstr Surg* 1997;99(7):1858–1867.
16. Lin P-Y, Chiang Y-C, Hsieh C-H, Jeng S-F. Microsurgical replantation and salvage procedures in traumatic ear amputation. *J Trauma* 2010;69(4):E15–E19.
17. Nath RK, Kraemer BA, Azizzadeh A. Complete ear replantation without venous anastomosis. *Microsurgery* 1998;18(4):282–285.
18. Shelley OP, Villafane O, Watson SB. Successful partial ear replantation after prolonged ischaemia time. *Br J Plast Surg* 2000;53(1):76–77.
19. Talbi M, Stussi JD, Meley M. Microsurgical replantation of a totally amputated ear without venous repair. *J Reconstr Microsurg* 2001;17(6):417–420.
20. Trovato MJ, Agarwal JP. Successful replantation of the ear as a venous flap. *Ann Plast Surg* 2008;61(2):164–168.
21. Wong W, Wilson P, Savundra J. Total ear replantation using the distal radial artery perforator. *J Plast Reconstr Aesthet Surg* 2011;64(5):677–679.
22. James NJ. Survival of large replanted segment of upper lip and nose. Case report. *Plast Reconstr Surg* 1976;58(5):623–625.
23. Hirasé Y, Kojima T, Hayashi J, Nakano M. Successful upper labial replantation after 17 hours of ischemia: case report. *J Reconstr Microsurg* 1993;9(5):327–329.
24. Baj A, Beltramini GA, Laganà F, Giannì AB. Microsurgical upper lip replantation: a case report. *J Oral Maxillofac Surg* 2010;68(3):664–667.
25. Taylor H, Andrews B. Lip replantation and delayed inset after a dog bite: a case report and literature review. *Microsurgery* 2009;29(8):657–661.
26. Seki JT, Haugen C. Lip Reconstruction. In Weinzweig J (ed). *Plastic Surgery Secrets*. Philadelphia: Hanley & Belfus, 1999, pp. 211–215.
27. Duroure F, Simon E, Fadhul S, et al. Microsurgical lip replantation: evaluation of functional and aesthetic results of three cases. *Microsurgery* 2004;24(4):265–269.
28. Schubert W, Kimberley B, Guzman-Stein G, Cunningham BL. Use of the labial artery for replantation of the lip and chin. *Ann Plast Surg* 1988;20(3):256–260.
29. Hendrick RGJ, Tiwari P. Successful replantation of upper lip avulsion injury using an arterialized venous anastomosis. *Plast Reconstr Surg* 2012;130(4):628e–629e.
30. Wong SS, Wang ML. Successful replantation of an bitten-off lower lip: case report. *J Trauma* 1999;47(3):602–604.
31. Crawford CR, Hagerty RC. Survival of an upper lip aesthetic complex using arterial reanastomosis only. *Ann Plast Surg* 1991;27(1):77–79.
32. Holtje WJ. Successful replantation of an amputated upper lip. *Plast Reconstr Surg* 1984;73(4):664–668.
33. Liliav B, Zaluzec R, Hassid VJ, et al. Lip replantation: a viable option for lower lip reconstruction after human bites, a literature review and proposed management algorithm. *J Plast Reconstr Aesthet Surg* 2012;65(7):e197–e199.
34. Walton RL, Beahm EK, Brown RE, et al. Microsurgical replantation of the lip: a multi-institutional experience. *Plast Reconstr Surg* 1998;102(2):358–368.
35. Venter TH, Duminy FJ. Microvascular replantation of avulsed tissue after a dog bite of the face. *South Afr Med J* 1994;84(1):37–39.
36. Jeng SF, Wei FC, Noordhoff MS. Successful replantation of a bitten-off vermilion of the lower lip by microvascular anastomosis: case report. *J Trauma* 1992;33(6):914–916.
37. Jeng SF, Wei FC, Noordhoff MS. Replantation of amputated facial tissues with microvascular anastomosis. *Microsurgery* 1994;15(5):327–333.
38. Husami TW, Cervino AL, Pennington GA, Douglas BK. Replantation of an amputated upper lip. *Microsurgery* 1992;13(3):155–156.
39. Davis C, Armstrong J. Replantation of an amputated tongue. *Plast Reconstr Surg* 2001;108(5):1441–1442.
40. Egozi E, Faulkner B, Lin KY. Successful revascularization following near-complete amputation of the tongue. *Ann Plast Surg* 2006;56(2):190–193.
41. Kim JS, Choi TH, Kim NG, et al. The replantation of an amputated tongue by supermicrosurgery. *J Plast Reconstr Aesthet Surg* 2007;60(10):1152–1155.
42. Agur AMR, Dalley AF (eds). *Grant's Atlas of Anatomy*, 13th ed. Baltimore: Lippincott Williams & Wilkins, 2012, pp. 888.
43. Park C, Lineaweaver WC, Rumly TO, Buncke HJ. Arterial supply of the anterior ear. *Plast Reconstr Surg* 1992;90(1):38–44.
44. Bauer BS, Fortes P. Ear reconstruction. In Weinzweig J (ed). *Plastic Surgery Secrets*. Philadelphia: Hanley & Belfus, 1999, pp. 207–211.
45. Yuksel E, Weinfeld A, Shenaq S. Reconstruction of the oral cavity. In Weinzweig J (ed). *Plastic Surgery Secrets*. Philadelphia: Hanley & Belfus, 1999, pp. 215–221.
46. Buncke GM. Replantation and revascularization. In Mathes SJ (ed). *Plastic Surgery*, vol. 8: *The Hand and Upper Limb, Part 2*, 2nd ed. Philadelphia: Saunders, 2005, pp. 565–585.

47. Baj A, Beltramini G, Lagana F, et al. Amputation trauma of the face: surgical techniques and microsurgical replantations. *Acta Otorhinolaryngol Ital* 2009;29(2):92–96.
48. Buntic RF, Buncke HJ. Replantation and revascularization. In Weinzweig J (ed). *Plastic Surgery Secrets*. Philadelphia: Hanley & Belfus, 1999, pp. 513–516.
49. Grabb WC, Dingman RO. The fate of amputated tissues of the head and neck following replacement. *Plast Reconstr Surg* 1972;49(1):28–32.
50. Jones NF. Replantation in the upper extremity. In Thorne CH, Bartlett SP, Beasley RW, et al (eds). *Grabb & Smith's Plastic Surgery*, 6th ed. Baltimore: Lippincott Williams & Wilkins, 2007, pp. 868–883.
51. Pederson WC. Principles of microvascular surgery. In Wolfe S, Hotchkiss R, Pederson W, Kozin S (eds). *Green's Operative Hand Surgery*, 6th ed. Philadelphia: Elsevier, 2010, pp. 1553–1584.
52. Wilson GR, Jones BM. The damaging effect of smoking on digital revascularisation: two further case reports. *Br J Plast Surg* 1984;37(4): 613–614.
53. Chang LD, Buncke G, Slezak S, Buncke HJ. Cigarette smoking, plastic surgery, and microsurgery. *J Reconstr Microsurg* 1996;12(7):467–474.
54. Mladick RA, Horton CE, Adamson JE, Cohen BI. The pocket principle: a new technique for the reattachment of a severed ear part. *Plast Reconstr Surg* 1971;48(3):219–223.
55. Juri J, Irigaray A, Juri C, et al. Ear replantation. *Plast Reconstr Surg* 1987;80(3):431–435.
56. Buntic RF, Brooks D. Standardized protocol for artery-only fingertip replantation. *J Hand Surg Am* 2010;35(9):1491–1496.
57. Daane SP. Leeches. In Weinzweig J (ed). *Plastic Surgery Secrets*. Philadelphia: Hanley & Belfus, 1999, pp. 439–441.

CHAPTER 30

Three-Dimensional Modeling in Head and Neck Reconstructive Surgery

Roman J. Skoracki and Matthew M. Hanasono

Advances in imaging, rigid fixation, and microvascular free tissue transfer of bone and composite tissues have greatly increased our ability to reconstruct complex congenital, traumatic, and oncologic defects of the facial skeleton. Nevertheless, complex reconstructions for these defects remain among the most difficult and arduous surgeries. Failure to precisely restore the height, width, and projection of the facial skeleton can be aesthetically and functionally devastating given its critical role in supporting the soft tissues of the face as well as in respiration, speech, swallowing, and mastication. Finding methods to improve the accuracy and speed of these procedures represents a major challenge to surgeons performing head and neck reconstruction.

COMPUTER-AIDED DESIGN SOFTWARE

Three-dimensional reformatting of sequential planar images, such as those acquired by fine-cut computed tomography (CT), has become routine practice to assist in the visualization, orientation, and diagnosis of various traumatic and disease processes that affect the craniofacial skeleton. In addition to producing three-dimensional computer representations of the facial skeleton, computer-aided design (CAD) software can be used to manipulate these images to "virtually" perform resections and reconstructions to assist with planning the actual surgery (1,2). Medical CAD packages, which were initially engineered for applications in neurosurgery and radiation therapy, that simplify such manipulations are now commercially available from a number of vendors for various applications in congenital craniofacial surgery, orthognathic surgery, dental implant surgery, and head and neck reconstructive surgery (3).

Computed tomography data are saved in Digital Imaging and Communications in Medicine (DICOM) format files and then exported to CAD software. The software then reassembles the two-dimensional images into a three-dimensional representation that can be rotated and viewed from any angle and digitally manipulated as the user desires. When parts of the facial skeleton are severely distorted or misaligned, such as by tumor, trauma, or prior surgery, CAD software can "erase" these parts and replace them with idealized parts, for example, by creating a mirror image of the normal side.

Next, a reconstruction can be planned using CAD software. In microvascular reconstructive surgery, a virtual fibula free flap can be shaped to create a symmetric and orthognathically optimal reconstruction in which the occlusal plane of the reconstructed mandible or maxilla matches the opposing native occlusal plane. Reconstructions can be checked from multiple angles to verify that they are accurate. The original skeleton or an idealized version of the original skeleton can also be translucently overlaid onto the reconstructed skeleton to verify that the reconstruction accurately restores the premorbid facial morphology. Osseointegrated implant placement for dental prosthetic retention can also be virtually planned.

Other uses of CAD software in reconstructive surgery include creation of patient-specific implants (4). Patient-specific implants have been commercially made of titanium, acrylics, ceramics or polyetheretherketone (PEEK, a thermoplastic) for missing craniofacial bones, most commonly, of the calvarium (5,6). These implants are most useful when the exact dimensions of the defect are already known and have been imaged because intraoperative contouring, although still possible, takes away from the time savings associated with customization. Thus, they are mostly used for delayed reconstruction. Additionally, preformed titanium mesh plates have been created using CAD software from a composite of normal orbital data (Synthes, Paoli, PA) (3).

RAPID PROTOTYPE MODELING

Advances in computer technology have resulted not only in the ability to produce three-dimensional virtual representations of the facial skeleton but also to create physical models using special printers that use serial material deposition to construct a three-dimensional object as a stack of slices, a technique known as rapid prototype modeling (RPM) (7–9). This technique, originally developed for industrial applications, usually involves either a powder substrate that is bound by selective application of glue or a polymer liquid that is cured by a laser, a technique known as stereolithography. These methods result in a physical model within minutes to hours, depending on the size of the model being built and the material used. Polymer acrylic models have the advantage of being sterilizable using gas sterilization, facilitating their use intraoperatively. Additionally, metal models can be built by melting particles together with an electron beam (electron beam melting) or a laser (selective laser sintering). Selective laser sintering is a process that is also used in the creation of models made from plastic, ceramics, or glass.

Rapid prototype modeling was first used in reconstructive surgery to provide added information in surgical treatment planning for orthognathic, congenital, and traumatic craniofacial deformities using osteotomies and rigid fixation (8–11). RPM has been shown to be highly accurate when compared with the actual skeleton, with an error of approximately 1.5 mm to as little as 0.016 mm, although, just as in CT imaging, some very thin, delicate structural detail can be lost because of partial volume-averaging artifacts (12,13). Such losses, occurring mainly in the regions of the orbital floors or walls of the paranasal sinuses, can be minimized by obtaining CT slices less than 1.5 mm in thickness; however, for some applications, such detail is not necessary and exposes the patient to unnecessary radiation.

In orthognathic, congenital, and posttraumatic patients, models of the affected facial skeleton give the surgeon a greater understanding of the three-dimensional nature of the deformity or anticipated defect. Tactile representation of the facial skeleton provides additional data for surgical planning, for example, for designing corrective osteotomies and the vectors needed in distraction osteogenesis. In addition, osteotomies and fixation can be performed on the model as a presurgical practice run in the laboratory setting to help ensure optimal outcomes.

More recently, several reports have shown that this technology is useful in planning head and neck reconstruction with vascularized bone flaps (14–18). In these cases, models are made of the virtually reconstructed facial skeleton, including the bony free flap reconstruction designed using CAD software. Beyond surgical planning, however, rapid prototype models can be created and used as templates to bend titanium hardware used for flap fixation during or before surgery (19–21). In addition to facial skeletal models, computer-generated custom cutting guides can be manufactured using RPM technology to help make osteotomies at the appropriate angles and lengths to precisely match the virtual plan, saving operative time and increasing reconstructive accuracy. Future applications might include a role in tissue engineering, in which the rapid prototype model is used to create a custom scaffold for tissue-engineered bone (13).

STEREOTACTIC NAVIGATION

Image-guided intraoperative stereotactic navigation now has a long history of use in neurologic and sinonasal surgery (22,23). More recently, stereotactic navigation has been used in craniofacial surgery to verify correct positioning of the reconstructed orbital wall after surgery for trauma (24) and in oncologic surgery to verify that the resection in patients with maxillofacial fibrous dysplasia results in symmetry with the normal contralateral side (2). In microvascular reconstructive surgery, the same stereotactic navigation systems used for neurologic and sinonasal surgery can be used to assist with difficult insetting of free flap constructs, particularly when access is limited and accurate positioning is crucial.

All stereotactic navigation systems incorporate a computer to track the location of instruments and the patient in space. Four different tracking systems have been developed, including optical, electromagnetic, electromechanical, and ultrasonographic (3). Optical tracking systems are currently the most commonly used and may be classified as active or passive. Active tracking systems use infrared light-emitting diodes (LED's) attached to the patient and the surgical instruments. As long as the LEDs stay within the line of sight of a digital camera, the location of the instrument and the patient can be accurately presented on the computer monitor. In passive tracking systems, reflective spheres rather than LEDs bounce infrared light back from an emission source to a receiver. Both the emitter and the receiver are located within the camera unit.

All navigation systems require performing a registration process to accurately define the location of the patient. Before the start of surgery, fiducial markers placed on various points of the patient's face are identified with a navigation probe, allowing the system to integrate x, y, and z coordinates on the patient with x', y', and z' coordinates on the images loaded into the navigation system workstation. These images are from scans (either CT or magnetic resonance imaging) obtained with the patient wearing fiducial markers before the surgery. During this registration process, either a headset or a navigation array replaces the fiducial markers. The headset is convenient and noninvasive but usually minimizes access to the midface and orbits. The navigation array allows free movement of the head during surgery without the need for repeating the registration process but must be rigidly fixed to the patient's head by means of small incisions and screw placement into calvarial bone. Accuracy after registration is usually within about 1 mm (25). Some navigation systems, such as StealthStation (Medtronic-Xomed, Jacksonville, FL) or VectorVision (BrainLab, Munich, Germany), allow for a markerless registration technique called surface matching in which a registration probe pointer is placed at multiple facial landmarks and correlated on the scan to the same anatomic site. This provides the navigation system with a contour map of the head. The computer workstation then quantifies the registration error as an index for the accuracy of the matching procedure between the surgical surface anatomy and the computer display. Generally, the greater the number of landmarks used and the thinner and less mobile the soft tissue envelope, the more accurate the registration. Surface matching is usually more time consuming but noninvasive and does not require an additional CT scan with fiducial markers.

Some CAD programs (e.g., Surgi Case CMF, Materialise, Leuven, Belgium) allow conversion of the virtually altered images back to DICOM format files. These files can then be combined with the preoperative CT data and uploaded into the navigation system central processing unit (CPU). During surgery, the location of the real-world reconstruction can be compared with the planned position of the virtual reconstruction. This allows the surgeon to verify that the position of the free flap construct matches the planned position. In facial reconstructions, malposition of a vascularized bone flap by as little as a few millimeters can result in malocclusion or orbital malposition, as well as distortion of facial landmarks, although this can be camouflaged by soft tissues or later contouring to some extent.

INDICATIONS

We believe that the strongest indications for use of virtual planning with CAD software and RPM to assist with microvascular free flap mandibular reconstruction are in patients with missing, fractured, or distorted mandibles. In these cases, the original architecture of the mandible is not easy to visualize, and accurate bending of titanium plates and contouring of the flap may be difficult or impossible. Also, in very extensive defects, virtual planning allows a preoperative estimate of the length of linear bone needed to reconstruct the mandible. For near-total mandibular defects, these measurements are helpful in verifying that the amount of fibular bone is adequate to reconstruct the defect. If the segmental defect is longer than the length of the available fibula, redesigning the reconstruction by setting the mandible back or considering a second flap or graft is an option before committing to intraoperative osteotomies.

For less experienced surgeons, preoperative virtual planning and RPM may be useful for the majority of reconstructions to visualize the defect and make the surgery more straightforward. The use of cutting guides also streamlines the process of making osteotomies. This is especially true of defects that include the anterior curvature of the mandible or the angle, ramus, and condyle. In these cases, virtual planning and use of a rapid prototype model saves time because of the relative complexity of free flap shaping to accommodate multiple curves and angles as well as the need for multiple osteotomies. Virtual planning and RPM is probably least useful, particularly in experienced hands, for small mandibular defects of the body, which are relatively straight and require few, if any, osteotomies to reconstruct.

We use virtual planning and RPM for nearly all midfacial reconstructions in which the use of bony free flaps is planned (26). In addition to planning and shaping the vascularized bone flap, we find that models are very useful when extensive use of titanium or bone grafts is needed, particularly around the orbit to shape hardware accurately. Stereotactic navigation is very useful to confirm positioning in midfacial reconstruction, particularly when access is limited because of minimal or no facial incisions. Unlike the mandible, which is well exposed through the neck, access to the midface is limited even when the upper lip has been split and a lateral rhinotomy incision has been made. With stereotactic navigation, however, even extensive maxillectomy defects can often be reconstructed accurately without facial incisions through a transoral approach alone (26).

TECHNIQUE: MANDIBULAR RECONSTRUCTION

Vascularized bone flaps are the gold standard for reconstructing most mandibular defects, and excellent aesthetic and functional results are routinely achieved. Although nearly all bony free flaps have been described for use in mandibular reconstruction, the fibula free flap is the preferred flap in most centers because of its long usable length, reliability, relative ease of harvest, and good-quality bone stock for placement of osseointegrated implants (27). Because of this, current CAD software is adapted toward use of the fibula flap for mandibular reconstruction, although in theory, the principles of virtual planning and RPM can be applied to any type of vascularized bone flap.

A virtual digital three-dimensional model of the facial skeleton, including not only the mandible but also the midface is first created using fine-cut (≤1.5 mm) axial CT data saved in DICOM format (Figure 30-1). Next, the reconstruction is planned by osteotomizing a fibula free flap on a virtual computer platform using CAD software specifically designed for this purpose (e.g., Surgi Case CMF) to match the contours of the mandibular segment that is absent or will be resected (Figure 30-2). The patient's own fibula may be used if a lower extremity CT scan is performed and imported as DICOM files. Otherwise, a standardized virtual fibula may be used.

The extent of the resection is estimated based on preoperative imaging and discussion with the resecting surgeon. The virtual reconstruction is adjusted as necessary so that the outer (lateral and inferior mandibular borders) contour of the mandible is restored and the reconstructed mandibular occlusal plane aligns with the maxillary dentition. The fibula is oriented such that the peroneal vessels assume a lingual position. In this case, the lateral surface of the fibula becomes the external (buccal-labial) surface of the new mandible.

We prefer to harvest fibula osteocutaneous free flap from the side that is contralateral to the side of the planned recipient vessels based on the shape of the fibula and the location of the cutaneous perforators, which emerge from the peroneal vessels along the posterior border of the bone. In this orientation, the perforators will emerge from the pedicle superiorly, so that the skin paddle can be used to reconstruct an intraoral defect. For reconstruction of an extraoral defect, the ipsilateral fibula is selected so that the perforators emerge inferiorly after the flap is inset. After a preliminary virtual reconstruction is created using the CAD software, the planned fibula free flap is checked to make sure it adequately restores the lower facial shape and aligns with the maxillary occlusion by rotating and reviewing it relative to the midfacial skeleton in multiple planes, and it is adjusted as necessary.

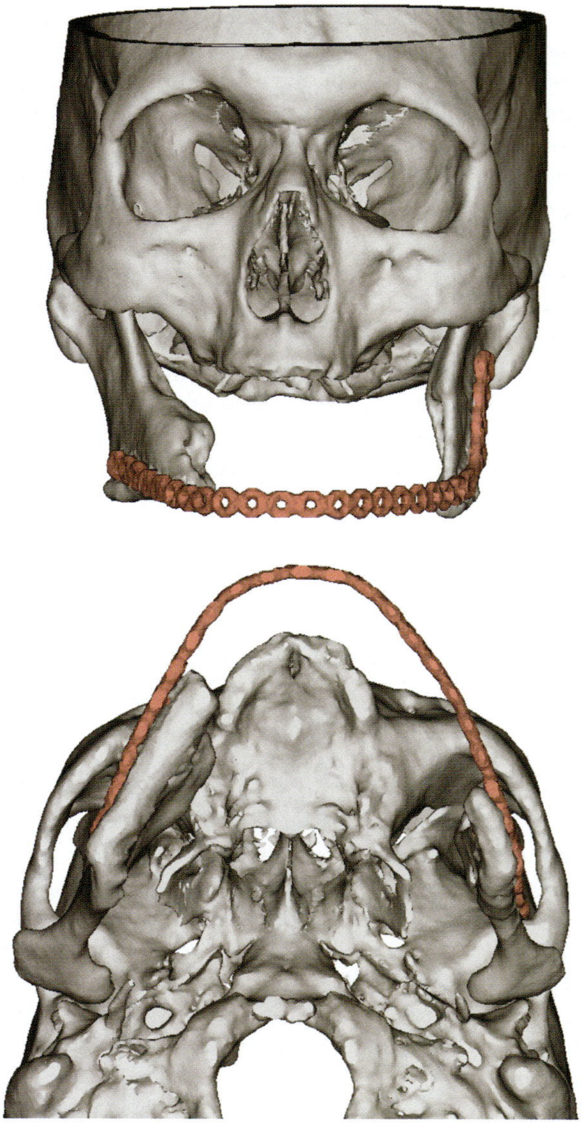

FIGURE 30-1 Three-dimensional computed tomography reconstruction of a patient who presented for delayed reconstruction after a segmental mandibulectomy for an ameloblastoma that was initially reconstructed with a titanium plate alone. Conventional fibula shaping can be difficult in the absence of the native mandible.

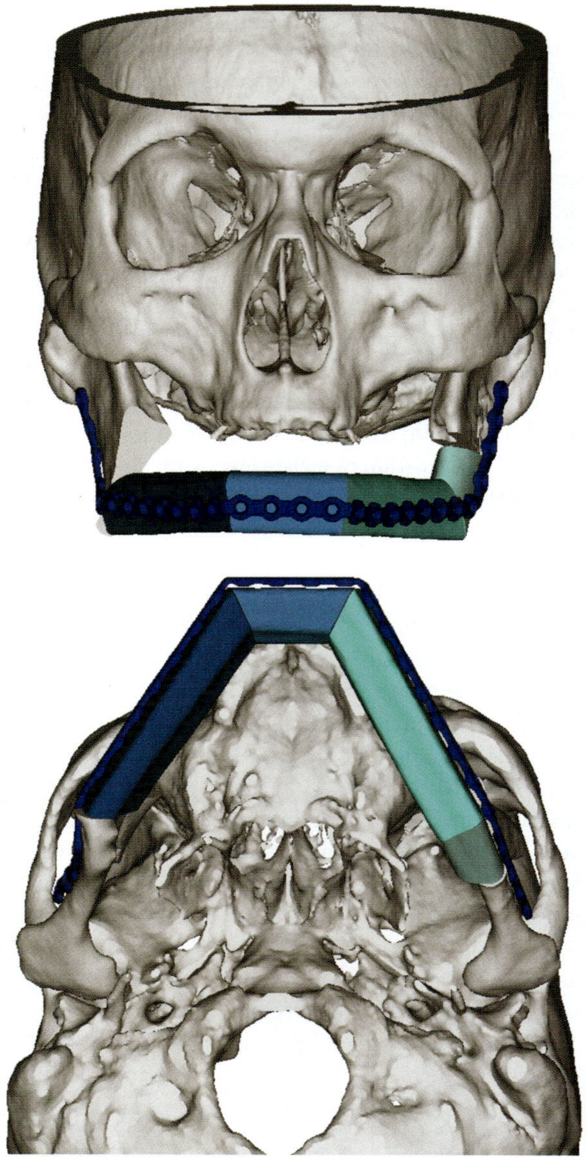

FIGURE 30-2 Preoperative virtual reconstruction with a fibula free flap extending from the right mandibular angle to the left mandibular ramus generated using computer-aided design software.

Acrylic physical models are then created using RPM technology. The models are sterilized before use in surgery for intraoperative use. Titanium plates are then bent to match the contours of the fibula and adjoining facial bones on the rapid prototype model, either before or during the surgery, by a second team, if possible, to save operative time (Figure 30-3). We prefer 2.0-mm locking reconstruction plates, although others prefer miniplates, which provide adequate stability. Occasionally, we find it helpful to have models of both the mandible in its normal unreconstructed state (or digitally restored to normal if parts were distorted or missing preoperatively) as well as in its reconstructed form, incorporating a shaped fibula flap, to refer to as a reference in case the extent of the resection changes during the surgery and the reconstruction needs to be adjusted accordingly.

Custom cutting guides are also manufactured using the same RPM process to assist in making the osteotomies needed to shape the fibula bone (Figures 30-4). During surgery, the cutting guide is temporarily fixed to the harvested fibula bone using 10-mm monocortical screws, and a reciprocating saw blade is inserted into slots in the cutting guide to make osteotomies at the precise angles and lengths required to replicate the virtual plan (Figure 30-5). Rigid fixation using the prebent titanium plate or plates is then performed (Figure 30-6). The flap is then inset and revascularized in the standard manner. Cutting guides intended to fit along the contours of the mandible to guide the mandibulectomy can also be manufactured to further increase the precision and accuracy of the reconstruction (Figure 30-7). A representative result after delayed near-total mandibular reconstruction is shown in Figure 30-8.

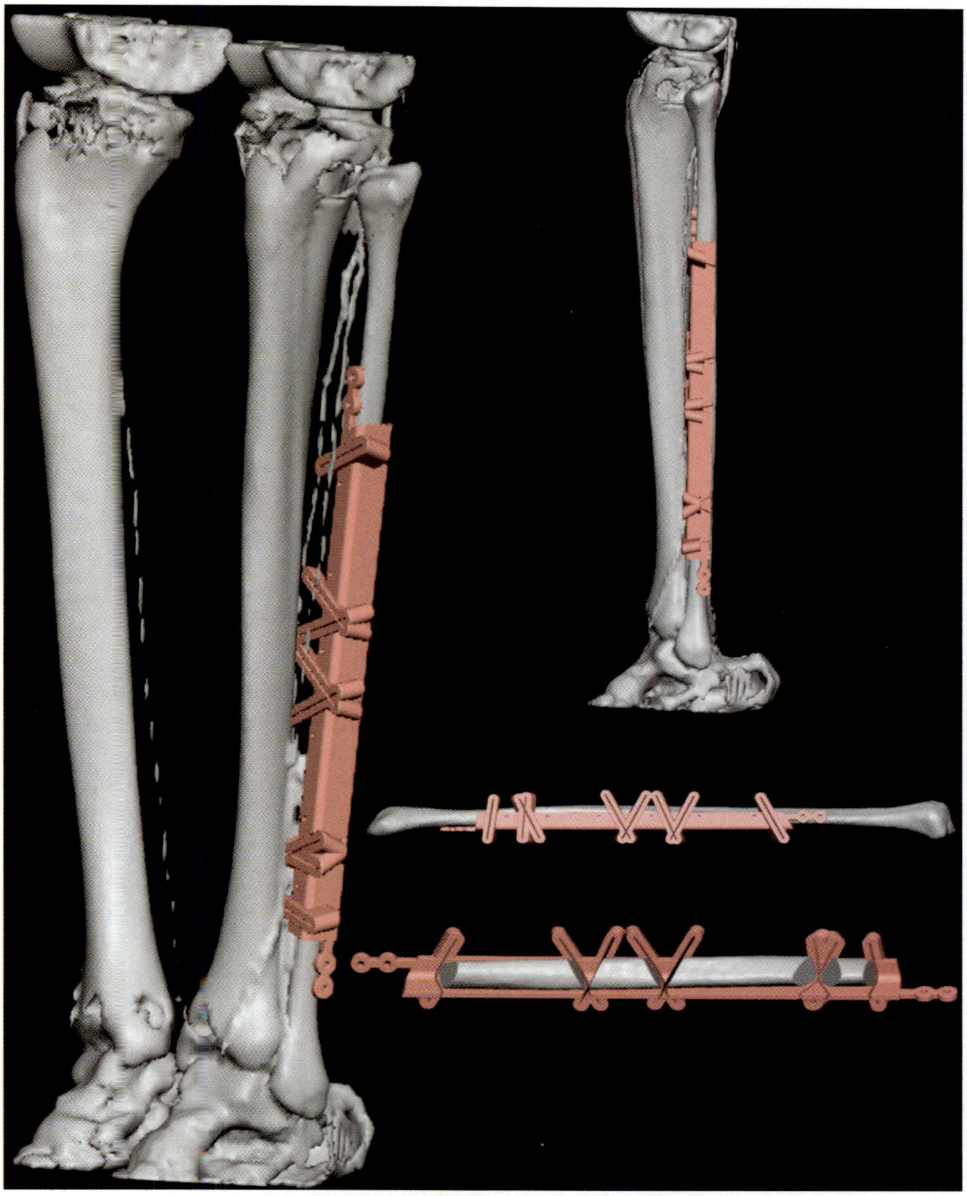

FIGURE 30-3 Rapid prototype model of the mandible incorporating the planned fibula free flap reconstruction. A titanium reconstruction plate was bent according to the model before surgery to save operative time.

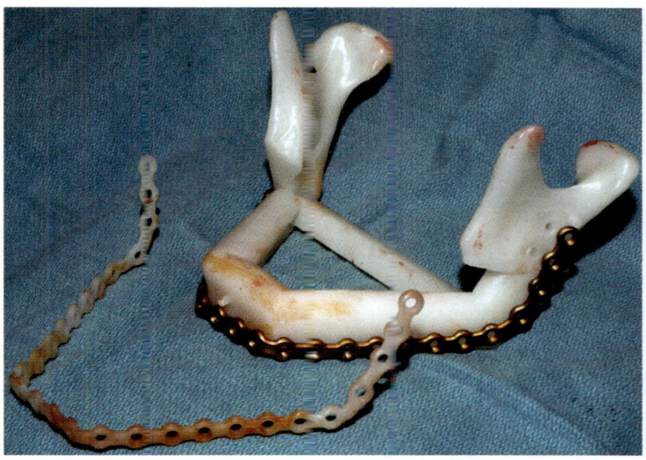

FIGURE 30-4 Computer-generated cutting guides can be designed to make osteotomies at the precise angles and lengths required to duplicate the virtually planned fibula free flap reconstruction.

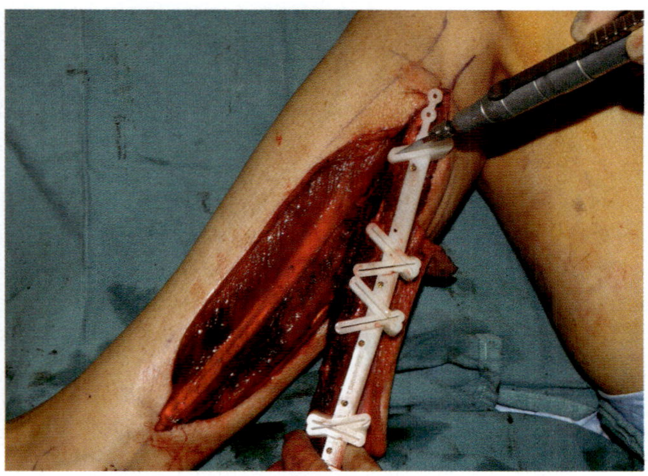

FIGURE 30-5 A cutting guide made using rapid prototype modeling technology assists in making the appropriate fibular osteotomies with a reciprocating saw.

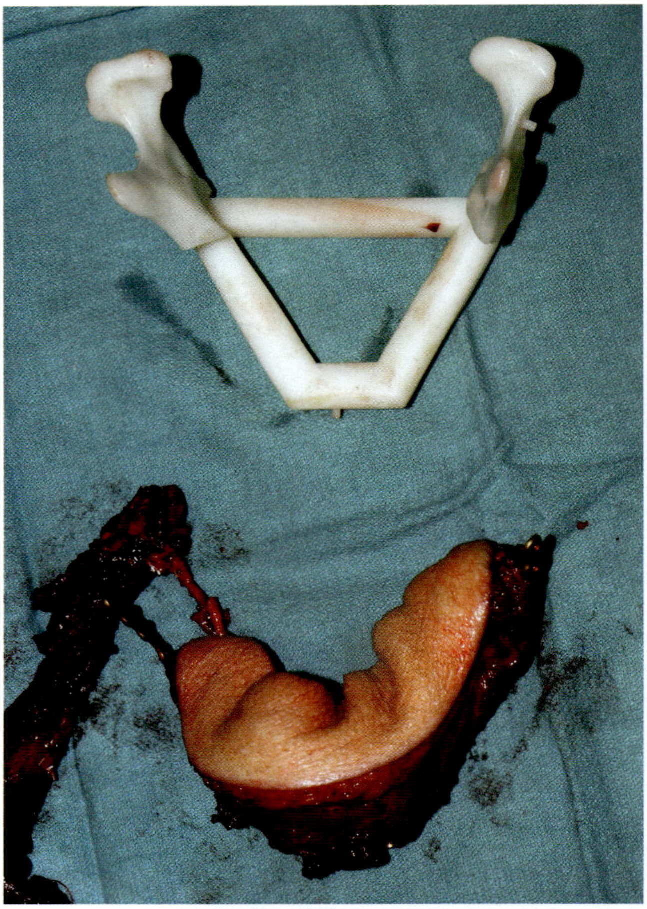

FIGURE 30-6 The actual fibula osteocutaneous free flap next to the rapid prototype model.

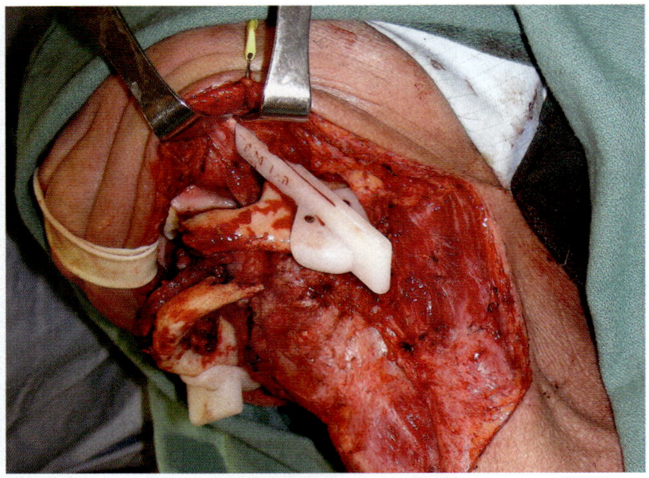

FIGURE 30-7 Mandibular cutting guides, made using rapid prototype modeling technology, in place before making osteotomies in a patient with a pathologic mandibular fracture caused by osteoradionecrosis.

TECHNIQUE: MIDFACE RECONSTRUCTION

Midfacial reconstruction is arguably an even greater challenge than mandibular reconstruction because of the complex three-dimensional shape of the maxillae, and many different techniques have been tried. Unlike mandibular reconstruction, no single reconstructive option has been adopted as a gold standard. Prosthetic obturators are satisfactory for some defects but have several drawbacks and are often unstable in larger defects (28,29). For defects limited to the posterolateral maxilla or central hard palate, soft tissue flaps may be adequate (30,31). However, for extensive defects, particularly those involving the anterior maxilla, vascularized bone flaps are needed to restore midfacial height, width, and projection, as well as provide a firm surface for mastication and accommodate osseointegrated implant placement for dental restoration (32,33).

Virtual planning using CAD software allows the surgeon to shape vascularized bone flaps to best reconstruct the complicated shape of the midface. Before this technique, our results with vascularized bone flap reconstruction were less favorable, particularly when soft tissue atrophy after radiation revealed irregular contours from inaccurately or nonanatomically placed bone. Accuracy in the placement of the flap, in addition to fixation of its osteotomized parts, is very important. In this limited space, inaccuracies of a few millimeters can have severe functional and aesthetic consequences. However, because of more limited exposure, flap inset and fixation is more difficult than in most mandibular reconstructions. Because of this, stereotactic navigation is also used to verify accurate positioning of the free flap construct.

Various vascularized bone flaps, including the iliac crest, scapula, radial forearm, and fibula free flaps, have been described in various configurations and orientations (34–38). We have found that the fibula free flap in a configuration that resembles the Greek letter omega in the transverse plane for a bilateral reconstruction and a half or "hemi-omega" for a unilateral reconstruction recapitulates the shape of the midface best and supplies adequate bone stock for osseointegrated implant dental restoration (see Figure 30-8) (39). When reconstructing bilateral maxillectomy defects, the lateral portions of the "omega" re-create the malar regions, and the central ("curved") portion restores the maxillary alveolus. In this configuration, the lateral surface of the fibula bone is used to restore the vertical maxillary height, measured from the orbital rim to the plane of the hard palate, by orienting it such that it faces anteriorly on the face. The peroneal vessels assume a posterior position facing the maxillary sinus. The portion of the fibula free flap that replaces the anterior maxillae is inset at the vertical level of the resected alveolus, rather than at the level of the dentition, to provide room for an implant-retained dental prosthesis. A slight downward angulation of the portion of the fibula used to re-create the anterior maxillae is usually desirable to fully restore vertical facial height. The leg that is ipsilateral to the side of the planned microvascular anastomosis (again, the side with the larger defect or better recipient vessels) is selected for fibula osteocutaneous free flap harvest so that the skin paddle can be used to restore the palate.

As with mandibular reconstruction, a digital three-dimensional model of the facial skeleton is first created using fine-cut CT data. Next, the reconstruction is planned by virtually osteotomizing a fibula free flap to match the contours of the midfacial bones that are absent or will be resected. The virtual reconstruction is adjusted such that all midfacial prominences

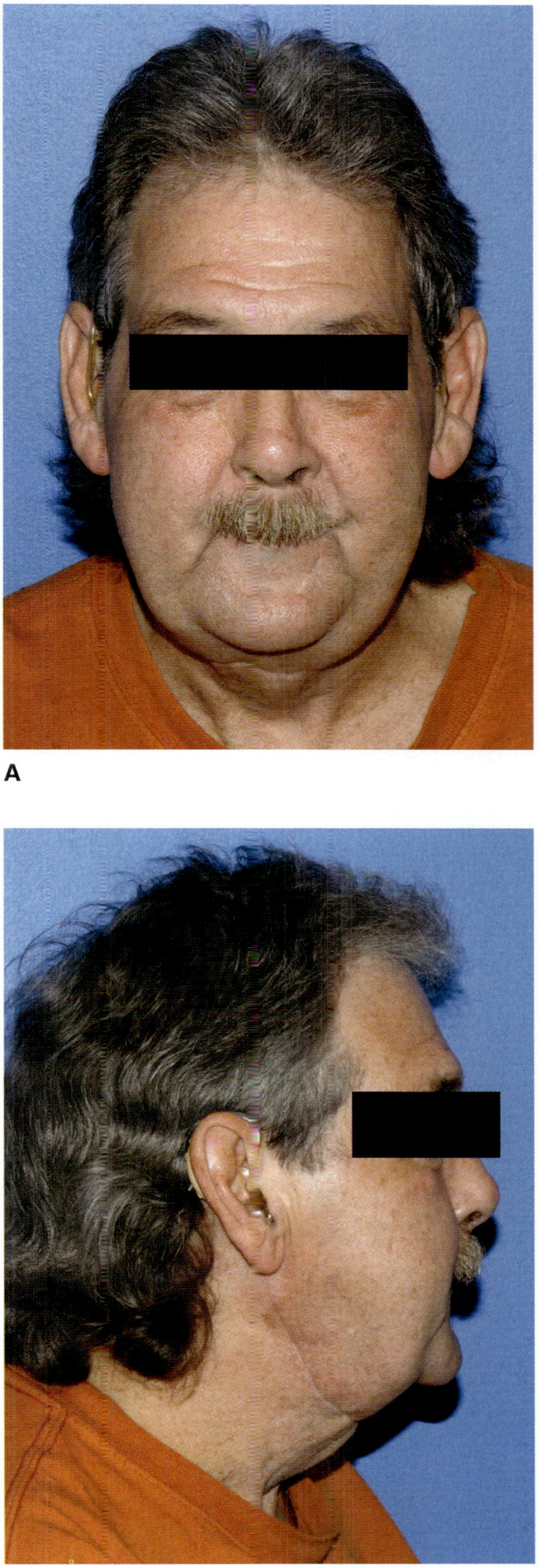

A

B

FIGURE 30-8 Postoperative result after the virtually planned mandibular reconstruction: anterior (**A**) and lateral (**B**) views. Osseointegrated implants were placed 3 months after the initial surgery.

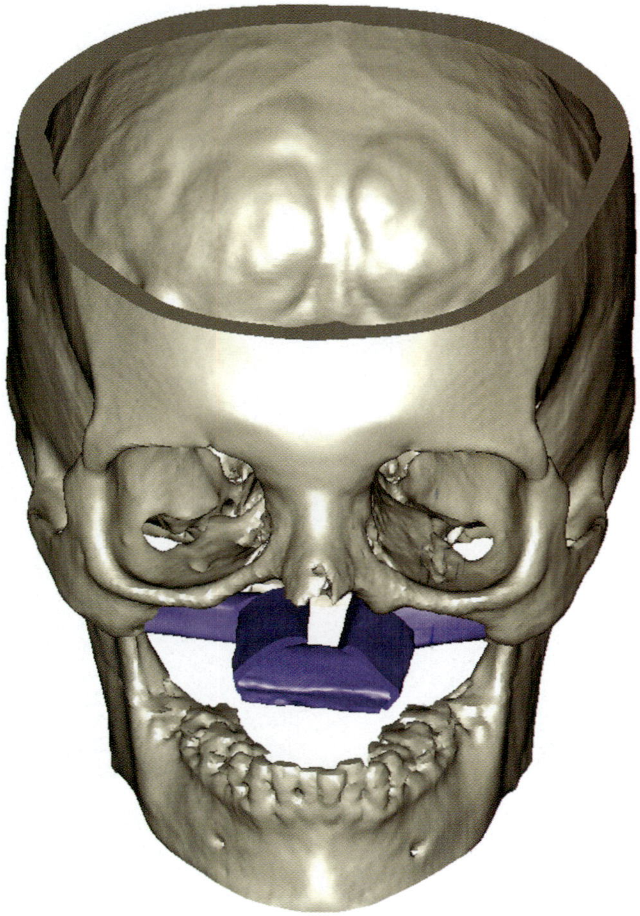

FIGURE 30-9 Preoperative virtual reconstruction with a fibula flap to restore the shape of the midfacial skeleton in a patient with squamous cell cancer of the hard palate.

are restored and the reconstructed maxillary occlusal plane aligns with the mandibular dentition. Sterilizable rapid prototype models of the reconstructed midface and computer-generated cutting guide are then printed (Figure 30-9).

Closing wedge osteotomies using the computer-generated cutting guide are performed on the fibular bone with a reciprocating saw, as in mandibular reconstruction. The plate is secured to the flap by locking screws placed unicortically through the fibular bone. Generally, two to three screw holes are available to secure each fibular segment. In our experience, 14 to 16 cm of bone length is typically needed to reconstruct a bilateral maxillectomy defect. Therefore, the entire fibular length, sparing only 5 to 7 cm distally and 5 to 7 cm proximally, is initially harvested, and the proximal bone is then trimmed to maximize vascular pedicle length.

Some flexor hallucis longus muscle is usually included with the flap to obliterate the maxillary sinus cavity and provide adequate soft tissue around the vascular pedicle to prevent its desiccation. The orientation of the skin paddle depends on the location of its perforator blood supply and may be longitudinally or transversely oriented in relation to the long axis of the fibula. As with mandibular reconstruction, we usually use a 2.0-mm locking reconstruction plate for fixation, although smaller plates or multiple plates also provide adequate stability. The lateral portions of the reconstruction plate must be long

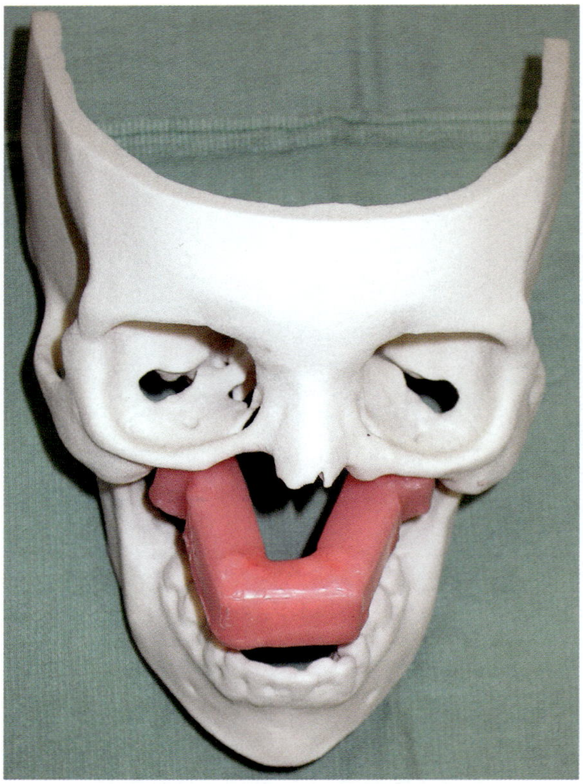

FIGURE 30-10 An early rapid prototype model of the midface based on the virtual fibula free flap reconstruction.

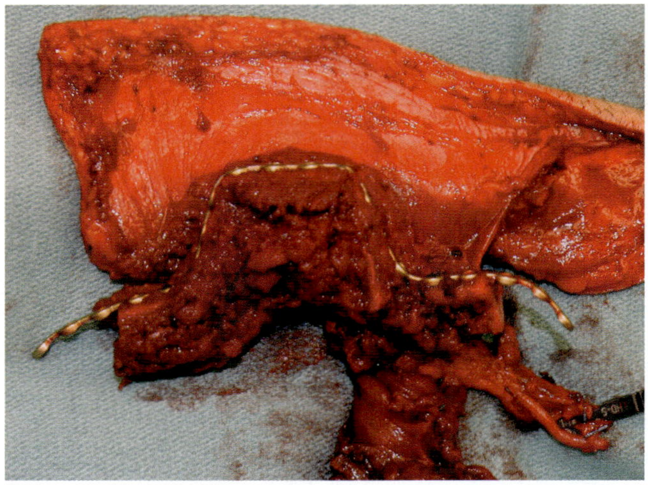

A

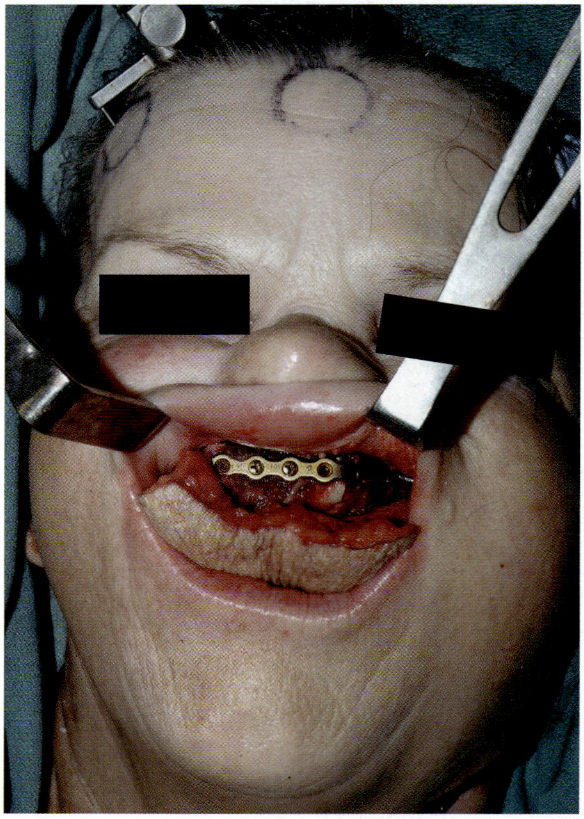

B

FIGURE 30-11 (**A**) An intraoperative photograph of a fibula osteocutaneous free flap shaped according to the virtual plan in order to restore a bilateral maxillectomy defect. (**B**) The flap being inset into the midfacial defect. The skin paddle is used to close the palatal defect.

enough to allow two- or three-screw fixation to the remaining zygomatic bones laterally.

When the orbital floor is resected, we reconstruct it separately from the rest of the maxilla. When postoperative radiation is anticipated, the orbital floor is reconstructed with autologous bone grafts; otherwise, titanium mesh is used. Whenever possible, we use fibula bone that would otherwise be discarded from the proximal flap to avoid creating a second donor site in the iliac or calvarial regions. The orbital floor reconstruction can be shaped based on the native orbit before its resection, if present. If the orbit has been destroyed by disease or is distorted because of an exophytic tumor, it is often helpful to have a second rapid prototype model bearing the premorbid or virtually restored orbits. Titanium hardware or mesh can be bent on the model to accurately reconstruct the orbital bones (Figure 30-10).

Insetting the bony free flap following osteotomies and rigid fixation with titanium plates is performed before microvascular anastomosis (Figure 30-11). The upper lip is usually split, and a lateral rhinotomy incision is usually made to perform the maxillary resection. An infraorbital extension to the incision (Weber-Fergusen approach) is not performed unless absolutely necessary because of the risk for postoperative ectropion. If the resection does not require them, we do not make any additional facial incisions to inset the fibula flap. However, insetting can be challenging through relatively limited incisions, and proper positioning is critical to restore facial symmetry as well as to reestablish the maxillary occlusal plane.

As mentioned, we employ stereotactic navigation in these cases to confirm the position of the free flap intraoperatively. When stereotactic navigation is planned, another head and neck CT scan is obtained with the patient wearing adhesive fiducial markers placed on the forehead before surgery. Because these fiducial markers must be in the same locations at the time of surgery to register with the stereotactic navigation device, the CT scan is performed the day before surgery, and the patient is instructed not to remove the fiducials before surgery. Before surgery, CT data are imported into the navigation system workstation as are the processed images, which include the virtual fibula reconstruction created during the planning session.

Registration is typically performed before complete prepping and draping using a rigidly fixed array. During surgery, after the fibula free flap has been inset, its actual position, indicated by the tip of the navigation probe, is compared with the intended position of the virtual fibula flap, whose position is shown on the navigation system monitor in axial, coronal, and sagittal views (Figures 30-12 and 30-13). The flap is rigidly fixed when its position matches the position of the fibula in the virtual plan. Revascularization of the free flap is then performed. A representative result is shown in Figure 30-14.

Vessel Anastomoses

For both mandibular and midfacial reconstruction, we prefer to use the facial blood vessels as recipients when available because of their proximity and their good caliber match to the peroneal blood vessels. For the midface, a subcutaneous tunnel through the cheek is made to the recipient blood vessels, which

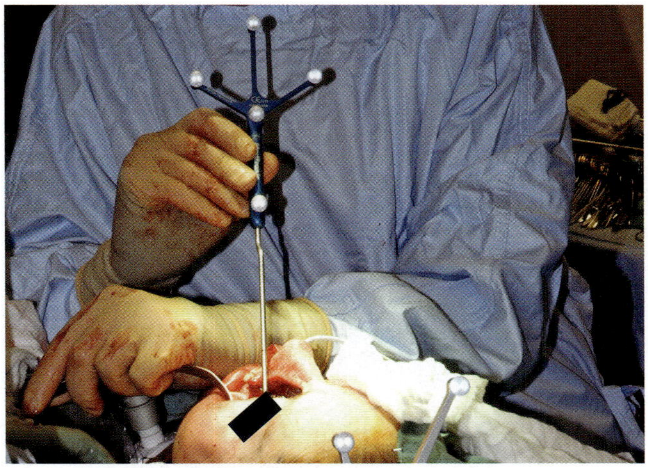

FIGURE 30-12 Confirmation of the positioning of the fibula osteocutaneous free flap after insetting using stereotactic navigation. The handheld probe tip is visualized on the navigation system monitor. Note the sensor array that is rigidly fixed to the calvarium that maintains registration with the navigation system even when the patient's head is moved.

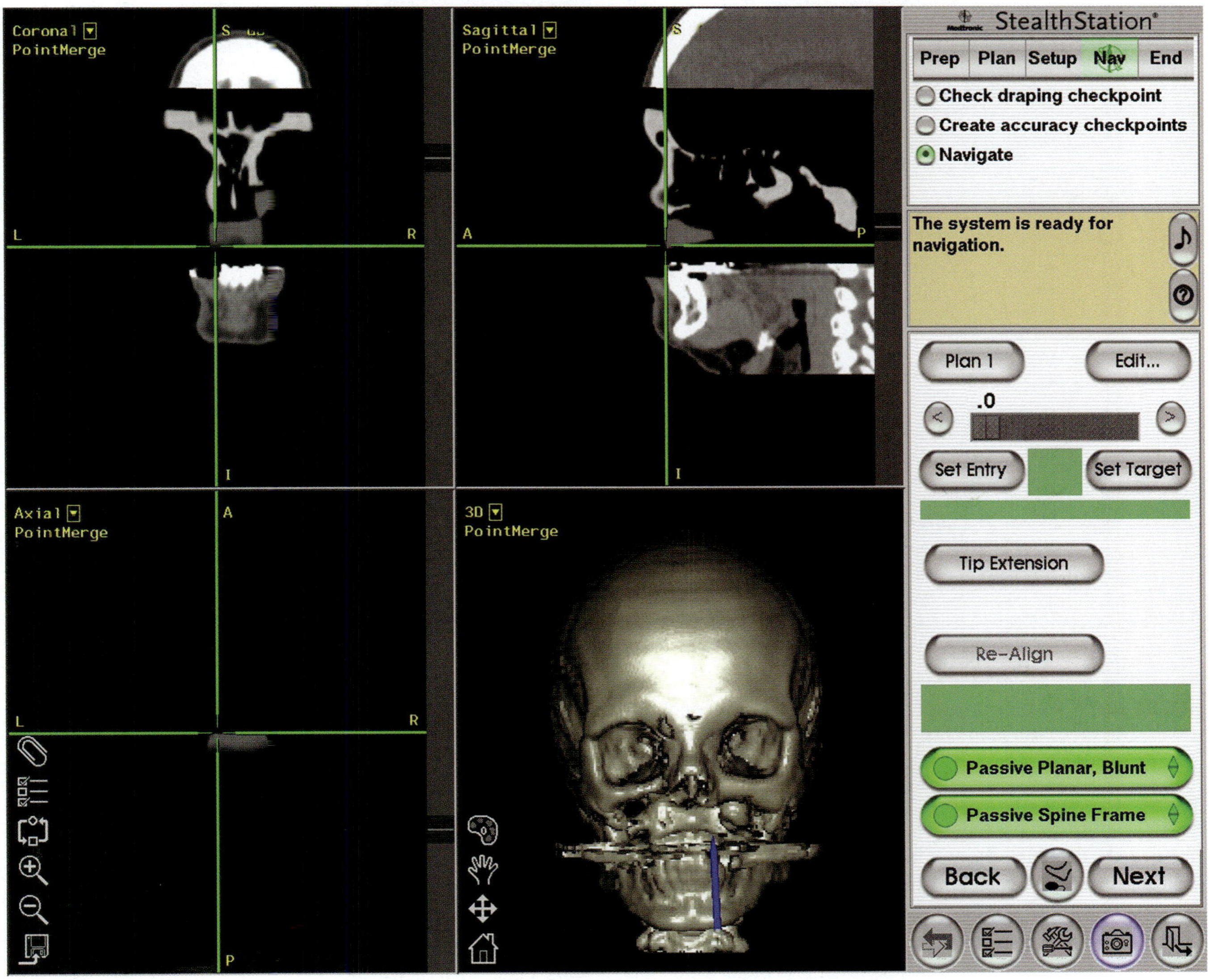

FIGURE 30-13 Stereotactic navigation allows the actual position of the probe tip (green cross) to be shown in the axial, coronal, and sagittal planes on images that include the virtually planned reconstruction to verify accurate positioning of the free flap.

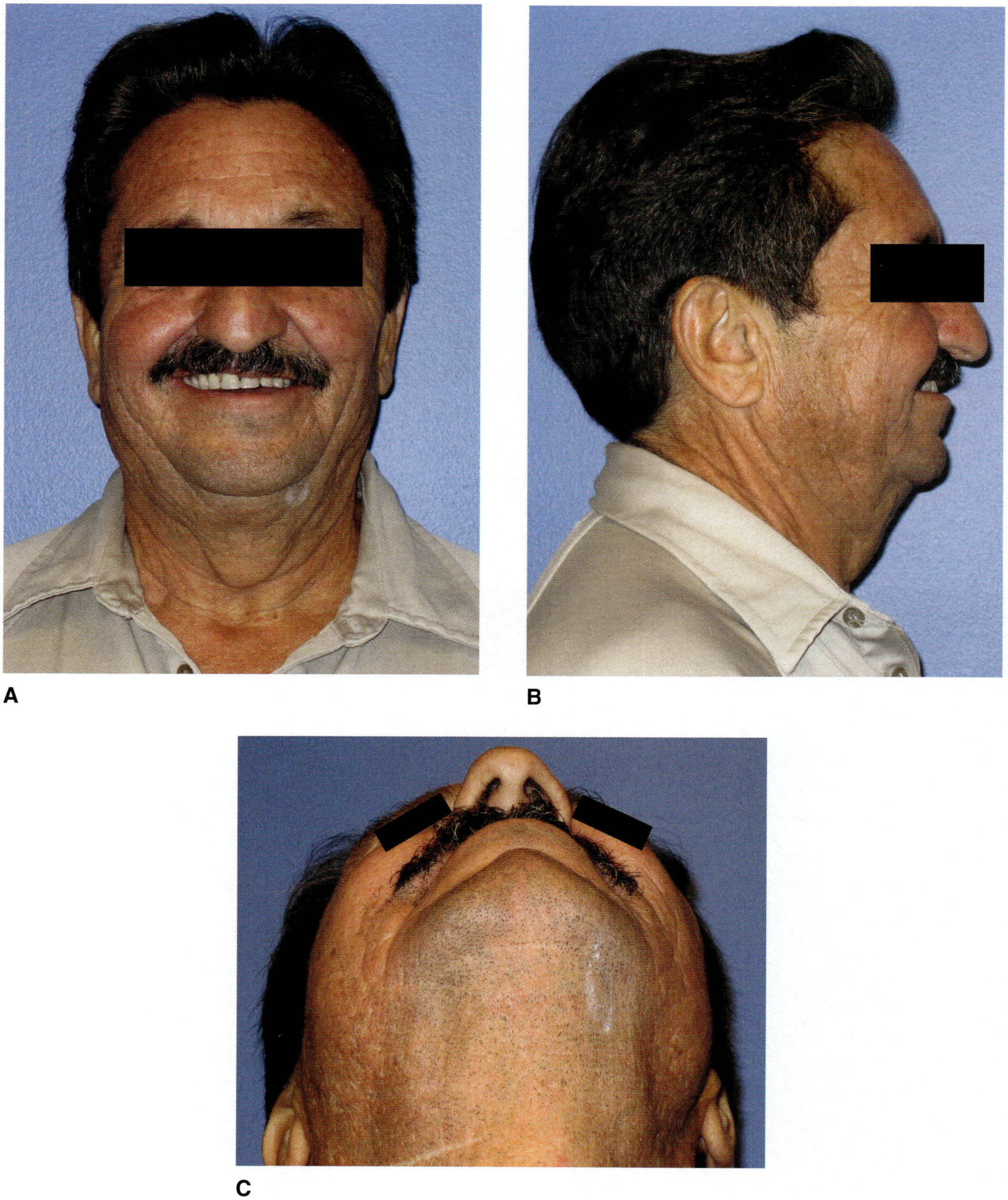

FIGURE 30-14 Postoperative result after the virtually planned midfacial reconstruction using stereotactic navigation for flap positioning: anterior (**A**), lateral (**B**), submental (**C**) and views.

are prepared through a separate submandibular incision before flap pedicle division. Bony and skin paddle insetting of the mandible can usually be performed before or after microvascular anastomosis. Especially in midfacial reconstruction, it is often safest to perform at least part of the inset before the vessel anastomoses to prevent tension on the pedicle while the flap is being manipulated. After the flap is rendered ischemic, the posterior skin paddle edge is first approximated to the remaining palate (usually the cut edge of the soft palate), and the bony component of the flap is secured to the zygomatic bones laterally via the reconstruction plate. When stereotactic navigation is used, the position of the free flap is verified and adjusted as necessary at this point. The microvascular anastomoses are then performed, and the remainder of the skin paddle is inset. Vein grafts are used if necessary to reach the recipient vessels.

POTENTIAL COMPLICATIONS

Potential complications are the same as for other mandibular and maxillary reconstructions. Malocclusion should be decreased based on more precise planning and fibula free flap shaping with osteotomies and plate fixation. One common problem, particularly in secondary reconstructions, is having inadequate labial tissue, resulting in obliteration of the gingivolabial sulcus. Without a satisfactory gingivolabial sulcus, the lip appears shortened, and if the dentition is restored by an implant or adhesive retained prosthesis, the teeth are excessively prominent. This is particularly a problem in delayed midfacial reconstruction when the upper lip contracts in the absence of maxillary bone. One way we have addressed this is to lengthen the upper lip with nasolabial flaps or a second skin paddle of the fibula free flap.

SECONDARY SURGERY

Dental restoration with osseointegrated implants is considered as early as 3 months after fibula free flap reconstruction. However, we do not routinely perform implant placement in patients who receive postoperative radiation therapy because of concern for complications, such as osteoradionecrosis (40,41). Others have successfully done so, sometimes incorporating hyperbaric oxygen therapy in an effort to theoretically reverse some of the deleterious effects of radiation on tissue vascularity (42,43). Alternately, osseointegrated implants can also be placed at the time of the initial free flap reconstruction (44). It appears that implants placed before radiation have a lower rate of complications, including implant failure, bony exposure, osteoradionecrosis, and fracture, at least in some series. In patients with a thick fibula free flap skin paddle, thinning of subcutaneous fat is usually performed simultaneously with implant placement to better accommodate a dental prosthesis.

RESULTS AND OUTCOMES

Virtual planning of the resection and reconstruction allows for the most accurate restoration of mandibular and midfacial shape using flaps and grafts, particularly when the facial skeleton has been distorted by exophytic tumor growth or destroyed by disease or prior surgical resection. In these situations, plates are not readily bent to fit the preresection anatomy intraoperatively, potentially resulting in inaccurate reconstruction and extended operative time because of trial and error. Visualizing the reconstruction superimposed on the preresection mandible or maxilla or in comparison with the normal side and the opposing occlusal surface is extremely helpful in designing the bony osteotomies needed to configure the fibular flap such that the facial shape and correct occlusion are restored. To evaluate the accuracy of the reconstructions, postoperative three-dimensional CT images may be superimposed on preoperative three-dimensional CT reconstructions. Excellent concordance in shape and positioning has been noted (Figure 30-15).

Dental rehabilitation in addition to bony and soft tissue reconstruction completes mandibular and midfacial restoration, both functionally and aesthetically. Patients who undergo osseointegrated implant-retained dental restoration are more likely to tolerate a regular mechanical diet. Patients with sufficient

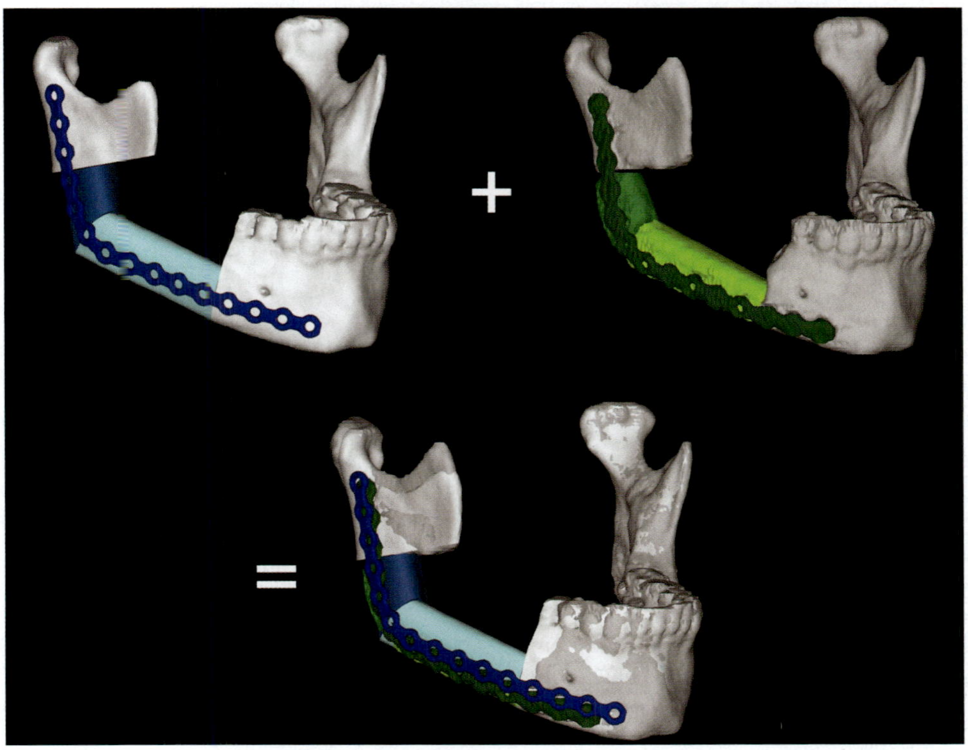

FIGURE 30-15 The virtually planned fibula flap superimposed on a three-dimensional computed tomography reconstruction of the actual fibula flap obtained after surgery shows very good concordance.

remaining dentition may be able to retain a conventional denture successfully without osseointegrated implant fixation. However, in those with more extensive defects or without adequate remaining dentition to anchor a denture or prosthesis, osseointegrated implants are usually required for dental restoration.

Our experience and the experience of others is that there is an operative time savings associated with this technique. Prebending hardware and use of the cutting guides to simplify osteotomies can make surgery faster, particularly in larger defects in which multiple osteotomies are needed. Additionally, the preoperative planning that occurs can often increase the surgeon's efficiency during surgery by improving surgical decision making and reducing trial and error during fibular harvest and shaping.

Medical models are also useful as a communication tool between the resecting surgeon and the reconstructive surgeon and as a teaching tool for the patient as well as surgical trainees. Early in our experience, models were made in house using proprietary software and a rapid prototype printer. Because of the time and computer expertise needed for this process and the limited availability of such software and hardware at various centers, virtual planning and RPM were not practical to routinely incorporate into the reconstructive surgery workflow. However, now, high-quality, sterilizable models can be designed and manufactured commercially and customized to the specifications of the surgeon via interactive web conferencing. Therefore, the protocol we describe can be used on a widespread basis from nearly anywhere in the world with Internet access.

There are some disadvantages to virtual planning and RPM. One drawback of virtual planning and RPM is the time that is needed to plan and create the models. Even using a commercial source for the virtual planning and RPM still requires approximately 30 minutes of web conference discussion to perform the planning and occasionally a second session to finalize the plans. Models need a modest amount of time to be manufactured and shipped as well. Costs may also be a disadvantage, depending on whether the patient or a third-party payor is willing to reimburse the reconstructive center for the creation of the model. However, based on our experience, we believe that the time and cost spent performing the virtual reconstruction and creating the rapid prototype models is offset by the operative time savings and increased accuracy of the reconstructive results, particularly for more complex defects as discussed earlier.

The registration process and placement of the navigation array in stereotactic navigation also adds to the operating time, averaging approximately 15 minutes at the start of the case. Use of the navigation system to confirm positioning takes an additional 5 to 10 minutes, provided major adjustments do not need to be made. We believe that the additional operative time is offset by the added confidence in flap positioning, which is very difficult to correct secondarily when bony healing has taken place and has major aesthetic and functional consequences. Use of the navigation system has allowed us to avoid making additional facial incisions, sometimes even performing the surgery entirely transorally.

Perhaps the greatest limitation we have encountered in virtual planning and RPM is the potential for the extent of resection to change based on unanticipated disease progression or microscopically positive margins necessitating additional resection at the time of surgery. A change in the extent of resection may reduce the usefulness of this technique by requiring additional bone length or osteotomies as well as altering the shape of the titanium plate, potentially increasing operative time and decreasing the accuracy of the reconstruction as it deviates from the preoperative plan. Because of this possibility, close communication with the resecting surgeon is mandatory. Use of recent CT scans is indicated to make the most accurate virtual plan and model. In our experience, it is often useful to tend toward modest overestimation of the defect because the plate cutting guides can still be useful even if a small amount of the fibula needs to be cut or burred back. Alternately, the native mandible resection can be enlarged, or, as we prefer, a notch can be cut into the native mandible, not unlike a tongue and groove joint design, to accommodate the slightly long fibular segment, increasing the stability of the joint and maximizing bony contact surface area while preserving the alveolar surface.

ACKNOWLEDGMENTS

The authors would like to thank Mr. Andrew M. Christensen and Ms. Katie A. Weimer of Medical Modeling, Inc., for their invaluable assistance with the material presented in this chapter.

REFERENCES

1. Saigal K, Winokur RS, Finden S, et al. Use of three-dimensional computerized tomography reconstruction in complex facial trauma. *Facial Plast Surg* 2005;21:214.
2. Murray DJ, Edwards G, Mainprize JG, Antonyshyn O. Advanced technology in the management of fibrous dysplasia. *J Plast Reconstr Aesthet Surg* 2008;61:906.
3. Bell RB. Computer planning and intraoperative navigation in cranio-maxillofacial surgery. *Oral Maxillofac Surg Clin North Am* 2010; 22:135.
4. Chang S, Liao YF, Hung LM, et al. Prefabricated implants or grafts with reverse models of three-dimensional mirror-image templates for reconstruction of craniofacial abnormalities. *Plast Reconstr Surg* 1999;104:1413.
5. Dean D, Min KJ, Bond A. Computer aided design of large format prefabricated cranial plates. *J Craniofac Surg* 2003;14:819.
6. Hanasono MM, Goel N, Demonte F. Calvarial reconstruction using polyetheretherketone (PEEK) implants. *Ann Plast Surg* 2009;62:653.
7. Sinn DP, Cello JE, Miles BA. Stereolithography for craniofacial surgery. *J Craniofac Surg* 2006;17(5):869
8. Sailer HF, Haers PE, Zollikofer CPE, et al. The value of stereolithographic models for preoperative diagnosis of craniofacial deformities and presurgical planning. *Int J Oral Maxillofac Surg* 1998;27:327.
9. Kermer C, Lindner A, Friede I, et al. Preoperative stereolithographic model planning for primary reconstruction in craniomaxillofacial trauma surgery. *J Craniomaxillofac Surg* 1998;26:136.
10. James WJ, Slabbekoorn MK, Edgin WA, et al.Correction of congenital malar hypoplasia using stereolithography for presurgical planning. *J Oral Maxillofac Surg* 1998;56:512.
11. Park GC, Wiseman JB, Clark WD. Correction of congenital microtia using stereolithography for surgical planning. *Plast Reconstr Surg* 2000;105:1444.
12. Choi JY, Choi JH, Kim NK, et al. Analysis of errors in medical rapid prototype models. Int. *J Oral Maxillofac Surg* 2002;31:23.
13. Chang PS, Parker TH, Patrick CW Jr, Miller MJ. The accuracy of stereolithography in planning craniofacial bone replacement. *J Craniofac Surg* 2003;14:164.
14. Ueda KM, Tajima SM, Oba SM, et al. Mandibular contour reconstruction with three-dimensional computer-assisted models. *Ann Plast Surg* 2001;46:387–393.

15. Eckardt A, Swennen GR. Virtual planning of composite mandibular reconstruction with free fibula bone graft. *J Craniofac Surg* 2005;16:1137–1140.
16. Lee JW, Fang JJ, Chang LR, Yu CK. Mandibular defect reconstruction with the help of mirror imaged coupled with laser stereolithographic modeling technique. *J Formos Med Assoc* 2007;106:244–250.
17. Kernan BT, Wimsatt JA. Use of a stereolithography model for accurate, preoperative adaptation of a reconstruction plate. *J Oral Maxillofac Surg* 2000;58:349.
18. Juergens P, Krol Z, Zeilhofer HF, et al. Computer simulation and rapid prototyping for the reconstruction of the mandible. *J Oral Maxillofac Surg* 2009;67:2167.
19. Cohen A, Laviv A, Berman P, et al. Mandibular reconstruction using stereolithographic 3-dimensional printing modeling technology. *Oral Surg Oral Med Oral Pathol Oral Radiol Endod* 2009;108:661.
20. Levine JP, Hirsch DL, Bastidas JA, et al. Importance of computer-aided design and manufacturing technology in the multidisciplinary approach to head and neck reconstruction. *J Craniofac Surg* 2010;21:1277.
21. Hirsch DL, Garfein ES, Christensen AM, et al. Use of computer-aided design and computer-aided manufacturing to produce orthognathically ideal outcomes: a paradigm shift in head and neck reconstruction. *J Oral Maxillofac Surg* 2009;67:2115.
22. Golfinos JC, Fitzpatrick BC, Smith LR, Spetzler RF. Clinical use of a frameless stereotactic arm: results of 325 cases. *J Neurosurg* 1995;83:197.
23. Roessler K, Ungersboeck K, Dietrich W, et al. Frameless stereotactic guided neurosurgery: clinical experience with an infra-red based pointer device navigation system. *Acta Neurochir (Wien)* 1997;139:551.
24. Gellrich NC, Schramm A, Hammer B, et al. Computer-assisted secondary reconstruction of unilateral posttraumatic orbital deformity. *Plast Reconstr Surg* 2002;110:1417.
25. Strong EB, Rafii A, Holhweg-Majert B, et al. Comparison of 3 optical navigation systems for computer-aided maxillofacial surgery. *Arch Otolaryngol Head Neck Surg* 2008;134:1080.
26. Hanasono MM, Jacob RF, Bidaut L, et al. Mid-facial reconstruction using virtual planning, rapid prototype modeling, and stereotactic navigation. *Plast Reconstr Surg* 2010;126:2002–2006.
27. Frodel JL Jr, Funk GF, Capper DT, et al. Osseointegrated implants: a comparative study of bone thickness in four vascularized bone flaps. *Plast Reconstr Surg* 1993;92:449.
28. Brown JS, Rogers SN, McNally DN, Boyle M. A modified classification for the maxillectomy defect. *Head Neck* 2000;22:17.
29. Okay DJ, Genden E, Buchbinder D, Urken M. Prosthodontic guidelines for surgical reconstruction of the maxilla: a classification system of defects. *J Prosthet Dent* 2001;86:352.
30. Cordeiro PG, Santamaria E, Kraus DH, et al. Reconstruction of total maxillectomy defects with preservation of the orbital contents. *Plast Reconstr Surg* 1998;102:1874.
31. Cordeiro PG, Santamaria E. A classification system and algorithm for reconstruction of maxillectomy and midfacial defects. *Plast Reconstr Surg* 2000;105:2331.
32. Genden EM, Okay D, Stepp MT, et al. Comparison of functional and quality-of-life outcomes in patients with and without palatomaxillary reconstruction: a preliminary report. *Arch Otolaryngol Head Neck Surg* 2003;129:775.
33. Moreno M, Skoracki RJ, Hanna EY, Hanasono MM. Microvascular free flap reconstruction versus palatal obturation for maxillectomy defects. *Head Neck* 2010;32:860.
34. Nakayama B, Matuura H, Ishihara O, et al. Function reconstruction of a bilateral maxillectomy defect using a fibula osteocutaneous flap with osseointegrated implants. *Plast Reconstr Surg* 1995;96:1201.
35. Futran ND, Haller JR. Considerations for free-flap reconstruction of the hard palate. *Arch Otolaryngol Head Neck Surg* 1999;125:665.
36. Brown JS, Jones DC, Summerwill A, et al. Vascularized iliac crest with internal oblique muscle for immediate reconstruction after maxillectomy. *Br J Oral Maxillofac Surg* 2002;40:183.
37. Chang DW, Langstein HN. Use of the free fibula flap for restoration of orbital support and midfacial projection following maxillectomy. *J Reconstr Microsurg* 2003;19:147.
38. Genden EM, Wallace D, Buchbinder D, et al. Iliac crest internal oblique osteomusculocutaneous free flap reconstruction of the postablative palatomaxillary defect. *Arch Otolaryngol Head Neck Surg* 2001;127:854.
39. Hanasono MM, Skoracki RJ. The omega-shaped fibula osteocutaneous free flap for reconstruction of extensive midfacial defects. *Plast Reconstr Surg* 2010;125:160e.
40. Roumanas E, Markowitz BL, Lorant JA, et al. Reconstructed mandibular defects: fibula free flaps and osseointegrated implant. *Plast Reconstr Surg* 1997;99:356.
41. Teoh KH, Huryn JM, Patel S, et al. Implant prosthodontic rehabilitation of fibula free-flap reconstructed mandibles: a Memorial Sloan-Kettering Cancer Center review of prognostic factors and implant outcomes. *Int J Oral Maxillofac Implants* 2005;20:738.
42. Niimi A, Ueda M, Keller EE, Worthington P. Experience with osseointegrated implants placed in irradiated tissues in Japan and the United States. *Int J Oral Maxillofac Implants* 1998;13:407.
43. Brogniez V, Lejuste P, Pecheur A, Reychler H. Dental prosthetic reconstruction of osseointegrated implants placed in irradiated bone. *Int J Oral Maxillofac Implants* 1998;13:506.
44. Chang YM, Santamaria E, Wei FC, et al. Primary insertion of osseointegrated dental implants into fibula osteoseptocutaneous free flap for mandible reconstruction. *Plast Reconstr Surg* 1998;102:680.

CHAPTER 31

Maxillary Reconstruction

Branko Bojovic, Amir H. Dorafshar, and Eduardo D. Rodriguez

BRIEF HISTORY OF CONVENTIONAL OPTIONS

In the last third of the 20th century, several advances in craniofacial surgery improved functional and aesthetic outcomes. First, novel surgical approaches to the craniofacial skeleton were developed to afford safe and predictable access to remote areas. Second, the structural pillars of the face responsible for maintaining height, width, and projection were defined and first applied to facial trauma reconstruction. Third, early restoration of hard and soft tissue craniofacial defects was shown to prevent involutional scar contracture. Last, the introduction of microsurgical techniques has facilitated predictable coverage of complex craniofacial defects. These developments have routinely been applied to the mandible and nose, but sheer momentum has led to their becoming the standard of care for the periorbital and midface regions as well.

Although it seems intuitive that these principles would transcend mandibular defects and be applied to the remaining facial skeleton, there has been significant reluctance to replace composite periorbital and midface regions with vascularized bone. Although microvascular soft tissue flaps may provide adequate volume, unsupported replacement without a bony framework can result in tissue descent and inadequate facial projection. Conventional bone grafts have been combined with soft tissue flaps, but nonvascularized bone undergoes partial to subtotal resorption and may not provide a foundation for osseointegrated prostheses.

Posttraumatic, high-energy defects of the midface can be challenging to reconstruct because they involve extensive composite tissue loss and result in significant permanent functional and cosmetic deformity. These injuries require replacement of the bony framework, external soft tissue, and intraoral mucosa.

The majority of maxillary defects are composite, involving the skin, skeleton, and mucosa. Successful reconstruction restores facial projection and lays the foundation for endosseous dental rehabilitation by replacing the buttresses, resurfacing the external and internal soft tissue lining, limiting oronasal fistulae, and restoring the alveolar ridge. Strict adherence to these principles limits unfavorable outcomes, including gross deformity, poor facial projection, incoherent speech, and oral incompetence.

The history of maxillary reconstruction closely parallels advances made in the field of plastic surgery. Prosthetic obturation is one of the earliest reconstructive tools and is still used today (1). Local flaps, including cervical, forehead, temporalis, and distant tubed flaps, combined with interposed nonvascularized autologous bone grafts (i.e., rib, cranium, and ilium) allow restoration of the skeleton and soft tissue envelope (2–5). These techniques, however, are plagued by gradual bone graft resorption, creating the need for additional reconstruction (Figure 31-1).

The introduction of free tissue transfer techniques in the 1970s—specifically, composite vascularized bone flaps—addressed this problem and provided a more enduring solution for composite maxillary defects. In addition, vascularized bone flaps provided a sound foundation for the final component of maxillary rehabilitation: the osseointegrated implant (6). Local skin flaps and nonvascularized bone grafts have been used for reconstruction, but bony resorption and the associated soft tissue collapse limit long-term viability. There is extensive literature on maxillary reconstruction using vascularized bone flaps after tumor extirpation; however, additional literature continues to be added on the use of composite free tissue transfer for high-energy posttraumatic maxillary defects. Recently, a classification scheme and treatment algorithm has been developed for traumatic maxillary defects (7).

FREE FLAPS AVAILABLE FOR RECONSTRUCTION

Nowadays, microvascular free tissue transfer techniques are preferred over pedicled flaps in major head and neck reconstruction (8). Earlier, the combination of pedicled flaps with interposed nonvascular bone grafts was considered the gold standard in the

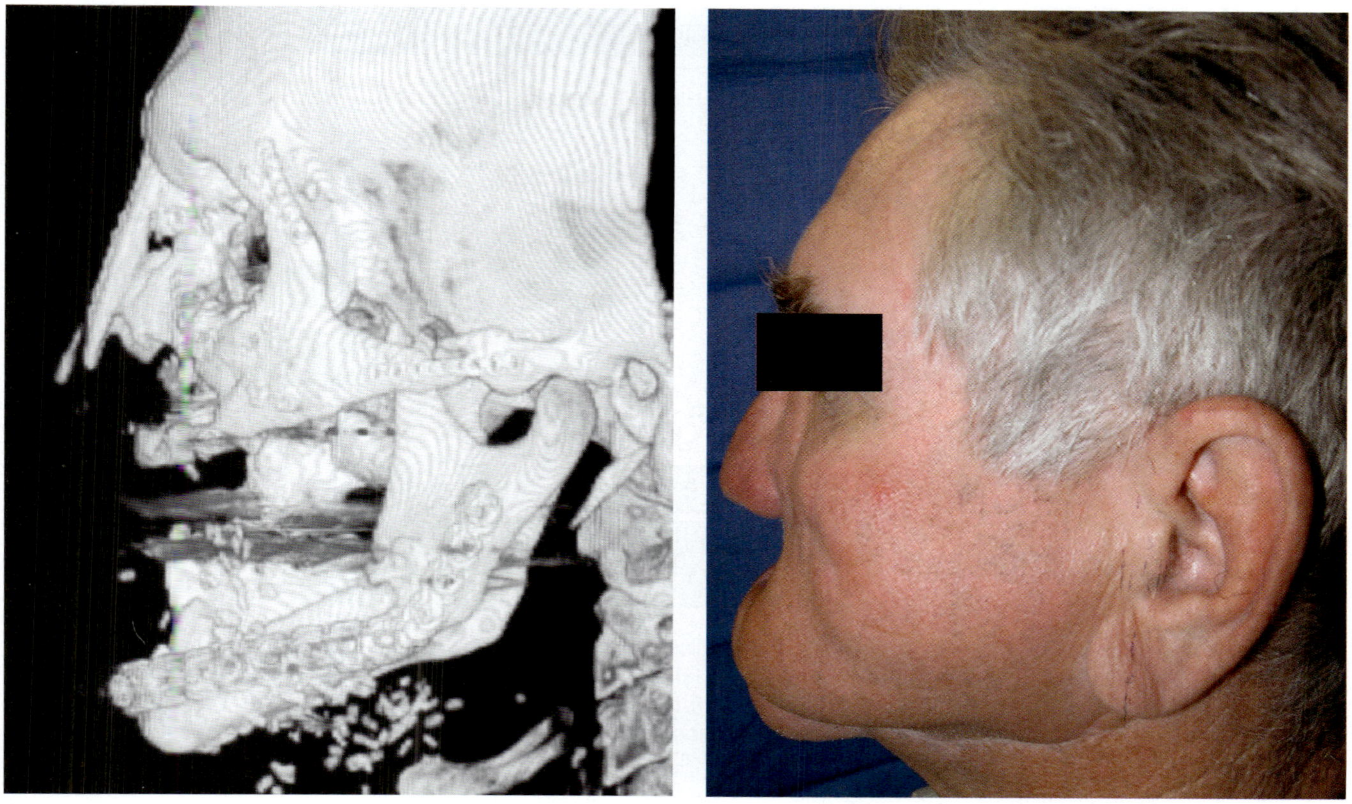

A B

FIGURE 31-1 Ten years before presentation, the patient's maxilla was reconstructed with a nonvascularized rib graft. The bone has resorbed, resulting in hard and soft tissue collapse.

management of acute high-energy midfacial injuries (2,9). Unfortunately, the long-term durability of this method is unreliable because the bone grafts undergo partial or subtotal resorption and require future augmentation with additional bone (9). Nonvascularized bone grafts may remain an option for the management of small bone defects surrounded by well-vascularized soft tissue (10). However, extensive maxillary trauma, such as injuries produced by high-energy ballistic weapons, is associated with deficient vascularized soft tissue and extensive bone loss and is thus less amenable to a nonvascularized bone graft (2,11). Free omental and muscle flaps were originally advocated because of their ability to obliterate dead space and provide vascularized coverage of nonvascularized bone (12). Presently, composite vascularized bone flaps are the gold standard.

The four major sources of vascularized bone routinely used for craniofacial reconstruction include the fibula, ilium, radius, and scapula. Each source of bone has its own limitations. With respect to dental rehabilitation with osseointegrated implants, the final goal in maxillary reconstruction, the fibula and iliac crest reliably provide adequate bone width and height as opposed to the scapula and radius (13).

The choice of osseous flap for maxillary reconstruction depends on recipient site requirements in terms of skin, bone, volume, and pedicle length as well as the availability of donor flaps. A well-designed fibular or iliac crest flap is ideal. Furthermore, a classification of maxillary defects has been devised that focuses on the essential maxillary functional subunits that require replacement and is purposely related to the selection of either the fibula or iliac crest free flaps for reconstruction (Figures 31-2 and 31-3) (7). When the maxilla is missing, the inferior orbital rim and contiguous malar prominence must also be replaced for a number of reasons. First, autogenous bone or a titanium mesh plate is necessary for eventual stabilization of the orbital floor defect. Second, when both the nasomaxillary and zygomaticomaxillary buttresses are damaged or absent, the newly reconstructed rim will provide a site of fixation for the neoalveolus. Third, the malar prominence defines the width and projection of the midface and its reconstruction is essential for optimal aesthetic outcomes.

OUTLINE OF THE INDICATIONS FOR THE SPECIFIC FLAPS THAT ARE DESCRIBED IN THIS CHAPTER

An algorithm that advocates vascularized composite tissue with either fibula or iliac crest flaps for all reconstructions is our preferred approach. These flaps are tailored based on the missing subunits—alveolus, orbital rim, or malar prominence. Our algorithm is different from previous ones in that it is based on functional and aesthetic structures rather than patterns of defects after tumor ablation. An ascending order of reconstructive complexity is therefore outlined in which a type I defect has a unilateral dentoalveolar defect, a type II defect is missing the inferior orbital rim in addition to having the dentoalveolar defect, a type III defect involves bilateral maxillary dentoalveolar loss, and a type IV defect involves bilateral maxillary dentoalveolar loss and

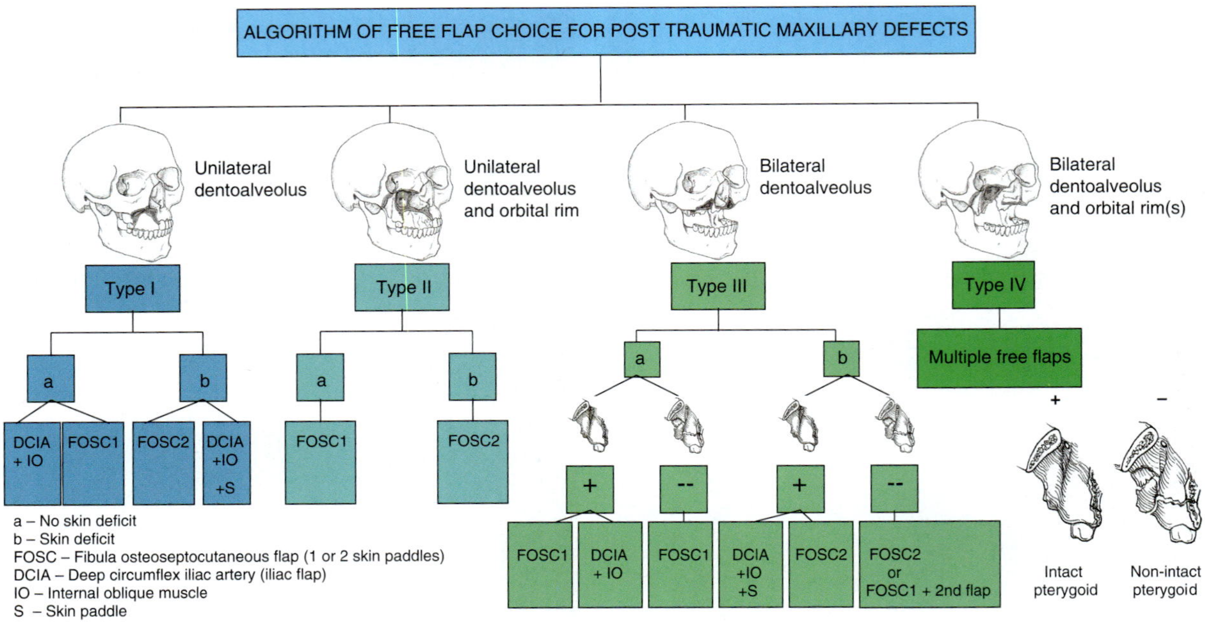

FIGURE 31-2 Algorithm of free flap choice for posttraumatic maxillary defects. a, no skin deficit; b, skin deficit; DCIA, deep circumflex iliac artery (iliac flap); FOSC, fibula osteoseptocutaneous flap (one or two skin paddles); IO, internal oblique muscle; S, skin paddle. (Reproduced with permission from Rodriguez, ED, Martin, M, Bluebong-Langner, R, et al. Microsurgical reconstruction of posttraumatic high-energy maxillary defects: establishing the effectiveness of early reconstruction. *Plast. Reconstr. Surg.* 120: 7, 2007.)

at least one orbital rim. The presence or absence of facial skin is denoted by the letters *a* and *b*, respectively. A modifier is included in the classification that indicates the presence (+) or absence (–) of a posterior point of fixation (pterygomaxillary buttress) and that affects the choice and complexity of fixation. Mucosal lining defects are intentionally not included in the classification because they are assumed to be present in all cases. The presence or absence of the globe is not included in the algorithm because we believe that optimal restoration of the periorbital area, whether provided by soft tissue reconstruction or prosthetic replacement, requires reconstruction of normal facial dimensions and an architecturally sound orbital rim.

When embarking on microsurgical reconstruction, the fibula osteoseptocutaneous flap is ideal for bilateral maxillary defects, given its long pedicle length. Although the iliac crest flap has been used for bilateral defects, in our experience, it is best suited for unilateral defects requiring a shorter pedicle length. The fibula flap may be harvested with a generous skin paddle to serve for both internal lining and external cover. In the case of the iliac crest flap, a skin paddle is less ideal, given its own thickness and the obligatory muscular cuff required to carry it. Instead, a portion of the internal oblique muscle is incorporated for intraoral lining. This muscle ultimately atrophies and mucosalizes over time.

PREPARATION OF RECIPIENT SITE—DEBRIDEMENT, RECIPIENT VESSELS, NERVES, AND BONY DEFECTS

In contemplating reconstruction, one must recognize that it may not be possible to do so in a single stage. This is especially so in patients with acute high-energy traumatic injuries because of the nature of the injury and the delayed progression of the full effects of tissue crush, ischemia, and cavitation (14). Such patients require early skeletal and soft tissue stabilization followed by serial debridements of nonviable tissue before pursuing microsurgical reconstruction. When embarking on microsurgical reconstruction, either the fibula flap (peroneal artery) or the iliac crest flap (deep circumflex iliac artery) can be harvested, depending on the type of bony defect, pedicle length required, and donor site availability.

Extensive preoperative planning is critical to achieve intraoperative success. To determine the operative plan, facial anthropometrics are assessed, including facial thirds, facial fifths, and facial and dental midlines, and upper and lower incisor show at rest and when smiling. Precise analysis of dimensions can be obtained using current clinical photographs, preinjury clinical photographs, dental impressions, and three-dimensional computed tomography (CT). If maxillofacial osteotomies are to be performed, bite registration, facebow transfer, and lateral and posteroanterior cephalograms are helpful in guiding the position of the skeletal pillars and occlusion. The relationship of the maxilla to the mandible in centric occlusion should be recorded and mounted on an articulator. Dental models and a three-dimensional CT scan provide information regarding dimensions of the soft and hard tissue defects, location of fistulas, and deficient alveolar dimensions. Preoperative computerized surgical planning may predict accurate placement of osteotomies and fixation, thereby expediting surgical care and limiting anesthesia morbidity.

For high-energy wounds of the midface, aggressive debridement followed by early reconstruction with plating, local flaps, or microsurgical tissue transfer is advocated. Earlier reconstruction (within 2 weeks), before scar contracture, facilitates dissection of anatomic planes, allowing more precise alignment of skeletal structures while maintaining adequate volume of the

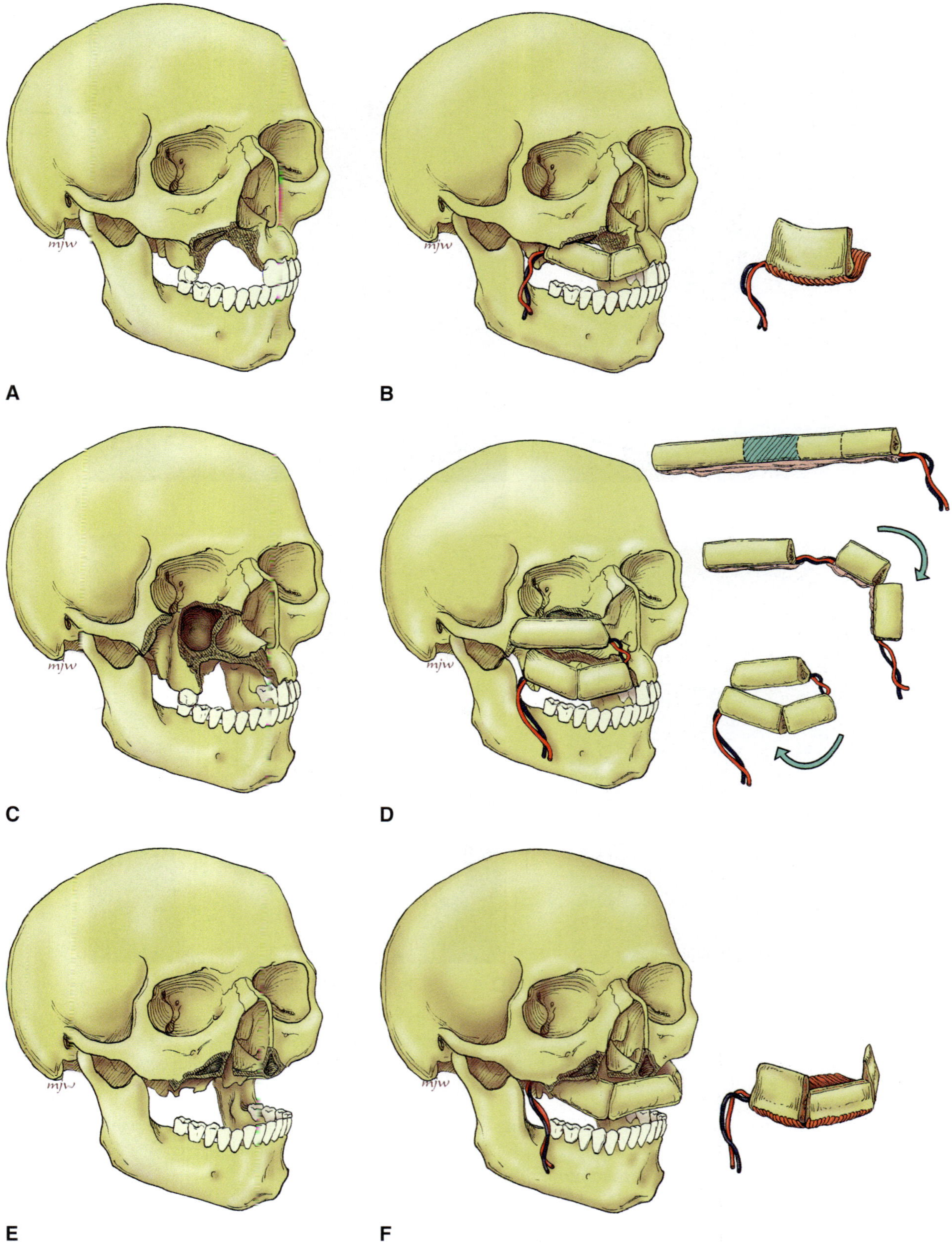

FIGURE 31-3 Illustrations of reconstructed defects. (**A** and **B**) Class I defect reconstruction with either a fibula or an iliac crest flap. (**C** and **D**) Class II defect reconstruction with a fibula flap. (**E** and **F**) Class II defect reconstruction with either a fibula or an iliac flap. Illustrations of reconstructed defects. (*Top*) Class I defect reconstruction with either a fibula or iliac crest flap. (*Center*) Class II defect reconstruction with a fibula flap. (*Bottom*) Class II defect reconstruction with either a fibula or iliac flap. (Reproduced with permission from Rodriguez, ED, Martin, M, Bluebond-Langner, R, et al. Microsurgical reconstruction of posttraumatic high-energy maxillary defects: establishing the effectiveness of early reconstruction. *Plast. Reconstr. Surg.* 120: 7, 2007.)

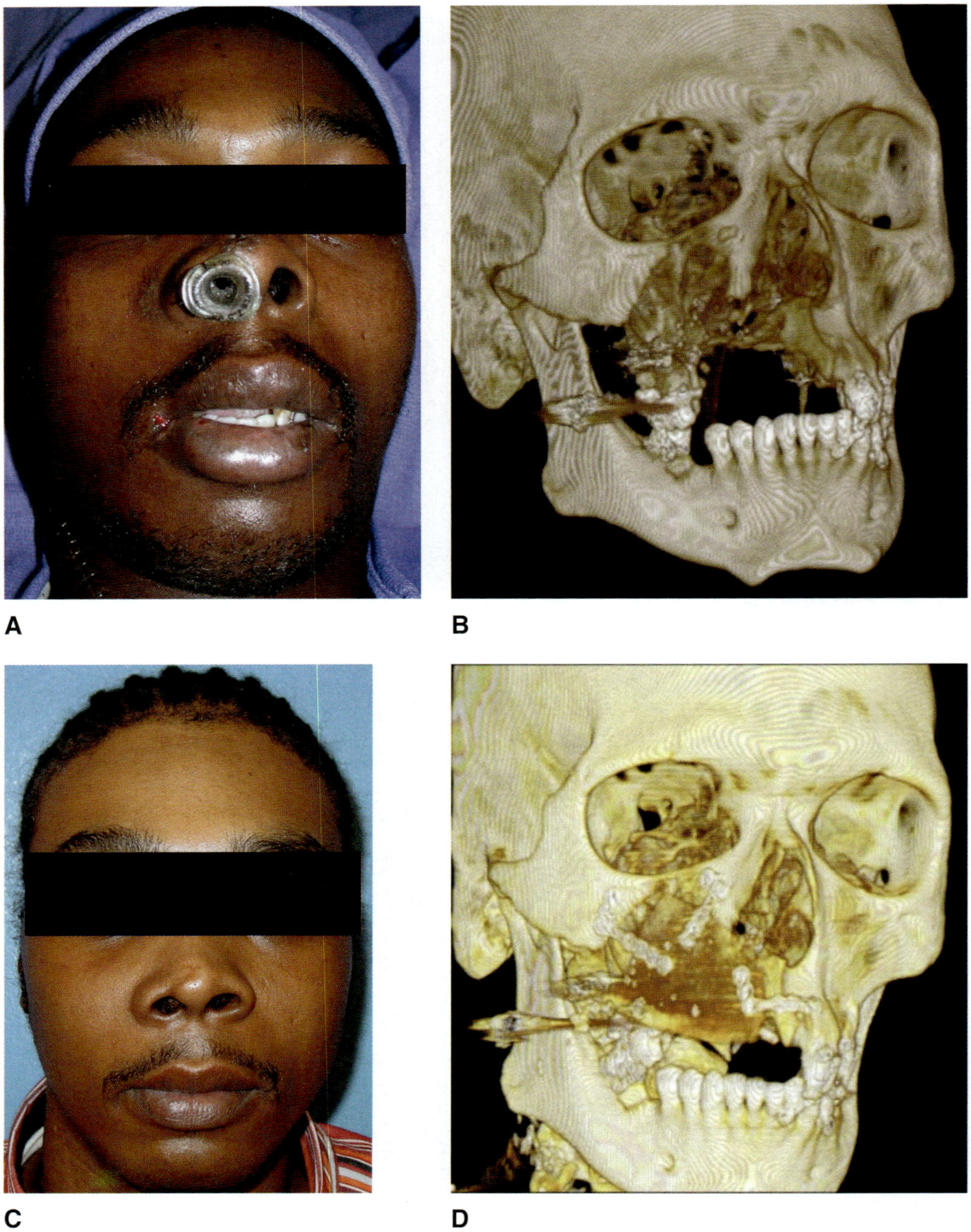

FIGURE 31-4 (**A**) Preoperative clinical photograph and (**B**) three-dimensional computed tomography (CT) scan of a right type Ia(+) maxillary defect caused by a gunshot wound. (**C**) Postoperative clinical photograph and three-dimensional CT scan. (**D**) 1 year after immediate reconstruction with a free iliac bone flap. There was no contracture of the soft tissue envelope. (Reproduced with permission from Robertson, BC, Manson, PN. High-energy ballistic and avulsive injuries. A management protocol for the next millennium. *Surg Clin North Am.* 79:6, 1999.)

soft tissue envelope during the acute phase of wound healing (Figure 31-4) (9).

In our experience, delayed reconstructions are more difficult, less accurate, and more time consuming. The defect must be recreated, scar tissue removed, and multiple osteotomies made to realign the distorted skeleton and reexpand the soft tissue envelope, ultimately producing suboptimal results (Figure 31-5).

Preoperative assessment of the donor vessels (i.e., superficial temporal, facial, and external carotid vessels) may be performed clinically by observation, palpation, and pencil Doppler, paying close attention to lacerations, incisions, contusions, hematomas, edema, and scarring. Potential tissue donor regions must also be evaluated. Preoperative lower extremity angiography is not routinely indicated before harvesting a fibula flap: however, it may be beneficial (15).

Preference is given to dissection of the donor vessels first followed by exploration of the defect and finally free flap harvest. This approach allows precise determination of the types and quantity of tissue and the pedicle length required. If external skin coverage is not required, the maxillary defect may be exposed by means of an intraoral approach, avoiding additional facial incisions. Defining the defect can be demanding in a patient presenting for secondary reconstruction, given dense scar tissue, debris, and obscured tissue planes. After precisely defining the composite tissue requirements and the location of

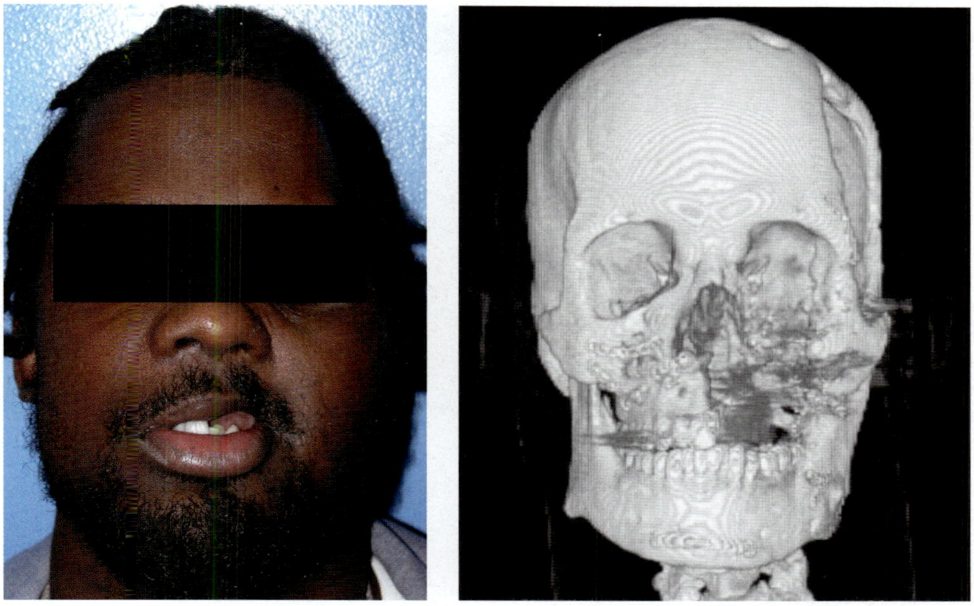

A B

FIGURE 31-5 Clinical photograph (A) and three-dimensional computed tomography scan (B) depicting a left type IIa(+) maxillary defect with involution and contracture of the soft tissue envelope resulting in vertical dystopia and loss of facial projection.

the recipient vessels, a second team may proceed with the flap harvest. It is at this time that corrective maxillofacial osteotomies and fixation may be performed. A coronoidectomy is routinely carried out to prevent flap interference and pedicle obstruction during mandibular excursion.

INSET OF FLAP: BONY FIXATION, SCULPTING OF FLAP, AND SO ON

The fibula can be harvested as an osteoseptocutaneous flap with a large, reliable skin paddle. It has a predictably long vascular pedicle and minimal donor site morbidity and allows a two-team approach. Up to 26 cm of long, straight bone may be harvested, and multiple osteotomies can be performed without embarrassing the vascular supply, allowing the fibula to be accurately shaped to match any contour defect (16). A portion of flexor hallucis longus or soleus muscle may be included with the flap to obliterate dead space. In addition, the fibula provides excellent bone stock to support osseointegrated implants and is the only bone flap that allows bicortical purchase during implant placement (13). Approximation of the posterior compartment musculature appears to preserve power of great toe flexion. All of these features make the fibula flap a versatile and reliable option in maxillary reconstruction.

The iliac crest flap was popularized by Urken et al. for mandibular reconstruction (17) and subsequently used by Brown et al. for maxillary reconstruction, achieving excellent orofacial rehabilitation (18,19). Ample height for osseointegrated implants, cheek projection, and orbital reconstruction can be obtained by harvesting this flap well into the pelvis (13). Furthermore, this flap has a rich supply of cancellous bone and high-quality bone stock, allowing for satisfactory placement of osseointegrated implants. The orientation of the iliac flap is versatile and allows it to fill both high and low defects. The internal oblique muscle is used to line the nasal and oral cavity. Over 2 to 3 weeks, the muscle contracts and epithelializes, precluding the need for later debulking as in skin paddle–based flaps (19,20).

A 2.0-mm titanium miniplate template is contoured preoperatively based on dental models of remaining dentoalveolus and three-dimensional stereolithographic models of the facial skeleton. It is sterilized and used intraoperatively to design flap dimensions and facilitate flap inset (Figure 31-6). This method minimizes warm ischemia time by guiding the location of osteotomies and allows for in situ semirigid stabilization. The pterygoid plates serve as the posterior stops for the neomaxilla. This method ensures a proper interarch relationship between the maxilla and mandible for eventual dental rehabilitation as well as an additional point for bone healing. Ostectomies are routinely limited to the region of the canine because it serves as the pivot point for the dentoalveolus. Watertight, layered repair of tissue planes is crucial to avoid fistula formation, flap dehiscence, and infection.

Recently, we have started the routine use of preoperative three-dimensional computer planning using CT scan data to fabricate individualized templates for donor flap osteotomies based on reconstructed anatomic models. In addition, this has greatly assisted in preoperative planning and streamlined the way in which these cases are planned and executed.

Finally, flap inset must be done such that there are no points of internal or external compression on the pedicle or the site(s) of anastomoses. This cannot be emphasized strongly enough. We take great care and pay meticulous attention to this aspect of flap inset, making certain there is generous room for the pedicle in any subcutaneous tunnels dissected and that these tunnels are neither actively bleeding nor oozing blood so that there is minimal chance of hematoma formation and subsequent pedicle compression. Additional time spent on this aspect of dissection and flap inset is well worth it based on our experience.

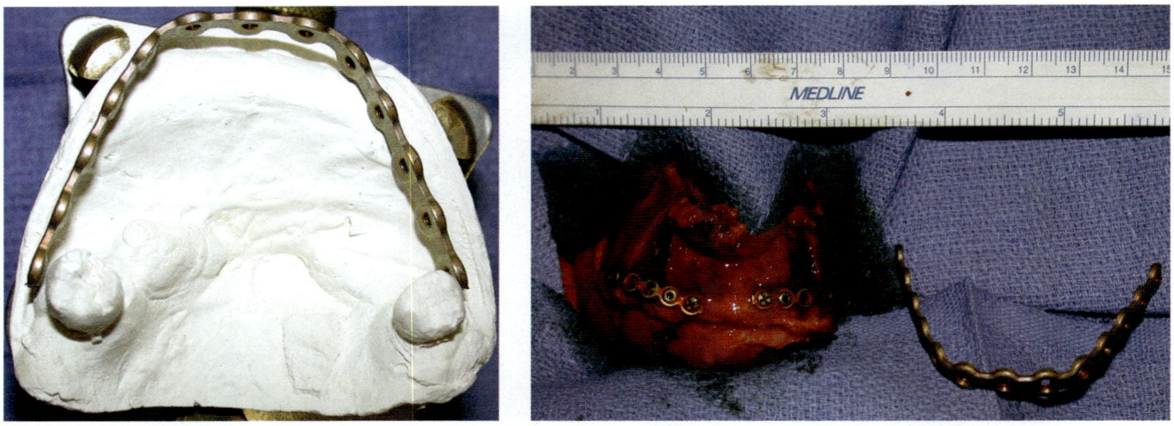

A B

FIGURE 31-6 A 2.0-mm reconstruction plate template is used to facilitate a bilateral maxillary reconstruction. (**A**) Plate is bent to a dental impression. (**B**) Bone graft is osteotomized to fit the curvature of the plate.

VESSEL ANASTOMOSES

Our preferred recipient vessels are to the superficial temporal or facial vessels, usually on the ipsilateral side of the reconstruction (Figures 31-7 to 31-9). Our preference is to do anastomoses in and end-to-end fashion when possible using 9-0 interrupted nylon. Venous coupler usage is at the discretion of the operating surgeon, but we generally prefer to hand sew the venous anastomosis if possible.

NERVE REPAIRS

To date, we have not performed any nerve coaptations to provide improved function or sensation. In our opinion, the additional time added to allow for donor and recipient site nerve dissection as well as nerve microsurgical nerve coaptation is not justified for a minimal chance of protective sensation to the maxillary reconstruction site. The anterior floor of mouth and tongue is another matter.

POSTOPERATIVE MONITORING

Routine postoperative monitoring takes place in the postanesthesia care unit (PACU) monitored by a team of nurses and support staff familiar with microsurgical reconstructive cases. The duration of stay before transfer to an intensive care unit or inpatient floor is based on the patient's condition and reconstructive complexity, but typically a period of 12 to 24 hours in the PACU is appropriate. In some institutions, a designated unit that cares for free tissue transfer patients exists, and these patients are taken directly there from the operating room. In those patients in whom airway stability is a concern because of potential edema and proximity to the oral or nasal cavity,

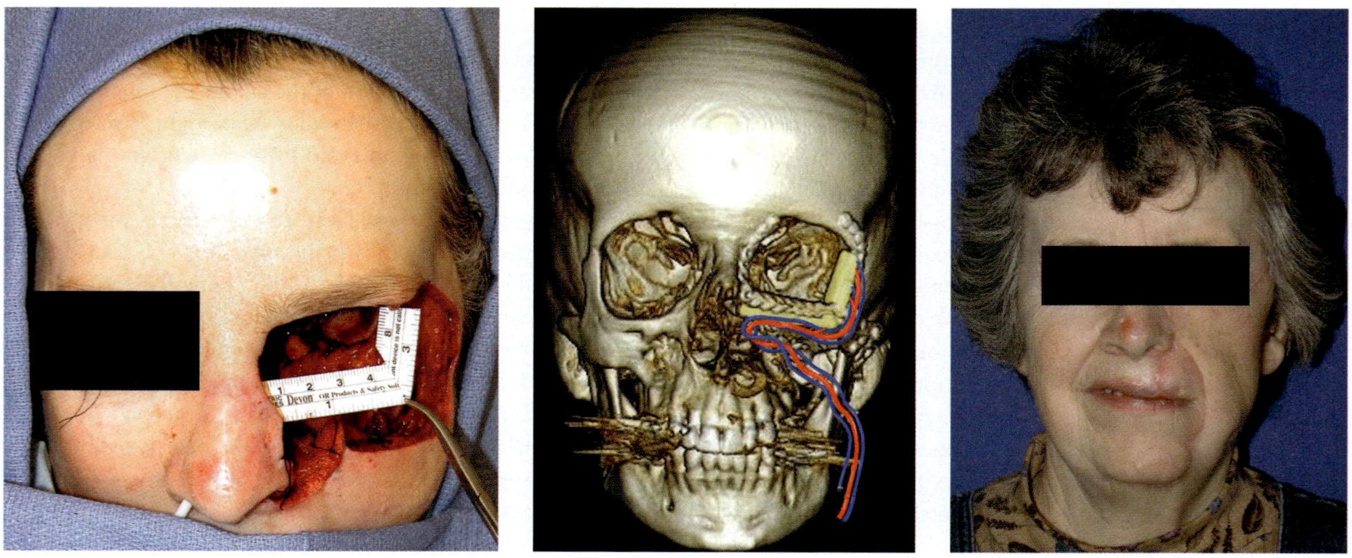

A B C

FIGURE 31-7 A 61-year-old woman with aggressive basal cell carcinoma requiring orbital exenteration with removal of the medial, inferior, and lateral orbital walls as well as the medial maxilla. The defect was obliterated, and the orbital rims (lateral and inferior) were restored with a single osteotomy free fibula osteoseptocutaneous flap. (**A**) Defect after bony and soft tissue resection. (**B**) Postoperative three-dimensional computed tomographic scan showing osteotomized fibula used to reconstruct the defect with the course of its vascular pedicle superimposed. (**C**) Postoperative result.

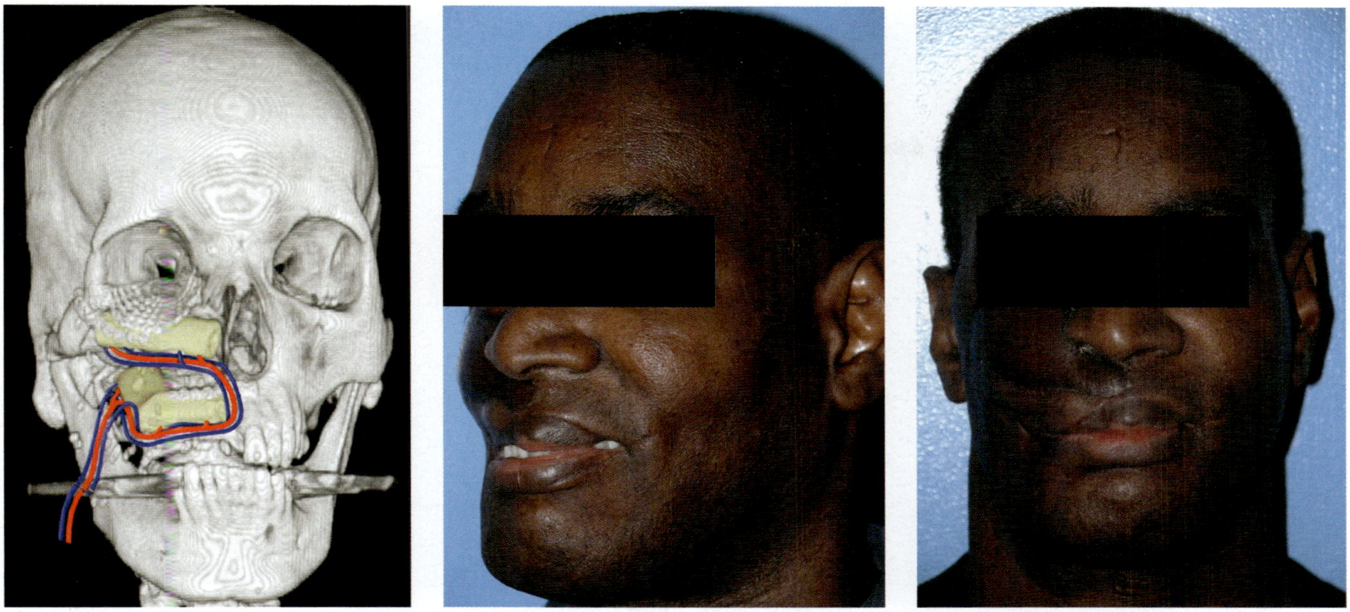

A B C

FIGURE 31-8 A 42-year-old man with a missing inferior orbital rim and maxillary dental alveolus after a motor vehicle collision. He had undergone prior attempts at reconstruction with a rectus abdominis and radial forearm free flap. However, this failed to correct the enophthalmos and did not provide a platform for dental rehabilitation. The orbital rim and hemi-maxilla were reconstructed with a single free fibula osteoseptocutaneous flap including two osteotomies. (**A**) Postoperative three-dimensional computed tomographic scan showing osteotomized fibula with the course of its vascular pedicle superimposed. (**B**) Postoperative left oblique view. (**C**) Postoperative frontal view.

extubation should be carefully coordinated with the anesthesiologist. In our experience, the first 24 to 48 hours appears to be the most critical with regards to vascular thrombosis, airway complications, and the need for emergency reoperation for flap rescue or salvage. We therefore leave patients intubated for 48 hours, allowing for the diminution of edema and bloody nasal airway secretions as well as to expedite operative care in patients returning to surgery.

We typically do not use implantable or external Doppler devices but do use traditional clinical examination as well as adjunctive external pencil Doppler probes for frequent flap monitoring at the sites of anastomoses as well as available exposed surfaces on the flaps themselves. Close postoperative monitoring of fluid balance, urine output, and blood pressure is mandatory and must not be understated or underestimated. Any need for vasopressor therapy in case of hemodynamic lability must be cleared with the surgical team because our preference is to avoid vasopressors perioperatively when at all possible. The reason for this is the danger of peripheral vasoconstriction causing a thrombogenic low flow state at the vascular anastomoses.

Close attention to the creation of a comfortable and watertight flap inset is vital. Open (e.g., Penrose) or closed (e.g., Blake) drainage is used to prevent any restrictive fluid collections or other compression of the flap or pedicle. We prefer not to use dressings on the head and neck, and the avoidance of any additional restrictive materials (e.g., oxygen masks, tracheotomy ties, nasal canula) is essential. A technically well-executed operation may be ultimately compromised by a casual lack of attention to seemingly trivial details in the immediate postoperative period.

POTENTIAL COMPLICATIONS

Complex maxillary reconstruction requires careful planning to ensure predictable results. Variables to consider when planning the operation include date and mechanism of injury (high or low energy), associated injuries, age, physical condition, nutritional status, comorbidities, and previous operative interventions (21). All can affect donor site selection.

Disadvantages of the iliac crest flap include the bulk associated with its obligatory muscle cuff and thick subcutaneous layer as well as its short pedicle (4–5 cm), making it problematic in small defects and when the facial vein and artery are inadequate (18,19). Donor site morbidity is comparable in both fibula and iliac crest flaps (22). Specifically, fibula flap donor sites have a slightly higher incidence of overall complications with reduced power and reduced sensation distal to the flap harvest site. In addition, clawing of the great toe is described. Iliac crest flap donor sites are very painful but have slightly less overall donor site morbidity. However, they do have a significant incidence of hernia or bulge on late follow-up evaluation (22). When selecting a donor site, we consider first concomitant injuries that may limit available tissue, the need for dental rehabilitation, and finally the dimensions of the bone defect. We do not consider the donor site deficit.

In conclusion, free tissue transfer for treatment of high-energy facial trauma is reserved for severe cases with significant bone and soft tissue loss. At our institution, this algorithm is applicable only to a fraction of patients with severe facial injuries (~0.1%). Although these cases are rare, proper initial treatment is critical. In our experience, tremendous amounts of time

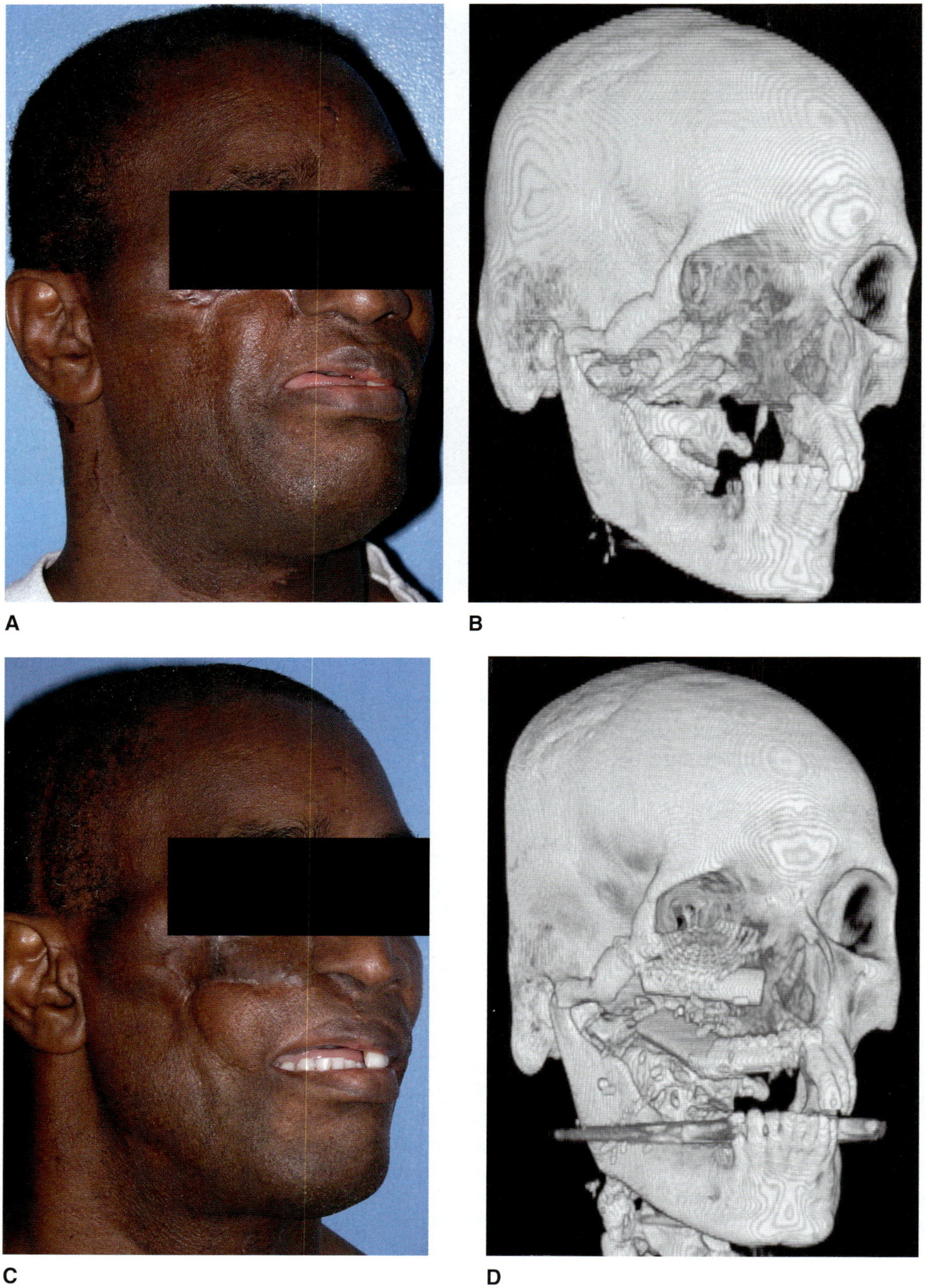

A B C D

FIGURE 31-9 The patient in Figure 31-8. (A) Clinical photograph and preoperative three-dimensional computed tomography (CT) scan (B) demonstrating a right type IIb(+) defect. (C) Clinical photograph and postoperative three-dimensional CT scan (D) 6 months after reconstruction with a single free fibula osteoseptocutaneous flap.

and effort have been spent correcting inadequate reconstructions that collapsed over time.

OUTLINE OF ANTICIPATED SECONDARY SURGERY

Many patients undergo revisions of secondary procedures. Achieving an optimal result is critical in trauma patients because they are generally young, without comorbidities and have long life expectancies. The goal of the first phase of reconstruction is to restore the skeletal anatomy and deliver adequate or, perhaps, abundant soft tissue bulk that can be contoured or rearranged at a later date. In the second phase, the bone and soft tissue are contoured, and the position of the eyelids and the nose are addressed. We have found that type II and presumably type IV deformities often require additional soft tissue augmentation in the periorbital and malar regions.

Patients who undergo delayed reconstruction before definitive microsurgical intervention have typically already had prior attempts at reconstruction using local, distant, or even free musculofascial flaps combined with nonvascularized bone grafts. The first step is to recognize that in such individuals' collapse of the bony architecture and disfiguring soft tissue contracture will necessitate formal reconstruction with recreation of the defect, accurate reconstruction of the facial skeleton, and the provision of a soft tissue envelope with adequate volume. Revisionary surgery in this context is surgery that follows adequate reconstruction according to these principles. Therefore, secondary surgery after a definitive microsurgical reconstruction may be considered part of the natural progression toward obtaining a "perfect" result rather than merely surgery for complications or to correct an unsatisfactory outcome. This should be discussed with all patients as part of the preoperative visit(s) as well as during the informed consent process.

Additional consideration must be given to close collaboration with our dental colleagues regarding dental rehabilitation after definitive microsurgical maxillary reconstruction has been satisfactorily completed. Osseointegrated implant placement should be closely planned and coordinated so as to optimize the rehabilitative process.

In addition, one must recognize that there will likely be the need for further sculpting procedures as mentioned earlier. These may include soft tissue cheek augmentation using fat grafting techniques or additional free tissue transfer, soft tissue debulking procedures, the possible need for distraction and stabilization of the neomaxilla, and osseous contouring of the neomaxilla following hardware removal.

RESULTS AND OUTCOMES

Our results are highlighted in Figures 31-8 to 31-11.

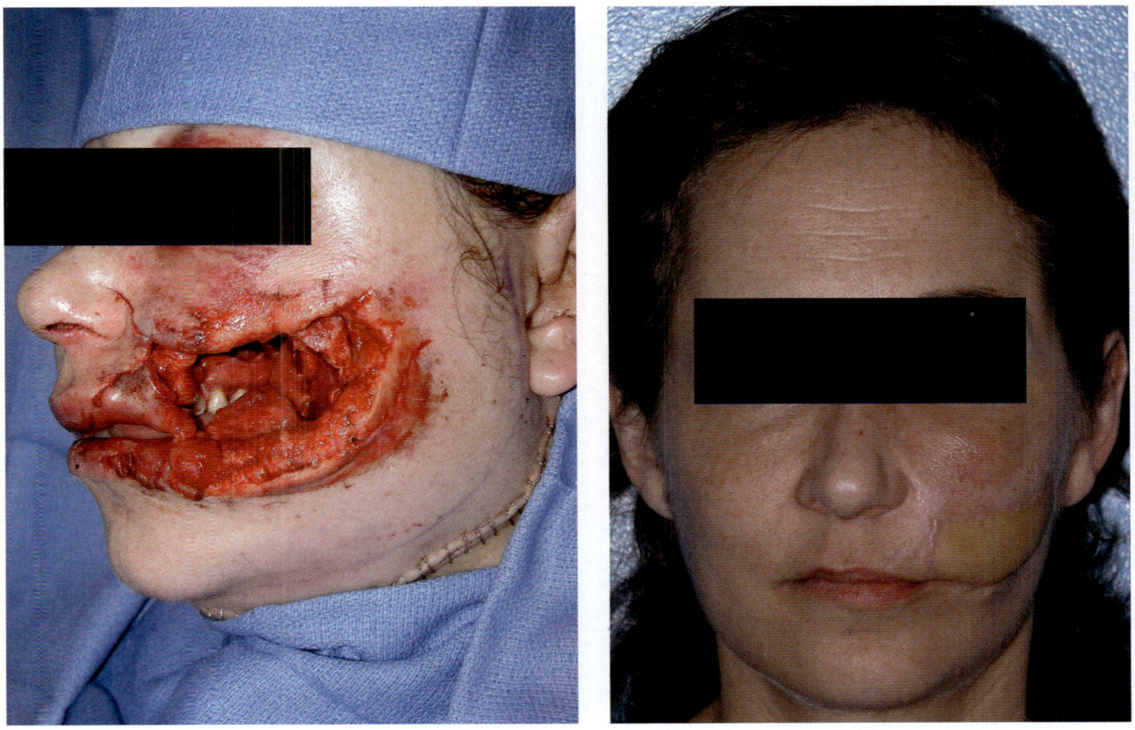

A B

FIGURE 31-10 (A) Right maxillary type Ib(+) defect from a gunshot wound. (B) Immediate reconstruction with a free iliac crest musculocutaneous flap. There is no contracture of the soft tissue envelope.

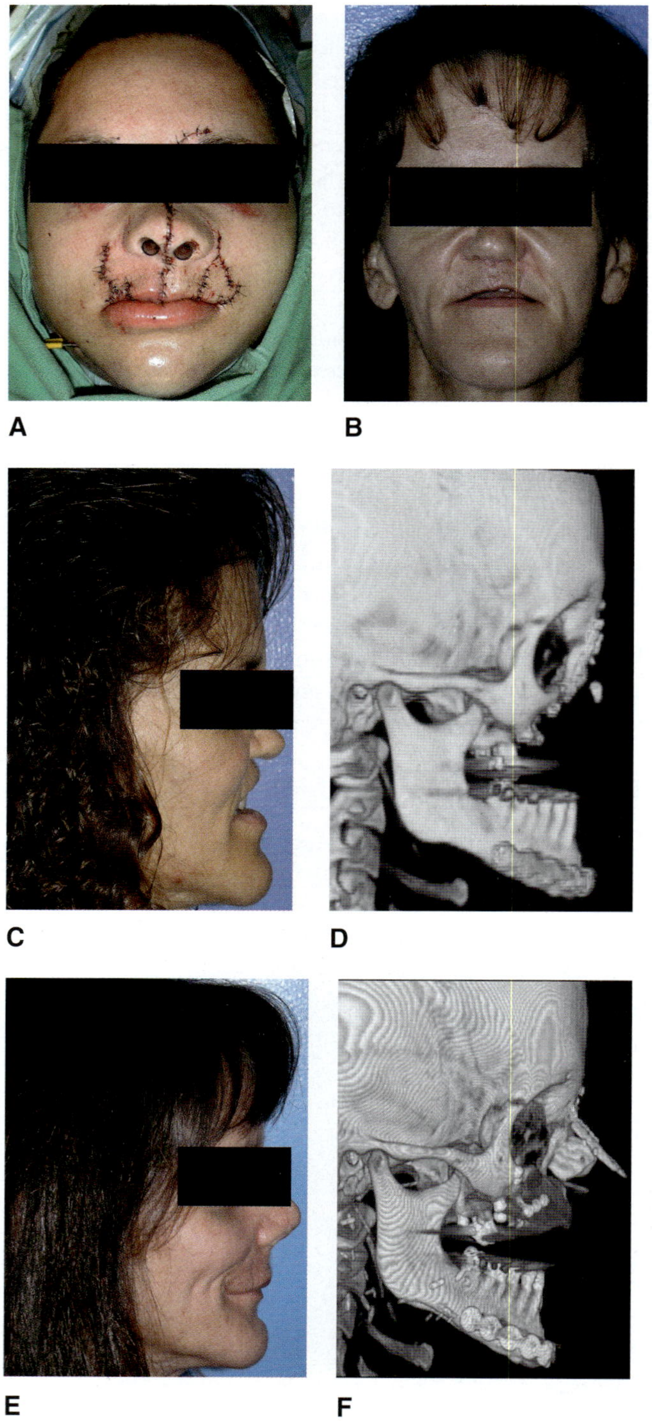

FIGURE 31-11 (A) A 40-year-old woman who sustained a self-inflicted submental midline gunshot wound after immediate soft tissue only reconstruction. (B) Three months after injury, there is total midface collapse because of lack of midface skeletal support. (C) Preoperative clinical photograph and (D) three-dimensional computed tomography (CT) scan of a type IIIa(+) maxillary defect. (E) Postoperative clinical photograph and (F) three-dimensional CT scan 1 year after free iliac crest with an internal oblique muscle flap.

REFERENCES

1. Genden EM, Okay D, Stepp MT, et al. Comparison of functional and quality-of-life outcomes in patients with and without palatomaxillary reconstruction: a preliminary report. *Arch Otolaryngol Head Neck Surg* 2003;129:775.
2. Gruss JS, Antonyshyn O, Phillips JH. Early definitive bone and soft-tissue reconstruction of major gunshot wounds of the face. *Plast Reconstr Surg* 1991;87:436.
3. Edgerton MT Jr, Zovickian A. Reconstruction of major defects of the palate. *Plast Reconstr Surg* 1956;17:105.
4. Miller TA. The Tagliacozzi flap as a method of nasal and palatal reconstruction. *Plast Reconstr Surg* 1985;76:870.
5. Campbell H. Reconstruction of the left maxilla. *Plast Reconstr Surg* 1948;3:66.
6. Branemark PI. Osseointegration and its experimental background. *J Prosthet Dent* 1983;50:399.
7. Rodriguez ED, Martin M, Bluebong-Langner R, et al. Microsurgical reconstruction of posttraumatic high-energy maxillary defects: establishing the effectiveness of early reconstruction. *Plast Reconstr Surg* 2007;120:7.
8. Genden EM, Higgins K, Urken ML. The role of pedicles flaps in a microvascular world. *Semin Plast Surg* 2003;17:3.
9. Robertson BC, Manson PN. High-energy ballistic and avulsive injuries. A management protocol for the next millennium. *Surg Clin North Am* 1999;79:6.
10. Muzaffar AR, Adams WP Jr, Hartog JM, et al. Maxillary reconstruction: functional and aesthetic considerations. *Plast Reconstr Surg* 1999;104:7.
11. Rohner D, Jaquiery C, Kunz C, et al. Maxillofacial reconstruction with prefabricated osseous free flaps: a 3-year experience with 24 patients. *Plast Reconstr Surg* 2003;112:3.
12. Suominen E, Tukiainen E. Close-range shotgun and rifle injuries to the face. *Clin Plast Surg* 2001;28:2.
13. Frodel JL Jr, Funk GF, Capper DT, et al. Osseointegrated implants: a comparative study of bone thickness in four vascularized bone flaps. *Plast Reconstr Surg* 1993;92:449.
14. Bartlett CS. Clinical update: gunshot wound ballistics. *Clin Orthop* 2003;408:28.
15. Lutz BS, Wei FC, Ng SH, et al. Routine donor leg angiography before vascularized free fibula transplantation is not necessary: a prospective study in 120 clinical cases. *Plast Reconstr Surg* 1999;103:121.
16. Yim KK, Wei FC. Fibula osteoseptocutaneous free flap in maxillary reconstruction. *Microsurgery* 1994;15:353.
17. Urken ML, Buchbinder D, Constantino PD, et al. Oromandibular reconstruction using microvascular composite flaps: report of 210 cases. *Arch Otolaryngol Head Neck Surg* 1998;124:46.
18. Brown JS. Deep circumflex iliac artery free flap with internal oblique muscle as a new method of immediate reconstruction of maxillectomy defect. *Head Neck* 1996;18:412.
19. Brown JS, Jones DC, Summerwill A, et al. Vascularized iliac crest with internal oblique muscle for immediate reconstruction after maxillectomy. *Br J Oral Maxillofac Surg* 2002;40:183.
20. Kakibuchi M, Fujikawa M, Hosokawa K, et al. Functional reconstruction of maxilla with free latissimus dorsi-scapular osteomusculocutaneous flap. *Plast Reconstr Surg* 2002;109:1238.
21. Dolin J, Scalea T, Mannor L, et al. The management of gunshot wounds to the face. *J Trauma* 1992;33:508.
22. Rogers SN, Lakshmiah SR, Narayan B, et al. A comparison of the long-term morbidity following deep circumflex iliac and fibula free flaps for reconstruction following head and neck cancer. *Plast Reconstr Surg* 2003;112:1517.

CHAPTER 32

Mandibular Reconstruction

James Sanger and J. Brian Boyd

Defects of the mandible frequently result in significant oral cavity morbidity. Loss of mandible continuity causes the remaining segments to become unstable. Unopposed muscle pull results in collapse toward the defect (Figure 32-1). If teeth remain, the shift of the remaining mandible segments causes loss of occlusal alignment, leading to abnormal wear patterns and accelerating dental caries. In patients with cancer, teeth are often removed before or at the time of mandible resection because edentulation is required for postoperative radiation therapy. Because of the instability and deformity, dentures can rarely be fitted. These changes limit mastication, which adversely affects nutritional intake.

Most mandible defects are accompanied by soft tissue defects, and reconstruction of the soft tissue in these composite defects is as important as restoration of bony continuity for optimum function and aesthetics. Loss of the oral lining contributes to the collapse deformity. Other adverse consequences of inadequate oral lining include decreased tongue mobility and a deficient sulcus. Tongue mobility is important for speech, manipulation of food, and control of saliva. An inadequate sulcus may contribute to oral incontinence, or "drooling." Intraoral soft tissue deficits also contribute to aesthetic defects, especially when dentition is not restored and the lower lip collapses and becomes retruded. External defects of the cheek or chin complicate mandible reconstruction and must be successfully addressed to obtain a good, functional result. Large unreconstructed anterior defects, also known as the "Andy Gump," deformity are especially devastating (Figure 32-2). The combined effects of intraoral functional loss and external deformity contribute to social isolation and depression, further reducing quality of life.

The goals of bony mandible reconstruction are to recreate a stable mandibular arch with normal joint mechanics and to set the stage for dental rehabilitation. Composite resections additionally require soft tissue reconstruction that minimizes external defects while restoring a sensate floor of the mouth, tongue mobility, and oral competence. A one-stage restitution of both form and function is paramount in maximizing the quality of life in patients whose life expectancies may be poor (1).

CLASSIFICATION OF MANDIBULAR AND ASSOCIATED SOFT TISSUE DEFECTS

Classification of both bone and soft tissue defects is helpful in selecting the best flap, comparing the results of different techniques, and developing algorithms to aid others in the management of these difficult cases.

Defects can be classified based on anatomy as well as function and aesthetics. Boyd et al. (2) classified bony defects simply on whether the missing segment is anterior or lateral and whether the segment includes a condyle or not (Figure 32-3). Epithelial defects are recorded as skin (s), mucosa (m), or both (sm). Briefly, the H segment is a lateral segment of mandible with a condyle attached, and the L segment is one without a condyle. Both can be of any length. The C segment is the anterior portion of the mandible containing canine and incisor teeth.

This classification system is predicated on the ease by which free microvascular bone transfers can reconstruct large or small defects, the length of the graft per se no longer affecting difficulty or outcome. The three issues that do increase the difficulty of mandibular reconstruction and potentially affect the quality of the final result are the essence of the system. These are:

1. Resection of the condyle
2. Resection of the anterior C segment
3. Resection of skin, mucosa, or both

Resection of a condyle means that some form of temporomandibular joint reconstruction must be carried out. This adds complexity and will be discussed later. Complex "through-and-through"

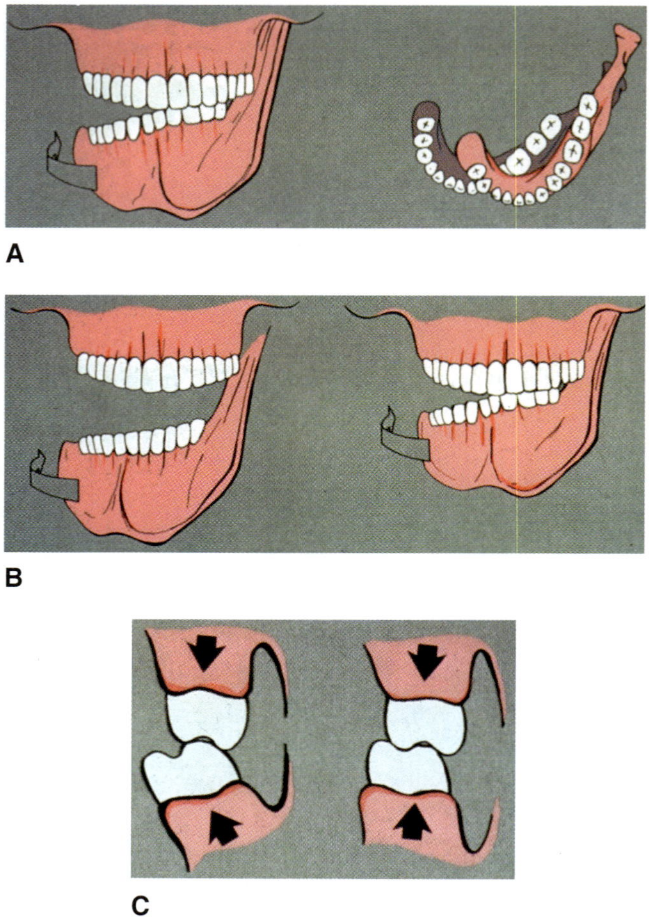

FIGURE 32-1 (A) and (B) After resection of a lateral segment of mandible, instability results in both collapse and rotation of the mandible posteriorly and superiorly. The mandible shifts toward the affected side. (C) The remaining mandibular teeth become canted inward, resulting abnormal wear patterns and caries.

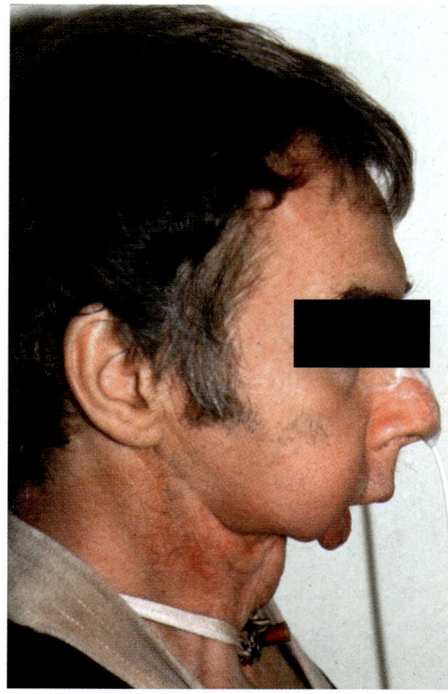

FIGURE 32-2 The "Andy Gump" deformity after resection of the anterior segment without reconstruction. The patient loses oral continence and drools when he eats. It also adversely affects speech and appearance, causing the person to become a recluse.

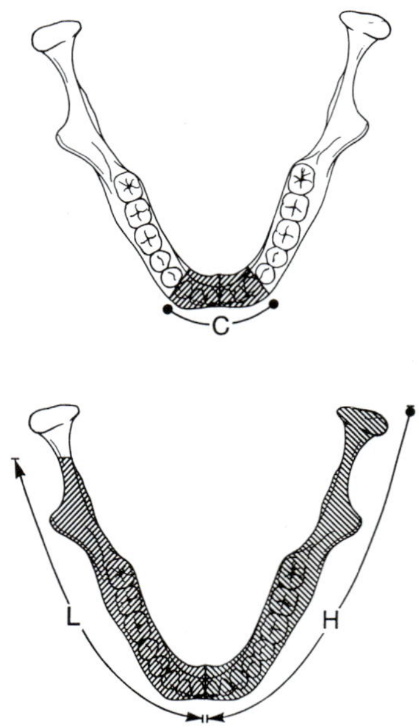

FIGURE 32-3 Diagram explaining the HCL classification. Anterior segments include both canine and incisor teeth and are designated by the letter C. Lateral defects of any size *without* the condyle are designated L. An L defect can extend into part of the central segment but does not include the condyle. If the condyle is included with any part of the lateral defect, the defect is designated as H. Using combinations of these designations, bony defects can be classified into one of eight possible categories. A lateral defect that extends to include the opposite canine is designated as LC, and a defect that includes the condyle and extends to the opposite angle of the mandible is an HCL defect. The addition of a mucosal defect is denoted by the letter c, a skin defect by the letter s, a through-and-through defect by the letters mc, and a bone-only defect by the letter o. (Reproduced with permission from Boyd JB, Gullane PJ, Rostein LE, et al: Classification of mandibular defects. *Plast Reconstr Surg* 92:1266,1993.)

or "full-thickness" defects require the reconstruction of skin as well as mucosa. As we shall see, this can necessitate two skin paddles or a second flap. Loss of the anterior (C) segment results in the detachment or partial resection of mouth-opening muscles, including the digastrics, the geniohyoids, and the mylohyoids. If not reattached to the reconstruction, these muscles attach themselves to adjacent soft tissues and pull them off the anterior arch, producing a condition known as "lip and chin ptosis" (Figure 32-4). The unopposed mouth-closing muscles, the medial pterygoid and the masseter, rotate the mandible upward, exacerbating this effect.

Using combinations of the H, C, and L designations, bony defects can be classified into one of eight possible groups. A lateral defect that extends to include the opposite canine is designated as LC, and a defect that includes the condyle and extends to the opposite angle of the mandible is an HCL defect.

Unfortunately, with the exception of benign dental tumors or limited traumatic or infection-related lesions, most bony defects do have accompanying soft tissue deficits, and these often have more impact on functional and aesthetic outcome than does the bone loss itself.

More complicated systems to classify the soft tissue component exist (3,4). For reconstructive purposes, the oral cavity can

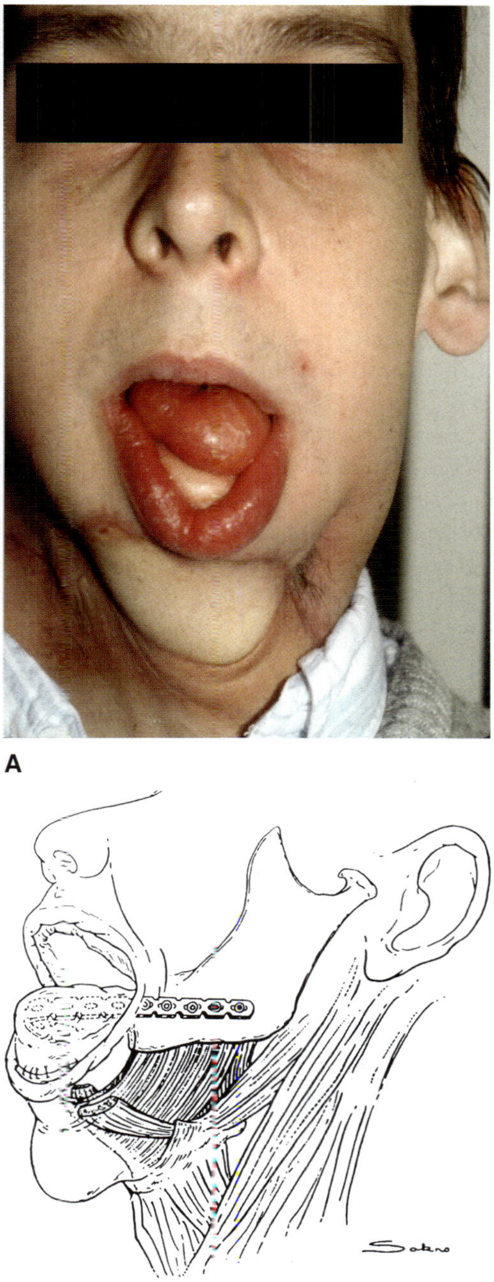

A

B

FIGURE 32-4 (A) and (B) Lip and chin ptosis after anterior mandibular and floor of mouth resection. The soft tissues (lip and chin) have been pulled off the anterior mandibular arch by the detached submental mouth-opening muscles, and the masseter and the medial pterygoid try to compensate, actually exacerbating the problem by rotating the mandible upward. The patient has a functional Andy Gump deformity. It is vital to (re)attach the soft tissues of the chin to the reconstructed anterior mandible. (Reproduced with permission from Boyd JB, Gullane PJ, Rostein LE, et al. Classification of mandibular defects. *Plast Reconstr Surg* 92:1266,1993.)

be divided into 10 functional units: oral sphincter, lingual and buccal sulci, alveolar ridges, floor of mouth, mobile tongue, base of tongue, tonsillar pillars, soft palate, hard palate, and buccal mucosa. Bone defects can exist with any one, but more frequently combinations, of these units. In general, the more contiguous units involved, the greater is the functional deficit for any given bone defect. Because there are so many possible combinations, the application of these classification schemes, although comprehensive and descriptive, is impractical because it gives rise to hundreds or thousands of possibilities.

Likewise, the TNM classification system (5) is unhelpful in classifying the reconstructive challenge. Most patients have T3 or T4 lesions. However, the resulting defect and the reconstructive needs of a T4 lesion in the anterior floor of mouth involving the anterior mandible and lip will be radically different from a T4 lesion of the tongue base, mandibular angle, and tonsillar pillar. Traumatic injuries are even more difficult to classify. The HCL classification, although simple, can often fall short in estimating the size, extent, and degree of difficulty in reconstructing the intraoral component. Although it helps with flap selection, the surgeon needs to assess each defect and then translate that into an operative plan that takes advantage of the options currently available to maximize functional and aesthetic outcomes.

RECONSTRUCTION OF MANDIBLE DEFECTS

Without Bone

In patients who have short lateral or posterior defects and who may have a poor outlook because of their age, general condition, or extent of disease, the application of a heavy-duty reconstruction plate without bone may restore mandibular support and facial symmetry and provide adequate reconstruction provided well-vascularized lining is supplied. Generally, the plate is covered by either a pedicled musculocutaneous or muscle flap, such as the pectoralis major, or a free flap such as the radial forearm or lateral thigh flap, to prevent its exposure (6,7). A 5% failure rate—as defined by plate removal—may be expected; however, the technique is not indicated for anterior (C-containing) defects, where there is a 35% incidence of failure. Plates are generally removed for exposure or fracture, the latter resulting from torque stress (8).

An alternative to this approach is to perform a soft tissue reconstruction for posterior defects and ignore the bony loss (9). The disadvantage of this is that the patient will certainly develop malocclusion (if he or she has teeth), caries, facial asymmetry, and occlusal tilt (see Figure 32-1). We believe that the addition of the plate in these individuals with posterior bony defects adds very little time to the procedure, is associated with a low failure rate, and is well worth the effort.

With Bone

It is not the purpose of this chapter to provide an extensive review of the evolution of bone grafting in mandibular reconstruction, interesting though it may be. However, we should pause to contemplate the stepwise improvements in technique, the failures, the prolonged hospitalizations, the chronic complications, the professional rivalries, and even the fatalities that have led us to where we are today.

Even in the best of hands, nonvascularized bone grafting had an unacceptably high failure rate when any degree of contamination was present (10–15). Such contamination is the norm in composite resections. Precise mandibular shaping led to improved results, and the techniques described by Manchester still have application in microsurgical reconstruction (16,17). Staged procedures were advocated to minimize the risk of infection and "dives" in hyperbaric oxygen used to improve revascularization (18,19). Today conventional bone grafting retains a place in noncontaminated and nonirradiated wounds when the bone gap is 6 cm or less (20). The 6-cm figure is actually derived from extensive orthopedic literature on bone grafting to the extremities, so its use in mandibular reconstruction may be considered somewhat arbitrary.

Pedicled osteomusculocutaneous flaps (21–25) represent a halfway house in the evolution of mandible bone grafting. Although they provided vascularized bone, tethering limited bone, and soft tissue positioning, bone stock was weak, osteotomies were difficult, and their vascularity was suspect. They are seldom used today.

Free vascularized bone grafts heal like a fracture rather than undergoing "creeping substitution" which is the fate of conventional bone grafts (26), in which prolonged revascularization exposes the grafts to infection, resorption, structural failure, and exposure, particularly in irradiated or scarred beds. In addition to living bone, the vascularized bone graft can carry soft tissue for lining, skin cover, or bulk replacement and the reconstruction can be completed safely in one stage without the need for hyperbaric oxygen, prolonged hospitalization, or deforming regional flaps.

There are a number of free vascularized bone flap options for reconstruction of the mandible. Most flaps can be harvested with skin or muscle to provide oral lining or external cover. Each flap has its own strengths and relative weaknesses; no one flap is superior in all aspects. Careful evaluation of the defect and potential donor sites dictates which flap is selected.

For major defects, the fibula (27), scapula (28), and iliac crest (29) free flaps are most often used. For lesser defects, the radial forearm (30), second metatarsal (31), or (rarely) rib (32) may be satisfactory. However, in practice, the fibula is used in more than 80% of cases. The relative strengths and weaknesses of these different flaps as well as the basic flap circulation will be discussed. Technical details of flap elevation are dealt with elsewhere in this text.

Fibula

The fibula is an outstanding source of vascularized bone. The peroneal artery and its venae comitantes provide large-caliber vessels that are ideal for microsurgery. Up to 25 cm of bone can be harvested. The fibula is the only vascularized bone flap that can be used reliably for a subtotal mandibular reconstruction (Figure 32-5). A skin paddle may be transferred with the bone based on either septocutaneous or musculocutaneous perforators. These are usually Dopplered along the posterior margin of the fibula near the junction of the middle and distal thirds of the bone. With two or more perforators, it may be possible to design two separate skin paddles. The positions of the perforators are confirmed during the dissection. Multiple osteotomies can be made without adversely affecting circulation to the bone. Use of the fibula for mandibular reconstruction is shown in Figures 32-5 and 32-6. Either the lateral sural cutaneous nerve (LCSN) (Figure 32-7) or the *recurrent branch* of the superficial peroneal nerve (RSPN), whichever is dominant in providing sensory innervation to the skin island, can be coapted to the lingual or mental nerve to restore sensation to the reconstructed oral lining (33,34). This is most advantageous when the mucosal or skin defect involves the tongue, anterior floor of the mouth, or lower lip, where the presence of sensation is intrinsic to function.

The fibula is currently the most frequently used flap due to its ease of elevation, reliability, and minimal long-term donor morbidity. If the skin paddle is greater than 5 cm in width, primary closure is difficult, and skin grafting is usually required. Minor wound healing problems are common but have little effect on ambulation over time. Simultaneous dissection permits the fibula to be raised while a second team completes the resection and prepares the neck. As a major leg vessel is sacrificed, its use is contraindicated in vasculopaths. Provided the posterior tibial and dorsalis pedis pulses are present, there is little chance of vascular compromise. Preoperative angiography is generally not needed but should be obtained if there is suspicion of occlusive disease. The height of the fibula is adequate for placement of osseointegrated implants but is often less than the native mandible.

Scapula

The scapular osteocutaneous flap has the unique advantage in mandibular reconstruction that the skin paddle(s) can be oriented independently from the axis of the bone. The circumflex scapular artery emerges through the triangular space formed by the long head of the triceps, teres major, and teres minor muscles. At the point where the vessel exits from this space, branches supply the lateral border of the scapula. The vessel arborizes into fasciocutaneous branches, and the skin paddle can be designed horizontally (scapular) or vertically (parascapular). If needed, two separate paddles are elevated, one for intraoral reconstruction and one for external skin replacement. Up to 14 cm of well-vascularized bone, which can undergo osteotomies for contour, is available (Figure 32-8).

The main disadvantage of the scapular flap is the need to place the patient in the lateral position, making it very difficult to elevate the flap while the ablation takes place. This factor prolongs the operation. In secondary reconstructions, simultaneous preparatory dissection of the neck is often possible. Early postoperative physical therapy prevents shoulder contractures. The scapula is not of uniform thickness along its border, and the bone is not always adequate for osseointegrated implants.

Iliac Crest

Mandibular reconstruction using nonvascularized iliac crest grafts has been well demonstrated by Manchester (16,17). Taylor and associates (35,36) introduced the groin osteocutaneous flap based on the deep circumflex iliac vessels (Figure 32-9). These vessels perfuse the bone and send perforating vessels through the external oblique muscle to the overlying skin. Up to 15 cm of bone and skin paddles of 10 cm by 30 cm may be transferred on the deep iliac circumflex vessels. The natural curve of the iliac crest lends itself to reconstruction of hemimandibular defects if the ipsilateral crest is harvested. For shorter defects, either side may be used. Anterior defects require

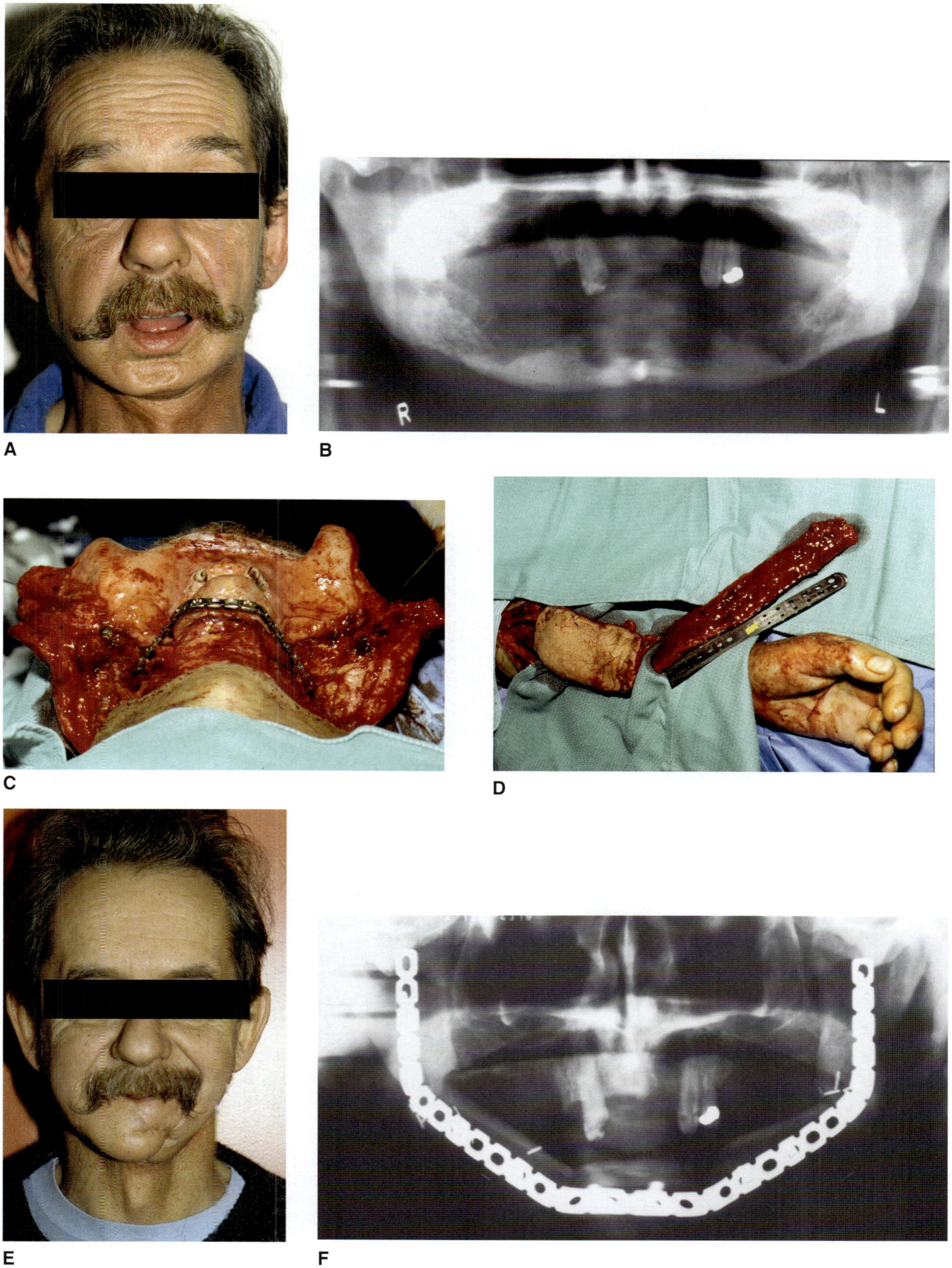

FIGURE 32-5 Subtotal mandibular reconstruction using a fibula flap. (A) and (B) Preoperative photograph and Panorex of a 62-year-old man with osteoradionecrosis of the mandible. (C) Defect spanned by a reconstruction plate that was temporarily removed to permit resection of the bone. (D) Reconstruction of bone and oral lining was performed using a fibula and a radial forearm flap connected in series (flow-through). (E) and (F) Result 12 months later.

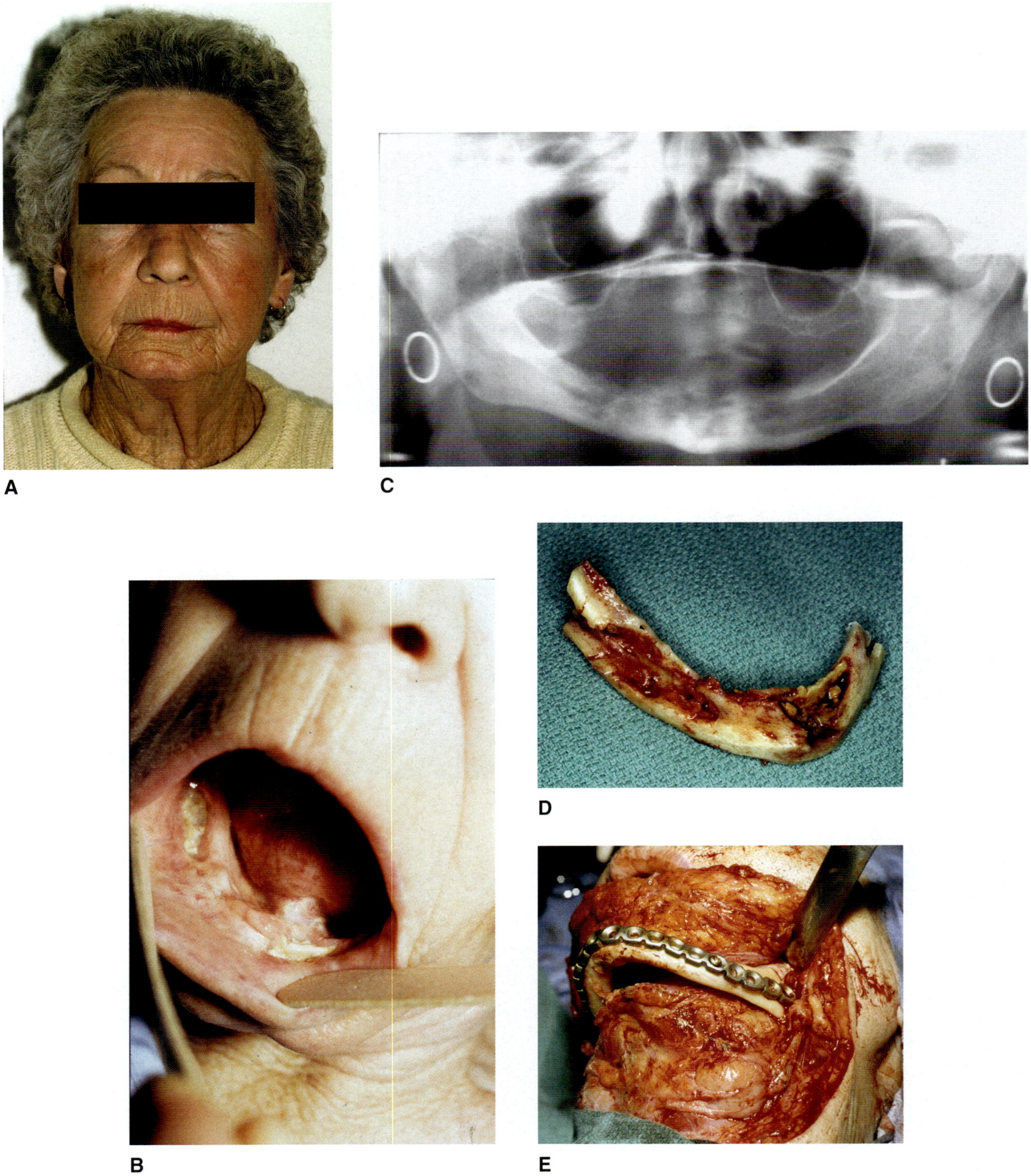

FIGURE 32-6 Use of an osteocutaneous fibula flap. (A) and (B) A 64-year-old woman with osteonecrosis of the mandible. (C) and (D) Panorex and resected mandible showing osteoradionecrosis. (E) A reconstruction plate is conformed to the shape of the mandible before its resection. Drill holes and temporary screws are placed in the remaining mandibular fragments to aid their accurate positioning on either side of the bone graft.

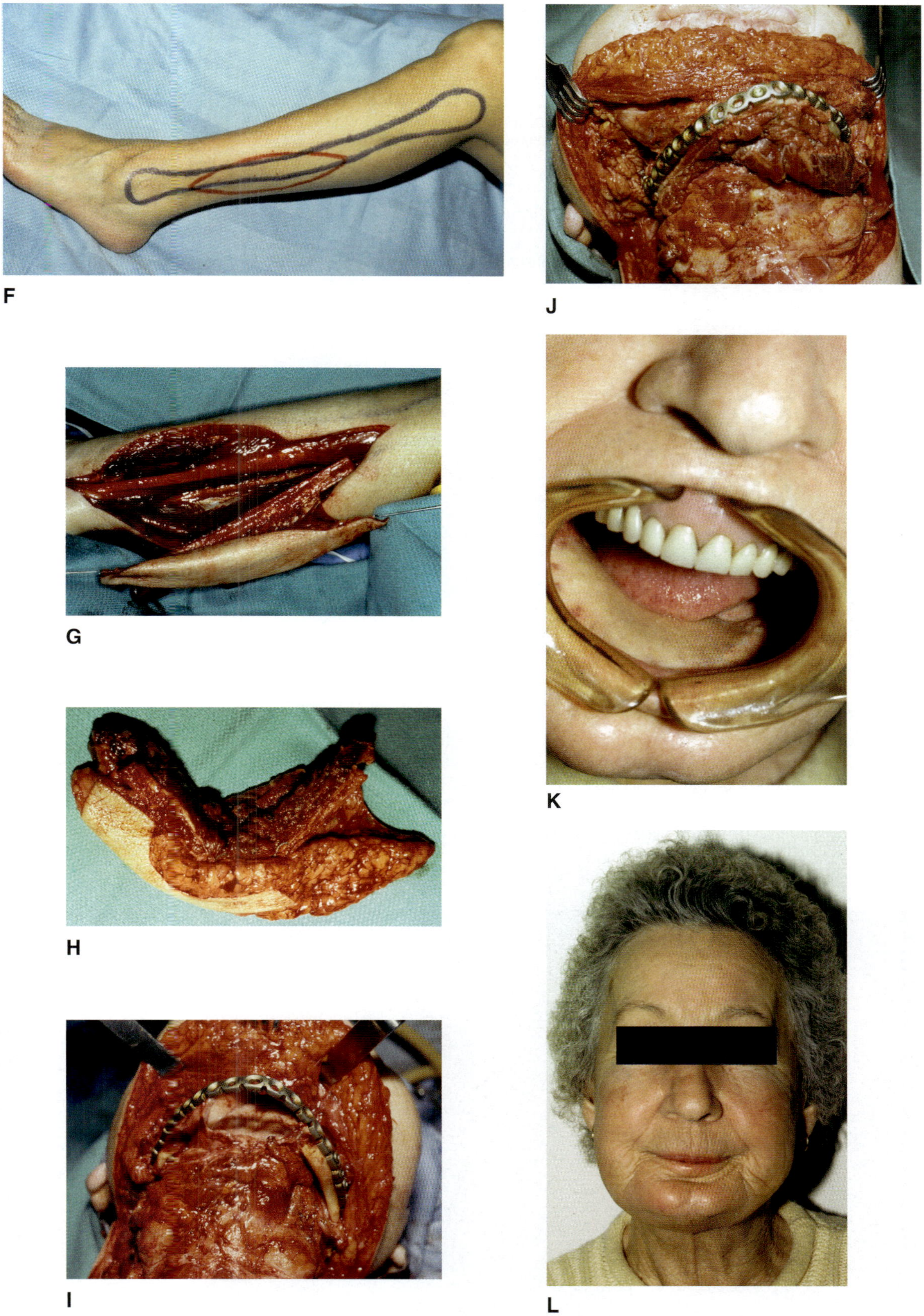

FIGURE 32-6 (*Continued*) (F) The skin island is positioned over a Doppler signal, roughly at the junction of the lower and middle thirds of the leg. (G) The fibula flap is isolated on its pedicle. (H) The graft is shaped with two closing wedge osteotomies, loosely held together by interosseous wires. The reconstruction plate is reapplied after the bone resection (I). The flap is fitted within it (J) and held with unicortical screws. (K) and (L) The final result at 7 months. Note that the intraoral flap will have to be replaced by a skin graft to facilitate osseointegrated dental implants. Also note that the height of the fibula is somewhat less than the native mandible.

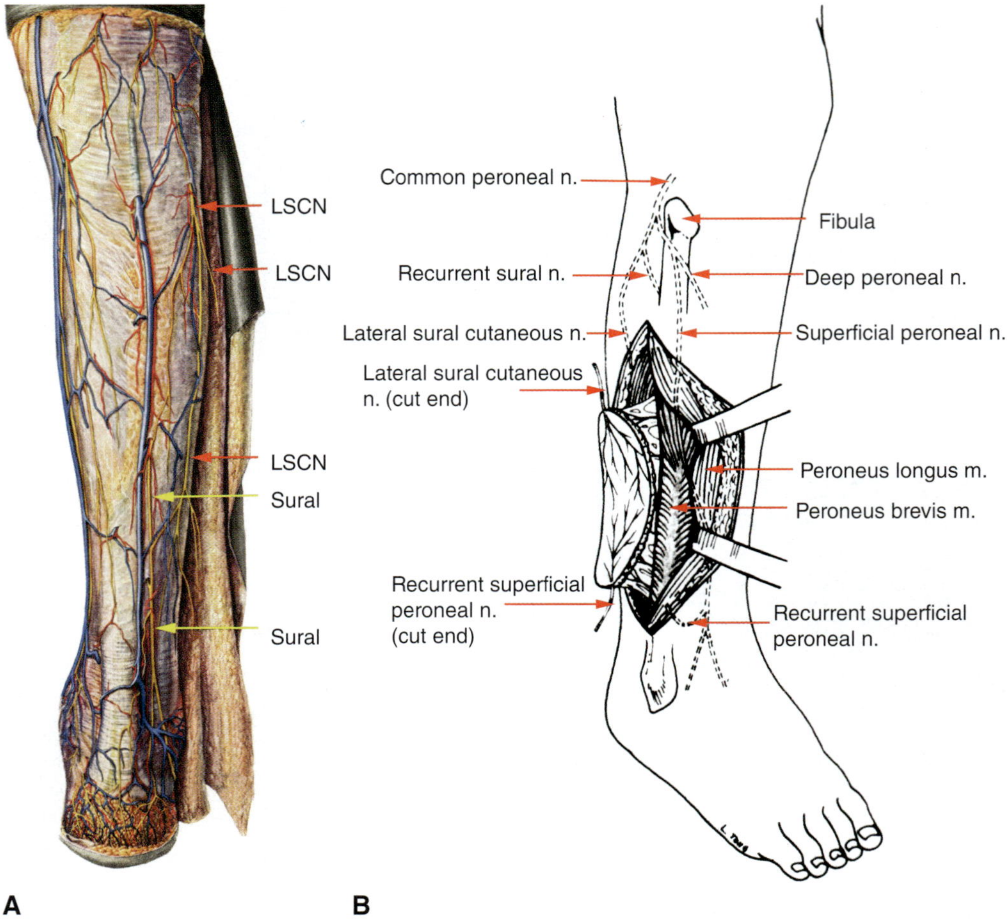

FIGURE 32-7 The lateral sural cutaneous nerve (LSCN) supplies the entire lateral aspect of the leg overlapping an area supplied by the recurrent superficial peroneal nerve (RSPN). m, muscle; n, nerve. (Reproduced with permission from Atlas of Topographical and Applied Human Anatomy. W.B. Saunders Company; 2nd revised edition October 1, 1979. © Elsevier. Elsevier.)

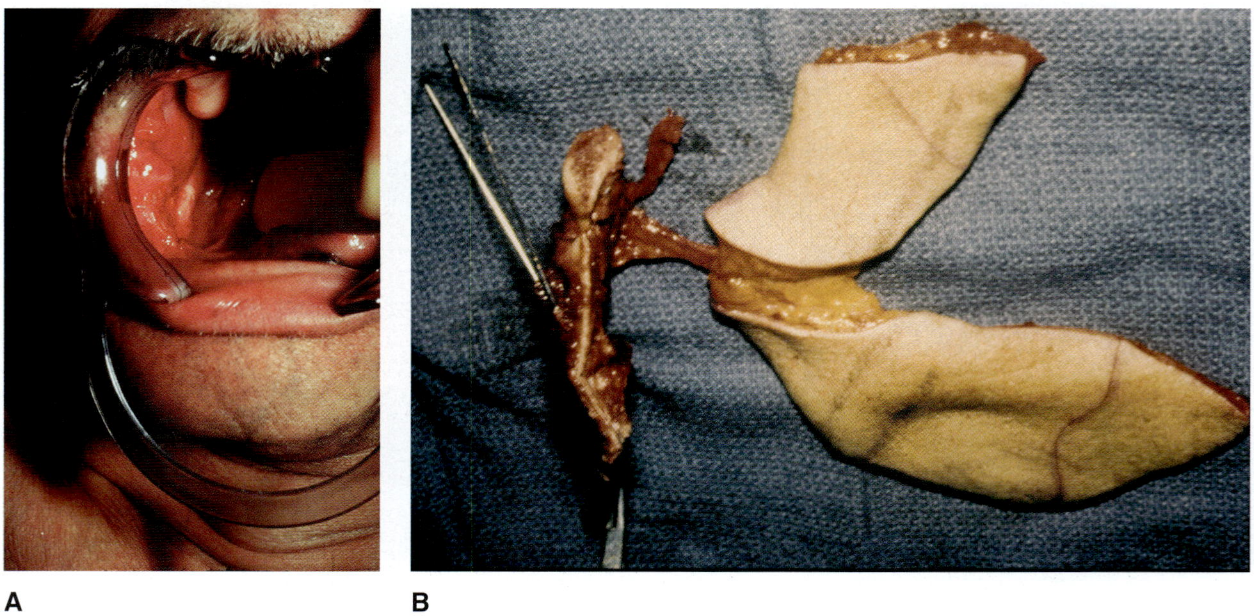

FIGURE 32-8 Scapula bipaddle osteocutaneous flap. (**A**) Through-and-through right cheek lesion consisting of a squamous cell cancer originating in the cheek mucosa and invading the mandible and skin. (**B**) Double paddle osteocutaneous flap with bone osteotomized to replicate resected mandible and two independent skin paddles. (Reproduced with permission from Dr. J. Banis, Louisville, KY.)

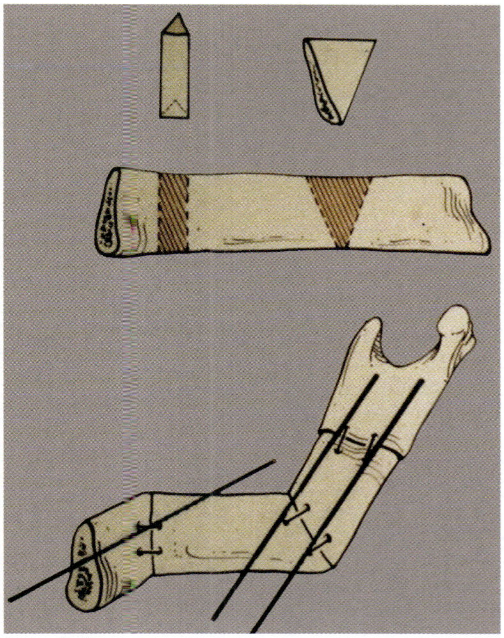

C

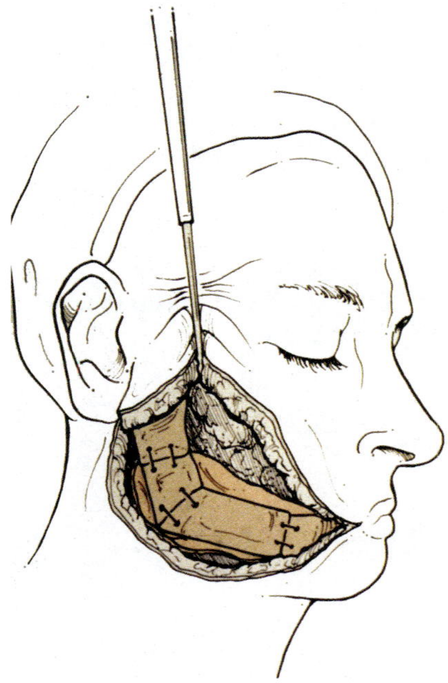

D

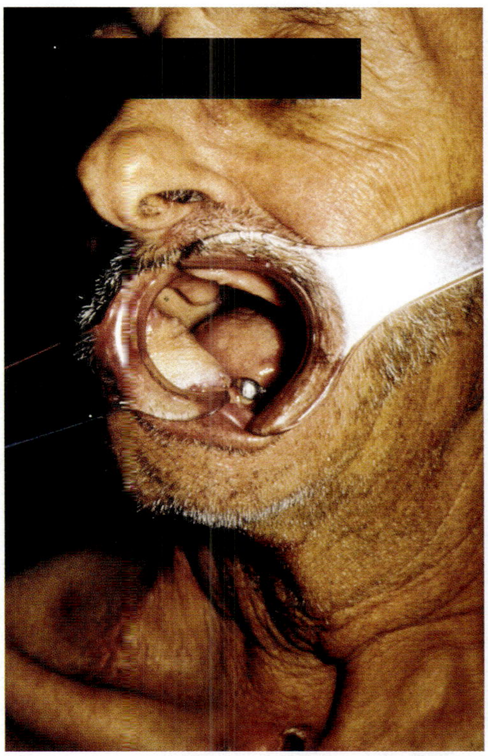

E

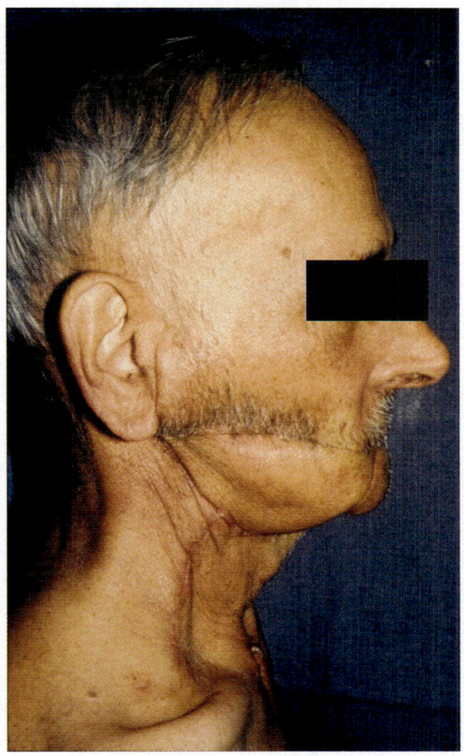

F

FIGURE 32-8 *(Continued)* (**C**) and (**D**) Diagram of the bony reconstruction showing osteotomies. (**E**) and (**F**) Final result, intraoral and lateral. (Reproduced with permission of Dr. J. Banis, Louisville, KY.)

osteotomies for contour, and care should be taken to preserve the inner periosteum and muscle cuff. The outer cortex may be removed or contoured with a burr without adversely affecting bone perfusion. To preserve hip contour, it is possible to harvest the internal table, leaving the outer cortex in situ (37).

The flap may be elevated simultaneously while another team prepares the neck. The main drawback of the iliac crest osteocutaneous flap is the bulk of its skin paddle and the bulky "obligatory" muscle cuff. It is poorly suited for intraoral use. Because it lies on the lateral surface of the crest, the skin is best suited for reconstruction of cheek, neck, or chin defects. If used intraorally, the paddle should be brought over, rather than under, the mandible to prevent tension on the cutaneous perforator vessels; however, this adds bulk to the cheek and may be frankly impossible to perform because of tethering and lack of room. Minor degrees of skin necrosis are common. As an

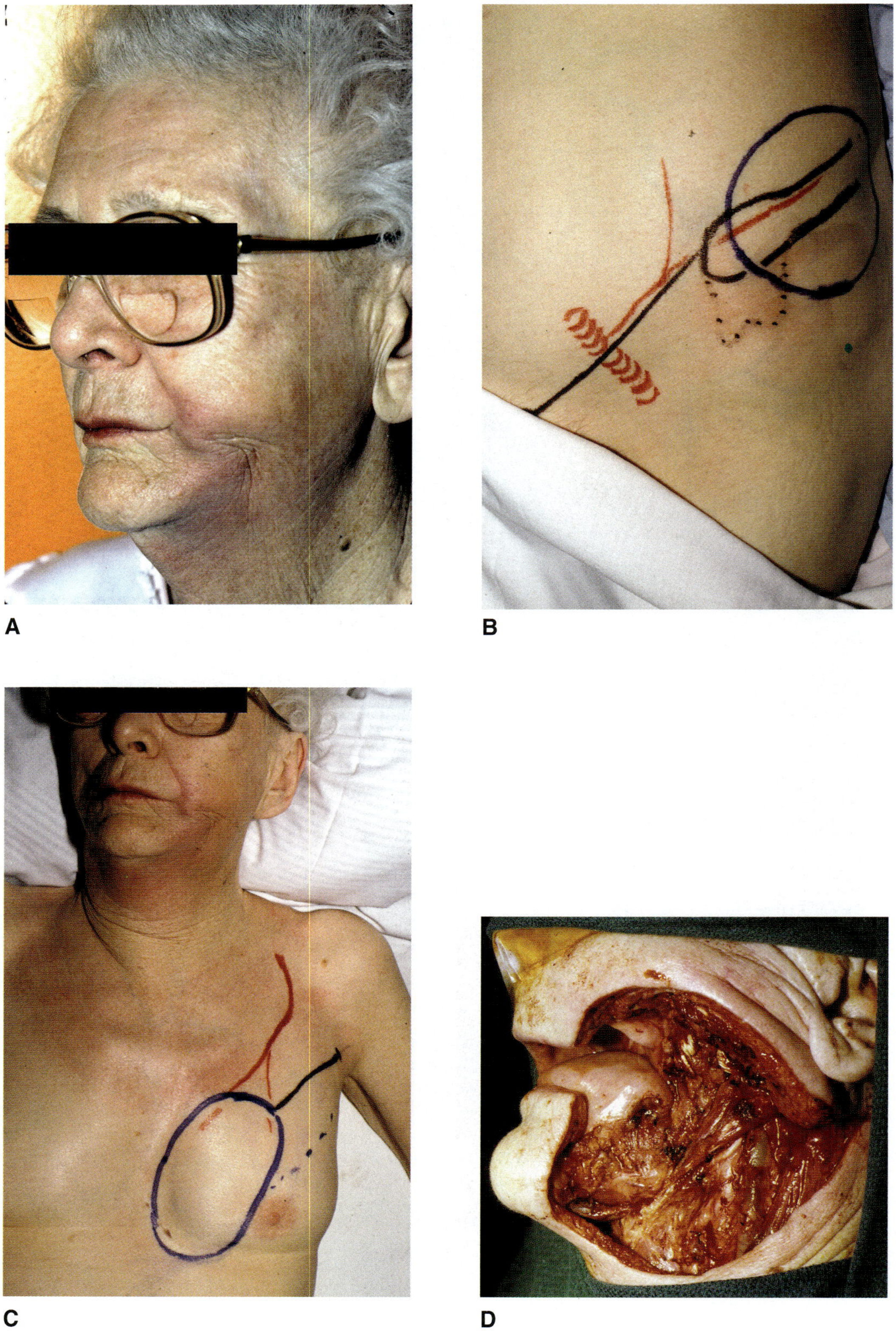

FIGURE 32-9 Iliac crest osteocutaneous flap used to reconstruct a full-thickness defect involving skin, mandible, and mucosa of the right cheek. Use of the skin paddle of the iliac crest is ideal for the external defect because it lies external to the normal curvature of the bone. Intraoral use of the skin flap is problematic (see text). An accessory flap, here the pectoralis major, reconstructs the oral lining. However, second free flaps such as the radial forearm or the anterolateral thigh flap may be used depending on requirements, availability, body habitus, and individual preference. (**A**) Before surgery, the mucosal squamous cell cancer has penetrated the mandibular body and can be seen to be involving the skin (**B**) The ipsilateral iliac crest flap is designed with an external paddle. (**C**) A pectoralis flap is outlined on the chest. (**D**) The composite defect.

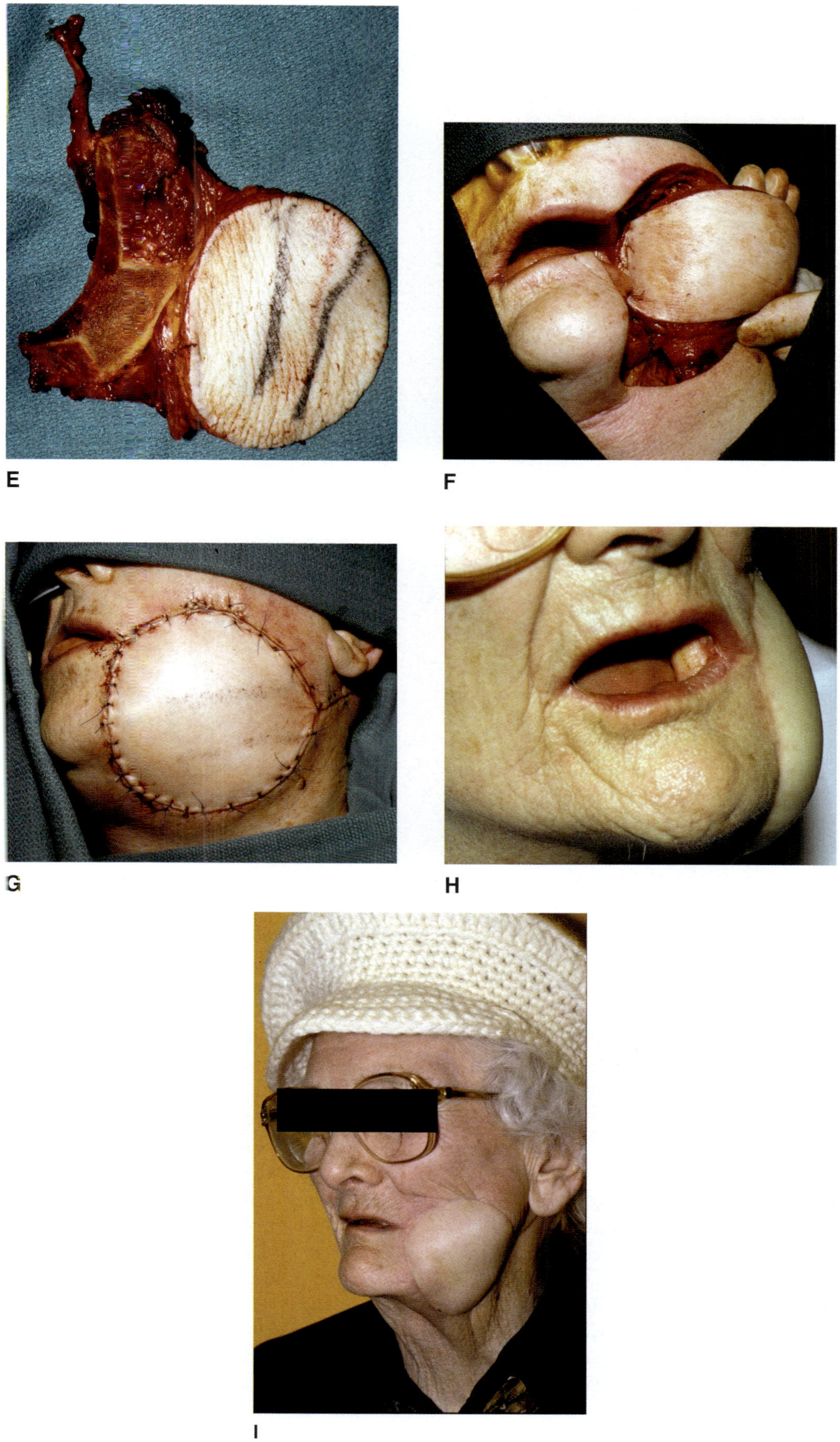

FIGURE 32-9 (*Continued*) (E) The iliac crest osteocutaneous free flap. Part of the outer cortex has been removed to improve contour. (F) The revascularized flap. (G) End of the procedure. (I) and (J) Six-month result.

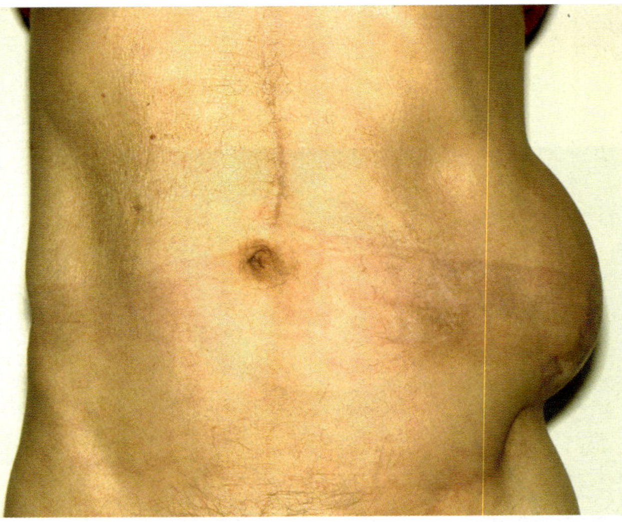

FIGURE 32-10 Hernia after the harvest of an iliac crest osteomuscular flap with internal oblique muscle paddle.

alternative, a paddle of internal oblique muscle can be harvested with the flap and skin grafted (or left to mucosalize) to provide thin oral lining (38). The muscle flap is based on the ascending branch of the deep circumflex iliac artery and vein. Atrophy of the muscle results in a thin layer of tissue adherent to the bone graft, which provides an excellent surface for dentures. Harvesting a large flap of internal oblique muscle increases the potential for hernia, so closure of the abdominal wall must be secure (Figure 32-10).

Because the skin paddle is bulky and recovery may be prolonged with a distinct potential for hernia formation, the flap is infrequently used when intraoral lining is required. Of all the bone flaps, it provides the best height. Furthermore, in patients with occlusive vasculature disease of the legs, it remains an excellent alternative to the fibula. In primary dental or osteogenic tumors that require bone-only flaps (Figures 32-11 and 32-12), it offers an aesthetically superior donor site as well as an anatomically exact replacement of the hemimandible without the need for osteotomies (39). Finally, the iliac crest may be used as a "combined flap" without its skin paddle. A fasciocutaneous flap such as the radial forearm flap is chosen for mucosal replacement. The effect is to minimize intraoral bulk while minimizing the chance of hernia at the donor site.

Radial Forearm

The radial forearm is an excellent source of thin, potentially sensate skin for head and neck reconstruction, but its bony component is limited to short, straight defects, usually of the body or ascending ramus. Osteotomies are avoided, if possible. The flap is perfused by the radial artery and drained by its venae comitantes or the cephalic vein. A rich plexus of fasciocutaneous vessels arises from the artery in the intermuscular septum between the brachioradialis and the flexor carpi radialis. Large, potentially sensate osteocutaneous flaps, including most of the forearm skin, can be raised if the radial half of the origin of the flexor pollicis longus, on which the radial vessels lie, is maintained between the radial vessels and the periosteum of the proposed radial graft. Distal to the attachment of the pronator teres, up to 10 cm of bone may be harvested as far as the insertion of the brachioradialis into the radial styloid.

Immobilization for 8 to 12 weeks in a long arm cast reduces the risk of fracture, although some have advocated primary bone grafting and plating the defect to reduce the period of immobilization and decrease the risk of fracture (40). Osteotomies must be done with care to avoid disturbing the periosteal vessels (Figure 32-13).

The main advantage of the flap is that the cutaneous paddle is large and thin and may be made sensate. The upper limb rarely has clinically significant atherosclerosis. Vessel caliber and pedicle length are excellent. Sacrifice of the radial artery when the ulnar artery is patent has not proved to be a problem.

Skin is often hairy in Whites, which can be a source of complaint when the flap is used intraorally. In some cases, the hair disappear as a result of radiation or metaplasia, but this is not universal. The aesthetic defect in the forearm is noticeable and may be diminished by closure with ulnar transposition flaps or by tissue expansion. Skin grafting of the fascia while on the forearm, with subsequent transfer of a hairless forearm flap, is possible but not commonly performed (41). Partial necrosis and delayed healing of the skin graft at the donor site are common. The main disadvantages of the osteocutaneous forearm flap in mandibular reconstruction are that the bone length and height are short and that the potential for osteotomies is limited. For this reason, we prefer to limit its use to short, straight segmental defects in patients who do not require the positioning of osseointegrated implants in the graft itself (Figure 32-14).

Second Metatarsal

In most people, the dorsalis pedis artery gives rise to the first dorsal metatarsal artery. The latter vessel arises between the heads of the intraosseous muscles where it courses between the first and second metatarsal bones toward the toes. It gives off small vessels to the overlying skin, to the periosteum of the second metatarsal bone, and to direct cortical branches to the bone. The dorsalis pedis flap may be transferred as a cutaneous or osteocutaneous unit. Venous drainage consists of paired venae comitantes, which accompany the dorsalis pedis artery. If a skin paddle is harvested, the superficial veins that drain the skin may be anastomosed to recipient vessels to ensure adequate outflow.

The skin of the dorsum of the foot is thin, pliable, and relatively hairless. Similar to the skin of the forearm, the skin of the dorsum of the foot is ideal for reconstruction of the floor of the mouth. The superficial peroneal nerve innervates this skin, and the potential for a sensate intraoral flap is an added advantage. An average of 6 cm of bone can be transferred. Because the metatarsal artery receives periosteal and direct cortical branches at both ends, a single osteotomy is easily made without interrupting circulation to the bone. This flap has been particularly useful for short defects involving the anterior segment in which one closing wedge osteotomy made in the metatarsal bone reestablishes chin projection (Figure 32-15). It is also useful for short defects of the body or ascending ramus.

However, the use of the metatarsal in mandibular reconstruction is largely historical because of the availability of superior alternatives with more acceptable donor sites.

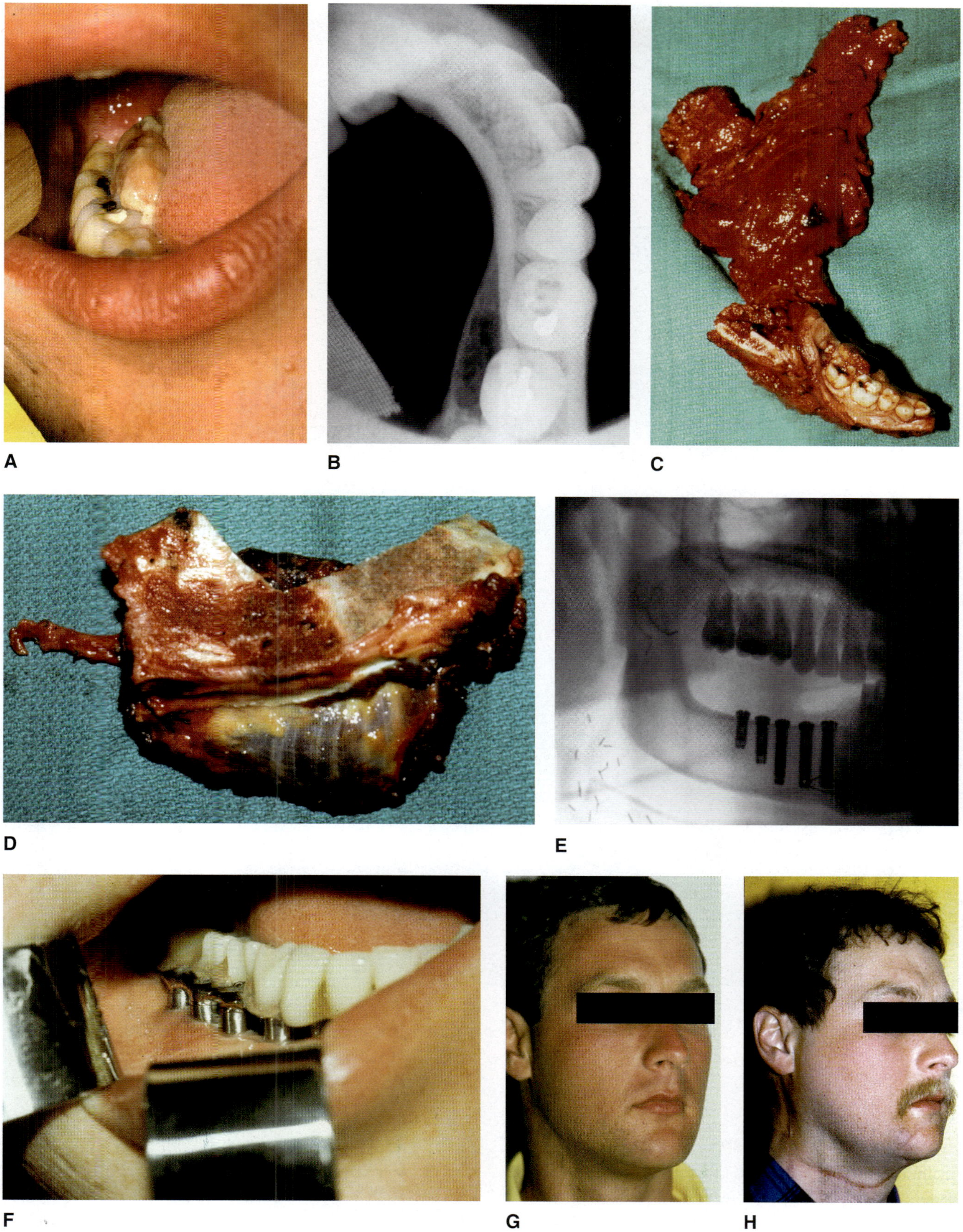

FIGURE 32-11 (A) and (B) A 2[illegible]-year-old man with a chondrosarcoma of the mandible presenting with an intraoral mass. (C) and (D) Composite resection and iliac crest graft with large internal oblique cuff to fill the dead space in the neck. (E) and (F) The iliac crest is an ideal host for osseointegrated implants. (G) and (H) Pre- and postoperative views at 6 months.

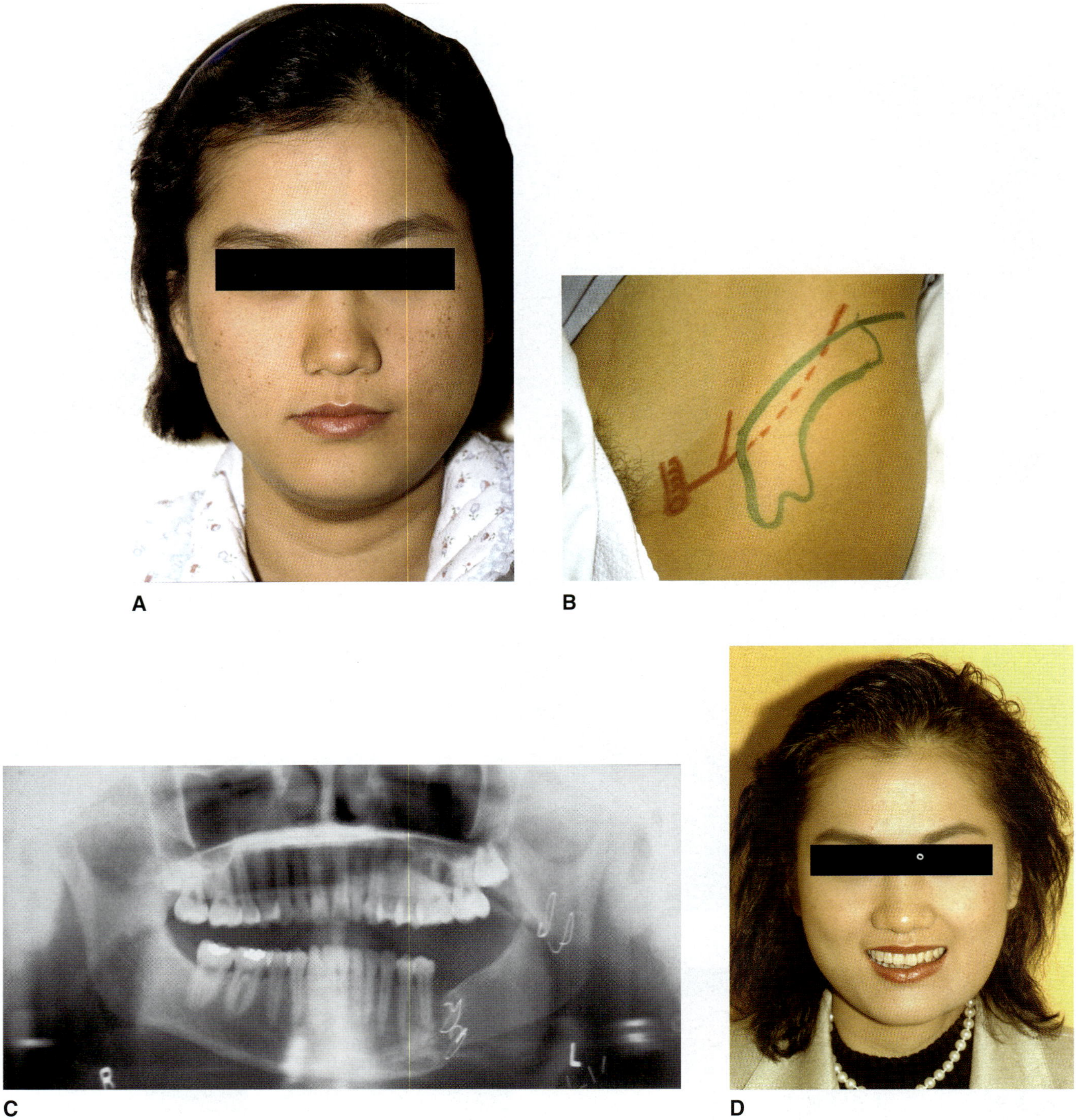

FIGURE 32-12 (A) and (B) A 22-year-old patient with adenocarcinoma. (C) and (D) L-shaped defect reconstructed with bone-only iliac crest.

Tibial–Dorsalis–Pedis Flap

Finally, the tibia–dorsalis–pedis (TDP) osteocutaneous free flap has recently been used for oromandibular reconstruction (42) and is described elsewhere in this text. The flap consists of a unicortical tibial bone graft centered on the middle third of the anterolateral surface of the tibia, elevated on the anterior tibial artery, and incorporating the dorsalis pedis skin flap. This unit has two distinct advantages over the fibula: a bone "height" similar to the mandible and a thin, supple skin paddle, which may be reinnervated and is almost completely independent of the bone. Furthermore, osseointegration is easy with the excellent bone stock. Because it is new, the role that this flap will play in oromandibular reconstruction awaits peer evaluation.

Combined Flaps

Two free flaps may be combined to reconstruct a composite defect (43,44). Although in most cases reconstruction of a composite defect by a single microvascular osteocutaneous or

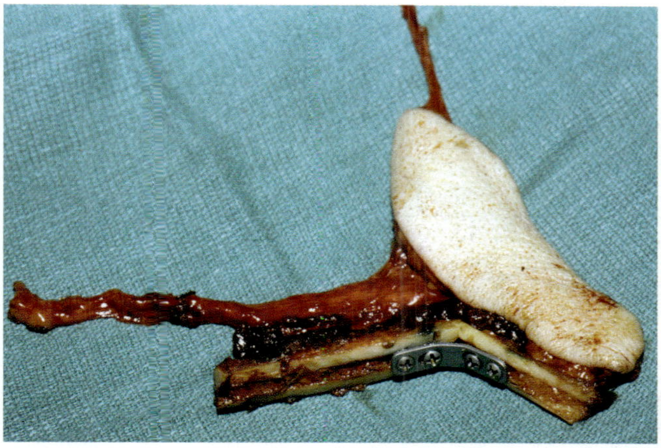

A

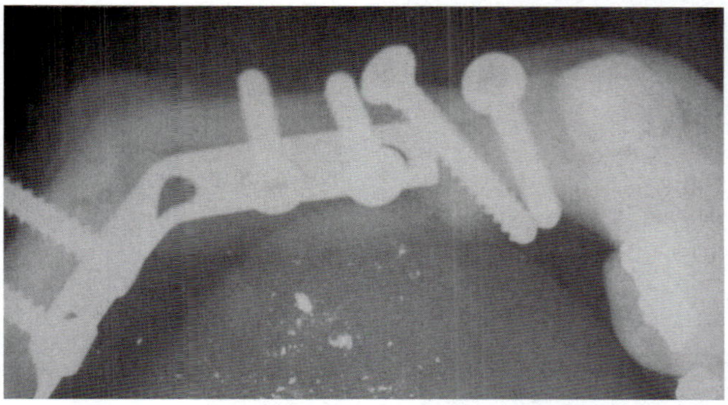

B

FIGURE 32-13 (A) and (B) Although not recommended, it is possible to osteotomize a radial bone graft and achieve bony union.

osteomuscular flap is adequate, there are occasions when combining two flaps is necessary or results in a better reconstruction. Extremely large "through-and-through" or "full-thickness" defects in which skin, bone, and oral lining all require reconstruction is one indication. A relative indication is to produce a better functional and aesthetic result by taking advantage of a flap's strength while eliminating some of its weaknesses. Combining a fibula or iliac crest flap with a soft tissue flap such as the radial forearm, ulnar forearm, or anterolateral thigh (ALT) flap are the most commonly used double-flap options (see Figure 32-5). The thick and bulky skin paddles associated with the iliac crest and scapular flaps are often unsatisfactory in the oral cavity, and their potential for reinnervation is questionable. The skin overlying the fibula is often thin but hairy, and the skin paddle must be centered over the distal leg, which may restrict its intraoral positioning. The skin paddle of the iliac crest is extremely bulky and unsuitable for intraoral use. By contrast, the radial forearm flap provides a large, thin, pliable skin paddle but limited bone. Even in obese patients, the volar forearm skin is thin. When the lateral antebrachial cutaneous nerve (LABC) is joined to the lingual or mental nerve, recovery of useful intraoral sensation is possible. The ALT flap (44) is another excellent flap for soft tissue reconstruction when used in combination with a vascularized bone flap. The ALT flap is unique in that two or at times three separate skin or adipofascial, musculocutaneous, or muscle segments can be independently oriented and transferred on a single vascular pedicle—the lateral circumflex femoral artery. Similar to the radial forearm flap, the ALT flap can be sensate if the lateral femoral cutaneous nerve is anastomosed to a recipient sensory nerve (45). Depending on reconstructive needs, the flap may include either or both of the descending and lateral branches of the lateral circumflex femoral vessels.

With the exception of the scapular osteocutaneous flap, skin paddle orientation in osteocutaneous free flaps parallels the bone. At times, independent orientation of the skin paddle in another direction is critical, as in a defect that extends onto the palate or in a combined skin and oral lining defect. In these situations, combined flaps offer a more functional reconstruction. In Whites, thigh subcutaneous fat is often too thick, but aggressive primary thinning is possible as long as a cuff of fat is preserved surrounding the vessel as it penetrates the fascia (46).

Simultaneous combined transfer may result in reduced overall donor site morbidity. For example, harvesting a significant piece of bone with the radial forearm flap is difficult and requires postoperative immobilization of the arm because the osteotomy predisposes the radius to fracture (47). Harvesting a large skin paddle with the fibula requires skin grafting and has the potential for pain and delayed healing. Harvesting the fibula as a bone-only flap and combining it with a fasciocutaneous flap allows immediate ambulation and decreased leg morbidity, although two dissections are required (see Figure 32-5). In the case of the radial forearm flap, an aesthetic defect occurs because skin grafting the donor site is invariably needed. On the other hand, the ALT donor site can often be closed directly, giving a superior aesthetic result. The main disadvantage of combined flaps is increased operating time, although this may be mitigated by a two-team approach.

Finally, flaps may be combined sequentially when a single recipient vessel in the neck is used and the second flap is revascularized by the distal end of the pedicle of the first flap. For example, the fibula flap can be combined with a cutaneous flap in which the distal peroneal vessels are anastomosed to the skin flap pedicle (see Figure 32-5). The skin flap then serves to monitor the circulation of both flaps. Although this has application in the infrequent case when recipient vessels are limited, it has the potential disadvantage that both flaps could be lost if there is thrombosis at the recipient vessel in the neck. Moreover, insetting of the two flaps is easier when the pedicles are independent. For these reasons, flaps are rarely connected "in series."

TIMING OF RECONSTRUCTION: IMMEDIATE AS OPPOSED TO DELAYED RECONSTRUCTION

In the past, many surgeons favored delayed reconstruction of mandibular defects. This preference was based on poor patient prognosis and unsatisfactory success rates with nonvascularized bone grafts or osteomusculocutaneous pedicled flaps. With better local control and high success rates currently achieved with vascularized bone grafts, immediate reconstruction has become the norm. Immediate reconstruction has several advantages:

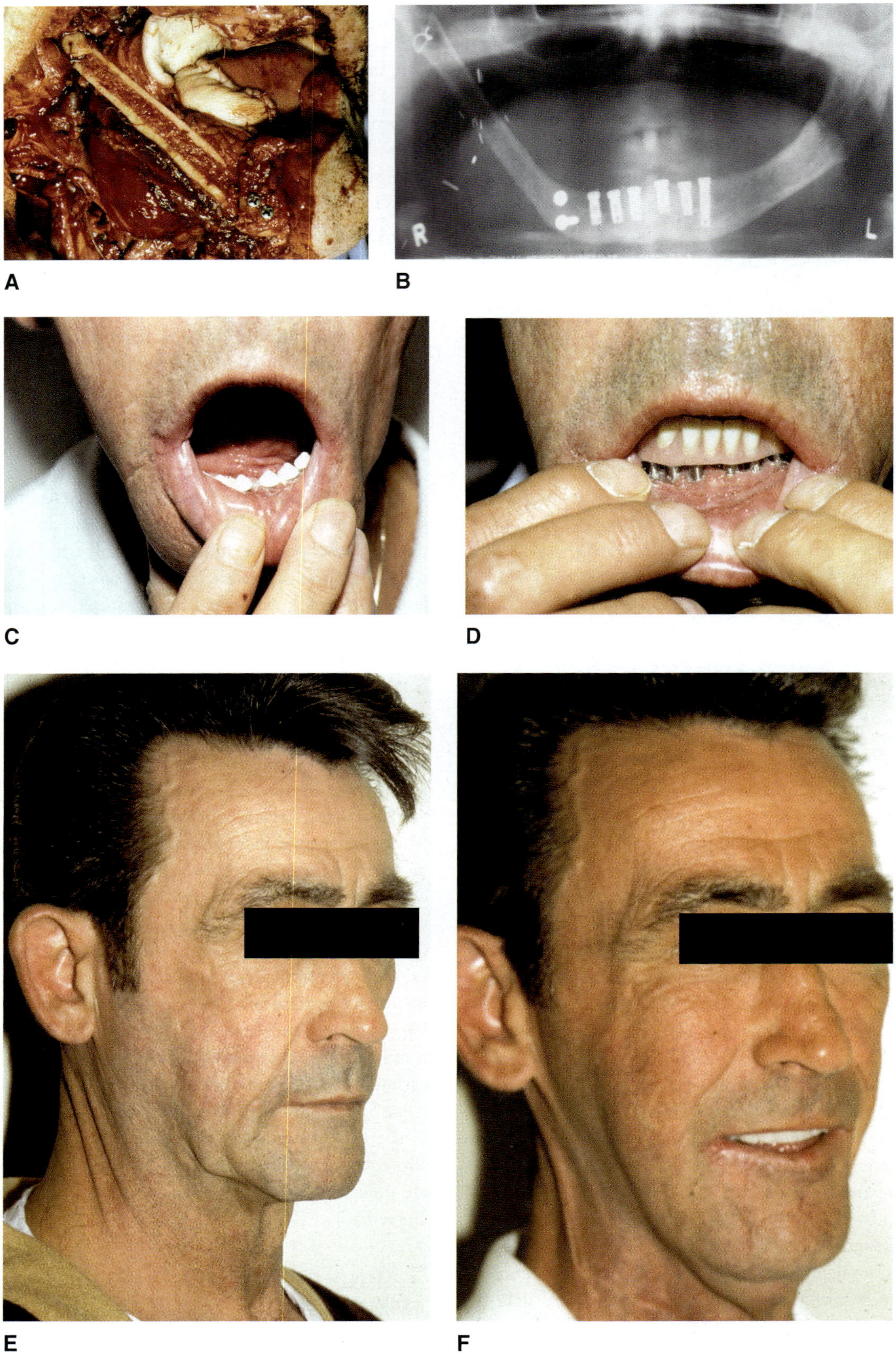

FIGURE 32-14 (A) Radial bone grafts are best for lateral reconstructions when osteotomies are not required. (B) to (D) Osseointegrated implants may be placed in adjacent bone. (E) and (F) Pre- and postoperative views. There is some flattening of the cheek because of the straight-shot reconstruction performed. This was thought to be acceptable in this patient in whom function was the paramount consideration.

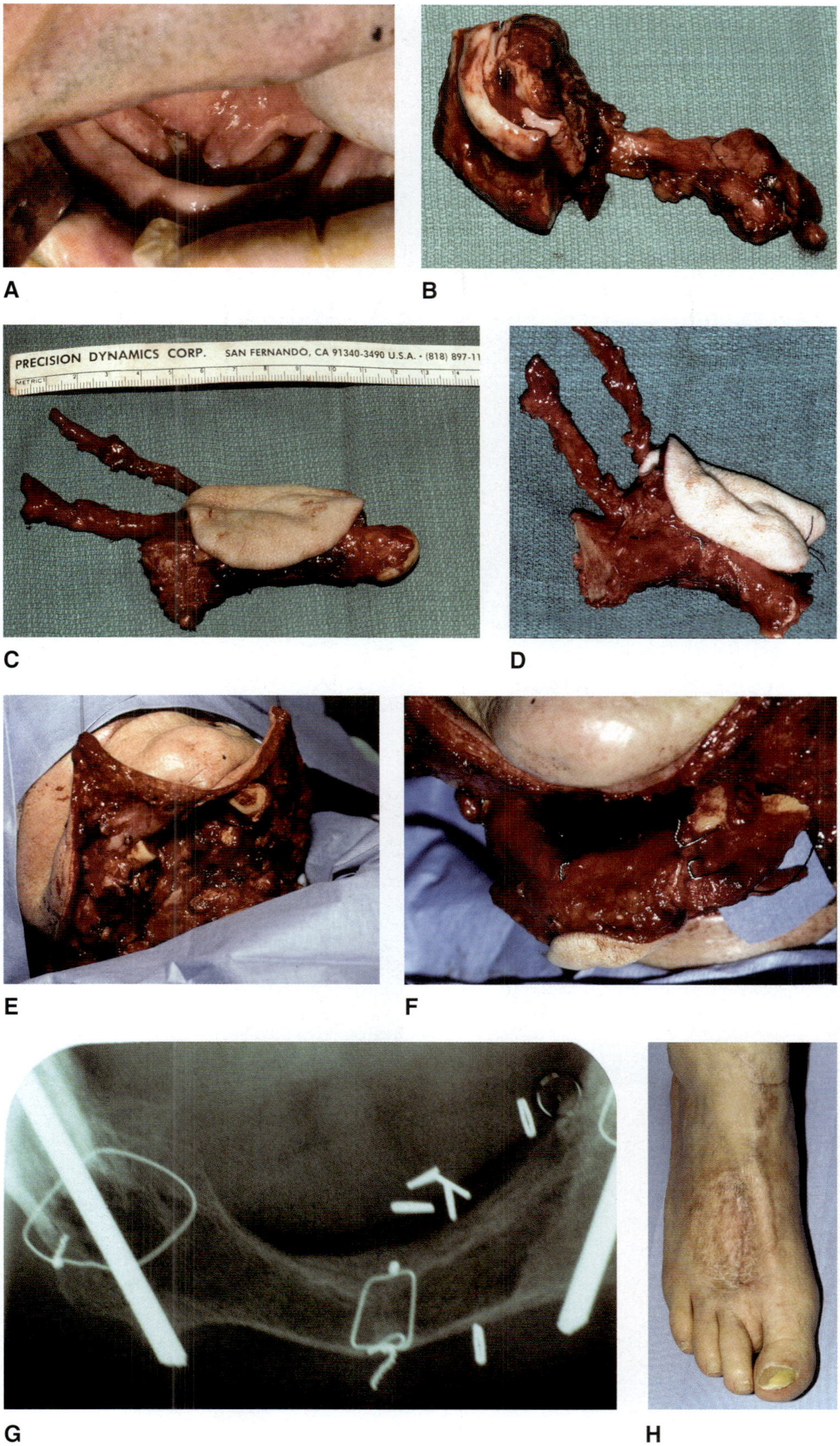

FIGURE 32-15 (A) and (B). Squamous cell carcinoma invading anterior alveolus and floor of the mouth before and after composite resection. (C) and (D) Second metatarsal osteocutaneous flap before and after closing-wedge osteotomy. (E) and (F) The anterior defect is reconstructed with the osteotomized metatarsal. (G) and (H) At 6 months, there is radiographic bony union, and the foot has healed.

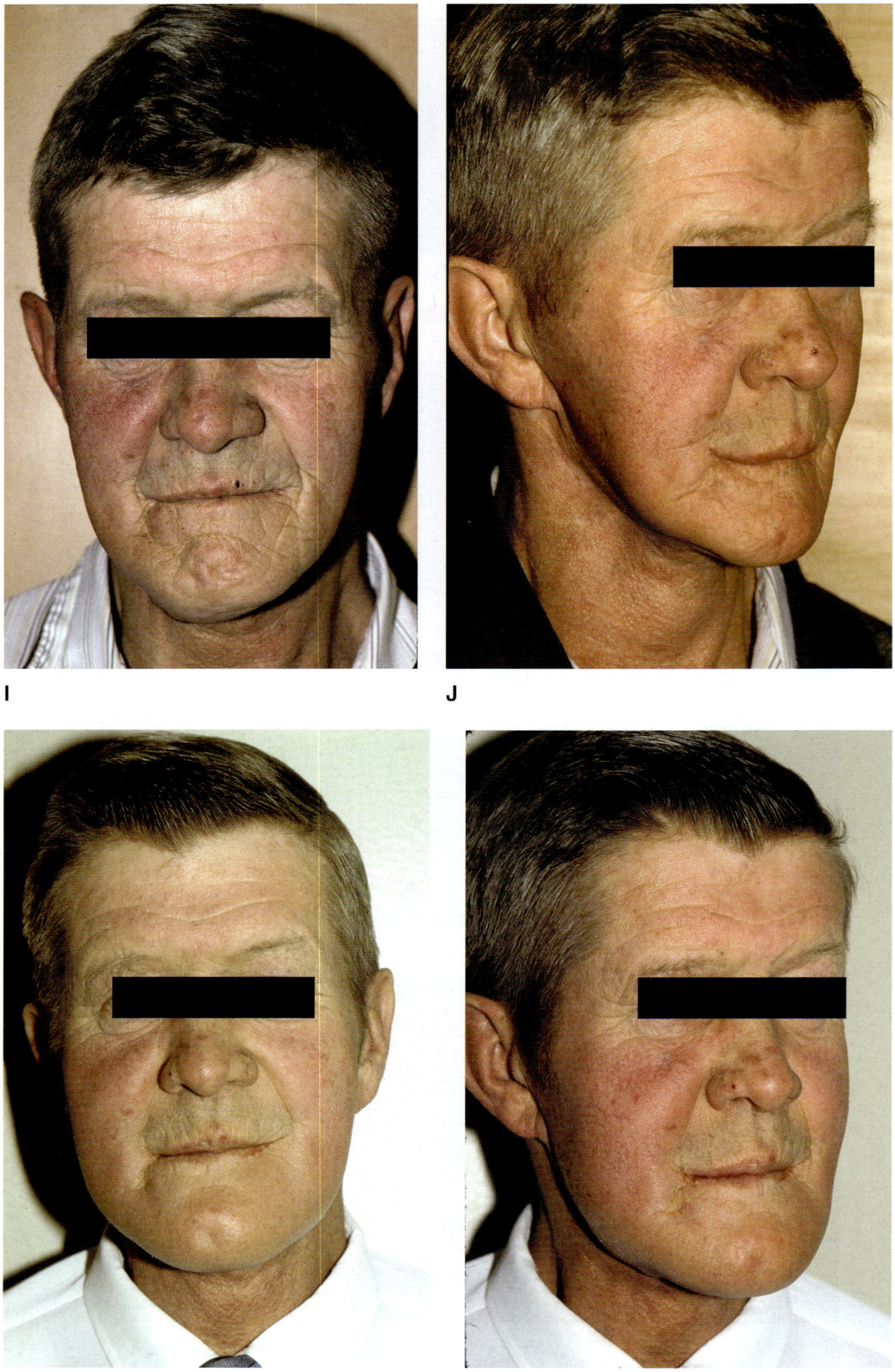

I J K L

FIGURE 32-15 (*Continued*) (I) and (J) Preoperative photos, frontal and right oblique. (K) and (L) Postoperative photos, frontal and right oblique.

- Reconstruction at the time of ablation or after resection for osteoradionecrosis is easier than if done later because no soft tissue contraction has occurred.
- Exposure of the vessels is optimal. There is no fibrosis that follows secondary scarring caused by surgical intervention.
- With the resection of most primary lesions, the surrounding tissues and recipient vessels are not damaged by radiation.
- In recurrent tumors or when radiation therapy has failed, exposure of the vessels is still better than at a delayed second operation.
- With immediate reconstruction, soft tissue contracture caused by a lack of bony support is avoided.
- Primary reconstruction avoids potential damage to the facial nerve during dissection of the proximal fragment of mandible.

One disadvantage of immediate reconstruction is increased operative time. However, this is minimized by a two-team approach and in any case is shorter than that required for two separate procedures. Another is the potential effect of postoperative radiation on the graft itself. Obliterative arteritis involving the pedicle or the interosseous vessels can adversely affect the success rate of osseointegrated implants (48).

In delayed reconstruction, great care must be taken to release all contracted tissues. Wide dissection of neck flaps and elevation of muscular attachments to the mandible are necessary to free the collapsed segments. Division of the coronoid process to release it from a contracted temporalis muscle is often necessary to bring the posterior mandibular segment into proper alignment. Rigid fixation is necessary to hold the alignment after the mandible has been brought into position. With few exceptions, the oral lining must be replaced in delayed reconstruction to release the tongue completely and provide an adequate sulcus to direct the flow of saliva. Reconstruction of neck and cheek skin may also be needed. The amount of lining required is frequently underestimated before surgery. Soft tissue replacement is as important as restoration of bony continuity. Areas of "dead space" behind reconstructed bony arches can lead to contractures postoperatively—as air is absorbed—and produce severe secondary deformities of both soft tissue and bone (Figure 32-16). This may be avoided by incorporating muscle or fat in the flap, which then may act as a "filler," thereby avoiding a dead space.

PLANNING

Preoperative planning using three-dimensional radiographic modeling has revolutionized mandibular reconstruction. Preoperative planning will be discussed in a separate chapter. However, several principles will be enumerated here.

1. Plate bending: When the tumor does not penetrate or distort the lateral mandibular cortex, a reconstruction plate can be bent to conform to the native mandible just before its resection. Drill holes are placed through it into the segments of the mandible to be left behind. The plate and screws are then removed and the resection carried out. When the hardware is replaced, the mandibular fragments are automatically in correct alignment. The bone flap may then be fitted to the defect.

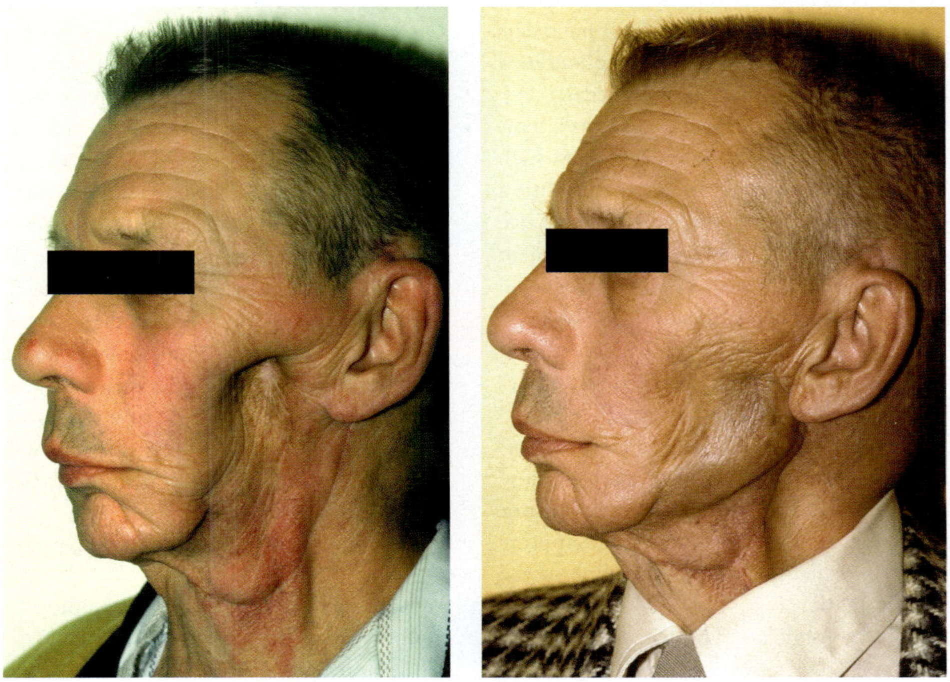

A B

FIGURE 32-16 (A) and (B) Severe soft tissue collapse after an unreconstructed left-sided composite resection. It was improved functionally and aesthetically using an iliac crest free flap, but the dissection was complicated because of the previous surgery and scarring. Problems included a difficult dissection of the facial nerve and the upward rotation of the posterior mandibular fragment.

2. Plate modeling: Where the lateral cortex is breached, as in a through-and-through defect or when the mandible has become expanded with, for example, an ameloblastoma, plate bending is not feasible. In such cases, three-dimensional modeling can be performed from fine-cut computed tomography (CT) scans. The destroyed mandibular cortex is mirror imaged from the normal side, and a reconstruction plate is produced to span the proposed defect. We prefer to request a plate that would go from condyle to condyle and then cut off the portion that is not required. This allows for a "change of plan" on the part of the ablative surgeon.
3. Bone and osteotomy modeling: Fitting a bone graft to the inside of a prebent plate can be difficult and time consuming, particularly with regard to fitting the graft flush with the cut edges of the mandibular fragments and with itself at osteotomy sites. With an increased number of osteotomies, this is particularly challenging. It is now possible to perform computer-aided modeling not only to produce an appropriate reconstruction plate but also to produce jigs for the bony resection and for the osteotomies in the bone graft itself. Using these means, an extremely accurate, shaped bone graft may be produced that will exactly fit the defect with all the cut bony surfaces coming together flush. The fibula lends itself to this technique. Modeling in preoperative planning will be discussed in detail elsewhere in this text.

BONY FIXATION

Stable fixation, accurate alignment, and good apposition are all important for bone healing both at the osteotomy sites and at the graft's junction with native mandible. If the mandibular fragments cannot be held in their anatomical positions by the means outlined earlier, external fixation before resection may be considered.

External fixation with biphase devices can be used as a temporary measure when delayed reconstruction is necessary, such as in blast injuries, or while awaiting pathologic confirmation of resection margins. External fixation can be very effective when using an iliac crest graft. However, it would remain in place until bony union occurred. Because it is not rigidly stable, external fixation is most effective when sufficient teeth are present that the patient can also be placed in intermaxillary fixation (IMF). However, external fixation is rarely used nowadays because of the excellent rigid alternatives available.

Plating systems are now routinely used in mandible reconstruction. Reconstruction plates were discussed earlier. Because the plate is applied to the outer surface, it may be prominent or palpable, sometimes producing a slightly prognathic appearance or a mild contour abnormality where the outline of the plate can be seen through the skin.

Another type of plate is the miniplate. This has the advantage of simple application between each osteotomy or osteosynthesis site. Each is sequentially fixed. The technique places more demand on the surgeon to correctly shape the mandible and maintain a proper occlusal relationship but allows for easier adjustment of segments. The resected segment of mandible, a cadaver mandible, or a computer-generated model can serve as a guide while shaping. Because of their thinness, miniplates are not prominent and are rarely palpable. They work well in dense cortical bone such as the fibula or radius but tend to loosen in bones with a higher cancellous content such as the iliac crest and scapula.

Temporary intraoperative IMF is useful with either type of plate application but is especially important if miniplates are used. The IMF is released at the end of the procedure unless the condyle has been replaced, when we prefer 2 to 3 weeks of immobilization to allow a "scar capsule" to form, which keeps the new condyle seated in the temporomandibular fossa. Bony union rates are comparable with both techniques and are at least 95% (49).

Accurate contouring of the graft is important for many reasons. To promote healing, a large area of bone-to-bone contact is best, and the precise fit of the segments to each other, especially if miniplates are used, contributes to stability. Contour defines the aesthetic result. The position of the angle and inferior border of the mandible are critical for an aesthetically pleasing reconstruction. Finally, accurate contour and solid bony union will give the best functional result, both for temporomandibular joint mechanics and for dental rehabilitation.

RECONSTRUCTION OF LATERAL DEFECTS

The location of the defect determines the type of osteotomies used. Lateral defects, including the ascending ramus, are easier to reconstruct than anterior defects. Posterior to the C segment, there is a slight curvature to the body but none to the ascending ramus, and the need for osteotomies is reduced. In general, it is rare for the condyle to be excised and an H defect to be created. The residual height of the condylar-bearing fragment plus a short segment of the graft establishes the ascending ramus. Its size can easily be measured from the resected segment or computer-generated models in immediate reconstructions. In delayed reconstruction, a computer-manufactured model partially "mirror imaged" from the normal side is useful. *The angle at which this bone segment meets the next segment of graft that will reconstruct the body defines the mandibular angle.* This must be precise for an optimal aesthetic outcome. It is important to recognize that the angle is part of a three-dimensional structure in which it and the posterior portion of the mandibular body lie more lateral to the midline than the anterior portion. The body has a slight curve but usually two straight bone segments with one osteotomy can give a reasonable contour. The osteotomy has to be adjusted in two planes to obtain the correct shape. Failure to recreate this dimension results in a flattened appearance of the cheek (see Figure 32-14F).

RECONSTRUCTION OF ANTERIOR DEFECTS

Anterior defects require careful planning to reproduce the chin contour. Two closing-wedge osteotomies are made and are adjusted to give a proper three-dimensional reconstruction. With the exception of the iliac crest, the bony height of the graft is usually less than that of the mandible (see Figure 32-6L). The graft segments are best aligned to the inferior border of the mandible because this defines chin projection and external contour.

If later dental rehabilitation is considered, this height deficiency can usually be compensated for by the prosthesis.

The width of the chin is carefully measured, and the osteotomies are planned so the central bone segment is midline. With this essentially reconstructing the chin point—which normally protrudes beyond the alveolus—it is anatomically incorrect to insert dental implants into it. However, an iliac crest graft may be angled backward so that its upper border lies in the correct position or a double-barreled fibula graft used for the anterior mandible, the upper segment lying posterior to the lower (50) and receiving the implants. More simply, laterally placed implants can support an anterior bridge in the normal alveolar position posterior to the new chin point.

As in lateral defects, the osteotomy should result in maximum bone-to-bone contact when miniplates are used. Three bone segments are generally needed to span a molar-to-molar defect. Miniplates are placed both across the anterior and inferior borders of the segments. Temporary IMF is very helpful. In edentulous patients or those with inadequate residual teeth, it is easy to misalign the bone segments because of the action of those unopposed muscles remaining after resection. However if a reconstruction plate is used, the anterior border of the plate defines the chin contour. Closing-wedge osteotomies are made to bring the segments into contact with the plate as well as with each other. If small gaps remain, bone graft can be added. As mentioned earlier, if the plate was prebent before resection, occlusion will be normal once it is reapplied, giving this method an advantage over miniplates.

When the iliac crest is used and the graft is taken from the ipsilateral hip, the natural shape and curve of the body and ascending ramus are achieved without osteotomy—rather like in the Manchester repair—with the crest forming the lower border of the mandible with the anterior superior iliac spine defining the angle. One or two closing-wedge osteotomies anteriorly permit the graft to reach the contralateral parasymphyseal region. A burr can be used to further contour the graft. The superior height of the iliac graft is an advantage for anterior and body contour as well as implant placement. However, the cancellous bone does not hold miniplate screws well. If a reconstruction plate is not used, cancellous screws and a larger plate are preferred.

RECONSTRUCTION OF THROUGH-AND-THROUGH DEFECTS

Full-thickness defects represent a major challenge in mandibular reconstruction. The appearance of external scars with skin paddles differing in color and texture from native facial skin adversely affects aesthetic appearance. To this may be added the unwelcome aesthetic and functional disabilities of major lower lip resection and facial paralysis when full-thickness excision of the cheek removes muscles of facial expression. It is quite wrong to compare the results of one center where full-thickness reconstruction is common with those of another, where it is rare. The importance of the HCL (ms) classification system as a means of comparing outcomes cannot be overemphasized.

The primary issue with through-and-through defects is the provision of a second skin paddle to facilitate a two-surface repair. Difficulties can arise when the skin paddles are tethered to one another as well as to the bone graft, as is often the case. Careful reverse planning is necessary, but plans can be thrown out the window if more tissue is excised than expected. There are a number of ways of providing two skin paddles:

1. Use a single skin paddle and divide it in two by deepithelializing an intervening strip of skin (Figure 32-17).
2. Use a flap with two separate pedicles bearing independent skin paddles (see Figure 32-8).
3. Use a flap with multiple skin islands, each based on one or more perforators from the main vascular system (radial forearm, fibula) (51) (Figure 32-18).
4. Use a second flap to reconstruct either the skin or the mucosa (see Figure 32-9). This may be pedicled (pectoralis major musculocutaneous flap, supraclavicular artery island flap, deltopectoral flap) or free (radial forearm flap, ALT flap).

Of the techniques listed, the *least* satisfactory is the deepithelialized strip method because it severely limits the independence of the two flaps, can never contribute to the height of the lower lip, and with external rotation can lead to severe deformities of the mouth. Option three involves some tethering, necessitating careful planning.

TEMPOROMANDIBULAR JOINT RECONSTRUCTION

Although resection of the condyle is seldom necessary, reconstruction of the temporomandibular joint presents a special challenge. With just the condyle and neck remaining, the proximal end of the bone graft may be fixed to the neck with an interosseous wire and a good functional result anticipated. Transplantation of the condyle onto the graft with miniplate fixation has been described following the creation of an H defect. Of course, this is predicated on noninvolvement of the condyle in the tumor process. However, if not involved, why destroy joint integrity by resecting it? Despite this quibble, the functional results of condyle transplantation in joint reconstruction appear to be excellent (52).

If the condyle is not available, several methods have been used successfully. The reconstructed ascending ramus may be suspended from the zygomatic arch with a heavy, nonabsorbable suture, and fascia can be interposed to prevent bony union. An awl is used to pass the suture around the zygomatic arch. A "functional nonunion" results. To provide better jaw mechanics, joint reconstruction using autogenous or prosthetic material may be carried out. Nonvascularized rib grafts, in which the cartilage at the costochondral junction is contoured to fit the fossa, can be secured directly to the reconstruction plate with the use of screws or miniplates. Postoperative immobilization for 4 to 6 weeks or mobilization with intermaxillary elastics is recommended to prevent displacement of the graft. Retention of the articular disk significantly improves functional outcome, protects against ankylosis, and resists upward displacement of the new condyle.

Several different reconstruction plates are available with metallic condylar heads. The metallic condylar head is secured directly to the plate or the graft. When a metallic prosthesis is

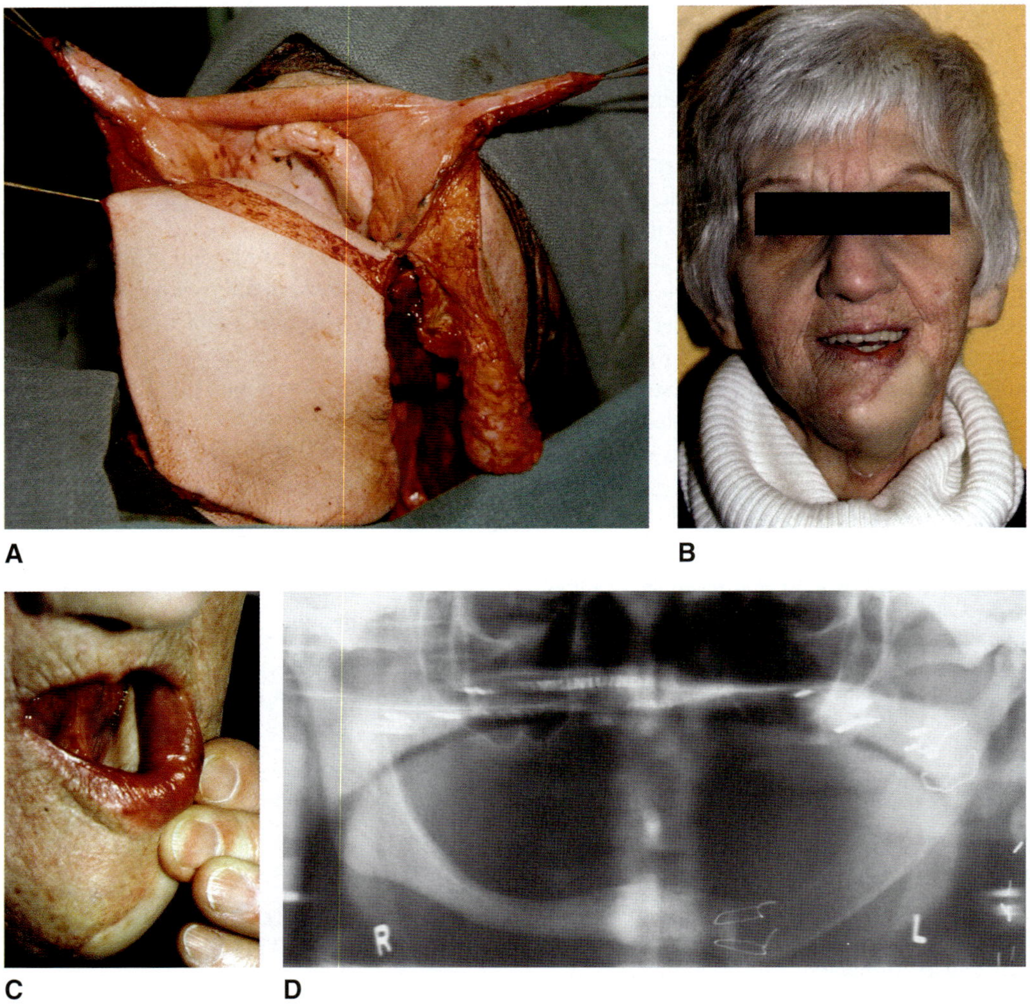

FIGURE 32-17 One means of providing closure of both oral mucosa and skin in through-and-through defects is by dividing a single skin paddle in two by a deepithelialized strip. (**A**) An iliac crest skin paddle is used for both lining and skin cover in a full-thickness defect after excision of a radiation-induced squamous cell carcinoma. (**B**) to (**D**) Postoperative result at 6 months.

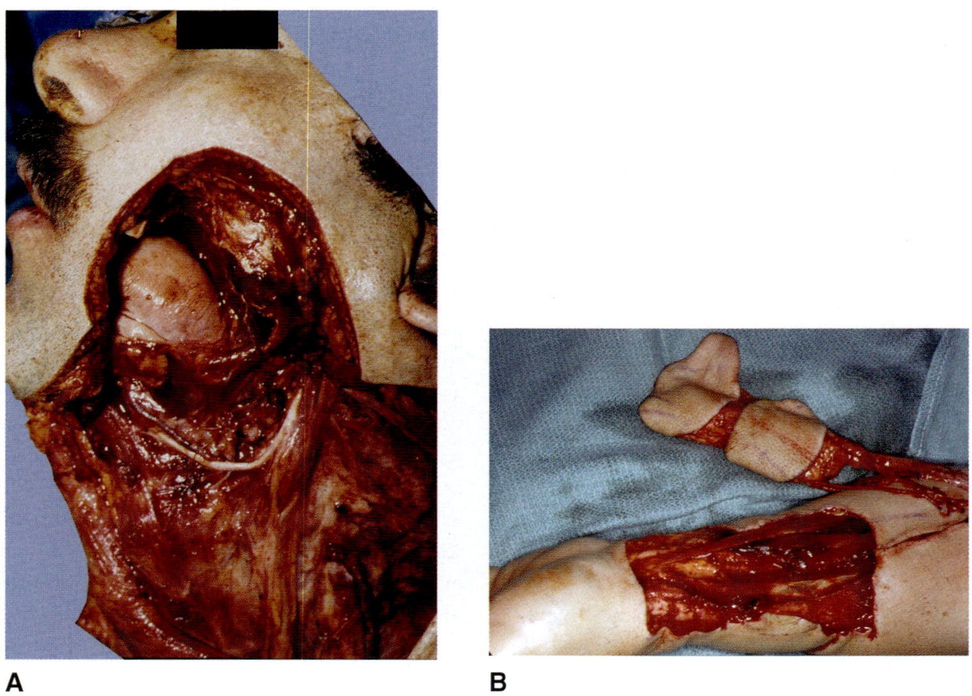

FIGURE 32-18 Another means of providing closure of both oral mucosa and skin in through-and-through defects is by using two separate skin paddles, each raised on separate perforators from the main vascular axis of the flap. Both the radial forearm and fibula flaps have this option. (**A**) A full-thickness defect consisting of bone, mucosa, and skin after resection of an invasive squamous cell carcinoma originating in the buccal mucosa of the left cheek. (**B**) Two independent skin paddles are elevated as part of a radial forearm osteocutaneous flap.

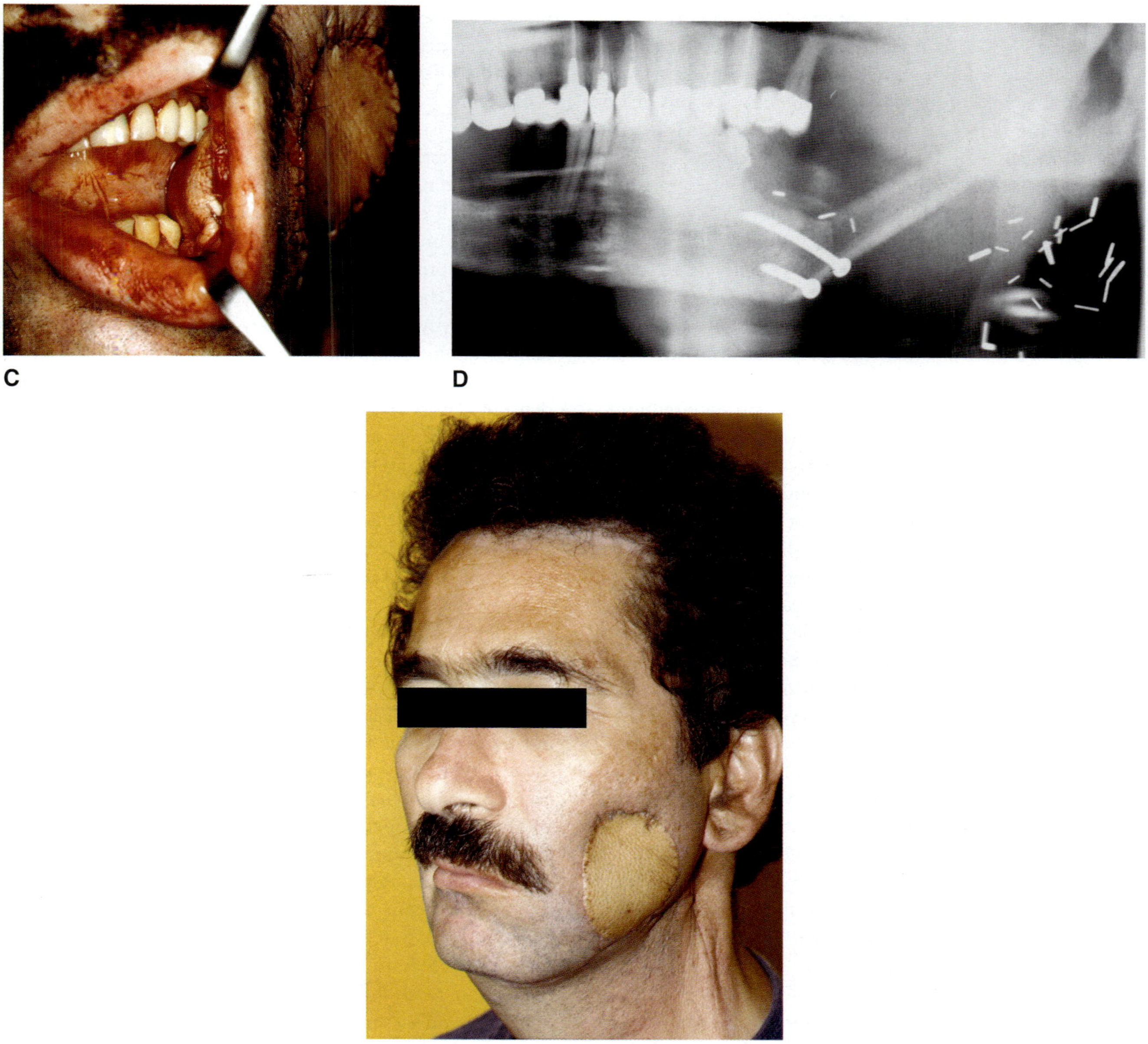

FIGURE 32-18 (*Continued*) (**C**) Postoperative view of both skin paddles at the termination of surgery. (**D**) and (**E**) Result at 6 months. Note that full-thickness reconstructions can never match the aesthetics of simpler bone and mucosa reconstructions because of the poor color match of exposed skin paddles; more extensive scarring; and, in this case, facial nerve injury.

attached to the end of a reconstruction plate, we tend to leave the ascending ramus unreconstructed by bone, terminating the fibula used for the horizontal ramus at the angle. The reasons are:

1. Plates used alone posteriorly have a low failure rate (8).
2. There is minimal biomechanical difference between reconstructing 1.5 cm of posterior ramus (condyle and neck) versus 4 cm (condyle, neck, and ascending ramus).
3. Using fibula for the ascending ramus in an LCL defects puts its pedicle in a disadvantageous position for accessing the neck vessels.
4. One osteotomy less needs to be carried out, saving time.

Reconstruction of the joint improves stability. Lateral deviation with opening and instability when closing are both decreased. Joint reconstruction is particularly worthwhile when dental rehabilitation is anticipated. It should be noted, however, that with the tissue contraction that follows radiotherapy, there have been cases when metallic condylar prostheses have been forced into the middle cranial fossa (53). Retention of the articular disk whenever possible is highly recommended because it may help prevent ankylosis as well as cranial penetration.

SELECTION OF RECIPIENT VESSELS AND NERVES

Preoperative assessment of the neck includes palpation of the carotid vessels and auscultation for bruits. If there is a history of cerebral ischemia or if abnormalities are noted on physical examination, an arteriogram is obtained. Magnetic resonance arteriography (MRA) is preferred over conventional arteriograms because of a lower complication rate secondary to the low dye load used. For most primary tumor resections or isolated traumatic defects, arteriography of the neck is seldom indicated because multiple recipient vessels are present. Arteriography is useful in patients with blast injuries, recurrent tumor, or a history of high dose irradiation.

With whatever flap is chosen, vessel selection and flap orientation must take into account how the pedicle will lie so that it does not kink or become compressed yet remains long enough to access the recipient vessels and facilitate a comfortable anastomosis. Most often, the ipsilateral neck vessels are used, especially during immediate reconstruction, because they are easily accessible. Previous radiation is not a contraindication in vessel selection (54). Examination of the branches of the external carotid artery almost always yields a satisfactory recipient artery. When dissecting around the external carotid artery, the hypoglossal nerve should be identified and protected. The superior thyroid artery is easily accessible and usually anastomosed close to its origin for maximum diameter and because it tends to be tortuous as it proceeds toward the thyroid gland. The lingual and facial arteries have excellent diameters and lengths but may be somewhat difficult to access because the bone graft often overlies them. The main trunk of the external carotid artery is almost always available for end-to-end or end-to-side anastomoses even in delayed reconstructions or recurrent or previously irradiated cases. Another alternative in these patients is the use of vessels in the opposite neck. Careful planning and orientation of the graft so the pedicle is anterior will usually prevent the need for vein grafts. In heavily irradiated necks, especially with recurrent disease, transverse cervical vessels have been shown to be reliable recipient vessels that are easily accessed. Vein grafts are rarely needed.

Venous access is usually not a problem because there are many veins in the upper neck that drain into the internal jugular system, especially those from the facial vein. The external jugular vein is of good caliber and, with the cooperation of the ablative surgeon, can be safely preserved during most neck dissections. Vein couplers are generally used for venous anastomosis to decrease operative time and arguably improve the patency rate. Because the internal jugular vein is now rarely taken in neck dissections, it is also an excellent recipient vessel for an end-to-side anastomosis. In difficult cases, the cephalic vein can be divided in the arm and pedicled on its point of penetration through the clavipectoral fascia to easily reach the neck (54).

REINNERVATION OF SOFT TISSUE FLAPS

In composite deficits in which the anterior floor of mouth, lower lip, or tongue is reconstructed, it is desirable to reinnervate the skin flap to help with speech, oral continence, and general masticatory function. Although some spontaneous sensory recovery may be expected after several years, the limited life expectancy of patients with stage IV oral cancer may preclude these individuals from ever returning to the normal social functions of everyday life. However, it has been shown that excellent functional recovery may be achieved in as little as 6 months when the flaps have been reinnervated (55).

To reinnervate the skin paddles of osteocutaneous flaps, the sensory nerve supply must be known and deliberately preserved during harvesting. The nerve "pedicle" should be long enough to reach the recipient nerve, in this case either the lingual or mental, both of which should be labeled at the time of resection. Nerve anastomosis adds little time to the procedure and may be performed under loupe magnification. Obviously, flaps used in the cheek, the roof of mouth, the posterior regions of the oral cavity, and the oropharynx benefit much less from reinnervation.

What does this reinnervation consist of? It has been shown that the sensory recovery, by all objectively measurable sensory parameters (except taste), is not significantly different from the preexisting sensation on the opposite (nonoperated) side. Furthermore—and more surprisingly—the resulting sensation is superior to that on the skin paddle in its native site *before* elevation. The mechanism for this "sensory upgrading" is unknown, but it has been postulated that the higher sensory acuity of the recipient nerve is responsible (55). For this reason, the lingual and mental nerves, with their larger cortical representation, are preferred over, say, the greater auricular or other cutaneous branches of the cervical plexus.

Radial forearm and fibula flaps have identifiable cutaneous nerves suitable for reinnervation (the LABC nerve in the former; the LSCN and RSPN in the latter). However, whenever cutaneous flaps are combined with osseous flaps in complex reconstructions, the possibility exists to reinnervate the cutaneous component, whether it be the ulnar forearm (medial antebrachial cutaneous nerve), the ALT (lateral femoral cutaneous nerve), or the lateral arm (inferior lateral cutaneous nerve of the arm) flap. Improved intraoral sensation contributes to better manipulation of the food bolus, prevention of drooling, and improved speech. Anatomical details of and elevation these innervated flaps are discussed elsewhere in this text.

POSTOPERATIVE MONITORING

Most vascular complications occur in the first 72 hours after flap transfer. During this period, flap checks are performed hourly. The majority of flaps have a cutaneous component that may be monitored by capillary refill, color, and turgor as well as by pencil Doppler. The Doppler is used to record arterial signals from a perforator, or sometimes the main vessel, marked with a 5-0 suture on the skin paddle immediately after surgery. A suture is also placed in the neck skin over the draining vein—frequently the external jugular—just inferior to the incision. A loud venous signal indicates good perfusion, but care must be taken to differentiate this signal from that from adjacent veins such as the internal jugular. In bone-only flaps, pedicle monitoring such as this is the only option aside from implantable probes.

After the third day, flap checks are reduced to every 4 hours. A change in the skin paddle or loss of signal prompts immediate reexploration.

COMPLICATIONS

Patients undergoing mandible reconstruction often have significant comorbidities, most frequently of a cardiopulmonary nature. Careful screening, preoperative medical optimization, and precise intraoperative fluid management reduce the incidence of postoperative problems. Full prophylaxis against thromboembolic disease is routinely given—in our case, intermittent calf compression, TED (thromboembolism-deterrent) stockings, and subcutaneous low-dose heparin.

Patients with posterior mandible defects, especially when combined with partial or total glossectomy, may undergo severe swelling with potential compromise of the airway. In these patients and those who need postoperative IMF, a tracheostomy should be done at the time of reconstruction. In composite mandibular reconstruction, a tracheostomy is always a safe option.

Agitation in the postoperative period can be a sign of pulmonary or cardiac problems. In patients undergoing cancer resections, there is a high incidence of alcohol abuse. Delirium tremens, which is a potentially fatal complication, should be included in the differential diagnosis and, if present, treated appropriately.

Although microvascular flap transfer in reconstruction of the mandible has a success rate of about 95%, the surgeon must be prepared for vascular complications that could result in flap loss. Arterial and venous complications are more frequent in irradiated patients and those undergoing surgery for recurrent disease or osteoradionecrosis (54). Careful inspection of recipient vessels for atherosclerotic plaques or choosing a vessel outside the main radiation field will decrease the chance for thrombosis. The surgeon should plan the position of the pedicle as it leaves the graft so it lies without kinking or compression. Fortunately, disruption of the vascular suture line with resultant bleeding is rare, but when it does occur, it is usually associated with intraoral fistula. Pressure should be carefully applied to the neck, and the patient should immediately be returned to the operating room for revision of the anastomosis.

Venous thrombosis occurs with about the same incidence as arterial thrombosis. Congestion of the skin paddle should prompt urgent reexploration. Whenever possible, two flap veins are anastomosed to decrease the chance of venous congestion. Revision with anastomosis to a different vein or end to side to the internal jugular vein is nearly always possible. The external jugular and, in rare cases, the cephalic vein are other recipient vessels that can be used for salvage.

Partial or total loss of the skin paddle of an osteocutaneous flap can occur even though the bone is viable. This is usually secondary to tension or twisting of the paddle as it is inset; and is best avoided by choosing a skin paddle that is the appropriate size and shape. Partial skin paddle loss is most likely to happen with the iliac crest and to a lesser degree with fibular skin paddles because the orientation is obliged to parallel the bone. This is a disadvantage when the lining defect is large or more transverse, extending onto the palate or retromolar trigone. In these cases, a second cutaneous flap is of value. The scapular flap or combined flaps have a definite advantage over other options because they can be harvested with one or two skin paddles that can be orientated independently from the bony component.

Orocutaneous fistulas can occur in the early or late postoperative periods. When they occur in the immediate postoperative period, they can lead to infection and produce bleeding or thrombosis at the anastomosis. Meticulous closure of intraoral soft tissue and adequate replacement of lining are keys to prevention. With posterior soft tissue defects such as tongue base or retromolar trigone lesions, swallowing puts additional stress on suture lines. Reexploration with multiple-layer repair and suction drains to divert any saliva is indicated. If inadequate soft tissue is present, an additional flap may be needed. When closure is not feasible, a *controlled fistula* is created by running a suction drain from the oral defect through the neck to the skin surface, avoiding vital structures such as the anastomosis and the great vessels of the neck. Late fistulas are less likely to cause vascular complications but should be treated because they can lead to osteomyelitis or resorption of graft segments or infections of the plate. Biopsy of the fistula tract is recommended to exclude persistent tumor as the cause of failed healing.

SECONDARY SURGERY

Few patients require secondary procedures on the mandible if the initial procedure is well planned and executed. Bone grafting for a nonunion at an osteotomy site or junction of the graft with the mandible is sometimes advisable, particularly if dental implants are anticipated. When reconstruction plates are used, fibrous unions are well tolerated. Removal of a reconstruction plate for improvement of contour may enhance the aesthetic outcome if the plate is prominent or contributes to a prognathic look.

The most common elective procedure after mandible reconstruction is dental rehabilitation with osseointegrated implants. Although implant placement at the time of bone grafting is possible (56), *we prefer* to do this as a secondary procedure (see Figures 32-11 and 32-14). A preoperative consultation with a prosthodontist is paramount in obtaining the best result. Vestibuloplasty is a common procedure in preparation for dental restoration. It is important that the skin over the reconstructed alveolar ridge is thin and adherent to the bone for placement of the dental prosthesis and for prevention of infection around the support structure. Skin paddles of the various bone flaps, including the typically thin radial forearm, are too bulky and unstable; they are usually replaced by split-thickness grafting directly onto the periosteum of the reconstructed alveolar ridge before implant exteriorization.

DENTAL REHABILITATION

Ideally, vascularized bone grafting should not be considered the end point in mandible reconstruction. Anatomic restoration of mandibular contour should allow later dental rehabilitation. Great strides have been made in the ability to restore dentition to patients who have had resection for cancer even when radiation is used. Conventional dentures can be fitted in a small percentage of patients with reconstruction of an adequate sulcus and alveolar ridge (see Figure 32-17). In patients with some remaining dentition, a skilled prosthodontist may be able to fashion a prosthesis that is supported by the residual teeth. A removable denture or bridge can be constructed in smaller gaps between teeth, but the prosthesis must be fixed directly to the teeth even when few teeth remain. This is precarious in teeth that have been irradiated, and meticulous hygiene and follow up are essential.

Satisfactory restoration of dentition most often requires placement of osseointegrated implants (see Figures 32-11 and 32-14). Osseointegration is defined as a direct structural and functional connection between ordered, living bone and the surface of a load-carrying implant. The implant consists of an anchorage unit made of a titanium alloy with an external threaded screw that is tapped flush into the bone. It also has internal threads to support prosthesis. At the time of installation, a thin cap is placed over the unit to prevent growth of bone into the internal threads, and the mucosa or skin flap is closed over the implant, which is flush with the bone. Over the next 6 to 12 months, osseointegration around the external threads of the implant occurs. Exteriorization of the implant to the oral cavity is accomplished at a second operation. The mucosa is opened and the cap removed. An abutment cylinder, attached to the implant, penetrates the mucosa and provides the intraoral attachment for the denture prosthesis. After a healing period of several weeks, during which the mucosal or graft epithelium attaches to the cylinder, the denture fixture can be placed by a prosthodontist.

Dental restoration improves function during eating and speech. There is also a significant aesthetic improvement from the support provided by dentures to the lower lip. The collapsed lower lip in edentulous patients contributes to an aging face. Patients receive a major psychological benefit from the combined functional and aesthetic improvements seen with dental restoration.

OUTCOMES

With careful preoperative planning and meticulous attention to detail, mandible reconstruction can be done satisfactorily in even the most difficult situations. Current flap transfer success rates in mandible reconstruction are 95% or better (57–60). The quality of the reconstruction depends on proper contouring of the bone for function and aesthetics, and on adequate soft tissue reconstruction because most defects are composite in nature. Results are best with smaller lateral (L, H, C, LC, HC) defects and worse with larger anterior (LCL, LCH, HCH) defects. Results are worse with large skin (s) or mucosal (m) defects and particularly with through-and-through defects (see Figure 32-18).

Oral intake is improved after mandible reconstruction. Mandibular continuity improves mastication, and adequate soft tissue reconstruction results in better manipulation of the food bolus and improved swallowing. Studies show that about 45% of patients resume a normal diet. Most of these are lateral or hemimandibular reconstructions. An additional 45% can take a soft diet with the majority having had anterior defects. Another 5% are able to tolerate a liquid diet, and only 5% require tube feeding (60).

Speech is also a beneficiary of mandible and soft tissue reconstruction. Results are worse with anterior defects and increasing amounts of tongue resection and, to a lesser degree, floor of mouth resection. Adequate replacement of the oral floor lining so that tongue mobility is restored is paramount. Reinnervation of the skin flap may enhance speech as well as food manipulation. After mandible reconstruction, Cordeiro and coworkers reported that speech was normal in 36%, near normal in 27%, intelligible in 28%, and unintelligible in 9% (60).

From an aesthetic standpoint, the outcome is heavily dependent on the magnitude of the resection, the presence or absence of radiation damage, and the HCL classification. As mentioned earlier, large anterior resections are more difficult to reconstruct than small lateral ones. Good aesthetic results are therefore harder to achieve. Furthermore, anterior resections can often involve much of the lower lip, the need for reconstruction of which negatively influences the aesthetic appearance. Loss of the central segment (C) can also result in lip and chin ptosis unless the soft tissues of the chin are firmly reattached to the osseous reconstruction. Lip and chin ptosis is a *functional* Andy Gump deformity with disastrous social and cosmetic consequences (2).

Adequate reconstruction of the oral lining results in improved tongue function and enhances chances for dental restoration. Psychological benefits of successful mandible reconstruction are immeasurable, particularly if dental rehabilitation is complete.

REFERENCES

1. Boyd JB, Morris S, Rosen IB, et al. The through-and-through oromandibular defect: rationale for aggressive reconstruction. *Plast Reconstr Surg* 1994;93:44.
2. Boyd JB, Gullane PJ, Rostein LE, et al. Classification of mandibular defects. *Plast Reconstr Surg* 1993;92:1266.
3. Urken ML, Weinberg H, Vickery C, et al. Oromandibular reconstruction using microvascular composite free flaps. Report of 71 cases and a new classification scheme for bony, soft tissue, and neurologic defects. *Arch Otolaryngol Head Neck Surg* 1991;117:733.
4. Yousif NJ, Matloub HS, Sanger JR, Campbell B. Soft-tissue reconstruction of the oral cavity. *Clin Plast Surg* 1994;21:15.
5. Deschler DG, Day T (eds). TNM Staging of Head and Neck Cancer/Neck Dissection Classification, 3rd ed, 2008. http://www.entnet.org/mktplace/NeckDissection.cfm?CFID=40777697andCFTOKEN=73269208.
6. Gullane PJ, Holmes. Mandibular reconstruction. New concepts. *Arch Otolaryngol Head Neck Surg* 1986;112:714.
7. Boyd JB, Mulholland S, Davidson J, et al. The free flap and plate in oromandibular reconstruction: long term review and indications. *Plast Reconstr Surg* 1995;95:1018.
8. Boyd JB, Mulholland S, Davidson J, et al. The free flap and plate in oromandibular reconstruction: long term review and indications. *Plast Reconstr Surg* 1995;95:1018.
9. Mosahebi A, Chaudhry A, McCarthy CM, et al. Reconstruction of extensive composite posterolateral mandibular defects using nonosseous free tissue transfer. *Plast Reconstr Surg* 2009;124:1571.
10. Millard DR, Garst WP, Campbell RC, et al. Composite lower jaw reconstruction. *Plast Reconstr Surg* 1970;46:22.
11. Benoist M. Experience with 220 cases of mandibular reconstruction. *J Maxillofac Surg* 1978;6:40.
12. Terz JJ, Bear SE, Brown PW, et al. An evaluation of the wire mesh prosthesis in primary reconstruction of the mandible. *Am J Surg* 1978;135:825.
13. Adamo AK, Szal RL. Timing, results, and complications of mandibular reconstructive surgery: report of 32 cases. *J Oral Surg* 1979;37:755.

14. Lawson W, Loscalzo L, Baek SM, et al. Experience with immediate and delayed mandibular reconstruction. *Laryngoscope* 1982;92:5.
15. Albert TW, Smith JD, Everts EC, et al. Dacron mesh tray and cancellous bone in reconstruction of mandibular defects. *Arch Otolaryngol Head Neck Surg* 1986;112:53.
16. Manchester WM. Immediate reconstruction of the mandible and temporomandibular joint. *Br J Plast Surg* 1965;18:291.
17. Manchester WM. Some technical improvements in the reconstruction of the mandible and temporomandibular joint. *Plast Reconstr Surg* 1972;50:249.
18. Marx RE. Mandibular reconstruction. *J Oral Maxillofac Surg* 1993;51:466.
19. Carlson ER, Marx RE. Part II. Mandibular reconstruction using cancellous cellular bone grafts. *J Oral Maxillofac Surg* 1996;54:889.
20. Foster RD, Anthony JP, Sharma A, et al. Vascularized bone flaps versus non-vascularized bone grafts for mandibular reconstruction: an outcome analysis of primary bony union and endosseous implant success. *Head Neck* 1999;21:66.
21. Cuono CB, Ariyan S. Immediate reconstruction of a composite mandibular defect with a regional osteomusculocutaneous flap. *Plast Reconstr Surg* 1980;65:477.
22. Panje W, Cutting C. Trapezius osteomyocutaneous island flap for reconstruction of the anterior floor of the mouth and the mandible. *Head Neck Surg* 1980;3:66.
23. Green MF, Gibson JR, Bryson JR, et al. A one-stage correction of mandibular defects using a split sternum pectoralis major osteo-musculocutaneous transfer. *Br J Plast Surg* 1981;34:11.
24. Barnes DR, Sisson GA, Pecaro B, et al. Immediate reconstruction of mandibular defects with a composite sternocleidomastoid musculoclavicular graft. *Arch Otolaryngol* 1981;107:711.
25. Maruyama Y, Urita Y, Ohnishi K. Rib-latissimus dorsi osteomyocutaneous flap in reconstruction of a mandibular defect. *Br J Plast Surg* 1985;38:234.
26. Doi K, Tominaga S, Shibata T. Bone grafts with microvascular anastomoses of vascular pedicles: an experimental study in dogs. *J Bone Joint Surg Am* 1977;59:809.
27. Hidalgo DA. Fibula free flap: a new method of mandible reconstruction. *Plast Reconstr Surg* 1989;84:71.
28. Swartz WM, Banis JC, Newton ED, et al. The osteocutaneous scapular flap for mandibular and maxillary reconstruction. *Plast Reconstr Surg* 1986;77:530.
29. Daniel RK. Mandibular reconstruction with free tissue transfers. *Ann Plast Surg* 1978;1:346.
30. Soutar DS, Widdowson WP. Immediate reconstruction of the mandible using a vascularized segment of radius. *Head Neck Surg* 1986;8:232.
31. Duncan MJ, Manktelow RT, Zuker RM, et al. Mandibular reconstruction in the radiated patient: the role of osteocutaneous free tissue transfers. *Plast Reconstr Surg* 1985;76:829.
32. Serafin D, Georgiade NG. Microsurgical composite tissue transplantation. *Ann Surg* 1978;187:620.
33. Boyd JB, Caton AM, Mulholland RM, et al. The sensate fibula osteocutaneous flap: neurosomal anatomy. *J Plast Reconstr Aesth Surg* 2013;66(12):1688–1694.
34. Boyd JB, Caton AM, Mulholland RM, Granzow JW. The sensate fibular osteoneurocutaneous flap in oromandibular reconstruction: clinical outcomes in 31 cases. *J Plast Reconstr Aesth Surg* 2013;66(12):1695–1701.
35. Taylor GI, Townsend P, Corlett R. Superiority of the deep circumflex iliac vessels as the supply for free groin flaps. *Plast Reconstr Surg* 1979;64:595.
36. Taylor GI, Townsend P, Corlett R. Superiority of the deep circumflex iliac vessels as the supply for free groin flaps. Clinical work. *Plast Reconstr Surg* 1979;64:745.
37. Shenaq SM. Refinements in mandibular reconstruction. *Clin Plast Surg* 1992;19:809.
38. Urken ML, Vickery C, Weinberg H, et al. The internal oblique-iliac crest osseo-myocutaneous free flap in oromandibular reconstruction. Report of 20 cases. *Arch Otolaryngol Head Neck Surg* 1989;115:339.
39. Boyd JB. Mandibular reconstruction in the young adult using free vascularized iliac crest. *Microsurgery* 1988;9:141.
40. Sidebottom AJ, Allen PE, Hayton M, et al. Management of the radial composite donor site: an orthopedic opinion. *Br J Oral Maxillofac Surg* 1999;37:213.
41. Moore MH, Sinclair SW, Blake GB. The hairless osteotomized radial forearm flap. *Plast Reconstr Surg* 1985;76:301.
42. Mulholland RS, Tanna N, Boyd JB. Introducing the tibial-dorsalis pedis osteocutaneous shin flap: a new option for oromandibular reconstruction. *Plast Reconstr Surg* 2013;132(4):611e–620e.
43. Sanger JR, Matloub HS, Yousif NJ. Sequential connection of flaps: a logical approach to customized mandibular reconstruction. *Am J Surg* 1990;160:402.
44. Wei FC, Celik N, Chen HC, et al. Combined anterolateral thigh flap and vascularized fibula osteoseptocutaneous flap in reconstruction of extensive composite mandibular defects. *Plast Reconstr Surg* 2002;109:45.
45. Kimata Y, Uchiyama K, Ebihara S, et al. Comparison of innervated and non-innervated free flaps in oral reconstruction. *Plast Reconstr Surg* 1999;104:1307.
46. Kimura N, Satoh K. Consideration of a thin flap as an entity and clinical applications of the thin anterolateral thigh flap. *Plast Reconstr Surg* 1996;97:985.
47. Timmons MJ, Missotten FE, Poole MD, et al. Complications of radial forearm flap donor sites. *Br J Plast Surg* 1986;39:176.
48. Granström G, Tjellström A, Brånemark PI. Osseointegrated implants in irradiated bone: a case-controlled study using adjunctive hyperbaric oxygen therapy. *J Oral Maxillofac Surg* 1999;57:493.
49. Boyd JB, Mulholland RS. Fixation of the vascularized bone graft in mandibular reconstruction. *Plast Reconstr Surg* 1993;91:274.
50. Chang YM, Wallace CG, Tsai CY, et al. Dental implant outcome after primary implantation into double-barreled fibula osteoseptocutaneous free flap-reconstructed mandible. *Plast Reconstr Surg* 2011;128:1220.
51. Daya M. Peroneal artery perforator chimeric flap: changing the perspective in free fibula flap use in complex oromandibular reconstruction. *J Reconstr Microsurg* 2008;24(6):413–418.
52. Hidalgo DA. Condyle transplantation in free flap mandible reconstruction. *Plast Reconstr Surg* 1994;93:770.
53. Driemel O, Braun S, Müller-Richter UD, et al. Historical development of alloplastic temporomandibular joint replacement after 1945 and state of the art. *Int J Oral Maxillofac Surg* 2009;38:909.
54. Mulholland S, Boyd JB, McCabe S, et al. Recipient vessels in head and neck microsurgery: radiation effect and vessel access. *Plast Reconstr Surg* 1993;92:628.
55. Boyd JB, Mulholland S, Gullane P, et al. Lateral antebrachial cutaneous neurosome flaps in oral reconstruction: are we making sense? *Plast Reconstr Surg* 1994;93:1350.
56. Urken ML, Buchbinder D, Weinberg H, et al. Primary placement of osseointegrated implants in microvascular mandibular reconstruction. *Otolaryngol Head Neck Surg* 1989;101:56.
57. Takushima A, Harii K, Asato H, et al. Mandibular reconstruction using microvascular free flaps: a statistical analysis of 178 cases. *Plast Reconstr Surg* 2001;108:1555.
58. Haughey BH, Wilson E, Kluwe L, et al. Free flap reconstruction of the head and neck: analysis of 241 cases. *Otolaryngol Head Neck Surg* 2001;125:10.
59. Podrecca S, Salvatori P, Squadrelli Saraceno M, et al. Review of 346 patients with free-flap reconstruction following head and neck surgery for neoplasm. *J Plast Reconstr Aesthet Surg* 2006;59:122.
60. Cordeiro PG, Disa JJ, Hidalgo DA, et al. Reconstruction of the mandible with osseous free flaps: a 10-year experience with 150 consecutive patients. *Plast Reconstr Surg* 1999;104:1314.

CHAPTER 33

Microsurgical Reconstruction of the Scalp and Skull

Reza Jarrahy and Neil F. Jones

FUNCTIONAL ANATOMY

Comprehensive anatomical studies of the scalp are well described elsewhere and are beyond the focus of this chapter. However, certain aspects of scalp anatomy that are relevant to free flap reconstruction merit attention here.

Anatomy

A thick layer of skin covers the most superficial layer of the scalp. The thickness of the cutis allows for harvest of split-thickness skin grafts that can be used for coverage of limited defects or local flap donor sites. The density of the scalp limits its elasticity, yet the loose layer of areolar tissue deep to the galea allows for smooth gliding of the scalp over the deeper tissues, particularly in the temporal areas. Dissection in this layer along with scoring of the overlying galea helps provide greater mobilization of these scalp flaps. In addition, the galea and the pericranium can each be raised as distinct vascularized flaps to cover exposed calvarial bone or assist with dural repair in full-thickness defects.

Vascular Supply

The scalp is richly supplied by the paired terminal branches of the external carotid system, including the superficial temporal, postauricular, and occipital vessels. These vascular pedicles can provide adequate recipient vessels for microsurgical anastomoses. Large scalp flaps should be based on at least one of these major branches. Successful scalp replantation can be accomplished with anastomosis of only one of these arteries (1).

Cranial Vault

Exposed cranial bone requires vascularized soft tissue coverage to prevent desiccation and potential infection. The calvarium is composed of inner and outer cortices that envelop a vascularized network of trabecular bone, the diploe. Removal of the outer table of the cranial vault to expose raw bleeding bone can sometimes provide a more suitable wound base for skin graft or flap coverage.

CONVENTIONAL OPTIONS FOR SCALP RECONSTRUCTION

The paradigm of the "reconstructive ladder" is perhaps more aptly applied to reconstruction of the scalp than to any other anatomical region of the human body. An open scalp wound with vascularized tissue at its base can be allowed to heal by secondary intention. Simple scalp defects of small surface area can be closed directly. When direct closure is not possible nor a more extensive reconstructive procedure advisable, a skin graft or allograft matrix can be used to cover a wound with a granulating base. Larger defects can be covered with local flaps of hair-bearing scalp. Regional flaps, including pedicled trapezius, deltopectoral, and latissimus flaps, can be recruited to cover defects when local tissues are insufficient or of poor quality.

However, despite the availability of increasingly complex surgical options, some surgeons argue that in the setting of scalp reconstruction, especially in the presence of composite defects of scalp and skull, the traditional paradigm should be replaced with the model of the "reconstructive elevator" (2). Failure of more conservative approaches can lead to serious infection and significant neurologic morbidity. In this model, reconstructive options start with the most comprehensive strategies to avoid potential complications, and the free flap becomes an attractive first-line therapy.

Nevertheless, the lower rungs of the reconstructive ladder for the scalp should not yet be relegated to the ranks of surgical procedures that are of historical interest only. Without an available microsurgeon or the resources needed to deliver the necessary perioperative care to a free flap candidate, the more traditional means of scalp coverage serve as useful surgical options.

Secondary Intention

Wounds that have a base of vascularized tissue can be allowed to heal spontaneously with local wound care. A vacuum-assisted closure (VAC) device may increase the rate of healing. Exposed calvarium devoid of pericranium, however, is unlikely to heal and requires some intervention. Drilling the outer table of the calvarium to the level of the diploe to expose healthy bleeding bone or recruiting adjacent galeal or pericranial flaps, can facilitate wound closure in these situations (3).

Primary Closure

Small defects of the scalp may be closed directly by mobilization and approximation of the wound edges. Although there is no standard size limitation to this approach, numerous authors have reported success with primary closure of wounds up to 3 cm (4). The elasticity of the scalp is limited, but its mobility can be improved by dissection in the loose areolar layer between the galea and the pericranium and by scoring of the galea parallel to the axis of the defect.

Skin Grafts, Allografts

Split-thickness skin grafting is a viable option for coverage of scalp defects in patients who may not be good candidates for major reconstructive procedures, including patients with major medical comorbidities. Because of its thick dermal layer, the scalp itself can serve as an excellent donor site for a split-thickness skin graft. The base of the wound must contain vascularized tissue. As described earlier, drilling the outer table or covering exposed calvarium with pericranial or galeal flaps can make a wound more hospitable to grafting. The obvious disadvantages of skin grafting include the need for a donor site and the resultant contour irregularities and alopecia associated with a graft. In addition, the long-term results of skin grafting have been shown to be suboptimal (5). Allograft dermal regeneration matrices may be associated with improved aesthetic and functional outcomes. These two options, however, will result in areas of alopecia that may not be conducive to hair transplantation.

Scalp Flaps

Defects that are too large to close primarily yet limited enough in scope and complexity to render a free flap unnecessary are appropriately covered with full-thickness scalp flaps. Smaller defects may be addressed with single or opposing rotation, transposition, or advancement flaps. These flaps should be based on one of the major paired arterial branches that supply the scalp. Scoring of the galea may decrease closing tension and extend the length of the raised flaps (6). Defects of larger surface area may require multiple flaps, as described by Orticochea (7). They are particularly useful for reconstruction of anterior and occipital defects, with more limited application to the parietal and vertex areas. These three- and four-flap reconstructions often require skin grafting of donor sites; the pericranium should therefore be left intact at the sites of flap harvest.

Tissue Expansion

Expansion of the normal scalp surrounding a scalp defect is an effective yet relatively inefficient method of reconstruction. It is particularly useful in cases in which reconstruction can be staged, such as in the setting of a scalp burn that has previously been covered with a skin graft with suboptimal results or in the primary excision of giant benign nevi. The ability to recruit flaps of hair-bearing scalp makes expansion an attractive option, as the outcome from expander-based reconstruction may provide the best aesthetics of any available surgical technique. Intraoperative expansion may also be used, but the additional tissue recruited by creep is limited. Expansion of previously irradiated tissues yields unsatisfactory results (8). In the setting of a primary extirpation that leaves a significant full-thickness scalp defect with or without a calvarial component requiring expedient closure, expansion of the surrounding scalp is typically not an option (9). If tissue expansion is considered, a coordinated multidisciplinary plan must be devised in advance.

INDICATIONS FOR FREE FLAP COVERAGE OF THE SCALP

In the modern era, advanced microsurgical techniques are being increasingly used as primary therapeutic options. Expertise in the design and transfer of flaps that are customized to address the reconstructive and aesthetic needs of any given defect is available at most major tertiary and quarternary care referral centers. It is important, however, for reconstructive surgeons who are skilled in microsurgery to be fully aware of the resources available to them at their institutions, including access to all necessary intraoperative material needs and perioperative monitoring equipment, as well as to anesthesiologists and nurses experienced in the perioperative care of microsurgical patients (10).

Extensive or complex defects of the scalp that are not amenable to coverage with local or regional flaps should be reconstructed with free flaps (Figures 33-1 to 33-3). Relative indications include the presence of residual scalp tissues that are in suboptimal condition, such as traumatized, irradiated, or otherwise poorly vascularized tissue. Some authors have related the magnitude of the defect to the need for free flap coverage (2,11). A staging system has been proposed to systematically categorize patients that would most benefit from free tissue transfer (4), but currently there is no uniformly accepted indication based on defect size. Exposure of vital intracranial contents that cannot be covered by other means strictly mandates free flap reconstruction. Free tissue transfer provides the ability to recruit large blocks of homogeneous or composite tissues that have the ability to conform to the convex surface of the cranial vault, provide protection for deeper structures during adjuvant radiotherapy, and yield acceptable cosmetic results. Regardless of defect size, microsurgical reconstruction has proven to be an effective means of addressing scalp defects of oncologic, traumatic, or congenital origin particularly in the presence of underlying osteomyelitis or osteoradionecrosis (12).

Contraindications to microsurgical free flap scalp reconstruction are few and include poor general medical condition of

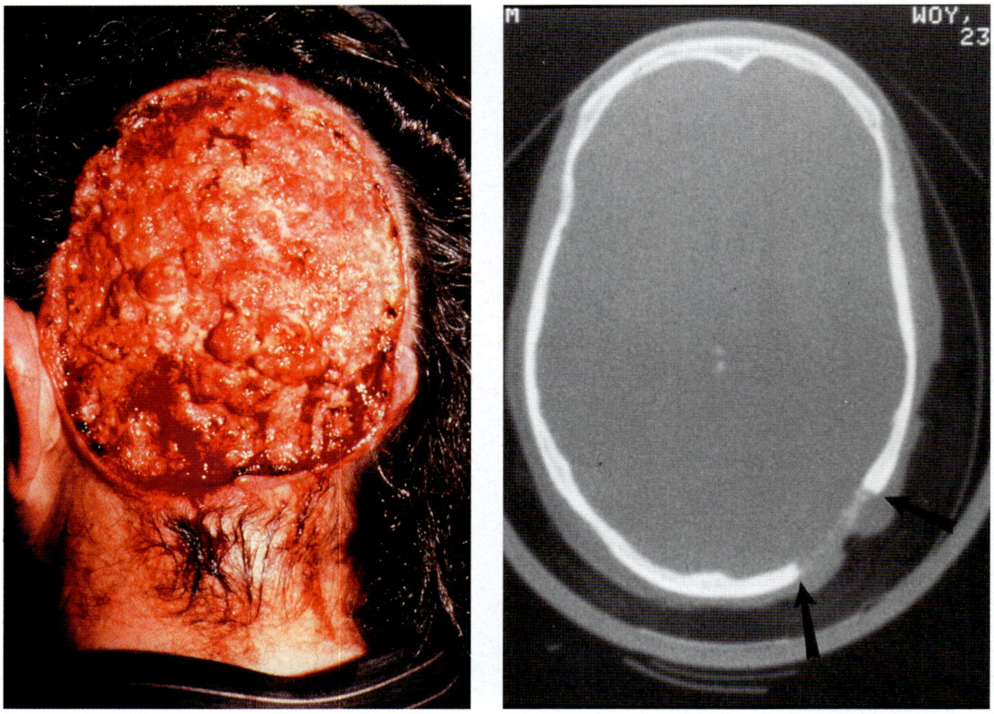

A B

FIGURE 33-1 Extensive neglected basal cell carcinoma of the posterior scalp (**A**) with invasion through both the inner and outer tables of the skull on computed tomography (**B**).

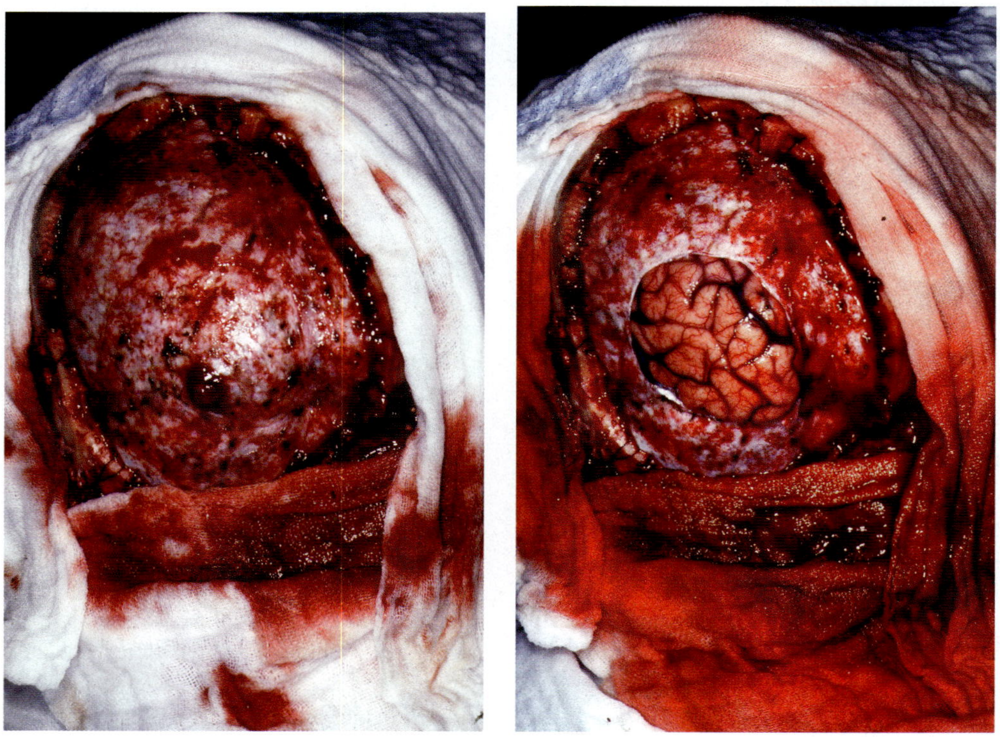

A B

FIGURE 33-2 Craniectomy revealed a nodule of basal cell carcinoma on the dura (**A**), which required excision of the dura (**B**). The dural defect was reconstructed with a fascia lata graft.

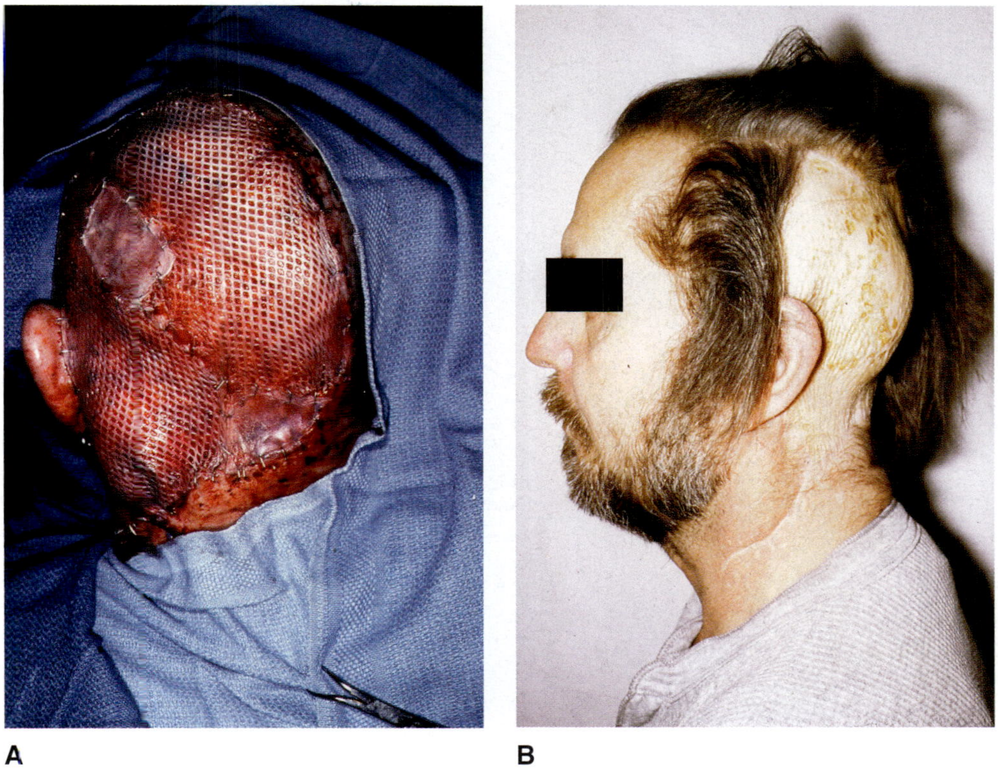

FIGURE 33-3 (A) The composite soft tissue and bone defect of the posterior scalp and skull was reconstructed with a latissimus dorsi muscle flap covered by a meshed split-thickness skin graft but without any bony reconstruction. (B) The result 9 years after surgery.

the patient, lack of appropriate recipient vessels, and absence of any of the necessary perioperative resources enumerated above.

OPTIMAL FREE FLAPS FOR SCALP RECONSTRUCTION

A myriad of options are available to microsurgeons tasked with free flap coverage of scalp defects. The choice of flap must be tailored to the individual patient and must take into consideration the specific functional and aesthetic goals of the reconstruction. Moreover, not only must the flap be designed to address the three-dimensional complexity of the defect, but surgical planning must also address the fourth dimension of time: the surgeon must predict how the anatomy and appearance of the transferred flap will evolve, and plan accordingly at the initial operative procedure. Failure to do so can result in flap "failure" by way of recurrence of the original defect or an unacceptable cosmetic result.

Following the reconstructive axiom of Sir Harold Gillies to "replace like with like," scalp defects should be reconstructed with donor scalp, even those that call for free tissue transfer. The ideal free flap replacement for a large segment of missing scalp is that same missing tissue, which is often available in total or subtotal scalp avulsion. If the traumatically absent scalp is appropriately preserved and recipient vessels are accessible, replantation of the scalp can be performed with a single pedicle anastomosis with excellent results (13). Although few patients have isogeneic donors available, free scalp transfer between identical twins has been described (14). Although these are relatively unique circumstances, numerous excellent flap choices have been described to provide surgeons with an extensive armamentarium for microsurgical reconstruction. Which flaps are "optimal" continues to be debated: to some degree, a number of different flaps can be used to cover any given defect. The choice of flap, then, depends on numerous factors, including the size and complexity of the defect, the intended recipient vessels, the required length of the vascular leash, and intraoperative positioning. The most favorable flap is the one that best addresses the reconstructive needs of the patient in the least burdensome manner, coupled with the lowest donor site morbidity and the most consistent success. Perhaps the most important considerations are the surgeon's preference, experience, and comfort level with a particular technique.

Latissimus Dorsi Flap

The latissimus dorsi is arguably the greatest "workhorse" flap used for scalp reconstruction. The potential size of the flap allows for total or subtotal coverage of the cranial vault (11). The length and caliber of the vascular pedicle typically permit direct and compatibly sized anastomoses to the superficial temporal vessels without the need for interpositional vein grafts (15).

The latissimus dorsi flap can be raised as a muscle or myocutaneous flap. The somewhat predictable branching pattern of the thoracodorsal pedicle allows for splitting of the muscle (16), which provides the opportunity to create a flap with dimensions

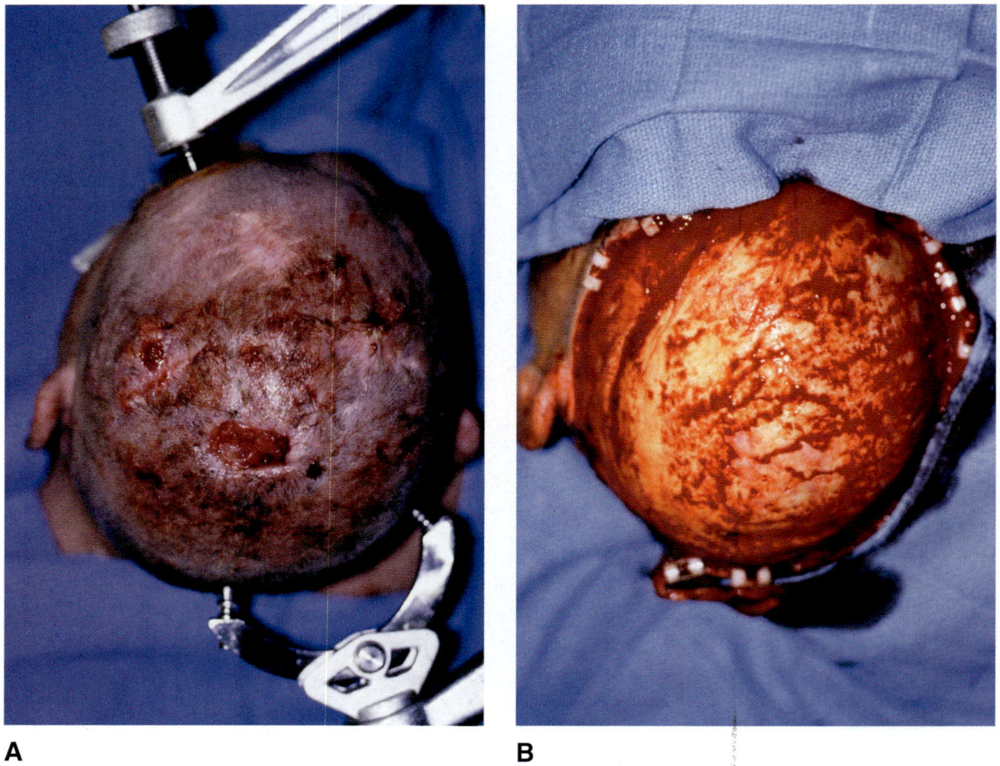

FIGURE 33-4 Multiple squamous cell carcinomas invading the scalp of an immunosuppressed heart transplant patient (**A**) requiring total resection of the scalp and pericranium (**B**).

that specifically match the anatomy of the defect. The versatility of the latissimus dorsi is further enhanced by the vascular anatomy it shares with the serratus anterior flap, the scapular and parascapular fasciocutaneous flaps, and the lateral scapular bone flap (17). When an extensive defect requires a flap with maximal surface area or extra volume, the latissimus may be raised along with the serratus anterior muscle based on the serratus branch of the thoracodorsal system (11) (Figures 33-4 to 33-6). Care must be taken in this circumstance to preserve the long thoracic nerve and some of the slips of the serratus to prevent winging of the scapula. Composite reconstructions are possible with the elevation of vascularized rib grafts in continuity with either a latissimus flap alone or a combined latissimus–serratus flap (18,19).

The latissimus dorsi free flap tends to atrophy with time, particularly when the nerve is not transferred with the muscle, which is almost always the case in the setting of scalp reconstruction. This can be advantageous because the thickness of the

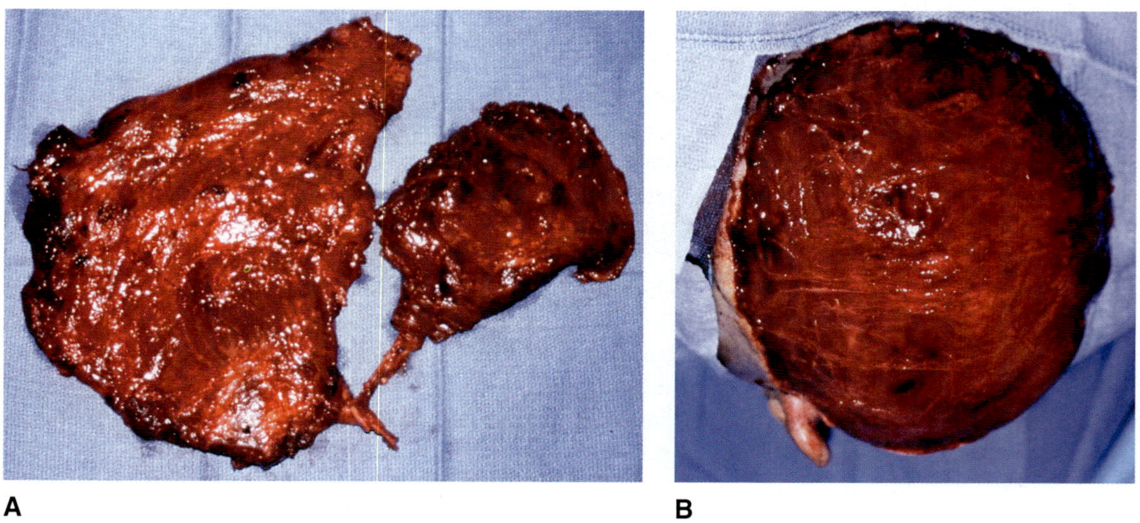

FIGURE 33-5 (**A**) and (**B**) The total scalp defect was reconstructed with combined latissimus dorsi and serratus anterior muscle flaps based on the subscapular artery.

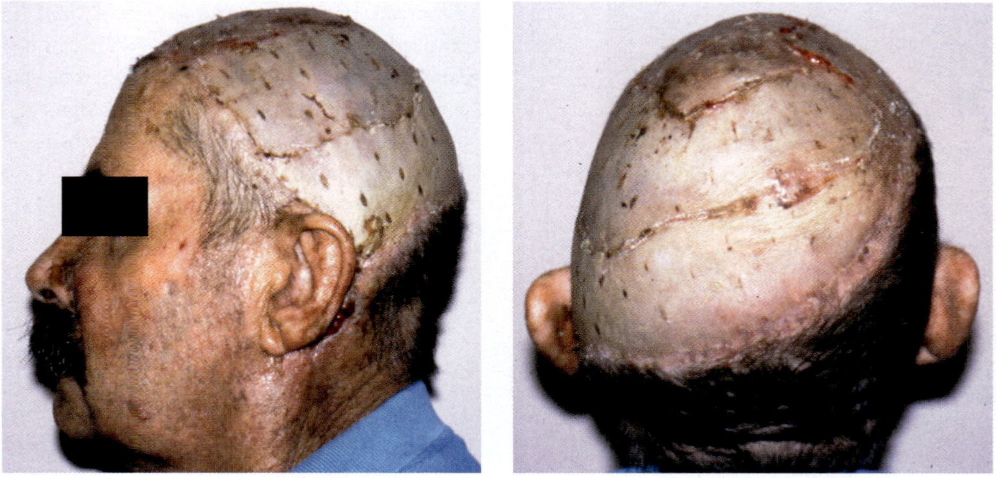

A B

FIGURE 33-6 (A) and (B) Early postoperative result of the total scalp reconstruction with combined latissimus dorsi and serratus anterior muscle flaps covered with a nonmeshed split-thickness skin graft.

atrophied flap may approach that of the native scalp and lead to an exceptional cosmetic result (11) (Figures 33-7 and 33-8). However, excessive thinning may lead to secondary exposure of the reconstructed defect and need for additional coverage.

Disadvantages to the use of this flap include donor site morbidity, such as unsightly scarring and a high risk of seroma formation. In addition, the need for decubitus positioning to elevate the flap may preclude the ability of two surgical teams to work simultaneously to harvest the flap and to perform the index procedure on the scalp, cranial vault, or intracranial cavity in preparation for flap inset.

Rectus Abdominis Flap

The rectus flap provides advantages that are similar to the latissimus dorsi: it can be elevated as a muscle or musculocutaneous flap depending on the architecture of the defect, it has a predictable and reliable blood supply that yields a pedicle of adequate length for microsurgical anastomosis; atrophy of the muscle flap subsequent to its transfer produces a thickness that approaches the native scalp and therefore an acceptable aesthetic outcome; and, especially in its muscle sparing and perforator-based incarnations, leaves minimal donor site morbidity (20). Equally important is the fact that it can be raised simultaneously with excision of the primary lesion and preparation of the recipient site. Whether designed in a vertical or transverse orientation, the overlying skin, subcutaneous tissue, and fascia may be incorporated for use in complicated defects requiring volume fill (20,21).

Despite these advantages, the rectus flap is limited by its size. Unlike the latissimus, the size of the flap precludes its use in subtotal or larger scalp defects, and it cannot be raised as a

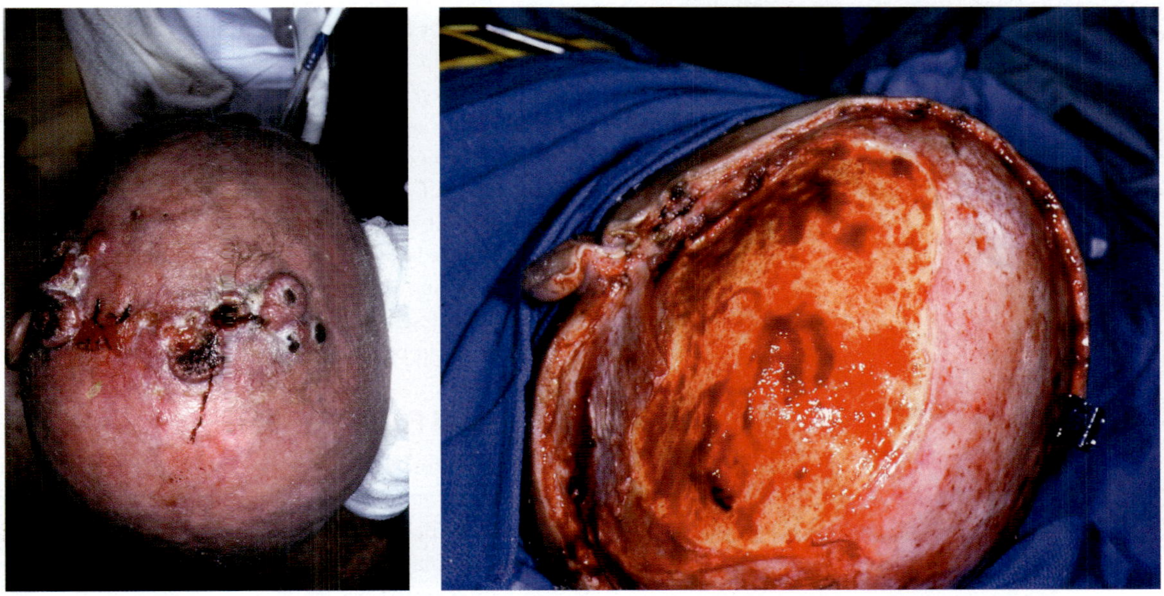

A B

FIGURE 33-7 Multiple squamous cell carcinomas of the scalp (A) treated by resection of almost three quarters of the scalp and removal of the outer table over the left half of the skull (B).

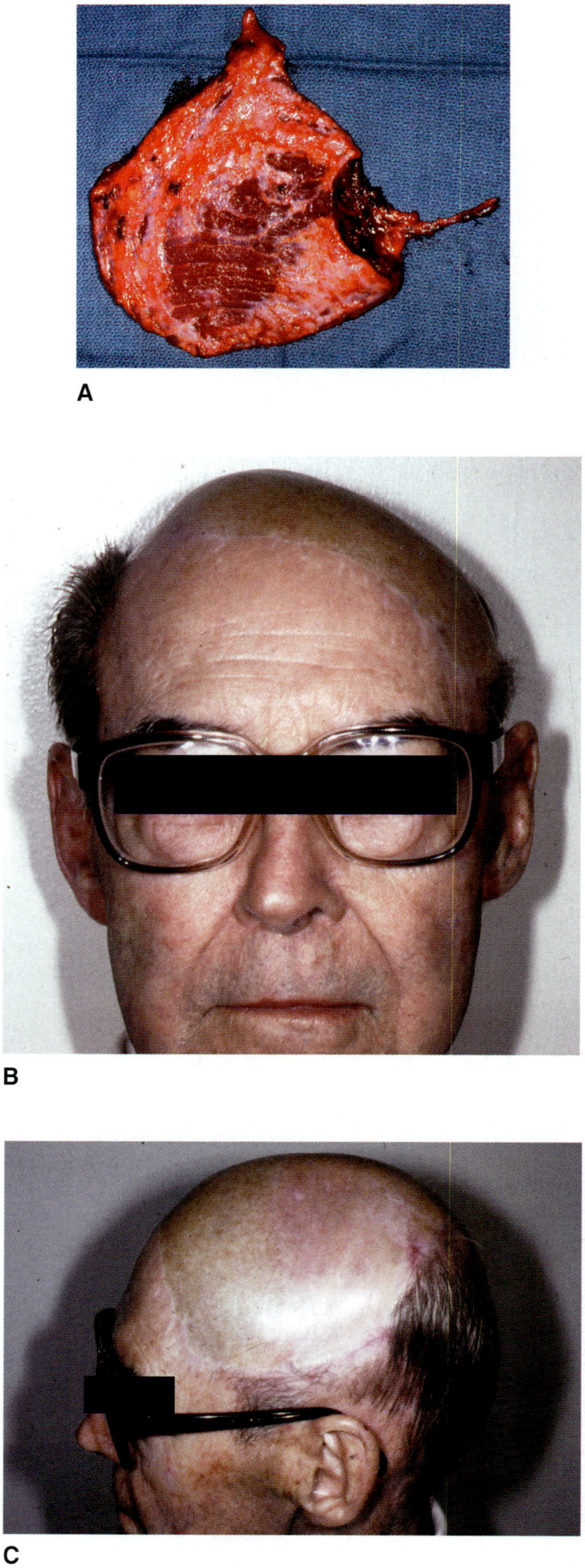

FIGURE 33-8 This was reconstructed with a free latissimus dorsi muscle flap that was tangentially thinned on its outer surface and covered with a nonmeshed split-thickness skin graft (A) with satisfactory aesthetic appearance 1 year after surgery (B and C).

composite flap to incorporate vascularized bone for composite calvarial reconstruction. Moreover, it can be excessively bulky, particularly in obese patients (2). The possible donor site sequelae of abdominal weakness, bulge, or hernia formation should also be considered when choosing this flap for scalp reconstruction (12). The deep inferior epigastric artery perforator (DIEP) flap variation addresses some of the shortcomings of the rectus muscle and myocutaneous flaps by providing a flap of greater surface area that is associated with less abdominal wall morbidity.

Anterolateral Thigh Flap

The anterolateral thigh (ALT) flap offers numerous advantages in the setting of scalp reconstruction, including the ability to harvest a large cutaneous area, long vascular pedicle vessels of appropriate size and acceptable donor site morbidity (22). In composite defects that involve absence of the dura, the fascial component of the ALT flap can be used as a vascularized fascial graft for dural reconstruction, with limited risk of subsequent cerebrospinal fluid (CSF) leak (23). The flap can also be safely raised with an extended skin paddle to address larger defects (24). The volume of the flap may be primarily modified by removing the deep fascia and subcutaneous fat when less bulk is needed or by retaining a cuff of muscle when more volume is required. "Chimeric" flaps have also been described, in which the ALT is raised with surrounding soft tissues that are nourished by the lateral femoral circumflex artery system, depending on the requirements of the reconstruction (22). The ability to raise the ALT as a perforator flap, myocutaneous flap, vastus lateralis muscle flap, sensate flap, deepithelialized skin flap, or flow-through flap provides tremendous versatility (25). Furthermore, the flap is harvested in the supine position, allowing for resection of the scalp and preparation of recipient vessels with simultaneous flap elevation. In hirsute individuals, the ALT also provides hair-bearing coverage for reconstructed scalp wounds, although the quality and density of the hair are noticeably different from the native scalp.

Donor site morbidity can pose an issue in cases when large flaps are harvested and the thigh wounds cannot be closed primarily. The anatomy of the major vascular pedicle and the musculocutaneous and septocutaneous perforators associated with the ALT may be inconsistent, making identification and dissection of these vessels tedious. However, variations in the course of the lateral circumflex femoral artery and its ascending, transverse, and descending branches to facilitate this dissection have been described (26). With experience, successful pedicle dissection can be consistently performed.

Radial Forearm Flap

The radial forearm flap is yet another fasciocutaneous option for scalp reconstruction. It has the benefit of a long and reliable vascular pedicle supplying a constant anatomic territory. The venous drainage of the free flap, either by the paired venae comitantes or the basilic or cephalic veins, enables the surgeon to choose vessels that have optimal size match with the recipient vessels. The ability to incorporate the lateral or medial antebrachial cutaneous nerves provides for sensate flap transfer.

The thin and pliable quality of the flap provides an appropriate color and texture match, particularly for defects involving the forehead and temporal areas. There is potential for single-stage reconstruction of composite defects with incorporation of a segment of the radius in an osteocutaneous flap (27). It is relatively straightforward to elevate the radial forearm flap with the patient in the supine position, allowing simultaneous work to be performed on the scalp.

Size limitations of the flap have been addressed by preexpansion, although this is not entirely without risk, and patient compliance during the expansion process is required (27). With appropriate planning and successful execution, expansion may treble the size of the flap (28). However, when large flaps are raised, a large skin graft for coverage of the donor site on the anterior surface of the forearm becomes necessary. This is conspicuous and has the potential for hypertrophic scar formation and adhesion to the underlying flexor tendons. Suprafascial elevation of the flap has been shown to improve the appearance of the grafted donor site (29). Technical adjustments can be made in the design of the flap to minimize flap width, thereby facilitating direct closure of the donor site, but still allow for manipulation of the flap to cover sizable defects (30).

Scapular and Parascapular Flaps

The shared vascular anatomic system that feeds the scapular, parascapular, latissimus, and serratus flaps translates clinically into a versatility in flap design that is unrivaled elsewhere in the body. The subscapular system provides flaps of diverse tissue type, large surface area, and significant volume that can be raised individually or en bloc on a single vascular pedicle (31). The independent vascular branches that supply the components of the subscapular system provide great mobility to the individual flaps relative to each other, enabling flap designs that can address any variety of three-dimensional reconstructive challenges, including composite defects requiring soft tissue and bone replacement (31). The ability to dissect a long pedicle of large caliber that will supply all of the various components of the subscapular system is yet another advantage (32).

The scapular flap can be elevated as an isolated fasciocutaneous or osteocutaneous flap in an expedient and safe manner because of its reliable vascular anatomy (33). A bone flap of up to 14 cm in length—which is amenable to osteotomy—can also be raised with the fasciocutaneous component of the flap, allowing for composite reconstruction of skull and scalp defects with a single flap (34). The parascapular flap, based on the descending branch of the circumflex scapular artery, can also incorporate a portion of the scapula bone of similar dimension. The cutaneous territory of the flap can also be preexpanded to yield greater flap dimension (34). The pedicle length and vessel caliber of both these flaps can be increased by proximal dissection from the major branches that supply them to the feeding subscapular vessel. If a thinner flap is desired, a perforator flap based on the circumflex scapular artery is also an option; studies have demonstrated the reliable vascular anatomy that is associated with successful elevation of these flaps (35). Both flaps, including fasciocutaneous and osteocutaneous permutations, have been shown to produce minimal functional deficit to the shoulder girdle (36).

Contraindications to the use of the scapular or parascapular flaps include prior extensive axillary or dorsal surgery, where the vascular anatomy may have been compromised (37). One major disadvantage to the fasciocutaneous flaps of the subscapular system is their location: patient repositioning must almost always be performed to access the subscapular region after preparation of the scalp recipient site. Some believe that the parascapular flap provides advantages over the scapular flap in this regard because of the ability to raise the flap with only partial rotation versus full lateral decubitus positioning (38). Both the scapular and parascapular flap donor sites may be unsightly if large flaps requiring skin graft coverage of secondary defects are harvested.

Omentum

The omental free flap was the first microsurgical flap described for the coverage of large defects of the scalp and skull (39). It can be raised on a single gastroepiploic vascular pedicle of generous length (40). The large surface area of the omentum, similar to the latissimus, allows for coverage of total or near-total scalp defects. The pliable nature of the tissue imparts perhaps its greatest versatility in conforming to irregularly shaped defects or those that require volumetric filling (see Figures 33-11D and 33-11E). The omentum can be folded, pleated, corrugated, or layered (39,40). Attention must be given to the status of the pedicle during such manipulation to avoid vascular compromise. The rich blood supply of the omentum and its unique immunologic properties allow it to maximally revascularize neighboring tissues—including skin and bone grafts—and resist infection while enhancing wound healing in irradiated or infected fields.

The abdominal harvest can either be performed by an open or endoscopic approach (41). However, the fine technique necessary to elongate the pedicle may be difficult to execute laparoscopically, mandating an open approach. Opening of the intraabdominal cavity potentially exposes the patient to additional morbidity. Reported complications from omental harvest have included laparotomy wound infection, gastric outlet obstruction, hemorrhage, and wound dehiscence (40).

The availability of muscle, musculocutaneous, and fasciocutaneous flaps that have greater structural integrity and lower morbidity associated with the donor site only make the omentum attractive as a primary option when these alternative flaps are not available or when it would offer an advantage because of an extremely large defect size, three-dimensional complexity of the defect, or severe radiation injury to surrounding tissues.

NEUROSURGICAL CONSIDERATIONS

Successful management of complex head and neck malignancies, particularly those involving the scalp and underlying skull, is predicated upon successful multidisciplinary collaboration between multiple surgical services. Specifically, head and neck oncologists and neurosurgeons should have "jurisdiction" over the resection component of the procedure, including the magnitude of the potential craniectomy, striving for complete three-dimensional resection (21). The microsurgeon, in turn, must communicate with the resection team and appropriately plan for a flap of adequate dimension and tissue quality to reconstruct the anticipated defect. Of paramount importance in this dialogue is determining the risk of recurrence of the malignancy.

Whenever preoperative radiographic or clinical evidence indicates involvement of the underlying calvarium by a scalp cutaneous malignancy (see Figures 33-1B and 33-2A), a traumatic defect, or a congenital deformity, neurosurgical consultation should be obtained. Similarly, secondary reconstruction of a full-thickness scalp defect that includes missing skull bone should be planned with neurosurgical consultation. Several questions arise in these scenarios: Should missing dura be replaced? If so, with what? Should a cranioplasty be performed in the acute setting or secondarily? What materials are best suited to the osseous reconstruction? What type of soft tissue coverage is necessary for the cranioplasty? Each question offers the opportunity for debate; there are no widely accepted standards. Microsurgeons must base their management plans on general principles, clinical acumen, the individual circumstances surrounding each case, and the input of their neurosurgery colleagues.

Dural Repair

Numerous autologous, xenographic and alloplastic materials are available for repair of the dura. The ideal dural graft should be inert, elastic, durable, biocompatible, readily available, and inexpensive. Common choices include pericranium, galea, temporalis fascia, tensor fascia lata, bovine pericardium, and collagen. Engineered nanoscale solutions are also being developed for this purpose (42).

The primary indication for dural repair in the setting of complex scalp and skull reconstruction is to prevent CSF leak (see Figure 33-2B). Partial-thickness defects of the dura mater that show no signs of CSF leak do not strictly require grafting. Small tears can be suture repaired and covered with fibrin glue. The ultimate decision should be made in conjunction with the neurosurgeon at the time of surgery. Consideration should be given to the nature of the defect and the quality of the surrounding tissues, as well as the planned reconstruction. In the setting of an infected or irradiated wound bed, for example, a vascularized fascial graft incorporated into an ALT free flap might be a better option for dural repair than nonvascularized autologous tissue or alloplastic materials (23,43).

Cranioplasty

Not all patients with a full-thickness skull defect require a cranioplasty (43). Small defects with supple and stable overlying soft tissue coverage can be safely managed in an expectant manner (9). Larger defects have been shown to alter regional CSF and cerebral blood flow, resulting in cognitive deficits and other potential symptoms referred to collectively as the "syndrome of the trephined" (44). However, there is no commonly accepted standard for defect size that would dictate the use of a cranioplasty over observation, despite the availability of diagnostic modalities that may be used to identify patients who would potentially benefit from cranioplasty (45) (Figures 33-9 to 33-13).

The list of materials that have been successfully used for cranioplasty is a lengthy one. Until tissue-engineered solutions are readily available, the fundamental choice is between autologous and alloplastic materials. Vascularized bone grafts that are incorporated into free latissimus flaps, scapular/parascapular flaps, or radial forearm flaps are an excellent source of autologous bone, as described previously. The most common sources for nonvascularized autologous bone graft are the calvarium, ribs, ilium, and tibia (46) (see Figure 33-11A to 33-11C). In the setting of a traumatic or hemorrhagic craniectomy where a decompressive craniectomy may be needed, the neurosurgeon may store the removed cranial bone in the patient's subcutaneous tissue or in cryopreservation units for use in secondary reconstruction. Autologous bone grafts serve as osteoconductive lattices, allowing for migration of surrounding bone cells into the defect and subsequent deposition of mineralized tissue. The ultimate "survival" of the graft (or more precisely, its replacement with *de novo* bone formation) provides a distinct

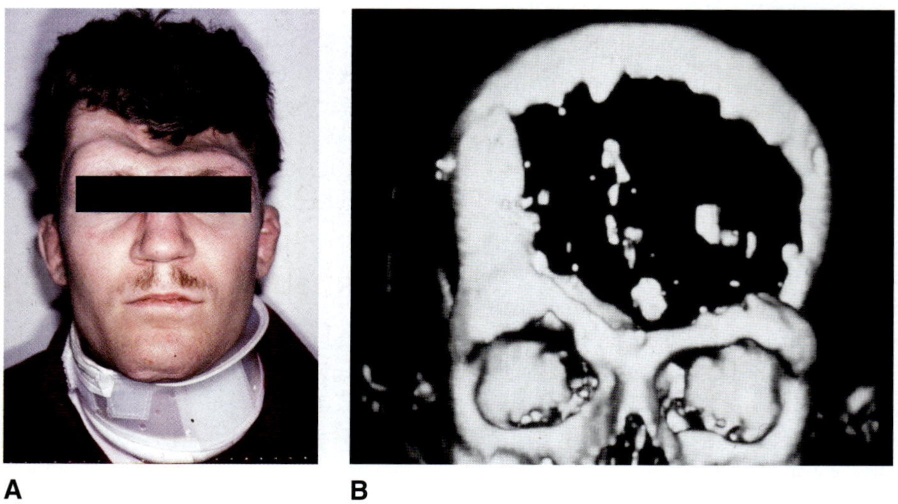

FIGURE 33-9 Frontal photograph (A) and three-dimensional computed tomography reconstruction (B) of a massive gunshot wound to the left frontal skull.

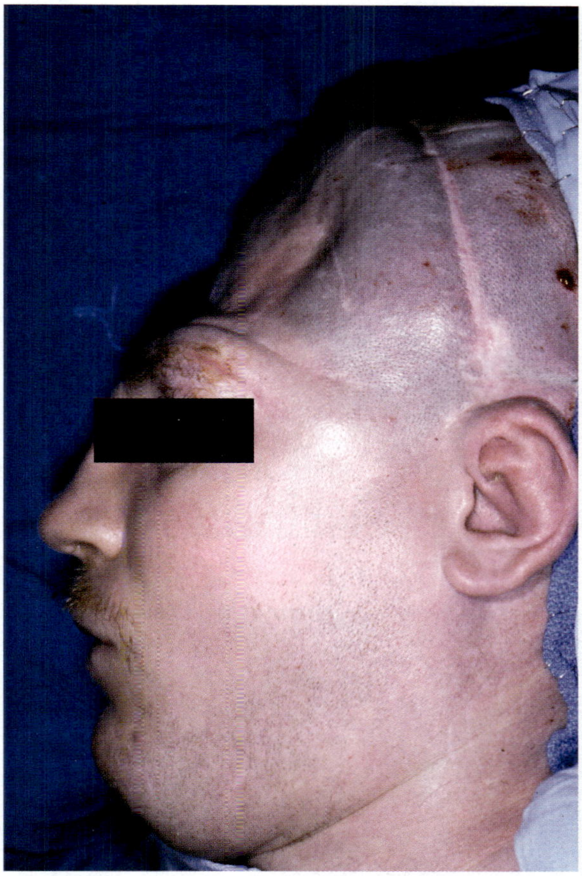

A

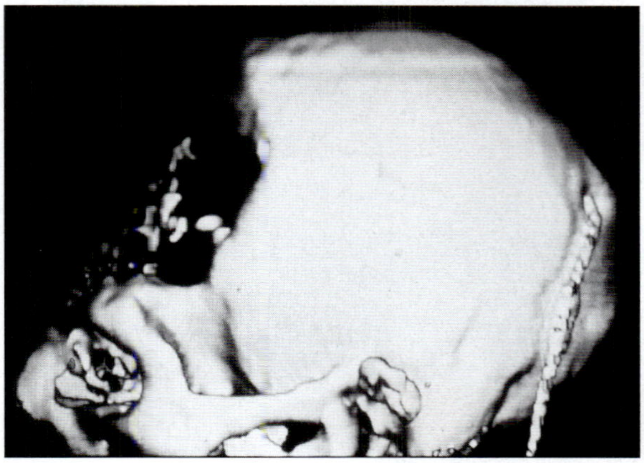

B

FIGURE 33-10 Lateral photograph (**A**) and three-dimensional computed tomography reconstruction (**B**) of the massive gun shot wound to the left frontal skull.

advantage over alloplastic material that is never incorporated. Detractors of autologous bone grafting often cite longer surgical time, added pain and discomfort, and donor site morbidity as reasons to avoid this strategy. Those who are well trained in these techniques, however, are likely to disagree.

The most commonly used alloplastic materials are metal, acrylic, calcium phosphate, or polymers (47). The primary benefit to these materials is that they are readily available "off the shelf." Each has the potential for customization to suit the needs of each individual patient. Stereolithographic mapping of the cranial defect with computed tomography can be used to prefabricate implants (48). Moreover, methylmethacrylate and viscous hydroxyapatite cements can be molded at the time of surgery to accurately conform to the architecture of the defect (Figures 33-14 and 33-15). Recently, various uniplanar and bilaminate resorbable and nonresorbable composites have been introduced to the market for this indication. Some of these are being used in conjunction with tissue engineering solutions, including incorporation of stem cells or potent growth factors, such as bone morphogenetic protein (49).

This decision on which type of material to use in cranioplasty and when to perform the reconstruction is ultimately left up to the discretion of the surgical team, and is largely subject to a personal bias based on the surgeon's training and experience. Any combination of soft tissue flaps and structural reconstructive components can be used. The choice should not be strictly arbitrary, however; several principles apply to the decision-making process, particularly with regard to the timing of bone reconstruction. Primary one-stage full-thickness reconstruction, including replacement of resected scalp, skull, and dura, can be safely performed in both pediatric and adult patient populations (21). In fact, the ability to effectively and aesthetically cover a large, complex defect in a single operative procedure is the overwhelming benefit of microsurgical reconstruction, compared with more traditional techniques. However, no attempt at primary calvarial reconstruction should be made in the setting of an oncologic resection when there is a reasonable suspicion that oncologic margins may be positive (see Figures 33-1 to 33-3). It is also reasonable to postpone a cranioplasty in elderly patients with aggressive tumors and poor overall prognoses, who are undergoing palliative coverage procedures, when there is a significant risk of short-term mortality from the disease process.

Unfavorable soft tissue conditions, including a history of infection or radiation of the defect site, warrant a strong consideration for delayed cranioplasty. The placement of any alloplastic material or large nonvascularized bone graft into an acutely infected field should be strongly discouraged. The delay between resolution of the infectious process and insertion of an implant or bone graft is debatable but may last up to one year. A shorter interval may be possible when autologous bone cranioplasty is planned, but stable soft tissue coverage over a healthy defect site is a prerequisite before attempted secondary reconstruction. Large bony defects that have been complicated by significant infection or irradiation can be appropriately and perhaps optimally reconstructed with vascularized bone grafts included as part of composite free flap coverage (18,47). Nonvascularized autologous bone covered by free muscle flaps, however, have also been successfully used to cover radiated wounds, as have free muscle flaps in combination with alloplastic material (50,51) (see Figures 33-14 and 33-15).

CHOICES OF RECIPIENT VESSELS

For microsurgical scalp reconstruction, the optimal recipient vessels are those that are located in or near the operative field, are of adequate caliber to match the diameters of the flap

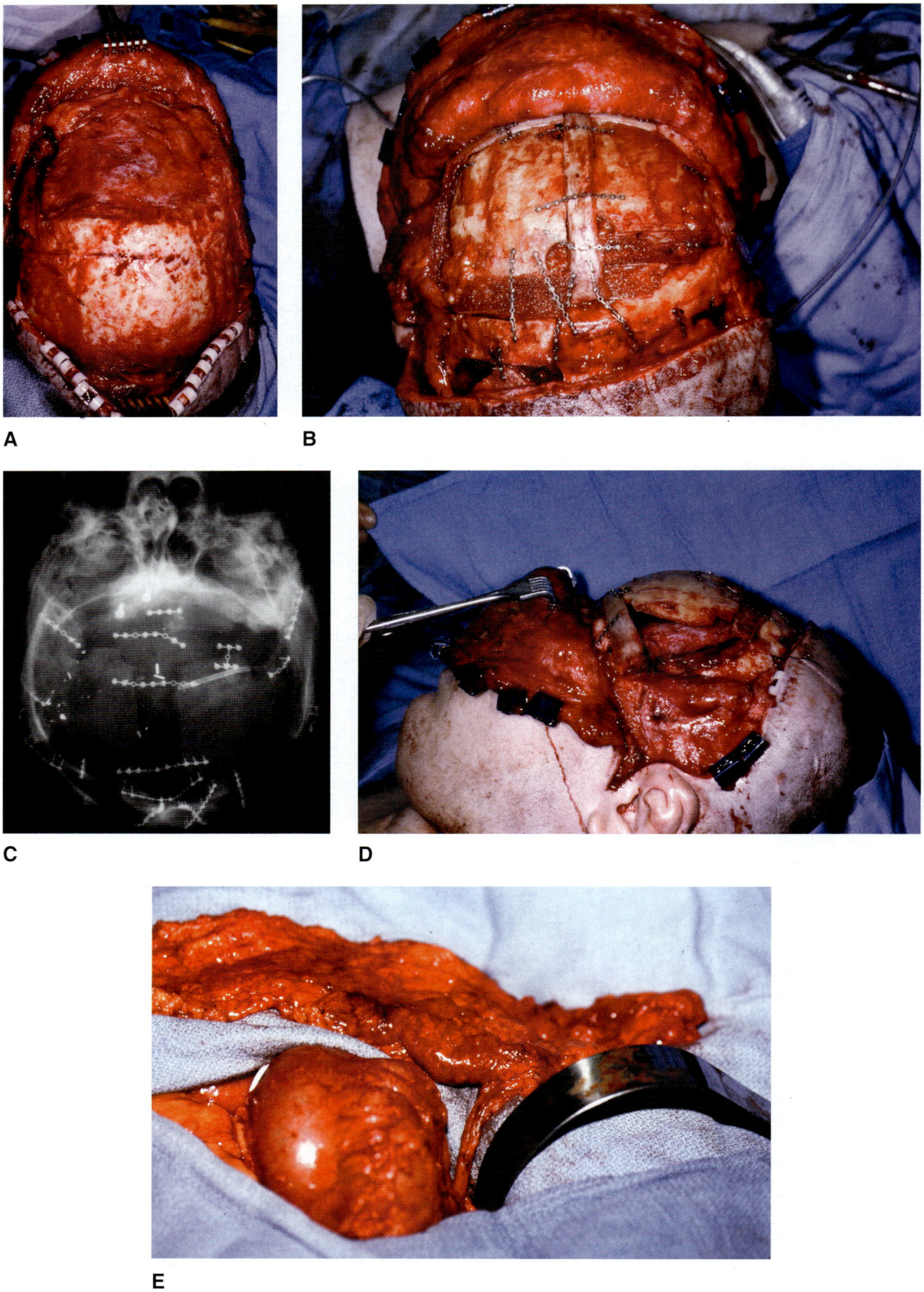

FIGURE 33-11 The frontal skull defect (A) was reconstructed with split rib grafts to reconstruct the fronto-orbital bar and a sagittal strut, with the remainder of the bony defect reconstructed with split calvarial bone grafts, all fixed with miniplates (B and C). This then left a dead space between the reconstructed frontal skull and the dura over the frontal lobes (D), which was filled with a free omental flap based on the right gastroepiploic artery (E) to prevent any intracranial infection or abscess formation.

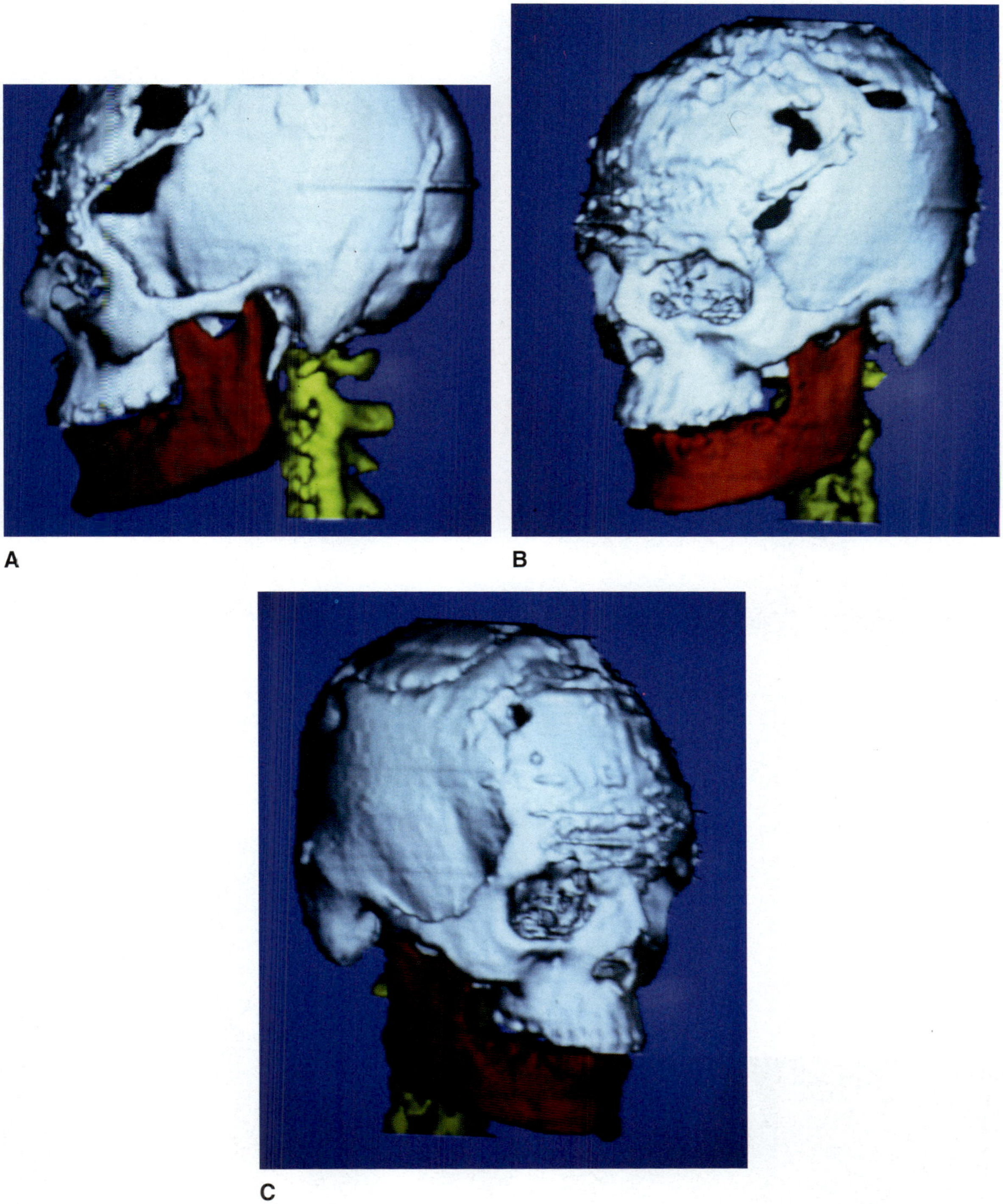

FIGURE 33-12 Left lateral (A), left oblique (B), and right oblique (C) three-dimensional computed tomography reconstructions of the bony reconstruction of the frontal skull.

pedicle vessels, and have not been compromised by the primary disease process or adjuvant therapies, such as radiation. Moreover, because the scalp reconstruction patient population is often an elderly one, vessels that are more resistant to atherosclerosis are preferable.

The primary recipient vessels for most surgeons are the superficial temporal artery and vein. The superficial temporal artery and vein are readily accessible in the preauricular and temporal regions, making them ideal for anterior and lateral defects. The artery has been shown to be minimally atherosclerotic in older patients, and the vein has been described to have a consistently adequate diameter (15). Dissection of the superficial parotid gland to gain more proximal access to either vessel with a larger caliber may be indicated. Occipital vessels have been used for anastomosis of scalp free flaps and are particularly useful for posterior defects, but vessel size and venous caliber in particular may be problematic.

When the paired major vessels of the scalp are not available or inappropriately sized, the external carotid and internal or external jugular systems provide a number of options for

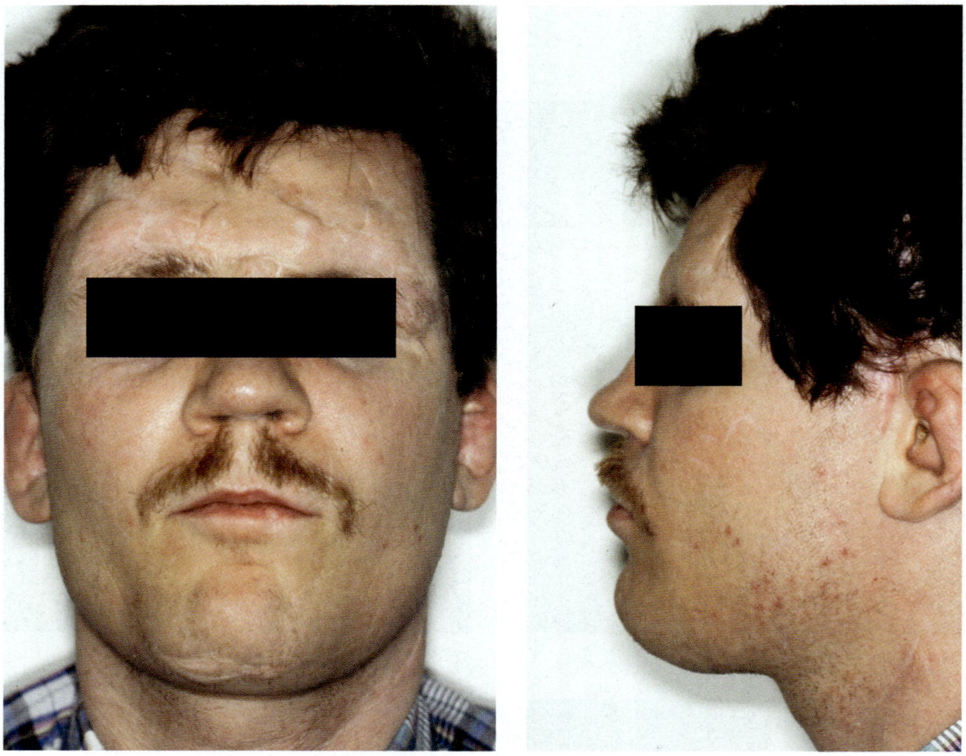

A B

FIGURE 33-13 Frontal (A) and lateral (B) photographs 1 year after surgery of the bony reconstruction of the frontal skull and obliteration of the dead space with a free omental flap. The patient did not develop any cerebrospinal fluid leak, extradural abscess, or intracranial abscess.

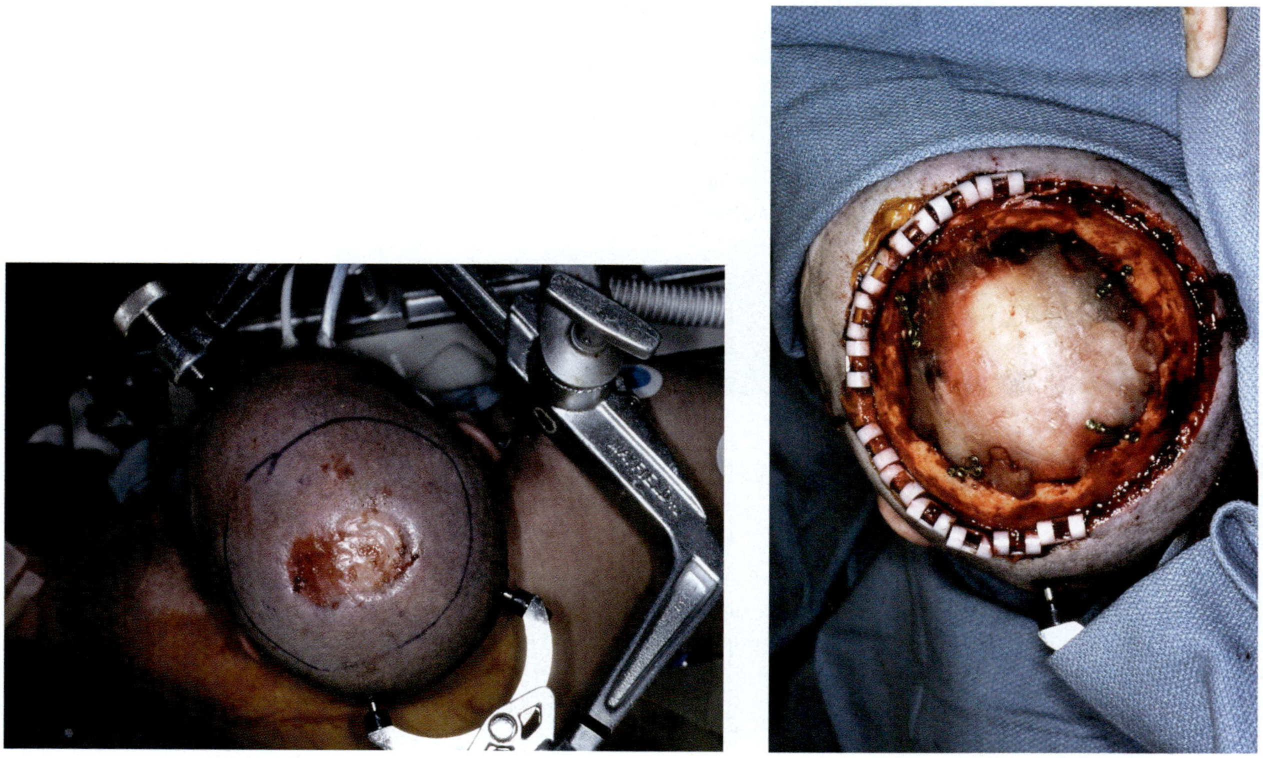

A B

FIGURE 33-14 Recurrent squamous cell carcinoma previously treated by excision and skin grafting and radiation therapy, now requiring radical excision of the vertex of the scalp (A) and immediate reconstruction of the craniectomy defect with methylmethacrylate cranioplasty fixed with miniplates (B).

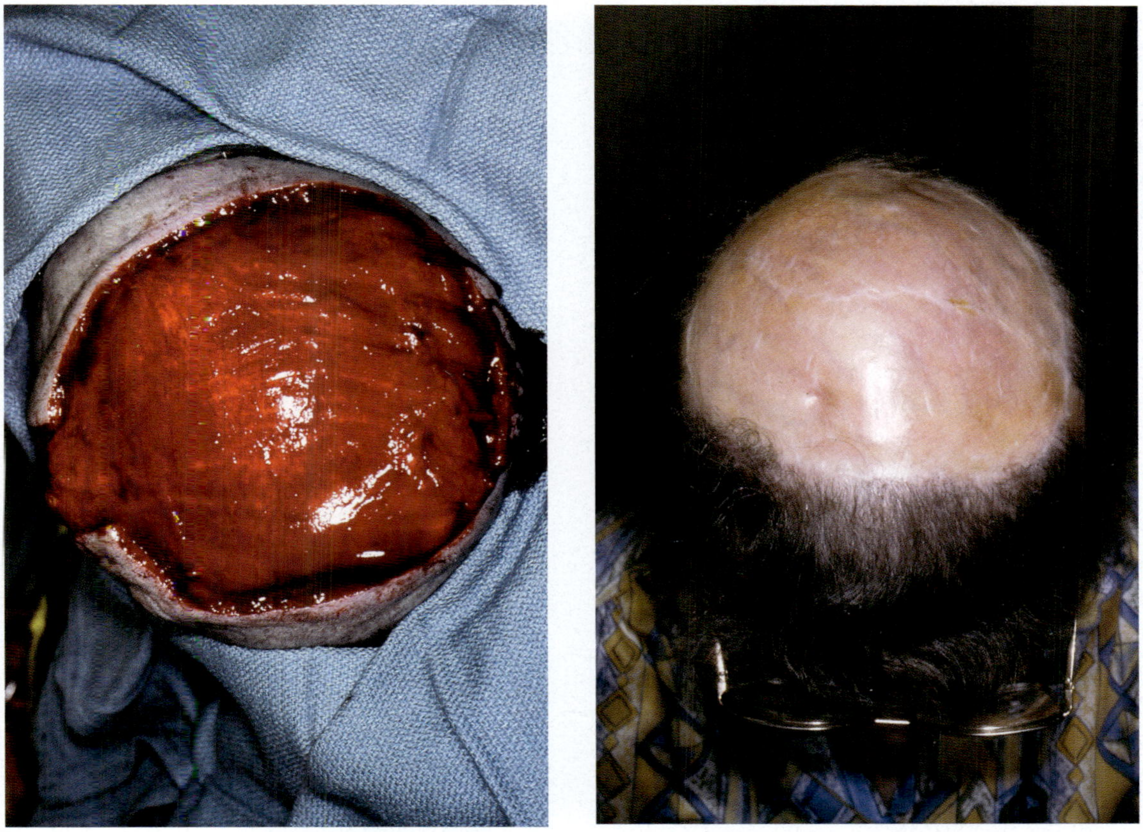

A B

FIGURE 33-15 Despite previous radiation therapy, immediate skull reconstruction with a methylmethacrylate cranioplasty could be performed because of reliable soft tissue coverage with a free latissimus dorsi muscle flap (**A**) and a nonmeshed split-thickness skin graft, preventing infection and providing an acceptable cosmetic appearance 1 year after surgery (**B**).

recipient vessels. Various descriptions have suggested the use of the external carotid artery proper, as well as its facial, lingual, and superior thyroid branches (21). The internal and external jugular veins have been successfully used as recipient vessels, as have branches of these systems (15,21). Although using recipient vessels in the neck does not necessarily mandate the use of interposition vein grafts, it does, however, increase the possibility that vein grafting will be required to reestablish flow to the flap. Moreover, prior irradiation to the neck may preclude the use of distal branches, requiring vein grafting to connect the flap pedicle to more distant better quality recipient vessels. The use of interposition vein grafts has been identified as a significant factor contributing to flap-related perioperative complications and flap loss (21). Flap options based on pedicle length and recipient vessels should be carefully considered during the planning process.

Alternatively, an arteriovenous (AV) loop can be constructed either before or at the time of resection by anastomosing a long vein graft between a branch of the external carotid system and the internal or external jugular veins

FLAP INSET AND SCULPTING

When insetting the flap, primary consideration must be given to the three-dimensional architecture of the defect, the optimal flap orientation needed to address this architecture, and the relationship of the flap pedicle to the recipient vessels when the flap is placed in this orientation. Numerous general principles and specific techniques that apply to the various flaps have been described that facilitate obtaining the best fit with the lowest chance of vascular compromise.

Flap Bulk

When muscle flaps are used, a larger flap than is seemingly necessary should be elevated and transferred to allow for the greater surface area needed to drape the flap over the convexity of the skull, and to provide for tension-free closure of soft tissues over the pedicle. Excess tissue will also permit mobility of the flap if secondary advancement is required and provides greater protection in the setting of adjuvant radiotherapy. If after these considerations are made, the flap is still thought to be too large, primary debulking of the muscle can be performed at the time of harvest and inset (11). Great care must be taken to preserve the integrity of the vascular pedicle. The latissimus can be tangentially excised at its thickest point near its tendon and proximal to the entry of the thoracodorsal pedicle. Denervated muscle flaps are expected to undergo atrophy with the passage of time and residual bulk can be refined secondarily after the muscle has atrophied.

Muscle flaps are commonly used without their associated cutaneous paddles. Split-thickness skin grafting of a latissimus dorsi or rectus abdominis muscle flap results in an acceptable contour and color match relative to the surrounding scalp (11). The best results are obtained with unmeshed sheet grafts that are quilted to the underlying flap (52) (see Figure 33-8). Myocutaneous flaps typically have a suboptimal aesthetic result due to color and contour irregularities. They may be beneficial, however, if extra bulk is needed to fill a voluminous defect or if a skin paddle is needed for flap monitoring. The cutaneous monitoring portion of the flap can be removed later and replaced with a skin graft after the need for monitoring is complete.

Depending on the specific donor site, fasciocutaneous flaps may be excessively bulky, requiring aggressive primary or secondary thinning. The amount of debulking necessary is largely determined by the site of reconstruction: whereas thin fasciocutaneous flaps such as the radial forearm flap are most appropriate for forehead and temporal defects, composite defects of the vertex or occiput can accommodate a thick ALT flap (9). Thin and pliable flaps can be folded to accurately adapt to the anatomy of the defect (30).

Pedicle Issues

Intramuscular dissection of the thoracodorsal vessels in a latissimus flap can lengthen the pedicle length but should be undertaken with extreme care. Use of the superficial temporal vessels effectively lengthens the pedicle of any flap used for scalp reconstruction by minimizing the distance from donor to recipient vessels, but dissection of the parotid gland may be necessary to achieve this goal (15). If the flap pedicle is passed through a subcutaneous tunnel to reach the recipient vessels, the galea should be widely undermined and scored to prevent compression. Alternatively, the intervening scalp between the pedicle and recipient site can be incised or excised.

For each specific flap, the pedicle can be dissected more proximally to produce a longer vascular pedicle. For latissimus flaps raised with or without scapular or parascapular components, dissecting the pedicle back to the origin of the subscapular artery from the axillary artery significantly increases the length and may decrease the need for vein grafting. Similarly, the radial artery can be dissected all the way back to its origin from the brachial artery (21).

Flap Orientation

Composite flaps, such as those derived from the subscapular system, should be designed and inset based on specific templates of the defect. Initial design of the flap should optimize the arc of rotation that each of its individual components has relative to the others. The individual components of the flap should be manipulated to address the specific areas they are intended to cover. Dural reconstruction should be water tight and reinforced with fibrin tissue glue. The bony component of the flap should be rigidly fixed to the surrounding calvarium with titanium plates and screws; the edges of the bone flap should be apposed to the native skull without gaps to allow for osteosynthesis. This principle of fixation applies to nonvascularized bone grafts and alloplastic materials as well. The soft tissue component should be inset without tension along its suture line and to cover the pedicle. "Vest-over-pants" closure has been described for muscle flaps to prevent wound dehiscence and calvarial exposure and to produce an optimal contour around the margin of the inset.

Patient Positioning and Dressings

Head dressings that provide uniform gentle compression can be used to support the flap and serve as bolsters for skin grafts. Postoperatively, the patient should lie with the head of the bed elevated between 45 to 90 degrees with rolls or pillows placed on either side of the head to prevent neck rotation. If these maneuvers are not adequate to prevent compression of the flap whether the patient is awake or asleep, a halo should be placed to immobilize the head and keep the flap protected from compression (53).

OUTCOMES

Success rates in microsurgical reconstruction of the scalp are excellent. As with all technically challenging surgical procedures, greater experience should predict a lower rate of overall surgical complications (54). In the modern microsurgical era, the challenge to the surgeon is not to simply execute the reconstructive procedure but to design the most appropriate flaps for the most complex defects and to achieve results that are both functionally and aesthetically optimal.

Surgical Complications

Recent series of microsurgical reconstructions of the scalp consistently show high flap survival rates (20). This collective experience includes the full spectrum of flap options, defect complexity, donor and recipient vessel choices, stages of malignant disease, and adjuvant therapies. Major and minor complications rates in these series, however, have been significant, ranging up to 59% in one report (9). The differentiation between what qualifies as a major versus a minor complication varies among authors, but documented morbidities include partial flap necrosis, wound infection or breakdown, hematoma, seroma, secondary calvarial exposure requiring additional free flap or local flap coverage, tumor recurrence requiring additional reconstructive procedures, poor skin graft "take" requiring revision, and calvarial bone graft or alloplast infection (2,9,11,18,25,30,43,47,52). Radiation therapy, previous scalp surgery, chemotherapy, and CSF leak may contribute to an increased risk in postoperative complications. As discussed earlier, the use of vein grafts is associated with a higher flap complication rate (21).

Donor Site Complications

Seroma and wound dehiscence are the most commonly observed donor site complications seen after harvest of latissimus dorsi musculocutaneous and scapular flaps. Hematoma and skin graft breakdown are also complications associated with the latissimus dorsi muscle flap (2). Dehiscence and skin graft loss are potential complications of ALT donor sites.

Medical Complications

Despite evidence that microsurgical reconstruction in older patient populations can be performed safely (55), elderly patients who present with advanced malignancies of the scalp are at particular risk for perioperative morbidity because of their often poor medical status and debilitated state. Perioperative mortality is a significant concern in this patient population (4). Moreover, advanced disease puts these patients at risk for mortality from recurrent disease, and their poor general medical condition accounts for significant morbidity and mortality (2,4,12,13,43).

Esthetic Results

Although functional restoration remains the primary goal of microsurgical scalp reconstruction, the desire for an aesthetic result should also influence surgical planning. Attempts should be made to tailor the flap choice to match the color and contour of the native surrounding scalp. With attention to detail in flap selection, design, and surgical technique, aesthetic outcomes can be good or excellent in almost all cases (30). Overall aesthetic results have been rated better for scalp versus forehead reconstruction, with a suggestion that muscle flaps covered with nonmeshed split-thickness skin grafts have a more acceptable appearance than fasciocutaneous flaps (21,52) (see Figure 33-8).

SUMMARY

Microsurgical reconstruction of the scalp is a safe and effective technique to address the broad spectrum of oncologic, traumatic, and congenital defects. Flap choice should be determined by the surface area and complexity of the defect. Total scalp defects would benefit from a combined latissimus and serratus muscle flap; large surface area defects may be covered by a latissimus muscle flap or an ALT flap; and moderate-sized defects of the frontal scalp or forehead are best reconstructed with a radial forearm or scapular flap. A full-thickness scalp and skull defect can be covered in a single stage with an appropriately designed composite flap. Cranioplasty using autologous bone or alloplastic substrate can be performed at the time of soft tissue coverage if wound conditions are suitable. Excellent aesthetic outcomes can be achieved with careful planning and refined surgical techniques. In many cases, microsurgical reconstruction of the scalp can be considered as the primary reconstructive option for patients with locally advanced disease.

REFERENCES

1. Kim JT, Kim YH, Yang EZ, Kim JB. Total scalp replantation—salvage following prolonged ischaemia with poor prognostic factors. *J Plast Reconstr Aesthet Surg* 2010;63(11):1917–1920.
2. Labow BI, Rosen H, Pap SA, Upton J. Microsurgical reconstruction: a more conservative method of managing large scalp defects? *J Reconstr Microsurg* 2009;25(8):465–474.
3. Lee S, Rafii AA, Sykes J. Advances in scalp reconstruction. *Curr Opin Otolaryngol Head Neck Surg* 2006;14(4):249–253.
4. Beasley NJ, Gilbert RW, Gullane PJ, et al. Scalp and forehead reconstruction using free revascularized tissue transfer. *Arch Facial Plast Surg* 2004;6(1):16–20.
5. Jensen F, Petersen NC. Repair of denuded cranial bone by bone splitting and free-skin grafting. *J Neurosurg* 1976;44:718.
6. Raposio E, Santi P, Nordstrom REA. Effects of galeostomies on scalp flaps. *Ann Plast Surg* 1998;41:17.
7. Orticochea M. Four-flap scalp reconstruction technique. *Br J Plast Surg* 1967;20:159.
8. Boyd JB. Tissue expansion in reconstruction. *South Med J* 1987;80(4): 430–432.
9. Hussussian CJ, Reece GP. Microsurgical scalp reconstruction in the patient with cancer. *Plast Reconstr Surg* 2002;109(6):1828–1834.
10. Singer JB, Gulin SP, Needham CW. Microvascular free-flap reconstruction of a large defect of the scalp. Experience in a community hospital. *Conn Med* 1990;54(2):56–58.
11. Jones NF, Hardesty RA, Swartz WM, et al. Extensive and complex defects of the scalp, middle third of the face, and palate: the role of microsurgical reconstruction. *Plast Reconstr Surg* 1988;82(6):937–952.
12. Lutz BS, Wei FC, Chen HC, et al. Reconstruction of scalp defects with free flaps in 30 cases. *Br J Plast Surg* 1998;51(3):186–190.
13. Alpert BS, Buncke HJ Jr, Mathes SJ. Surgical treatment of the totally avulsed scalp. *Clin Plast Surg* 1982;9(2):145–159.
14. Buncke HJ, Hoffman WY, Alpert BS, et al. Microvascular transplant of two free scalp flaps between identical twins. *Plast Reconstr Surg* 1982;70(5):605–609
15. Hansen SL, Foster RD, Dosanjh AS, et al. Superficial temporal artery and vein as recipient vessels for facial and scalp microsurgical reconstruction. *Plast Reconstr Surg* 2007;120(7):1879–1884.
16. Elliott LF, Raffel B, Wade J. Segmental latissimus dorsi free flap: clinical applications. *Ann Plast Surg* 1989;23:231.
17. Aviv JE, Urken ML, Vickery C, et al. The combined latissimus dorsi-scapular free flap in head and neck reconstruction. *Arch Otolaryngol Head Neck Surg* 1991;117(11):1242–1250.
18. Seitz IA, Adler N, Odessey E, et al. Latissimus dorsi/rib intercostal perforator myo-osseocutaneous free flap reconstruction in composite defects of the scalp: case series and review of literature. *J Reconstr Microsurg* 2009;25(9):559–567.
19. Lee JW, Hsueh YY, Lee JS. Composite skull and dura defect reconstruction using combined latissimus dorsi musculocutaneous and serratus anterior muscle-rib free flap coupled with vascularized galea transfer: a case report. *Microsurgery* 2010;30(8):632–635.
20. Wax MK, Burkey BB, Bascom D, Rosenthal EL. The role of free tissue transfer in the reconstruction of massive neglected skin cancers of the head and neck. *Arch Facial Plast Surg* 2003;5(6):479–482.
21. Jones NF, Johnson JT, Shestak KC, et al. Microsurgical reconstruction of the head and neck: interdisciplinary collaboration between head and neck surgeons and plastic surgeons in 305 cases. *Ann Plast Surg* 1996;36(1): 37–43.
22. Wei FC, Jain V, Celik N, et al. Have we found an ideal soft tissue flap? An experience with 672 anterolateral thigh flap. *Plast Reconstr Surg* 2002;109:2219–2226.
23. Heller F, Hsu CM, Chuang CC, et al. Anterolateral thigh fasciocutaneous flap for simultaneous reconstruction of refractory scalp and dural defects. Report of two cases. *J Neurosurg* 2004;100:1094–1097.
24. Mosahebi A, Disa JJ, Pusic AL, et al. The use of the extended anterolateral thigh flap for reconstruction of massive oncologic defects. *Plast Reconstr Surg* 2008;122(2):492–496.
25. Lutz BS. Aesthetic and functional advantages of the anterolateral thigh flap in reconstruction of tumor-related scalp defects. *Microsurgery* 2002;22(6):258–264.
26. Choi SW, Park JY, Hur MS, et al. An anatomic assessment on perforators of the lateral circumflex femoral artery for anterolateral thigh flap. *J Craniofac Surg* 2007;18(4):866–871.
27. Kobienia BJ, Migliori M, Schubert W. Preexpanded radial forearm free flap to the scalp. *Ann Plast Surg* 1996;37(6):629–632.
28. Masser MR. The preexpanded radial free flap. *Plast Reconstr Surg* 1990;86(2):295–301.
29. Lutz BS, Wei FC, Chang SC, et al. Donor site morbidity after suprafascial elevation of the radial forearm flap: a prospective study in 95 consecutive cases. *Plast Reconstr Surg* 1999;103(1):132–137.
30. Mateev MA, Beermanov KA, Subanova LK, et al. Shape-modified method using the radial forearm perforator flap for reconstruction of soft-tissue defects of the scalp. *J Reconstr Microsurg* 2005;21(1):21–24.
31. Germann G, Bickert B, Steinau HU, et al. Versatility and reliability of combined flaps of the subscapular system. *Plast Reconstr Surg* 1999;103(5):1386–1399.
32. Valentini V, Gennaro P, Torroni A, et al. Scapula free flap for complex maxillofacial reconstruction. *J Craniofac Surg* 2009;20(4):1125–1131.
33. Moukarbel RV, White JB, Fung K, et al. The scapular free flap: when versatility is needed in head and neck reconstruction. *J Otolaryngol Head Neck Surg* 2010;39(5):572–578.

34. Wehage IC, Fansa H. Complex reconstructions in head and neck cancer surgery: decision making. *Head Neck Oncol* 20118;3(1):14.
35. Dabernig J, Ong KO, McGowan R, et al. The anatomic and radiologic basis of the circumflex scapular artery perforator flap. *Ann Plast Surg* 2010;64(6):784–788.
36. Roll C, Prantl L, Feser D, et al. Functional donor-site morbidity following (osteo-) fasciocutaneous parascapular flap transfer. *Ann Plast Surg* 2007;59:410–414.
37. Robb GL. Free scapular flap reconstruction of the head and neck. *Clin Plast Surg* 1994;21(1):45–58.
38. Kucera Marcum K, Browne JD. Parascapular free flaps in skin malignancies. *Laryngoscope* 2011;121(3):533–540.
39. McLean DH, Buncke HJ Jr. Autotransplant of omentum to a large scalp defect, with microsurgical revascularization. *Plast Reconstr Surg* 1972;49(3):268–274.
40. Hultman CS, Carlson GW, Losken A, et al. Utility of the omentum in the reconstruction of complex extraperitoneal wounds and defects: donor-site complications in 135 patients from 1975 to 2000. *Ann Surg* 2002;235(6):782–795.
41. Kamei Y, Torii S, Hasegawa T, et al. Endoscopic omental harvest. *Plast Reconstr Surg* 1998;102:2450–2453.
42. Kurpinski K, Patel S. Dura mater regeneration with a novel synthetic, bilayered nanofibrous dural substitute: an experimental study. *Nanomedicine (Lond)* 2011;6(2):325–337.
43. McCombe D, Donato R, Hofer SO, Morrison W. Free flaps in the treatment of locally advanced malignancy of the scalp and forehead. *Ann Plast Surg* 2002;48(6):600–606.
44. Granthan E, Landis H. Cranioplasty and the post- traumatic syndrome. *J Neurosurg* 1947;5:19–22.
45. Isago T, Nozaki M, Kikuchi Y, et al. Sinking skin flap syndrome: a case of improved cerebral blood flow after cranioplasty. *Ann Plast Surg* 2004;53(3):288–292.
46. Tessier P, Kawamoto H, Matthews D, et al. Taking long rib grafts for facial reconstruction—tools and techniques: III. A 2900-case experience in maxillofacial and craniofacial surgery. *Plast Reconstr Surg* 2005;116 (5 suppl):38S–46S.
47. Baumeister S, Peek A, Friedman A, et al. Management of postneurosurgical bone flap loss caused by infection. *Plast Reconstr Surg* 2008;122(6): 195e–208e.
48. Dean D, Min KJ, Bond A. Computer aided design of large-format prefabricated cranial plates. *J Craniofac Surg* 2003;14(6):819–832.
49. Thesleff T, Lehtimäki K, Niskakangas T, et al. Cranioplasty with adipose-derived stem cells and biomaterial. A novel method for cranial reconstruction. *Neurosurgery* 2011;68(6):1535–1540.
50. Stueber K, Salcman M, Spence RJ. The combined use of the latissimus dorsi musculocutaneous free flap and split-rib grafts for cranial vault reconstruction. *Ann Plast Surg* 1985;15(2):155–160.
51. Ueda K, Oba S, Omiya Y, Okada M. Cranial-bone defects with depression deformity treated with ceramic implants and free-flap transfers. *Br J Plast Surg* 2001;54(5):403–408.
52. Chang J, Jones N. Muscle free flaps with full-thickness skin grafting: improved contour over traditional musculocutaneous free flaps. *Microsurgery* 2001;21(2):70–73.
53. Wooden WA, Curtsinger LJ, Jones NF. The four-poster halo vest for protection of a microvascular free-tissue transfer to the scalp. *Plast Recontr Surg* 1995;95:166–167.
54. Disa JJ, Pusic AL, Hidalgo DH, et al. Simplifying microvascular head and neck reconstruction: a rational approach to donor site selection. *Ann Plast Surg* 2001;47:385–389.
55. Shestak KC, Jones NF, Wu W, et al. Effect of advanced age and medical disease on the outcome of microvascular reconstruction for head and neck defects. *Head Neck* 1992;14(1):14–18.

CHAPTER 34

Skull Base Reconstruction

Eldon Mah, Christine B. Novak, Toni Zhong, and Stefan O.P. Hofer

Extirpation of tumors located in the skull base may result in significant functional and aesthetic consequences to the patient and complex three-dimensional defects that can present a surgical reconstructive challenge. The risk of potential life-threatening complications as a result of failed reconstruction adds to the complexity. The management of patients with skull base tumors has improved with the use of multidisciplinary surgical and medical teams and improved surgical techniques, diagnostic radiology, and ancillary services.

In the past, management of patients with skull base tumors was limited by the lack of reliable reconstructive options. The advent of free tissue transfer has positively changed the outcome of surgical reconstruction, particularly for complex skull base defects. The ability to transfer a large amount of healthy well-vascularized tissue to match any defect has significant advantages over pedicled or local flaps in skull base reconstruction (1–6). Successful reconstruction requires an understanding of the anatomical defect, realistic reconstructive goals, appropriate selection of the reconstructive method, and a multidisciplinary team approach (7).

BRIEF HISTORY OF SKULL BASE RECONSTRUCTION

Because of limited surgical options in the early 20th century, skin grafts were often used for reconstruction of skull base defects (8–10). Placement of the skin graft directly onto the dura or the cranium often resulted in failure of this repair. The temporalis muscle flap was described for reconstruction in the orbital region by Golovine (11) and then Gillies (12). Thomson described the use of the ipsilateral forehead flap for this type of orbital reconstruction (13). The temporalis and pericranial flaps were used for small defects in the skull base (14–16). Before the advent of free tissue transfers, large, complex defects were limited by the availability of large pedicled flaps in the skull base region. Flaps such as the pectoralis major, the latissimus dorsi, the sternocleidomastoid, and the trapezius were used for larger defects; however, their reach was limited and most of their bulk consumed in their transposition.

The introduction of free tissue transfer has improved outcomes for patients with head and neck cancer and particularly with surgical management of skull base tumors (3). Outcomes after free tissue transfer for reconstruction of skull base defects have improved with a reduction in morbidity and perioperative complications despite having to manage increasing numbers of large and complex skull base tumors (7,14,17). Free tissue transfer provides the unique ability to bring in well-vascularized tissue for the reconstruction of large complex skull base defects. Because the free flap is not attached to a pedicle, a free tissue transfer can be precisely tailored to the defect and varying flap designs constructed.

ANATOMY AND CLASSIFICATION OF SKULL BASE DEFECTS

A thorough understanding of the anatomic region and defect and the relationship to surrounding structures is essential for successful skull base reconstruction. The skull base is formed by the anterior, middle, and posterior cranial fossae intracranially. The orbital roof, sphenoid sinus, nasopharynx, and infratemporal fossa form the extracranial components. The anterior fossa of the skull base is formed by the bony structures of the ethmoid (anterior and cribriform plate), the sphenoid (lesser wings), and the jugum sphenoidale. The middle fossa is bordered by the sphenoid (body and greater wing), temporal pyramid (anterior surface), and components of the temporal squama. The posterior fossa is formed by the clivus, occipital bone, and the pyramid of the temporal bone.

Classification

Several classification systems have been described to categorize skull base tumors and to assist with the selection of clinical treatment and reconstructive needs (18–20). Jones et al. in their description classified the skull base into the anterior, middle, and posterior cranial fossae (20). Jackson and Hide divided the skull base into anterior, posterior-anterior, posterior-central, and posterior-posterior based on surgical reconstruction requirements (19). A three-region classification system was introduced by Irish et al. in a review of the treatment of 77 patients with skull base tumors (18). The skull base was divided into three regions according to tumor anatomic position, tumor growth patterns, and surgical approach. Region I tumors include those that arise from the sinuses, orbit, maxilla, maxillary antrum, midfacial skin, and other local anterior structures and extend to the anterior cranial fossa. Tumors commonly originating in this region include adenocarcinoma, squamous cell carcinoma, adenocystic carcinoma, and basal cell carcinoma. Region I also includes tumors that arise from or extend down the clivus to the foramen magnum because these tumors are approached anteriorly and behave like anterior skull base tumors. As reported by Irish et al. and Chang et al., the majority of skull base tumors arise in this region (18,21). Region II tumors arise laterally and primarily involve the infratemporal and pterygopalatine fossa with extension into the middle cranial fossa. The boundaries of the middle cranial fossa extend from the posterior aspect of the orbit to the posterior aspect of petrous temporal bone. Vital anatomical structures pass through this region, including the internal carotid artery, maxillary nerve branches, mandibular nerve branches, and facial nerve. Common tumors found in region II include basal cell carcinoma, as well as middle ear and invasive parotid tumors. Region II tumors have the highest incidence of dural involvement (43%) compared with regions I and III.

Region III tumors arise from within or around the temporal bone, including the ear and parotid, with intracranial extension to involve the posterior cranial fossa or middle cranial fossa. Structures encountered in the resection of these tumors include the glossopharyngeal nerve, the vagus nerve, and the internal jugular vein. Tumors in region III are most frequently squamous cell carcinoma and glomus tumors.

SURGICAL RECONSTRUCTION

The principles for head and neck reconstruction are to provide optimal function and cosmesis while providing soft tissue coverage and structural support. The additional considerations for reconstruction in the skull base are to reestablish orbital and oral cavities and to restore facial symmetry and appearance. Because of the location of the skull base and the proximity to vital structures, the reconstruction focuses on the prevention of life-threatening central nervous system (CNS) complications. The selection of surgical reconstruction must include strategies to minimize perioperative complications, maintain a watertight dural repair, separate the CNS from the naso-oropharynx, and obliterate dead spaces (Table 34-1).

TABLE 34-1 Goals of Skull Base Reconstruction

1. Water tight dural repair
2. Separation of central nervous system from nasopharynx
3. Obliteration of dead space
4. Reestablish orbital and oral cavities
5. Restore facial symmetry and appearance

Surgical Approaches

The surgical approach selected for excision of skull base tumors depends on tumor pathology, defect size, and location. Clear preoperative planning, which includes a multidisciplinary team of surgeons, radiologists, anesthesiologists, oncologists, and other health care professionals, is necessary. In general terms, region I tumors (anterior skull base) typically require an anterior approach with lateral rhinotomy or maxillotomy combined with a coronal incision and frontal craniotomy. A partial or total maxillectomy, frontal sinus resection, and orbital exenteration may also be required. For region II, the tumor is exposed laterally through an infratemporal or transtemporal approach, which requires a hemicoronal incision with either a preauricular or retroauricular extension. Mandibulectomy or mandibulotomy (lateral or anterior) may be required to increase exposure in an infratemporal approach. Region III tumors require a transtemporal approach with a total or partial lateral temporal resection.

Reconstructive Surgery

Because of the various locations and complexities of the defects after tumor ablation, there is no single reconstruction option acceptable for all skull base defects. Successful reconstruction requires the selection of the most reliable option in consideration of the defect (size, location, breach of dura) and patient factors (comorbidities, age, tumor pathology, previous radiotherapy, available donor sites). Because postoperative complications can be devastating both in terms of morbidity and mortality, the selection of reconstruction should also be in consideration of the option with the least likelihood of perioperative complications. Microsurgical free tissue transfer has dramatically changed and improved the scope of reconstructive practice in skull base surgery.

Skull base tumors in different regions have slightly different reconstructive requirements and available options. Region I defects usually involve an anterior base of skull bony defect, a dural defect, a varying sized dead space from maxillectomy with or without orbital exenteration, a loss of nasal mucosa, and a loss of external skin. Reconstruction requires a reliable dural repair and a flap that can fill the dead space while providing adequate mucosa and skin coverage. Bony defects of the skull base usually do not require bony reconstruction and in most cases can be adequately supported with soft tissue. Region II and III skull base resections can also result in bony and dural defects. Skin loss tends to be more extensive, but the degree of soft tissue or dead space tends to be less. The facial nerve may also be sacrificed with tumor resection, and reconstruction may be necessary.

Flap Reconstruction Options

Flap selection is made with consideration of the complexity of the defect and patient factors. For smaller defects, reconstruction using local flaps such as the pericranial flap or temporalis muscle flap may be satisfactory. However, for large complex defects, our preference is to use a free tissue transfer in the appropriately selected patient. By introducing reliable, well-vascularized tissue, which can be tailored to any defect size and position, a free tissue transfer provides is an excellent reconstructive option for large or complex defects. Our preference for the most commonly used local flaps (temporalis muscle flap, pericranial flap) and free flaps (rectus abdominis, anterolateral thigh [ALT], radial forearm, latissimus dorsi) in skull base reconstruction are reviewed.

Local Flaps

Temporalis Muscle Flap

Historically, the temporalis muscle flap was used to provide either an additional support to dural repairs with a pericranial flap or to provide a small amount of vascularized tissue for the repair. The temporalis muscle flap is based on the deep temporal arteries and retains a limited role in reconstruction of the skull base. If the skull base defect is located in the lateral region of the anterior cranial fossa, the temporalis muscle can be used. However, it is difficult to reliably transpose this flap medially because of compromised vascularity which may result in flap necrosis or wound dehiscence. The flap has a small arc of rotation, thin muscle bulk, and considerable donor site morbidity, and as such, the application is restricted in the skull base. If the vascularity to this flap is preserved after tumor resection, the temporalis muscle flap may be useful for small defects in the anterolateral skull base region.

Pericranial Flap

The pericranial flap can provide good soft tissue coverage in patients with a relatively small defect that is located in the midline of the skull base. This flap is based anteriorly on the supratrochlear and supraorbital vessels. The pericranium can be harvested with or without the galea, and the flap may be draped over the bony defect and secured with sutures. This thin flap can be used for small defects in the central skull base to obliterate the nasofrontal duct, wrapped around a bone graft, or used to reinforce dural repairs (15,16,22).

Pedicled Flaps

Pectoralis Major Musculocutaneous Flap

The pectoralis major musculocutaneous flap was described in 1979 by Ariyan and has been widely used in head and neck reconstruction before the advent of microsurgical free tissue transfer (23,24). It is based on the pectoral branch of thoracoacromial artery, and it can reach to level of the zygomatic arch. Therefore, this flap is rarely used in skull base reconstruction, and in most cases, it has been replaced with a free tissue transfer. It is often difficult to mobilize the flap sufficiently to fully obliterate the dead space in anterior skull base defects and provide adequate support to the brain and dura. The distal part of the flap is also the least reliable part with respect to vascularity, yet it is the distal aspect that is often the most critical for a successful reconstruction. In some cases of lateral skull base tumors (regions II and III), this flap may reach the defect and provide sufficient bulk for the reconstruction. However, a pedicled pectoralis major flap would be considered only in patients who are not candidates for a free tissue transfer or as a secondary reconstructive procedure.

Free Tissue Transfers

Rectus Abdominis Flap

For region I defects, the rectus abdominis flap is the workhorse flap in skull base reconstruction. It has reliable anatomy, a long pedicle length, and an adequate pedicle size. This flap may be harvested either as a musculocutaneous unit or using only the muscle. It offers a large amount of well-vascularized tissue bulk to obliterate the dead space and to provide structural support. The abdominal skin can be used to provide coverage for skin, nasomucosal, or palatal defects. If the orientation of the defect is appropriate, separate skin islands with deepithelialized bridges can be designed to provide simultaneous reconstruction of more than two epithelial linings, such as for the mucosal surface and external skin. Because a two-team approach can be used, operative time is decreased, and patient repositioning is not needed for flap harvest. The major limitation of the rectus abdominis flap is that, depending on the patient's habitus, it can sometimes be too bulky for the defect. In such cases, it is best to trim the most distal part of the flap because it is also the least reliable in terms of vascularity. In patients who are morbidly obese, the rectus flap with skin paddle may not be the best choice because of the flap characteristics and donor site morbidity. In these cases, alternative free flaps should be considered.

Anterolateral Thigh Flap

First described by Song and colleagues, the ALT flap is a fasciocutaneous flap based on the descending branch of lateral circumflex femoral artery perforators (25). It has become the flap of choice for many soft tissue defects because it offers a large amount of fasciocutaneous tissue, a moderately long pedicle, and minimal donor site morbidity (26–31).

In the skull base, the ALT flap is more commonly used for defects in regions II and III. These defects often require a large amount of skin coverage and a relatively small amount of bulk, making the ALT flap a good selection (Figure 34-1). The skin paddle of the flap can be harvested much larger than the surface area of the actual defect, and then it can then be partially deepithelialized and folded for added bulk. Increased volume can also be added by taking part or all of the vastus lateralis muscle (Figure 34-2). The deep fascia in the ALT flap is much thicker than that of the radial forearm flap and can be used as an additional vascularized fascial layer to further strengthen the dural seal. The deep fascia of the flap may also be used to suspend it onto the bone or deep fascia of the scalp to minimize drooping. Strips of the tensor fascia lata may also be taken and used as a static sling in cases when the facial nerve was sacrificed. The flap can also be thinned peripherally

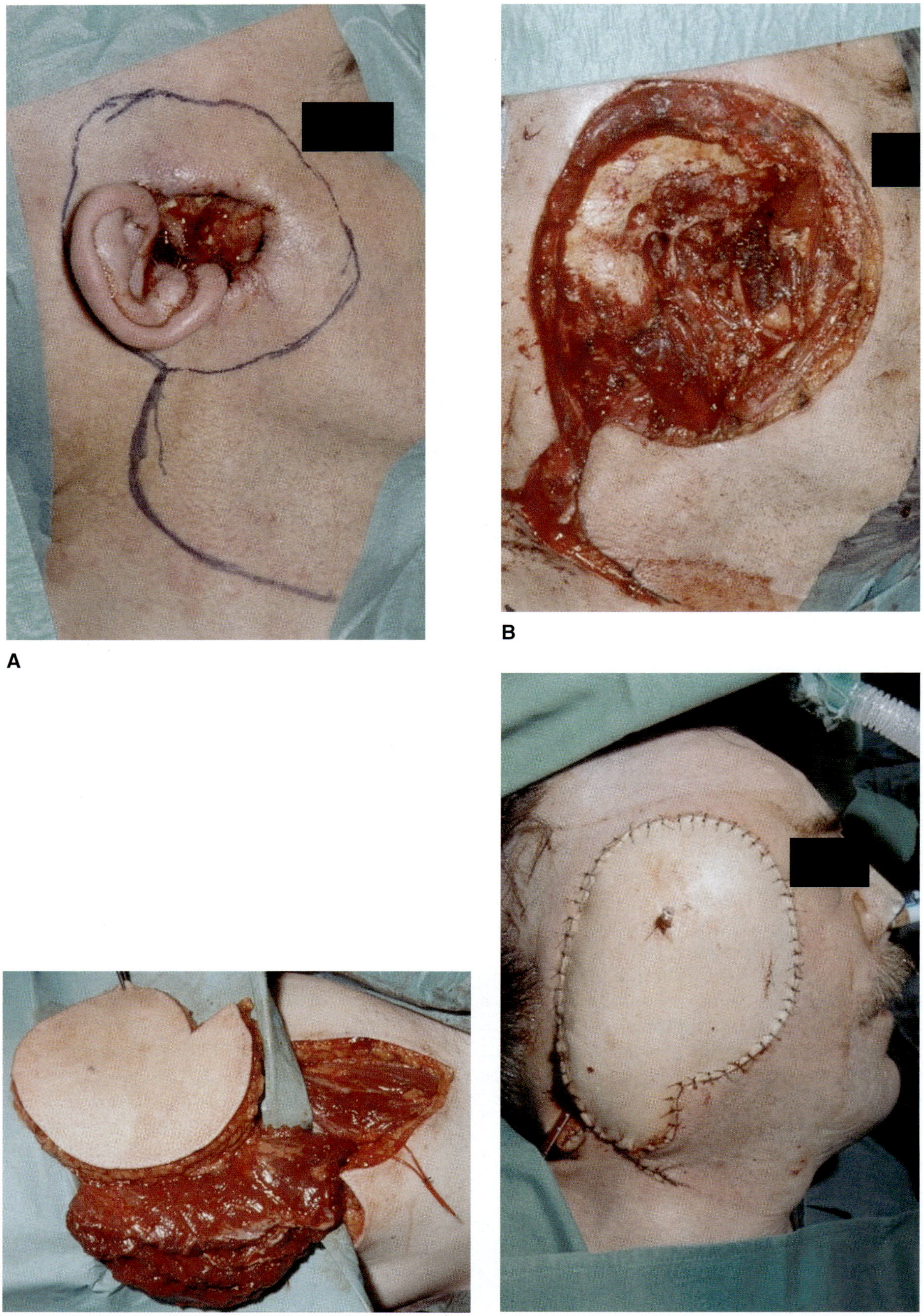

A

B

C

D

FIGURE 34-1 (A) This 47-year-old man had a diagnosis of a basal cell carcinoma. (B) After tumor extirpation with clear margins, the defect is shown. (C) An anterolateral thigh free flap was used for the reconstruction, which provided ample soft tissue for this complex defect. (D) The inset free flap.

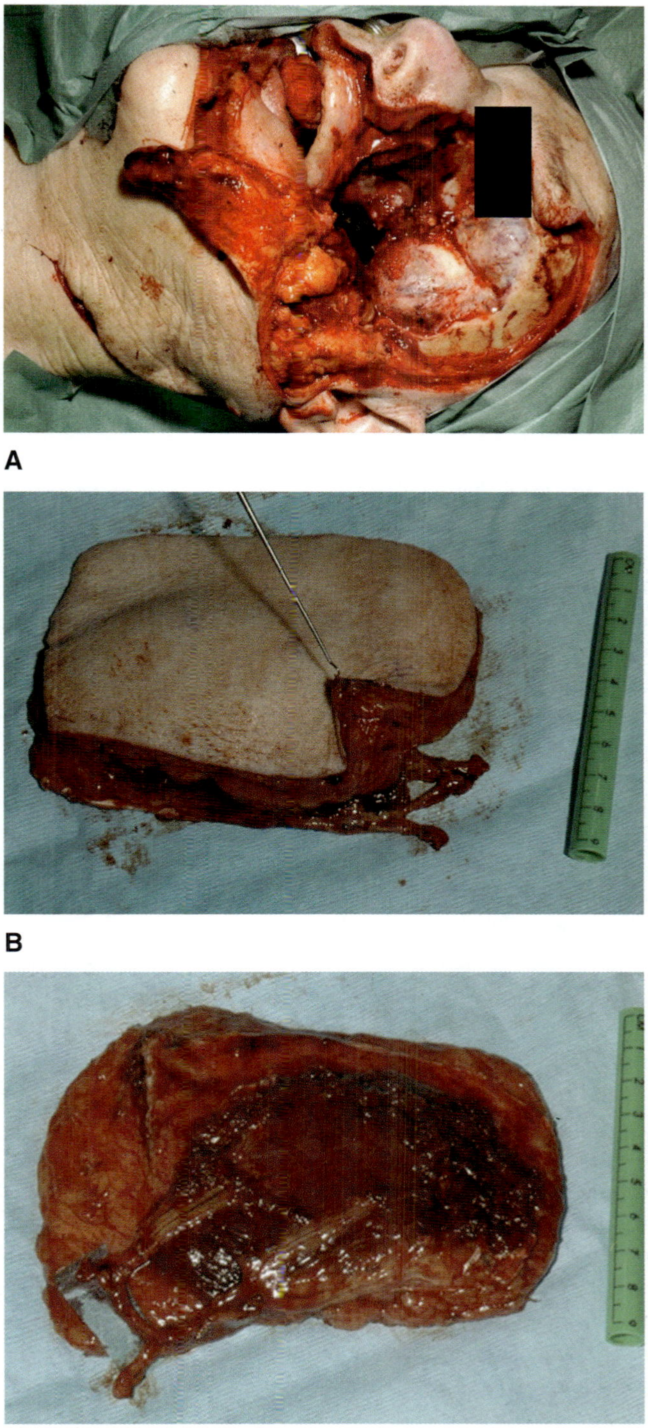

A

B

C

FIGURE 34-2 (A) After excision of a squamous cell carcinoma in a 61-year-old woman, a very large complex defect is shown. (B) The anterolateral thigh flap can provide a large volume of soft tissue with the addition of part or all of the vastus lateralis muscle if required. (C) The flap can also be deepithelialized to meet the reconstructive needs.

to provide better contour during inset. The ALT flap allows the use of a two-team approach without the need for patient repositioning to harvest the flap. Donor site morbidity is relatively low, and in many cases, the donor site can be closed primarily (30).

The ALT flap can also be used for region I defects, but it is probably not as malleable as a muscle flap to fill in three-dimensional dead space. Depending on the site of the skin perforators, pedicle length may also be a limitation. Although the ALT flap anatomy and harvesting techniques are well described, the vascular anatomy can be variable (32). If the perforator follows an extensive intramuscular course, the dissection is more difficult compared with the rectus abdominis flap or radial forearm flap. Some advocate harvesting a section of the vastus lateralis to ensure fasciocutaneous vascular supply and to provide additional bulk for filling.

Radial Forearm Flap

The radial forearm flap is a thin, pliable flap and has some use in the reconstruction of smaller defects in regions II and III. This free flap is based on the radial artery and is a reliable free tissue transfer with an acceptable donor site morbidity (30,33–36). The lack of bulk and size of the radial forearm flap are major limitations for use with skull base reconstruction. It is, however, useful for small defects that do not require much dead space obliteration, particularly when local tissue is unavailable because of resection or previous radiation.

Latissimus Dorsi Musculocutaneous Flap

The latissimus dorsi flap is based on the thoracodorsal artery. This free flap, which can be harvested as a muscle or musculocutaneous flap, has a long pedicle length and can provide a large amount of muscle to obliterate the dead space if needed and provide support to the dural repair. Based on the same vascular axis, a chimeric flap can be harvested to include muscle, fascia, skin, and bone to address extensive defects. One of the major limitations with this flap is the need to reposition the patient for flap harvest; thus, the latissimus dorsi free flap is not routinely used for skull base reconstruction.

OPERATIVE CONSIDERATIONS AND TECHNIQUES

Several technical aspects of skull base reconstruction require special attention to minimize the likelihood of perioperative complications and reduce morbidity.

Recipient Site Preparation

Successful reconstruction requires adequate preparation of the recipient site. At most centers, skull base tumor surgeries are performed with a two-team approach (resection and reconstruction). The final extent of the defect, surrounding structures involved, availability of recipient vessels, distance to recipient vessels, and positions of critical structures preserved such as the facial nerve are aspects to consider. Although careful preoperative planning is necessary for selection of the best reconstructive option, final assessment of the defect after tumor ablation frequently leads to some minor changes in the flap design or reconstructive plans.

Meticulous hemostasis should precede all recipient site preparation. For free tissue transfer, the selection of the recipient vessels depends on the site of the defect and length of the free flap pedicle. Consideration must also be given to prior surgical or radiation treatment that may compromise the vessels in the skull or neck region (37). For region I tumors, common recipient arteries are the superficial temporal artery and neck vessels, such as the facial artery (38). The facial vessels may be accessed through an incision below the mandibular margin. Careful identification of the marginal mandibular branch is necessary in this approach. If upper neck vessels, such as the facial or superior thyroid vessels, are unavailable, the pedicle should be extended and the transverse cervical vessels should be considered.

For most region II or III defects, a number of vessels are available in the neck, including the facial artery, superior thyroid artery, and lingual artery. The choice is based on the vessel size match, pedicle length, and desired position of the pedicle. Similarly, there are numerous recipient vein choices; the internal jugular vein is preferable either as an end-to-end anastomosis to its branches or end to side to the vein itself. The external jugular vein can be used but may not be available because of sacrifice in case of a neck dissection.

Successful microsurgical vascular anastomosis requires meticulous and precise operative technique. Careful positioning of the pedicle to avoid tension, twisting, or kinking of the vessels is crucial. The venous anastomosis is performed first with a venous coupler end to end, or handsewn in an end-to-side fashion. The arterial anastomosis is usually performed in an end-to-end fashion using either 8-0 or 9-0 nylon sutures.

Dural Reconstruction

In cases in which the dura has been breached, a successful reconstruction requires a watertight dural closure to prevent a cerebrospinal fluid (CSF) leak and potential life-threatening complications. Historically, reconstruction of dural defects with skin grafts resulted in a high incidence of postoperative complications and reconstructive failure (8).

The selection of the reconstructive option to repair the dura depends in part on the size and complexity of the defect. Small dural defects may be closed primarily, ensuring a watertight seal. Nonvascularized fascial grafts such as deep temporal fascia can be used for smaller defects or a tensor fascia lata graft for larger defects. The fascial graft is tacked under the edge of dural defect and sutured carefully in place. Artificial patches such as the NeuroPatch (B. Braun Melsungen AG, Melsungen, Germany) are also available. In some cases, it may be possible to use a second layer of fascial graft that is overlapped against the primary repair and secured with fibrin glue for additional support. Local vascularized tissue such as a pericranial flap or temporalis flap may also be used for this second layer of support.

For small midline or anterior skull base defects, by providing a vascularized fascial layer over the dural repair, the pericranial flap has shown to markedly reduce the incidence of CSF leaks (4). For defects located more anterolaterally in the skull base, the temporalis muscle flap is suitable, provided that the vascularity has not been sacrificed during resection.

In large, complex skull base defects in which the dura has been breached, a free tissue transfer is preferred. This provides adequate vascularized tissue to repair the dura and obliterate the dead space. Suspension sutures can be used to maintain the position of the flap and ensure maximum contact between the vascularized tissue and the dural repair. These sutures are often placed through drill holes in the surrounding bone to provide additional support to the repair, strengthen the seal, and minimize dead space.

Bony Reconstruction

If bony reconstruction is considered, attention should be given to patients who may need postoperative radiation. Avascular bone should be avoided in skull base reconstruction when radiotherapy is contemplated because it is associated with an increased risk of infection or osteoradionecrosis. In case bony support is needed, vascularized bone or an inert metal, such as titanium are preferred. Titanium mesh is an inert material that does not preclude postoperative radiologic assessments such as computed tomography (CT) or magnetic resonance imaging (MRI) and can provide rigid structural support (39). In most cases, sufficient soft tissue can be introduced to the skull base, thereby eliminating the need for bony reconstruction while achieving the reconstructive needs.

Facial Nerve Reconstruction

Facial nerve impairment can result as a consequence of skull base tumor growth, pathology, or resection. Morbidity associated with facial palsy may be substantial, and if possible, reconstruction of the facial nerve function and facial symmetry should be performed (40). If the facial nerve is transected or segmentally resected, direct microsurgical repair or nerve graft should be performed at the end of the reconstruction provided proximal and distal nerve stumps are available. If a direct nerve repair cannot be achieved without tension, then a nerve graft should be used. Common nerve graft donor sites include the sural nerve, the lateral femoral cutaneous nerve (if an ALT was harvested), the medial or lateral antebrachial cutaneous nerve, or the greater auricular nerve (often at the inferior end of the region II or III defects). The selection of donor nerve depends on the length of the deficit, the number of cable grafts needed, and the available donor sites. The effects of postoperative radiation do not appear to adversely affect nerve regeneration; therefore, immediate facial nerve reconstruction should always be considered (41–43). In a retrospective analysis of 44 patients who underwent facial nerve grafting after skull base tumor resection, 30 patients required postoperative radiation therapy (44). The authors reported favorable function with a House-Brackman grade II or III in 83% of patients. When the proximal facial nerve is not available, secondary facial reanimation options such as free muscle transfer innervated by cross-facial nerve grafts (or the masseteric nerve), hypoglossal jump, or static slings can be considered (45,46).

Postoperative Monitoring

Postoperative systemic monitoring, which includes blood pressure, heart rate, oxygen saturation, respiratory rate, urine output, and fluid balance, is important. Neurologic assessment and the Glasgow Coma Scale (GCS) should be part of the routine systemic assessment. Changes in the GCS score may be secondary to pneumocephalus, subdural hematoma, or meningitis. Routine postoperative investigation should include a full blood count, urea and creatinine, and electrolytes. Some neurosurgical centers advocate postoperative CT of the brain.

If a free flap reconstruction was used and an external skin paddle is accessible, capillary return, color, and temperature should be monitored. Occasionally, a perforator to the skin paddle may be audible with a handheld Doppler. If the flap is buried or not accessible, Doppler of the pedicle distal to the anastomosis may be useful. However, care should be taken to ensure that there is no other vessel in the vicinity, which may create a false signal.

A multidisciplinary team involved with postoperative care will minimize perioperative complications.

Complications

Early complications in patients after skull base reconstruction include wound infection, hematoma, flap loss (total or partial), CSF leak, cranial nerve injury, pneumocephalus, seizure, and meningitis. Late complications include delayed wound healing, soft tissue fibrosis or atrophy, bony instability, diplopia, ectropion, enophthalmos, and orbital dystopia. In a multicenter retrospective review, the significant predictors for overall postoperative complications were the presence of dural invasion, the presence of brain involvement, prior radiation, and medical comorbidity (17).

The most common complication related to skull base reconstruction is infection related to the wound. Because of the location of the skull base, infections require early intervention to avoid fatal CNS consequences. Prophylactic antibiotics are often instituted in operative cases that include a breach of the oral or nasal cavities during surgery.

To avoid flap failure or necrosis, close monitoring of the arterial and venous vessels is necessary. Prompt treatment of vascular compromise is critical to restore good flow to the flap and avoid the complications associated with flap failure. Initial treatment of venous congestion may include leech therapy; if unsuccessful, operative investigation may be necessary to regain vascular integrity and flow.

The occurrence of CNS-related complications such as CSF leak, meningitis, or abscess ranges from 4.4% to 23% (7,17). One multicenter international review showed no difference in complication rate between free flap and pedicled flap reconstruction; however, this study was limited by study design (retrospective historical review), and no consideration was given to the factors related to the complexity of the defect (17). Studies by Neligan et al. and Califano et al. reported a significant decrease in CNS-related complications with the use of free tissue transfer (1,3). Jackson et al. reported a marked reduction in the incidence of CSF leaks with the use of pericranial flaps (47). To minimize the likelihood of a CSF leak and the associated perioperative complications, a watertight dural seal is imperative, and this is best achieved with careful closure of the dural repair and use of vascularized tissue in cases that require reconstruction. For small CSF leaks, nonoperative treatment such as head elevation and avoidance of Valsalva maneuvers may be successful. However, in some cases, a lumbar drain or operative procedures may be required.

Outcomes of Skull Base Reconstruction

The treatment of complex defects in the skull base using free tissue transfer has improved outcome in these patients. Neligan et al. reported on the changing trend of skull base reconstructive surgery and increased use of free tissue transfers (3). Chiu et al. reported on 70 patients who underwent free flap reconstruction for an anterior or middle skull base tumor (48). In the majority of cases, the rectus abdominis was used for the reconstruction. There were no flap failures, and there were five CSF leaks (7%), which resolved without operative intervention. One patient died after the development of an intracranial abscess. Teknos et al. reviewed 35 patients with skull base tumors who underwent free flap reconstruction (5). The rectus abdominis flap was used in 20 cases, and there were 43 reported complications and two deaths. Complications were reportedly higher in patients who had previous radiotherapy treatment. Weber et al. reviewed 38 patients after skull base reconstruction using free tissue transfer (6). The radial forearm flap was used in 25 cases and the rectus abdominis flap in 12 cases. Complications included flap loss ($n = 3$), partial flap necrosis ($n = 2$), and CSF leaks ($n = 3$), and two patients died in the early postoperative period. Chang et al. reviewed 77 patients after skull base tumor ablation and reconstruction; the overall survival rate was 77% at a 2-year follow-up (21). Free tissue transfer was performed in 52 patients with three total flap losses. Califano et al. reviewed 135 patients with anterior skull base reconstruction (1). This series showed a change in reconstructive procedures to more free tissue transfers in the more recent period. There were no flap losses and similar rates of complications despite the increased complexity of skull base defects. The difficulty with interpreting many of these studies collectively is the relatively small sample size at each institution and diverse tumor characteristics (location, pathology, reconstruction). In a collaborative review of 17 centers, Patel et al. summarized the results from 1307 patients who underwent surgery for malignant skull base tumors. The postoperative mortality rate was 4%, and with a median follow-up period of 2 years, the recurrence-free survival rate was 53%. However, this study was a retrospective report and includes patients treated from 1956 to 2000, thus representing a changing medical and surgical approach to treatment of patients with skull base tumors. Overall, many of the studies that report outcomes after skull base reconstruction are limited by small sample size, diverse skull base tumor pathology and location, various methods of reconstruction and perioperative care, and lack of valid reliable outcome measures. It is therefore difficult to compare outcome among studies. However, the trend appears to have expanded the surgical management to include previously inoperable tumors, and this is at least partly due to advances in microsurgical free flap surgery.

CONCLUSION

Progress in skull base tumor ablation has resulted in smaller surgical defects and thus changed the reconstruction requirements. With future innovation and development of endoscopic and robotic surgery, imaging, radiotherapy, and early tumor detection, this specialty will continue to evolve and improve patient outcomes. Skull base reconstruction is technically challenging, and successful surgical management of these patients requires a multidisciplinary team approach, careful preoperative planning, meticulous surgical technique, and multifaceted perioperative care.

REFERENCES

1. Califano J, Cordeiro PG, Disa JJ, et al. Anterior cranial base reconstruction using free tissue transfer: changing trends. *Head Neck* 2003;25:89–96.
2. Mulholland RS, Boyd JB, Irish J, et al. Flap selection in cranial base reconstruction—local, pedicled or free? *Plast Surg Forum* 1993;62: 265–266.
3. Neligan PC, Mulholland RS, Irish J, et al. Flap selection in cranial base reconstruction. *Plast Reconstr Surg* 1996;98(7):1159–1166.
4. Palme CE, Irish JC, Gullane PJ, et al. Quality of life analysis in patients with anterior skull base neoplasms. *Head Neck* 2009;31:1326–1334.
5. Teknos TN, Smith JC, Day TA, et al. Microvascular free tissue transfer in reconstructing skull base defects: lessons learned. Laryngoscope 2002;112:1871–1876.
6. Weber SM, Kim JH, Wax MK. Role of free tissue transfer in skull base reconstruction. *Otolaryngol Head Neck Surg* 2007;136:914–919.
7. Patel SG, Singh B, Polluri A, et al. Craniofacial surgery for malignant skull base tumors. *Cancer* 2003;98(6):1179–1187.
8. Ketcham AS, Hoye RC, Van Buren JM, et al. Complications of intracranial facial resections for tumors of the paranasal sinuses. *Am J Surg* 1966;112(4):591–596.
9. Parson H, Lewis JS. Subtotal resection of the temporal bone for cancer of the ear. *Cancer* 1954;7:995–1001.
10. Ward GE, Loch WE, Lawrence W. Radical operation for carcinoma of the external auditory canal and middle ear. *Am J Surg* 1951;82:169–178.
11. Golovine SS. Procede de cloture plastique de l'orbite apres l'exenteration. *Arch d'Opthalmol* 1898;18:679–682.
12. Gillies HD. *Plastic Surgery of the Face*. London: Oxford University Press, 1920.
13. Thomson HG. Reconstruction of the orbit after radial exenteration. *Plast Reconstr Surg* 1970;45(2):119–123.
14. Neligan PC, Boyd JB. Reconstruction of the cranial base defect. *Clin Plast Surg* 1995;22(1):71–77.
15. Noone MC, Osguthorpe JD, Patel S. Pericranial flap for closure of paramedian anterior skull base defects. *Otolaryngol Head Neck Surg* 2002;127(6):494–500.
16. Price JC, Loury M, Carson B, Johns ME. The pericranial flap for reconstruction of anterior skull base defects. *Laryngoscope* 1988;98: 1159–1164.
17. Ganly I, Patel SG, Singh B, et al. Complications of craniofacial resection for malignant tumors of the skull base: report of an International Collaborative Study. *Head Neck* 2005;27:445–451.
18. Irish J, Gullane PJ, Gentili F, et al. Tumors of the skull base: outcome and survival analysis of 77 cases. *Head Neck* 1994;16(1):3–10.
19. Jackson IT, Hide TAH. A systematic approach to tumors of the base of the skull. *J Maxillofac Surg* 1982;10(2):92–98.
20. Jones NF, Schramm VL, Sekhar LN. Reconstruction of the cranial base following tumour resection. *Br J Plast Surg* 1987;40(2):155–162.
21. Chang DW, Langstein HN, Gupta A, et al. Reconstructive management of cranial base defects after tumor ablation. *Plast Reconstr Surg* 2001;107:1346–1355.
22. Scher RL, Cantrell RW. Anterior skull base reconstruction with the pericranial flap after craniofacial reconstruction. *Ear Nose Throat J* 1992;71(5):210–212.
23. Ariyan S. The pectoralis major myocutaneous flap. A versatile flap for reconstruction of the head and neck. *Plast Reconstr Surg* 1979;63:73–81.
24. Ariyan S. Further experiences with the pectoralis major myocutaneous flap for the immediate repair of defects from excisions of head and neck cancers. *Plast Reconstr Surg* 1979;64:605–612.
25. Song YG, Chen GZ, Song YL. The free thigh flap: a new free flap concept based on the septocutaneous artery. *Br J Plast Surg* 1984;37(2):149–159.
26. Kimata Y, Uchiyama K, Ebihara S, et al. Anterolateral thigh flap donor-site complications and morbidity. *Plast Reconstr Surg* 2000;106(3): 584–589.
27. Koshima I, Fukuda H, Yamamoto H, et al. Free anterolateral thigh flaps for reconstruction of head and neck defects. *Plast Reconstr Surg* 1993;92(3):421–428.
28. Koshima I. Free anterolateral thigh flap for reconstruction of head and neck defects following cancer ablation. *Plast Reconstr Surg* 2000;105(7): 2358–2360.
29. Lipa JE, Novak CB, Binhammer PA. Patient-reported donor site morbidity following anterolateral thigh free flaps. *J Reconstr Microsurg* 2005;21(6):365–370.
30. Novak CB, Lipa JE, Noria S, et al. Comparison of anterolateral thigh and radial forearm free flap donor site morbidity. *Microsurgery* 2007;27: 651–654.
31. Shieh SJ, Chiu HY, Yu JC, et al. Free anterolateral thigh flap for reconstruction of head and neck defects following cancer ablation. *Plast Reconstr Surg* 2000;105:2349–2357.
32. Wong CH, Wei FC. Anterolateral thigh flap. *Head Neck* 2010;32:529–540.
33. Bardsley AF, Soutar DS, Elliot D, Batchelor AG. Reducing morbidity in the radial forearm flap donor site. *Plast Reconstr Surg* 1990;86(2):287–292.
34. Brown MT, Couch ME, Huchton DM. Assessment of donor-site functional morbidity for radial forearm fasciocutaneous free flap harvest. *Arch Otolaryngol Head Neck Surg* 1999;125(12):1371–1374.
35. Evans GR, Schusterman MA, Kroll SS, et al. The radial forearm flap for head and neck reconstruction: a review. *Am J Surg* 1994;168:446–450.
36. Lutz BS, Wei FC, Chang S, et al. Donor site morbidity after suprafascial elevation of the radial forearm flap: a prospective study in 95 consecutive cases. *Plast Reconstr Surg* 1999;103(1):132–137.
37. Wong KK, Higgins KM, Enepekides DJ. Microvascular reconstruction in the vessel-depleted neck. *Curr Opin Otolaryngol Head Neck Surg* 2010;18:223–226.
38. Nahabedian MY, Singh N, Deune EG, et al. Recipient vessel analysis for microvascular reconstruction of the head and neck. *Ann Plast Surg* 2004;52(2):148–155.
39. Badie B, Preston JK, Hartig GK. Use of titanium mesh for reconstruction of large anterior cranial base defects. *J Neurosurg* 2000;93:711–714.
40. Myckatyn TM, Mackinnon SE. The surgical management of facial nerve injury. *Clin Plast Surg* 2003;30:307–318.
41. Brandt K, Evans GRD, Ang KK, et al. Postoperative irradiation: are there long-term effects on nerve regeneration? *J Reconstr Microsurg* 1999;15(6): 421–425.
42. Evans GRD, Brandt K. Peripheral nerve regeneration: the effects of postoperative irradiation. *Plast Reconstr Surg* 2003;112:2023–2024.
43. Gullane PJ, Havas TJ. Facial nerve grafts: effects of postoperative irradiation. *J Otolaryngol* 1987;16:112–115.
44. Leonetti JP, Anderson DE, Marzo SJ, et al. Intratemporal grafting of the facial nerve following lateral skull base tumor resection. *Skull Base* 2007;17:181–186.
45. Manktelow RT, Tomat LR, Zuker RM, Chang M. Smile reconstruction in adults with free muscle transfer innervated by the masseter motor nerve: effectiveness and cerebral adaptation. *Plast Reconstr Surg* 2006;118:885–899.
46. Manktelow RT. Free muscle transplantation for facial paralysis. *Clin Plast Surg* 1984;11(1):215–220.
47. Jackson IT, Marsh WR, Hide TAH. Treatment of tumors involving the anterior cranial fossa. *Head Neck* 1984;6(5):901–913.
48. Chiu ES, Kraus DH, Bui DT, et al. Anterior and middle cranial fossa skull base reconstruction using microvascular free tissue techniques. Surgical complications and functional outcomes. *Ann Plast Surg* 2008;60:514–520.

CHAPTER 35

Microsurgical Reconstruction of the Nose

Robert L. Walton and Thomas Willson

HISTORY OF CONVENTIONAL NASAL RECONSTRUCTION

Rhinoplasty and nasal reconstruction have origins in ancient India, when amputation of the nose was often used as punishment in women for adultery (1). The highly visible deformity resulting from amputation of the nose was a strong impetus for innovation in nasal reconstruction. It was quickly recognized that grafts alone were inadequate. For reconstruction of large, composite defects, well-vascularized flaps, having their own blood supply, were essential. The first detailed description of a nasal reconstruction appears to be the repair of an amputated nose with a forehead flap in the Sushrutas Samhita (circa 600–800 BC), commonly known as the Indian method (2). Although there are subsequent reports of early Greeks and Romans using the forehead skin and soft tissue for nasal reconstruction, it was not until much later that the forehead flap came to prominence in Europe. The French used cheek tissues. The Italians, such as the Branchas of Sicily in the mid-15th century, used arm flaps for nasal reconstruction, as documented and popularized by Gaspare Tagliacozzi in 1597 (3). One of the first introductions of the Indian method of reconstruction to the Western world was a report in a London magazine in 1794 in which a central forehead flap was used to reconstruct the mutilated nose of a driver of the English army whose nose and one of his hands were amputated in India as a penalty of war (4). Joseph Carpue's subsequent report of a midline forehead flap in 1816 appears to be pivotal for the application of this technique in Europe (5).

Early attempts to reconstruct the nose focused on using flaps to restore the most obvious defect, the missing nasal skin cover. As experience evolved, however, it soon became apparent that when the nasal lining was missing or not restored, the nasal reconstruction fared rather poorly. By the early 20th century, surgeons came to realize that in addition to the external covering, a functional, stable reconstruction required a multilaminate approach, including the restoration of the nasal lining and support of the three-dimensional nasal construct with rigid grafts of bone, cartilage, or both (6,7). Over the next 50 years, a number of practitioners attempted to address these important aspects of nasal reconstruction, and their approaches were carefully reviewed and synthesized by VP Blair in 1946 (8). Blair is largely credited with the concept of promoting the restoration of all the components of the missing nose, including the use of a forehead flap for skin cover in conjunction with a well-vascularized lining and bone and cartilage for structural support. The tenets laid down by Blair remain the basis for modern nasal reconstruction. In modern times, Burget and Menick have advanced this approach to nasal reconstruction by artistically meshing the elements of flap design and structural support with nasal subunit anatomy to achieve aesthetic results heretofore unattainable (9–11). When applied to the management of partial nasal defects, this subunit approach has come to be recognized as the "gold standard" in nasal reconstruction.

HISTORY OF MICROSURGICAL NASAL RECONSTRUCTION

For total and subtotal nasal defects, however, the traditional approaches described earlier often fell short of projected goals owing to the sheer dimensions of the total and subtotal nasal defects as well as the relative paucity of available local facial tissues for use to reconstruct these defects. Moreover, large nasal defects reconstructed using local tissues were frequently compromised by the lack of functional nasal airways.

The use of tissues remote to the face for reconstruction of large nasal defects grew exponentially as a result of World War II. The tissues were initially delivered to the facial site by means of large or small random tube pedicle flaps that required multiple surgical stages and were fraught with complications (12). With the advent of applied microsurgical techniques in reconstructive surgery in the mid 1970s, sporadic accounts of microsurgical transfer of remote tissues for nasal reconstruction were reported (13,14). Typically, relatively bulky, reliable flaps, such as the scapular flap, would be microsurgically transferred "en masse" to the nasal site, and over several subsequent surgical debulking interventions, these bulky free flaps were gradually rendered to the desired shape. Remote flaps used for external nasal coverage were soon recognized to be inferior in quality to the forehead or facial skin because they lacked appropriate skin texture and color. And it is largely for this reason that the Indian forehead flap survived as the preferred flap for restoration of external nasal coverage.

Over the past 15 years, further experience with free tissue transfer for nasal reconstruction has resulted in numerous improvements in both design and application (15–21). This has allowed for nasal reconstruction to become a realistic goal in patients whose nasal and adjacent facial defects previously precluded functional and esthetic reconstruction. These advances can be attributed to an improved knowledge of functional nasal anatomy, flap vascular anatomy unique to specific territories, and a fundamental appreciation of how these flap soft tissues could be surgically modified and articulated at the nasal site. Importantly, we have learned that remote flap tissues cannot withstand excessive kinking or twisting to the extent tolerated by well-vascularized facial soft tissues. Reconstruction of the nasal lining and adjacent nasal soft tissues has emerged as the most important application of free flaps in the restoration of large nasal defects. Indeed, the restoration of the nasal lining and its composite elements of vestibule, floor, columella, and adjacent cheek or lip have come to represent the keystone of complex nasal reconstruction. In addition, free flaps have promoted the restoration of a functional nasal airway as an integral part of the total or subtotal nasal reconstruction, a goal not previously attainable.

This chapter reviews our current strategies for use of free tissue transfers in the reconstruction of total and subtotal nasal defects.

INDICATIONS FOR MICROSURGICAL NASAL RECONSTRUCTION

Although standard nasal reconstructive techniques use local or regional tissues and autologous cartilage grafts to replace and support a component part or aesthetic subunit, excessive tissue loss such as that encountered in total and subtotal nasal defects exceeds the dimensions and capabilities of available local tissues, dramatically increasing the complexity of the reconstruction. Microsurgical transfer of tissues remote to the nasal site provides the surgeon a unique means for addressing the tissue deficit without sullying local tissues, thereby preserving facial anatomy, function, and aesthetics. Microsurgical reconstruction of the nose is generally directed toward restoring the critical nasal base and lining, allowing for preservation and utilization of the central forehead tissues for restoration of the external nasal cover owing to its color and texture that closely replicates that of the native nose.

CLASSIFICATION OF THE NASAL DEFECT

Evaluation and classification of the nasal defect are important for operative planning as well as for outcomes analysis; therefore, considerable effort should be expended to correctly identify the full extent of the deformity in a logical, stepwise fashion. In general, nasal defects can be categorized as total, subtotal, heminasal, lining only, and isolated columella defects (Figure 35-1). In brief, total defects include the entire composite nose, including the nasal bones, and lining elements. Subtotal defects involve composite defects that may include all or portions of the lining, cartilage, external cover, bony radix, and so on, constituting 50% to 75% of the nose and including defects on both sides of the nose. Heminasal defects involve all or composite portions of only one side of the nose. Lining-only defects involve primarily the lining and supporting cartilaginous structures of the middle nasal vault, septum, and tip of the nose but not the external native skin cover. As the name implies, Columellar defects involve composite loss of all or portions of the columella and membranous septum. Frequently, the nasal defect may also include defects of the upper lip, cheek, and maxilla, complicating the requirements for reconstruction. These adjacent defects should be classified as component addenda of the primary nasal defect.

APPROACH TO THE COMPOSITE DEFECT

Evaluation of the Nasal Defect

The approach to management of total and subtotal nasal defects marries the microsurgical stage(s) with the standard approach to aesthetic reconstruction using structural elements of cartilage and bone and a paramedian forehead flap. In most cases, the microsurgical component of the reconstruction is used for restoration of the nasal lining elements and any adjacent defects of the upper lip and cheeks (Figure 35-2). These are the base elements of the reconstruction. Analysis of the defect must therefore take into consideration what will be required for restoration of the base elements (Figure 35-3).

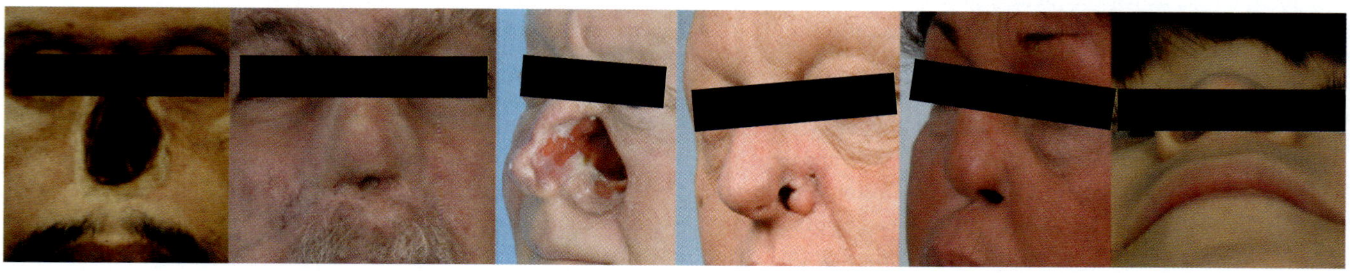

FIGURE 35-1 Classification of nasal defects. From left: total, subtotal, heminasal, partial, lining only, and isolated columellar.

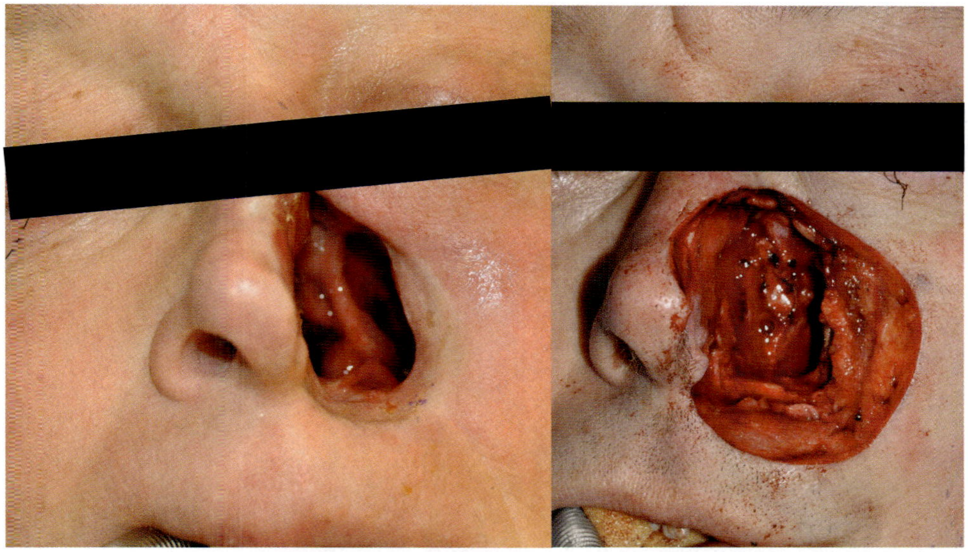

FIGURE 35-2 Preparation of the nasal defect. The microsurgical component of the reconstruction is used for restoration of the nasal lining elements and any adjacent defects of the upper lip and cheeks. (**A**) A composite, heminasal defect is shown 1 year after resection of cancer and postoperative radiation therapy. (**B**) Preparation of the defect involves resection of the previous skin graft and scar, returning the adjacent soft tissues to their correct anatomic position.

Additionally, if previous skin grafts have been used for closure of the original wounds and if these have been subsequently radiated (particularly the nasal floor), consideration should be given to removing the radiated skin graft and replacing it with a well-vascularized, nonradiated flap.

Initial examination will give the examiner a clue as to what will be required for the reconstruction. The precise sizes, shapes, and orientation of the various elements are determined during surgery when the defect is rendered near to its original dimensions and templates of the base and lining elements to be reconstructed are fabricated. In some cases when the cheek or lip defects are excessively large, a separate free flap may be required.

The Nasal Base

The nose rests on the face on a platform or nasal base provided by structural elements of the piriform aperture and maxilla, bony floor, and the adjacent soft tissues of the cheek and upper lip. Restoration of these elements is an essential prerequisite to total and subtotal nasal reconstruction. Without a nasal base, the reconstruction will have inadequate support and fall short of achieving both functional and aesthetic goals.

Nasal Lining

A second key element is the nasal lining, which together with the nasal base provides the basic foundation for the nasal reconstruction (Figures 35-4 and 35-5). The nasal lining is composed of the floor, the vestibule, and the columellar elements. It was recognized early that unlined flaps for nasal reconstruction did not permit stability of nasal shape and form over time, and nasal airway function was compromised. Historically, the majority of techniques used to create a lining in a nasal reconstruction focused on the transfer of available local tissues, including internal nasal lining flaps and local skin flaps. For large defects, local flaps proved to be simply insufficient to meet the demands of the reconstruction. Additionally, local flaps, particularly those involving the remnant nasal lining, frequently resulted in partial obstruction of the nasal airway by virtue of their bulk and

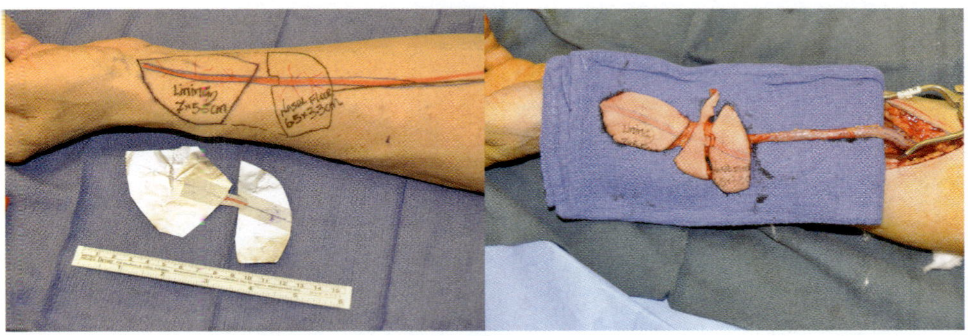

FIGURE 35-3 Rendering of defect and design of flap elements. (**A**) The design elements are duplicated onto foil templates, which are aligned to the radial vascular pedicle in the forearm. (**B**)

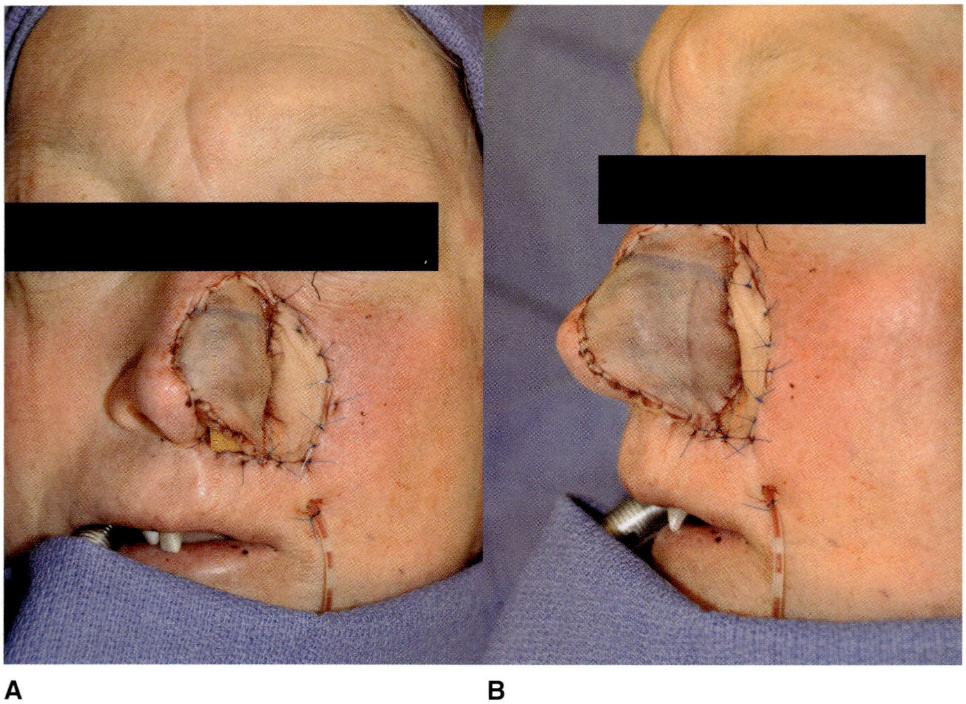

FIGURE 35-4 (A) and (B) Flap inset at the facial site. Full-thickness skin grafts are used to temporarily close the exposed undersurface of the lining flaps.

transfer to the site of deficiency within the confines of the limited nasal airway space. Because of the considerable latitude afforded by free flaps in providing the requisite, precise dimensions of area, shape, and volume, the use of free flaps for restoration of the nasal lining has resulted in a paradigm shift in total and subtotal nasal reconstruction that addresses both form and function as a collective goal.

All or portions of these lining elements may be missing, and each must be included in the reconstructive plan. For total and subtotal defects, the lining elements are configured and aligned

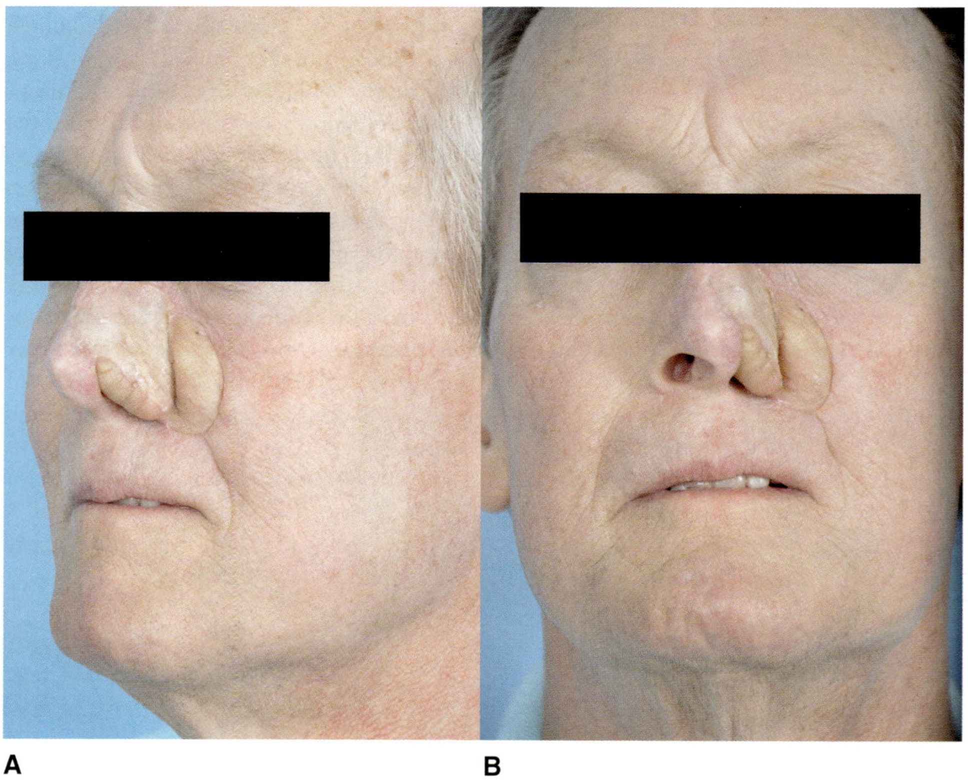

FIGURE 35-5 (A) and (B) Healed free flaps before second stage operation. Note restoration of the nasal base, vestibular lining, and adjacent soft tissue defects.

anatomically at the nasal site and joined with the nasal base elements to provide the foundation for the structural support and external cover. The importance of these base and lining elements in achieving a successful nasal reconstruction cannot be overemphasized.

For isolated nasal lining defects such as in the cocaine-injured nose or deformities arising from systemic disorders such as Wegener's granulomatosis, pemphigus, or leprosy, flap planning is approached differently than for total or subtotal defects. In these cases, computer imaging is used to visualize the dimensions of the contracted nasal vestibule and bony landmarks of the piriform aperture, bony pyramid, nasal floor, and nasal spine. Using archive high-resolution, facial computed tomography (CT) scans, the normal or optimal nasal dimensions are predicted, and from these, a forearm flap is designed that will duplicate the desired dimensions of the missing nasal lining elements. Computer imaging has proved to be an invaluable tool in the preoperative planning for reconstruction of lining defects. By avoiding a "blind" approach to the design of the missing nasal lining elements, computer imaging allows the reconstructive surgeon much latitude for configuration of a flap design that precisely fulfills the objectives of the reconstructive effort while avoiding situations of flap deficiency or excess.

In distinction to the reconstruction of total and subtotal nasal defects, microsurgical flaps used for reconstruction of nasal lining–only defects are performed in staged fashion because of the imperative for ultra thin lining elements that can only be effected through sequential surgical delay.

Structural Support

Millard promoted the use of integral structural grafts in reconstructive nasal surgery to maintain the shape and dimension of the soft tissues, a principle extrapolated and refined by Burget and Menick (7,11) Fundamental differences exist in the skeletal requisites for support in the native nose and the structural elements necessary to effect a stable nasal reconstruction. In the native nose, the nasal bones provide for rigid stability of the nasal root, and the upper lateral and lower lateral cartilages articulate with each other, allowing for considerable mobility and flexibility while retaining the three-dimensional configuration of the soft tissues they support. After trauma or surgical amputation, simple anatomic replacement of a missing structural part is inadequate for maintenance of nasal shape. The forces of scarring and wound contracture that follow any reconstructive effort necessitate the use of a rigid skeletal framework in both anatomic and nonanatomic fashion to render a stable nasal form. Diminished mobility of the reconstructed nose is an unavoidable consequence of this approach, albeit an acceptable trade-off for achieving three-dimensional stability over time.

In nasal reconstruction, ear and rib cartilage grafts and bone grafts are used to replace missing anatomic structural elements such as the nasal bones and alar cartilages (Figure 35-6). Nonanatomic grafts are needed to support the alar rims and to render aesthetic form, especially in the nasal tip and alar areas. Use of existing native nasal cartilages can be an effective adjunct for providing skeletal support for the reconstruction. Support of the nasal midline may be nicely achieved through the use of nasal septal pivot flaps or free septal cartilage grafts for dorsal support. Pivoted nasal septal flaps are based on the septal branch of the superior labial artery, which enters the base of the septum anteriorly near the nasal spine (22). The composite septal–mucosal flap is back cut posteriorly and then pivoted anteriorly and secured to the remaining septum to restore the dorsal support for the middle nasal vault. Although structurally important in the native nose, the septum proper is not generally considered a major element of the reconstructive effort. If the septum is compromised, dorsal grafts configured as an "L" strut, and cantilever grafts are used for midline nasal support. Cantilever grafts are articulated with and supported by the remaining nasal bone at the radix. They extend to the nasal tip without columellar support. These grafts are usually derived from calvarial bone because of its resiliency, hardness, and resistance to resorption. Despite the advantages of the calvarial graft, however, cantilever grafts are inherently unstable and may collapse at the level of the nasal tip because of lack of columellar support. More structural stability to the reconstruction is provided by the use of an integrated dorsal and columellar support (L-strut) and is the preferred method. This can be achieved through articulation of a nasal dorsal graft with a columellar strut or using an integrated "L"-configured graft of cartilage or bone.

Missing anatomic support structures such as the lower lateral cartilages are replaced as nasal sidewall grafts made from templates rendered in the surgical setting. Nonanatomic supportive grafts such as a columellar strut or nasal tip grafts (or both) are used to provide support and to effect certain desired nuances of tip shape and projection. Small, matchstick-sized, rim cartilage batten grafts can be used to provide support for the alar rims to maintain shape, correct alar rim notching, and stifle alar collapse during inspiration.

Materials for Support The materials used to provide rigid support in nasal reconstruction are primarily autogenous cartilage and bone. Prosthetic materials carry an unacceptably high complication rate in the nose. Bone grafts, either from the iliac crest or calvarium, may be used for the nasal dorsum or sidewall, but these are difficult to harvest, and iliac crest grafts are especially prone to resorption.

Autologous cartilage is a far more versatile graft material. Auricular cartilage harvested from the conchal bowl provides elastic fibrocartilage that approximates the size and shape of the native, curved lower lateral cartilages. But the small volume and weak, pliable nature of the alar cartilage limits its application in nasal reconstruction. The nasal septum provides high-quality, strong hyaline cartilage, but the septum may be unusable as a donor site in cases of nasal reconstruction or provide inadequate volume of graft material for the reconstruction. Rib cartilage is the favored graft material in nasal reconstruction and complex secondary rhinoplasty because of the quality and volume of graft available. The "floating" twelfth rib is commonly used for support in the ala and tip. For total and subtotal defects, the fifth or sixth costal cartilages are optimal for providing sufficient graft material for the dorsum, columella, sidewalls, and ala combined. These grafts are harvested through a split rectus

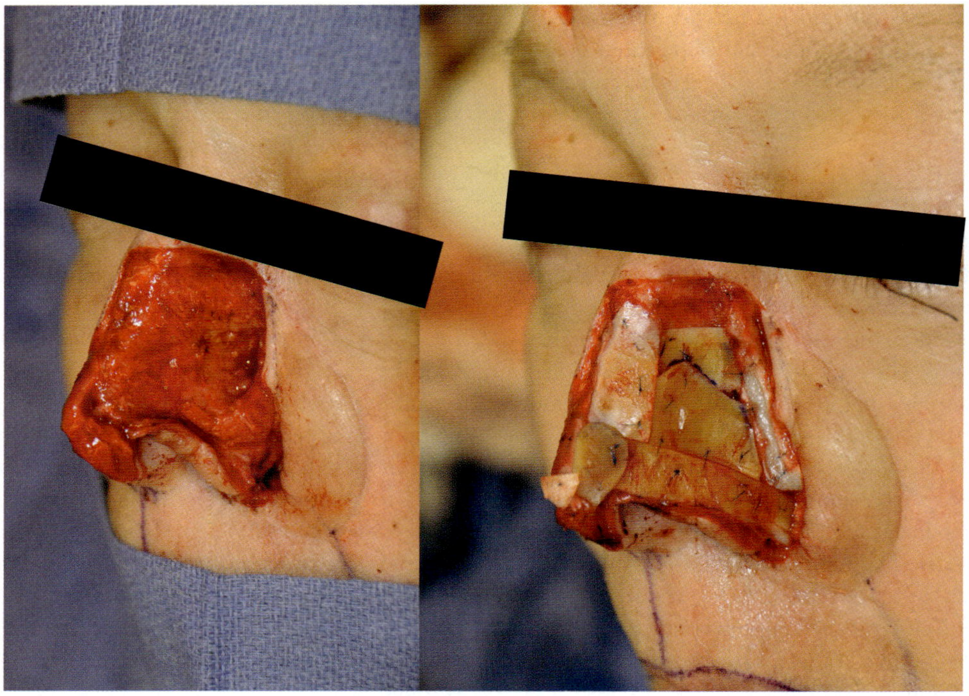

A B

FIGURE 35-6 Second stage operation. (A) The covering skin grafts are removed from the vestibular elements, which are then debulked of fat to the subdermis, preserving the vascular pedicle. (B) A cartilage framework consisting of a dorsal graft, columellar strut, alar grafts, sidewall grafts, and tip graft is fabricated from costal cartilage and inset using fine monofilament sutures.

muscle approach using subperichondrial dissection. After harvest, it is helpful to insert a small 19- to 20-gauge catheter in the wound bed for postoperative delivery of bupivacaine for pain control.

After harvest, the costal cartilage must be carved with care because it has a unique tendency to warp. Costal cartilage will warp away from the edge on which it is cut, especially if the uncut side is the outermost layer of the graft with or without attached perichondrium. To avoid warping of the graft, the concept of carving the graft with a balanced, cross-sectional area has been introduced (23). To understand this concept, it is useful to consider the cartilage graft as having a pressurized stromal core that is restrained by an outer cortex and perichondrial lining. Removal of the restraining forces (cortex and lining) on one side of the graft will result in expansion of the unrestrained core with bending or warping of the graft. To avoid this problem, the graft, to be straight, must be carved so that the core and restraining forces are equal on all sides. Alternatively, costal cartilage graft warping can be stifled by the placement of selected permanent mattress sutures as described by Gunter and coworkers (24). These sutures can also be used to effect a desired curvature to a graft that is stable over time and have proven utility in all types of nasal surgery. Alternatively, the warping phenomenon of costal cartilage can be used to advantage to create a curved surface in the construct such as the ala.

In elderly patients, autogenous rib cartilage may be calcified and brittle and crack when manipulated. These grafts are frequently inadequate for use in nasal reconstruction. As an alternative to autologous cartilage grafts in elderly patients, cadaver costal cartilage grafts can be used. The utility of these grafts appears to relate to the method in which they are preserved following harvest. We have found that lyophilized, irradiated cartilage grafts are prone to softening and resorption over time and are generally unsuitable for use in nasal reconstruction. When irradiated and preserved in saline, however, cadaver rib cartilage allografts are suitable alternatives to autologous cartilage grafts in patients older than 60 to 70 years of age (25). This cartilage is rendered acellular with radiation and has been successfully used in rhinoplasty. Although concerns for infectious sequelae from the donor and increased resorption compared with autologous cartilage have not been substantiated in most studies, the long-term stability of cadaver cartilage allografts over time remains unproved.

All nonvascularized bone and cartilage grafts have the potential for resorption. The small size and generally high success rate of nonvascularized grafts in nasal reconstruction render the need for a microsurgically augmented graft rare. We have used vascularized bone or cartilage grafts in problematic cases such as repeated infection of nonvascularized grafts in a heavily irradiated setting (25). Because of their propensity for infection and extrusion, alloplastic materials are rarely used for structural support in nasal reconstruction.

Bone grafts are used infrequently in total or subtotal nasal reconstruction because of their rigidity. However, they have particular utility in the restoration of the bony nasal pyramid in total nasal reconstructions. Calvarial bone grafts are generally preferred because of their durability and resistance to resorption. Occasionally, vascularized rib and scapular bone grafts have

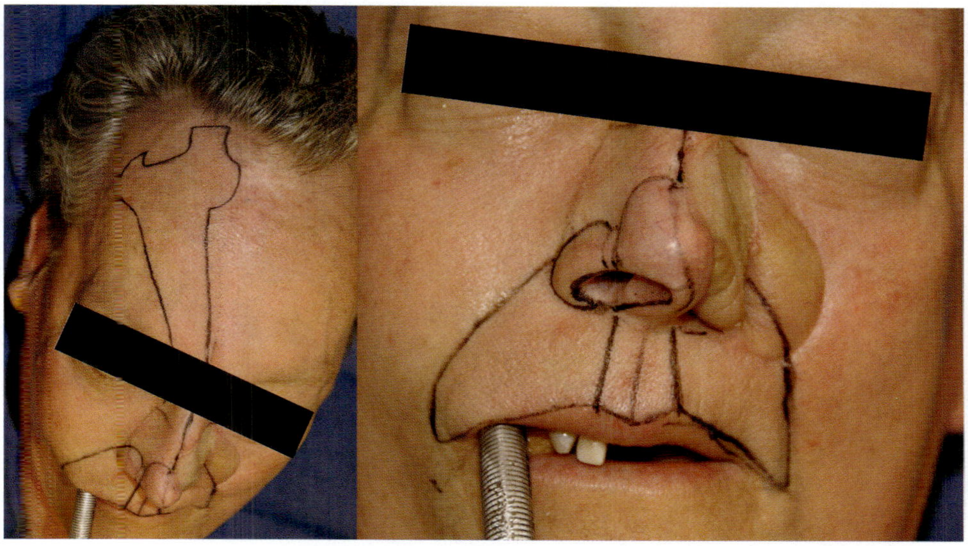

A B

FIGURE 35-7 (A) and (B) Design of the forehead flap. The template for the forehead flap is based on the opposite normal nose if available. For total and subtotal defects, the flap template is based on a clay model using a plaster moulage of the patients face and nasal defect.

been used to provide dorsal support in complex total and subtotal nasal reconstructions.

External Cover

In most cases, the external nasal cover is provided by a paramedian forehead flap, owing to its excellent color match, texture, reliability, and acceptable donor site deformity (Figures 35-7 to 35-10). In certain situations, however, the forehead is unavailable because of prior trauma such as burn or surgical injury, necessitating the use of an alternative donor site for the external cover (Figure 35-11).

In an otherwise unsullied face, use of a flap above the clavicle provides for optimal color match in the reconstruction. Unfortunately, flaps in this area are not anatomically well defined and, as free flaps, tend to be thick with short vascular pedicles. Khouri, Mathy and Pribaz, and others have described the design and use of delayed, engineered, pedicled flaps from the neck or supraclavicular region for use in reconstructing the external soft tissue envelope of the nose and cheek (26,27).

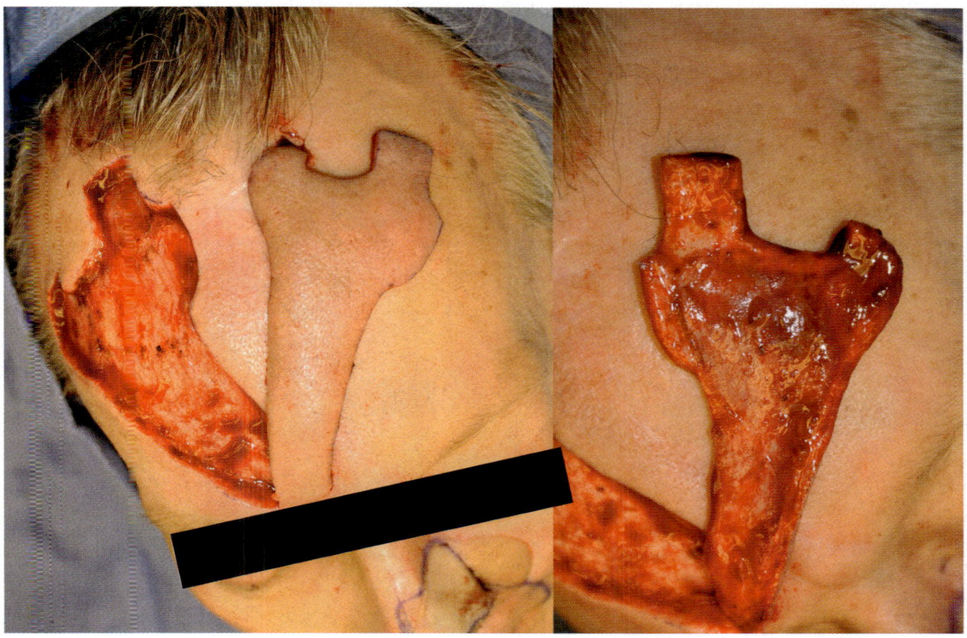

A B

FIGURE 35-8 Forehead flap elevation. (A) The forehead flap is elevated above the level of the forehead periosteum to the level of the medial brow and then in the subperiosteal plane to optimize inclusion of the supratrochlear branches. (B) The distal aspect of the forehead flap is debulked of frontalis muscle and fatty subcutaneous tissue, preserving the longitudinal veins.

SECTION 2

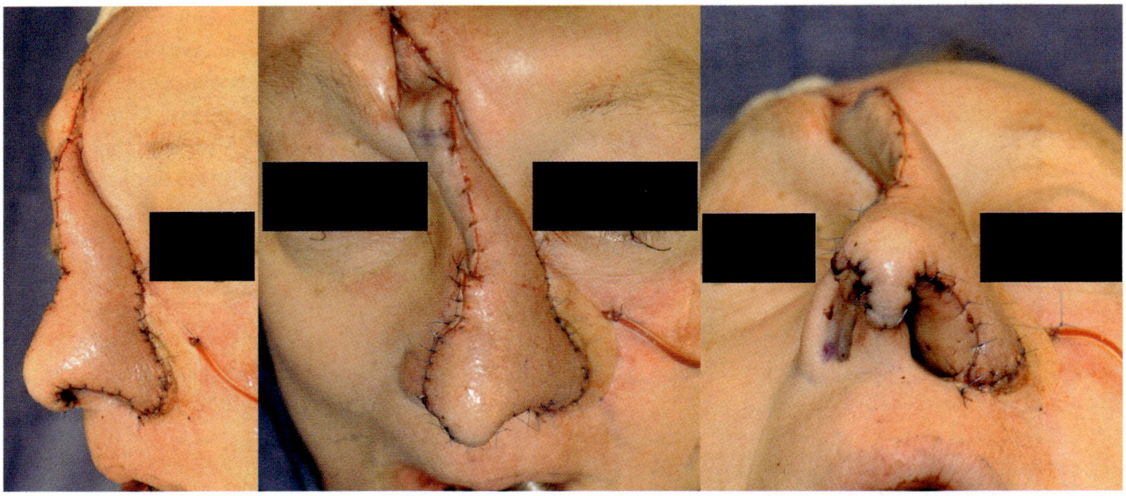

A B C

FIGURE 35-9 (A) to (C) Forehead flap inset.

These flaps require several surgical interventions to establish a reliable blood supply. They also tend to be rather rigid, bulky, and prone to venous congestion after transfer.

In burn patients and in patients having multiple facial trauma requiring skin grafts or flaps, the face is a mosaic of different colors as a result of the variable pigmentation characteristics unique to each body donor site. In these cases, color match of the external nasal flap is less problematic. Because of its reliability, thinness, and ease of harvest, we prefer the radial forearm flap, when available, for restoration of the external nasal cover. Alternative flaps include the deltoid, scapular, and anterior lateral thigh (ALT) flaps. The relative large dimensions and complex configuration of the caudal end of the external nasal cover make it somewhat risky for transfer without surgical delay. In several of our patients, partial loss of an alar or columellar element has been encountered after immediate flap elevation and transfer. This problem can be avoided by a simple surgical delay in which the complex, convoluted borders of the flap are surgically rendered and undermined to assure uniform vascularity.

An adjunct for improving the coloration of the external nasal lining flap is epidermal overgrafting (28). This technique involves deepithelizing the external nasal lining flap and resurfacing it with a thin, split-thickness, scalp epidermal graft.

Neurorrhaphy for restoration of sensibility in the external cover and nasal lining flaps is not generally performed. These flaps regain variable levels of sensibility over time, presumably by sensory nerve branch ingrowth from the adjacent facial soft tissues. Although aesthetic restoration and establishment of functional airways constitute the first priorities in nasal reconstruction, restoration of protective sensibility might be considered a valuable adjunct toward achieving an optimal outcome. Although we have not pursued this option, the potential for restoration of sensibility is available in most of the flaps used to reconstruct the nose. In the forehead flap, branches of the supratrochlear and supraorbital nerves are available for coaptation. In the radial forearm flap, branches of the medial and lateral antebrachial cutaneous nerves, the dorsal sensory branch of the radial nerve, and the sensory branch of the musculocutaneous nerve are all potential conduits for providing sensibility

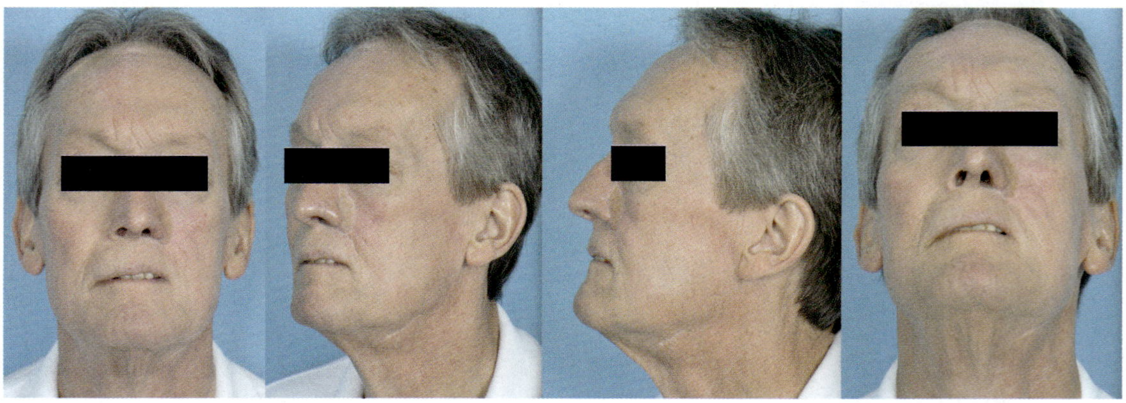

A B C D

FIGURE 35-10 Completed reconstruction of heminasal defect. (A) to (D) The patient is shown 12 months after surgery. From the time of cancer presentation to completion of the reconstructive effort, a total of 30 months transpired. Twelve months of observation for cancer recurrence was allowed from the time of cancer resection and radiation therapy before reconstruction.

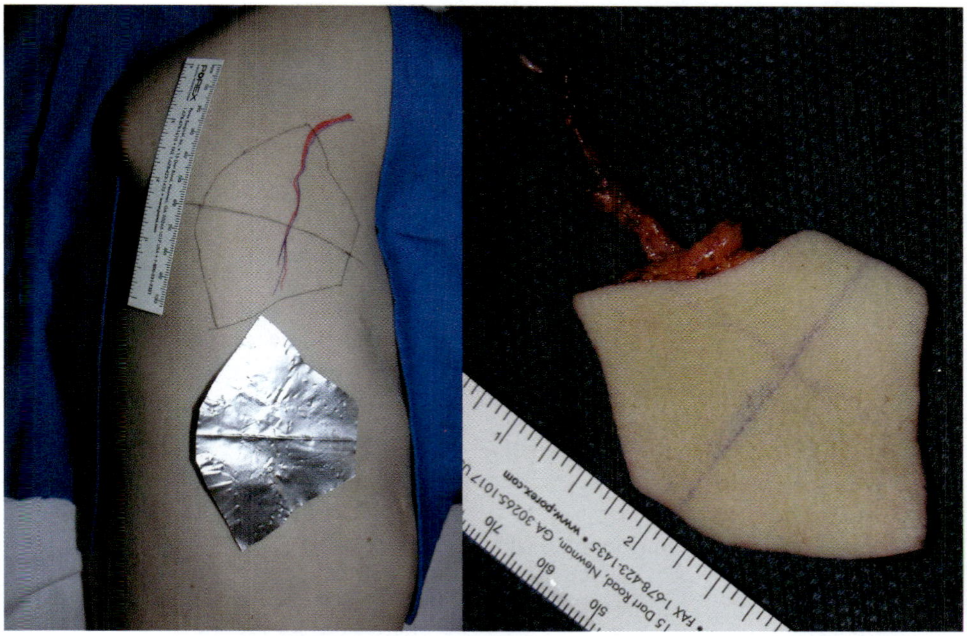

A B

FIGURE 35-11 (A) and (B) Parascapular flap used for external nasal cover.

to the flap. The recipient nerve to be used, in most cases, would be a branch of the infraorbital nerve.

Staging of the Reconstruction

Nasal reconstruction consists of a staged sequence of specific interventions that logically follow a preordained agenda, assuming successful completion of each prior procedure. Similar to the construction of a building, nasal reconstruction begins first with the establishment of a foundation that includes the nasal base and the lining elements. This is followed by fabrication and placement of the structural support and external nasal cover. The last procedures involve shaping or rendering the nose to its final size, form, and proportion with particular attention given to the airways and to rendering the delicate contours and deflections that define the nasal aesthetic. The procedures are spaced at regular intervals with 2 to 3 months between the microsurgical transfer and the forehead flap and then 4 to 8 weeks between each contouring procedure to the final division and inset of the forehead flap. The total time commitment for completion of the reconstruction is 9 to 12 months, which underscores the need for patient commitment to the reconstructive effort. Although many seek one- or two-staged approaches to nasal reconstruction, this is somewhat unrealistic for total and subtotal defects, at least given our current approach to management.

Patient Issues

Patient Selection

In most large medical centers throughout the world, microsurgery has become a routine adjunct in the reconstruction of complex deformities. Most centers have a dedicated facility and nursing support to conduct these procedures safely and efficiently. Success in elective microsurgical free tissue transfer today can be expected to exceed 95% in all age groups. Patient selection plays a significant role in determining a successful outcome. Clearly, patient morbidity and complication rates are increased in patients having underlying systemic disease and dysfunction. Hypertension, heart and lung disease, kidney disease, and diabetes mellitus are all associated with increased complication rates and flap failure rates, and these risks should be carefully weighed against the potential benefits of microsurgical transfer. Interestingly, patient age does not appear to directly relate to success or failure in free tissue transfers (29).

For patients who have significant facial defects and significant systemic disease, alternative therapy such as rehabilitation with a prosthesis may be the most appropriate approach to management. The ability and willingness of a patient to undergo numerous operative procedures to achieve an aesthetic and functional result must also be taken into consideration. Microsurgical nasal reconstruction involves many surgical interventions that incur time away from friends and loved ones, recuperation, pain, donor site morbidity, and so on. Patients who have unrealistic expectations about the process or who are unreliable and noncompliant to the reconstructive plan should be offered alternative solutions to reconstructive surgery.

In children, the selection process is relatively easy because these patients generally do not have systemic disease. Although the blood vessels in children are relatively small, they are nevertheless unsullied by vascular disease. We have performed microsurgical nasal reconstruction in children as young as age 4 years without a problem. These reconstructions grow as the child grows but not to the extent seen in normal nasal growth and development. In some patients, a second reconstruction may be necessary as the child grows into adolescence. With few exceptions, children adapt quite well to the reconstructive process.

FREE FLAPS USED IN NASAL RECONSTRUCTION

Nasal Base and Lining

Radial Forearm Flap

The radial forearm flap is considered the workhorse flap for reconstruction of the nasal base and lining owing to its consistent anatomy, large vessel size, thinness, and ability to be partitioned into multiple islands that can be articulated anatomically to restore selected elements (30). The radial forearm flap may be used for external nasal cover in the absence of suitable forehead tissue.

The flap is based on multiple small perforating branches from the radial artery. The primary venous drainage of the flap is via the paired venae comitantes coursing with the radial artery. Contrary to popular opinion, the cephalic vein is a secondary conduit as evidenced by its sparse branching in the volar forearm.

For nasal reconstruction, the flap is harvested in the suprafascial plane. It can be designed and transferred acutely or delayed depending on the location and size of the nasal defect. In the acute setting, the flap can be thinned extensively using operative magnification with care taken to avoid injury to the subdermal plexus.

Before harvest, an Allen's test is used to check the adequacy of ulnar arterial inflow to the hand after occlusion of the radial artery inflow. Clinical experience suggests that prior catheterization of the radial artery compromises flap perfusion even years later, and this constitutes a relative contraindication to the use of the flap, particularly in the setting of multiple island flaps.

The donor site defect on the volar forearm is closed with a full-thickness skin graft harvested from the inguinal region. The full-thickness skin graft provides for excellent coverage of the forearm that is supple, pliable, and stable over time. The forearm donor site scar remains a permanent visible sequela to the reconstructive effort. Although tolerated well by most patients, a few have objected to the appearance of the donor site scar, necessitating surgical revision for improvement.

The Scapular and Parascapular Flap

The scapular and parascapular flaps have been used occasionally for provision of nasal cover in the absence of a suitable forehead or radial forearm flap (31,32) (see Figure 35-11). In Whites, the scapular flap skin color is generally quite pale compared with the adjacent facial skin, making it a relatively poor color match.

The scapular and parascapular flaps are based on the major branches of the circumflex scapular artery, which emerges from the "triangular space" on the back adjacent the lateral edge of the scapula. Classified as fasciocutaneous flap, the major vessels course superficial to the thoracolumbar fascia of the back. The flap is insensate. The vascular anatomy of the flap is fairly consistent. The arterial vessel size is 1.2 to 2.0 mm diameter, and the pedicle length averages 3 to 6 cm in length. The flap is aligned to one of its major branching vessels that has been previously identified by Doppler. Elevation is relatively straightforward and quick. In obese patients, identification of the vascular pedicle can be problematic and requires careful dissection. Flap thickness is quite variable and relates to overall body habitus. The flap cannot be thinned acutely without compromising its vascular supply. Double island configurations of the flap are feasible when based on the scapular and parascapular vascular systems.

The relatively short vascular pedicle length may be problematic, particularly when attempting to establish venous outflow. The relative paucity of large-sized venous conduits in the perinasal vicinity frequently necessitates use of interposition vein grafts to access the facial, external jugular, or superficial temporal systems. The location of the flap on the back complicates positioning for recipient and donor site preparation. In the ideal situation, the patient may be positioned in the lateral decubitus position, providing for simultaneous access to both the face and back; this may prove to be awkward, however, for final inset of the flap. The donor site is closed primarily. The resulting scar is cosmetically quite acceptable with no functional deficits.

Indications for the scapular flap are primarily external cover and to provide bulk for adjacent cheek and upper lip defects. Because of its thickness, the flap is not generally used for nasal lining. Even when used for external cover, debulking procedures are necessary to achieve final size, shape, and contour.

Other Flaps

Although the radial forearm flap is the preferred flap for microsurgical reconstruction of the nasal lining, one occasionally encounters situations in which the flap is unavailable such as in a previously traumatized forearm or when a radial forearm flap has been used for reconstruction of another site. In these cases, alternative flaps are used. The choice of flap in these cases will depend on donor site availability and the requisites for reconstruction. The ALT flap is quite useful because it has a long vascular pedicle with large-diameter vessels, it can be elevated in a multi-island configuration, and it can be aggressively thinned without a surgical delay. Other options include the superficial inferior epigastric, deltoid, and lateral arm flaps (33–35). These flaps are particularly useful for reconstruction of the external nose, although they require secondary thinning in most cases. Also, the pedicle length of these flaps may be insufficient to reach the facial vessels through a subcutaneous tunnel, necessitating the use of interposition vein grafts.

Pribaz and Falco described a composite crus of superior helix flap based on the auricular branch of the superficial temporal artery for reconstruction of the alar rim (36). This flap has undergone a number of modifications over the years and has found limited use in the reconstruction of isolated alar rim defects.

For isolated columellar and membranous septal defects, the first dorsal metacarpal island flap has proved quite useful owing to its consistent anatomy, thinness, and modest donor site deformity and morbidity (37) (Figure 35-12). With the possible exception of the deltoid flap, the above-mentioned flaps, if used for restoration of the external nose, will exhibit poor color match to the surrounding facial tissues. This problem is less of an issue in patients of color and in burn patients when there has been extensive facial grafting. In Whites, color match discrepancies can

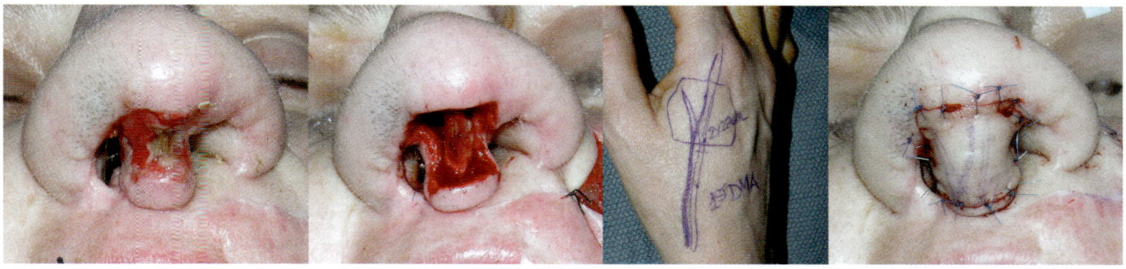

A B C D

FIGURE 35-12 Isolated columellar defect. (**A**) Columellar necrosis encountered during subtotal nasal reconstruction. (**B**) Debrided columella defect. (**C**) A first dorsal metacarpal island free flap was used to reconstruct the columella defect. Vascular repairs were performed to the pedicle of a previous radial forearm flap used for restoration of the nasal lining. (**D**) Flap inset.

be improved by performing scalp epidermal overgrafting of the nasal flap after its transfer inset, and final contouring at the nasal site.

Prelaminated Flaps Prelamination of flaps involves pretransfer grafting of various supporting (cartilage or bone) or lining elements (skin or mucosa) onto the native flap. Prelamination of free flaps has proved to be a promising technique for total nasal lining reconstruction (26,27). First introduced by Pribaz and Fine, prelamination allows for fabrication of the composite tissue layers unique to a particular reconstruction and remote to the reconstructive site (38). In the nose, prelamination has been used primarily for reconstruction of the nasal lining in which precise configuration and integration of the various elements with intrinsic cartilaginous support provides excellent, three-dimensional stability for noses in which the cartilage infrastructure is absent. Additionally, prelamination allows for the fabrication of flaps that are composed of only skin for lining, cartilage, and a thin layer of fascia. These ultra-thin flaps are occasionally used for restoring functional airway conduits without compromising nasal or facial aesthetics.

Use of prelamination increases the number of operative interventions that are required to complete the nasal reconstruction. Additionally, we have found that the unpredictable nature of wound healing, tissue contraction, cartilage warping, and so on inherent to prelamination can adversely influence the outcome of these types of reconstructions. To minimize these adverse effects, it is important to assure that cartilage grafts used in prelamination are configured with a balanced cross-sectional area and that wounds heal by primary intent.

The choice of a prelaminated construct versus an immediate geometrically configured and defatted free flap depends on the local conditions of the nasal site, the urgency of the reconstruction, and the available donor site anatomy. For example, prelamination may have certain advantages in reconstructing defects involving the nasal lining only when access is limited and the local tissues are compromised by prior cocaine injury or disease. By fabricating the three-dimensional nasal lining structures remote to the face as one vascularized unit, the process of flap transfer and inset is made much easier. Additionally, surgical access to the confined nasal lining site is less problematic.

Engineered and Prelaminated Flaps In certain situations, traditional flaps may be unavailable or unsuitable for microsurgical transfer and reconstruction such as in obese patients. In these cases, the shear thickness of the subcutaneous elements of the flap makes them unsuitable for reconstruction (see Figure 35-12). Also, debulking of a thick flap may invoke considerable risk for jeopardizing its blood supply. Flap engineering is used in these cases to provide a means for overcoming these anatomic and physiologic limitations. Although there are many types of engineered flaps, most involve the creation of a functional blood supply to selected tissues targeted for reconstruction (26,38). For example, in an obese patient, one might transplant a dissected vascular pedicle from an intermuscular septum to the subdermal region to create a vascularized skin graft that could be used for reconstruction of the nasal lining (Figure 35-13). The primary flap can be prelaminated with various tissues (skin or mucosa) or structural components (bone or cartilage) and configured anatomically to

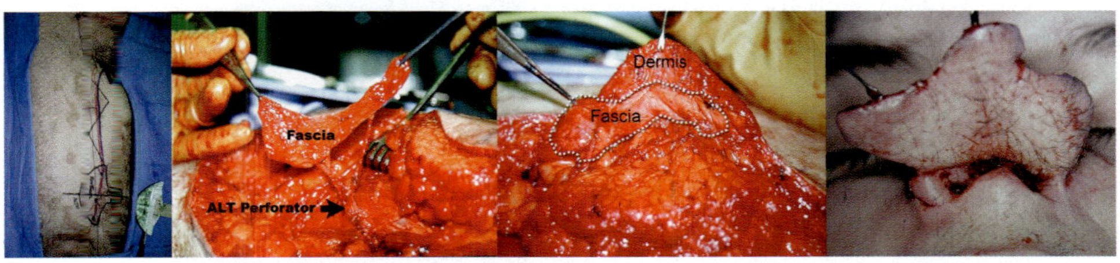

A B C D

FIGURE 35-13 Engineered free flap. Four-extremity amputee with subtotal nasal loss. Thick fatty subcutaneous tissue precluded use of the anterolateral thigh flap for vestibular lining. An engineered flap based on the anterior lateral thigh (ALT) perforators was fabricated. (**A**) Flap template designed over ALT perforators. (**B**) ALT perforators isolated to the attached deep fascia. (**C**) The perforator–fascia composite is sewn to the undersurface of the dermis of overlying skin template. (**D**) The engineered flap is shown revascularized at the nasal site.

suit the needs of the reconstruction. Engineered flaps involve multiple stages that include identification and transplantation of a functional vascular pedicle to the target tissue site, prelamination, configuration, and subsequent delay procedures to grow a functional blood supply. The final result is never as pristine or as supple as a thin radial forearm flap. Engineered flaps tend to be stiff and friable and are prone to venous congestion and persistent edema after microsurgical transfer. After healing and maturation at the recipient site, however, these flaps become quite thin and appear to "shrink wrap" to the underlying cartilaginous or bony framework. As well, both prelaminated and engineered flaps may change considerably over time, and this unpredictable aspect of behavior constitutes their most undesirable feature.

As with prelamination, flap engineering expands the dimensions of the microsurgeon's tool chest to address the demands imposed by unique reconstructive challenges.

External Cover Flaps

The color match and texture of flaps harvested from sites remote to the face are poor compared with facial tissues, and this has greatly limited the application of remote free flaps for use as external cover in nasal reconstruction. Additionally, the robust blood supply of facial tissues compared with distant tissues enables them to endure the surgical thinning and manipulations necessary to achieve a refined and aesthetic result in nasal reconstruction. Remote tissues simply do not tolerate this degree of thinning without undue vascular compromise. Although we have used free flaps for external nasal reconstruction, we have limited this practice to patients in whom the forehead was simply not available, such as in patients with extensive facial burns. The forehead flap has unsurpassed superiority for nasal cover reconstruction, affording an ideal color and textural match in a flap with a robust vascular supply, and we preferentially use it for this purpose.

PREPARATION OF THE RECIPIENT SITE

Microsurgical reconstruction of the nasal lining is usually performed in the delayed setting for both traumatic and postcancer excision defects, the latter preferably after a period of observation for cancer recurrence (see Figure 35-2). In both instances, the defect margins and any skin graft scars are resected to recreate the original defect. A template of the defect is made of foil and then enlarged 2 to 3 mm on all sides to allow for primary flap contraction (see Figure 35-3). If multiple flap islands are required, these are articulated with sterile tapes to replicate the radial vascular pedicle. The flap island templates are then arranged anatomically to ensure proper alignment and to avoid kinking of the vascular pedicle. After the flap design is set and confirmed, the template is oriented to the radial vascular pedicle, and flap harvest begins under tourniquet control (see Figure 35-3).

Preparation of the Recipient Vessels

The facial artery and vein are preferred recipient vessels. These can be easily palpated on the mesial edge of the mandibular notch along the lower border of the mandible. Confirmation of the location and course of the facial vessels is performed with a Doppler. A 2.5-cm skin incision is made approximately 1 cm below and parallel to the inferior margin of the mandible directly over the facial vessels. Dissection extends through the subcutaneous tissues to the muscle fibers of the platysma. The subcutaneous dissection is then extended over the platysma superiorly and inferiorly to facilitate exposure of the facial vessels. Small vascular branches coursing from the muscle to the overlying skin are cauterized with a bipolar electrocautery. The pulsating facial vessels can be seen or palpated lying directly beneath the platysma. The fibers of the platysma, which course obliquely from posterior to anterior, are then teased apart to reveal the underlying facial vessels. The muscle incision is extended superiorly and inferiorly, and the subplatysmal plane is dissected to facilitate exposure. The edges of the incised muscle are then tacked to the skin edges with fine silk sutures to isolate exposure of the facial vessels. The facial artery follows a serpentine course from the neck to the cheek. It is dissected over a distance of 2 to 3 cm and secured with a vessel loop. The facial vein can usually be found deep and posterior to the artery. After dissection, it is also secured with a vessel loop to allow easy retrieval for performance of the vascular repairs. The vessels are prepared using operative magnification. A subfascial tunnel is then created from the surgical defect site to the facial vessel site using blunt scissors dissection followed by progressive cervical dilators. It is through this tunnel that the vascular pedicle of the flap will eventually be delivered after the flap is transferred to and positioned at the nasal site. After the tunnel is created, a #32 French chest tube is placed in the tunnel to serve as a low-friction conduit for passage of the vascular pedicle. This is kept in position for a short period of time to compress any small vascular branches that may have been cut during dissection of the tunnel (Figure 35-14).

After harvest of the forearm flap, the end of the dangling pedicle of the flap is directed toward the nasal end of the transcheek chest tube, which is cut flush with the level of the nasal wound bed. With gentle irrigation using lactated Ringer's solution (LRS), the vascular pedicle is sluiced through the transcheek tube using light suction from the opposite end. This technique is atraumatic and avoids twisting of the pedicle within

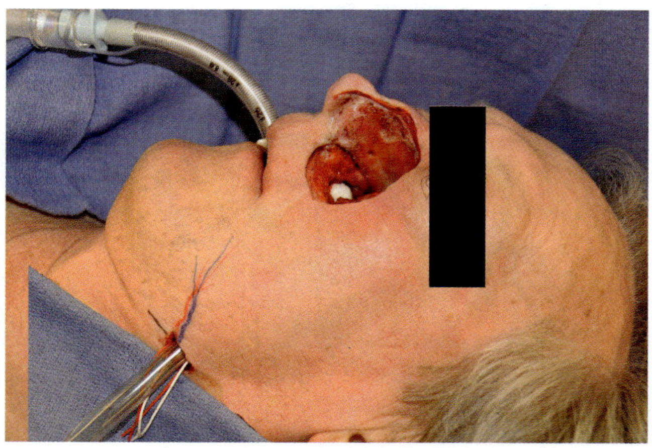

FIGURE 35-14 Chest tube conduit for atraumatic delivery of the vascular pedicle.

the tunnel and avulsing branch clips or ligatures that have been placed on the vessel wall. After the end of the pedicle appears at the facial vessel site, the chest tube is gently withdrawn.

Performance of the Vascular Anastomoses

After delivery of the flap pedicle through its cheek tunnel, vascular repairs are performed in end-to-end fashion between the facial artery and vein and the flap pedicle. Before commencement of the vascular repairs, the flap is temporarily secured to the nasal site with sutures to avoid inadvertent dislodgement. The flap is then covered with a moist sponge and towel for protection as attention is directed toward the facial anastomotic site at the cheek margin. Both vena comitantes of the flap pedicle are used when present to assure unrestricted outflow from the flap. The vena comitantes are coapted in a double-barrel fashion using horizontal mattress sutures that evert the intima on the shared side. The joined vena comitantes are then anastomosed to the open end of the efferent facial vein.

Vascular repairs are routinely performed with 10-0 nylon suture in interrupted fashion. During performance of the microvascular anastomoses, heparinized LRS (50,000 U/50 cc) is used topically for irrigation. No systemic anticoagulants are used before, during, or after the vascular repairs.

After completion of the vascular anastomoses, 2% lidocaine is applied topically to the perianastomotic site just before release of the vascular clamps. Flap perfusion is then observed for 20 minutes to assure adequacy of inflow and outflow. Look for pulsations of the flap artery beneath the flap island at the nasal site as confirmatory evidence that there is no kinking of the pedicle and that the cheek tunnel does not compress vascular inflow or outflow. The flap islands should exhibit bright pink coloration with 2-second capillary refill. Purple staining (back bleeding) of the flap edges or rapid refill may herald venous congestion and warrant a second look at the vascular repair site. Using the strip or flicker test, venous outflow should be confirmed before closure of the vessel access site.

INSET OF THE FLAP

After assuring that the vascular perfusion of the flap is satisfactory, the flap is then inset at the nasal site (see Figure 35-4). If multiple islands are used, these are articulated anatomically and then coapted to each other as dictated by the requirements of the reconstruction. The vestibular lining and floor elements are inset to the nasal mucosal edges using everting sutures of 5-0 chromic catgut. Care is taken to assure eversion of the coapted flap and mucosal edges to avoid fistula formation and to provide a watertight seal for cartilage grafts if these are used. The flap edges abutting the facial skin are coapted with fine absorbable dermal sutures (5-0, 6-0 polydioxanone) and fine percutaneous polypropylene sutures, which are removed after 5 to 7 days.

The undersurface of the vestibular element of the nasal lining flap will need to be temporarily closed with a skin graft in the interim between free flap transfer and application of the external cover flap, which is usually a forehead flap. To stifle shrinkage of the nasal lining flap, small temporary struts composed of cadaver cartilage allograft are placed along the exposed undersurface of the vestibular lining element in both longitudinal and transverse directions (Figure 35-15). These are secured with 6-0 polydioxanone sutures with care taken to avoid compression of the vascular pedicle. After placement of the cartilage allograft struts, the flap undersurface is closed with a full-thickness skin graft harvested from the inguinal region. The skin graft is secured to the flap edges with fine chromic catgut sutures. It is helpful to place a small #19 butterfly vacutainer drain beneath the skin graft to facilitate coaptation of the graft to the wound bed. The drain is removed after 5 to 7 days.

DRESSINGS

After the flap inset has been completed, the facial incision sites are dressed with antibacterial ointment (mupirocin), and a petrolatum-impregnated, nonadherent dressing is applied to the nasal skin graft site for protection. The vascular access site is closed with skin tapes. A large, 1-in-wide tape is placed on the cheek skin overlying the course of the vascular pedicle from the nasal site to the mandibular jaw line with a penned warning of "NO PRESSURE" to avoid inadvertent interventions by paramedical personnel during the postoperative period.

The forearm donor site is closed with a full-thickness skin graft harvested from the lower abdomen or inguinal region. The graft is secured with a tie-over stent dressing, and the hand and forearm are wrapped in a bulky fluff gauze dressing secured with an ACE bandage. Full-thickness skin grafts provide excellent coverage for the volar forearm donor site

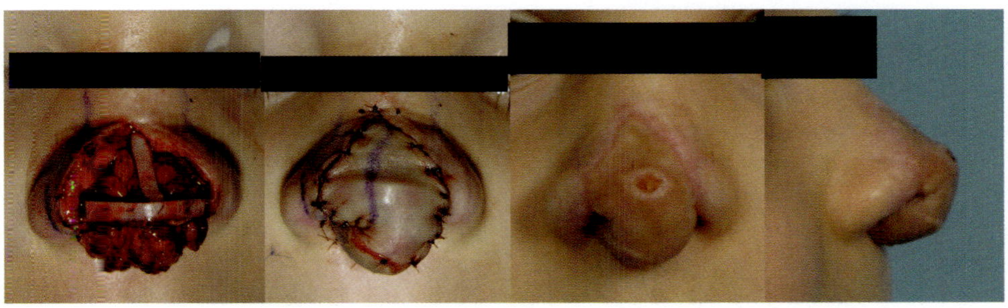

A B C D

FIGURE 35-15 Application of cadaver cartilage allograft. (**A**) Allograft applied to undersurface of the vestibular free flap to stifle flap contraction during the interim between microvascular flap transfer and forehead flap. (**B**) A full-thickness skin graft is used to close the wound. Graft survives by "bridging" over the cartilage. (**C**) Healed skin graft before removal and forehead flap. (**D**) Note maintenance of flap length and tip projection.

owing to their pliability, minimal tendency to contract, and resistance to shear. The patient is instructed to keep the donor arm elevated above the level of the heart but is free to move the arm overhead to range the shoulder and elbow joints, thereby stifling their tendency to stiffness. Arm slings are avoided. When in bed, the patient elevates the donor arm on a soft pillow.

Before the patient leaves the operating room (OR), the arterial and venous signals in the flap are confirmed by Doppler. This site is generally located at the upper aspect of the nasolabial crease where the vascular pedicle exits the cheek tunnel and courses beneath the floor or vestibular elements of the lining flap. This site is identified for the nursing staff with a fine 6-0 polypropylene epidermal suture, which is removed before the patient's discharge from the hospital.

POSTOPERATIVE CARE

The flap is observed closely for the first 48 hours after surgery because this is the critical period during which most thromboses occur. It is important to have a nursing staff familiar with postoperative monitoring of free flaps attending the patient at all times during this period. For nasal free flaps especially, the surgeon should meet with the nursing staff and residents in the monitoring unit in the immediate postoperative period to point out the important visual aspects of the flap in situ and to confirm location of the Doppler assessment site.

It is important to be quite compulsive about the various adjuncts used for patient care such as the use of ambient oxygen delivery systems. Circumferential neck straps and facemasks should be avoided because these can impair flow through the vascular pedicle. Use of mist humidification can be problematic because the evaporating mist may cool the flap and excite a vasoconstrictive response. If ambient humidification is to be used, it should be heated to minimize the propensity for flap cooling, and the surgical and nursing staff should fastidiously monitor this.

With small, potato chip–sized flap elements, it is often quite difficult for the uninitiated to discern the native cutaneous portions of the free flap from those parts that are covered by full-thickness skin graft. As the flap circulation stabilizes, the once pink blush of the skin islands pales, making the distinction between skin island and skin graft more difficult. A flashlight shone on the nasal free flap will quickly allow for assessment of flap perfusion. Avoid use of LED flashlights because these tend to reflect a false coloration of the flap that can be confusing to the less experienced members of the team. Gentle stroking of the flap skin island with a Q-Tip should reveal the tell-tale capillary refill. Flap monitoring is performed by visual inspection of the flap elements for color, capillary refill, and flap turgor and by Doppler assessment of arterial and venous flow. We generally perform flap checks hourly for the first 24 hours after surgery and then every 2 hours for the second 24-hour period.

After 48 hours, the patient is transferred from the monitoring unit to the surgical floor, where flap monitoring is performed every 4 hours. The patient is allowed to ambulate at this time as well. Discharge from the hospital is on the third or fourth day after surgery.

SUBSEQUENT STAGES IN THE RECONSTRUCTION

After microsurgical reconstruction of the nasal lining and base elements, the nasal site is prepared to host the standard nasal reconstructive effort. Descriptions of aesthetic nasal reconstruction are available in several excellent publications by Menick and Burget (9–11). The patient generally returns 8 to 10 weeks later to begin reconstruction of the structural support and final external cover (see Figure 35-10). It is during these series of interventions that special effort is made to achieve refinement and aesthetic form in the reconstruction. For total and subtotal defects, the skin grafts covering the lining elements are removed, and the flaps are debulked of fat to the subdermis. This debulking renders the vestibular and columellar elements to dimensions that provide for adequate dermal perfusion but are thin enough so as to not obstruct the nasal airway. Debulking is generally performed under operative magnification to preserve the subdermal vascular plexus. The main radial vascular pedicle is preserved but skeletonized. Meticulous hemostasis is used with a fine bipolar electrocautery to minimize damage to the vascular bed.

After the debulking procedure, the skeletal elements are constructed. This structural layer serves two general purposes. The first is to provide support for the lining elements to prevent their collapse and create and maintain a functional nasal airway. The second is to provide a scaffold upon which the external cover flap may rest, giving it aesthetic proportion, form, and stability. As noted earlier, the structural elements supporting the nasal dorsum, columella, nasal sidewalls, ala, and nasal tip are generally fabricated from costal cartilage. These elements are assembled in sequence with the dorsum and columella elements placed first to establish the appropriate relationships of nasal height, length, and projection. The columellar strut is carved to angle approximately 15 to 20 degrees cephalad to duplicate the normal angle of the columella. This graft is anchored to the nasal spine through an intraoral, labiogingival sulcus incision. The dorsal graft is anchored to the nasal bone remnant(s) with a through-and-through suture or screw fixation. The columella strut and dorsal grafts are joined using a tenon-mortise articulation secured with fine monofilament sutures. We have found that temporary stabilization of the cartilage grafts with fine needles facilitates precise placement of the supporting sutures. Next, the nasal sidewalls are carved using foil templates. These grafts are secured to the dorsal graft superiorly and the maxillary or piriform aperture soft tissues inferiorly with fine mattress sutures of polypropylene or polydioxanone. In this fashion, the nasal pyramid is rendered stable. The alar support grafts are placed along the caudal edge of the nasal lining flap. The base end of the rim graft is seated against the nasomaxillary buttress of the maxilla through a bluntly dissected soft tissue tunnel. The nasal tip end of the alar rim graft is anchored to the dorsal graft at the point of juncture of the columella strut. Here the grafts arc slightly above the projection point of the dorsal graft. Again, temporarily anchoring of the grafts in position with fine 25-gauge straight needles facilitates suture placement. The nasal lining flap is tacked to the undersurface of the alar and sidewall cartilage grafts with fine 6-0 polydioxanone sutures with care taken to avoid tension that might compromise the dermal circulation of the lining flap. The tip graft is placed last between the crura of the alar rim grafts. In some reconstructions, conchal cartilage may be harvested to provide support for the alar rims. These grafts tend to be somewhat flimsy and are reserved for partial tip reconstructions or in secondary revisions, when they are placed to improve nasal tip definition with little requirement for structural support.

After fabrication and installation of the nasal structural elements, the external nasal cover is applied. The forehead flap is the flap of choice for external cover. It is extremely important that the flap is carefully designed to assure its adequate size and ability to extend to the most distal parts of the reconstruction without tension (contralateral alar base and base of columella). To eliminate dead space, we prefer the use of small butterfly drains on each side of the nasal reconstruction to occlude the lining and external cover flaps to the framework, creating a unified multilaminate construct.

COMPLICATIONS

As with any surgical endeavor, and particularly in complex reconstructions of the nose, complications in microsurgical reconstruction of the nose can and do occur. Most are avoidable with careful preoperative planning and meticulous surgical execution. Complications can be grouped into two general areas, flap ischemia or necrosis and infection.

Flap Ischemia or Necrosis

Complications with use of the radial forearm flap are few as this is a very robust flap with large-caliber vessels and an infinite assortment of configurations and applications. Be especially wary of using the radial forearm flap if prior catheterization of the radial artery has been performed even if the Allen's test demonstrates robust perfusion via both radial and ulnar systems. We have found that prior catheterization of the radial artery can damage the fine perforators of the radial system and compromise perfusion of the normal radial forearm territory. Inasmuch as the radial forearm flap for nasal reconstruction is harvested above the level of the forearm fascia, the dependence of flap perfusion on the fine, wispy perforators from the radial artery assumes utmost importance.

When using the flap around hardware, one must be cognizant of the fact that hardware can very quickly occlude the pedicle with normal postoperative flap swelling. Judicious placement of the pedicle away from any restricting hardware or bone grafts will serve to avoid constriction of the pedicle and prevent middle-of-the-night phone calls. If the pedicle is designed to lie toward the edge of the flap, as is often the case in nasal lining reconstruction, it is often helpful to delay this type of flap to optimize its perfusion before transfer.

In total and subtotal nasal reconstructions when multiple islands of the radial forearm flap are articulated anatomically as elements representing the nasal floor, vestibule, columella, and so on, kinking of the vascular pedicle is a defined risk. Therefore, extra care must be exercised in designing how the flap elements articulate with each other so as to avoid sharp angles or folds that may result in twisting or kinking of the pedicle. Here the adage "measure twice, cut once" rings quite true. It is useful to include a 3- to 5-mm gap between the islands to allow for some pedicle slack as the islands articulate into position at the nasal site. To facilitate skin flap island alignment, we design the flap "string of pearls" using foil templates interconnected with 0.5-in strips of paper tape and then articulate these anatomically to observe and adjust pedicle placement, allowing for the smoothest, unsullied pedicle transition from island to island.

After initial vascular repairs, if the flap islands appear congested or poorly perfused, one should assume that there is a technical problem with the pedicle. It is either twisted or kinked at the nasal site or restricted within the cheek tunnel. This will likely not improve unless intervention is undertaken to remedy the problem; wishful thinking will not save the day. It is important not to leave the OR until and unless the all components of the nasal lining flap are warm and pink with good capillary refill and a bounding pulse evident in the pedicle at the nasal site.

Partial or complete necrosis of any element of the lining free flap, although rare, constitutes a major complication that must be dealt with expeditiously. Allowing for demarcation and healing by secondary intent simply promotes induration, contraction, and fibrosis at the nasal site, which will undoubtedly compromise the final aesthetic and functional result. In the unusual circumstance, well-vascularized local tissues may be available for use as flaps to replace the necrotic element(s). In most cases, however, the availability of local tissues for this purpose is limited, and another free flap will be required. After it has been determined that additional tissue will be required to replace the necrotic elements, surgical intervention should not be delayed. The exact dimensions of the necrotic or missing elements should be carefully measured and templates made to allow for selection of the appropriate flap. Usually these are very small flaps (potato chip size) that can be harvested from the dorsal hand (first dorsal metacarpal system), circumflex scapular system, superficial inferior epigastric system, deep inferior epigastric perforator system, or opposite radial forearm (see Figure 35-15). In nearly every instance, these flaps can be repaired to the previous vascular pedicle of the original radial forearm free flap in end-to-side fashion so as to not adversely impact the perfusion of the original nasal free flap.

Infection

Infection in total and subtotal nasal reconstructions can have devastating consequences. Two conditions that most often contribute to the development of infection in nasal reconstruction are partial or complete necrosis of the nasal lining and prior irradiation of the nasal site. Both conditions can lead to dehiscence of the nasal lining. Infection is most always the result of nasal lining dehiscence in the presence of necrosis and or radiation injury with subsequent exposure of the recently placed cartilage and bone grafts to the mucous and bacterial flora of the internal nose. This underscores the vital importance of a well-vascularized, intact nasal lining in securing a successful total or subtotal nasal reconstruction.

When an infection is noted, it should be dealt with expediently with formal exploration and treatment in the OR setting. All necrotic nasal lining tissues should be debrided, and if possible, the nasal lining defect should be closed without tension. If cartilage or bone grafts were placed at the most recent surgery, consideration should be given to their removal. This situation constitutes a double-edged sword, however, because removal of the supporting cartilage or bone grafts will ultimately result in contraction of both the nasal lining as well as the external cover flap. Some surgeons advocate leaving the grafts in place and allowing the infection to smolder until it "burns itself out," thinking that preservation of the underlying support will stifle the soft tissue contraction (39). Later, after the wounds have healed, the wound is reexplored, and fresh cartilage grafts are inserted to provide for additional support and to replace grafts that have resorbed or softened as a result of the infection.

Alternatively, in selected cases in which infection is manifest within 3 to 7 days after surgery, after repair of the nasal lining, the recently placed cartilage grafts are retained but treated with continuous, culture-specific antibiotic irrigation provided by through-and-through nasal irrigation catheters (40) (Figure 35-16). The irrigation is continued for 5 to 6 days, and then the catheters are removed. Using this approach, most infections can be successfully resolved, and the supporting cartilage and bone grafts can be retained without subjecting the soft tissues to the chronic inflammation, fibrosis, and contraction that follow a conservative approach as outlined earlier. With irrigation, total elimination of bacteria from the wound is probably unrealistic because bacteria remain within the cartilage and bone grafts subclinically. In these cases, we have favored delayed removal (after 2–3 months) of the affected structural grafts and regrafting with fresh cartilage and bone.

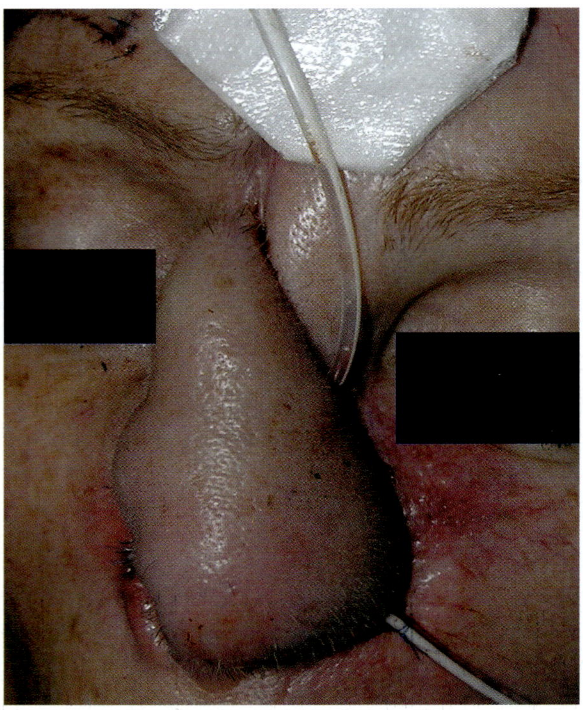

FIGURE 35-16 Use of intranasal antibiotic irrigation catheter to salvage a post-operative nasal infection during subtotal nasal reconstruction.

If the infection has been smoldering for more than 5 days, it is probably wise to remove the infected cartilage and bone grafts; repair the lining defect; and institute continuous, culture-specific antibiotic irrigation provided by through-and-through nasal irrigation catheters to sterilize the wound. After resolution of the infection and healing and softening of the nasal soft tissues, regrafting is performed, usually within 6 weeks. The important tenets here are early intervention, aggressive treatment of the infection, and obtaining a healed wound.

SECONDARY SURGERY

With the exception of perhaps the external ear, lips, and eyelids, aesthetic reconstruction of the nose is perhaps one of the most technically challenging problems in reconstructive surgery. The surgeon must have a keen eye for aesthetics that embraces the requisites of proportion, contour, color, and texture in the context of ethnicity and sex of the patient. The surgeon must also appreciate the importance of the nasal airway, nasal breathing, and physiology as integral components of the reconstructive effort. These two elements, aesthetics and function, must be maximized using all the tools of the reconstructive trade. These must embrace a profound understanding of wound repair, a thorough schooling in flap anatomy and physiology, a technically precise surgical approach, an appreciation of the requisites for nasal reconstruction, and a commitment to perfection.

This brings us to the question, "When is the reconstruction finished?" The answer to this question is not easy and may differ considerably from surgeon to surgeon and patient to patient. In Gary Zukav's *The Dancing Wu Li Masters*, a book offering a mystical interpretation of quantum physics, it is proposed that physicists (*Wu Li*) rarely achieve perfection in their pursuit of mathematic solutions; rather, they "dance with perfection," hence "Dancing Wu Li" (41). As nasal reconstructive surgeons, we too can be perceived to "dance with perfection" through our relatively crude interventions to achieve an ideal.

Our surgical interventions are staged; we modify a little bit here, a little bit there, shepherding the result closer to the desired form. After each surgical intervention, we wait to see what effects the variables of wound repair will exert on our surgical efforts: how will the tissues heal, how much scar will form, will the wound contract, will there be resorption of the cartilage grafts? And then we intervene, again "dancing with perfection."

So, the corollary to our question becomes "When do we do secondary revisions in nasal reconstructive surgery?" The topic of secondary revisions has never been adequately addressed in any aspect of reconstructive surgery. For the nose, explaining all circumstances in which secondary surgery would be performed in the context of nasal reconstruction could probably fill a book. That said, one might categorize secondary surgery of the nose after nasal reconstruction into two general areas: nasal appearance and airway obstruction.

Secondary Revision to Improve Nasal Appearance

As Dr. Gary Burget has often mused, "a reconstructed nose is not a nose. It is a composite of skin, flaps, cartilage, and bone that is rendered by the surgeon to look like a nose" (42). Indeed, a reconstructed nose is not a nose. Its shape was not genetically predetermined to be a nasal shape; its support cartilages are sculpted from rib or ear and forced to assume a certain configuration by sutures or carving. The new nasal lining is not ciliated mucosa but rather squamous epithelium. The tissues transplanted to the nasal site do not behave as native nasal tissues and are subject to the unpredictable ravages of wound repair, contraction, resorption, remodeling, and aging. These forces have considerable impact on the outcomes of our surgical efforts to achieve refinement in nasal reconstruction and often result in distortion of the nasal shape that detracts from the final result. It is often said that a nasal reconstruction will look its best at about 12 to 24 months after completion of the reconstruction (43). After this time, the reconstruction may change as a result of cartilage resorption, tissue thinning, and aging. Thus, secondary revisions in nasal reconstruction generally address the unpredictable changes in the hard and soft tissues used for the reconstruction. Most often the revision will address asymmetry of the nasal tip or contouring or repositioning of the nasal ala. Small slices or diced autologous banked costal cartilage can be placed through small, discreet incisions to add volume and improve contour. If more definition is required, such as in the alar crease, the surgeon may debulk the fat beneath the crease and place quilting sutures to further enhance the declivity. Occasionally, a simple z-plasty might be used for correction of notching of the alar rim or nostril apex.

Secondary Revision to Improve the Patency of the Nasal Airway

Early in our reconstructive efforts in total and subtotal nasal reconstruction, we encountered a relatively high incidence of airway obstruction. This has been remedied by a better understanding of flap design and placement combined with the liberal use of supporting framework to maintain configuration of the nasal airway and stifle soft tissue contraction. Contracted nasal airways cause significant morbidity in terms of patient discomfort and the maintenance of normal nasal and sinus physiology. This perhaps constitutes the most problematic issue in secondary nasal revision surgery in total and subtotal nasal reconstruction. In general, a contracted nasal airway requires more lining soft tissue. Extensive excision of the contracted vestibular soft tissues is essential for establishing a functional nasal airway. Depending on the size and location of the airway obstruction, this is followed by immediate resurfacing with a stented full-thickness skin graft, a free composite ear cartilage graft, or a free flap. Use of nasal airway stents to treat nasal airway constriction is an older approach that should be condemned because it simply does not work and is very uncomfortable for the patient.

CLINICAL CASES

Figures 35-17 to 35-23 provide clinical cases for microsurgical reconstruction of the nose.

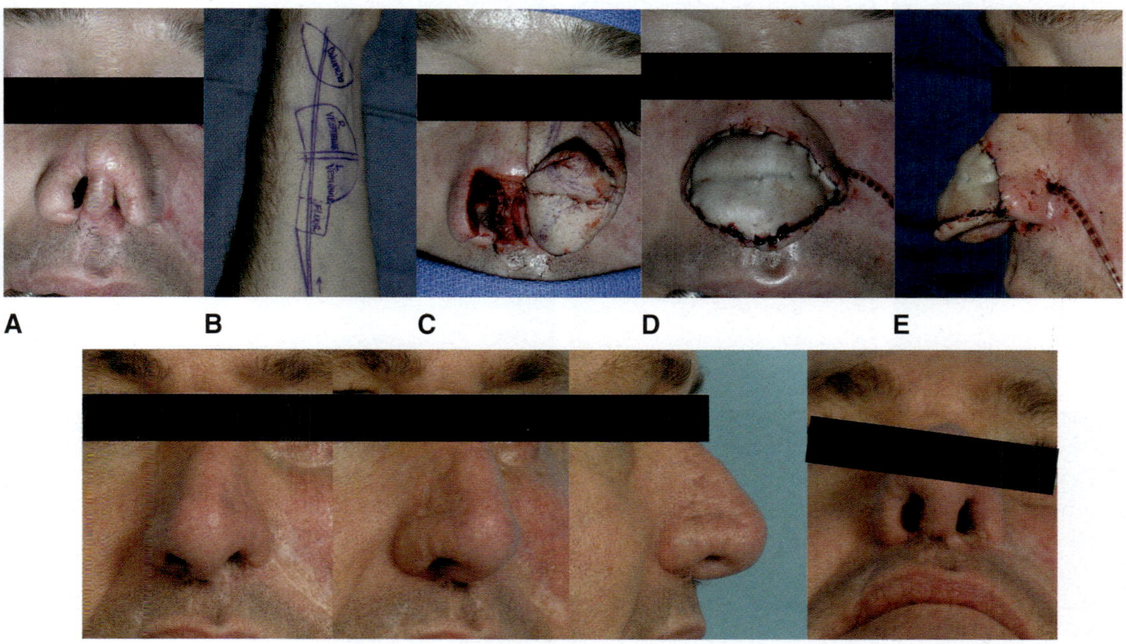

A B C D E F G H I

FIGURE 35-17 (A) to (I) Clinical case of subtotal nasal loss after a high-velocity gunshot wound. A two-island radial forearm flap was used for restoration of the vestibular lining and membranous septum.

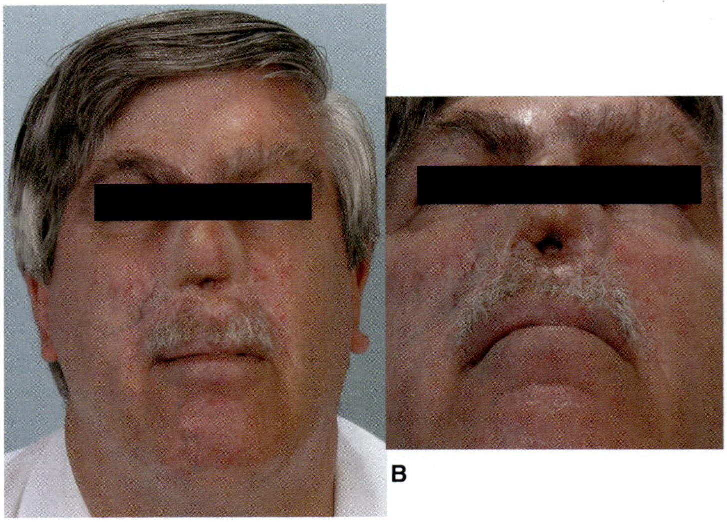

A B

FIGURE 35-18 (A) and (B) Posttraumatic subtotal nasal loss after a blast injury. The patient had undergone more than 20 prior surgeries to reconstruct his nose.

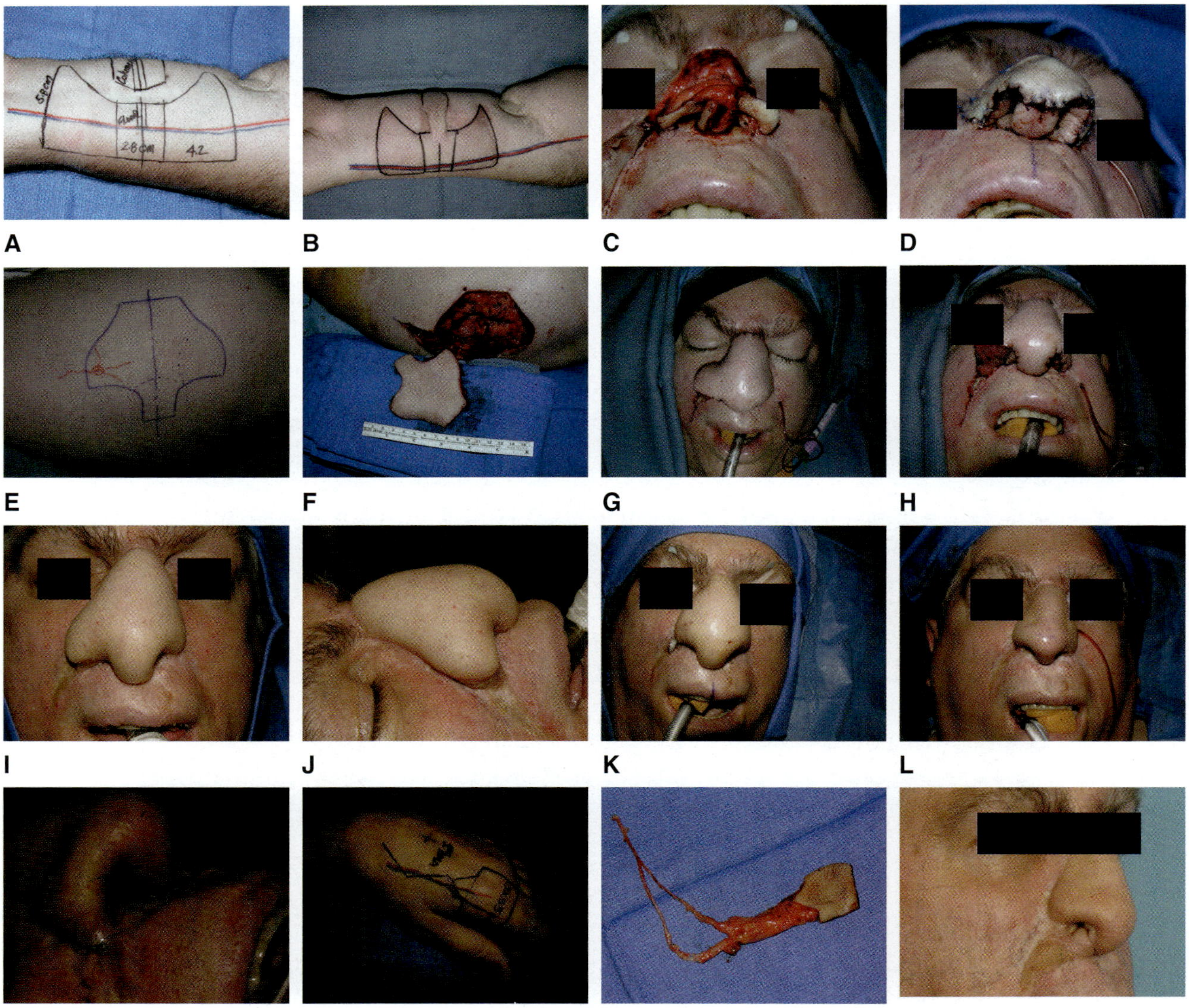

A B C D E F G H I J K L M N O P

FIGURE 35-19 (A) to (P) Post traumatic, subtotal nasal loss after a blast injury. Reconstruction was accomplished using a radial forearm flap for nasal lining, a free deltoid flap for the external nasal cover, and a first dorsal metacarpal flap for closure of a columellar defect.

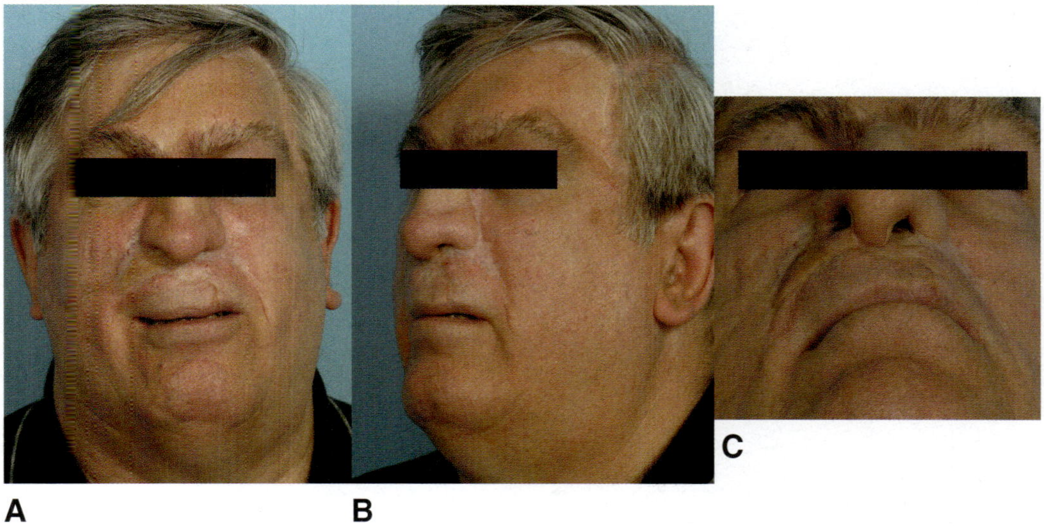

FIGURE 35-20 (A) to (C) Posttraumatic subtotal nasal loss after a blast injury. The patient is shown 12 months after completion of the reconstruction.

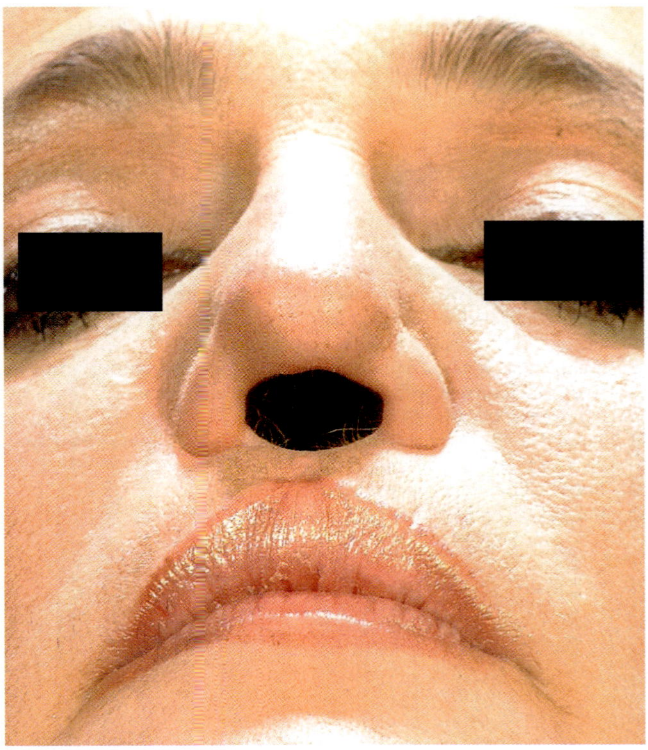

FIGURE 35-21 Drug induced nasal deformity. Presenting with loss of the nasal lining and columella.

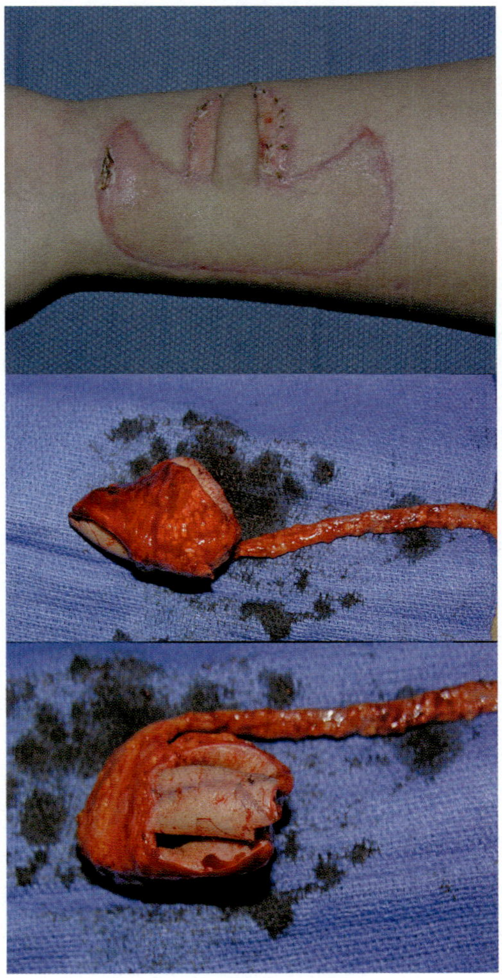

FIGURE 35-22 Drug induced nasal deformity. Nasal lining was reconstructed utilizing the "bat-flap" design on the radial forearm. This flap was used to restore the nasal floor, vestibular lining, and columella.

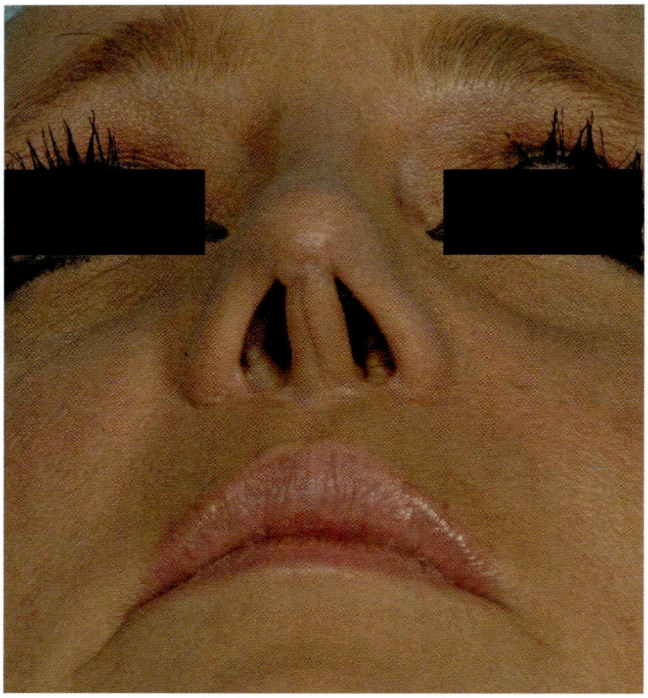

FIGURE 35-23 Drug induced nasal deformity. The patient is shown 12 months following reconstruction of the nasal lining with a radial forearm free "bat" flap.

REFERENCES

1. Whitaker IS, Karoo RO, Spyrou G, Fenton OM. The birth of plastic surgery: the story of nasal reconstruction from the Edwin Smith papyrus to the twenty-first century. *Plast Reconstr Surg* 2007;120(1):327–336.
2. From the *Sushruta Samita*, circa 600 BC. Translated from the Sanskrit and published by K.K.L. Bhishagratna, Calcutta, 1907.
3. Gnudi MT, Webster JP. *The Life and Times of Gaspare Tagliocozzi, Surgeon of Bologna, 1545–1599.* New York: H. Reichner, 1950.
4. *Gentleman's Magazine.* London, October 1794, p. 891.
5. Carpue JC. *An Account of Two Successful Operations for Re-storing a Lost Nose from the Integuments of the Forhead.* London: Longman, Hurst, Rees, Orme & Brown, 1816.
6. Keegan DF. *Rhinoplastic Operations, with a Description of Recent Improvements in the Indian Method.* London: Balliere, Tindall, and Cox, 1900.
7. Millard DR Jr. Total reconstructive rhinoplasty and a missing link. *Plast Reconstr Surg* 1966;37:167.
8. Blair VP, Byars LT. Hits, strikes and outs in the use of pedicle flaps for nasal restoration or correction. *Surg Gynecol Obstet* 1946;82:367–385.
9. Burget GC. Aesthetic restoration of the nose. *Clin Plast Surg* 1985;12(3):463–480.
10. Burget GC, Menick FJ. The subunit principle in nasal reconstruction. *Plast Reconstr Surg* 1985;76(2):239–247.
11. Burget GC, Menick FJ. Nasal reconstruction: seeking a fourth dimension. *Plast Reconstr Surg* 1986;78(2):145–157.
12. Gilles HD, Millard DR. *The Principles and Art of Plastic Surgery.* Boston: Little Brown & Company, 1957.
13. McCraw JB, Furlow LT. The dorsalis pedis arterialized flap: a clinical study. *Plast Reconstruct Surg* 1975;55(2):177–185.
14. Shaw WW. Microvascular reconstruction of the nose. *Clin Plast Surg* 1981;8(3):471–480.
15. Brent B, Upton J, Acland RD, et al. Experience with the temporoparietal fascial free flap. *Plast Reconstr Surg* 1985;76(2):177–188.
16. Swartz WM. Microvascular approaches to nasal reconstruction. *Microsurgery* 1988;9:150–153.
17. Pribaz JJ, Falco N. Nasal reconstruction with auricular microvascular transplant. *Ann Plast Surg* 1993;31(4):289–297.
18. Beahm EK, Walton RL, Burget GC. Free first dorsal metacarpal artery flap for nasal lining. *Microsurgery* 2005;25(7):551–555.
19. Walton RL, Burget GC, Beahm EK. Microsurgical reconstruction of the nasal lining. *Plast Reconstr Surg* 2005;115(7):1813–1829.
20. Burget GC, Walton RL. Optimal use of microvascular free flaps, cartilage grafts, and a paramedian forehead flap for aesthetic reconstruction of the nose and adjacent facial units. *Plast Reconstr Surg* 2007;120(5):1171–1207.
21. Menick FJ, Salibian A. Microvascular repair of heminasal, subtotal, and total nasal defects with a folded radial forearm flap and a full-thickness forehead flap. *Plast Reconstr Surg* 2011;127(2):637–651.
22. Burget GC, Menick FJ. Nasal support and lining: the marriage of beauty and blood supply. *Plast Reconstr Surg* 1989;84(2):189–202.
23. Peer LA. Cartilage grafting. *Br J Plast Surg* 1954;7(3):250–262.
24. Gunter JP, Clark CP, Friedman RM. Internal stabilization of autogenous rib cartilage grafts in rhinoplasty: a barrier to cartilage warping. *Plast Reconstr Surg* 1997;100(1):161–169.
25. Strauch B, Wallach SG. Reconstruction with irradiated homograft costal cartilage. *Plast Reconstr Surg* 2003;111(7):2405–2411; discussion 2412–2413.
26. Khouri RK, Ozbek MR, Hruza GJ, Young VL. Facial reconstruction with prefabricated induced expanded (PIE) supraclavicular skin flaps. *Plast Reconstr Surg* 1995;95(6):1007–1015.
27. Mathy JA, Pribaz JJ. Prefabrication and prelamination applications in current aesthetic facial reconstruction. *Clin Plast Surg* 2009;36(3):493–505.
28. Cohn AB, Walton RL. Immediate autologous breast reconstruction using muscle sparing TRAM flap with superficial epigastric system turbocharging: a salvage option. *Ann Plast Surg* 2006;22(3):153–156.
29. Chick L, Walton RL, Colen L. Free flaps in the elderly. *Plast Reconstr Surg* 1992;90:87–94.
30. Walton RL. *The Radial Forearm Flap. Expert Commentary in Reconstructive Surgery: Anatomy, Technique, and Clinical Applications.* Zenn MR, Jones NF, eds. St. Louis: Quality Medical Publishing, 2012.
31. Burget GL, Panje WR, Krause CJ. Nasofacial defect following fibrosarcoma excision and radiotherapy. *Head Neck Surg* 1988;10(5):350–356.
32. Angrigiani C, Grilli D. Total face reconstruction with one free flap. *Plast Reconstr Surg* 1997;99(6):1566–1575.
33. Koshima I, Hosoda M, Moriguchi T, et al. Three-dimensional combined flaps for reconstruction of complex facial defects following cancer ablation. *J Reconstr Microsurg* 13(2):73–80; discussion 80–81,1997.
34. Zhou LY, Cao YL. Clinical application of the free flap based on the cutaneous branch of the acromiothoracic artery. *Ann Plast Surg* 1989;23(1):11–16.
35. Yamamoto Y, Minakawa H, Sugihara T, et al. Facial reconstruction with free-tissue transfer. *Plast Reconstr Surg* 1994;94(3):483–489.
36. Pribaz JJ, Falco N. Nasal reconstruction with auricular microvascular transplant. *Ann Plast Surg* 1993;31(4):289–297.
37. Beahm EK, Walton RL, Burget GC: Free dorsal metacarpal artery flap for nasal lining. *Microsurgery* 2005;25(7):551–555.
38. Pribaz JJ, Fine NA. Prefabricated and prelaminated flaps for head and neck reconstruction. *Clin Plast Surg* 2001;28(2):261–272.
39. Burget GC. Personal communication, 2010.
40. Walton, RL, Wu LC, Beahm EK: Salvage of infected cartilage grafts for nasal reconstruction with a through-and-through irrigation system. *Ann Plast Surg* 2005;54(4):445–449.
41. Zukav G: *The Dancing Wu Li Masters: An Overview of the New Physics.* New York: William Morrow, HarperCollins, 1979.
42. Burget GC. Personal communication, 1997.
43. Burget GC. Personal communication, 2007.

CHAPTER 36

Intraoral Reconstruction

J. Brian Boyd

Microvascular intraoral reconstruction is required when conventional methods are impractical, hazardous, suboptimal, or simply impossible (1). It goes without saying that simpler methods are preferred when all else is equal, yet the peculiar local features of the oral cavity, the diseases that affect it, and the treatments that it receives frequently necessitate microvascular techniques (2–4).

The complex overlapping functions of the oral cavity—speech, taste, chewing, swallowing, maintenance of oral competence, and breathing—rarely have to be addressed together, but the loss of even one of these functions is potentially catastrophic to the patient's quality of life. Their preservation, whenever possible, should be the goal of the reconstructive surgeon.

The anatomy of the oral cavity follows its function. Significant anatomical regions from a reconstructive viewpoint are as follows:

1. Lips
2. Gums
3. Mandible
4. Teeth
5. Floor of the mouth and tongue
6. Cheeks
7. Palate
8. Oropharynx

Because of the intimate relationship between the mandible and the oral mucosa of the gums, diseases that affect the mandible often affect the oral cavity, and those that affect the gums involve the mandible at a very early stage. Reconstruction of the mandible will be addressed in another chapter, as will the associated dental reconstruction and rehabilitation.

HISTORY OF CONVENTIONAL OPTIONS

The Lips

The function of the lips is multifaceted and difficult to reproduce with any reconstructive technique. Apart from acting as a sensate dam to provide oral continence, the lips aid in the articulation of sounds, produce an airtight seal to facilitate swallowing, play a major role in facial expression, and participate in the intimate display of affection.

Up to one quarter of the lip in young individuals and one third of the lip in elderly adults may be reconstructed by direct approximation with excellent results. Larger defects of up to 50% may be repaired using an Abbe (5) or Eslander flap (6) from the opposite lip. The use of these flaps is still appropriate for the indications given. The Karapandzic technique (7) rotates the orbicularis and overlying skin around the oral commissures. The muscle is detached from its peripheral attachments (later to be resutured), and the motor and sensory nerves are preserved. Function is thus theoretically preserved. It can be used partial defects in the upper and lower lips and has even been described for total lip reconstruction. However any lip-sharing procedures for defects greater than 50% effectively result in microstomia, which presents functional problems with speech, eating, oral hygiene, cosmesis, and the insertion and removal of dentures.

The recruitment of cheek skin and mucosa in the form of bilateral Gillies (8) or Webster (9) flaps can provide more lip length for larger defects but often at the expense of further facial scarring, microstomia, occasional oral incontinence, and musculosensory denervation.

The Gums

The mucosa directly applied to the alveolar processes and through which the teeth emerge is adherent to bone, immobile, highly sensate, replete with mucous glands, devoid of subcutaneous fat, and very difficult to replicate. However, exposed bone in the mouth, whether it is hard palate, anterior maxilla, or mandible, tends to become epithelialized from the periphery of the wound, provided the wound is stable—not part of a sinus or fistula—and the bone is undamaged by radiation, trauma, or infection. Thus, in the case of small defects, the gum mucosa may replicate itself, or to put it a different way, the bone may "mucosalize."

Reconstruction is usually indicated when both mandible and mucosa have been resected or where an incontinuity neck dissection leads to a communication between the oral cavity and neck. A watertight seal is vital to protect the soft tissues and great vessels of the neck from saliva, ingested food, and other oral contents. The corrosive effect of digestive enzymes coupled with infection from bacterial contamination and the presence of particulate foreign matter can lead to cellulitis, fistulae, wound dehiscence, abscess formation, or even fatal carotid blowout.

Reconstruction of the gums frequently takes place as part of an oromandibular reconstruction, which is dealt with in another chapter. However, from time to time, soft tissue reconstruction of the gum area is performed without mandibular resection or perhaps after a marginal mandibulectomy. The history of gum reconstruction is not easy to separate from that of oral lining in general. Over the years, the whole panoply of plastic surgery techniques has been applied to this purpose. Small areas of exposed bone may be left to epithelialize provided they do not communicate with the neck. Larger areas with an associated neck dissection require a flap. In the past, local tongue flaps (10) have been used but always at the risk of uncertain viability, wound breakdown, and decreased oral function. Regional pedicled transfers such as nasolabial flaps (11–13), facial artery musculomucosal (FAMM) flaps (14), and submental island pedicled flaps based on an anterior branch of the facial artery (15,16) have proved useful and are still used in replacing oral lining in smaller anterior defects. Forehead flaps, pedicled on the anterior branch of the auriculotemporal artery (17), date back to the time of Gillies and are also used occasionally, although distal viability can be unpredictable. The total forehead donor defect replaced by a single sheet skin graft looks much more acceptable than one would expect. Certainly, the need for Botox is eliminated. The temporalis muscle flap (18), by contrast, has excellent vascularity and may be used for intraoral reconstruction in many locales. It mucosalizes and atrophies over 4 to 6 weeks, giving a stable platform through which to insert osseointegrated implants.

Other regional flaps used for larger defects include the deltopectoral flap (19), the pectoralis major musculocutaneous (20), and the supraclavicular fasciocutaneous (21) flaps. Unlike pure muscle flaps, none of these options replicates the anatomic features of gum mucosa. However, by making a good seal and providing epithelium, they permit healing and avoid loss of function (speech, oral continence, mouth opening, and so on) caused by tethering. However, if osseointegrated implants (22) are planned, it is unwise to insert them through thick cutaneous flaps such as these. Excessive motion between a "wobbly" skin flap and a rigid titanium post leads to infection around the points where the attachments pass through the epidermis. It is much more effective to remove the skin at a later stage and apply a split-thickness skin graft to the periosteum of the mandibular or maxillary remnant or reconstruction. Such a graft becomes, like the gum mucosa or a mucosalized muscle flap, adherent to the bone and provides an ideal epithelial surface through which to insert osseointegrated dental implants (Figure 36-1).

Floor of the Mouth and Tongue

Because of the close functional and anatomical interrelationship between tongue and floor of mouth in handling food and saliva, together with the importance of sensation to these vital structures, they will be considered together. This is appropriate because a reconstructive surgeon is rarely presented with a solitary defect of either; tumors in the floor of mouth frequently invade the tongue and vice versa. To preserve function and maintain the quality of life, it is highly desirable that the tongue remains free and mobile as much as possible. Often when there has been a partial resection of tongue and adjacent floor of the mouth, there is a temptation to use the tongue remnant to close the floor of mouth defect. This should be resisted at all costs because the resulting tethering will adversely affect speech, chewing, and even oral hygiene. Rather, the floor of mouth should be adequately reconstructed by thin, supple tissue that permits movement and does not infringe on the tongue's activity.

Small defects of the tongue may be sutured or even skin grafted. However, even moderate composite defects communicating with a neck dissection generally need a flap. The same local and regional flaps mentioned under gum reconstruction have been used and are still used extensively, particularly for smaller defects.

The importance of a watertight seal remains the major consideration when reconstructing tongue and floor of mouth defects. The problem with many of the cutaneous and musculocutaneous pedicled flaps is that the blood supply to a portion of the skin paddle may be tenuous, leading to intraoral breakdowns and possible fistula formation. A major advantage of free tissue transfer is the excellent vascularity of the skin; it reliably produces primary wound healing.

Cheeks

Reconstruction of the cheeks as part of facial reconstruction will be considered elsewhere. As part of intraoral reconstruction, the cheeks are often neglected. This is presumably because of the tendency of isolated mucosal defects in the cheek to "mucosalize" spontaneously. For small defects, this is helpful, but for larger ones, there is often an associated shortening of the tissues that assists healing but at the expense of contracture and trismus. Skin grafts and local and regional flaps have been used in cheek reconstruction and still retain a place to prevent distortion and functional loss. However, when extensive floor of mouth defects are associated with adjacent cheek defects, it is often expedient to design the skin flap in such a way that part of it may be used to line the cheek at the same time.

As mentioned, exposed muscle flaps have been shown to mucosalize inside the mouth and have been used as a substitute for skin as part of complex oromandibular reconstruction (23). Again, although adequate in the short term, there is a danger of trismus and functional loss if the reconstructed mucosal area is extensive. However, if the muscle flap is only

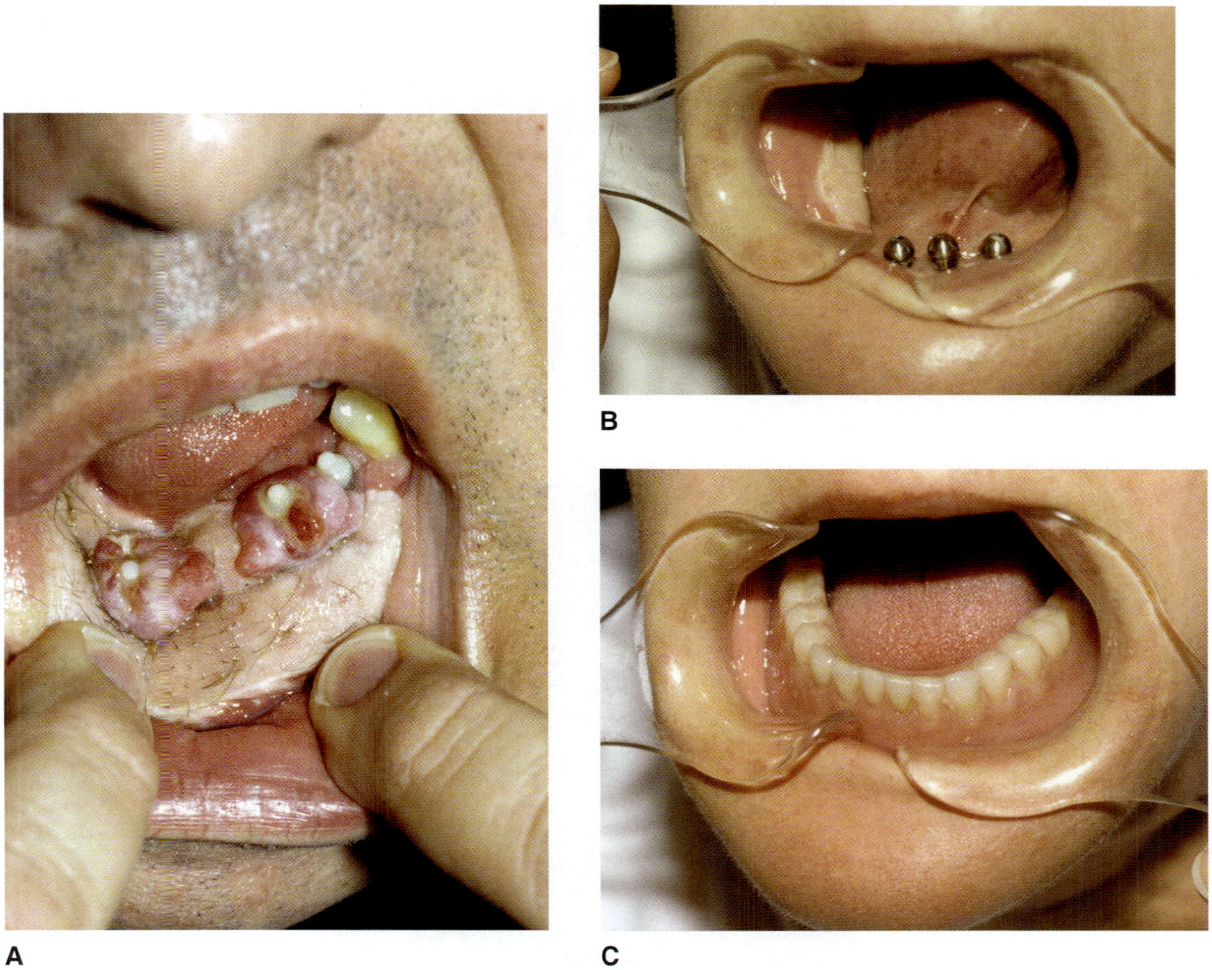

FIGURE 36-1 (A) Granulation tissue around osseointegrated implants as a result of placing them through a cutaneous lining flap. (B) Successful osseointegrated implants placed through a skin graft. (C) Prosthesis securely in place.

used to cover exposed bone, then contractures are unlikely (Figure 36-2).

Palate

Oral malignancies and gunshot trauma—self-inflicted or otherwise—can severely damage the hard and soft palates with disastrous results for speech and mastication. Isolated defects or fistulae in the palate have been handled by standard craniofacial techniques for many years. Such techniques often follow initial stabilization of the wound and involve septal mucosal flaps, turnover flaps from the edge of the wound, mobilization of the entire palatal mucosa (as for a primary palate repair), tongue flaps, and the use of superiorly based pharyngeal flaps.

Unfortunately, the defects produced by penetrating trauma or large tumor resections often exceed the reconstructive capacity of local flaps such as these. Regional and distal pedicle flaps have been used alone or in combination with a local method with some success. One method involves the use of the temporalis muscle as a pedicled flap (24–27). The zygomatic arch is osteotomized in two places so the muscle can be mobilized out of the temporal fossa. The bone segment is replaced and plated after transfer. The muscle may be split into thirds and only the posterior two thirds transferred for a better donor site appearance. A coronoidectomy is occasionally necessary to gain length (~4 cm). Mucosalization and atrophy of the muscle work in favor of an excellent result. The donor defect is moderately severe but is improved when the muscle transfer is partial, and can be corrected at the time of harvest by a temporal fossa cranioplasty. Flaps derived from the shoulder and chest have also been used. The disadvantages of such flaps, which include scarring and marginal perfusion, have been mentioned already. However, the risk of leakage of oral contents into the neck is not generally a major issue with reconstruction of defects in the roof of the mouth.

When palatal defects are in continuity with excisions in the cheeks or floor of mouth, it is often possible to extend the flap used to reconstruct these areas onto the palatal surface of the oral cavity and provide closure there, too. However, most regional cutaneous or musculocutaneous flaps are too bulky for primary palatal repair. More commonly, the palatal wound is allowed to heal and the exposed bone mucosalize. After the tissues have stabilized, the patient is fitted with a palatal obturator to permit him or her to speak and eat normally. Often this is all that is required.

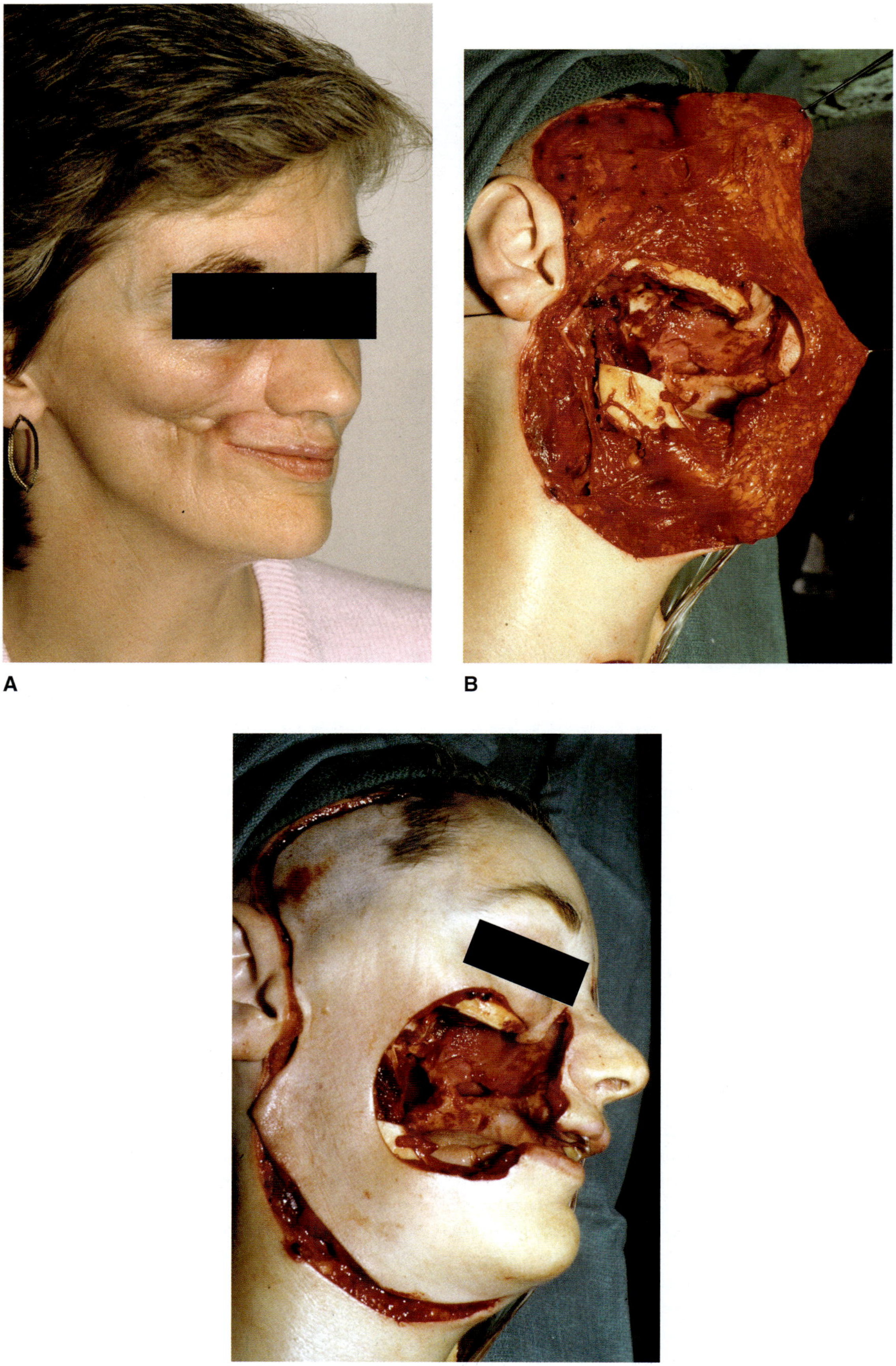

A B C

FIGURE 36-2 A recurrent adenocarcinoma involving the skull base, mandible, cheek, and oral lining. (A) Preoperative image. (B) After wide resection. (C) The cheek flap back in place.

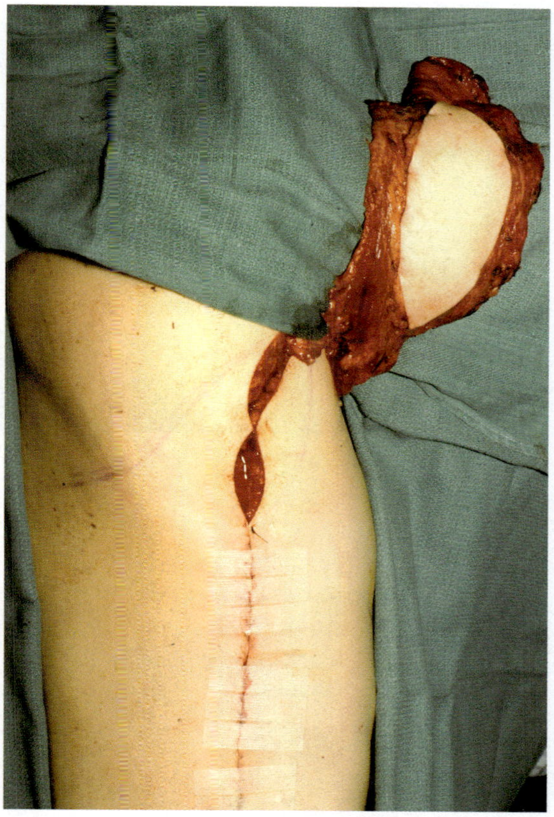

D

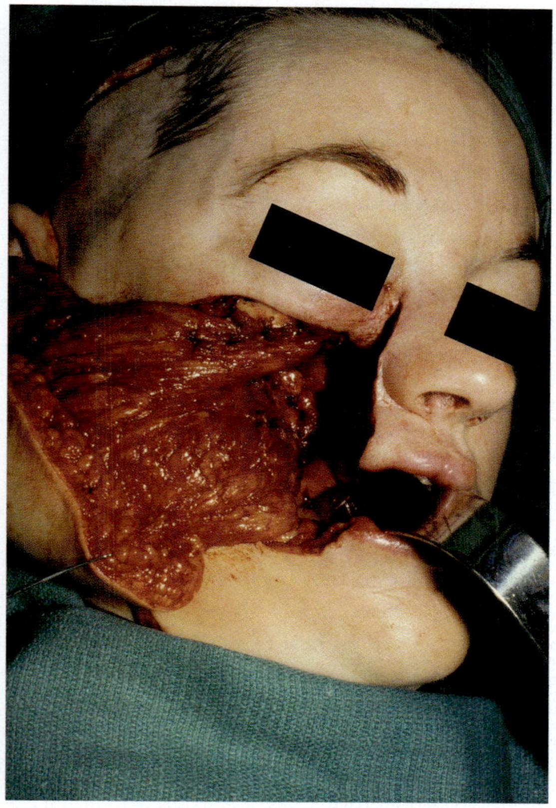

E

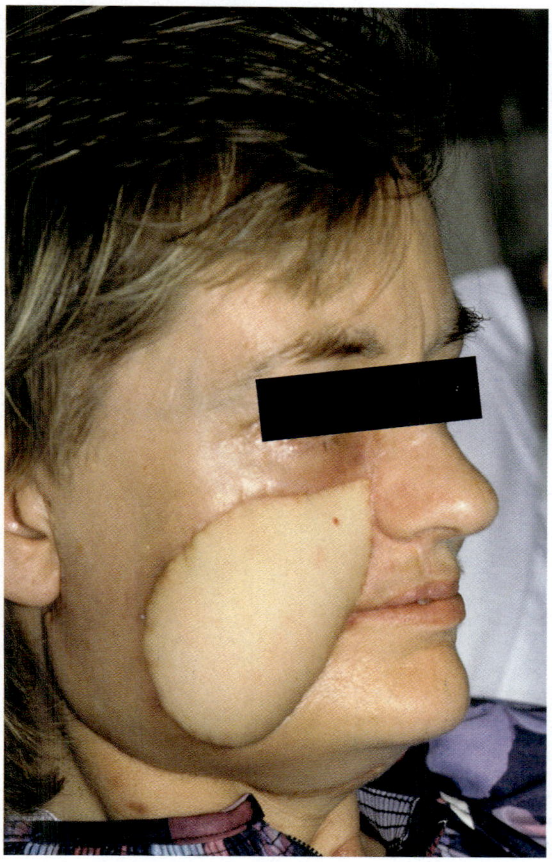

F

FIGURE 36-2 (*Continued*) (D) Elevation of the latissimus musculocutaneous flap. (E) Muscle used to seal off the skull base and line the cheek. (F) Short-term postoperative result.

When the palate has been resected as part of a major anterior skull base excision, its reconstruction is usually tied in with reconstruction of the maxillary and skull base defect (28). This has been handled in various ways, either by designing a skin flap with multiple skin paddles (29), one of which forms the palatal surface, or by filling the whole defect with a muscle flap and suspending it aloft by either a dental plate or a sheet of Alloderm. In a matter of weeks, the exposed muscle in the roof of the mouth will have mucosalized (30). However, skull base reconstruction is discussed elsewhere.

Oropharynx

Oropharyngeal defects rarely exist in isolation. They are most commonly part of a defect produced by resection of tumors of the posterior tongue or floor of mouth. Alternatively, they are sometimes part of a pharyngeal resection for tumors of the larynx or laryngopharynx. Historically, they have been reconstructed as a single defect using the same flap. In the case of oral lesions invading the oropharynx, deltopectoral and pectoralis major flaps have been used and are still the first choice in many centers. The supraclavicular artery flap (Figure 36-3) works reasonably well and has the advantage of having a closer point of rotation. Gastric pull-up (31) operations have been used for pharyngeal defects but are not so reliable when these defects extend as high as the nasopharynx.

FREE FLAPS FOR INTRAORAL RECONSTRUCTION

These free flaps include:

1. Radial forearm flap (32)
2. Ulnar forearm flap (33)
3. Anterolateral thigh (ALT) flap (34,35)
4. Rectus abdominis flap (36)
5. Dorsalis pedis flap (37,38)
6. Latissimus dorsi (39)
7. Osteocutaneous flaps as part of oromandibular reconstruction (discussed elsewhere)
   a. Fibula (40,41)
   b. Iliac crest (42)
   c. Scapula (43)
   d. Radius (44)
   e. Tibia (45)

INDICATIONS FOR SPECIFIC FLAPS

Many clinical scenarios necessitate free flap intraoral reconstruction, and many of them have been alluded to already. However, it is impossible to describe every possible defect where this surgery is indicated. Nevertheless, in this discussion of the major situations encountered and the methods of dealing with them, it is hoped that a general set of principles will become apparent and that these might then be applied to conditions and combinations of conditions not yet encountered.

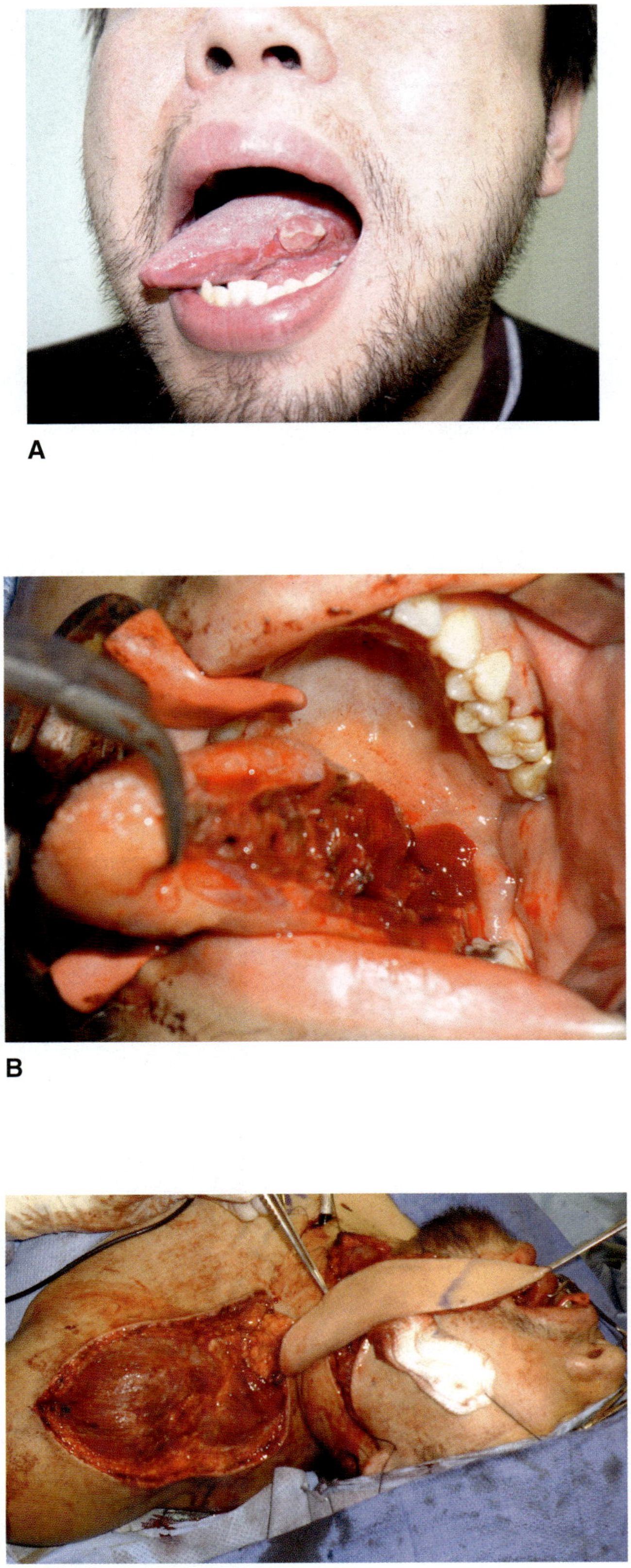

A

B

C

FIGURE 36-3 Oropharyngeal defect repaired using a supraclavicular island flap based on a specific branch of the transverse cervical artery. (**A**) The lesion occupied the left side of the tongue, adjacent floor of mouth, and oropharynx. (**B**) Anterior portion of the defect after excision of the tumor. (**C**) Supraclavicular island fasciocutaneous flap elevated and rotated. The tunneled portion will be deepithelialized.

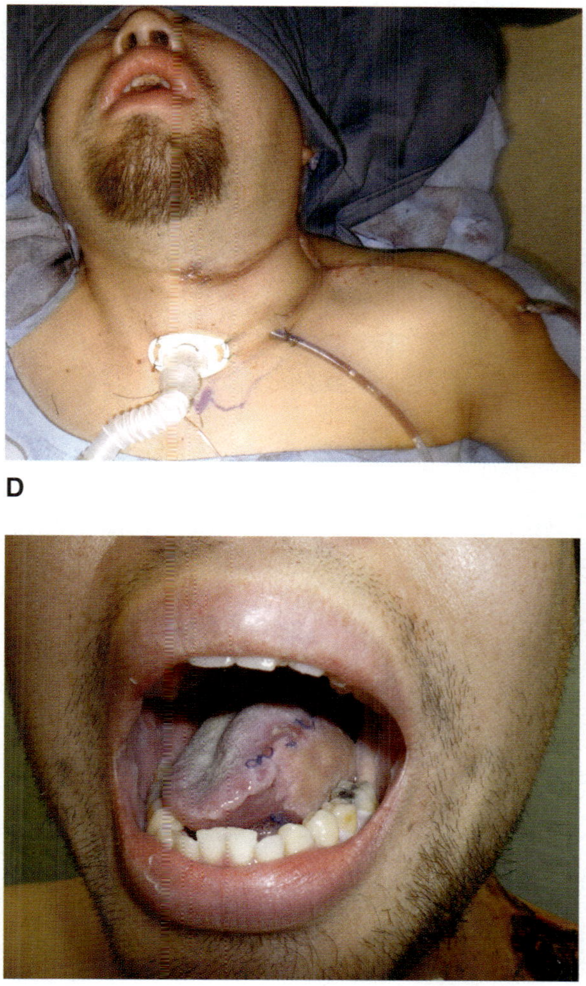

FIGURE 36-3 (*Continued*) (D) The donor site is closed directly. (E) Postoperative view.

The Lips

The use of microvascular transfer, specifically an innervated radial forearm flap, is an elegant way to reconstruct the whole aesthetic unit of the lower lip (46) using sensate tissue without adding further scars to the face (Figure 36-4). Because of the utility of conservative methods for defects of 50% or even more, microvascular transfer has its best indication when the deficiency is total or subtotal. The upper lip (47) may be reconstructed by the same means (Figure 36-5).

The radial forearm flap combines thinness, reinnervation potential and a contained palmaris longus tendon for lip suspension (see Figure 36-4). Some surgeons might prefer the ulnar forearm flap, which shares much of the anatomy, on the basis of its scar being less conspicuous. However, the skin flap for a total lip reconstruction occupies most of the anterior wrist and distal forearm, whichever is selected, the cosmetic result being equally suboptimal.

The other vital component in lower lip reconstruction is the maintenance of a soft tissue "dam." The palmaris longus tendon—used as a sling—replaces the orbicularis muscle of the lower lip and is included within the forearm flap, thus

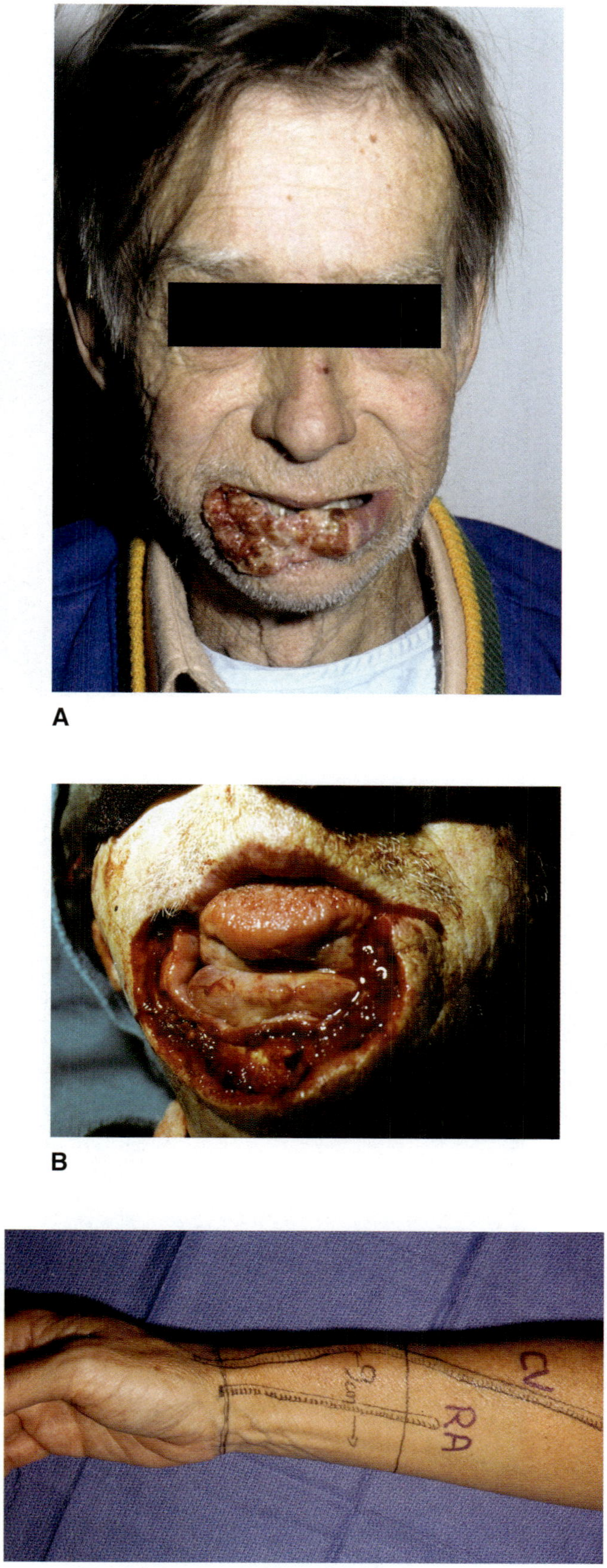

FIGURE 36-4 Lower lip reconstruction using an innervated and suspended radial forearm flap (A) and (B) The lower lip was completely resected for an advanced squamous cell carcinoma. (C) The radial forearm donor site centered over the palmaris tendon.

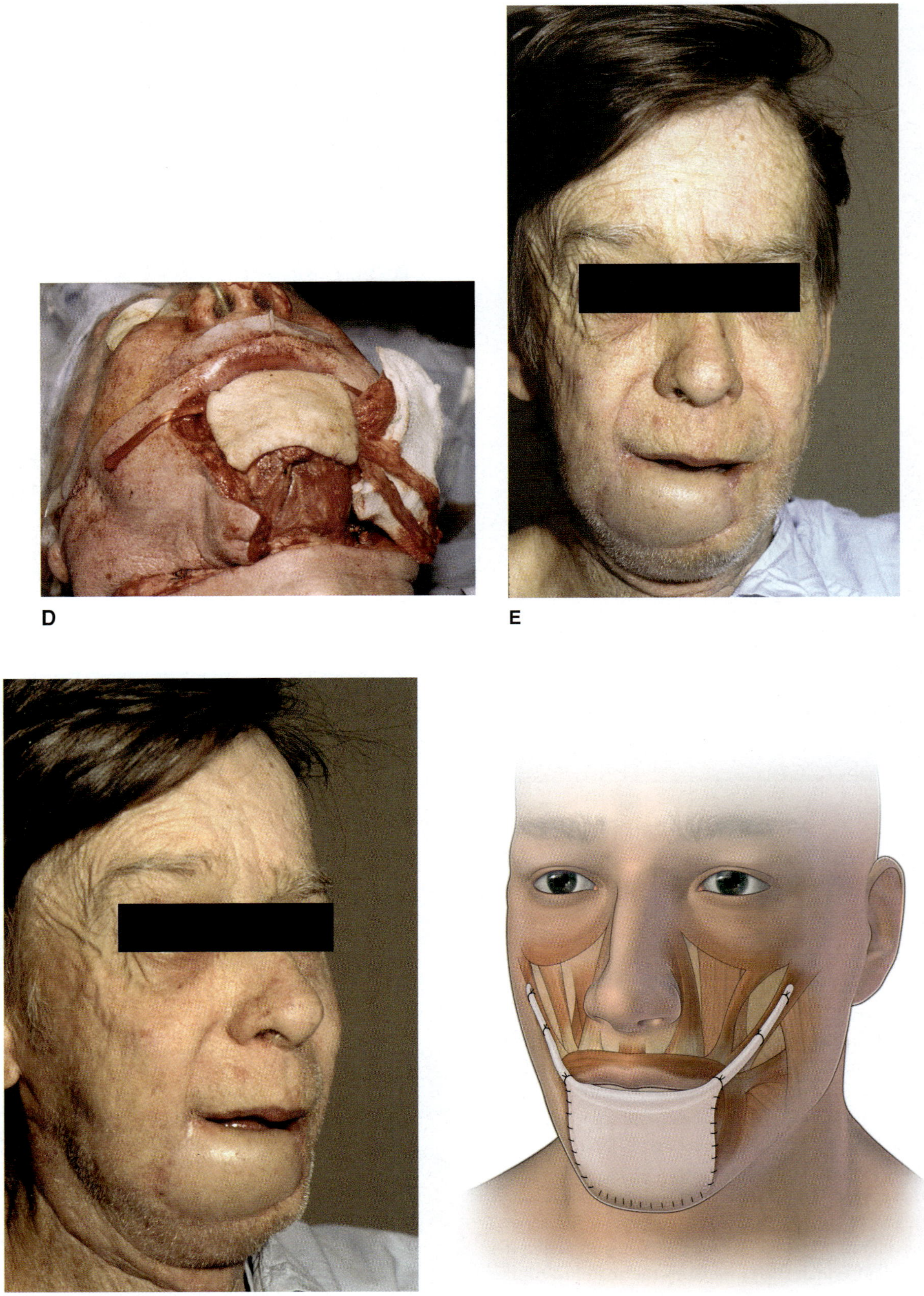

D E F G

FIGURE 36-4 *(Continued)* (D) The lateral antebrachial cutaneous nerve was anastomosed to one mental nerve and the medial antebrachial cutaneous nerve to the other. (E) and (F) The final result at 6 months. (G). Method of tendon suspension. The palmaris is fixed at each modiolus and then to the zygomaticus major at two points in each cheek. Nonabsorbable sutures are used. For access, an incision is made in the nasolabial fold and another parallel to it between the nasolabial fold and the zygoma.

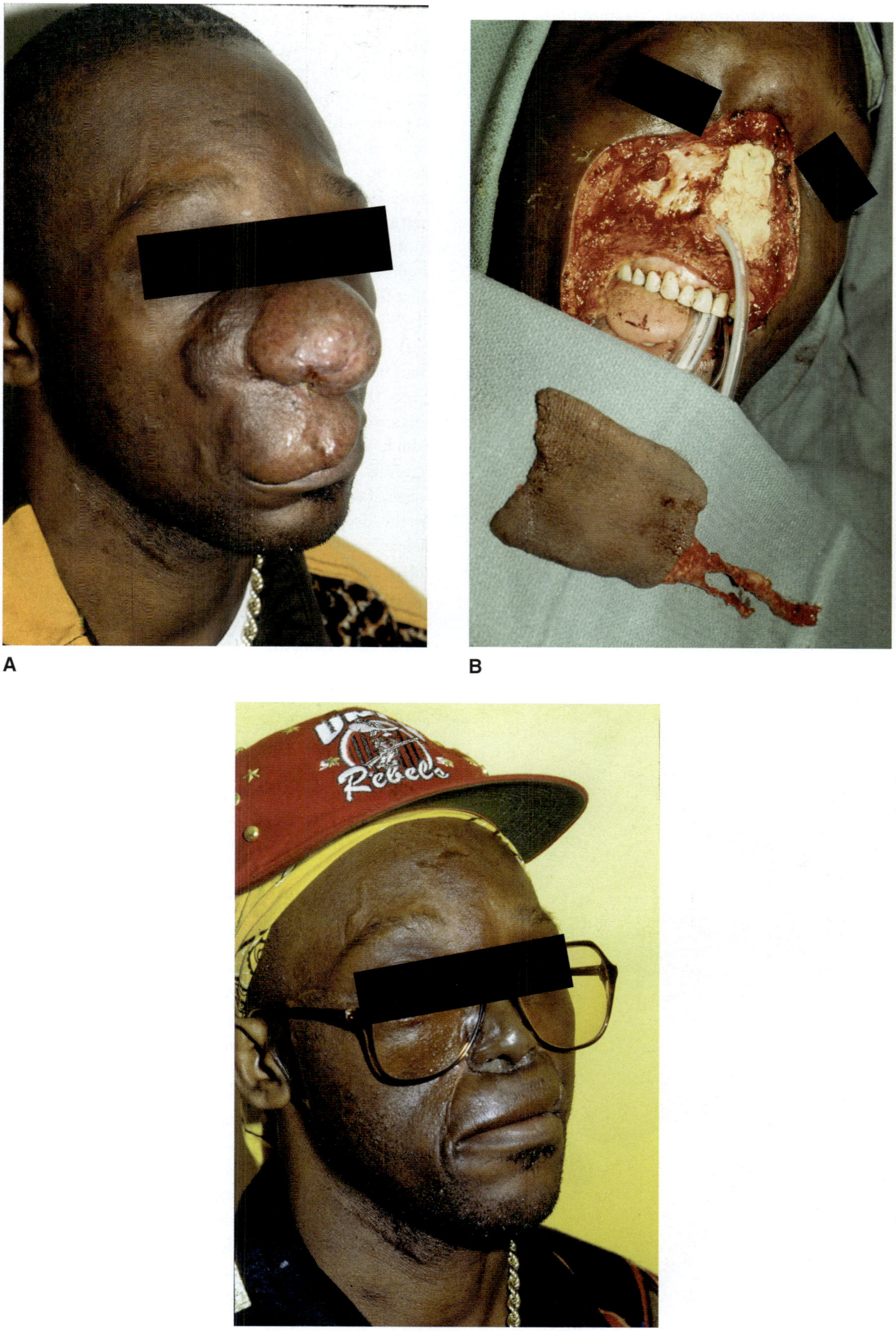

FIGURE 36-5 (A) to (C) A patient with an arteriovenous malformation involving his central face. After radical excision, the upper lip was reconstructed using a folded radial forearm flap. Suspension was not necessary. The flap was reinnervated using the infraorbital nerve on the right side. A delayed nasal reconstruction was planned, but the patient preferred to use a prosthesis.

becoming a "vascularized tendon graft." Fixation of the tendon graft should be multifocal to eliminate slippage and to tie it into the muscles of facial expression, specifically, the zygomaticus major (see Figure 36-4G). It is sutured to each modiolus under moderate tension using nonabsorbable 4:0 mattress sutures and then to the zygomaticus major at two points in each cheek, small incisions being made for the purpose. It is inadvisable to fix it to bone because all movement would be thereby abolished. Some surgeons have advocated reconstruction of the red lip using tongue flaps (48). However, the oral component of the flap often "mucosalizes," making this step redundant (Figure 36-6).

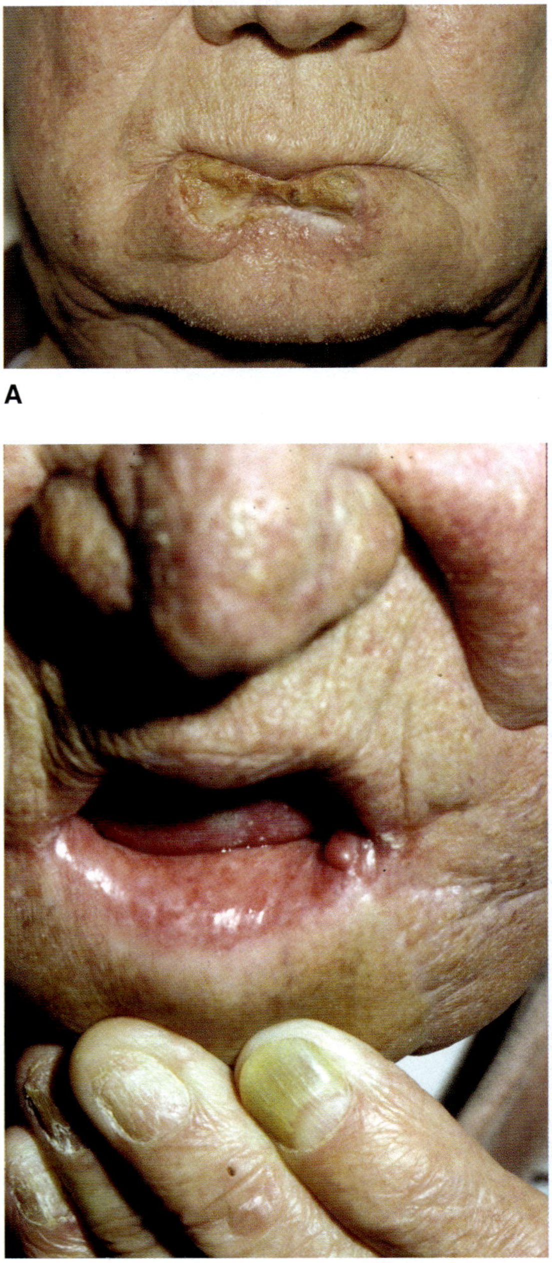

A

B

FIGURE 36-6 (A) Squamous cell carcinoma of the lower lip. (B) Subtotal reconstruction using an innervated, folded, and suspended radial forearm flap. Note the "mucosalization" along the lip line.

Composite Defects

The most frequent condition in most head and neck centers is the composite defect in which a squamous cell carcinoma arises in the floor of mouth and invades the mandible. Reconstruction of oromandibular defects are handled elsewhere, but a few principles should be noted as they apply to the intraoral component. It is probably true that osteocutaneous flaps are selected more for the bony requirement than for the mucosal replacement. For example, the fibula, as well as being the best all-round flap, is unparalleled in its ability to reconstruct angle-to-angle defects. Its skin paddle, although not as thin and pliable as either forearm flap, can still be reinnervated and is vastly superior to that associated with the iliac crest or scapula, both of which can be rather bulky. It follows that when the mandible is not reconstructed or is reconstructed simply by a plate, then the best option for oral lining will come from the forearm. The iliac crest has an extremely bulky skin paddle, which is difficult to use intraorally because it lies external to the natural curvature of the bone. If mucosa is required, then the internal oblique muscle can be taken on the ascending branch of the deep circumflex iliac artery, sutured into the mucosal defect, and allowed to epithelialize. Although the unosteotomized iliac crest makes an excellent hemimandible, this must be weighed against the increased risk of donor site bulge or hernia when the internal oblique is taken in this way. Certainly, for bone-only reconstruction of the hemimandible, the iliac crest still leads the pack. Unfortunately, nowadays, few surgeons are familiar with it. The fibula can certainly be made to serve adequately.

The scapula osteocutaneous flap is an excellent option for oromandibular reconstruction, particularly for through-and-through defects, because two independent paddles of skin may be obtained. In emaciated individuals (many patients with oral cancer are emaciated), these are thin enough to provide a good functional mucosal replacement. However, they cannot be reinnervated, and the repositioning of the patient required for elevation—and again for insetting—presents significant hurdles for the reconstructive team.

The radial forearm osteocutaneous flap is an excellent solution for small straight lateral defects of bone and mucosa. The problem is obviously the risk of radial fracture. This is rare if the surgeon is in the habit of doing the operation week in and week out. However, there are now few such individuals, since the fibula is used in 90% of cases.

Finally, the tibia–dorsalis–pedis (TDP) osteocutaneous free flap has recently been used for oromandibular reconstruction (45) and is described elsewhere in this text. The flap consists of a unicortical tibial bone graft centered on the middle third of the anterolateral surface of the tibia, elevated on the anterior tibial artery, and incorporating the dorsalis pedis skin flap. This unit has two distinct advantages over the fibula: a bone "height" similar to the mandible and a thin, supple skin paddle, which may be reinnervated, and is almost completely independent of the bone. Furthermore, osseointegration is easy with the excellent bone stock. Because it is new, the place that this flap will play in oromandibular reconstruction awaits peer evaluation.

Selection and design of the skin flap as well as its orientation to the attached bone and its final positioning in the mouth are of vital importance. To obtain the best possible result, it is useful to know *in advance* what size the defect will be and how many surfaces it will involve. Some head and neck surgeons are good at estimating this; unfortunately, others are not. Even with the best, microscopic spread of disease is often detected on frozen section, and wider excisions than expected are frequently encountered. A full head and neck examination and reference to a computed tomography scan will certainly be helpful but unfortunately not definitive. Prior knowledge permits the reconstructive surgeon to harvest a flap with the appropriate dimensions simultaneously with the ablation. When the estimate remains indefinite, then larger skin flaps need to be take taken "just in case" the defect has been underestimated. Reducing the size of a skin paddle after it has been raised can prove tricky and occasionally dangerous.

Through-and-Through Defects

Generally, the biggest challenges are *through-and-through* defects in which mucosa, skin, and often the mandible are all required. Two flaps are occasionally necessary, although many free flaps can carry two separate skin islands (Figure 36-7). Free tissue transfer, preferably using a reinnervated flap, is still the best replacement for anterior floor of mouth, lip, and tongue defects with or without a bony component. Thinness and pliability together with the capacity for reinnervation make the forearm flaps a popular choice for this task. However, the donor scar bothers many patients as well as physicians and has led to the development of the *thinned* ALT flap (49). The donor site of the ALT flap is often closed directly without a skin graft and is more readily concealed. Reinnervation is possible using the lateral sural cutaneous nerve (lateral cutaneous nerve of the thigh).

Palatal Reconstruction and Cheek Reconstruction

In palatal defects, as well as cheek defects, reinnervation of the flap used in reconstruction is not so important because these regions play a lesser role in mastication, speech, and oral continence. However, it is advisable to use thin flaps that do not physically intrude into the oral cavity where excessive bulk and redundancy might interfere with normal function. Although a dental plate with an obturator will often be sufficient to close large palatal defects; in younger patients, a definitive closure may be preferable to avoid the necessity of wearing a lifelong prosthesis. The cutaneous skin paddle of the flap selected for oromandibular reconstruction may close adjacent palatal defects resulting from large composite resections.

For isolated palatal defects, small forearm flaps permit primary closure of the donor site and an excellent cosmetic outcome. In reconstruction of the palate, a pathway needs to be tunneled through the cheek to bring the vascular pedicle to either the facial or the temporal vessels for microvascular anastomosis (Figure 36-8). A two-layer closure is desirable but not

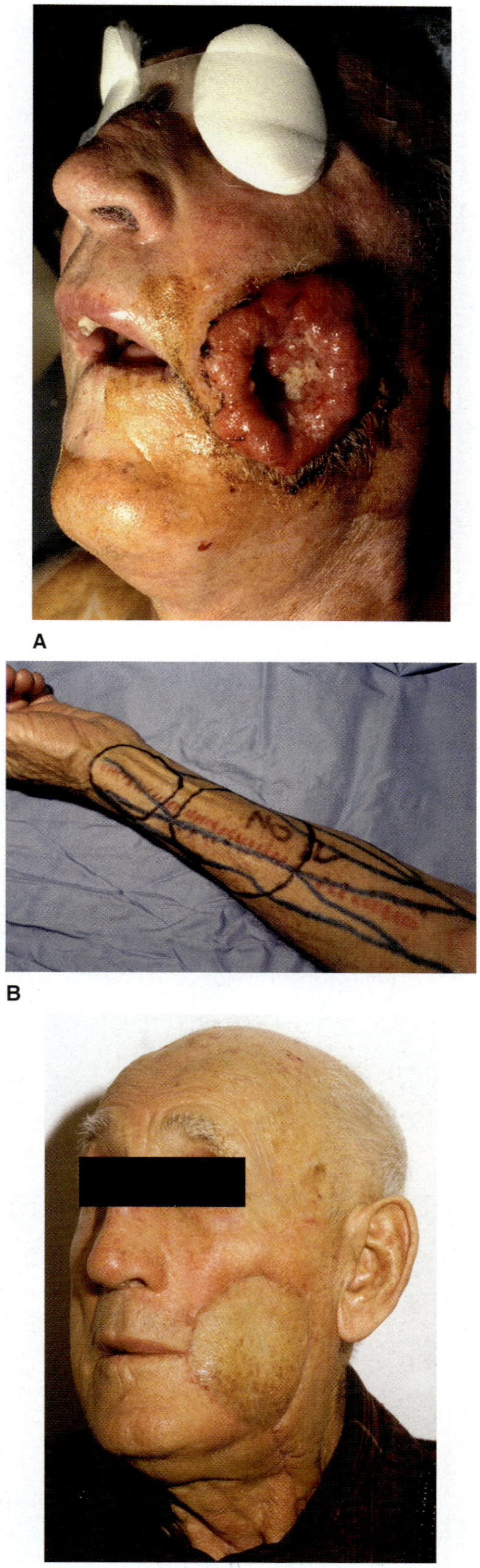

A B C

FIGURE 36-7 Through-and-through defect reconstructed using a radial forearm flap with two skin islands. (A) Exophytic low-grade squamous cell carcinoma involving cheek skin and mucosa but sparing the mandible. (B) Double-paddle radial forearm flap. (C) Postoperative image at 1 month. The distal pedicle was used for mucosal replacement and the proximal one for skin cover.

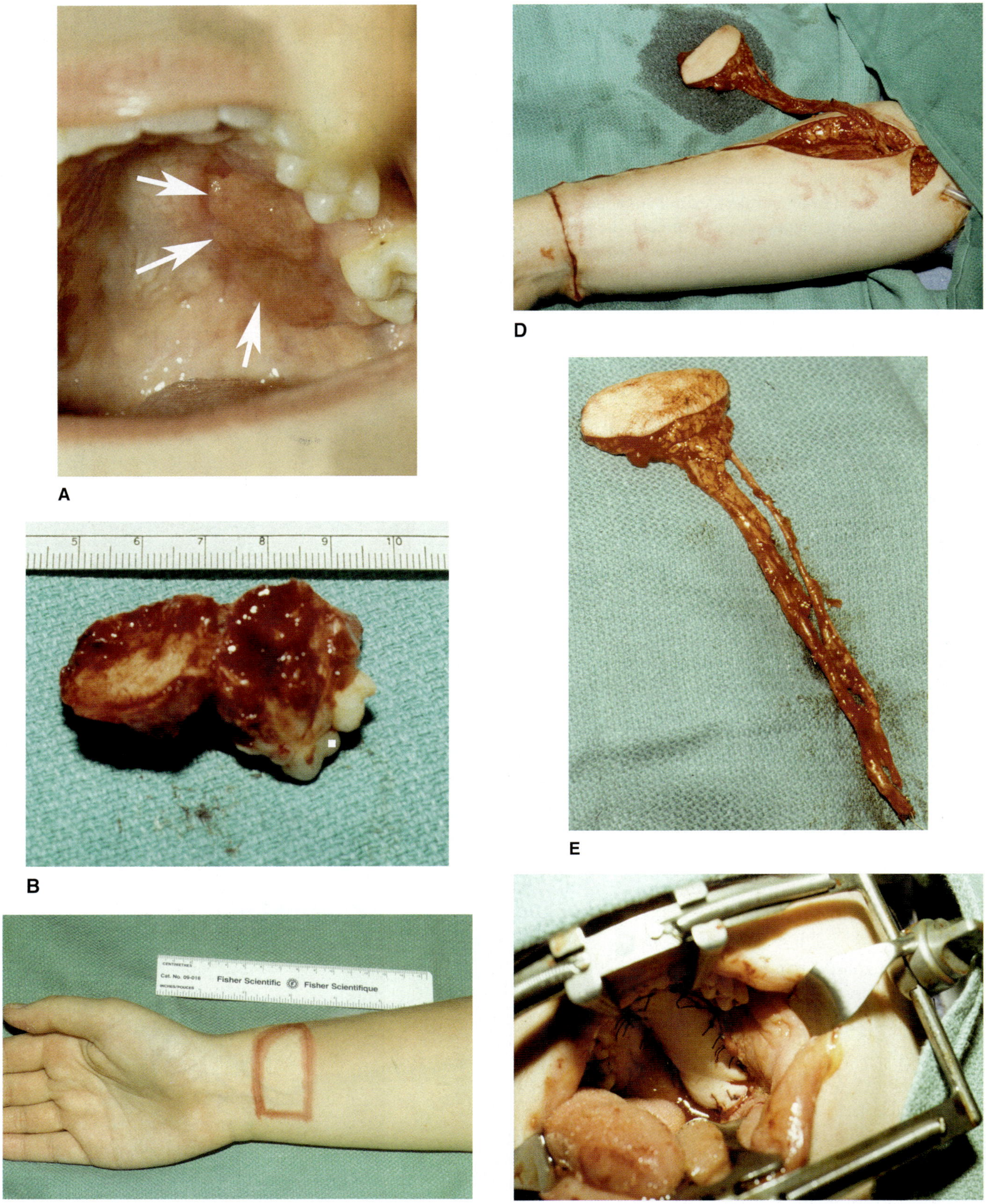

FIGURE 36-8 Palatal repair using a radial forearm flap with primary closure of donor site. (**A**) Malignant salivary gland tumor arising in palatal mucosa in a 26-year-old woman. (**B**) Excised specimen consisting a portion of the palate and adjacent alveolar ridge. (**C**) Small radial forearm flap designed on the thinnest skin of the anterior wrist. (**D**) The defect closed primarily using an ulnar based rotation flap. (**E**) Flap elevated on a long pedicle that may be used to access vessels in the neck, in this case the facial artery and vein. (**F**) Defect repaired and the flap revascularized.

essential, provided the flap overlaps the adjacent hard palate. Double-paddle forearm flaps have been used but are generally too bulky. However, septal mucosal flaps, superiorly based pharyngeal flaps, or adjacent turnover flaps (in a delayed setting) may be considered for the nasal layer when adequate overlap is not possible. Other thin free flaps such as the dorsalis pedis or a thinned anterolateral free flap can work well, depending on the patient's constitution and the surgeon's preference.

Palatal defects that are part of larger maxillary or skull base injuries are dealt with elsewhere.

Tongue and Floor of Mouth

A significant advantage of free tissue transfer is the possibility of reinnervation by anastomosing of a sensory nerve serving the skin flap to the stump of the lingual or mental nerves in the recipient site (see Figure 36-4). As mentioned earlier, sensory recovery is most important in the areas of the tongue, floor of mouth, and lower lip (50). Innervated tissue in these sites is not only the best protection against drooling but also greatly improves oral hygiene and facilitates mastication, thereby enhancing the quality of life. Flaps that best lend themselves to reinnervation include the fibula flap, the lateral thigh flap, and both forearm flaps (Figure 36-9). The recipient nerve is preferably the lingual in end-to-end fashion, but an end-to-side fashion may be adequate if the nerve has not been divided. The mental nerve may also be considered as a recipient, particularly for lower lip reconstruction. The efficacy of reinnervating intraoral flaps has been questioned (51), but it has clearly been shown that the acuity of sensation restored in this way not only resembles that of the recipient site but also is superior to the flap's sensation in its native site before elevation and transfer. In other words, the sensory acuity of a reinnervated flap depends more on the recipient than on the donor nerve (48). This process is termed *sensory upgrading*.

Although the medial antebrachial (MABC) and lateral antebrachial cutaneous (LABC) nerves share the innervation of the anterior wrist, there is considerable overlap, and it has been shown that full sensation may be regained by using the LABC nerve alone (52). In dissecting out the nerve, it is vital to first identify it in the proximal forearm where it lies medial to and in the same plane as the cephalic vein. It is seldom more than 1 cm from this vessel, although it can lie volar or dorsal to it. As it travels distally, it breaks up into smaller branches before entering the proximal border of the flap. By maintaining connective tissue around these branches, the integrity of the nerve may be preserved.

Small defects of the tongue may be sutured or skin grafted as long as tethering is not produced. Hemitongue and some partial

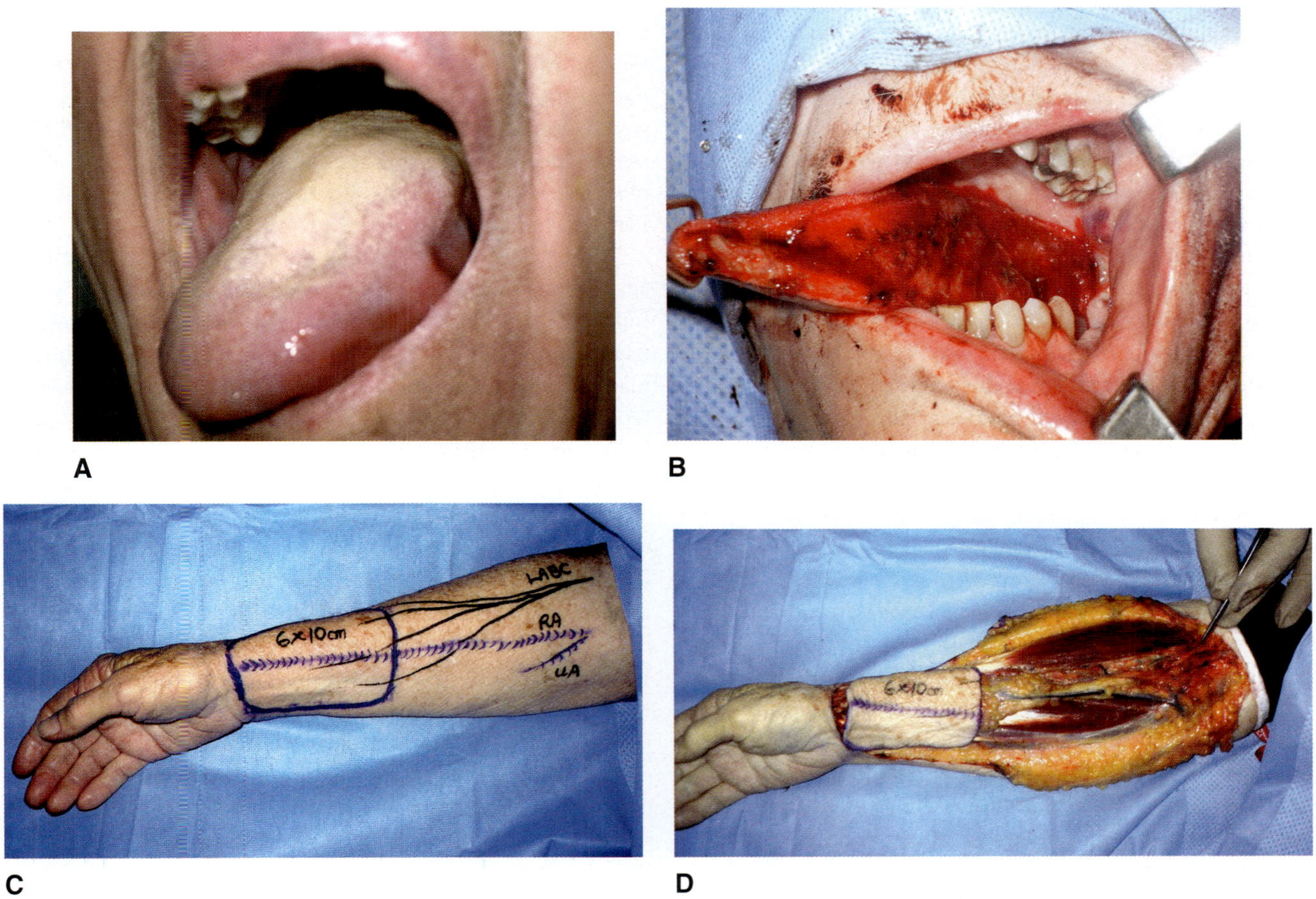

FIGURE 36-9 An innervated radial forearm flap used for hemitongue reconstruction. (A) The patient presents with an indurated ulcer on the left lateral tongue. It was biopsied as squamous cell carcinoma. (B) A hemitongue resection was carried out in addition to a left neck dissection. (C) and (D) The lateral antebrachial cutaneous nerve (LABCN) is identified proximally in the forearm, where it lies deep and usually on the medial side of the cephalic vein. If it is necessary to use the medial antebrachial cutaneous nerve (MABCN), this structure may be found close to the basilic vein.

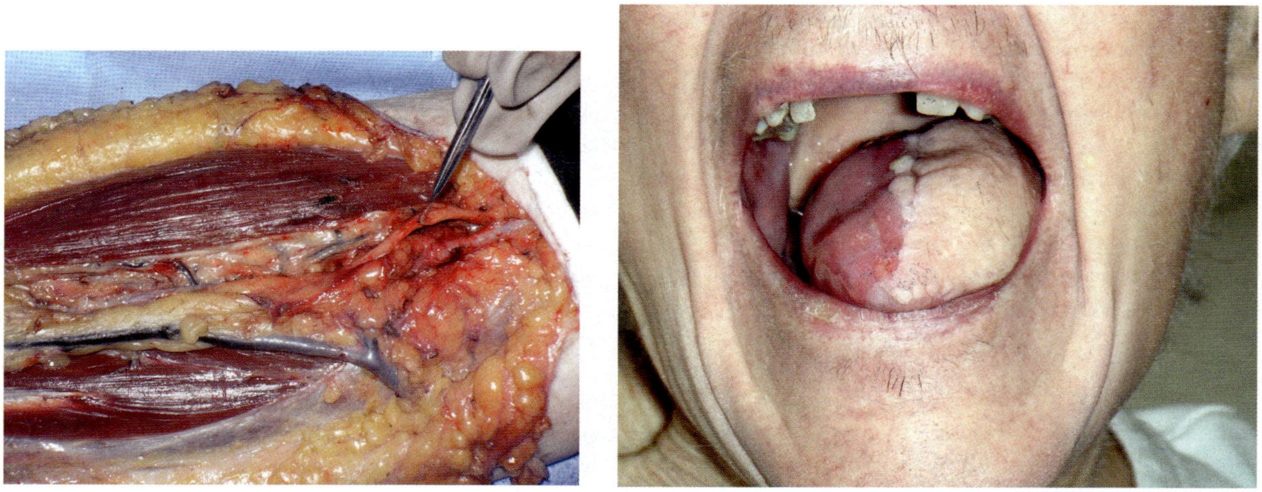

E F

FIGURE 36-9 (*Continued*) (**E**) The LABC nerve is a fairly large structure in the proximal forearm. It is dissected distally, and its branches are preserved as they enter the proximal border of the flap. (**F**) The tongue reconstruction. Excellent sensation may be anticipated in 6 to 9 months if the LABC is sutured to the divided stump of the lingual nerve.

tongue defects are ideally reconstructed using an innervated forearm fasciocutaneous flap, the relatively small bulk of the flap being adequate for the purpose. Reconstruction of total and subtotal tongue and defects is more controversial. Some argue that total glossectomy patients should have a concomitant laryngectomy to prevent aspiration. In this case, virtually any cutaneous free flap (or cutaneous component of an osteocutaneous flap when there is also a mandibular defect) would be suitable. However, current concepts envisage the creation of a "neotongue" with a bulky flap. This enables articulation with the palate to facilitate swallowing and speech. Furthermore, a prominent neotongue funnels food and saliva into the lateral gutters during swallowing to minimize aspiration. Suitable flaps for this purpose are the rectus abdominis (53) and latissimus dorsi (54) musculocutaneous flaps and the ALT perforator flap (55). Deep inferior epigastric artery perforator flaps have also been used (56).

Haughey used the latissimus dorsi musculocutaneous flap (57), reinnervating the muscle by joining the thoracodorsal to the hypoglossal nerve. The muscle is oriented transversely suspended to the skull base and forming a dynamic sling for the sagitally positioned skin paddle, which constitutes the tongue proper. The neotongue thus actively articulates with the roof of the mouth and aids in speech as well as swallowing. Others have described using transverse gracilis (58), rectus abdominis (59), and ALT musculocutaneous flaps (60), also with motor function. However, the author of the last citation, in an excellent review (61), concluded: "A review of the literature and our own experience does not seem to show substantial advantages of functional muscle for tongue reconstruction." Suspension of the larynx to the mandible with heavy static sutures (62) helps prevent aspiration and may be superior to attempts at restoring muscle function.

In optimizing the function of the reconstructed tongue, the provision of sensation would appear to be of more benefit. The innervated radial forearm flap is capable of achieving near normal oral sensation; however, although adequate for a hemitongue, it lacks the requisite bulk for a total or subtotal reconstruction. The rectus abdominis is bulky, but its segmental nerves are 70% motor, resulting in suboptimal sensory recovery (63). A better choice is the ALT flap, which can be harvested with the lateral sural cutaneous nerve, a purely sensory nerve. Yu has shown that not only do the patients regain sensation superior to that in the donor site, but they also have improved swallowing and overall patient satisfaction (60). He sutures the upper part of the flap to the gingival and pharyngeal mucosa, as one would expect. However, an inferior extension is deepithelialized, folded forward, and secured to the inferior arch of the mandible via drill holes so as to reconstruct the floor of mouth. Laryngeal suspension is also used.

It is a feature of total tongue reconstruction that an initially adequate neotongue will shrink over time, resulting in a loss of function. Muscular atrophy—in the case of musculocutaneous flaps—and the effects of postoperative radiation are mainly to blame. Some initial overcorrection is therefore acceptable, and fat grafting may be considered later.

As part of oromandibular reconstruction, it is also possible to reinnervate the cutaneous component of an osteocutaneous flap and provide improved oral function. As mentioned before, this is particularly advantageous with defects in the anterior floor of mouth, lower lip, and tongue. The innervation of the forearm flaps has already been discussed, and they have indeed been used as innervated flaps for composite reconstruction. However, because of the forearm bone's insufficiency and the risk of fracture at the donor site, the fibula is generally preferred over the radius for bony replacement. Sensation to most of the skin of the lateral leg is supplied from the lateral sural cutaneous nerve (64), a branch of the lateral peroneal (65,66), and the *recurrent branch* of the superficial peroneal nerve (RSPN), a branch of the superficial peroneal nerve (65). This LSCN is easily identified approximately 2.5 to 5.0 cm behind the center of the fibula head. From here, the nerve may be dissected distally until it enters the proximal border of the skin paddle and then used as the "donor" sensory nerve when the fibula osteocutaneous flap is transferred (Figure 36-10). The RSPN

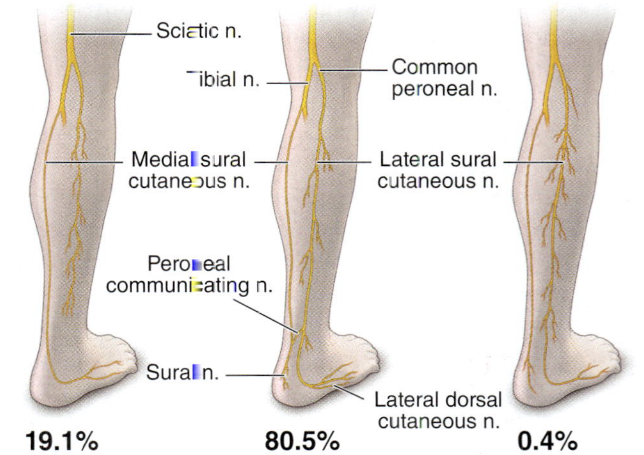

A

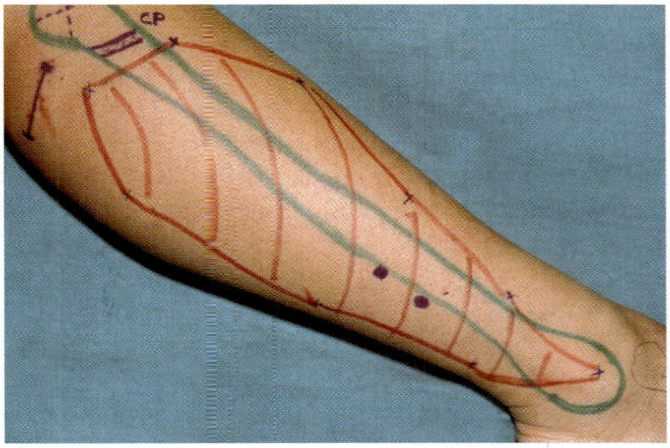

B

FIGURE 36-10 Location of LSCN and functional neurosome. (**A**) Drawing of the anatomic variations of the sural nerve (aka medial sural cutaneous nerve) after Huelke (64). It is the lateral sural cutaneous nerve that innervates the cutaneous of the fibula flap. n, nerve. (**B**) A horizontal line can be drawn from a point 2 cm to a point 5 cm posterior to the midpoint of the fibula head. The lateral antebrachial cutaneous nerve (LABC) lies within this area. If a block is produced by the injection of a local anesthetic solution, a large area of numbness (marked green) is produced. This is the "neurosome" of the LABC.

branches off the superficial peroneal nerve 8 cm proximal to the lateral malleolar tip (range, 4.2–10.5 cm). From here, the RSPN travels horizontally or slightly distally for approximately 3 to 5 cm before coursing superiorly to innervate the cutaneous tissue of the distal, lateral calf (63). The skin of the lateral calf thus has a dual, overlapping innervation supplied by the LSCN and the RSPN. One or other of these nerves may be dominant, and the dominant one should be selected for neurorrhaphy. Selective nerve blocks are used to determine dominance preoperatively (63).

Pharyngeal Reconstruction

Alternatives for pharyngeal reconstruction are free jejunal transfers (67) or tubed cutaneous flaps such as the radial forearm (68) and ALT (69). However, pharyngeal reconstruction will be formally dealt with elsewhere.

Isolated oropharyngeal defects, when they occur, are amenable to closure using the regional flaps mentioned earlier. It is in this relatively rare scenario that in the future minimal access surgery may have a part to play if a free flap were selected.

PREPARATION OF THE RECIPIENT SITE

In cases of major tumor ablation, much of the recipient site has been exposed and to some degree prepared. When looking at a defect in the oral lining, it is important to identify its mucosal perimeter. This should be a continuous line of divided mucosa that rejoins itself after passing around and delineating the excision. It will not be a simple circle but rather a complex shape, frequently doubling back and at times plunging deeply into the pharynx. Nevertheless, the entire circuit of cut mucosal edge should be identified and each portion assessed for suture placement. Ragged, devascularized, and torn borders should be excised. Sometimes the divided mucosa passes onto the gums, lying very close to mandibular bone. In such cases, the periosteum, together with the mucosa, should be elevated off the underlying hard structures to obtain a cuff of tissue that will take a suture. Occasionally, bone will protrude and impinge on the prospective closure. It is reasonable to remove small spikes of bone with a rongeur to prevent them from intruding on the suture line.

When a neck dissection has been performed, recipient vessels are usually visible. Head and neck surgeons knowledgeable about microsurgery will preserve the external jugular vein while leaving the major branches of the external carotid artery intact and often the internal jugular vein as well. Vessels are selected on the basis of their proximity, diameter, and ease of access for the vascular pedicle of the flap. Radiated vessels can usually be used without problems (70). The branches of the external carotid artery are convenient recipient vessels, and it is quite reasonable to use the *external* carotid artery itself in end-to-end manner when a larger diameter is required. Use of the facial artery is common. It sometimes helps to dissect it to its origin to increase pedicle length. Division of the posterior belly of the digastric muscle facilitates this exposure. Both the internal jugular vein and the external carotid artery can be used in an end-to-side manner if necessary.

In cases when there are no available veins left in the neck, it is possible to divide the cephalic vein in the arm and dissect it cranially to the point where it pierces the clavipectoral fascia. Thus, a long recipient vein, unaffected by radiotherapy or a neck dissection, is available for direct usage or for the construction of an A-V loop (70). In the presence of a tracheostomy, the anterior jugular vein should only be selected as a recipient with extreme caution. There is a chance that it may have been tied off, the tracheostomy tube flange may impinge upon it, or contamination from the stoma may result in thrombosis.

When a neck dissection has not taken place, then deep vessel access becomes more difficult, but vessel availability is better. The external jugular vein remains the first choice for venous drainage and is easily located because it can be palpated through the skin. It is found below the mandibular angle deep to platysma. The external carotid artery is approached directly by dissecting medially close to the anterior border of the sternocleidomastoid muscle. Occasionally, it is feasible to access the facial artery and vein as they cross the body of the mandible. They are exposed via a submandibular incision in which the marginal mandibular branch of the facial nerve is identified a finger's breadth below the mandibular body, deep to the platysma and usually superficial to the facial vein; it is thereby safeguarded. The superficial temporal vessels are available in the immediate preauricular area. These vessels, although convenient, are often small. However, they are useful recipients in isolated reconstructions of the upper buccal cavity. When a radical neck dissection has been performed, these vessels are likely to have been ligated proximally and should not be used. Occasionally, the vein is too small to use, and the cephalic vein may be turned up as described earlier.

Crossing to the opposite side of the neck is occasionally necessary when the ipsilateral vessels have been damaged by previous surgery or severe radiation. Careful planning is required, not only in flap selection but also in positioning the skin paddle so as to obtain maximal usable pedicle length. Vein grafts are occasionally needed.

INSET OF THE FLAP

The flap is sutured into position before definitive bony fixation so that full access to the posterior limit of the defect may be achieved. Before this is done, the bone may be temporarily fitted in place to make sure that there will be no orientation problems. Closure is performed using a single horizontal mattress layer of 3:0 Vicryl. Because of the potentially catastrophic consequences of a leak, the closure must be watertight. The surgeon should be aware of the size and circumference of the flap so he or she can adjust the spacing of sutures to best accommodate it to the defect. If the flap is much larger than the defect, it should be trimmed to avoid the functional loss that would result in cramming too much bulk into the mouth.

In cases of total or subtotal tongue reconstruction, the floor of mouth must be reconstructed as part of the repair. As mentioned above, the inferior third of the flap may be deepithelialized, rotated forward, and fixed to the lower border of the anterior mandibular arch using drill holes and nonabsorbable sutures as mentioned earlier. This stabilizes the floor of the mouth.

ANASTOMOSES

After the intraoral suturing is complete, the neuroanastomosis is performed followed by the microanastomoses of the vessels. Nerve anastomosis is preferably to a divided stump of the lingual nerve for tongue and lateral floor of mouth reconstructions. However, if the lip or anterior floor of mouth is being reconstructed, the mental nerve is preferred. When these nerves remain undivided, then an end-to-side anastomosis can be contemplated, but the quality of sensation will be less (71). Sensory recovery will also be suboptimal when other somatic sensory nerves of the head and neck, such as the greater auricular or branches of the cervical plexus, are used. These nerves have a smaller cortical representation on the sensory homunculus, and this, it is believed, results in a poorer sensory recovery.

Vascular anastomoses are routine. The artery is sutured using standard microvascular techniques while the veins may be joined using a coupler. Frequently, the veins exceed the diameter of the largest coupler and must be sutured conventionally. When closing the wound, kinks in the vessels must be avoided, and drains should be positioned without impingement on the vascular pedicle, the recipient vessels, or the anastomoses. Finally, tracheostomy ties should be avoided to limit external compression of the vessels; the flanges of the tube should be simply sutured to the skin in the anterior neck.

POSTOPERATIVE MONITORING

Intraoral flaps can be difficult to monitor directly, particularly when they lie posterior in the mouth and when the jaw has been reconstructed. Nevertheless, observations on the capillary return of the flap are extremely useful and should be performed if at all possible. Doppler readings from perforators on the flap or the vascular pedicle in the neck are reasonably reliable and can be performed percutaneously by the nursing staff.

Other than that, the implantable laser Doppler has its adherents (72), and tissue oxygen saturation (StO_2) probes (73) are being adapted for intraoral use. Flap monitoring is discussed more fully elsewhere.

POTENTIAL COMPLICATIONS

The vascular complications associated with microvascular surgery in general apply to free flaps used for intraoral reconstruction. Venous or arterial occlusion can occur because of kinking, hematoma, or infection. Close monitoring facilitates early and aggressive take-back—the only hope of rescue.

If an intraoral flap is lost either because of unrecognized vascular compromise or after multiple take-backs with anastomotic revisions, then—as with any surgery—a "plan B" must be available. Plan B may consist of a second free flap or, if not practical, a regional pedicled flap such as a pectoralis musculocutaneous flap or a supraclavicular artery fasciocutaneous flap. The aim of the second flap is to seal the oral cavity and protect the great vessels of the neck.

Leaks from the intraoral suture line may produce inflammation and infection within the soft tissues of the neck. This, in turn, can lead to fistula formation, vascular thrombosis, and loss of the flap. Leaks should also be treated aggressively with exploration, wound toilet, and the insertion of a drain to create a "controlled" fistula remote from the microvascular repairs or major neck vessels. Antibiotic cover and tube feeds should also be used.

Hair growth within the mouth is common when the patient is hirsute, particularly when a radial forearm flap is used in the reconstruction. An advantage of the ulnar forearm flap is that it is less hairy. Oddly, hair is more a "cosmetic" than a functional problem. Often the hair disappears with time, either as a result of postoperative radiation or because of spontaneous epithelial metaplasia.

Bulky, nonsensate tissue used for intraoral reconstruction may interfere with speech, mastication, and swallowing. Failure in planning, constitutional factors, and poor flap selection may all contribute to an excess of tissue. Local excisions at a later stage (6 months) may remedy the situation to some extent.

If osteointegrated implants are inserted through skin flaps used for oral lining, the excessive movement around each pin can lead to infection and the formation of granulation tissue at the abutment (see Figure 36-1). Stripping the flap from the prospective alveolar ridge and replacing it with a skin graft before fitting the posts may avoid this complication. The mucosalization of exposed muscle flaps provides an excellent covering through which to insert osseointegrated implants. A skin graft is much less mobile and mimics gum mucosa more closely.

SECONDARY SURGERY

In general, primary definitive reconstruction is the goal after major head and neck cancer ablation. Secondary surgery is avoided if at all possible. The reason is that the 5-year survival rate is relatively poor, and it is highly desirable that the patient be allowed to spend his or her remaining days at home rather than in repeated admissions to the hospital for staged procedures. Nevertheless, although usually unplanned, secondary surgery may be required.

In the previous section, situations were outlined in which secondary surgery is required to deal with complications, and, of course, if a one-stage reconstruction is planned, then most secondary surgery is essentially surgery for complications.

When a total lower lip has been reconstructed with a radial forearm flap, it sometimes happens that the contained tendon graft becomes loose, and its suspensory function diminishes. The resulting oral incontinence usually necessitates a second tendon or fascial graft with multipoint fixation to the zygomaticus major muscles as well as to the oral commissures.

Poor function may necessitate debulking of tissues and scar releases. Flaps covering bone may be removed and replaced with skin grafts to facilitate osseointegrated implants. Secondary surgery may be required at donor sites for delayed wound healing, neuroma formation, tendon exposure, seroma, and hernia.

Other revisionary surgery concerning the osseous component of osteocutaneous flaps is dealt with in the chapter on mandibular reconstruction.

RESULTS AND OUTCOMES

Historically, the survival rate of free flaps used in the head and neck is well over 90% (74–79). However, the patient may not be cured of the disease and frequently experiences functional and aesthetic disabilities as a result of both the resection and the reconstruction. Many individuals succumb to their disease within a few years or even months. The extent of the disease, the volume of the resection, the location of the defect, the quality of the reconstruction, the incidence of complications, and the presence of comorbidities all influence residual function. Success may be measured by the quality of life remaining irrespective of its duration. Markers positively influencing the quality of life include:

1. Living at home
2. Living independently
3. Not tube dependent
4. Ability to eat in public
5. Ability to eat, taste, chew, and swallow
6. Ability to hold an intelligible conversation
7. Physical acceptance

Studies have shown better function when the tongue is reconstructed with a free flap as opposed to a pedicled musculocutaneous one (80). The capability of performing reconstructions in one stage has been greatly facilitated by microsurgery. It follows that the number of days spent at home will be increased as a result.

When it comes to oral function, it is fair to say that whatever remains after the resection is enhanced by the use of a thin, well-tailored flaps. Such flaps permit movement of the residual oral structures, which will enhance mastication, oral continence, and speech. Acceptably thin flaps include radial and ulnar forearm flaps; the thinned ALT flap; the skin component of a fibula flap; and, perhaps, the dorsalis pedis flap. However, in obese patients and in cases when the flap has not been tailored to the defect, bulk can still present a problem, resulting in restriction of movement, difficulty chewing, a "hot potato" voice, eversion of the lower lip, and oral incontinence.

As mentioned earlier, the sensory recovery after the reinnervation of a radial forearm flap used for intraoral reconstruction approaches normal and exceeds the sensory discrimination of the same tissue in the forearm before it is raised. Histologic differences between innervated and noninnervated radial forearm flaps have even been identified (81). The use of innervated flaps in critical areas (tongue, anterior floor of mouth) has been shown to enhance the quality of life by improving the awareness of saliva and food particles. This decreases pooling, aids oral hygiene, and facilitates oral continence and mastication. However, to date, there is little evidence that sensate flaps enhance speech.

Although the volume of tongue base resection plays an important role in the development of aspiration, free flap reconstruction does not seem to palliate the effect of the loss of functional tongue base volume, as regards swallowing-related quality of life (82).

There has been great progress in intraoral reconstruction over the past 30 years. Much of this has come in the train of microsurgical advances. As we fine tune our techniques, outcome studies become vital in the consolidation and extension of our knowledge for the benefit of our patients.

REFERENCES

1. Soutar DS, McGregor IA. The radial forearm flap in intraoral reconstruction: the experience of 60 consecutive cases. *Plast Reconstr Surg* 1986;78:1–8.
2. Acland RD, Flynn MB. Immediate reconstruction of oral cavity and oropharyngeal defects using microvascular free flaps. *Am J Surg* 1978;136:419–423.
3. Zuker RM, Rosen IB, Palmer JA, et al. Microvascular free flaps in head and neck reconstruction. *Can J Surg* 1980;23:157–162.
4. Urken ML, Buchbinder D, Weinberg H, et al. Functional evaluation following microvascular oromandibular reconstruction of the oral cancer patient: a comparative study of reconstructed and non-reconstructed patients. *Laryngoscope* 1991;101:935–950.

5. Abbe R. A new plastic operation for the relief of deformity due to double harelip. *Plast Reconstr Surg* 1968;42(5):481–483.
6. Estlander JA. A method of reconstructing loss of substance in one lip from the other lip. *Arch Klin Chir* 1872;14:622–631. (Reprinted in English: *Plast Reconstr Surg* 1968;42:361–366.)
7. Karapandzic M. Reconstruction of lip defects by local arterial flaps. *Br J Plast Surg* 1974;27:93–97.
8. Gillies HM. *Principles and Art of Plastic Surgery.* Boston: Little Brown, 1957, pp. 507–508.
9. Webster JP. Crescentic peri-alar cheek excision for upper lip flap advancement with a short history of upper lip repair. *Plast Reconstr Surg (1946)* 1955;16:434–464.
10. Conley JJ, DeAmesti F, Pierce MK. The use of tongue flaps in head and neck surgery. *Surgery* 1957;41:745–751.
11. Thiersch C. Verschluß eines Loches im harten Gaumen durch die Weichteile der Wange. *Arch Heilk* 1868;9:159–162.
12. Esser JF. Deckung von Gaumendefekten mittels gestielter Naso-Labial-Hautlappen. *Dtsch Zschr Chir* 1918;147:128–135.
13. Varghese BT, Sebastian P, Cherian T, et al. Nasolabial flaps in oral reconstruction: an analysis of 224 cases. *Br J Plast Surg* 2001;54:499–503.
14. Pribaz J, Stephens W, Crespo L, et al. A new intraoral flap: facial artery musculomucosal (FAMM) flap. *Plast Reconstr Surg* 1992;90:421–429.
15. Hurwitz DJ, Rabson JA, Futrell JW. The anatomic basis for the platysma skin flap. *Plast Reconstr Surg* 1983;72:302–314.
16. Coleman JJ 3rd, Jurkiewicz MJ, Nahai F, et al. The platysma musculocutaneous flap: experience with 24 cases. *Plast Reconstr Surg* 1983;72:315–323.
17. McGregor IA. The temporal flap in intra-oral cancer: its use in repairing the post-excisional defect. *Br J Plast Surg* 1963;16:318–335.
18. Bradley P, Brockbank J. The temporalis muscle flap in oral reconstruction. *J Maxillofac Surg* 1981;9:139–145.
19. Bakamjian VY, Long M, Rigg B. Experience with the medially based deltopectoral flap in reconstructuve surgery of the head and neck. *Br J Plast Surg* 1971;24:174–183.
20. Ariyan S. The pectoralis major myocutaneous flap. A versatile flap for reconstruction in the head and neck. *Plast Reconstr Surg* 1979;63:73–81.
21. Chen WL, Zhang DM, Yang ZH, et al. Extended supraclavicular fascio-cutaneous island flap based on the transverse cervical artery for head and neck reconstruction after cancer ablation. *J Oral Maxillofac Surg* 2010;68:2422–2430.
22. Brånemark PI, Hansson BO, Adell R, et al. Osseointegrated implants in the treatment of the edentulous jaw. Experience from a 10-year period. *Scand J Plast Reconstr Surg* 1977;16(suppl):1–132.
23. Urken ML, Vickery C, Weinberg H, et al. The internal oblique-iliac crest osseomyocutaneous free flap in oromandibular reconstruction. Report of 20 cases. *Arch Otolaryngol Head Neck Surg* 1989;115:339–349.
24. Koranda FC, McMahon MF, Jernstrom VR. The temporalis muscle flap for intraoral reconstruction. *Arch Otolaryngol Head Neck Surg* 1987; 113:740.
25. Breidahl AF, Morrison D, Donato RR, et al. A modified surgical technique for temporalis transfer. *Br J Surg* 1996;49:46–51.
26. Browne JD, Holland BW. Combined intraoral and lateral temporal approach for palatal malignancies with temporalis muscle reconstruction. *Arch Otolaryngol Head Neck Surg* 2002;128:531.
27. Michaelidis IG, I Hatzistefanou IM. Functional and aesthetic reconstruction of extensive oral ablative defects using temporalis muscle flap: a case report and a sort review. *J Craniomaxillofac Surg* 2011;39:200–205.
28. Cordeiro PG, Santamaria E. A classification system and algorithm for reconstruction of maxillectomy and mid-facial defects. *Plast Reconstr Surg* 2000;105:2331–2346; discussion 2347–2348.
29. Earley MJ. Primary maxillary reconstruction after cancer excision. *Br J Plast Surg* 1989;42:628–637.
30. Gullane PJ, Lipa JE, Novak CB, et al. Reconstruction of skull base defects. *Clin Plast Surg* 2005;32:391–399, vii.
31. Silver CE. Gastric pull-up operation for replacement of the cervical portion of the esophagus. *Surg Gynecol Obstet* 1976;142:243–245.
32. Song R, Gao Y, Song Y, et al. The forearm flap. *Clin Plast Surg* 1982;9: 21–26.
33. Lovie MJ, Duncan GM, Glasson DW. The ulnar artery forearm free flap. *Br J Plast Surg* 1984;37:486–492.
34. Luo LS. A new free skin flap—anterolateral femoral flap—its anatomy and clinical application [article in Chinese]. *Zhonghua Zheng Xing Shao Shang Wai Ke Za Zhi* 1985;1:50–52.
35. Song YG, Chen GZ, Song YL. The free thigh flap: a new free flap concept based on the septocutaneous artery. *Br J Plast Surg* 1984;37:149.
36. Taylor GI, Corlett RJ, Boyd JB. The versatile deep inferior epigastric (inferior rectus abdominis) flap. *Br J Plast Surg* 1984;37:330–350.
37. McCraw JB, Furlow LT Jr. The dorsalis pedis arterialized flap. A clinical study. *Plast Reconstr Surg* 1975;55:177–185.
38. Leeb DC, Ben-Hur N, Mazzarella L. Reconstruction of the floor of the mouth with a free dorsalis pedis flap. *Plast Reconstr Surg* 1977;59: 379–381.
39. Bunkis J, Mulliken JB, Upton J, et al. The evolution of techniques for reconstruction of full-thickness cheek defects. *Plast Reconstr Surg* 1982;70:319–327.
40. Hidalgo DA. Fibula free flap: a new method of mandible reconstruction. *Plast Reconstr Surg* 1989;84:71–79.
41. Peterson RA, Ellenberg AH, Carroll DB. Vermilion flap reconstruction of bilateral cleft lip deformities (a modification of the Abbé procedure). *Plast Reconstr Surg* 1966;38(2):109–115.
42. Taylor GI, Townsend P, Corlett R. Superiority of the deep circumflex iliac vessels as the supply for free groin flaps. Clinical work. *Plast Reconstr Surg* 1979;64:745–759.
43. Swartz WM, Banis JC, Newton ED, et al. The osteocutaneous scapular flap for mandibular and maxillary reconstruction. *Plast Reconstr Surg* 1986;77:530–545.
44. Soutar DS, Scheker LR, Tanner NS, et al. The radial forearm flap: a versatile method for intra-oral reconstruction. *Br J Plast Surg* 1983;36:1–8.
45. Mulholland RS, Tanna N, Boyd JB. Introducing the tibial-dorsalis pedis osteocutaneous shin flap: a new option for oromandibular reconstruction. *Plast Reconstr Surg* 2013;132(4):611e–620e.
46. Sadove RC, Luce EA, McGrath PC. Reconstruction of the lower lip and chin with the composite radial forearm-palmaris longus free flap. *Plast Reconstr Surg* 1991;88:209–214.
47. Takada K, Sugata T, Yoshiga K, et al. Total upper lip reconstruction using a free radial forearm flap incorporating the brachioradialis muscle: report of a case. *J Oral Maxillofac Surg* 1987;45:959–962.
48. Serletti JM, Tavin E, Moran SL, et al. Total lower lip reconstruction with a sensate composite radial forearm-palmaris longus free flap and a tongue flap. *Plast Reconstr Surg* 1997;99(2):559–561.
49. Loreti A, Di Lella G, Vetrano S, et al. Thinned anterolateral thigh cutaneous flap and radial fasciocutaneous forearm flap for reconstruction of oral defects: comparison of donor site morbidity. *J Oral Maxillofac Surg* 2008;66:1093–1098.
50. Boyd B, Mulholland S, Gullane P, et al. Reinnervated lateral antebrachial cutaneous neurosome flaps in oral reconstruction: are we making sense? *Plast Reconstr Surg* 1994;93:1350–1359; discussion 1360–1362.
51. Netscher D, Armenta AH, Meade RA, et al. Sensory recovery of innervated and non-innervated radial forearm free flaps: functional implications. *J Reconstr Microsurg* 2000;16:179–185.
52. Boyd JB, Kim SS, Granzow J, et al. Documenting the density of innervation in a sensate radial forearm flap based on the lateral antebrachial cutaneous nerve. *Plast Reconstr Surg* 2009;123:216e–217e.
53. Lyos AT, Evans GR, Perez D, et al. Tongue reconstruction: outcomes with the rectus abdominis flap. *Plast Reconstr Surg* 1999;103(2): 442–447; discussion 448–449.
54. Howaldt HP, Bitter K. Total tongue replacement by a microsurgical latissimus dorsi transplant. *Fortschr Kiefer Gesichtschir* 1990;35:53–54.
55. Koshima I, Fukuda H, Yamamoto H, et al. Free anterolateral thigh flaps for reconstruction of head and neck defects. *Plast Reconstr Surg* 1993;92:421–428; discussion 429–430.
56. Koshima I, Hosoda M, Moriguchi T, et al. New multilobe "accordion" flaps for three-dimensional reconstruction of wide, full-thickness defects in the oral floor. *Ann Plast Surg* 2000;45:187–192.
57. Haughey BH. Tongue reconstruction: concepts and practice. *Laryngoscope* 1993;103:1132–1141.
58. Yousif NJ, Dzwierzynski WW, Sanger JR, et al. The innervated gracilis musculocutaneous flap for total tongue reconstruction. *Plast Reconstr Surg* 1999;104:916–921.
59. Yamamoto Y, Sugihara T, Furuta Y, et al. Functional reconstruction of the tongue and deglutition muscles following extensive resection of tongue cancer. *Plast Reconstr Surg* 1998;102:993–998; discussion 999–1000.
60. Yu P. Reinnervated anterolateral thigh flap for tongue reconstruction. *Head Neck* 2004;26:1038–1044.
61. Yu P, Robb GL. Reconstruction for total and near-total glossectomy defects. *Clin Plast Surg* 2005;32:411–419.
62. Weber RS, Ohlms L, Bowman J, et al. Functional results after total or near total glossectomy with laryngeal preservation. *Arch Otolaryngol Head Neck Surg* 1991;117:512–515.
63. Kimata Y, Uchiyama K, Ebihara S, et al. Comparison of innervated and noninnervated free flaps in oral reconstruction. *Plast Reconstr Surg* 1999;104:1307–1313.
64. Huelke DF. The origin of the peroneal communicating, nerve in adult man. *Anat Rec* 1958;132:81–92.

65. Boyd JB, Caton AM, Mulholland RM, et al. The sensate fibula osteocutaneous flap: neurosomal anatomy. *J Plast Reconstr Aesth Surg* 2013;66(12):168[illegible]–1694.
66. Wei FC, Chuang SS, Yim KK. The sensate fibula osteoseptocutaneous flap: a preliminary report. *Br J Plast Surg* 1994;47:544–547.
67. Berger A, Tizian C, Hausamen J, et al. Free jejunal graft for reconstruction of oral, oropharyngeal, and pharyngoesophageal defects. *J Reconstr Microsurg* 1984;1:83–94.
68. Anthony JP, Singer MI, Mathes SJ. Pharyngoesophageal reconstruction using the tubed free radial forearm flap. *Clin Plast Surg* 1994;21:137–147.
69. Murray DJ, Novak CB, Neligan PC. Fasciocutaneous free flaps in pharyngolaryngo-oesophageal reconstruction: a critical review of the literature. *J Plast Reconstr Aesthet Surg* 2008;61:1148–1156.
70. Mulholland S, Boyd JB, McCabe S, et al. Recipient vessels in head and neck microsurgery: radiation effect and vessel access. *Plast Reconstr Surg* 1993;92:628–632.
71. Santamaria E, Wei FC, Chen IH, et al. Sensation recovery on innervated radial forearm flap for hemiglossectomy reconstruction by using different recipient nerves. *Plast Reconstr Surg* 1999;103:450–457.
72. Paydar KZ, Hansen SL, Chang DS, et al. Implantable venous Doppler monitoring in head and neck free flap reconstruction increases the salvage rate. *Plast Reconstr Surg* 2010;125:1129–1134.
73. Keller A. A new diagnostic algorithm for early prediction of vascular compromise in 208 microsurgical flaps using tissue oxygen saturation measurements. *Ann Plast Surg* 2009;62:538–543.
74. Rosen IB, Manktelow RT, Zuker RM, et al. Application of microvascular free osteocutaneous flaps in the management of post-radiation recurrent oral cancer. *Am J Surg* 1985;150:474–479.
75. Schusterman MA, Miller MJ, Reece GP, et al. A single center's experience with 308 free flaps for repair of head and neck cancer defects. *Plast Reconstr Surg* 1994;93:472–478; discussion 479–480.
76. Urken ML, Weinberg H, Buchbinder D, et al. Microvascular free flaps in head and neck reconstruction. Report of 200 cases and review of complications. *Arch Otolaryngol Head Neck Surg* 1994;120:633–640.
77. Jones NF, Johnson JT, Shestak KC, et al. Microsurgical reconstruction of the head and neck: interdisciplinary collaboration between head and neck surgeons and plastic surgeons in 305 cases. *Ann Plast Surg* 1996;36: 37–43.
78. O'Brien CJ, Lee KK, Stern HS, et al. Evaluation of 250 free-flap reconstructions after resection of tumours of the head and neck. *Aust N Z J Surg* 1998;68:698–701.
79. Hidalgo DA, Disa JJ, Cordeiro PG, et al. A review of 716 consecutive free flaps for oncologic surgical defects: refinement in donor site selection and technique. *Plast Reconstr Surg* 1998;102:722–732; discussion 733–734.
80. Su WF, Hsia YJ, Chang YC, et al. Functional comparison after reconstruction with a radial forearm free flap or a pectoralis major flap for cancer of the tongue. *Otolaryngol Head Neck Surg* 2003;128:412–418.
81. Katou F, Shirai N, Kamakura S, et al. Intraoral reconstruction with innervated forearm flap: a comparison of sensibility and reinnervation in innervated versus noninnervated forearm flap. *Oral Surg Oral Med Oral Pathol Oral Radiol Endod* 1995;80:638–644.
82. Hartl DM, Dauchy S, Escande C, et al. Quality of life after free-flap tongue reconstruction. *J Laryngol Otol* 2009;123:550–554.

CHAPTER 36

CHAPTER 37

Oropharyngeal Reconstruction

Steven Lo and Hung Chi Chen

INTRODUCTION

Indications for Surgery

Reconstruction of the laryngopharyngeal tract remains one of the most challenging areas of head and neck surgery, with complication rates far exceeding those of other sites (1). But conversely, it also remains one of the most stimulating and innovative areas of reconstructive surgery, with techniques recently described for applications as diverse as functional restoration of voice and extra-anatomic diversion of the food bolus in recalcitrant aspiration.

Pharyngeal tumours present late because they are relatively asymptomatic and therefore have a concomitantly poor prognosis. About 75% present at stage III and IV and have a 5-year survival rate of 17% to 35% which is independent of treatment modality (2). Given that chemoradiotherapy has similar survival rates and locoregional control to surgery, the popularity of radical surgery has declined in recent years (3,4). However, there are a number of caveats to nonsurgical therapy despite the perceived advantages of laryngeal preservation and avoidance of surgical risk.

First, the failure rate of definitive chemoradiotherapy at 5 years is up to 50% (5). Secondary surgery after failed radiotherapy is more challenging, with some studies indicating an increase in flap failure rate and significantly higher stricture and fistula rates (6,7). Second, larynx preservation does not necessarily equate to a functioning larynx. A recent systematic review concluded that voice and speech impairment after definitive radiotherapy, although generally better than after laryngectomy, is difficult to quantify because of inconsistent outcome measurements (8). Similarly, preservation of the pharyngeal tract is not synonymous with the ability to swallow or tolerate a normal oral diet. Irradiated hypopharyngeal tumours are more likely to result in dysphagia than those involving the larynx or oropharynx, with up to 12% having silent aspiration (9). A more favorable result may be possible with surgical reconstruction of isolated hypopharyngeal tumours. Notwithstanding these concerns, more recent data comparing salvage reconstruction after laryngopharyngectomy with jejunal flaps do not appear to show a significant difference in complications whether with or without preoperative radiotherapy (10).

Goals of Surgery

In those deemed appropriate for surgery, the goals in pharyngeal reconstruction are specific for hollow viscus reconstruction with the addition of the specialized functions of speech and swallowing. As with any hollow viscus surgery, fistulas and strictures are innate problems and must be addressed in both the surgical design and the subsequent complication management. Other outcomes are nonspecific and are as per other sites of reconstruction such as flap necrosis, wound infection, early wound healing to expedite radiotherapy, and operative mortality.

There are therefore three primary goals in pharyngeal reconstruction: (1) restoration of swallowing allowing normal oral diet and freedom from feeding tubes, (2) the avoidance of hollow viscus complications such as fistula and stricture, and (3) restoration of intelligible speech after laryngopharyngectomy. The first two goals are eminently realistic, but the third is continually evolving and remains one of the "holy grails" of head and neck reconstruction.

HISTORY OF PHARYNGEAL RECONSTRUCTION: TRADITIONAL METHODS OF RECONSTRUCTION

Introduction

The history of pharyngeal reconstruction reflects many of the revolutionary advances in plastic surgery itself, with the evolution from skin flaps through to axial pattern flaps and the first reported attempt at a free flap by Seidenberg in 1959. There have been four main phases in the evolution of pharyngeal reconstruction. The first phase was in addressing the problem of vascularity of random skin flaps, first solved by the axial pattern deltopectoral flap. The second problem was in reducing reconstructions to a single stage, initially solved with the introduction of the pectoralis major flap. The third phase involved addressing fistula, stricture, and poor vascularity. This still remains something of a challenge but has improved immeasurably with the use of free vascularized tissue transfers. The fourth phase is our current era, with pharyngeal reconstruction no longer simply concerned with simple passive conduit reconstruction but now attempting more specialized functional reconstructions such as restoration of voice and surgical diversion for aspiration. It should be noted that throughout the evolution of pharyngeal reconstruction, there have been two parallel approaches, with either the skin flap approach or the enteric approach. This dichotomy still exists today, and strong advocates can be found for both techniques.

Skin Flaps

Multistaged Skin Flap Procedures: Late 19th Century to 1979

Random Cutaneous Flaps Historically, local skin flaps were used for attempts at hypopharyngeal reconstruction from the end of the 19th century. These entailed multiple stages, prolonged hospitalizations, and ultimately poor functional outcomes (11). In the early 20th century Gillies described the use of multistaged "waltzing" pedicled flaps taken from a remote site such as the abdomen to the arm and finally to the pharynx. With treatment spreading over several months and with some patients dying before final completion of surgery, it was remarked that the treatment was sometimes worse than the disease itself. Although shorter two-stage flaps were described, such as the Wookey cervical flap, these were random pattern flaps and therefore were associated with high rates of wound complication, especially after radiotherapy (12).

Axial Flaps In 1965, Bakamjian described the deltopectoral flap (13). This revolutionized hypopharyngeal reconstruction as it offered the first axially vascularized flap. This was conceptually important for two reasons. First, it allowed a greater amount of tissue to be transferred, and second, the perforating vessels were protected from the site of surgery and radiotherapy. Although axial pattern flaps provided the possibility of reliable soft tissue transfer, distal flap hypovascularity was still a problem. Furthermore, although it was still a multistaged procedure, it could be performed and completed in two stages within 1 month. First, an end-to-end proximal pharyngeal anastomosis and an end-to-side distal anastomosis was created, with the thoracic esophagus joined to the seam of the DP flap. The DP flap thus acted as a controlled salivary fistula. The second stage was performed at 4 weeks with division of the DP flap and closure of the distal end of the DP flap.

Single-Stage Skin Flap Procedures: 1979 Onward

Pectoralis Major Musculocutaneous Flaps In 1979, Ariyan described the pectoralis myocutaneous flap (14). This was the first major technical advance over the multistaged procedures because it allowed transfer of a reliable flap that could be done in a single stage. This not only saved in hospital stay and the tedium of controlled fistulae but also expedited oral intake and postoperative radiotherapy. Although revolutionary at the time, the pectoralis major musculocutaneous flap has since fallen out of favor as a first-line treatment because of increased complication rates compared with free flaps.

Pedicled Enteric Flaps

Traditionally, pedicled enteric flaps such as the gastric transposition (15) have not been able to reconstruct extensive hypopharyngeal segments, partly because of difficulties in reach but also in vascularity. Furthermore, they have been associated with relatively high mortality rates related to extensive thoracic and intraabdominal dissection, with reviews indicating a mortality rate of up to 9% in early series (2). More recently, pedicled enteric flaps with distal revascularization have been used for extensive combined hypopharyngeal and thoracic esophageal lesions, either alone or in combination with a free flap for pharyngeal reconstruction (16).

RECONSTRUCTIVE MICROSURGERY IN HYPOPHARYNGEAL RECONSTRUCTION

Introduction

The advent of free flap reconstruction has enabled single-stage reconstructions with a concomitant reduction in hospital stay and the ability to expedite postoperative radiotherapy. Furthermore, they have drastically reduced morbidity from fistula, stricture, and partial necrosis. They have now replaced pedicled flaps as the first-line choice for hypopharyngeal reconstruction in most centers, with pedicled flaps such as the pectoralis major relegated to a role in salvage surgery. More recently, functional free flaps have also been described to produce the voice.

Free Enteric Flaps

Jejunum

Enteric free flaps preceded fasciocutaneous free flaps by nearly 2 decades. Although it is widely acknowledged that Seidenberg described the first free jejunum flap in 1959, the patient died, and it was not until 1961 that the first successful case was reported (17,18). Jejunum is one of the most established flaps for hypopharyngeal reconstruction, with more than 1000 cases in the literature. Fistula and stricture rates are relatively low, but there are some functional concerns regarding "wet"-sounding speech because of mucus as well as lack of a stiff resonator and dysphagia because of hyperperistalsis. We will review outcomes later.

Gastro-omental Flaps

Baudet described the gastro-omental flap in 1979, and being well vascularized, it has a role in salvage surgery. However, the published case series are relatively small (19).

Free Fasciocutaneous Flaps

Radial Forearm Flap

The radial forearm free flap (RFFF) was initially described by Yang in 1981, and its use as for intraoral reconstruction was popularized by David Soutar in Canniesburn (20,21). A systematic review of pharyngeal reconstructions with the RFFF indicated relatively high complication rates with fistula in 27% of cases and stricture in 30% of cases (2). This may be attributable to a limited amount of tissue available for tubing, which may contribute to stricture, lack of a robust secondary waterproofing layer, and the insufficiency of the flap volume to obliterate dead space.

Anterolateral Thigh Flap

The anterolateral thigh (ALT) flap was first described by Song and coworkers in 1984 (22). It has been popularized in recent years by Peirong Yu at the MD Anderson Cancer Center (23,24). In a review article, 79-100% of patients resumed their normal diet and 90-100% attained their preoperative speech, with fistula and stricture rates of 6% and 13% respectively (2). There are a number of perceived advantages of the ALT over the RFFF; there is an abundant amount of skin, fascia, and muscle (if vastus lateralis is included) that allows versatility in planning; increased width at the pharyngeal and esophageal anastomoses; waterproofing via a layered fascial closure; and dead space obliteration. Although there is some concern regarding tubing in overweight patients, the flaps can be thinned. Also, by creating a tongue-shaped anastomosis, the overall circumference is increased, and stricture formation is reduced (Figure 37-1).

A number of technical points are worth highlighting in the successful application of the ALT flap in hypopharyngeal reconstruction (23). The skin flap should have a width of 9.4 cm, allowing a 3-cm-diameter tubed neopharynx, equivalent to the native esophageal width. The inclusion of two perforators allows flexibility in design, permitting a second skin paddle for monitoring or external skin reconstruction (e.g., a tracheal stomatoplasty). To reduce the risk of stricturing, the proximal end of the flap is left "spatulated" at its junction with the base of tongue. To widen the esophageal end, a 1.5-cm longitudinal split in the esophagus is performed. This also helps to prevent esophageal spasm. The fascia is subsequently tubed to provide a second waterproofing layer (Figure 37-2).

Earlier series describe the use of externalized strip of deepithelialized skin used as a monitoring paddle, but this resulted in a high fistula rate (23). Subsequent series describe the use of monitoring with an implantable Doppler probe or external device or use of a second skin paddle (which may be used adjunctively for skin neck resurfacing) (Figures 37-3 and 37-4).

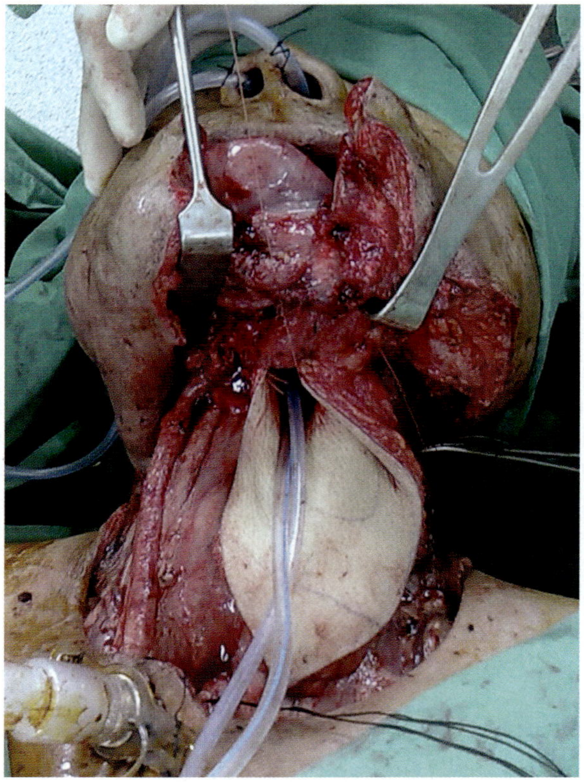

FIGURE 37-1 Anterolateral thigh flap in situ over two large-bore nasogastric tubes. The proximal pharyngeal anastomosis is "tongue" shaped to reduce stricturing.

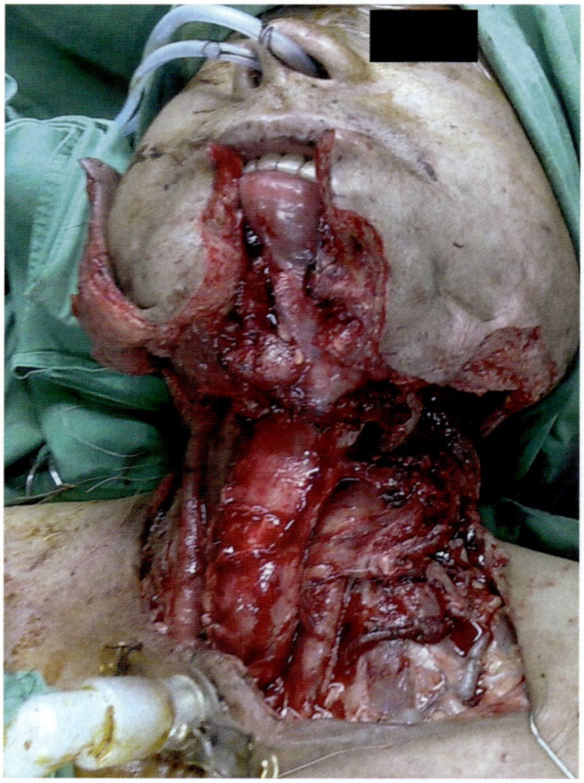

FIGURE 37-2 Anterolateral thigh flap tubed and a second waterproofing layer is performed by suturing the fascia longitudinally and to the pharyngeal and esophageal anastomoses. The recipient vessels are the transverse cervical vessels, visible on the patient's left.

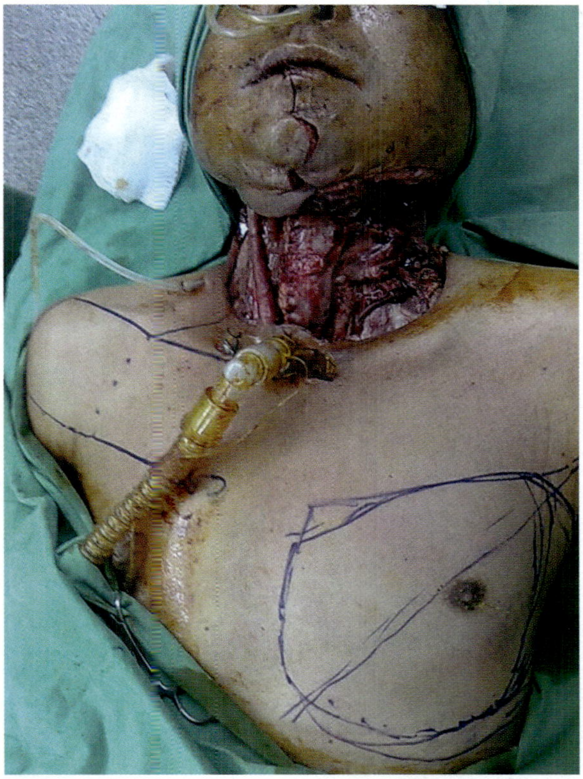

FIGURE 37-3 Coverage of external defect with pectoralis major and deltopectoral flaps.

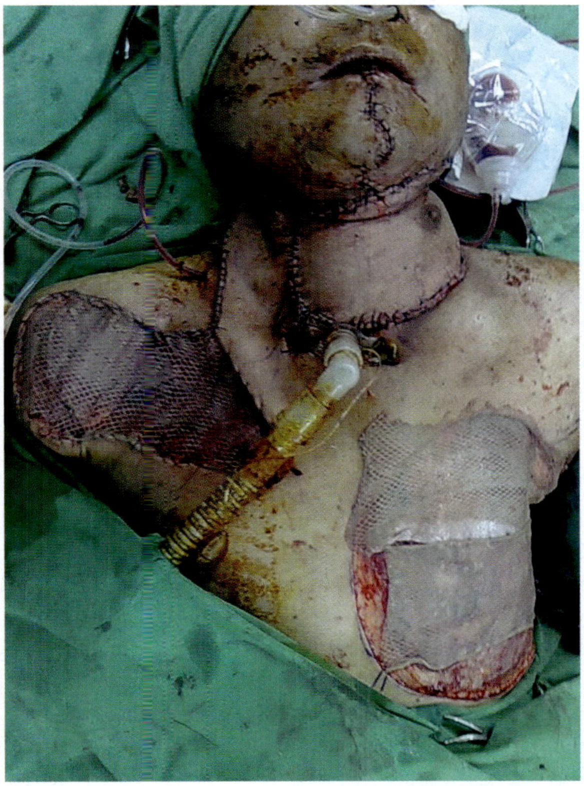

FIGURE 37-4 Inset of pedicled flaps. The pectoralis major muscle is sutured around the proximal and distal anastomoses to close off dead space and reduce the risk of fistulae.

ADVANCED FUNCTIONAL RESTORATION USING RECONSTRUCTIVE MICROSURGERY

Introduction

Functional free flap transfers are now a reality in pharyngeal reconstruction. We describe a number of techniques used in our unit that allow restoration of voice after laryngopharyngectomy and diversion of the food bolus in cases of recalcitrant aspiration.

Ileocolic Transfer for Voice Restoration

The essential component of surgical voice reconstruction is creation of a conduit between the tracheal air source and the neopharynx, which we term the "voice tube." This can be constructed in three ways: with ileum via the ileocolic valve, with a segment of jejunum, or with a rolled skin flap. We describe the ileocolic transfer below, but the general principles apply in the other techniques (25,26) (Figures 37-5 to 37-10).

The postoperative regimen for voice reconstruction patients is as follows. Usually we let the patients eat at 3 weeks. Then they are sent for adjuvant radiotherapy, chemotherapy, or both when indicated. If they do not need radiotherapy or chemotherapy, we start training of voice at 2 months to not disrupt the internal plication of the ileocaecal valve by commencing too early. The time required to achieve good voice production varies with individual patients. One of the factors in this is the length of the tracheal stump above the tracheostomy itself because patients who have a preserved length of tracheal stump generally start speaking early and achieve good voice (usually couple of months). In the absence of a tracheal stump above

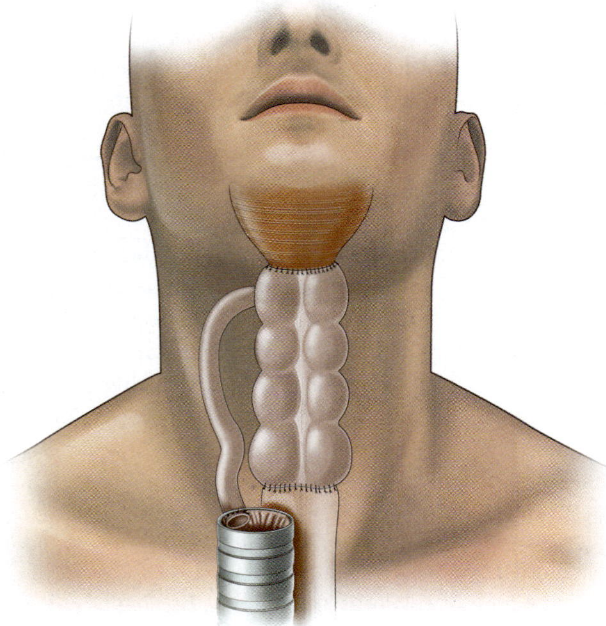

FIGURE 37-5 Illustration of ileocaecal segment with ileum anastomosed to the tracheal stump and the ascending colon as the neopharyngeal conduit. The ileocaecal valve acts as a one-way valve but also as part of the vibratory production for voice in addition to the flap walls themselves.

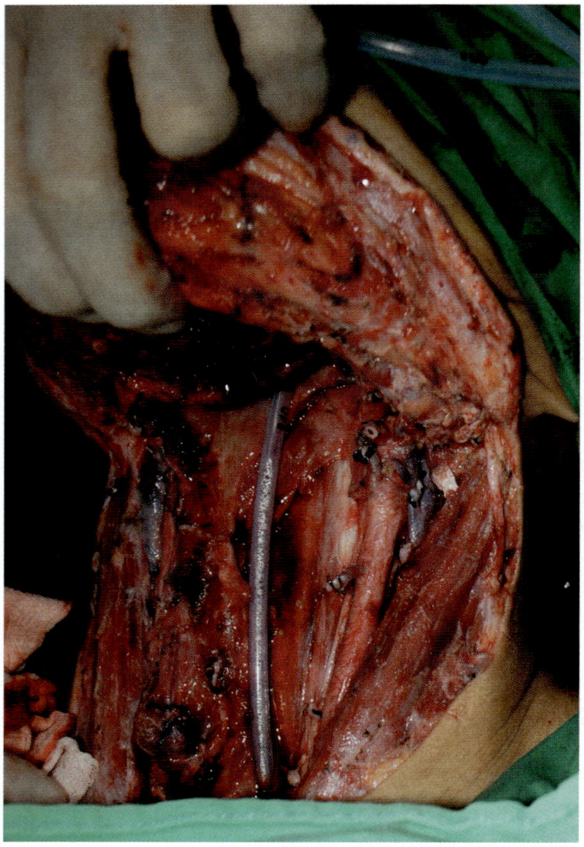

FIGURE 37-6 Circumferential hypopharyngeal defect.

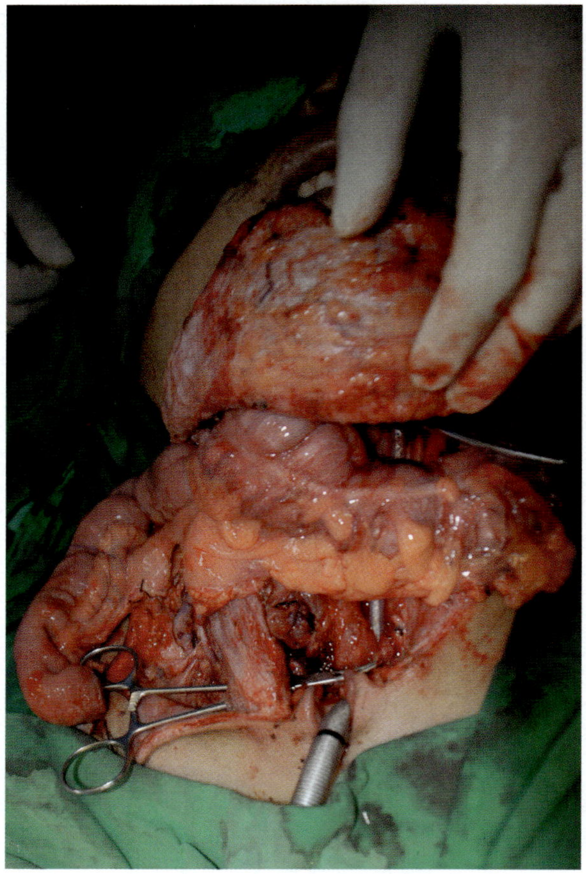

FIGURE 37-7 Ileocolon segment in situ. The colon is on the left and the ileum on the right, with the ileocaecal valve superior. The colon is used as the pharyngeal conduit, and the ileum acts as the voice tube. Note that the ileocaecal valve is narrowed by plication (not shown). The sternocleidomastoid muscle is shown over the artery clip and will be divided to allow inset of the ileal segment.

the tracheostomy, the ileum segment has to be sutured to the sidewall of the trachea, and the patient may need a "voice hood" (a skin flap to facilitate digital obstruction of the tracheostomy) to obtain a good voice. These patients generally take 6 months to obtain a good voice. However, we are becoming more and more proficient in the inset of the voice tube and creation of the voice hood, and in recent years, almost all patients can speak very well.

Diversion Loop Technique

Recalcitrant aspiration is an uncommon but debilitating condition, not only resulting in recurrent aspiration pneumonia but also depriving the patient the joy of eating. We have developed a technique that allows an extra-anatomic bypass of the normal route of swallowing, named the "diversion loop" (27). There are a number of indications for diversion loop, including:

1. Corrosive injury with dysfunction of epiglottis (partial destruction with fibrosis or complete destruction of the epiglottis)
2. Dysfunction of epiglottis and pharynx because of radiation therapy for head and neck cancers
3. Central nervous system (CNS) diseases resulting in dysfunction of the pharynx and choking (e.g., cerebrovascular accident or other CNS diseases resulting in functional problems of cranial nerves IX and X)
4. Ablative surgery of laryngeal tumors with dysfunction of epiglottis, resulting in choking
5. Collapse of mandible, resulting in retrusion of tongue and inability to swallow
6. Rare case: violent use of voice (e.g., in psychiatric disorder) causing inflammation around the larynx and epiglottis, frequent choking, and cessation of eating even when inflammation is over

Diversion loop is a two-stage operation. In the first stage, the patient is prepared in a supine position. The following should be done: (1) release of neck contracture, (2) right DP flap for creation of a tunnel for pharyngostomy, (3) finding proper recipient vessels for anastomoses of jejunal flap at left neck, and (4) division of the cervical esophagus. A free jejunal flap about 20 cm in length is harvested via a midline laparotomy. It is transferred to left side of the neck with anastomoses of vessels. The distal end of the jejunal flap is anastomosed to the distal end of cervical esophagus, and its proximal end is left open outside the skin, waiting for the second-stage inset to the left buccogingival sulcus. The postoperative care is the same as other free jejunal flap transfer. The patient is put in the microsurgical

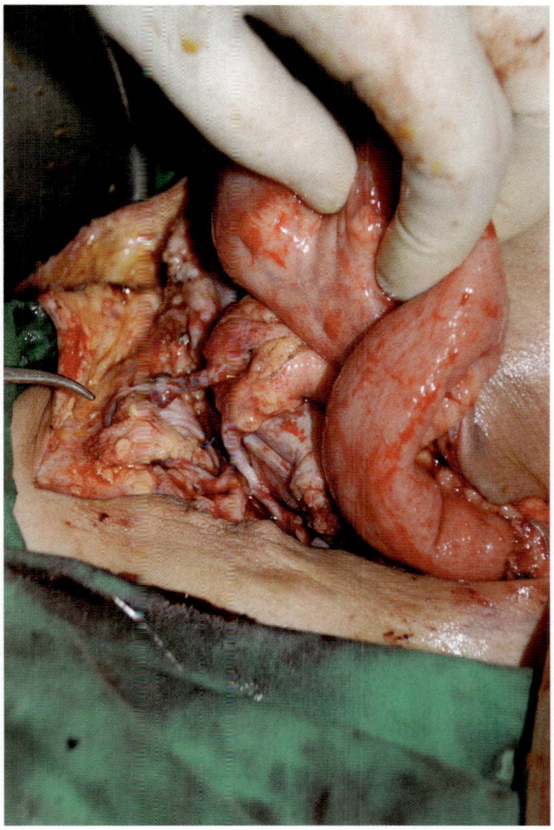

FIGURE 37-8 Anastomosis of the ileocaecal vessels.

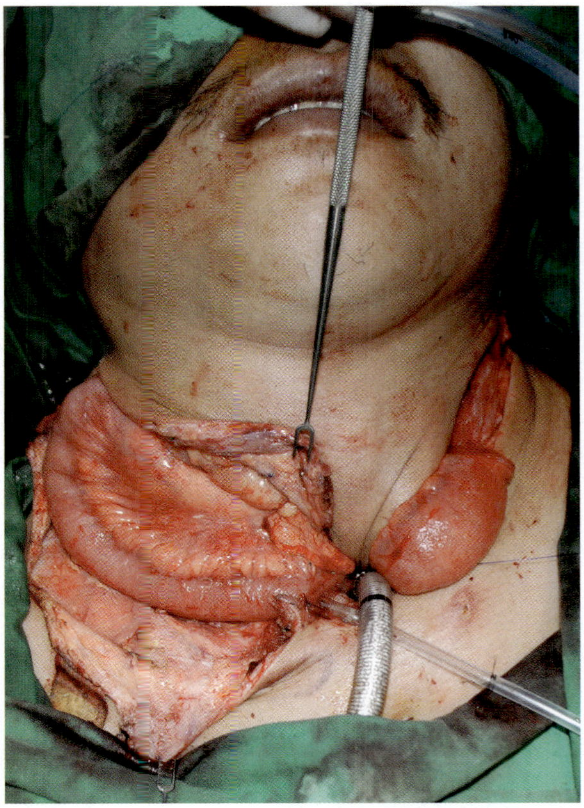

FIGURE 37-9 The ileal segment is split into two on the mesentery, with the segment on the patient's left acting as an external monitor. The ileum segment on the right is the voice tube and is inset into the tracheal remnant where possible, although here it is situated in the skin immediately adjacent.

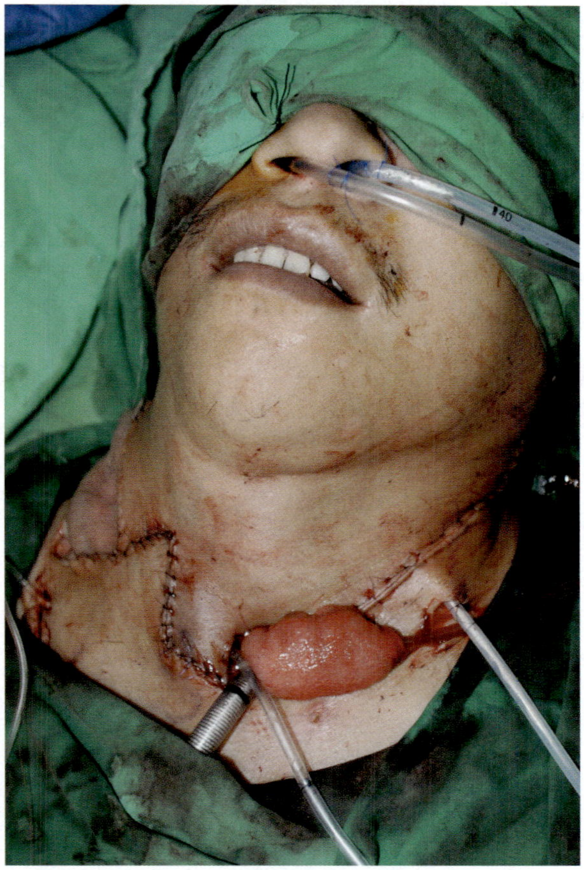

FIGURE 37-10 If the skin flaps cannot close the wound without tension, the ileal neo-voice tube is skin grafted. Both the voice tube and monitoring segment have drainage tubes to allow collection of secretions.

intensive care unit for 1 or 2 days and is sent to the ordinary ward after stabilization of the cardiopulmonary condition.

The second-stage operation is carried out 3 weeks later. The proximal end of the previous jejunal flap is dissected out. A tunnel is prepared over the periosteum of the left mandible. In this procedure the left marginal mandibular branch of the left facial nerve and left mental nerve should be dissected and preserved. An aperture is made at the left buccogingival sulcus. The proximal end of the jejunal flap is passed through the prepared tunnel to be anastomosed to the oral mucosa at left buccogingival sulcus. Two stent tubes are inserted through the orifice at the buccogingival sulcus to prevent stricturing.

Two weeks later when the wounds are healed, the patients are allowed to eat from the left buccogingival sulcus. They start with a liquid diet and gradually advance to a semisolid and solid diet, depending on the progress of their training. All of them are able to take a semisolid diet smoothly without choking. Initially, some of the food may go astray to the pharynx and then come out from the pharyngostomy. However, none of them need the pharyngostomy eventually. They can even cope with saliva in the night that would have previously caused them to wake with nocturnal choking.

We have primarily performed this for dysfunction of the epiglottis or pharynx secondary to radiotherapy. Originally, this was performed as a single-stage procedure, but in three cases, necrosis of the proximal jejunal segment occurred, thought to be due to postoperative swelling against the mandible. It is now our preference to perform this as a staged procedure, with the proximal jejunal segment kept percutaneous initially and tunneled over the mandible in the second stage. Of the 27 cases we have performed thus far, all patients have been able to successfully take oral feeding via the diversion loop between approximately 3 to 5 months after surgery, and they can all take a semisolid diet. Only one patient still requires occasional tube feeding (Figures 37-11 to 37-19).

CLASSIFICATIONS AND ALGORITHMS FOR PHARYNGEAL DEFECTS

A number of classifications exist, and the main differences in the reconstructive algorithms are based on a preference for ALT or jejunum for circumferential defect reconstruction.

University of Toronto, Patel et al 2010 (2)

1. ALT
2. RFFF
3. After failed chemoradiotherapy: gastro-omental flap

Memorial Sloan Kettering, Disa et al 2003 (7)

Type I: partial defects less than 50% circumference—RFFF

Type II: circumferential (or >50% circumference): jejunum (Note that Peirong Yu, also at MD Anderson Cancer Center, has published widely on the use of ALT as the first choice for circumferential defects.)

Type III: longitudinal defects (extensive involving multiple anatomic levels, including the hypopharynx, oropharynx, floor of mouth): rectus abdominis myocutaneous flap

Type IV: extension to thoracic esophagus: gastric pull-up

China Medical University Hospital, Taiwan. Chen et al 2010 (25)

It is important to consider the primary defect not simply as a hollow conduit reconstruction. We therefore compartmentalize the primary defect as three separate problems: the conduit, the functional restoration, and the external cover. Furthermore, although not popularized yet in the Western world, we make extensive use of nonprosthetic surgical voice reconstruction and diversion loop techniques. Our algorithm for secondary defect reconstruction after fistula and stricture is covered later (Figure 37-20).

TECHNICAL DETAILS AND ADJUNCTIVE MEASURES

Recipient Vessels in Pharyngeal Reconstruction

A general principle in all of head and neck reconstruction is that with an abundance of vessels, the choice is somewhat opportunistic—whatever is left and has adequate outflow and

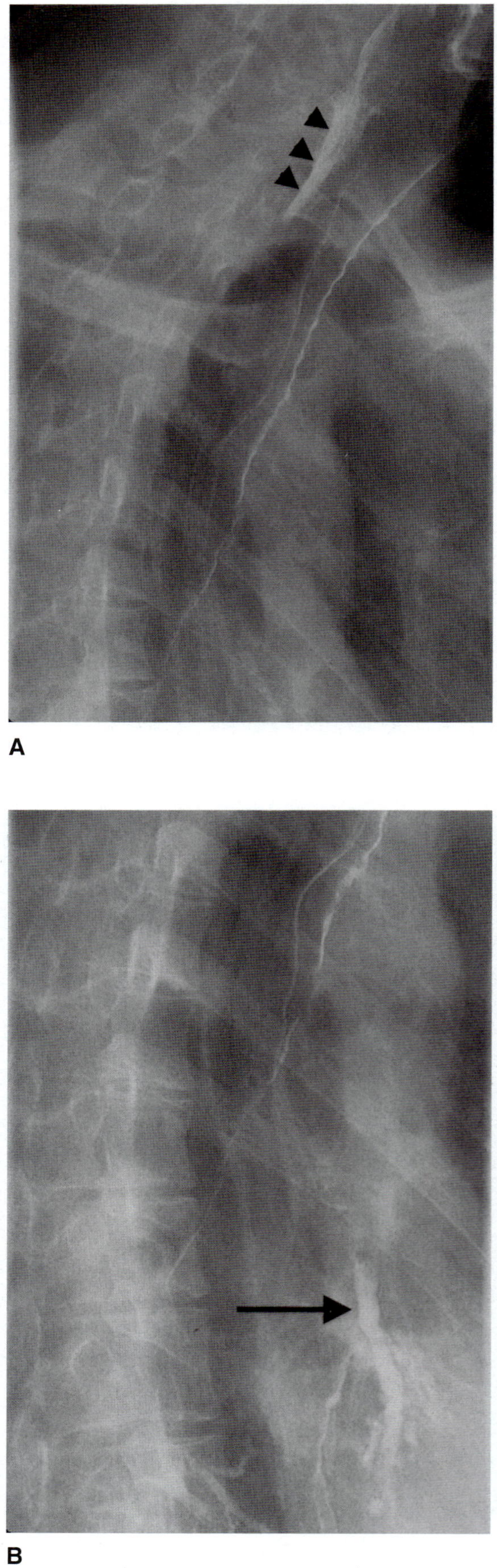

FIGURE 37-11 (A) The small arrowheads indicate laryngeal penetration by contrast. (B) The long single arrow indicates contrast aspiration in the bronchial tree

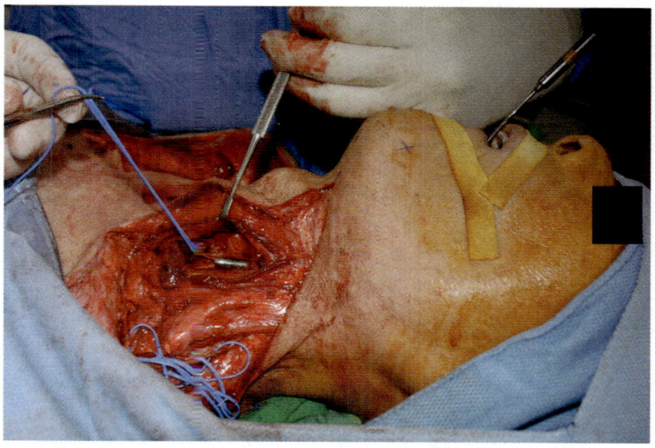

FIGURE 37-12 Patient with recurrent aspiration after radiotherapy. The metal probe is passed from the mouth to an opening at the pyriform sinus for creation of the salivary bypass (pharyngostomy).

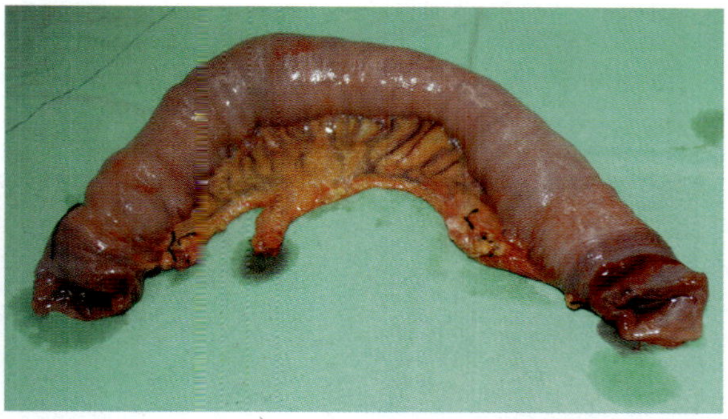

FIGURE 37-13 Jejunal segment taken with the second arterial arcade.

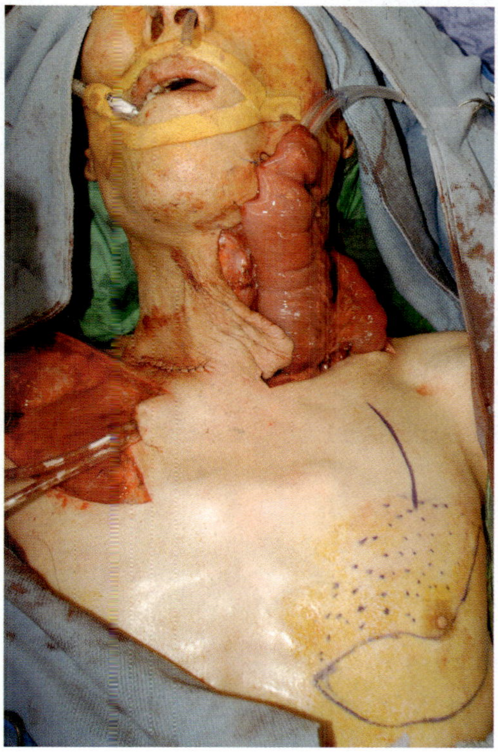

FIGURE 37-14 Jejunum in situ with microvascular anastomoses to transverse cervical vessels. Pharyngostomy is created with a tubed deltopectoral flap.

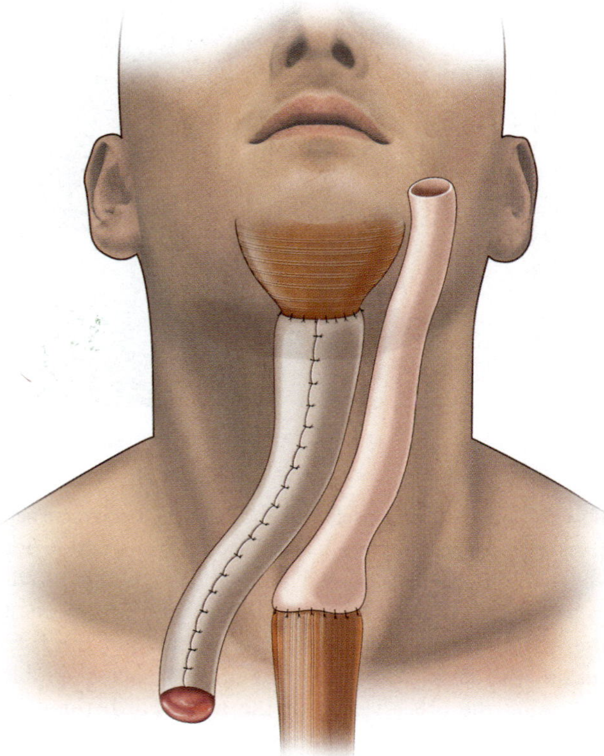

FIGURE 37-15 Illustrative representation of Figure 37-14. The deltopectoral pharyngostomy is shown on the patient's right, and the jejunum diversion segment is on the left.

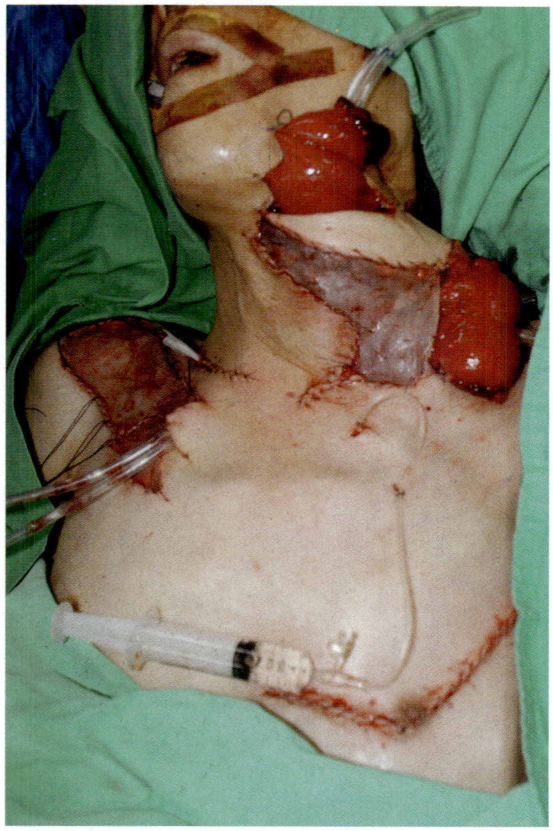

FIGURE 37-16 Jejunum covered in pectoralis major flap and temporary externalization of the jejunum superiorly. A monitoring segment of jejunum is visible inferiorly.

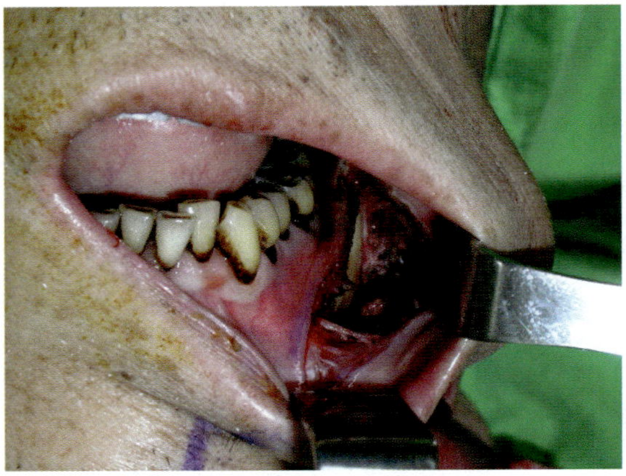

FIGURE 37-17 Second stage: the inferior gingivobuccal sulcus neostoma is created.

inflow can be used. Our preferred choice is the transverse cervical vessels because they are usually spared from radiotherapy and previous neck dissections. The superior thyroid is also usually available. It is our preference to avoid end-to-side anastomoses to the great vessels of the neck because of the risk of avulsion with neck turning. This is not an inherent problem when using the other vessels of the neck. Furthermore, the lingual artery should be avoided if other vessels are available because it puts the vascularity of the tongue at risk. It should also be noted that in free jejunal flap transfer, the mesenteric artery and vein cannot be dissected widely; therefore, the recipient vessels should be in relatively close apposition, except for the use of the external jugular vein in which a long recipient vein can be dissected and brought adjacent to the recipient artery. The ALT and RFFF artery and vein are easily separated and can be anastomosed in different locations.

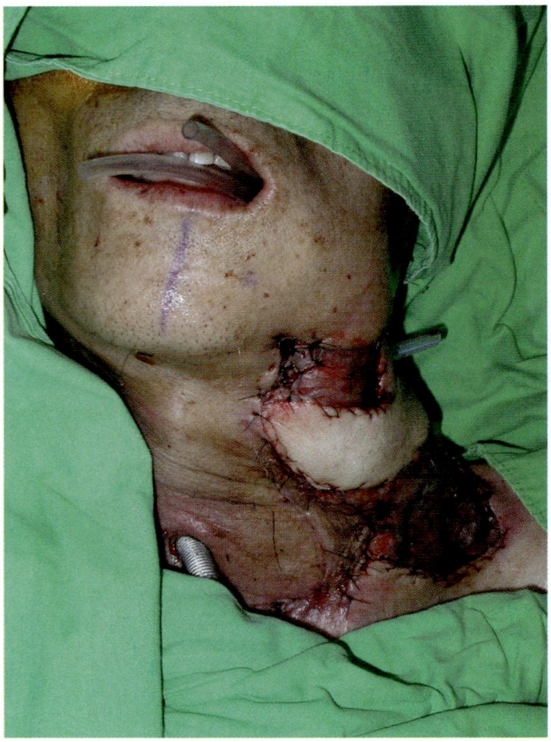

FIGURE 37-18 The exteriorized proximal jejunal segment is tunneled and sutured to the gingivobuccal sulcus.

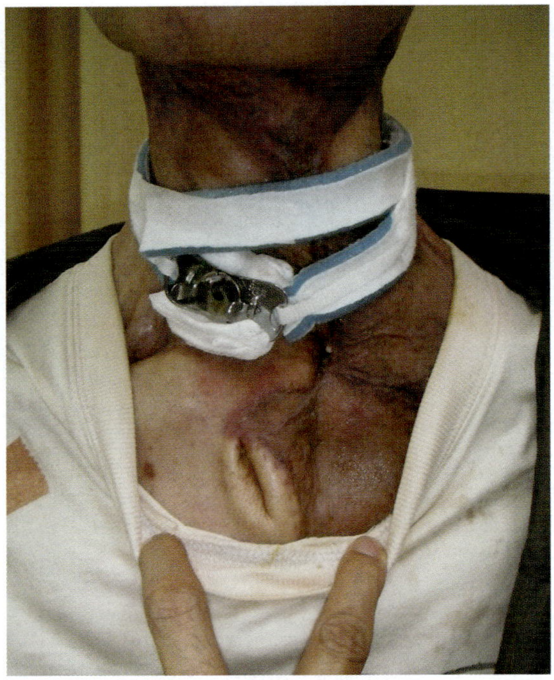

A

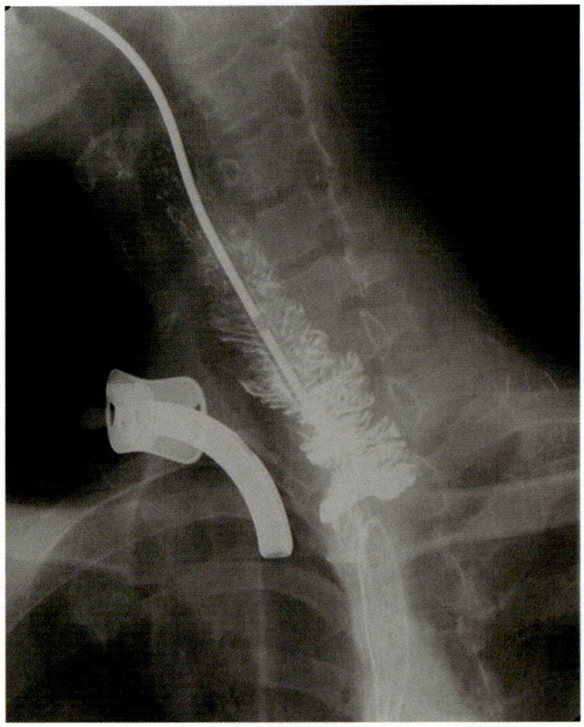

B

FIGURE 37-19 (**A**) The patient is able to take 500 mL of liquid through the diversion loop in 10 minutes. There are minimal salivary secretions from the esophagostomy. (**B**) Contrast filling of diversion loop segment.

Flap Monitoring

Flap monitoring is especially difficult with buried flaps. For the jejunum, we use a combination of externalized monitoring segment and transcutaneous Doppler. The implantable Doppler probe has been used in some units but is not always reliable because of numerous other vessels in the neck and problems

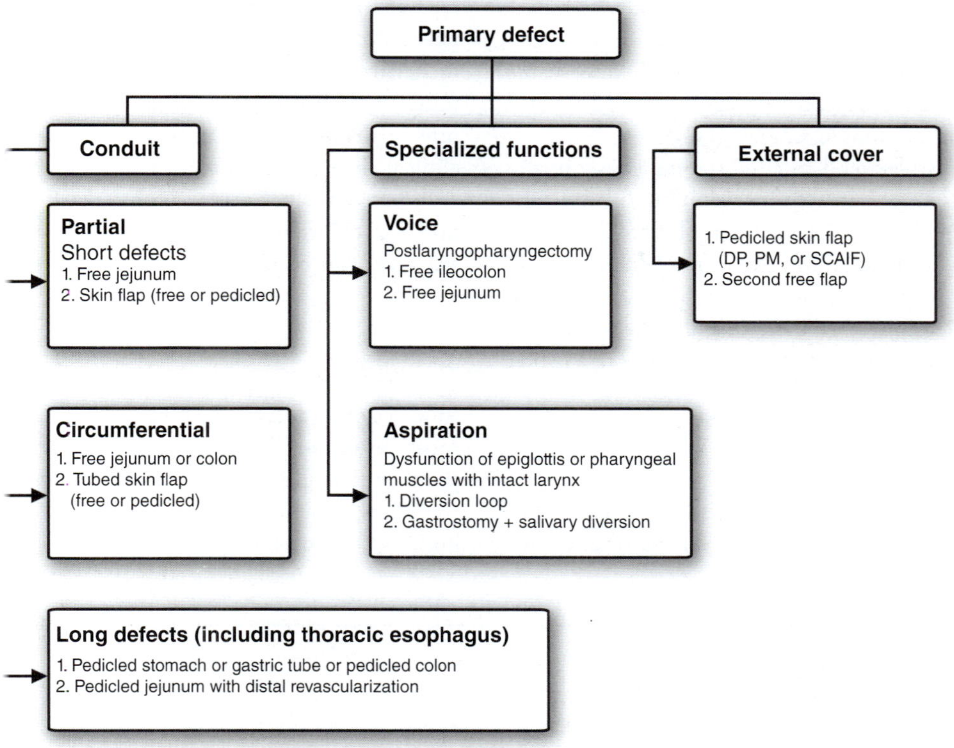

FIGURE 37-20 China Medical University Hospital algorithm for primary defects. First and second choice options for each defect are noted in the boxes below. DP, deltopectoral flap; PM, pectoralis major flap; SCAIF, supraclavicular artery island flap.

with false-negative explorations (23). We have occasionally encountered late failures (latest at 17 days) with jejunal flap and therefore leave the monitoring segment until at least day 17.

With the ALT free flap, monitoring with handheld Doppler is relatively straightforward if the cutaneous perforator is placed anteriorly so that it can be detected beneath the skin neck flaps. We prefer to listen to both the arterial and venous signals.

Salivary Diversion Tubes

Salivary diversion tubes such as the Montgomery tube serve to stent the neopharynx but also to protect the anastomotic suture lines from saliva. These are generally recommended when performing ALT pharyngeal reconstruction.

Gastrografin Studies

Gastrograffin swallow can be performed to exclude occult fistula, traditionally at 2 weeks, and if a leak is found, the patient is kept NPO (nil per os) and the Gastrografin repeated 2 weeks later. When no leak is demonstrated, then a liquid diet is commenced for 2 days before advancing to regular diet. Not all centers perform this routinely, and an evaluation at MD Anderson Cancer Center found it to be relatively unreliable (28).

Voice Restoration by Tracheoesophageal Puncture

Voice reconstruction is performed in our unit with the nonprosthetic voice reconstruction techniques described earlier. Tracheoesophageal puncture (TEP) is the current technique of choice in most other centers and is best performed as a secondary procedure. Although it is possible to do this as a primary procedure, it is associated with a higher complication rate.

MANAGEMENT OF COMPLICATIONS

Introduction

Any hollow viscus reconstruction, such as hypopharyngeal reconstruction and hypospadias, carries with it two particular complications—those of stricture and fistula. Speech and oral feeding will be covered later under Outcomes. Overall hypopharyngeal reconstruction complication rates are higher than in other aerodigestive tract sites at 30% versus 8% (1). Furthermore, preoperative radiotherapy has been shown to be a significant factor leading to increased complications in hypopharynx reconstruction (7).

Fistula

Fistula formation has been one of the defining problems of hypopharyngeal reconstruction ever since they were first attempted and has been investigated extensively. There are a number of characteristics of fistula formation, which tend to differ between jejunum and fascial flap reconstructions. Fistulae are more common at the proximal anastomosis in jejunum reconstructions than with ALT (50% vs. 25%) because the ALT can be shaped to allow widening at the tongue base. The bulk of the fascial flap also enables filling in of the proximal dead space. Leaks occur at the proximal and distal ends in fascial flaps rather than along the longitudinal suture line (23). One also cannot be complacent with fascial flaps because fistulae can occur late in fascial flaps, on average on day 32 in ALT and on day 16 in the jejunum (23,29).

Despite all this, fistulae tend to close spontaneously in the vast majority of cases. About 75% of jejunum fistulae heal spontaneously, taking about 7.4 weeks to heal on average, which may delay radiotherapy (28). Preoperative radiotherapy reduces the chance of spontaneous healing to 46% (29). ALT fistulae appear to heal quicker (<30 days), and some authors do not delay adjuvant radiotherapy even in the presence of a fistula (24) (Figure 37-21).

Stricture

There are no standard clinical parameters for postreconstructive strictures, and this may reflect the variable stricture rates reported in the literature. One definition that has been proposed is clinical dysphagia confirmed by endoscopic findings of narrowing to less than 10 mm (23). In this study it was found that all clinically significant strictures were less than 10 mm in diameter, with those greater than 10 mm being subclinical. It is important to exclude other causes of dysphagia such as redundancy of the reconstructed segment and synchronous or recurrent tumors. With fasciocutaneous free flaps, strictures can become evident at a late stage, even years after surgery.

Dysphagia

All cases of dysphagia must be investigated for synchronous or recurrent tumor. Dysphagia unrelated to stricture or tumor is a problem that appears to be unique to enteric flaps. This can be secondary to redundancy of the jejunal segment (resulting in kinking), hyperperistalsis, or dyscoordinated peristalsis.

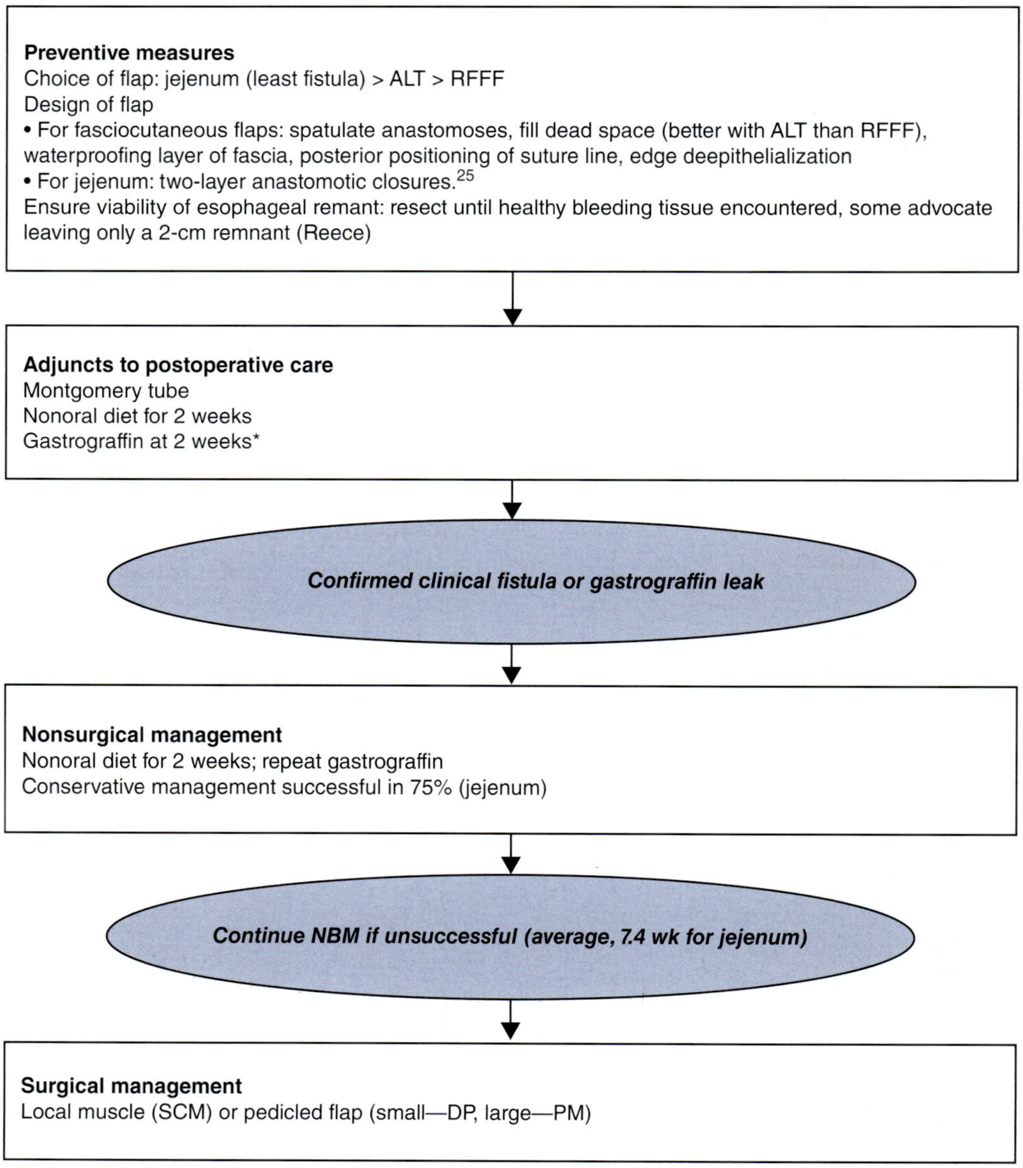

FIGURE 37-21 Algorithm of secondary defects: management of fistulae. Asterisk indicates that traditionally, Gastrografin has been performed at 2 weeks, but this is not compulsory. ALT, anterolateral thigh; DP, deltopectoral flap; PM, pectoralis major; RFFF, radial forearm free flap; SCM, sternocleidomastoid muscle.

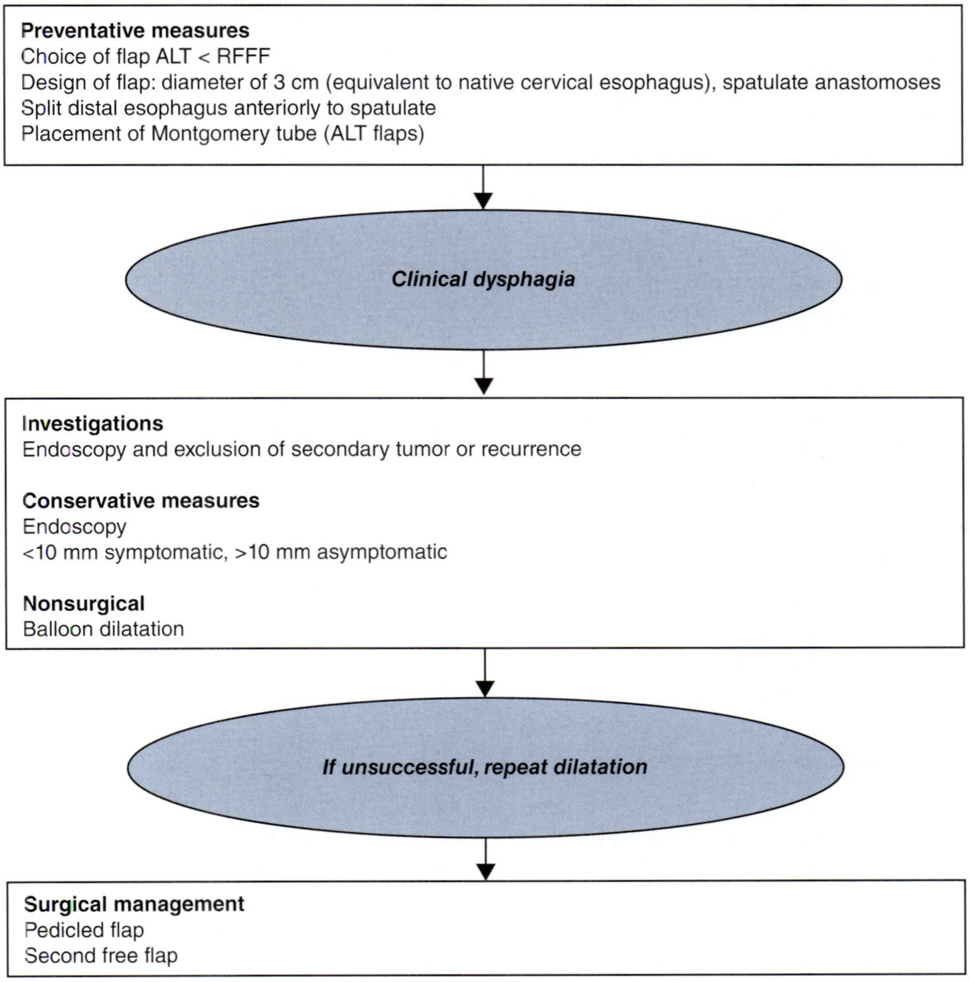

FIGURE 37-22 Algorithm for management of stricture/dysphagia. ALT, anterolateral thigh; RFFF, radial forearm free flap.

Whereas redundancy may require segmental shortening, hyperperistalsis is left to improve expectantly (30) (Figure 37-22).

OUTCOMES IN PHARYNGEAL RECONSTRUCTION

Outcomes in the Literature

Outcomes in hypopharyngeal reconstruction can be divided into complications related to hollow viscus reconstruction (fistula and stricture) and outcomes related to restoration of specialized functions (speech and swallowing). Evidence in the literature largely comes from retrospective case series and systematic reviews, with no randomized controlled trials or true meta-analyses published. It is therefore impossible to say with conviction which reconstructive technique provides the optimum outcomes in hypopharyngeal reconstruction even though many authors would attempt to suggest otherwise.

Areas that continue to evoke controversy include which flap is best for circumferential defects and what is the most appropriate method of voice reconstruction. We review the evidence for this below, but ultimately, given the paucity of high-level evidence (level I or II, Oxford Centre for Evidence Based Medicine), it may come down more to surgical preference and experience.

Circumferential Defects

Circumferential defects appear to pose a quite different challenge to partial defects. The remnant of the cervical esophagus in partial defects appears to obviate many of the complications related to stricture and fistula formation, possibly by providing a zone of compliance. There are proponents to be found for both free and pedicled ALT and jejunum flaps, and ultimately, it may be a matter of surgeon preference and surgical experience rather than any true demonstrated superiority of one flap over another in the literature. Indeed, the larger published series may often be a reflection of single surgeon's skill rather than the flap itself. Yu describes his reduction in complications with his later series of ALT flaps.

There is no single flap that encapsulates the optimum characteristics of low rates of fistula and stricture, with excellent functional restoration. Flaps with a low fistula rate such as jejunum have a poorer functional outcome in terms of speech rehabilitation and vice versa for ALT flaps. The trend in many centers towards using rolled ALT flaps may also reflect a reluctance by plastic surgeons to enter the abdomen or difficulties with general surgical colleagues who may not understand fully the delicate tissue handling required for jejunal flaps.

Free Flap versus Pedicled Flap

There is not much dispute in the major cancer centers that free flaps are superior to pedicled flaps in hypopharyngeal reconstruction, with flaps such as the PM relegated to a role in salvage surgery. Chepaha (level III evidence) compares the PM with free flap reconstruction and makes a strong case for the avoidance of PM in primary reconstruction of the pharynx (1). This paper found a complication rate of 57% with PM versus 21% with free flaps and a gastrostomy-dependent rate of 42% versus 16%. However, this group is a heterogenous mix of all sites of resection and does not involve solely the hypopharynx. There are, however, some authors who continue to advocate the primary use of the PM flap, such as Spriano and coworkers (level IV evidence), using a modification of Fabiano's method and reporting a fistula rate of 13% (31).

Enteric (Jejunum) versus Fasciocutaneous Flap (ALT Flap or RFFF)

An area of greater controversy is whether jejunum or fasciocutaneous flaps is superior for circumferential pharyngeal reconstruction. Strong advocates are found on both sides, and comparisons in the literature are not always justified. Our own preference is to use the jejunum for reconstruction.

Noncomparative Case Series (Level IV Evidence)

There are many cases series with large patient numbers for jejunum flaps with relatively consistent results for fistula and stricture. When fasciocutaneous flaps were first reported, they were generally small numbers with higher complication rates. More recent data suggest similar complication outcomes.

In 2008, Murray and coworkers reviewed a number of series of fasciocutaneous free flaps in the literature, including 242 RFFF and 67 ALT flaps (32). This makes a strong argument for use of fasciocutaneous flaps in terms of low complications and better functional outcomes than jejunum. This noted a stricture rate of 16.1% and fistula rate of 13%. An oral diet was possible in 94% (of which 75% regained full normal diet), and 88.5% of those who had TEP performed regained "functional" speech.

In 2003, Disa and coworkers described his experience with 52 RFFF, 90 jejunum, and 23 rectus flaps (7). However, this is a noncomparative case series because only the jejunum flaps were used for circumferential defects, with the RFFF and rectus used for partial defects. The jejunum flaps had a stricture rate of 7% and fistula rate of 10%. A total of 64% returned to an oral diet. Both the RFFF and rectus flaps had a significantly lower fistula rate of 0% to 1% which is more likely a reflection of the partial defect reconstruction than the choice of flap.

Chang and coworkers conducted one of the largest retrospective case series of 168 jejunum flaps, with a fistula rate of 13.7% (29).

Retrospective Comparative Reviews (Level III Evidence) There are few single center comparative reviews in the literature. Yu and coworkers compare 26 ALT with 31 jejunum reconstructions for circumferential hypopharyngeal defects (24). There were fewer fistulae in the jejunum group with 3% versus 8% for ALT and higher strictures rates with 19% versus 15% for ALT flaps. Neither of these reached statistical significance. Speech rehabilitation was with the TEP in approximately one third of patients, and of those patients with TEP, only 22% in the jejunum achieved intelligible speech versus 89% for the ALT ($P<0.01$). Swallowing was noted to be significantly better in the ALT group with 95% regaining total oral diet versus 65% for jejunum ($P<0.01$). But complete reliance on tube feeding was 4% and 8%, respectively, which was not significant. Twelve percent of the jejunum flaps also developed dysphagia secondary to hyperperistalsis, but the patients were able to take a soft diet. It should be noted that a direct comparison of these outcomes should be taken with caution because in this series, it compares a single author's experience in ALT (Yu) with the experience of multiple jejunum surgeons.

Systematic Reviews (Level III Evidence) The most recent systematic review of multiple comparative case series is by Patel and coworkers in (2). In this paper, 1018 jejunum flaps are reviewed from eight papers, indicating a mortality rate of 3%, fistula in 12%, and stricture in 10%. Functional outcomes are not clearly defined, but an oral diet in 85% and speech in 60% to 66% (from two papers only) are reported. Sixty cases of RFFF are reviewed from four papers, with a mortality rate of 0%, fistula in 27%, and stricture in 30%. Oral diet was achieved in 91% to 100% and speech in 75% to 93%. Fifty-two cases of ALT from three papers are reported, with a mortality rate of 0%, fistula in 6%, stricture in 13%, oral diet in 79% to 100%, and speech in 90% to 100%. This systematic review concludes in favor of the ALT over jejunum in terms of functional outcomes, as is the overall trend in the literature. However, with reported numbers of more than 1000 cases for jejunum in this systematic review versus 52 for ALT flaps and the absence of any level I or II evidence, this must be interpreted with some caution.

ALT Flap versus RFFF

The general consensus from the literature is that the ALT flap is first-line choice over the RFFF for circumferential defects. The stricture and fistula rate of the RFFF are consistently worse than for the ALT flap, partly because of limitations of tubed flap size but also because of technical aspects such as lack of bulk for dead space obliteration and fascia for a waterproofing layer. There is little doubt, however, that the RFFF is the ideal flap for partial defects.

Functional Outcomes

Introduction

Although the most obvious and concrete outcome in head and neck cancer is disease-free survival and a low mortality rate, it should be remembered that hypopharyngeal cancer can be physically, emotionally, and socially isolating. All efforts should be made to address the functional outcomes of total oral diet and restoration of natural speech because these greatly enhance quality of life issues and enable the patient to cope better with potentially terminal disease.

Swallowing and Oral Diet Outcomes

Oral diet and swallowing is an essential component of quality of life and should not be viewed simply as the intake of calories and nutrition, something that can be easily accomplished with tube feeding. Furthermore, deglutition is a complicated process, and the hypopharynx does not simply function in isolation as a passive conduit. The tongue is the key component in food bolus propulsion and may contribute to swallowing difficulties after tongue base resection or hypoglossal nerve damage. Sensation and proprioceptive feedback may also be impaired. Avoidance of aspiration must be considered in concert with swallowing, and resuspension of the hyoid should be performed when necessary. Resistant cases of feed aspiration may require resorting to tube feeding or the technique of diversion loop we have described.

Voice and Speech Restoration Outcomes

One of the main challenges in laryngopharyngectomy is the restoration of pleasant, intelligible speech and thereby enhancement of quality of life. The approaches to this can be nonsurgical such as electrovibrator and esophageal speech or surgical such as prosthetic devices (TEP) and neolarynx flap techniques.

Nonsurgical options include the electrolarynx and esophageal speech. The electrolarynx creates an unpleasant, nonhuman sound, which in itself is stigmatizing. Esophageal speech has relatively poor success rates, with only about 30% patients able to achieve useful esophageal speech, which in itself is limited to short bursts of four to six words during each insufflation.

Surgical options include prosthetic options such as TEP and nonprosthetic options, including ileocolon voice reconstruction. In the Western world, TEP is the gold standard for voice restoration. A number of studies appear to indicate superior results with ALT versus jejunum flaps, with jejunum flaps additionally providing a poor vibrator and giving a "wet"-sounding speech (33,34). Fluent TEP speech has been reported between 78% and 89% with ALT and between 22% and 25% with jejunum (24,35). However, speech therapy may help in the long term with jejunum TEP speakers (36).

The role of nonprosthetic voice restoration with ileocolon flaps is emerging, with work ongoing in our unit. The advantages of native voice reconstruction are the avoidance of prosthetic material and associated risks of infection, dislodgement, encrustation, and continual prosthesis replacement. We have thus far performed ileocolon voice reconstruction in 72 patients, with approximately one third excellent (anyone can understand), one third good (family and friends can understand), and one third fair to poor (this generally includes patients with recurrence who had to resume chemoradiotherapy or those were noncompliant with voice physiotherapy) (Chen 2011, unpublished) (Table 35-1).

SUMMARY

Pharyngeal reconstruction is one of the most challenging areas of head and neck reconstruction in terms of the complications related to hollow viscus reconstruction such as fistula and stricture and also in terms of functional restoration of swallowing and voice. We have presented our algorithm for primary defect reconstruction and our algorithms for management of secondary defects, including stricture and fistula. Although outcomes in the literature are emerging that appear to favor the ALT as the first-line choice for circumferential reconstruction, this must be tempered with the realization that reported numbers of cases are still far less than for the jejunum, which remains a tried and tested method of reconstruction. Furthermore, there is no level I or II evidence to suggest which is the ideal surgical reconstruction. The frontiers of hypopharyngeal reconstruction include restoration of voice with vascularized flaps and techniques of diversion of the pharyngeal tract for aspiration.

REFERENCES

1. Chepeha DB, Annich G, Pynnonen MA, et al. Pectoralis major myocutaneous flap vs revascularized free tissue transfer: complications, gastrostomy tube dependence, and hospitalization. *Arch Otolaryngol Head Neck Surg* 2004;130(2):181–186.
2. Patel RS, Goldstein DP, Brown D, et al. Circumferential pharyngeal reconstruction: history, critical analysis of techniques, and current therapeutic recommendations [review]. *Head Neck* 2010;32(1):109–120.
3. Bourhis J, Overgaard J, Audry H, et al. Hyperfractionated or accelerated radiotherapy in head and neck cancer: a meta-analysis. *Lancet* 2006;368(9538):843–854.
4. Pignon JP, Bourhis J, Domenge C, et al. Chemotherapy added to locoregional treatment for head and neck squamous-cell carcinoma: three meta-analyses of updated individual data. MACH-NC Collaborative Group. Meta-Analysis of Chemotherapy on Head and Neck Cancer. *Lancet* 2000;355(9208):949–955.
5. Zelefsky MJ, Kraus DH, Pfister DG, et al. Combined chemotherapy and radiotherapy versus surgery and postoperative radiotherapy for advanced hypopharyngeal cancer. *Head Neck* 1996;18(5):405–411.
6. Khouri RK, Cooley BC, Kunselman AR, et al. A prospective study of microvascular free-flap surgery and outcome. *Plast Reconstr Surg* 1998;102(3):711–721.
7. Disa JJ, Pusic AL, Hidalgo DA, et al. Microvascular reconstruction of the hypopharynx: defect classification, treatment algorithm, and functional outcome based on 165 consecutive cases. *Plast Reconstr Surg* 2003;111(2):652–660; discussion 661–663.
8. Jacobi I, van der Molen L, Huiskens H, et al. Voice and speech outcomes of chemoradiation for advanced head and neck cancer: a systematic review. *Eur Arch Otorhinolaryngol* 2010;267(10):1495–1505.
9. Carrara-de Angelis E, Feher O, et al. Voice and swallowing in patients enrolled in a larynx preservation trial. *Arch Otolaryngol Head Neck Surg* 2003;129(7):733–738.
10. Kadota H, Fukushima J, Nakashima T, et al. Comparison of salvage and planned pharyngolaryngectomy with jejunal transfer for hypopharyngeal carcinoma after chemoradiotherapy. *Laryngoscope* 2010;120(6):1103–1108.
11. Mikulicz J. Ein fall von resection des carcinomatosen eosophagos mit plastichem ersatz des excidirten stuckes. *Prager Medizinische Wochenschrift* 1886;11:93–97.
12. Wookey H. The surgical treatment of carcinoma of the hypopharynx and the oesophagus. *Br J Surg* 1948;35(139):249–266.
13. Bakamjian VY. A two-stage method for pharyngoesophageal reconstruction with a primary pectoral skin flap. *Plast Reconstr Surg* 1965;36:173–184.
14. Ariyan S. The pectoralis major myocutaneous flap. A versatile flap for reconstruction in the head and neck. *Plast Reconstr Surg* 1979;63(1):73–81.
15. Ong GB, Lee TC. Pharyngogastric anastomosis after oesophago-pharyngectomy for carcinoma of the hypopharynx and cervical oesophagus. *Br J Surg* 1960;48:193–200.
16. Chana JS, Chen HC, Sharma R, et al. Microsurgical reconstruction of the esophagus using supercharged pedicled jejunum flaps: special indications and pitfalls. *Plast Reconstr Surg* 2002;110(3):742–748.
17. Seidenberg B, Rosenak SS, Hurwitt ES, et al. Immediate reconstruction of the cervical esophagus by a revascularized isolated jejunal segment. *Ann Surg* 1959;149(2):162–171.
18. Roberts RE, Douglass FM. Replacement of the cervical esophagus and hypopharynx by a revascularized free jejunal autograft. Report of a case successfully treated. *N Engl J Med* 1961;264:342–344.
19. Baudet J. Reconstruction of the pharyngeal wall by free transfer of the greater omentum and stomach. *Int J Microsurg* 1979;1:53–59.
20. Yang GF, Chen B, Gao Y, et al. Forearm free skin flap transplantation. *National Medical Journal of China* 1981;61:139–142.

TABLE 37-1 Summary of Flap Options and Outcomes (Using Highest Available Level of Evidence)

Flap	Advantages	Disadvantages	Fistula and Stricture Rates	Swallowing	Speech
Radial forearm free flap	Long pedicle Good speech Easy to raise	Increased fistula rates Poor donor site Too narrow to make same width as native hypopharynx	Fistula, 27% Stricture, 30% (level III, Patel and coworkers [2])	"Oral diet," 91%–100% (level III, Patel and coworkers [2])	75%–93% (level III, Patel and coworkers [2])
Jejunum	Decreased fistula rates Reliable: >1000 cases in literature	Wet speech Hyperperistalsis dysphagia	Fistula, 12% Stricture, 10% (level III, Patel and coworkers [2])	"Oral diet," 85% (level III, Patel and coworkers [2])	60%–65% (level III, Patel and coworkers [2])
PM	Easy to perform Does not require microsurgery	High complication rates Poor donor site, particularly in women	Fistula, 13%–63% Stricture, 5%–75% (level IV, Spriano and coworkers [31] in discussion by Reece [31])	"Regular" diet, 33%–100% (level IV, Spriano and coworkers [31]) Gastrostomy dependent, 42% (level III, Chepaha and coworkers [1])	
Anterolateral thigh	Flexibility of design Can include VL for dead space obliteration Fascia for waterproofing Good TEP speech	Technically more difficult to raise Potential for late fistulae	Fistula, 6% Stricture, 13% (level III, Patel and coworkers [2])	"Oral diet," 79%–100% (level III, Patel and coworkers [2])	90%–100% (level III, Patel and coworkers [2])

TEP, tracheoesophageal puncture; VL, vastus lateralis muscle.

21. Soutar DS, Scheker LR, Tanner NS, et al. The radial forearm flap: a versatile method for intra-oral reconstruction. *Br J Plast Surg* 1983;36(1):1–8.
22. Song YG, Chen GZ, Song YL. The free thigh flap: a new free flap concept based on the septocutaneous artery. *Br J Plast Surg* 1984;37(2):149–159.
23. Yu P, Robb GL. Pharyngoesophageal reconstruction with the anterolateral thigh flap: a clinical and functional outcomes study. *Plast Reconstr Surg* 2005;116(7):1845–1855.
24. Yu P, Lewin JS, Reece GP, Robb GL. Comparison of clinical and functional outcomes and hospital costs following pharyngoesophageal reconstruction with the anterolateral thigh free flap versus the jejunal flap. *Plast Reconstr Surg* 2006;117(3):968–974.
25. Chen HC, Tang YB, Chang MH. Reconstruction of the voice after laryngectomy [review]. *Clin Plast Surg* 2001;28(2):389–402.
26. Chen HC, Patel H, Chen YC, et al. Talking jejunum: a new, safe technique for voice reconstruction using free-jejunum transfer. *Plast Reconstr Surg* 2003;111(1):336–340.
27. Chen HC, Chana JS, Chang CH, et al. A new method of subcutaneous placement of free jejunal flaps to reconstruct a diversionary conduit for swallowing in complicated pharyngoesophageal injury. *Plast Reconstr Surg* 2003;112(6):1528–1833.
28. Cordeiro PG, Shah K, Santamaria E, et al. Barium swallows after free jejunal transfer: should they be performed routinely? *Plast Reconstr Surg* 1999;103(4):1167–1175.
29. Chang DW, Hussussian C, Lewin JS, et al. Analysis of pharyngocutaneous fistula following free jejunal transfer for total laryngopharyngectomy. *Plast Reconstr Surg* 2002;109(5):1522–1527.
30. Nakamura T, Inokuchi K, Sugimachi K. Use of revascularized jejunum as a free graft for cervical esophagus. *Jpn J Surg* 1975;5(2):92–102.
31. Spriano G, Pellini R, Roselli R. Pectoralis major myocutaneous flap for hypopharyngeal reconstruction. *Plast Reconstr Surg* 2002;110(6):1408–1413; discussion 1414–1416.
32. Murray DJ, Novak CB, Neligan PC. Fasciocutaneous free flaps in pharyngolaryngo-oesophageal reconstruction: a critical review of the literature. *J Plast Reconstr Aesthet Surg* 2008;61(10):1148–1156.
33. Robb GL, Lewin JS, Deschler DG, et al. Speech and swallowing outcomes in reconstructions of the pharynx and cervical esophagus. *Head Neck* 2003;25(3):232–244.
34. Ahmad I, Kumar BN, Radford K, et al. Surgical voice restoration following ablative surgery for laryngeal and hypopharyngeal carcinoma. *J Laryngol Otol* 2000;114(7):522–525.
35. Lewin JS, Barringer DA, May AH, et al. Functional outcomes after circumferential pharyngoesophageal reconstruction. *Laryngoscope* 2005;115(7):1266–1271.
36. Benazzo M, Bertino G, Lanza L, et al. Voice restoration after circumferential pharyngolaryngectomy with free jejunum repair. *Eur Arch Otorhinolaryngol* 2001;258(4):173–176.

CHAPTER 38

Soft Tissue Augmentation of the Face

Summer E. Hanson and John W. Siebert

CONVENTIONAL TREATMENT OPTIONS

Several techniques have been described to address soft tissue defects of the face secondary to congenital anomalies, traumatic defects, and a variety of other pathologies. Microsurgical correction of facial contour deformities illustrates the evolution of surgical techniques to address facial asymmetry. Among the surgical options are fat grafting, injectable fillers, tissue expansion, bone and cartilage grafting, dermal and fat grafting, local flaps, and microvascular free tissue transfer. Fat grafting and injectable fillers are often considered for secondary procedures after local or regional flaps or free tissue transfer. Autologous fat grafting has been used for decades to address not only areas of soft tissue paucity but scar or contracted soft tissue as well; however, transferred adipocytes are highly sensitive to ischemia, and given the nature of tissue encountered in disease such as hemifacial atrophy and linear scleroderma, avascular grafts are likely to resorb (1).

The defects addressed with free flaps are typically too large or complex to be amenable to fillers—synthetic or autologous—or local flaps such as temporalis muscle, superficial temporal fascia, or superficial musculoaponeurotic system (SMAS)–platysmal composite flaps. The senior author (JWS) has performed several hundred microvascular free tissue transfers to correct facial contour irregularities. Over the past 2 decades, one's approach to correcting such facial asymmetry has evolved from filling in the obvious defect to placing emphasis on the esthetic component of facial reconstruction.

FREE FLAPS AVAILABLE FOR RECONSTRUCTION

A variety of free tissue transfers have been described for facial contour or asymmetry correction. The most commonly used flaps include parascapular and scapular flaps, superficial inferior epigastric artery (SIEA) flaps, deep inferior epigastric perforator (DIEP) flaps, or anterolateral thigh (ALT) flaps (2–4). Although less commonly cited in the literature, free omentum, gracilis, and transverse rectus abdominus myocutaneous (TRAM) flaps have been used as well (5). In the authors' opinion, only fasciocutaneous free flaps should be considered as potential donors for facial reconstruction unless a bone component is needed. These types of flaps offer reliable, long-term results. Muscle or myocutaneous flaps are less desirable from an aesthetic standpoint because of the bulk of the tissue and unpredictable atrophy of the muscle overtime. Alternatively, a recent extension of the perforator flap techniques is the free-style flap, which allows for designing a flap of nearly any cutaneous paddle based on arterial inflow or Doppler signals (6), depending on the soft tissue needs. The authors' preferred choice for facial contour is the parascapular flap or inframammary extended circumflex scapular (IMECS) modification in most cases (7).

INDICATIONS

Free tissue transfer has been used to address any subtle facial contour deformity not amenable to correction with local or regional tissue rearrangement. The facial contour challenges particularly amenable to microsurgical reconstruction include hemifacial microsomia, hemifacial atrophy or collagen vascular disorders, facial trauma or palsy, vascular or lymphatic malformations, sequelae of radiation or other treatment of tumors, traumatic defects, and other congenital facial anomalies (5).

When evaluating potential donor sites for facial soft tissue correction, it is important to consider the defect in three dimensions and the components necessary for reconstruction. The authors prefer a customized flap based on the circumflex scapular system with dorsal thoracic fascial extensions that can be thinned or folded upon itself to provide variability in the soft tissue augmentation. Similarly, the ALT offers a thick, reliable adipofascial flap for soft tissue reconstruction; however, in our experience, the branching pattern of the pedicle is not as robust or extensive as the circumflex scapular artery (CSA), limiting the extent of the fascial components. An SIEA flap may be suitable for a defect requiring skin in addition to soft tissue without the need for extended fascia for augmentation. The SIEA flap may be limited by pedicle length, restricting the three-dimensional inset of the flap. Free TRAM offers a considerable amount of bulk and unreliable atrophy of the rectus muscle, as well as the possibility of neurotization of the transferred muscle from underlying normal facial musculature, producing asymmetry with facial expression.

PREPARATION OF RECIPIENT SITE

Facial contour irregularities are marked preoperatively with the patient in the upright position. Facial moulage has been reported in other series (8); however, the authors do not routinely use this in their preoperative planning. Markings are made to identify the soft tissue defects in three dimensions (Figure 38-1). Areas requiring more bulk or less depth are marked differently, and a two-dimensional template can be made, although this is not necessary with experience. The flap size, including skin paddle and fascial extensions to correct subtle irregularities, is determined and outlined on the donor site. The authors generally prefer a fasciocutaneous free flap based on the circumflex scapular system because of the robust branching pattern to all segments of the fascia and cutaneous components, as well as the ability to tailor the flap based on the dorsal thoracic fascia to accommodate subtle deficiencies around the forehead, orbit, nose, and upper lip (Figure 38-2).

The recipient site of the face should be addressed through a limited preauricular rhytidectomy incision. We find that the limited preauricular incision allows for adequate exposure of the soft tissue with an inconspicuous scar. Additionally, when the superficial temporal vessels are being used, as in most of our cases, this allows exposure for end-to-end anastomosis. An incision at the neck can be used for an alternative inflow, such as the facial or superficial thyroid, or additional venous outflow. If vascularized bone to the mandible is required, a separate, Risdon-type incision on the neck is often necessary for bony fixation.

The recipient site is prepared in a subcutaneous facelift plane and carried out beyond the limits of the soft tissue defects as determined by the preoperative markings. To fully address the three-dimensional deficiency, the facial flap is routinely raised throughout the cheek to the inferior and lateral orbital rims, above the zygomatic arch, extending to the temporal area, across the forehead, onto the nose, and across the midline of the upper lip and chin as needed.

In addition to soft tissue deficiency, positional asymmetry may be addressed simultaneously as needed. Dissection across the lip and adjacent oral commissure may be used to lengthen a deficient upper lip. The alar–facial junction may be repositioned through deep dissection at the piriform aperture with additional tissue support to build up the alar base in an anteroposterior direction. Similarly, release of a tethering tissue deficiency at the base of the ear may allow for repositioning and additional support, eliminating the need for secondary otoplasty. In our experience, the dissection is carried out at least 1 cm beyond the marked defects, into normal skin and subcutaneous tissue, to allow for redraping and to yield a natural-appearing contour.

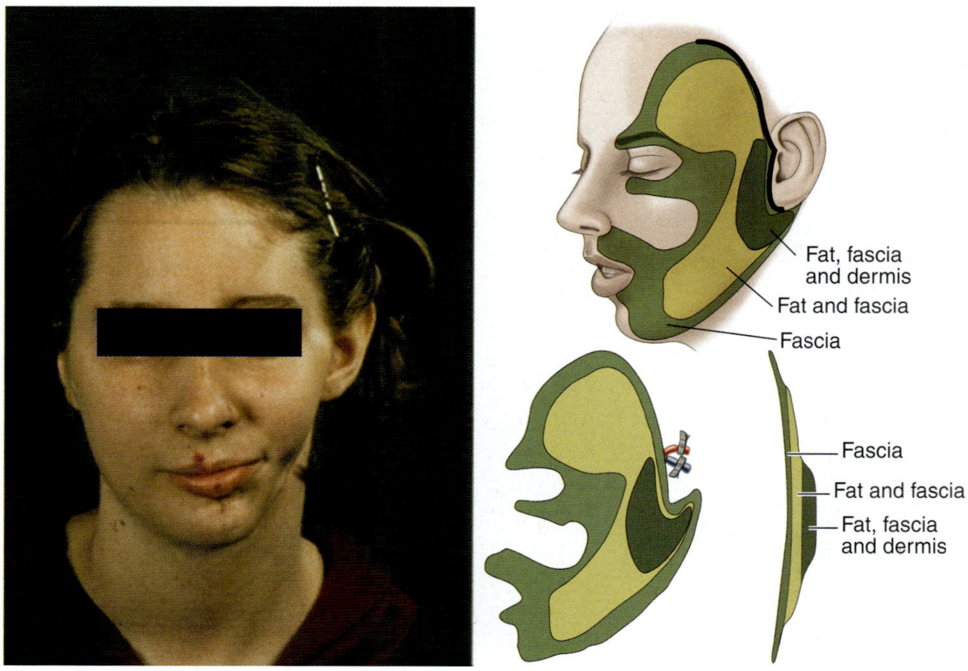

A B

FIGURE 38-1 A 17-year-old young woman with left-sided hemifacial atrophy. (A) Preoperative frontal view. A left-sided parascapular flap is planned. (B) Corresponding line drawing the extent of atrophy and the proposed soft tissue requirements for reconstruction. The customized flap in the frontal and cross-sectional views. Note the possible variations in flap thickness depending on the tissue used: fascia alone; folded fascia; fat and fascia, or fat, fascia and dermis.

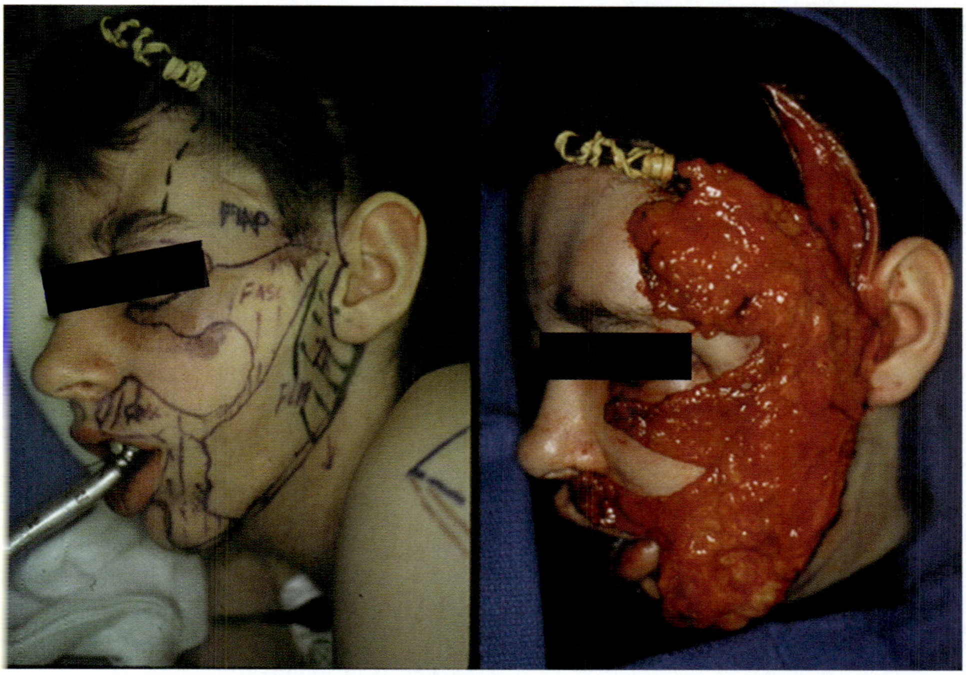

A B

FIGURE 38-2 (A) Left anterior oblique photograph of the patient in Figure 38-1 demonstrating left-sided facial atrophy. The markings correspond to tissue requirements. (B) Photographic appearance of customized flap after sculpting before inset.

VESSEL ANASTOMOSES

The recipient vessels most commonly used in our experience are the superficial temporal artery (STA) and vein in an end-to-end fashion. These are easily identified through the preauricular incision (Figure 38-3) and offer favorable positioning of the flap with the central zone in the cheek where the depth of deficiency is often the greatest and allows for fascial extensions to be tailored across the forehead, temple, alar–facial junction, lip, and chin (see Figure 38-2). If the STA is not adequate, a proximal branch from the external carotid is selected, such as the facial, superior thyroid, or transverse cervical arteries, again in an end-to-end fashion. If the paired recipient vein is not adequate for venous outflow, alternative options include transposition of the posterior auricular end-to-end, the external jugular end-to-end, or the internal jugular end-to-side. Vein graft is used liberally as needed. Microvascular anastomoses are performed venous followed by arterial to prevent engorgement with interrupted 9-0 or 10-0 nylon. Rarely is a venous coupler used in facial reconstruction because of the thin vessel wall found especially in the superficial temporal vein.

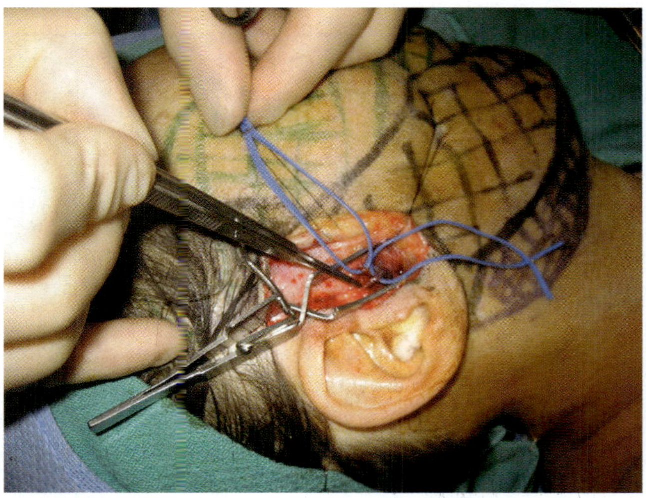

FIGURE 38-3 Right lateral photograph of the superficial temporal artery and vein accessed through a preauricular incision. These vessels can be dissected proximal toward the parotid gland to achieve more length and vessel diameter.

INSET OF FLAP

After the microvascular anastomoses are complete, the flap is laid out across the face. The depth and fascial requirements are confirmed based on preoperative markings. The skin paddle is almost always deepithelialized, if not completely removed, and contoured to accommodate areas of the face that transition from more to less soft tissue requirements. This ensures a natural-appearing facial contour. The flap is positioned with the dermal side superficial. The free flap is stretched out to maximal dimensions when insetting. A skin island is used only if there is undue tension with primary closure of the preauricular incision, as in the case of prior irradiation. The flap is secured in place near the anastomoses, being careful not to compress the vessels, with buried absorbable suture, as well as with nonabsorbable suture to the periosteum of the orbital rim and zygoma to prevent downward shift. Nylon is used for fixation of the boundaries of the flap, with the suture brought through the skin and tied over bolsters of petroleum gauze (Figures 38-2, 38-3, and 38-7). A 10-Fr Blake suction drain is placed with the tip at the inferiormost portion of the flap and brought out the scalp. The drain is usually removed at postoperative day 1 or 2. Bolsters and preauricular sutures are removed at 7 days after surgery. A Doppler is used to confirm both arterial and venous signals for postoperative monitoring.

In our experience, although the tissue requirements are variable across defects, we have found that more tissue is required for the malar region than initially suspected. The fascial extensions or flap itself may be folded over on itself for more depth. Alternatively, less tissue than initially suspected is usually required almost everywhere else, especially at the jawline. It is important to interdigitate the borders of the free flap with normal tissue at the outskirts of the subcutaneous dissection and advance the flap into this normal transition zone farther than one might expect. This allows for the most natural-appearing contour and accounts for some tissue laxity with time or inevitable contracture and pullback with healing.

POSTOPERATIVE MONITORING

A skin paddle is generally not used for monitoring unless it is needed to relieve tension on the flap at the time of closure. All flaps are monitored by Doppler analysis of the arterial and venous signals. We do not routinely use tissue oximetry because the flap is almost always buried. Additionally, we have not found the implantable Doppler device to be advantageous. Postoperative anticoagulation varies; our patients receive a daily aspirin during the first month after free tissue transfer.

POTENTIAL COMPLICATIONS

Complications in free tissue transfer for facial reconstruction include hematoma, vascular thrombosis, partial or total flap loss, wound breakdown, infection, and donor site wound complication. In general, these complications are rare (3,8,9). Revision procedures are expected in such complex reconstructions.

SECONDARY SURGERY

With the evolution of microsurgical techniques and focus on the aesthetic outcomes of facial reconstruction, additional ancillary procedures are expected and discussed as such preoperatively. The timing of revision procedures is beginning at 6 months after the free tissue transfer to allow for resolution of all edema. Debulking of the flap can be performed at this time. With the circumflex scapular or parascapular flaps, liberal debulking or tailoring can be performed at the initial transfer except in the area of the vascular pedicle; however, further refinements can be expected to achieve optimal contour. Unilateral defects often present a bigger challenge than bilateral defects in terms of final outcome and symmetry (10). Flap revisions can be approached through the same preauricular incision, and the subcutaneous plane is elevated. This incision is converted to a retrotragal incision at the time of revision. Common secondary procedures include advancement or rotation–advancement or tissue turnover or transposition to accommodate areas where more or less soft tissue is needed after the initial postoperative period.

Secondary or ancillary cosmetic procedures can be used to achieve optimal results. The adipofascial flap may be treated similar to the SMAS–platysma, and we have often used aggressive SMASectomy with resuspension as in a modified facelift. Autologous fat grafting is used to address small defects, contracture, or tethering, particularly for subtleties of the lip or nasal ala. Additionally, standard blepharoplasty, nasalplasty, browpexy, otoplasty, and genioplasty have been performed in select cases.

RESULTS AND OUTCOMES

The evolution of microsurgical techniques, from bulky myocutaneous flaps to perforator flaps and customized adipofascial flaps, mirrors the evolving approach of the microsurgeon to facial reconstruction, particularly in asymmetry or soft tissue augmentation. Free tissue transfer has many therapeutic advantages compared with other approaches in long-term outcomes and stability (9). Our experience includes nearly 400 microvascular free flaps for facial reconstruction related to congenital or acquired defects, some with more than 20 years of follow-up (2,9,11–13). The authors prefer a customized parascapular or IMECS flap to address contour irregularities and soft tissue defects (Figures 38-4 and 38-5), although we have included SIEA (Figures 38-6 and 38-7), DIEP, and myocutaneous flaps. Subjectively, all patients had improved outcomes in terms of their soft tissue contour, tone, color, and symmetry. Twenty-five patients had bilateral deformities, as in Figures 38-5 and 38-7 (10). The unplanned reoperation or reexploration rate in our series is less than 5% for hematoma or suspected vascular thrombosis and total flap loss occurring in one patient 2 weeks after surgery when he smoked heavily. Combining standard facial aesthetic techniques with secondary procedures will further enhance results.

Inigo and colleagues have described their experience with facial reconstruction in patients primarily with Romberg's disease treated with free groin flap, rectus abdominus, latissimus dorsi, and scapular flaps, all with excellent results (3,14). Similarly, Nasir et al. reported their favorable experience with fasciocutaneous

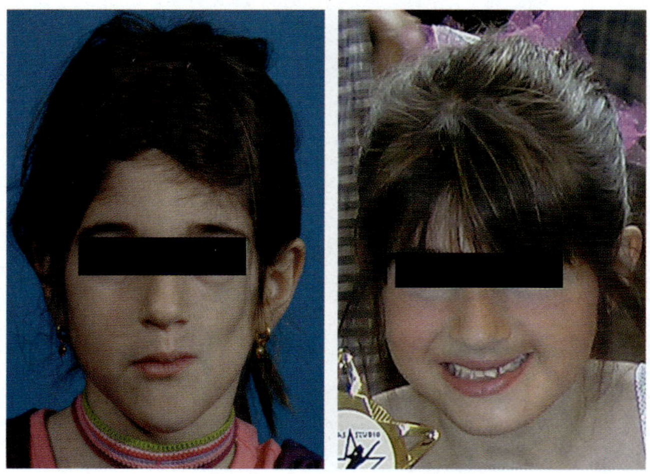

A B

FIGURE 38-4 A 5-year-old girl with left-sided hemifacial atrophy. (A) Preoperative frontal view. (B) Postoperative frontal view 2 years after parascapular free tissue transfer.

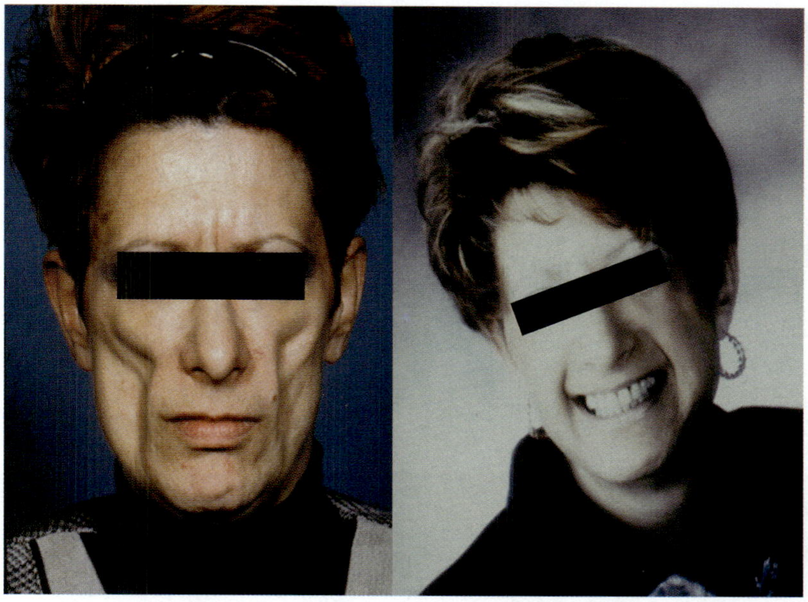

A B

FIGURE 38-5 A 48-year-old woman with severe bilateral facial atrophy. (A) Preoperative frontal view. (B) Postoperative frontal view 2 years after bilateral customized inframammary extended circumflex scapular free tissue transfer. Secondary procedures included a modified upper facelift. Note the natural-appearing animation of the face with smiling despite bilateral subcutaneous free flaps. (Reproduced with permission from Siebert JW, Longaker MT. Aesthetic facial contour reconstruction with microvascular free flaps. *Head Neck Reconstr* 2001;28(2):361.)

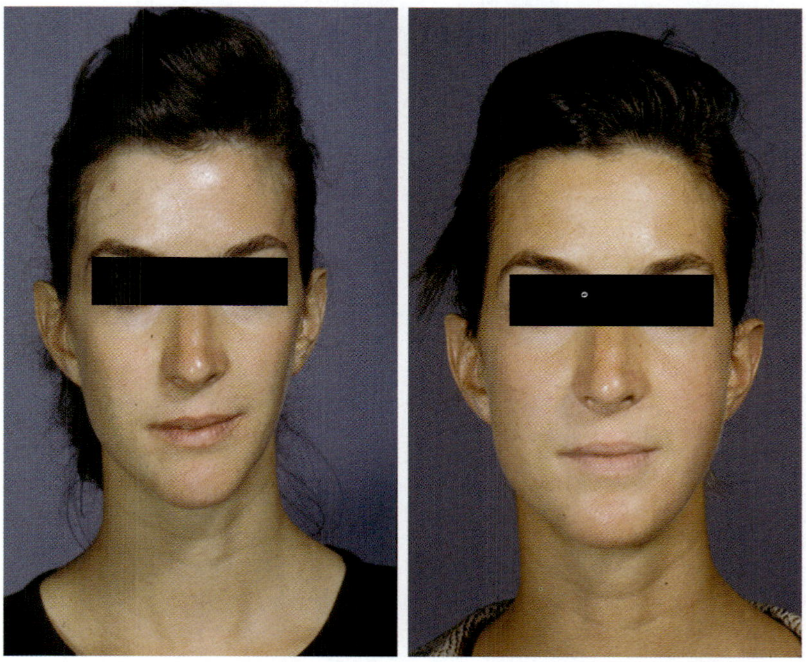

A B

FIGURE 38-6 A 25-year-old woman with left-sided craniofacial microsomia who had previously undergone a LeFort I and sagittal split osteotomies with subsequent soft tissue deficiency of the left side. (A) Preoperative frontal view. (B) Postoperative frontal view 2 years after reconstruction with superficial inferior epigastric free flap augmentation. Secondary procedures included a modified midface lift. (Reproduced with permission from Saadeh PB, Chang CC, Warren SM, et al. Microsurgical correction of facial contour deformities in patients with craniofacial malformations: a 15-year experience. *Plast Reconstr Surg* 2008;121(6):368e–378e.)

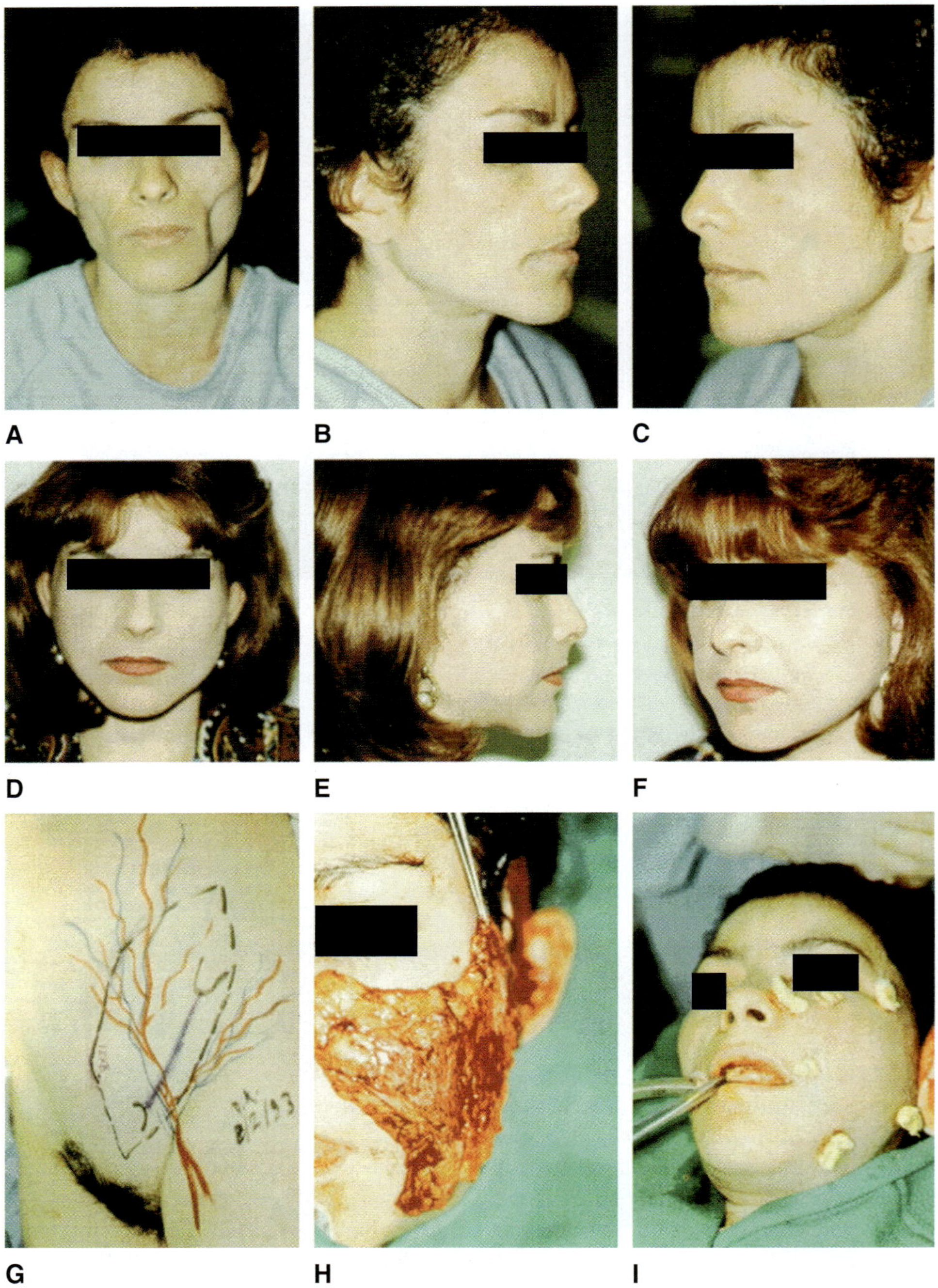

FIGURE 38-7 A 28-year-old woman with systemic lupus erythematous (**A**) Preoperative frontal view demonstrating severe bilateral facial atrophy and accelerated facial aging. (**B**) Preoperative right lateral oblique view. (**C**) Preoperative left lateral oblique view. (**D**) Postoperative frontal view at 20 months after bilateral free tissue transfer with superficial inferior epigastric flaps. Secondary procedures included modified upper facelift. (**E**) Postoperative right lateral view at 20 months after reconstruction. (**F**) Postoperative left lateral oblique view at 20 months after reconstruction. (**G**) Intraoperative photograph demonstrating left superficial inferior epigastric (SIE) flap design. (**H**) Intraoperative photograph of flap draped across the left face after sculpting before flap inset. (**I**) Immediate intraoperative result after SIE free tissue transfer to the left face with tie-over bolsters for fixation and draping of the flap. (Reproduced with permission from Longaker MT, Flynn A, Siebert JW. Microsurgical correction of bilateral facial contour deformities. *Plast Reconstr Surg* 1996;98(6):951–957.)

groin flaps supplied by the superficial circumflex iliac artery (SCIA) or the superficial inferior epigastric artery (SIEA) in four patients (15), and Vaienti and colleagues discuss excellent outcomes with parascapular flap reconstruction combined with autologous fat transfer in four patients (16). The face is not only the most prominent visible part of one's body but is also responsible for conveying emotion, sense, and communication. Facial deformity, whether from a congenital anomaly, traumatic defect, disease process, or treatment, has implications for psychosocial function and patient well-being. The primary requirements of the tissue selected for transfer in facial reconstruction and soft tissue augmentation are that (1) it is malleable for contouring and inset, (2) it undergoes minimal change over time, and (3) it is similar to the unaffected subcutaneous tissue in pliability and texture (Figure 38-8). The goal of facial reconstructive surgery is to restore both form and function to as close to normal as possible.

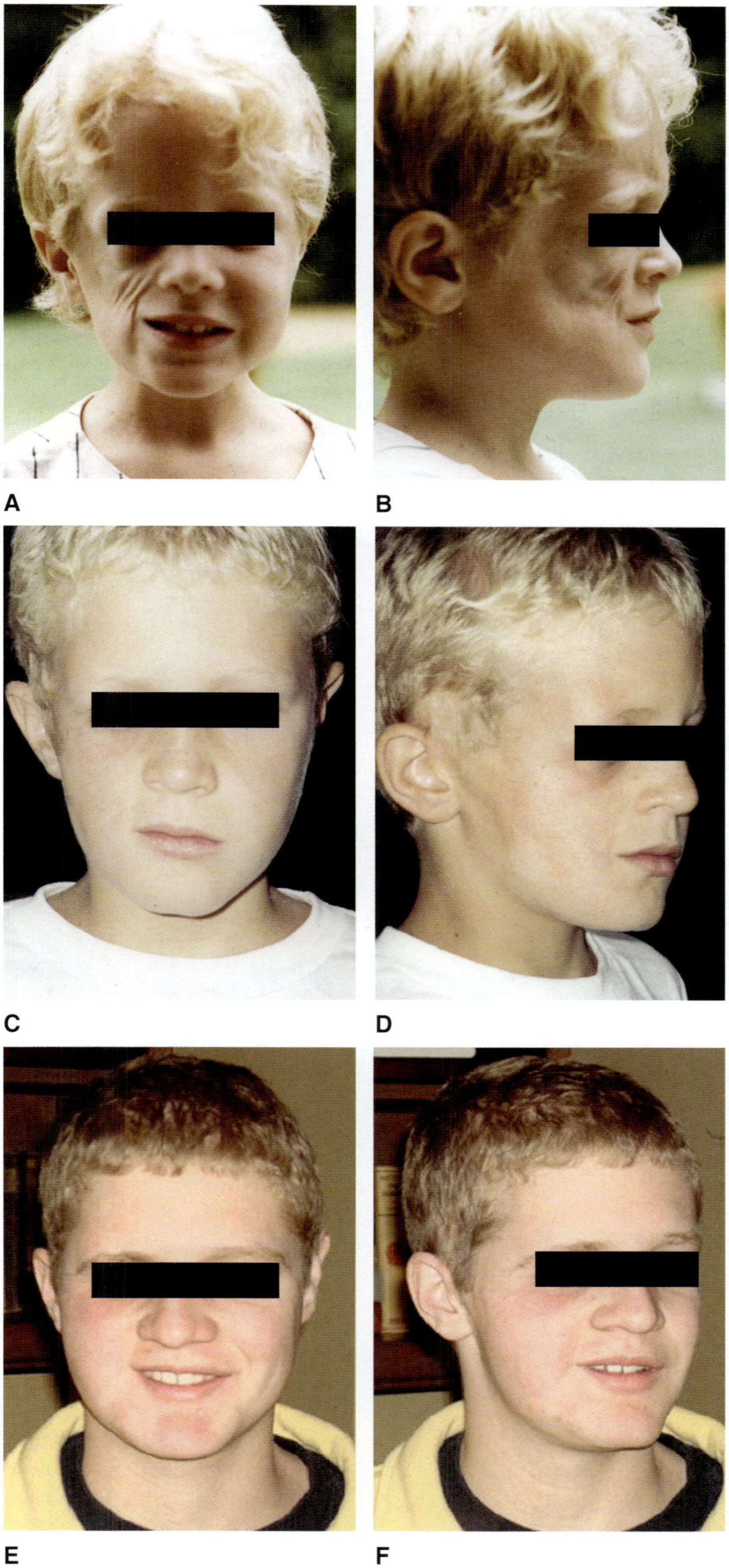

FIGURE 38-8 A 4-year-old boy with severe right-sided facial atrophy. (**A**) Preoperative frontal view. (**B**) Preoperative right lateral view. (**C**) Postoperative frontal view 6 years after free tissue transfer with a right sided parascapular flap. (**D**) Postoperative right lateral view 6 years after reconstruction. (**E**) Postoperative frontal view 20 years after reconstruction. (**F**) Postoperative right lateral view 20 years after reconstruction. Note the long-term stability and predictability with free tissue transfer.

SECTION 2

REFERENCES

1. Coleman SR. Facial recontouring with lipostructure. *Clin Plast Surg* 1997;24(2):347–367.
2. Longaker MT, Siebert JW. Microvascular free-flap correction of severe hemifacial atrophy. *Plast Reconstr Surg* 1995;96(4):800–809.
3. Inigo F, Jimenez-Murat Y, Arroyo O, et al. Restoration of facial contour in Romberg's disease and hemifacial microsomia: experience with 118 cases. *Microsurgery* 2000;20(4):167–172.
4. Agostini T, Agostini V. Adipofascial anterolateral thigh free flap for hemifacial atrophy. *Acta Otorhinolaryngol Ital* 2009;29(2):103–107.
5. Siebert JW, Anson G, Longaker MT. Microsurgical correction of facial asymmetry in 60 consecutive cases. *Plast Reconstr Surg* 1996;97(2): 354–363.
6. Wallace CG, Wei FC. The current status, evolution and future of facial reconstruction. *Chang Gung Med J* 2008;31(5):441–449.
7. Siebert JW, Longaker MT, Angrigiani C. The inframammary extended circumflex scapular flap: an aesthetic improvement of the parascapular flap. *Plast Reconstr Surg* 1997;99(1):70–77.
8. Upton J, Albin RE, Mulliken JB, Murray JE. The use of scapular and parascapular flaps for cheek reconstruction. *Plast Reconstr Surg* 1992;90(6):959–971.
9. Saadeh PB, Chang CC, Warren SM, et al. Microsurgical correction of facial contour deformities in patients with craniofacial malformations: a 15-year experience. *Plast Reconstr Surg* 2008;121(6):368e–378e.
10. Longaker MT, Flynn A, Siebert JW. Microsurgical correction of bilateral facial contour deformities. *Plast Reconstr Surg* 1996;98(6):951–957.
11. Longaker MT, Siebert JW. Microsurgical correction of facial contour in congenital craniofacial malformations: the marriage of hard and soft tissue. *Plast Reconstr Surg* 1996;98(6):942–950.
12. Siebert JW, Longaker MT. Salvage reconstruction of an extensive facial deformity due to congenital giant hairy nevus. *Plast Reconstr Surg* 1998;102(7):2414–2419.
13. Saadeh P, Reavey PL, Siebert JW. A soft-tissue approach to midfacial hypoplasia associated with Treacher Collins syndrome. *Ann Plast Surg* 2006;56(5):522–525.
14. Inigo F, Rojo P, Ysunza A. Aesthetic treatment of Romberg's disease: experience with 35 cases. *Br J Plast Surg* 1993;46(3):194–200.
15. Nasir S, Aydin MA, Altuntas S, et al. Soft tissue augmentation for restoration of facial contour deformities using the free SCIA/SIEA flap. *Microsurgery* 2008;28(5):333–338.
16. Vaienti L, Soresina M, Menozzi A. Parascapular free flap and fat grafts: combined surgical methods in morphological restoration of hemifacial progressive atrophy. *Plast Reconstr Surg* 2005;116(3):699–711.

CHAPTER 39

Free Flaps for Burns of the Face and Neck

Rodney K. Chan and Julian J. Pribaz

The opinions or assertions contained herein are the private views of the authors and are not to be construed as official or as reflecting the views of the Department of the Army or the Department of Defense.

FACE AND NECK BURN RECONSTRUCTION

Head and neck burns present substantial challenges to the reconstructive surgeon. The basic goals of reconstruction are restoration of appearance (symmetry, contour, color, texture) and function (mobility, sensation, and facial expression). In the face, aesthetics is of utmost importance, but in the neck, mobility (full neck flexion and extension) takes on higher priority.

Historically, skin grafting done acutely for coverage or subacutely for the correction of functional contractures has afforded reasonable results in limited burns of the face (1,2). However, few patients achieve satisfactory results when burns involve more than one subunit or deeper facial structures (3). Burn reconstructive surgeons often have to resort to other rungs on the reconstructive ladder to transfer composite tissue. Although these theoretically can include local flaps, regional flaps, and tissue expanded flaps, they are often not available because of collateral damage (4).

A few centers have recently achieved the ultimate in replacing "like" tissue with "like" tissue through composite tissue allotransplantation (CTA) (5–8) and have given hope to some severely burned patients. However, there are several reasons that burn patients might not be the ideal population for facial transplantation aside from the obvious lack of donors and the downsides of immune suppression. Anecdotal reports suggest increased alloantibodies from multiple sensitizing events such as the use of allografts and the need for multiple transfusions, resulting in a more difficult cross-match (9). Furthermore, burns that destroy only superficial soft tissue, sparing the underlying musculature and bony skeleton, might not be the ideal candidates for CTA. Therefore, face transplantations might be best reserved for patients with more extensive destruction, including the muscle and the underlying bony support. At this time, the risks of the transplantation procedure are substantial and may be best reserved for patients with these combined soft tissue losses, in particular extensive muscle loss, loss of the oral commissures, eyelids, and bony support.

Free flaps for burn facial reconstruction have lagged behind that for other causes such as trauma and cancer. Published literature is limited to case reports or small case series. Harii and Ohmori reported the first free flap for burn reconstruction in 1975 (10), and Rose reported use of a sculpted free scapular flap in 1995 (11). In 1997, Angrigiani reported a total face resurfaced using bilateral scapular free flaps (12). The criticisms of this 1997 report highlight some of the challenges of utilizing free flaps for burn facial reconstruction (13).

Free flaps have inherent drawbacks. They are time consuming and technically demanding and require an experienced team. Furthermore, there is a perception that local donor vessels might be inadequate and result in additional microsurgical difficulties. In actuality, the vessels deep to the muscles are usually spared and healthy. Head and neck free flaps have a 5% failure rate, and some surgeons believe that loss of the free flap might be akin to taking two steps back with the additional loss of the excised scarred skin (14). Some argue that facial resurfacing using free flaps leads to a masklike appearance. The transmission of facial animation is blunted by the presence of thick subcutaneous fat, and multiple debulking operations are frequently needed (15). However, patients with deep facial burns often already have scarred facial musculature, and their expressions are frozen even when resurfaced with just a thin skin graft. Finally, finding a free flap donor site can be a challenge, especially in a burn survivor who has sustained a large burn. The ideal tissue is thin, pliable, and large enough for subunit facial resurfacing.

Although there are many hurdles why free flaps are not widely adopted, there are also reasons why they should be given some consideration. First, full-thickness burns by definition involve loss of full-thickness skin. It is sound surgical principle to replace all the tissues lost, including epidermis, dermis and subcutaneous fat (16). This represents the best chance for restoring normal facial skin quality. Replacement of only the epidermis and some dermis with a split-thickness skin graft or even a full-thickness skin graft is insufficient to reproduce the elasticity, suppleness, and resilience of normal facial skin. According to Rose, "even in optimal circumstances, [full thickness skin grafts] will never mimic the normal skin perfectly and they often yield flat, adynamic facies with corrugated, thick surface texture" (11).

With improved understanding of perforator anatomy and advances in flap prefabrication (17,18), prelamination (18–20), preexpansion (21), chimeric flaps (22), and super thin flaps (16), free flaps in selected cases are the best option for facial burn reconstruction. This selection of flaps has given reconstructive surgeons more choices with better color match, appropriate thickness, and improved texture.

Regardless of the choice of reconstruction, an accurate diagnosis of the deformity and an appraisal of the missing parts are essential. This is particularly challenging in burn reconstruction because there is not often a physical deficit, at least not until an adequate excision or release has been performed. The deformity is compared with what is considered the "perceived normal." If the deficit is unilateral, the best guide is a comparison with the opposite side. With more extensive defects when both sides are involved, a consideration of baseline appearance as seen on an old photograph may serve as a guide to reconstruction. However, realistic goals must be set from the start as to what might be achievable with the reconstruction. When considering a free flap for burn reconstruction, a thorough investigation into the history of the patient, in particular the operations and flaps that were previously used, paying close attention to the remaining donor vessels in the head and neck is needed (15). This also includes examination of all potential donor sites, including adjacent burns and distant sites. Areas that have previously been skin grafted might not be appropriate for facial skin resurfacing but also should not be immediately excluded as areas of potential flap harvest (23). Preoperative photograph is mandatory.

Finally, it is important to formulate a comprehensive treatment plan based on the diagnosis. This is presented to the patient and family with a timetable of reconstruction, emphasizing that the sequences are designed not to burn future bridges and that flexibility is necessary. A good rapport with the patient and his or her family is as important as the reconstructive plan. Rarely are one or two operations enough to achieve the result that the patient is looking for.

FREE FLAPS FOR RECONSTRUCTION

Parrett et al. reviewed our institution's experience with free flap for cervicofacial burns in their 17-year experience from 1989 to 2005 (15). Thirty-six flaps were performed in 32 patients with cervicofacial burns with the majority being flame burns (30) and the minority (two) being electrical burns. The sites of involvement are distributed as follows: the neck (13) and face or scalp (23). The indications are 20 for severe contractures and scarring and 16 from exposed bone and cartilage.

Multiple flaps are possible, and flap selection is based on suppleness, color, thickness, and size. Generally, fasciocutaneous flaps are considered first because musculocutaneous flaps can rarely achieve the proper thickness. They are also thinner, more elastic, and more easily contoured. The addition of tissue expansion before flap harvest also allows for additional flap thinning and delay before transfer. Fifteen flaps were expanded before transfer. The free flaps most frequently used were the anterolateral thigh (ALT) flap (31%) and scapular–parascapular flap (31%) followed by the radial forearm flap (17%). Other flaps that were used include latissimus, rectus, dorsalis pedis, groin, and lower abdominal fasciocutaneous flaps. Debulking and secondary operations are common, and the patient should be advised from the initial consultation.

Fourteen flaps were prefabricated; one was prelaminated. Prelamination and prefabrication are necessary when donor options are scarce and composite reconstruction is needed. Prefabrication in our experience has also resulted in thin flaps not requiring additional debulking (nine of 14 or 64% did not require additional debulking).

INDICATIONS FOR FREE FLAPS IN FACE AND NECK BURN RECONSTRUCTION

There are three general reasons for free flap reconstructions of the face and neck after burn. The first is coverage of exposed cartilage or bone, which is an absolute indication for flap coverage. As reconstructive surgeons, we are now less frequently consulted during the acute admission of a facial burn, except when grafting is not possible. However, we should still be aware of the treatment necessary to achieve the most optimal outcome (24). Reconstructive surgeons are often consulted when the burn is deep and involves the underlying bony and cartilaginous skeleton. In these cases, flap coverage is warranted. It is important to first establish the bony platform and then perform the soft tissue reconstruction. Although it is tempting to use local flaps as first-line options for coverage, it is wise to consider their use for secondary resurfacing because they usually have the best color and texture match for facial skin.

The second reason is extensive and often recurrent neck flexion contractures. These are usually treated with scar release or excisions followed by skin grafting as a first line. Skin grafts can work well but often require prolonged immobilization and pressure and often not aesthetically pleasing. Furthermore, involuntary movement of the thyroid cartilage, especially in men, results in nonuniform graft take and recontractures. Skin grafts applied onto the platysma muscle can also lead to hypertrophic scarring from muscle contraction. When contractures are recurrent or after multiple failed reconstructions, it is appropriate to consider use of a free flap. Defects more than two thirds of the anterior neck require distant tissue and are usually not amenable to local flaps. Free flaps provide full-thickness skin and subcutaneous tissue, with improved aesthetics and better resurfacing than skin grafts. In addition, mobility is greatly enhanced with free flaps. However, their thickness can blunt the cervicomental and the mandibulomental angles, and they routinely require thinning procedures. The treatment of choice is a large, thin flap that covers the entire exposed neck when a shirt is worn. Our preference is the parascapular flap, but when that is unavailable, an expanded free groin flap or the prefabricated thigh flap maybe considered.

The third indication is failure of skin grafting of the face. Despite multiple revisions, these patients have continued contraction, hypertrophic scarring, or wound breakdown. As expected, the majority of flaps for full or partial facial resurfacing were secondary procedures performed after initial treatments have failed despite allowing time for graft maturation and physical therapy maximization. Most of the patients in this category had severe hypertrophic scarring or had poor results because of grafting, sometimes over exposed bone.

PUBLISHED EXPERIENCE

Published works on the use of free flaps for head and neck burn reconstruction are mostly limited to case reports or small case series. Rose reported his experience with 18 patients over 8 years. His strategy focuses on the primary enhancement of aesthetic appearance. He judged the criteria for success as (1) an undistracted "normal" look at conversational distance, (2) facial balance and symmetry, (3) distinct aesthetic units fused by inconspicuous scars, (4) "doughy" skin texture, and (5) dynamic facial expression. He preferred the use of forearm skin for chin, lip, and neck reconstruction; scapular for cheek and malar reconstruction; forehead for nose; and temporoparietal fascia for scalp and ear reconstructions. He had one complete flap loss early on in his series. Although most patients have achieved near normal appearance with make-up in social settings at conversational distance, he believed that microvascular free tissue transfer in aesthetic restoration of the burned face has not gained acceptance based on criticisms for abnormal color match, bulkiness and masking of facial expressivity. He has tried to overcome these criticisms through a combination of prepatterned flaps of entire facial subunits, extensive intraoperative tailoring, and cosmetic camouflage with make-up. Other critics of his work have argued that his patients are so camouflaged that it is difficult to judge the results of the reconstruction.

In our experience, we have treated the face and neck differently, stressing the importance of aesthetics in the face but emphasizing mobility for the neck. In the neck, the treatment of choice is a large, thin flap that covers the entire exposed neck when a shirt is worn. Our preference is the parascapular flap (case 1) or the ALT flap. However, the lateral thigh is often the choice of skin graft donor site and is often scarred. For that reason, even though the parascapular flap has the probable disadvantage of requiring position changes, it has assumed a prominent role in face and neck burn reconstruction. If these sites are unavailable, however, an expanded free groin flap or dorsalis pedis flap maybe used.

Not infrequently, none of these donor site are available, and prefabrication is used to bring an exogenous blood supply to an area that otherwise does have not an axial pattern pedicle. Prefabrication was used in two general settings. First, prefabrication was done at a distant site where a patient has no local option and no distant fasciocutaneous flap option. The descending branch of the lateral femoral circumflex was the preferred pedicle, and even in deep burns to the thigh, the vessel is usually spared (case 2). This can be similarly done in the lower abdomen with prefabrication using the deep inferior epigastric pedicle (case 3).

The second scenario for prefabrication is when a flap of similar texture and color is needed and local tissue is prefabricated when known axial flaps were not available. The lower neck and scalp are turned into donor sites by free pedicle transfer, allowing secondary transfer for facial reconstruction (case 4).

Our preference for facial reconstruction is to replace the entire subunit with a large expanded scapular–parascapular flap. Even for bilateral facial reconstruction, a unilaterally expanded flap is generally sufficient (case 5). When a multifaceted defect exists, especially when the central third of the face is involve, prelamination can be very helpful (case 6). Similar to the neck, prefabrication can also be used to create flaps with the best color match or texture (cases 7 and 8).

EXAMPLES OF NECK AND FACE BURN RECONSTRUCTION USING FREE FLAPS

Examples of these flaps are given in Figures 39-1 to 39-8.

SECONDARY REVISIONARY SURGERY

Multiple operations are often required to achieve a finally acceptable outcome. Essentially, all patients need revision. This is discussed in detail with the patient from the start and the plan modified on an "as needed" basis. Realistic goals need to be communicated. Depending on the complexity of reconstruction, the number of secondary revisions necessary ranges from two or three for relatively simple reconstructions to exceeding 20 to 30 for more complex defects.

The types of secondary revisions are unique to each reconstruction and to each patient. In general, the secondary procedures are aimed at restoring contour. Some principles that are observed in secondary facial reconstructions are (25):

1. Restore to their normal location uninjured or partially injured anatomical features.
2. Release scar contractures, especially around the oral commissures and the mobile parts of the face.
3. Recreate the subunits of the face by placing the scars along the natural crease lines, which often involve putting scars on the flap. Restoring the contour may involve direct thinning of tissue, debulking or augmenting soft facial parts with dermis fat grafts, or autogenous fat grafting (26,27). Local subcutaneous tissue rearrangement to re-create the peaks, valleys, and creases are often needed. Restoration of contour is more important than the presence of scars.
4. Use local flap options with better color and texture match as advancement or transposition flaps to provide better cutaneous coverage of deepithelialized, previously placed distant free flaps.

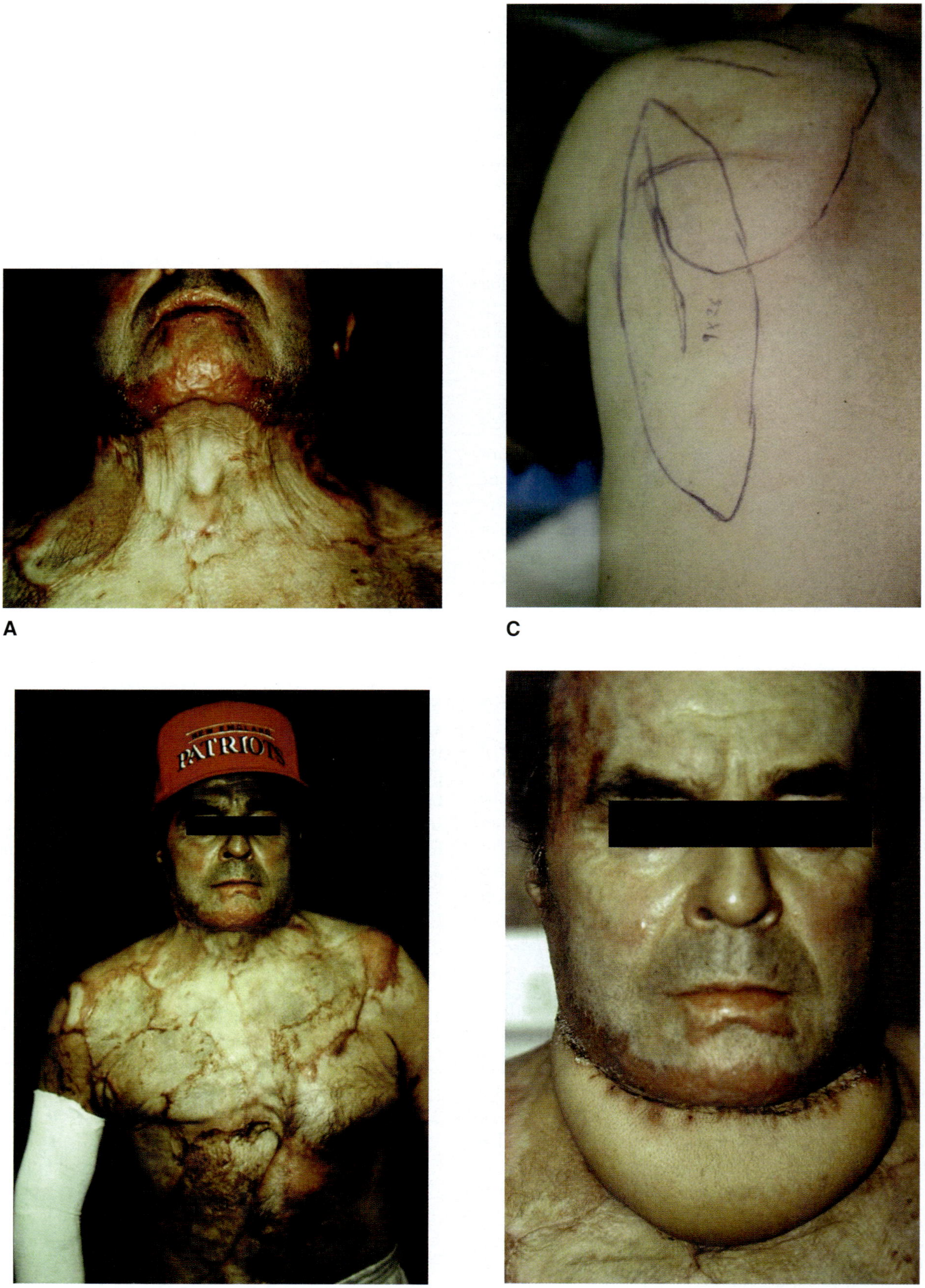

A C B D

FIGURE 39-1 Neck reconstruction with a free parascapular flap. A 45-year-old man with extensive burn scars of the neck and anterior torso. He has had multiple prior grafts on his anterior torso. (**A** and **B**) He has a severe neck contracture limiting extension. (**C** and **D**) His neck was released and covered with a parascapular flap, inset like a sling. Patients are warned ahead of time that the initial appearance of the neck will be very bulky.

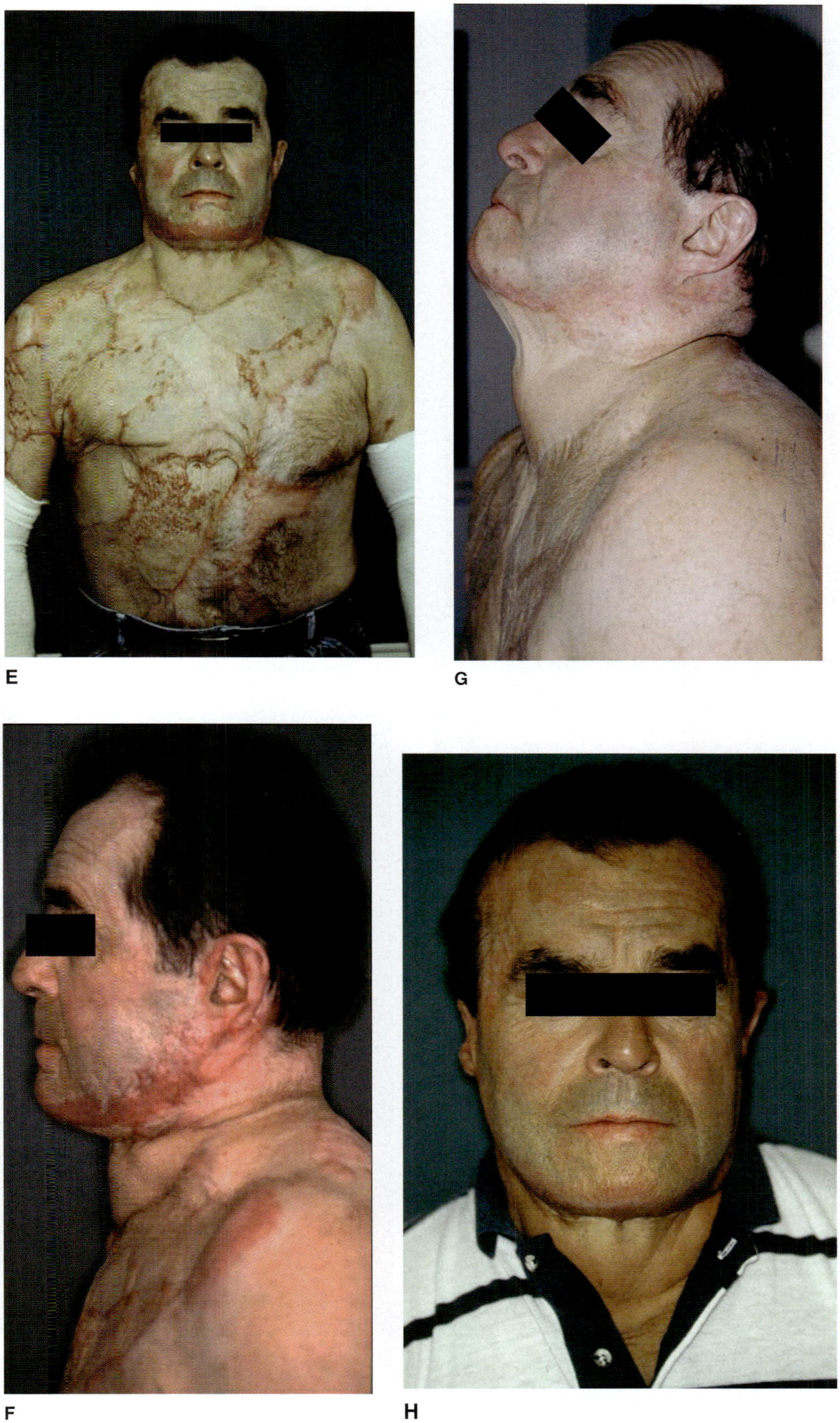

FIGURE 39-1 (*Continued*) (E to H) The flap required one debulking procedure, and the patient has a good outcome with full mobility of his neck.

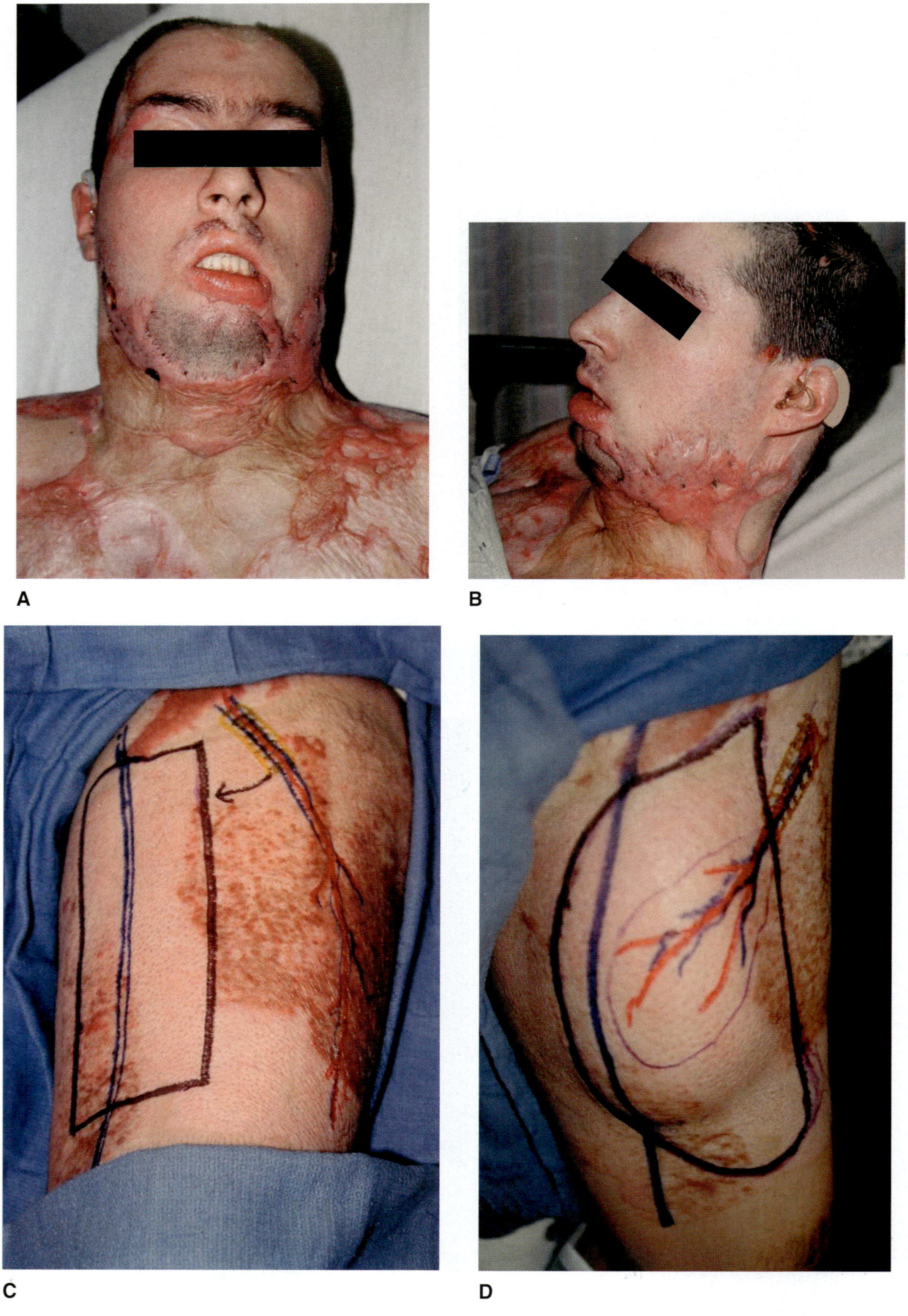

FIGURE 39-2 Neck and jawline reconstruction with a prefabricated thigh flap. (**A** and **B**) Burn patient with severe neck contracture. The lateral thigh is scarred from a previous skin graft harvest. (**C**) However, the medial thigh skin was spared, and design of the locally transposed pedicle of the descending branch of the lateral circumflex femoral vessels to prefabricate the medial thigh skin flap was performed over a tissue expander. (**D**) The patient is shown before the flap transfer during the second stage of prefabrication, with the transposed pedicle over the medial thigh skin flap, expanded and prefabricated with a reliable blood supply.

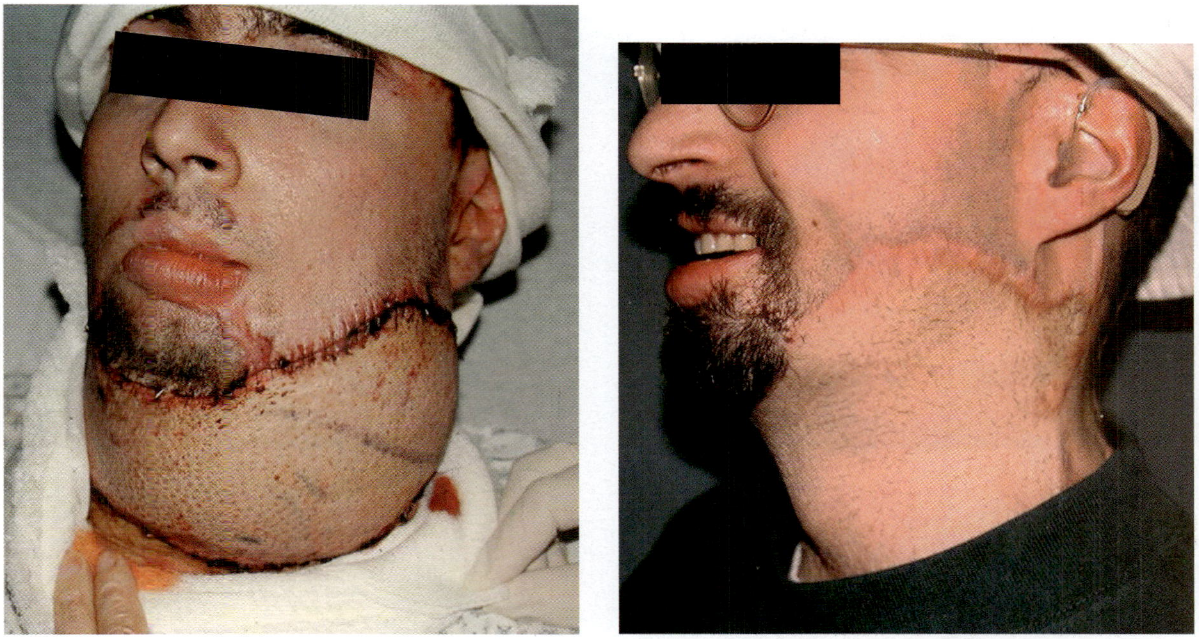

E F

FIGURE 39-2 (*Continued*) (**E**) Early postoperative result after microvascular transfer of the prefabricated tissue. (**F**) Appearance at long-term follow-up (17).

5. Use local specialized flaps (e.g., hair-bearing flaps) to reconstruct specific subunits previously covered by large distant flaps. These are also used to help break up scars and create an allusion of a more normal appearance. Successful facial reconstructions, especially in men, also need to recognize the pattern of hair growth, particularly in the sideburn and beard areas, to maintain symmetry. This is also true for eyebrow reconstruction. The temporal scalp, frontal scalp, and submental region all can give satisfactory results (28). The frontal scalp can be transferred using the supratrochlear artery and the submental region can be transferred on the submental branch of the facial artery, but these donor areas may not be available. Temporal scalp skin contains an abundance of hair follicles, although it may need implantation of a heterotopic vessel as a first stage reconstruction (prefabrication). Finally, follicular hair grafting should also be considered.
6. If local flaps are not available to improve the color mismatch of distant flaps, consider the use of thin split-thickness skin grafts harvested from the scalp as overgrafts to resurface these areas after deepithelialization of the existing flap (29).
7. Consider functional restoration of absent muscles of facial expression, especially for restitution of a smile and

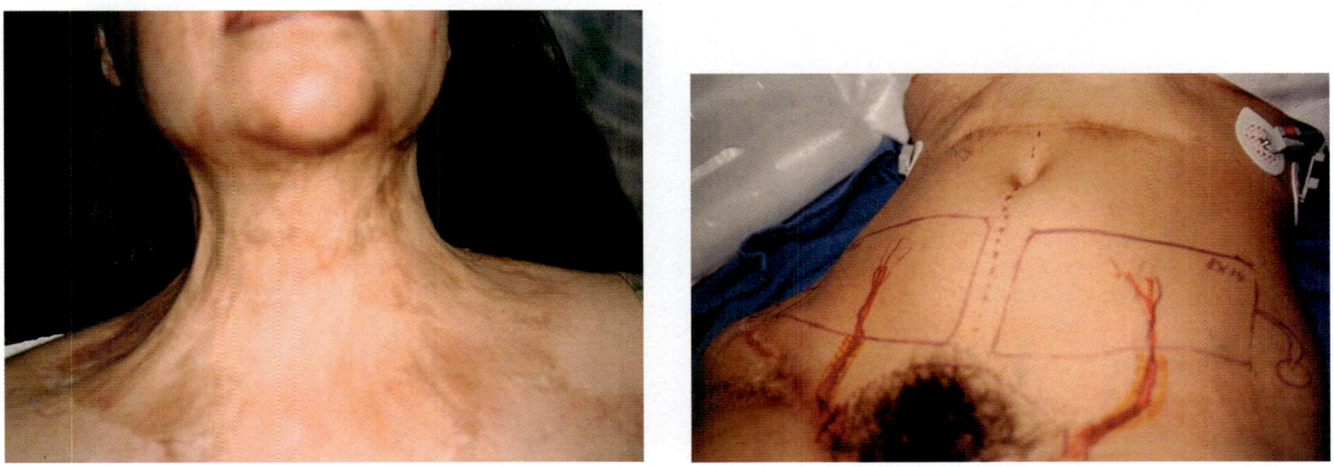

A B

FIGURE 39-3 Neck reconstruction with a prefabricated lower abdominal flap. (**A**) A 32-year-old woman presented with severe neck contractures 2 years after extensive head, neck, and chest chemical burns. (**B**) She had past skin grafts to her neck and has had multiple full-thickness grafts harvested from her thighs, groin, epigastrium, and back, severely limiting her donor sites.

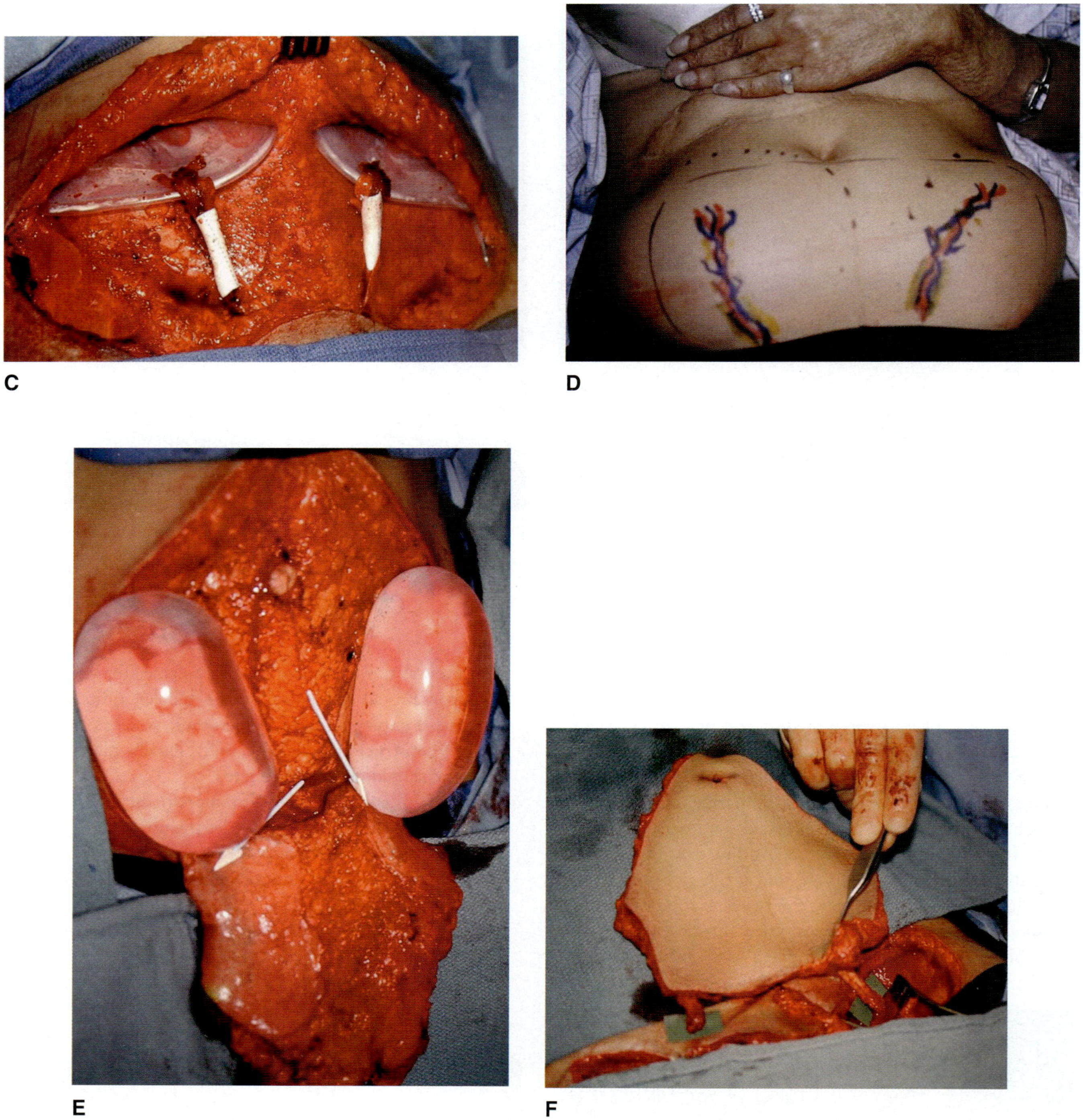

FIGURE 39-3 (*Continued*) (**D** and **E**) In the first stage of reconstruction, a lower abdominal fasciocutaneous flap was prefabricated with local transfer of bilateral deep inferior epigastric pedicles and placement of tissue expanders below the pedicles. Performing an expanded deep inferior epigastric perforator flap was out of the question because the expansion would destroy the perforators. Ten weeks later, she underwent excision of the neck scars, leaving a 16 x 22 cm defect. A microvascular transfer of the prefabricated, double-pedicle abdominal flap (**E** and **F**) was then performed to the neck.

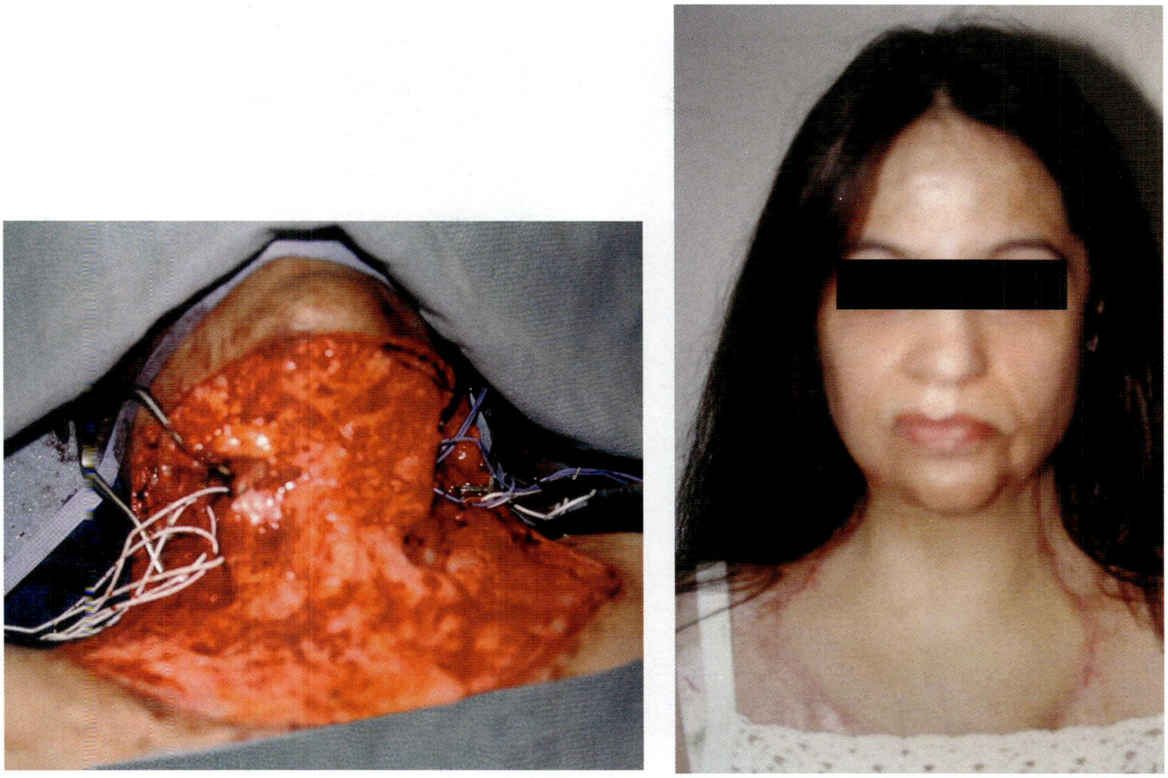

G H

FIGURE 39-3 (*Continued*) G). The flap survived, and the patient underwent two subsequent defatting procedures to decrease bulk (H) (15).

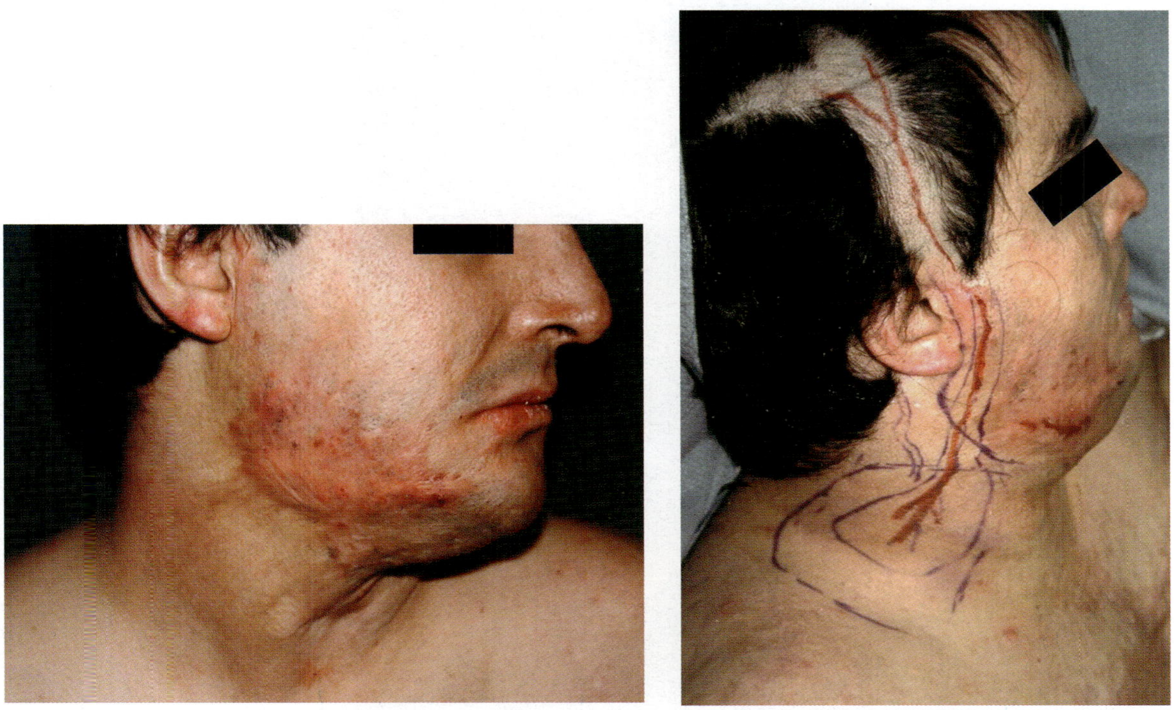

A B

FIGURE 39-4 Cheek reconstruction with a prefabricated supraclavicular flap. Prefabrication can be used to import thin, color- and texture-matched tissue into highly visible facial defects. (A) A 25-year-old man with a hypertrophic burn scar involving his right cheek and mandibular skin. In addition to aesthetic concerns, the patient complained of recurrent folliculitis within the scar that frequently required medical intervention. (B) A prefabricated flap of thin, color- and texture-matched skin was designed for eventual resurfacing of the affected area. Supraclavicular skin is axialized by pretransfer implantation of the superficial temporal vessels and its vascularized temporoparietal fascia. The vascular pedicle and fascia turned 180 degrees and fed under a preauricular skin bridge into the supraclavicular area.

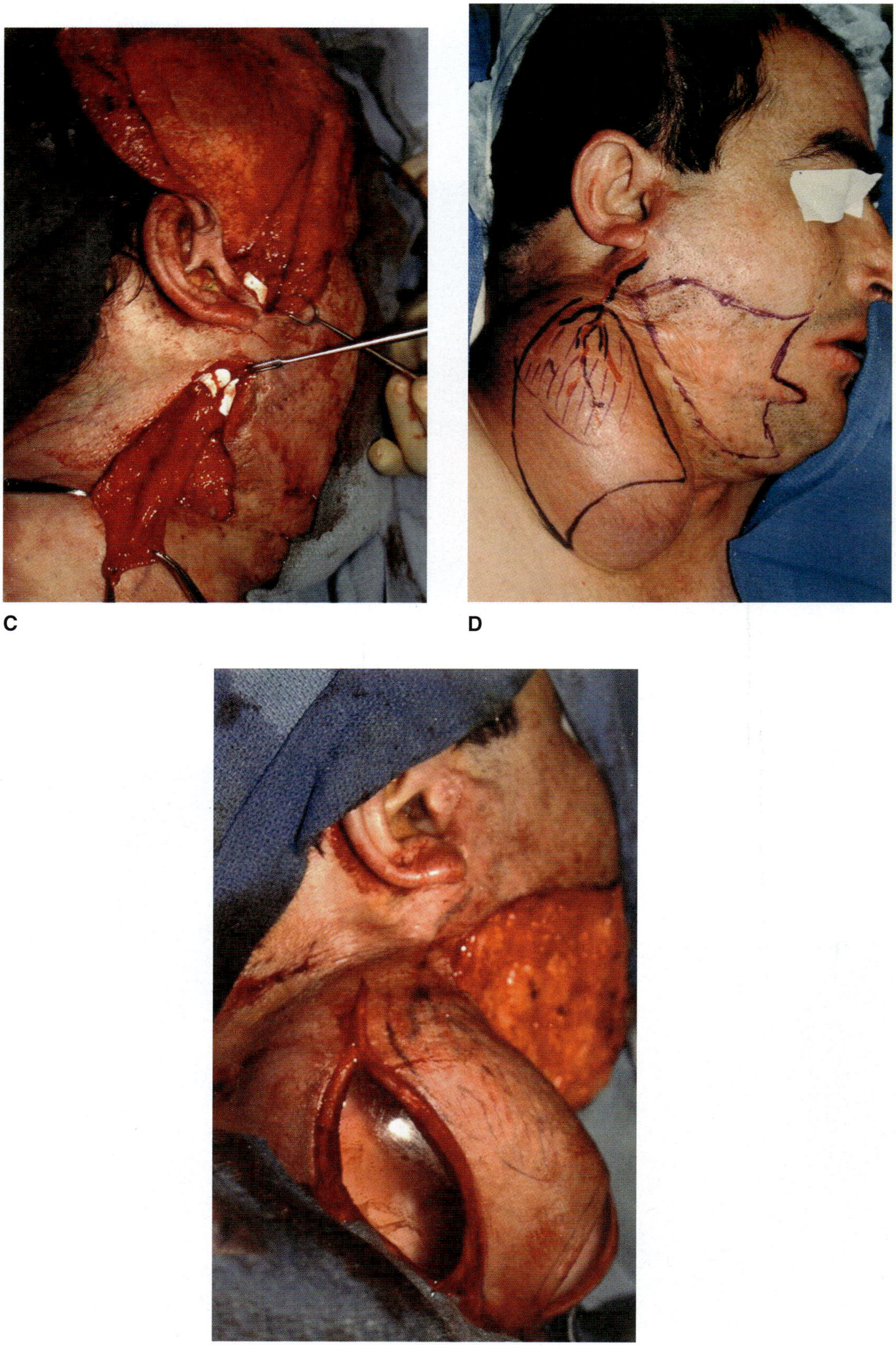

C D E

FIGURE 39-4 (*Continued*) (**C**). A thin Gore-Tex sleeve was placed around the proximal segment of this vascular bundle to facilitate its dissection at the subsequent stage of flap transfer. The distal end of the pedicle and its fascia were implanted directly underneath skin and over a minimally preinflated tissue expander. Expansion was initiated on postoperative week 1 and continued weekly for 8 weeks. At postoperative week 8, the hypertrophic skin was excised, and the prefabricated supraclavicular skin was elevated (**D** and **E**). The donor area was closed primarily with minimal cervical advancement, and the prefabricated skin was transposed into the facial defect.

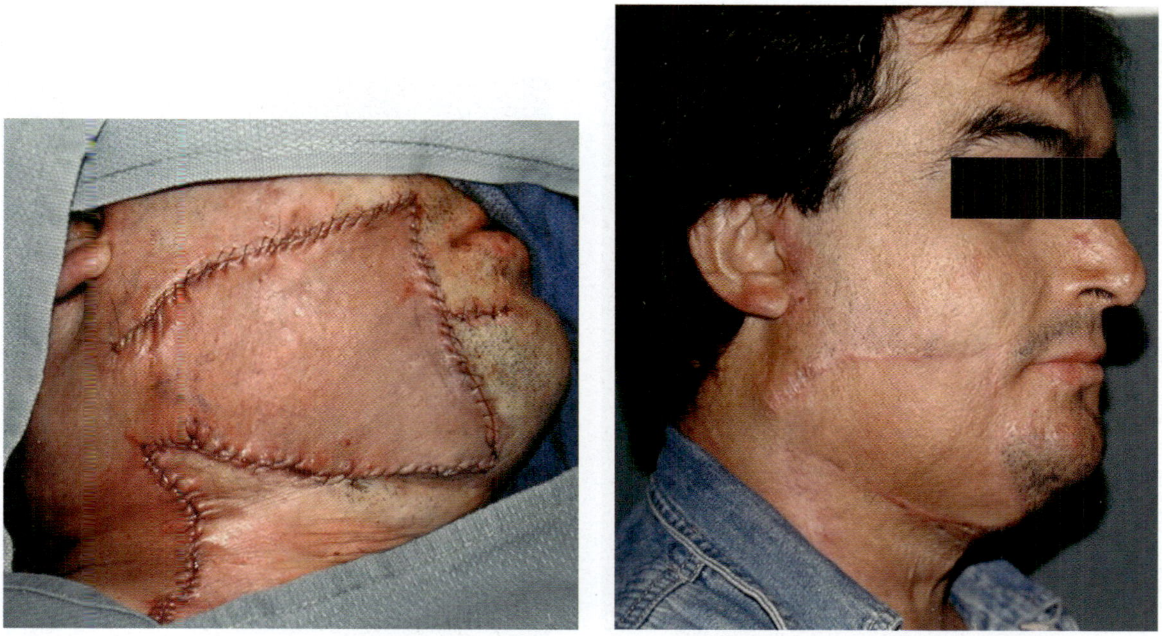

F G

FIGURE 39-4 (*Continued*) (F). Note that flap perfusion is based almost entirely on the implanted superficial temporal system at this point, which could be demonstrated as a persistently strong pulse by Doppler examination. Trace venous congestion that was present immediately after transfer resolved spontaneously within 72 hours. (G) The 3-month postoperative result demonstrates a satisfactory aesthetic facial reconstruction.

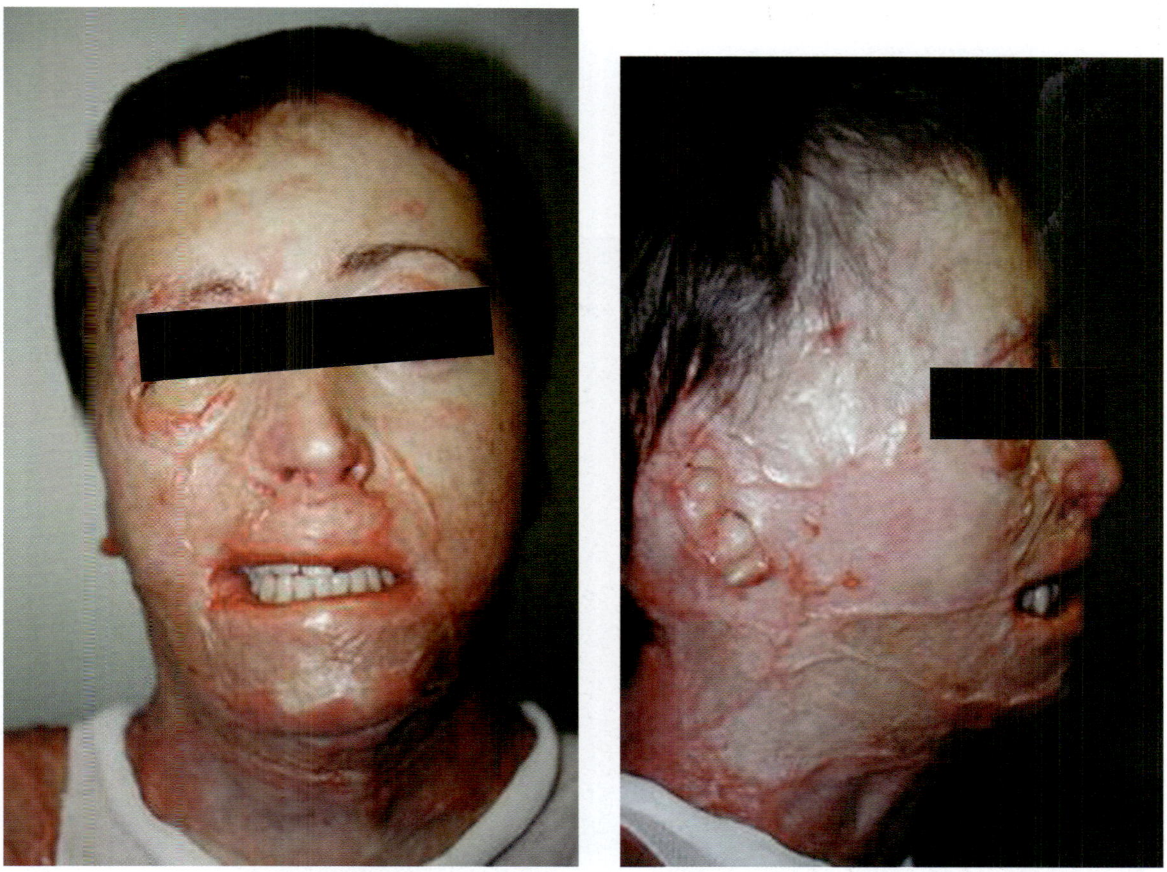

A B

FIGURE 39-5 Full facial reconstruction with an expanded scapular–parascapular flap. A 23-year-old woman with a history of extensive burn and multiple facial skin grafts and releases who now desires better texture and uniformity. (A and B) She has a loss of normal nasal and facial contours from contractures of the face and nose.

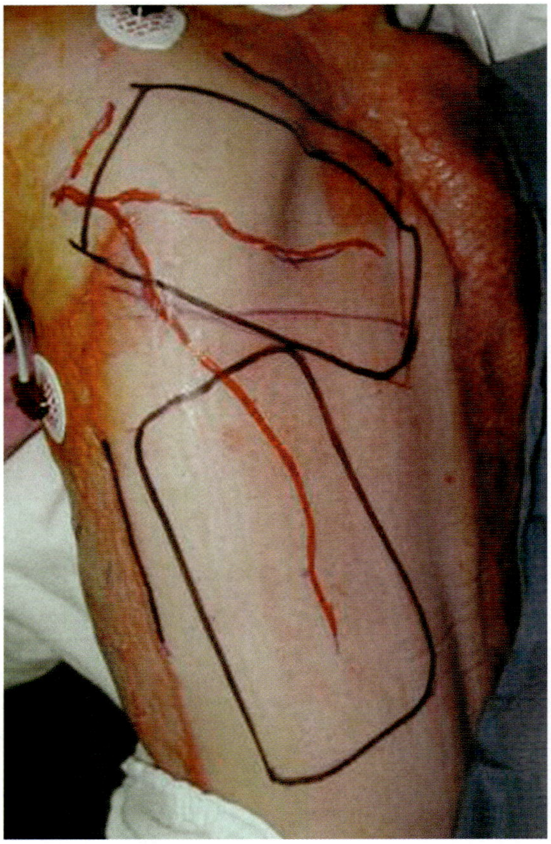

C

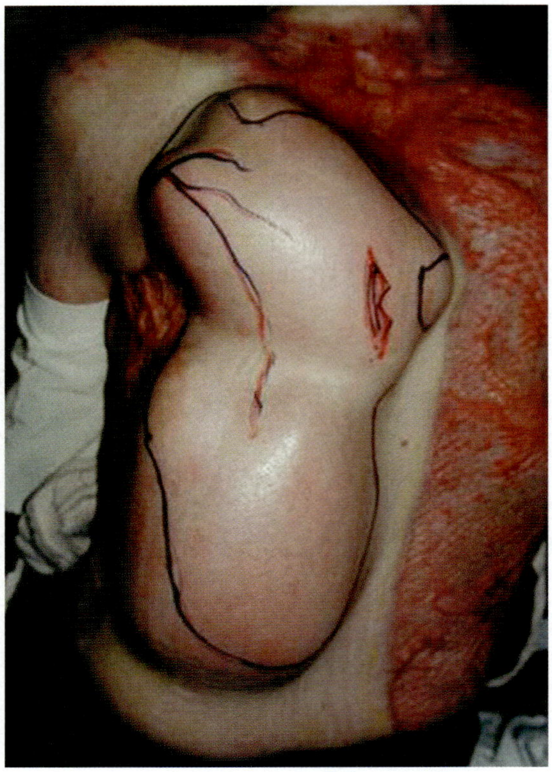

D

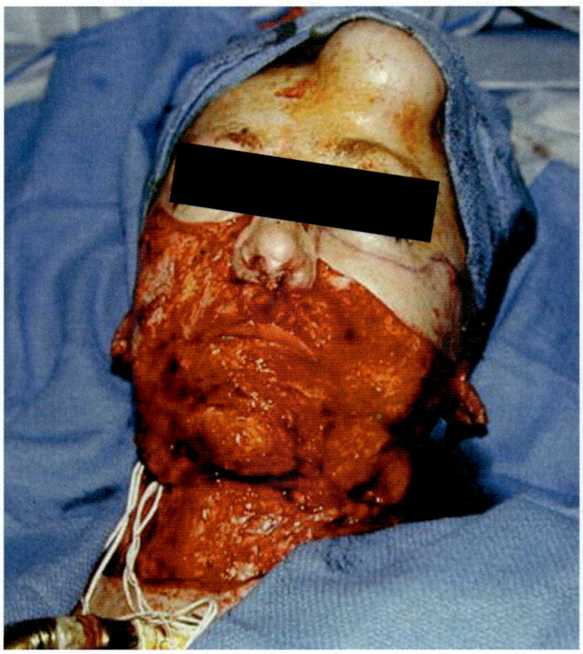

E

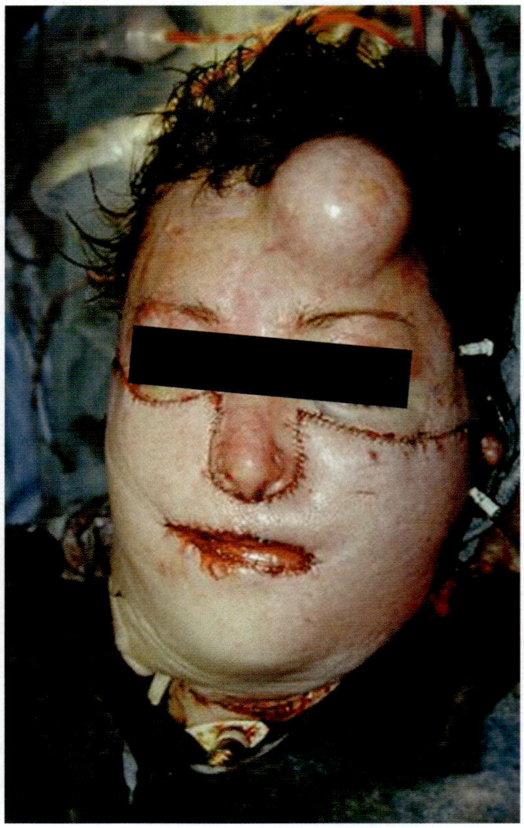

F

FIGURE 39-5 *(Continued)* (C and D) Facial resurfacing using an expanded free scapula–parascapula free flap was designed and outlined. (E) After expansion, hypertrophic burn scar was excised from her face and neck. (F) She is seen immediately after free tissue transfer.

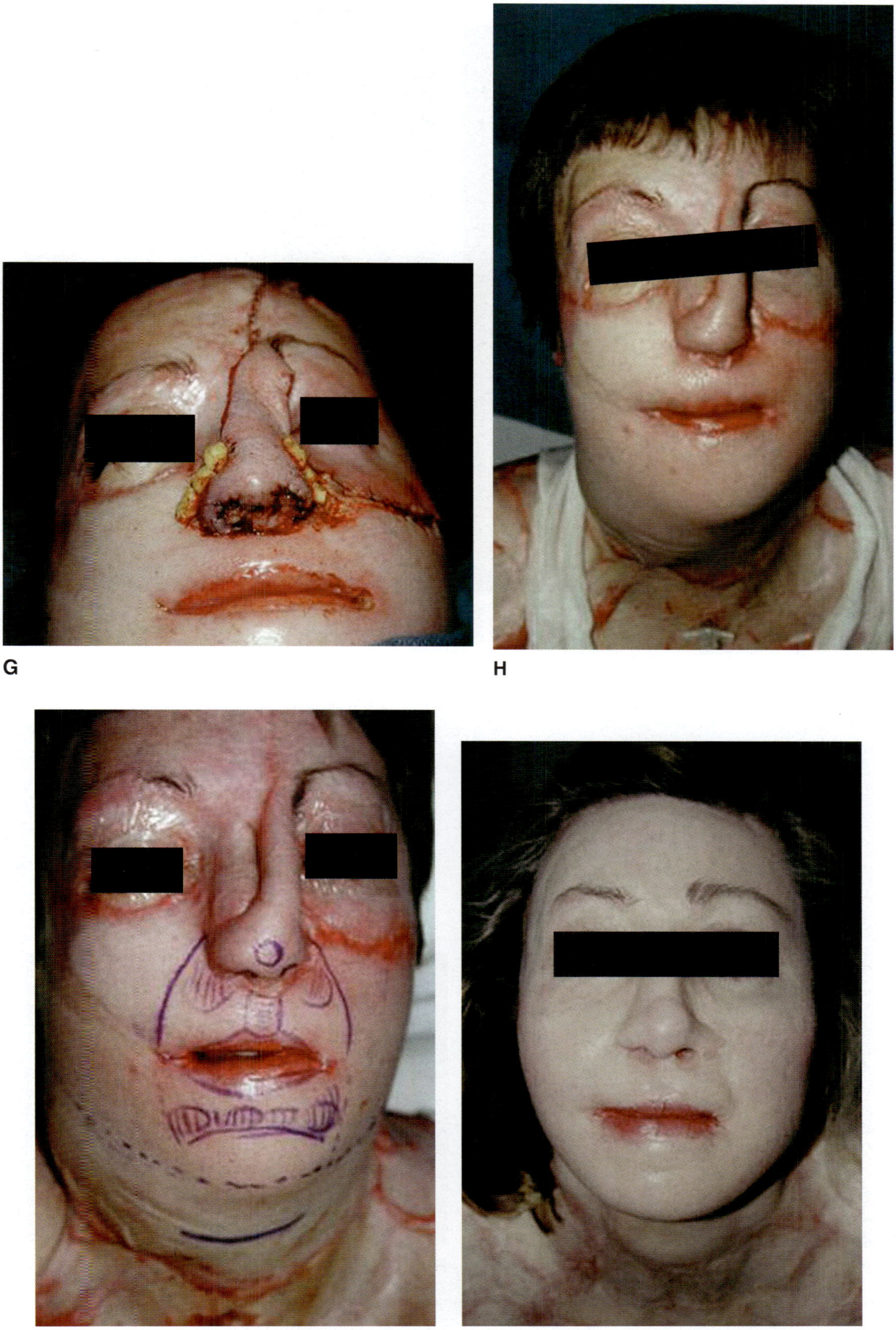

G H I J

FIGURE 39-5 (*Continued*) (G) Expanded forehead flap was used for nasal resurfacing. (H) She is seen after healing of her free flap, which still lacks normal facial creases and contours. (I) Facial aesthetic units were re-created through debulking and placement of scars in lines of natural creases to re-create lines of the cheek, the philtrum, upper lip, and chin through subcutaneous sculpting and turn-over flaps. (J) Resurfacing of unstable skin has achieved a more uniform appearance to her face and neck.

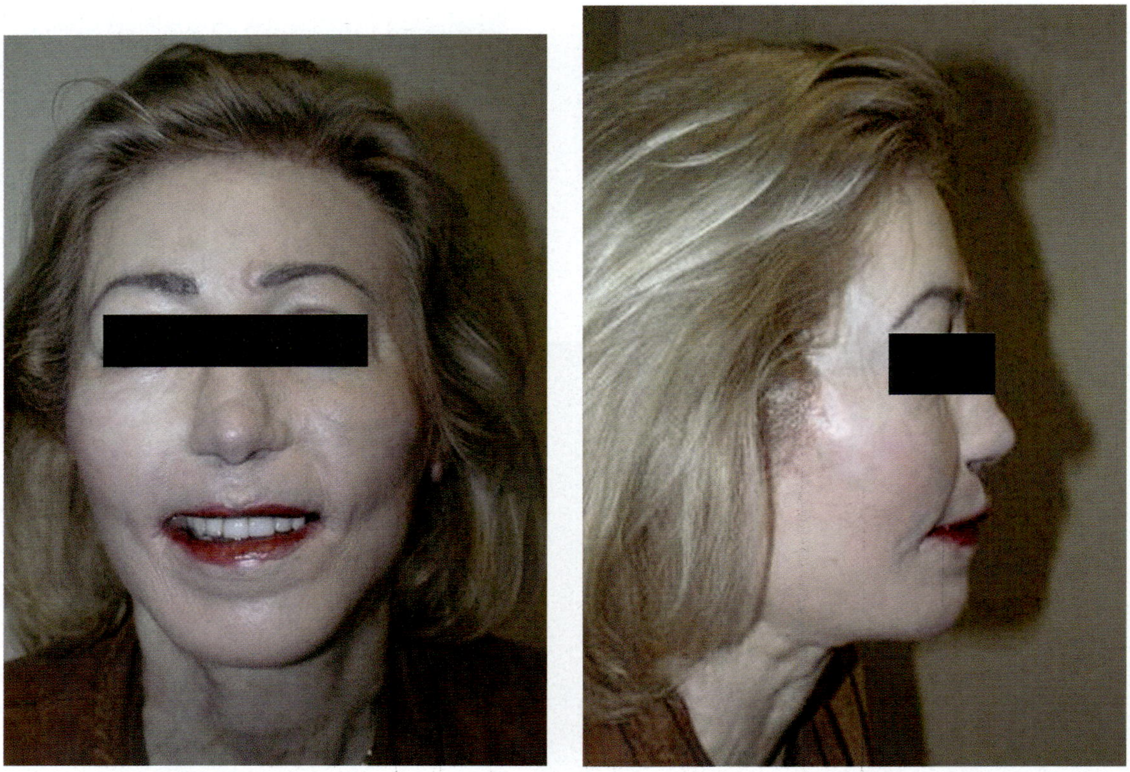

K L

FIGURE 39-5 (*Continued*) (**K**) and (**L**) Fifteen-year follow-up.

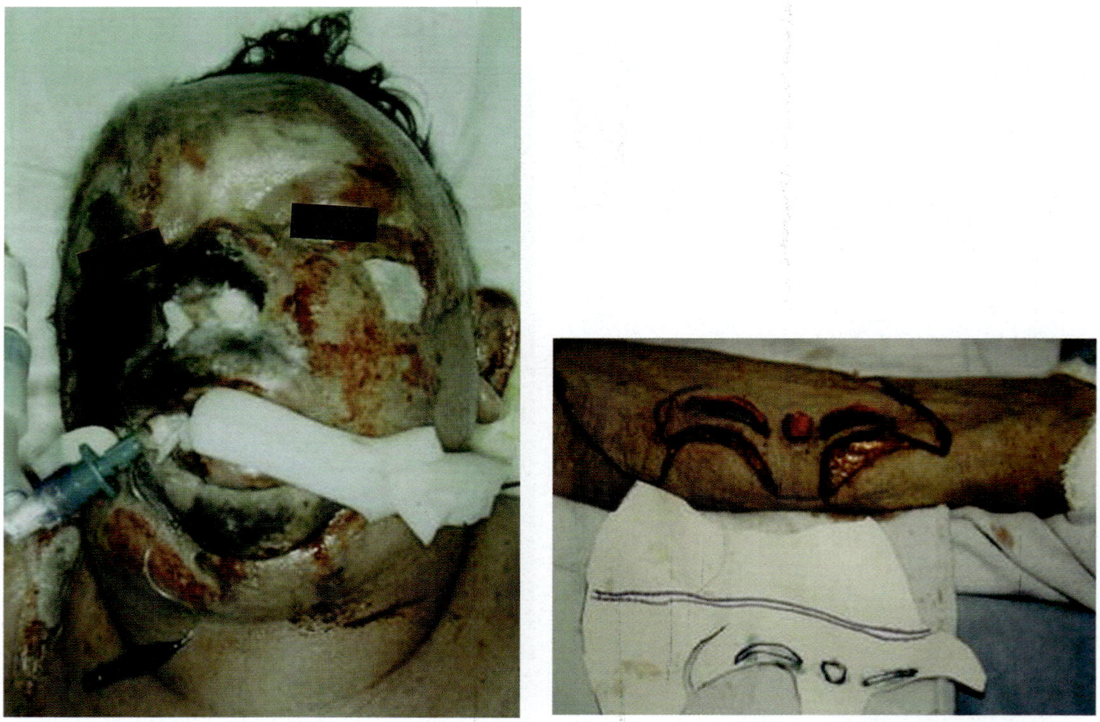

A B

FIGURE 39-6 Acute facial reconstruction with a prelaminated flap. An elderly man presented with a severe facial burn in an occupational accident that resulted in extensive full-thickness thermal injury to the nose, right cheek, lower eyelid, and upper lip (**A**). Burn debridement resulted in loss of the distal subunits of his nose and full-thickness cutaneous loss of the nasal dorsum, right cheek, and upper lip, with exposed bone and cartilage. A template was used to plan a composite reconstruction of the patient's central face within the vascular territory of his nondominant radial forearm (**B**). The design of the prelaminated flap on the right forearm shows the pattern and cartilage grafts to be inserted into the flap for neonasal vestibular lining and tip structure. Tie-over bolsters and internal splints were used to reinforce tip shape during initial healing.

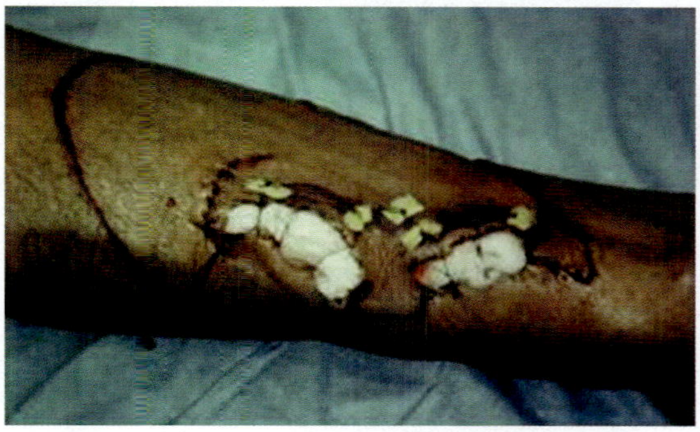

C

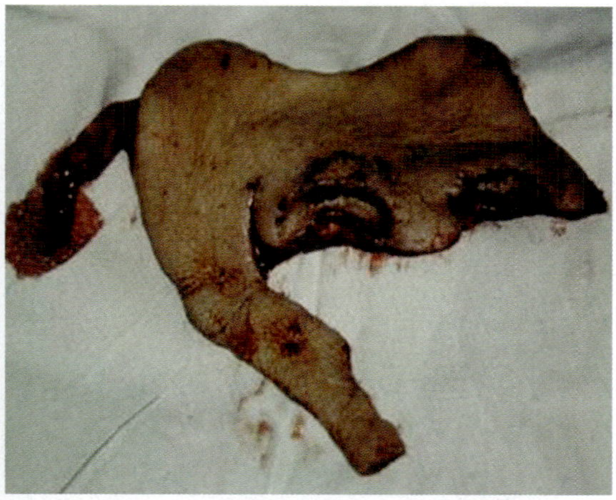

D

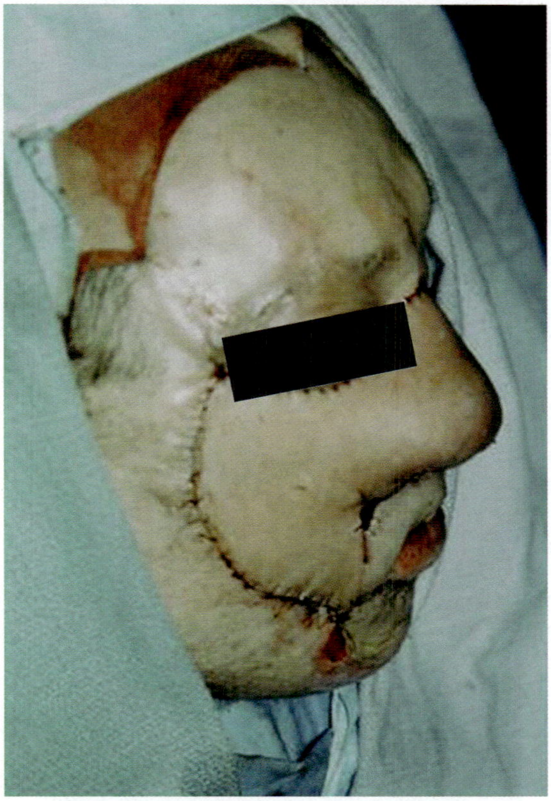

E

FIGURE 39-6 (*Continued*) (**C**) Harvested prelaminated flap done 3 weeks later on its native radial pedicle is seen (**D**). The prelaminated flap was inset after microvascular transfer and the use of local turn in flaps of his residual dorsal nasal skin as lining (**E**). Appearance of the patient 6 months after surgery after minor revision performed to deepen the nasal labial fold, creating distinct cheek and lip subunits through subcutaneous sculpting.

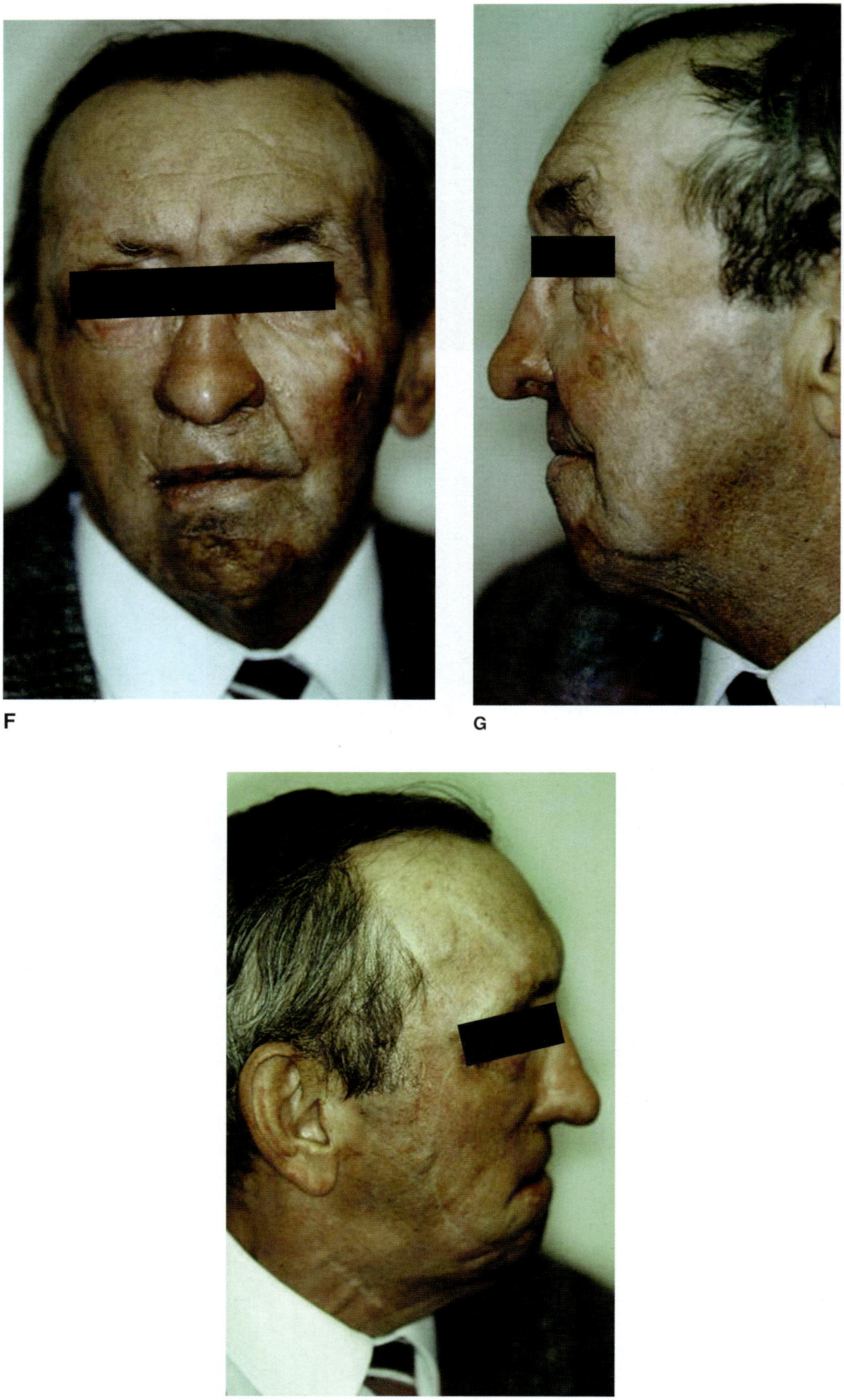

F G H

FIGURE 39-6 *(Continued)* (F to H). This example demonstrates how the use of prelamination can lead to an acceptable aesthetic reconstruction of a patient's extensive thermal burn (17,18).

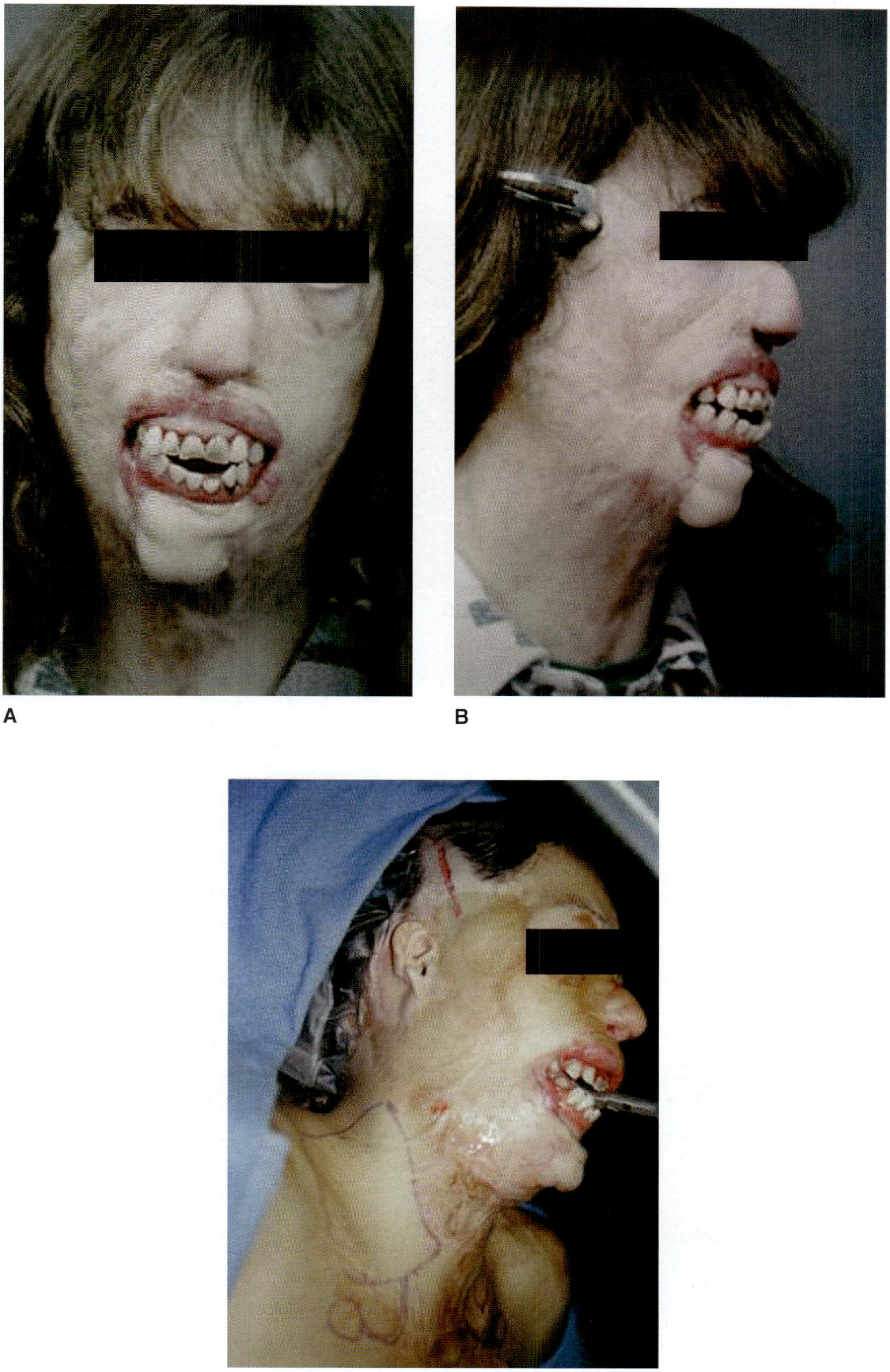

FIGURE 39-7 Full facial reconstruction with conventional free flap and prefabricated flaps. A 16-year-old girl with severe facial burns from a hot oil spill as a baby. (A and B) Her initial reconstruction with staged tube pedicle flap from her groin for nose and chin reconstruction were unfortunately inadequate to give her oral competence and facial expression.

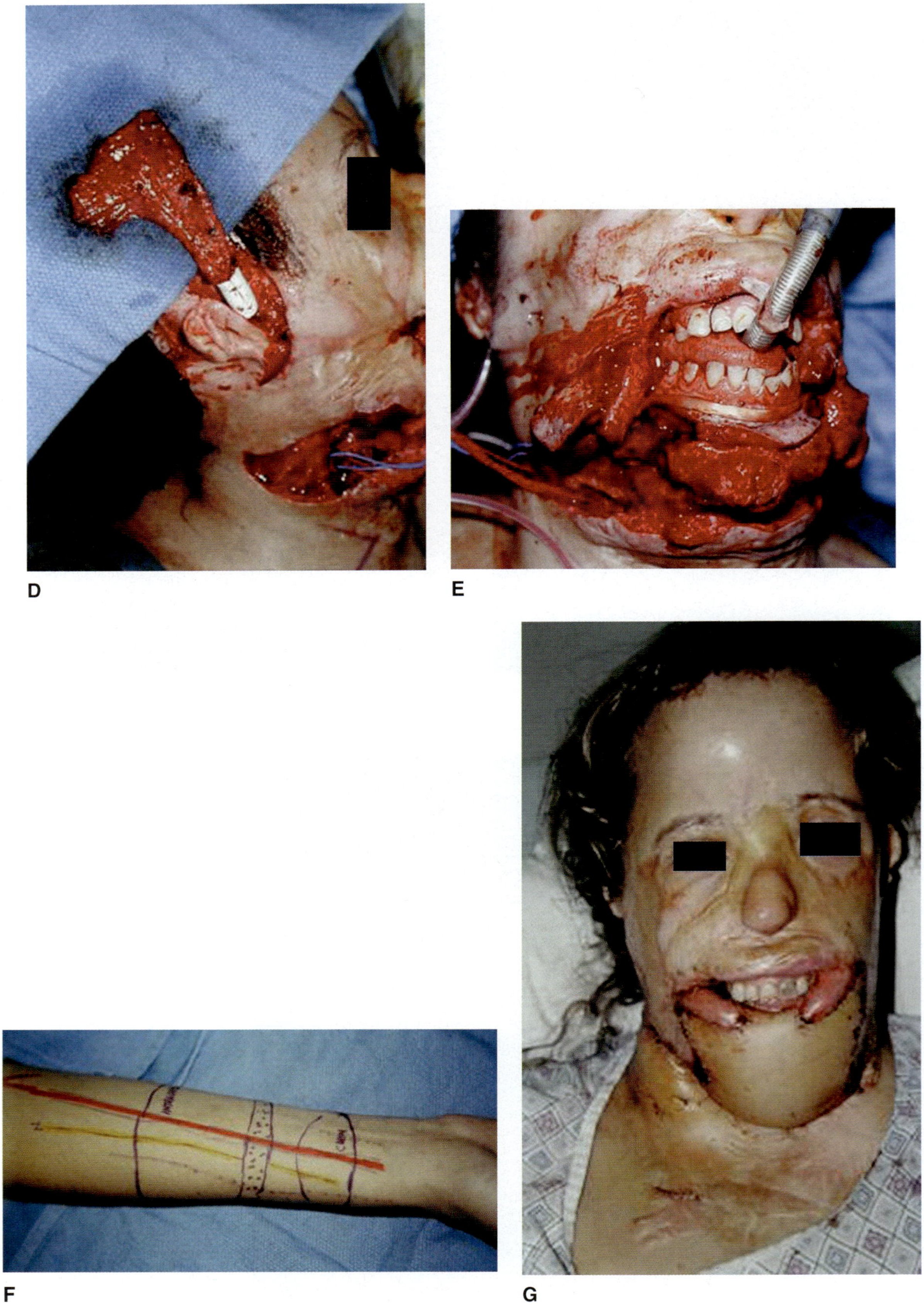

FIGURE 39-7 *(Continued)* (D and E) At the first stage, right neck skin is prefabricated using pedicled temporal parietal fascia flap over a tissue expander for upper lip reconstruction. (E and F) The lower lip and chin was reconstructed with free folded radial forearm flap and bilateral facial artery musculomucosal flaps. (G) Her interim appearance with diminished lower incisor show is already evident. Tissue expander was placed under forehead flap for nasal reconstruction. At the second stage, her upper lip was reconstructed with the prefabricated expanded pedicle neck flap.

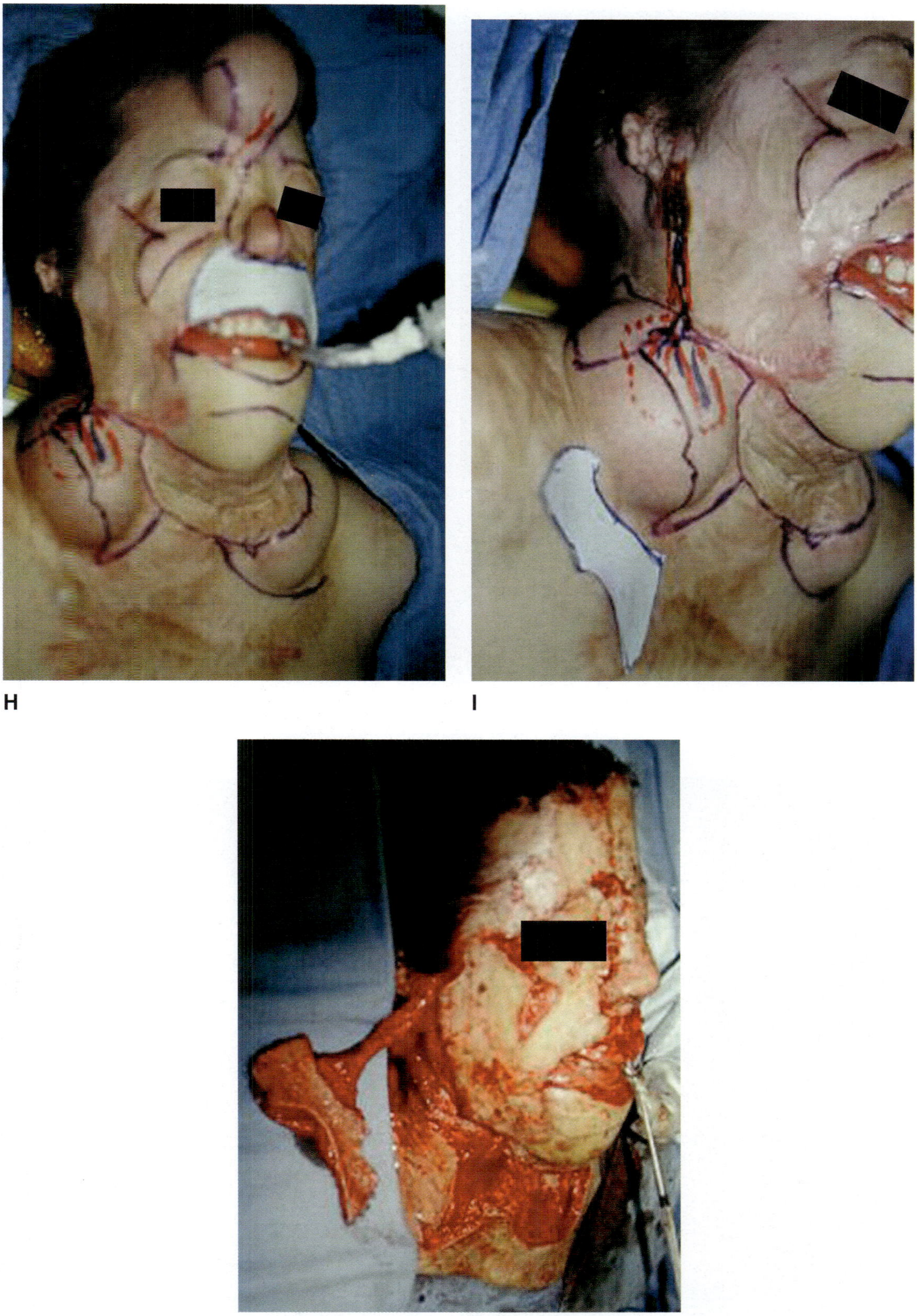

H I J

FIGURE 39-7 *(Continued)* (H and I) Template of the upper lip defect is seen and the course of the transposed pedicle outlined. (J) Her nose was reconstructed with the expanded forehead flap over lining flaps and cartilage grafts.

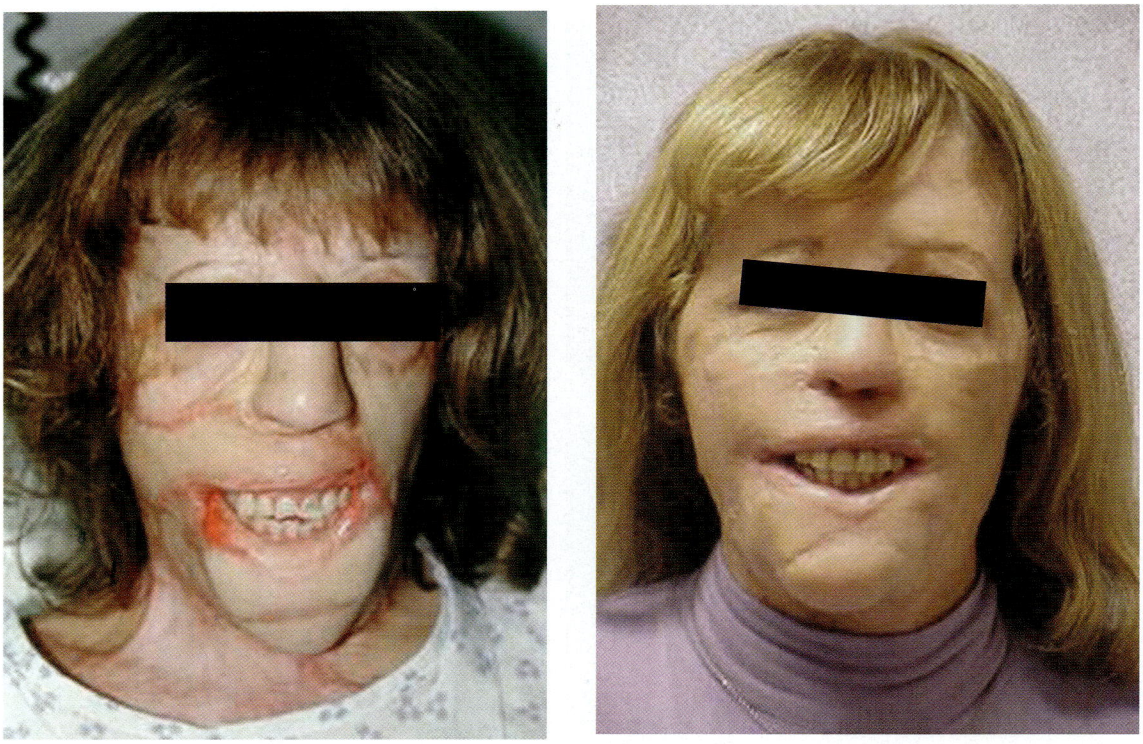

K L

FIGURE 39-7 *(Continued)* (**K**) She was seen 3 months after surgery with lower lip sagging. Dynamic temporalis muscle slings were designed to support her lower face and lips (not shown). (**L**) A satisfactory outcome is achieved 2 years after her initial presentation. She has achieved oral competence and improved nasal aesthetics (15).

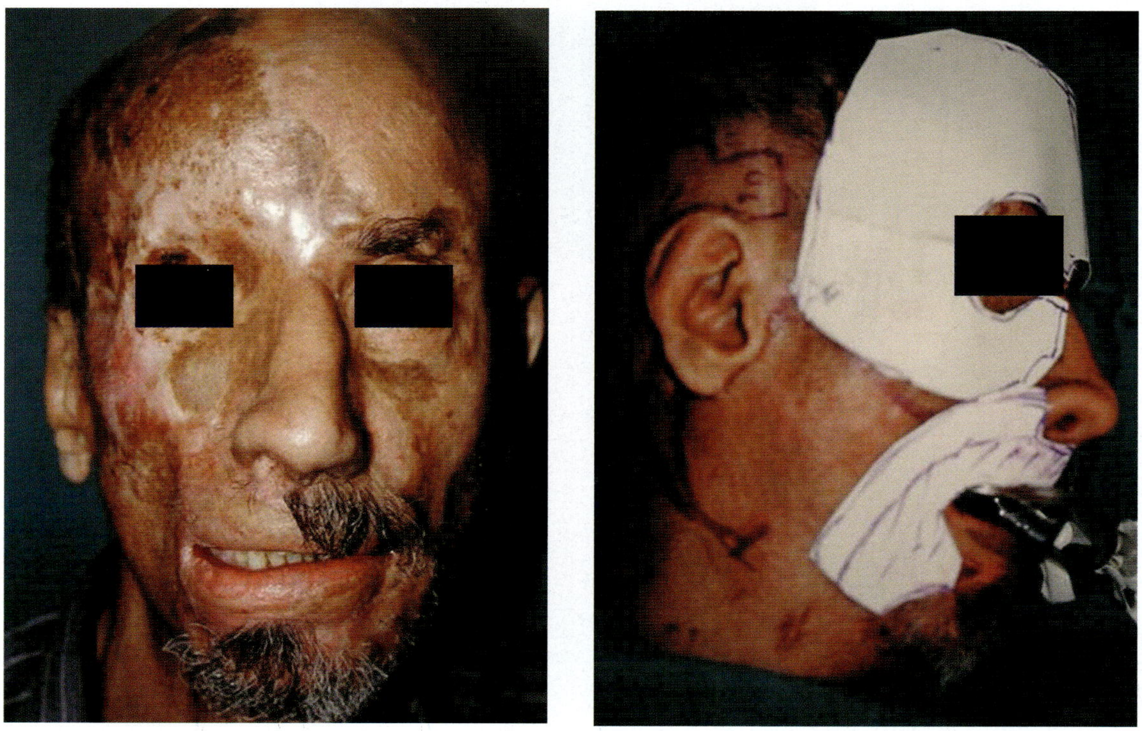

A B

FIGURE 39-8 A bomb victim with severe facial burns 5 years before presentation. (**A**) He had absent right eye and has undergone multiple skin grafts directly over bone to his right face, resulting in contraction, hypertrophic scarring, and skin breakdown. He also had absent right perioral and cheek facial hair. He desired to have his right cheek reconstructed, in particular in the area of his mustache and beard. In the first stage, the unstable burn scars over the right periocular area were replaced with a free parascapular flap. A template of the proposed defect was made (**B**) and transposed onto the back in the parascapular flap territory.

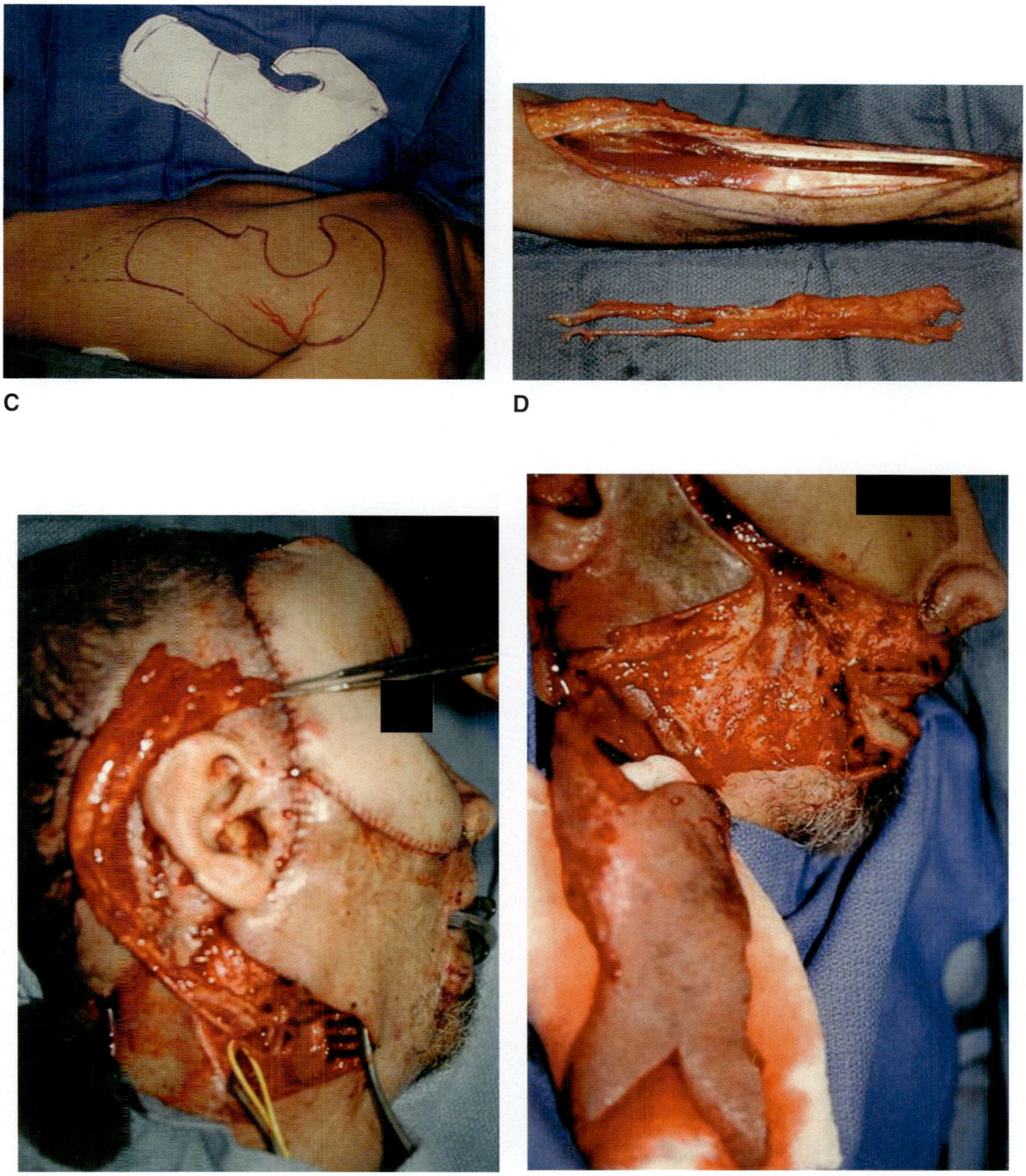

C D E F

FIGURE 39-8 (*Continued*) (C). A free parascapular flap was transferred to the right face and forehead. To transfer hair-bearing skin to the right cheek and perioral area, a free radial forearm fascial flap was transferred to the postauricular area for prefabrication (D). Alternate donor sites of hair-bearing skin were not available other than the temporal scalp. However, the temporal skin cannot be easily pedicled to reach the desired location because the superficial temporal artery was damaged. Therefore, prefabrication is planned to bring an axial blood vessel to transport this area of hair-bearing skin. A radial forearm fascial flap was used as a free pedicle and tunneled beneath the temporal scalp and laid over a tissue expander (E). In addition, the parascapular free flap was seen already inset into the forehead and orbit defect to resurface the unstable skin. Eight weeks later, the prefabricated flap over the tissue expander is ready for transfer and the right mustache and beard area scar was excised, and transfer of the prefabricated hair-bearing flap from the right postauricular region was performed (F). Intraoperative dissection of the prefabricated flap raised based on its implanted pedicles is seen.

SECTION 2

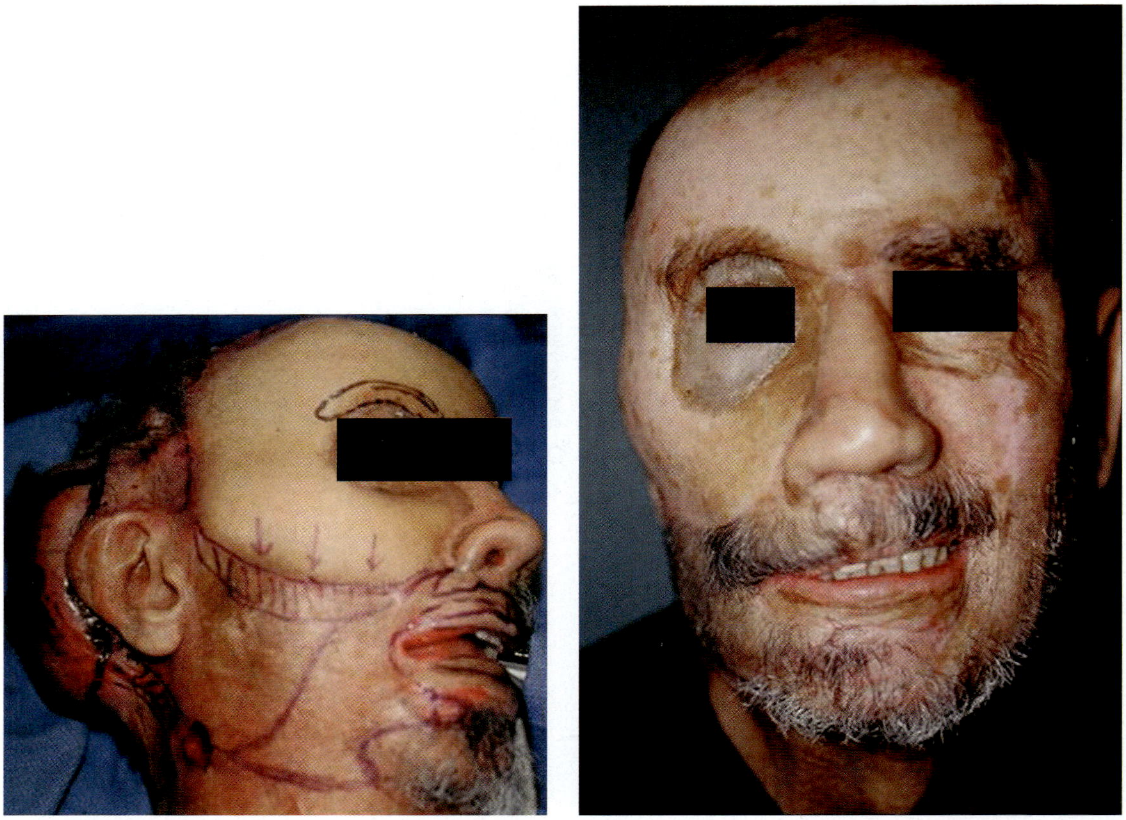

FIGURE 39-8 (*Continued*) (**G**) The flaps survived, and the patient returned for minor debulking of the flaps, a fascial sling, a right eye prosthesis, and eyebrow hair grafts. (**H**) Nine months later, the prefabricated flap has good hair growth (17).

adequate closure of the eyelids and mouth. The options of free muscle transfer, with and without nerve grafts or local or regional muscle transfers of functioning muscle, can all be considered (30).

8. Consider supplemental prosthetic reconstruction of nonreconstructable parts (e.g., orbital and ear prostheses).

CONCLUSION

Deep burns to the head and neck are challenging during the acute period and continue to be a challenge years after the burn. The late effects of burn injury to the head and neck present as functional impairments and poor cosmesis. Free flaps represent one of many different approaches to facial skin resurfacing among skin grafts, local flaps, regional flaps, and tissue expansion, which all need to be taken into consideration. Secondary operations for debulking are common, and many patients require multiple operations over many years to achieve what some would consider a marginally acceptable outcome. Sometimes these patients are done with their operation not because they are fully satisfied with their results but because they are burned out from their multiple operations spread out over a decade. Ultimately, the patients need to be counseled from the start that their appearance will never be back to normal because the only tissue that can truly replace facial soft tissue is facial soft tissue. Flaps and grafts come close but are never exactly the same. To that end, advances in CTA and immune tolerance might one day make this a reasonable option for these patients, especially if an experienced burn reconstructive surgeon deems that even after years of revisions, an optimal result is not possible. As such, local, regional, and free flap options might actually become "lifeboats".

REFERENCES

1. Achauer BM. Reconstructing the burned face. *Clin Plast Surg* 1992;19(3):623–636.
2. Cole JK, Engrav LH, Heimbach DM, et al. Early excision and grafting of face and neck burns in patients over 20 years. *Plast Reconstr Surg* 2002;109(4):1266–1273.
3. Chai J, Song H, Sheng Z, et al. Repair and reconstruction of massively damaged burn wounds. *Burns* 2003;29(7):726–732.
4. Gahhos FN, Ariyan S, Cuono CB, Arons MS. Burn wound excision and local flap closure. *Ann Plast Surg* 1985;14(6):535–540.
5. Devauchelle B, Badet L, Lengele B, et al. First human face allograft: early report. *Lancet* 2006;368(9531):203–209.
6. Guo S, Han Y, Zhang X, et al. Human facial allotransplantation: a 2-year follow-up study. *Lancet* 2008;372(9639):631–638.
7. Lantieri L, Meningaud JP, Grimbert P, et al. Repair of the lower and middle parts of the face by composite tissue allotransplantation in a patient with massive plexiform neurofibroma: a 1-year follow-up study. *Lancet* 2008;372(9639):639–645.
8. Siemionow M, Papay F, Alam D, et al. Near-total human face transplantation for a severely disfigured patient in the USA. *Lancet* 2009;374(9685):203–209.
9. Meningaud JP, Benjoar MD, Hivelin M, et al. The procurement of total human face graft for allotransplantation: a preclinical study and the first clinical case. *Plast Reconstr Surg* 2010;126(4):1181–1190.
10. Harii K, Ohmori K. Free groin flaps in children. *Plast Reconstr Surg* 1975;55(5):588–592.

11. Rose EH. Aesthetic restoration of the severely disfigured face in burn victims: a comprehensive strategy. *Plast Reconstr Surg* 1995;96(7): 1573–1585; discussion 1586–1577.
12. Angrigiani C, Grilli D. Total face reconstruction with one free flap. *Plast Reconstr Surg* 1997;99(6):1566–1575.
13. Latifoglu O, Ayhan S, Atabay K. Total face reconstruction: skin graft versus free flap. *Plast Reconstr Surg* 1999;103(3):1076–1078.
14. Kroll SS, Schusterman MA, Reece GP, et al. Timing of pedicle thrombosis and flap loss after free-tissue transfer. *Plast Reconstr Surg* 1996;98(7): 1230–1233.
15. Parrett BM, Pomahac B, Orgill DP, Pribaz JJ. The role of free-tissue transfer for head and neck burn reconstruction. *Plast Reconstr Surg* 2007;120(7):1871–1878.
16. Gao JH, Ogawa R, Hyakusoku H, et al. Reconstruction of the face and neck scar contractures using staged transfer of expanded "super-thin flaps." *Burns* 2007;33(6):760–763.
17. Guo L, Pribaz JJ. Clinical flap prefabrication. *Plast Reconstr Surg* 2009;124(6 suppl):e340–e350.
18. Mathy JA, Pribaz JJ. Prefabrication and prelamination applications in current aesthetic facial reconstruction. *Clin Plast Surg* 2009;36(3): 493–505.
19. Pribaz JJ, Fine NA. Prelamination: defining the prefabricated flap—a case report and review. *Microsurgery* 1994;15(9):618–623.
20. Pribaz JJ, Weiss DD, Mulliken JB, Eriksson E. Prelaminated free flap reconstruction of complex central facial defects. *Plast Reconstr Surg* 1999;104(2):357–365; discussion 366–357.
21. Hallock GG. Preexpansion of free flap donor sites used in reconstruction after burn injury. *J Burn Care Rehabil* 1995;16(6):646–653.
22. Baumeister S, Koller M, Dragu A, et al. Principles of microvascular reconstruction in burn and electrical burn injuries. *Burns* 2005;31(1): 92–98.
23. Pribaz JJ, Pelham FR. Use of previously burned skin in local fasciocutaneous flaps for upper extremity reconstruction. *Ann Plast Surg* 1994;33(3): 272–280.
24. Engrav LH, Heimbach DM, Walkinshaw MD, Marvin JA. Excision of burns of the face. *Plast Reconstr Surg* 1986;77(5):744–751.
25. Pribaz JJ, Chan R. Secondary Facial Reconstruction. In *Plastic Surgery* 3rd ed, Neligan P, Gurtner G, Warren R, Rodriguez E, Song D, Grotting J, Chang J, Losee J, and van Beek A (eds). Elsevier, London 2010.
26. Erol OO. Facial autologous soft-tissue contouring by adjunction of tissue cocktail injection (micrograft and minigraft mixture of dermis, fascia, and fat). *Plast Reconstr Surg* 2000;106(6):1375–1387; discussion 1388–1379.
27. Moseley TA, Zhu M, Hedrick MH. Adipose-derived stem and progenitor cells as fillers in plastic and reconstructive surgery. *Plast Reconstr Surg* 2006;118(3 suppl):121S–128S.
28. Ridgway E, Pribaz J. Reconstruction of male hair bearing facial regions. *Plast Reconstr Surg.* 2011;127(1):131–411.
29. Walton RL, Cohn AB, Beahm EK. Epidermal overgrafting improves coloration in remote flaps and grafts applied to the face for reconstruction. *Plast Reconstr Surg* 2008;121(5):1606–1613.
30. Chan R, Bojovic B, Talbot S, Weiss D, Pribaz J. Lower lip suspension using bilateral temporalis muscle flaps and fascia lata grafts. *Plast Reconstr Surg* 2012;129(1):119–122.

CHAPTER 40

Facial Reanimation in Children and Adults

Gregory H. Borschel, Adel Fattah, Ralph Manktelow, and Ronald M. Zuker

Facial paralysis is a complex clinical problem with functional, psychological, and aesthetic components. The facial nerve is responsible for the tone and dynamic activity that are vital to ocular protection, nasal airflow, articulation of speech, and oral continence. Loss of frontalis activity can lead to eyebrow ptosis with consequent limitation of the superior visual field. Reduced tone in the orbicularis oculi can create a lagophthalmos partly caused by eyelid retraction (as levator palpebrae superioris overcomes resting orbicularis tone) and partly caused by lower eyelid atonicity with subsequent paralytic ectropion. In more severe cases, this can lead to corneal exposure; ulceration; and, if untreated, blindness. The loss of resting tone in the midface leads to ptosis of the cheek tissues, further reducing lower eyelid support and exacerbating the lagophthalmos. Paralysis of the orbicularis oris and perioral muscles can lead to difficulty in articulation and affect oral continence, with patients becoming too self-conscious to eat in public.

Although functional impairment is a significant issue, mimetic activity is essential for normal social interaction with those perceived as "different," who experience ridicule at the hands of their peers and become socially withdrawn. The nonverbal communication conveyed by facial expression is essential in normal social engagement, and a spontaneous dynamic smile is critical for such communal interaction. As a result, restoration of facial nerve function is able to achieve great psychosocial benefit in addition to solving the specific functional issues that arise. After permanent injury to the facial nerve, the aim of reconstruction is therefore not only to restore function but also to re-create the smile.

CLASSIFICATION

The causes of facial palsy are myriad, and a comprehensive classification based on clinical presentation has been designed (1). It may be congenital or acquired, unilateral or bilateral, partial or complete. In addition, it may be classified by site of damage to the nerve (intracranial, temporal, or extracranial) and the etiology specified (trauma, tumor, infection, toxic, idiopathic, iatrogenic).

Congenital paralysis is present at birth and affects 2% of live births (2). It is thought to be caused by compression of the nerve by the sacral prominence in utero or by instrumentation, the blades of delivery forceps exerting pressure over the facial nerve. The nerve is especially vulnerable in early life because the cartilaginous portion of external acoustic meatus is immature and shallow, exposing the facial nerve to surface pressure. The most common presentation is a panfacial paralysis caused by injury to the proximal portion of the nerve. The next most common form is that which affects the mandibular division, which causes the lower lip to ride up because of paralysis of the lip depressors. Congenital paralysis may also be syndromic, the most common cause being hemifacial microsomia in which all tissues of the face may be affected, including both the facial nerve and facial musculature. In the authors' experience, unilateral paralysis in the pediatric population is congenital in two thirds of cases and acquired in the remaining third. Of the latter, half are caused by intracranial tumors, and half caused by extracranial trauma such as resectional surgery for a cystic hygroma (macrocystic lymphatic malformation of the neck). Acquired bilateral palsy is rare and may be caused by bilateral skull base trauma or intracranial tumors, typically in the brainstem. Bilateral congenital palsy is more commonly caused by Möbius syndrome (Figure 40-1), affecting one in 200,000 live births. It involves the sixth and often other cranial nerves and is associated with limb and pectoral defects (3). Such palsies are challenging to correct because of the paucity of reconstructive options given that these children lack both facial nerve and facial musculature, necessitating microvascular transfer of muscle and careful choice of recipient nerve.

Overall, the most common cause of facial paralysis is Bell's palsy, an idiopathic condition thought to be of viral etiology from which 50% of patients recover fully, but 10% are left with

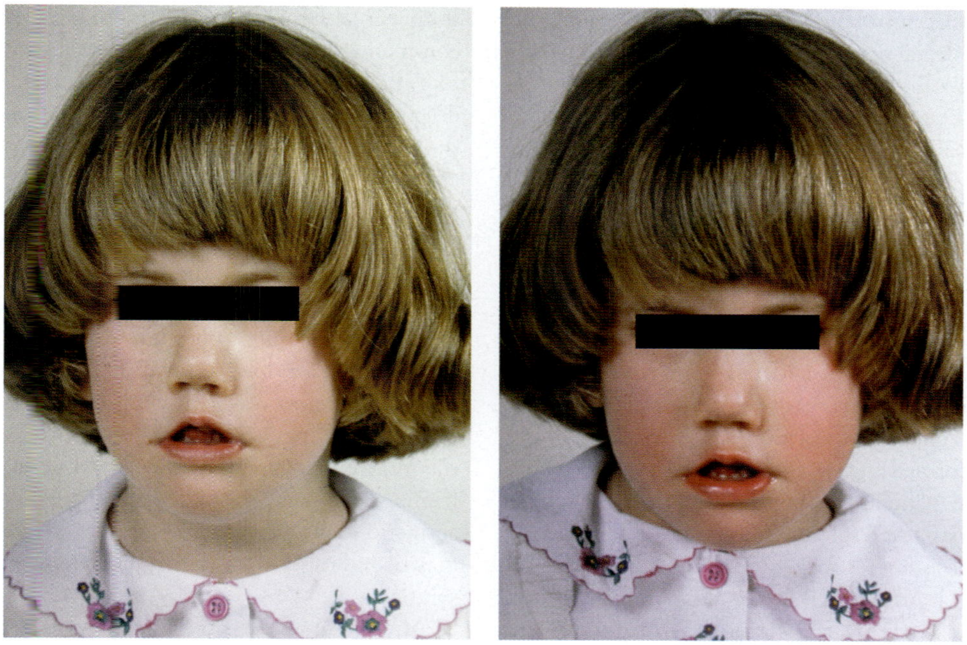

A B

FIGURE 40-1 Mobius syndrome. (A) At rest. (B) Attempted smile. (Reproduced with permission from Zuker RM, Goldberg CS, Manktelow RT. Facial animation in children with Möbius syndrome after segmental gracilis muscle transplant. *Plast and Reconstr Surg* 2000;106:1.)

a severe residual deficit (Figure 40-2). In children, as mentioned, trauma and tumor are the most common causes of acquired palsy, with blunt cranial base trauma capable of producing bilateral facial nerve damage. In adults, the tumors classically involved in facial nerve dysfunction are parotid neoplasms and acoustic neuromas. In children, they are more likely to be ependymomas or medulloblastomas. Parotid masses are uncommon in the young.

ASSESSMENT

The strategy for restoration of function begins during the consultation when the physician, the patient, and the patient's family address the primary concerns and define the common objectives for treatment while considering: "Are these achievable muscle-specific goals?" The therapeutic plan depends on numerous factors, including the cause of facial nerve injury, the deficit (partial or complete, unilateral or bilateral), the prognosis for recovery, and the time elapsed since the injury.

The history should include the mechanism and time since the injury because both will give clues as to the presence or absence of a proximal facial nerve stump or viable facial musculature. These are key factors in formulating a reconstructive plan because attempts to reinnervate facial musculature after 18 to 24 months of denervation are unlikely to succeed. If the injury is partial, one must determine which muscle groups are involved and whether function has been regained, is still improving, or has reached a plateau. Thereafter, the history focuses on functional deficits, working down the face: eyebrow ptosis with limitation of superior visual field, ocular surface symptoms, nasal

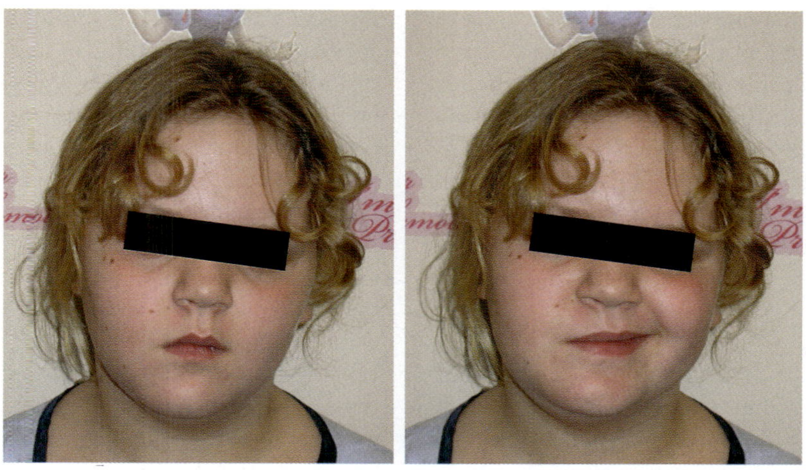

A B

FIGURE 40-2 Unilateral Bell's palsy. (A) At rest. (B) With smile. Note the hypertonicity as well as decreased movement on the involved right side.

airflow issues, and speech and masticatory problems. Speech can be impacted with bilabial plosives such as /b/ and /p/ being particularly affected. Furthermore, food may be pocketed in the buccal sulcus, making dental hygiene difficult to maintain. Finally, a frank discussion regarding the aesthetic and psychological issues raised by the condition should be documented. For example, eyebrow ptosis may impart an unhappy countenance to the patient, affecting relationships and career prospects.

Examination is directed at determining surgical problems that can be corrected and anticipating issues that could be worsened by poorly planned surgery. Again, from above down, eyebrow ptosis and dermatochalasis are documented. Lagophthalmos and Bell's phenomenon are noted, as are corneal abrasions, ectropion, and tear pooling. A snap test of the lower eyelid is performed to assess tone. Care should be taken when operating on patients lacking a Bell's phenomenon or exhibiting a poor snap test result. Such patients are at particular risk of corneal exposure after surgery around the eyelids, and one should consider lubrication, eyelid support procedures, careful follow–up, and even a temporary tarsorrhaphy if there is concern of postoperative exposure. Nasal airflow is assessed with a Cottle's test, and an intranasal inspection is performed to exclude fixed structural causes of nasal airflow obstruction. Cheek ptosis is evaluated, and the mouth is examined to determine the position at rest and while the patient is smiling. The degree of tooth show is specifically evaluated, as is the vector of the smile (see later discussion). Drooping of the upper lip, the degree of vermillion eversion, the position of the nasolabial crease, and the excursion of the angle of the mouth are all recorded (4). The facial nerve is carefully examined on both sides as are other potential donor nerves, including the trigeminal nerve (muscles of mastication), the spinal accessory nerve, and the hypoglossal nerve. Synkinesis, the simultaneous contraction of two or more groups of muscles that do not normally contract together, should be documented. Synkinesis is thought to occur by the misdirected regrowth of axons from the site of injury forming aberrant connections with the denervated musculature. The most common types are simultaneous eye closure with smiling (5), eyebrow wrinkling when the mouth is moved (6), and grimacing when the eyes close. Photographs and videos are important records and should be taken at rest, normal smile, full smile, eyebrows raised, eyes open, and eyes closed. This allows evaluation of the efficacy of procedures at each stage of the treatment pathway. Specific electrophysiological investigations are of limited use clinically but may be useful for research purposes. Facial palsy is a multidisciplinary effort, and the expertise of other medical specialties, including ophthalmology, otolaryngology, and neurosurgery, together with input from allied health care professionals such as psychologists and speech therapists are the key to a successful outcome

TREATMENT OPTIONS FOR FACIAL PALSY

Numerous surgical and nonsurgical options exist for the treatment of facial paralysis, and they may be classified as static or dynamic. Different combinations of treatments can be used to tackle the different clinical presentations of facial palsy. Nonetheless, the primary objective is protection of the ocular sphincter, although exposure of the globe in children is not as common as in adults. However, some cases may remain refractory to lubrication and if ocular surface symptoms persist despite maximal conservative measures, then a surgical solution should be sought. Treatment of the paralyzed upper eyelid with a gold weight is one of the most commonly used methods to achieve corneal protection secondary to lagophthalmos. Lower eyelid paralytic ectropion or oculopalpebral diastasis may equally lead to corneal exposure, scleral show, tear pooling, and epiphora. Treatment of such horizontal lower eyelid laxity requires a tensioning procedure in the form of a canthopexy, canthoplasty, or lower eyelid fascial sling, respectively, for increasing degrees of severity. It is important to avoid intervening too soon because eyelid laxity evolves over time, and surgical intervention should be reserved until the full extent is manifest. Permanent tarsorrhaphy is avoided because of the cosmetic deformity that results, but temporary tarsorrhaphy may be indicated as an urgent procedure pending a permanent solution.

After ocular protection is achieved, a number of static procedures can be used for the other facets of facial palsy. Browpexy is an effective method for dealing with limitation of upper field of view and is of most value in older adults in whom brow ptosis is a more significant issue. Unilateral palsy may cause a difference in eyebrow height of 12 mm, and a direct brow lift is the best method to deal with such a large discrepancy. This involves a "melon-slice" excision of the skin and frontalis muscle just above and parallel to the upper border of the affected eyebrow. If the incision is placed along the first line of hair follicles, the scar is usually less noticeable. The excision of frontalis provides a reliable correction with minimal recurrence, but overcorrection is required and is actually beneficial if the normal side is quite active during facial expression. Open brow lifts may be performed through coronal or hairline incisions and can be augmented by suspending the brow with fascial grafts from the temporal fascia or frontal bone. Although the scar is concealed, the lift (acting at a distance from the required site) may not be adequate. The authors have little experience with endoscopic browpexy, but the amount of lift using this technique may be similarly insufficient for a unilateral facial palsy.

To tackle the problems of the nose, mouth, and midface, the aim is to lift the midface to provide lower eyelid support, lift the angle of the mouth, open the nasal valve(s), and restore facial symmetry at rest. Fascia lata and palmaris tendon slings have been used to suspend the face after being secured at various points around the commissure, cheek, and nasal base and suspended from the deep temporal fascia. We have found the Buck-Gramcko tendon weaving forceps especially good for attaching the tendon to the oral commissures. Fascia lata harvest may result in unsightly bulges as muscle herniates through the defect, and the palmaris tendon is absent in 10% of the population. To circumvent donor site complications, Gore-Tex (polytetrafluoroethylene [PTFE]) slings have been tried but have resulted in unacceptable inflammatory reactions in the authors' hands. A different approach using subperiosteal, superficial musculoaponeurotic system (SMAS), and sub-orbicularis oculi fat (SOOF) (7) facelifts have been used to achieve a similar result. Such techniques are successful at restoring facial symmetry at rest and may help oral symptoms such as speech and drooling by tensioning the lower lip to some degree. For some patients who only request symmetry at rest and are not concerned with dynamic movement, such static procedures will serve them well. However, these procedures do not *reanimate* the face and cannot provide the patient with the ability to smile or produce facial expressions.

To address this, a number of regional muscle flaps have been used to try to provide a dynamic component to the reconstruction. These have been used for many years and use muscles of trigeminal innervation that can be transposed to act upon the oral commissure. Gillies (8) first described a retrograde temporalis flap in which the origin of the temporalis muscle was lifted from the temporal fossa, reflected over the zygomatic arch, and lengthened using strips of fascial graft to reach the oral commissure. A number of modifications have been proposed to avoid the problems with this technique. Reflecting a portion of the deep temporal fascia in an anterograde direction before raising the muscle can obviate the need for fascial extensions. The cosmetic deformity created by the temporal hollowing can be addressed by leaving behind the anterior portion of muscle (9) or filling the defect with a MEDPOR (high-density porous polyethylene) implant or stacked MERSILENE (polyethylene terephthalate) mesh. Alternatively, the insertion of temporalis can be detached from the coronoid process of the mandible and passed to the angle of the mouth with fascial grafts as an anterograde transfer (10). Labbé and Huault (11) have modified the anterograde temporalis transfer by osteotomy of the zygomatic arch for access and significant release of the temporalis origin, allowing it to slide forward and increase the reach of the tendon to the mouth. The tendon is passed through the buccal fat pad, allowing a more natural gliding, and is secured to the modiolus via an intraoral incision.

Another muscle of mastication used is the masseter (9), which is detached from the lower border of the mandible and transposed anteriorly to reach the upper and lower lips. The dissection should proceed with caution on the posterior surface to preserve the motor nerve to masseter. A good static control of the mouth can be achieved with the masseter, but it lacks sufficient force and excursion to produce a full smile, and the vector of pull is too lateral for a natural one. Critics of such transpositions suggest that the excursions produced are little better than static support.

Muscle transpositions that lack spontaneity as smiling then require an often unrelated action (e.g., clenching teeth). But with practice, patients can activate the muscle without moving their jaws and may achieve a natural-appearing smile. However, if one muscle is used in more than one area of the face, then mass action is inevitable. More sophisticated transpositions using the anterior belly of digastric to recreate lip depressor function have been reported in which a cross-face nerve graft is used in conjunction with muscle transposition to achieve a more natural reanimation (12).

STRATEGIES FOR FACIAL REANIMATION

In contrast to regional flap transposition, reanimation involves the restoration of neural control to denervated facial musculature or to imported muscle in order to restore spontaneous dynamic smile to the face while maintaining resting symmetry. These advantages have led reanimation to become the standard of care in the majority of cases. In adopting this strategy, two basic criteria need to be considered. The first is whether the reconstruction should be based on the facial nerve or another cranial nerve (13). Reanimation based on the facial nerve can be ipsilateral or contralateral depending on the presence of an ipsilateral nerve stump. If neither facial nerve is available for use, another cranial nerve must be selected to provide motor innervation. Second, the requirement for muscle transplantation depends on the viability of the facial musculature. After denervation, the muscles begin to degenerate but may remain viable for up to 12 to 24 months and may be suitable for reanimating by nerve grafting alone during that time. After 24 months, they are deemed to be irreversibly atrophic and require a free muscle transfer to replace their function.

Early nerve injuries in which the facial musculature is viable and there is an ipsilateral nerve stump have the greatest potential for a satisfactory recovery. Direct repair gives good results and is indicated in a clean wound. By contrast, in a heavily contaminated wound, delayed repair is preferred. In such a case, the nerve ends are tagged with a nonabsorbable suture to facilitate their identification at a subsequent procedure. In injuries that have been sutured without identifying the nerve injury, the best results are obtained with early exploration because this minimizes the degree of postinjury retraction of the nerve ends, thereby reducing the need for an interposition nerve graft. Furthermore, early exploration allows for accurate identification of the distal nerve ends using intraoperative nerve stimulation and reduce the mismatching of branches with subsequent synkinesis. With time, the distal branches become difficult to find because they become refractory to nerve stimulation. If primary repair creates tension on coaptation, then nerve grafting is mandatory. Success depends on the relative number of proximal axons, the potential for regeneration through the graft, a perfect technical repair, and the status of the facial muscles. The greater the number of proximal axons, the greater is the chance of a more powerful functional recovery. It takes approximately 1 month for axons to cross the suture line. Thereafter the rate of axon growth across a nerve graft is approximately 1 mm/day, and although the length of the nerve graft does not affect the result, the diameter and number of reinnervating axons does (14). The most commonly used nerve grafts include the greater auricular nerve, branches of the cervical plexus, and the sural nerve. The former two have the benefit of being locally available, and thus no further incisions are required. However, we prefer the sural nerve because it affords a two-team approach with minimal sensory deficit and scarring.

In the absence of an ipsilateral facial nerve stump, the best way to restore spontaneous dynamic smile to the paralyzed side of the face is to use the contralateral intact facial nerve. To achieve this, the authors prefer to use a cross facial nerve graft. Multiple techniques and methods of cross-face nerve grafting have been described (9,15–17), but the principles remain the same. A sural nerve graft is used to relay the activity of the contralateral facial nerve to viable ipsilateral facial musculature. After the injured side has been explored and distal nerve stump(s) have been identified, they are tested by intraoperative nerve stimulation to determine which muscle groups they control. This is carefully noted, and attention is turned to the contralateral side to identify similar branches. The basis of the technique rests on the knowledge that the facial muscles are innervated by multiple braches of the facial nerve and that each of the nerve branches can innervate multiple muscles; thus, ample nerve supply is retained on the donor side when sacrificing even large branches from this overlapping network of innervation. The appropriate branches are divided, and the nerve graft is used to direct regenerating axons from the contralateral nerve to the ipsilateral muscles. This takes from 6 to 9 months, during which time the muscle may further atrophy. To maintain the viability of the facial muscles, the "babysitter" concept (18) was proposed to use a cranial nerve transfer to more rapidly reinnervate the facial muscles (there being a shorter distance for axons to travel) while awaiting the axons to grow through the cross-face nerve graft. This is a two-stage procedure in which the first operation involves the cross-facial nerve graft and a hypoglossal–facial transfer. The cross-facial nerve graft is coapted to the donor facial nerve and then tunneled across the midline and banked in the temporal region. Under the same anesthetic, a short nerve graft is used to connect the distal stump of the injured facial nerve to the hypoglossal or masseteric nerves. By 2 to 3 months, the muscle will contract in response to activation of the donor cranial nerve. About 6 to 9 months later, when a Tinel sign indicates regeneration across the cross-face graft, a second procedure coapts the banked end of that graft to the facial nerve distal to the previous neurorrhaphy. Within 3 to 6 months, coordinated facial nerve motion will begin and in time will take over from the cranial nerve transfer. If motion from the cranial nerve transfer remains noticeable, this neurorrhaphy can be transected.

Cross-facial nerve grafting requires a functioning contralateral facial nerve, and it cannot be applied to cases of bilateral facial palsy or other situations in which the contralateral facial nerve is unavailable. In these instances, an alternative donor nerve must be identified. Such cranial nerve transfers have been used for more than 50 years and can provide a powerful source of innervation for viable facial musculature or free muscle flaps. Their advantages such as good muscle tone and symmetry at rest are counterbalanced by drawbacks such as uncoordinated movements when the cranial nerve is activated and loss of donor nerve function. The most commonly transferred nerve is the hypoglossal nerve, which can cause synkinetic facial motion in response to tongue actions and ipsilateral atrophy of the tongue musculature. End-to-side neurorrhaphy limits loss of donor activity, and such a "mini-hypoglossal transfer" may be indicated as a "babysitter" (18). The authors' preference is to use the motor nerve to masseter, and we have demonstrated that in children and adults, it provides a symmetric smile with excellent muscle transplant excursion in response to biting. Furthermore, the degree of cortical plasticity prevalent in children leads to more than half of the patients being able to smile spontaneously without consciously biting to activate the motor nerve to the masseter (13,19,20). The motor nerve to the masseter is a purely motor branch of the mandibular division of the trigeminal nerve arising in the infratemporal fossa. The nerve runs on the deep surface of masseter for some distance before it begins to arborize into the muscle substance. It is a powerful source of innervation that is located close to the operative field and is an excellent size match for branches of the facial nerve. Additionally, in our experience, there is virtually no functional deficit when this nerve is used; we believe that the other muscles of mastication and possibly more proximal nerve branches to the masseter maintain normal jaw movement.

If there is no viable facial musculature, then cross-facial nerve grafting and cranial nerve transfers can be coupled with free muscle transfer to reanimate the face. Indeed, combinations of all the therapeutic modalities outlined earlier (conservative, static, dynamic, and so forth) can be used to formulate an individualized treatment strategy with which to achieve the best result for each individual patient.

FREE FLAP OPTIONS

The first attempts at free muscle transfer involved the free grafting of muscles to the face (21). Although histologically shown to survive, their function was unpredictable, and free microvascular transfer of muscle flaps quickly superseded their use. Tamai et al. (22) demonstrated the survival and function of transferred muscle in an animal model, and Harii et al. (23) presented the first free gracilis transfers for facial paralysis with good functional results. One major advantage of free muscle transfer is that it allows for "free-style" positioning of the muscle to reproduce the appropriate smile vector for each individual. In addition, one may adjust the dimensions and tension on the muscle flap to maximize excursion and improve the contour of inset. Since the concept of free functioning muscle transfer was introduced, numerous authors have tried to find the optimal donor muscle. The ideal muscle would be small, able to be divided into multiple slips with adequate excursion, have a long neurovascular pedicle, and leave no functional deficit. No muscle truly fulfills these criteria, but many options have been described, including the latissimus dorsi (LD; 24), pectoralis minor (25), and extensor digitorum brevis (EDB; 26).

The EDB appears to be an ideal muscle for transfer, being flat, with four tendons that can be inserted into various parts of the face and minimal or no functional donor deficit. However, results of transfer were discouraging; in one study (27), only 50% of patients achieved a symmetrical smile with the remaining patients having little or no movement. O'Brien (28) had similarly discouraging results when compared with his free gracilis transfers, and the use of this muscle is now obsolete. In contrast to the flat EDB, the LD is a large, powerful muscle with independent fascicular territories, allowing for the transfer of multiply innervated muscle segments on a single vascular pedicle (24). Thus, two cross-face nerve grafts can used to innervate two independent muscle territories within the LD flap when each cross-face nerve graft is coapted to the appropriate fascicle of the thoracodorsal nerve. Some authors prefer the LD as the single-stage reconstruction of choice for bilateral facial palsy in Möbius syndrome (29). Although an attractive idea, the LD muscle is very bulky in the face, and the proximity of the harvesting surgical team to the recipient site team together with the need to harvest the muscle with the patient supine make it a challenging procedure from an organizational point of view. This difficulty of applying a two-team approach also applies to the pectoralis minor muscle flap. The pectoralis minor flap is a flat muscle that can be inset without bulkiness to the face and minimal donor deficit with a well-hidden scar. It would seem an excellent flap for facial reanimation; however, it is realistically a single-team procedure with longer operating times. Furthermore, the vascular anatomy of the pedicle can be variable (30,31).

We prefer to use a segmental dissection of the gracilis muscle for a number of reasons. Similar to many of the other muscles, the gracilis muscle is functionally redundant; it has a constant anatomy and straightforward dissection (unlike the pectoralis minor), and the nerve is purely motor (unlike that of EDB). It does not require patient repositioning for harvest and has lesser bulk than LD. Furthermore the segmental dissection (32) allows one to control the volume of muscle harvested so that fullness to the cheek is minimized. Finally, a two-team approach is both time and cost effective.

ANATOMY OF THE FACE

The face may be considered to be composed of five layers: skin, subcutaneous fat, SMAS, innominate "sub-SMAS" fascia, and facial nerve. There has been argument whether these layers are continuous across the face and temporal region. This debate is hampered by the widely varying nomenclature used by different authors, but a standardized nomenclature and description aids understanding of the region (33). Mitz and Peyronie (34) described the SMAS layer and found it to be in continuity with the frontalis and platysmal layers. It is thickest in the parotid and masseteric area and continues forward as a rarified layer over the facial muscles with the facial nerve lying deep to it. The only structures passing through the SMAS are fine sensory nerve branches and extrinsic lip-elevating muscles as they reach their cutaneous insertions via the retinacula cutis. Below the SMAS is a layer of innominate fascia, which lies over the parotid gland posteriorly and continues anteriorly over the parotid duct, transverse facial vessels, and facial nerve branches. The floor of this space is the masseteric fascia that extends caudally from the zygomatic arch periosteum over the surface of the masseter muscle.

The parotid gland extends inferiorly from the zygomatic arch with the inferior pole siting in the interval between the mastoid process and the angle of the mandible, enveloped in the SMAS-derived parotid fascia. Stensen's duct emerges from its anterior border and runs along the middle third of a line between the tragus and a point midway between the ala and oral commissure. The parotid gland contains a number of important structures, the deepest being the external carotid artery, which gives branches within the substance of the parotid gland to emerge superiorly as the superficial temporal artery and anteriorly as the transverse facial artery (from the superficial temporal). These are notable in that they and their concomitant veins may be used as recipient vessels for microvascular anastomosis. The superficial temporal artery emerges from the parotid and passes superiorly over the zygomatic arch under the temporoparietal fascia to supply the scalp. Here it is vulnerable to injury, and it is important during the surgical approach to preserve the vessel in case it may be required later. The transverse facial artery runs inferior to the zygomatic arch and superior to the parotid duct on the surface of the masseter muscle and anastomoses with branches of the facial artery in the medial cheek. The facial artery is a branch of the external carotid in the neck and enters the face by winding around the lower border of the mandible at the anterior border of the masseter muscle to head toward the angle of the mouth proceeding toward the nasal base deep to the zygomaticus muscles. Branches of the facial nerve cross the artery in the face, and the anterior facial vein runs posterior to the artery and may be separated from it by a considerable interval. These vessels are our preferred recipient vessels for free muscle transfer, but we have experienced occasions in which the anterior facial vein has been absent, in which case a larger than usual transverse facial vein has bailed us out.

ANATOMY OF THE FACIAL NERVE

The seventh cranial nerve has an intracranial, temporal, and extracranial course. The intracranial course is the journey the nerve makes from the brain to the internal auditory meatus. Thereafter, its course through the temporal bone is convoluted and closely related to the semicircular canals of the inner ear. It passes through the middle ear to finally exit at the stylomastoid foramen to ramify on the face and supply the mimetic muscles from their deep surface with the exception of buccinator, levator anguli oris, and mentalis, which are innervated from their superficial surfaces. Most pertinent to this chapter, the extracranial course will be considered in more detail.

The facial nerve exits the stylomastoid foramen, turns superficially, and immediately enters the substance of the parotid gland, where it is classically described as dividing into five branches: the temporal (frontal), zygomatic, buccal, mandibular, and cervical. Davis et al. (35) described numerous branching patterns of the facial nerve; however, this is of limited use surgically because of the variability of the anatomy. In practice, they comprise five variably interconnected groups of branches hereafter referred to as divisions. The nerve usually divides into upper (temporal) and lower (cervical) trunks at first, from which the divisions arise and anastomose with each other to a greater or lesser degree within the substance of the parotid; the frontal and mandibular divisions show little interconnection with the zygomatic and buccal divisions that lie between them. By contrast, branches of the zygomatic and buccal divisions are so highly interconnected that some would describe them as a zygomaticobuccal group. Despite the variability of the anatomy, some general anatomical landmarks should be set forth.

The temporal division of the facial nerve exits from the upper pole of the parotid gland and becomes superficial, plastered onto the underside of the temporoparietal fascia and lying immediately under the subcutaneous fat of the temple region. The course of the nerve is along a line drawn from 0.5 cm below the tragus to 1.5 cm (a finger's breadth) above the eyebrow. At the lateral margin of frontalis, the nerve, or more accurately, its branches, pass deep to frontalis and orbicularis oculi, which they innervate, eventually reaching the glabella region to supply the depressors of the brow.

The mandibular division leaves the lower portion of the parotid gland and swings down below the body of the mandible only to recross it anteriorly to supply the muscles of the lip and chin. Cadaveric dissection and nerve stimulation studies in vivo demonstrate that the nerve always comprises at least three major branches that run on the undersurface of the platysma and superficial to the facial vessels (36). The branch to the depressor anguli oris is the largest and runs just above the body of the mandible before ascending sharply to enter the deep surface of the muscle. Superior to this, one or two branches also run above the body of the mandible to supply platysma, risorius, orbicularis oris, and co-innervate depressor anguli oris. The inferiormost branch to depressor labii inferioris and mentalis is located at a variable distance 1 to 2 cm below the mandible (9) with some branches supplying platysma.

The cervical division exits the inferior pole of the parotid gland below the angle of the mandible and deep to platysma, innervating this muscle at the junction between its upper and middle thirds (12). The complex innervation of the platysma illustrates a multiple branching and overlapping pattern of innervation that is actually most developed between the zygomatic and buccal divisions of the facial nerve.

The zygomatic division leaves the upper anterior portion of the parotid gland to run just inferior the zygomatic arch immediately deep to the SMAS to innervate the elevators of the upper lip and lower portion of orbicularis oculi. Inferior to the zygomatic division, branches from the buccal division exit the anterior border of the parotid gland and run inferior to Stensen's duct and on the surface of the buccal fat pad deep to the now-thin SMAS layer to supply the muscles of the mouth and cheek. Both divisions have a highly overlapping distribution that affords division of one or more branches without weakness; this premise constitutes the basis for cross-facial nerve grafting.

Despite the numerous studies of facial nerve anatomy, it may be more practical to consider the facial nerve as consisting of physiological and functional components that do not always correlate to textbook anatomical distributions of branches but instead relate to muscular groups and actions. Multiple branches distal to the parotid are exposed, and controlled intraoperative stimulation of each one is carried out to identify its functional contribution to facial animation. The divisions from which these branches originate are unimportant, but the information obtained is vital in the formulation of a surgical strategy.

ANATOMY OF THE FACIAL MUSCLES

There are 23 pairs of facial muscles, 18 of which convey facial expression together with the solitary orbicularis oris. The frontalis muscle is the anterior belly of the occipitofrontalis muscle that spans the scalp; it is a sheet of muscle 1 mm thick and 5 to 6 cm wide. The origin is from an intermediate tendon, termed the *galea aponeurotica*, and the muscle passes forward and merges with the fibers of orbicularis and attaches both to the supraorbital ridge via the periorbital septum (37) and to the dermis through multiple fibrous septae (38). It provides tone and is an elevator of the brow; loss of function causes ptosis of the brow and exacerbates dermatochalasis of the upper eyelids. The orbicularis oculi muscle overlies the frontalis and forms the sphincter of the eye, consisting of orbital and palpebral portions. The orbital portion begins at the medial palpebral raphe, a fibrous interdigitation of the orbicularis fibers, and winds around the rim of the orbit without being interrupted laterally. It lies superficial to zygomaticus, levator labii superioris, and levator labii alaeque nasi and receives multiple motor branches from the frontal and zygomatic divisions of the facial nerve that enter its deep surface 3 to 4 mm inside its lateral border. The orbital portion of the orbicularis oculi enacts powerful voluntary eyelid closure. In contrast, the palpebral portion is involved in gentle eyelid closure and has an elaborate arrangement of muscle fibers suspended between the medial and lateral canthi that are divided into the preseptal and pretarsal portions. Both take origin from the medial canthus and pass laterally across the eyelid; whereas the preseptal muscle fibers interdigitate laterally to form the lateral palpebral raphe, the pretarsal fibers form the lateral canthus proper and turn deeply into the orbit to attach to Whitnall's tubercle inside the orbital rim. In this manner, the eyelid remains apposed to the curved surface of the globe (39). As the muscle fibers of the palpebral portion contract, they affect eyelid closure by shortening the length of muscle between the canthi. The mechanism is similar to that of stretching an elastic band between two pegs except that rather than moving the pegs apart, the band itself actively tightens.

The mimetic musculature of the mouth is complex and important to understand because an appreciation of the contributions of the many muscles to the movement of the lips aids design for smile reconstruction. These muscles can be divided into elevators, depressors, and the solitary orbicularis oris sphincter, which acts as an antagonist to the other groups (40). The orbicularis is a large, circular muscle that constitutes the bulk of the lip, being closely attached to the skin peripherally. A detailed anatomic and electrophysiologic study (41) demonstrated that it consists of a deep sphincteric portion and a superficial part that relates to facial expression and the precise movements needed to coordinate speech. The sphincteric portion is partly derived from buccinator and has horizontal fibers that lie close to the mucosal surface, which act to close the mouth with a scissor-like action. In addition, the pars marginalis is derived from the deep part and creates the eversion of the vermillion and definition of the white roll. In contrast, the superficial portion, commensurate with its role in facial expression and articulation receives contributions from the lip elevators and depressors and inserts into the skin over the lips. In the upper lips, this insertion is bilaminar, with long and short fibers creating the contralateral and ipsilateral philtral columns, respectively.

The depressor anguli oris; depressor labii inferioris; and to a lesser extent, platysma are the depressors of the lower lip. The mentalis is the deepest muscle of the lower lip muscles but acts as an elevator by virtue of its superior bony origin from the mandible at the level of the incisor roots and insertion onto the skin of the chin prominence. Contraction of these muscle fibers serves to draw the chin prominence superiorly, wrinkling the chin. The depressor labii inferioris arises from the mandible just behind and inferior to the mental foramen and passes medially and superiorly augmenting the orbicularis while attaching to the vermillion and skin of the lip through fibrous septae. This arrangement serves to draw the lower lip down and evert the vermillion as if one was displaying the lower teeth. Overlying this is depressor anguli oris that arises from the lower border of the mandible and inserts into the modiolus to pull the angle of the mouth downward and lateral.

The elevators of the lip are those responsible for smile, which together with the depressors and orbicularis act in a coordinated fashion to create facial expression and articulate speech. The main elevators consist of the levator labii superioris, levator anguli oris, and zygomaticus major. The zygomaticus major arises from the zygoma just anterior to the zygomatico-temporal suture; here it is deep and covered by the orbital part of orbicularis and zygomaticus minor. It passes to the angle of the mouth to contribute to the modiolus, a fibrous structure at the commissure formed by contributions from levator anguli oris, risorius, buccinators, orbicularis oris, and depressor anguli oris muscles. The remaining portion of zygomaticus major blends with the insertion of levator labii superioris, which arises from the infraorbital margin and descends to partly insert around the alar crease and partly into the underside of orbicularis oris with its deepest fibers contributing to the modiolus. The levator anguli oris arises from the anterior face of the maxilla and runs vertically downward in the canine fossa to insert into the modiolus.

The interplay between the orbicularis, the elevators, and the depressors of the lips creates a unique smile configuration in each individual. Rubin (42) grouped the various smiles into three classes: the "Mona Lisa" smile in which the corners of the mouth are pulled upward and laterally by zygomaticus major followed by contraction of the levators to expose the upper teeth. The "canine smile" is the reverse order, in which the upper lip elevators draw the lip in an upward vector to expose the canines followed by zygomaticus motion to draw the angles of the mouth up and out. Last is the "full denture smile" in which the upper lip elevators, zygomaticus, and depressors act in unison to display the upper and lower teeth. Establishing the individual's smile type and defining the landmarks that portray that smile are key to surgical planning. No less important is the determination of the vector of muscle excursion, together with the precise insertion points around the mouth that will create a natural facial movement and nasolabial crease definition.

PLANNING SMILE RECONSTRUCTION WITH FREE SEGMENTAL GRACILIS TRANSPLANTATION

By analyzing the smile on the normal side, the appropriate vector of lip and commissure excursion can be projected. However, we have found that great care in the positioning of anchoring sutures and inset of the muscle flap are also critical in achieving a dynamic spontaneous and symmetrical smile. The importance of this step cannot be overestimated.

As noted earlier (42), there are distinct types of smile in which the commissures and upper and lower lips play a greater or lesser role in creating the smile. Indeed, there is great individual variation in the shape and symmetry of the smile in nonparalyzed individuals (4). The easiest method to assess a patient's smile is to carefully inspect the smile on the normal side; the vector of movement at the commissure and upper lip should be noted. The greatest amount of movement is at the oral commissure—roughly 40 degrees from the horizontal—together with a vertical movement of the upper lip. Surgeons should concentrate efforts in reproducing this movement; otherwise, inadequate incisor show will result, and the upper lip will appear to sag (4). In patients with long-standing palsy, there may be a degree of facial scoliosis, which may lead to the unaffected side having distorted or exaggerated movements. Nonetheless, it remains the best indicator of the patient's premorbid smile. In addition to observing movements of the lips, one should also scrutinize the face globally, noting the symmetry and position of the nasolabial creases, the degree of bulk in the malar region, and to what the degree the eyes close and brows move during normal and "full" smile. Appreciation of these smaller details allows for a more complete recreation of a "smiling face" by careful planning of adjuvant surgical procedures rather than by simply creating an isolated smiling mouth with the free muscle transfer alone.

In addition to the qualitative assessment, one may measure the movement with a transparent ruler and a protractor to quantify specific parameters. This can be done in the clinic by hand or based on photographs or video films (4,20). Most recently, three-dimensional video analysis has been used to evaluate outcomes of surgery (43), but such methods are more useful for research than for preoperative planning. Immediately before surgery, the dominant vector of the smile is marked on the cheek, as is the nasolabial crease of the normal side. A symmetrical nasolabial crease is then marked on the affected side to guide insertion of a free muscle transfer (Figure 40-3). In the case of bilateral facial palsy, especially congenital forms such as Möbius syndrome, landmarks such as the nasolabial creases are not present, and the surgeon needs to carefully estimate the position of the new nasolabial crease.

FIRST-STAGE PROCEDURE: CROSS-FACE NERVE GRAFT

The patient is positioned supine on the operating table with the neck slightly extended and turned away from the side of the operation. An orotracheal intubation is performed with a "south-facing" midline oral right angle endotracheal tube. This is used to allow the movements of the face in response to nerve stimulation to be visualized while permitting easy access to the upper buccal sulcus through which the nerve graft will be banked. The face is prepared with nonalcoholic povidone–iodine solution with care taken to protect the eyes with lubricating ointment and taping the eyelids closed. At the same time, the second surgical team prepares the donor site for the nerve harvest.

Facial Dissection

The face is infiltrated with a 1:400,000 dilution of epinephrine in saline to promote hemostasis and aid dissection; no local anesthesia is used because this will interfere with nerve stimulation.

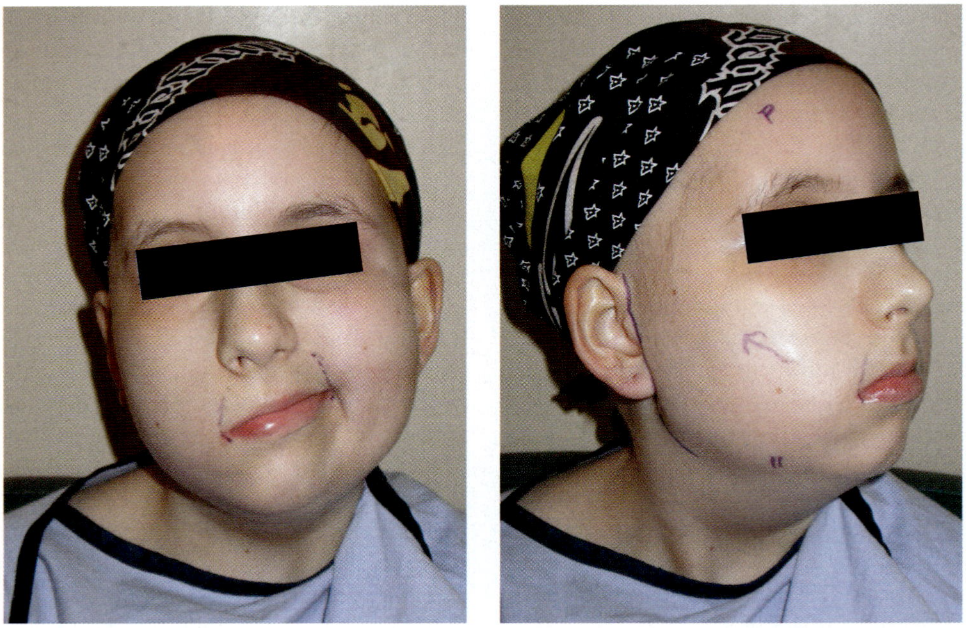

A B

FIGURE 40-3 Preoperative markings. (**A**) The nasolabial crease is marked on the normal side first and then transposed to the contralateral side. (**B**) The arrow denotes the primary vector of the patient's smile. The pulsation of the facial artery is palpated at the lower border of the mandible and marked with short parallel lines. The full extent of the preauricular incision is marked. P indicates the side on which the muscle transplant is to be performed.

The preauricular incision begins at the temple 1 to 2 cm above the zygomatic arch, runs in front of the tragus, and at the lobule of the ear curves behind the angle of the mandible for a short distance toward the submandibular gland, ending in a neck crease. The incision is made with a scalpel, and a subcutaneous dissection is performed over the surface of the parotid fascia until the anterior border of the parotid gland is reached. Traction on the skin flap posteriorly with a Maxwell or rake retractor, together with countertraction by the assistant's fingers on the cheek, maintains tension in the flap and facilitates dissection. The plane of dissection is immediately above the parotid fascia, leaving a decent layer of fat on the underside of the facelift flap. Care is taken to avoid exposure of dermis, which can later adhere to the muscle flap, causing tethering and dimpling of the skin when the muscle contracts. The thickness of the flap should also be even to avoid postoperative contour irregularities and can be judged by palpation at regular intervals or transilluminating the flap with the operating lights.

At the anterior border of the parotid gland, the dissection is deepened through the SMAS to expose the facial nerve branches as they emerge from the gland sitting in facial fat and covered by the innominate fascia. They are systematically identified and can be dissected in a retrograde fashion to find size-matched donor branches. The key to success of this procedure is to functionally match the donor nerve action to the intended target to create symmetrical conjugate animation. Careful nerve stimulation identifies nerve branches that activate the appropriate actions with minimal collateral movement. A nerve "map" is recorded, attributing specific actions to the branches of the nerve that have been identified and temporarily tagged with vessel loops. These can then be used to drive equivalent actions on the paralyzed side of the face if connected to an appropriate motor via a cross-face nerve graft. Ideally, two or more branches are found that perform the same function so that one branch remains on the normal side and the largest and most powerful branch is used to power the contralateral side. For example, to reconstruct the smile, two branches that activate the zygomaticus in a similar fashion on the donor side should be found; one remains to motor the unaffected side, and the other can be divided and used to power the muscle transfer on the contralateral side. For consistent results during this stage, we use a microbipolar stimulator with a variable voltage and frequency control (Neurosign 100, Spring Gardens, UK) because in our experience, the disposable nerve stimulators can be of variable efficacy, often producing tetanic muscle contraction. Facial nerve mapping identifies which nerve branches stimulate the orbicularis oculi, lip elevators, and lip retractors. Nerve branches that produce an isolated smile upon stimulation are selected (Figure 40-4). It is sometimes difficult to find "smile" branches that do not produce orbicularis oculi contraction, but there are usually two to four branches that activate the zygomaticus without eye movement.

After the appropriate donor branches are selected, a subcutaneous tunnel is made from one side of the face toward the mouth by blunt dissection. A hemostat is passed from the facial dissection toward the upper lip in the subcutaneous plane, and an incision in the upper buccal sulcus on the opposite, affected, side is made to meet the tips of the hemostat. This creates a tunnel that will allow the nerve graft to span the distance between the facial nerve dissection and the upper lip region

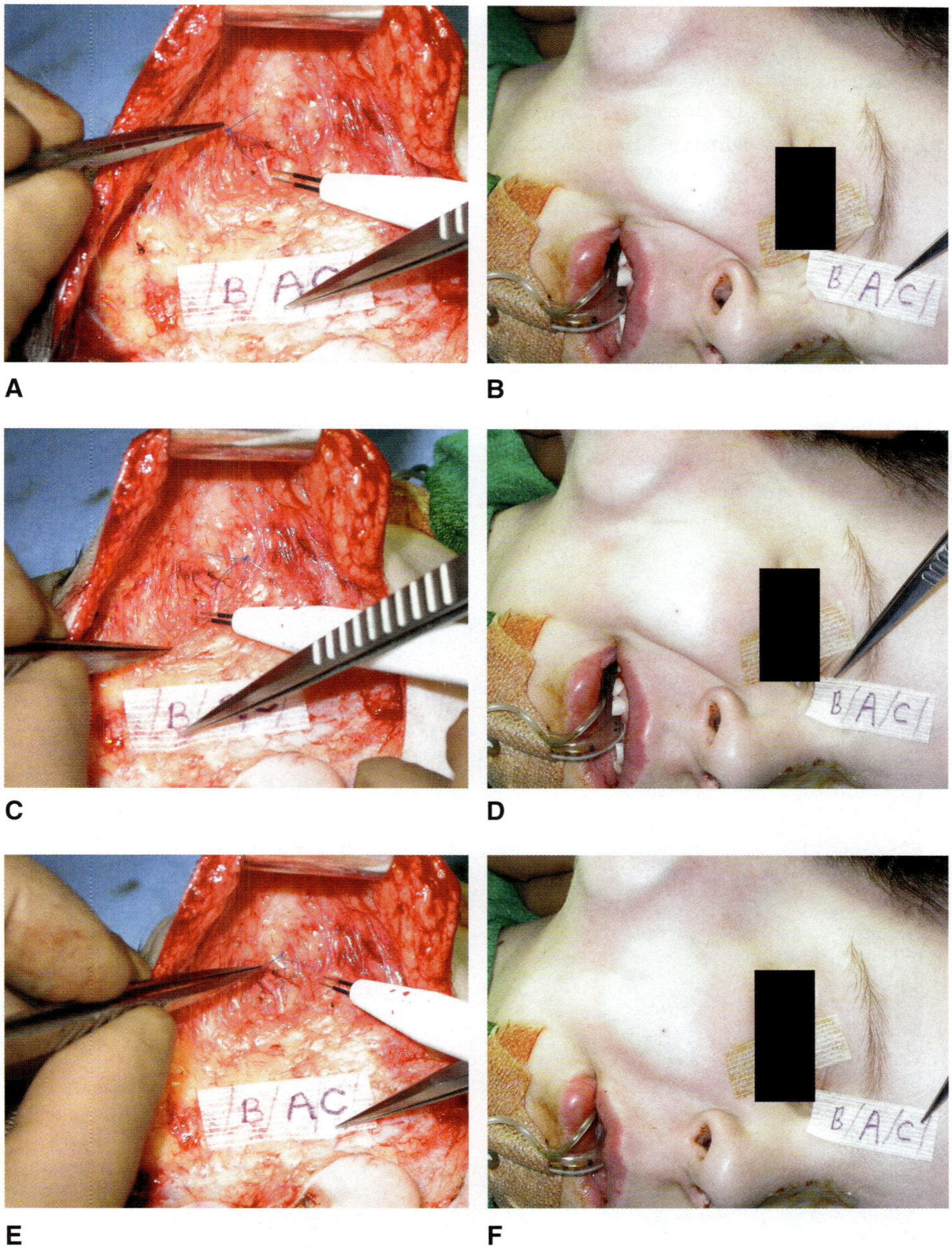

FIGURE 40-4 Nerve mapping. Three branches of the facial nerve have been dissected; designated B/A/C from superior to inferior. Branch A is retracted with a Prolene suture. (**A**) A bipolar stimulator is used to activate the nerve branch. (**B**) The consequence of the stimulation is manifest by facial movement. Stimulation of A causes activation of zygomaticus and levator labii superioris and levator labii superioris alaeque nasi. (**C**) and (**D**) Stimulation of B activates zygomaticus without stimulation of lip levators. (**E**) and (**F**) Stimulation of C does not create a smile. Therefore, branch B is selected as a motor for cross-face nerve graft.

where the graft end will be banked ready for coaptation to the gracilis nerve at the second-stage procedure.

Nerve Harvest

A second surgical team performs harvest of the sural nerve while the facial dissection is underway. The sural nerve is a branch of the tibial nerve arising at the popliteal fossa that runs distally in a subfascial plane between the two heads of the gastrocnemius muscle, eventually passing subcutaneously down toward the lateral aspect of the heel, where it supplies sensation to the lateral portion of the heel and foot as far as the base of the fifth toe. It is joined in the distal third of the leg by a communicating branch from the common peroneal nerve (44). We harvest the *proximal* portion of this nerve to minimize donor morbidity while obtaining an even-diameter graft with a high neuronal content and a perfect size match to receive the facial nerve branches. With the patient supine on a beanbag, the knee is flexed, the hip is adducted, and a sterile thigh tourniquet is inflated after limb elevation but not exsanguination. A small transverse incision is made in the midline of the calf 4 cm below the popliteal crease. The incision is deepened through the fat to expose the deep fascia into which a cautious transverse incision is made. This is carefully opened, and the sural nerve is identified. The sural nerve should lie between the two heads of gastrocnemius and may appear quite superficial, the short saphenous vein lying medial to the nerve. After being identified, the nerve can be dissected proximally with care toward the popliteal fossa where it joins the tibial nerve. The popliteal artery and vein are at risk, especially in young children, so dissection should proceed under direct vision. The proximal end of the nerve is divided, and a nerve stripper used to harvest the nerve in a minimal access fashion. The free proximal end of the nerve is placed through the eye of stripper, and with a steady, firm action the stripper can be passed distally, freeing the nerve from the surrounding tissue. At the point where the nerve emerges from the deep fascia and the peroneal communicating branch joins it, the stripper often meets resistance. Here, the second transverse incision can be made, the distal end of the nerve divided, and the graft retrieved. In this way, greater than 12 cm of nerve can be harvested via two small incisions in the leg, and this is of sufficient length for use in a free muscle transfer (Figure 40-5). A longer length is required for a full cross-face nerve graft, in which instance, the full length of the nerve is taken using three or more stair-stepped incisions. Here, the nerve is not divided at the junction with the peroneal communicating branch; instead, the communicating branch is transected and the stripper replaced around the nerve, which is now in a suprafascial plane. The stripper is passed distally with the same action as earlier and should reach as far as the ankle. A transverse incision is made posterior to the lateral malleolus, and the distal end of the nerve is found. The nerve is retrieved and dissected as far distally as possible until it begins to ramify. At this point the nerve is divided, retrieved and wrapped in damp gauze until required. Of note, some centers harvest the sural nerve with the patent prone, which is easier in larger individuals but precludes a two-team approach.

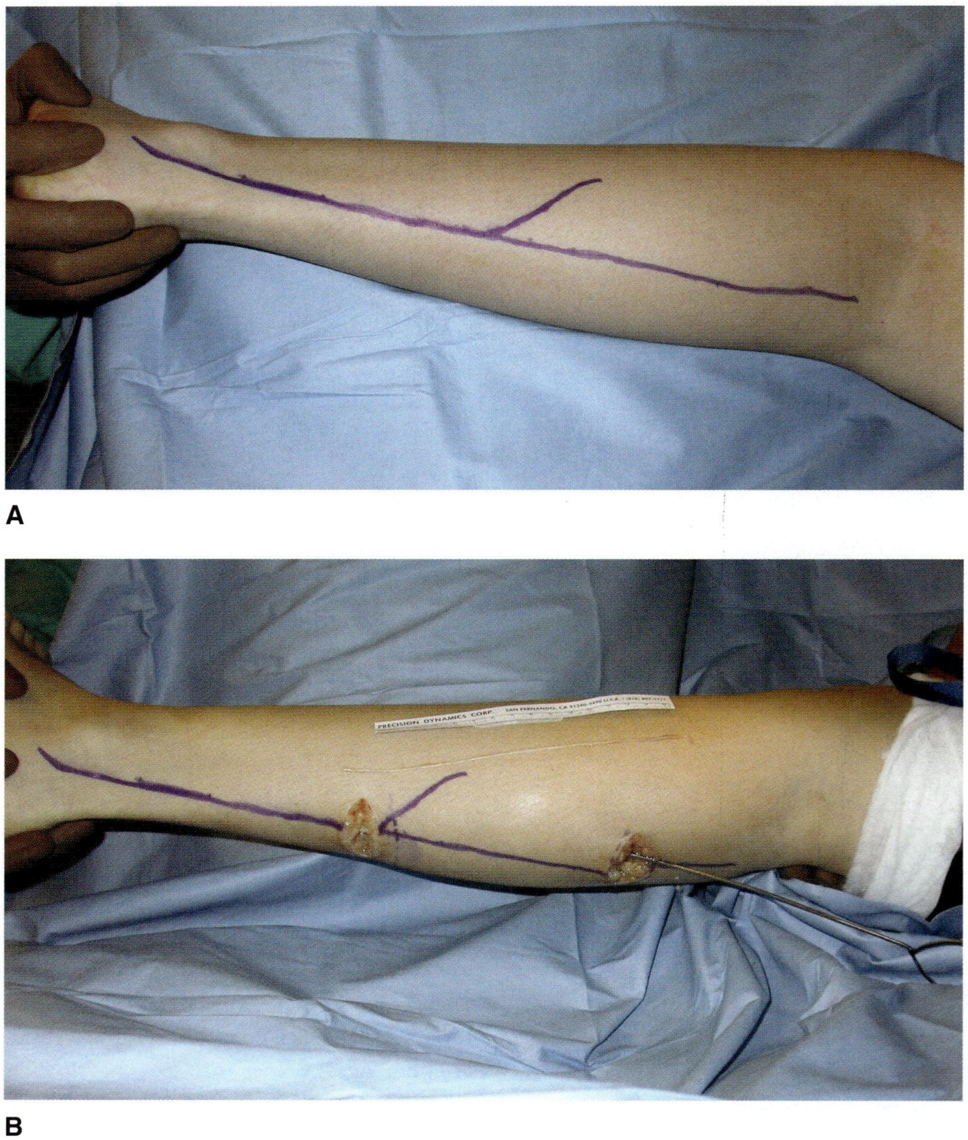

FIGURE 40-5 Harvest of the sural nerve. (A) The course of the nerve is marked with the sural communicating branch heading laterally. (B) Through two incisions, the nerve is harvested with the nerve stripper (seen emerging from the proximal incision). Approximately 12 cm of nerve was harvested while the sural communicating branch was preserved to minimize the sensory deficit following harvest.

Inset of the Cross-Facial Nerve Graft

When the facial dissection is complete and the nerve harvested, the nerve can be carefully threaded through the subcutaneous tunnel to the upper buccal sulcus to allow for a tension-free, precise coaptation using the operating microscope (Figure 40-6). The distal end of the nerve in the upper buccal sulcus is tagged using a colored nonabsorbable suture and tacked to the alar base of the affected side to facilitate identification and retrieval at the second stage. The proximal end of the nerve is coapted to the donor nerve as described in the neurorrhaphy section (Figure 40-7). When complete, hemostasis is secured, and the wounds are closed. The patient recovers overnight at 45 degrees and is allowed to mobilize as tolerated the next day. The patient is discharged as soon as he or she is well and is reviewed in the clinic on a regular basis to clinically monitor signs of axonal growth along the nerve graft using Tinel's sign.

Cross-Face Nerve Grafting to Viable Facial Musculature in One Stage

If performing a cross-face nerve graft to reinnervate viable facial musculature without free muscle transfer, the above procedure is performed with some modifications. A longer length of sural nerve is harvested as described earlier. This may be microdissected

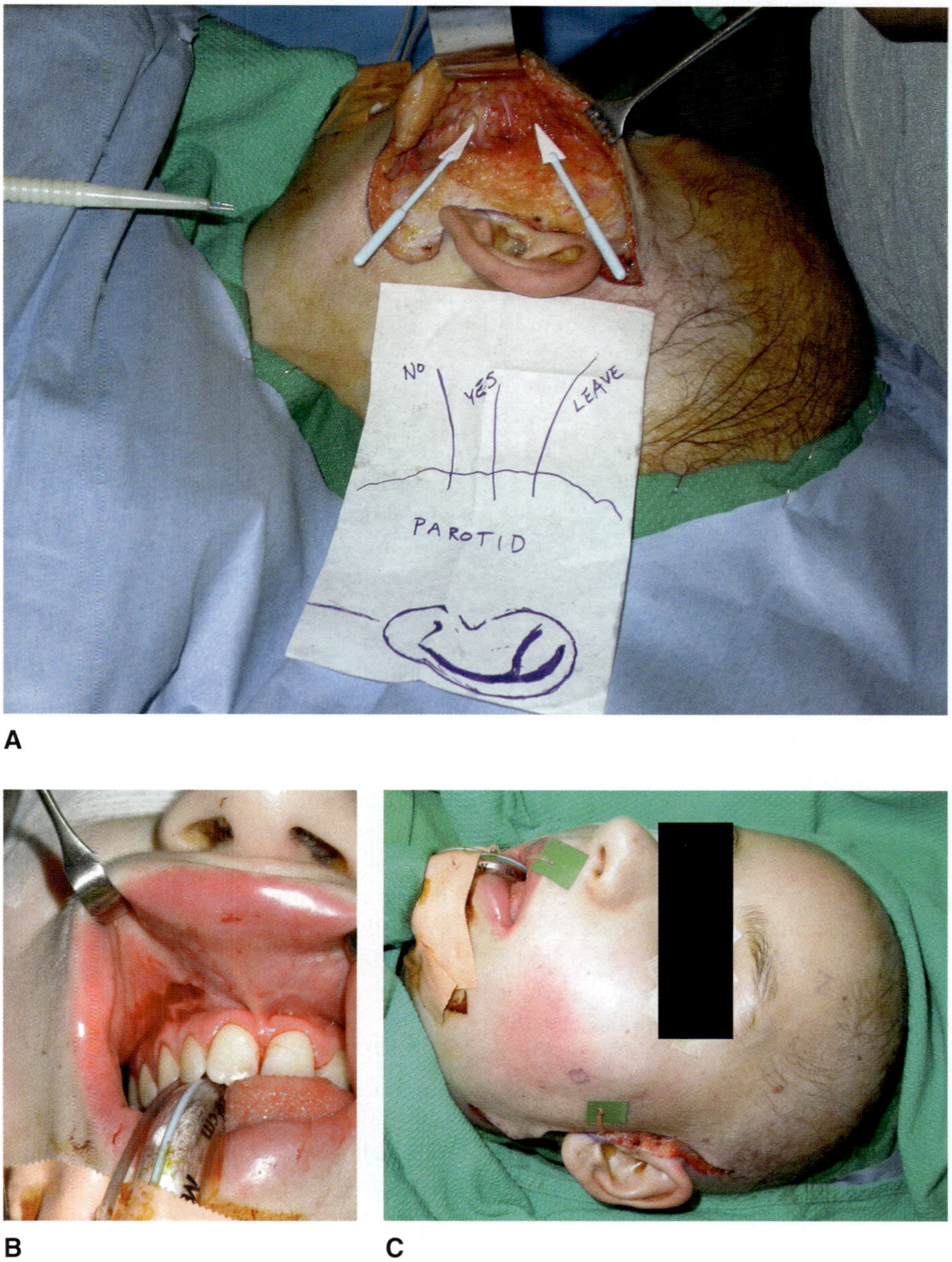

FIGURE 40-6 Inset of cross-face nerve graft. (A) The intraoperative diagram following nerve mapping denotes which branch is to be coapted to the nerve graft. (B) The buccal incision. The nerve graft will be threaded from the facial dissection to be banked at the level of the canine tooth via this incision. (C) The nerve graft in situ before coaptation of the proximal end to the selected branch of the facial nerve.

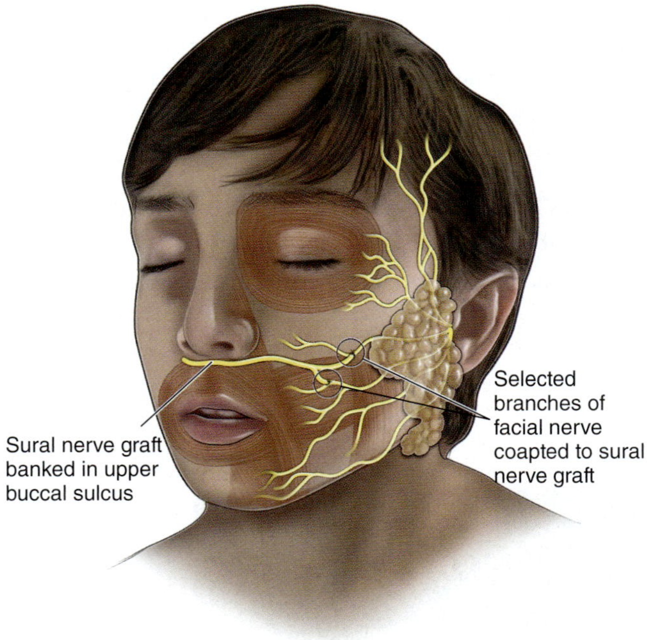

FIGURE 40-7 Schematic of the cross-facial nerve graft in position.

under the operating microscope into two fascicular groups to perform more than one cross-face graft (e.g., between upper and lower divisions of the facial nerve). However, the distance over which this may be possible may be limited by crossover between fascicles. A facial dissection and nerve exploration is also performed on the paralyzed side to identify branches that functionally match the donor nerves. These matched branches are then joined via the cross-face nerve graft. The axons may take 6 to 9 months to grow across the graft, and thus a "babysitter" procedure may be indicated to maintain muscle function. In this instance, the motor nerve to masseter can be dissected and anastomosed to the distal stumps of the paralyzed side while awaiting axonal regrowth across the sural nerve graft. A second-stage procedure is then performed to coapt the cross-face nerve graft to the distal stumps as described earlier.

SECOND-STAGE PROCEDURE: FREE MUSCLE TRANSFER

The timing of the second procedure is usually 6 to 9 months after the cross-face nerve graft. The patient is reviewed in the clinic to monitor axonal regrowth by Tinel's sign. When there is an indication that the growth has reached the end of the nerve graft, surgery is scheduled.

The patient set up is the same as for the first-stage procedure except that a nasotracheal intubation is performed with the tube secured to the membranous septum with a 2-0 silk suture and passed superiorly to allow unfettered access to the face. Great care is taken to avoid pressure on the alar rim by the tube, and it is carefully splinted away from this structure by a combination of padding on the forehead and by suturing the tube to the scalp to prevent the weight of the respiratory circuit's pulling the tube cephalically against the nostril.

A two-team approach is used: one team to perform the facial recipient site dissection and a second team to harvest the gracilis muscle. The facial dissection is performed on the affected side in a similar fashion to the first-stage procedure. However, it extends farther toward the oral commissures and into the upper and lower lips. The aim is to identify the sinewy material around the oral commissure that will readily accept heavy #1 or #2 Vicryl (Ethicon) sutures that are used to secure the muscle flap to the commissure. Sutures are inserted into the upper lip and commissure, and if there is a static ptosis of the lower lip, sutures may be positioned here to elevate and correct this. The positioning of these sutures is a critical portion of the operation and makes the difference between a natural-appearing smile and a contrived "pull" on the commissure. It is important to try to create a nasolabial crease that is symmetrical; by placing traction on the sutures in the appropriate vector, the smile can be evaluated on the operating table (Figure 40-8). The depth of suture placement is important because placing the sutures too superficial causes lip eversion and a snarl, and deep insertion causes lip inversion. The technique of establishing the correct level is to carry out the dissection immediately superficial to the musculature at the corner of the mouth. The heavy Vicryl sutures are then used in mattress fashion to suture the anterior end of the muscle graft down to the underlying facial muscles and modiolus. In the upper lip, the dissection is extended to the alar base and ipsilateral philtral ridge.

One can appreciate that careful preoperative evaluation of the landmarks and vector of the smile outlined earlier are important in fine tuning the surgical maneuvers to create a natural result. Bulkiness of the reconstruction is one of the most common postoperative complaints. To address this, defatting of the facelift flap and removal of the buccal fat pad can be performed at this time. However, care must be taken not to expose the dermis because this might adhere to the underlying muscle graft, causing tethering and dimpling when the muscle contracts.

The facial vessels are most easily identified at the anterior inferior border of the masseter muscle and are followed superiorly toward the nasal ala whereupon they may be divided and brought down into the wound for anastomosis. Likewise, via a buccal incision, the end of the cross-face nerve graft is identified and retrieved. The neuroma at the end is excised, and if required, a sample of the nerve can be sent for frozen section analysis to confirm adequate numbers of axons in the graft. The facial dissection and upper buccal sulcus incisions are connected by blunt dissection as described earlier.

Flap Elevation

The gracilis is harvested through a longitudinal incision on the medial thigh overlying the axis of the muscle. The line begins proximally midway between the pubic tubercle and ischial tuberosity lying just behind the palpable tendinous border of adductor longus and extends distally toward the insertion on the upper medial tibia. The incision is approximately 10 cm in length and is made down to and through the deep fascia onto the gracilis muscle. In the loose areolar plane between the muscle and the deep fascia, blunt dissection proceeds to free the

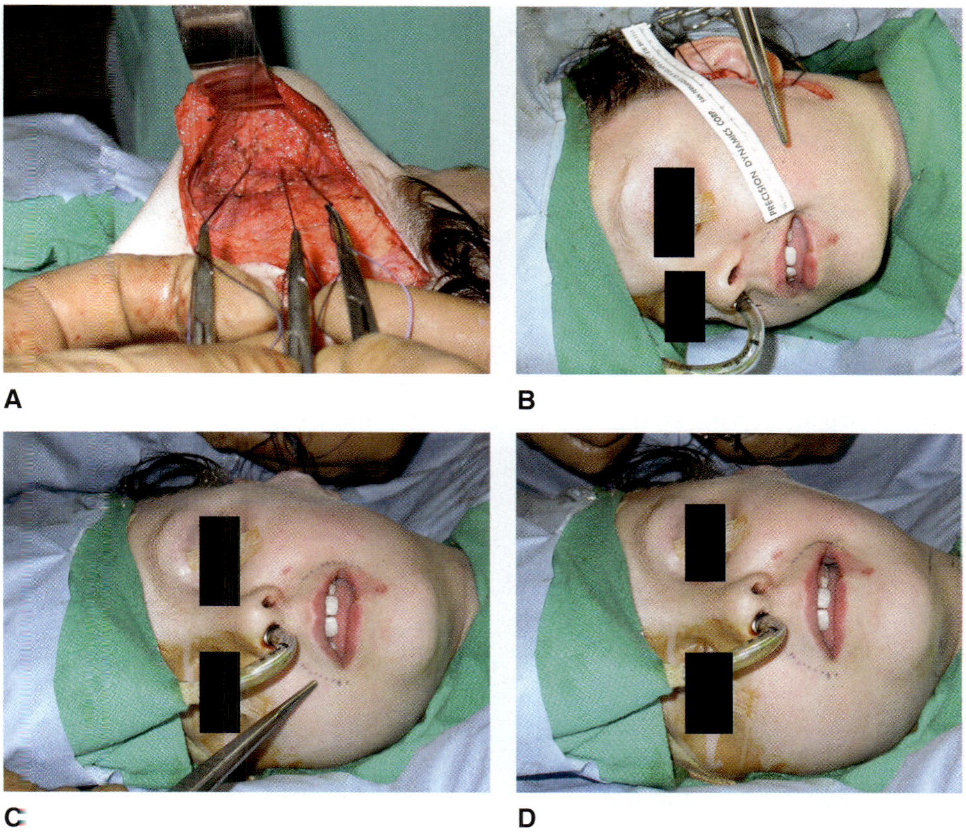

FIGURE 40-8 Placement of anchoring sutures to the commissure. (A) View through the facial dissection demonstrating the heavy Vicryl sutures placed in the fibrous tissue at the commissure. The plane of this is on the superficial surface of the facial musculature. (B) The positioning of these sutures is critical, and light traction can be placed on the sutures to measure the length of gracilis required. (C) View of the face at rest with sutures in place. The instrument points to the normal nasolabial crease. (D) Traction on the sutures in the vector that the flap will be inset recreates a smile. Assessment at this crucial stage allows for repositioning of sutures if necessary to minimize lip eversion or inversion and create a more natural smile.

anterior border of the muscle from the deep fascia to identify the dominant vascular pedicle. It emerges between adductor longus anteriorly and adductor magnus posteriorly to enter the lateral posterior surface of gracilis roughly 8 cm below the pubis. A skin perforator emerging form the superficial surface of the muscle often corresponds to the position of the pedicle. Two centimeters proximal in the same plane lies the nerve to gracilis that courses downward and medially, bisecting the right angle the vascular pedicle makes with the muscle. After the neurovascular structures are identified and protected, the muscle is circumferentially dissected free of its fascial sheath. The pedicle is dissected as far as possible toward the parent structures of its constituents (obturator nerve and profunda femoris vessels). The adductor longus can be retracted to facilitate the dissection, which is carried out as proximal as possible to maximize pedicle length. To reduce bulk in the recipient site (i.e., the face), the muscle is split along the length of the fibers so as to harvest only the anterior one-third to half of the muscle. This provides sufficient motor power without exacerbating asymmetry in the face. Thus, the anterior third of the muscle is now isolated on a neurovascular pedicle and attached to the pubis and tibia at either end. Although the muscle can be split longitudinally without concern, on occasion the vascular pedicle enters the muscle in the middle of its deep surface. In this situation, it may be necessary to remove a portion of the anterior and posterior muscle, preserving the middle part on the neurovascular pedicle.

The next step is to judge the length of muscle required. After the facial dissection is complete and the commissural sutures are in place, the distance from the commissure to the deep temporal fascia is measured, and the position of the recipient vessels is noted. The muscle flap is then designed such that the required length plus 1 cm at either end is harvested, with the neurovascular structures in the appropriate position to facilitate anastomosis. After the planning for the length and orientation of the muscle flap is complete, the distal end of the muscle is divided, and a row of mattress sutures is inserted to act as brace against which the anchoring sutures may be placed reducing the risk of the sutures "cheese wiring" through the muscle (19). Thereafter, the origin of gracilis is divided and the proximal row of brace sutures placed while the flap remains perfused via the pedicle. After this is completed and the recipient site is ready to receive the flap, the pedicle can be divided the flap removed and the donor defect closed (Figure 40-9). The deep fascia is sutured to avoid unsightly bulging of the remaining gracilis or other adductor muscles through the defect. A layered closure is performed with absorbable sutures and a light dressing

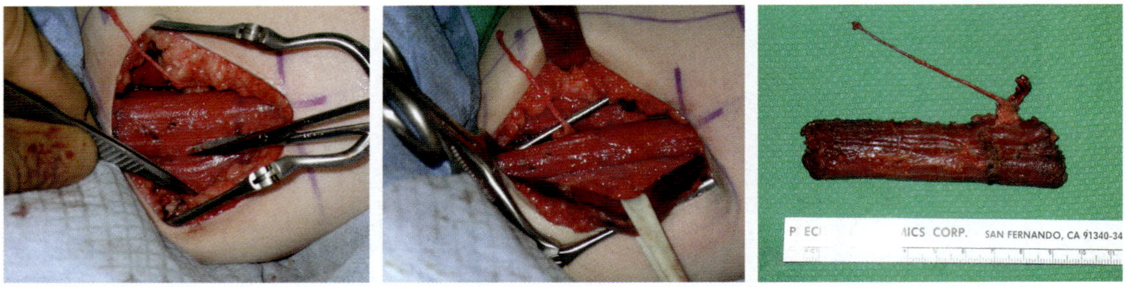

A B C

FIGURE 40-9 Segmental harvest of the gracilis muscle transplant. (A) The gracilis muscle is about to be split to create the segmental flap. Just beyond the tips of the scissors lies a constant vessel that runs toward the posterior portion of the muscle that will be left behind. This vessel is ligated. (B) The nerve to gracilis is observed passing upward in the photograph. Below this, the gracilis has been split into two portions; the posterior portion is being retracted by a silicone loop and will remain in situ. The anterior part will be harvested for transplant. (C) The muscle harvest is completed. In this case, a 9-cm length of muscle was required for a child. The shorter vascular pedicle is seen on the right emerging from the anterior border with the longer nerve to gracilis.

applied; we do not routinely use a drain. The scar does spread with time, but because it lies on the medial aspect of the thigh, it is reasonably well hidden, and no patients have complained about it.

Flap Inset

At the recipient site, the muscle is orientated with the pedicle deep and angled toward the facial vessels. The commissural anchoring sutures are secured to the muscle behind the row of mattress sutures, and the flap is draped in the appropriate vector with the other end tacked onto the deep temporal fascia to secure the muscle in place. The position is then adjusted to allow access to the vessels on the underside, and the neurovascular structures are aligned and positioned ready for anastomosis. The nerve to gracilis is positioned toward the upper lip and tunneled through to reach the end of the sural nerve graft in the upper buccal sulcus (Figure 40-10). Wet gauze is placed over the nerve ends to prevent them from drying out, and vessel anastomosis is performed before neuroanastomosis to minimize ischemic time.

Vessel Anastomoses

The surgeon and assistant sit on either side of the head, while the microscope support comes in from the top of the patient and is set at 45 degrees to allow both surgeons to sit comfortably (Figure 40-11A). Under the microscope, the recipient vessels are cleaned of adventitia and the tunica intima inspected. Loose clot is removed with heparinized saline irrigation, and the vessel flow is checked by releasing the clamps and observing the spurt. Invariably, the facial vessels demonstrate good flow. However, there are instances in which the facial vessels are unavailable for anastomosis. In this case, the superficial temporal vessels, exposed during the dissection, can be divided cephalad in the temple and carefully turned down to reach the muscle flap. Another option is the transverse facial vessels adjacent to the parotid duct; the position of these vessels is convenient for anastomosis to the flap. We have observed that on occasions when the anterior facial vein is small, an unusually large transverse facial vein is present. A standard microvascular anastomosis is performed with 9-0 or 10-0 sutures. We do not use anticoagulants during or after the surgery under normal circumstances.

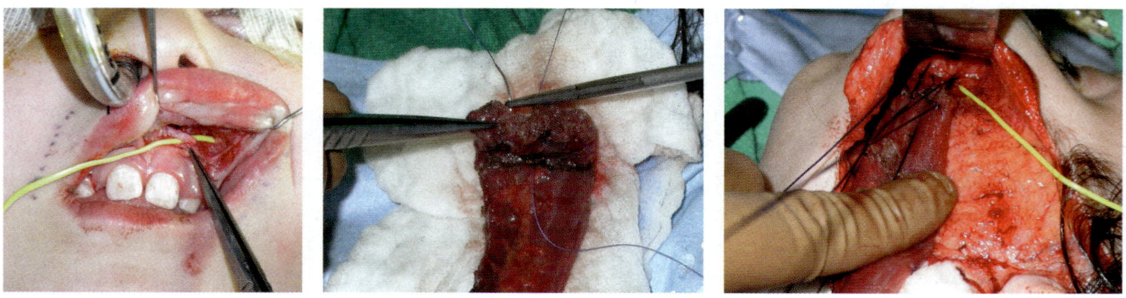

A B C

FIGURE 40-10 Inset of flap to the commissure. (A) The buccal sulcus incision is reopened, and the tagged end of the banked nerve graft is retrieved from the alar base. The yellow silicone loop passes from the facial dissection through a subcutaneous tunnel to the buccal incision. This is the path along which the motor nerve to gracilis will be passed to reach the site of coaptation. (B) After a row of bracing mattress sutures has been placed at each end of the flap, the commissural sutures are passed into the substance of the muscle behind the mattress sutures. (C) The gracilis transplant is then "parachuted" along the commissural anchoring sutures into position. Note how the anchoring sutures pass through the muscle substance behind the row of mattress sutures. When the commissural attachment is complete, the motor nerve to gracilis is passed via the tunnel (marked by the yellow silicone loop) to the buccal incision. The other end of the flap is tacked into place to establish stability while the vascular anastomosis and neurorrhaphy are performed.

When anastomosis is complete, an Acland test is performed to confirm patency, the muscle is inspected for bleeding to confirm restoration of the microcirculation, and attention is turned to the neurorrhaphy.

Neurorrhaphy

After perfusion is restored, precise coaptation of the nerve is performed in the buccal sulcus with the operating microscope. The quality of the neurorrhaphy is critical to maximize the number of axons reaching the muscle transfer. This is made easier by a good size match between the sural nerve and nerve to gracilis, thereby minimizing axonal loss at the neurorrhaphy (Figure 40-11). A completely tension-free epineurial repair is performed with 9-0 nylon microsutures. After they are completed, the nerve is returned to the incision, where it may be tacked by the epineurium to muscle in the deeper portion of the wound. The wound is then irrigated with warm saline and the oral mucosa closed in a watertight fashion with absorbable sutures.

To complete the procedure the muscle needs to be formally inset along the vector that was determined at pre-operative planning. The tension is adjusted such that there is symmetry of the commissures on table and then formally secured to the deep temporal fascia (Figure 40-12), body of the zygoma, or preauricular fascia in a fashion similar to that at the commissure. The muscle is spread out over the fascia before being secured, and it should course below the malar prominence to avoid excessive bulk in the malar area. Hemostasis is achieved, and the wound is rinsed with warm saline. The skin flap is replaced and closed with absorbable sutures over a Penrose drain that exits through a stab incision behind the ear. A blunt mouth hook is used to take the tension off the flap insertion during the initial postoperative period to limit the risk of sudden movements displacing

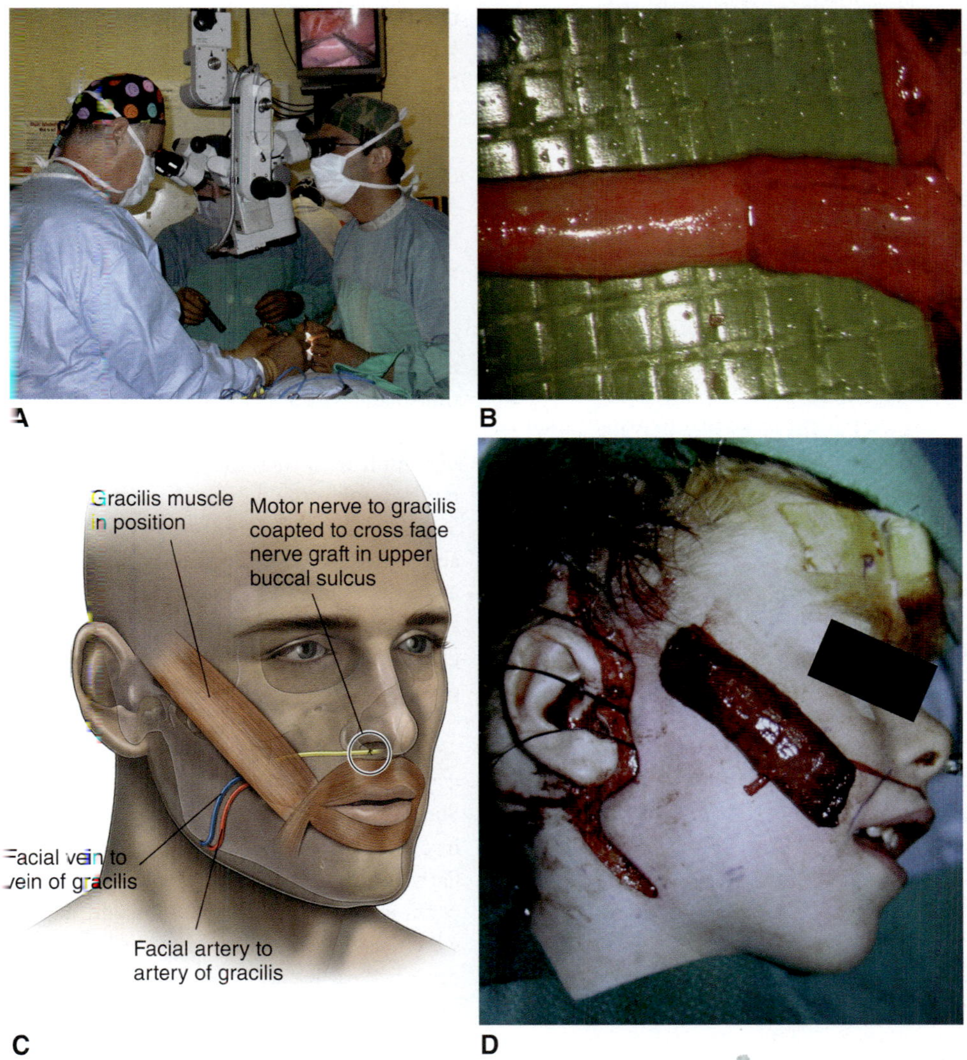

FIGURE 40-11 Neurorrhaphy. (A) For vascular anastomosis and neurorrhaphy, the microsurgeon and assistant sit either side of the head in comfortable operating positions. (B) The coaptation is performed in the buccal sulcus. Note the excellent size match between sural nerve graft and motor nerve to gracilis. (C) Diagrammatic representation of the orientation of the muscle flap and the scheme of anastomosis and neurorrhaphy. (D) Intraoperative photograph demonstrating the vector of the gracilis muscle. The pedicle is seen emerging at the inferior border of the muscle, and the motor nerve to gracilis is observed traversing the upper lip. The anchoring sutures are seen issuing from the preauricular incision.

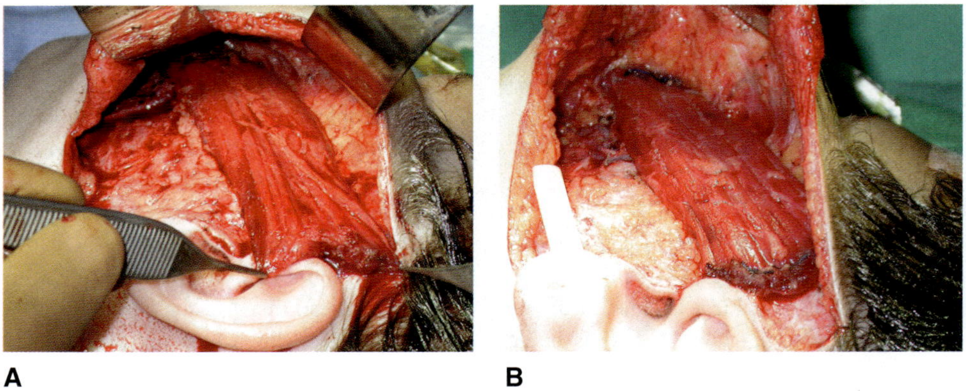

FIGURE 40-12 Final inset of the gracilis. (A) The vector of the muscle and the degree of tension are checked. (B) When the correct tension and vector are set, the muscle is secured to the deep temporal fascia using anchoring sutures is the same fashion as at the commissure.

the muscle or avulsing the pedicle. This hook is prepared by an occupational therapist from thermoplastic material and is sutured to the scalp with silk sutures via an elastic band in such a manner as to stabilize the oral commissure to the temporal region without excessive tension or pressure.

Postoperative Monitoring

Postoperatively, standard free flap precautions are maintained; a warm, well-hydrated, and pain-free patient provides an optimal milieu for the muscle flap. Perioperative prophylactic antibiotics are used, the patient is propped up at 45 degrees, and gentle mobilization is started after the first postoperative day. Mobility is gradually increased, the drain is removed on day 3, and the patient is usually discharged after 5 days. The mouth hook is removed at 10 days, and the patient is advised to avoid caffeine and contact with the operative site for 6 weeks.

There is regular follow-up in the clinic, and by 5 or 6 months, evidence of innervation is usually evident, and a program of strengthening and biofeedback exercises is initiated to improve excursion and control of the muscle. These are carried out in front of a mirror to allow the patient to visually assess the degree of movement and optimize the chance of achieving a symmetrical smile. We advise our patients to practice for 5 minutes two or three times a day to improve strength of contraction, excursion, and symmetry. An example of pre- and postoperative results with a free gracilis transplant and cross-face nerve graft is presented in Figure 40-13.

BILATERAL CASES AND MÖBIUS SYNDROME

The procedure discussed is our standard for reanimation of a unilateral facial palsy, but bilateral facial palsy requires a modified technique because there is no functional facial nerve to share. In the authors' practice, this is most commonly encountered in Möbius syndrome or in patients with brainstem tumors that have been resected. In such instances, an alternate donor nerve such as the hypoglossal or motor nerve to masseter is required. We have found the hypoglossal nerve unsatisfactory because the power generated with an end-to-side neurorrhaphy is insufficient to drive muscle transplants. Additionally, in patients with cranial nerve palsies affecting the lower cranial nerves, the sacrifice of the hypoglossal nerve may lead to worsening of speech. We therefore prefer to use the motor nerve to masseter to innervate the muscle transplants (Figure 40-14). This nerve runs anteriorly and inferiorly on the deep surface of the masseter muscle and can be identified with the help of a nerve stimulator at a point 1 cm below the zygomatic arch and 3 cm anterior to the tragus. A short transverse incision is made just below the zygomatic arch to reach the masseter, and then a muscle-splitting approach can be used to find and follow the course of the nerve. When it begins to branch, the nerve can be divided and reflected up into the operative field. Being a purely motor nerve, it provides powerful innervation to the muscle transplant with the additional benefit that the nerve to gracilis may be shortened, thereby reducing the time taken for reinnervation to 2 to 3 months. For bilateral reconstructions, we perform each muscle transplant as a separate procedure at least 3 months apart. In this way, we are able to assess the location and vector of the smile and try to match this on the contralateral side. Figure 40-15 shows the result of bilateral smile reconstruction using motor nerve to masseter, demonstrating the great excursion produced by this powerful nerve and the independent activity of the two sides.

SECONDARY SURGERY

Successful muscle transfer achieves spontaneous dynamic smile in one or two procedures, but revisionary surgery is often palliative rather than curative. A number of issues can lead to patients requesting further procedures, the most common of which is the increased facial bulk on the operated side. As described earlier, segmental muscle transfer, removal of the buccal fat pad, and thinning of the facelift flap can all minimize the appearance of fullness to the cheek. Nonetheless, patients may request further recontouring of the face. This is a difficult problem, necessitating dissection in a scarred environment with the risk of damage to the pedicle and innervation of the flap. When the muscle is exposed, shaving of the surface of the muscle can be performed with a blade. Because the pedicle and nerve supply to the flap lie on the deep surface, this is the safest option.

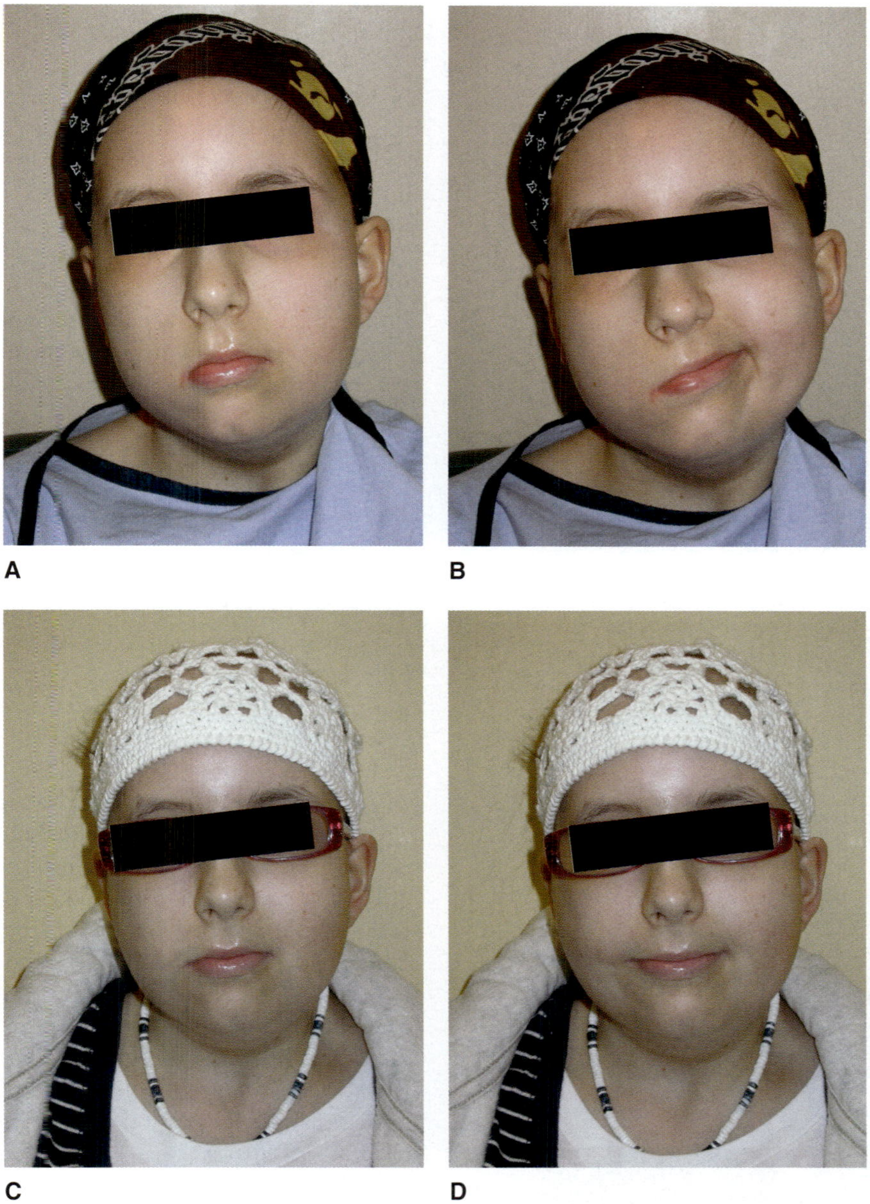

FIGURE 40-13 Results of reconstruction with gracilis muscle transplant and cross-face nerve graft. This young woman had a medulloblastoma removed at age 15 years with subsequent right facial nerve palsy. Reconstruction was performed 2 years after resection. Preoperative photographs at rest (**A**) and smiling (**B**). Postoperative photographs at rest (**C**) and smiling (**D**).

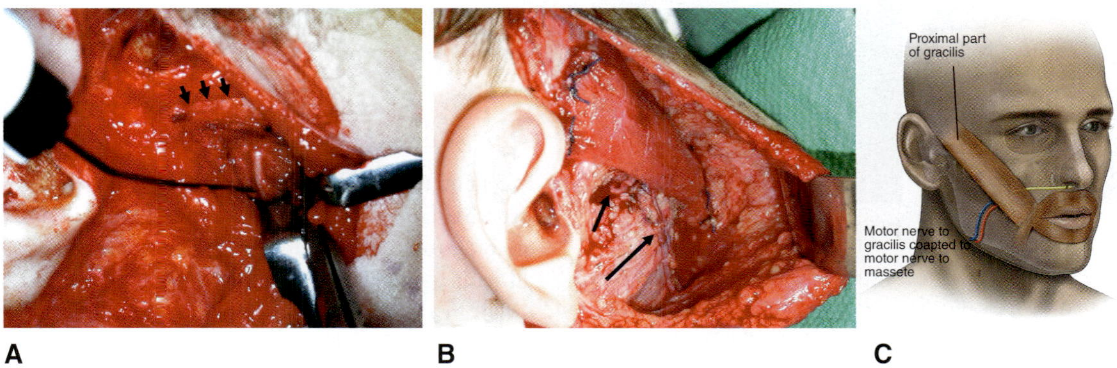

FIGURE 40-14 Inset of the flap when using the motor nerve to masseter. **A.** The nerve runs anteriorly and inferiorly on the deep surface of the masseter muscle. The muscle fibers of the masseter are split, and with the help of a nerve stimulator, the motor nerve is found approximately 3 cm in front of the tragus and 1 cm below the zygomatic arch. The stimulator is pointing at the nerve, and arrows delineate the upper border of the zygomatic arch. (**B**) Intraoperative photograph demonstrating the vector of the muscle and the anchoring sutures at either end. The motor nerve to masseter is sitting at the inferior border of the muscle flap (short black arrow), and the vessels are situated more anteriorly where the anastomosis is performed (long black arrow). (**C**) Diagrammatic representation of the orientation of the muscle flap and the scheme of anastomosis and neurorrhaphy.

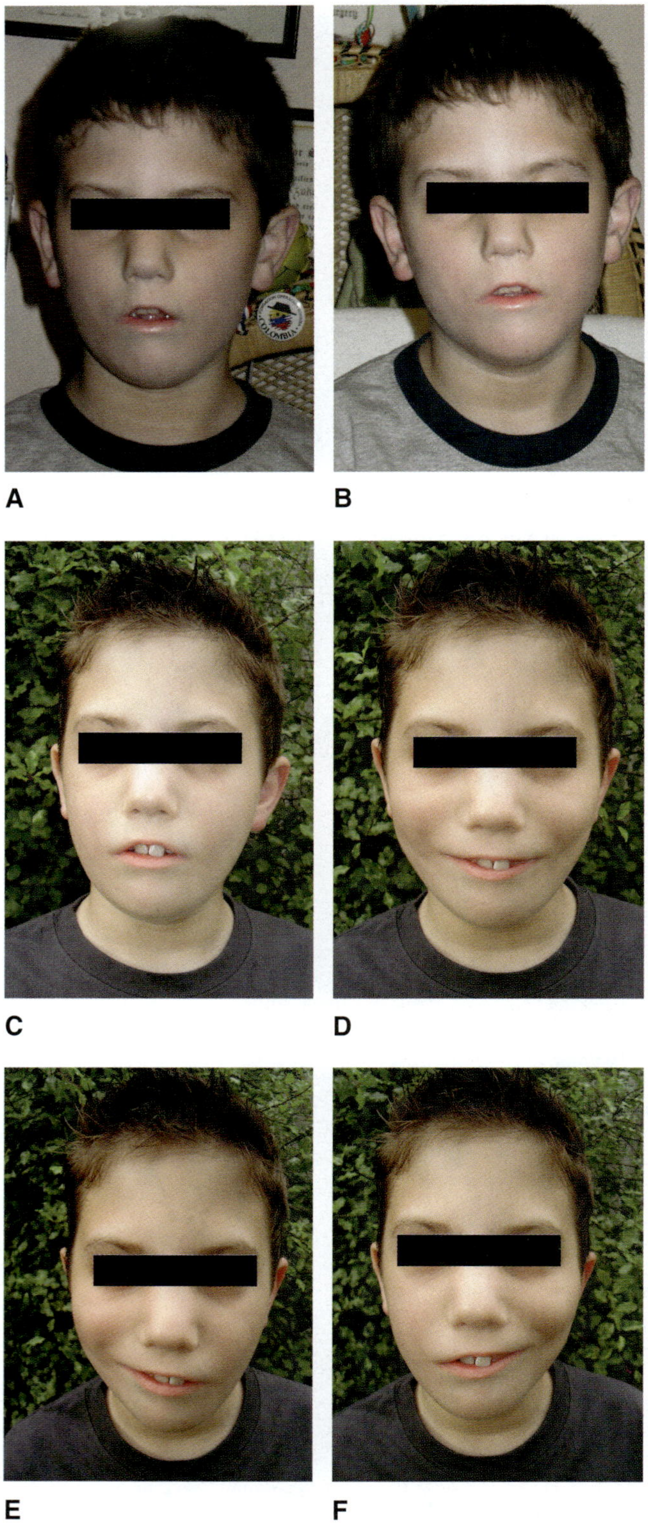

FIGURE 40-15 Bilateral smile reconstruction for Möbius syndrome using motor nerve to masseter. Preoperative photographs at rest (A) and attempted smile (B). Postoperative photographs at rest (C) and bilateral smile (D). Right (E) and left (F) smiles are independent and demonstrate a good excursion (compare with Figure 40-13).

Free muscle transplantation has an intrinsic problem: a single muscle with only one vector is used to replicate the action of numerous smaller muscles that act in different directions. Thus, the planning and positioning of the muscle is extremely important. Failure of planning may easily lead to asymmetry of smile, and moreover, displacement or detachment of the muscle flap can lead to ineffective contractions. In such scenarios, there may be an indication to reexplore the reconstruction, which may be a hazardous endeavor, and all the more reason to take great care securing the muscle flap definitively during the primary procedure. If the muscle is too tight, it may be released from its origin and allowed to slide toward the mouth. If poor excursion is an issue, there are few options. Open reinsertion can be performed, or the commissure may be reconnected to the muscle by tendon grafts, but this may leave the commissure tight or distorted. When an attempt is made to reposition the flap, the amount of excursion is often reduced, and the likelihood of successfully recreating true symmetry is low. Others have suggested using the temporalis regional transfer to "patch" the reconstruction (45).

It may be necessary to repeat the muscle transplantation, and if the cause of failure is not clear, it may be wise to use an alternate nerve to power the transplant (e.g., using the motor nerve to masseter after a failed cross-face nerve graft). The risks of revision transplantation are higher because the procedure is performed in a scarred bed reusing the previous recipient vessels. However, it may be useful in selected patients. Whatever the proposed procedure, a frank and open discussion with the patient is advisable to manage expectations.

After cross-facial nerve grafting, or nerve transfer to a distal facial nerve stump, synkinesis may occur; for example, the patient may involuntarily close the eyelids when smiling. This is due to regenerating axons reaching unintended targets and can be effectively reduced with injection of botulinum toxin (Botox; Allergan, Irvine, CA) into the appropriate muscle. In a similar fashion, asymmetry at rest or during smile, most commonly caused by paralysis of the depressor anguli oris, can be treated with Botox to the contralateral active muscle to achieve symmetry. Such strategies are temporary but have the advantage that if the results are unacceptable, an irreversible change will not have been produced.

RESULTS AND OUTCOMES

Excellent results have been achieved with the current reconstructive toolbox (Figures 40-16 and 40-17), but we still are unable to achieve a perfect smile. For example, it is particularly difficult to achieve a natural-looking superior part to the nasolabial crease. On the other hand, commissure excursion has been improved with experience by optimizing fixation, muscle length, and tension to gain maximal force of contraction. A number of studies have shown superior outcomes for smile reconstruction by free muscle transfer, but it has been found that a greater number of secondary procedures may be needed to achieve such good results. Nonetheless, such secondary surgery significantly improved outcomes that were rated better by independent observers (46).

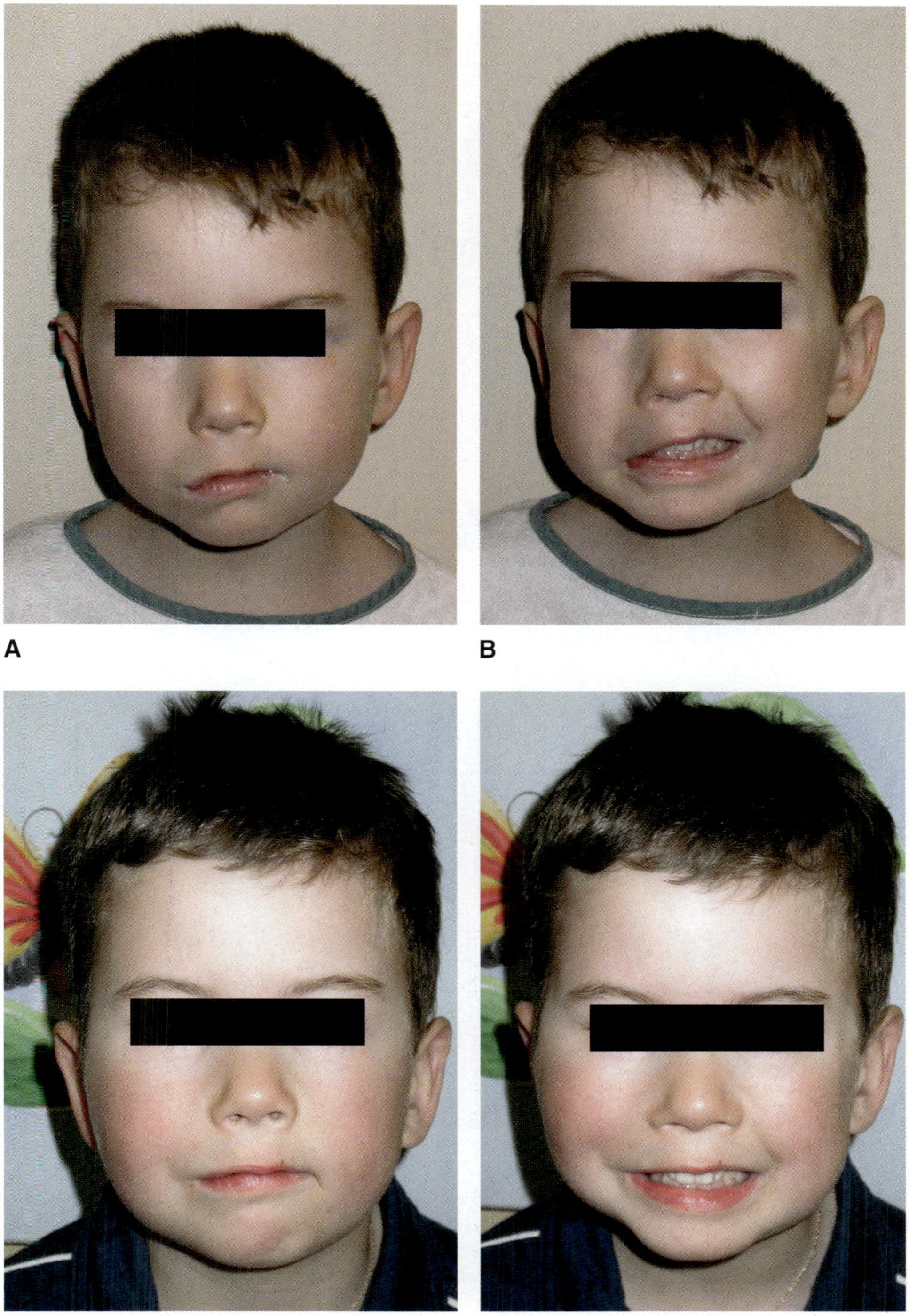

FIGURE 40-16 Smile reconstruction for unilateral Möbius syndrome. Preoperative photographs at rest (A) and attempted smile (B). Postoperative photographs at rest (C) and smiling (D).

A number of free muscle transplant and motor nerve combinations have been used, but there is little literature that directly compares different reconstructive methods. For example, no study published directly compares pectoralis minor and gracilis muscle transplants, but a comparison of cross-facial nerve grafting with motor nerve with masseter transfer has been performed (20). A cross-face nerve graft with mini-gracilis transfer was shown to achieve 50% of the excursion of the unaffected side with excellent resting tone and a pleasing smile that is totally spontaneous. On the other hand, the use of the motor nerve to masseter achieved an excursion within 2 mm of the normal side and was especially effective for addressing lower lip incompetence and improving bilabial plosive production. Forty-five muscle transfers in 27 adult patients were analyzed, and it was determined that muscle weight was a factor in muscle excursion (13). The greater excursion may also be due to the fact that the masseter is much larger than the muscles of facial expression, and the

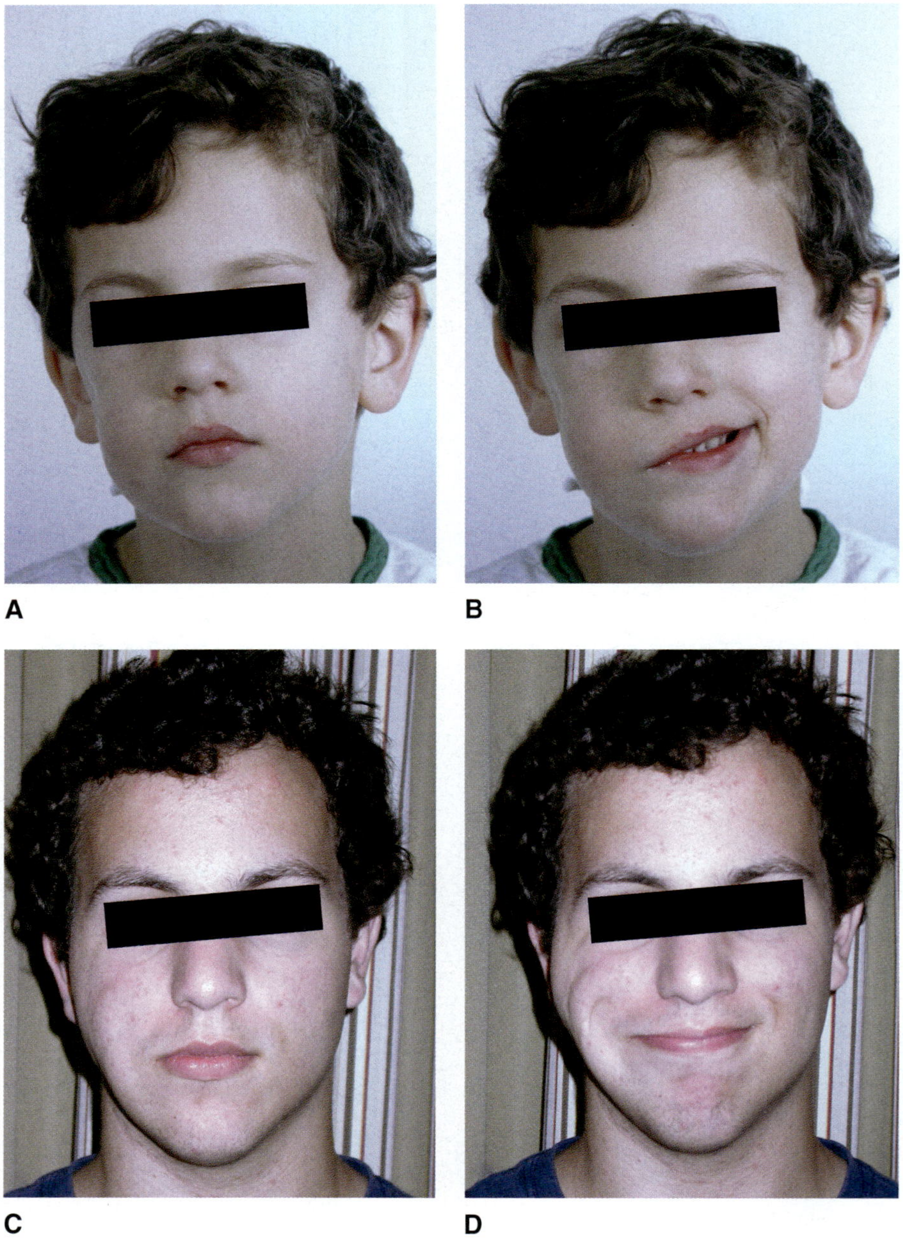

FIGURE 40-17 Smile reconstruction of right unilateral facial palsy. This boy had a rhabdomyosarcoma of the right cheek resected at age 2 years with necessary sacrifice of the facial nerve. He presented at age 6 for reconstruction, which required a free muscle transplant. To achieve a symmetrical smile, a cross-face nerve graft was used to power the muscle from the contralateral facial nerve. Preoperative photographs at rest (**A**) and attempted smile (**B**). Postoperative photographs taken at age 16 years at rest (**C**) and smiling (**D**).

innervation to this may be a more powerful stimulus than branches of the facial nerve. It is likely that fewer motor fibers reach the muscle along a cross-face nerve graft compared with the number of motor fibers in the nerve to masseter. This could be the reason for reduced excursion. However, the greater excursion when the masseter nerve was used was achieved at the expense of total spontaneity because activation of the masseteric nerve requires a biting action. In the review, it was thought that spontaneity more than made up for reduced excursion.

Although activation of the masseteric nerve requires biting, Manktelow et al. (13) demonstrated that more than 50% of patients demonstrated a cortical plasticity that resulted in a spontaneous smile. Most interestingly, a questionnaire found that 85% had learned to smile without biting, and 89% of patients reported the ability to produce a spontaneous smile; this occurred most or all of the time in 37%. Cortical plasticity is thought to be responsible, and although the exact mechanism remains to be elucidated, it is suggested that cortical connections form between the biting and smiling areas, permitting a spontaneous smile. A key determinant of success was the use of biofeedback exercises in which visual feedback reinforces the learning process. Neurosurgical dogma holds that older individuals are less likely to be successful in cortical reorganization. It is suggested that advanced age renders the patient incapable of cortical plasticity and that less complex strategies should therefore be used in this population. However, age was not found to limit the development of a spontaneous smile in this study. Notably, children were found to be able to undergo such cortical reorganization even when they did not comply with their biofeedback exercises (47,48). In this series of 32 children, pectoralis minor or gracilis free muscle transfer was associated with good outcomes that continued to improve years after the primary surgery as determined by independent observer-rated scales and electromyographic (EMG) analysis. Similarly, in adults the long-term outcomes of smile reconstruction were better more than 2 years after reconstruction demonstrated by increased motor unit recruitment on EMG (49). This is in keeping with the authors' experience as well.

When considering these reported outcomes and selecting a recipient nerve, it is important to ascertain from the patient what his or her reconstructive goals are. If the patient is very keen to achieve spontaneous smile and is willing to undergo two procedures, then a cross-face nerve graft and free muscle transfer is a good option. In contrast, if the patient requires a more powerful smile, is not demanding of spontaneity, and would like a single procedure, then reinnervation by the masseteric nerve may be more appropriate.

CONCLUSIONS

Facial palsy inflicts major morbidity, and reconstruction is aimed at addressing functional, aesthetic, and psychological issues. The reconstructions are static or dynamic with free muscle transfer able to provide a true facial reanimation. Careful assessment of the deficit and the needs of the patient are required to plan a cohesive reconstructive strategy. A number of critical points need to be considered when performing free muscle transfer: The innervation for the transplant should be chosen with care by meticulous nerve mapping of the contralateral facial nerve, or if this is unavailable, a powerful motor such as the ipsilateral masseteric nerve should be used. The bulk of the muscle transfer should be minimized; we use segmental transfer of the gracilis together with buccal fat pad excision and facelift flap defatting to address this. Positioning of the sutures at the commissure has a direct impact on the subsequent aesthetic result, and great attentiveness to detail at this stage is a vital part of the procedure. Similarly, the vector of muscle placement determines the type of smile the patient will possess, and accurate preoperative planning with precise inset can achieve excellent results. Complications comprise excess bulk, muscle malposition, and excess or inadequate movement. These are extremely difficult to correct and can be avoided with forethought and meticulous technique.

REFERENCES

1. Westin LM, Zuker RM. A new classification system for facial paralysis in the clinical setting. *J Craniofac Surg* 2003;14:672.
2. Falco NA, Eriksson E. Facial nerve palsy in the newborn: incidence and outcome. *Plast Reconstr Surg* 1990;85:1.
3. Zuker RM, Manktelow RT. A smile for the Möbius syndrome patient. *Ann Plast Surg* 1989;22:188.
4. Paletz JL, Manktelow RT, Chaban R. The shape of a normal smile: implications for facial paralysis reconstruction. *Plast Reconstr Surg* 1994;93:784.
5. Guerrissi JO. Selective myotomy for post paretic facial synkinesis. *Plast Reconstr Surg* 1991;87:459.
6. Neely JG. Computerized quantitative dynamic analysis of facial motion in the paralyzed and synkinetic face. *Am J Otol* 1992;13:97.
7. Horlock N, Sanders R, Harrison DH. The SOOF lift: its role in correcting lower facial asymmetry in patients with partial facial palsy. *Plast Reconstr Surg* 2002;109:839.
8. Gillies H. Experiences with fascia lata grafts in the operative treatment of facial paralysis. *Proc R Soc Med* 1934;27:1372.
9. Baker DC, Conley J. Regional muscle transposition for rehabilitation of the paralyzed face. *Clin Plast Surg* 1979;6:317.
10. McLaughlin CR. Surgical support in permanent facial paralysis. *Plast Reconstr Surg* 1953;11:302.
11. Labbé D, Huault M. Lengthening temporalis myoplasty and lip reanimation. *Plast Reconstr Surg* 2000;105:1289.
12. Terzis JK, Kalantarian B. Microsurgical strategies in 74 patients for restoration of dynamic depressor muscle mechanism: a neglected target in facial reanimation. *Plast Reconstr Surg* 2000;105:1917.
13. Manktelow RT, Tomat LR, Zuker RM, et al. Smile reconstruction in adults with free muscle transfer innervated by the masseter motor nerve: effectiveness and cerebral adaptation. *Plast Reconstr Surg* 2006;118:885.
14. MacQuillan A, Grobbelaar A. Functional muscle transfer and the variance of reinnervating axonal load: part I. The facial nerve. *Plast Reconstr Surg* 2008;121:1570.
15. Anderl H. Reconstruction of the face through cross-face nerve transplantation in facial paralysis. *Eur J Plast Surg* 1973;2:17.
16. Fisch U. Facial nerve grafting. *Otolaryngol Clin North Am* 1974;7:517.
17. Scaramella LF. Anastomosis between two facial nerves. *Laryngoscope* 1975; 85:1359.
18. Terzis JK, Tzafetta K. The "babysitter" procedure: minihypoglossal to facial nerve transfer and cross-facial nerve grafting. *Plast Reconstr Surg* 2009;123:865.
19. Zuker RM, Goldberg CS, Manktelow RT. Facial animation in children with Möbius syndrome after segmental gracilis muscle transplant. *Plast Reconstr Surg* 2000;106:1.
20. Bae YC, Zuker RM, Manktelow RT, Wade S. A comparison of commissure excursion following gracilis muscle transplantation for facial paralysis using a cross face nerve graft versus the motor nerve to masseter. *Plast Reconstr Surg* 2006;117:2407.
21. Thompson N. Autogenous free grafts of skeletal muscle. A preliminary experimental and clinical study. *Plast Reconstr Surg* 1971;48:11.
22. Tamai S, Komatsu S, Sakamoto H, et al. Free muscle transplants in dogs with microsurgical neurovascular anastomoses. *Plast Reconstr Surg* 1970;46:219.
23. Harrii K, Ohmori K, Torii D. Free gracilis muscle transplantation, with microneurovascular anastomosis for the treatment of facial paralysis. *Br J Plast Surg* 1980;33:202.
24. Mackinnon SE, Dellon AL. Technical considerations of the latissimus dorsi muscle flap: a segmentally innervated muscle transfer for reanimation. *Microsurgery* 1988;9:36.
25. Harrison DH. The pectoralis minor vascularised muscle graft for the treatment of unilateral facial palsy. *Plast Reconstr Surg* 1985;75:206.
26. O'Brien BM. *Microvascular Reconstructive Surgery*. London: Churchill Livingstone, 1977.
27. Mayou BJ, Watson SJ, Harrison DH, et al. Free microvascular and microneural transfer of the extensor digitorum brevis muscle for the treatment of unilateral facial palsy. *Br J Plast Surg* 1981;34:362.
28. O'Brien BM, Franklin JD, Morrison WA. Cross-face nerve grafts and microneural free muscle transfer for long established facial palsy. *Br J Plast Surg* 1980;33:202.
29. Woolard ACS, Harrison DH, Grobbelaar AO. An approach to bilateral facial paralysis. *J Plast Aesthet Reconstr Surg* 2010;63:1557.
30. Manktelow RT. The pectoralis minor vascularised muscle graft for the treatment of unilateral facial palsy. Discussion. *Plast Reconstr Surg* 1985;75:214.
31. MacQuillan A, Horlock N, Grobbelaar A, et al. Arterial and venous anatomical features of the pectoralis minor muscle flap pedicle. *Plast Reconstr Surg* 2004;113:872.
32. Manktelow RT, Zuker RM. Muscle transplantation by fascicular territory. *Plast Reconstr Surg* 1984;73:751.
33. Accioli de Vasconcellos JJ, Britto JA, et al. The fascial planes of the temple and face; an en bloc anatomical study and a plea for consistency. *Br J Plast Surg* 2003;56:623.
34. Mitz V, Peyronie M. The superficial musculoaponeurotic system (SMAS) in the parotid and cheek area. *Plast Reconstr Surg* 1976;58:80.

35. Davis RA, Anson BJ, Budinger JM, et al. Surgical anatomy of the facial nerve and parotid gland based upon a study of 350 cervico-facial halves. *Surg Gynaecol* 1956;102:385.
36. Nelson DW, Gingrass RP. Anatomy of the mandibular branches of the facial nerve. *Plast Reconstr Surg* 1979;64:479.
37. Moss CJ, Mendelson BC, Taylor GI. Surgical anatomy of the ligamentous attachments in the temple and periorbital regions. *Plast Reconstr Surg* 2000;105:1475.
38. Knize DM. An anatomically based study of the mechanism of eyebrow ptosis. *Plast Reconstr Surg* 1996;97:1321.
39. Muzzaffar AR, Mendelson BC, Adams WP Jr. Surgical anatomy of the ligamentous attachments of the lower lid and lateral canthus. *Plast Reconstr Surg* 2002;110:873.
40. Freilinger G, Gruber H, Happak W, et al. Surgical anatomy of the mimic muscle system and the facial nerve: importance for reconstructive and aesthetic surgery. *Plast Reconstr Surg* 1987;80:686.
41. Nicolau PJ. The orbicularis oris muscle: a functional approach to its repair in the cleft lip. *Br J Plast Surg* 1983;36:141.
42. Rubin LR. The anatomy of a smile: its importance in the treatment of facial paralysis. *Plast Reconstr Surg* 1974;53:384.
43. Frey M, Giovanoli P, Gerber H, et al. Three-dimensional video analysis of facial movements: a new method to assess the quantity and quality of the smile. *Plast Reconstr Surg* 1999;104:2302.
44. Ortiguela ME, Wood MB, Cahill DR. Anatomy of the sural nerve complex. *J Hand Surg Am* 1987;12:1119.
45. Terzis JK, Olivares FS. Mini-temporalis transfer as an adjunct procedure for smile restoration. *Plast Reconstr Surg* 2009;123:533.
46. Terzis JK, Olivares FS. Secondary surgery in adult facial paralysis reanimation. *Plast Reconstr Surg* 2009;124:1916.
47. Lifchez SD, Matloub HS, Gosain AK. Cortical adaptation to restoration of smiling after free muscle transfer innervated by the nerve to masseter. *Plast Reconstr Surg* 2005;115:1472.
48. Terzis JK, Olivares FS. Long-term outcomes of free-muscle transfer for smile restoration in children. *Plast Reconstr Surg* 2009;123:543.
49. Terzis JK, Olivares FS. Long-term outcomes of free-muscle transfer for smile restoration in adults. *Plast Reconstr Surg* 2009;123:877.

CHAPTER 41

Face Transplantation

Maria Siemionow and Can Ozturk

The human face has a complex functional structure that includes not only four of the five main sensorial organs of the body (ears, eyes, nose, and tongue) but also essential properties for personal identity and social interaction. Until recently, the functional and aesthetic outcomes after reconstruction of complex composite facial defects have been generally less than optimal because of the unique characteristics of facial structures, such as texture, contour, and an individual anatomical configuration that cannot be reproduced by conventional reconstructive options.

Such options include primary closure, skin grafting, local flaps, tissue prelamination or prefabrication, distant flaps, tissue expansion, and free tissue transfers (1–6). Primary closure and local flaps are ideal surgical methods with good functional and aesthetic outcomes in mild to moderate defects without extensive tissue loss. Skin grafting is the preferred reconstruction method of moderate size skin defects after burns. However, poor color match, secondary deformities caused by graft contracture, and applicability to surface defects only limit its indications to selected cases. Tissue prelamination and prefabrication are used for the reconstruction of complex, unique, partial facial defects such as nasal tip or eye socket defects. Tissue expansion is an ideal reconstruction method for moderate to large skin defects with good aesthetic and functional outcomes as long as there is enough normal facial skin adjacent to the defect to expand. The preferred method for reconstruction of moderate to large complex skin, soft tissue, mucosa, and bone defects is single or combined free flaps, which include anterolateral thigh (ALT), radial forearm, groin, scapular, parascapular, latissimus dorsi, serratus anterior, rectus abdominis, gracilis, fibula, and iliac crest flaps. Finally, for a selective group of trauma patients, replantation of the missing parts or tissues provides the best functional and aesthetic outcome. If these conventional reconstructive options fail or do poorly, then facial allotransplantation may be considered as the last option for facial reconstruction.

In November 2004, the senior author (MS) was granted the world's first institutional review board (IRB) approval for human face transplantation (7). One year later, on November 27, 2005, French surgeons Devauchelle and Dubernard performed the first partial facial composite tissue allotransplantation (CTA) in Amiens, France (8). Thus, face transplantation became a clinical reality as a new reconstructive option for severely disfigured patients. To date, 13 partial and total facial CTAs have been performed worldwide, including in France (7), Spain (3), the United States (2), and China (1) (7–18). However, even though face transplantation presents a unique reconstructive option for patients with extensive and complex facial defects, it is still considered experimental because long-term outcomes need to be studied before it will be considered standard of care. In this chapter, we summarize our current knowledge and experience with human face transplantation.

INDICATIONS

Patients with severe facial disfigurement, including congenital and acquired deformities and diseases, are potential candidates for face transplantation. The indications include trauma (e.g., animal attacks, electrical or fall injuries, explosions, ballistic injuries, and burns), tumor resections, and congenital deformities. Traumatic facial injury was the main indication for clinical facial CTA in eight of 13 (61%) patients, with five of these being shotgun blast injuries, two animal attacks, and one injury from a fall (7–9,11–13,18). The other indications were congenital deformities: neurofibromatosis in three of 13 (23%) patients, burn injuries in one of 13 (8%) patients, and acquired facial deformity after cancer treatment in one of 13 (8%) patients (10,14–17). The male-to-female ratio of facial CTA was 11 to 2, and all donors were gender matched. Whereas osteomyocutaneous components were included in eight of the 13 facial allotransplantations, the other five were myocutaneous allografts. As of November 2010, two patients—one from

China, the other from France—have died, at 2 years and at 2 months after surgery, respectively, because of transplant-related complications (14,19). Currently, the overall survival rate is 11 of 13 (85%).

INSTITUTIONAL REVIEW BOARD PROTOCOL

The world's first IRB protocol approval, for face transplantation, was granted to the Cleveland Clinic in 2004 (7). Based on our experience, obtaining IRB approval is a complicated and detailed process. In the facial transplantation literature, there are few publications explaining the optimal sequence and steps for developing an IRB-approved face transplant protocol (20,21).

In their articles, Siemionow and Gordon have described recommendations for developing an IRB protocol and approval process (20,21). The first step is establishing a facial transplant team consisting of reconstructive microsurgeons, transplant surgeons, infectious disease specialists, immunologists, psychiatrists, social workers, and media coordinators. Requirements for a face transplantation program include obtaining IRB approval, appropriate funding, organ procurement organization (OPO) approval, patient recruitment, informed consent, optimal donor–recipient matching, outlining face transplantation procedure, graft surveillance protocol, physical rehabilitation, and functional assessment. The facial transplant protocol that should be submitted to the IRB includes details of the three main phases of face transplantation (pretransplant, peritransplant and posttransplant); the donor and recipient consent forms; and the scientific descriptions of experimental, cadaver, and clinical studies. The team leader often participates in meetings with IRB members explaining protocol and answering questions. Based on these meetings, revisions and amendments to the protocol are made. Obtaining initial IRB approval for face transplantation took us about 2 years; however, now that more face transplants have been performed, and many institutions have IRB-approved protocols for both hand and other CTAs, the approval process should be expedited for those seeking it (20,21).

PROCUREMENT OF THE DONOR FACE

Facial allograft procurement from a donor face is a race against time. Because of the unstable metabolic and hemodynamic condition of the donor, excessive blood loss or a delay in timing of the procedure can cause failure to recover the essential solid organs (e.g., kidney, liver, heart), which would be ethically unacceptable. To prevent this, training of face transplant team members using cadaver models and performing facial allograft procurement based on the patient's facial defect in a series of mock transplantations helps in orchestrating the timing, sequence and role of each team member. Mock transplantation not only helps minimize surgical mistakes, but also facilitates close cooperation between surgical team members before the procurement procedure is carried out for real.

The different types of face transplantations include partial, near-total, and total face transplants (Figure 41-9). Partial face transplantation is divided into upper, middle, and lower face, but it may combine one or more of these anatomic regions (Figures 41-1 to 41-6, and 41-9). The allograft may include skin, subcutaneous tissue, muscle, or bone in any combination. The missing parts or subunits of facial tissue will differ in each patient. Thus, the anatomic and technical idiosyncrasies have to be considered in each case, as discussed in published experimental and cadaver studies (22–30).

General Principles of Facial Allograft Procurement

Most of the donors are heart-beating, brain-dead, intubated donors; however, in cases where the heart is not beating, more pressure will be put on the transplant team members as they race against ischemia time (9,17). The first step in case of a heart-beating donor is the establishment of donor life support by performing a tracheostomy.

Template Outline

After stabilization of cardiopulmonary functions by the anesthesia team, the skin incision borders are outlined with a colored surgical pen. The precise design of the facial incisions is based on the recipient's requirements. The outline of the defect is transferred to a Silastic sheet, a piece of silence cloth, or a sterile green towel that serves as a reverse template for the surgeon in planning the exact amount of facial tissue to be taken from the donor.

Neck Vessel Dissections

After subcutaneous infiltration of saline solution with 0.5% lidocaine and 1/200 epinephrine, the skin incision begins around the outlined template. However, if the template does not cover the neck region, it is strongly recommended to extend the skin incision over the neck to facilitate dissection of the vascular pedicles. Soft tissue dissection of the facial flap is performed in the subplatysmal plane over the neck and continues in a caudal to cranial direction to expose the major vascular arterial and venous pedicles and their branches. The external carotid artery and its branches (superficial temporal, facial, and maxillary arteries); the internal, external, and anterior jugular veins; the thyro-linguo-facial trunks; and the concomitant veins of the arteries are identified and tagged using vessel loops in the region lying between the cricoid cartilage, the angle of the mandible, and the base of the skull. However, it may be necessary to extend the vessel dissections more proximally as far as the bifurcation of the common carotid and subclavian arteries to create long vascular pedicles.

Nerve Dissections

The great auricular and lesser occipital nerves are both transected on the lateral edges of sternocleidomastoid (SCM) muscles and are incorporated into the graft. The facial nerve trunks are located by bilateral standard parotidectomy approaches and are identified at their exit from the stylomastoid foramen. The dissection of the nerves continues distally between the superficial and deep parotid lobes, where the individual branches can be identified and elevated with the flap.

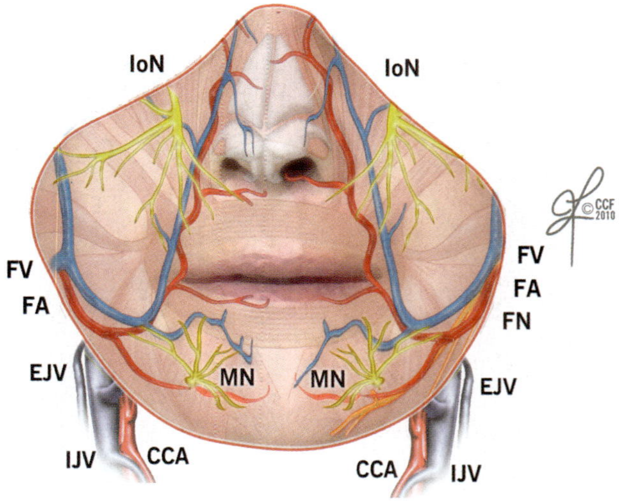

FIGURE 41-1 Partial middle and lower face transplant including myocutaneous components based on the first French facial transplant patient. (For details, see Table 41-3, patient 1.) CCA, common carotid artery; EJV, external jugular vein; EMA, external maxillary artery; FA, facial artery; FV, facial vein; FN, facial nerve; IJV, internal jugular vein; IaN, inferior alveolar nerve; IoN, infraorbital nerve; LN, lingual nerve; MN, mental nerve; SoN, supraorbital nerve. (Reprinted with permission, Cleveland Clinic Center for Medical Art & Photography © 2009-2010. All Rights Reserved.)

Special care is taken to identify and preserve the marginal mandibular branch, which passes just below the angle of the mandible. Anterior to the parotid along the mandibular border, the dissection changes to a subperiosteal plane so as to identify the mental nerve exiting the mandible from the mental foramen. A sagittal split mandibular osteotomy should be performed if greater nerve length (mental plus inferior alveolar nerve) is required (22). Alternatively, the canal can be drilled out for the same purpose. If required, the hypoglossal and the lingual nerves may also be included in the transplant if the tongue or anterior floor of the mouth is part of the donor tissue. The supraorbital, supratrochlear, and infraorbital branches of trigeminal nerves are identified at the supraorbital and infraorbital foramina. Osteotomies are performed if necessary to release the nerves from the orbital rims and facilitate their proximal dissection.

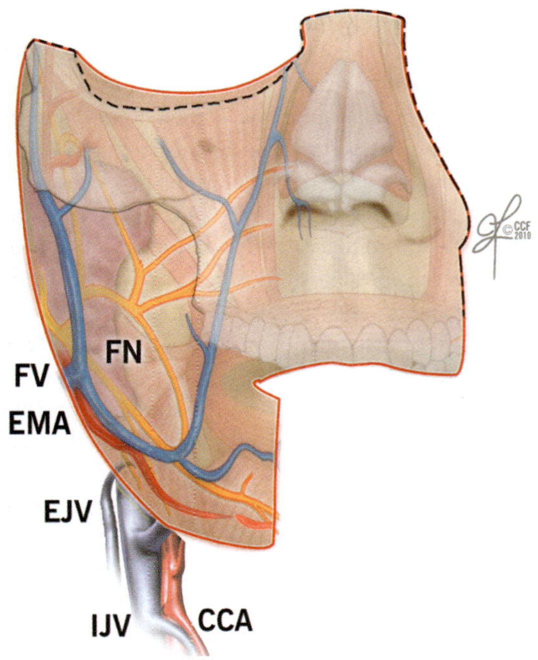

FIGURE 41-2 Partial midface transplant including osteomyocutaneous components based on the Chinese facial transplant patient. (For details, see Table 43, patient 2. See Figure 41-1 for abbreviations.) (Reprinted with permission, Cleveland Clinic Center for Medical Art & Photography © 2009-2010. All Rights Reserved.)

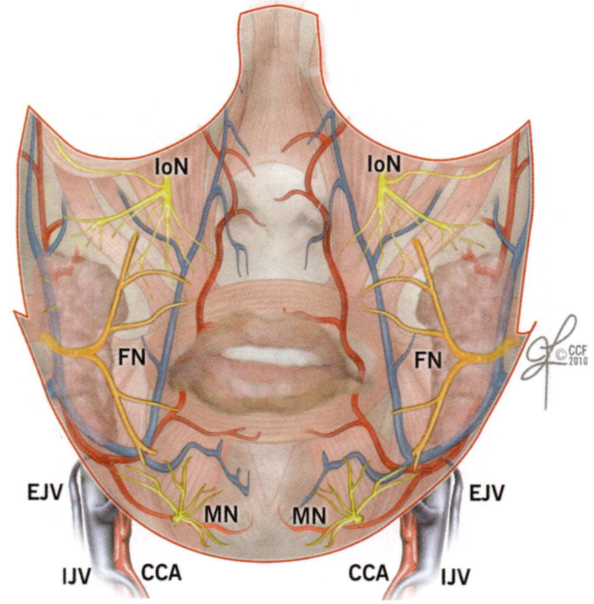

FIGURE 41-3 Partial middle and lower facial transplant including myocutaneous components based on the second French facial transplant patient. (For details, see Table 41-3, patient 3. See Figure 41-1 for abbreviations.) (Reprinted with permission, Cleveland Clinic Center for Medical Art & Photography © 2009-2010. All Rights Reserved.)

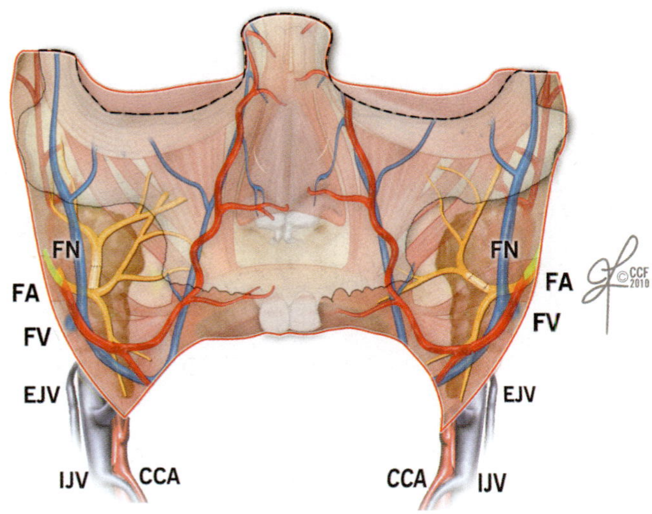

FIGURE 41-4 Near-total facial transplant including osteomyocutaneous components based on the first American facial transplant patient. (For details, see Table 41-3, Patient 4. See Figure 41-1 for abbreviations.) (Reprinted with permission, Cleveland Clinic Center for Medical Art & Photography © 2009-2010. All Rights Reserved.)

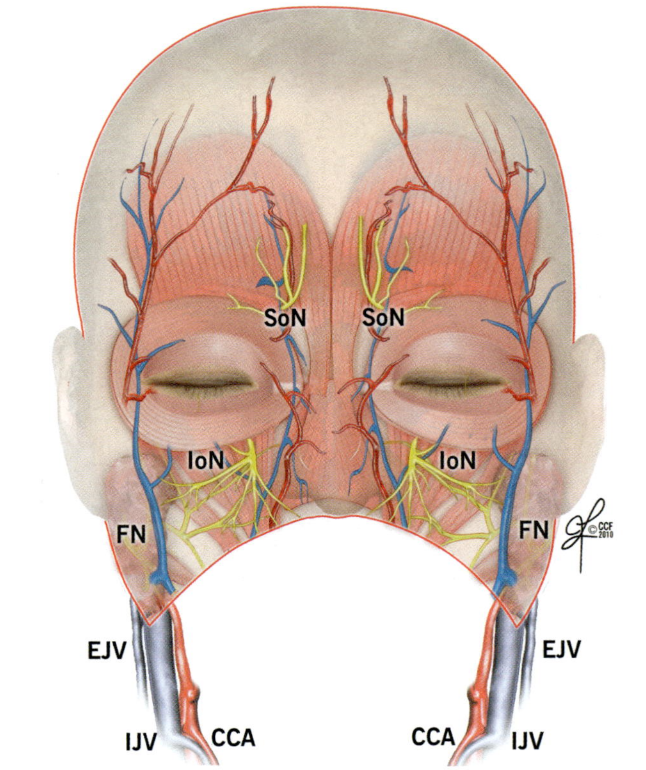

FIGURE 41-5 Partial upper and middle facial transplant including myocutaneous components based on the fourth French facial transplant patient. (For details see, Table 41-3, patient 6. See Figure 41-1 for abbreviations.) (Reprinted with permission, Cleveland Clinic Center for Medical Art & Photography © 2009-2010. All Rights Reserved.)

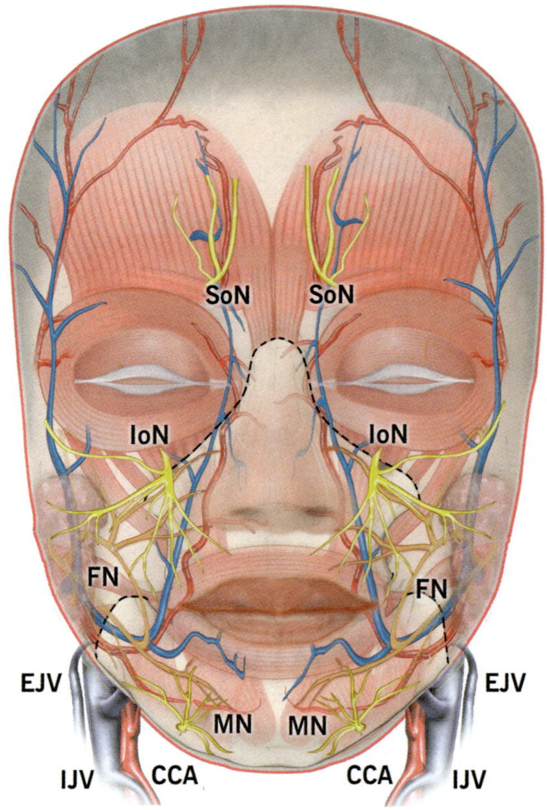

FIGURE 41-7 Total facial transplant including osteomyocutaneous components based on the third Spanish facial transplant patient. (For details, see Table 41-3, patient 12. See Figure 41-1 for abbreviations.) (Reprinted with permission, Cleveland Clinic Center for Medical Art & Photography © 2009-2010. All Rights Reserved.)

Bone Osteotomies

Osteotomies are planned with the aid of a three-dimensional skull model reverse engineered from a fine-cut computed tomography (CT) scan of the recipient's head (computer-aided design and computer-aided manufacturing [CAD-CAM]). The defect itself can be then modeled and will serve as a template for bone harvest. Donor bone is taken using standardized Le Fort bone cuts according to what is needed. If there is a requirement for any part of a facial bone, then that whole bone is taken. Trimming is performed during the actual transfer. Osteotomies may be placed at the zygomatic arch, the lateral orbital rim, the nasofrontal suture, and the pterygomaxillary junctions for a full midface. The superior orbital rim may be included if needed. If the pattern is more similar to a Le Fort II, then the most lateral osteotomies will pass through the inferior orbital rims and the zygomatico-maxillary sutures to free up the central midface.

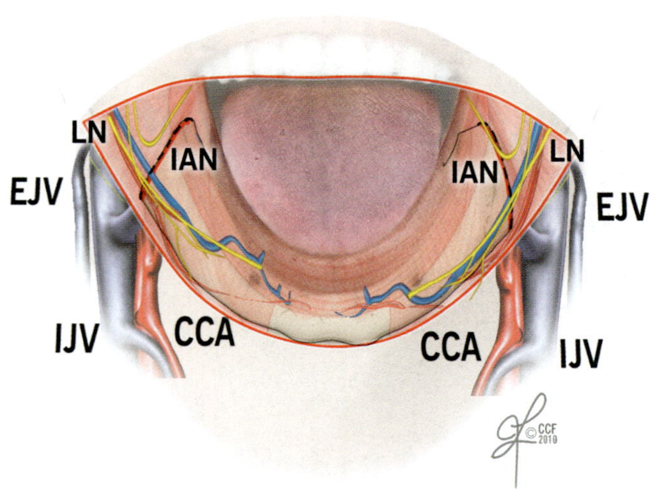

FIGURE 41-6 Partial lower face transplant including osteomyocutaneous components and tongue based on the first Spanish facial transplant patient. (For details, see Table 41-3, patient 9. See Figure 41-1 for abbreviations.) (Reprinted with permission, Cleveland Clinic Center for Medical Art & Photography © 2009-2010. All Rights Reserved.)

Applying downward pressure on the alveolar segment of the maxilla fractures the posterior ethmoids and completes the separation of the maxillofacial bones from the skull base. However, final mobilization of the craniofacial skeleton is only accomplished after transection of the attached muscles, intraoral mucosa, and buccal fat pad.

If required, the entire mandible, complete with articular condyle, is included in the flap without performing osteotomies. The mobilization of the bone is accomplished by transecting the temporalis, both pterygoids, the geniohyoid, mylohyoid, and the digastric muscles. Attachments to the tongue may be maintained if the tongue is to be included and divided if it is not. In the latter case, a lingual mucosal cuff should be tailored to the recipient site. For partial mandible

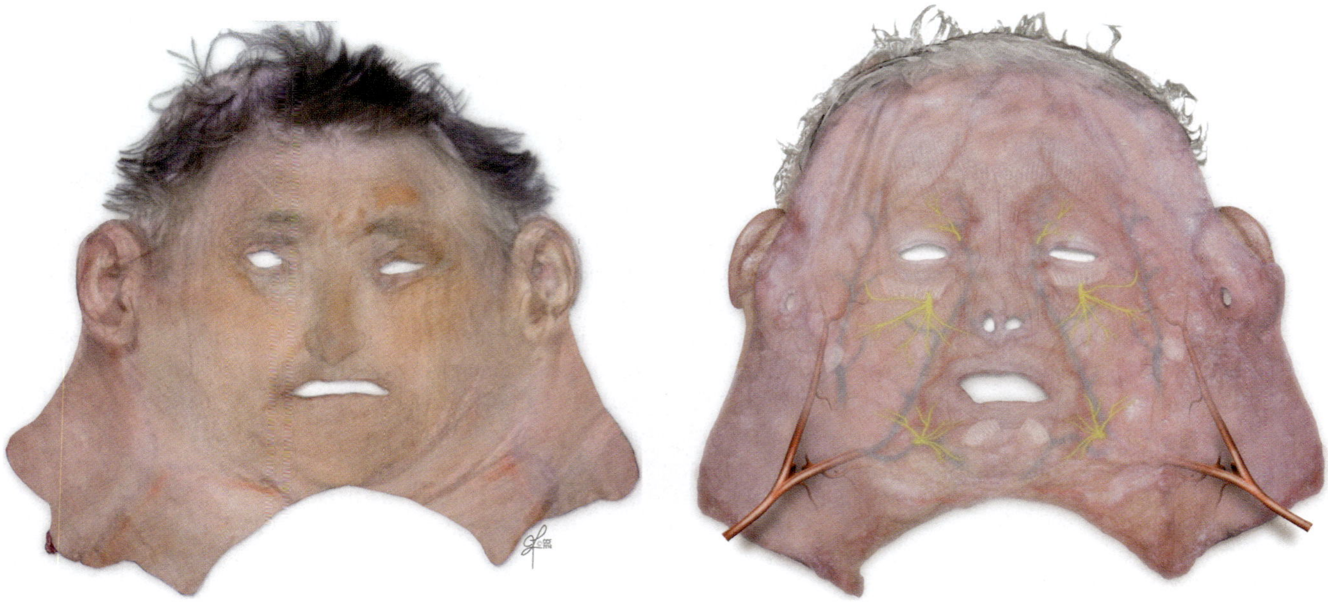

A B

FIGURE 41-8 Anterior (A) and posterior (B) views of a total face and scalp transplant including skin and subcutaneous tissue components based on cadaver studies (25). (Reprinted with permission, Cleveland Clinic Center for Medical Art & Photography © 2009-2010. All Rights Reserved.)

requirements, mandibular osteotomies are performed paying special attention to the preservation of the mental and inferior alveolar nerves.

Facial Allograft Detachment and Transfer

As a final step, detachment of the flap is performed by clamping and transection of the bilateral vascular pedicles. From this point, the ischemia time is recorded. The facial allograft is either not perfused, in the case of a short ischemia time, or when longer periods are anticipated, is perfused by heparinized saline or University of Wisconsin (UW) solution. It is then covered with cold saline–soaked gauze and wrapped in a sterile towel. For transportation, this should be sealed in a watertight plastic bag and placed in a sterile container containing ice.

Principles of Partial Face Transplantation

Upper Face Transplantation (Figure 41-5)

The approach to upper face procurement starts with either a bicoronal or a frontal hairline incision depending on the recipient defect. Dissection continues in the subgaleal plane of the scalp but enters the subperiosteal plane from the frontal region to the level of zygomatic arch, superior orbital rim, and nasofrontal suture. The supraorbital and supratrochlear nerves are isolated at the exit of their foramina (if present), and bone osteotomies may be required to extend the length of the nerves as previously described. After transection of the nerves, subperiosteal dissection extends over the anterior zygoma and periorbital area. The periorbital dissection proceeds over the medial and lateral canthal regions, where the medial and lateral canthal

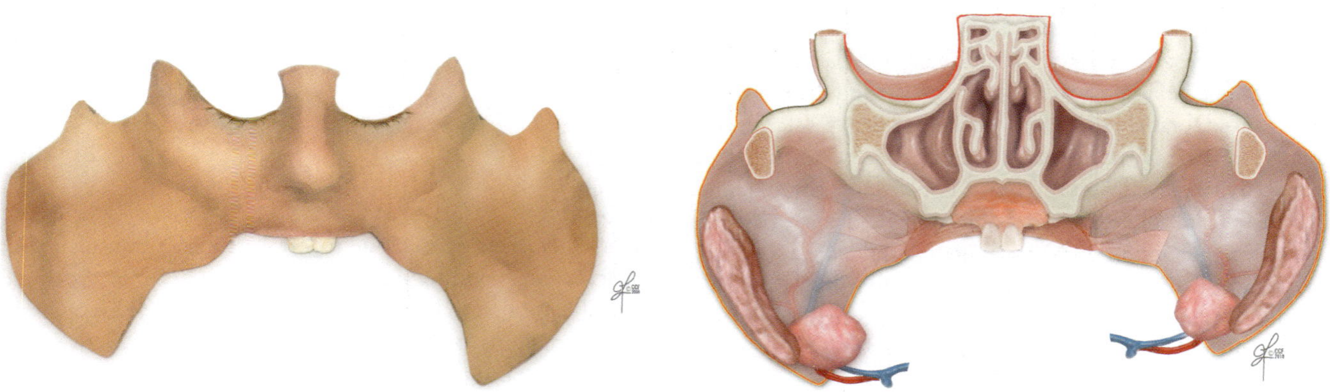

A B

FIGURE 41-9 Anterior (A) and posterior (B) views of recovery of the midface including the Le Fort III midfacial skeleton, zygoma, maxilla with teeth, nasal cartilage, parotid glands, lower eyelids, nose, upper lip, and facial arteries and veins based on the first American facial transplant patient. (For details, see Table 41-3, patient 4.) (Reprinted with permission, Cleveland Clinic Center for Medical Art & Photography © 2009-2010. All Rights Reserved.)

ligaments are tagged by suture. Upper and lower conjunctival incisions are performed circumferentially at the tarsal margins to release the eyelids and incorporate them into the flap. Using this approach, the frontal bones, supraorbital rims, zygomatic bones, lacrimal glands, and lacrimal ducts can be included into the allograft according to the requirements of the recipient.

The next step is the inferior incision, which begins around the anterolateral neck and extends to the angle of the mandible and the preauricular region. The external carotid artery and its branches (superficial temporal, posterior auricular, and facial arteries) are identified and isolated. The internal, external, and anterior jugular veins as well as the thyrolinguofacial trunk are similarly handled.

After completion of upper and lower incisions the entire upper face graft is detached and prepared for transplantation as already described.

Midface Transplantation (Figures 41-1, 41-2, 41-4, and 41-9)

Depending on specifics of the facial defect, different midface transplantation options are available. The "golden triangle" of the nose, upper lip and eyelids or the lower and/or upper lips and chin can be selectively harvested. Grafts can be expanded bilaterally to the temporal hairline and preauricular region creating facial transplant of a much larger surface area. A midface transplantation involving the lower eyelids would start at the temporal hairline, extend horizontally to the lateral canthus, and pass through the depth of the lacrimal sac as far as the medial canthus. The two sides would be linked by an incision across the nasal bridge. This represents the upper border of the skin incision of the midface graft. The inferior incision would be tailored to the defect but, if limited to the midface, would pass from the angle of the mandible—at the lower end of a preauricular incision—to the lateral commissure of the mouth. The dissection, isolation, and transection of the vascular pedicles are as described earlier.

After the vascular dissections are completed low in the neck to obtain maximal pedicle length, a subplatysmal flap is carried superolaterally to identify the parotid glands and link up with the facial nerve dissections, which have essentially split each gland into superficial and deep lobes. The facial nerve is elevated together with the superficial lobe of the parotid, leaving the deep lobe behind, the nerve ultimately being divided at the stylomastoid foramen as it exits the skull. At this level, the deep branch of the internal maxillary artery can be identified or ligated by incising the temporomandibular joint from behind. The superficial temporal vessels are visualized and preserved (14). After transection of the facial nerve trunk at the stylomastoid foramen, dissection continues inferomedially to the submandibular gland level, including the facial nerve branches and the superficial lobe of the parotid gland, Stenson's duct, and all facial nerve branches in the flap. Preservation of the facial artery is critical for survival of the midfacial graft. Thus, the superficial lobe of the parotid gland as well as the entire submandibular gland are included into the flap not only to keep the vascular flow intact but also to protect the facial nerve branches from damage (22). Superiorly, by transection of the orbital septum over the infraorbital rim, the infraorbital nerve is identified at its foramen. The length of the nerve can be extended by osteotomy of the infraorbital bone and can be followed through the inferior orbital fissure and foramen rotundum, if required.

The Le Fort I, II, III and hemimaxillary osteotomies are performed as described earlier. Transverse and lateral nasal osteotomies are performed to separate the nasal framework from the adjacent structures. Then the upper lateral cartilages and nasal soft tissues are elevated together with the adjacent septal cartilaginous framework. The upper and lower gingivobuccal mucosa is incised and the tissues elevated to connect with the peripheral dissections described above. The lips, vermillion, and intraoral mucosa are included as required.

Lower Face Transplantation (Figures 41-3 and 41-6)

For lower face procurement, the incision begins at the level of the suprasternal notch and extends to the anterior edges of the SCM muscles. Transverse division of the SCM muscles, with care to preserve the external jugular veins, exposes the sheath of the common carotid artery and internal jugular vein. The subplatysmal dissection then extends cranially toward the styloid process for identification and ligation of the small vascular branches. The lingual and facial arteries are the main vascular source for the lower facial segments, and great care must be taken to preserve them during dissection. The larynx, with attached muscle groups, is easily identified and transected around the hyoid bone level. The lingual nerve is dissected and transected proximally after the larynx has been separated. The hypoglossal nerves are identified by dissection of the mylohyoid and digastric muscles. At each mandibular border in the region of the notch, the submandibular gland, with a cuff of distally oriented mandibular periosteum and masseter muscles, should be included in the allograft to minimize the risk of injury to facial vessels and the marginal mandibular branch of the facial nerve (31). Either the entire mandible or just a segment of it is included in the flap as required, and the hypoglossal and mental nerves are taken following their isolation as described earlier. At the medial edge of the masseter and buccinator muscles, access to the intraoral mucosa can be achieved via subperiosteal dissection around the mandible. The tongue, hard palate, alveolar ridge, lower lips, and perioral facial muscles remain attached to the facial allograft based on the extent of the recipient requirements.

Principles of Facial Subunit Transplantations

Currently, there is only one report on subunit transplantation that includes partial scalp and ear allograft (32). However, functional subunits such as the auricle, nose, lips, and eyelids are considered to represent the next step in reconstructive facial transplantation.

Scalp Transplantation

There are rich intervascular connections between scalp arteries. Based on cadaver studies and clinical reports, a single external carotid artery is adequate for the vascularization of the entire scalp graft. The superficial temporal artery and vein are the preferred vessels for maintaining the blood supply of the frontal and temporal scalp regions, but blood flow of occipital part of the scalp is supplied by the posterior auricular and occipital arteries with concomitant veins. The subperiosteal dissection is quick and safe at the anterior part of the scalp; however, from the vertex to the occipital region, the dissection of the occipital arteries through the occipital muscles and osteofibrous tunnels is the most challenging part of the harvesting process (14). A scalp graft based on superficial temporal arteries and veins is ready for transplantation after a relatively simple dissection.

Ear Transplantation

The external ear has a unique composition consisting of cartilage covered with thin skin. For ear procurement, the circular skin incision begins at the preauricular area and curves to the posterior aspect of the auricle at the inferior border of the earlobe. The subcutaneous dissection continues in an anterosuperior direction. The great auricular nerve and the auricular branches of the superficial temporal, posterior auricular arteries, and external jugular vein are identified and included into the graft. However, in their anatomical study, Ulusal et al. emphasized, using a dye injection method, that neither the superficial temporal artery nor the posterior auricular artery alone was adequate to homogenously stain the entire auricle (33). Based on this study, the inclusion of the external carotid artery as the donor vessel and preservation of these two branches in the flap is recommended. The soft tissue dissection continues with detaching the posterior auricular muscles and auditory canal from the mastoid fascia and temporal bone. The auricular graft, based on the external carotid artery and external jugular vein, is then harvested and ready for transplantation. Sensation is restored by coaptation of the greater auricular nerve.

Nose Transplantation

The nose, because of its critical function, central location, and aesthetic significance, is potentially an important subunit transplant. Its blood supply is maintained by the ophthalmic, angular, and superior labial arteries and their branches, and the venous return is provided by concomitant veins. For the feasibility of future vascular anastomosis, special attention should be given to isolation and dissection of these small vessels.

Nasal unit harvesting begins with skin incisions at the nasofrontal junction, passing down the side of the nose and ending at the alar base and columella. The soft tissue dissection continues in a cranial to caudal direction with or without detachment of the upper lateral and lower lateral cartilages from the underlying nasal bone. A sagittal saw is used to cut the nasal bones. The cartilaginous septum with overlying nasal mucosa is transected from the junction of the bony septum cranially and from the maxillary crest caudally. Finally, the lower part of the nose consisting of the nasal tip, alar lining, and columella with the septal cartilaginous framework is detached from the underlying muscles and soft tissues. After dissection, the nasal subunit, including facial artery branches and concomitant veins, is ready for transplantation.

Eyelid Transplantation

One of the most challenging transplants is the eyelid subunit because of the complex function and delicate structure of muscles responsible for upper and lower eyelid movements and the need for the maintenance of eyelid symmetry. The arterial blood supply of the upper and lower eyelids comes primarily from the branches of the ophthalmic artery (medial palpebral and lateral lacrimal arteries). These two branches anastomose through the tarsal arcades. However, the greater amount of blood flow comes from the medial canthal region, and it is critical to maintain vessel integrity during vessel dissection.

Bilateral skin incisions are made over the medial and lateral canthal regions. The canthal tendons are tagged by suture and are released from the surrounding soft tissue and muscles. The skin incisions are positioned according to the recipient requirements. Upper and lower conjunctival incisions are performed near the reflection of the membrane onto the globe, leaving the tarsal plate and eyelids intact. The lower eyelid dissection continues deeply through the orbital septum. Once divided, the infraorbital rim is exposed, and the infraorbital nerve is visualized. At the upper border, the supraorbital nerve is dissected in a similar manner and is left attached to the upper eyelid flap with or without the lacrimal glands and ducts. After completion of dissection, the eyelid graft, including the ophthalmic artery and concomitant veins, is ready for transplantation.

Lip Transplantation

The other challenging allograft subunit is the lip. This is the most difficult defect to reconstruct by conventional means because no matching tissues are available in the body for lip reconstruction. Achieving a normal lip appearance with restoration of normal oral muscle symmetry and function is the goal of this facial subunit transplantation. A lack of motor recovery may result in lip asymmetry, loss of labial competence, and other functional disabilities, and a failure of sensory recovery would lead to drooling and further social inhibition.

The composite lip graft consists of skin, vermillion, intraoral mucosa, perioral muscles (orbicularis oris, zygomatic major et minor, levator anguli oris, levator labii superior, depressor anguli oris, depressor labii inferior), facial nerve branches (buccal and marginal nerves), and vascular pedicles based on the facial vessels. These should be carefully dissected from the underlying maxillofacial skeleton, taking special care to preserve the Modiolus, which is the chiasma of the perioral muscles, for proper functioning. The upper and lower lips are vascularized by the superior and inferior labial arteries, with concomitant veins. However, utilization of their parent (facial) vessels adds length to the pedicles for flexibility and maximizes the diameter of the donor vessels for reliable and secure anastomosis. The proper reinsertion of the perioral muscles, with the remaining stumps of the recipient muscles, is essential for adequate lip motion.

PREPARATION OF THE RECIPIENT FACE

The recipient patient should undergo preoperative imaging to analyze the details of the facial defect and determine the required structures for allotransplantation. The preoperative imaging studies include CT scan, CT angiography (mapping of the vessels), magnetic resonance imaging of the head and neck, and carotid Doppler studies.

The recipient surgery begins with bilateral neck skin incisions and is followed by the identification and preparation of the appropriate recipient arteries and veins. In some cases, this step takes a long time because significant scarring and fibrosis of the soft tissues can make it difficult to find the vessels. The common carotid artery and its branches (external carotid and internal carotid); the internal, external, and anterior jugular veins; and the retromandibular veins are dissected and tagged with vessel loops for end-to-end or end-to-side vessel anastomosis. After confirmation of suitable tissues being available from the donor, the next step is the excision of those portions of the facial tissues that will be electively excised to accommodate the graft. These may consist of skin and underlying soft tissue, as well as previously transferred flaps, grafts, implants, and even hardware such as plates and screws. The recipient motor and sensory nerves and their branches are located and dissected to obtain sufficient length for proper nerve coaptation. Intraoperative nerve stimulation is useful in identifying the hypoglossal nerve and the individual facial nerve branches. It may be necessary to perform an internal neurolysis to gain adequate nerve length. After meticulous hemostasis, the recipient defect is ready for donor allograft inset.

FACIAL ALLOGRAFT INSET

The insetting of a facial allograft containing bone components begins with osteosynthesis, which takes place before microvascular anastomosis. Excess craniofacial bones are removed by an oscillating saw and are trimmed to allow a precise fit and inset. The craniofacial skeletal components (frontal bone, maxilla, orbital rim, zygoma, and mandible) are rigidly fixed with titanium plates, screws, and occasionally wires. It is important to accurately stabilize the bone components for proper facial projection and dental occlusion. Thus, the composite tissue graft is secured for microvascular reconstruction. Additionally, for the prevention of mucoceles, sinus infections, and infectious complications, which may cause sepsis and death under immunosuppression treatment, removal or stripping of the donor sinus mucosa and obliteration of the frontal sinus may be considered.

Conventional microvascular techniques are used during anastomosis, and an end-to-end repair is preferred in most cases. After the first arterial repair is completed, the microsurgical clamps are released before completion of other vessel anastomosis. This minimizes ischemia time, which is important not only for muscle function but also because a longer ischemia time may play a role in graft rejection and failure (34). Generally, the ischemia time should not exceed 3 hours. After all of the vascular anastomoses are completed and adequate perfusion of the facial graft is provided, additional plates and screws may be applied to complete rigid stabilization of the maxillofacial skeleton.

After reperfusion is established, repair of motor and sensory nerves is completed. The coaptation of nerve ends is performed using standard epineural repair and fibrin glue if indicated. However, in some cases, donor nerve grafts may need to be used to bridge unplanned gaps between donor and recipient nerve ends (7). As mentioned previously, osteotomies are useful in mobilizing, gaining better access, and obtaining greater length in the recipient as well as the donor nerves.

Finally, attachment of muscle, the periorbita, skin, soft tissue, and intraoral mucosa is performed with interrupted sutures. Overall skin closure should be tension free. A light, absorbent dressing may be applied.

Monitoring for tissue viability and anastomotic patency is performed as for any exposed free flap and may vary from center to center. In addition to clinical assessment, it may include pencil Doppler to detect signals from perforating vessels or to record flow in the vascular pedicles; it may include probes such as the Vioptix that monitor tissue oxygenation directly below the surface, and it may include laser Doppler flow probes placed directly around draining veins. This is carried out on a more or less continuous basis, but, in addition, the flap is monitored for signs of rejection such as erythema, edema, blistering, and so on every day by an experienced team member. As with any microsurgical procedure, if a vascular complication occurs in the early posttransplant period, the flap may be salvageable after rapid diagnosis and take-back. In the event of facial allograft failure caused by technical problems or acute graft rejection, the facial CTA must be removed and the defect restored by application of autologous skin grafts or free flaps. This "plan B" must be established before the initial transplant.

IMMUNOSUPPRESSION PROTOCOLS

Previous reports on composite tissue allotransplantations have confirmed that, currently, there is no standard immunosuppressive protocol accepted by most CTA centers. Each center has reported different induction and maintenance therapy protocols (7–10,14,34,35) (Table 41-1). The most common regimen for face transplantation is based on kidney transplantation protocols and includes standard induction therapy with antithymocyte globulin (ATG) followed by triple maintenance therapy consisting of Tacrolimus (FK506), mycophenolate mofetil (MMF), and prednisone. This regimen has also been successfully used on more than 40 clinical cases of hand transplantation patients, with minimal toxicity (36). Additionally, donor-derived bone marrow cell infusions aimed at establishing chimerism and tolerance induction have been clinically introduced to prevent acute graft rejection (35). Signs of graft rejection are monitored clinically by macroscopic observation and by taking routine biopsies from skin and mucosa.

COMPLICATIONS

In the early posttransplant period, the main surgical complications include failure of the arterial or venous anastomosis, which can occur with any microsurgical procedure. The multiplicity of vessels used should minimize this risk, however. Wound dehiscence, stenosis of the glandular or lacrimal ducts, ectropion, ptosis, malunion or nonunion of the transplanted facial bones, and graft failure are possible surgical complications that may occur in the early or late periods of the posttransplant phase. Additionally, these patients may require secondary

TABLE 41-1 Immunosuppressive Protocol Details of Facial Transplant Patients

Patient	Induction Immunosuppressive Protocol	Maintenance Protocol	Acute Rejection Episodes	Rescue Therapy
Patient 1, 38 y, female Amiens, France, 2005	ATG (1.25 mg/kg/d × 10 d) Tacrolimus (10–15 ng/mL) MMF (2 g) Prednisolone (250 mg d 1, 100 mg d 2, 60 mg for 10 d)	Tacrolimus (10–15 ng/mL) Sirolimus (8–12 ng/mL started 11 mo after surgery) MMF (2 g/d) Prednisolone (25 mg/ d) Bone marrow infusion on POD 4 and 11	Two episodes POD 18 and 214 (erythema and edema on oral mucosa and skin) Grades I–II	1. Rejection Dose increase in • Tacrolimus • MMF • Prednisone Clobatesol ointment, prednisone mouthwashes • Methylprednisolone (3 × 1000 mg) 2. Rejection Methylprednisolone (3 × 750 mg) Clobatesol, tacrolimus ointments, prednisone mouthwashes Prednisolone(50 mg × 10 d; then 5 mg × 8 wk) ECP started at 10 mo after transplant
Patient 2, 30 y, male Xian, China, 2006	Tacrolimus (25 ng/mL) MMF (500 mg) Prednisolone (25 mg) Methylprednisolone (1 g) Humanized IL-2 receptor monoclonal antibody (50 mg)	Tacrolimus (10–25 ng/mL) MMF (taper dose) Prednisolone (taper dose; stopped after 22 mo) Humanized IL-2 receptor monoclonal antibody (50 mg on POD 15 and 30)	Three episodes 3, 5 and 17 mo after transplantation Grades I–II	1. Rejection Dose increase in tacrolimus (15–25 ng/mL) 2. Rejection Methylprednisolone pulse therapy Prednisolone 3. Rejection Dose increase in • Tacrolimus
Patient 3, 29 y, male Paris, France, 2007	Antilymphocyte serum (1.25 mg/kg/d × 10 d) Tacrolimus (10–13 ng/mL) MMF (2 g) Prednisone (500 mg d 1, 250 mg d 2, 120 mg d 3, 60 mg for 7 d)	Tacrolimus (8–10 ng/mL) MMF (2 g/d) Prednisolone (10 mg/d)	Two episodes POD 28 and 64 Grades I–II	1. Rejection Prednisolone (60 mg/d) 2. Rejection Prednisolone (500 mg × 3 d) Antilymphocyte serum (1 mg/kg × 1 wk) ECP started at 3 mo after surgery
Patient 4, 45 y, female Cleveland, OH, 2008	Rabbit ATG (1.2 mg/kg/d × 3 d) Methylprednisolone (1000 mg/d 1) Tacrolimus (12–15 ng/mL × 3 mo) MMF Prednisone	Tacrolimus (10–12 ng/mL) MMF (stopped at 6 mo after surgery) Prednisone 10 (mg/d)	Two episodes POD 47 and 459 Grades 0–I	Methylprednisolone (1000 mg × 1 d)
Patient 6, 37 y, male Paris, France, 2009	ATG Tacrolimus MMF Prednisone	No available data	No available data	No available data

ATG, antithymocyte globulin; ECP, extracorporeal photopheresis; IL, interleukin; MMF, mycophenolate mofetil; POD, postoperative day.

surgeries, including scar revisions, graft debulking, and suspension procedures, to remove soft tissue excess and to keep the facial graft properly suspended.

Graft rejections and opportunistic infections are other expected complications, similar to those reported in solid organ transplantation. However, acute graft rejection rates are higher than with solid organ transplants, most likely because of high antigenicity of the oral mucosa and skin (37,38). In the literature, facial transplant recipients were reported to have had at least one acute graft rejection episode that was reversed by adjusting the dose of immunosuppressive therapy, administering a bolus of steroids (methylprednisolone), or by introduction of extracorporeal photochemotherapy (ECP) to the treatment protocol (7–10,34,35) (see Table 41-1). Hyperacute and chronic rejections have not been reported yet. This may be due to a relatively short posttransplant follow-up period since the first face transplant was reported or perhaps due to early detection and treatment of acute graft rejections (39,40).

In addition to standard antibacterial medication, the prophylaxis protocol for cytomegalovirus (ganciclovir followed by valganciclovir), herpes simplex virus, (acyclovir), and pneumocystis jiroveci (trimethoprim–sulfamethoxazole) is recommended after a facial allotransplantation procedure. In the early posttransplant period, infections are generally related to the surgical procedure; however, opportunistic infections, which occur later, are usually due to immunosuppressive treatment. The incidence of infection is high in CTA recipients. The primary cause is the requirement of adequate immunosuppressive treatment to prevent skin rejection (40). Despite the death of one patient (Table 41-2, patient 6) because of a fatal *Pseudomonas aeruginosa* infection 2 months after facial transplantation, other reported infections were treated successfully by systemic or local antibiotics and antiviral medications (7–10,14,19,35) (see Table 41-2).

Kidney toxicity, new-onset diabetes mellitus, hypertension, severe rhabdomyolysis, Cushing's syndrome, avascular necrosis, hematologic problems (e.g., transient leucopenia, thrombocytopenia, anemia), malignancies, and death are the other serious complications that can be seen during posttransplant follow-up (7–10,16,19,35,40). Finally, the systemic complications associated with face transplantations are fewer and less toxic than these observed in solid organ transplants. This may be due to the absence of preexisting life-threatening diseases and morbidities of face transplant recipients when compared with solid organ recipients.

POSTOPERATIVE REHABILITATION AND PSYCHIATRIC EVALUATION

The postoperative rehabilitation starts with facial reeducation therapy or speech therapy. The therapy sessions continue daily for the first 2 to 3 months after transplant, twice or three times per week for another 6 months, and at least once a week for another year. The progression of motor and sensory recovery of the facial allograft is measured objectively by functional magnetic resonance imaging, electroneuromyographic (EMG) studies, volumetric analysis, temperature testing, two-point discrimination testing, and Semmes-Weinstein monofilament tests. Additionally, facial functions, including smiling; blinking; mimicry; eyelid closing; and ability to smell, masticate, and swallow, are evaluated by professional teams regularly and documented by serial photography and video recording (21).

The psychiatrist belonging to the transplant team should visit the patient daily, for 1-hour sessions, during the first 4 to 6 weeks after the transplant and then once a month (or more as needed) thereafter during the first year. Psychiatric evaluation involves various assessment tools, which are implemented at each visit, and these include Rosenberg's self-esteem scale, perception of teasing scale, and physical appearance state. According to the literature, facial transplants are reported as being well accepted psychologically by the patients (21).

CLINICAL RESULTS AND OUTCOMES

As of November 30, 2010, two scalp transplantation and 13 facial allotransplantation cases have been performed worldwide (7–18,32,41). The anatomical and technical details are presented in Table 41-3. The first successful scalp transplantation was an isotransplantation between identical twins without use of any immunosuppression therapy and was performed by Buncke and colleagues in 1982 (41). In 2005, Jiang and colleagues performed the second scalp transplantation, including bilateral ears, in a 72-year-old male patient, for reconstruction of a wide scalp defect (32). The triple immunosuppressive drug regimen, including MMF, prednisone, and Zenapax, was given to the patient, with no signs of rejection, during the 4-month posttransplant follow-up period.

On November 27, 2005, in Amiens, France, Devauchelle and Dubernard performed the world's first partial facial allotransplantation in a 38-year-old woman with a soft tissue defect of the central face area caused by a dog bite (8). In addition to the facial allograft transfer, a radial forearm flap from the same donor (a 46-year-old brain-dead woman) was transferred to monitor the immunological response of the grafts and was aimed at diminishing damage, caused by repeated skin biopsies, to the facial allotransplant. The surgery time was 15 hours, and the ischemia time was 230 minutes. The immunosuppressive protocol and postoperative complications are described in Tables 41-1 and 41-2. ECP treatment was given to the patient at 10 months after transplantation to prevent the recurrence of graft rejection. Functional outcome by the end of the first week confirmed that the patient was eating and drinking almost normally. It was reported that sensitivity to light touch, heat, and cold had returned to normal at 6 months. However, motor recovery was slower than sensory recovery, and labial contact, with complete mouth closure, was not seen until 10 months after the transplant (8,35) (see Table 41-3). The pronunciation of words beginning with P and B had improved by the end of the third month. Normal mastication of food was seen at 6 months. Eight months after transplantation, the patient had a successful surgical operation for stenosis of Stenson's duct. The patient returned to a normal social life by the end of postoperative week 12. Psychological acceptance of the graft improved over time. At the end of 18 months, the patient was satisfied with the final aesthetic and functional outcomes (8,35).

On April 13, 2006, Guo et al. performed the second partial facial allotransplantation, in Xian, China (9). The recipient was

TABLE 41-2 Details of Prophylaxis Protocols and Postoperative Complications in Facial Transplant Patients

Patient	Prophylaxis Protocol	Infectious Complications	Other Complications
Patient 1, 38 y, female Amiens, France, 2005	Cytomegalovirus • Gancylovir (10 mg/kg/ 5 d) • Valgancyclovir (900 mg/d 5 mo) *Pneumocystis jiroveci* pneumonia • Trimethoprim–sulfamethoxazole (400 mg/d 4 mo) Amoxicillin–clavulanate (3 g/10 d) • Aspirin • Heparin	HSV type I (POD 185) • Treatment: valacyclovir and topical acyclovir cream Molluscum contagiosum virus (POD 214) • Treatment: curettage	Renal failure • Serum creatinine from 0.6–1.5 mg/dL • Treatment: decreasing tacrolimus, adding sirolimus Thrombotic microangiopathy • Thrombocytopenia, hemolytic anemia, acute renal failure, hypertension) • Treatment: tacrolimus and sirolimus stopped, fresh-frozen plasma infusion, and immunoglobulin
Patient 2, 30 y, male Xian, China, 2006	• Ceftizoxime (3 × 2 g/2 wk) • Vancomycin (2 × 1 g/4 d) • Metronidazole • Acyclovir • Allicin • Glucurolactone (protect liver) • Omeprazole, famotidine • Human immunoglobulin	None reported	New-onset diabetes mellitus • Treatment: insulin, repaglinide, and metformin hydrochloride tablets. Death (2 y after transplant)
Patient 3, 29 y, male Paris, France, 2007	Cytomegalovirus • Valgancyclovir (900 mg/d 6 mo) *Pneumocystis carinii* pneumonia • Trimethoprim–sulfamethoxazole (400 mg/d 6 mo) Syphilis • Phenoxymethylpenicillin (2 × 3, 000, 000 IU/15 d)	Cytomegalovirus • Valganciclovir-resistant on POD 64 • Treatment: foscarnet 8 g/d 2 mo)	Transient steroid-induced confusion Treatment: chlorpromazine 25–50 mg/5 d
Patient 4, 45 y, female Cleveland, OH, 2008	Cytomegalovirus • Gancylovir (10 mg/kg/d 8 wk) • Valgancyclovir (2 × 900 mg/d 5 mo) *Pneumocystis jiroveci* pneumonia • Trimethoprim–sulfamethoxazole (160 mg/800 mg)	None reported	Transient leucopenia • Treatment: ganciclovir, lowering MMF dosage (first episode), leukocyte growth factor (second episode)
Patient 6, 37 y, male Paris, France, 2009	None reported	*Pseudomonas aeruginosa* (POD 15, multidrug resistant) • Treatment: triple antibiotic regimen was unsuccessful	Death (2 mo after transplant)

HSV, herpes simplex virus; MMF, mycophenolate mofetil; POD, postoperative day.

TABLE 41-3 Anatomical and Surgical Details of Facial Transplant Patients

	Patient 1, 38 y, Female Amiens, France, 2005	Patient 2, 30 y, Male Xian, China, 2006	Patient 3, 29 y, Male Paris, France, 2007	Patient 4, 45 y, Female Cleveland, OH, 2008	Patient 5, 28 y, Male Paris, France, 2009	Patient 6, 37 y, Male Paris, France, 2009
Type of CTA	Partial myocutaneous	Partial osteomyocutaneous	Partial myocutaneous	Near-total osteomyo-cutaneous	Partial osteomyo-cutaneous	Partial myocutaneous
CTA design	Partial nose, cheek, oral and nasal mucosa, and total upper and lower lips	Right zygoma with lateral orbital wall, upper lip, nose, parotid gland and masseter, and intraoral mucosa	Upper and lower lips, chin, cheeks, nose, bilateral parotid glands, parotid ducts, and intraoral mucosa	Le Fort III midfacial skeleton, total infraorbital floor, bilateral zygoma, lower eyelids, nose, anterior maxilla with teeth, anterior hard palate, alveolus, upper lip, parotid glands, and intaroral mucosa	Cheek, nose, parotid glands and ducts, upper and lower lips, premaxilla, chin, and intraoral mucosa	Entire scalp with bilateral ears, forehead, lower eyelids, nose, bilateral cheeks, parotid glands and parotid ducts, and intraoral mucosa
Vessel and nerve repair	Bilateral facial arteries and veins Bilateral infraorbital and mental nerves Left mandibular branch of facial nerve	Right external maxillary artery and anterior facial vein Right facial nerve not well coapted	Bilateral external carotid arteries and thyrolingofacial trunks Bilateral facial, infraorbital, and mental nerves (mental nerves not coapted)	Bilateral common facial arteries, left external jugular, posterior facial, and right facial veins Bilateral facial nerve repair with nerve grafts	Bilateral external carotid arteries, external jugular veins, and thyrolinguofacial trunk Bilateral facial nerves	Bilateral external carotid arteries and thyrolinguofacial trunks Bilateral facial, supraorbital, and infraorbital nerves
Nerve recovery	Light touch (10 wk) Temperature (6 mo) Eat and drink (1 wk) Labial contact (6 mo) Chin and nose pyramidal muscle motion (12 mo) Smile (14–18 mo)	Light touch (3 mo) Temperature (8 mo) Unable to smile completely Facial nerve not functional Eat, drink and talk normally	Light touch (3 mo) Temperature (3 mo) Eat and speak (10 d) Orbicularis oris and oculi voluntarily contract (6 mo) Spontaneous mimicry (9 mo) Trigeminal and facial motor function (12 mo)	Smell (2 d) Light touch (5 mo) Temperature (5 mo) Upper lip occlusion Facial mimicry Eat and drink from a cup	None reported	None reported

TABLE 41-3 Anatomical and Surgical Details of Facial Transplant Patients

	Patient 7, 59y, Male Boston, MA, 2009	Patient 8,33 y, Male Paris, France, 2009 (13,45)	Patient 9, 42 y, Male Valencia, Spain, 2009 (17,45)	Patient 10, 27 y, Male Amiens, France, 2009 (18,45)	Patient 11, 34 y, Male Sevilla, Spain, 2010 (16,45)	Patient 12, 30 y, Male Barcelona, Spain, 2010 (12,44,45)	Patient 13, 35 y, Male Paris, France, 2010 (15,45)
Type of CTA	Partial osteomyo-cutaneous	Partial osteomyo-cutaneous	Partial osteomyo-cutaneous	Partial osteomyo-cutaneous	Partial myo-cutaneous	Total osteomyo-cutaneous	Total myocutaneous
CTA design	Nose, upper lip, bilateral cheek, bilateral parotid ducts, maxilla with teeth and palate, and intraoral mucosa	Maxilla, mandible, nose, bilateral cheek, upper and lower lip, and intraoral mucosa	Mandible, bilateral partial cheek, lower lip, chin, tongue, and intraoral mucosa	Mandible, nose, upper and lower lips, and chin	Partial nose, bilateral cheek with parotid gland, upper and lower lip, chin, and intraoral mucosa	Forehead, lower eyelids, bilateral orbital floor, nose, zygoma, cheek, maxilla with teeth, palate, intraoral mucosa, lips, and mandible	Forehead, bilateral ears, upper and lower eyelids with lacrimal glands and ducts, nose, cheeks, parotid glands and ducts, upper and lower lips, and intraoral mucosa
Vessel and nerve repair	Left external carotid, right facial arteries, bilateral facial veins Bilateral facial, infraorbital, and buccal sensory nerves	Bilateral external carotid arteries, external jugular veins, and thyrolingofacial trunk Bilateral facial nerves	Left CCA, right ICA, bilateral external jugular veins, and right internal jugular vein Bilateral hypoglossal, inferior alveolar, lingual, and unilateral cervicofacial nerves	Bilateral facial arteries and veins Bilateral facial, infraorbital, and mental nerves	Bilateral external carotid arteries and internal jugular veins Bilateral facial, infraorbital, and mental nerves	Bilateral external carotid arteries and external jugular veins, unilateral anterior jugular and retromandibular veins Bilateral facial, supraorbital, infraorbital, and mental nerves	Bilateral external carotid arteries, external jugular veins, and thyrolinguofacial trunk Bilateral facial, supraorbital, infraorbital, and mental nerves
Nerve recovery	None reported	None reported	None reported	None reported	None reported	None reported	None reported

CCA, common carotid artery; CTA, composite tissue allotransplantation; ICA, internal carotid artery.

a 30-year-old male patient who had a soft tissue and bony defect of the midface caused by a bear attack. Sensory recovery was similar to the first case. However, because the quality of the facial nerve coaptation was poor, the function of the facial muscles remained poor, and the patient was unable to smile completely or symmetrically. The functions of eating, drinking, and speech were normal (see Table 41-3). Two additional operations were performed under local anesthesia to improve facial appearance. These operations included debulking of the graft, correction of deviation of the mouth using local flaps, and repair of a right orbital floor deformity with an autologous cartilage graft (9). The patient was satisfied with the functional and aesthetic results but gave up taking the immunosuppressive drugs and died 2 years after surgery because of transplant-related complications (19).

Lantieri et al. performed the third facial transplantation in Paris, France, on January 21, 2007 (10). The recipient was a 29-year-old male patient with neurofibromatosis type I who had a plexiform neurofibroma that infiltrated and disfigured the middle and lower parts of his face. After debulking of the tumor, the final defect included all of the soft tissues and skin below the zygomatic arch. The CTA inset and microsurgical repair of the arteries and nerves were managed as described here, but the submental nerves were not coapted because each recipient nerve had been transected at the submental foramen during surgery (10,31). The donor nerves were merely positioned near the foramina in the hope of eliciting neurotrophism. The immunosuppressive therapy is summarized in Table 41-2. In addition, ECP treatment, which has an immunomodulatory affect, was introduced as a prophylactic treatment for the prevention of rejection episodes. The patient had revisionary surgery for correction of a right eyelid deformity and dental restoration with implants 10 months after facial transplantation. EMG findings confirmed that motor reinnervation of the facial and trigeminal nerves had begun with voluntary contraction in the bilateral orbicularis oris and left orbicularis oculi muscles by the end of the sixth month and improved function over the first year after transplant (see Table 41-3). The authors commented that the procedure had an excellent psychological effect on the patient; he had acquired a job and a normal social life, which he had not had before transplantation (10).

The fourth facial allotransplantation was performed in our department at the Cleveland Clinic, in Ohio, on December 9, 2008 (7). The recipient was a 45-year-old woman with a midface defect after a shotgun blast. She had 23 reconstructive procedures previously, resulting in inadequate function, poor aesthetic outcome, and extensive donor site morbidity from the use of autologous tissues. The facial CTA design is shown in Figure 41-9. The major anatomical deficits of the recipient's face were complete absence of the nose, maxilla, zygoma, and orbital rims bilaterally; loss of midfacial soft tissues and orbicularis oris muscle function; oral commissure droop; loss of the right eye and a facial nerve deficit with complete loss of the midface division; and paresis of its lower divisions (Figure 41-10). The functions of eating, drinking, mastication, and speech were impaired.

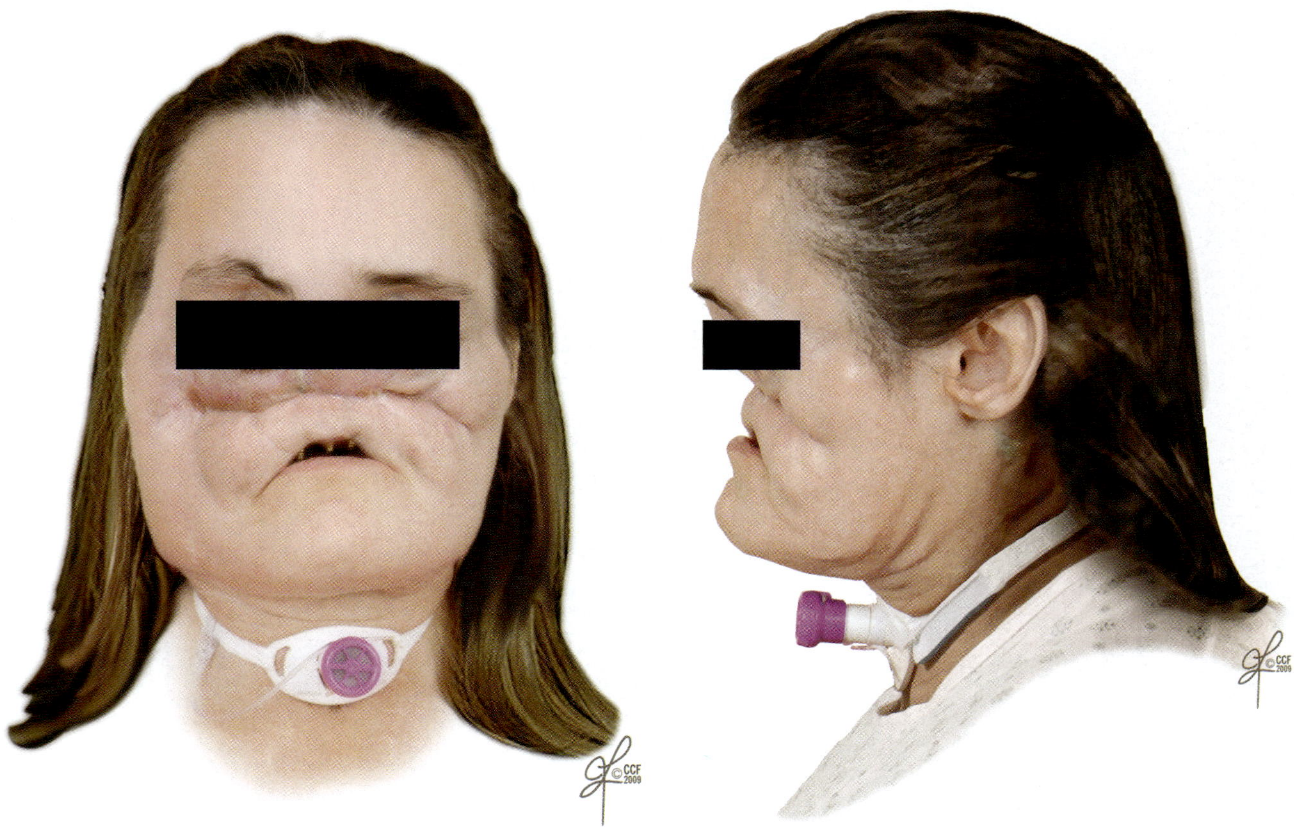

A B

FIGURE 41-10 Anterior (**A**) and lateral (**B**) views of the Cleveland Clinic patient's facial defect before facial transplantation indicating severe midfacial defects with a missing nose, lower eyelids, and upper lip. (For details, see Table 41-3, patient 4.) (Reprinted with permission, Cleveland Clinic Center for Medical Art & Photography © 2009-2010. All Rights Reserved.)

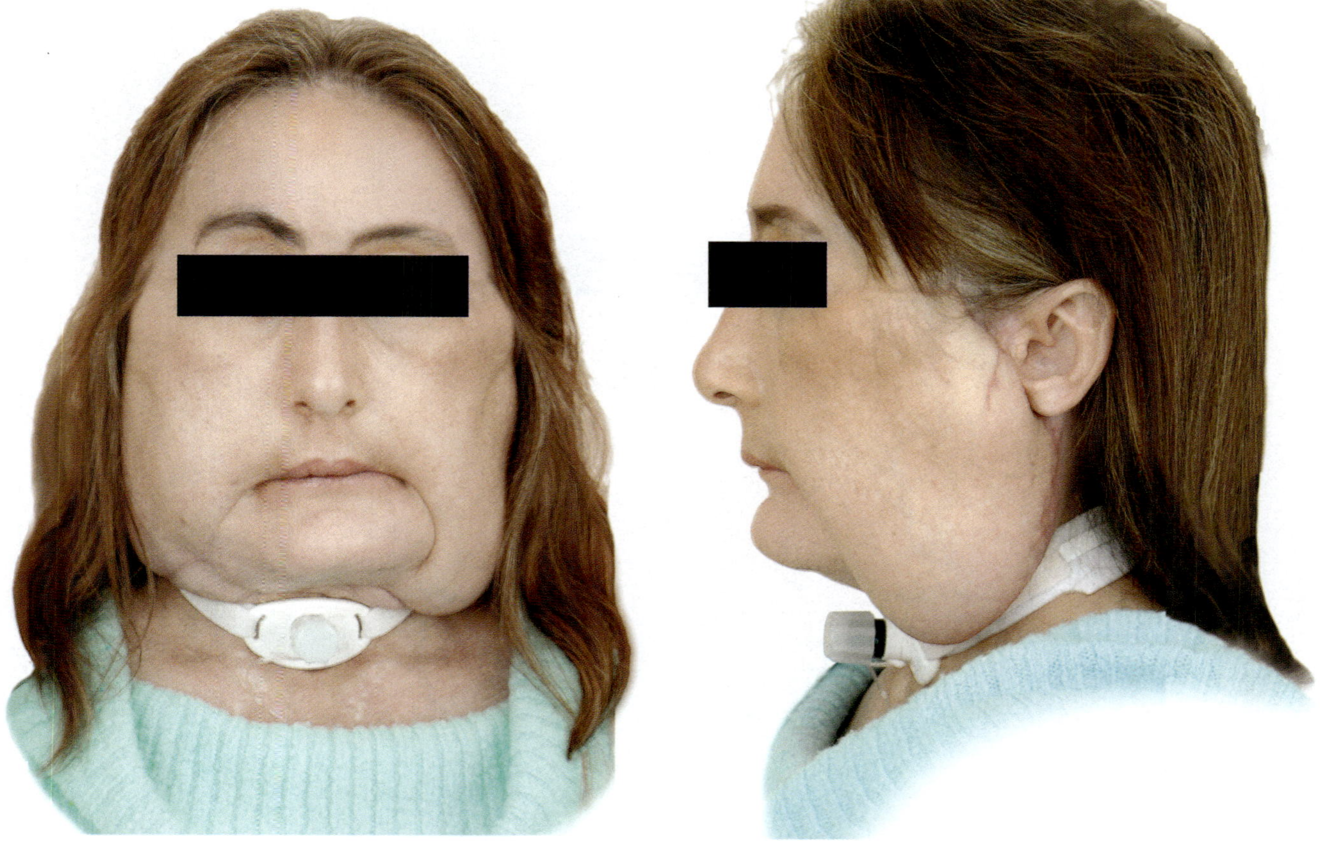

A B

FIGURE 41-11 Anterior (A) and lateral (B) views of the Cleveland Clinic patient's face after facial allotransplantation demonstrating reconstruction of the facial defect with restoration of the nose, upper lip, and lower eyelids. (For details, see Table 41-3, patient 4.) (Reprinted with permission, Cleveland Clinic Center for Medical Art & Photography © 2009-2010. All Rights Reserved.)

Additionally, she was receiving parenteral nutrition via an epigastric tube and had a tracheostomy tube for breathing. The patient had no surgical complications after the facial transplantation except for delayed wound healing (Figure 41-11). After resolution of facial edema and swelling, residual tissue bulk and skin redundancy were removed by a secondary surgery 18 months after the transplant (Figure 41-12). Postoperative rehabilitation began 48 hours after transplantation and continued daily for the first 6 weeks and then three times per week during the follow-up period. Sensory discrimination returned to the entire face and was confirmed by the presence of 7-mm 2-point discrimination at the end of 8 months; however, motor recovery of the functions of smile, pucker, repose, and upper lip occlusion improved after 1 year, as expected. The patient was able to breathe through her nose, smell, taste, eat, drink, demonstrate improved speech, convey satisfaction with her facial appearance, and regain self-confidence (see Table 41-3) (7,42,43).

The fifth and sixth facial transplantation cases were performed by Lantieri et al. in Paris in March and April 2009 (13,14). The fifth patient was a 28-year-old man who had a partial myocutaneous defect involving the lower part of his face caused by a shotgun blast injury (13,19). The sixth case was a 37-year-old male patient who had extensive burn sequelae in his face; both upper extremities had been amputated, also because of the burn injury (13,14). Facial and concomitant bilateral upper extremity allotransplantation was performed from two donors. The whole face, including both ears and scalp, was harvested followed by removal of those parts such as the lips and chin, which were not included in the transplant (see Table 41-3). According to the authors, they prefer this "en bloc" harvesting technique for reconstruction of partial facial defects to decrease the surgery time for graft procurement and to prevent tissue injury (14). However, they experienced two very challenging technical problems during the facial allograft procurement. One was during the dissection of the temporal pedicle around the temporomandibular joint, and the other one was the dissection of the occipital pedicle from its fibrous tunnel. The anastomosis of a single external carotid artery seemed sufficient for maintaining the arterial blood flow to the whole facial flap; however, bilateral external carotid artery anastomoses were performed to eliminate potential vascular problems. The authors suggest that choosing the external carotid artery rather than a more peripheral vessel for arterial anastomosis is the best option because it has a large diameter and a long pedicle (14). The immunosuppression therapy was similar to the previous cases (see Table 41-1). On day 15, the patient had a multidrug-resistant *P. aeruginosa* infection with swelling of the face and left hand allografts. The dose of immunosuppression was reduced, and triple antibiotic treatment was started.

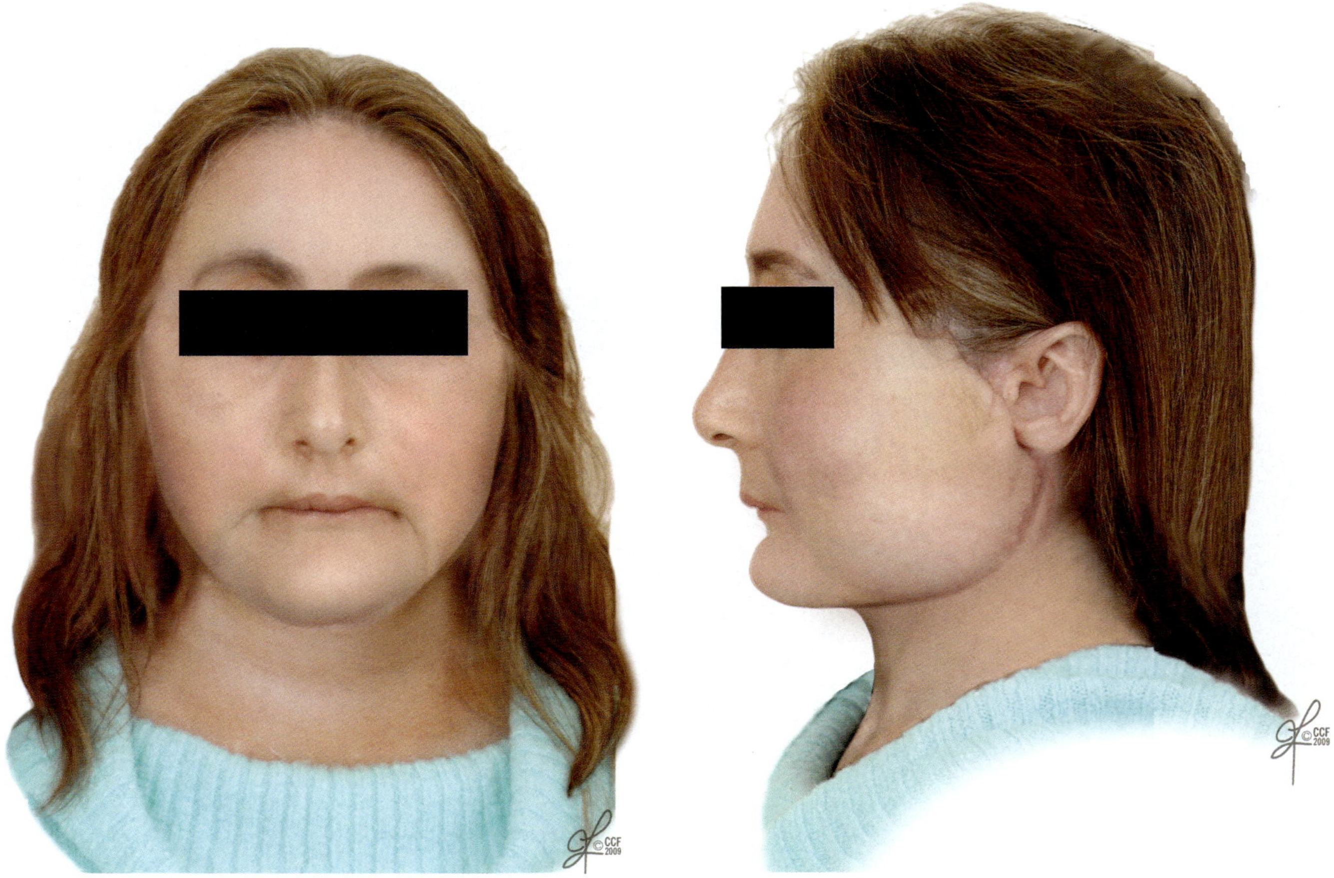

A B

FIGURE 41-12 Anterior (**A**) and lateral (**B**) views of the computer-generated image of Cleveland Clinic patient's face demonstrating satisfactory aesthetic outcome after revision surgery at 18 months after transplantation. (For details, see Table 41-3, patient 4.) (Reprinted with permission, Cleveland Clinic Center for Medical Art & Photography © 2009-2010. All Rights Reserved.)

However, the infection progressed, and the patient died 2 months after transplantation despite several surgical procedures for debridement of the infected tissues and tissue necrosis (see Table 41-2). Autopsy showed that the vascular anastomoses were patent, and there was no sign of graft rejection. The authors concluded that the long surgery time, as well as the fact that multiple surgeons were involved in this combined transplantation case, could have contributed to an increased risk of infection (14).

Pomahac et al. performed the world's seventh facial allotransplantation in Boston, Massachusetts, in April 2009 (11). The recipient was a 59-year-old male patient who had a midfacial defect caused by an electrical injury (see Table 41-3). The authors suggested that the facial artery alone can supply blood flow to the maxilla and zygoma; therefore, it is important to harvest the maxilla and overlying soft tissues to maintain the viability of the bone segment. Otherwise, the maxilla is dependent on an endosteal supply from the maxillary arteries (11).

The world's eighth face transplantation was performed by Lantieri in Paris, France, in 2009 (13). Between 2009 and 2010, the following four cases were performed by Cavadas in Valencia, Spain; Gomez-Cia in Sevilla, Spain; Barret in Barcelona, Spain; and Dubernard in Amiens, France (12, 16–18). The important highlights were the first facial CTA to include the tongue (performed by Cavadas) and the first near-total facial allotransplantation (performed by Barret), which included the entire face except for the lacrimal glands and ducts (12,17). Gomez-Cia et al. performed face transplantation in a 35-year-old patient with neurofibromatosis type I (see Table 41-3). After transplant, severe rhabdomyolysis was observed (16). Suspicion of rhabdomyolysis began with the observation of dark urine with positive heme dipstick and was confirmed by elevated creatine kinase serum levels, to a peak of 31,081 IU/L, 48 hours after surgery. According to the authors, this was due to prolonged surgery with mild hypothermia, electrolyte disorders, drug interactions, or gram-negative bacteremia (16). The patient was treated with forced alkaline diuresis and fluids.

According to early reports on the Barcelona case, the surgeons had first connected the donor's facial allograft to the recipient's femoral artery to check the vascular perfusion of the donor tissues. After 45 minutes, when graft perfusion was confirmed, the recipient's facial tissues were removed (12). The patient had two venous thromboses 3 days after transplant. Rehabilitation therapy is still in progress, but the patient has gained sensory recovery in most of his facial allograft, and some motor function of the facial muscles has returned (44). In June 2010, Lantieri et al. performed a full facial allotransplantation in France (see Table 41-3) (15,45). This time, the facial allograft consisted of the entire face, including the lacrimal glands and ducts. This was the last face transplant case performed in 2010.

CONCLUSION

Despite its immunologic side effects and life-threatening complications, face allotransplantation has opened a new field in reconstructive plastic surgery. Its future will be enhanced by the development of less toxic immunosuppressive drugs and therapies, as well as by the implementation of facial subunit transplantation, so that a much larger population of facially disfigured patients may be helped.

REFERENCES

1. Erol OO. The transformation of a free skin graft into a vascularized pedicled flap. *Plast Reconstr Surg* 1976;58:470–477.
2. Khouri RK, Upton J, Shaw WW. Prefabrication of composite free flaps through staged microvascular transfer: an experimental and clinical study. *Plast Reconstr Surg* 1991;87:108–115.
3. Mathy JA, Pribaz JJ. Prefabrication and prelamination applications in current aesthetic facial reconstruction. *Clin Plast Surg* 2009;36:493–505.
4. Menick FJ. Facial reconstruction with local and distant tissue: the interface of aesthetic and reconstructive surgery. *Plast Reconstr Surg* 1998;102:1424–1433.
5. Stamatopoulos C, Panayotou P, Tsirigotou S, et al. Use of free flaps in the aesthetic reconstruction of face and neck deformities. *Microsurgery* 1992;13:188–191.
6. Cheng K, Zhou S, Jiang K, et al. Microsurgical replantation of the avulsed scalp: report of 20 cases. *Plast Reconstr Surg* 1996;97:1099–1106; discussion 1107–1098.
7. Siemionow M, Papay F, Alam D, et al. Near-total human face transplantation for a severely disfigured patient in the USA. *Lancet* 2009;374:203–209.
8. Devauchelle B, Badet L, Lengele B, et al. First human face allograft: early report. *Lancet* 2006;368:203–209.
9. Guo S, Han Y, Zhang X, et al. Human facial allotransplantation: a 2-year follow-up study. *Lancet* 2008;372:631–638.
10. Lantieri L, Meningaud JP, Grimbert P, et al. Repair of the lower and middle parts of the face by composite tissue allotransplantation in a patient with massive plexiform neurofibroma: a 1-year follow-up study. *Lancet* 2008;372:639–645.
11. Pomahac B, Lengele B, Ridgway EB, et al. Vascular considerations in composite midfacial allotransplantation. *Plast Reconstr Surg* 2010;125:517–522.
12. Eaton L. Spanish doctors carry out first transplantation of a full face. *BMJ* 2010;340:c2303.
13. Lantieri L, Grimbert P, Meningaud JP, Bellivier F. Face transplantation outcomes: Feasibility, reproducibility and efficacy. In *Paper presented at: 21st Annual Meeting of the European Association of Plastic Surgeons,* Manchester, UK, May 27–30, 2010.
14. Meningaud JP, Benjoar MD, Hivelin M, et al. The procurement of total human face graft for allotransplantation: a preclinical study and the first clinical case. *Plast Reconstr Surg* 2010;126:1181–1190.
15. MSNBC. Doctors perform face transplant with eyelids, July 8, 2010. http://www.msnbc.msn.com/id/38144667
16. Hinojosa Perez R, Porras Lopez M, Escoresca-Ortega AM, et al. Severe rhabdomyolysis after allogeneic transplantation of facial structures: a case report. *Transplant Proc* 2010;42:3081–3082.
17. Cavadas P. Clinical update & update on hand and face transplant outcomes. *American Society for Reconstructive Transplantation 2nd Biennial Meeting.* Chicago, November 18–20, 2010.
18. Morelon E, Testelin S, Petruzzo P, et al. New partial face allograft transplantation: report on first six months. *Paper presented at: American Society for Reconstructive Transplantation 2nd Biennial Meeting.* Chicago, November 18–20, 2010.
19. Gordon CR, Siemionow M, Papay F, et al. The world's experience with facial transplantation: what have we learned thus far? *Ann Plast Surg* 2009;63:572–578.
20. Siemionow M, Gordon CR. Overview of guidelines for establishing a face transplant program: a work in progress. *Am J Transplant* 2010;10:1290–1296.
21. Siemionow MZ, Gordon CR. Institutional review board-based recommendations for medical institutions pursuing protocol approval for facial transplantation. *Plast Reconstr Surg* 2010;126:1232–1239.
22. Siemionow M, Papay F, Kulahci Y, et al. Coronal-posterior approach for face/scalp flap harvesting in preparation for face transplantation. *J Reconstr Microsurg* 2006;22:399–405.
23. Siemionow M, Agaoglu G. The issue of "facial appearance and identity transfer" after mock transplantation: a cadaver study in preparation for facial allograft transplantation in humans. *J Reconstr Microsurg* 2006;22:329–334.
24. Siemionow M, Unal S, Agaoglu G, et al. A cadaver study in preparation for facial allograft transplantation in humans: part I. What are alternative sources for total facial defect coverage? *Plast Reconstr Surg* 2006;117:864–872; discussion 873–865.
25. Siemionow M, Agaoglu G, Unal S. A cadaver study in preparation for facial allograft transplantation in humans: part II. Mock facial transplantation. *Plast Reconstr Surg* 2006;117:876–885; discussion 886–878.
26. Baccarani A, Follmar KE, Baumeister SP, et al. Technical and anatomical considerations of face harvest in face transplantation. *Ann Plast Surg* 2006;57:483–488.
27. Baccarani A, Follmar KE, Das RR, et al. A pilot study in sub-SMAS face transplantation: defining donor compatibility and assessing outcomes in a cadaver model. *Plast Reconstr Surg* 2007;119:121–129.
28. Wang HY, Li QF, Zheng SW, et al. Cadaveric comparison of two facial flap-harvesting techniques for alloplastic facial transplantation. *J Plast Reconstr Aesthet Surg* 2007;60:1175–1181.
29. Follmar KE, Baccarani A, Das RR, et al. Osteocutaneous face transplantation. *J Plast Reconstr Aesthet Surg* 2008;61:518–524.
30. Banks ND, Hui-Chou HG, Tripathi S, et al. An anatomical study of external carotid artery vascular territories in face and midface flaps for transplantation. *Plast Reconstr Surg* 2009;123:1677–1687.
31. Meningaud JP, Paraskevas A, Ingallina F, et al. Face transplant graft procurement: a preclinical and clinical study. *Plast Reconstr Surg* 2008;122:1383–1389.
32. Jiang HQ, Wang Y, Hu XB, et al. Composite tissue allograft transplantation of cephalocervical skin flap and two ears. *Plast Reconstr Surg* 2005;115:31e–35e; discussion 36e–37e.
33. Ulusal BG, Ulusal AE, Lin JY, et al. Anatomical and technical aspects of harvesting the auricle as a neurovascular facial subunit transplant in humans. *Plast Reconstr Surg* 2007;120:1540–1545.
34. Hui-Chou HG, Nam AJ, Rodriguez ED. Clinical facial composite tissue allotransplantation: a review of the first four global experiences and future implications. *Plast Reconstr Surg* 2010;125:538–546.
35. Dubernard JM, Lengele B, Morelon E, et al. Outcomes 18 months after the first human partial face transplantation. *N Engl J Med* 2007;357:2451–2460.
36. Petruzzo P, Lanzetta M, Dubernard JM, et al. The international registry on hand and composite tissue transplantation. *Transplantation* 2008;86:487–492.
37. Kanitakis J, Jullien D, Petruzzo P, et al. Clinicopathologic features of graft rejection of the first human hand allograft. *Transplantation* 2003;76:688–693.
38. Lee WP, Yaremchuk MJ, Pan YC, et al. Relative antigenicity of components of a vascularized limb allograft. *Plast Reconstr Surg* 1991;87:401–411.
39. Vasilic D, Alloway RR, Barker JH, et al. Risk assessment of immunosuppressive therapy in facial transplantation. *Plast Reconstr Surg* 2007;120: 657–668.
40. Pushpakumar SB, Barker JH, Soni CV, et al. Clinical considerations in face transplantation. *Burns* 2010;36:951–958.
41. Buncke HJ, Hoffman WY, Alpert BS, et al. Microvascular transplant of two free scalp flaps between identical twins. *Plast Reconstr Surg* 1982;70:605–609.
42. Alam DS, Papay F, Djohan R, et al. The technical and anatomical aspects of the world's first near-total human face and maxilla transplant. *Arch Facial Plast Surg* 2009;11:369–377.
43. Siemionow MZ, Papay F, Djohan R, et al. First U.S. near-total human face transplantation: a paradigm shift for massive complex injuries. *Plast Reconstr Surg* 2010;125:111–122.
44. Eaton L. First patient to receive complete face transplant can leave hospital. *BMJ* 2010;341:c4088.
45. Siemionow M, Ozturk C. An update on facial transplantation cases performed between 2005–2010. *Plast Reconstr Surg* 2011;128(6):707e–720e.

SECTION 3

THE TRUNK

CHAPTER 42

Vascular Imaging and Mapping in Breast Reconstruction

Risal Djohan, Cemile Nurdan Ozturk, and Robert Lohman

VASCULAR IMAGING AND MAPPING IN BREAST RECONSTRUCTION

Patients undergoing mastectomy have many reconstructive options. Autologous tissue is often preferred because a more natural-appearing breast can be created. When using autologous tissue, complication rates are generally low, and patient satisfaction high. Although the short-term cost of prosthetic breast reconstruction is less (1), the long-term expenses associated with autologous tissue reconstruction are similar to, or less than that of implant reconstruction, and the potential for long-term implant complications is eliminated. In the 1980s, the transverse rectus abdominis musculocutaneous (TRAM) flap was introduced for use in autologous breast reconstruction. This flap, supplied by the superior epigastric vessels, was rotated from the abdomen and tunneled beneath the intervening tissue to reconstruct the breast. Today, the abdomen still remains the most common donor site for breast reconstruction. However, the techniques of flap elevation and transfer have evolved considerably. Contemporary breast reconstruction frequently uses perforator flaps to transfer skin and subcutaneous fat to the chest while preserving the rectus abdominus muscle and fascia in situ. The perforators are supplied by the deep inferior epigastric vessels, which are usually anastomosed at the recipient site to the internal mammary or thoracodorsal vessels using microvascular techniques. Perforator flaps are reliable; allow for a considerable degree of flexibility in the shape and position of the breast mound; and have the benefit of minimal donor site morbidity, especially in the setting of bilateral breast reconstruction.

The initial step in performing a perforator flap, whether pedicle or free, involves identifying the best large perforator or an adequate number of suitably sized smaller perforators to perfuse the flap without zones of ischemia. The size, location, and course of these vital perforators can be complex and unpredictable. Because of this, vascular imaging and mapping can play an important role in flap design for perforator breast reconstruction. Whereas the term *vascular mapping* refers to the identification of the availability and topographic anatomy of a vessel (a perforator in this instance) or vessels, *vascular imaging* concerns the various methods used to obtain these "maps." Preoperative vascular imaging can be used to identify the location and anatomic course of the perforators, enabling the flap to be designed around the most robust ones. An understanding of the anatomic location and course of the perforators preceding surgery also helps facilitate dissection during the operation. *Intraoperative* mapping can also play a role in perforator selection. It allows a surgeon to validate the design of a flap in real time. Superfluous perforators, as well as those that are critical to the perfusion of the flap, can be identified. The superfluous perforators can be sacrificed as they exit the anterior rectus sheath, thus minimizing unnecessary dissection and the risk of donor site morbidity while the surgeon's efforts are critically focused on the perfusion of the flap. After the flap has been transferred to the chest, both intraoperative mapping and imaging can be used to identify potential problems such as kinks or external compression of the vascular pedicle, as well as areas of ischemia in the flap. Intraoperative mapping might also be useful in evaluating the condition of mastectomy skin flaps so that potentially necrotic skin may be excised. Identification of these problems is vitally important to avoid early complications such as partial or total flap loss and unplanned reoperation, as well as late complications such as ischemic fat necrosis that can delay healing and lead to poor aesthetic outcomes.

The technology for vascular mapping and imaging has developed rapidly and in parallel with the increasing popularity of

SECTION 3

TABLE 42-1 Characteristics of Imaging Modalities

Features	HHD	CDU	CTA	MRA	ICG-A	NIRS
Preoperative imaging	+	+	+	+	+	–
Intraoperative imaging	+	–	–	–	+	+
Three-dimensional imaging	–	+	+	+	–	–
Radiation exposure	–	–	+	–	–	–
Invasiveness	–	–	+	+/–	+	–
Reproducibility	–	–	+	+	–	–
Information on regional anatomy	–	+	+	+	–	–
Accuracy	+	++	++++	+++	++	+
Practicability	+	–	+	+	–	+
High costs	–	–	+	++	++	+

CDU, color duplex ultrasound; CTA, computed tomography angiography; HHD, handheld Doppler; ICG-A; indocyanine green angiography; MRA, magnetic resonance angiography; NIRS, near-infrared spectrophotometry.

perforator flaps for breast reconstruction. Currently, several different modalities are commercially available that can provide surgeons with a detailed knowledge of topography at the flap harvest site and help to evaluate perfusion of the flap both before and after transfer. There are unique strengths and weaknesses associated with each of these methods, which are summarized in Table 42-1. Used either individually or in concert, the various techniques of vascular imaging and mapping can facilitate flap preparation while potentially reducing postoperative complications.

The primary purpose of preoperative mapping is to define the relevant vascular anatomy to facilitate an expedient and safe operation. Without preoperative mapping, the surgeon is blind to vascular anomalies until the operation is well underway. If the surgeon is aware of the vascular anatomy ahead of time, a more complete operative plan can be developed, which results in more carefully targeted dissection. Although preoperative mapping usually implies an evaluation of perforators at the donor site, the same techniques can also be used to investigate recipient vessels (2). This is especially useful in situations in which previous chest irradiation or operations have occurred in the chest before reconstruction.

Common methods of preoperative perforator mapping include use of handheld Doppler, color-flow ultrasonography, and conventional angiography, as well as computed tomography (CT) and magnetic resonance angiography (MRA).

Preoperative planning is especially important for perforator flaps because of the variability of the anatomy as well as the complexity of the dissection. Without it, the surgeon must decide, rapidly, which perforators are important for perfusion of the flap. To do this requires more dissection than that required when the position of the dominant perforators is already known. Furthermore, imaging also reveals the location, course, and arborization pattern of the main axial vessels. With this knowledge, the surgeon can make reasonable predictions about which perforators will be critical for flap perfusion and which ones will be superfluous. Preoperative imaging also provides information about other aspects of the abdominal wall, such as hernias, or rectus diastasis, which might complicate flap preparation (3). The investigation may also be performed in combination with a survey for recurrence or metastases as part of the oncologic evaluation.

Without preoperative imaging, the surgeon has no option but to explore most or all of the perforators for the best combination of vessels. This process can be time consuming and may result in inadvertent injury or vasospasm to the fragile vasculature. It can initiate a self-reinforcing feedback loop that actually increases the difficulty of the operation. Preoperative imaging can drive the course of the operation in the opposite direction: it is likely to shorten the operative time and minimize dissection at the donor site. Rozen et al. showed that patients who underwent computerized tomography angiography (CTA) before abdominal perforator flap surgery had fewer flap and donor site complications (4). Patients who underwent preoperative imaging experienced less flap loss, less fat necrosis, and less abdominal weakness. The best outcomes in breast reconstruction occur when the flaps are well perfused, when there is minimal disruption of muscle and the donor site, and when the motor nerves are preserved. Preoperative imaging allows the surgeon to select larger but fewer perforators, thus minimizing injury to the underlying muscle and nerves.

METHODS OF PREOPERATIVE MAPPING

Handheld Doppler Ultrasonography

The oldest and most basic tool for perforator mapping is the handheld Doppler probe. This device has been in clinical use for more than 40 years and is commonplace among most plastic surgeons (5). This is an inexpensive, noninvasive, simple, and effective technique to identify perforators under the skin paddle before the operation starts. Furthermore, it is highly portable and almost universally available. Handheld Doppler is used in the preoperative setting to mark the location of perforating vessels on the skin paddle, but it can also be used intraoperatively to follow the course of an intramuscular vessel.

A variety of commercially available handheld Doppler probes are available. Standard ultrasound frequencies for these probes are 8 and 10 MHz, allowing the signal to penetrate 20 and 15 mm deep to the surface, respectively (6). The angle of insonation should be perpendicular to the vessel of interest. It may be necessary to change the angle of insonation by adjusting the position of the probe to find the loudest signal. The loudest signals typically correlate with the largest perforators; these points are marked on the skin with a small suture or indelible marker. It is important to realize that pressure from the Doppler probe may occlude flow in the underlying perforator, and in most circumstances, the probe should only lightly rest on the surface of the flap.

Although handheld Doppler is easy to use, the audible output can be difficult to interpret for a number of reasons, one of them being that no actual image of the underlying vessels is created. Handheld Doppler cannot be used to determine the caliber of the perforators and is ineffective in predicting where the perforators exit the fascia and enter the skin paddle. Handheld Doppler also cannot be used to distinguish between the perforators and the main axial vessel deep to them. Furthermore, its accuracy is also dependent on thickness of subcutaneous tissue (7). In heavier patients, handheld Doppler cannot be used to locate vessels within or deep to the rectus abdominis muscle before surgery.

Another problem with handheld Doppler lies with the fact that it is quite sensitive in identifying pulsatile blood flow, but it is not very specific (3,8–10). Thus, the number of false-positive signals is high. Giunta et al. reported a false positivity rate of 47.6 percent in their series, a significantly high rate, which he attributed to devicès ability to detect very small vessels (8). These smaller perforators, although audible with handheld Doppler, may not be able to support a perforator-based flap. It can also be difficult to distinguish between dominant perforators that must be preserved and superfluous perforators that can be sacrificed. A superficially located main vessel may also potentially confound the process of locating the perforators. Therefore, handheld Doppler is more reliable for cases such as a superior gluteal artery perforator (SGAP) flap, where the perforators are crossing the muscle fascia almost perpendicularly (3).

Handheld Doppler provides, then, only a limited amount of information about the location of the perforators and essentially no information about the quality of the perforators. In patients with straightforward anatomy, handheld Doppler can be used as the primary method of mapping (6). However, during dissection of the flap, the surgeon is advised to initially leave a substantial margin of tissue around the Doppler signal because there can be a wide variation between the point where the perforator exits the fascia and the point where the signal was marked on the skin paddle. Although handheld Doppler facilitates the intraoperative location of vessels and allows for some degree of preoperative mapping, it should not be used as the only method of evaluation in more complex cases. For obese patients who have had prior abdominal operations or inconclusive signal interpretation, more definitive techniques for perforator mapping should be considered, and handheld Doppler should only be used as an adjunctive technique.

Color Duplex Ultrasonography

As with handheld Doppler, color duplex ultrasonography also uses a crystal to generate an ultrasonic signal to locate blood vessels. The hardware and software used by the color duplex system is more complex, more expensive, and is not as widely available. However, the color duplex system addresses many of the shortcomings of handheld Doppler. Transducers are available that can identify vessels within and deep to the rectus abdominus muscle. A colorized image of the vessels is created that displays the location of the perforators and axial vessels, as well as the direction of flow and flow velocity within them (Figure 42-1). Color duplex ultrasonography has greater sensitivity and specificity than handheld Doppler (3,11,12). Furthermore, it can also be used to evaluate the diameter of the perforators and estimate hemodynamic characteristics such as flow, volume, and velocity. This powerful tool has the ability to identify the dominant perforator supplying a flap (3,9,13,14). Additionally, color-flow duplex imaging provides detailed information about the three-dimensional course of perforators, as well as any segments of reduced flow, stenosis, or occlusion (3,15). This information is especially valuable when the perforators or the inferior epigastric vessels themselves may have been injured by previous surgery or trauma (14).

Despite its potential advantages, use of color-flow duplex ultrasonography has not become the dominant method of perforator mapping, mainly because of the complexity in completing an examination and interpreting the results. Even in the hands of a skilled technologist, it can take up to 1 hour to complete an examination. Interpretation of the results requires a physician who is both familiar with vascular imaging and has some knowledge of the specifics of perforator flap surgery. Furthermore, plastic surgeons often find it difficult to interpret the images, which limits the usefulness of these pictures in the operating room.

Very few operating rooms have the capability for intraoperative color-flow scanning, and real time imaging is almost

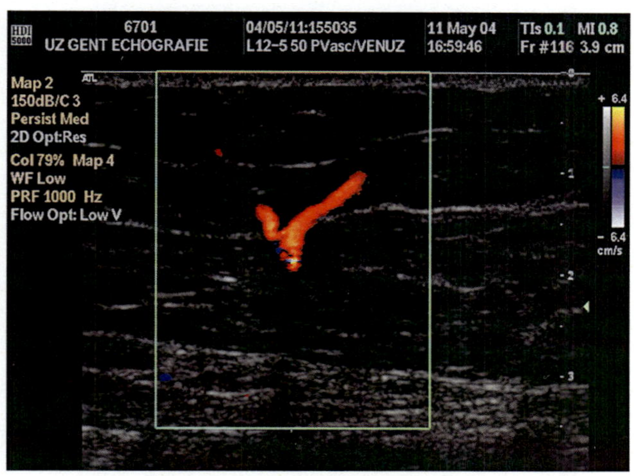

FIGURE 42-1 The perforator is clearly visible with color duplex ultrasonography. (Courtesy of Philip Blondeel.)

never performed. Color-flow duplex mapping has largely been supplanted by CTA and magnetic resonance angiography (MRA) but is still indicated when these techniques are contraindicated or unavailable.

Computed Tomography Angiography

Computed tomography angiography rapidly became the preferred method of preoperative imaging for perforator flaps after the technique was introduction by Masia et al. in 2006 (2,10). Advances in CT currently allow for high-resolution cross-sectional images to be spaced 1 mm apart. Software can then be used to reconstruct these images in multiple different planes. A typical study takes 5 to 10 minutes (actual image acquisition, 10–12 seconds) to complete (9,10). A bolus of iodinated contrast medium is injected intravenously at a rate of 4 mL/sec and 1-mm or thinner image slices are generated depending on the CT scanner used (6,9). These scans are then reformatted into multiple-view reconstructions using commercially available software. Selective contrast injection into the deep inferior epigastric vessels is used to highlight the axial vessels and the perforators.

Computed tomography angiography is highly accurate and provides anatomic detail that is superior to color duplex ultrasonography as reported by several authors (12,16–18). Using CTA, the location, size, and course of the perforators, as well as branching patterns of main axial vessels can be effectively demonstrated (10,16,18) (Figure 42-2). Even vessels as small as 0.3 mm can be visualized (19). CTA has most commonly been used to evaluate the abdominal wall donor site in preparation for deep inferior epigastric perforator (DIEP) flaps. It has proven particularly useful because of the anatomic variability of the inferior epigastric vessels and their perforators.

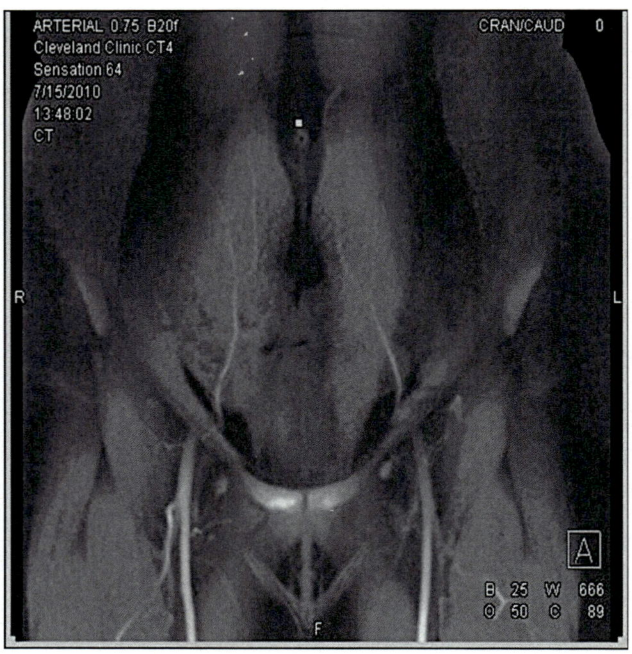

FIGURE 42-2 The branching pattern of the deep inferior epigastric artery can be clearly visualized with computed tomography angiography.

Interpretation of the results is fairly straightforward, and there is little interobserver variability. The radiology report usually includes the location and diameter of suitable perforators in each hemiabdomen. The locations where the perforators emerge from the fascia are reported as coordinates relative to the umbilicus. Additional information about the arborization pattern of perforators in subcutaneous fat, the intramuscular course of the perforators (short vs. long), and branching patterns of the main pedicle can be easily seen on the actual CTA scan. Digital or printed copies of the studies can be brought to the operating room for reference during surgery, and findings can be correlated with handheld Doppler.

Potential disadvantages of CTA include the need for contrast injection, radiation exposure, and the relatively high cost. The radiation dose is similar to that of a conventional abdominal CT (10,12) but can be decreased by limiting the study to the area between the origin of deep inferior epigastric arteries and a level 4 cm superior to the umbilicus (2,9). No useful perforators are present above to this level, and imaging there adds no value to the study. A small dose of contrast (100–150 cc of iodinated contrast medium) is used. Allergic reactions to contrast are possible with any dose, and CTA is contraindicated for patients with a history of iodine-based contrast allergy. In a well-hydrated patient with no history of preexisting renal disease or diabetes, there is essentially no risk to the kidneys. It is true that CTA is expensive. A typical study, including interpretation, cost about $400 in 2010 (2,12). However, CTA may be cost effective if the information it provides leads to shorter operative time, reduced complications, and reduced length of stay in the hospital for the patient (4,10).

Magnetic Resonance Angiography

Magnetic resonance angiography is another powerful imaging tool, which makes use of a strong magnetic field and radio waves. Ionizing radiation is not required. In response to these conditions, hydrogen nuclei from the patient emit a signal. Variations in these signals are then used to generate a high-resolution image. MRA is particularly useful for imaging changes in blood flow. Although most MRA studies involve the administration of non–iodine-based contrast mediums, in some situations, the need for contrast material may be eliminated completely (20,21). Although MRA is a promising technique, it has not proven consistently useful for imaging vessels smaller than 1 mm, such as perforators (19). Although some authors have been able to accurately identify perforators in the abdominal wall (20–22), others have been less successful and believe that CTA is more useful for imaging small vessels (11,19,23,24). Some of these discrepancies may result from the wide variety of equipment and scanning protocols used by various authors. It is often difficult for patients to hold still during MRA studies, which generally require more time than CTA. Thus, MRA is more often limited by motion artifact. Other factors that can limit MRA image quality include imperfect fat suppression and inferior spatial resolution; the latter is more likely the result of a weak magnet or other hardware or software issues. However, inferior spatial resolution may not be the cause of poor images per se (19,20,25). Furthermore, MRA cannot be used in patients with certain metal implants and pacemakers. Patients who are claustrophobic or sensitive to loud noises may have difficulty completing the examination without sedation. As with CTA, MRA is expensive; in 2010, a typical preoperative study cost about $600 (2,19).

Currently, MRA is still under investigation an investigational tool for perforator mapping. The evolution and refinement of hardware, software, scanning protocols, and contrast material continue rapidly (2,25). Some centers report satisfactory results, but others have found the technique less useful.

TECHNIQUES FOR EVALUATING INTRAOPERATIVE PERFUSION

Fluorescent Angiography with Indocyanine Green

Although color-flow duplex ultrasonography, CTA, and MRA proved useful in determining information about the location and course of blood vessels in the flap, they do not provide any information about actual perfusion of the flap. One technique useful to evaluate perfusion is laser-assisted indocyanine green imaging. This method was initially used for angiography of retina, which then followed by its use to evaluate perfusion of pedicle flaps and vascular anastomoses in cardiovascular surgery in the late 1990s. Holm et al. used this method to monitor free flaps starting in 2002 (26). The commercially available system is known as SPY Elite® (LifeCell Corporation, a division of KCI).

Its principle is somewhat similar to standard angiography except fluorescent dye is injected rather than iodine contrast solution, and no radiation is required. Indocyanine green dye is administered through a peripheral venous catheter. Light from an overhead laser (at near infrared wavelength of 805 nm) excites the dye, and a camera then captures the image, which is manipulated using proprietary software. The camera then records a cinegraphic image for up to 4 minutes, which is saved to a hard drive. It is possible to image the flap several times during the operation because multiple injections of dye are possible, up to a maximum of 5 mg/kg (27). The half-life of indocyanine green injected in this manner is 3 to 4 minutes (26). The laser penetrates about 2 to 3 mm deep to the surface of the skin, and the image is a composite of the tissue in that region.

Laser-assisted indocyanine green imaging contributes three general types of information. It provides live documentation of blood flow in the pedicle and across the microvascular anastomoses. Areas of stenosis, occlusion, and other technical problems can easily be demonstrated (27–31). In addition, the skin paddle can be evaluated to gather information about global perfusion of the flap (Figure 42-3). Zones of ischemia and hypoperfusion can be identified and excised as needed after transfer of the flap. In this manner, flap design can be validated during the operation, which may limit problems with fat or skin necrosis after surgery. After the flap has been transferred, indocyanine green imaging can also be used to identify venous congestion. Under normal conditions, the dye is expected to wash out of the flap after 3 to 4 minutes. A final image of the flap is made 4 to 5 minutes after the last dye injection. Any dye remaining in the skin paddle at that time is very suggestive of venous congestion.

Another potential application of laser assisted indocyanine green imaging is functional perforator mapping just before surgery and to aid with perforator selection during surgery. Recent modifications in the image processing software allow the device to construct a perfusion map of the flap, which highlights areas of increased tissue oxygenation (Figure 42-4). The perforators appear as a "fluorescent blush" on the skin (see Figure 42-3A). Using this map, the skin incision can be adjusted to ensure that areas of maximal perfusion, which correspond to the perforators,

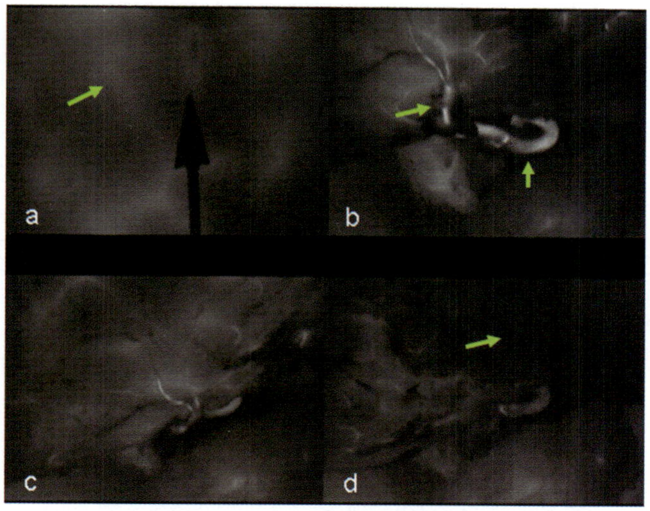

FIGURE 42-3 (A) Fluorescence blush (green arrow) on the DIEP skin paddle shows perforator location. (B) Pedicle (arrow, right) and perforator (arrow, left) on the undersurface of the flap. (C) Undersurface of a well perfused flap. (D) Dark area (arrow) without fluorescence represents hypoperfusion.

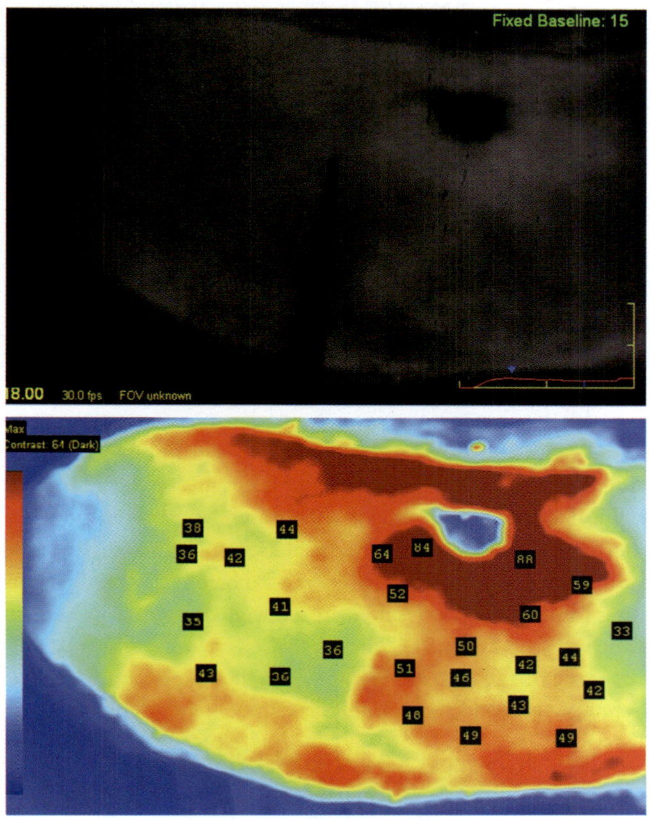

FIGURE 42-4 The correlation of fluorescence with color perfusion topography.

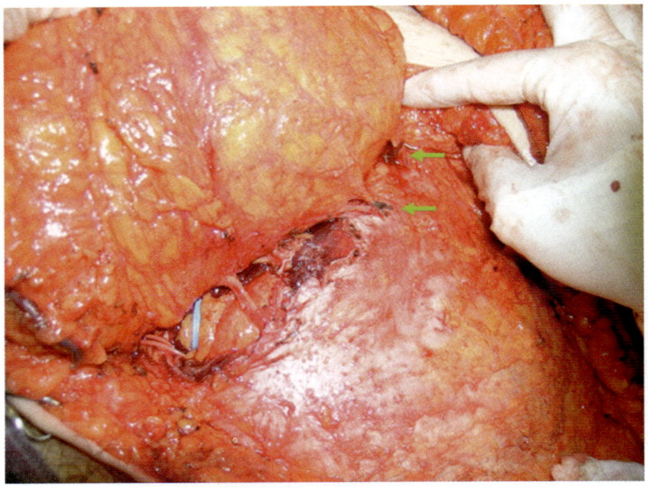

FIGURE 42-5 Some of the perforators are temporarily clamped (arrows) to see perfusion on the remaining perforator.

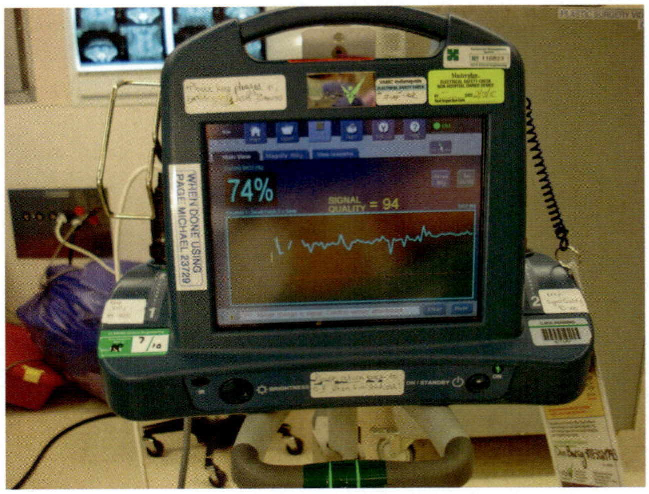

FIGURE 42-6 The near-infrared spectrophotometry monitor showing oxygenation of flap.

are included with the skin paddle (27,29,31). During the elevation of a DIEP flap, indocyanine green dye studies can be used to determine which row of perforators (or group of perforators) makes the most significant contribution to perfusion of the flap. This can be done by applying microvascular clamps to the perforators the surgeon is considering sacrificing (Figure 42-5). After the clamps have been applied, a bolus of dye is administered, and the flap is then imaged. If there is no change in perfusion of the flap, then the clamped perforators can be divided without concern for ischemia. However, if imaging shows areas of hypoperfusion after the clamps are applied, the corresponding perforator should not be divided. This method can systematically identify the dominant perforator to the flap and potentially minimize the number of perforators that must be dissected during preparation of the flap (29).

Although rare, hypersensitivity to indocyanine green dye has been reported, and a small test dose is recommended before administration of a full dose. A drawback of this method is that the system is somewhat cumbersome to use. The camera must be positioned immediately overhead from the tissue to be imaged. Fluorescent signals arising from tissue that are not parallel to the face of the camera give the false impression of greatly reduced perfusion. Also, the camera must be positioned approximately 30 cm away to generate an accurate image (30). The fluorescence captured by the camera arises from the most superficial 2 to 3 mm of the flap. However, the system can be used to image multiple different types of tissue and is not just restricted to skin. Clinical studies have shown indocyanine green imaging can effectively identify areas of critical ischemia and anastomotic problems that can be successfully revised before leaving the operating room. This has resulted in reduced complication rates in some settings (27,30,31). These benefits may offset the relatively high cost of the system. However, further experience with the technique is needed so that its role can be better defined.

Near-Infrared Spectrophotometry

Near-infrared spectrophotometry (NIRS) is another method to measure tissue oxygenation. A probe is used to emit near-infrared light into the tissue. The infrared light is either absorbed by chromophores in the tissue or scattered. A portion of the scattered light is reflected to the sensor, which uses proprietary software to convert this signal to data about tissue oxygenation status. NIRS allows for noninvasive assessment of tissue oxygenation as it changes in real time. The data are then plotted over time on a computer display. NIRS is most commonly used in plastic surgery for postoperative flap monitoring (ViOptix, Fremont, CA) (Figure 42-6). Another commercially available system is Spectros, T-Stat VLS Tissue Oxymeter (Spectros Corp., Portola Valley, CA), which is marketed as a tool to monitor perfusion and relatively sensitive in detecting tissue ischemia. A similar spot tissue oxygenation monitoring system is called InSpectra monitor (Hutchinson Technology Inc, Hutchinson, MN), which is marketed as a device designed to monitor perfusion in critically ill patients. There is considerable variation in baseline values for tissue oxygenation (32), and there can also be considerable regional variation in values for the same patient. Therefore, spot values can be difficult to interpret, and most authors emphasize the importance of trends in tissue oxygenation over time (32,33). A rapid decline of 20% or greater from initial baseline, sustained for half an hour, is considered to be a sign of acute critical ischemia (32). When used as a monitoring technique, tissue oxymetry is useful for identification of compromised flaps. Problems at either the arterial or venous anastomosis or because of other factors such as external compression cause a rapid fall in tissue oxygen levels. This often occurs before changes in Doppler signals or the clinical appearance of the flap (33–35).

In addition to postoperative monitoring, NIRS can be used to identify functionally important perforators. Initially, a baseline value for tissue oxygenation is obtained. Then microvascular clamps are applied to perforators the surgeon is considering ligating. After allowing the flap to equilibrate for 2 to 3 minutes, tissue oxygenation is reassessed. It is important to measure the tissue oxygen levels in the same location. If there is no reduction in tissue oxygenation, the perforators can be ligated without risk of ischemia. However, if tissue oxygenation falls by more than 20%, the perforator in question should probably be preserved. More work is needed to determine if there is an absolute value for tissue oxygenation that is associated with critical ischemia and if patterns of changes in oxygenation are associated with specific injuries.

MAPPING AND PERFORATOR SELECTION IN PERFORATOR FLAPS

Flap Selection

Most flaps used for microvascular breast reconstruction come from the abdomen. The abdomen usually provides an adequate volume to reconstruct both breasts if needed. The texture of the soft tissue is similar to that of the native breast, and the skin quality is usually adequate (36). Preoperative imaging of abdomen contributes invaluable information to the surgeon. It is possible learn about the size and quality of the perforators, as well as to evaluate the superficial and deep inferior epigastric vessels (Figure 42-7). With this information in hand, the surgeon can decide about the relative merits of a TRAM, a DIEP, or a superficial inferior epigastric artery (SIEA) flap for a given patient or if an abdominal flap is contraindicated altogether. Preoperative imaging will alert the surgeon to the possibility of situations such as rectus diastasis or hernias, which could complicate preparation of the flap. Furthermore, preoperative imaging can help the surgeon determine which half of the abdomen to use for unilateral breast reconstruction, which row of perforators is dominant, and where the largest perforators are located within a given row. This is especially useful if the patient is obese or has undergone previous abdominal surgery in which the perforators may have been injured or if they are encased in scar tissue. Under these conditions, the results of preoperative imaging can influence the decision about which flap to use for breast reconstruction.

The DIEP Flap

In the axial CTA view, the deep inferior epigastric artery (DIEA) can be seen to travel in a cephalad direction from its origin from the external iliac artery. After passing though preperitoneal tissue, it enters the rectus abdominis muscle from its lateral side and travels either deep to or within the muscle. Typically, the artery bifurcates inferior to the umbilicus to give rise to a medial and lateral branch from which spring the medial and lateral row perforators, respectively. Superior to the umbilicus, the DIEA anastomoses with the superior epigastric artery, which is itself derived from the internal mammary artery. CTA is used to image the vessels from the point of their origin to a level about 4 to 5 cm above to the umbilicus (10). DIEP (and SIEA) flaps are usually designed inferior to this level. Branching patterns in the DIEA pedicle (see Figure 42-2) and the presence of a potentially useful SIEA are noted (Figure 42-8). Special attention is paid to the location, number, diameter, and rectus sheath exit points of the perforators, as well as their course outside the muscle. A virtual coordinate system, with the umbilicus at its center, a y-axis running in the superior/inferior direction, and an x-axis running transversely is used to describe the location of these perforators (Figure 42-9). The position of the perforators, as measured in centimeters from the umbilicus, is plotted along these axes. The diameter of the perforators is also noted. While this information is reported by the radiologist, it is important for the surgeon to review the study to become familiar with the three-dimensional anatomy of the vessels. At the time of surgery, the position of the largest perforators is confirmed using handheld Doppler and is marked on the skin with respect to the umbilicus.

DIEA perforators are quite variable. They often exit at the tendinous inscriptions, travel directly under the rectus abdominis

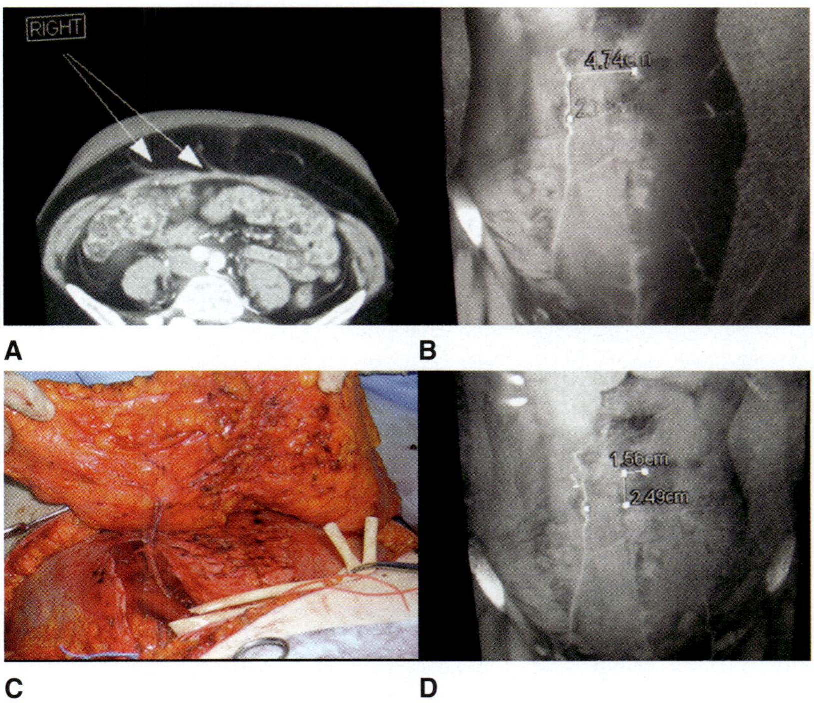

FIGURE 42-7 The computed tomography angiography images correlate accurately with intraoperative findings. (A) The perforator vessels are seen on the CTA as they exit the fascia (arrows). (C) The intraoperative view of the same perforators. (B, D) The coordinates of the perforator vessels in relation to umbilicus are marked on CTA.

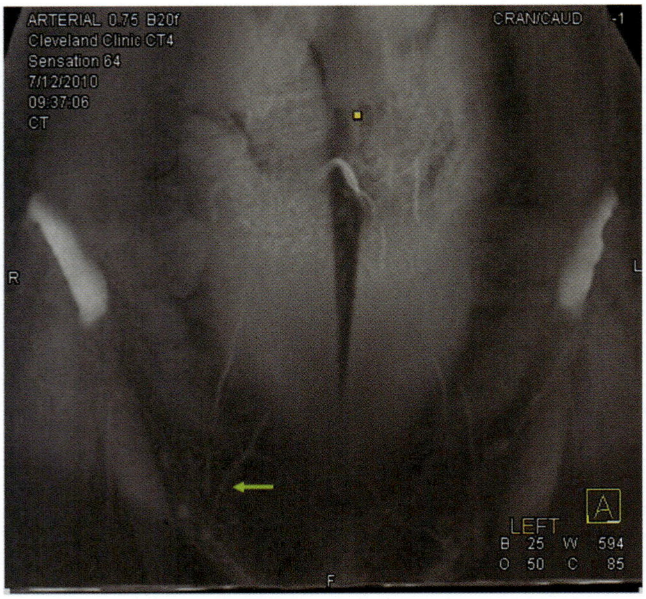

FIGURE 42-8 The superficial inferior epigastric artery (arrow) can be usually identified.

sheath for variable distances, traverse rectus muscle at different angles, and can course around the medial edge of the muscle without ever penetrating it. An ideal DIEA perforator has been described as having the following attributes: large diameter (>1 mm), located near the center of the flap, a short intramuscular course, a broad subcutaneous branching pattern to supply a large segment of skin, and a long subfascial course without adhering to the tendinous inscriptions (2,4) (Figure 42-10). Preoperative imaging with CTA or MRA can be used to identify perforators with these characteristics and help the surgeon focus dissection on the most promising vessels with minimal morbidity to the rectus muscle. Communication between superficial and deep venous networks is also desirable to prevent problems related to venous drainage; however, this is not so easy to visualize. A single large perforator or several perforators may be used to supply the flap. The ideal number of perforators is not known and probably varies from case to case depending on the diameters of the perforators themselves. However, donor site morbidity increases with a more extensive dissection, (2,16,36), and it is therefore most desirable to dissect "just enough" perforators—ideally, a single perforator—to adequately perfuse the flap without including superfluous vessels. Intraoperative perfusion studies help the surgeon to safely arrive at this endpoint. In most cases, for a unilateral DIEP flap, a medial row perforator will provide sufficient perfusion on both sides of midline. The use of medial perforators also allows an easier dissection without the concern of injuring the motor nerve branches that innervate the rectus muscle laterally. However, when bilateral reconstruction is planned, a lateral perforator may be preferred to maximize perfusion at the most lateral zones of the flaps (37).

The SIEA Flap

The SIEA flap is not a popular choice among autologous reconstruction options because of its variable anatomy with relatively smaller vessel caliber. If a SIEA flap is to be harvested, the skin island should be positioned somewhat inferiorly to the skin paddle of a DIEP flap. This improves the likelihood that the flap will be well perfused and appropriately drained by the SIEV (36,38). The larger periumbilical perforators, which are critical to perfusion of the DIEP flap, are not included with the SIEA flap. Preoperative imaging plays an important role here because it is possible to visualize SIEA or SIEV, including its position and diameter, with CTA (18,36,39). An SIEA flap may be considered if the artery visualized on the CTA is greater than 1.5 mm in diameter (35,39). Alternatively, the skin paddle can be designed overlying both the SIEA territory and the DIEP territory. The final decision between the two flaps is then made based on the results of intraoperative perfusion studies. Holm et al. suggested this strategy because of the variable patters of perfusion noted in SIEA flaps. Tailoring the shape of the skin paddle based on results of perfusion studies ensures that the flap is well perfused. If the SIEA skin paddle is not well perfused or appears congested, the DIEP flap is selected instead (40). Even if the SIEA is not clearly visible on the CTA, most surgeons would still make an attempt to find the vessels along

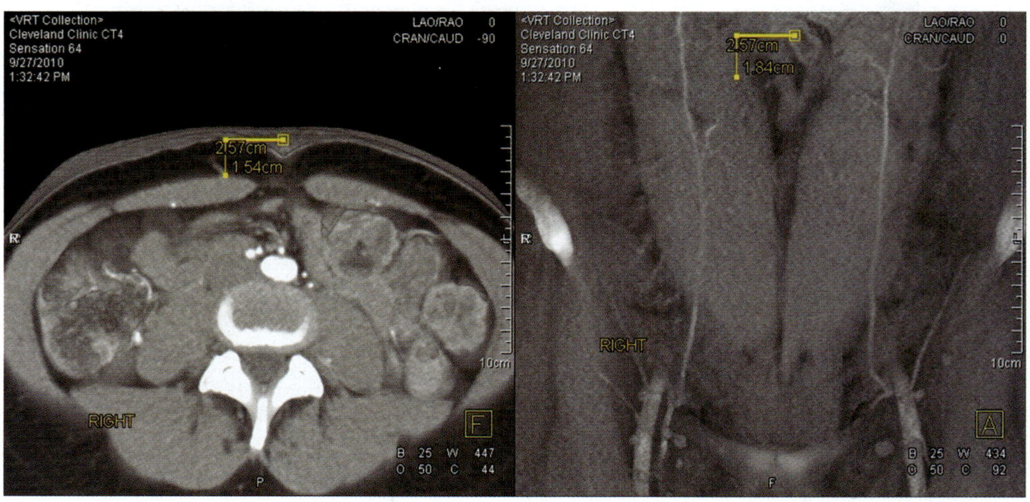

FIGURE 42-9 Coordinates are marked on axial and coronal sections.

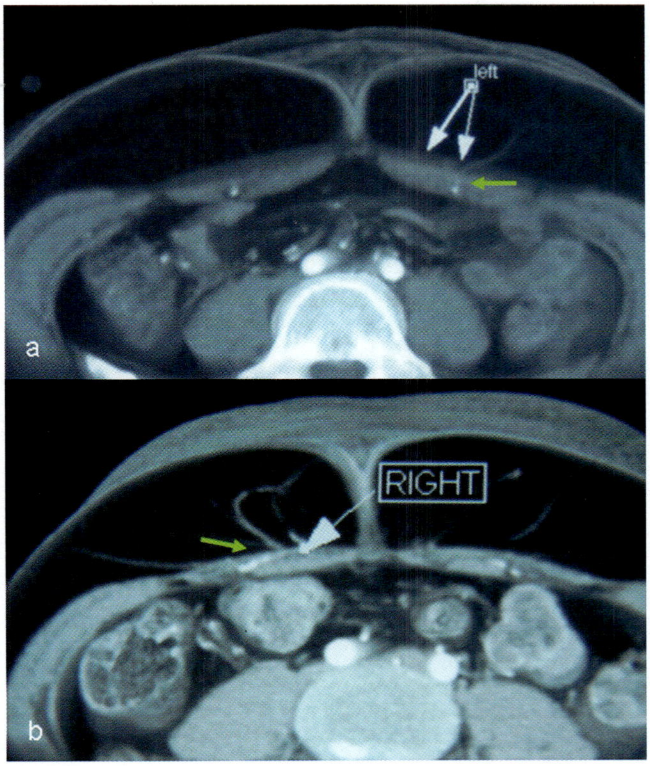

FIGURE 42-10 (**A**) An ideal perforator (arrow) that is in a central location and has very short intramuscular course. (**B**) A good size perforator (arrow) but with a long intramuscular course.

the lower abdominal incision. A good-caliber superficial vein is almost always saved as a backup in case there is venous outflow insufficiency from the deep venous system.

Other Perforator Flaps

After a partial mastectomy, regional pedicled perforator flaps may be suitable for reconstruction, depending on the location and size of the defect. The thoracodorsal artery perforator (TAP) flap makes use of a skin paddle centered over the latissimus muscle and is perfused by a single large perforator from the thoracodorsal system. In breast reconstruction, this flap is indicated for superolateral, inferolateral, and inferomedial defects (41). The location of the perforator can be predicted using handheld or color-flow Doppler. Design can be validated during surgery using either indocyanine green or tissue oxymetry. We are not aware of surgeons using CTA or MRA to image this flap preoperatively. Another choice for lateral defects is the lateral intercostal artery perforator (LICAP) flap. This flap uses a skin paddle supplied by a perforator located between the fourth and eighth intercostal arteries. As with the TAP flap, there is little reported experience with preoperative imaging of this flap, but intraoperative mapping proves useful in assessing the perfusion for the skin flap as it is prepared (36,42).

The SGAP flap uses a skin paddle at the buttocks and is supplied by perforators from the superior gluteal artery. This flap is indicated for patients who desire autologous reconstruction and are in need of a large flap when the abdomen is not available as a donor site. The medial perforators have a relatively short course; however, the lateral perforators travel obliquely through the muscle, thereby yielding more length. (25). Dissection can be tedious, but preoperative mapping with CTA or MRA may facilitate dissection and help in selection of the dominant perforator (25,43).

Another option for reconstructing the breast in patients with unsuitable abdominal tissue as donor site is transverse upper gracilis (TUG) or transverse myocutaneous gracilis (TMG) free flap. This flap can provide a sufficient tissue from the medial upper thigh with a relatively hidden scar with minimal or no functional deficit on the donor site. The criticism on this flap is the modest volume of reconstruction and potential donor site wound complication (44,45). We have so far not used any means of preoperative radiographic imaging or mapping in planning the surgery, but the use of an indocyanine green perfusion study could help in determining the estimated location of the potential perforators identified as "blush" spots in the proposed flap design.

CONCLUSION AND FUTURE

The goals of preoperative imaging and intraoperative mapping are to provide a roadmap that facilitates planning, to minimize dissection and morbidity at the donor site, to ensure that the flap is well perfused, and to reduce long-term complications such as fat necrosis. Furthermore, it is important to use imaging and mapping techniques that minimize costs as well as the risk of side effects. Currently, the most accurate imaging methods are CTA and MRA. MRA has great potential in becoming the method of choice if the image quality can be improved. Efforts to improve image quality and resolution while reducing the need for radiation and toxic contrast are likely to dominate work in this area in the near future. Functional mapping using techniques such as NIRS and indocyanine green are in their infancy. Both systems are currently somewhat expensive and cumbersome to use. However, they also show promise because they allow flap design to be validated in real time based on accurate information about perfusion and oxygenation. As these imaging and mapping technologies develop, the outcomes of perforator flaps will continue to improve.

ACKNOWLEDGMENT

Special thanks to Nirmala Ramanth for assistance in editing.

REFERENCES

1. Spear SL, Mardini S, Ganz JC. Resource cost comparison of implant-based breast reconstruction versus TRAM flap breast reconstruction. *Plast Reconstr Surg* 2003;112:101.
2. Rozen WM, Garcia-Tutor E, Alonso-Burgos A, et al. Planning and optimising DIEP flaps with virtual surgery: the Navarra experience. *J Plast Reconstr Aesthet Surg* 2010;63:289–297.
3. Blondeel PN, Beyens G, Verhaeghe R, et al. Doppler flowmetry in the planning of perforator flaps. *Br J Plast Surg* 1998;51:202.
4. Rozen WM, Anavekar NS, Ashton MW, et al. Does the preoperative imaging of perforators with CT angiography improve operative outcomes in breast reconstruction? *Microsurgery* 2008;28:516.
5. Aoyagi F, Fujino T, Ohshiro T. Detection of small vessels for microsurgery by a Doppler flowmeter. *Plast Reconstr Surg* 1975;55:372.
6. Smit JM, Klein S, Werker PM. An overview of methods for vascular mapping in the planning of free flaps. *J Plast Reconstr Aesthet Surg* 2010;63:e674.

7. Yu P, Youssef A. Efficacy of the handheld Doppler in preoperative identification of the cutaneous perforators in the anterolateral thigh flap. *Plast Reconstr Surg* 2006;118:928.
8. Giunta RE, Geisweid A, Feller AM. The value of preoperative Doppler sonography for planning free perforator flaps. *Plast Reconstr Surg* 2000;105:2381.
9. Mathes DW, PC. Current techniques in preoperative imaging for abdomen-based perforator flap microsurgical breast reconstruction. *J Reconstr Microsurg* 2010;26:3.
10. Masia J, Clavero JA, Larranaga JR, et al. Multidetector-row computed tomography in the planning of abdominal perforator flaps. *J Plast Reconstr Aesthet Surg* 2006;59:594.
11. Tsukino A, Kurachi K, Inamiya T, Tanigaki T. Preoperative color Doppler assessment in planning of anterolateral thigh flaps. *Plast Reconstr Surg* 2004;113:241.
12. Rozen WM, Ashton MW. Improving outcomes in autologous breast reconstruction. *Aesthetic Plast Surg* 2009;33:327.
13. Chidyllo SA, Jacobs JS. The application of duplex ultrasonography in the preoperative evaluation of patients prior to TRAM flap reconstruction. *Plast Reconstr Surg* 1993;92:174.
14. Hallock GG. Doppler sonography and color duplex imaging for planning a perforator flap. *Clin Plast Surg* 2003;30:347.
15. Dominici C, Pacifici A, Tinti A, et al. Preoperative and postoperative evaluation of latissimus dorsi myocutaneous flap vascularization by color flow duplex scanning. *Plast Reconstr Surg* 1995;96:1358.
16. Masia J, Kosutic D, Clavero JA, et al. Preoperative computed tomographic angiogram for deep inferior epigastric artery perforator flap breast reconstruction. *J Reconstr Microsurg* 2010;26:21.
17. Scott JR, Liu D, Said H, et al. Computed tomographic angiography in planning abdomen-based microsurgical breast reconstruction: a comparison with color duplex ultrasound. *Plast Reconstr Surg* 2010; 125:446.
18. Rozen WM, Phillips TJ, Ashton MW, et al. Preoperative imaging for DIEA perforator flaps: a comparative study of computed tomographic angiography and Doppler ultrasound. *Plast Reconstr Surg* 2008;121:9.
19. Rozen WM, Stella DL, Bowden J, et al. Advances in the pre-operative planning of deep inferior epigastric artery perforator flaps: magnetic resonance angiography. *Microsurgery* 2009;29:119.
20. Greenspun D, Vasile J, Levine JL, et al. Anatomic imaging of abdominal perforator flaps without ionizing radiation: seeing is believing with magnetic resonance imaging angiography. *J Reconstr Microsurg* 2010;26:37.
21. Masia J, Kosutic D, Cervelli D, et al. In search of the ideal method in perforator mapping: noncontrast magnetic resonance imaging. *J Reconstr Microsurg* 2010;26:29.
22. Newman TM, Vasile J, Levine JL, et al. Perforator flap magnetic resonance angiography for reconstructive breast surgery: a review of 25 deep inferior epigastric and gluteal perforator artery flap patients. *J Magn Reson Imaging* 2010;31:1176.
23. Chernyak V, Rozenblit AM, Greenspun DT, et al. Breast reconstruction with deep inferior epigastric artery perforator flap: 3.0-T gadolinium-enhanced MR imaging for preoperative localization of abdominal wall perforators. *Radiology* 2009;250:417.
24. Rozen WM, Stella DL, Phillips TJ, et al. Magnetic resonance angiography in the preoperative planning of DIEA perforator flaps. *Plast Reconstr Surg* 2008;122:222e.
25. Alonso-Burgos A, Garcia-Tutor E, Bastarrika G, et al. Preoperative planning of DIEP and SGAP flaps: preliminary experience with magnetic resonance angiography using 3-tesla equipment and blood-pool contrast medium. *J Plast Reconstr Aesthet Surg* 2010;63:298.
26. Holm C, Tegeler J, Mayr M, et al. Monitoring free flaps using laser-induced fluorescence of indocyanine green: a preliminary experience. *Microsurgery* 2002;22:278.
27. Pestana IA, Coan B, Erdmann D, et al. Early experience with fluorescent angiography in free-tissue transfer reconstruction. *Plast Reconstr Surg* 2009;123:1239.
28. Lee BT, Matsui A, Hutteman M, et al. Intraoperative near-infrared fluorescence imaging in perforator flap reconstruction: current research and early clinical experience. *J Reconstr Microsurg* 2010;26:59.
29. Matsui A, Lee BT, Winer JH, et al. Image-guided perforator flap design using invisible near-infrared light and validation with x-ray angiography. *Ann Plast Surg* 2009;63:327.
30. Newman MI, Samson MC. The application of laser-assisted indocyanine green fluorescent dye angiography in microsurgical breast reconstruction. *J Reconstr Microsurg* 2009;25:21.
31. Komorowska-Timek E, Gurtner GC. Intraoperative perfusion mapping with laser-assisted indocyanine green imaging can predict and prevent complications in immediate breast reconstruction. *Plast Reconstr Surg* 2010;125:1065.
32. Keller A. Noninvasive tissue oximetry for flap monitoring: an initial study. *J Reconstr Microsurg* 2007;23:189.
33. Colwell AS, Wright L, Karanas Y. Near-infrared spectroscopy measures tissue oxygenation in free flaps for breast reconstruction. *Plast Reconstr Surg* 2008;121:344e.
34. Keller A. A new diagnostic algorithm for early prediction of vascular compromise in 208 microsurgical flaps using tissue oxygen saturation measurements. *Ann Plast Surg* 2009;62:538.
35. Repez A, Oroszy D, Arnez ZM. Continuous postoperative monitoring of cutaneous free flaps using near infrared spectroscopy. *J Plast Reconstr Aesthet Surg* 2008;61:71.
36. Hamdi M, Van Landuyt K, Van Hedent E, Duyck P. Advances in autogenous breast reconstruction: the role of preoperative perforator mapping. *Ann Plast Surg* 2007;58:18.
37. Bailey SH, Saint-Cyr M, Wong C, et al. The single dominant medial row perforator DIEP flap in breast reconstruction: three-dimensional perforasome and clinical results. *Plast Reconstr Surg* 2010;126:739.
38. Hamdi M, Blondeel, PN. The superficial inferior epigastric artery flap in breast reconstruction. In Spear S (ed). *Surgery of the Breast, Principles and Art.* Philadelphia: Lippincott Williams and Wilkins, 2006, p. 873.
39. Fukaya E, Kuwatsuru R, Iimura H, et al. Imaging of the superficial inferior epigastric vascular anatomy and preoperative planning for the SIEA flap using MDCTA. *J Plast Reconstr Aesthet Surg* 2011;64:63–68.
40. Holm C, Mayr M, Hofter E, et al. Interindividual variability of the SIEA Angiosome: effects on operative strategies in breast reconstruction. *Plast Reconstr Surg* 2008;122:1612.
41. Hamdi M, Van Landuyt K, Hijjawi JB, et al. Surgical technique in pedicled thoracodorsal artery perforator flaps: a clinical experience with 99 patients. *Plast Reconstr Surg* 2008;121:1632.
42. Hamdi M, Van Landuyt K. Pedicled perforator flaps in breast reconstruction. In Spear S (ed). *Surgery of the Breast, Principles and Art.* Philadelphia: Lippincott Williams and Wilkins, 2006, p. 833.
43. LoTempio MM, Allen RJ. Breast reconstruction with SGAP and IGAP flaps. *Plast Reconstr Surg* 2010;126:393–401.
44. Fattah A, Figus A, Mathur B, Ramakrishnan V. The Transverse myocutaneous gracilis flap: technical refinements. *J Plast Reconstr Aesthet Surg* 2010;63:305–313.
45. Vega S, Sandeen S, Bossert R, Perrone A, Ortiz L, Herrera H : Gracilis Myocutaneous Free Flap in Autologous Breast Reconstruction. *Plast Reconstr Surg* 2009;124:1400.

CHAPTER 43

Breast Reconstruction: Free Transverse Rectus Abdominus Myocutaneous Flaps

Babak J. Mehrara and Christina Y. Ahn

BRIEF HISTORY OF CONVENTIONAL OPTIONS: PEDICLED TRAM AND BIPEDICLE TRAM

Hartrampf and colleagues described the pedicled transverse rectus abdominus myocutaneous (TRAM) flap in 1982 (1). This technique gained rapid acceptance and has become widely used for breast reconstruction. In fact, because of the versatility of the TRAM flap, relative ease of dissection, and excellent outcomes that can be expected from this operation, the pedicled TRAM flap remains a workhorse for breast reconstruction. Even today the pedicled TRAM flap is the most commonly performed autologous tissue transfer used for breast reconstruction. Technical modifications of this procedure have been described over the years to improve blood supply (e.g., bipedicled TRAM, midabdominal TRAM), decrease abdominal wall morbidity (e.g., muscle sparing pedicled TRAM), and improve breast shape (e.g., ipsilateral vs. contralateral pedicled TRAM).

Outcomes after pedicled TRAM and microsurgical TRAMs have also been compared in a variety of studies (2,3). Unfortunately, these studies are for the most part case series or other retrospective studies; therefore, high-level scientific studies comparing these outcomes are lacking. In general, however, most studies have shown that microsurgical TRAM flap procedures have decreased abdominal wall complications, decreased fat necrosis and partial flap loss, and possibly improved breast aesthetics (4). In addition, in experienced hands, microsurgical TRAM flap procedures have very low total flap loss rates (<1%) that compare favorably with those reported for pedicled TRAM variants (4,5).

FREE TRAM FLAPS FOR BREAST RECONSTRUCTION

Many variations of the microsurgical TRAM flaps have been described and reflect the evolution of this technique from its initial description as a pedicled flap. The goal has been to decrease potential donor site morbidity while maintaining the excellent vascular supply of abdominal tissues to provide a natural breast reconstruction. In general, variations of the TRAM flap can be most simply classified based on the amount of muscle that is harvested with the flap. Although the term *free TRAM flap* is used in general terms to describe any microsurgical TRAM flap transfer, most authors use this term for a TRAM flap that includes the entire width of the rectus muscle encompassing both the medial and lateral rows of perforators arising from the deep inferior epigastric system (Figure 43-1). The term *muscle-sparing TRAM* (msTRAM) is used to describe flaps in which a portion of the muscle is harvested together with the flap. Nahabedian et al. further categorized msTRAM based on the region of muscle harvested with the flap; lateral, central, or medial portions of the muscle correspond to the terms MS-1, MS-2, and MS-3, respectively (6). Although useful for categorization, the functional significance of this classification has yet to be proven. Perforator flaps, also referred to as deep inferior epigastric perforator (DIEP) flaps as popularized by Allen and Treece, refer to flaps transferred without any rectus muscle (7). In these flaps, the vessels are harvested by dissection through or around the rectus muscle, leaving the bulk of the muscle intact. A classification system enabling precise description of the dissection techniques for DIEP flaps has not been described and would be useful for comparison of abdominal outcomes

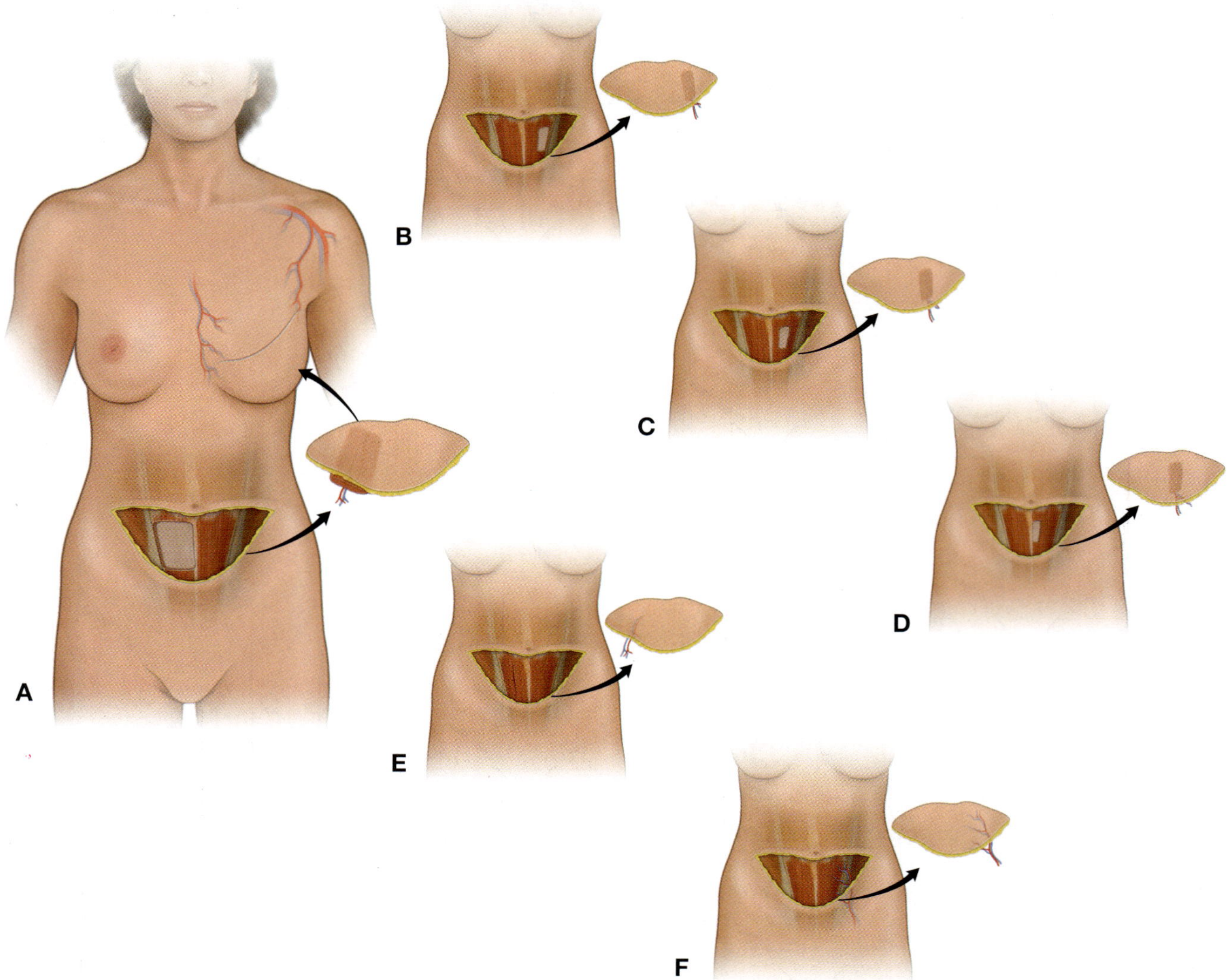

FIGURE 43-1 Schematic drawing of various types of free transverse rectus abdominus myocutaneous (TRAM) flaps: free TRAM (**A**), MS-1 TRAM (**B**), MS-2 TRAM (**C**), MS-3 TRAM (**D**), deep inferior epigastric perforator flap (**E**), and superficial inferior epigastric artery and vein flap (**F**).

comparing traditional flaps with perforator flaps. This statement is based on the fact that intuitively more damage and denervation occurs in a scenario in which perforators are dissected through a long intramuscular course compared with periumbilical perforators (i.e., septocutaneous, which commonly encircle the muscle, thereby minimizing muscle injury during harvest). The superficial inferior epigastric artery (SIEA) flaps are based on the superficial epigastric vessels and therefore do not require incision of the anterior abdominal wall fascia or rectus muscle. Perforator flaps are covered in more detail in other sections of this book.

INDICATIONS AND TIMING

The free TRAM (fTRAM) or msTRAM flaps are indicated for breast reconstruction after mastectomy or partial mastectomy, acquired absence or deformity of the breast after trauma radiation or complications of cosmetic breast procedures, or congenital absence of the breast. These flaps are also useful for reconstruction of contour deformities and chest wall coverage.

The fTRAM or msTRAM flaps can be performed either at the time of mastectomy (immediate reconstruction) or in a delayed manner even years after mastectomy. Immediate reconstruction is, in general, simpler to perform, particularly if skin-sparing mastectomy is performed because the flap is used primarily as a filler, and the natural contours of the breast are maintained (Figure 43-2). Care must be taken to evaluate skin flaps to determine if they are viable after mastectomy and before deepithelization of the TRAM flap skin paddle. Occasionally, this may be performed in a delayed manner with a planned return to the operating room.

Delayed breast reconstruction with the TRAM flap is performed by recreating the mastectomy defect and separating the breast skin from the underlying pectoralis major muscle. If an implant is present, then the implant and implant material are removed, the mastectomy defect is recreated, and the pectoralis major muscle is placed back on the chest wall in its normal

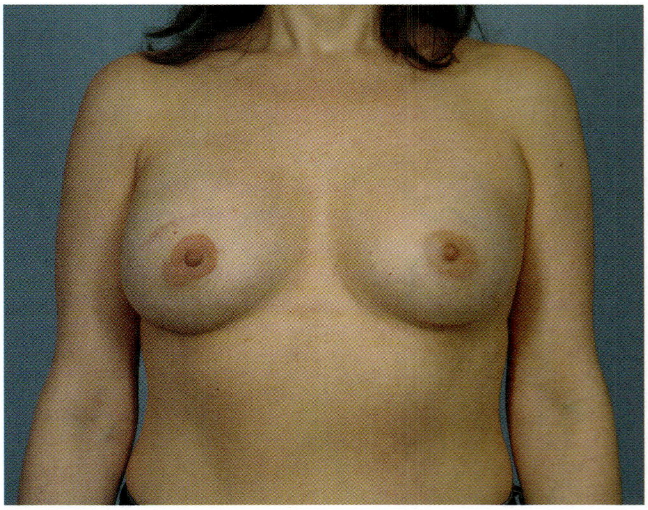

FIGURE 43-2 Case example of immediate right breast reconstruction with a free MS-2 TRAM flap after areola-sparing mastectomy. Note maintenance of breast contours and minimal scarring.

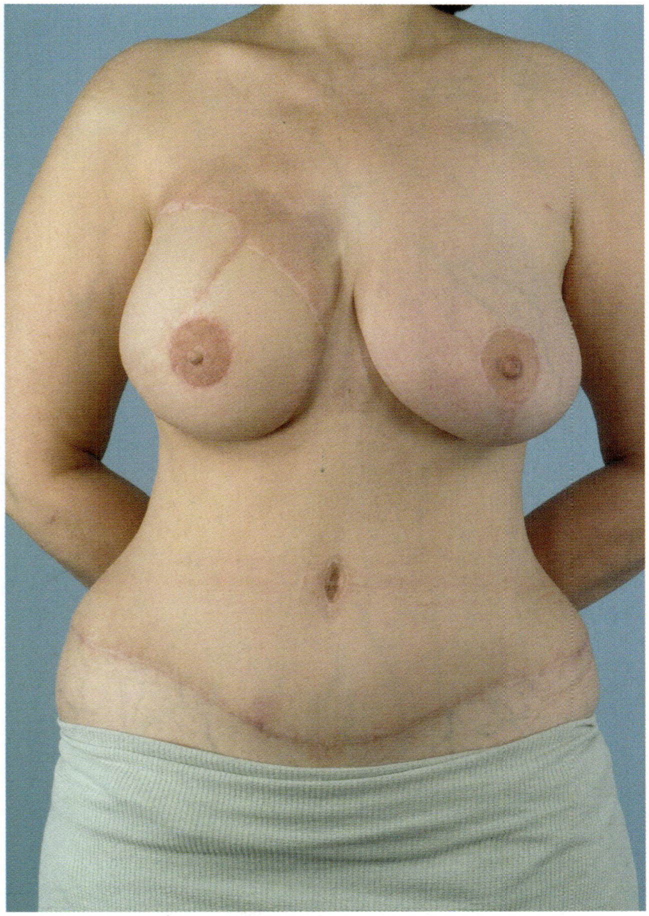

FIGURE 43-3 Case example of delayed right breast reconstruction with a free transverse rectus abdominus myocutaneous (TRAM) flap. Note the excellent breast shape but conspicuous scarring. Placement of the TRAM flap skin paddle to replace the inferior mastectomy skin minimizes the appearance of the scar.

anatomic position. Excessively thick capsules can be removed to release scar contracture. Delayed breast reconstruction with the fTRAM flap can result in excellent cosmetic outcomes. However, larger TRAM flap skin paddles are necessary to make up for the breast skin lost as a result of mastectomy and contracture, resulting in a perception of larger or longer scars by patients. Placing the abdominal skin paddle on the inferior aspect of the reconstructed breast minimizes this effect (Figure 43-3).

The timing of autologous breast reconstruction in patients who require (or may require) postoperative adjuvant radiation has been debated. Some authors have reported favorable outcomes in these cases and do not consider postoperative radiation a contraindication to immediate reconstruction with fTRAM flaps. In contrast, other centers have reported high rates of fibrosis and fat necrosis as a result of postoperative radiation and recommend delayed reconstruction with TRAM flaps if postoperative radiation is necessary. A simple solution to this conundrum may be placement of a tissue expander to maintain the breast contours and limit mastectomy skin flap loss followed by exchange of the tissue expander for a TRAM flap at an appropriate time (i.e., after completion of radiation; Figure 43-4). Long-term comprehensive studies comparing outcomes and patient satisfaction in these scenarios have not been performed and would be helpful.

PREPARATION OF DONOR AND RECIPIENT SITE

Flap markings for the fTRAM and msTRAM are similar with the skin paddle marked on the lower abdominal area. Handheld Doppler can be used to mark skin perforators and the position of the SIEA and superficial inferior epigastric vein (SIEV). The upper portion of the flap marking should include the region around the umbilicus as the majority of perforators arising from the deep inferior epigastric muscle exit and enter the subcutaneous tissues in this region. The lower abdominal incision is determined based on the abdominal tissue laxity with care taken to avoid excessively tight closure.

After skin incision, the upper abdominal flap is elevated to the level of the xiphoid centrally in the middle two thirds and the costal margins laterally to preserve vascular supply. The inferior skin incision is then performed, and the lower skin flap is minimally undermined to avoid pulling the mons pubis superiorly with wound closure. Care is taken to identify and preserve the superficial epigastric vessels (particularly the vein) in the subcutaneous tissues of the lower skin flap. These vessels are very superficial deep to the dermis and dissected for a length of 4 to 6 cm to enable microsurgical anastomosis if the flap is venous congested after anastomosis of the deep system.

Flap dissection begins from lateral to medial to expose the lateral row perforators arising from the inferior epigastric vessels (Figure 43-5). For bilateral reconstructions, the flap is bisected, and medial row vessels are identified. For unilateral reconstructions, the umbilicus is dissected, preserving its vascular supply to the stalk. The flap dissection is performed superiorly and inferiorly to dissect the medial row perforators. After the perforators in the medial and lateral rows of both flaps are dissected, the surgeon selects the flap based on the size of perforators as

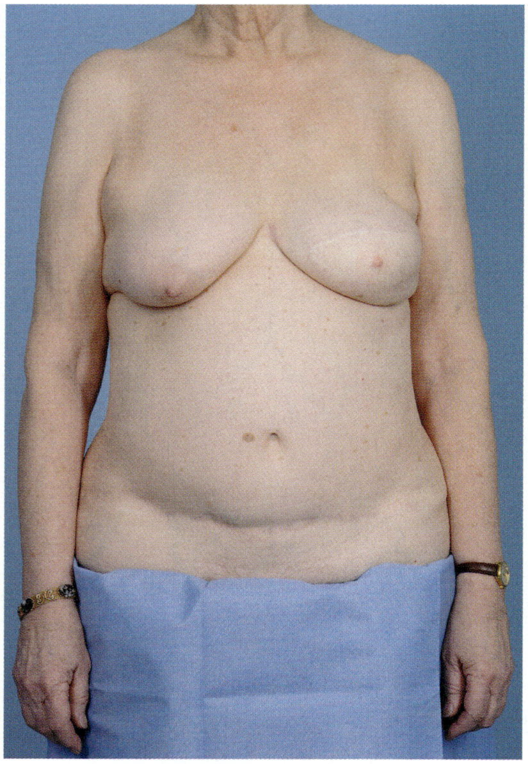

FIGURE 43-4 Case example of left breast reconstruction after temporary tissue expander placement and conversion to free MS-2 transverse rectus abdominus myocutaneous flap. Results after 2-year follow-up and nipple areola reconstruction are shown.

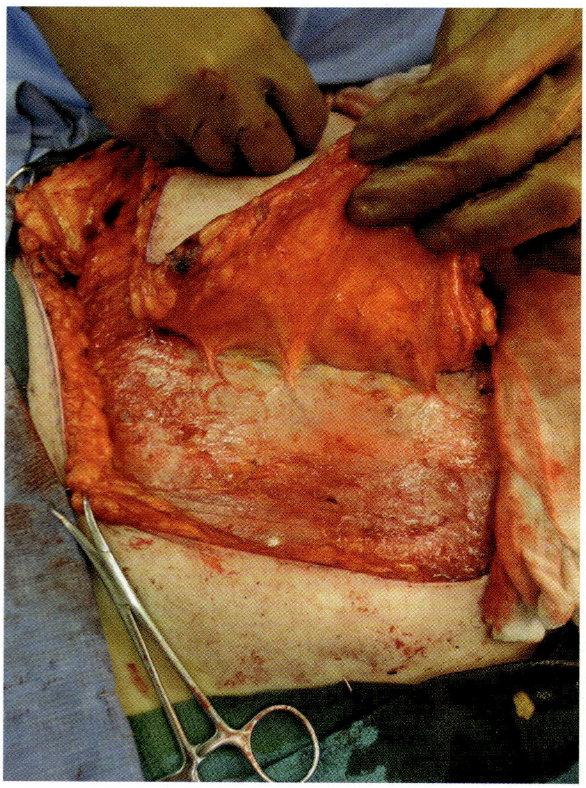

FIGURE 43-5 Lateral to medial dissection of the transverse rectus abdominus myocutaneous flap. Lateral row perforators have been completely dissected to facilitate fascial incision.

well as reconstructive needs. The anterior rectus sheath is incised with care taken to preserve as much fascia as possible while avoiding injury to the perforating vessels. Ideally, dissection should be performed to enable primary closure of the fascia. Usually, 1 cm of the fascia is taken. In some circumstances, small perforators may be sacrificed if sufficient vessels are present to preserve fascia for primary closure and to avoid malposition of the umbilicus.

The portion of muscle to be harvested is exposed by minimal fascial dissection, and the muscle inclusive of the perforators is harvested. Generally, this is done by incising the muscle in the direction of its fibers approximately 1 cm lateral to the lateral row and 1 cm medial to the medial row. The inferior dissection continues until the main medial row branch is identified and the muscle is transected. If possible, the lower intercostal nerves are preserved. The upper muscle segment is then transected, and the superior epigastric vessels are ligated.

The flap is elevated from superior to inferior, and the perforating vessels arising from the main pedicle to the fascia or muscle are identified and ligated. Pedicle dissection proceeds to the take-off of the vessels from the external iliac artery and vein, and the deep inferior epigastric vessels are separated and prepared for later ligation. It is important to assess the flap zone vascularity at this point before ligation. The pedicle is ligated after the recipient vessels are dissected and made ready for microvascular anastomosis. Both the pedicle and recipient vessels are marked on its anterior surface using methylene blue ink to facilitate microsurgical anastomosis and prevent inadvertant twisting of the pedicle.

Preparation of the recipient site is usually performed simultaneously as flap dissection. Historically, most surgeons used the thoracodorsal vessels for microsurgical anastomosis of free TRAM flaps. This was based on the fact that many patients who underwent mastectomy had simultaneous axillary lymph node dissection, thereby exposing these vessels in the surgical field. However, with the advent of sentinel lymph node dissection, fewer women had axillary lymph node dissection, and in some instances, some patients required reoperation for lymph node dissection at a later time, thereby exposing microvascular anastomoses in the axilla to the risk of inadvertant injury. These factors, together with limitations in insetting of the flaps and occasional compression of anastomoses in the axilla, particularly in obese patients, has led many surgeons to use the internal mammary vessels for microsurgical TRAM flap reconstruction (4).

In immediate mastectomy reconstruction, exposure of the thoracodorsal or mammary vessels is simple and can be performed expeditiously. However, in delayed reconstruction, previously scarred axilla exposure can be challenging. Dissection starts by incising the clavipectoral fascia and identifying the latissimus dorsi muscle. This is safer if the dissection is started high in the axilla before the thoracodorsal neurovascular bundle enters the latissimus muscle proximal to the serratus branch. The intercostobrachial nerve and long thoracic nerve are preserved during the dissection. The vessels are carefully dissected to their subscapular vessel origin and separated from the thoracodorsal nerve, which is usually anterior and medial to the vessels in the high axilla. The anastomosis is performed just superior to the take off of the serratus branch in an end-to-end fashion.

The serratus branch is preserved to maintain the option of latissimus flap transfer (via retrograde flow through the serratus branch) if it becomes necessary at a later date. The thoracodorsal nerve is transposed posterior to the thoracodorsal vessels at the time of anastomosis to prevent vascular pedicle compression.

A number of techniques have been described for dissection of the internal mammary vessels. Although perforating vessels from the internal mammary vessels can be used on occasion, usually the artery in these perforators is too small for an end-to-end anastomosis to the inferior epigastric artery. Most authors expose the vessels between the second-third or third-fourth ribs. The muscle can simply be split over the rib to expose the selected interspace. Alternatively, a small superiorly based pectoralis flap can be elevated to expose the appropriate interspace (8). This technique enables wide exposure of the vessels, thereby facilitating anastomosis. In addition, this technique is associated with decreased contour deformities in the medial portion of the breast arising from rib resection for exposure of the vessels. The internal mammary vessels are localized with a handheld Doppler and then exposed in the interspace by removing the overlying intercostal muscles in that region. Typically, a portion of muscle measuring 1.5 cm is removed to expose the vessels. Care must be taken to avoid avulsion of branches arising from these vessels and perforating the intercostal muscles. If the interspace is too small for adequate microanastomosis or there is venous branching, then a portion of the rib can be removed to improve exposure and facilitate anastomosis to a larger vein.

VESSEL ANASTOMOSES

In most cases, the internal mammary vessels are adequate for microsurgical transfer. The artery on both sides is usually 2 to 3 mm in diameter with high flow. The right-sided vein is in most cases appropriate for microsurgery with a diameter of 2.5 to 3.5 mm (9). The left internal mammary vein can on occasion (10%–15%) be too small for microsurgical anastomosis, particularly if it has branched (9). Typically, branching occurs at the level of the third or fourth ribs; however, occasionally the branch point is higher, thereby complicating anastomosis because of the presence of two small veins. In general, size mismatch of more than 2:1 should be avoided if at all possible (4). Venous anastomosis in most instances is performed using the microvascular coupler after the appropriate size has been determined. The arterial anastomosis can also be performed using the coupler (10,11); however, most authors prefer to use suture anastomosis (9.0 nylon).

INSET OF THE FLAP: SCULPTING OF THE FLAP

After completion of the microsurgical anastomosis, the pectoralis muscle is closed to cover the defect created by intercostal muscle resection (8). A space of 1 cm is left for the vessels to exit and care is taken to avoid kinking or twisting of the pedicle. The rectus muscle can be sutured to the pectoralis muscle to maintain its position in a favorable direction and prevent pulling, twisting, or redundant kinking of the pedicle. Care should be taken, however, to avoid injury to the main pedicle or perforating vessels. A limited deepithelization is performed based on skin requirements. In addition, perfusion of the flap is assessed to ensure adequate flow. Usually, the portions of the flap most distal to the deep inferior epigastric vessels (i.e., zone 4) are removed to avoid fat necrosis. If additional flap thinning is required, then the sub-Scarpa fat component can be removed because perfusion to this area occurs via the subdermal plexus.

Insetting of the flap is performed after the completion of the microanastamosis with care taken to avoid twisting, kinking, or traction. The orientation that the flap is inset into the breast defect is determined based on reconstructive needs and the quality of perforating vessels present. A vertically oriented flap is, in general, best used for narrow or tall breasts or if ptosis is required to match the contralateral breast (Figure 43-6). A horizontally oriented flap is generally best for wide breasts (e.g., in obese patients) because this orientation uses the length of the TRAM flap to recreate the width of the breast. If the thoracodorsal artery and vein are used as recipient vessels, then a flap based on the ipsilateral (i.e., same side as the reconstruction) deep inferior epigastric vessels will assume a vertical orientation when inset. In contrast, a flap based on the contralateral deep inferior epigastric vessels will assume a more horizontal orientation when inset. The laterality of the flap is less critical in cases in which the internal mammary vessels are used because the location of these flaps facilitates flap placement.

Insetting is initiated in the inferior, medial portion of the breast and continued superiorly to recreate the medial portion of the breast. The inferior portion of the TRAM flap is then inset into the lower portion of the breast. The flap is medialized as necessary to create more ptosis or projection. In addition, the flap can be folded upon itself in a limited fashion to increase ptosis and projection. After the inferior portion is inset, the upper portion of the flap is inset into the mastectomy defect by suturing Scarpa's fascia to the muscle or to the edge of the mastectomy defect. The tail of the flap is sutured to the tail of Spence to avoid contour deformities in this region. Before final, insetting of vascular pedicle is inspected again, and flap perfusion is reassessed. The final deepithelization is performed, the skin paddle is inset, and a cutaneous Doppler stitch is placed to facilitate postoperative monitoring. Drains are placed well away from the vascular pedicle and anastomosis, and care is taken to avoid compression of the flap with the drain.

POSTOPERATIVE MONITORING

Postoperative monitoring is most commonly performed using frequent physical examinations and Doppler ultrasonography. Capillary refill and color are examined carefully. Doppler ultrasonography evaluation should be performed by experience observers to ensure presence of a biphasic sound pattern. Temperature monitoring is also used by some authors because it has been shown to be an early predictor of venous thrombosis (12). A number of new technologies have been reported, including laser Doppler, perfusion scanning, and oxygen monitoring; however, these techniques usually require trained staff and expensive equipment. In addition, the clinical utility

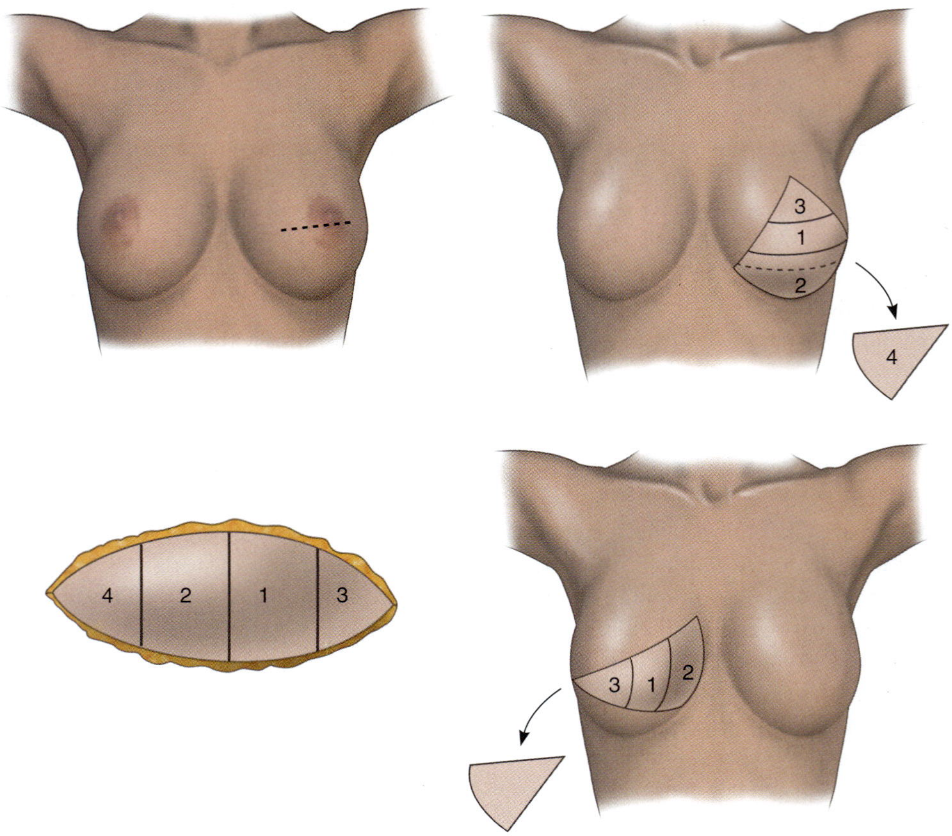

FIGURE 43-6 Schematic of vertical (**A**) and horizontal (**B**) orientation of the flap.

of these measures has not been definitively proven in randomized clinical trials. As a result, these methods are in most cases experimental and not widely adopted.

Patients are kept warm and well hydrated to avoid vascular spasm. Some authors recommend limiting caffeine or chocolate for the same reasons. Pressure on the microsurgical site is also avoided, and patients are discouraged from extreme ranges of motion and/or wearing bras and tight-fitting garments for 2 to 4 weeks after surgery. Blood pressure monitoring is performed to ensure adequate perfusion pressures. Patients with a history of hypertension should take their medications; however, specific lower limits to hold the medication is provided to avoid inadvertent hypotension postoperatively.

The highest risk of microvascular complications is within the first 24 hours of surgery; therefore, patients are most carefully monitored during this time period (13). Usually, flaps are monitored every 15 to 30 minutes for the first 6 hours, then every 30 minutes to 1 hour for the next 6 hours, and then hourly for the next 24 hours. After this time, flaps can be safely monitored every 2 to 4 hours. Most patients are discharged home after 3 to 5 days and instructed to monitor the color and temperature of their flap reconstructions at home.

COMPLICATIONS

Complications arising after microsurgical TRAM flap procedures can be categorized in a variety of ways. Early complications are thought to occur within 30 days of surgery, and late complications occur later. Complications can also be divided into recipient, donor, or systemic sites and further classified as minor or major complications.

A recent review of nearly 1200 free tissue transfers (including nearly 1000 free TRAMs) demonstrated an overall complication rate of 27.8% with roughly equal distribution of early (17.3%) and late (15.3%) complications (4). The majority of complications were minor (21.7%), requiring either no intervention or a minor intervention (e.g., oral antibiotics). The overall fat necrosis rate in this study was 11.2%; however, most fat necrosis cases were minor (<3 cm^2; 5.8%) and were excised at the time of secondary revision. Reported rates of fat necrosis after free TRAM flap reconstruction vary widely in the literature primarily because of the lack of a uniform definition of this complication (4). Some studies report fat necrosis rates without reporting criteria used in its definition. Others use the criteria of "clinically significant" or "radiologically noted." Infections and wound healing complications at the donor or recipient sites occurred in 11% of patients and usually resolved with conservative management.

Abdominal wall complications (hernia or bulge) also occur after free TRAM flap procedures. The rates of abdominal complications after free TRAM flap procedures are variable depending on their definition, however, in general, most cases report hernia rates of less than 5% and bulge rates of less than 10% (4,14–16). A variety of techniques have been described to minimize this complication, including the use of inlay or only mesh, Alloderm, and other prosthetic materials. Minimizing fascial harvest and injury during dissection may be helpful in this regard; however, prospective clinical trials are lacking. Similarly, comparisons of the various techniques such as mesh or Alloderm have not been performed in a randomized manner. Not surprisingly, previous abdominal surgery location and abdominal incision are major risk factors for this complication (4). In addition, obesity and a history of smoking increase the rates of abdominal wall complications particularly skin slough. In these situations, the rates of wound healing complications may be minimized with limited skin flap undermining.

Abdominal wall weakness is also a potential complication of free TRAM flap procedures (4,16). The exact rates or the effect of these operations on the abdominal wall strength remain unknown; however, several studies have demonstrated increased weakness after bilateral transfer compared with unilateral procedures (17,18). In addition, a number of studies have attempted to examine outcomes with pedicled TRAMs compared with free TRAMs with variable results. Although some authors have reported excellent abdominal wall integrity with pedicled TRAMs (15,19), in general, most studies have shown improved objective and subjective measures of abdominal wall function after free TRAM flap procedures.

Spear and colleagues reported the incidence of altered abdominal wall sensibility after TRAM flaps in a small cohort (25 patients) compared with normal volunteers demonstrating a statistically significant decrease in TRAM flap patients even as long as 2 years after surgery (20). The functional and subjective significance of this finding is unknown but deserves additional study.

Transient brachial plexus injuries after free TRAM flap procedures have been reported in a small number of patients (1%) (4). These injuries are traction injuries resulting from abduction of the arm either at the time of mastectomy or reconstruction. Care must be taken to minimize abduction of the shoulder beyond 90 degrees for extended periods of time. We have previously reported the use of the Omni retractor to facilitate exposure of axillary vessels (21). This technique was associated with a decreased incidence of brachial plexus injury possibly by improving exposure without the need for excessive arm abduction.

Major complications after free TRAM flap procedures are relatively rare. Mehrara et al. reported a rate of 7.7% in their review of 1200 free tissue transfers for breast reconstruction (21). This rate included total flap loss (0.4%), partial flap loss (2.2%), arterial thrombosis (0.8%), venous thrombosis (0.8%), and hematoma (1.6%). Severe systemic complications were rare (<1%) and included congestive heart failure (0.8%), sepsis (0.1%), and intestinal compartment syndrome (0.1%). Similar rates of major complications have been reported in other large series of breast reconstructions with free TRAM flaps (22).

Deep vein thrombosis (DVT) is a potential complication of any prolonged procedure. The incidence of this complication is increased in cancer patients. Therefore, steps should be taken to reduce the incidence of this complication in patients who undergo TRAM flap reconstruction. These steps include intraoperative compression devices and postoperative anticoagulation strategies. A review of 225 consecutive TRAM flap patients by Lemaine et al. demonstrated DVT formation in 3.4% of patients screened with duplex ultrasonography before discharge (23). There were no cases of pulmonary embolus in this study; however, this complication has been reported after TRAM flaps. Therefore, vigilance is required in assessing patients postoperatively to diagnose and initiate treatment in a timely manner.

The major risk factors for complications after TRAM flap procedures are similar to most surgical procedures and include obesity, smoking, and previous surgery (4). This analysis is often difficult to perform, however, because of a significant interaction between risk factors and the limits of univariate and multivariate analyses. Obesity is associated with increased rates of fat necrosis, wound healing complications, and abdominal wall problems (more than threefold increase) (4). Similarly, prior abdominal surgery increases the risk of abdominal wall laxity or hernia most likely as a result of additional injury or devascularization of the abdominal fascia.

SECONDARY SURGERY

Secondary procedures are routinely performed after TRAM flap reconstruction and include shaping procedures, contralateral symmetry procedures, and nipple areola reconstruction. The timing of these procedures is variable and determined by adjuvant therapy necessary (e.g., chemotherapy or radiation), local healing, and patient desires. Usually, most secondary procedures are delayed for 3 to 6 months to allow complete healing of the flap and resolution of postoperative edema. At this time, shaping procedures such as breast lifts, revision of inframammary fold, and contour deformities are performed using standard techniques. Reduction can also be simply performed either by direct excision or, more commonly, using liposuction. Liposuction of the flap is safe and well tolerated. However, in these situations, significant undermining or flap dissection should be deferred to avoid ischemic complications. Aggressive flap revision of radiated flap is not recommended because it may further compromise the vascularity and result in contraction deformity. In rare cases, augmentation of the flap can also be performed to improve symmetry. This may be done either with placement of implants or tissue expander implant placement depending on the size of implant necessary. Augmentation is performed in a similar manner as conventional breast augmentation usually with subpectoral placement of the implant. The subpectoral location decreases risk of injury to the pedicle vessels and, in our experience, decreases contour deformities that may occur after subflap insertion of the implant. With the recent advancement in fat grafting technique, microfat grafting can be used to augment volume and correct depression contour deformities.

Contralateral breast procedures are performed using standard techniques, including mastopexy, reduction, and augmentation. Symmetry is improved in these cases if the patient is evaluated in the sitting position in the operating room. Careful positioning and collaboration with anesthesia colleagues is necessary for this evaluation.

Nipple areola reconstruction is performed using either local tissues (e.g., C-V flap) and nipple areola tattoo or local tissues with full-thickness skin grafting (e.g., skate flap) for areola

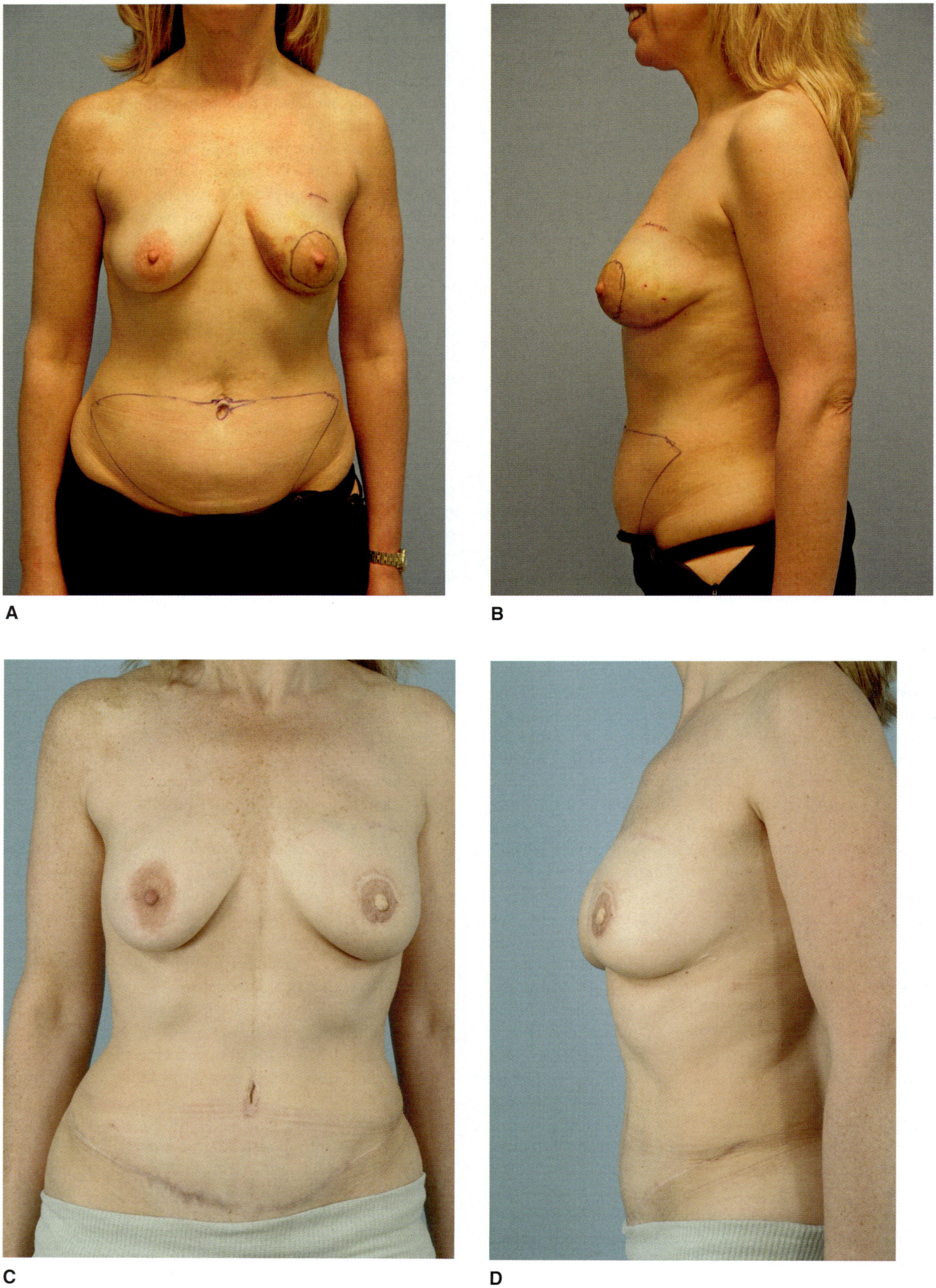

FIGURE 43-7 Preoperative (A, B) and 2 year postoperative (C, D) views of case 1.

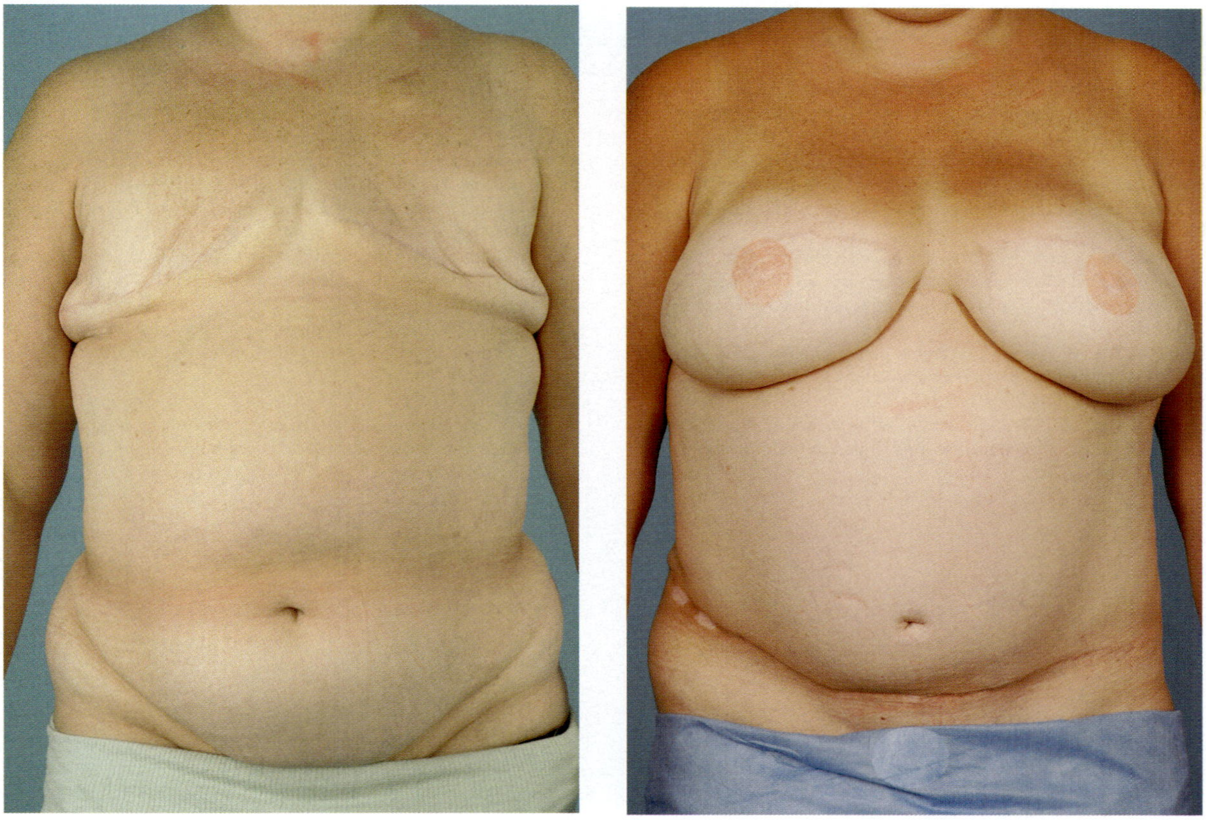

A B

FIGURE 43-8 Preoperative (**A**) and 3-year postoperative (**B**) views of case 2.

reconstruction. Both techniques are highly successful with good cosmetic outcomes. Selection of technique is based on tissue availability, patient desires, and color of the areola. Symmetrical nipple reconstruction is often facilitated with preoperative marking of the patient in the standing position while wearing a bra.

CASE EXAMPLES

Case 1

The patient was a 47-year-old woman with ductal carcinoma in situ of the left breast who underwent a left skin–sparing mastectomy and immediate reconstruction with a free MS-2 free TRAM flap. Preoperative and 2-year postoperative views are shown after nipple and areola reconstruction with a skate flap and full-thickness skin graft (Figure 43-7).

Case 2

The patient was a 43-year-old woman with stage IIb breast cancer who underwent bilateral mastectomy and delayed reconstruction with free MS-2 bilateral TRAM flaps. Preoperative and 3-year postoperative views are shown after nipple reconstruction, nipple areola tattoo, and liposuction of the mons pubis (Figure 43-8).

REFERENCES

1. Hartrampf CR, Scheflan M, Black PW. Breast reconstruction with a transverse abdominal island flap. *Plast Reconstr Surg* 1982;69:216–225.
2. Moran SL, Serletti JM. Outcome comparison between free and pedicled tram flap breast reconstruction in the obese patient. *Plast Reconstr Surg* 2001;108:1954–1960; discussion 1961–1952.
3. Larson DL, Yousif NJ, Sinha RK, et al. A comparison of pedicled and free tram flaps for breast reconstruction in a single institution. *Plast Reconstr Surg* 1999;104:674–680.
4. Mehrara BJ, Santoro TD, Arcilla E, et al. Complications after microvascular breast reconstruction: experience with 1195 flaps. *Plast Reconstr Surg* 2006;118:1100–1109; discussion 1110–1101.
5. Chen CM, Halvorson EG, Disa JJ, et al. Immediate postoperative complications in diep versus free/muscle-sparing tram flaps. *Plast Reconstr Surg* 2007;120:1477–1482.
6. Nahabedian MY, Momen B, Galdino G, Manson PN. Breast reconstruction with the free tram or diep flap: patient selection, choice of flap, and outcome. *Plast Reconstr Surg* 2002;110:466–475; discussion 467–476.
7. Allen RJ, Treece P. Deep inferior epigastric perforator flap for breast reconstruction. *Ann Plast Surg* 1994;32:32–38.
8. Mosahebi A, Da Lio A, Mehrara B. The use of a pectoralis major flap to improve internal mammary vessels exposure and reduce contour deformity in microvascular free flap breast reconstruction. *Ann Plast Surg* 2008;61:30–34.
9. Mehrara BJ, Santoro T, Smith A, et al. Alternative venous outflow vessels in microvascular breast reconstruction. *Plast Reconstr Surg* 2003;112: 448–455.
10. Spector JA, Draper LB, Levine JP, Ahn CY. A technique for atraumatic microvascular arterial coupling. *Plast Reconstr Surg* 2007;119:1968–1969.
11. Spector JA, Draper LB, Levine JP, Ahn CY. Routine use of microvascular coupling device for arterial anastomosis in breast reconstruction. *Ann Plast Surg* 2006;56:365–368.

12. Khouri RK, Shaw WW. Monitoring of free flaps with surface-temperature recordings: is it reliable? *Plast Reconstr Surg* 1992;89:495–499; discussion 492–500.
13. Bui DT, Cordeiro PG, Hu QY, et al. Free flap reexploration: indications, treatment, and outcomes in 1193 free flaps. *Plast Reconstr Surg* 2007;119:2092–2100.
14. Momeni A, Kim RY, Heier M, et al. Abdominal wall strength: a matched-pair analysis comparing muscle-sparing tram flap donor-site morbidity with the effects of abdominoplasty. *Plast Reconstr Surg* 2010;126: 1454–1459.
15. Ascherman JA, Seruya M, Bartsich SA. Abdominal wall morbidity following unilateral and bilateral breast reconstruction with pedicled tram flaps: an outcomes analysis of 117 consecutive patients. *Plast Reconstr Surg* 2008;121:1–8.
16. Nahabedian MY. Secondary operations of the anterior abdominal wall following microvascular breast reconstruction with the tram and diep flaps. *Plast Reconstr Surg* 2007;120:365–372.
17. Kroll SS, Schusterman MA, Reece GP, et al. Abdominal wall strength, bulging, and hernia after tram flap breast reconstruction. *Plast Reconstr Surg* 1995;96:616–619.
18. Selber JC, Fosnot J, Nelson J, et al. A prospective study comparing the functional impact of siea, diep, and muscle-sparing free tram flaps on the abdominal wall: part II. Bilateral reconstruction. *Plast Reconstr Surg* 2010;126:1438–1453.
19. Chun YS, Sinha I, Turko A, et al. Outcomes and patient satisfaction following breast reconstruction with bilateral pedicled tram flaps in 105 consecutive patients. *Plast Reconstr Surg* 2010;125:1–9.
20. Spear SL, Hess CL, Elmaraghy MW. Evaluation of abdominal sensibility after tram flap breast reconstruction. *Plast Reconstr Surg* 2000;106: 1300–1304.
21. Mehrara BJ, Santoro T, Smith A, et al. Improving recipient vessel exposure during microvascular breast reconstruction. *Ann Plast Surg* 2003;51: 361–365.
22. Chang DW, Reece GP, Wang B, et al. Effect of smoking on complications in patients undergoing free tram flap breast reconstruction. *Plast Reconstr Surg* 2000;105:2374–2380.
23. Lemaine V, McCarthy C, Kaplan K, et al. Venous thromboembolism following microsurgical breast reconstruction: an objective analysis in 225 consecutive patients using low-molecular-weight heparin prophylaxis. *Plast Reconstr Surg* 2011;127(4):1399–1406.

CHAPTER 44

Breast Reconstruction: Clinical Utilization of the Deep Inferior Epigastric Perforator Flap

Joshua Fosnot and Joseph M. Serletti

Despite many advances in the detection and treatment of breast cancer over the years, mastectomy continues to play a significant role in the management of this disease. Breast reconstruction remains a vital component of the treatment of and recovery from the resultant defect. Although alloplastic techniques of reconstruction using expander and implants remain more common for the restoration of a breast mound, autologous reconstruction has become increasingly popular and, when done well, offers the opportunity for a more natural and aesthetically pleasing result. Autologous reconstruction has gone through an evolution over the years. Although pedicled latissimus dorsi musculocutaneous flaps offer the ability to transfer healthy autologous tissue to the breast, more often than not, implants are still required for adequate volume restoration. This led to the increased popularity of pedicled transverse rectus abdominis myocutaneous (TRAM) flaps initially described by Hartrampf in 1982 (1). Although the pedicled TRAM is still used today, at high-volume centers, it has been completely replaced by the free TRAM or deep inferior epigastric perforator (DIEP) flap based on the deep inferior epigastric vessels. The free flap has the added benefit of a more robust blood supply as well as significantly less donor site morbidity because of muscle and fascia preservation. As microsurgery has become routine, many surgeons have become more comfortable with harvesting the abdominal flap on one or two perforators, allowing for complete preservation of the rectus musculature.

It is important to recognize the different options when abdominal integument is harvested. Complete muscle harvest with the flap (MS [muscle sparing]-0) is more invasive than taking only half the muscle (MS-1) or a small portion of the muscle (MS-2). A true DIEP flap, in which all of the muscle is spared (MS-3), offers the least invasive option based on the deep inferior epigastric vessels; however, it is more technically demanding with an increased risk of microvascular ischemia resulting in fat necrosis long term (2). Ideally, in raising the DIEP flap, the muscle fibers are temporarily splayed apart to allow for removal of the inferior epigastric vessels and selected perforators (Figure 44-1). Proponents of this technique suggest that it results in less postoperative pain, shorter hospitalization, a more prompt recovery, and little or no functional deficit in the abdominal donor site (3). Because this flap relies on one or two perforators, it may be less suitable for high-risk patients. For the purpose of this chapter, we will refer to the DIEP flap quite broadly because not all patients' anatomies allow for complete muscle-sparing techniques.

INDICATIONS AND PATIENT EVALUATION

The Initial Consult: General Considerations

A breast cancer patient seeking reconstruction from a plastic surgeon presents at varying stages of the treatment of her disease, often with varying levels of understanding of the types of reconstruction available. It is important to take the time with each patient to describe the options fully, listen to the patient's wishes and expectations, and formulate a plan for moving forward. Breast reconstruction is not a simple procedure and can result in complications, making an open dialogue paramount to avoiding untoward outcomes and disappointment with the final result. Many women present predisposed to the notion that implants are bad, stemming from concerns about foreign bodies and an historical fear of implants being associated with cancer. No studies have found a link between implants and systemic illness. These patients should be counseled on the safety and benefits of expander and implant reconstruction regardless of their initial preconceptions because a patient's initial understanding is often inadequate to make an educated decision. Expander and implant reconstruction may provide excellent results, lacks donor site morbidity, and is more appropriate in specific circumstances.

That being said, autologous reconstruction offers the unique ability to replace "like with like," which leads to improved overall and long-term patient satisfaction in most patients.

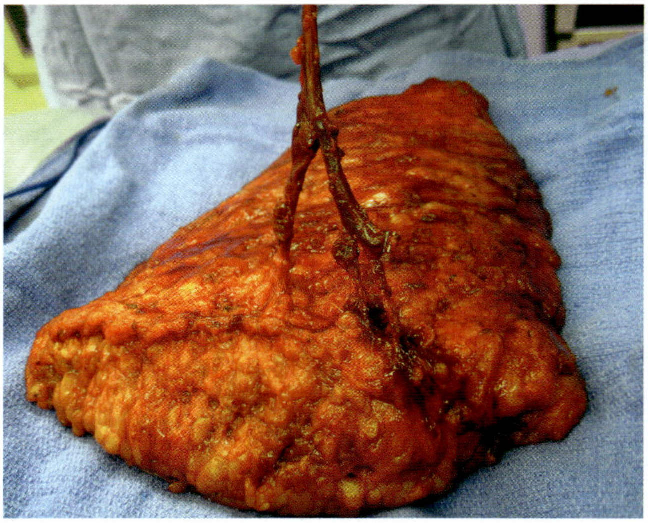

FIGURE 44-1 After completion of a deep inferior epigastric perforator (DIEP) harvest, one or two perforators are typically dissected, resulting in a flap with a pedicle devoid of any fascia or muscle. This is an example of a two-vessel DIEP in which all muscle was spared.

Autologous reconstruction is particularly beneficial in unilateral reconstruction to create lasting symmetry. Over time, an implant-based reconstruction tends to behave differently than the normal contralateral breast, resulting in different degrees of ptosis. This is ameliorated by autologous tissue reconstruction, which behaves more similar to native tissue. In addition, autologous reconstruction is not associated with some of the long-term complications in alloplastic reconstruction such as implant infection, extrusion, rupture, and capsular contracture. In addition, once reconstructed, patients need not worry about having to have implant exchanges, which on average occur every 10 years.

Assessing Your Patient's Risk

Patient comorbidities play a critical role in the likelihood of complications and should be recognized before undertaking any operation. Although smoking and obesity have repetitively been implicated as independent risk factors for wound complications such as wound infection, mastectomy flap necrosis, abdominal flap necrosis, and fat necrosis, these are not considered contraindications to free flap breast reconstruction (4). Conversely, many have shown free flap reconstruction to be safe in the obese, comorbid diseased, or elderly populations (5,6).

Although not necessarily an absolute contraindication, a hypercoagulable state does place a patient at higher risk for thrombosis during free flap reconstruction. Patients should be asked specifically about a history of deep vein thrombosis (DVT), multiple miscarriages, and pulmonary embolism (PE), as well as family history of DVT, PE, stroke, or genetic diseases such as factor V Leiden. Although no studies definitively support the practice, if patients are willing to accept an increased risk of flap failure and wish to proceed, more aggressive anticoagulation should be considered postoperatively. Although our success rate in these patients is 80%, one cautionary observation is that when these flaps thrombose, there is essentially a 0% salvage rate (7,8). In our practice, we offer free flap reconstruction if the patient accepts the higher risk but rarely offer attempts at heroic salvage in the event of a postoperative thrombosis.

Prior surgical history is important to ensure that the inferior epigastric pedicle or the perforators have not been sacrificed. A previous inguinal hernia or paramedian incision may have transected the inferior vessels, making a DIEP based on the pedicle on that side impossible. Even a laparoscopic puncture for an oophorectomy can damage the DIEA. A prior abdominoplasty is generally considered an absolute contraindication to a DIEP given the transection of all central perforators. A prior coronary artery bypass graft may make the internal mammary (IM) vessels unavailable or undesirable for recipients of a free flap. In such a case, the viability of the thoracodorsal system should be affirmed.

Timing and Adjuvant Therapy

Breast reconstruction may be performed at the same time as mastectomy or at a later date in delayed fashion. Although delayed reconstruction generally should not be performed until several months after mastectomy, there is no temporal limitation. In fact, many patients opt for reconstruction 10 or 15 years after cancer treatment. The benefit of immediate reconstruction is multifactorial. First, the native skin envelope can be preserved if the oncologic surgeon is comfortable performing a skin-sparing or nipple-sparing mastectomy. As a result, the cutaneous component of the DIEP flap is often only a small, natural-appearing circle used to replace the lost nipple–areolar complex. Second, the native skin at the time of mastectomy tends to be more pliable and predictable than that used in delayed reconstruction when new skin flaps are raised from a previously operated, often irradiated field. Because of the resultant discrepancy of skin quality between reconstructed and normal breasts in a unilateral delayed reconstruction, there is a tendency for asymmetry in the long term. Third, symmetry is easier to obtain because of the unaltered native inframammary fold (IMF) position in immediate reconstruction. In delayed reconstruction, the new IMF must be approximated either by comparison to the contralateral breast or by the impression left by a well-fitting brassiere. Although this does not usually result in any noticeable problems, it does introduce more unpredictability. Last, immediate reconstruction allows for completion of two major operations at one time. This efficiency should not be minimized because breast cancer patients often navigate a long journey to complete their treatment. In the end, whether immediate or delayed, long-term outcomes remain excellent. An important point to make to patients who seek unilateral reconstruction is that after the abdominal donor site is used, this cannot be used again in the future; therefore, prophylactic mastectomy on the contralateral side should at least be discussed at the time of preoperative evaluation and a recent normal mammogram documented on the contralateral side as well.

Although many women with breast cancer undergo chemotherapy, it does not appear to play a significant role in increasing complications in breast reconstruction (4). It is prudent, however, to avoid operations while the patient is actually taking chemotherapy to allow for normal wound healing. Radiation therapy, on the other hand, can have a significant deleterious effect on autologous reconstruction. The use of radiation therapy for the treatment of breast cancer is increasing, and although plastic surgeons have no control over its utilization, they do have control over the timing of reconstruction in relation to planned postmastectomy radiation therapy. Whether administered before or after reconstruction, radiation therapy leads to decreased overall aesthetic outcomes (9,10). Fat necrosis, volume loss, and asymmetry are also more likely in flaps that are subjected to irradiation. Although there is some literature to suggest that radiation field design may be compromised by breast reconstruction, to date there are no reports of higher recurrence rates or worse oncologic outcomes in women who receive adjuvant radiation therapy after breast reconstruction (11). Although aesthetically patients may benefit from delaying reconstruction until after any radiation therapy is complete, this must be balanced with the ability to forgo a second major operation with immediate reconstruction. In addition, previously irradiated recipient vessels are associated with increased technical challenges as well (12). Ultimately, timing is more a matter of creating an open dialogue between the patient and surgeon than hard and fast rules. In our practice, we have migrated over time to increasingly encourage patients toward delayed reconstruction if postoperative radiation therapy is likely.

Imaging

Little in the way of preoperative imaging is necessary before proceeding for reconstruction, although this statement is admittedly controversial in perforator flaps. Some authors conclude that preoperative Doppler or computed tomography (CT) angiography is important to identify the perforator vessels when performing a DIEP flap (13,14). Although imaging may make the surgeon more comfortable that a large perforator is available and in the end may shorten operating room time, it is unclear whether the added risk and expense of contrast-enhanced CT has any significant impact on patient outcome or overall expenditure. Preoperative imaging for DIEP flaps is dealt with elsewhere in this volume.

TECHNICAL PEARLS

Technical harvest of a DIEP flap is discussed elsewhere in this book; however, we outline below a few technical steps we use in our practice.

Recipient Site

The axilla is fairly well exposed during a modified radical mastectomy, making the thoracodorsal system useful as a recipient site; however, in most circumstances, the IM vessels have become the primary recipient site for free flap breast reconstruction. Outcomes between the two recipient sites have proven to be similar and the IM site allows for more medial positioning of the flap, leading to improved symmetry and aesthetics (15). In addition, using the IM avoids having to access the axilla in a simple mastectomy and avoids the risk of injury in cases in which reoperating in the axilla for further nodal resection is possible at a later date. The IM system also requires less pedicle length compared with the thoracodorsal, which is particularly helpful in short pedicles such as those found in other free autologous methods such as transverse upper gracilis and superior or inferior gluteal flaps.

The IM vessels are first approached by separating the fibers of the pectoralis muscle overlying the third costal cartilage. The perichondrium is incised along the midanterior surface from the junction of the sternum to 1 to 2 cm medial to the costochondral junction. The perichondrium is separated off of the cartilage, although complete separation of the posterior perichondrium can be difficult and is unnecessary. Next, a rongeur is used to remove the cartilage. The posterior perichondrium is incised lateral to the IM vessel and reflected lateral to medial. Care must be taken to avoid transection of the small intercostal vessel branches coming off of the IM system. After the vessels are identified and separated from the IM lymphatics, the length of dissection is increased by dividing the intercostal musculature from the top of the fourth rib to the bottom of the second rib; this is done by staying lateral to the IM vessels. The second costal cartilage can be removed to reach a larger diameter vein if needed. Compared with most other recipient vessels throughout the body, the IM artery is more susceptible to injury and thrombosis during its dissection. Minimal use of vascular forceps is recommended. The IM vein tends to be larger on the right side than on the left side. After fully dissected, the IM artery and vein are divided at the level of the third rib. The free flap is temporarily positioned to allow easy performance of the anastomoses. The artery is typically handsewn with 8-0 or 9-0 nylon. The vein is usually amenable to use of the coupler device (Figure 44-2).

Flap Inset

At the end of a long case, the surgeon must maintain focus and resolve for insetting the flap because this is paramount to creating

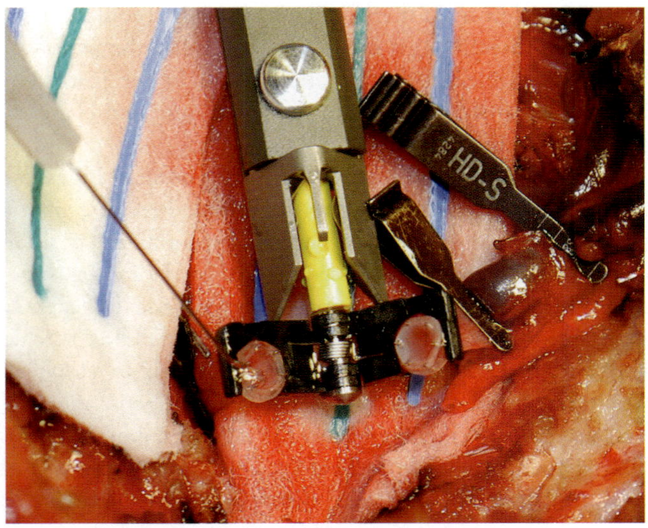

FIGURE 44-2 For venous anastomoses, the coupler device offers a fast and reliable alternative to handsewing the vein. The coupler can be sized and used on veins of various calibers. We have not had reliable success with coupling arterial anastomoses. This is likely attributable to the thicker arterial wall and more dynamic nature of the artery compared with the vein.

an aesthetically pleasing result. Ultimately, this is the most important factor leading to a satisfied patient. A decision as to whether to use an ipsilateral or contralateral free flap has usually been made preoperatively based on the shape of the contralateral breast, the timing of reconstruction, and the planned recipient vessels. In general, when the thoracodorsals are used, a narrow ptotic breast is reconstructed with an ipsilateral flap that has been rotated 90 degrees with the umbilicus positioned in an inferomedial orientation. As a result, the height of the free flap design thus corresponds to the width of the base of the breast mound. To increase projection, the base may be folded over upon itself. A less ptotic but wide breast is reconstructed with a contralateral free flap with the flap rotated approximately 140 degrees such that the lateral aspect of the initial flap design becomes the tail of the neobreast mound. This may be rotated up to 180 degrees for increased width. If the IM vessels are used, the concept is the same except that the exact opposite is performed—whereas a contralateral flap is used for a narrow, pendulous breast, an ipsilateral flap is used to construct a wider breast mound.

After the anastomosis is complete and orientation established, the buried portions of the flap are deepithelialized. The goal is to remove the epidermis and a portion of the dermis; however, care should be exercised not to injury the subdermal vascular plexus, which likely helps with more uniform perfusion of the edges of the flap. It is important to plan which portions of the flap are deepithelialized. One must always be cognizant of the amount of flap skin needed to ensure proper closure of the recipient skin defect created by the mastectomy. In most cases of skin-sparing mastectomy, the only exposed free flap skin after insetting is that occupying the site of the excised NAC. In delayed reconstruction, often there is a need to resect additional native skin during chest wall flap elevation. The breast surgeon may have excised a large skin ellipse with the mastectomy specimen. In addition, the skin may be inadequate for use as an envelope because of shrinkage and scarring from prior radiation therapy. This defect must therefore be replaced by the skin of the free flap. Generally, it is safe to deepithelialize the periphery of the flap while still on the abdomen or before inset. The final deepithelialization occurs after final inset and is greatly facilitated by this maneuver.

Inset should be performed in an upright position if possible as this helps to properly position the flap and recreate what a patient will see in a mirror. We begin by securing the position of the superomedial flap. This is followed by the medial, superior, and last the IMF position. Scarpa's fascia is generally secured to the pectoralis fascia with 2-0 Vicryl. These stitches need not be incredibly tight because this may lead to peripheral flap ischemia and pockets of fat necrosis. The superior aspect of the flap is secured in a manner to recreate the tail of the breast mound directed toward the shoulder. The inferolateral aspect of the breast should be suspended superiorly to avoid a square or boxy appearance of the mound. Last, the skin of the lateral chest wall often benefits from being tacked back down to the underlying muscle fascia. This helps eliminate dead space but also helps define the lateral aspect of the breast mound. Drains are always left in place. The skin is then closed in standard fashion.

Abdominal Closure

After the free flap is harvested, a fascial defect will have been created in the lower abdominal wall. Depending on the amount of fascia sacrificed, various techniques may be used for closure. For instance, a MS-3 or MS-2 flap typically has a very small resultant fascial defect that may be closed primarily without tension. This is one of the benefits of a DIEP flap—easier abdominal wall closure. An MS-1 or MS-0 defect, on the other hand, may preclude apposition of the free fascial edges. In this case, mesh in routinely used. Polypropylene mesh remains the most common subtype used for fascial closure in a clean wound. It is permanent with incredible tensile strength. Unfortunately, the same qualities that give it durability also make it stiff and unnatural. Acellular dermal matrix (human, porcine, or bovine) is one of many "biosynthetic" meshes that proponents argue are less prone to infection and result in a more natural contour. Alloderm (Lifecell Corporation, Branchburg, NJ) has been used successfully in free TRAM reconstruction; however, the long-term results of abdominal wall integrity after biosynthetic mesh implantation remain to be seen. To date, no prospective studies have compared results of abdominal wall closure techniques to guide an evidence-based closure algorithm. The abdominal donor site is closed in a manner similar to that of an aesthetic abdominoplasty. We routinely use the use of a temporarily implanted pain catheter.

POSTOPERATIVE CARE

Our practice pattern is to continue Doppler checks every hour for the first 48 hours and then every 2 hours until discharge, which typically is postoperative day (POD) 3 or 4. It has been shown that the faster a patient with a thrombosis returns to the operating room for exploration, the higher the likelihood of salvage. Monitoring is performed by nurses familiar with managing free flaps. Pain control is best managed with a patient-controlled analgesic pump for the first 48 hours at which point patients can usually be converted to an oral regimen. The patient remains on nothing by mouth status until the morning of POD 1, at which point they start clear liquids and are advanced as tolerated. As for activity, patients are encouraged to get out of bed to a chair on POD 1 and to fully ambulate on POD 2 at which point the Foley catheter is removed. Sequential compression devices are placed preoperatively and are continued postoperatively while the patient is in bed until discharge.

Anticoagulation remains a controversial subject in free flap breast reconstruction. At our institution, all surgeons prescribe subcutaneous heparin before and immediately after surgery both for DVT prophylaxis and to maintain a mildly hypocoagulable state after microanastomosis. The use of aspirin varies, with the goal of decreasing the thrombosis rate without adding additional risk of hematoma postoperatively. The significance of aspirin's effect on either outcome remains unclear (16).

The patient is discharged home usually with a visiting nurse to help with drain management. The drains are removed in the office over the next 1 to 2 weeks, usually when the output of each is less than 30 cc/day. Over the next several weeks, the patient is instructed to slowly increase activity but generally should avoid lifting for 6 weeks after surgery.

Patients should be instructed to follow up regularly with their medical and surgical oncologists. In unilateral reconstruction, patients will need to continue routine mammography of the contralateral breast as well as continue bilateral self-examination. Unfortunately, both systemic metastatic disease and local recurrence do occur after mastectomy and reconstruction. Patients should be instructed to continue self-examination of the reconstructed breast. Although fat necrosis can be mistaken for a neoplastic lesion, biopsy should be considered if a new mass is present. Mammography of the reconstructed mound has been shown to be less sensitive for picking up malignant lesions compared with the native breast; however, cases have been reported in which calcifications have been identified that are not otherwise palpable on examination. Currently, routine mammography of the reconstructed breast mound is not considered standard of care.

COMPLICATIONS

A broad category of wound complications may arise, including seroma, delayed wound healing, hematoma, and mastectomy skin flap necrosis. As a whole, the noninfectious wound complications may be as high as 28% to 43%; however, most of the time, these heal without intervention or long-term sequelae (17). Wound infection occurs in 3.5% to 9.5% of patients but is usually limited to simple cellulitis and is easily treated with antibiotics. Vascular complications such as thrombosis or ischemia may lead to flap loss or fat necrosis; however, complete flap loss is rare. Close observation of these flaps is paramount in the immediate postoperative period because arterial or venous thrombosis can be salvaged with rapid surgical intervention.

Because of the microvascular anastomosis and operative manipulation, the artery and vein are both subject to thrombosis (Figure 44-3). In a review of the most recent 700 free TRAM flaps performed at our institution, 2.7% experienced an intraoperative arterial thrombosis, 0.3% an intraoperative venous thrombosis, 0.9% a postoperative arterial thrombosis, and 0.9% a postoperative venous thrombosis. Of the intraoperative thromboses, none resulted in eventual flap loss. Of the delayed arterial thromboses, 66.7% of the flaps were salvaged by returning to the operating room, but only 50% of the delayed venous thromboses were salvaged. Clearly, delayed thromboses confer a more clinically detrimental outcome. In addition, unrecognized or delayed recognition of a thrombosis likely contributes to flap loss; therefore, close observation of these flaps is paramount in the immediate postoperative period. Venous congestion after surgery can be treated with leach therapy; however, sudden changes in flap character or Doppler signal warrant exploration. Once in the operating room, the flap is explored through the same incision and the pedicle should be fully reexplored and managed according with standard microvascular techniques for reestablishing flow. The pedicle usually requires a completely new anastomosis.

Donor site morbidity is an unfortunate downside of autologous reconstruction not seen with expander and implant reconstruction. Hernias may require reoperation for repair.

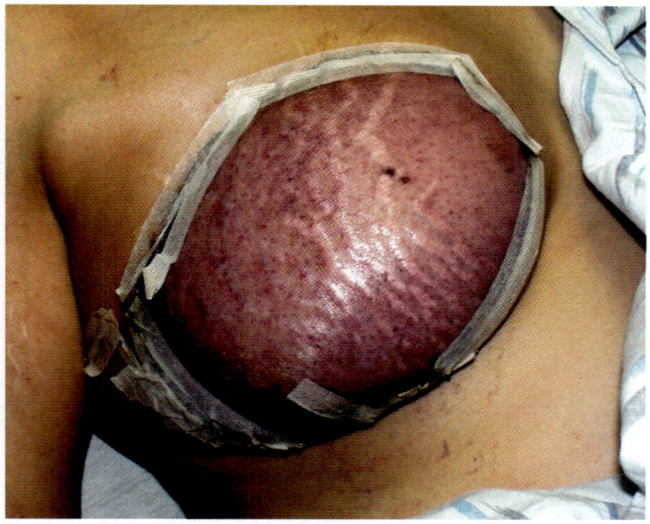

FIGURE 44-3 This patient underwent unilateral free flap breast reconstruction and was discharged home only to return with a blue and swollen flap. This is the classic finding of venous thrombosis which in this case was salvaged with reexploration and vein grafting.

In addition, after manipulation of the abdominal wall, many patients may experience a permanent decrease in abdominal wall strength. A hot topic in autologous reconstruction remains the relative risks and benefits of free TRAM and muscle-sparing free TRAM compared with more technically challenging muscle-preserving procedures such as the superficial inferior epigastric artery (SIEA) or DIEP flaps. The proponents of the DIEP and SIEA group believe that sparing the rectus muscle leads to less donor site morbidity such as weakness or hernia formation with little downside. The competing argument is that the blood supply to a perforator flap or SIEA may be less robust, leading to increased flap complications and increased incidence of fat necrosis. In addition, it remains unclear as to the significance of the donor site morbidity on patient functionality and satisfaction (3,18,19). Although debate will likely continue, our interpretation of the existing data is that sparing muscle and fascia will lead to decreased abdominal wall morbidity over time; however, this must be weighed against a higher flap complication rate in procedures such as the DIEP and SIEA.

OUTCOMES

The mastectomy defect can be devastating both physically and psychologically. Numerous studies have documented significant improvement in self-confidence and mental health after breast reconstruction. Although not routinely done, efforts to reestablish innervation to free flaps has been shown to improve patient satisfaction overall. No one procedure outshines another in all circumstances; however, certain patients clearly benefit from careful procedural selection. In the end, the overall plan for reconstruction must be the result of an open dialogue between surgeon and patient, one that ultimately involves listening and education.

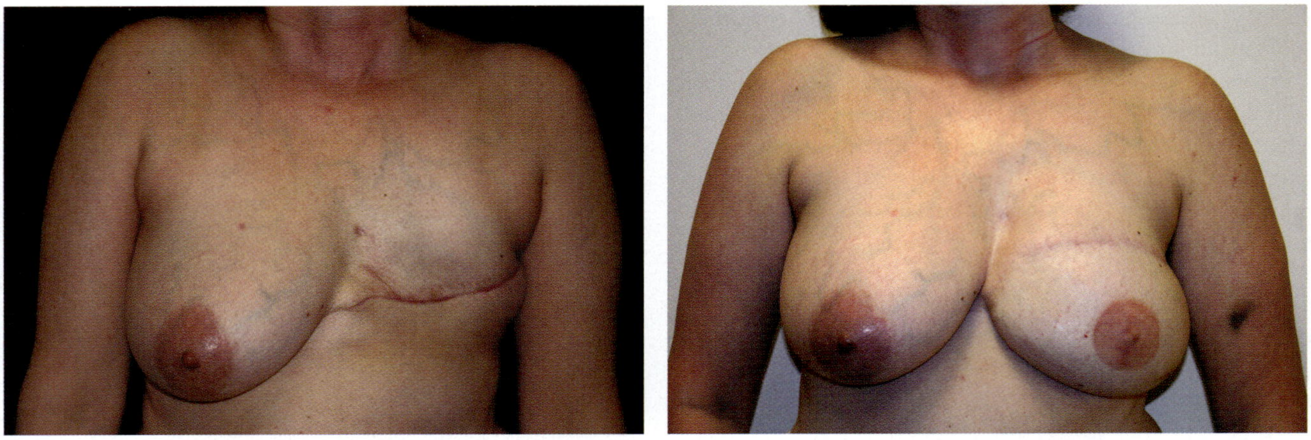

A B

FIGURE 44-4 Preoperative (A) and 6-month postoperative (B) photographs of a patient who underwent left delayed unilateral breast reconstruction with a deep inferior epigastric perforator flap. She has completed nipple areolar reconstruction and tattooing for color.

Aesthetic complications should be discussed with the patient preoperatively. These include breast mound asymmetry, contour irregularities, contracture and volume loss related to radiation or fat necrosis, poor wound healing, and scaring. With proper planning, these setbacks can be ameliorated with revisionary surgery such as scar revision, liposuction, breast reduction, mastopexy, implant augmentation, and newer techniques such as fat grafting for contour irregularities. Proper counseling of patients preoperatively is, as mentioned, imperative because accurate expectations will most often yield the greatest patient satisfaction. Figures 44-4 through 44-6 demonstrate examples of DIEP breast reconstruction and the resultant donor site defect.

SECONDARY SURGERY

Although some patients will undergo free flap reconstruction and never require further surgery, it is not uncommon for patients to require minor revisionary surgery. In general, we prefer to wait until the completion of any adjuvant therapy before embarking on secondary surgery. For contour irregularities and small size discrepancies, fat grafting is a powerful tool. Although the ideal method of fat harvest and processing remains controversial, most would agree that multiple aliquots of small amounts of refined fat has a high take rate in the reconstructed breast and can make a substantial difference. Although large-volume fat grafting for augmentation is possible, this is not a modality used commonly. Conversely, liposuction can easily decrease volume in oversized areas of the reconstructed breast mound. Because the flap is all fat, liposuction can remove a large amount of fat in a short amount of time; therefore, a surgeon must exercise caution and not be too aggressive. For larger changes in volume, breast implants can be inserted. For this, we generally recommend placing the implant in a subpectoral position to avoid any risk to the undersurface of the flap and its pedicle. The last tool commonly used is flap repositioning. In the event that the mound is malpositioned, this

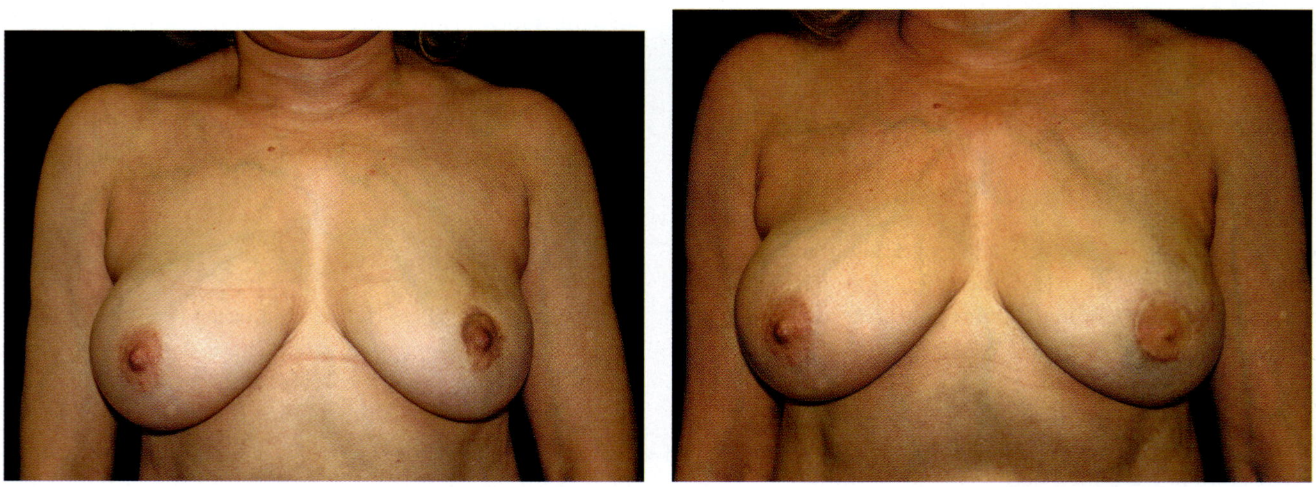

A B

FIGURE 44-5 Preoperative (A) and 6-month postoperative (B) photographs of a patient who underwent immediate left unilateral breast reconstruction with a deep inferior epigastric perforator flap. She has completed nipple areolar reconstruction and tattooing for color. Note in this skin-sparing mastectomy, far less free flap skin is needed compared with the delayed reconstruction in Figure 44-4, which makes the scars much less conspicuous.

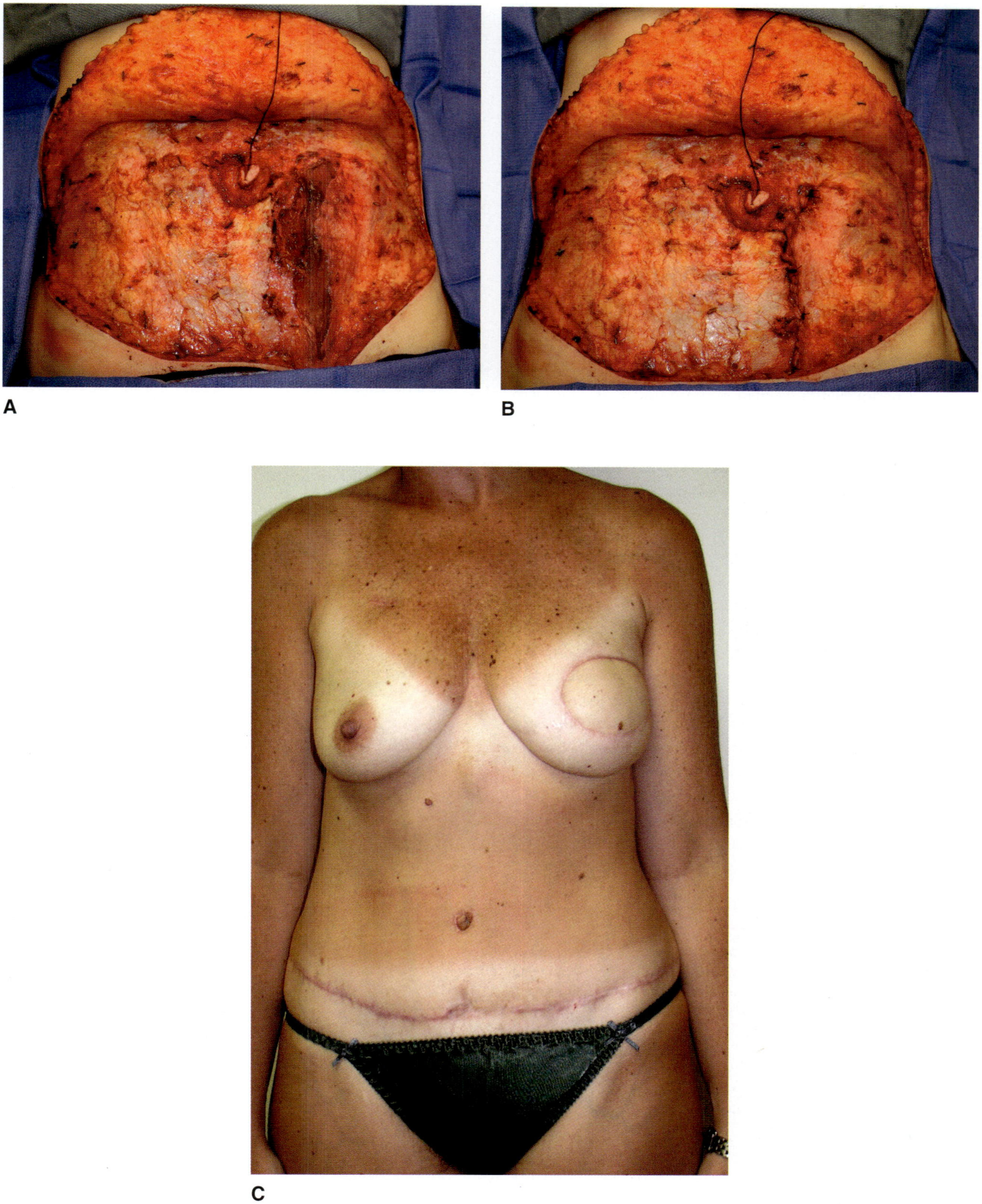

FIGURE 44-6 In this deep inferior epigastric perforator flap harvest (A), all of the fascia and muscle are spared, resulting in a straight-line closure of the anterior fascia without the need for mesh (B). (C) A typical example of the donor site scar.

can be corrected using common plastic surgical techniques of mastopexy and reduction or can be corrected via existing surgical scars, flap undermining, and mound repositioning.

Last, nipple areolar reconstruction constitutes a significant psychological step toward the final completion of the breast reconstruction process in women. The history of nipple reconstruction follows a similar timeline as autologous reconstruction, having been around for years and having undergone many permutations. Techniques used in the past have included grafting from skin, buccal mucosa, labia minora or majora, thigh, buttocks, groin, upper eyelids, or earlobes. Although the technique varies, the principles remain the same: to provide color, texture, size, and projection that are all in line with the patient's aesthetic wishes. The most common method used today consists of local skin flap rearrangement to create texture and projection followed by tattooing for color. NAC reconstruction in most cases is performed more than 3 to 4 months after mound reconstruction. This allows for complete healing of the flap and ensures stable mound symmetry, which is a key prerequisite before recreating a NAC. Immediate NAC recreation at the time of flap has been reported but is far less common.

CONCLUSION

Although breast reconstruction has changed over the years, the general principles of creating an aesthetically pleasing, subtle, natural-appearing mound that holds up over time remains constant. Fortunately, free flap reconstruction offers the ability to more reliably create a long-lasting reconstruction with high reproducibility and patient satisfaction. Although some surgeons advocate a DIEP in all patients with an abdominal donor site, one must be cognizant that sacrificing muscle on occasion to ensure good flap perfusion in a safe manner should never be considered a failure. In the end, women are in search of a soft reconstruction without complications. The abdominal donor site, whether used as a muscle-sparing free TRAM, DIEP, or SIEA, offers an opportunity to deliver great results to a broad spectrum of patients.

REFERENCES

1. Hartrampf CR, Scheflan M, Black PW. Breast reconstruction with a transverse abdominal island flap. *Plast Reconstr Surg* 1982;69(2):216–225.
2. Man L-X, Selber JC, Serletti JM. Abdominal wall following free TRAM or DIEP flap reconstruction: a meta-analysis and critical review. *Plast Reconstr Surg* 2009;124(3):752–764.
3. Wu LC, Bajaj A, Chang DW, Chevray PM. Comparison of donor-site morbidity of SIEA, DIEP, and muscle-sparing TRAM flaps for breast reconstruction. *Plast Reconstr Surg* 2008;122(3):702–709.
4. Selber JC, Kurichi JE, Vega SJ, et al. Risk factors and complications in free TRAM flap breast reconstruction. *Ann Plast Surg* 2006;56(5):492–497.
5. Fischer JP, Nelson JA, Sieber B, et al. Free tissue transfer in the obese patient: an outcome and cost analysis in 1258 consecutive abdominally based reconstructions. *Plast Reconstr Surg* 2013;131(5):681e–692e.
6. Nelson JA, Fosnot J, Selber JC, et al. Age and abdominal wall strength: assessing the aging abdominal wall after autologous breast reconstruction. *Microsurgery* 2013;33(1):14–23.
7. Wang TY, Serletti JM, Cuker A, et al. Free tissue transfer in the hypercoagulable patient: a review of 58 flaps. *Plast Reconstr Surg* 2012; 129(2):443–453.
8. Mirzabeigi MN, Wang T, Kovach SJ, et al. Free flap take-back following postoperative microvascular compromise: predicting salvage versus failure. *Plast Reconstr Surg* 2012;130(3):579–589.
9. Rogers NE, Allen RJ. Radiation effects on breast reconstruction with the deep inferior epigastric perforator flap. *Plast Reconstr Surg* 2002;109(6): 1919–1924; discussion 1925–1926.
10. Williams JK, Carlson GW, Bostwick J 3rd, et al. The effects of radiation treatment after TRAM flap breast reconstruction. *Plast Reconstr Surg* 1997;100(5):1153–1160.
11. Kronowitz SJMD, Robb GLMD. Radiation therapy and breast reconstruction: a critical review of the literature. *Plast Reconstr Surg* 2009; 124(2):395–408.
12. Fosnot J, Fischer JP, Smartt JM Jr, et al. Does previous chest wall irradiation increase vascular complications in free autologous breast reconstruction? *Plast Reconstr Surg* 2011;127(2):496–504.
13. Masia J, Kosutic D, Clavero JA, et al. Preoperative computed tomographic angiogram for deep inferior epigastric artery perforator flap breast reconstruction. *J Reconstr Microsurg* 2010;26(1):21–28.
14. Giunta RE, Geisweid A, Feller AM. The value of preoperative Doppler sonography for planning free perforator flaps. *Plast Reconstr Surg* 2000;105(7):2381–2386.
15. Serletti JM, Moran SL, Orlando GS, Fox I. Thoracodorsal vessels as recipient vessels for the free TRAM flap in delayed breast reconstruction. *Plast Reconstr Surg* 1999;104(6):1649–1655.
16. Fosnot J, Jandali S, Low DW, et al. Closer to an understanding of fate: the role of vascular complications in free flap breast reconstruction. *Plast Reconstr Surg* 2011;128(4):835–843.
17. Mehrara BJ, Santoro TD, Arcilla E, et al. Complications after microvascular breast reconstruction: experience with 1195 flaps. *Plast Reconstr Surg* 2006;118(5):1100–1109; discussion 1110–1111.
18. Selber JC, Fosnot J, Nelson J, et al. A prospective study comparing the functional impact of SIEA, DIEP, and muscle-sparing free TRAM flaps on the abdominal wall: part II. Bilateral reconstruction. *Plast Reconstr Surg* 2010;126(5):1438–1453.
19. Selber JC, Nelson J, Fosnot J, et al. A prospective study comparing the functional impact of SIEA, DIEP, and muscle-sparing free TRAM flaps on the abdominal wall: part I. unilateral reconstruction. *Plast Reconstr Surg* 2010;126(4):1142–1153.

CHAPTER 45

Breast Reconstruction: Gluteal Artery Perforator Flaps

Joshua Louis Levine, Julie Vanille Vasile, David Todd Greenspun, Maria M. LoTempio, and Robert Johnson Allen

The gluteal area has long been an outstanding choice for autologous perforator flap breast reconstruction. An adequate volume of tissue can be found from the superior or inferior buttock to reconstruct appropriately sized breasts in most patients. The abdomen is considered the first choice of donor tissue for breast reconstruction. However, gluteal tissue is an excellent alternative in patients for whom an abdominal flap (deep inferior epigastric perforator [DIEP] flap) may not be the best option.

BRIEF HISTORY

Fujino et al. were the first to use the gluteal area, in the form of a myocutaneous free flap, to reconstruct a breast in 1975 (1). Le Quang introduced the inferior gluteus myocutaneous free flap in 1980 (2). The superior gluteal myocutaneous free flap for breast reconstruction was further developed and popularized by Shaw in 1983 (3). Paletta et al. further developed the inferior gluteal myocutaneous free flap for breast reconstruction in 1989 (4). In 1993, Koshima et al. were the first to describe local transposition of gluteal flaps, based on perforating vessels without the underlying gluteus muscle, to heal sacral decubitus wounds (5). Allen et al. first described the use of free gluteal artery perforator (GAP) flaps to transfer gluteal tissue without sacrificing the gluteus muscle for breast reconstruction in 1993 (6). The inferior gluteal artery perforator (IGAP) flap was further refined by designing the flap in the inferior gluteal crease in 2004 by Allen et al. (7).

INDICATIONS

The gluteal region should be considered for any patient interested in autologous breast reconstruction. The abdomen is the first choice donor site whenever it is available. However, there are increasing circumstances in which abdominal tissue is not available or not the best option. Common indications for gluteal flap breast reconstruction are insufficient abdominal tissue, prior abdominoplasty, extensive abdominal liposuction, failed abdominal flap, pear-shaped habitus (greatest volume of fat distributed on the buttocks), or patient preference. In very thin patients, and especially in bilateral breast reconstruction, the abdomen may not provide enough volume for two reasonable breast reconstructions. The buttock is a natural area of fat deposition in most women and can usually be used to make reasonable-sized breasts in even the most athletic patient (7,8). Also, sometimes a patient does not want a long scar across her front and would prefer a scar that she does not have to see in the mirror daily. Gluteal flaps have the advantage of providing adequate tissue for breast reconstruction while hiding the scar behind the patient.

SUPERIOR VERSUS INFERIOR GLUTEAL ARTERY PERFORATOR FLAP

Indications for choosing a superior gluteal artery perforator (SGAP) or IGAP flap are based on each individual patient's preference and anatomy. A patient's preference toward a SGAP or IGAP flap is influenced by the advantages and disadvantages of each gluteal flap procedure. The scar from an SGAP flap can be covered by a bathing suit, but the scar is located in a more prominent position on the buttock. In addition, harvesting an SGAP can disturb the superior fullness of the buttock, causing unfavorable flattening of this area. Conversely, the scar from an IGAP flap can be located in a less prominent area of the buttock in the inferior gluteal crease. In addition, an IGAP flap may remove the "saddle bags," commonly an area of abundant fat deposition in women, without disturbing the aesthetic unit of the buttock (7). A disadvantage of the IGAP flap is that the lateral portion of the scar can be visible in a bathing suit and sometimes the inferior gluteal crease can be distorted or shifted cephalad or caudal. Contrary to previous reports, the sciatic nerve has never been injured with an IGAP flap and is never exposed during dissection of the flap (8). Rarely, temporary paresthesias can occur if the posterior femoral cutaneous nerve is stretched during harvest of an IGAP flap (9).

Anatomic considerations on the decision to choose an SGAP or IGAP flap are based on a patient's distribution of fat on the buttock and location of the most favorable vessels in the buttock. Cross-sectional preoperative gluteal imaging with intravenous (IV) contrast has been immensely helpful with the latter. We use magnetic resonance angiography (MRA) preoperatively to view the gluteal vessels because of the lack of radiation exposure and iodinated contrast. On occasion, we have switched the preoperative plan from a SGAP flap to an IGAP flap and vice versa based on the vascular anatomy in the planned donor site (10).

CONTRAINDICATIONS

Liposuction is considered a contraindication to perforator flap surgery because it can disrupt the fine vascular connections at the capillary level. If the area of liposuction was confined to only a portion of the buttock, sometimes a gluteal flap can be designed on a vessel in the nonoperated area. Copies of previous operative reports and preoperative imaging can be helpful in this regard (11,12).

A 10-year review of perforator flap breast reconstruction with DIEP flaps clearly showed that chemotherapy, abdominal scars, diabetes, and advanced age alone did not affect the surgical outcome of perforator flap breast reconstruction (13). The results of this study are also applicable to gluteal perforator flap breast reconstruction. Obesity increases wound healing complications but is not a contraindication if the patient understands the risks. However, morbid obesity is a contraindication because of increased pulmonary complications. Smoking is a contraindication to all flap procedures, and we recommend to patients a 3-month period of abstinence from tobacco, but this period can be shortened in select cases. Radiation can cause fibrosis and damage to any type of breast reconstruction and may affect the recipient vessels in the chest. We recommend postponing breast reconstruction until 6 months after radiation is completed to allow inflammation to subside at the recipient vessels. Hypertension can be associated with increased complications, and we recommend medical consultation for good blood pressure control before surgery. Hematologic disturbances in a patient's clotting cascade require consultation with a hematologist for advice on perioperative management strategies and close follow-up in the postoperative period and may not be a contraindication in select cases.

LIMITATIONS

A technical consideration of using the gluteal region is that compared with the abdomen, gluteal fat may be more spongy and firm in some patients. Thus, it can be slightly less pliable in shaping the breast reconstruction. Also, the gluteal flap has a higher fat to skin ratio, and the amount of skin available may be less than that of an abdominal flap in some patients. This may pose limitations in radiated patients undergoing delayed reconstruction. These issues are usually minor and can be overcome with proper planning and realistic expectations. The major limitation is the extreme difficulty of the procedure. Of all perforator flaps used for breast reconstruction, most experienced surgeons agree that GAP flaps are the most technically challenging. Most surgeons offer GAP flap procedures one at a time, so that a staged reconstruction is done for a bilateral procedure. Bilateral simultaneous GAP flap breast reconstructions may also be done. It requires two experienced microsurgeons harvesting the gluteal flaps simultaneously, preferably at the same rate, and intraoperative repositioning of the patient twice (14,15).

PREOPERATIVE PLANNING

Gluteal artery perforator flap procedures take significant effort, patience, and stamina to perform successfully. Preoperative imaging is enormously helpful in hastening the procedure and reducing anxiety. We developed a MRA protocol for high-resolution cross-sectional imaging of the gluteal vasculature. Our protocol has been fine tuned over the years such that we consistently get extremely useful and reliable information. Knowledge of the best gluteal perforator location and its course helps to plan the best incision and dissection (10,16).

Surgical candidates for gluteal perforator flap breast reconstruction are imaged in the prone position with MRA. The radiologist identifies the diameter, location, and course of all large gluteal vessels. The locations of the vessels at the fascia level are determined at a perpendicular point on the skin surface in relation to a marker placed on the superior point of the gluteal crease. Figure 45-1 shows a mark placed on the superior point of the gluteal crease. The measurements in relation to the marker are taken along the curved skin surface of the prone buttock using three-dimensional reconstructed MRA images to yield the most accurate information. Figure 45-2 demonstrates an example of how the location of a GAP is measured on an MRA.

From the radiology report and by reviewing the MRA images, we choose the optimal vessels on each buttock. The foremost factors in determining the optimal vessel upon which to base a flap in order of importance are vessel diameter, length of pedicle, location at which a vessel enters the planned flap, and vessel arborization pattern within the subcutaneous fat. In this regard, a larger vessel diameter, pedicle of sufficient length for insetting, central location of the vessel on the flap, or pattern of

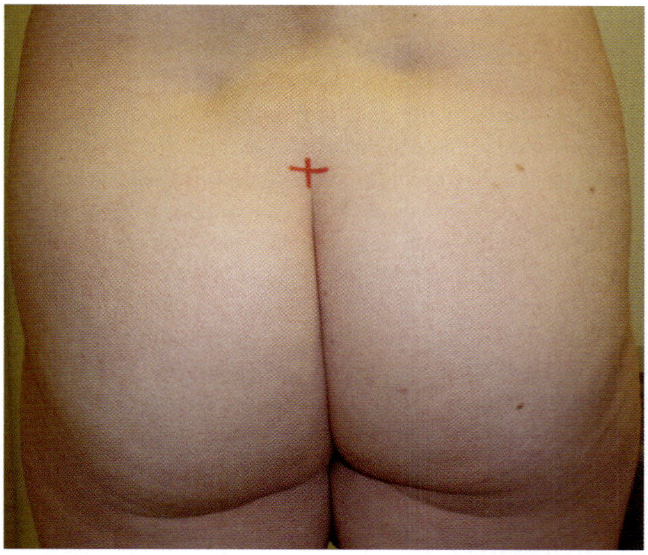

FIGURE 45-1 Photograph of the buttock with a mark placed at the superior point of the buttock crease. (Reproduced with permission from Vasile JV, Newman T, Rusch DG, et al. Anatomic imaging of gluteal perforator flaps without ionizing radiation: seeing is believing with magnetic resonance angiography. *J Reconstr Microsurg* 2010;26(1):47.)

arborization that suggests perfusion of the tissue to be transferred are all considered favorable. Vessels located laterally on the buttock produce longer pedicles, but if a vessel is located too laterally, it will be at the edge of the designed flap. An ideal vessel for insetting is one that will produce a pedicle length of between 8 to 10 cm. Special consideration in the selection of vessels is taken with bilateral gluteal flap procedures. To create symmetrical scars on the buttock, we try to select vessels that are located at a similar position on each buttock.

The course of a vessel is a secondary factor that influences vessel selection. If two vessels appear to be of similar size and both have equivalent vascular arborization patterns within the subcutaneous fat of the planned flap, then the vessel that can be dissected more easily or with the least trauma to the muscle is selected. Provided there is adequate length for insetting, a perforator with a more direct intramuscular course is favored because the dissection is usually technically easier, proceeds more quickly, and reduces trauma to the gluteal muscle. A septocutaneous branch of the superior gluteal artery, which travels around the gluteus muscles or between the gluteus maximus and medius muscles, may also be advantageous. However, sometimes the dissection can be tedious with gluteal septocutaneous vessels that are enveloped by thick fascia where they emerge laterally from the muscle (e.g., deep femoral artery branches).

In the office, on the day before the planned surgery, the locations of the optimal vessels selected on MRA are marked with indelible ink on the gluteal skin using measurements calculated from the MRA. A handheld Doppler is also used to confirm the locations of the perforators. The opportunity to plan and contemplate the details of the procedure is tremendously helpful. Ample time can then be taken in the office to design the flap skin pattern. An elliptical skin pattern is drawn to incorporate the selected vessels. The width of the ellipse varies based on the location of the selected vessels that are to be incorporated, the amount of skin required to reconstruct the breast, and the laxity of a patient's buttock skin. Typical flap widths used to be 8 to 10 cm. With the increased certainty of an adequate vessel, MRA enables us to design flaps with smaller skin patterns. For immediate reconstruction when extra skin is not needed, the skin paddle width can be 6 to 8 cm. Flap lengths can vary from 20 to 26 cm. A planned pattern of beveling of subcutaneous fat is outlined around the elliptical skin pattern based on tissue volume requirements to reconstruct the breast.

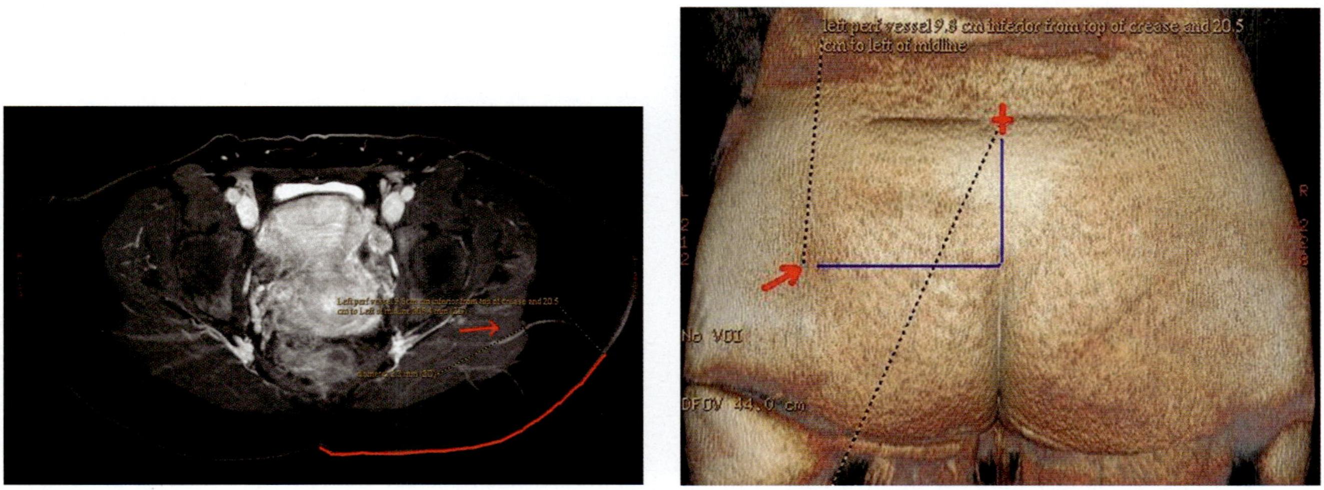

A B

FIGURE 45-2 (**A**). Axial magnetic resonance angiography (MRA) image. The gluteal perforator location is measured along the curved skin surface. The arrow points to the gluteal perforator. (**B**). Surface-rendered three-dimensional reconstruction MRA. The same perforator located on the buttock in reference to the top of the gluteal crease mark. (Reproduced with permission from Vasile JV, Newman T, Rusch DG, et al. Anatomic imaging of gluteal perforator flaps without ionizing radiation: seeing is believing with magnetic resonance angiography. *J Reconstr Microsurg* 2010;26(1):48.)

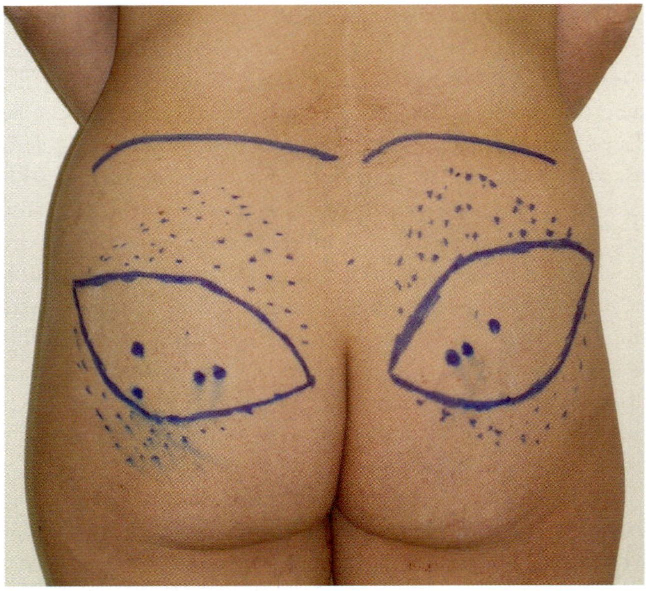

FIGURE 45-3 Photograph of bilateral superior gluteal artery perforator flaps designed using information from magnetic resonance angiography. Dotted markings show the planned harvest of subcutaneous fat.

An attempt is made to design flaps that will result in a scar that can be hidden under a bathing suit and that will result in symmetrical scars for bilateral gluteal flap procedures. A photograph is taken of the gluteal markings to bring to the operating room. Figure 45-3 shows photographs of a patient marked for bilateral SGAP flaps using information from MRA. Figure 45-4 shows photographs of bilateral IGAP flaps designed using information from MRA.

OPERATIVE PROCEDURE

Before the GAP flap procedure begins, a subcutaneous heparin injection is given, and sequential compressive devices are placed on the legs to prevent deep venous thrombosis. Standard anesthesia monitors are placed. An IV line is started, and a prophylactic dose of antibiotic is given. General anesthesia is administered, and a urinary catheter is inserted. Standard sterile antiseptic skin prep and draping is used. A team of two perforator flap microsurgeons operate simultaneously to maximize efficiency. The preparation of recipient vessels in the chest and the dissection of the gluteal vessels are performed with loupe magnification. The microscope is used for the anastomosis of the gluteal flap vessels to the chest vessels.

For a unilateral breast reconstruction, a gluteal flap is harvested from the same side of the body as the breast reconstruction. A patient is placed on a bean bag in the lateral decubitus position with appropriate padding of pressure points. The upper and lower extremities on the side of the breast reconstruction are prepped in the field. Figure 45-5 shows a patient prepared for a unilateral GAP flap. For immediate reconstruction, the mastectomy is performed in this position. Dissection of the recipient vessels in the chest and harvest of the gluteal flap proceed simultaneously. After the flap is harvested, the donor site is closed over a drain, and an occlusive dressing is applied. The patient is moved into the supine position for microsurgical anastomosis and flap insetting.

The sequence of the operation and patient positioning are different with a bilateral simultaneous breast reconstruction. The procedure begins with a patient placed supine for mastectomy and preparation of the recipient vessels on both sides of the chest simultaneously. The chest incisions are stapled closed temporarily, and an occlusive dressing is applied. The patient is moved into the prone position with adequate protection of the face and padding of pressure points. Bilateral gluteal flaps are harvested simultaneously by two microsurgeons. The gluteal incisions are closed over a drain, and an occlusive dressing is applied. The patient is returned to the supine position for microsurgical anastomosis and flap insetting.

Recipient Site

In delayed reconstruction, the recipient site is prepared by developing an appropriate pocket for the gluteal flap to rest in. The pocket is created by opening the space where the breast parenchyma was once located, under the subcutaneous tissue and overlying the pectoralis muscle. The most commonly used recipient vessels are the internal mammary vessels, which run parallel to the sternum and are located in a protected position under the ribs. These vessels are usually patent, and their medial location enables the flap to be inset medially where the volume of the flap is most needed. Near the sternum, the muscle fibers of the pectoralis muscle are separated at the intercostal space between the second and third or third and fourth ribs. Occasionally, adequately sized perforators from the internal mammary vessels can be used for anastomosis with the gluteal vessels. The perichondrium is elevated off the most medial portion of the ribs, and the most medial section of the intercostal muscle is resected. A pale yellow layer of fat containing the internal mammary vessels is located under the intercostal muscle and over the pleura. The internal mammary artery is accompanied by one or two veins. The vessels are dissected from the surrounding fat using bipolar cautery. Side branches of the vein are preserved distally to create a wider lumen in case of size mismatch with the gluteal vein. An intercostal space of 2 to 3 cm is usually sufficient to perform anastomosis. The edge of a rib or a portion of a rib may need to be rongeured off to achieve adequate room for anastomosis. The arterial size match is usually favorable if the GAP pedicle dissection was pursued all the way to the source vessel (SGA or IGA). If the pedicle was harvested before the larger artery, the pedicle vessel may be of smaller diameter. In this case, a better arterial size match may be achieved by using a perforating artery or branch off of the internal mammary artery. Alternative recipient vessels are the thoracodorsal or lateral thoracic vessels.

Donor Site

An incision is made along the planned skin pattern of the GAP flap. Subcutaneous fat is beveled to yield adequate volume and to obtain a more rounded flap for breast reconstruction. Figure 45-6 demonstrates beveling of the subcutaneous fat.

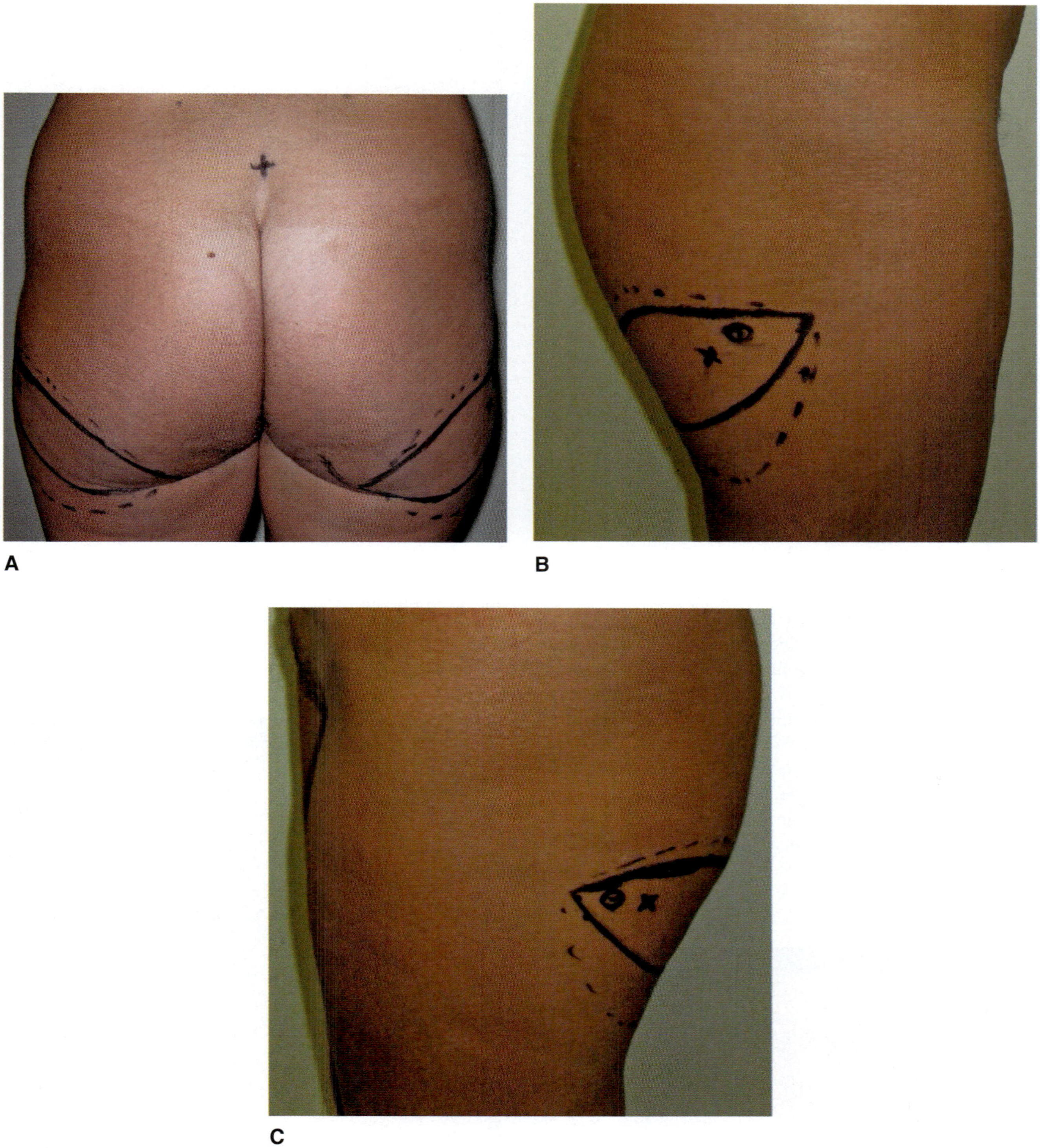

FIGURE 45-4 Photographs of bilateral inferior gluteal artery perforator flaps designed using information from magnetic resonance angiography. Planned harvest of subcutaneous fat is marked with dotted lines. (**A**) The posterior buttock. Flaps were positioned laterally to spare the cushioning fat medially. (**B**) The right lateral buttock. (**C**) The left lateral buttock. (Reproduced with permission from Vasile JV, Newman T, Rusch DG, et al. Anatomic imaging of gluteal perforator flaps without ionizing radiation: seeing is believing with magnetic resonance angiography. *J Reconstr Microsurg* 2010;26(1):51.)

The amount of beveling can be adjusted from the original markings based on the actual mastectomy specimen or implant. After the skin is opened, the flap is mobile, and the position of the marked Doppler signal may change with respect to its position as it emerges from the muscle. It is important to be aware of the original vessel position with respect to all the landmarks. The gluteal fascia is incised, and the flap is elevated from laterally to medially along the direction of the muscle fibers using bipolar cautery. Each muscle bundle should be completely uncovered to the extent of the entire field before moving to the next bundle. This results in a neat and predictable dissection, so that the perforators are easily visible when they emerge within

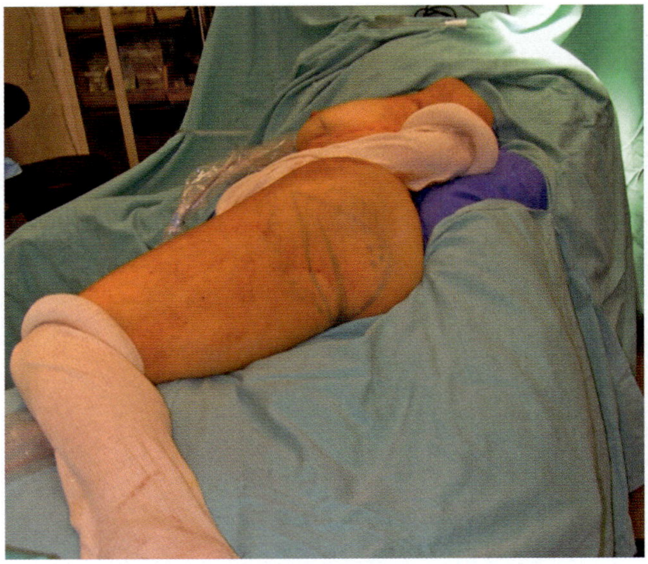

FIGURE 45-5 Photograph of the patient in the lateral decubitus position prepared for a unilateral gluteal artery perforator flap with the arm and leg sterile in the field.

the septum between two muscle bundles. Figure 45-7 is a photograph of a gluteal perforator emerging between two muscle bundles. When the best vessel identified on MRA is encountered, the septum is opened completely to the extent of the operative field. This technique is to avoid "getting in a hole." The dissection is very deep, and it is important to open the field as wide as possible to maximize visibility. Exposure is facilitated with deep self retaining retractors. If more than one perforator is being considered, each one should be fully visualized so that an appropriate decision can be made. Figure 45-8 is a photograph of an intramuscular gluteal perforator being dissected with wide exposure.

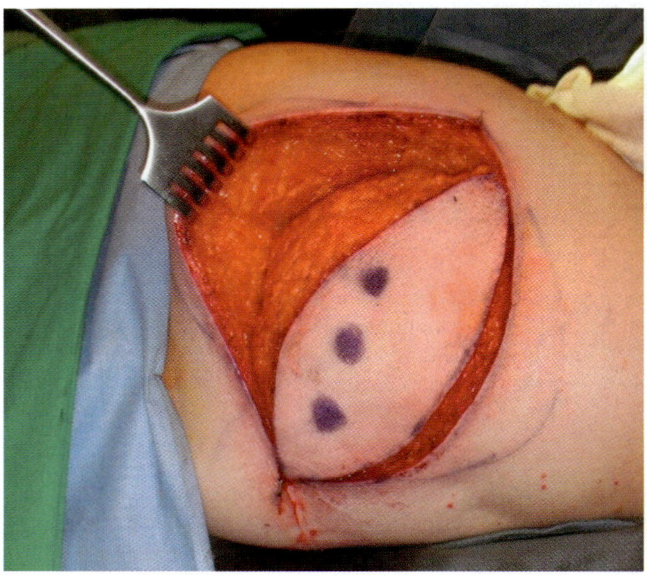

FIGURE 45-6 Photograph demonstrating beveling of the subcutaneous fat during dissection of a gluteal artery perforator flap.

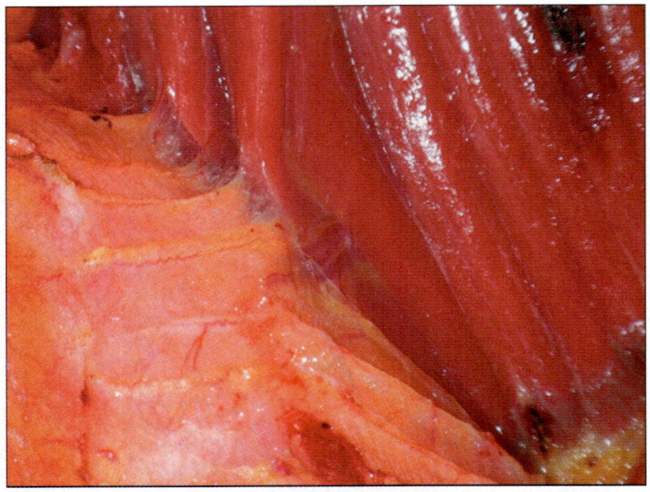

FIGURE 45-7 Photograph of a gluteal perforator emerging between two muscle bundles.

As dissection proceeds proximally toward the main superior or inferior gluteal artery trunk, multiple side branches are ligated, and vessel caliber increases. The pedicle is transected when an adequately sized artery is reached. Good retraction and exposure are of key importance in this dissection. In a SGAP flap dissection, a thick layer of posterior gluteal fascia is encountered. Figure 45-9 is a photograph of posterior gluteal

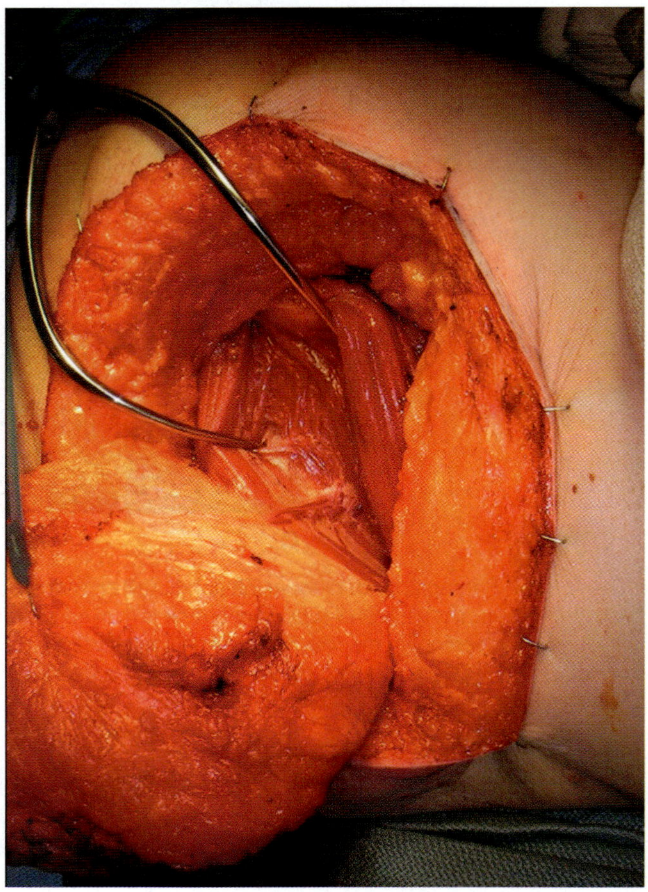

FIGURE 45-8 Photograph of an intramuscular gluteal perforator being dissected with wide exposure.

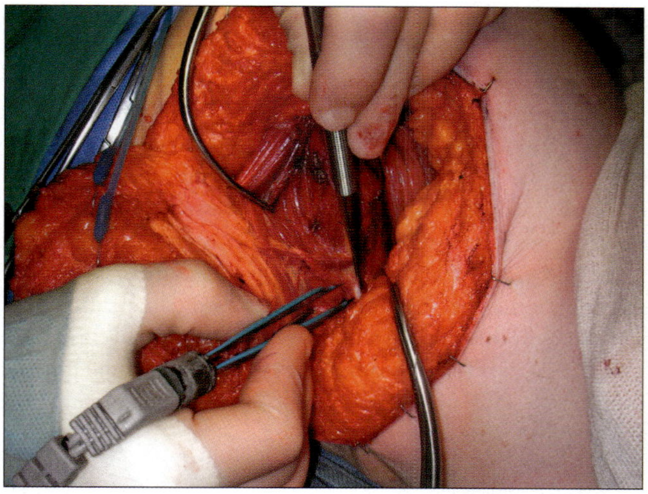

FIGURE 45-9 Photograph of posterior gluteal fascia encountered during a superior gluteal artery perforator flap dissection. Forceps and bipolar cautery instrument point to posterior gluteal fascia.

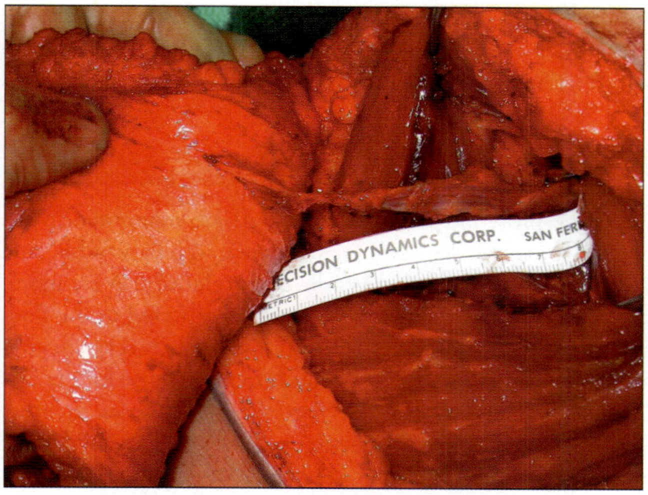

FIGURE 45-11 Photograph of a gluteal perforator dissection completed with adequate vessel length and caliber.

fascia seen during a SGAP flap dissection. This fascia layer does not exist in an IGAP flap dissection. At this level, multiple large, thin-walled venous branches are seen, called the "Medusa's head." The fascia must be opened widely to adequately dissect and ligate these venous branches. If the dissection can proceed past this obstacle, the painstaking effort is rewarded with a gluteal artery of larger diameter. Figure 45-10 is a photograph of a gluteal perforator dissected proximally to the source artery. If the pedicle is transected too early at the level of the perforator, the diameter of the artery will be less than 2 mm. If the dissection is continued more proximally and a cuff of gluteal artery is used, the diameter will be greater than 2 mm, resulting in an easier anastomosis. The diameter of the vein can be large and usually varies between 3 to 4.5 mm but can reach a diameter of 6 mm. Adequate vessel length is usually not a problem because a laterally located vessel is selected on MRA preoperatively.

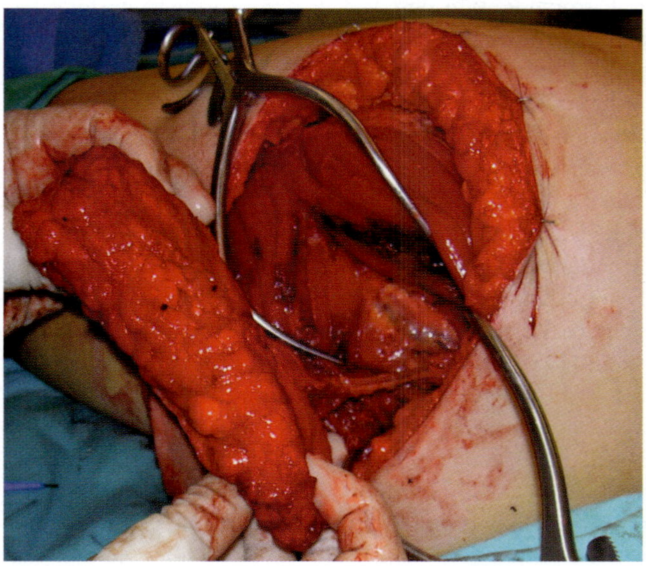

FIGURE 45-10 Photograph of a gluteal perforator dissected proximally after dissection and ligation of many venous branches.

Figure 45-11 is a photograph of a gluteal perforator dissection completed with adequate vessel length and caliber. An IGAP flap typically yields a longer pedicle of 8 to 11 cm compared with 6 to 8 cm with an SGAP flap. An IGAP flap dissection is very similar to a SGAP flap except the perforator length is usually much longer, and thus a longer dissection may be required to reach an artery of adequate diameter. If the posterior femoral cutaneous nerve is encountered, it is separated from the artery and preserved. The sciatic nerve is not encountered with an IGAP dissection. The donor site is closed over a drain using layers of interrupted absorbable sutures. Interrupted permanent sutures may be placed in the skin to reinforce wound closure but may be removed early. An occlusive dressing and a compressive garment are applied.

Anastomosis and Flap Insetting

The gluteal flap is brought to the chest, and care is taken to align the pedicle with the recipient vessels without a twist. In bilateral gluteal flap procedures, the decision of which flap to use at each recipient site (e.g., right gluteal flap to right chest or right gluteal flap to left chest) is determined by placing the gluteal flap into the recipient site pocket and observing the location of the pedicle entering the flap when the flap is optimally inset. The gluteal flap is temporarily sutured to the chest to prevent the flap from shifting and causing avulsion of the anastomosis. The veins are anastomosed first using a coupling device. A coupling device stents the veins open and is usually faster to use than sutures. The arteries are joined together with a handsewn anastomosis. The patency of the vein is checked by observing filling of the recipient vein proximal to the anastomosis. An arterial pulse and Doppler signal is checked in the distal pedicle. A Doppler signal of the GAP is confirmed on the skin, and a mark is applied. The color and capillary refill of the gluteal flap skin are checked. Excess flap skin is deepithelialized, and good flap bleeding is confirmed. The flap is inset over a drain using absorbable sutures. An island of gluteal flap skin is left visible for flap monitoring and can be used for future nipple reconstruction. A temperature strip is placed on the gluteal flap skin, and a control temperature strip is placed on the anterior chest. A supportive surgical bra is applied.

POSTOPERATIVE MONITORING

After the procedure, the patient's vitals are monitored in the recovery room. The color, temperature, capillary refill, and Doppler signal of the skin paddle of the gluteal flap are monitored every 15 minutes. The patient is transferred to the floor after awakening from anesthesia, and the flap checks are continued hourly and then every 2 hours by a 1:1 nurse for the first 24 hours. The frequency of flap checks decreases to every 4 hours until the patient is discharged. In select cases (e.g., the skin paddle Doppler signal must be located under the chest skin to optimize flap inset), continuous monitoring with a buried Doppler is used, but clinical flap checks remain our gold standard for monitoring flaps.

POSTOPERATIVE CARE

On the morning after the procedure, the surgical team advances the patient if the flap is well perfused. The IV fluids are discontinued, a regular diet is given for breakfast, the Foley catheter is removed, and the patient is out of bed to a chair with bathroom privileges. We have observed that patients with a perforator flap procedure have significantly less pain than those who have undergone a myocutaneous procedure. On the second postoperative day, the patient is ambulating into the hallways. On the third postoperative day, the patient is permitted to shower. The drain at the recipient can be removed if the output is less than 30 cc in 24 hours. On the fourth postoperative day, the patient is discharged on an oral antibiotic and ibuprofen. Most patients do not require a prescription for narcotic pain relief on discharge.

COMPLICATIONS

Complications unique to GAP flaps include those related to the donor site. To reduce the risk of a seroma at the donor site, closure of the buttock must be done with care to obliterate dead space. This can be difficult if significant beveling was used to maximize harvest volume and may require undermining of the buttock fat superiorly and inferiorly to mobilize this tissue for closure. A girdle is used to control swelling and to keep the dead space compressed, and donor site drains should be left in for a minimum of 2 weeks. The drains are removed only when output is less than 40 to 50 cc in 24 hours. When seroma formation occurs, it is managed by percutaneous aspiration in the office or with ultrasound-guided drainage by a radiologist. Persistent seromas may be managed by reinsertion of a drain.

Contour irregularities of the buttock are expected, and patients should be prepared for secondary procedures to improve the shape of the donor site. These procedures include dog-ear excision; liposuction of the lateral buttock, thighs, and posterior hip areas; and occasionally lipo-filling in the upper buttocks to restore volume. We have also used local flap mobilization to fill in upper buttock depressions.

Microsurgical complications are slightly more common with GAP flaps than with DIEP flaps. It is important to understand the limitations of the GAP pedicle and plan for potential challenges. If the SGAP pedicle is short (<6 cm), one may obtain more length on the internal mammary vessels by taking out a rib cartilage. It is also important to anticipate size discrepancies in both the artery and vein. If the pedicle artery is small in diameter, it may be better to find a perforating branch for anastomosis with the internal mammary. If the pedicle vein is large in diameter, it is helpful to find a branch point on the internal mammary vein to maximize the diameter of the recipient vessel and improve the size match.

SECOND STAGE

The second stage is an ambulatory procedure and usually is performed 2 to 3 months after the initial procedure. Adjustments are made to the reconstructed breast to try to improve symmetry. A nipple reconstruction may be needed from the flap skin paddle. An increasing number of patients in our practice are choosing nipple sparing mastectomy. In these patients, the gluteal flap skin that was left visible for flap monitoring is removed as early as the fourth postoperative day depending on the viability of the nipple. Adjustments to the donor site can also be performed, such as excision of a "dog ear" or liposuction to smooth the contour. The nipple and areola are tattooed about 6 weeks after the nipple reconstruction and can require two to three sessions because the tattoo pigment can fade.

LITERATURE REVIEW OUTCOMES

A review of 492 GAP flaps for breast reconstruction demonstrated that the incidence of complications was low (17). The overall take-back rate for vascular complications was 6%. Venous occlusion, accounting for 4%, was caused by mechanical kinking or twisting of the pedicle. Arterial issues requiring reanastomosis were observed in 2% of cases. The total flap failure rate was 2%. Donor site seroma occurred in 15% of patients, requiring aspiration, and 20% of patients required revision of the donor site at the second stage of breast reconstruction. The most common donor site revisions in SGAP patients are related to contour deformity of the upper buttock. These procedures include fat grafting, local flaps, and liposuction. The most common donor site revision for IGAP patients is contouring of the lateral trochanter fat with liposuction. Dog-ear revisions are also often done at the time of these revisions. GAP flaps for breast reconstruction had fat necrosis requiring revision at a rate of 8%. Breast flap asymmetry required fat grafting or revision in 10% of cases.

In an early series of 12 bilateral simultaneously performed SGAP flaps, the average operating time decreased from 10.3 hours to 8.7 hours with increased efficiency of the surgeons and support staff with the procedure and patient position changes (14). The average blood loss was 390 cc, and no flaps failed. There was one incidence of delayed donor site wound healing treated with conservative wound care. In a later series of

40 bilateral simultaneously performed SGAP flaps, the average operating time was 7.8 hours, average flap weight was 573 g, no flaps failed, and there was one seroma complication at the donor site (18).

In a series of 44 bilateral simultaneously performed in-the-crease IGAP flaps, average operating time was 9 hours; no flaps failed; there were two reoperations for venous congestion; one flap had partial fat necrosis; and there were two patients with delayed donor site healing, two patients with dehiscence of the donor site, and one patient with paresthesias that resolved (15). In the properly selected patient, bilateral simultaneously performed GAP flap can be an efficient and safe procedure.

CASES

Case 1 is a 54-year-old woman with a body mass index (BMI) of 25.5. The patient had a history of left ductal breast cancer and right lobular breast cancer, a bilateral mastectomy, chemotherapy, and failed implant reconstruction. The surgical history is significant for an emergency cesarean section through a midline abdominal scar. The patient desired bilateral C cup breast reconstruction but lacked the volume of abdominal fat to achieve her reconstructive goals. However, the patient had an ample volume of gluteal fat. The patient preferred a SGAP flap procedure so that the scar could be hidden below the bikini line. Figure 45-12 are photographs of the patient before and after surgery for bilateral simultaneous SGAP flaps.

Case 2 is a 47-year-old woman with a BMI of 18.2. The patient had a history of right lobular carcinoma in situ, atypical ductal hyperplasia, and multiple negative breast biopsies. The patient opted for bilateral mastectomies and immediate autologous reconstruction. She desired breasts larger than her current A cup but did not have enough abdominal tissue to meet her reconstructive goal. However, the patient had ample gluteal fat, with the greatest volume on her inferior buttock. Figure 45-13 is photographs of the patient before and after surgery for bilateral simultaneous in-the-crease IGAP flaps.

Case 3 is a 36-year-old woman with BRCA-positive breast cancer. The patient opted for bilateral nipple-sparing prophylactic mastectomy and immediate autologous reconstruction. She did not want a scar on her abdomen or upper buttock and chose bilateral IGAP flap breast reconstruction. Figure 45-14 is photographs of the patient before and after surgery for bilateral simultaneous in-the-crease IGAP flaps.

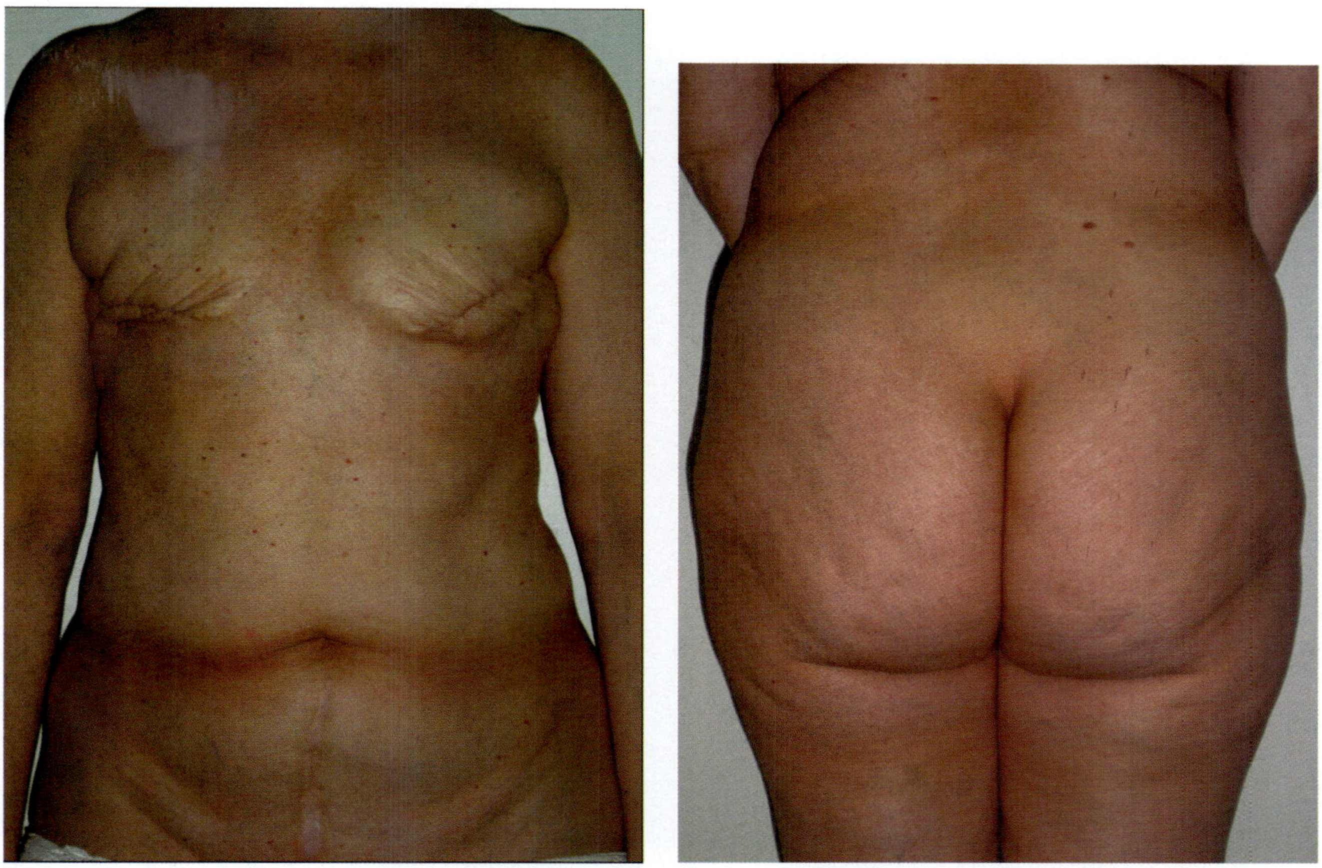

A B

FIGURE 45-12 A 54-year-old woman with history of bilateral breast cancer and mastectomies, failed implant breast reconstruction, a lower midline abdominal incision, and a lack of abdominal tissue to achieve her reconstructive goal of C cup breasts. The patient underwent bilateral simultaneous superior gluteal artery perforator flaps. (A). Photograph of the preoperative anterior view. (B) Photograph of the preoperative donor site showing ample gluteal fat volume.

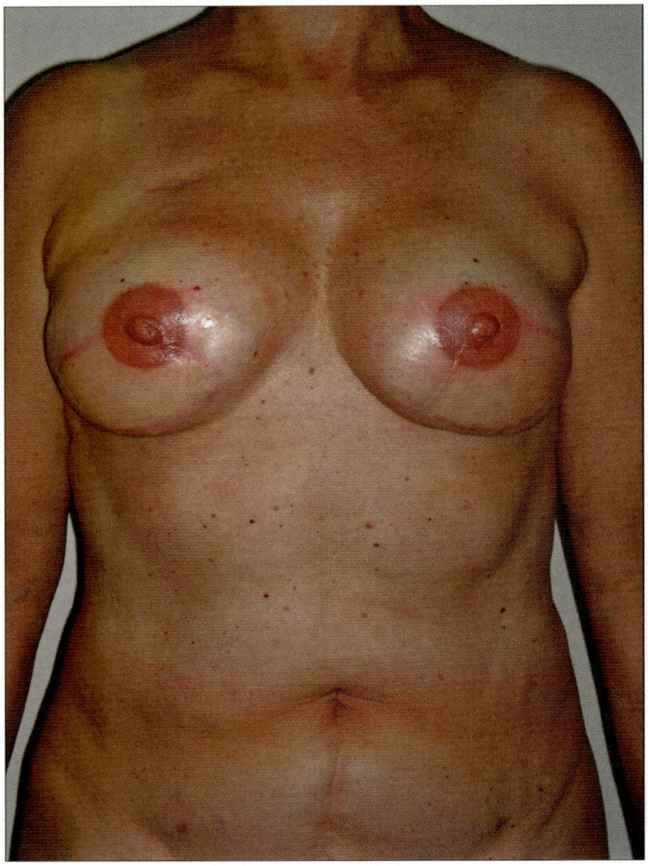

C

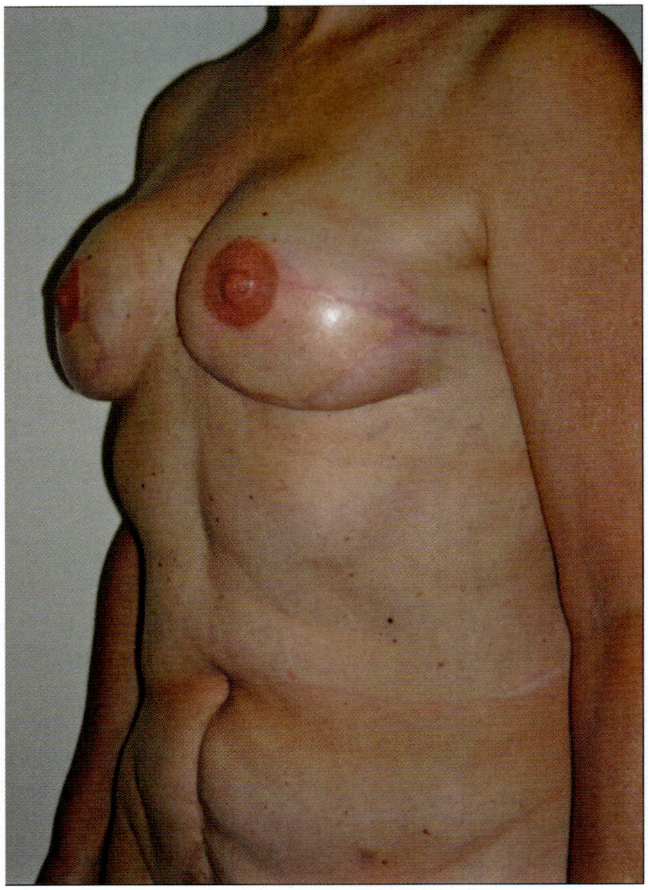

D

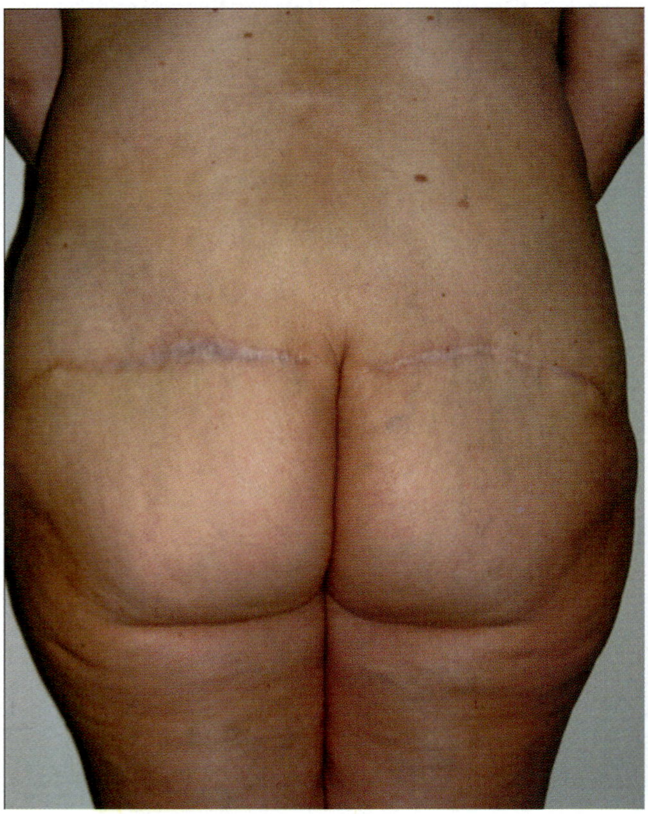

E

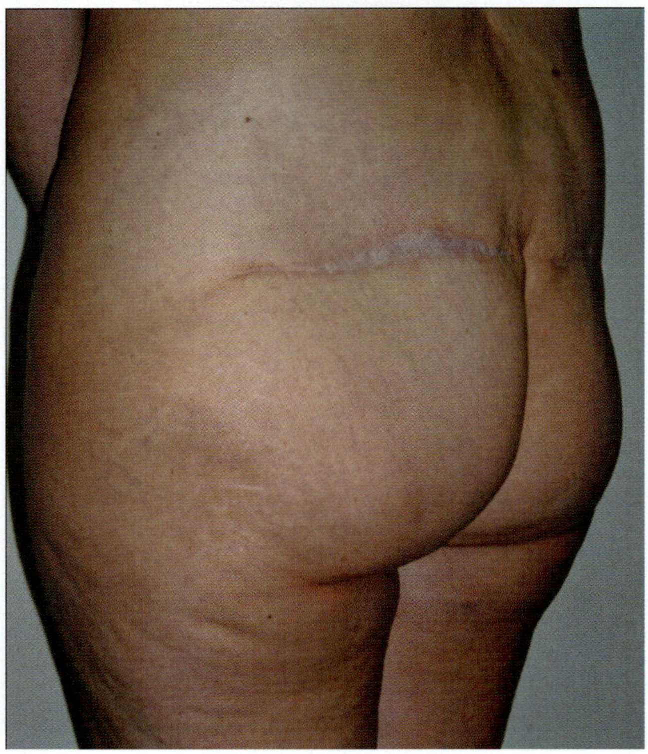

F

FIGURE 45-12 (*Continued*) (**C**) Photograph of the postoperative recipient site, anterior view. (**D**) Photograph of the postoperative recipient site anterior, oblique view. (**E**) Photograph of the postoperative donor site, posterior view. (**F**) Photograph of the postoperative donor site, posterior oblique view.

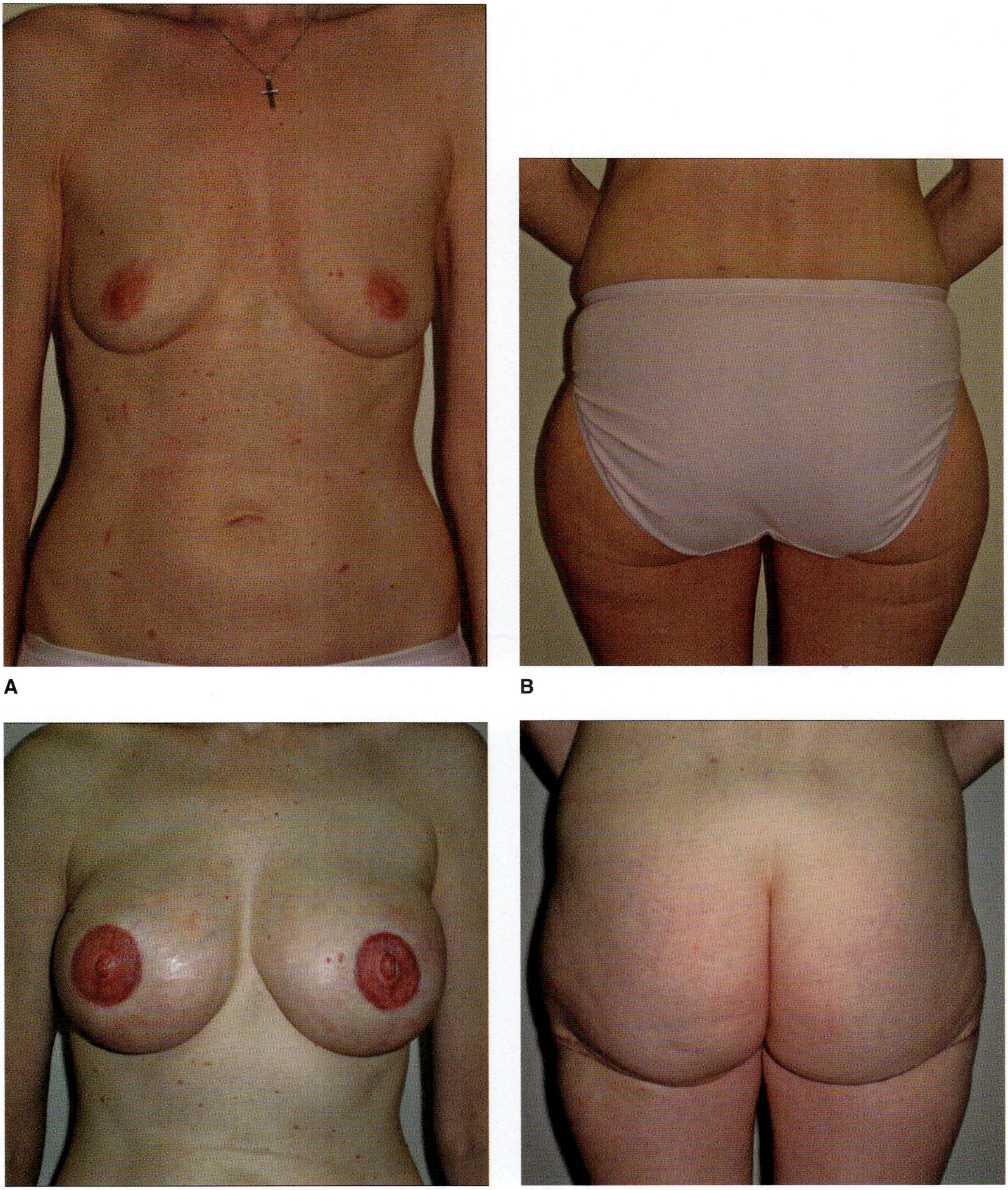

A B C D

FIGURE 45-13 A 47-year-old woman with a body mass index of 18.2, a history of right lobular carcinoma in situ and atypical ductal hyperplasia, multiple negative breast biopsies, and a lack of abdominal tissue to achieve her reconstructive goal of greater than A cup breasts. The patient underwent bilateral mastectomy and immediate reconstruction with bilateral simultaneous in-the-crease inferior gluteal artery perforator flaps. (**A**). Photograph of the preoperative anterior view. (**B**) Photograph of the preoperative donor site showing ample inferior gluteal fat volume. (**C**) Photograph of the postoperative recipient site. (**D**) Photograph of the postoperative donor site.

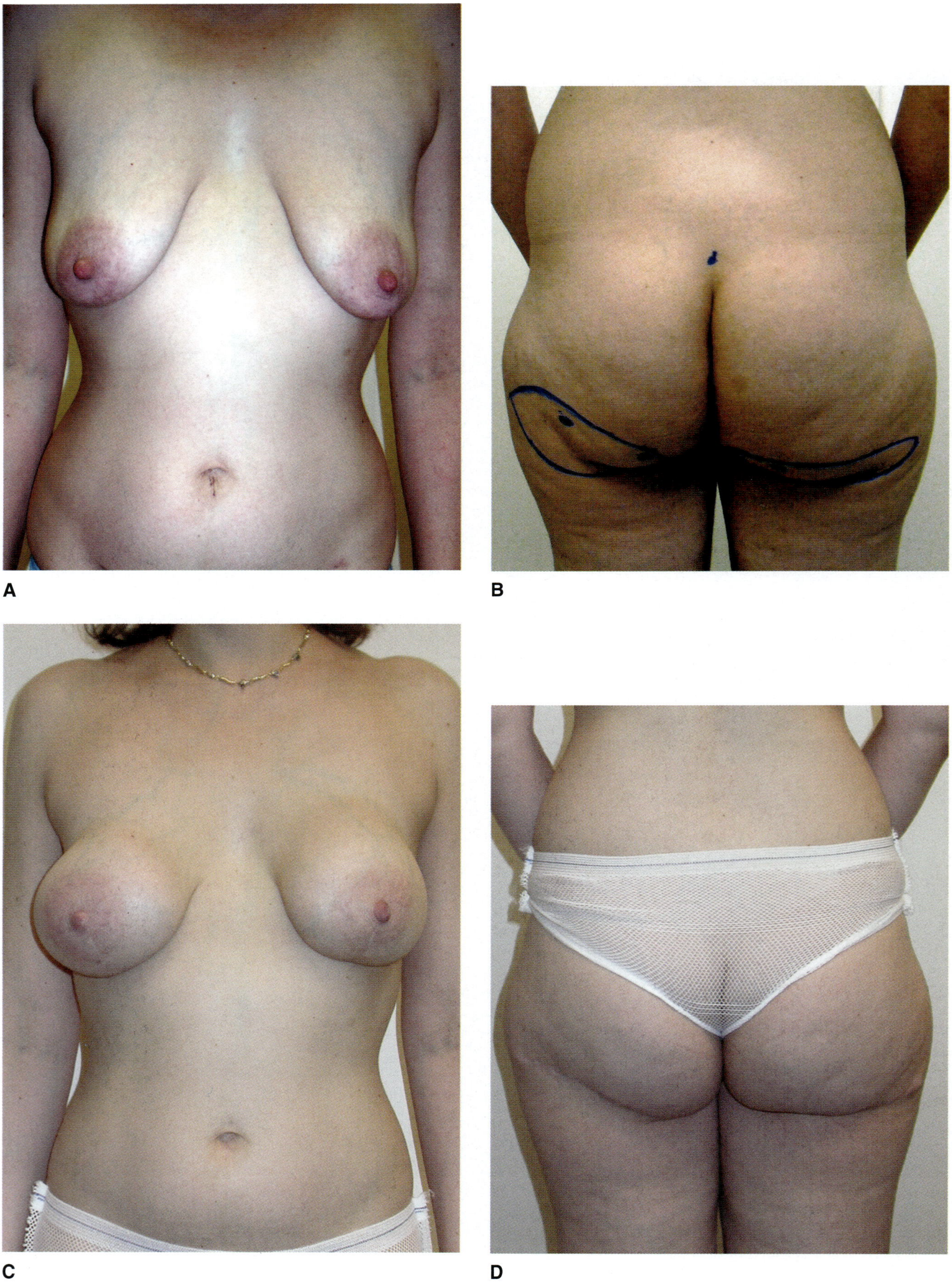

FIGURE 45-14 A 36-year-old woman with BRCA-positive breast cancer who did not want a scar on her abdomen. She underwent bilateral nipple-sparing prophylactic mastectomy and immediate reconstruction with bilateral simultaneous in-the-crease inferior gluteal artery perforator flaps. (A). Photograph of the preoperative anterior view. (B) Photograph of the preoperative donor site showing ample inferior gluteal fat volume. (C) Photograph of the postoperative recipient site. (D) Photograph of the postoperative donor site.

CONCLUSION

The GAP flap is an excellent alternative to the abdominal perforator flap for breast reconstruction. The high fat to skin ratio of gluteal flaps produce breasts with good projection, and the contour and scar at the donor site are usually good. Preoperative imaging has removed some of the stress from performing this challenging procedure. Accurate and advance knowledge of the caliber, location, and course of GAPs improves our ability to confidently select donor sites and design flaps and our efficiency in the planning and execution of the procedure.

REFERENCES

1. Fujino T, Harasina T, Aoyagi F. Reconstruction for aplasia of the breast and pectoral region by microvascular transfer of a free flap from the buttock. *Plast Reconstr Surg* 1975;56(2):178–181.
2. Le Quang C. Two new flaps developed from aesthetic surgery. II. The inferior gluteal flap. *Aesthetic Plast Surg* 1980;4:159.
3. Shaw WW. Breast reconstruction by superior gluteal microvascular free flaps without silicone implants. *Plast Reconstr Surg* 1983;72(4):490–501.
4. Paletta CE, Bostwick J 3rd, Nahai F. The inferior gluteal free flap in breast reconstruction. *Plast Reconstr Surg* 1989;84(6):875–883.
5. Koshima I, Moriguchi T, Soeda S, et al. The gluteal perforator-based flap for repair of sacral pressure sores. *Plast Reconstr Surg* 1993;91(4):678–683.
6. Allen RJ, Tucker C Jr. Superior gluteal artery perforator free flap for breast reconstruction. *Plast Reconstr Surg* 1995;95(7):1207–1212.
7. Allen RJ, Levine JL, Granzow JW. The in-the-crease inferior gluteal artery perforator flap for breast reconstruction. *Plast Reconstr Surg* 2006;118(2): 333–339.
8. Guerra AB, Metzinger SE, Bidros RS, et al. Breast reconstruction with gluteal artery perforator (GAP) flaps: a critical analysis of 142 cases. *Ann Plast Surg* 2004;52:118–125.
9. Heitmann C, Levine JL, Allen RJ. Gluteal artery perforator flaps. *Clin Plast Surg* 2007;34(1):123–130.
10. Vasile JV, Newman T, Rusch DG, et al. Anatomic imaging of gluteal perforator flaps without ionizing radiation: seeing is believing with magnetic resonance angiography. *J Reconstr Microsurg* 2010;26(1):45–58.
11. DeFrene B, Van Landuyt K, Hamdi M, et al. Free DIEAP and SGAP flap breast reconstruction after abdominal/gluteal liposuction. *J Plast Reconstr Aesthet Surg* 2006;59(10):1031–1036.
12. Greenspun D, Vasile J, Levine JL, et al. Anatomic imaging of abdominal perforator flaps without ionizing radiation: seeing is believing with magnetic resonance imaging angiography. *J Reconstr Microsurg* 2010;26(1): 37–44.
13. Gill PS, Hunt JP, Guerra AB, et al. A 10-year retrospective review of 758 DIEP flaps for breast reconstruction. *Plast Reconstr Surg* 2004;113(4): 1153–1160.
14. Guerra AB, Metzinger SE, Bidros RS, et al. Simultaneous bilateral breast reconstruction with superior gluteal artery perforator (SGAP) flaps. *Ann Plast Surg* 2004;53(4):305–310.
15. Levine JL, Miller Q, Vasile J, et al. Simultaneous bilateral breast reconstruction with in-the-crease inferior gluteal artery perforator flaps. *Ann Plast Surg* 2009;63(3):249–254.
16. Vasile JV, Newman TM, Prince MR, et al. Contrast-enhanced magnetic resonance angiography. *Clin Plast Surg* 2011;38(2):263–275.
17. LoTempio MM, Allen RJ. Breast reconstruction with SGAP and IGAP flaps. *Plast Reconstr Surg* 2010;126(2):393–401.
18. Dellacroce FJ, Sullivan SK. Application and refinement of the superior gluteal artery perforator free flap for bilateral simultaneous breast reconstruction. *Plast Reconstr Surg* 2005;116(1):97–103.

CHAPTER 46

Breast Reconstruction with Superficial Inferior Epigastric Artery Flaps

J. Brian Boyd

BRIEF HISTORY OF MICROVASCULAR BREAST RECONSTRUCTION

The use of pedicled musculocutaneous flaps from the abdomen for breast reconstruction dates from Drever (1) in the late 1970s, who described the vertical rectus abdominis musculocutaneous (VRAM) flap and later Hartrampf et al. (2) in the early 1980s, who described the transverse rectus abdominis musculocutaneous (TRAM) flap. The TRAM flap proved truly revolutionary in that the donor site resembled a cosmetic abdominoplasty with tight skin and a bikini-line scar—an aesthetic enhancement for many patients. Pedicled tissue transfers based on the superior epigastric system are still performed but have the disadvantage of weakening the abdominal wall, leading to bulges, hernias, discomfort, and functional loss (3–5). In many cases, the use of synthetic mesh is required for abdominal repair, and this has its own set of potential complications (6). Furthermore, the blood supply of the flap can be tenuous, skin survival uncertain, and fat necrosis common (7).

In an attempt to limit abdominal wall weakening and to augment the circulation in the transferred tissue, *free* TRAM flaps were developed (8,9). The circulation proved superior because the skin and subcutaneous tissue of the flap lay in the primary vascular territory of the deep inferior epigastric artery (DIEA), the vessel on which the flap was raised (Figure 46-1). A section of the rectus abdominis muscle was taken (usually the lower half) to safeguard the perforators from the DIEA. Yet a significant lower abdominal defect was created, still often requiring mesh closure. Free TRAM flaps quickly evolved into *muscle-sparing* free TRAM flaps (10) and ultimately deep inferior perforator (DIEP) flaps (11), each removing successively less rectus muscle and fascia, eliminating the need for mesh, and decreasing the incidence of hernias and bulges. Although harvesting a DIEP flap theoretically "spares" the entire rectus muscle, it still weakens it by direct injury because the muscle is split in the dissection of perforators with associated damage to its segmental nerve supply.

Notwithstanding the fact that the earliest free flaps were based on the superficial inferior epigastric artery (SIEA), the use of the SIEA flap in breast reconstruction is a relatively recent innovation (12–15). Its vascular territory overlaps and lies a little lateral to that of the DIEA (Figure 46-2), and its harvest involves no injury to the abdominal musculature. However, as we shall see, it is not always a practical alternative.

MAJOR FREE FLAPS AVAILABLE FOR BREAST RECONSTRUCTION

These flaps are:

- TRAM flap (8,9)
- Muscles-sparing free TRAM flap (10)
- DIEP flap (11)
- SIEA flap (12–15)
- Gluteal artery perforating (GAP) flaps (16,17)
- Transverse upper gracilis (TUG) flap (18,19)
- Deep circumflex artery flap (Reuben's) flap (20)

INDICATIONS FOR SUPERFICIAL INFERIOR EPIGASTRIC ARTERY FLAP BREAST RECONSTRUCTION

Because the anatomical location and the primary vascular territory of the SIEA flap lie somewhat lateral to the DIEA's, that portion of the SIEA flap crossing the midline is considered somewhat less reliable than the transmidline portion of

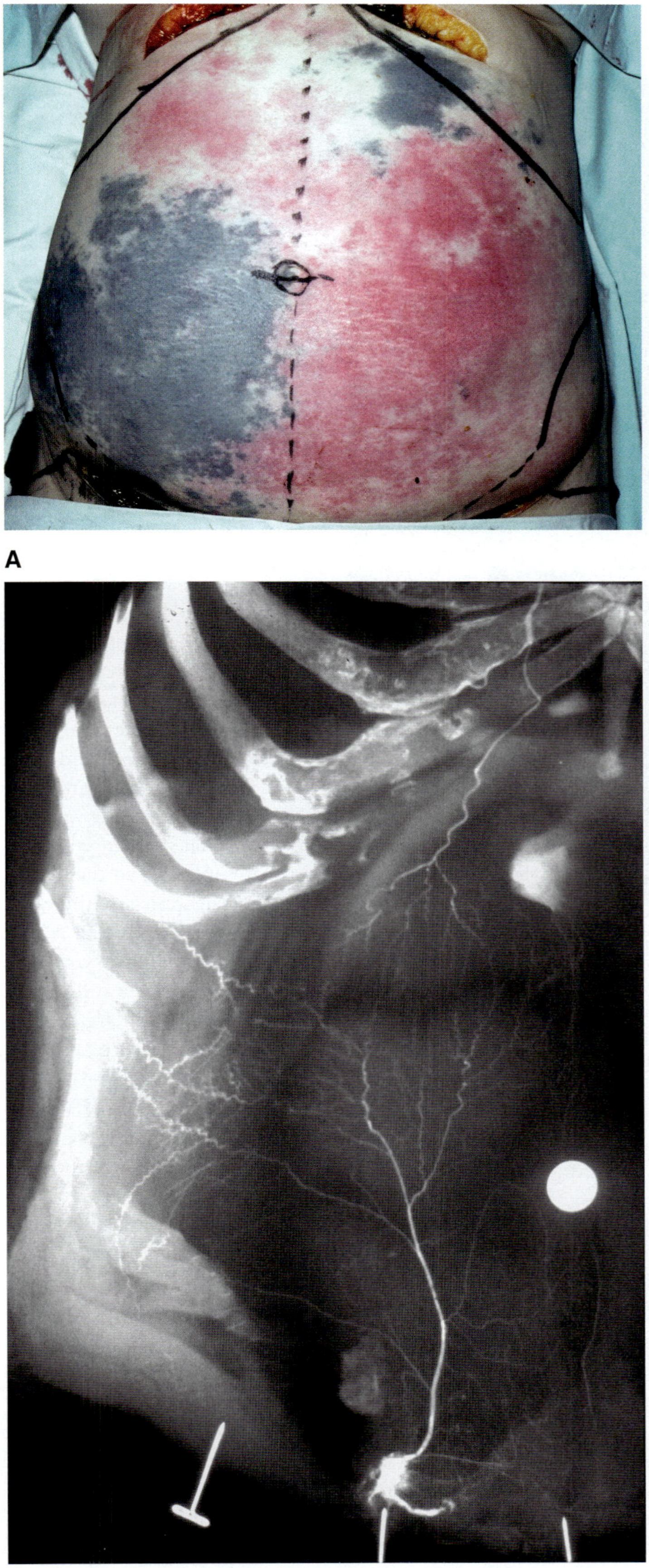

A

B

FIGURE 46-1 (A) "Harlequin" ink injection study on a fresh cadaver showing the vascular territories of the SEA and DIEA over the anterior abdominal wall. Note that the lower abdominal tissue (that which would be harvested as a TRAM or DIEP flap) lies entirely within the territories of the DIEA. Pedicled TRAM flaps are based on the SEA and rely on the (choke) interconnections between the two adjacent vascular territories. This makes the blood supply more tenuous. (B) Dye injection study of the DIEA and SEA with integument removed, showing their communicating "choke" vessels lying within the rectus muscle between the xiphisternum and umbilicus. Choke vessels also demarcate the boundary between the vascular territories of the intercostal vessels and both the SEA and the DIEA.

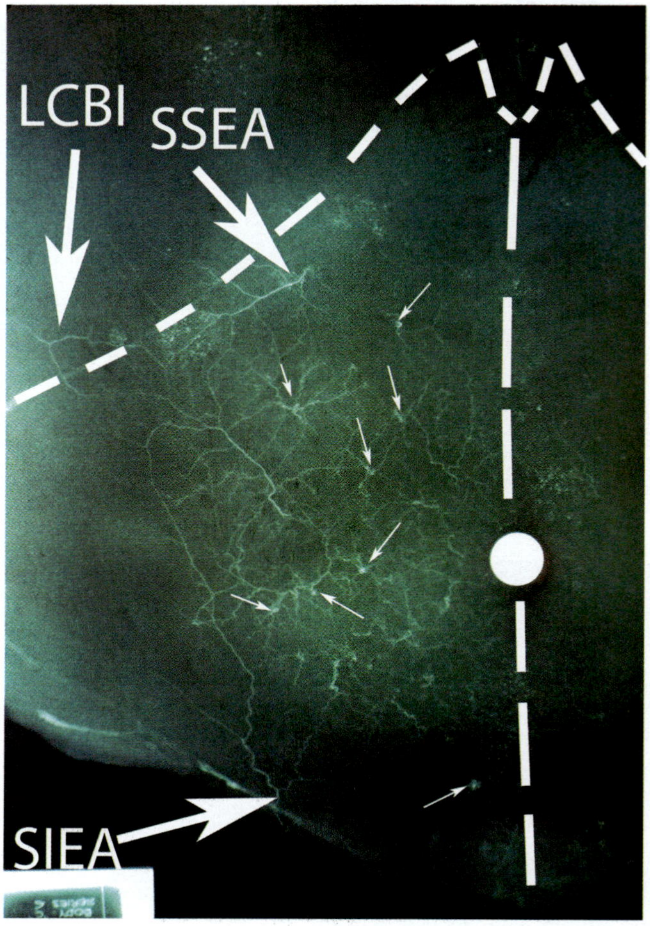

FIGURE 46-2 Dye injection study of the isolated integument from the Figure 46-1B specimen. The SIEA is shown contributing to a network of vessels over the anterior abdominal wall. This network communicates with a vessel that may be termed the superficial superior epigastric artery (SSEA), the lateral cutaneous branches of the intercostal arteries (LCBI), and perforators from DIEA and SEA (small arrows).

the DIEA. Depending on the patient's body habitus, this usually limits its use to smaller unilateral reconstructions or when a bilateral operation is required. Indeed, the technique is particularly appropriate for bilateral reconstructions when the potential for abdominal weakening is greater with other methods.

A number of surgeons who routinely perform autogenous breast reconstruction by free tissue transfer, particularly DIEP flaps, have developed algorithms regarding the use of SIEA flaps (14,15,21,22). These algorithms are mainly concerned with the size of the SIEA at the inferior margin of the flap. Two of the authors agree that an external diameter of 1.5 mm and a palpable arterial pulsation must be present. The third (22) also stipulates a palpable pulse but only requires the vessel to be 1.0 mm in diameter at the inferior border of the flap. Because the vessel often does not get very much larger when dissected to its origin, I agree with the recommendations of Arnez et al. (14,15) and Spiegel et al. (21). If the criterion of a 1.5-mm minimum diameter is adhered to, then one can expect to perform SIEA flaps in about 30% of patients. Less stringent requirements may increase the yield up to about 60%, possibly at the expense of a higher flap loss rate (21). The greatest diameter of the SIEA is at generally its origin from the femoral artery; however, its diameter as it enters the flap may be most critical. The entry point of the vessel into the edge of the flap makes it prone to kinking after the flap has been positioned and flow reestablished, a situation not shared with the DIEP flap when the pedicle enters from beneath.

Accordingly, the SIEA and superficial inferior epigastric vein (SIEV) should be thoroughly assessed both preoperatively using the pencil Doppler probe, as well as including it in any imaging studies being performed for perforators and by direct visualization and measurement at surgery. Frequently, a Pfannenstiel, appendectomy, or hernia scar will indicate preexisting damage to the vessel. It is often said that there is a reciprocal relationship between the number and size of DIEA perforators and the SIEA itself; however, although perhaps intuitive, this has not been substantiated scientifically.

Anatomically, the SIEA lies deep to Scarpa's fascia at the lower border of the flap, and the vein is usually described as medial to the artery and superficial to this fascia. Actually, the artery is accompanied by two tiny venae comitantes closely adherent to its wall. These often join and form a single vein that then enters the femoral vein in close proximity (usually inferior) to the origin of the SIEA from the femoral artery. Theoretically, this vein is really the SIEV. However, the much larger medial vein mentioned earlier, which often drains into the great saphenous vein and which is generally considered to be the SIEV, is the one that should be used (Figure 46-3). Its large diameter and excellent flow characteristics make it preferable to the tiny vessels accompanying the artery (Figure 46-4).

If the SIEA and SIEV meet the criteria mentioned earlier (14,15,21) when they are uncovered at the lower border of the transverse skin ellipse, then they should be dissected to their junction with their parent vessels before dividing any DIEP perforators. With the flap elevated on the SIEA pedicle and one or two DIEA perforators, the latter may be temporarily cross-clamped and the circulation assessed before finally electing to use the superficial system.

PREPARATION OF THE RECIPIENT SITE

The SIEA flap may be used both in primary and secondary breast reconstructions. Generally, the internal mammary vessels are preferred as recipients because the SIEA pedicle is relatively short. However, although the pedicle is indeed shorter than that of a DIEP flap, it is positioned at the border of the flap, but the DIEP flap's perforators enter the flap's undersurface. The result is that the shorter SIEA pedicle can extend farther from the margin of the flap than the longer DIEP pedicle, which uses part of its length simply to reach the flap's edge. The disadvantage of this arrangement is that there is less freedom to position the SIEA flap because its

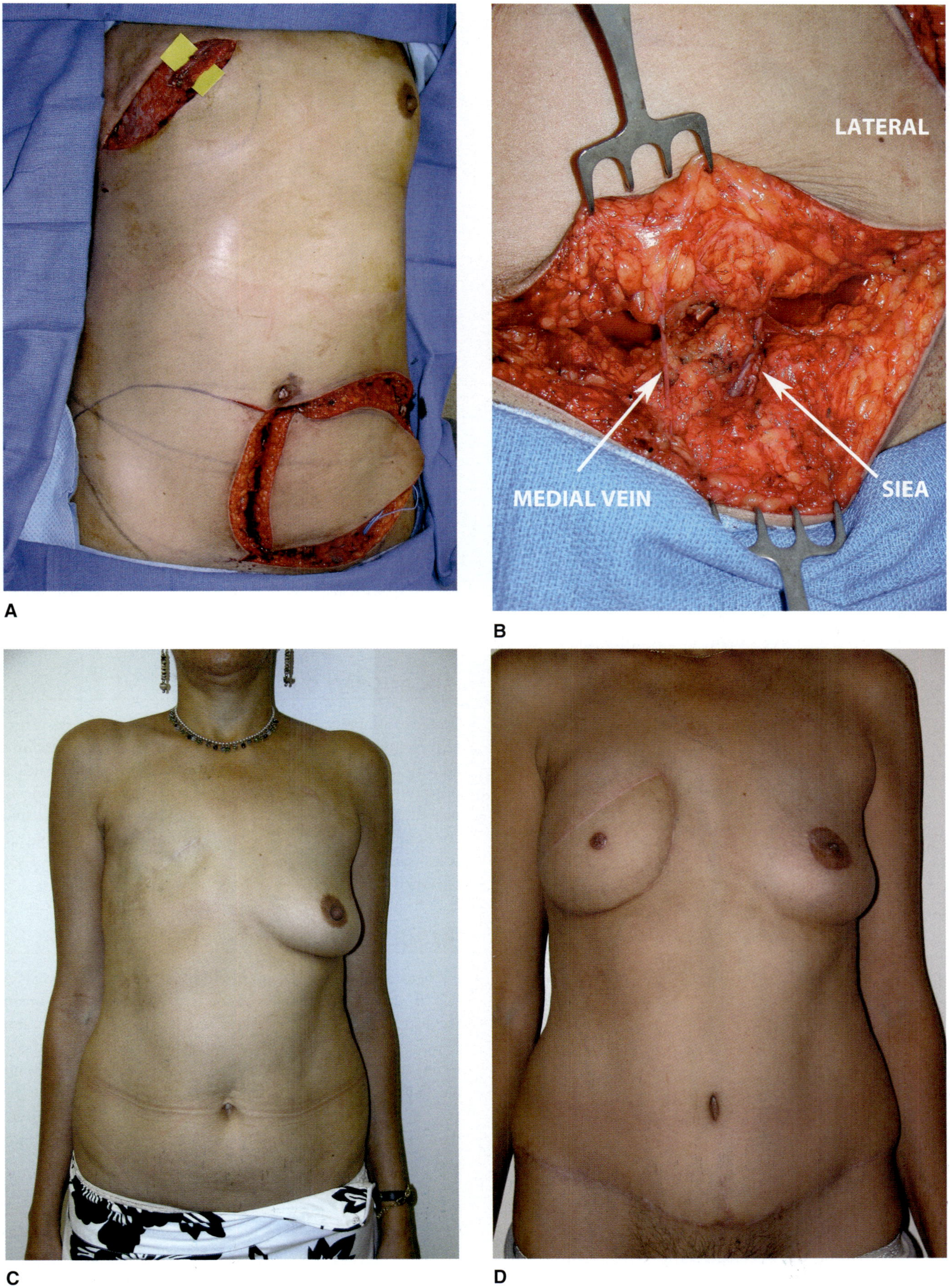

FIGURE 46-3 Right breast reconstruction using a left superficial inferior epigastric artery (SIEA) flap. (**A**) Right internal mammary vessels dissected endoscopically using a robotic device. Left-sided SIEA flap ready for harvest. (**B**) Close-up view of the inferior incision showing the SIEA vascular pedicle and a separate, large medial vein. This drains into the saphenous system and is usually the preferred vein for microanastomosis. Before (**C**) and after (**D**) photographs of the same patient. She has had a nipple-sparing procedure and awaits an areolar tattoo.

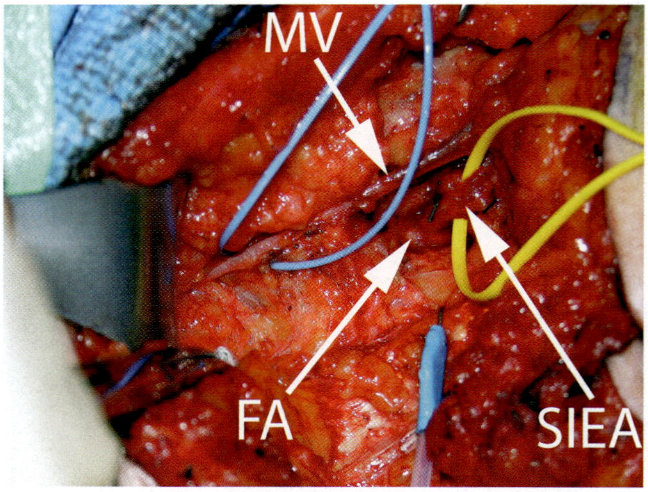

FIGURE 46-4 Left groin with a superficial inferior epigastric artery (SIEA) flap (and the patient's head) to the right. Operative dissection showing the left SIEA origin from the left femoral artery (FA) and the large medial vein (MV) draining into the saphenous system. Small venae comitantes accompany the artery and should be considered the true superficial inferior epigastric veins.

pedicle emerges from a specific point on the flap's border. This point must lie adjacent the recipient vessels. Conversely, the DIEP flap may, to some extent, be rotated without significantly shortening the pedicle's usable length. As with DIEP flaps, the SIEA flap is usually taken from the contralateral side and positioned with its lateral apex in the infraclavicular fossa and its paramedian border occupying the inframammary fold. This positions the tissue to the best anatomical advantage with the bulkiest portion inferior, giving the reconstructed breast a normal "teardrop" shape.

The recipient vessels are exposed at the level of the third rib. It is often possible to use the intercostal perforators, but if these are unsuitable, then the main internal mammary vessels may be accessed via the third interspace or through the bed of the third costal cartilage.

As an alternative, the thoracodorsal vessels are also usable. However, their use may preclude the use of the pedicled latissimus dorsi flap as a "lifeboat" if the flap fails or if another resection becomes necessary. To maintain the possibility of elevating the latissimus dorsi flap, the trunk of the thoracodorsal artery must only be used proximal to its serratus anterior branch. By leaving the latter intact, a communication is maintained between it and distal part of the thoracodorsal artery (the part that enters and supplies the flap) holding out the possibility of maintaining circulation via retrograde flow if the latissimus flap needs to be raised. However, it may not be entirely reliable; indeed, the use of the thoracodorsal pedicle as a recipient can still be problematic when definitive sections of a sentinel node biopsy prove positive, requiring the oncologic surgeon to perform a full nodal dissection during a second operation. The whole anastomosis is then at serious risk.

INSET OF THE FLAP, VESSEL ANASTOMOSES, AND POSTOPERATIVE MONITORING

Apart from the restrictions on flap positioning mentioned earlier, the insetting of an SIEA flap, the microvascular anastomoses, and the postoperative monitoring are exactly like that for a DIEP flap.

COMPLICATIONS

Although the SIEA is generally smaller than the DIEA, the anastomotic success rate in the two operations is not significantly different provided a conservative selection protocol has been observed before embarking on the SIEA operation (15,21). General complications are similar, but abdominal wall weakness is absent with the SIEA flap. However, it should be noted that as a rule, abdominal wall complications are rather uncommon with DIEP flaps. Postoperative recovery from SIEA flap involves much less muscle pain for obvious reasons.

SECONDARY SURGERY

Secondary surgery, similar to that after most breast reconstruction techniques, is usually performed between 3 and 6 months after the initial operation. However, there is no problem if it is postponed. It may consist of nipple reconstruction, balancing procedures, scar revisions, liposuction, fat injections, and abdominal recontouring. These operations and their timing are common to most autogenous breast reconstructions and are discussed elsewhere.

RESULTS AND OUTCOMES

As mentioned earlier, the anastomotic success rate for the SIEA flap is similar to other forms of free abdominal flap breast reconstruction. Operating time is less than with perforator flaps, and postoperative abdominal pain is less. The aesthetic results are also indistinguishable from other forms of abdominal flap breast reconstruction and have more to do with the craft of the surgeon and the condition of the patient's tissues than to the name of the artery feeding the flap (Figures 46-5 and 46-6).

Yet the advantages presented by the SIEA flap offer the microsurgeon an appealing option that he or she should consider whenever embarking on the elevation of an abdominal flap for breast reconstruction.

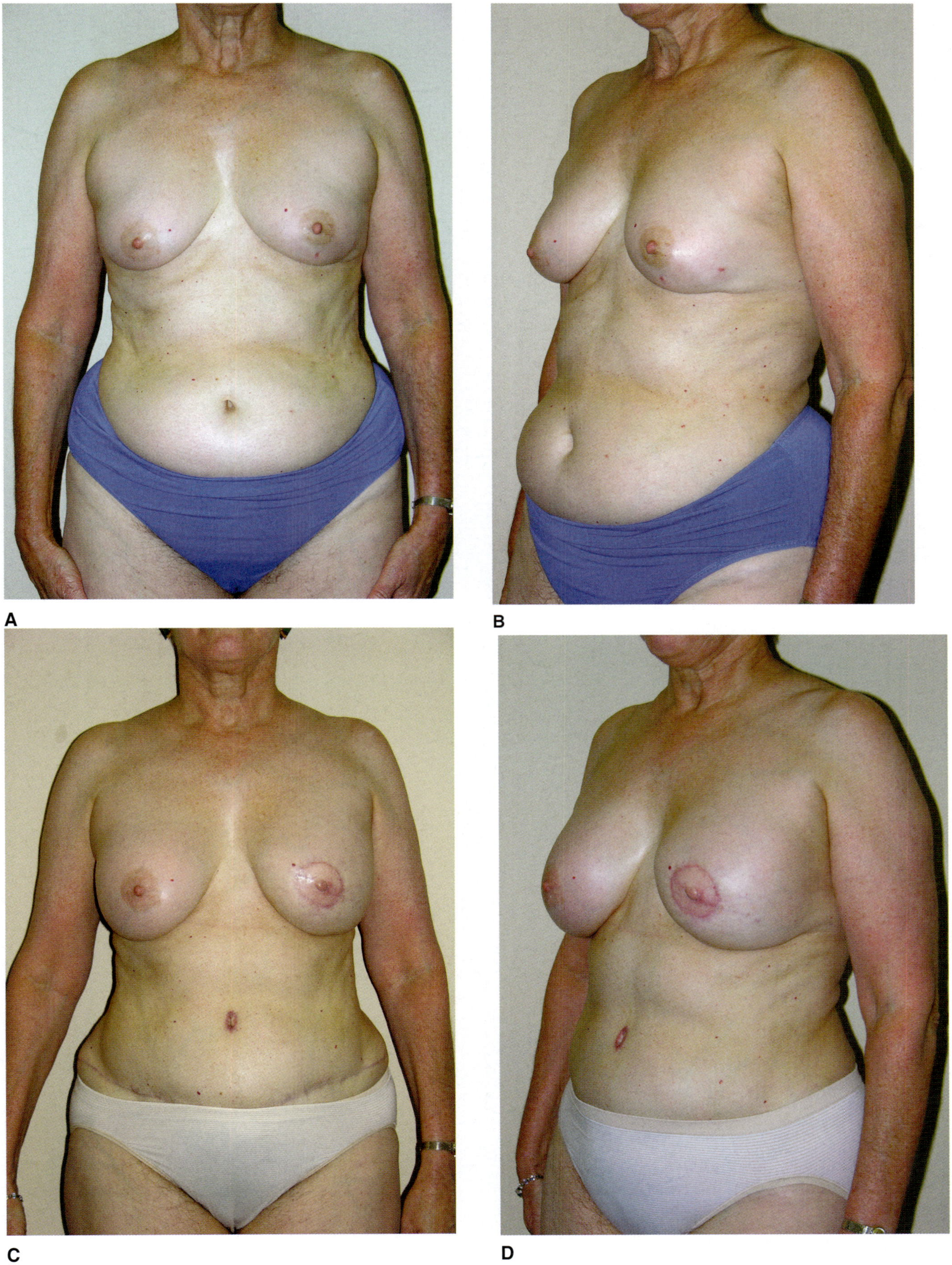

FIGURE 46-5 (A) and (B) Preoperative photographs of a patient undergoing a left-sided skin-sparing mastectomy and immediate reconstruction using an superficial inferior epigastric artery (SIEA) flap. (C) and (D) Postoperative images of the same patient after SIEA flap and nipple reconstruction.

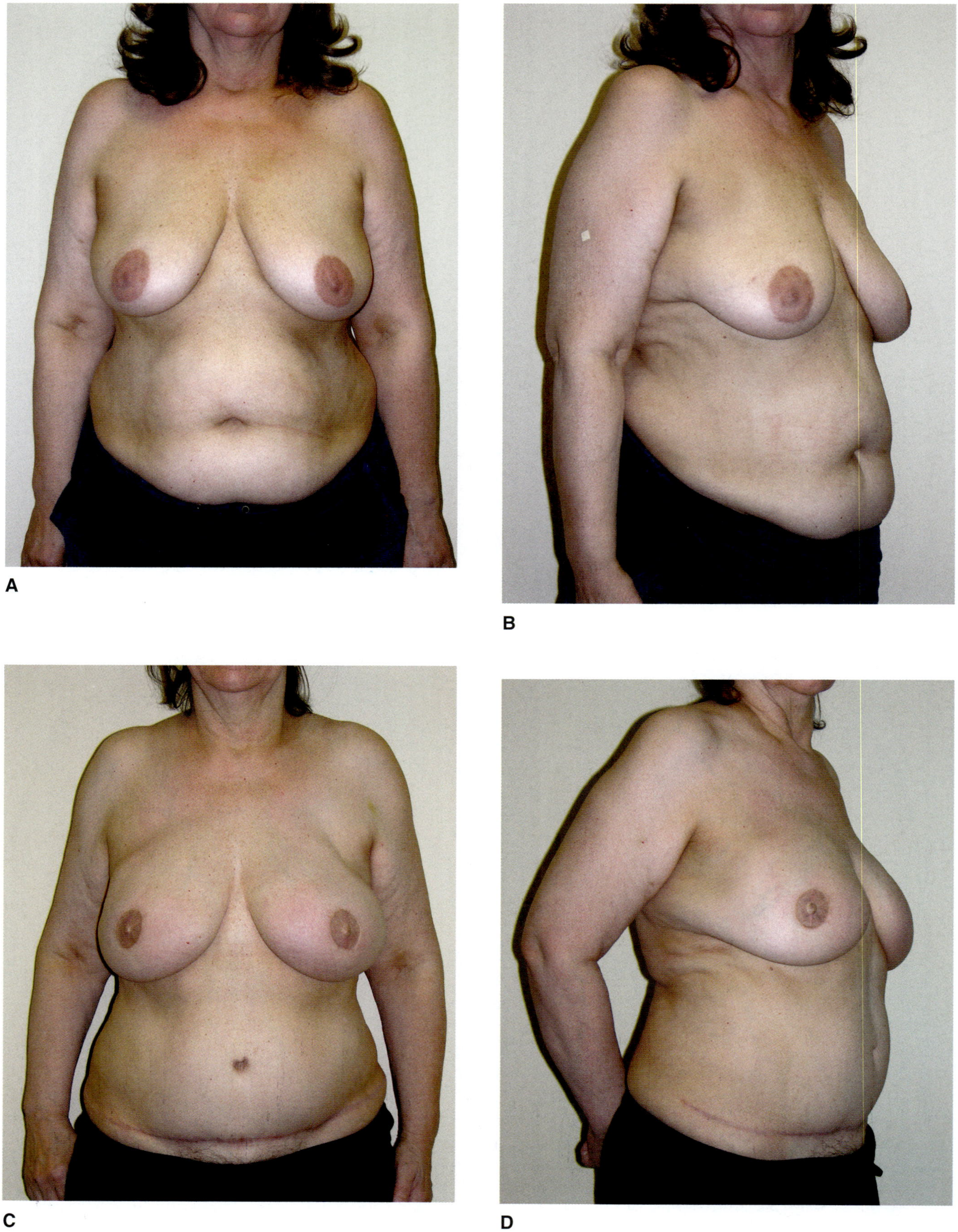

FIGURE 46-6 (A) and (B) Preoperative pictures of a patient undergoing a bilateral skin-sparing mastectomy and immediate reconstruction using superficial inferior epigastric artery (SIEA) flaps. (C) and (D) Postoperative images of the same patient after bilateral SIEA flap and nipple reconstruction.

REFERENCES

1. Drever JM. Total breast reconstruction with either of two abdominal flaps. *Plast Reconstr Surg* 1977;59:185–190.
2. Hartrampf CR, Scheflan M, Black PW. Breast reconstruction with a transverse abdominal island flap. *Plast Reconstr Surg* 1982;69:216–225.
3. Kroll S, Schusterman M, Reece G, et al. Abdominal wall strength, bulging, and hernia after TRAM flap breast reconstruction. *Plast Reconstr Surg* 1995;96:616–619.
4. Edsander-Nord A, Jurell G, Wickman M. Donor-site morbidity after pedicled or free TRAM flap surgery: a prospective and objective study. *Plast Reconstr Surg* 1998;102:1508–1516.
5. Feller AM. Free TRAM. Results and abdominal wall function. *Clin Reconstr Surg* 1994;21:223–232.
6. Fitoussi A, Laki F, Coutureau B et al. Management of donor-site synthetic mesh infection after TRAM flap breast reconstruction. *Plast Reconstr Surg* 2009;123:202e–203e.
7. Kroll S, Gherardini G, Martin J, et al. Fat necrosis in free and pedicled TRAM flaps. *Plast Reconstr Surg* 1998;102:1502–1507.
8. Holmström H. The free abdominoplasty flap and its use in breast reconstruction: an experimental study and clinical case report. *Scand Plast Reconstr Surg* 1979;13:423–427.
9. Arnez ZM, Smith RW, Eder E, et al. Breast reconstruction by the free lower transverse rectus abdominis musculocutaneous flap. *Br J Plast Surg* 1988;41:500–505.
10. Feller AM. Free TRAM. Results and abdominal wall function. *Clin Reconstr Surg* 1994;21:223–232.
11. Allen RJ, Treece P. Deep inferior epigastric perforator flap for breast reconstruction. *Ann Reconstr Surg* 1994;8:32.
12. Antia NH, Buch VI. Transfer of an abdominal dermo-fat graft by direct anastomosis of blood vessels. *Br J Reconstr Surg* 1971;24:15–19.
13. Taylor GI, Daniel RK. The free flap: composite tissue transfer by vascular anastomosis. *Aust N Z J Surg* 1973;43:1–3.
14. Arnez ZM, Khan U, Pogorelec D, et al. Breast reconstruction using the free superficial inferior epigastric artery (SIEA) flap. *Br J Plast Surg* 1999;52:276–279.
15. Arnez ZM, Khan U, Pogorelec D, et al. Rational selection of flaps from the abdomen in breast reconstruction to reduce donor site morbidity. *Br J Plast Surg* 1999;52:351–354.
16. Allen RJ, Tucker C Jr. Superior gluteal artery perforator free flap for breast reconstruction. *Plast Reconstr Surg* 1995;95:1207–1212.
17. Granzow JW, Levine JL, Chiu ES, Allen RJ. Breast reconstruction with gluteal artery perforator flaps. *J Plast Reconstr Aesthet Surg* 2006;59:614–621.
18. Arnez ZM, Pogorelec D, Planinsek F, Ahcan U. Breast reconstruction by the free transverse gracilis (TUG) flap. *Br J Plast Surg* 2004;57:20–26.
19. Schoeller T, Wechselberger G. Breast reconstruction by the free transverse gracilis (TUG) flap. *Br J Plast Surg* 2004;57:481–482.
20. Elliott LF, Hartrampf CR Jr. The Rubens flap: the deep circumflex iliac artery flap. *Clin Reconstr Surg* 1998;25:283.
21. Spiegel AJ, Khan FN. An intraoperative algorithm for use of the SIEA flap for breast reconstruction. *Plast Reconstr Surg* 2005;120:1450–1459.
22. Chevray PM. Breast reconstruction with superficial inferior epigastric artery flaps: a prospective comparison with TRAM and DIEP flaps. *Plast Reconstr Surg* 2004;114:1077–1083.

CHAPTER 47

Breast Reconstruction: Transverse Upper or Myocutaneous Gracilis Flaps

Thomas Schoeller and Georg M. Huemer

HISTORY OF CONVENTIONAL OPTIONS

Breast reconstruction with autologous tissue has evolved from pedicled tissue transfer, such as the latissimus dorsi flap (1) and the pedicled transverse rectus abdominis myocutaneous flap (2) to microsurgically transplanted tissue. There are several reasons for this shift. First, blood perfusion in free tissue transfer is usually better as long as there is no problem with the anastomosis. Second, flap insetting and shaping is easier, and there is more freedom with free flaps because there is normally no tethering due to the attached pedicle. Third, donor site morbidity is usually less when harvesting a free flap from a specific anatomic region compared with its pedicled variant.

The pedicled latissimus dorsi flap is one of the oldest methods for reconstruction of the breast mound and was described in 1896 by Tansini (3). It is usually combined with an implant to increase volume. Despite its continuing popularity, there are drawbacks such as problems related to the implant or the large scar on the back. One may argue that this combined modality shares the disadvantages of both autologous and prosthetic reconstruction. On the other hand, with the pedicled latissimus dorsi flap, there is no need for microsurgery. Nevertheless, there remains a certain amount of donor site morbidity with this flap (4).

LIST OF FREE FLAPS AVAILABLE FOR BREAST RECONSTRUCTION

Nowadays the so-called "gold standard" for breast reconstruction is the lower abdomen. Since the initial description of Hartrampf et al. (2) and Holmström (5), the flap has evolved from a pedicled variant via a free musculocutaneous flap (6) to a perforator flap (deep inferior epigastric perforator [DIEP]) (7). The DIEP flap has revolutionized autogenous breast reconstruction with regard to donor site morbidity and restoration of a natural-looking breast mound (8,9). However, there are certain clinical circumstances in which the lower abdomen is not the best option. Scars resulting from previous operations, such as Pfannenstiel or median laparotomy incisions, may have already disrupted or limited blood flow to the lower abdomen (10). Also, scars in a more remote site, such as long subcostal incisions, may interfere with uncomplicated donor site closure in the lower abdomen. This problem may be circumvented with rather tedious planning, but one has to consider if there is not a better suitable donor site in such a case (11). Other different donor areas are located in the gluteal region, namely the superior (SGAP) or inferior (IGAP) gluteal artery perforator flaps (12). Depending on the patient's anatomy, these flaps offer sufficient volume for reconstruction of small- to medium-sized breasts. However, the drawbacks of these flaps are: the occasionally troublesome perforator dissection; the inevitable need for intraoperative patient repositioning, and the rather conspicuous donor site scar (SGAP). Flaps such as the Rubens flap (13) or the anterolateral thigh flap (14) for breast reconstruction are mentioned somewhat anecdotally in the literature but do not have many adherents.

INDICATIONS

The transverse upper or myocutaneous gracilis (TUG or TMG) flap has recently become a popular secondary option for breast reconstruction. Although described by Yousif et al. as long ago as 1992, this useful flap became somewhat neglected in the ensuing years. The initial publication even contained a case of breast reconstruction. With the evolution of skin-sparing mastectomy, flap requirements changed. There was no longer any need for a large skin island but just moldable autologous filling material. Because the TMG flap has a relatively narrow (6–10 cm) but long skin island, immediate breast reconstruction after skin-sparing mastectomy is the primary indication for this flap. This is where all advantages of the TUG flap come into play: namely, a very inconspicuous donor site scar in the inguinal crease; a straightforward dissection of a reliable pedicle, and the possibility for a two-team approach in which the breast surgeon performs the oncologic resection while the reconstructive surgeon simultaneously harvests the (remote) flap. Donor site morbidity is confined to the scar because the loss of the muscle function or contour is negligible.

However, the TMG-flap is not limited to breast reconstruction after skin-sparing mastectomy. Secondary breast reconstruction can be performed in the appropriate patient just as with the gluteal flaps (SGAP or IGAP). In certain cases, a single breast mound can be reconstructed with a transfer of two TMG flaps. Nevertheless, one of the main strengths of this flap is in bilateral reconstruction. Both flaps can be harvested independently and transferred to the two recipient sites. We have used the flap very successfully not only in bilateral prophylactic skin-sparing mastectomy but also in bilateral secondary reconstruction cases.

Regarding patient selection, the ideal patient is slim with a full upper thigh and a flat abdomen who is undergoing skin-sparing mastectomy. The breast should be small to moderate in volume. Ideally, the patient should benefit aesthetically from a horizontal thigh lift, just as a DIEP flap patient would from an abdominoplasty. If the patient would profit equally from a thigh lift or an abdominoplasty, it is our preference to choose the TMG flap because of the easier dissection and the more hidden donor scar. A prerequisite, of course, is sufficient volume obtainable from the thigh for breast mound restoration. In rare exceptions, a bilateral TMG flap may be harvested for unilateral breast reconstruction if the lower abdomen donor site is precluded for any reason. However, this technically challenging operation has to be weighed against the risks of four microsurgical anastomoses and increased operative time.

PREPARATION OF RECIPIENT SITE

One of the main strengths of the TMG flap is immediate reconstruction after skin-sparing mastectomy. Typically, the nipple–areola complex (NAC) is excised together with all glandular tissue by the oncologic breast surgeon (Figure 47-1). After hemostasis is obtained, the second or third intercostal space is chosen for exploration of the internal mammary vessels. One can choose between the traditional removal of the costal cartilage to gain a wider exposure or use a muscle-splitting technique to preserve the costal cartilage (15). The internal mammary vessels are then prepared after isolating them just beneath the intercostal muscles (Figure 47-2).

HARVEST AND INSET OF THE FLAP

The anatomy of the gracilis flap is described earlier in this book in detail. However, there are some differences when raising the TMG flap that are worth mentioning. Exposure to the flap's pedicle starts with incising the transverse skin island.

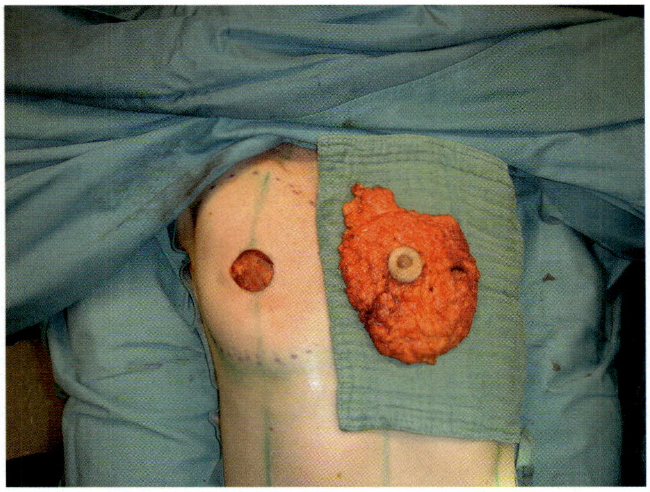

FIGURE 47-1 Typical operative site after skin-sparing mastectomy with complete removal of breast tissue, including the nipple–areola complex, in a medium-sized breast. This represents an ideal indication for immediate reconstruction with a transverse myocutaneous gracilis flap.

The anterior portion of the skin island is then lifted off the deep fascia with care taken to preserve the lymphatic tissue and saphenous vein in the inguinal triangle. When one encounters the belly of the adductor longus muscle, the deep fascia is included in the adipocutaneous portion of the flap. Dissection proceeds dorsally around the muscular belly of the adductor longus muscle until the main pedicle of the gracilis flap is seen. Preparation of the flap's pedicle is similar to the traditional gracilis muscle flap (see earlier chapter). After the pedicle is fully isolated, the posterior portion of the skin island is incised and elevated. The limitations of the size of the skin island have to be evaluated preoperatively in the standing position just as for a horizontal thigh lift. The usual width of the skin island is between 6 and 10 cm. After the skin island of the flap has been mobilized but is still broadly attached to the gracilis muscle via the deep fascia, the muscle is divided at its origin and the most

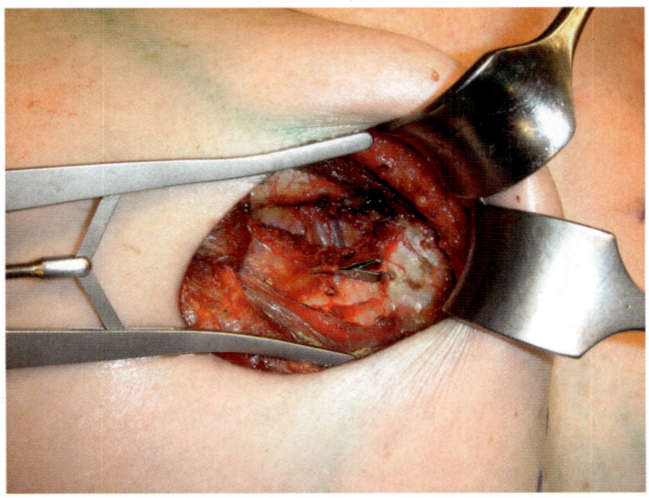

FIGURE 47-2 Even in skin-sparing mastectomies with removal of the nipple–areola complex only, sufficient exposure of the internal mammary vessels in either rib-sparing or rib removal fashion can be achieved. Here, an intercostal approach is shown.

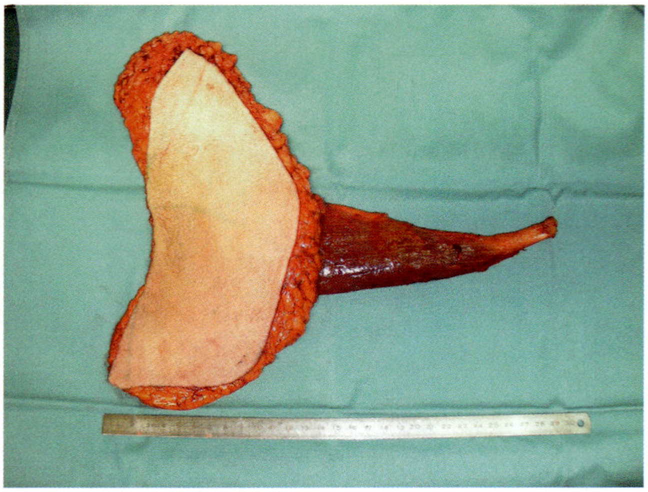

FIGURE 47-3 The harvested transverse myocutaneous gracilis flap with a large adipocutaneous portion. The dimension of the adipocutaneous portion depends on the individual anatomy of the patient, but the usual vertical dimension lies between 8 and 10 cm. In this case, the patient experienced massive weight loss and therefore such a voluminous skin island could be harvested without difficulty.

distal point that can be reached through the distal incision of the skin island. A separate incision over the gracilis tendon is not necessary. After complete flap harvest, the donor site is closed in layers similar to a horizontal thigh lift.

The flap is then shaped on a sterile side table according to the needs of the specific mastectomy defect (Figures 47-3 and 47-4). The spindle-shaped adipocutaneous portion of the flap is brought together at both ends to form a cone. Then the upper incision line

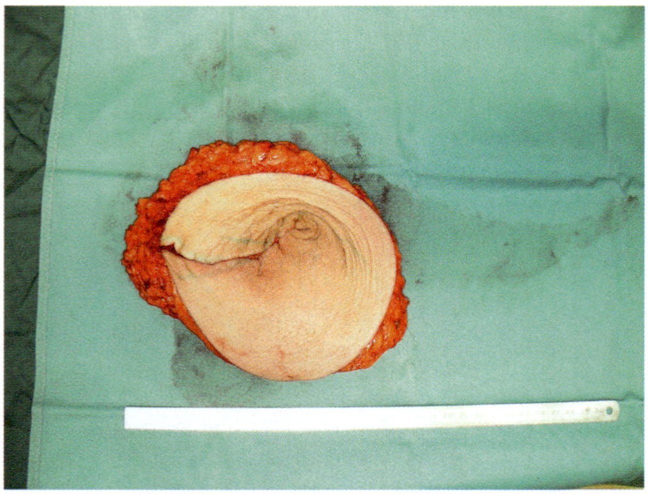

FIGURE 47-4 Shaping of the flap for ideal breast mound reconstruction begins on a sterile side table by "coning" of the skin island. Both endpoints of the inguinal edge of the skin island are sutured together, and the rest of the inguinal edges are closed subcutaneously. The flap is then brought to the recipient site, and the microvascular anastomoses are completed. Then the amount of missing skin at the recipient site is estimated, and the remaining area of the cutaneous surface of the flap is deepithelialized. Usually, the skin requirements of the flap are confined the removed nipple–areola complex; a little surplus of skin for immediate or late nipple reconstruction should be anticipated.

of the skin island is closed with resorbable sutures in a running fashion. The flap is now shaped in a three-dimensional manner to fill the envelope of the skin-sparing mastectomy defect.

VESSEL ANASTOMOSES

After transfer to the recipient site, the shaped flap is temporarily fixed on the chest wall to facilitate the microvascular anastomoses. We usually perform the arterial anastomosis in an end-to-side fashion with interrupted 8-0 or 9-0 nylon sutures, but the venous anastomosis is achieved with the microvascular coupler system (between 2.0 and 3.0 mm) in an end-to-end fashion. A single venous anastomosis is usually sufficient (16). A nerve repair for increased sensation of the reconstructed breast is not available for this type of flap. After adequate and stable perfusion of the flap is assured, the flap is detached from its temporary fixation and carefully inserted into the recipient site via the opening created by the previously excised NAC. Great care is taken not to injure the vascular pedicle. The amount of skin needed for the NAC defect is marked with a surgical pen, and the remaining skin of the flap is deepithelialized. According to the surgeon's preferences, the nipple can be reconstructed immediately at this point or deferred to a later stage. The skin wound is then closed in two layers with care taken to even out the levels of the skin between the breast envelope and the skin island of the flap.

POSTOPERATIVE MONITORING

The mode of postoperative monitoring the flap depends on the individual surgeon's preferences and most likely the availability of different monitoring devices. Because of the visible skin island of the flap, pure clinical monitoring is an easy and very effective approach. We routinely use a continuous tissue oxygen tension measurement device (Licox; Integra Life Sciences, Plainsboro, NJ) (17), but any other monitoring device, such as laser Doppler, will yield good results.

POTENTIAL COMPLICATIONS

The potential complications of this flap include the usual problems encountered with microvascular flap transfer, such as venous or arterial thrombosis at the anastomotic site, postoperative hematoma, or infection. Inadequate flap perfusion may also result in necrosis of the fat tissue of the adipocutaneous portion of the flap, which may be palpable. However, the intrinsic perfusion of the flap is usually very reliable so that if flap perfusion is stable and sufficient, a problem of fat necrosis is not likely.

The major concern at the donor site is wound dehiscence. This may be due to excessive tension as a result of an inadequate skin availability and tight closure or premature mobilization by the patient. The patient should be thoroughly informed about this potential risk and advised not to strain the affected leg too early. Usually, a 2- to 3-week period of limited movement should be sufficient. Other donor site complications or sequelae include postoperative hematoma, decreased sensibility on the medial aspect of the thigh, a visible indentation in the upper medial thigh and a caudal migration of the donor site scar. However, this can be managed by a surgical revision (18).

SECONDARY SURGERY

Secondary procedures after breast reconstruction with the TMG flap may include the following:

- Completion of NAC reconstruction: If the nipple is not reconstructed at the time as the immediate reconstruction, this can be performed in a delayed fashion. At the same time, the skin of the NAC can be tattooed as well. Various techniques for nipple reconstruction with local flaps are available in the literature; however, care has to be taken in designing the flap because there is an inherent scar present in the skin island of the TMG flap because of the closure of the skin paddle to from a cone (see earlier discussion).
- Lipofilling for volume enhancement of the whole breast or for contour irregularities just on the cranial edge of the flap to make a more harmonic blending in the "décolleté" region.
- Revision of the donor scar if there is a caudal migration or hypertrophic scarring present.

RESULTS AND OUTCOMES FROM THE LITERATURE

After performing more than 300 cases of various types of breast reconstruction with the TMG flap to date, we are convinced that this flap represents more than a second-line option in autologous breast reconstruction (19–21). As a result, several other groups have included this flap into their repertoire for microvascular breast reconstruction (22–24). Figures 47-5 and 47-6 present typical results of TMG flap breast reconstruction

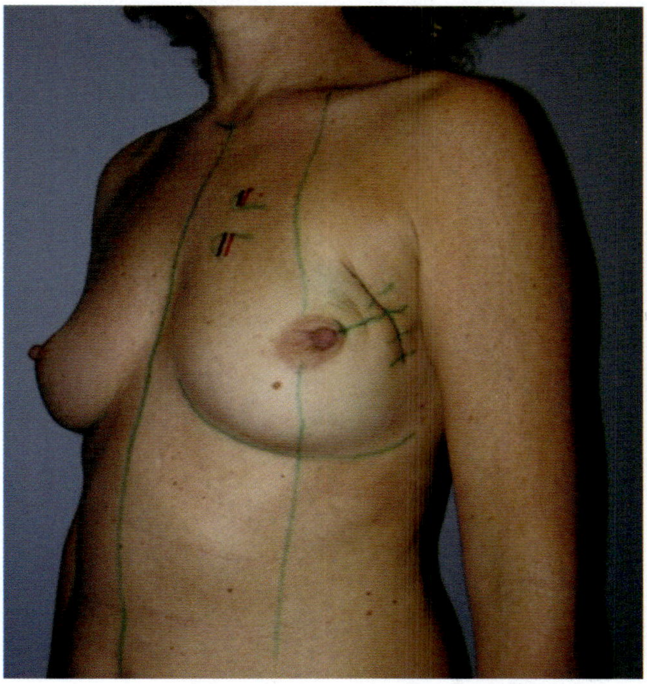

A

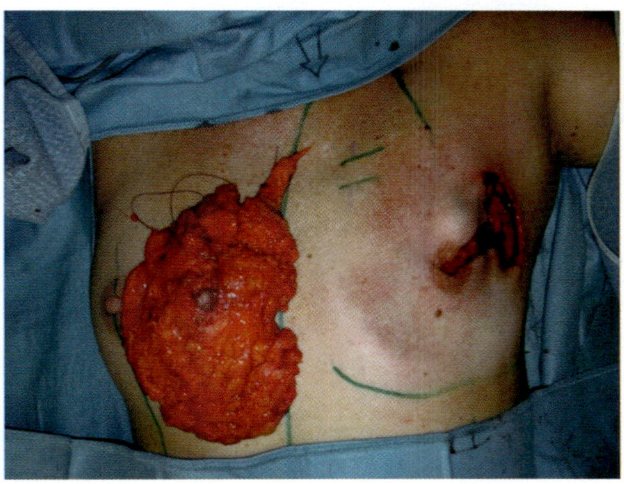

B

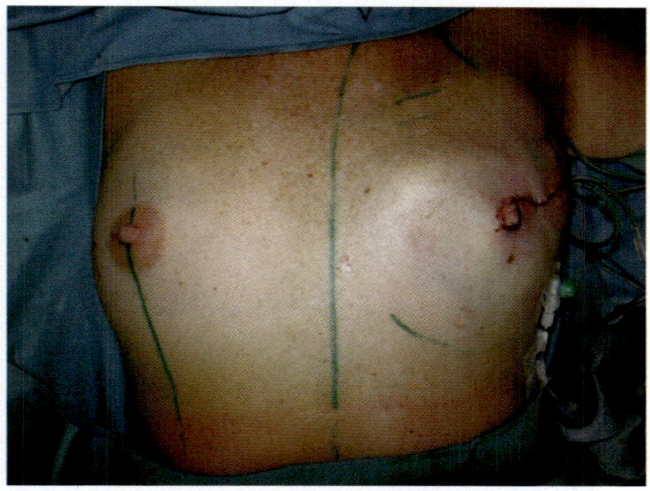

C

FIGURE 47-5 A unilateral breast reconstruction with a transverse upper gracilis (TUG) flap. A 38-year-old patient was diagnosed with ductal carcinoma in the upper lateral quadrant of the left breast. She had already undergone breast conservation therapy (BCT) with lumpectomy, the final histology revealing inadequate margins but a negative sentinel lymph node (**A**). The patient was scheduled for mastectomy and immediate reconstruction. A skin-sparing mastectomy was performed, and the initial defect from the BCT was re-created (**B**). A TUG flap was harvested from the contralateral thigh with a skin island measuring 18 × 10 cm. The donor site was closed primarily. The flap was connected to the internal mammary vessels after partial removal of the third rib and shaped as described in the text. The skin island was partially deepithelialized, and the initial skin defect of the BCT was reconstructed (**C**). The nipple was reconstructed concomitantly. At 3-month follow-up, the reconstructed left breast had good symmetry without any clinical signs of fat necrosis (**D**). In a secondary procedure, the skin island of the flap was completely deepithelialized and buried, and the areola was tattooed. At 18 months, the reconstructed breast appears very natural, although there is moderate scar hypertrophy (**E**). The donor site is concealed in the gluteal crease, and there is only minimal asymmetry from the rear view (**F** and **G**).

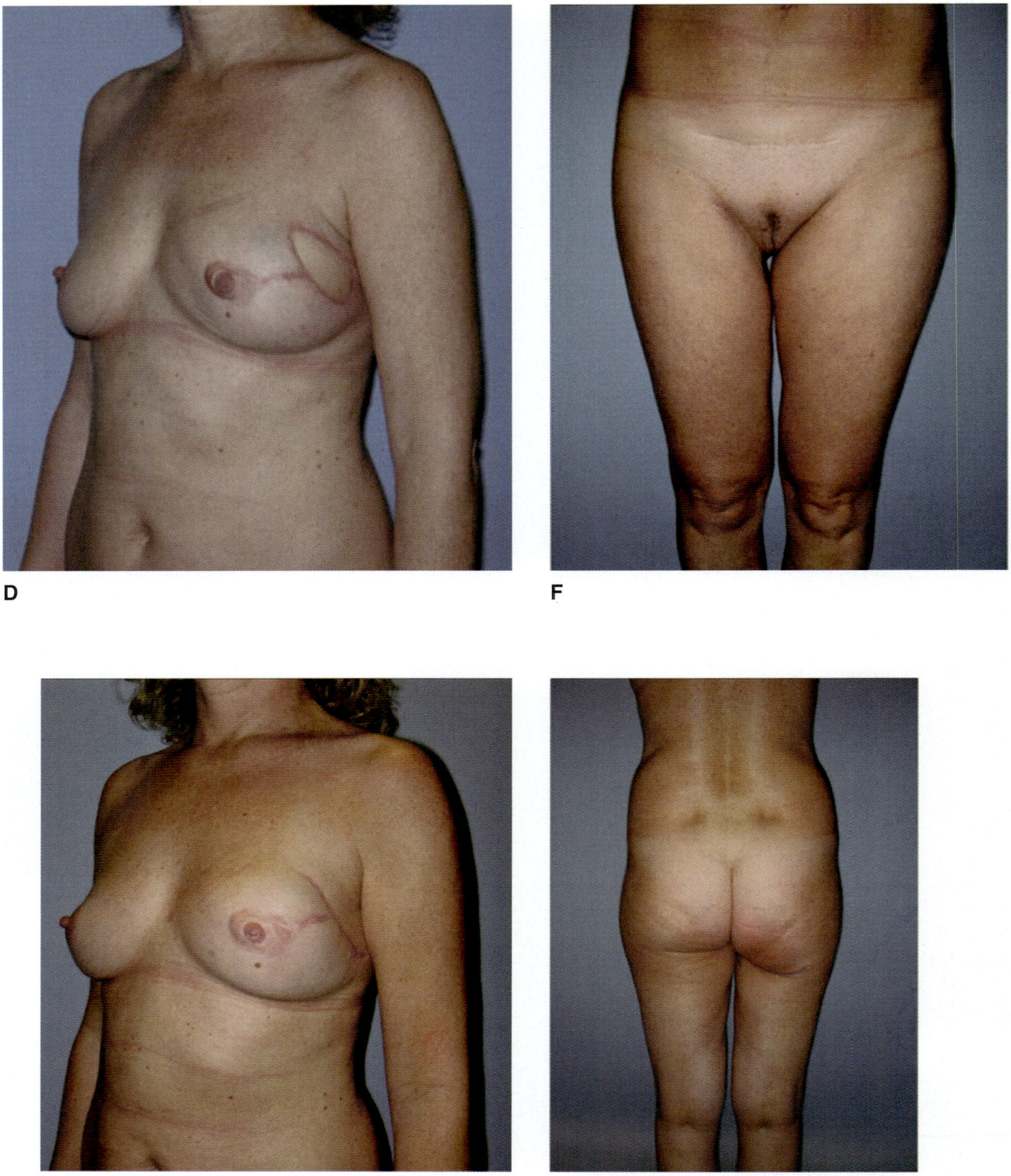

D F E G

FIGURE 47-5 *(Continued)*

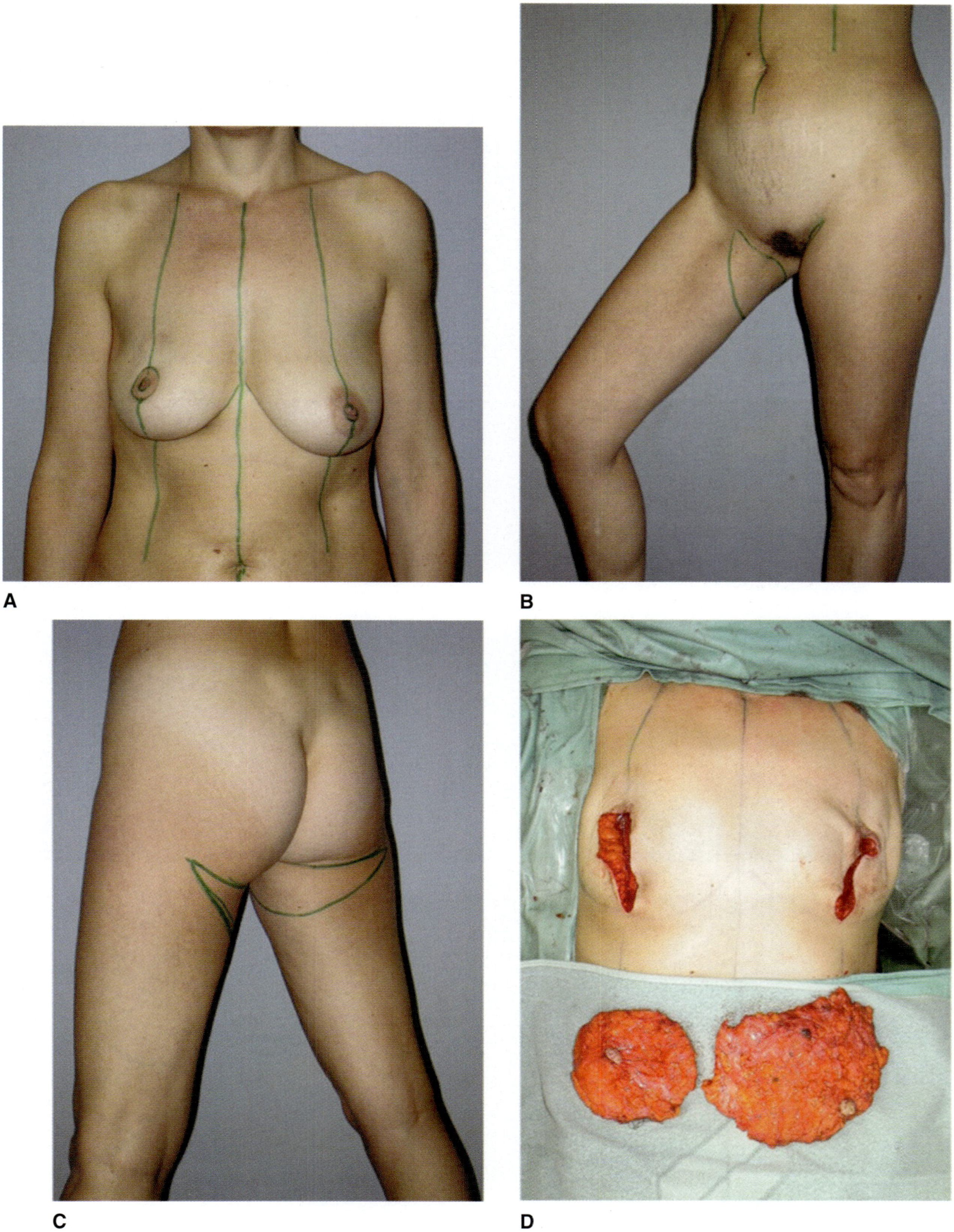

FIGURE 47-6 Bilateral breast reconstruction using transverse upper gracilis (TUG) flaps. A 42-year-old patient was scheduled for prophylactic bilateral skin-sparing mastectomy after prior breast conservation therapy on the right side (**A**). Preoperative skin markings for the skin islands of the TUG flaps are outlined on the thighs (**B** and **C**). The markings closely resemble those for a horizontal thigh lift, the vertical height lying between 8 and 12 cm, according to the patient's habitus. After completion of the bilateral mastectomy (**D**), both flaps are harvested (**E**). The adipocutaneous portion of a TUG flap greatly exceeds in volume the contained gracilis muscle, so there is only minor shrinkage of the flap in the long term (**F**). (**G**) The immediate postoperative result. (**H**) The 25-month follow-up. The donor site is very symmetrical and inconspicuous, particularly in bilateral cases such as this (**I** and **J**).

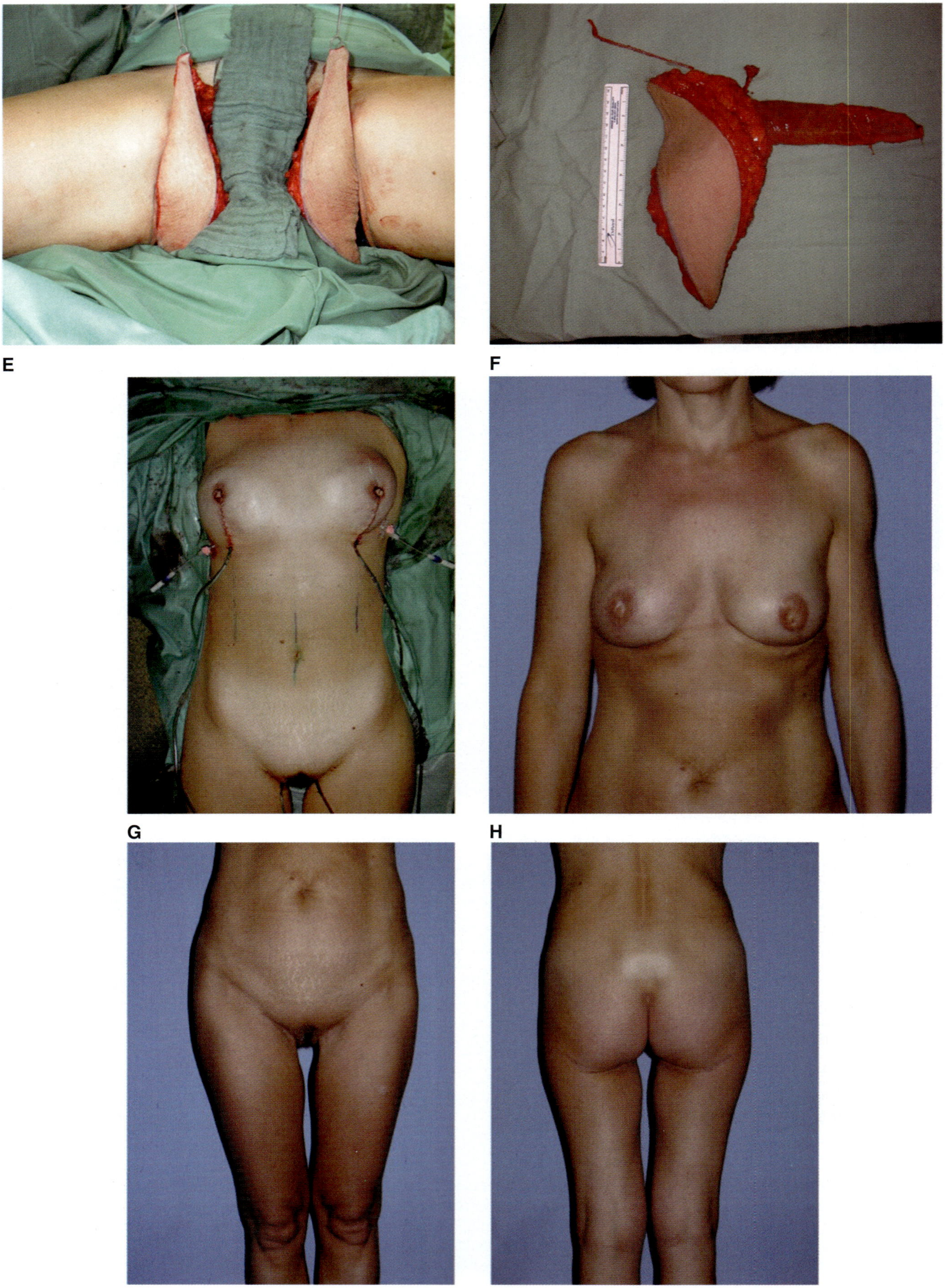

FIGURE 47-6 *(Continued)*

in various indications. The associated captions reflect the particular circumstances of each case.

REFERENCES

1. Bostwick J 3rd, Scheflan M. The latissimus dorsi musculocutaneous flap: a one-stage breast reconstruction. *Clin Plast Surg* 1980;7(1):71–78.
2. Hartrampf CR, Scheflan M, Black PW. Breast reconstruction with a transverse abdominal island flap. *Plast Reconstr Surg* 1982;69(2):216–225.
3. Tansini I. Nuovo processo per l'amputazione della mammaella per cancre. *Reforma Medica* 1896;12:3.
4. Adams WP Jr, Lipschitz AH, Ansari M, et al. Functional donor site morbidity following latissimus dorsi muscle flap transfer. *Ann Plast Surg* 2004;53(1):6–11.
5. Holmström H. The free abdominoplasty flap and its use in breast reconstruction. An experimental study and clinical case report. *Scand J Plast Reconstr Surg* 1979;13(3):423–427.
6. Arnez ZM, Bajec J, Bardsley AF, et al. Experience with 50 free TRAM flap breast reconstructions. *Plast Reconstr Surg* 1991;87(3):470–478.
7. Koshima I, Soeda S. Inferior epigastric artery skin flaps without rectus abdominis muscle. *Br J Plast Surg* 1989;42(6):645–648.
8. Blondeel PN. One hundred free DIEP flap breast reconstructions: a personal experience. *Br J Plast Surg* 1999;52(2):104–111.
9. Gill PS, Hunt JP, Guerra AB, et al. A 10-year retrospective review of 758 DIEP flaps for breast reconstruction. *Plast Reconstr Surg* 2004;113(4): 1153–1160.
10. Parrett BM, Caterson SA, Tobias AM, Lee BT. DIEP flaps in women with abdominal scars: are complication rates affected? *Plast Reconstr Surg* 2008;121(5):1527–1531.
11. Schoeller T, Wechselberger G, Roger J, et al. Management of infraumbilical vertical scars in DIEP-flaps by crossover anastomosis. *J Plast Reconstr Aesthet Surg* 2007;60(5):524–528.
12. LoTempio MM, Allen RJ. Breast reconstruction with SGAP and IGAP flaps. *Plast Reconstr Surg* 2010;126(2):393–401.
13. Elliott LF, Hartrampf CR Jr. The Rubens flap. The deep circumflex iliac artery flap. *Clin Plast Surg* 1998;25(2):283–291.
14. Rosenberg JJ, Chandawarkar R, Ross MI, Chevray PM. Bilateral anterolateral thigh flaps for large-volume breast reconstruction. *Microsurgery* 2004;24(4):281–284.
15. Darcy CM, Smit JM, Audolfsson T, Acosta R. Surgical technique: the intercostal space approach to the internal mammary vessels in 463 microvascular breast reconstructions. *J Plast Reconstr Aesthet Surg* 2011;64(1):58–62.
16. Hanasono MM, Kocak E, Ogunleye O, et al. One versus two venous anastomoses in microvascular free flap surgery. *Plast Reconstr Surg* 2010;126(5):1548–1557.
17. Wechselberger G, Rumer A, Schoeller T, et al. Free-flap monitoring with tissue-oxygen measurement. *J Reconstr Microsurg* 1997;13(2):125–130.
18. Huemer GM, Dunst KM, Schoeller T. Restoration of the gluteal fold by a deepithelialized skin flap: preliminary observations. *Aesthetic Plast Surg* 2005;29(1):13–17.
19. Wechselberger G, Schoeller T. The transverse myocutaneous gracilis free flap: a valuable tissue source in autologous breast reconstruction. *Plast Reconstr Surg* 2004;114(1):69–73.
20. Schoeller T, Huemer GM, Kolehmainen M, Otto-Schoeller A, Wechselberger G. A new "Siamese" flap for breast reconstruction: the combined infragluteal-transverse myocutaneous gracilis muscle flap. *Plast Reconstr Surg* 2005;115(4):1110–1117.
21. Schoeller T, Huemer GM, Wechselberger G. The transverse musculocutaneous gracilis flap for breast reconstruction: guidelines for flap and patient selection. *Plast Reconstr Surg* 2008;122(1):29–38.
22. Fansa H, Schirmer S, Warnecke IC, et al. The transverse myocutaneous gracilis muscle flap: a fast and reliable method for breast reconstruction. *Plast Reconstr Surg* 2008;122(5):1326–1333.
23. Vega SJ, Sandeen SN, Bossert RP, et al. Gracilis myocutaneous free flap in autologous breast reconstruction. *Plast Reconstr Surg* 2009;124(5): 1400–1409.
24. Saint-Cyr M, Shirvani A, Wong C. The transverse upper gracilis flap for breast reconstruction following liposuction of the thigh. *Microsurgery* 2010;30(8):636–638.

CHAPTER 48

Stacked Flaps in Breast Reconstruction

Charles Y. Tseng, Thomas Hayakawa, Edward W. Buchel, and Joan E. Lipa

A breast mound that appears and feels similar to the natural breast can be created from a patient's own tissues using a variety of flap designs. Microsurgical breast reconstruction has evolved toward techniques that harvest autologous tissue with minimal disruption of the muscle through which the blood supply passes, as observed in the evolution of flaps from the abdominal donor site: pedicled transverse rectus abdominis musculocutaneous (TRAM), free TRAM, muscle-sparing (MS-)TRAM, and deep inferior epigastric artery perforator (DIEP). Indeed, a more sophisticated understanding of vascular anatomy and technical expertise will continue to expand and refine the microsurgeon's armamentarium.

In general, the most natural-appearing breasts are reconstructed with autologous tissue from the lower abdominal donor site. For many patients, an aesthetically pleasing breast can be created with tissue from a single donor site, particularly if the patient is considering contralateral breast augmentation or reduction mammaplasty to improve symmetry. However, some patients who elect mastectomy and desire autologous tissue breast reconstruction may, at first glance, not necessarily be considered good candidates for this mode of reconstruction because of a thin body habitus. Often, these women are young, physically fit, and slim with medium or large breasts and are highly concerned about the aesthetic outcome. Alternatively, a midline abdominal scar limits the volume of tissue that can be transferred on a single vascular supply for a patient who is otherwise a good candidate for unilateral breast reconstruction from the abdominal donor site.

Similarly, patients who initially opted for alloplastic reconstruction because of body habitus but are later dissatisfied because of capsular contracture, asymmetry, or dynamic distortion with activation of the pectoralis major muscle may strongly desire revision breast reconstruction using autologous tissue techniques. In these patients, the disparity between body mass index and preoperative breast size can create a difficult problem for the plastic surgeon.

CONVENTIONAL OPTIONS

Unfortunately, the amount of abdominal tissue required to match a large contralateral breast in a thin patient cannot be transferred reliably on a single pedicle. In these difficult cases, the literature describes transfer of the entire lower abdominal flap using double pedicle TRAM flaps, double pedicle free MS-TRAM or DIEP flaps, and stacked pedicle TRAM flaps. Alternative techniques for large-volume breast reconstruction include hybrid procedures such as the latissimus dorsi musculocutaneous flap with a subpectoral implant or free-TRAM flap combined with a subpectoral implant.

A double pedicle TRAM flap consists of both the right and left superior epigastric pedicles enclosed within the rectus abdominis muscles to transfer the entire TRAM flap for reconstruction of one breast (1,2). The stacked pedicle TRAM flap consists of two single pedicle hemi-TRAM flaps raised simultaneously from each side of the abdomen. The pedicle flaps are stacked to increase the volume and projection of the reconstructed breast (3). In the stacked configuration, the base flap provides "filler" volume, and the layered flap supplies additional volume and skin replacement. The major disadvantage of these double pedicle designs is the donor site morbidity associated with sacrificing both rectus abdominis muscles.

In comparison, the double pedicle free MS-TRAM and DIEP flap involves both the right and left deep inferior epigastric (DIE) pedicles to transfer the entire lower abdominal flap for reconstruction of one breast. In the "supercharge" construct, the DIE pedicles are anastomosed to separate recipient vessels (i.e., thoracodorsal and internal mammary vessels) or anterograde and retrograde internal mammary vessels (4) (Figure 48-1). In the "turbocharged" construct (Figure 48-2A), the ipsilateral DIE pedicle is anastomosed to the internal mammary vessels, and the contralateral DIE pedicle is anastomosed to a large side branch of the main ipsilateral pedicle (Figure 48-2B) or to the superior continuation of the DIE

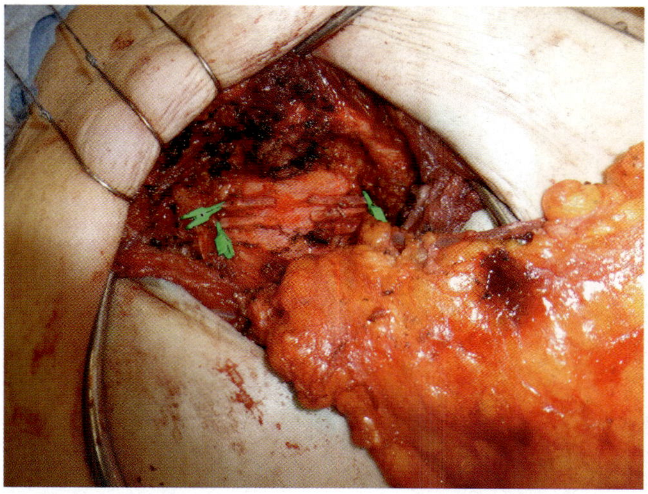

FIGURE 48-1 Dissection of internal mammary vessels with anterograde and retrograde flow. When the overlying costal cartilage is removed and the internal mammary recipient vessels are dissected out within the superior and inferior interspaces, there is sufficient length to allow for division of the vessels in the central portion of the dissected segment, thereby providing sufficient length in the two sets of recipient vessels for either turbocharged flap or stacked flap anastomoses.

vessels just beyond the junction with the superior-most perforator supplying the ipsilateral DIEP flap (Figure 48-2C) (4–6). When the superficial inferior epigastric vessels are suitable, a superficial inferior epigastric artery (SIEA) flap can be elevated in lieu of a DIEP or MS-TRAM flap. The potential disadvantage of these designs is that folding the flap onto itself can make it difficult to create an aesthetic breast mound and can lead to a squared-off appearance of the lower pole (7). However, the squared-off shape may still be appropriate to match the contralateral breast with a similar footprint (vertical height less than horizontal dimension) and conus (Figure 48-3). Furthermore, the turbocharged flap can be coned such that the lateral ends of the abdominal flap are brought together and oriented at the superior aspect of the reconstruction (8) (Figure 48-4). This brings the two pedicles into close proximity so that the anastomosis of one pedicle to a side branch of the other can be carried out on a back table. The resulting shape can mimic a ptotic breast and create a footprint with a long vertical dimension (Figure 48-5).

Hybrid techniques incorporating both expander/implant and autologous tissue techniques have also been described for patients with a thin body habitus (9). In these cases, the implant is placed in the subpectoral position to increase volume and projection, and the latissimus dorsi musculocutaneous flap or free-TRAM flap (anastomosed to the thoracodorsal recipient vessels) is used for skin replacement. However, augmentation of the reconstructed breast may not be acceptable to the patient who wants to avoid the use of alloplastic materials or risk the known complications of implant reconstruction, including rupture and capsular contracture.

Other proposed solutions include contralateral breast reduction. A decrease in breast size, however, may not be an acceptable alternative for a patient who wants to preserve her native breast volume, wishes to avoid scarring on the contralateral

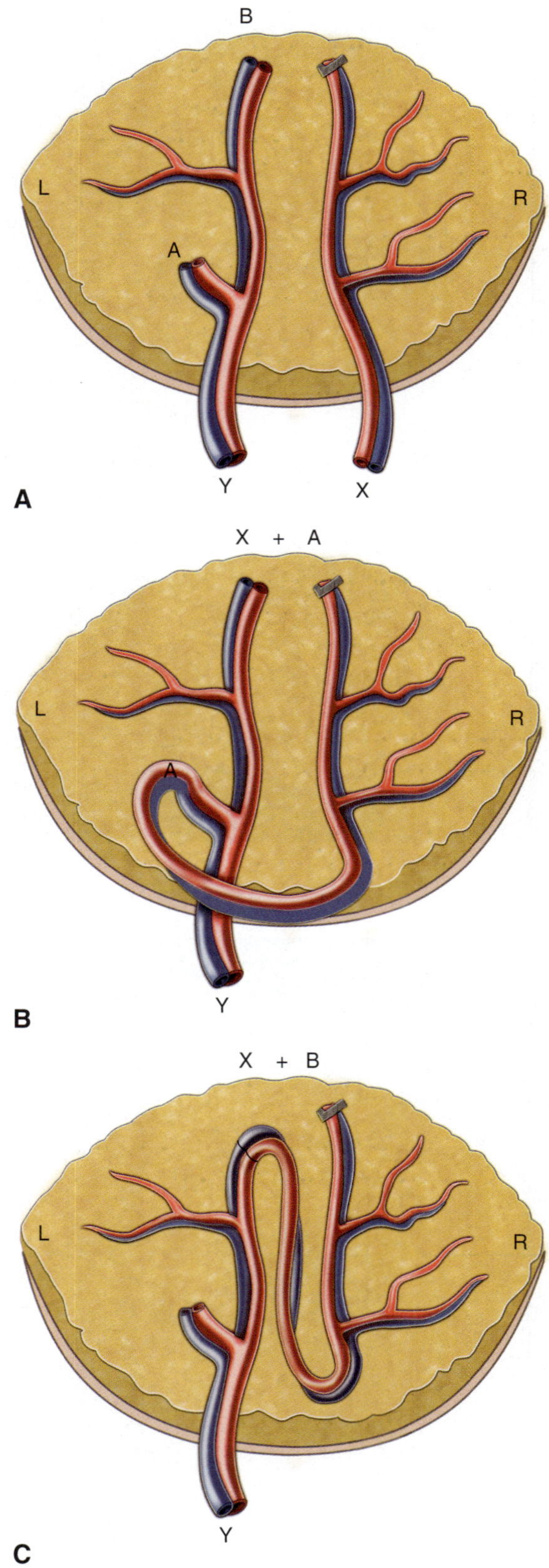

FIGURE 48-2 Turbocharged deep inferior epigastric artery perforator (DIEP) flap option. (**A**) DIEP flaps still connected in the midline are elevated. The undersurface of the flap is shown. DIEP pedicle X represents the pedicle that will be connected to the main DIEP pedicle, Y. A and B represent option for in series configurations where A is a side branch and B is the superior continuation of the main DIEP pedicle Y. (**B**) Pedicle X is anastomosed to the side branch A. (**C**) Pedicle X is anastomosed to the end of the contralateral pedicle, B.

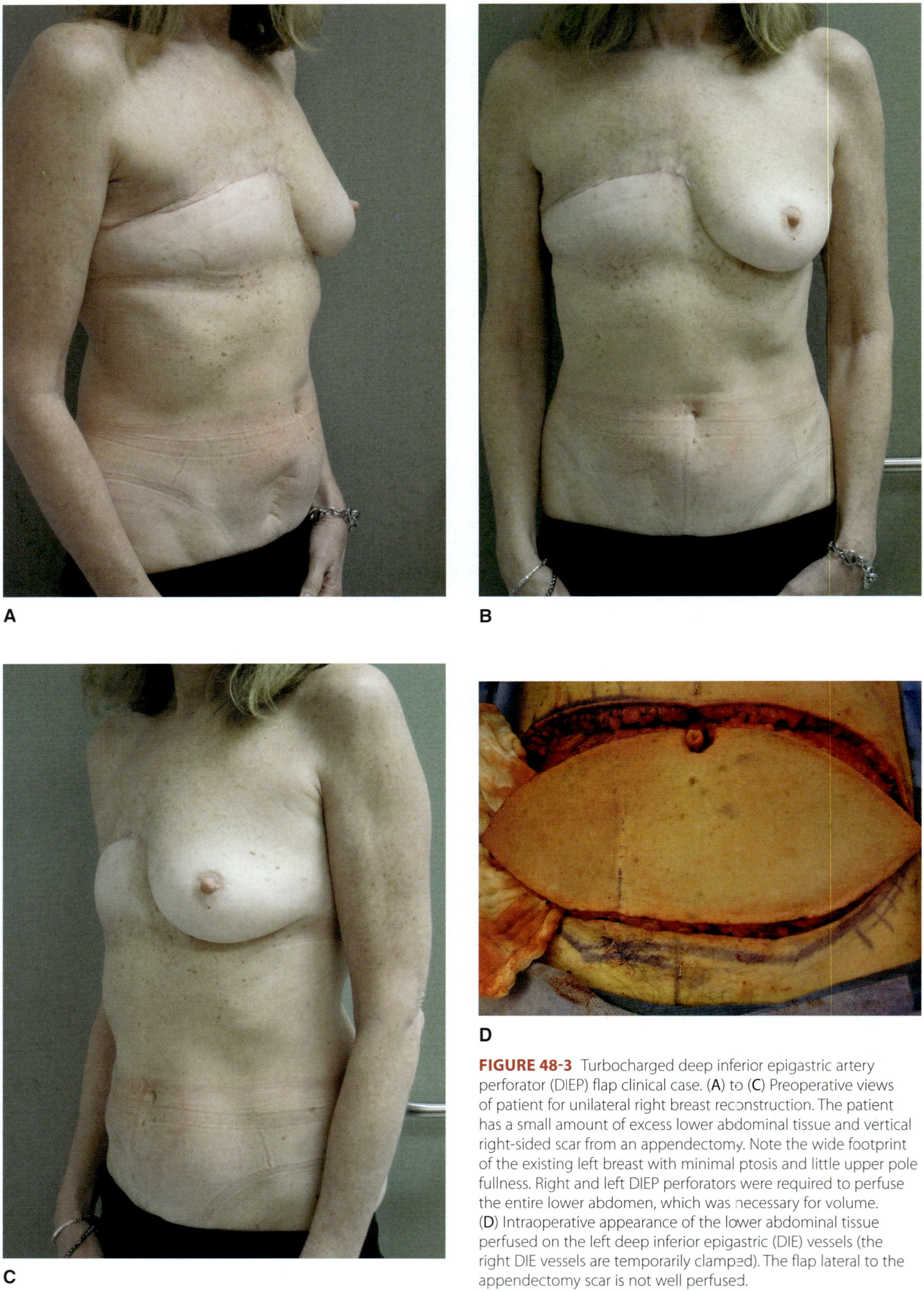

FIGURE 48-3 Turbocharged deep inferior epigastric artery perforator (DIEP) flap clinical case. (A) to (C) Preoperative views of patient for unilateral right breast reconstruction. The patient has a small amount of excess lower abdominal tissue and vertical right-sided scar from an appendectomy. Note the wide footprint of the existing left breast with minimal ptosis and little upper pole fullness. Right and left DIEP perforators were required to perfuse the entire lower abdomen, which was necessary for volume. (D) Intraoperative appearance of the lower abdominal tissue perfused on the left deep inferior epigastric (DIE) vessels (the right DIE vessels are temporarily clamped). The flap lateral to the appendectomy scar is not well perfused.

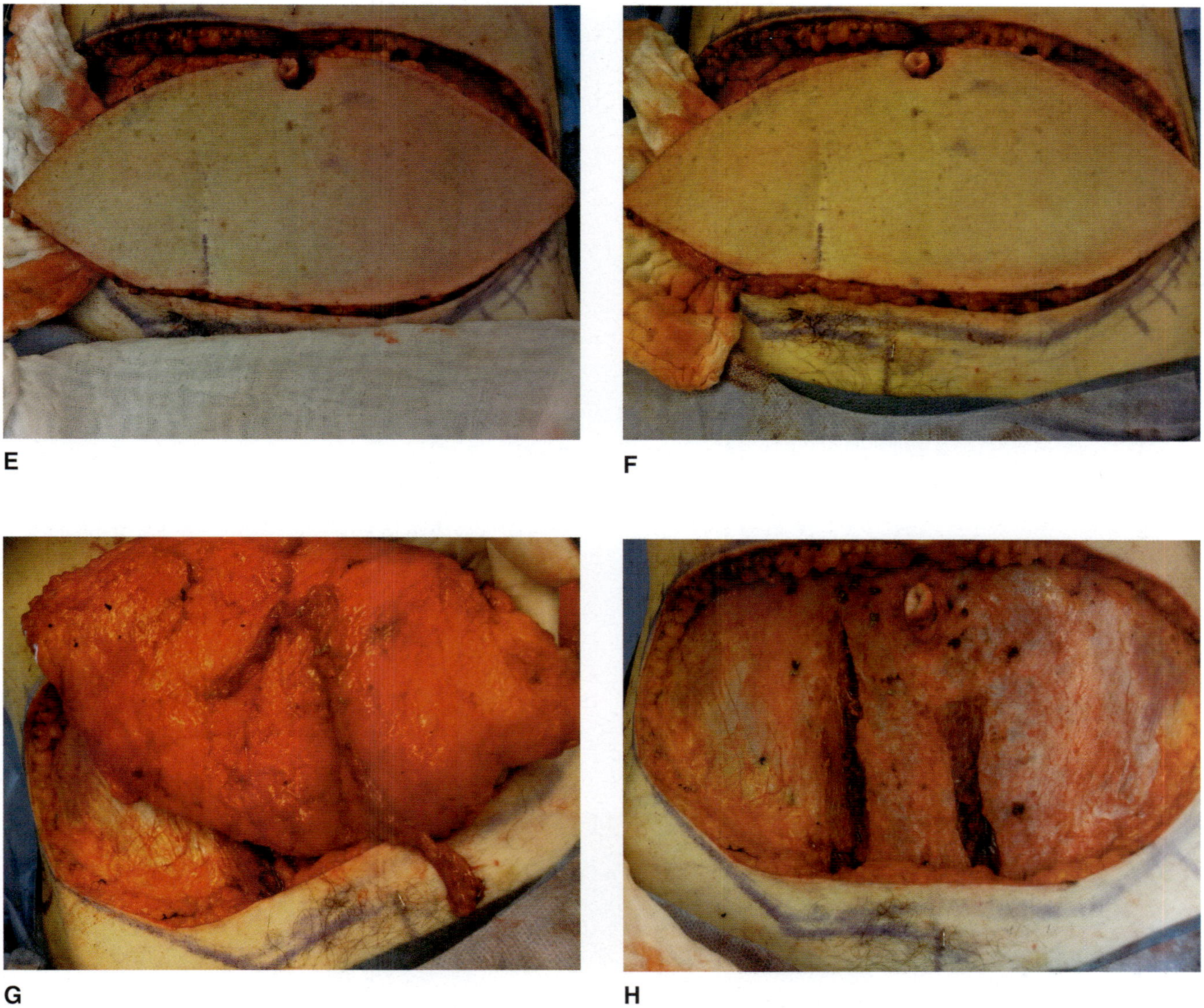

FIGURE 48-3 (*Continued*) (**E**) Intraoperative appearance of the lower abdominal tissue perfused on the right DIE vessels (the left DIE vessels are temporarily clamped). The flap lateral to the midline is not well perfused. (**F**) The entire lower abdominal flap is well perfused when both systems are supplying the flap. (**G**) Turbocharged flap. The right DIEP pedicle has been anastomosed to the superior continuation of the left DIEP pedicle on a side table before transfer to the recipient site. (**H**) The donor site before closure. There is preservation of the abdominal integrity.

breast, or wishes to avoid the associated potential risks of nipple–areola loss and changes in sensitivity.

THE STACKED FREE FLAP OPTION FOR BREAST RECONSTRUCTION

As more women elect bilateral mastectomy, the problem of autologous tissue reconstruction in the setting of inadequate donor site volume will become more common. In these situations, transferring multiple free flaps and insetting them in a stacked construct to increase overall breast volume and enhance breast mound projection can achieve larger volume unilateral or bilateral reconstruction.

For example, in unilateral reconstruction, the right and left hemi-DIEP flaps can be stacked atop one another to achieve more volume, projection, and shape so that the reconstructed breast mound can better match the native contralateral breast (7). In the case of bilateral reconstruction, flaps from multiple donor sites (i.e., DIEP or superior gluteal artery perforator [SGAP]) can be stacked atop one another to achieve more volume, projection, and shape than would be created with just one donor site. In both situations, the reconstruction utilizes the entire volume of tissue available at the donor site(s) and maintains the appeal of simultaneous abdominoplasty or circumferential body lift.

DONOR SITES AND FLAPS USED IN STACKED FREE FLAP BREAST RECONSTRUCTION

Lower Abdominal Flaps

Flap designs for the lower abdominal donor site highlight the evolution and sophistication of microsurgical technique. Hartrampf's introduction of the pedicled TRAM flap in 1982

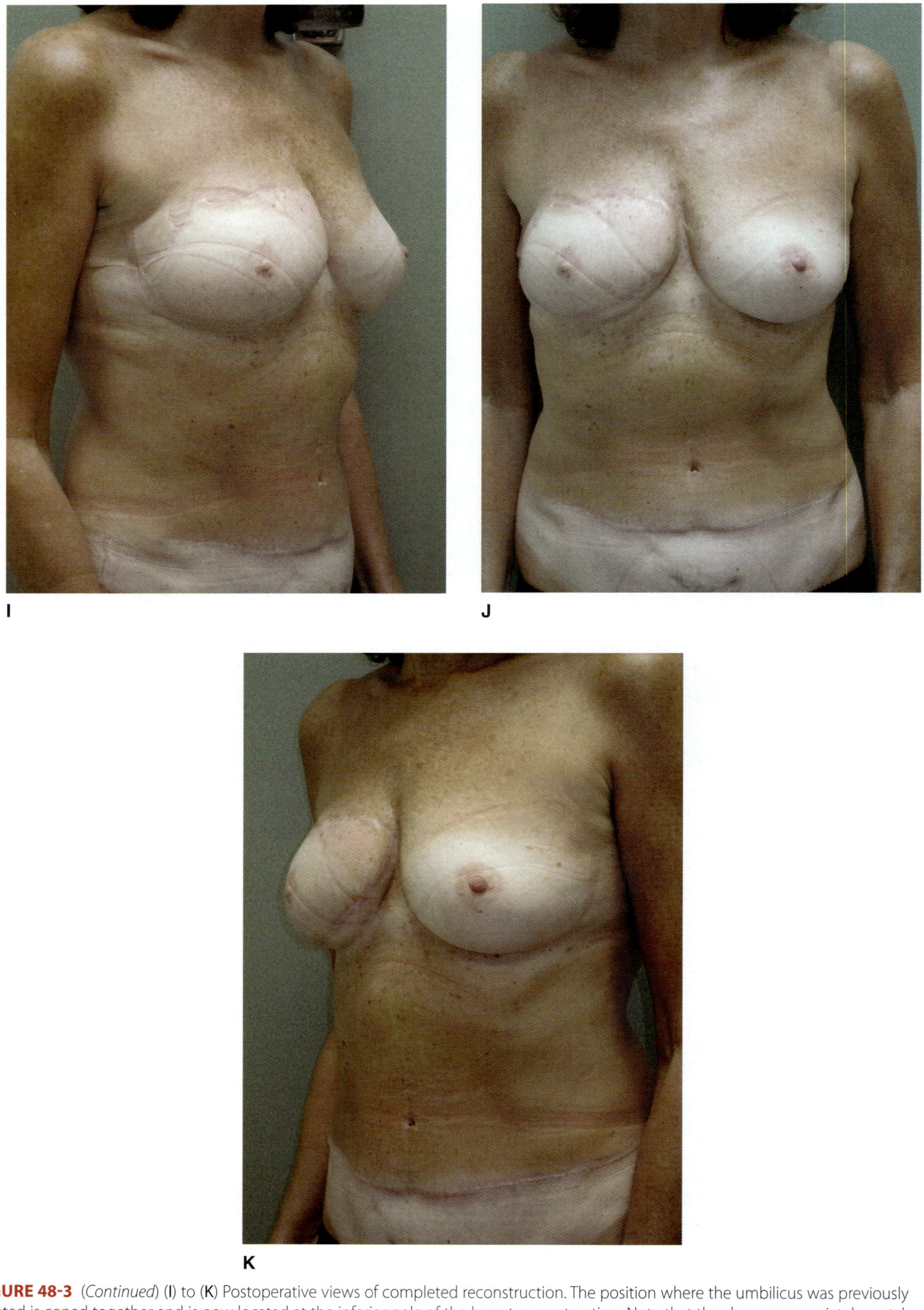

FIGURE 48-3 (*Continued*) (I) to (K) Postoperative views of completed reconstruction. The position where the umbilicus was previously located is coned together and is now located at the inferior pole of the breast reconstruction. Note that the shape appropriately matches the natural left breast.

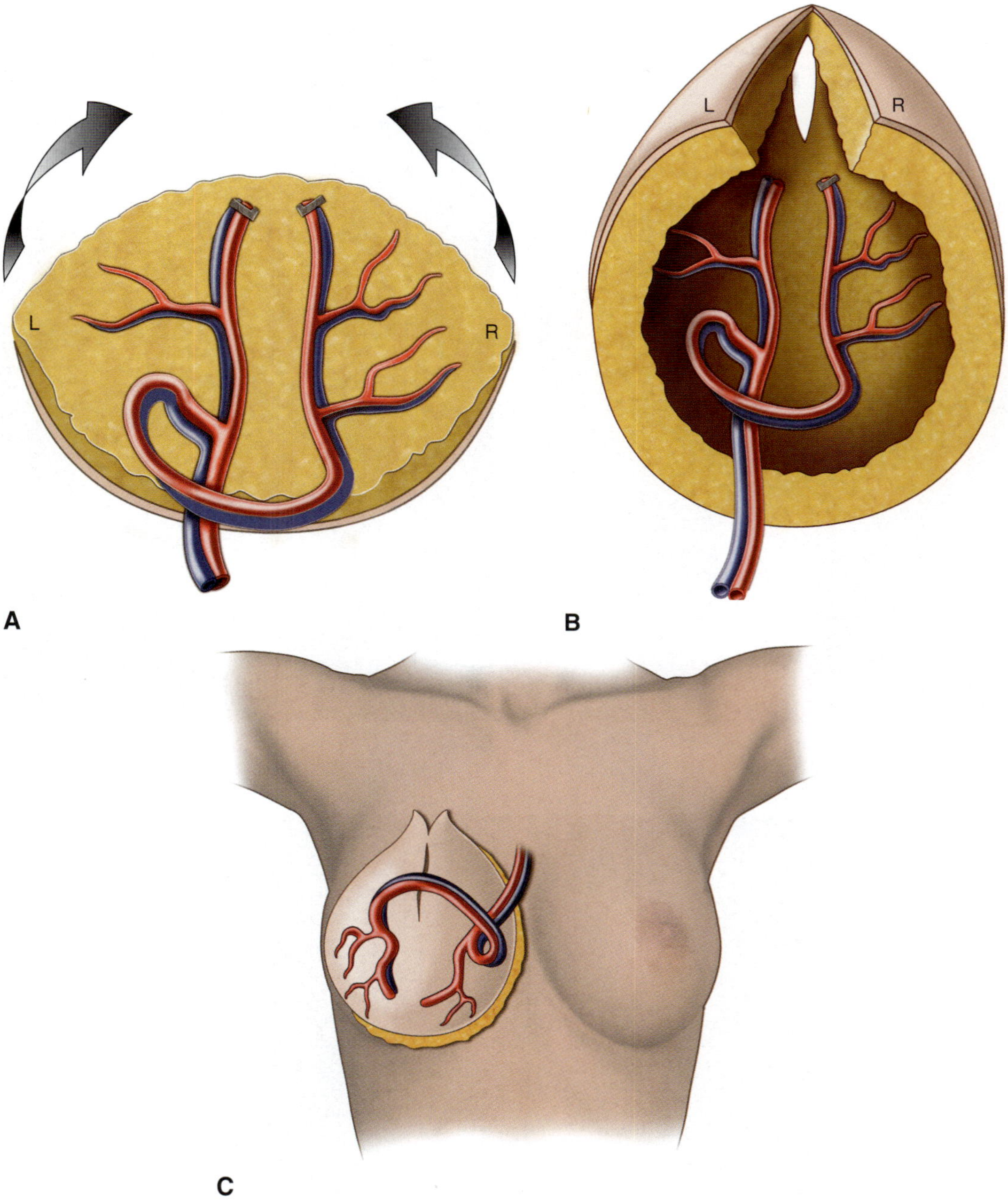

FIGURE 48-4 Coned turbocharged deep inferior epigastric artery perforator (DIEP) flap configuration. (**A**) Demonstration of flap shaping. The lateral ends of the abdominal flap are brought together, making a very long vertical dimension to the reconstructed flap. (**B**) Coning. The pedicles are brought in closer proximity. (**C**) Inset of the coned turbocharged flap. The lateral ends that were brought together are positioned superiorly.

ushered in the modern era of breast reconstruction. Further investigation into the vascular anatomy of this flap design revealed that the dominant arterial supply to the rectus abdominis muscle is the deep inferior epigastric artery (DIEA) (10,11).

The concepts of donor site muscle sparing were introduced with the "segmental" latissimus dorsi musculocutaneous and free-TRAM flaps (12,13). Koshima et al. refined this concept even further when they used the skin paddle overlying the rectus abdominis muscle for reconstruction of the mouth and groin (14). Their flap designs were based on a single periumbilical perforating vessel off the DIEA and composed of subcutaneous fat and skin only. Soon after, Allen and Treece performed the first DIEP flap for breast reconstruction by transferring the lower abdominal fat and skin from the same donor area of a TRAM flap while sparing the underlying rectus abdominis muscle (15).

The quest to minimize donor site morbidity has given rise to the development of the MS-TRAM and DIEP flap designs, each of which spares more muscle. Nahabedian et al. developed a classification system to describe the degree of sparing of the rectus abdominis muscle. MS-0 describes the sacrifice of the full-width (partial length) of the muscle; MS-1 describes the preservation of the lateral segment; MS-2 describes the preservation of the lateral and medial segments; and MS-3 refers to the preservation of all the rectus muscle, the equivalent of a DIEP flap (16).

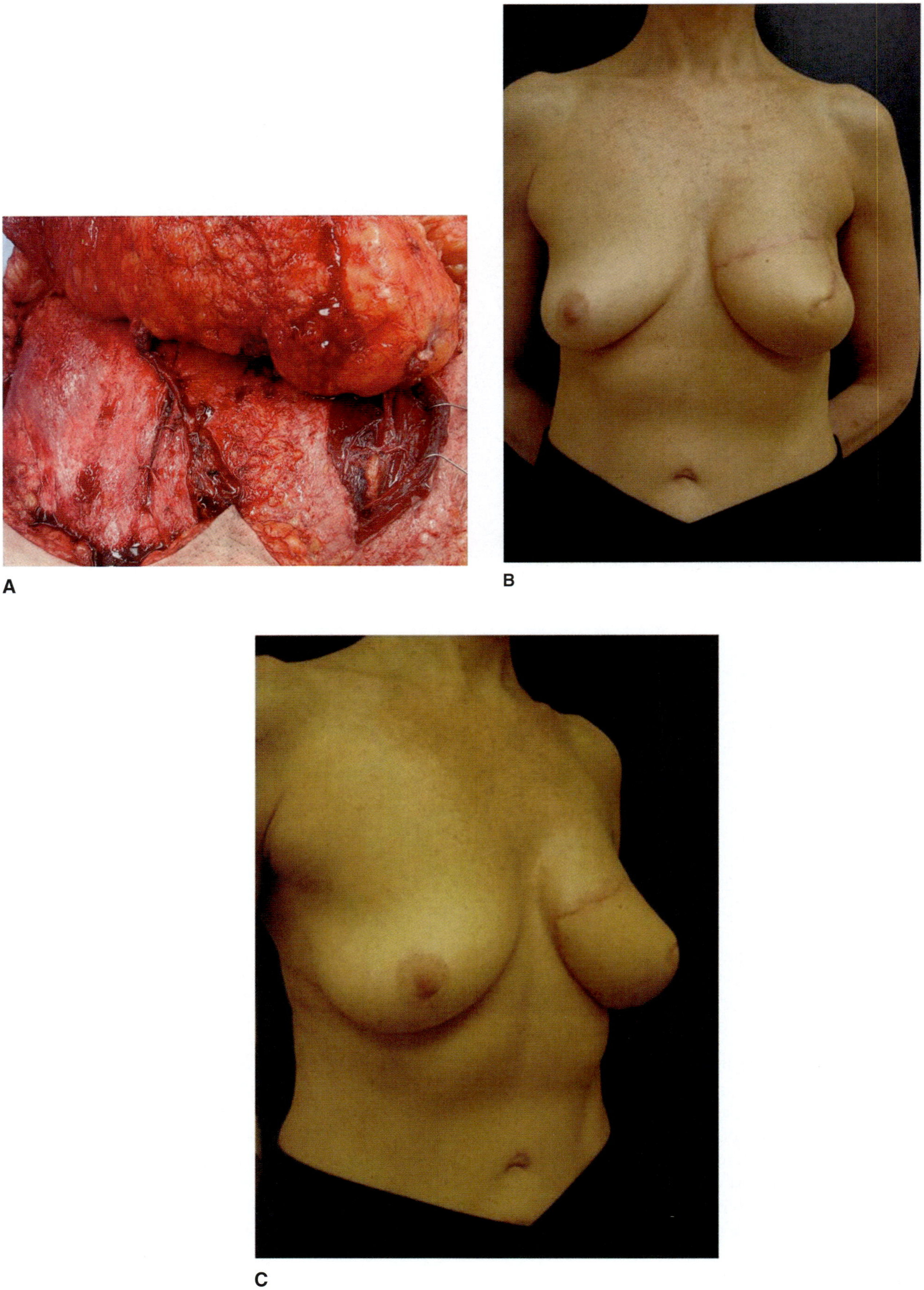

FIGURE 48-5 Clinical example of a coned turbocharged deep inferior epigastric artery perforator flap. (**A**) The dissected flap. The two pedicles are shown, with preservation of motor nerves to the rectus abdominis muscle. (**B**) and (**C**) Postoperative views. The lateral ends of the abdominal skin flap are positioned superiorly in this coned turbocharged construct. Excellent ptosis and conical shape have been achieved.

Deep Inferior Epigastric Artery Perforator Flaps

Many women with breast cancer who will have or have had mastectomies are potential candidates for DIEP flap breast reconstruction. Most patients will be of an age when they have excess fat and skin overlying the lower abdomen. The fat in this region is typically soft and easy to shape and therefore will most closely approximate the feel of a normal breast.

An absolute contraindication specific to the use of the lower abdominal tissues for breast reconstruction is prior abdominoplasty. Prior abdominal liposuction does not preclude DIEP flap elevation (17), but caution should be exercised to ensure proper preoperative and intraoperative perforator evaluation before committing to elevating the abdominal tissue as a DIEP flap in this situation. Active smoking within 4 to 6 weeks of planned surgery contributes to fat necrosis or partial flap loss, delayed wound healing, and random flap loss at both the mastectomy and abdominal donor sites.

Excellent state-of-the-art descriptions of DIEP flap elevation are included in this textbook. Readers are directed to these chapters for detailed descriptions of technique.

For all flaps, an ellipse is outlined on the lower abdomen that extends from the suprapubic crease inferiorly to just above the umbilicus superiorly and laterally to the anterior superior iliac spines. However, the amount of tissue that can be safely taken and still allow for closure of the donor site must be estimated. In unilateral or bilateral stacked flap breast reconstruction, the ellipse of tissue will be split down the midline or near the midline. Therefore, the surgeon must also estimate how much of the lower abdominal flap will be required for the base flap and layered flap. Each hemi-flap can be reliably transferred on a single adequately sized perforator from the medial or lateral row. An adequate perforator should have a vein greater than 1 mm in diameter where it is entering into the flap and a palpable or visibly pulsating artery. The fascia is opened and the dominant perforator(s) are then dissected through the muscle until adequate pedicle length of the DIE vessels is obtained.

The DIEP flap design is ideal for stacked flap reconstruction because complete muscle sparing and preservation of the motor nerves to each rectus abdominis muscle will significantly reduce donor site morbidity relative to free TRAM and MS-TRAM flap designs.

The DIEP flap has proven reliability and a low complication rate. In their experience, Allen's group report that 25% of flaps were based on one perforator, 50% on two perforators, and 25% on three or more perforators (18). In a 10-year retrospective review of 758 DIEP flaps by the same group, 6% of patients returned to the operating room for flap-related problems. Partial flap loss occurred in 2.5% of cases. Total flap loss occurred in fewer than 1% of all cases. Problems with the vein or venous anastomoses were nearly eight times more likely than problems with the artery or arterial anastomoses. Fat necrosis appeared in 13% of flaps. Seroma formation at the abdominal donor site occurred in approximately 5%. Abdominal hernia occurred in 0.7% of cases.

Nahabedian et al. reported their experience with the MS-2 TRAM and DIEP flaps. For MS-2 TRAM flaps, the complications included total necrosis in 1.8% of cases, fat necrosis 7.1%, venous congestion 2.7%, and abdominal bulge in 4.6% of unilateral reconstructions and 21% of bilateral reconstructions. In comparison, the DIEP flap group complications included total necrosis in 2.7% of cases, fat necrosis in 6.4%, and venous congestion in 4.5% and abdominal bulge rates of 1.5% after unilateral reconstruction and 4.5% after bilateral reconstruction (19).

Superficial Inferior Epigastric Artery Flaps

Although not a true perforator flap in the sense that the SIEA does not give off vessels that penetrate muscle or traverse a septum to supply overlying fat and skin, harvest of an SIEA flap precludes the need to open the anterior rectus sheath. Thus, breast reconstruction using the SIEA flap virtually eliminates donor site morbidity compared with DIEP flap harvest. There is no risk of a new abdominal hernia and even less abdominal pain compared with other abdominal flaps that require disruption of the anterior rectus sheath.

Despite these compelling advantages, several factors may preclude the SIEA flap from being deployed in stacked flap breast reconstruction. First, the SIEA flap is limited by variability in its vascular anatomy and skin territory. The SIEA and superficial inferior epigastric vein (SIEV) are inconsistently present in sufficient caliber to reliably support sufficient tissue for breast reconstruction. The SIEA is absent in approximately 35% to 51% of the population and is not suitable, mainly because of small diameter, in an additional 19% of cases (20). Compared with the DIEA (2–4 mm), the superficial artery is typically smaller (mean diameter, 1.1–1.6 mm), has a shorter pedicle length (mean, 7 cm), and is often size mismatched when anastomosed to the thoracodorsal, internal mammary, or DIEA recipients. Because the superficial vessels lie more lateral than the lateral row of rectus abdominis perforators and because they enter into the edge of the flap, insetting in the chest may be more difficult than the DIEP flap. Last, the SIEA and SIEV pedicle does not have large branch points to which a stacked flap can be anastomosed.

When the harvested SIEA flaps were based on arteries with diameters 1.5 mm or greater, reported complication rates included fat necrosis in 3.7%, partial flap loss in 3.7%, arterial thrombosis in 3.7%, and venous congestion in 3.7%. In contrast, when the harvested SIEA flaps included arteries with diameters less than 1.5 mm, reported complication rates included arterial thrombosis in 8.3%, total flap loss in 6.9% partial flap loss in 5.6%, and venous congestion in 1.4%. As would be expected, there were no complications with abdominal bulge or hernia (21).

Gluteal Artery Perforator Flaps

Just as the DIEP flap naturally evolved from the free TRAM and MS-TRAM predecessors, the SGAP and inferior gluteal artery perforator (IGAP) flaps have evolved from the superiorly or inferiorly based free gluteal musculocutaneous flap.

Terminal branches of the internal iliac artery, the superior and inferior gluteal arteries pass out of the pelvis above and below the piriformis muscle to supply the upper and lower halves of the gluteus maximus muscle, respectively. As the superior gluteal artery passes through the greater sciatic foramen, it divides into a superficial and a deep branch. The superficial branch supplies the gluteus muscle and sends perforating vessels that penetrate the muscle to supply the overlying subcutaneous fat and skin of the upper buttock. The inferior gluteal artery accompanies the greater sciatic nerve, the internal pudendal vessels, and the posterior femoral cutaneous nerve. It exits the pelvis caudal to the piriformis muscle and travels under the inferior portion of the gluteus maximus, giving off perforating vessels that penetrate the muscle to supply the overlying fat and skin of the lower buttock (22).

Whereas perforating vessels closer to the medial aspect of the buttock have relatively short intramuscular lengths, those located laterally must travel more obliquely through the muscle substance. Therefore, pedicles based on perforators to the lateral aspects of the skin paddle tend to be longer than those based on medial perforators. Compared with the course of the superior gluteal vessels, the course of the inferior gluteal vessels is more oblique through the gluteus maximus muscle. Hence, the IGAP pedicle has the potential to be longer than the SGAP pedicle (23). More importantly, the superior and inferior gluteal arteries and veins should be carefully dissected down to their takeoff from the internal iliac vessels to obtain adequate size match with the recipient internal mammary artery and vein (average diameter, 2.5–3.5 mm).

Patients ideally suited for GAP flap breast reconstruction include women who have more subcutaneous tissue in the buttock region than in the abdominal region. In addition, a younger patient with larger breasts and genetic risk factors predisposing to breast cancer who elects prophylactic bilateral mastectomy may lack sufficient abdominal tissue for bilateral reconstruction but may have enough tissue in the abdomen and buttock regions for stacked free flap bilateral breast reconstruction.

General advantages to GAP flap reconstruction include an associated body contouring procedure (modest buttock lift) at the same time as breast reconstruction. Furthermore, the flap designs result in a relatively shorter scar that can be well concealed by clothing or camouflaged in the natural body contours.

Unlike the soft and pliable tissues of the lower abdominal region, the gluteal subcutaneous fat is globular and supported by dense fibrous septa, making it firmer than abdominal fat. This gives it good projection for the relatively limited volume of tissue harvested but also makes it more difficult to shape into a breast mound. Thus, in stacked flap breast reconstruction, the GAP flap is more commonly used as the filler flap with the more pliable DIEP flap stacked on top to provide volume and skin replacement.

Absolute contraindications include prior gluteal surgery or buttock lift involving the donor site and active smoking. Relative contraindications include prior cosmetic liposuction of the gluteal donor site because of possible injury to the perforators. Caution should be exercised with proper preoperative radiologic imaging and intraoperative perforator evaluation.

Superior Gluteal Artery Perforator Flaps

The superior gluteal artery musculocutaneous flap has been used for autologous breast reconstruction but is associated with a difficult dissection and a short pedicle such that interposition vein grafts were often needed to reach the intended recipient vessels. In 1995, Allen et al. described the SGAP flap for breast reconstruction (24). Dissection of the perforating vessels out of the muscle yielded two key advantages over the original musculocutaneous predecessor. Specifically, dissection of the perforator vessels out of the muscle made dissection of the superior gluteal artery much easier and perhaps more important, resulted in a much longer pedicle such that microvascular transfer can be completed without the need for interposition vein grafting. Similar to the DIEP flap, no sacrifice of muscle is required.

Excellent state-of-the-art descriptions of SGAP flap elevation are included in this textbook. Readers are directed to these chapters.

Based on their 9-year experience with 142 GAP flaps, Allen's group suggest basing the flap on a single large perforator, if present, and adjusting the orientation of the typical oblique, superomedial-to-inferolateral skin paddle to a more horizontal design to reduce postoperative contour deformity and thereby place the scar in a more favorable position (22). They also suggest using perforators positioned laterally on the long axis of the flap to maximize pedicle length. Furthermore, the internal mammary vessels are the preferred recipients given the shorter pedicle length of the SGAP flap.

Reported complications included arterial and venous complication in 6%, donor site contour deformity requiring secondary correction in 4%, partial flap necrosis in 4%, donor site seroma in 2%, and donor site hematoma in 1% (22).

Inferior Gluteal Artery Perforator Flaps

Early experience with the inferior gluteal musculocutaneous flap and IGAP flap used an oblique, superolateral-to-inferomedial skin paddle. The literature describes significant donor site morbidity associated with this flap design. The most significant problems were postoperative lower extremity dysesthesia and pain syndromes (25).

Modification of the skin paddle design to a more horizontal skin paddle located just above and parallel to the gluteal crease resulted in a significant improvement in donor site morbidity. The flap is elevated in the subfascial plane and the perforators approached from lateral to medial. A single large perforator is typically used, but multiple perforators in the same plane of muscle splitting dissection can be incorporated into the flap. Limiting dissection over the sciatic nerve precludes sciatic nerve exposure and leaves a sufficient pat pad medially over the ischium reduces postoperative pain syndromes. The scar is hidden in the gluteal crease.

Transverse Myocutaneous Gracilis Flap

As an alternate flap for women who do not have an adequate volume of tissue in either the abdominal or buttock donor sites, the transverse myocutaneous gracilis (TMG) flap has been developed. Readers are directed to the description of the elevation of this flap in this textbook. Essential features include design of the flap medial to the femoral triangle and anterior dissection at the level of the superficial fascia to avoid complications of lymphedema and to preserve the great saphenous vein. Posteriorly, the limit of the flap is to the ischial tuberosity in the gluteal crease so that increased bulk in the flap is obtained by skewing the skin and subcutaneous paddle posterior to the axis of the gracilis muscle. Similarly, deep fat elevated inferior to the 8- to 10-cm skin paddle adds to the bulk. In unilateral reconstruction, the harvested TMG flap is typically coned for shaping. However, in the case of double (stacked) TMG flaps for unilateral reconstruction, the flaps are left without being coned and are positioned in a "ying-yang" configuration, with one pedicle reaching the internal mammary and the other pedicle reaching the thoracodorsal recipient vessels (26). This is different from the "filler" and "layered" flap configuration of stacked DIEP or DIEP–GAP flaps described below.

TECHNIQUES FOR STACKED FREE FLAP BREAST RECONSTRUCTION

As mentioned, stacked flap reconstruction is considered for patients who have inadequate abdominal or gluteal soft tissue volume for routine breast reconstruction or require larger volume or projection. These techniques can be applied to immediate or delayed reconstruction in patients being treated for cancer, prophylactic mastectomy, or failed implant reconstruction.

Patient evaluation begins with estimation of soft tissue volume at all available donor sites in relation to desired breast volume. When the estimated volume that can be reliably harvested from a single donor site is less than the desired final volume, stacked flap reconstruction should be considered. Particular consideration should be given to women who desire replacement of unsatisfactory implant reconstruction because the estimated volume is derived from the size of the existing implant plus overcorrection by 20% to account for the flattened thoracic platform. The potential donor sites are evaluated to determine which site or combination of sites will be used, with planning for recipient vessels and interflap anastomoses.

For unilateral reconstruction, the lower abdominal donor site is considered the first-line option. For bilateral reconstruction, the lower abdominal and SGAP donor sites are considered together because of the tissue requirement and the fact that the donor site combination effectively results in a circumferential body lift.

Although not necessary, computed tomography angiography can be used in the presurgical planning process to maximize accuracy of donor site markings, identify perforator vessel location, and plan the microsurgical anastomoses.

Unilateral Stacked Flap Reconstruction

The example of DIEP–DIEP flap reconstruction will be described here. Regardless of the flap combination (DIEP, SIEA, MS-TRAM, or bilateral TMG flaps), the principles are as described here.

1. Surgery begins with dissection of the DIEP flap contralateral to the breast being reconstructed. This will be the layered (superficial) flap that will have its skin island exposed in the final reconstruction.
2. The SIEA and SIEV are identified. If present, the SIEA and SIEV are dissected carefully and ligated just distal to the common femoral artery and vein.
3. As with standard DIEP flap dissection, the perforators emanating from the DIEA and DIEV are identified and dissected free of the surrounding fascia and muscle.
4. As the selected perforators are dissected free of the surrounding tissues, all large branches suitable for microsurgical anastomoses are carefully dissected for at least 2 cm and ligated (Figure 48-6).
5. As dissection proceeds, the surgeon creates a mental image of the possible vascular links as related to flap inset.
6. After the flap pedicle is dissected and isolated, attention is turned to the remaining hemiabdomen ipsilateral to the breast being reconstructed. The second DIEP flap is dissected in similar fashion to the first flap with preservation of the SIEA or SIEV and particular attention to preservation of the large branch points off the DIEA or DIEV that may be used for anastomoses if needed. This flap will become the buried (base) flap that will be deepithelialized.
7. The desired recipient vessels—the internal mammary artery and vein or thoracodorsal artery and vein—are exposed and prepared.
8. The lower abdominal flap is then split into two separate flaps. The flaps can be split near the midline or off center depending on the desired construct as related to breast shape and projection (Figure 48-7).
9. The ipsilateral flap is deepithelialized, inset dermal side down into the breast pocket, and anchored to the chest wall using absorbable suture. This flap is the base (buried) flap. The pedicle of the ipsilateral flap is carefully oriented for anastomosis to the most favorable branch point of the contralateral flap.
10. The contralateral flap is harvested, brought up to the chest wall and rotated 90 degrees. Microsurgical

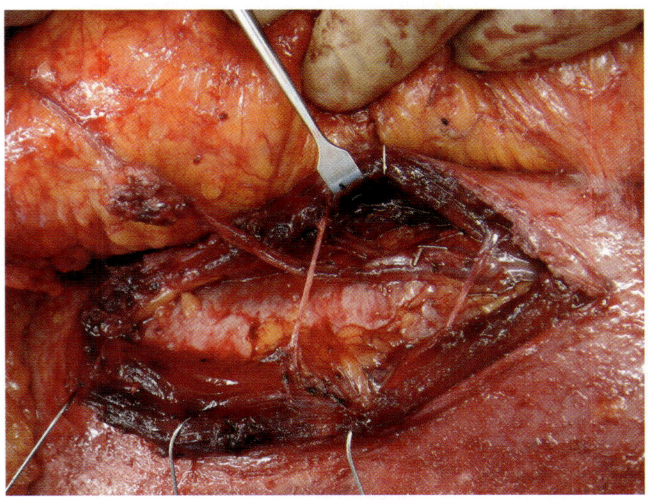

FIGURE 48-6 Side branch. After a suitable side branch of the deep inferior epigastric pedicle has been identified, at least a 2-cm length should be preserved before dividing it.

SECTION 3

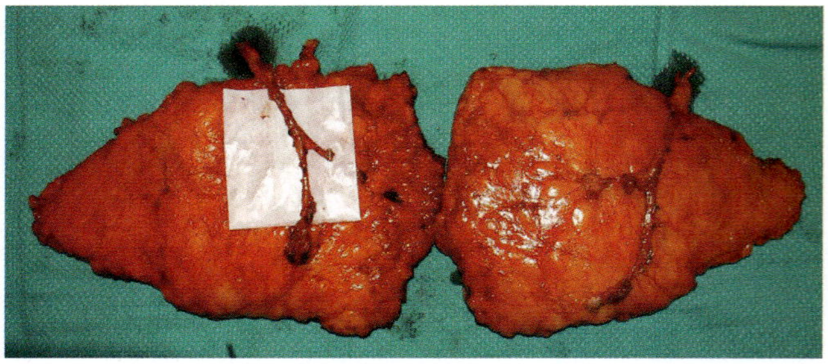

FIGURE 48-7 Bilateral deep inferior epigastric artery perforator (DIEP) flaps. Two DIEP flaps have been elevated. There is a suitable side branch that has been preserved on the flap shown on the left in order to perfuse the other flap.

anastomoses of the contralateral flap's DIEA and DIEV to the recipient internal mammary artery (IMA) and internal mammary vein (IMV) are completed.

11. After confirmation of arterial and venous flow through the contralateral (layered) DIEP flap, the ipsilateral (base) flap's DIEA and DIEV or SIEA and SIEV are anastomosed to the selected branch point of the contralateral flap pedicle. In this way, the contralateral and ipsilateral flaps are connected in series (Figure 48-8). Alternatively, the two flaps may be connected to separate recipient vessels, such as the anterograde and retrograde internal mammary vessels (Figure 48-9). This may be necessary when bilateral SIEA flaps are elevated because it is unlikely that there will be a side branch of sufficient caliber from the superficial system to connect the flap in series (Figure 48-10).
12. Alternatively, the flaps can be anastomosed to one another on a side table and then transferred en mass to the recipient site where microsurgical anastomoses of the DIEA and DIEV to the IMA or IMV is completed.
13. After confirmation of arterial and venous flow in both flaps, the contralateral flap is carefully layered atop the base flap and inset to avoid kinking, twisting, and other mechanical obstruction. The layered flap is deepithelialized as needed to match the skin defect, and the wound is closed. This is shown diagrammatically in Figure 48-11 and in a clinical example in Figure 48-12.

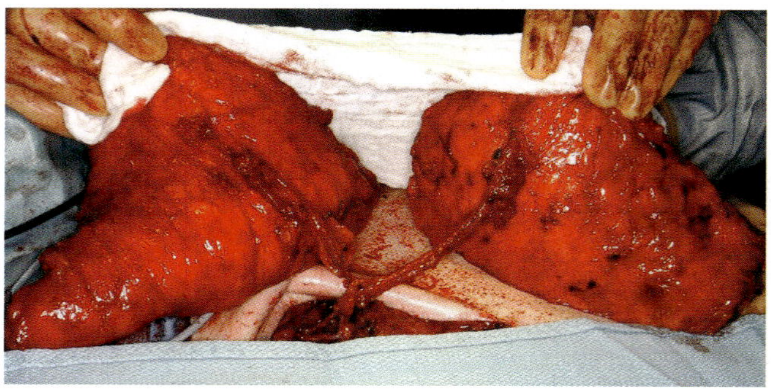

FIGURE 48-8 Stacked flaps at the recipient site. Microvascular anastomoses of the contralateral and ipsilateral flaps in series have been completed; one flap will become the base, and the other will be layered for external skin coverage.

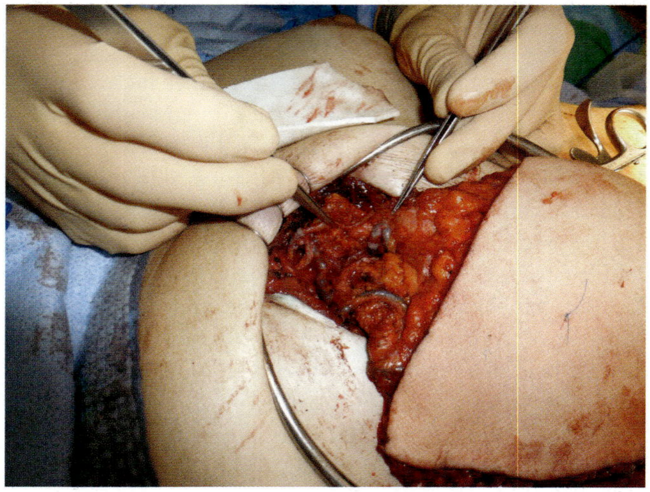

FIGURE 48-9 Stacked flaps ready for insetting. These are stacked superficial inferior epigastric artery flaps with the two flaps anastomosed to anterograde and retrograde internal mammary vessels ready for insetting and shaping.

Bilateral Stacked Flap Reconstruction

Bilateral DIEP and bilateral SGAP flaps are designed to mimic a body lift (27) (Figure 48-13). As with unilateral stacked flap breast reconstruction, the right and left hemiabdominal flaps are dissected with particular attention to preservation of the SIEA and SIEV, if present, and identification of all large branch points that might be used for flow-through anastomoses.

The example of DIEP and SGAP flap reconstruction will be described here. Regardless of the flap combination used, the principles described herein are the same for any flap combination. An IGAP or TMG flap can potentially be used in lieu of an SGAP flap.

1. The SGAP flap can be harvested using an incision that extends toward the planned abdominal donor site (similar to that used for circumferential lower body lift).
2. The perforators emanating from the gluteal muscle are identified. The selected perforators are carefully dissected away from the surrounding fascia and muscle.
3. Dissection continues through the deep gluteal fascia toward the takeoff of the gluteal artery and vein from the internal iliac artery and vein.
4. After adequate vessel caliber and pedicle length are obtained, the gluteal flap is harvested and passed off the field. The gluteal wounds are closed.
5. The patient is returned to the supine position and the DIEP flaps are harvested as described for unilateral flap reconstruction.
6. The recipient IMA and IMV vessels are exposed and prepared.
7. The ipsilateral SGAP flap is deepithelialized, inset dermal side down into the breast pocket, and anchored to the chest wall. The SGAP pedicle should be carefully oriented to optimize anastomosis to the selected branch point of the layered DIEP flap.
8. The contralateral DIEP flap is harvested and brought up to the chest wall. The DIEA and DIEV is anastomosed to the IMA and IMV.

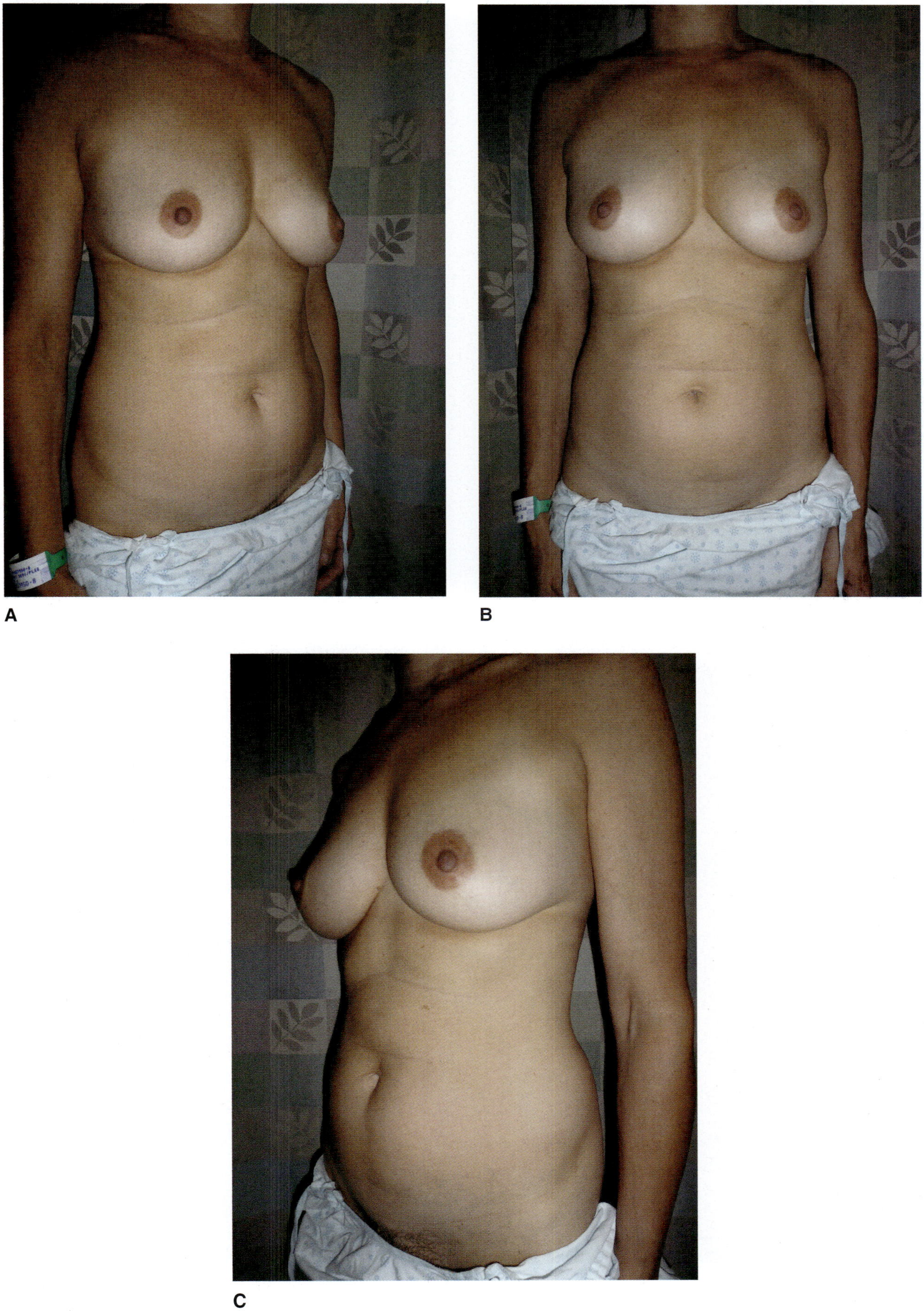

FIGURE 48-10 Stacked superficial inferior epigastric artery (SIEA) flaps in a clinical example. (**A**) to (**C**) Preoperative views of a patient for immediate right breast reconstruction. Stacked flaps are planned.

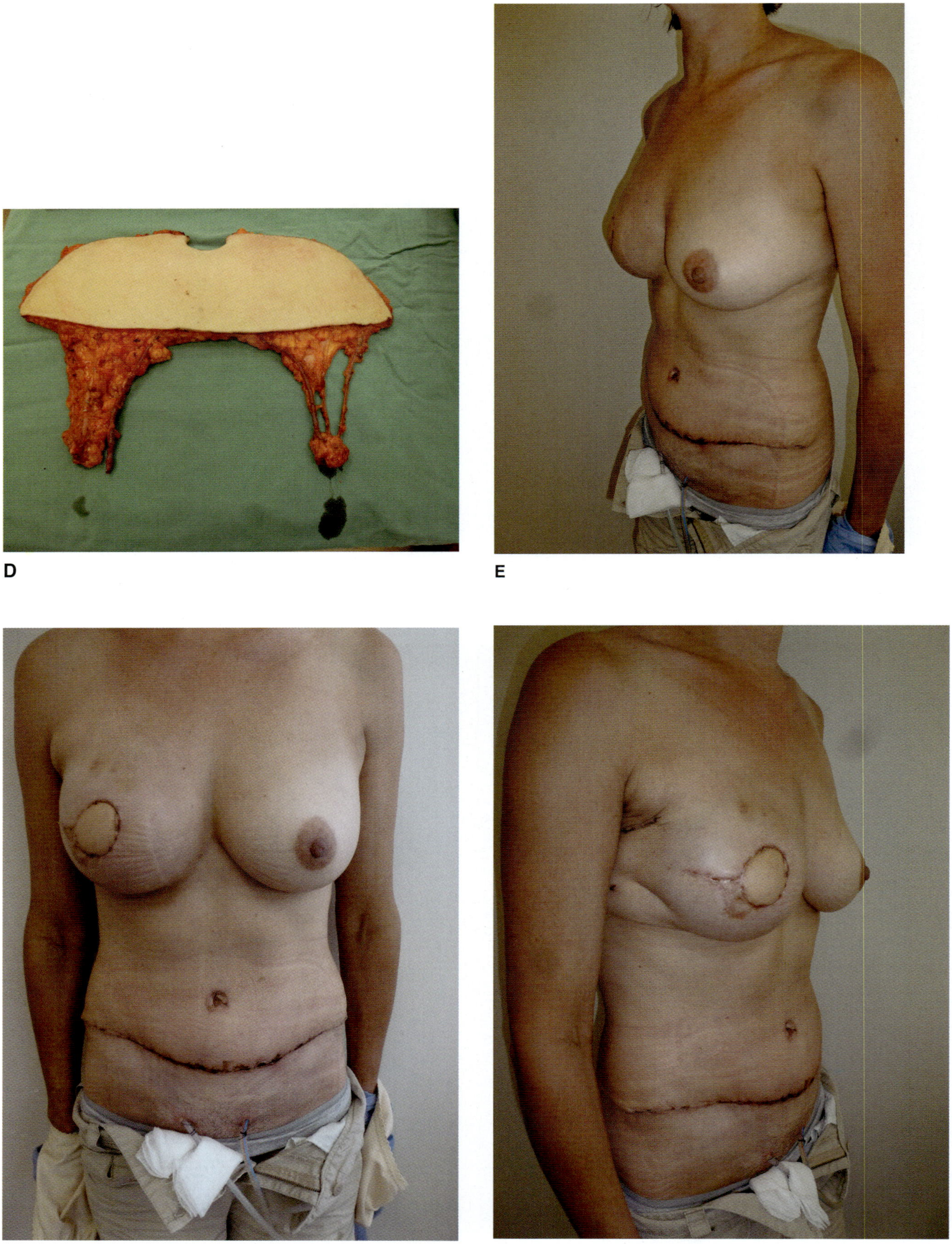

D E F G

FIGURE 48-10 (*Continued*) (**D**) Bilateral SIEA flaps have been elevated and are shown before being divided. (**E**) to (**G**) Postoperative views of the early stacked flap result.

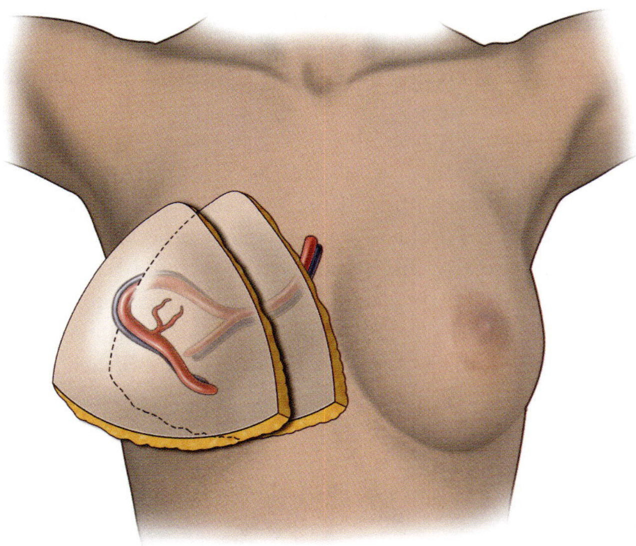

FIGURE 48-11 Stacked deep inferior epigastric artery perforator (DIEP) flap configuration. This diagram shows the manner in which the stacked flaps can be connected in series. In this case, the layered flap pedicle is anastomosed to the side branch of the base flap pedicle.

9. After confirmation of arterial and venous flow through the DIEP flap, the SGA and SGV are anastomosed to the selected branch point of the DIEA and DIEV pedicle.
10. After confirmation of arterial and venous flow through both flaps, the DIEP flap is layered atop the SGAP flap and carefully inset to avoid kinking, twisting, and other mechanical obstruction. The layered flap is deepithelialized to match the mastectomy skin defect, and the wound is closed.

POSTOPERATIVE FLAP MONITORING

Accurate postoperative flap monitoring is a critical factor to success in microsurgical breast reconstruction. Changes in perfusion must be recognized quickly for rapid assessment, exploration, and salvage.

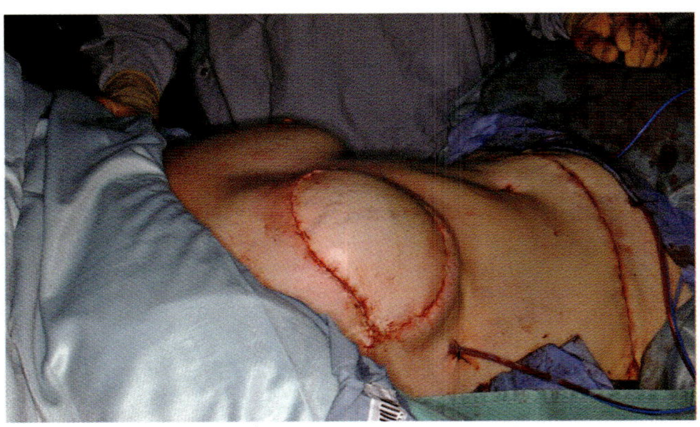

FIGURE 48-12 Stacked flap insetting. This is an on-table appearance of the stacked flaps after tailoring the flaps to achieve appropriate shaping and redraping of the mastectomy skin flaps. Good on-table projection is obtained.

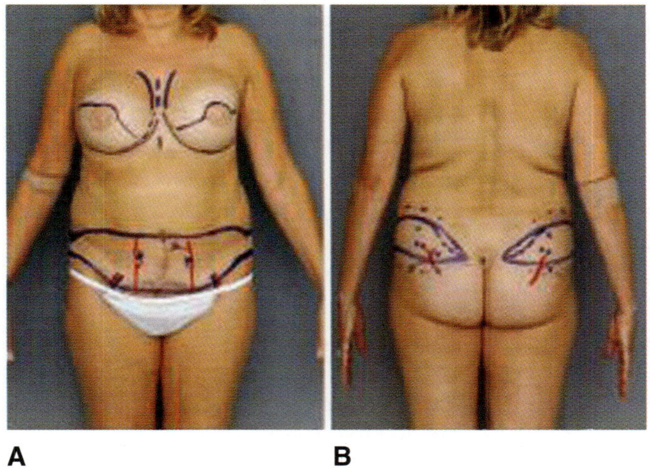

FIGURE 48-13 (A) and (B) Body lift design for a bilateral stacked flap reconstruction. The superior gluteal artery perforator flaps are marked to achieve elevation of the gluteal crease and extend from the lateral limits of the deep inferior epigastric artery perforator flap markings.

Clinical evaluation by an experienced microsurgeon is the gold standard but is heavily dependent on the experience of the evaluator to accurately evaluate flap color, capillary refill, and tissue turgor among other variables. Handheld Doppler probe monitoring is a simple adjunct. However, clinical evaluation of the buried base flap is not possible through these routine means. Therefore, other instruments and devices, including the Cook-Swartz implantable Doppler flow probe (Cook Medical, Bloomington, IN) and Gem Flow Coupler (Synovis Micro Companies Alliance, Inc., Birmingham, AL) devices have been developed and may be used to monitor flap circulation and serve as an adjunct to clinical examination.

STACKED FREE FLAP BREAST ARCHITECTURE AND SHAPE

Developing the blueprint for an aesthetically appealing stacked flap breast reconstruction is a combination of careful measurement and meticulous planning and requires understanding the important features of the native breast, including the footprint, the conus, and the skin envelope (28,29). The reconstruction of an appealing breast is a combination of artistic license and accurate execution of each step, including creating the breast footprint on the chest wall, placing and shaping the proper conus on the footprint, reestablishing arterial and venous perfusion to the flaps, and redraping the appropriate skin envelope over the conus.

The footprint is the interface of the posterior surface of the breast with the chest wall. It is outlined by the lateral mammary fold, the inframammary fold, the medial border of the sternum, and the curvilinear superior border (about two finger breadths below the clavicle). Unfortunately, the footprint is often altered or entirely obliterated during mastectomy. In breast reconstruction, the footprint defines the area of the chest on which the flaps will be stacked. Therefore, the footprint should be reestablished by suturing the affected borders back to the chest wall with particular reference to the preoperative markings or adjustments to match the contralateral breast footprint accordingly.

The conus is the volume, projection, and shape of the mammary gland. The naturally appearing breast is noticeably fuller in the lower pole than the upper pole. In profile view, the upper pole slopes gradually from its superior border down to the nipple, and the lower pole is full and rounded. In stacked flap breast reconstruction, the flaps should be oriented and inset such that the base flap provides some upper pole fill and the layered flap positioned on top to provide anteroposterior projection in the lower pole. The bulk of flap tissue should be situated in the lower pole—as illustrated in an anatomically shaped breast implant—with maximal projection at the anticipated site of the nipple–areola complex. The flaps are then sculpted to excise excess tissue, smooth the sharp edges, and camouflage any step-offs or transitions to produce a three-dimensional asymmetric conus.

The skin envelope is both the quantity and quality of breast skin that remains after mastectomy. After the flaps are positioned, perfused, and sculpted to the desired conus volume, projection, and shape, the breast skin is draped over the construct similar to a well-fitted brassiere. Attractive breast projection and shape result from the combination of the sculpted conus and the well-tailored skin envelope (29). Excess skin in the vertical and horizontal dimensions should be excised using standard mastopexy patterns to leave the exact amount of skin necessary to highlight the sculpted conus. The skin should not be overtightened to avoid flattening the breast mound or wound healing problems.

STACKED FREE FLAP PERFUSION AND CIRCUIT DESIGN

The reconstructive challenge to create an aesthetically appealing stacked flap breast reconstruction is made even more difficult when one also considers the vascular circuit required to perfuse two flaps.

In stacked flap breast reconstruction, the vascular circuit can be designed such that blood flows through each flap from two distinct and separate vascular systems, or the vascular circuit can be designed in series from one recipient vessel. As with electrical circuits, components connected in series are connected along a single path. Likewise, flaps connected in series are connected to each other so that blood circulates from one flap to the next.

Two different circuits can be created in which the flaps are perfused in series. First, the layered (exposed) flap can be anastomosed directly to the recipient vessels and the base (buried) flap connected to a large side branch of the layered flap's pedicle (as described in the technique section above). In this configuration, if there is a problem at the recipient vessel anastomoses, both the stacked flap and buried flap would be compromised and detected by the clinical appearance of the stacked flap. However, if there is a problem at the branch chain anastomoses, the base (buried) flap would be compromised, but this would not be visible on clinical examination. Therefore, an implantable Doppler device may be used to monitor perfusion to the buried flap in this design. The potential advantage of this circuit design is that the layered flap may be viable even if the buried flap is unsalvageable, in which case the reconstruction can be deemed successful by replacing the unsalvageable buried flap with an implant.

In contrast, the base (buried) flap can be anastomosed directly to the recipient vessels and the layered flap connected to a large side branch of the base flap's pedicle. In this configuration, if there is a problem at the recipient vessel anastomoses, both the buried flap and the layered flap would be compromised and detected by the stacked flap's clinical appearance (e.g., absent capillary refill, signs of venous congestion, or loss of Doppler signal). If there is a problem at the branch chain anastomoses, the layered flap would be compromised and would be similarly detected by its clinical appearance. The disadvantage of this design is that loss of the layered flap and its skin paddle may result in deficient skin for closure and a failed reconstruction.

If, alternatively, the flaps are connected to separate recipient vessels such as anterograde and retrograde internal mammary vessels or a combination of internal mammary and thoracodorsal vessels, then the survival of each flap is independent of the other. This technique of restoring vascularity to the flaps may be chosen in the event that there are no appropriate branching sites on one of the flaps to allow for an "in series" supply. Although using anterograde and retrograde flow of the internal mammary vessels would require dissection of only one set of recipient vessels, dissection of the thoracodorsal vessels would add to the operative time and may not allow for appropriate positioning of the GAP flap with its shorter pedicle. However, this is the preferred combination of recipient vessels as described for the double (stacked) TMG flap for unilateral reconstruction (25). When using two independent recipient vessels, the buried flap can only be monitored by an implantable device, but the layered flap can be monitored by clinical means.

POTENTIAL PITFALLS

Stacked flap breast reconstructions present technical challenges as result of their complexity in design. Despite Dellacroce et al.'s experience with 100% survival using stacked DIEP flaps, this is not always the case (7). As part of a series of 18 cases in which various strategies were used to maximize perfusion to the entire lower abdomen for unilateral breast reconstruction, six stacked flaps were used (30). Two flap failures occurred attributed to kinking of the layered flap pedicle as it descended over the edge of the filler flap. Conversely, when flaps were turbocharged and coned in six cases, there were no failures and no need for revisions. Therefore, in each case when one plans to increase the volume a breast reconstruction, one must assess and carefully select the technique that is anticipated to give a successful outcome.

Furthermore, in this series, there was one other case of a residual step deformity at the site of overlap of the two flaps despite intraoperative contouring and postoperative revision.

Although an "in series" vascular connection of the stacked flaps may be planned and desirable, this may not always be possible. In particular, the SGAP vein is often of a large caliber and may be an inappropriate size match to a branch of the DIEA pedicle. Therefore, the microsurgeon needs to be prepared for intraoperative changes in terms of recipient vessel choice.

As already alluded to, monitoring of the buried flap usually requires an implantable device.

DISCUSSION

Women seek autologous tissue reconstruction for a variety of reasons. One advantage is that autologous tissue reconstruction uses the most natural and durable material with which to recreate a breast. Certainly, the psychological power of immediate breast reconstruction combined with the bonus of an abdominoplasty or circumferential body lift appeals to many patients. As reconstruction becomes more common, greater attention is placed on optimizing breast aesthetics and improving symmetry between the native and reconstructed breast with regard to overall volume, shape, and projection.

At some point in their careers, every plastic surgeon will encounter the patient who desires autologous tissue breast reconstruction but has an inadequate amount of tissue at the donor site. When a single donor site cannot provide sufficient volume for unilateral or bilateral breast reconstruction using conventional methods, the stacked flap technique can achieve the desired soft tissue volume and projection with high success rates. The fundamental concept of stacked free flap breast reconstruction is to transfer any combination of flaps and configure them in a way that will realize more volume and projection than what might otherwise be attained using traditional breast reconstruction flaps.

REFERENCES

1. Ishii CH, Bostwick J, Raine TJ, et al. Double-pedicle transverse rectus abdominis musculocutaneous flap for unilateral breast and chest wall reconstruction. *Plast Reconstr Surg* 1985;76:901–907.
2. Wagner DS, Michelow BJ, Hartrampf CR. Double pedicle TRAM Flap for unilateral breast reconstruction. *Plast Reconstr Surg* 1991;88:987–997.
3. Spear SL, Travaglino-Parda RL, Stefan M. The stacked transverse rectus abdominis musculocutaneous flap revisited in breast reconstruction. *Ann Plast Surg* 1994;32:565–571.
4. Beahm EK, Walton RL. The efficacy of bilateral lower abdominal free flaps for unilateral reconstruction. *Plast Reconstr Surg* 2007;120:41–54.
5. Agarwal JP, Gottlieb LJ. Double pedicle deep inferior epigastric perforator/muscle-sparing TRAM flaps for unilateral breast reconstruction. *Ann Plast Surg* 2007;58:359–363.
6. Tseng CY, Lang PO, Cipriani NA. Pedicle preservation technique for arterial and venous turbocharging of free DIEP and muscle-sparing TRAM flaps. *Plast Reconstr Surg* 2007;120:851–854.
7. DellaCroce FJ, Sullivan SK, Trahan C. Stacked deep inferior epigastric perforator flap breast reconstruction: a review of 110 flaps in 55 cases over 3 years. *Plast Reconstr Surg* 2011;127:1093–1099.
8. Hayakawa T, Buchel E. *Maximizing Limited Abdominal Tissue in Free DIEP Breast Reconstruction.* Presented at the Annual Scientific Meeting of the American Society for Reconstructive Surgery, 2010.
9. Kronowitz SJ, Robb, GL, Youssef A, et al. Optimizing autologous breast reconstruction in thin patients. *Plast Reconstr Surg* 2003;112:1768–1778.
10. Taylor GI, Daniel RK. The anatomy of several free flap donor sites. *Plast Reconstr Surg* 1975;56:243–253.
11. Boyd JB, Taylor GI, Corlett R. The vascular territories of the superior epigastric and the deep inferior epigastric systems. *Plast Reconstr Surg* 1984;73:1–14.
12. Elliott LF, Raffel B, Wade J. Segmental latissimus dorsi free flap: clinical considerations. *Ann Plast Surg* 1989;23:231–238.
13. Feller AM. Free TRAM. Results and abdominal wall function. *Clin Plast Surg* 1994;21:232.
14. Koshima I, Moriguchi T, Soeda S, et al. Free thin paraumbilical perforator-based flaps. *Ann Plast Surg* 1994;32:12–17.
15. Allen RJ, Treece P. Deep inferior epigastric perforator flap for breast reconstruction. *Ann Plast Surg* 1994;32:32.
16. Nahabedian MY, Momen B, Galdino G, et al. Breast reconstruction with the free TRAM or DIEP flap: patient selection, choice of flap, and outcome. *Plast Reconstr Surg* 2002;110:466–475.
17. De Frene B, Van Landuyt K, Hamdi M, et al. Free DIEAP and SGAP flap breast reconstruction after abdominal/gluteal liposuction. *J Plast Reconstr Aesthet Surg* 2006;59:1031–1036.
18. Granzow JW, Levine JL, Chiu ES, et al. Breast reconstruction with the deep inferior epigastric perforator flap: history and an update on current technique. *J Plast Reconstr Aesthet Surg* 2006;59:571–579.
19. Nahabedian MY, Tsangaris T, Momen B. Breast reconstruction with the DIEP flap or the muscle-sparing (MS-2) free TRAM flap: is there a difference? *Plast Reconstr Surg* 2005;115:436–444.
20. Chevray PM. Breast reconstruction with superficial inferior epigastric artery flaps: a prospective comparison with TRAM and DIEP flaps. *Plast Reconstr Surg* 2004;114:1077–1083.
21. Spiegel AJ, Khan FN. An intraoperative algorithm for use of the SIEA flap for breast reconstruction. *Plast Reconstr Surg* 2007;120:1450–1459.
22. Guerra AB, Metzinger SE, Bidros RS, et al. Breast reconstruction with gluteal artery perforator (GAP) flaps. A critical analysis of 142 cases. *Ann Plast Surg* 2004;52:118–125.
23. Granzow JW, Levine JL, Chiu ES, et al. Breast reconstruction using perforator flaps. *J Surg Oncol* 2006;94:441–454.
24. Allen RJ, Tucker C. Superior gluteal artery perforator free flap for breast reconstruction. *Plast Reconstr Surg* 1995; 95:1207–1212.
25. Paletta CE, Bostwick J, Nahai F. The inferior gluteal free flap in breast reconstruction. *Plast Reconstr Surg* 1989;84:875.
26. Fattah A, Figus A, Mathur B, Ramakrishnan VV. The transverse myocutaneous gracilis flap: technical refinements. *J Plast Reconstr Aesthet Surg* 2010;63:305–313.
27. DellaCroce FJ, Sullivan SK, Trahan C, et al. Body lift perforator flap breast reconstruction: a review of 100 flaps in 25 cases. *Plast Reconstr Surg* 2012;129:551–561.
28. Blondeel PN, Hijawi J, Depypere H, et al. Shaping the breast in aesthetic and reconstructive breast surgery: an easy three-step principle. *Plast Reconstr Surg* 2012;123:445–462.
29. Blondeel PN, Hijawi J, Depypere H, et al. Shaping the breast in aesthetic and reconstructive breast surgery: an easy three-step principle. Part II—breast reconstruction after total mastectomy. *Plast Reconstr Surg* 2012;123:794–805.
30. Hayakawa T, Buchel E. *Maximizing Limited Abdominal Tissue in Free DIEP Breast Reconstruction.* Presented at the Annual Scientific Meeting of the American Society for Reconstructive Surgery, Boca Raton, Florida, 2010.

CHAPTER 49

Abdominal and Chest Wall Reconstruction

Lawrence J. Gottlieb and Aaron T. Pelletier

CLASSIFICATION OF DEFECTS REQUIRING ABDOMINAL AND CHEST WALL RECONSTRUCTION

There are many ways to classify abdominal and chest wall defects and deformities that may require reconstruction. These include classification by etiology, location, tissue layers involved, and whether or not there are physiologic consequences. Classification by etiology may be categorized as congenital or acquired. Acquired defects and deformities may have been caused by excision of tumor, severe soft tissue infection, trauma, radiation, or hernia. Classifications by topographic location have been proposed to help guide what flap may be available to use to close a particular defect in particular location or zone (1–4). Whatever the etiology or location, one must consider the size of the defect and the tissue layer(s) involved in a particular location. In full-thickness defects, one must determine if there is a true tissue deficit or just a loss of abdominal or chest wall integrity (i.e., hernia, sternal separation). The astute clinician will consider each of these categories and then individualize his or her treatment plan depending on comorbidities, age, lifestyle, status of disease, donor site scars, risk of morbidity, and resources available. Determination of whether any particular defect or deformity has or will cause a loss of functional and physiologic integrity will further guide reconstructive efforts.

INDICATIONS

Indications for abdominal and chest wall reconstruction include loss of structural integrity that may lead to functional and physiologic derangements, exposure of vital structures, loss of skin integrity, and contour abnormalities.

Structural Integrity

Loss of structural integrity of the abdomen generally refers to disruption or loss of fascial or myofascial units or their attachment to the ribs superiorly, pelvis inferiorly, or linea alba in the ventral midline. Loss of structural integrity of the chest wall generally refers to disruption or loss of ribs, sternum, or clavicle. Each of these losses can be replaced with prosthetic material, autologous tissue, allogeneic tissue, or a combination thereof. The prosthetic material can be subclassified as permanent, absorbable, or biologic. Autologous and allogeneic tissue may be subclassified as vascularized or nonvascularized tissue.

Physiologic Derangements

Whereas acute full-thickness disruption or loss of the abdominal wall may lead to evisceration, loss of structural integrity with an intact skin envelope will lead to hernia. Denervation of a portion of the abdominal wall will lead to laxity or bulging. Large hernia defects are generally at little risk for strangulation of bowel but may cause difficulty with bowel evacuation. Musculoskeletal imbalance of the trunk frequently manifests as back pain. If left unattended, a large hernia can lead to loss of domain and at times be so large that it affects basic activities of daily living. Denervation of the abdominal wall, although structurally intact, can be a vexing problem leading to unrelenting laxity and bulging (Figure 49-1). This is typically seen after tumor excision or extensive trauma in the lower anterolateral chest wall or upper lateral aspect of the abdomen as well as after long subcostal and flank incisions in which thoracoabdominal intercostal or subcostal nerves are divided. Functional loss or severe scarring and fibrosis of lateral abdominal wall musculature may also lead to progressive scoliosis.

Loss of structural integrity of the chest wall may lead to impaired respiratory function attributed to skeletal instability and paradoxical motion from a flail segment phenomenon. This seems particularly relevant to large anterior and lateral defects. It is generally accepted that structural restoration of the anterolateral thorax is necessary for a deficit of four or

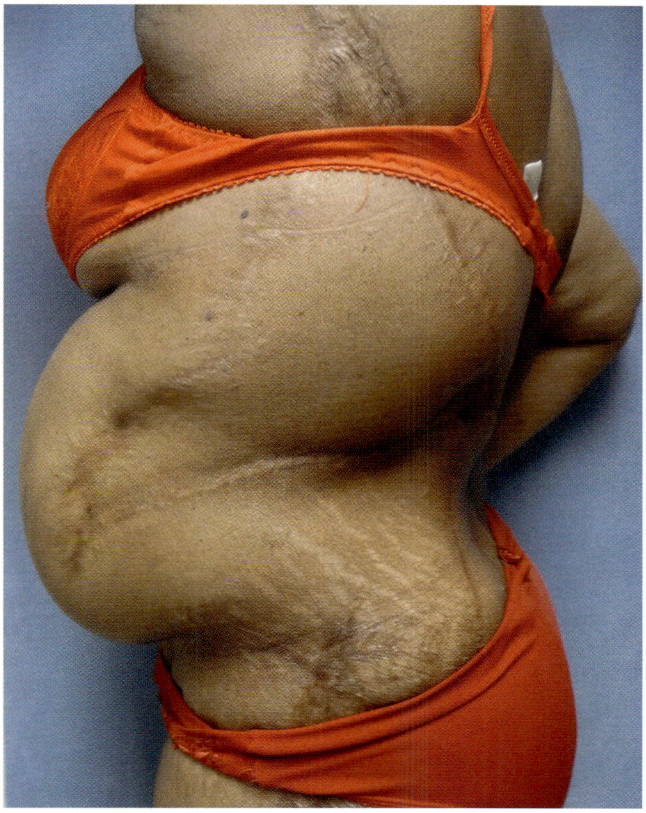

A

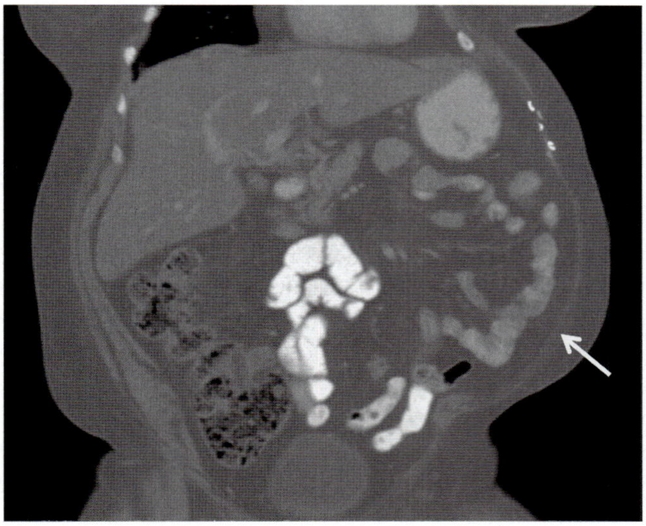

B

FIGURE 49-1 A 60-year-old woman who presented more than 20 years after full-thickness lower lateral chest wall and upper lateral abdominal wall resection with mesh closure and successful soft tissue closure. This resection lead to denervation and subsequent atrophy of the muscles on the left side of her abdomen (**A**). Coronal view of abdomen on computed tomography scan shows laxity with severe atrophy of left-sided abdominal wall musculature (arrow) (**B**).

more adjacent ribs or a defect greater than 5 cm (5,6). In addition to its role in respiratory mechanics, the bony anterior chest wall provides a rigid base for upper limb movement, and loss of chest wall skeletal stability may reduce shoulder girdle function.

Whether or not the loss of structural integrity of the abdominal or chest wall causes physiologic derangements is frequently related to the circumstances of the loss and whether or not there is underlying scar and fibrosis from infection, inflammation, or radiation. Acute loss of structural integrity such as from tumor extirpation, severe trauma, or acute disruption of a postsurgical closure in otherwise normal tissue may have far more severe physiologic effects than when the defect is more chronic, when inflammation, scarring, and effects of radiation provide some rigidity and stability. Interestingly, as scar matures, edema recedes, and the tissue softens, many patients who did not initially require structural support may show signs of physiologic impairment 6 to 18 months after surgery and may require secondary surgery to provide structural support.

CONVENTIONAL METHODS OF ABDOMINAL AND CHEST WALL RECONSTRUCTION

Most defects of the abdomen and chest can be closed or reconstructed with conventional methods. Full-thickness abdominal wall wounds can be closed with a skin graft (with or without an underlying absorbable mesh) with a planned hernia defect that could be repaired in a staged fashion. Although the epidermis of the skin graft can be removed by dermabrasion, if one waits 6 months, a loose areolar layer develops under the skin graft that makes excision relatively safe and straightforward (Figure 49-2). Partial-thickness defects of the abdominal or chest wall with a well-vascularized bed can generally be closed with a skin graft, but contour irregularities may be better treated with a local or regional flap either acutely or in a delayed fashion.

Soft Tissue Flaps

Although the use of skin flaps dates back to the earliest reported history of reconstructive surgery, one of the earliest recorded use of an axial pattern flap for abdominal wall reconstruction dates back to 1864 when Woods described closing an abdominal wall defect from extrophy of the bladder with bilateral groin flaps (7). The first description of the latissimus dorsi muscle flap used for chest wall reconstruction was reported by Tansini in 1906 (8), and Kanavel used the latissimus muscle to fill an empyema chest cavity in 1921 (9). Although Wangensteen described repairing complex hernias and other large defects of the abdominal wall with tensor fascia lata (TFL) flaps and pedicle muscle flaps to close persistent bronchopleural fistulas in the mid 1930s (10,11) and Webster described a long bipedicled thoracoepigastric flap based on named arteries in 1937 (12), the dominant method of reconstruction for defects throughout the body for the first half of the 20th century was the random pattern pedicle flap. The beginning of the modern era of the understanding and clinical transfer of vascularized tissue began with Bakamjian's description of the long paramedian perforators of the internal thoracic system in 1965 (13). It was not until 8 years later that we truly understood the clinical distinction of flaps based on a known axial blood supply and those based on random vessels with the important article by McGregor and Morgan (14). In the same year, Daniel and

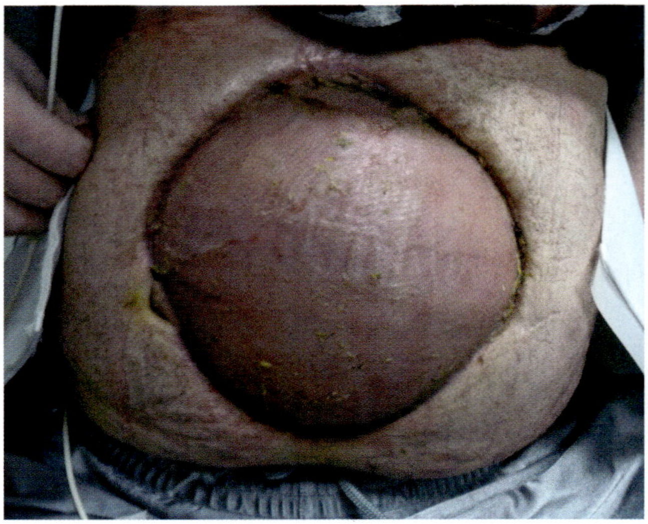

A

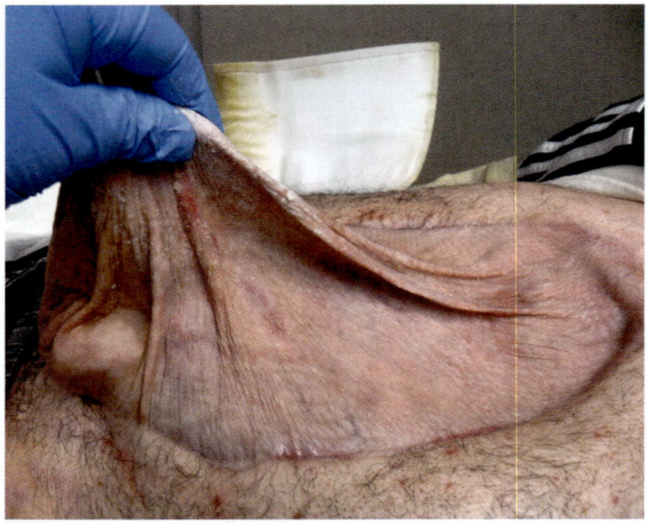

B

FIGURE 49-2 One month after abdominal wall closure with a skin graft placed on a granulating bowel (**A**). Six moths later, a loose areola layer develops, which allows elevation and safe excision of skin graft off the bowel (**B**).

Taylor elucidated the differences between direct cutaneous and musculocutaneous vessels (15) and reported the first clinical free flap (16), and McCraw and colleagues set the stage for widespread use of the musculocutaneous flap (17). Mathes and Nahai went on to popularize muscle and musculocutaneous flaps for reconstruction throughout the body (18). The extensive clinical experience of Arnold and Pairolero substantiated the advantages of muscle and omental flaps for chest wall reconstruction (19). In 1987, Taylor and Palmer brought all the anatomical knowledge of tissue circulation together in their three dimensional concept of tissue circulation that they called angiosomes (20). Although Manchot first described a detailed anatomic description of the blood supply to the skin throughout the body, including perforating vessels, in 1889 (20) and Fujino described the importance of perforator vessels for flap viability in 1967 (21), the first clinical use of a true perforator flap was not described until 1989 by Koshima and Soeda (22). Since that time, the perforator-based flap has become the standard of care to precisely reconstruct parts while limiting donor site morbidity (4).

Structural Integrity

Most incisional hernia defects in which no fascia was lost can be closed primarily (with or without prosthetic reinforcement) by meticulously dissecting each layer of the abdominal wall back to unscarred tissue. In vertical midline incisions, this closure may be facilitated with one of the many fascial releasing techniques described, the most popular being the components separation technique described by Ramirez and colleagues (23). However, components separation is frequently not an option in patients with transverse or subcostal incisions and is more difficult when there is extensive scarring from multiple previous operations. In addition, the components separation technique may lead to some unexpected consequences, including atrophy of the external oblique muscles (24).

Full-thickness abdominal wall defects in which there is a significant loss of fascia and muscle invariably require a "patch" to bridge the fascial defect. Fascia lata is the only available autologous tissue of adequate surface area and strength to accomplish this goal and has been the gold standard of structural support since the early 1900s (10). The limitations of using fascia lata are the requirement for a donor site incision with a closure that may require a skin graft if the skin paddle is greater than 8 cm wide as well as the fact that there is only a finite amount of material available. When harvested as a myofasciocutaneous flap based on the transverse or ascending branch of the lateral femoral circumflex (LFC) artery and vein, the distal end of the TFL flap frequently has a marginal or poor blood supply. Performing a delay procedure or including the descending branch of the LFC system in the flap design may obviate this and ensure a robust blood supply throughout the flap (Figure 49-3). In addition, to use its strength in an optimal way, the orientation of the fascia lata should be horizontal, which is difficult to accomplish, except in very low abdominal wall defects, unless it is detached and transferred as a graft or free flap.

In 1940, wire metallic mesh was used routinely, and by the late 1950s, synthetic meshes made of various plastic materials were introduced. In the 1990s, biologic materials came onto the market in an attempt to avoid or at least minimize many of the complications associated with synthetic materials, including fistula, infection, extrusion, and foreign body reaction. One of the earliest products used extensively for abdominal and chest wall reconstruction was human acellular dermal matrix. The concept behind this processed allogeneic material was that tissue ingrowth would gradually replace the bioprosthetic collagen with autologous collagen guided by the bioprosthetic matrices. Unfortunately, there are no data in humans showing that this remodeling is ever complete; moreover, the overwhelming evidence indicates that with ongoing remodeling, there seems to be a loss of integrity with resultant laxity and

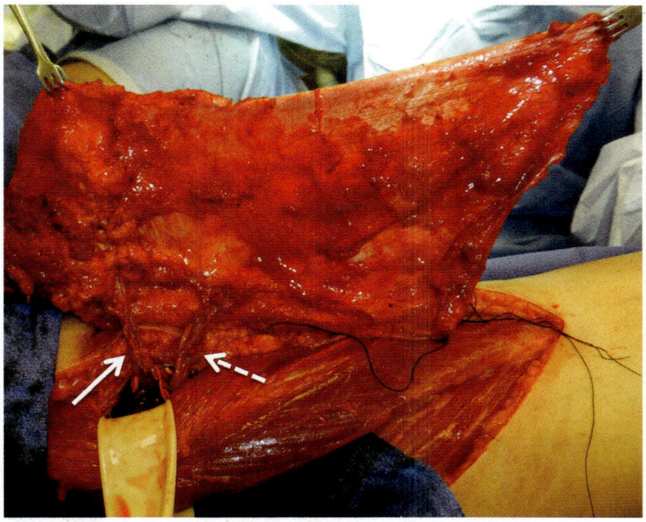

FIGURE 49-3 Tensor fascia lata flap based on transverse branch of lateral femoral circumflex vessels (solid arrow) and the descending branch (dashed arrow) provides a more robust blood supply to the distal portion of the flap than just using the transverse or ascending branch.

bulging of the abdominal wall (25,26). Newer porcine-based biologic prosthetic materials have been introduced in the past few years. However, here, too, there are no long-term data to definitively support a lower risk of laxity and bulging.

Providing structural integrity of the chest wall was described in the late 1940s with fascia lata grafts and split-rib grafts (27,28). Soon thereafter, similar prosthetics described above for abdominal reconstruction were introduced for chest wall reconstruction. In 1977, Eschapasse reported the use of a Marlex mesh–methylmethacrylate sandwich for chest wall stabilization (29). Although this was used successfully by many reconstructive surgeons, reports of patient discomfort, dislodgement, and extrusion led others to develop alternative techniques (29–31). Exposure and extrusion of prosthetic material in hostile wound environments from infection and severe radiation fibrosis stimulated others to pursue the transfer of vascularized bone for thoracic reconstruction. In the 1970s, 1980s, and 1990s, a number of techniques of transferring ribs were described using the vascular connections between them and overlying muscle flaps such as the pectoralis major, latissimus dorsi, and serratus anterior (32–37). All these procedures rely on the rib vascularity being derived from its muscle attachments. However, Schlenker and colleagues identified connecting vessels from the posterior intercostal vessels that extended directly into the undersurface of the latissimus muscle in dogs (38). Schmidt and Robson subsequently confirmed this finding intraoperatively in humans, showing interconnecting vessels between the latissimus branch of the thoracodorsal artery and vein and the lateral branch of the dorsal rami of the intercostals vessels (39). These discrete interconnecting vessels between the latissimus dorsi muscle and the intercostal vessels allow for independent movement of the rib and the muscle, enabling greater degree of freedom for insetting to complex defects (40). Initially, the use of this flap was primarily for microsurgical head and neck reconstruction but subsequently has been used in extremity and cranial reconstruction (41–43).

Our improved knowledge of tissue vascularity has led to the development of a plethora of local, regional, distant, and free flaps from the torso and extremities. Whether a skin, muscle, compound, chimera, or perforator-based flap is chosen, virtually all defects or deformities of the abdomen and chest wall can be reconstructed with autologous tissue. Because most defects of the abdomen and chest wall are amenable to pedicle flap reconstruction, the indication for a free flap is generally relegated to the rare situation in which a pedicle flap is unavailable, out of range, or insufficiently large or when the donor site morbidity of the pedicle flap outweighs its benefits. There are, however, several advantages of using a free flap, including freedom to harvest the exact tissue requirements from any place on the body; utilization of the healthiest blood supply of the flap; avoidance of limitations created by the pivot point of the pedicle; precision and ease of insetting; and the ability to align transferred tissue appropriately, whether it is vascularized bone for thoracic reconstruction or fascia or functional muscle in abdominal wall reconstruction. In making the decision to perform a free flap when a pedicled flap could "do the job," one needs to balance these potential advantages with a likely increase in operative time, the experience and technical expertise of the surgeon, and the relative risks of partial versus complete flap loss.

Finally, a select group of solid organ transplant patients may be candidates for abdominal wall vascularized composite allotransplantation (VCA) (44–46). This concept allows for transferring of vascularized tissue for structural support or cutaneous coverage without the need to alter immunosuppressive therapy. The VCAs have all the advantages of autologous flap transfer without any donor site morbidity or scars to the recipient. Although it is controversial whether or not it is reasonable to place a non–solid organ recipient on lifelong immunosuppression for abdominal or chest wall reconstruction, transplant patients already on immunosuppression may be candidates for abdominal or chest wall transplants, thereby avoiding an autologous donor site.

CHOICE OF FREE FLAP FOR ABDOMINAL AND CHEST WALL RECONSTRUCTION

The choice of free flap for abdominal and chest wall reconstruction depends on the size, depth, quality, and location of the defect; the health and lifestyle of the patient; the type of tissue component(s) needed; and perhaps most important, the goal(s) of the operation. Is the priority to close a wound, fill a space, protect a vital organ, restore functionality of a part, or some combination of these?

Although any free flap of the appropriate size and tissue components can be used for either abdominal or chest wall reconstruction, the most common free flaps used are harvested from the LFC system of the thigh, the subscapular system of the back, or the deep inferior epigastric (DIE) system of the abdomen. The choice may be predicated on tissue availability, intraoperative positioning, tissue component needed, and donor site morbidity. When a large amount of muscle is needed, flaps from the subscapular system can use the latissimus and serratus anterior muscles. The subscapular system can also provide vascularized bone (rib or scapula) if skeletal support is desired for thoracic reconstruction (Figure 49-4). Alternatively, flaps based on the DIE (Figure 49-5) or LFC system (Figures 49-6 and 49-7) can provide a large amount of skin for resurfacing. The thigh also offers the largest piece of strong autologous fascia in the body in the form of the fascia lata. Functional muscle is usually harvested from the back or thigh (47–49). The potential advantage of using innervated extraabdominal muscles for abdominal wall reconstruction is the reestablishment of tone and dynamic function. Functional reconstruction can balance abdominal wall musculature, avoiding strain on the back muscles and improving bowel evacuation. Although innervated muscle flaps may indeed provide a dynamic repair, they must be supplemented with fascia or prosthetic mesh to avoid laxity and bulging. Intrathoracic flaps may be required to fill space and provide vascularized coverage over vascular and bronchial stumps. When regional flaps are no longer available or not large enough to accomplish the goal, then intrathoracic free flaps are required. Typical flaps include contralateral latissimus or serratus muscles, rectus abdominus muscle, or omentum.

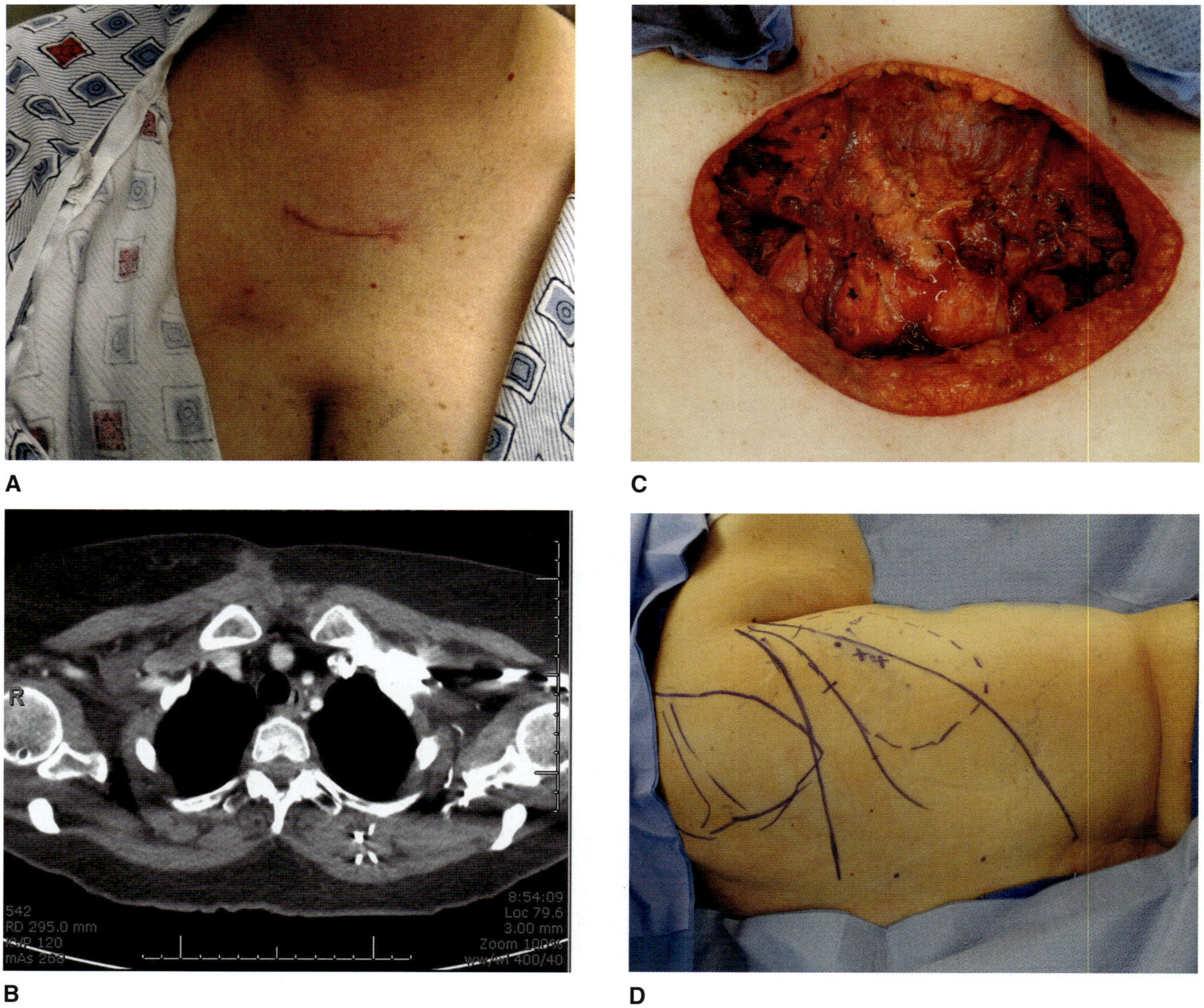

FIGURE 49-4 A 63-year-old woman with a high-grade myxofibrosarcoma of sterno-clavicular joint (A). Computed tomography scan showing tumor (B). After wide resection of tumor, manubrium, bilateral medial clavicles, and first ribs (C), the patient is repositioned to the lateral decubitus position (D) for harvesting a chimera flap including a latissimus myo-osseocutaneous component based on the thoracodorsal vessels with the seventh and ninth ribs (asterisk) attached via interconnecting vessels (dashed line) and a 4 x 6 portion of the scapula tip (curved arrow) based on the thoracodorsal's angular branch (straight arrow) (E). During back closure, the flap is kept cool in an ice slurry machine (F), and the patient is then turned back into the supine position. The flap is then inset with rigid interosseous fixation and microvascular anastomosis to the right internal mammary vessels (thick straight arrow) (G). The muscle and skin were then inset (H). Please note that osteosynthesis needs to be done with large plates to withstand the forces and torque placed on the clavicles. Initially, the left clavicular rib osteosynthesis was performed with a smaller plate that lead to fracture of the plate, necessitating exchange for a larger plate. Postoperative chest radiograph demonstrates the hardware required for a stable construct (I).

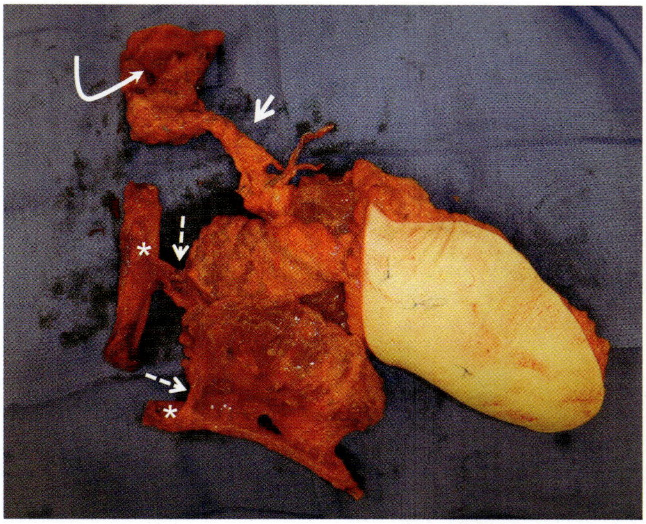

E

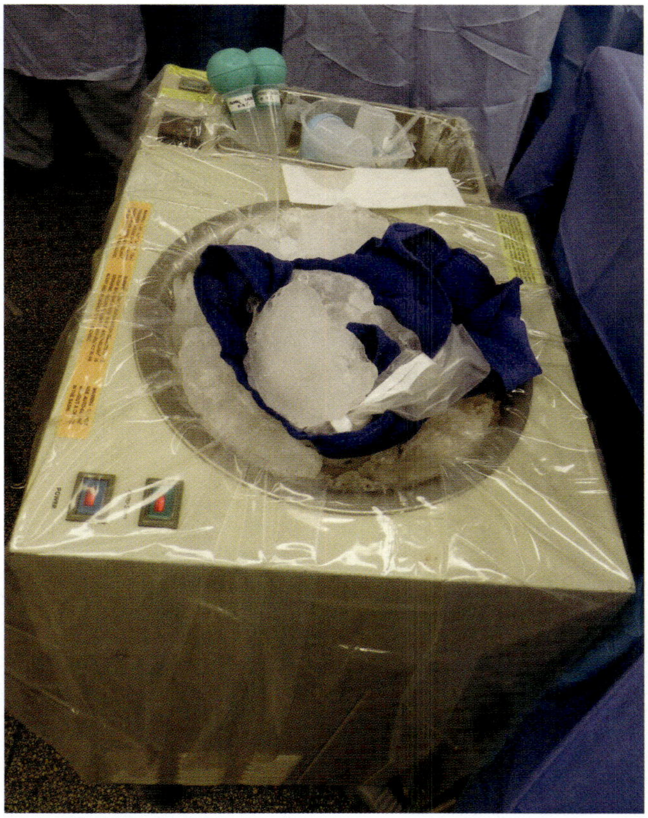

F

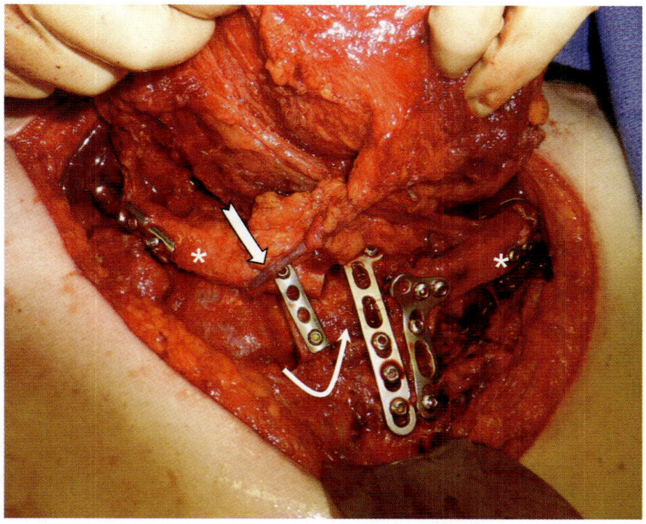

G

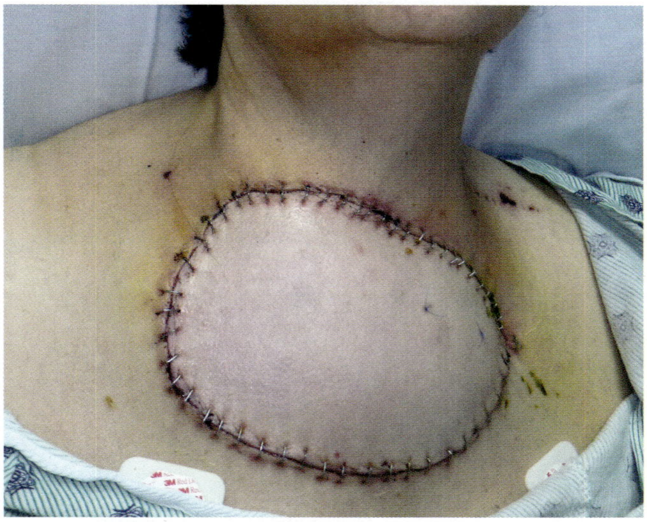

H

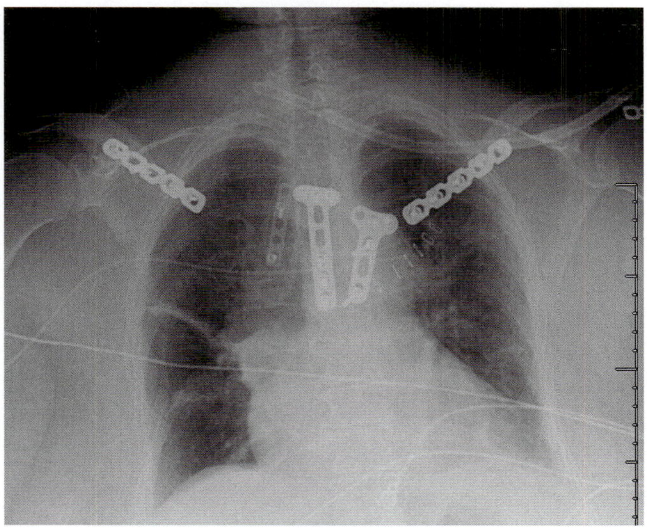

I

FIGURE 49-4 *(Continued)*

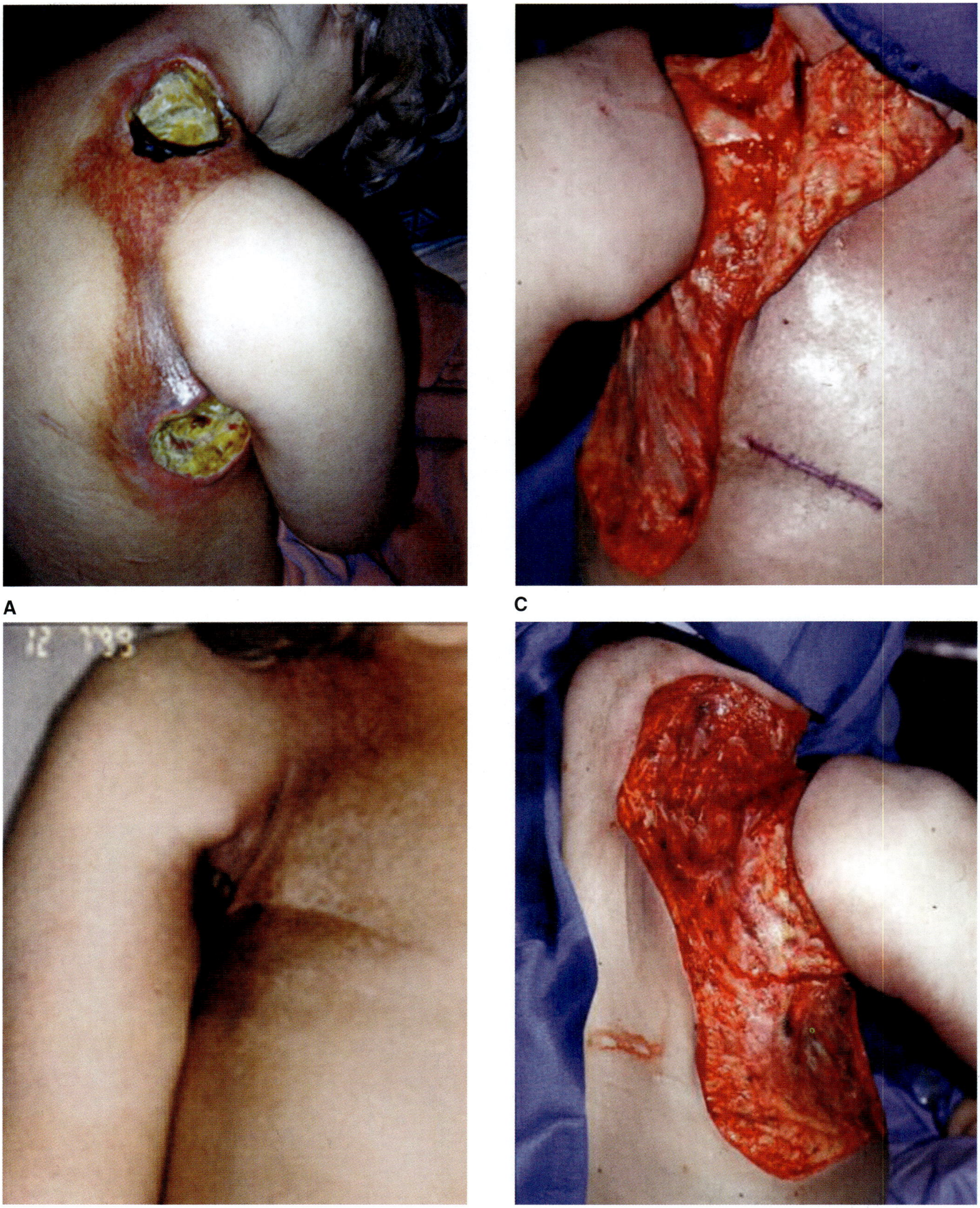

A B C D

FIGURE 49-5 A 57-year-old woman presented with an acute circumferential radiation injury and two extremely painful, infected, devitalized radiation ulcers (**A and B**). Treatment necessitated radical excision of infected ulcers and circumferential radiation damaged skin (**C**, anterior view; **D**, posterior view). An extended double-pedicle lower abdominal flap based on bilateral deep inferior epigastric perforator vessels was used to close the wound and minimize donor site morbidity (**E**). Microvascular anastomoses were performed to arm and neck vessels. Despite this long extended flap, circumferential closure could not be accomplished without using a latissimus myocutaneous flap posteriorly that was advanced in a V-Y fashion. Seen here 6 months after surgery (**F** and **G**).

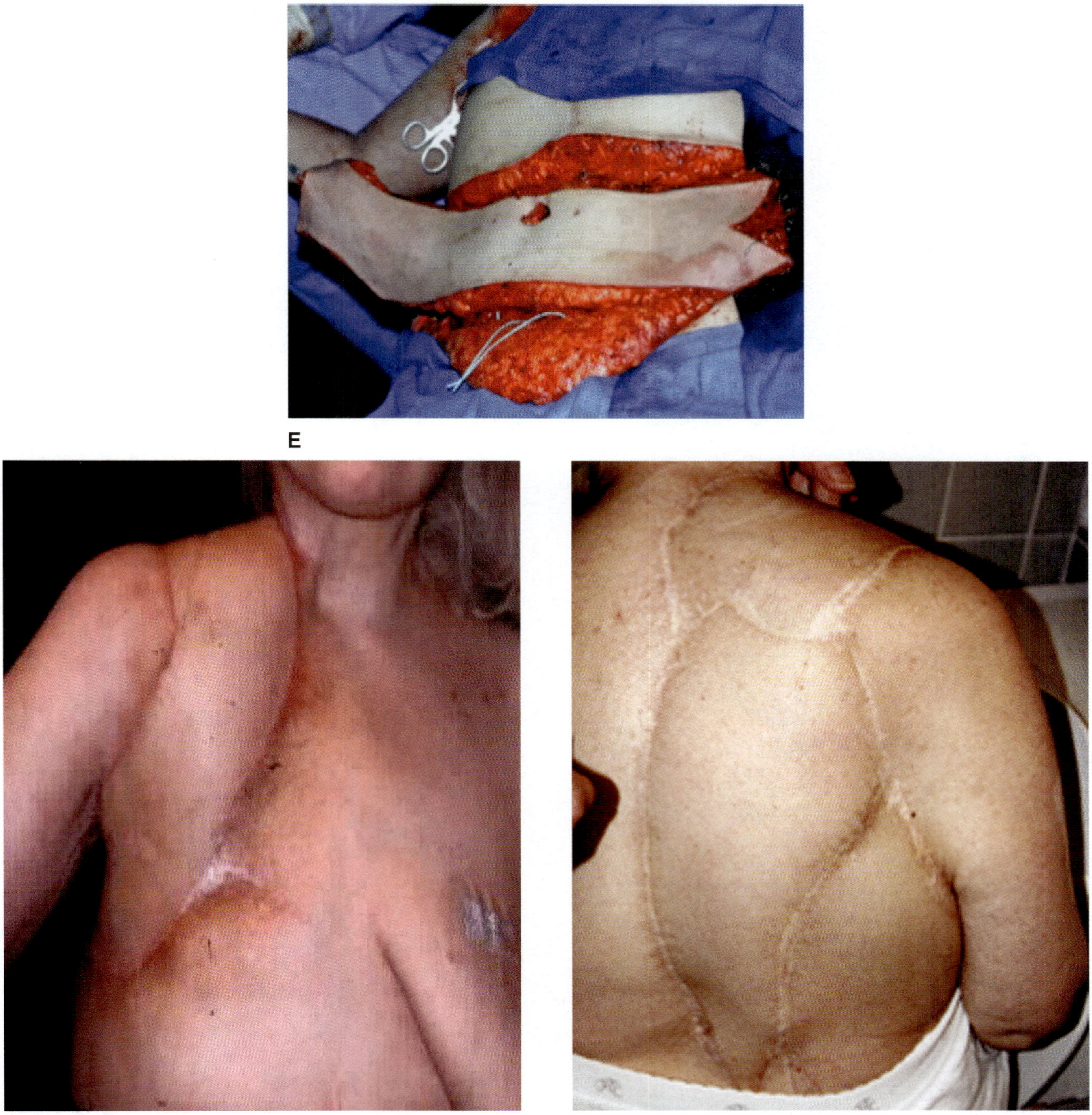

E

F

G

FIGURE 49-5 *(Continued)*

CONSIDERATIONS OF DESIGN AND CONSTRUCTION OF FLAPS FOR ABDOMINAL AND CHEST WALL RECONSTRUCTION

As with the choice of flaps, the design and construction of flaps for abdominal and chest wall reconstruction is predicated on reconstructive needs. If structural support is being provided by prosthetic material, most designs are quite straightforward, basically designing a well-vascularized soft tissue flap to protect the prosthesis and close the wound (Figure 49-8). However, in the setting of infection, radiation, or otherwise marginalized tissue, providing structural support with vascularized autologous tissue has a better chance for success, and this may require a more sophisticated design (Figure 49-9).

Before consideration of the design and construction of flaps, successful reconstruction requires adherence to the basic principles of reconstructive surgery. These include obtaining bacteriologic balance in infected wounds and debridement of as much necrotic scarred, radiated, and poorly vascularized tissue

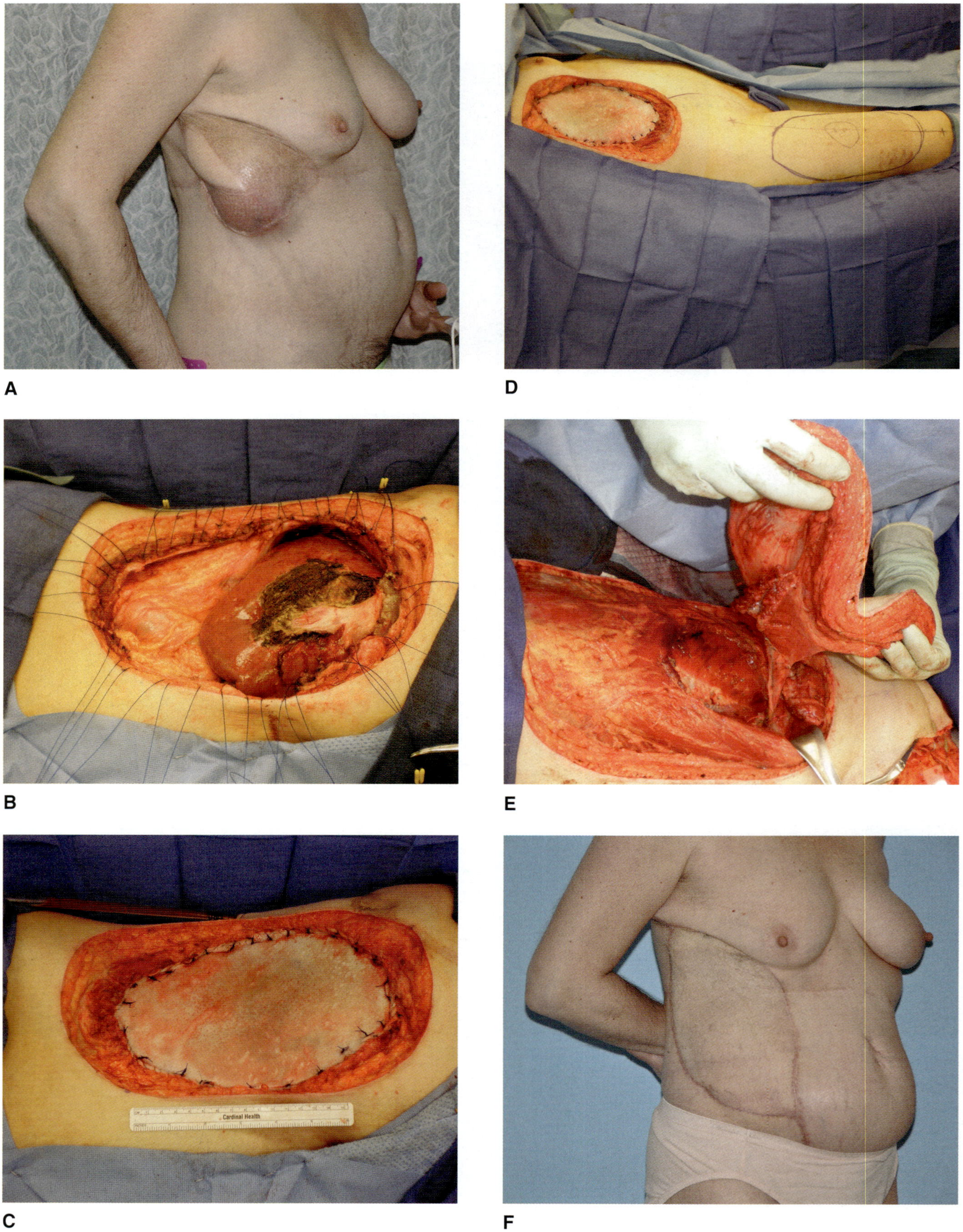

FIGURE 49-6 A 56-year-old woman with radiation resistant recurrent sarcoma of right lateral lower chest and upper abdomen. One year before, she had a resection and closure with a Gore-Tex patch and a contralateral fee latissimus dorsi musculocutaneous flap with microvascular anastomosis to the ipsilateral thoracodorsal vessels (**A**). Resection entailed the recurrent tumor and the previously transferred musculocutaneous flap (**B**). Structural support was provided by processed acellular porcine dermal matrix and supplemented by existing fibrosis from previous radiation and surgery (**C**). Soft tissue closure was provided by a free muscle sparing vastus lateralis musculocutaneous anterolateral thigh flap with microvascular anastomosis to the inferior epigastric vessels (**D** to **F**). Thigh donor site was closed with a contralateral split-thickness skin graft (**G**). (Case complements of Drs. David Song and Michelle Roughton.)

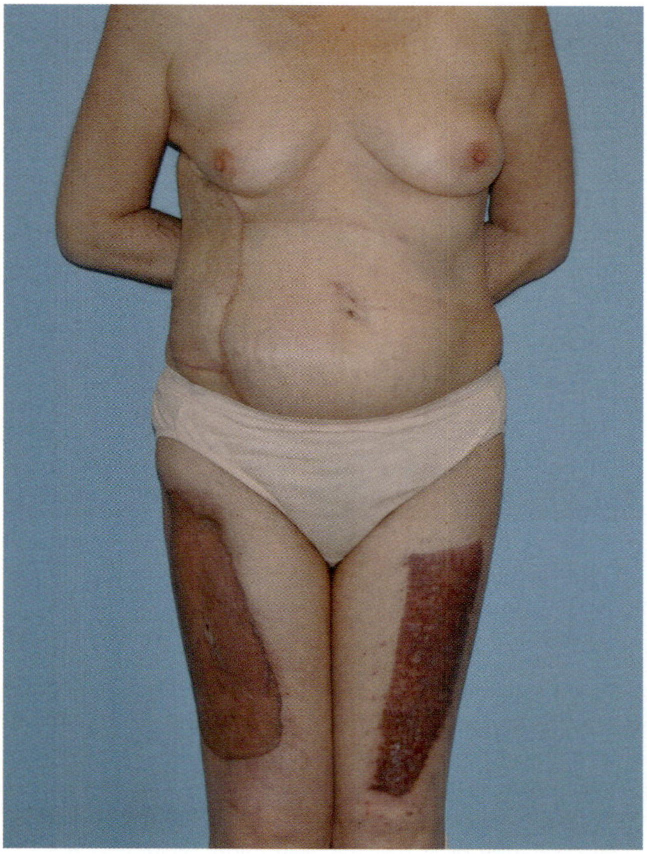

G

FIGURE 49-6 *(Continued)*

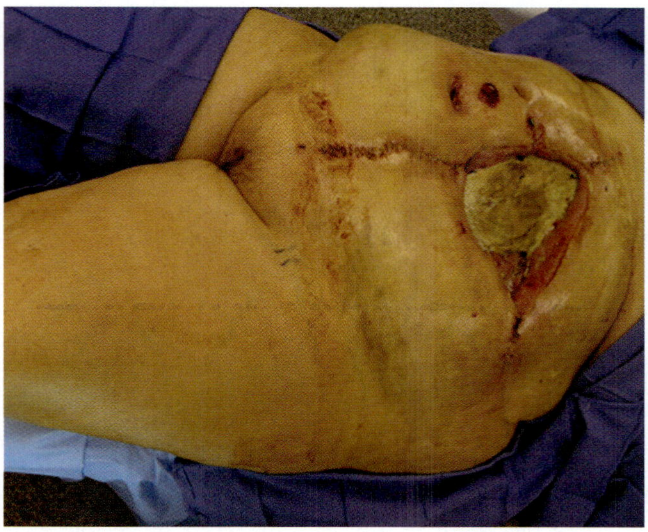

A

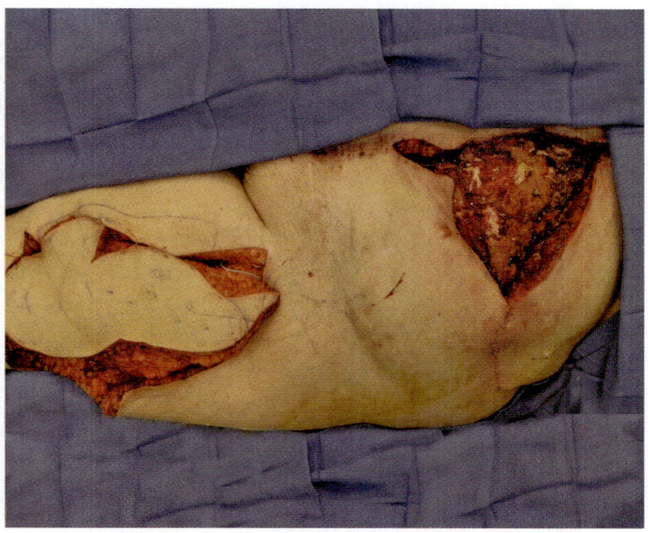

B

FIGURE 49-7 A 50-year-old woman with a chronic complex left upper quadrant (LUQ) abdominal defect with infected human acellular dermal matrix (**A**). After removal of the dermal matrix and debridement of wound, an extended anterior lateral thigh musculofasciocutaneous flap supplied by the descending and medial (innominate) branches of the LCF were harvested (**B**) and transposed to close the fascia and skin of the LUQ defect. The thigh donor site was closed with a perforator-based V-Y flap from the posterior lateral thigh circulation, avoiding the contour deficit of a skin graft (**C**).

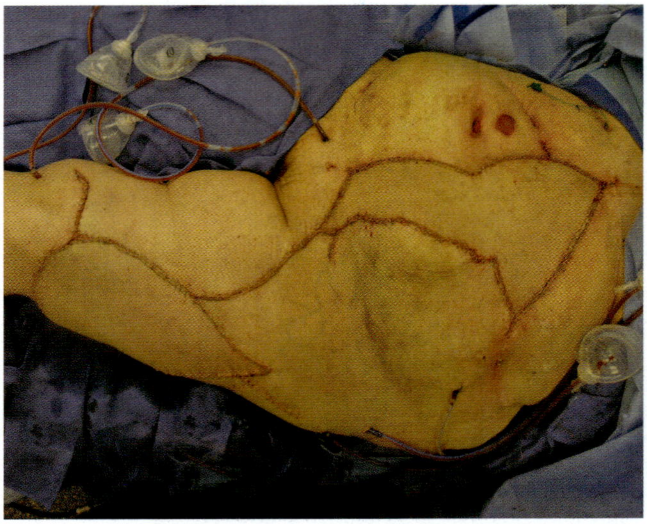

C

FIGURE 49-7 *(Continued)*

as possible. A comprehensive knowledge of anatomy and tissue vascularity is paramount in the design of successful flaps. The principles and concepts of angiosomes and perforasomes provide one with a general idea of how much tissue may be transferred from a single vascular source (50,51). In a compromised wound bed, such as with bacterial contamination or unresectable scar and fibrosis from radiation, a more robust blood supply is required to maximize success. These considerations may move the surgeon to convert a pedicled flap to a free flap so that the most robust blood supply (the primary angiosome) of a free flap is used rather than the distal and typically less vascularized portion of the pedicled flap. Another design change may be to dissect out a distal secondary pedicle to supercharge (or superdrain) the distal part of a flap, thereby improving its perfusion pressure or venous return.

Surface area requirements of a flap seem straightforward, and most surgeons use a template to be sure to end up with the most appropriate sized flap. In young athletic people with excellent skin elasticity, caution should be used when creating such templates. Elastic recoil of the skin can both enlarge the recipient site (after excision of surrounding scar) and decrease the surface area of a flap. More often than not, a flap cannot be stretched to its original dimensions without compromising circulation. In addition to surface area considerations, the thickness of the flap relative to the depth of the wound needs to be considered. Whereas a thin flap placed in a deep wound may produce a contour defect, a thick flap placed in a shallow wound bed may appear bulky and cause functional limitations. In either situation, the surface area required to adequately close the defect will be increased for tension-free inset. As such, use of a three-dimensional template is recommended to avoid this problem. Often it is necessary to choose or design a flap that can be thinned, at least around the periphery, to facilitate insetting.

The perforator flap concepts have taught us that most cutaneous flaps can be harvested without including muscle, thereby limiting donor site morbidity and allowing for more exacting dimensions and design. Muscle may be desirable to fill a dead space, resurface a wound, provide function if innervated, or simplify flap dissection. Noninnervated muscle will atrophy over time. This loss of volume needs to be considered in flap design. For functional muscle transfer, it is crucial to mark the resting tension before dividing the origin and insertion. In addition, the orientation of the muscle fibers should be aligned with the direction of the muscle being replaced.

Chimera flaps of the subscapular vascular system have the ability to provide vascularized bone, muscle, fascia, and skin that are especially useful in chest wall reconstruction when autologous tissue is desired. Chimera flaps, with each tissue component attached to a separate branch or perforating vessel of a main source vessel, allows for free independent placement of each component of the flap. Designing a chimera flap requires a sophisticated understanding of anatomy with the ability to deconstruct angiosomes into their component parts, all while appreciating how the tissue components may be rearranged into a three-dimensional construct.

In addition to determining the surface area, volume, and type of tissue to be included in the flap, the length of the vascular pedicle and length of each branch in a chimera or multipaddle flap need to be carefully assessed. Recipient vessels need to be prepared before the flap design is finalized. This allows for either a change in flap design to accommodate different recipient vessel location or harvest of vein grafts before the start of ischemia time. When dealing with long pedicles, multipaddle flaps, or long vein grafts, there is always a risk of twisting, which potentially compromises venous drainage. By marking one surface of the vessels in situ (after dissection but before division), subsequent twisting or kinking of the pedicle or vein graft can be recognized.

Contralateral free flaps for intrathoracic transfer can be a challenge and require careful planning to limit warm ischemia time during repositioning of the patient. After the thoracic surgeon has completed his or her part of the surgery, the recipient vessels should be assessed and prepared before changing positions. Wounds are usually covered with a sterile

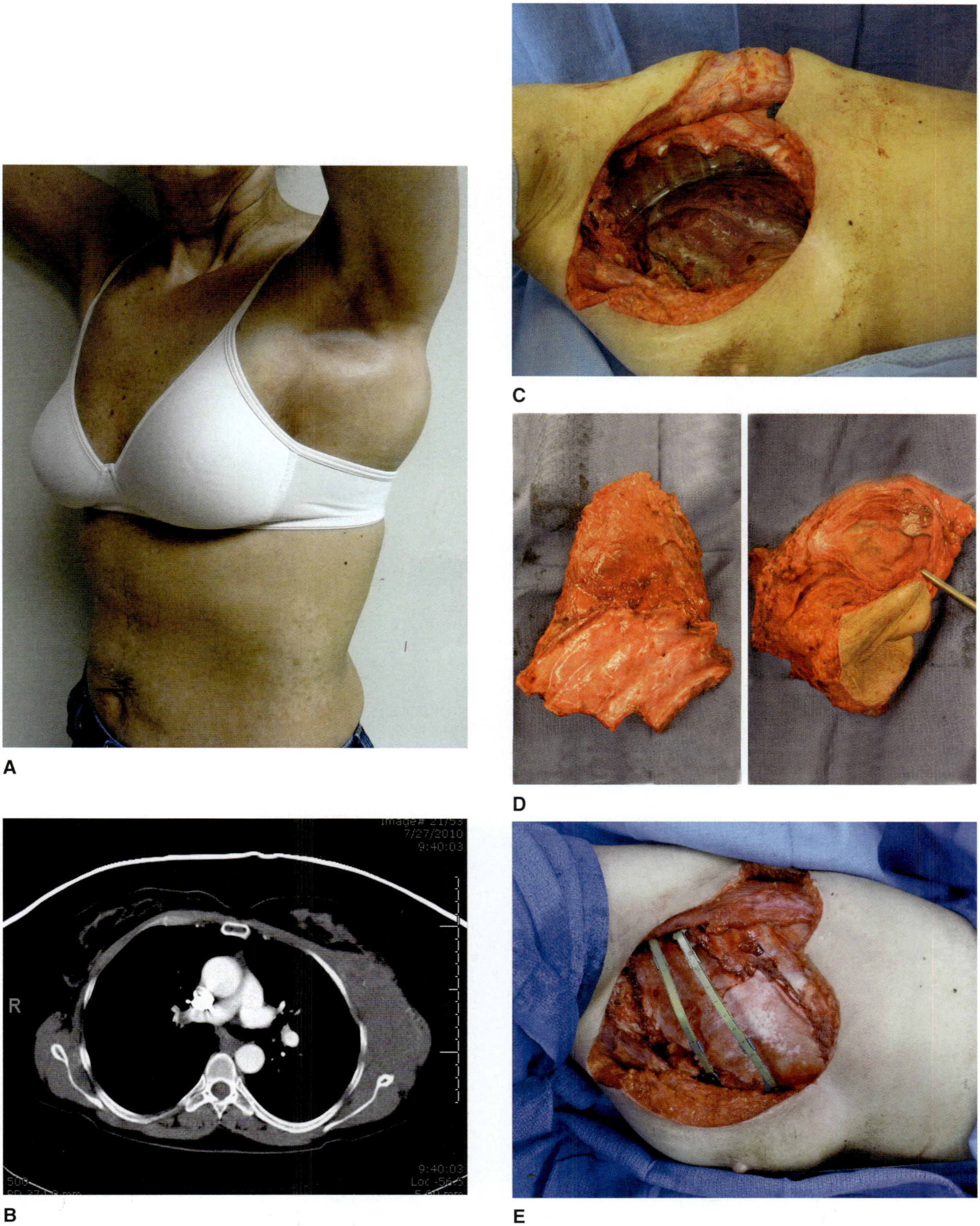

FIGURE 49-8 A 53-year-old woman with a radiation induced high-grade pleomorphic sarcoma of the left side of the chest wall (**A**). Computed tomography scan showing the tumor (**B**). After wide resection of tumor, four ribs, and the lateral edge of the scapula (**C** and **D**), structural integrity was reestablished with processed acellular porcine dermal matrix and titanium ribs (STRATOS-Strasbourg Thoracic Osteosyntheses System; MedXpert GmbH, Heitersheim, Germany) (**E**). Soft tissue was closed with a vertical rectus abdominus musculocutaneous flap with microvascular anastomosis to previously divided thoracodorsal vessels and a full-thickness skin graft, viewed here at 1 year after surgery (**F**). Chest radiograph demonstrating the titanium ribs (**G** and **H**).

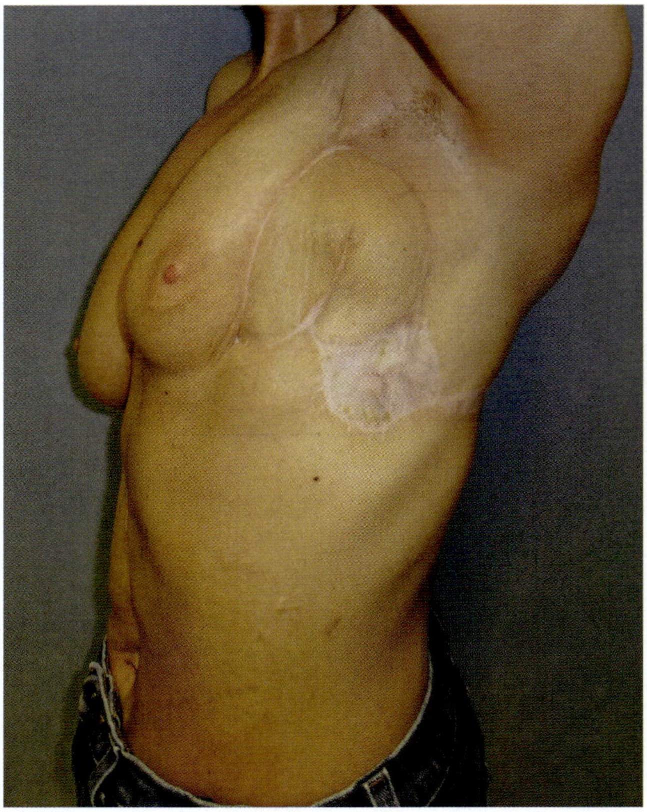

F

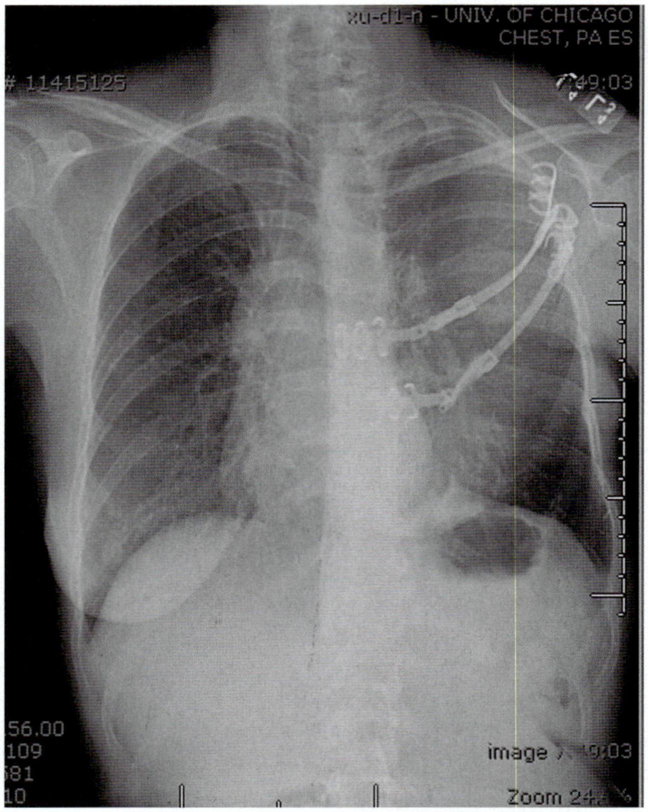

G

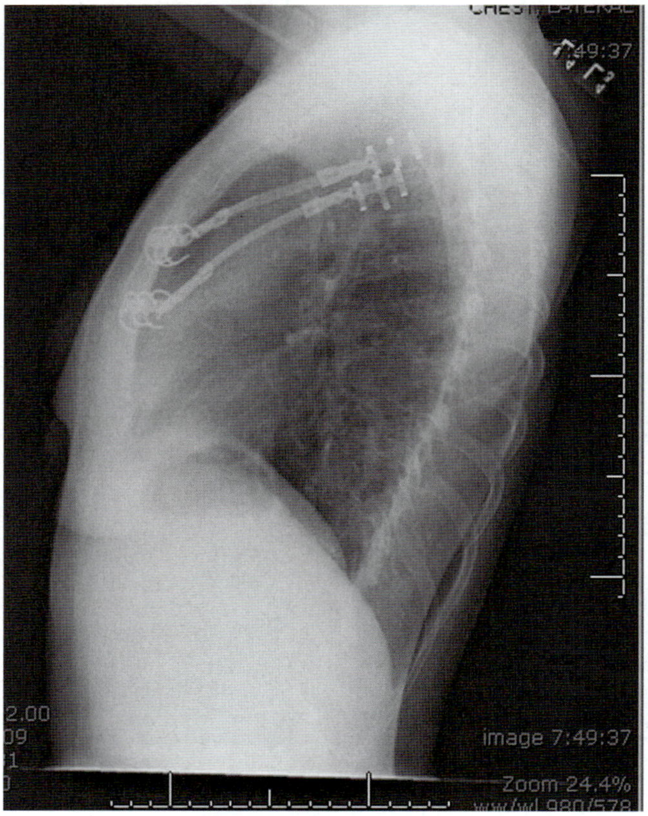

H

FIGURE 49-8 *(Continued)*

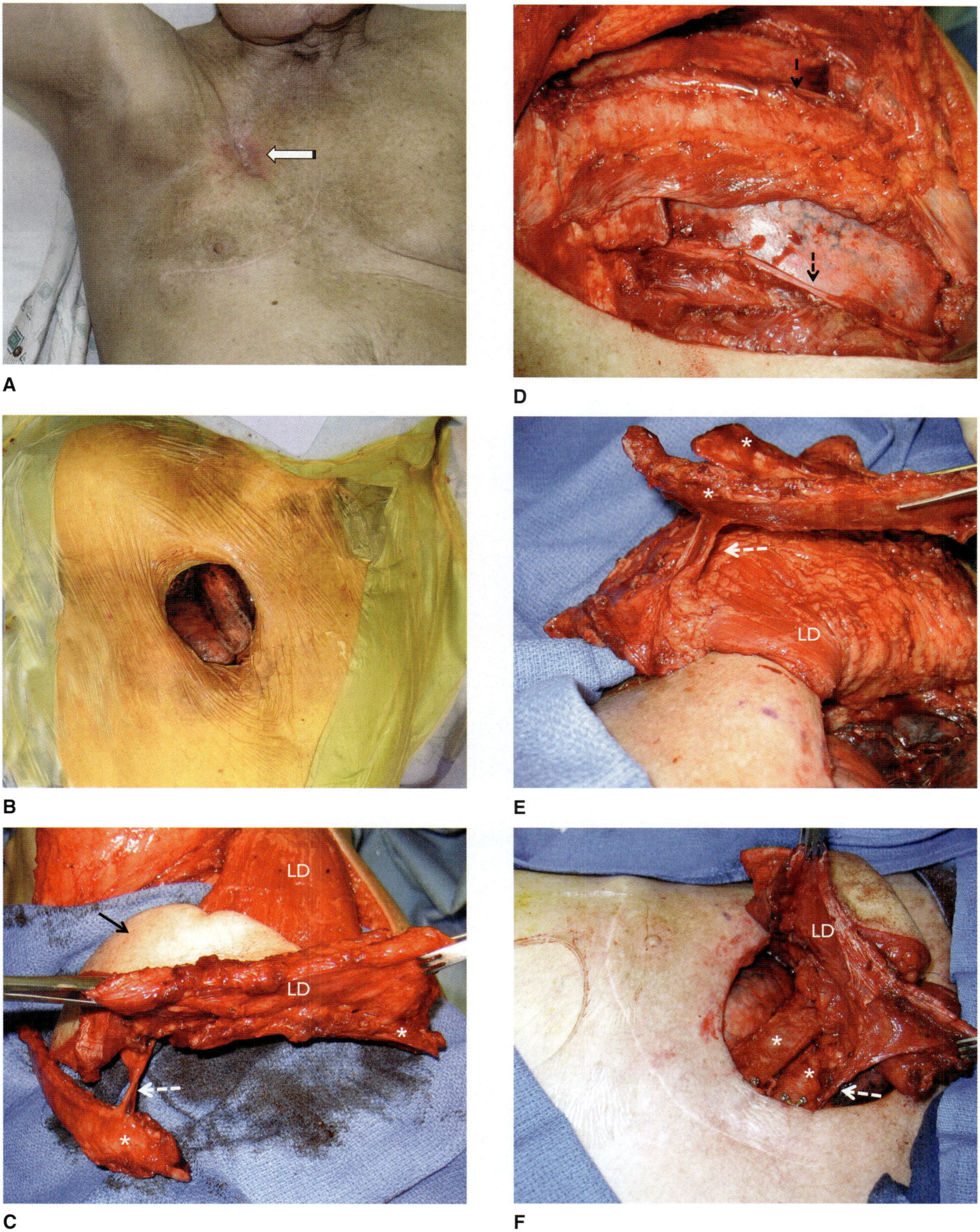

FIGURE 49-9 A 71-year-old man with a history of recurrent floor of mouth carcinoma presented with a metastatic focus of tumor in a right chest wall port site overlying the donor site of a pectoralis major myofascial flap. This was treated with chemoradiation, and he developed osteoradionecrosis of ribs 2 to 4 anteriorly, with osteomyelitis and a purulent draining cutaneous fistula (arrow) (A). Resection of all devitalized and infected tissue, including wedge resection of the right upper lobe of the lung, was performed (B). An ipsilateral pedicled latissimus myo-osseocutaneous (LMOC) flap (C) was raised (black arrow on skin paddle; LD, latissimus dorsi muscle). Notice the significant length of interconnecting vessel (dashed white arrow) to the eighth rib (white asterisk on both ribs). Intercostal nerves (dashed black arrows) were preserved in the donor site to minimize abdominal wall morbidity from denervation (D). The LMOC flap is transposed anteriorly, and the ribs are positioned into the skeletal defect independent of the muscle orientation and secured with rigid fixation (F). The latissimus muscle is then inset beneath surrounding skin (G), and the skin component of the flap is closed (H). The back donor site healed without complications (I).

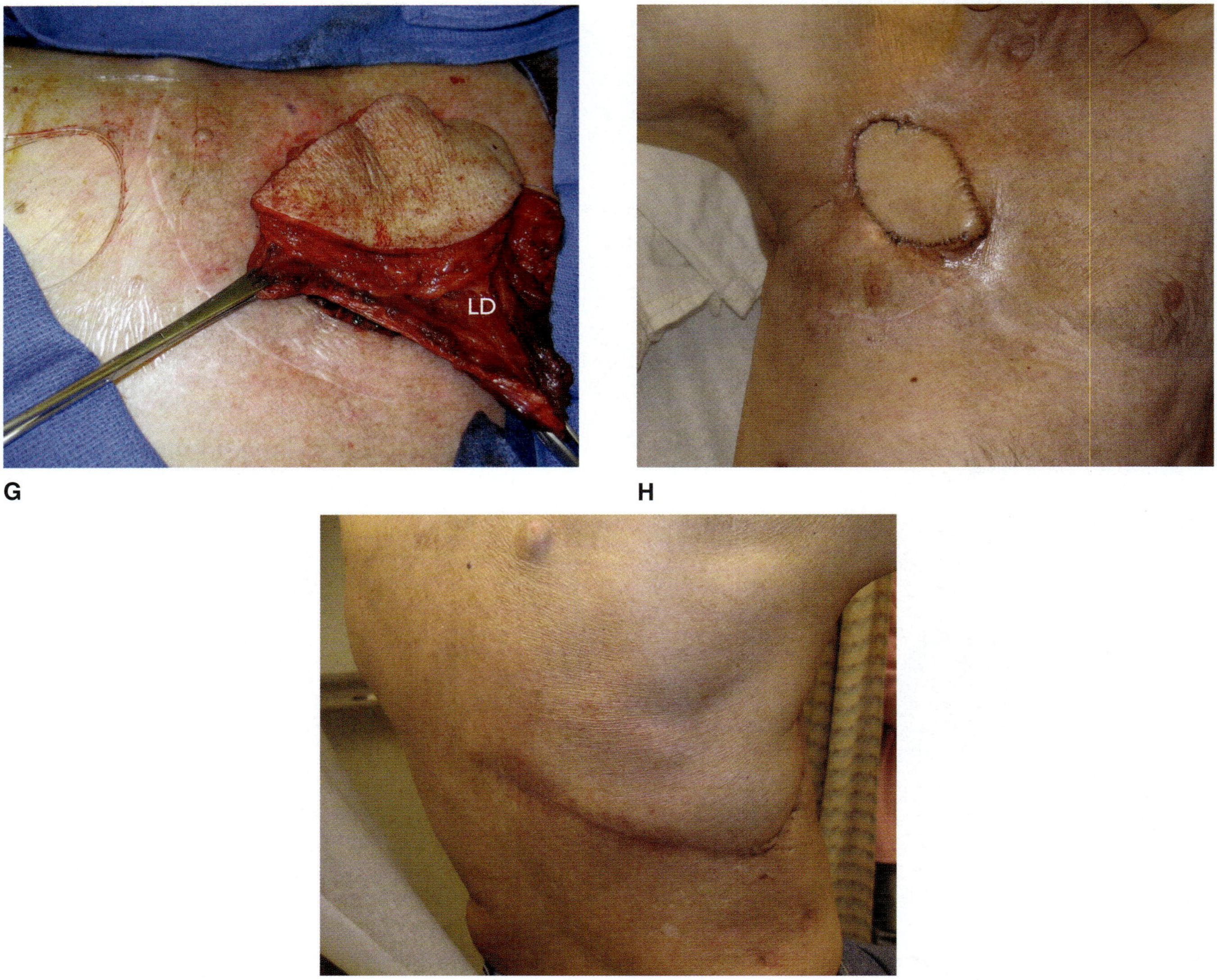

FIGURE 49-9 *(Continued)*

dressing, drapes are removed, the patient is turned to the opposite lateral decubitus position, and the contralateral chest wall is prepped. The flap is harvested, placed in a plastic bag, and submerged in an ice slurry machine to minimize warm ischemia time while the donor site is closed and the patient is placed back into the original position. After rechecking recipient vessel flow, the flap can then be removed from the ice slurry machine and inset and the microvascular anastomosis performed.

RECIPIENT VESSELS AND NERVES FOR ABDOMINAL AND CHEST WALL RECONSTRUCTION

The choice of recipient vessels is generally based on the proximity to the defect and the relative size and quality of the available vessels. Recipient vessels in the upper half of the chest and lower half of the abdomen are usually abundant. In the upper half of the chest, branches of the subscapular system are usually available as recipient vessels for intrathoracic, lateral, or posterolaterally placed flaps. The thoracoacromial, internal mammary, transverse cervical, or even intrathoracic vessels such as the innominate vein are usually available for anteriorly placed flaps. In the lower half of the abdomen, the iliac vessels or its branches, particularly the DIEs, are usually available as recipient vessels. Although there is more of a paucity of recipient vessels in the midtorso, occasionally, the internal mammary, superior epigastric, intercostal, or intraperitoneal (e.g., gastroepiploic, jejunal) vessels are available. However, it is common that free flaps in these locations require long vein grafts (52,53).

The intercostal nerves, subcostal nerves, and first lumbar nerves that contribute to the innervation of the anterior abdominal wall are available for neurorrhaphy if a sensate flap is desired or if a functional muscle transfer is to be done. These nerves run with their accompanying blood vessels in a neurovascular plane known as the transversus abdominis plane between the internal oblique muscle and the transversus abdominis muscle (54).

When working with a multidisciplinary team, the reconstructive surgeon should communicate with the extirpative surgeon to ensure critical vessels and nerves are preserved if possible and tagged (for potential nerve grafting) if unable to be preserved.

FLAP MONITORING IN ABDOMINAL AND CHEST WALL RECONSTRUCTION

Flap monitoring for abdominal and chest wall reconstruction is no different than for any other free flap. Clinical examination assessing color and temperature along with Doppler ultrasonography is usually adequate for skin flaps. It is more of a challenge to assess perfusion in muscle flaps with overlying skin grafts, especially venous drainage. Because of this, many surgeons include a skin paddle with their muscle flaps to facilitate postoperative monitoring. Intrathoracic flaps, without an external skin paddle, are usually monitored with an implantable Doppler probe. A variety of additional technologies and modalities are available to reconstructive microsurgeons for free flap monitoring. These include near-infrared spectroscopy, laser Doppler flowmetry, and microdialysis. Selection of these devices depends on type and location of flap, availability, surgeon experience, and preference. Their use is discussed in another chapter.

OUTCOMES AND RESULTS

Most free flaps reported in the literature demonstrate a high rate of success. Indeed, it is rare to see a clinical series involving free tissue transfers with negative results. In that most abdominal and chest wall reconstructions can be successfully performed with locoregional flaps, with or without the use of alloplastic material, most reports of free flap reconstruction describe very small series of a particular flap or innovation. Although free flaps tend to accomplish the goal set forth by the reconstructive surgeon, a litany of systemic complications are associated in these high-risk operations (see later discussion), especially when performed on sick patients with many comorbidities.

There will always be debate regarding success rates of particular procedures and techniques. This is especially true when evaluating the utility of prosthetic and alloplastic materials. One common scenario that has been thoroughly studied and seems to have consensus in the literature is midline abdominal hernia repair.

Illustrative case studies in abdominal and chest wall reconstruction are depicted in Figures 49-4 to 49-9.

COMPLICATIONS

Complications in abdominal and chest wall reconstruction may occur with the free tissue transfer itself, with the recipient or donor site, or with the patient in general. Arterial or venous thrombosis of a free flap requires prompt reexploration of the microvascular anastomoses and evaluation of the pedicle. Complete loss of a flap generally requires another flap. Partial loss of a flap covering a reasonably healthy wound bed can usually be managed with debridement and local wound care. However, even a small loss of a flap in a wound bed compromised by severe radiation injury can be devastating, leading to multiple potential wound healing issues, including a lack of adherence of the flap to the wound bed, progressive wound dehiscence, localized infection, and subsequent tissue loss. In addition, dead space, fluid collection, and especially infection adjacent to vascular structures put the vessels at risk for thrombosis or rupture.

If structural integrity was provided by a prosthesis, partial flap loss may lead to exposure and potential infection. Although biologic mesh seems to tolerate contamination better than prosthetic material, clinical infection typically mandates removal. Even if the biologic materials can be preserved after infection, long-term functional integrity is usually compromised, leading to bulging, laxity, or hernia formation.

A live flap does not necessarily translate into success. The recipient and donor sites may develop a hematoma, seroma, and infection. Wounds may separate or dehisce, and hernias may recur. The clinical effects of denervation may not be evident for many months. Skin grafts used to close donor sites may fail, and the donor site of the skin graft may get infected or demonstrate delayed healing. In chest wall reconstruction, hardware may fail or transferred bones may fracture. If ribs are harvested, there is the risk of pneumothorax. In functional abdominal wall reconstruction, neurotization of the transferred muscle may fail or be inadequate to provide appropriate tone, strength, or excursion. For all types of oncologic reconstruction, radiation therapy can compromise the durability of the reconstruction, and it is important to consider the potential need for such adjuvant therapy when developing a reconstructive plan.

Cardiopulmonary complications may occur with any surgery involving the abdominal and chest wall, including cardiac ischemia, arrhythmias, congestive heart failure, pulmonary edema, pulmonary embolism, and the requirement for prolonged intubation. Intraabdominal surgery risks bowel injury with subsequent peritonitis and enterocutaneous fistulae. Prolonged ileus plagues some patients, and all patients with intraperitoneal surgery are at risk for bowel adhesions, small bowel obstruction, and recurrent hernia. Tight closure of the abdomen or significant bowel edema after surgery puts the patient at risk for abdominal hypertension or abdominal compartment syndrome. One should be aware of changes in the peak pulmonary pressure throughout the operation, and bladder pressure should be measured after closure and monitored postoperatively. Other systemic complications may include deep vein thrombosis, electrolyte abnormalities, urinary tract infections, bleeding, sepsis, and multisystem organ failure.

REFERENCES

1. Hurwitz DJ, Hollins RR. Reconstruction of the abdominal wall and groin. In Cohen M (ed). *Mastery of Plastic and Reconstructive Surgery* vol. 2 ed. Boston: Little, Brown, 1994, pp. 1349–1359.
2. Mathes SJ, Steinwald PM, Foster RD, et al. Complex abdominal wall reconstruction: a comparison of flap and mesh closure. *Ann Surg* 2000; 232:586–596.

SECTION 3

3. Rohrich RJ, Lowe JB, Hackney FL, Bowman JL, Hobar PC. An algorithm for abdominal wall reconstruction. *Plast Reconstr Surg* 2000;105:202–216.
4. Hallock GG. A paradigm shift for soft-tissue coverage of the zones of the abdominal wall using perforator flaps. *Plast Reconstr Surg* 2012;130: 590–599.
5. Din AM, Evans GRD. Chest wall reconstruction. In McCarthy JB, Galiano RD, Boutros S (eds). *Current Therapy in Plastic Surgery.* Philadelphia: Saunders, 2006, p. 362.
6. Weyant MJ, Bains MS, Venkatraman E, et al. Results of chest wall resection and reconstruction with and without rigid prosthesis. *Ann Thorac Surg* 2006;81:279–285.
7. Boo-Chai K. John Wood and his contributions to plastic surgery: the first groin flap. *Br J Plast Surg* 1977;30:9–13.
8. Maxwell GP. Iginio Tansini and the origin of the latissimus dorsi musculocutaneous flap. *Plast Reconstr Surg* 1980;65:686.
9. Kanavel AB. Plastic procedures for the obliteration of cavities with non-collapsible walls. *Surg Gynecol Obstet* 1921;32:453.
10. Wangensteen OH. Repair of recurrent and difficult hernias and other large defects of the abdominal wall employing the ilio-tibial tract of fascia lata as a pedicled flap. *Surg Gynecol Obstet* 1934;59:766.
11. Wangensteen OH. The pedicle muscle flap in the closure of persistent bronchopleural fistulas. *J Thorac Surg* 1935;5:27.
12. Webster JP. Thoracic-epigastric tubed pedicles. *Clin North Am* 1937; 17:145.
13. Bakamjian VY. A two stage method for pharyngoesophageal reconstruction with a primary pectoral skin flap. *Plast Reconstr Surg* 1965;36:173.
14. McGregor IA, Morgan G. Axial and random pattern flaps. *Br J Plast Surg* 1973;26:202.
15. Daniel RK, Williams HB. The free transfer of skin flaps by microvascular anastomoses. *Plast Reconstr Surg* 1973;52:16.
16. Daniel RK, Taylor GI. Distant transfer of an island flap by microvascular anastomoses. *Plast Reconstr Surg* 1973;52:111.
17. McCraw JB. The recent history of myocutaneous flaps. *Clin Plast Surg* 1980;7:3.
18. Mathes SJ, Nahai F, eds. *Clinical Applications for Muscle and Musculocutaneous Flaps.* St. Louis: CV Mosby, 1979.
19. Arnold PG, Pairolero PC. Intrathoracic muscle flaps: an account of their use in the management of 100 consecutive patients. *Ann Surg* 1990; 211:656.
20. Taylor GI, Palmer JH. The angiosomes of the body. *Br J Plast Surg* 1987;40:130.
21. Fujino T. Contribution of the axial and perforator vasculature in circulation of flaps. *Plast Reconstr Surg* 1967;39(2)125–137.
22. Koshima I, Soeda S. Inferior epigastric artery skin flaps without rectus abdominis muscle. *Br J Plast Surg* 1989;42:645–648.
23. Ramirez OM, Ruas E, Dellon AL. "Components separation" method for closure of abdominal-wall defects: an anatomic and clinical study. *Plast Reconstr Surg* 1990;86:519–526.
24. Hicks CW, Krpata DM, Blatnik JA, et al. Long-term effect on donor sites after components separation: a radiographic analysis. *Plast Reconstr Surg* 2012;130(2):354–359.
25. Gaertner WB, Bonsack ME, Delaney JP. Experimental evaluation of four biologic prostheses for ventral hernia repair. *J Gastrointest Surg* 2007;11:1275–1285.
26. Lin SJ, Butler CE. Subtotal thigh flap and bioprosthetic mesh reconstruction for large, composite abdominal wall defects. *Plast Reconstr Surg* 2010;125(4):1146–1156.
27. Bisgard JD, Swenson SA. Tumor of the sternum: report of a case with special operative technique. *Arch Surg* 1948;56:570.
28. Campbell DA. Reconstruction of the anterior thoracic wall. *J Thorac Surg* 1950;19:456.
29. Lampl L Chest wall resection: a new and simple method for stabilization of extended defects. *Eur J Cardiothorac Surg* 2001;20:669–673.
30. Paris F, Blasco E, Tarazona V, et al. Total sternectomy for malignant disease. *J Thorac Cardiovasc Surg* 1980;80:459–462.
31. Coonar AS, Qureshi N, Smith I, et al. A novel titanium rib bridge system for chest wall reconstruction. *Ann Thorac Surg* 2009;87:e46–e48.
32. Ariyan S, Finseth FJ. The anterior approach for obtaining free osteocutaneous rib grafts. *Plast Reconstr Surg* 1978;62:676.
33. Serafin D, Riefkohl R, Thomas I, Georgiade NG. Vascular Rib-periosteal and osteocutaneous reconstruction of the maxilla and mandible: an assessment. *Plast Reconstr Surg* 1980;66:718.
34. Richards MA, Poole MD, Godfrey AM. The serratus anterior/rib composite flap in mandibular reconstruction. *Br J Plast Surg* 1985;38:466.
35. Ohsumi N, Simamoto R, Tsukagoshi T. Free composite latissimus dorsi muscle-rib flap not containing the intercostals artery and vein for reconstruction of bone and soft-tissue defects. *Plast Reconstr Surg* 1994;94:372.
36. Maruyama Y, Urita Y, Ohnishi K. Rib-latissimus dorsi osteomyocutaneous flap in reconstruction of a mandibular defect. *Br J Plast Surg* 1985;38:234.
37. Hirase Y, Kojima T, Kinoshita Y, et al. Composite reconstruction for chest wall and scalp using multiple ribs–latissimus dorsi osteomyocutaneous flaps as pedicled and free flaps. *Plast Reconstr Surg* 1991;187:555.
38. Schlenker JD, Indresano AT, Raine T, et al. A new flap in the dog containing a vascularized rib graft—the latissimus dorsi myoosteocutaneous flap. *J Surg Res* 1980;29:172.
39. Schmidt DR, Robson MC. One-stage composite reconstruction using the latissimus myoosteocutaneous free flap. *Am J Surg* 1982;144:470.
40. Yamamoto Y, Sugihara T, Kawashima K, Qi F. An anatomic study of the latissimus dorsi-rib flap: an extension of the subscapular combined flap. *Plast Reconstr Surg* 1996;98(5):811–816.
41. Pelissier P, Pistre V, Casoli V, et al. Reconstruction of short lower leg stumps with the osteomusculocutaneous latissimus dorsi-rib flap. *Plast Reconstr Surg* 2002;109:1013.
42. Nazerani S, Motabar AR. Reintroducing the latissimus-rib free flap as a long bone substitute in the reconstruction of lower extremity injuries. *Med J Islam Rep Iran* 2008;22:104.
43. Seitz, IA, Adler N, Odessey E, et al. Latissimus dorsi/rib intercostals perforator myo-osseocutaneous free flap reconstruction in composite defects of the scalp: case series and review of literature. *J Reconstr Microsurg* 2009;25:559.
44. Cipriani R, Contedini F, Santoli M, et al. Abdominal wall transplantation with microsurgical technique. *Am J Transplant* 2007;7:1304–1307.
45. Levi DM, Tzakis AG, Kato T, et al. Transplantation of the abdominal wall. *Lancet* 2003;361:2173–2176.
46. Agarwal S, Dorafshar AH, Harland RC, et al. Liver and vascularized posterior rectus sheath fascia composite tissue allotransplantation. *Am J Transplant* 2010;10:2712–2716.
47. Ninkovic M, Kronberger P, Harpf C, et al. Free innervated latissimus dorsi muscle flap for reconstruction of full-thickness abdominal wall defects. *Plast Reconstr Surg* 1998;101(4):971–978.
48. Koshima I, Moriguchi T, Inagawa K, et al. Dynamic reconstruction of the abdominal wall using a reinnervated free rectus femoris muscle transfer. *Ann Plast Surg* 1999;43(2):199–203.
49. Koshima I, Nanba Y, Tutsui T, et al. Dynamic reconstruction of large abdominal defects using a free rectus femoris musculocutaneous flap with normal motor function. *Ann Plast Surg* 2003;50(4):420–424.
50. Taylor GI, Corlett RJ, Dhar SC, Ashton MW. The anatomical (angiosome) and clinical territories of cutaneous perforating arteries: development of the concept and designing safe flaps. *Plast Reconstr Surg* 2011;127(4): 1447–1459.
51. Saint-Cyr M, Wong C, Schaverien M, et al. The perforasome theory: vascular anatomy and clinical implications. *Plast Reconstr Surg* 2009;124:1529–1544.
52. Earle AS, Feng L-J, Jordan RB. Long saphenous vein grafts as an aid to microsurgical reconstruction of the trunk. *J Reconstr Microsurg* 1990;6:165.
53. Reichenberger MA, Harenberg PS, Pelzer M, et al. Arteriovenous loops in microvascular free tissue transfer in reconstruction of central sternal defects. *J Thorac Cardiovasc Surg* 2010;140(6):1277–1283.
54. Rozen WM, Tran TMN, Ashton MW, et al. Refining the course of the thoracolumbar nerves: a new understanding of the innervation of the anterior abdominal wall. *Clin Anat* 2008;21:325–333.

CHAPTER 50

Perineal Reconstruction to Include Vaginal Reconstruction

Hooman Soltanian and Charles E. Butler

BACKGROUND

The indications for perineal and vaginal reconstruction include a wide spectrum of defects. The defects may be congenital, such as vaginal agenesis, or caused by trauma or by surgical extirpation of malignancies. By far, the largest numbers of perineal and vaginal reconstructions are performed after surgical resection of neoplasms.

The pelvic floor is the most inferior portion of the funnel-shaped pelvis and consists of several structures, including the pelvic diaphragm, lower urogenital tract, reproductive organs, rectum, and anal sphincter (Figure 50-1A) (1). The majority of the perineum's surface area is occupied by the urogenital and gastrointestinal tract openings. The bony walls of the pelvic outlet provide rigid structures that do not collapse after extirpation of the visceral contents; this can result in dead space (Figure 50-1B). The limited amount of redundant soft tissue in the perineal region renders the use of local tissue for reconstruction difficult, especially after extensive resection. The goal of perineal reconstructive procedures is to deliver well-vascularized soft tissue with adequate volume to obliterate any dead space, enable primary healing, and prevent perineal hernia/bulge.

Many of the complications after perineal tumor resection are related to the persistent noncollapsible bony dead space or closure of the perineal skin under tension. For example, persistent perineal sinus tracts develop after abdominoperineal resection (APR) for low rectal cancer in up to 30% of the cases (2). In fact, the benefits of muscle flaps for single-stage reconstruction of perineal defects are well established (3). In addition, high rates of postoperative complications are seen after APR when direct closure of perineal defects is done without using a flap (4). Another less common complication after APR is perineal herniation of viscera, which may require subsequent repair with a flap (5).

This chapter describes techniques used for perineal and vaginal reconstruction. Pedicled musculocutaneous and fasciocutaneous flaps are the workhorse flaps for perineal and vaginal reconstruction (6), but free tissue transfer has a role in certain cases.

VERTICAL RECTUS ABDOMINIS MUSCULOCUTANEOUS FLAP

The vertical rectus abdominis musculocutaneous (VRAM) flap is the most commonly used regional flap for coverage of the perineum, obliteration of pelvic dead space, and repair of partial or complete vaginal defects. The role of rectus abdominis flaps in reconstruction for perineal defects was first described in 1984 (7). The vascular pedicle for the VRAM flap is the deep inferior epigastric (DIE) vessels, which are relatively large and reliable. Because these vessels might have been injured by previous surgeries or the resection prompting reconstruction, it is important to assess the patency of the vessels before the dissection of the flap. VRAM flaps generally include the entire length of the rectus abdominis muscle with a variable-sized skin paddle overlying the muscle (Figure 50-2A). Depending on the size of the defect, the skin can be extended superiorly and laterally beyond the muscle to create an extended or oblique rectus flap (see Figure 50-2A) (8).

The extended VRAM (eVRAM) flap includes skin and subcutaneous fat extending superolaterally beyond the costal margin toward the axilla. The eVRAM flap has been shown to have reliable vascularity even to the flap tip and is valuable when greater flap reach or volume is required for pelvic or perineal reconstruction than is possible with a standard VRAM flap (9). If needed, a portion of the skin paddle can be tubed and used to construct a neovagina (Figure 50-2B and C).

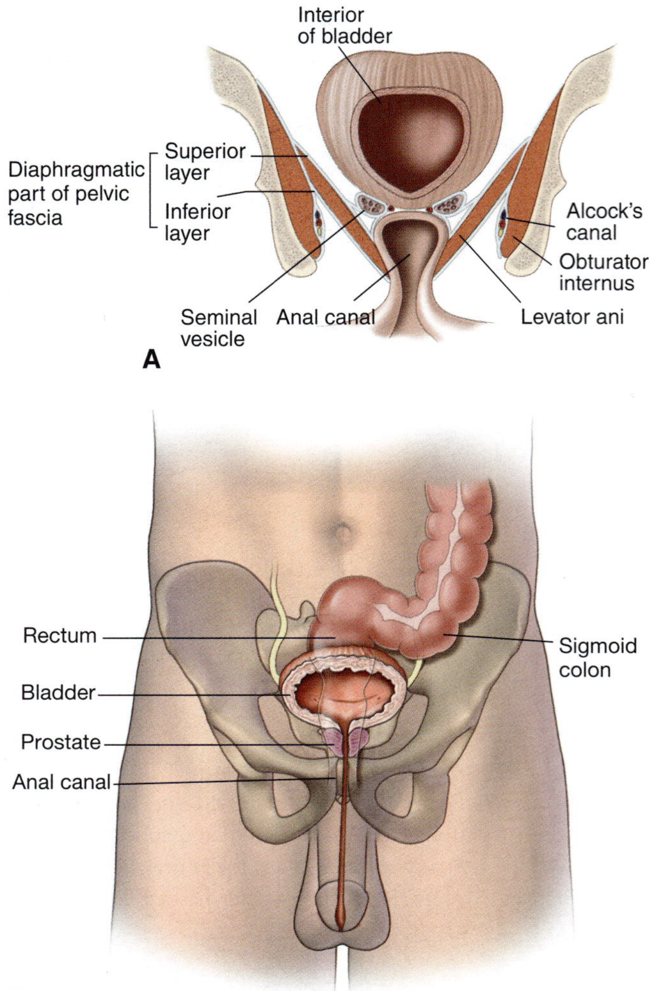

FIGURE 50-1 Cross-sectional anatomy of the pelvic floor demonstrating (**A**) the rigid walls of the pelvic outlet, the levator muscles and the orientation of the bladder and anus. (**B**) Anatomy of the gastrointestinal and urogenital organs in the pelvis.

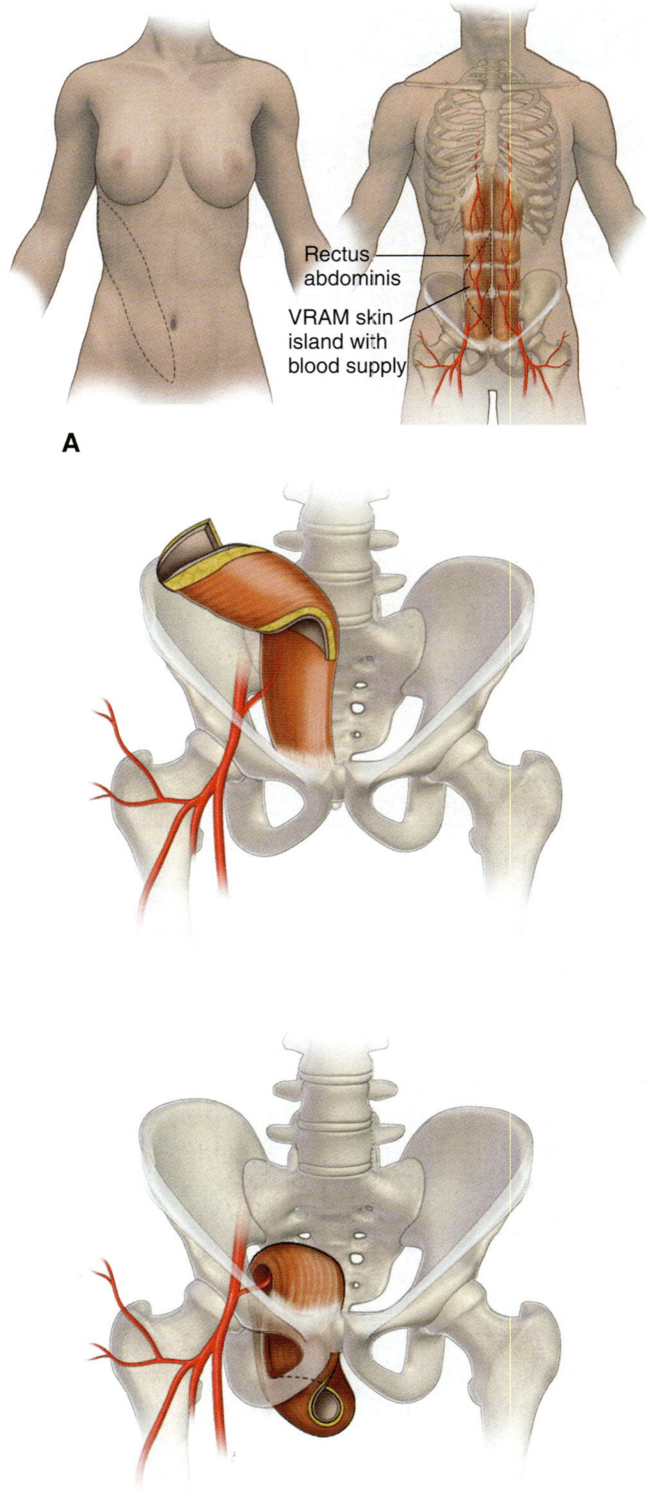

FIGURE 50-2 (**A**) Anatomic delineation of the rectus abdominis muscle and location of the deep inferior epigastric vessels (*left*). The skin flap design in an extended vertical rectus abdominis musculocutaneous (*right*). (**B**) Formation of a tube for vaginal reconstruction and transfer of the flap into the pelvic defect.

The VRAM flap can be harvested with fascia- and muscle-sparing techniques (10,11). When a fascia-sparing technique is used, the fascia medial to the medial perforators and lateral to the lateral perforators is saved (Figure 50-3). This technique results in less tension on the fascial closure. Ipsilateral component separation can also be used to reduce fascial closure tension and preclude the need to use surgical mesh. This technique has been shown to improve outcomes when VRAM donor site closure is tight (12). Fascia-sparing and component separation techniques can be combined to further reduce tension on the fascial closure. These techniques can reduce the potential for donor site complications, such as bulging and hernia formation.

Operative Technique

The VRAM flap is interpolated into the pelvis, and a section of the skin paddle is positioned at the perineal defect. The skin peripheral to the planned perineal skin paddle is deepithelialized and buried. The bulk of the muscle and subcutaneous tissue fills the pelvic dead space. The pelvic cavity and the perineal area should be drained with closed-suction drainage catheters to reduce the risk of fluid collections and subsequent wound healing complications.

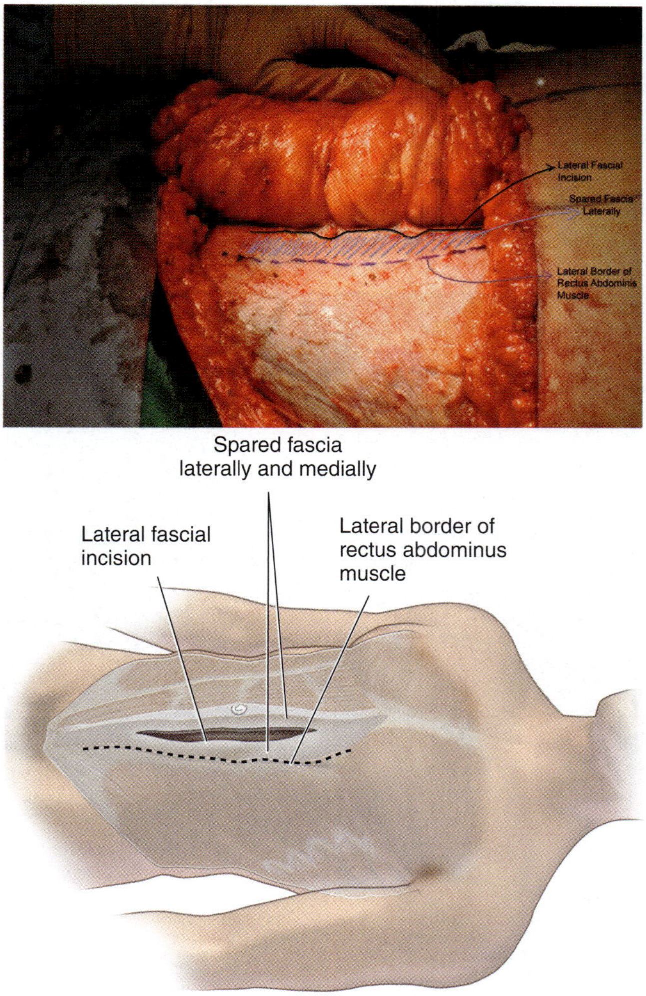

FIGURE 50-3 Demonstration of fascial-sparing vertical rectus abdominis musculocutaneous dissection. *Top,* Intraoperative visualization of the lateral row perforators. *Bottom,* Schematic depiction of the rectus abdominis sheath after harvest of the muscle and preservation of the majority of the anterior fascia.

Immediate perineal reconstruction with a VRAM flap has been shown to result in markedly less donor and recipient site morbidity than reconstruction with thigh-based flaps (4,13). In large series, the risk of total flap loss has been rather low (1.4%–2.2%), and the risk of abdominal wall complications has been reported to be approximately 5% (3).

In patients undergoing perineal reconstruction, the VRAM flap is often harvested from the right side because of the presence of a colostomy or ileostomy through the left rectus muscle. VRAM reconstruction begins with the marking of a large strip of skin overlying the width of the rectus muscle. The horizontal laxity and redundancy of the skin dictate how wide of a skin paddle can be harvested. The medial border of the skin paddle is the abdominal midline (see Figure 50-2B). The skin paddle is tapered superiorly and inferiorly to allow for closure with no significant dog ear. The skin paddle can extend vertically from the lower ribs to the pubis. If a very long flap reach or a large volume of tissue is required for reconstruction, an eVRAM flap is useful (12).

The laparotomy incision is made in the midline along the medial border of the skin paddle. The incision should be made on the side of the umbilicus ipsilateral to the flap. The midline incision extends through the subcutaneous layers down to the linea alba.

After the abdominal portion of the resection is completed, the remainder of the VRAM flap can be elevated. The lateral incision is made and taken down to the level of the external oblique muscle fascia. When a fascia-sparing technique is used, the skin and subcutaneous fat are dissected from lateral to medial until the lateral row of rectus perforators is visualized. The anterior rectus sheath is then incised along the perforators. Next, the rectus abdominis muscle is mobilized within the rectus sheath both medially and laterally. The muscle is transected superiorly at its origin from the costal margin. The skin and muscle are elevated out of the rectus sheath from superior to inferior. During this maneuver, the surgeon must take care to avoid trauma to the DIE vessels on the deep surface of the muscle. After the flap is mobilized inferiorly and inset, the anterior rectus sheath is repaired. The anterior rectus sheath consists of two distinct layers; these are more distinct below the arcuate line. The closure must include both layers with each bite of the sutures. If the fascial edges cannot be approximated without tension, an ipsilateral component separation can be performed to allow for medialization of the lateral portion of the rectus sheath.

The VRAM flap enters the peritoneal cavity through an opening in the inferomedial aspect of the rectus sheath. The opening must be of adequate size to avoid pressure on the pedicle. The flap is passed through the pelvis and exposed through the defect in the perineum. The attachment of the rectus muscle to the pelvic rim is usually maintained as added security to avoid undue tension on the pedicle. Before complete closure of the midline, the pedicle should be checked to assure proper location and orientation. The portion of the flap skin needed for coverage of the perineum and vaginal wall is marked. The flap is then returned into the peritoneum, the excess skin beyond the marking is deepithelialized, and the flap is advanced into its final position in the perineum. The flap is inset in multiple layers. A few interrupted sutures placed at the level of the pelvic entrance will position the flap at the pelvic floor defect and may decrease the risk of visceral herniation toward the perineum. A #19 closed-suction drainage catheter is placed above the pelvic entrance. The perineal defect is also closed in layers over drainage catheters. Finally, the skin on the flap donor site is advanced toward the midline, and the abdominal donor site is closed in layers over a drainage catheter.

When the patient is positioned in the lithotomy position at the beginning of the case, special attention must be paid to place the patient with the buttocks at the lower end of the operative table to allow access to the posterior perineal area. The patient's shoulders should be padded and secured to avoid gradual cranial movement when the patient is the Trendelenburg position on the operating table. For the closure of the posterior perineal area, the patient's legs are moved into the extreme lithotomy position. These maneuvers improve exposure.

GRACILIS FLAP

In 1976, McCraw et al. first described the use of the gracilis musculocutaneous flap for vaginal reconstruction (14). The gracilis muscle is supplied primarily by the ascending branch of the medial circumflex femoral artery, which is a branch of the deep femoral artery (Figure 50-4). The symphysis pubis and the medial femoral epicondyle are used as landmarks for myocutaneous flap design (Figure 50-5). For circumferential vaginal defects, bilateral flaps can be used; each flap provides half of the circumference of the reconstructed vagina (Figure 50-6). In patients whose ablative procedure does not require a laparotomy, such as in laparoscopy-assisted APR, the gracilis musculocutaneous flap may also be a valuable flap in reconstruction for perineal defects. There are data to show that use of an immediate gracilis flap in an irradiated

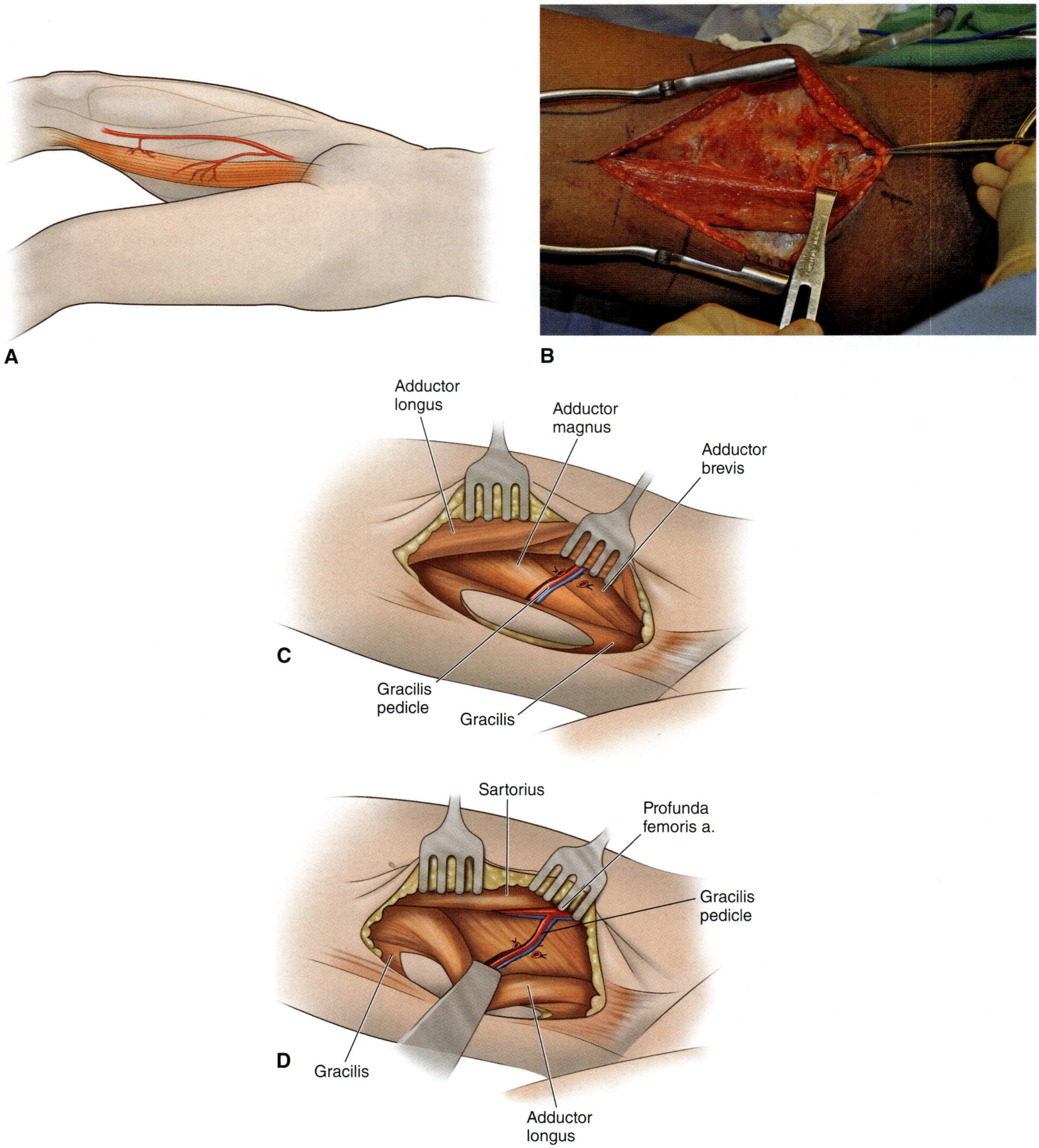

FIGURE 50-4 (A) Schematic delineation of the gracilis muscle and its blood supply. (B) Intraoperative visualization of the dominant and minor pedicle for the gracilis flap. (C) Dissection of the gracilis main pedicle under the adductor longus muscle. (D) Extension of the pedicle to the take off from the deep femoral vessels.

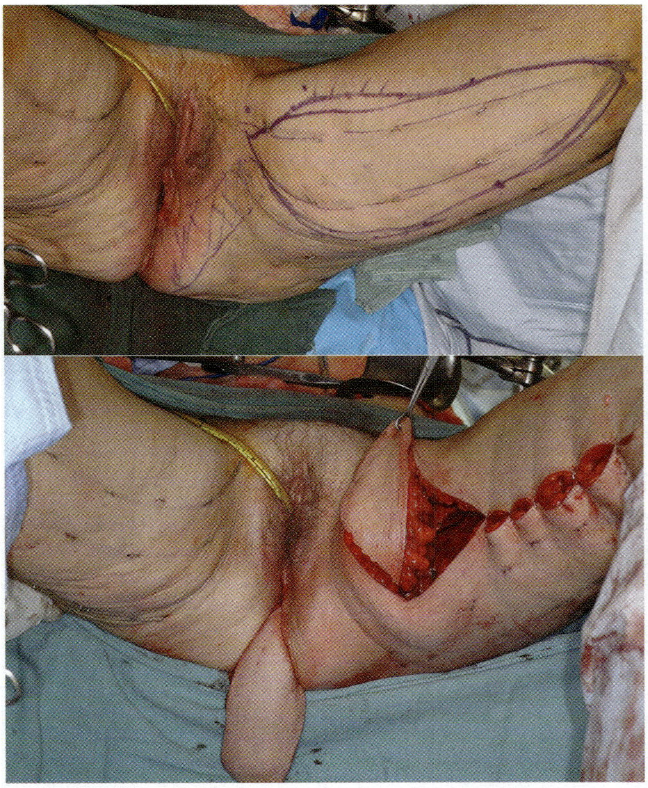

FIGURE 50-5 Markings for harvest and transfer of the gracilis flap (*top*). Transposition and Inset of the gracilis myocutaneous flap (*bottom*).

perineum after APR decreases the rate of postoperative complications (15).

The gracilis flap can also be used as a muscle-only flap. As a unilateral or bilateral muscle flap, the gracilis flap can be used to fill small- to moderate-sized pelvic dead space when additional skin is not needed. Gracilis muscle flaps can also be used to create a neoscrotum or repair vulvar defects (16). A gracilis flap is also a good choice for repair of persistent rectovaginal or rectovesical fistulas with or without the need for anal sphincteroplasty (Figure 50-7) (17).

Operative Technique

The landmarks for locating the gracilis muscle are the medial femoral condyle distally and the symphysis pubis superiorly. The skin incision should be made 2 to 3 cm posterior to the line connecting the two landmarks (see Figure 50-5). If a skin paddle is planned, the incision should be made first distally on the thigh. The medial thigh musculature has variable laxity and mobility. With the patient in stirrups and the lithotomy position, the muscle is usually displaced somewhat posteriorly. If the gracilis muscle's course is not easily discernible, it is advisable to make an incision distal to the proposed skin island close to the medial femoral epicondyle. The musculotendinous fibers of the gracilis muscle can be identified posterior to the fibers of the sartorius muscle and anterior to the fibers of the hamstring muscles. With the use of a clamp or a Penrose drain, the gracilis muscle is retracted distally, and its course along the medial aspect of the thigh is marked. The skin island can then be designed centered over the proximal third to half of the muscle. The saphenous vein is commonly located anterior to the incision and should be preserved if possible.

As the skin island is incised and separated from the surrounding tissue, the surgeon must take care to avoid any shearing motion between the muscle and the overlying skin and fat. The skin island can be secured to the muscle with interrupted sutures as the dissection progresses proximally.

The dominant neurovascular pedicle enters the gracilis muscle on its deep surface, approximately 10 cm inferior to the symphysis pubis, and passes posterior to the adductor longus muscle and anterior to the Adductor Magnus muscle (see Figure 50-4). After the pedicle is visualized, the dissection of the muscle can proceed more rapidly. The distal tendinous portion of the muscle is then transected, and the muscle is reflected superiorly. After the muscle and the skin island are completely free, a tunnel can be created from the gracilis compartment on the medial thigh to the defect in the perineum. The tunnel should be wide enough to allow easy passage of the flap. The proximal portion of the skin island may have to be deepithelialized if it will be buried. In obese patients, the thickness of the subcutaneous tissue may present a problem for the transfer of the flap through the subcutaneous tunnel and may require insetting the flap base into an incision between the donor and recipient defects.

In case of smaller perineal defects, unilateral or bilateral gracilis muscles can be used to fill the void in the lower pelvis without the need for additional skin. Gracilis muscle flaps can also be used for reconstruction of neoscrotum or vulvar defects (16). Gracilis muscle is also a good choice for repair of persistent rectovaginal or rectovesical fistulas with or without the need for anal sphincteroplasty (see Figure 50-7) (17).

If additional pedicle length is needed for insetting of the flap, further dissection of the vascular pedicle can be performed. Several muscular branches to the adductor muscles emanate from the gracilis pedicle. These branches can be ligated to allow for further rotation of the muscle. In extended dissection of the muscle, its pedicle can be followed to the profunda femoris vessels (see Figure 50-4C and D) (18).

The gracilis flap is next secured into the perineal defect in layers. If bilateral flaps are used to construct a neovagina, the skin island can be sutured together on one side (preferably the anterior aspect). Then the construct is inset in the location of the native vagina, and the closure of the posterior suture line is completed. It would be more difficult to rotate a completely formed neovagina into position in the pelvis. Inserting the flaps into position with one side still open is easier and less traumatic (see Figure 50-6).

Finally, the donor site is closed in layers over a closed-suction drainage catheter. The thigh is wrapped with an elastic bandage to control swelling and help reduce seroma formation.

PUDENDAL THIGH FLAP

The pudendal thigh fasciocutaneous flap, or Singapore flap, is a type A fasciocutaneous flap. Its main blood supply is through the internal pudendal artery. In 1989, Wee and Joseph first described the pudendal thigh flap for vaginal reconstruction (19). This relatively thin and pliable flap can also be used in

SECTION 3

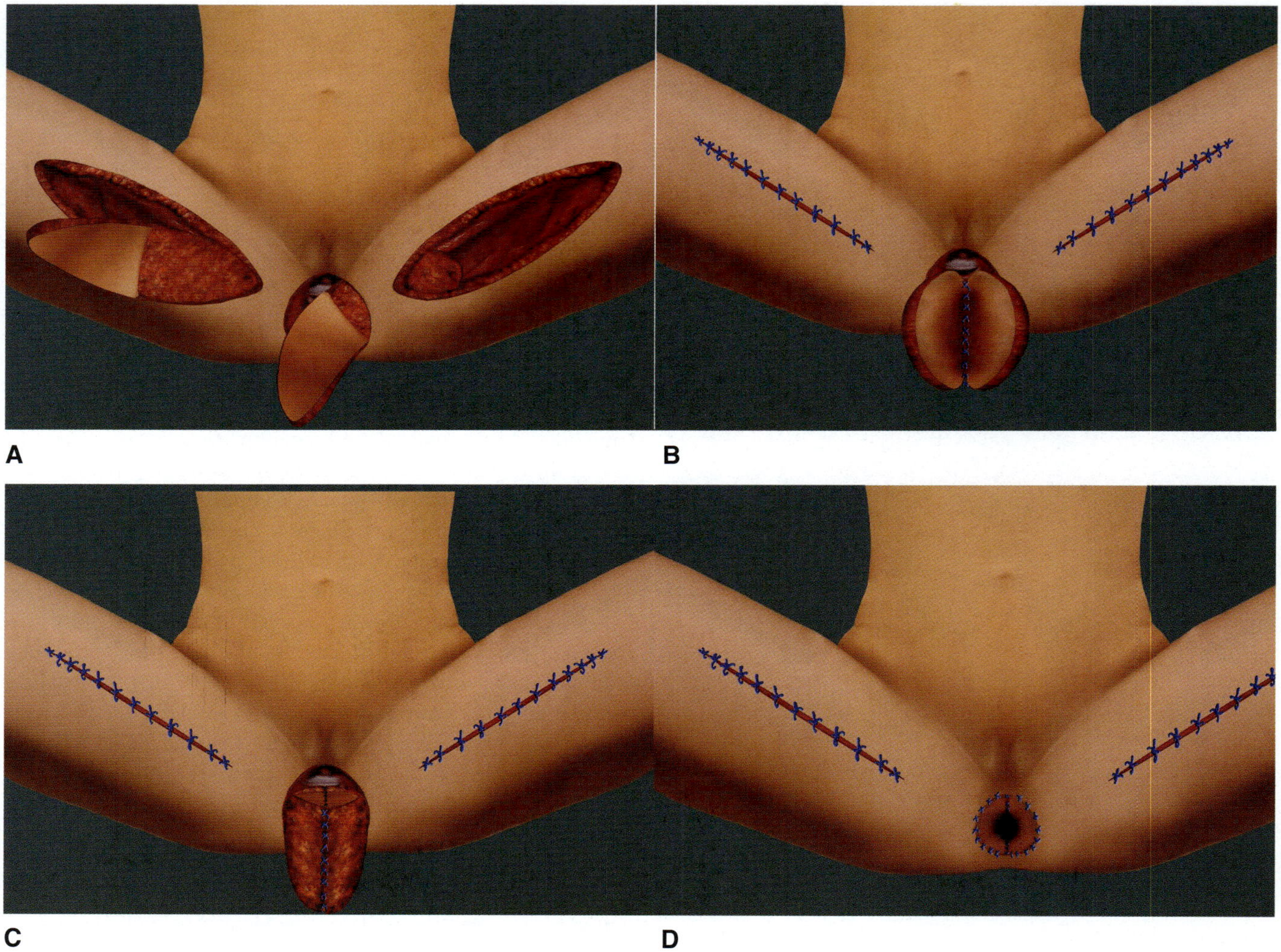

FIGURE 50-6 Bilateral gracilis flaps for vaginal reconstruction. (**A**) Harvest of the myocutaneous flaps and partial deepithelization for transfer into the perineal defect. (**B**) Transfer of both flaps and closure on one side. (**C**) Closure of the gracilis flaps on both sides and creation of a tubular structure. (**D**) Insertion of the construct into the vaginal defect and closure of the perineum.

perineal reconstruction. In the original description, the flap was designed as a fasciocutaneous island and passed under the labia majora into the vaginal defect (Figure 50-8). Woods et al. reported a modification of the Singapore flap for repair of total vaginal defects; the authors released the posterior aspects of the labia majora and used bilateral flaps without any tunneling under the labia (20).

The survival rate of the flap has been very variable, especially the apical region of the flap toward the femoral triangle (21,22). A recent study provided a more detailed understanding of the blood supply of this flap, and this knowledge may help surgeons improve the survival of the distal skin (23).

Operative Technique

The pudendal thigh flap is based posteriorly. It is designed lateral to the labia majora and the hair-bearing skin. Anteriorly, the flap extends into the femoral triangle. The flap is centered over the groin (see Figure 50-8) and has a width of approximately 6 cm at the base. Because the vascular supply is superficial to the fascia, the flap is dissected deep to the fascia to avoid injury to the vessels. The incision is made superiorly first and extended gradually toward the base of the flap. The posterior incision is made at the end and kept rather superficial. This incision makes the transposition into the perineal and vaginal area easier (see Figure 50-8). For circumferential reconstruction of the vagina, bilateral flaps have to be sutured together.

The flap is then transferred medially, either through a subcutaneous tunnel or open incision in the posterior aspect of the labia majora.

ANTEROLATERAL THIGH FLAP

The anterolateral thigh (ALT) flap was first described for clinical use in 1984 by Song et al. (24). Descending branches of the lateral circumflex femoral artery provide the main blood supply to this flap. The ALT flap has been used mainly as a free flap for soft tissue reconstruction in various areas, including the head and neck and extremities (Figure 50-9A).

The ALT flap can also be elevated as an island flap for repair of defects in the pelvic and perineal regions (25). The pedicle of the flap can be dissected to its origin from the deep femoral vessels and passed medially deep to the rectus femoris muscle to reach these defects (Figure 50-9B). For larger defects, additional

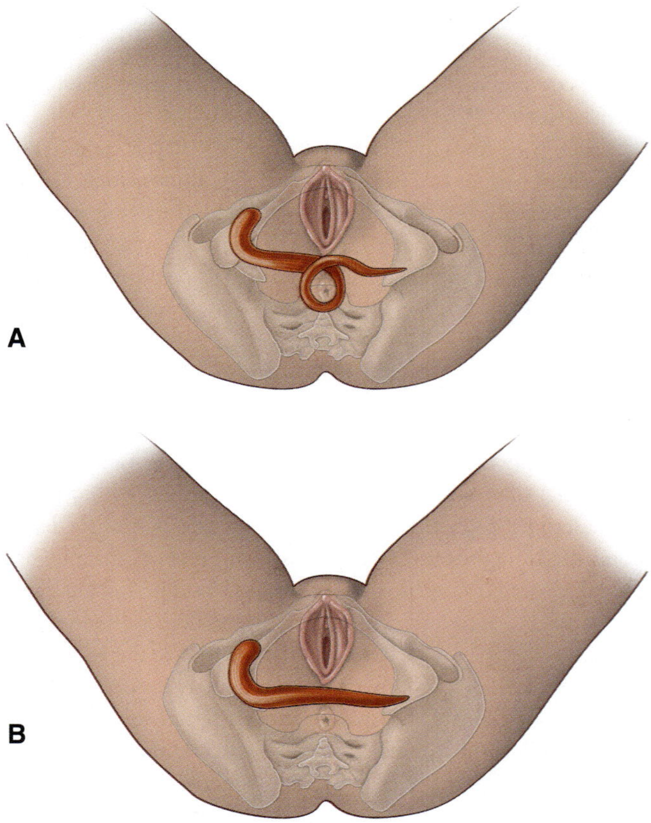

FIGURE 50-7 (**A**) Anal sphincter reconstruction with a unilateral gracilis muscle. (**B**) Interposition of the gracilis muscle for repair of a chronic rectovesical or rectovaginal fistula.

volume can be obtained by harvesting the ALT flap as a musculocutaneous flap, including a portion of the vastus lateralis muscle. For substantial but superficial defects of the vulva and perineum, the fasciocutaneous ALT flap is a good option, providing relatively thin, pliable, and well-vascularized tissue (26).

Operative Technique

The vascular supply enters the ALT flap on a line drawn from the anterior iliac spine to the lateral border of the patella. A handheld Doppler probe is useful for identifying the location of the perforators (see Figure 50-9A). The incision is made first proximally, and the dissection is carried down to the lateral edge of the rectus femoris muscle. The septum between the rectus femoris and vastus lateralis muscles is dissected carefully to visualize the perforators to the ALT flap. The ALT flap perforators are more commonly musculocutaneous perforators through the vastus lateralis muscle rather than septocutaneous perforators between the vastus lateralis and rectus femoris muscles. After the flap pedicle is identified, the remainder of the skin incision can be made and adjusted accordingly.

GLUTEAL THIGH FLAP

The gluteal thigh flap is a fasciocutaneous flap based on the descending branch of the inferior gluteal artery. In the 1981 description by Hurwitz et al., the proximal portion of the flap was raised as a musculocutaneous flap (27). Achauer et al.

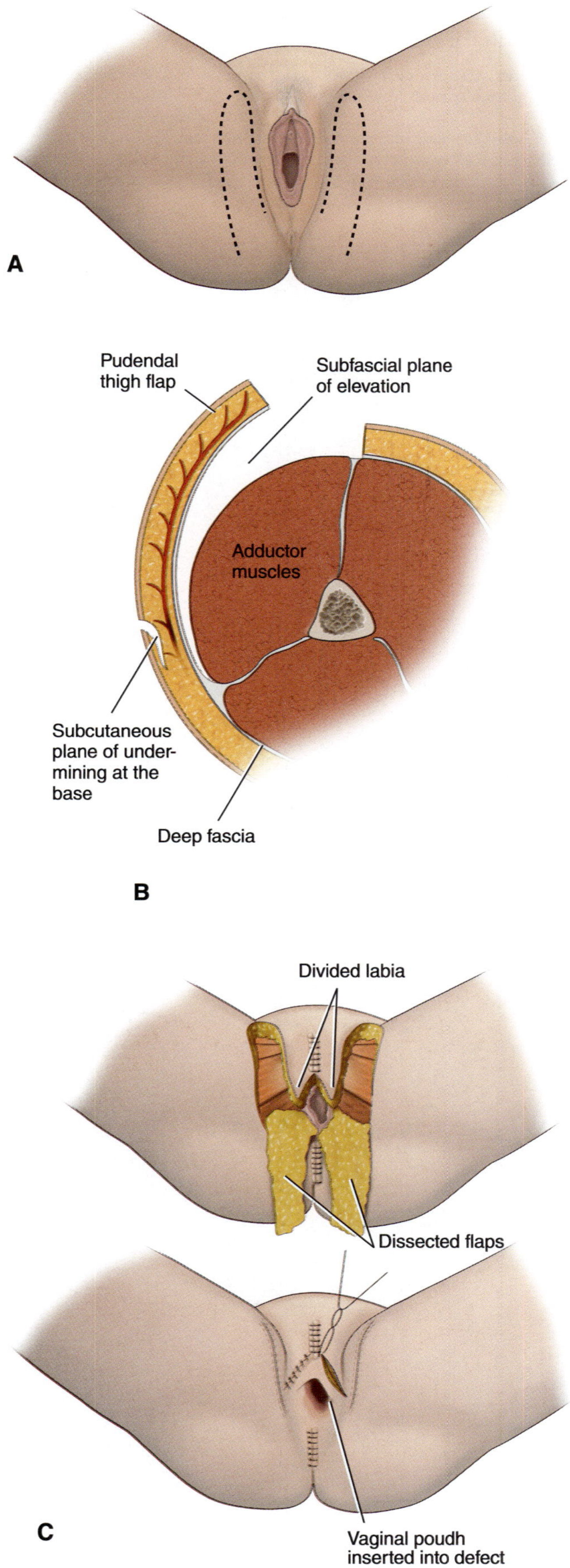

FIGURE 50-8 Singapore flap. (**A**) Flap design. (**B**) Plane of dissection for flap elevation. (**C**) Modified Singapore flap.

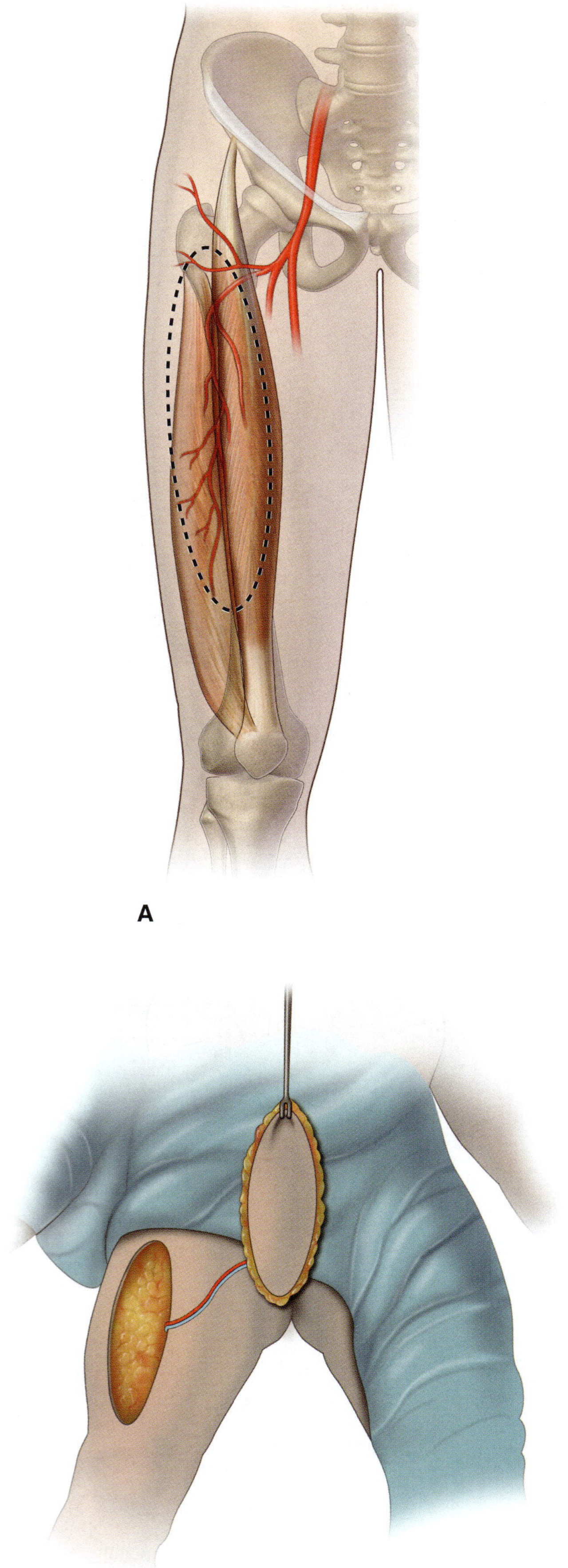

A

B

FIGURE 50-9 Anterolateral thigh flap: location and vascular supply.

described the first use of a posterior gluteal thigh flap for vaginal reconstruction (28). The posterior gluteal thigh flap can also be combined with other flaps and mesh to repair pelvic and vulvar defects (29).

When used in vaginal reconstruction, the flap is centered on the posterior thigh and can be sensate. The donor site is usually closed primarily, but if a wide flap is needed, the donor site may require a skin graft. The flap is transferred to the perineum through a subcutaneous tunnel. The buried portion of the flap is deepithelialized.

Operative Technique

The pedicle is located along a vertical line drawn from the midpoint between the femoral trochanter and the ischial tuberosity. The inferior gluteal artery can be mapped with a handheld Doppler probe. The flap is designed as a triangle based along the infragluteal crease. The dissection starts distally, just cranial to the popliteal fossa (Figure 50-10). The fasciocutaneous flap is elevated and centered along the descending pedicle. The course of the artery can be marked with the use of a handheld Doppler device. Proximally, the skin is incised and dissected superficially. The flap is then transferred to the perineal area through a subcutaneous tunnel, which should be inferior to the ischial tuberosity. The cutaneous nerve accompanies the vessels, so the flap can be harvested as a sensate flap.

The flap can be designed as an island on the mid to distal portion of the posterior thigh based on the inferior gluteal vessels, which travel under the gluteus maximus muscle. The subcutaneous tissue, including the neurovascular pedicle, is dissected superiorly toward the inferior gluteal vessels. The flap then can be tunneled to reach the vulvovaginal defect (30). The posterior thigh flap can also be combined with other flaps and mesh to reconstruct pelvic and vulvar defects (31).

GLUTEAL PERFORATOR FLAPS

Superior and inferior gluteal perforator flaps can be raised based on medial perforators and rotated into perineal and posterior vaginal defects (Figure 50-11) (31). These flaps remove the donor site from the primary operative site, so they are useful when stomas would interfere with flap harvest from the abdominal wall. V-Y advancement flaps can be based on the gluteal perforators to cover sacral and perineal defects (32,33). If the patient is in the prone position for the ablative portion of the procedure, the use of gluteal flaps obviates the need for repositioning.

OMENTAL FLAP

Omental tissue is relatively thin but very pliable and is predominantly supplied by the right and left gastroepiploic vessels. The entire omentum can be harvested based on one set of these vessels. Ligation of the left gastroepiploic and short gastric vessels allows for interpolation of the omentum into the lower abdominal and pelvic areas (Figure 50-12) (34). Internal dissection of the omentum into a "Y" or "W" configuration elongates the flap and allows for repair of smaller defects or a

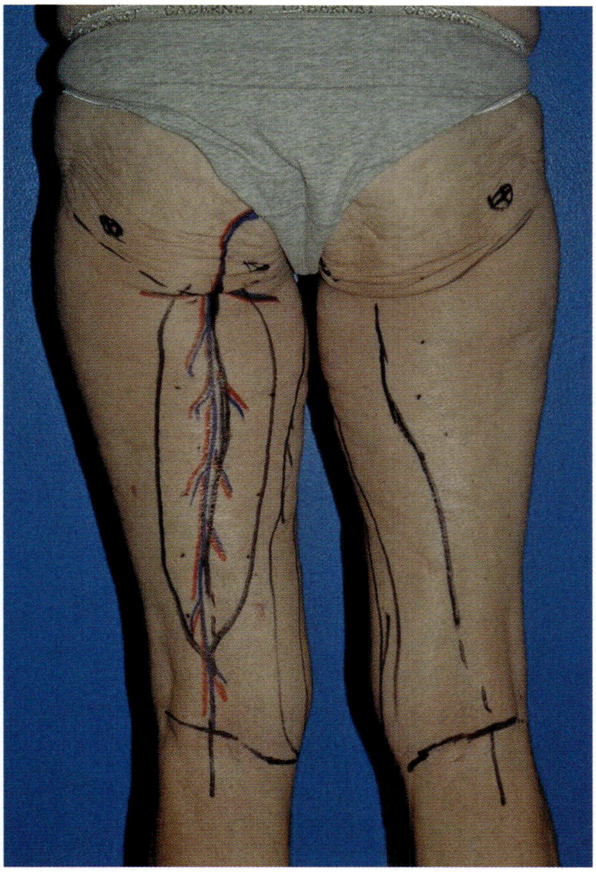

A

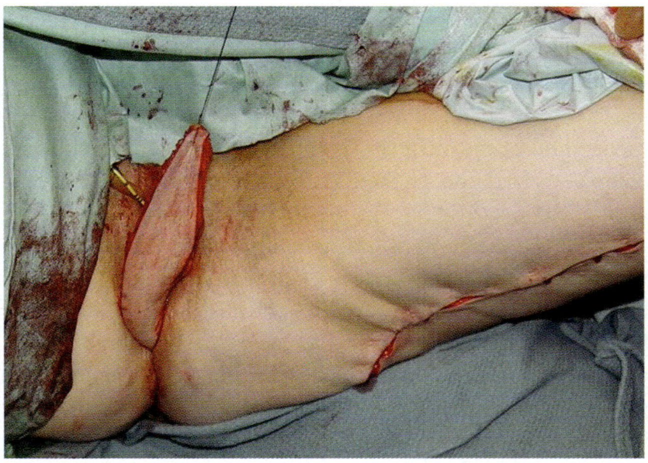

B

FIGURE 50-10 Gluteal thigh flap. (**A**) Location and flap design. (**B**) Elevation and transfer of the flap into a perineal defect.

persistent perineal sinus tract (2). A shortcoming of the omental flap is that it does not include a skin paddle.

MICROVASCULAR RECONSTRUCTION

Pedicled flaps are the mainstay of perineal and vaginal reconstruction. However, in cases of extensive defects or injury to the vascular pedicle of what would otherwise be the available pedicled flaps, microvascular tissue transfer may be an option.

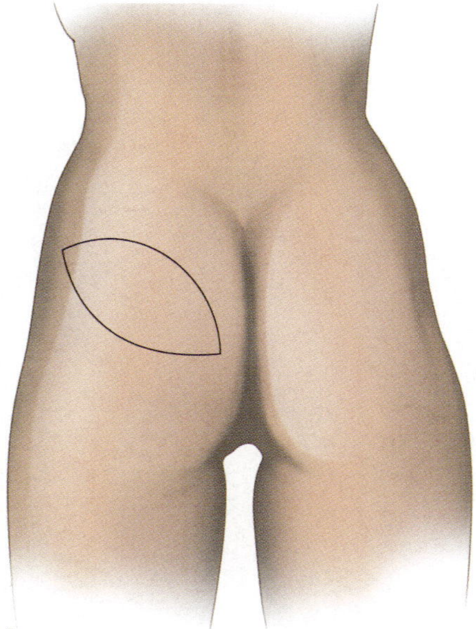

A

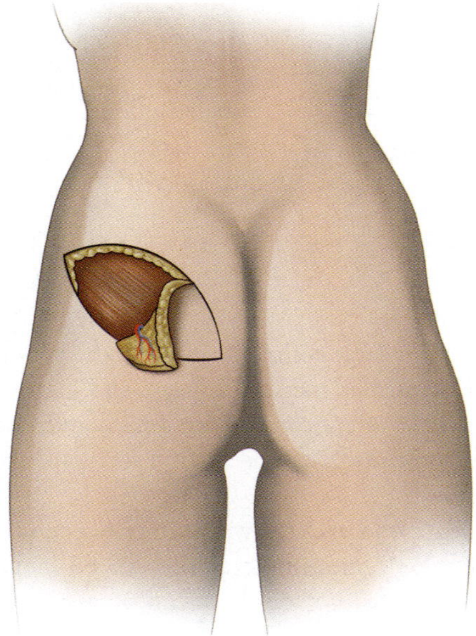

B

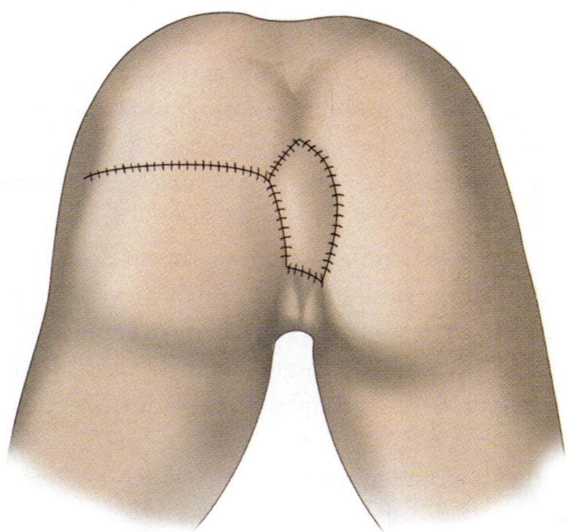

C

FIGURE 50-11 Gluteal flap. (**A**) Flap design for a posterior defect. (**B**) Flap elevation based on a superior gluteal artery perforator. (**C**) Flap inset and donor site closure.

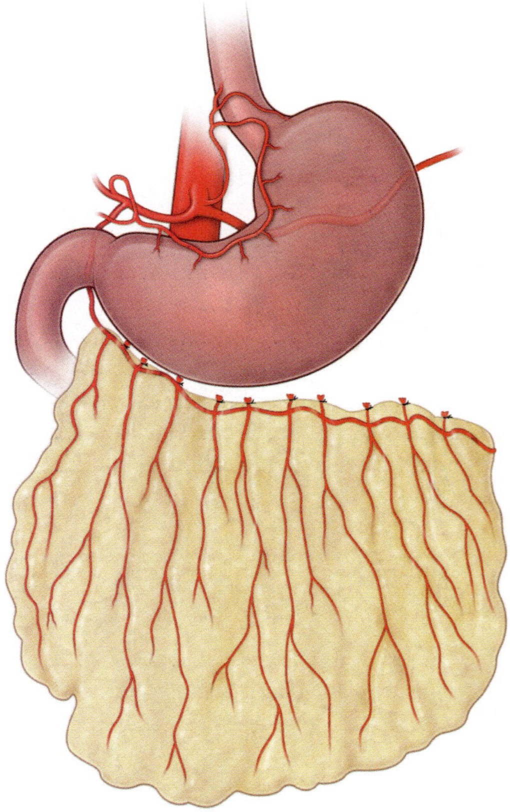

FIGURE 50-12 Omentum: anatomy and vascular supply.

There are no large recipient vessels in the perineal region for direct microvascular transfer. Instead, the intraperitoneal vessels, such as the inferior mesenteric vessels and vascular cascade within the omentum, can be used in free flap transfers to this region (35).

In patients who undergo wide tumor resection for low rectal cancer, a colonic mesenteric arcade can be mobilized during colon resection to provide the recipient vessels for free tissue transfer to repair perineal defects.

The gastroepiploic vessels have been used for more than a decade as recipient vessels for free tissue transfer in abdominal wall reconstruction (36). When used in perineal reconstruction, the omentum is divided along the right or left gastroepiploic vessels (37) to mobilize the omentum so that it can reach the pelvic region. The vascular cascade within the omentum can then be used as recipient vessels for microvascular anastomosis (38).

Even when the rectus abdominis muscles are not available for transfer to the perineum because of previous procedures or the presence of a stoma, the deep inferior mesenteric vessels may still be present and patent. In such cases, the DIE artery and veins can serve as recipient vessels for free tissue transfer (39).

Another alternative is the greater saphenous vein. This vein can be harvested distally while preserving its proximal connection to the femoral system. The distal end of the vein is then anastomosed to the superficial femoral artery or one of its branches, creating an arteriovenous (AV) fistula (Figure 50-13) (40). The resulting venous loop is tunneled to the perineal area and used as recipient vessels for a free flap. This technique requires only one additional anastomosis compared with typical arterial and venous vein grafting. The tissue transfer can be performed during the same procedure or in a delayed fashion (7–10 days later) to allow for maturation of the AV fistula. Other veins, such as the cephalic or lesser saphenous veins, can be used as traditional vein grafts to femoral vascular branches to provide adequate recipient vessels for free tissue transfer to the perineum.

For posterior perineal defects, the gluteal artery and vein can also serve as recipient vessels for free flap reconstruction (41).

Various flaps have been used for free tissue transfer to the perineum. The latissimus dorsi muscle, which is supplied by the thoracodorsal vessels, provides a large, versatile muscle flap with a relatively long, large-caliber pedicle (Figure 50-14) (34). The latissimus dorsi musculocutaneous flap can be used to repair a perineal defect that includes a skin deficit (35,41).The latissimus dorsi flap can be harvested endoscopically to reduce donor site morbidity (42).

Operative Technique for Vascular Anastomoses With an Arteriorvenous (AV) Loop

In free tissue transfer to the perineum, the anastomoses are performed with standard atraumatic microvascular techniques. Because of the potential for postoperative shifting of the abdominal contents in patients with perineal defects, the vascular pedicle has to be long enough to allow for movement of the tissues. The pedicle should not traverse open spaces, such as the pelvic inlet, to avoid tethering from the weight of the viscera when the patient is in an upright position.

The flap ischemia time should be kept to a minimum. The preparation of the recipient vessels should be performed before complete separation of the flap from its circulation if technically possible.

Patients undergoing free tissue transfer should receive a deep vein thrombosis prophylaxis as indicated. Their body temperature should be kept close to 37°C during surgery; an underbody warming blanket may be indicated because a large portion of the body is exposed in the surgical field. Throughout the procedure, normovolemia is maintained. This is especially important at the time of the microvascular anastomoses. An anastomotic coupler may be used for the venous anastomosis.

An implantable Doppler probe can be used to monitor buried flaps or those whose skin paddle is not easily accessible for monitoring.

In the immediate postoperative period, the patient should have complete bed rest in a bed with a fluidized mattress. The patient can be mobilized 24 to 48 hours after the surgery. During transfers in and out of bed, extreme caution must be used to avoid any undue tension on the perineal closure; the patient may need to be "log rolled" in and out of bed. Depending on the type of flap, a sitting regimen can be started 3 to 4 days after surgery, starting with short periods; a direct visual flap check must be made at the end of each sitting period. The flap perfusion should be checked before and after each major repositioning of the patient. An implantable Doppler

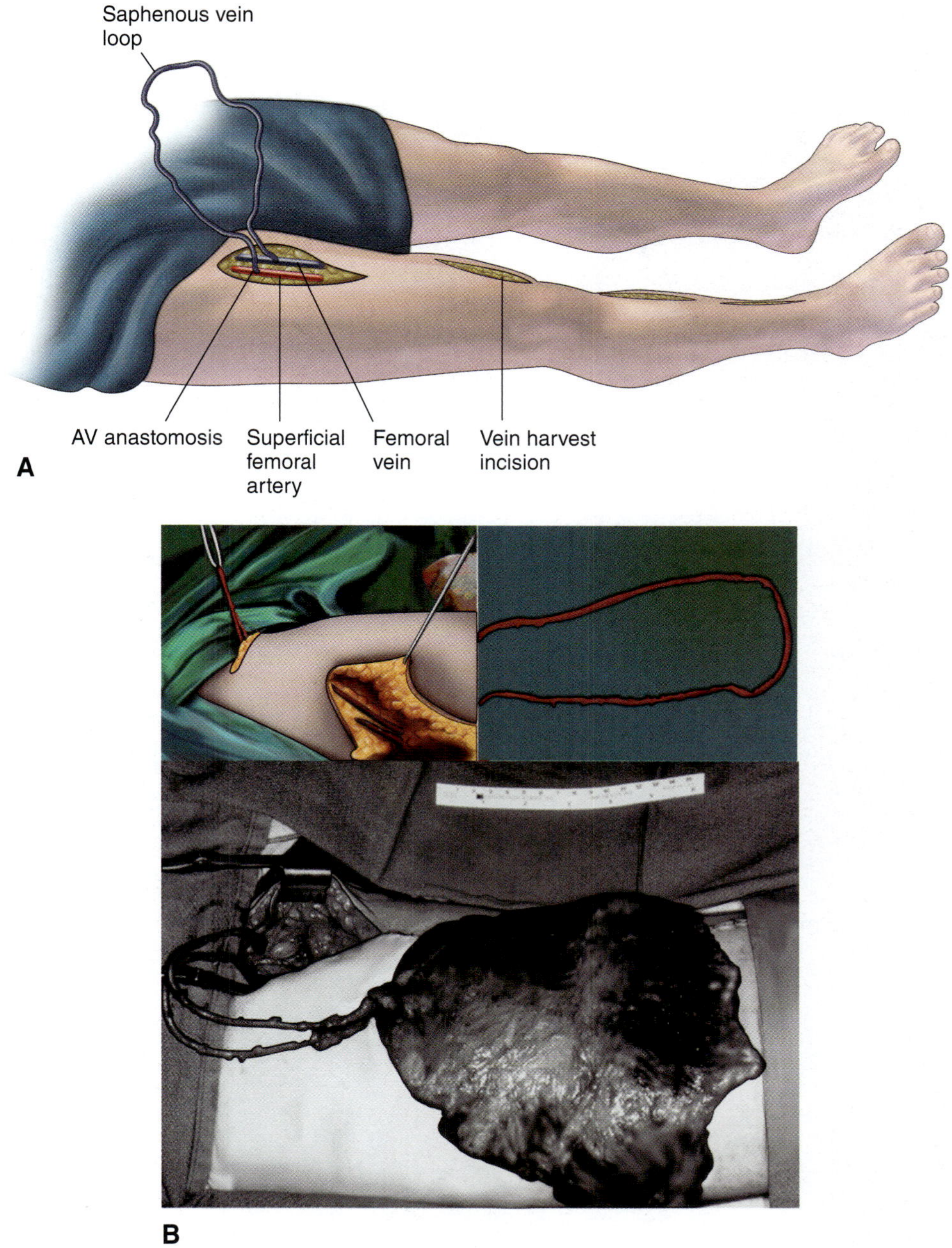

FIGURE 50-13 Saphenous vein loop for microvascular tissue transfer involves harvest of the greater saphenous vein from the ankle to sapheno-femoral junction and anastomosis to the superficial femoral artery system. (**A**) Saphenous vein loop transposed to the groin. (**B**) Free latissimus muscle connected to the saphenous vein loop.

provides continuous monitoring of the flap perfusion while the patient is in the sitting position.

VAGINAL RECONSTRUCTION

Vaginal reconstruction requires a relatively large epithelialized surface to create a tubular neovagina. Congenital vaginal defects are commonly repaired with local tissues. In many cases of vaginal agenesis, the local perineal tissue can be stretched and expanded over time to create a cavity resembling the normal vaginal vault (43).

In the late 1800s, Abbe described a method of surgically creating an opening in the perineum and covering it with a skin graft. When this technique is used, patients require use of dilators to avoid secondary stenosis.

When the vaginal defect results from resection or trauma, regional pedicled flaps, such as the Singapore and gracilis musculocutaneous flaps, can be used for vaginal reconstruction. Extirpation of colorectal and gynecologic tumors accounts for many cases requiring complex reconstruction of the perineum and vagina with regional and distant flaps. To further complicate these cases, many of the patients have received radiation to the perineum.

Cordeiro et al. proposed a classification system for acquired vaginal defects as a guide for treatment planning (44): anterior and lateral partial vaginal defects (type IA) (Figure 50-15) are repaired with a pudendal thigh flap. Posterior vaginal wall defects are repaired with a rectus abdominis flap. Circumferential defects of the upper two thirds of the vagina (type IIA) are repaired with tubed rectus abdominis flaps. Total circumferential

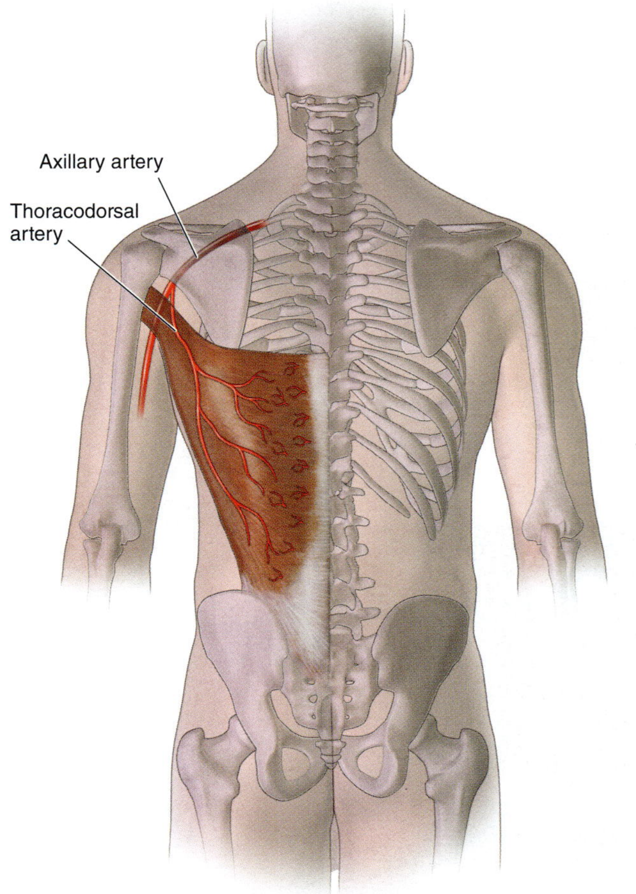

FIGURE 50-14 Latissimus dorsi muscle flap and its blood supply.

defects (type IIB) are repaired with bilateral gracilis or pudendal thigh flaps.

Various types of enteric, jejunal, and colon flaps can also be used for repair of a total vaginal defect (45).

FLAP INSET

Generally, flaps in the perineal and vaginal region are inset with layered closure. The bulk of the flap must be stabilized in the pelvis to avoid delayed descent and bulging of the perineum. Closure of the pelvic inlet reduces the risk of future herniation.

When a rectus abdominis flap is used for reconstruction of a circumferential vaginal defect, the flap is tubed before being inset in the pelvis. Before the abdomen is closed, the surgeon must assure that the vascular pedicle is not kinked or twisted.

Both peritoneal and perineal drains are used to assist with primary healing of the external incisions by preventing seepage of peritoneal fluid and seroma formation.

COMPLICATIONS

Potential complications related to perineal and vaginal reconstruction include bleeding, infection, seroma, delayed wound healing, and partial or complete flap loss. The type and extent of the complications may dictate whether the patient requires a return to the operating room. Problems with the perfusion of free flaps require urgent reoperation to increase the chance of flap salvage. Wound separation is common in the perineal region and can usually be successfully treated with dressing changes allowing

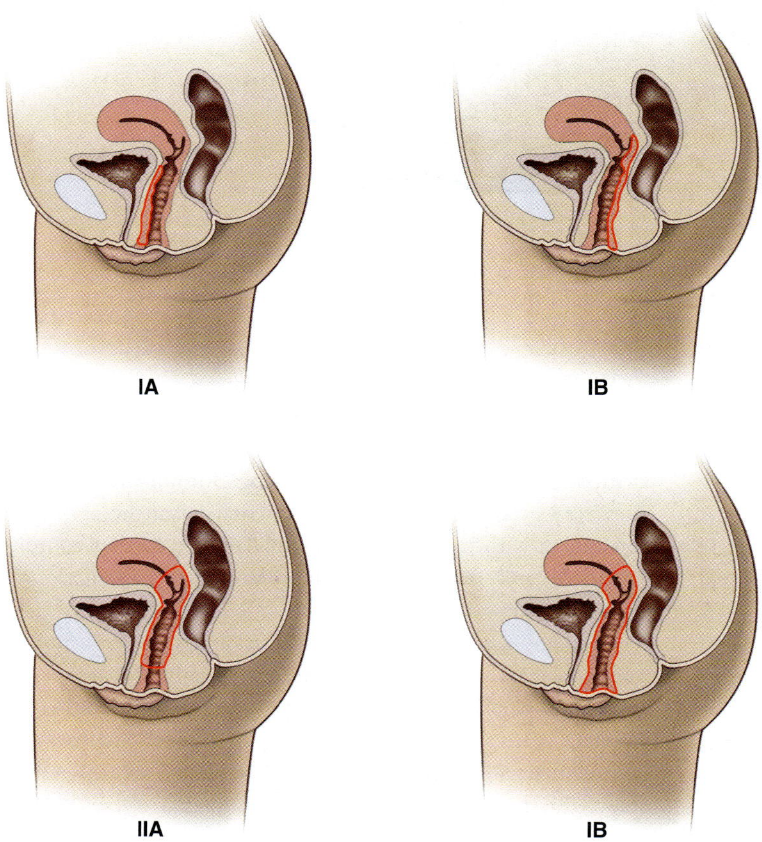

FIGURE 50-15 Cordeiro et al. (44) classification of vaginal defects.

healing by secondary intention. Partial skin-paddle flap necrosis can usually be tackled with debridement and flap readvancement. Some perineal wounds become chronic, particularly those that are large and have received previous radiotherapy. These wounds are often treated with negative-pressure wound therapy devices and occasionally require salvage free flap reconstruction.

REFERENCES

1. Ninkovic M, Dabernig W. Flap technology for reconstructions of urogenital organs. *Curr Opin Urol* 2003;13:483.
2. Lohsiriwat V. Persistent perineal sinus: incidence, pathogenesis, risk factors, and management. *Surg Today* 2009;39:189.
3. Nisar PJ, Scott HJ. Myocutaneous flap reconstruction of the pelvis after abdominoperineal excision. *Colorectal Dis* 2009;11:806.
4. Butler CE, Gundeslioglu AO, Rodriguez-Bigas MA. Outcomes of immediate vertical rectus abdominis myocutaneous flap reconstruction for irradiated abdominoperineal resection defects. *J Am Coll Surg* 2008;206:694.
5. Skipworth RJ, Smith GH, Anderson DN. Secondary perineal hernia following open abdominoperineal excision of the rectum: report of a case and review of the literature. *Hernia* 2007;11:541.
6. Buck DW, Khalifeh M, Redett RJ. Plastic surgery repair of abdominal wall and pelvic floor defects. *Urol Oncol* 2007;25:160.
7. Shukla HS, Hughes LE. The rectus abdominis flap for perineal wounds. *Ann R Coll Surg Engl* 1984;66:337.
8. Abbott DE, Halverson AL, Wayne JD, et al. The oblique rectus abdominal myocutaneous flap for complex pelvic wound reconstruction. *Dis Colon Rectum* 2008;51:1237.
9. Villa M, Saint-Cyr M, Wong C, et al. Extended vertical rectus abdominis myocutaneous flap for pelvic reconstruction: three-dimensional and four-dimensional computed tomography angiographic perfusion study and clinical outcome analysis. *Plast Reconstr Surg* 2011;127:200.
10. Campbell C, Butler CE. *Optimizing Surgical Outcome after Complex Reconstruction of Pelvic Cancer Defects with the Vertical Rectus abdominis Myocutaneous Flap.* ASPS Annual Scientific Meeting. Vol 126. Toronto, Canada, 2010, p. 79.
11. Weiwei L, Zhifei L, Ang Z, et al. Vaginal reconstruction with the muscle-sparing vertical rectus abdominis myocutaneous flap. *J Plast Reconstr Aesthet Surg* 2009;62:335.
12. Baumann DP, Butler CE. Component separation improves outcomes in VRAM flap donor sites with excessive fascial tension. *Plast Reconstr Surg* 2010;126:1573.
13. Nelson RA, Butler CE. Surgical outcomes of VRAM versus thigh flaps for immediate reconstruction of pelvic and perineal cancer resection defects. *Plast Reconstr Surg* 2009;123:175.
14. McCraw JB, Massey FM, Shanklin KD, et al. Vaginal reconstruction with gracilis myocutaneous flaps. *Plast Reconstr Surg* 1976;58:176.
15. Persichetti P, Cogliandro A, Marangi GF, et al. Pelvic and perineal reconstruction following abdominoperineal resection: the role of gracilis flap. *Ann Plast Surg* 2007;59:168.
16. Noack N, Spierer R. [Uni- and bilateral pedicled muscular gracilis flaps for reconstruction of the scrotum in Fournier's gangrene]. *Handchir Mikrochir Plast Chir* 2009;41(4):248–251.
17. Furst A, Schmidbauer C, Swol-Ben J, et al. Gracilis transposition for repair of recurrent anovaginal and rectovaginal fistulas in Crohn's disease. *Int J Colorectal Dis* 2008;23:349.
18. Ducic I, Dayan JH, Attinger CE, et al. Complex perineal and groin wound reconstruction using the extended dissection technique of the gracilis flap. *Plast Reconstr Surg* 2008;122:472.
19. Wee JT, Joseph VT. A new technique of vaginal reconstruction using neurovascular pudendal-thigh flaps: a preliminary report. *Plast Reconstr Surg* 1989;83:701.
20. Woods JE, Alter G, Meland B, et al. Experience with vaginal reconstruction utilizing the modified Singapore flap. *Plast Reconstr Surg* 1992;90:270.
21. Gleeson NC, Baile W, Roberts WS, et al. Pudendal thigh fasciocutaneous flaps for vaginal reconstruction in gynecologic oncology. *Gynecol Oncol* 1994;54:269.
22. Gleeson N, Baile W, Roberts WS, et al. Surgical and psychosexual outcome following vaginal reconstruction with pelvic exenteration. *Eur J Gynaecol Oncol* 1994;15:89.
23. Tham NL, Pan WR, Rozen WM, et al. The pudendal thigh flap for vaginal reconstruction: pptimising flap survival. *J Plast Reconstr Aesthet Surg* 2009;63:826.
24. Song YG, Chen GZ, Song YL. The free thigh flap: a new free flap concept based on the septocutaneous artery. *Br J Plast Surg* 1984;37:149.
25. Ng RW, Chan JY, Mok V, et al. Clinical use of a pedicled anterolateral thigh flap. *J Plast Reconstr Aesthet Surg* 2008;61:158.
26. Sun BD, Wu M, Shen K, et al. [Vulvar form reconstruction in extended radical vulvectomy of vulvar carcinoma]. *Zhonghua Fu Chan Ke Za Zhi* 2006;41:540.
27. Hurwitz DJ, Swartz WM, Mathes SJ. The gluteal thigh flap: a reliable, sensate flap for the closure of buttock and perineal wounds. *Plast Reconstr Surg* 1981;68:521.
28. Achauer BM, Braly P, Berman ML, et al. Immediate vaginal reconstruction following resection for malignancy using the gluteal thigh flap. *Gynecol Oncol* 1984;19:79.
29. Said HK, Bevers M, Butler CE. Reconstruction of the pelvic floor and perineum with human acellular dermal matrix and thigh flaps following pelvic exenteration. *Gynecol Oncol* 2007;107:578.
30. Rosen JM, Mo ST, Liu A. Experience with the island inferior gluteal thigh flap compared with other local flaps for the reconstruction of the pelvic area. *Ann Plast Surg* 1990;24:498.
31. Wagstaff MJ, Rozen WM, Whitaker IS, et al. Perineal and posterior vaginal wall reconstruction with superior and inferior gluteal artery perforator flaps. *Microsurgery* 2009;29:626.
32. Benito P, Garcia J, De Juan A, et al. Reconstruction of a perianal defect by means of a bilateral V-Y advancement flap based on the perforating arteries of the gluteus maximus shaped over a cicatricial area. *J Plast Reconstr Aesthet Surg* 2009;62:412.
33. Di Mauro D, D'Hoore A, Penninckx F, et al. V-Y Bilateral gluteus maximus myocutaneous advancement flap in the reconstruction of large perineal defects after resection of pelvic malignancies. *Colorectal Dis* 2008;11:508.
34. Mathes SJ, Nahai F. *Reconstructive Surgery: Principles, Anatomy, and Technique*, vol 1.St. Louis: Churchill Livingstone and Quality Medical Publishing, 1997.
35. Petrie N, Branagan G, McGuiness C, et al. Reconstruction of the perineum following anorectal cancer excision. *Int J Colorectal Dis* 2009;24:97.
36. Sekido M, Yamamoto Y, Sugihara T, et al. Microsurgical reconstruction of chest- and abdominal-wall defects associated with intraperitoneal vessels. *J Reconstr Microsurg* 1996;12:425.
37. Clement RW, Young VL, Marsh JL. Use of the greater omentum as a vascular supply for free-flap transfer. *Plast Reconstr Surg* 1984;74:131.
38. Koshima I, Nanba Y, Tutsui T, et al. Dynamic reconstruction of large abdominal defects using a free rectus femoris musculocutaneous flap with normal motor function. *Ann Plast Surg* 2003;50:420.
39. Penington AJ, Theile DR, MacLeod AM, et al. Free tensor fasciae latae flap reconstruction of defects of the chest and abdominal wall: selection of recipient vessels. *Scand J Plast Reconstr Surg Hand Surg* 1996;30:299.
40. Vogt PM, Steinau HU, Spies M, et al. Outcome of simultaneous and staged microvascular free tissue transfer connected to arteriovenous loops in areas lacking recipient vessels. *Plast Reconstr Surg* 2007;120:1568.
41. Miles WK, Chang DW, Kroll SS, et al. Reconstruction of large sacral defects following total sacrectomy. *Plast Reconstr Surg* 2000;105:2387.
42. Miller MJ, Robb GL. Endoscopic technique for free flap harvesting. *Clin Plast Surg* 1995;22:755.
43. Lesavoy MA. Vaginal reconstruction. *Urol Clin North Am* 1985;12:369.
44. Cordeiro PG, Pusic AL, Disa JJ. A classification system and reconstructive algorithm for acquired vaginal defects. *Plast Reconstr Surg* 2002;110:1058.
45. Emiroglu M, Gultan SM, Adanali G, et al. Vaginal reconstruction with free jejunal flap. *Ann Plast Surg* 1996;36:316.

CHAPTER 51

Penoscrotal Reconstruction

Stan Monstrey, Piet Hoebeke

INDICATIONS FOR PENOSCROTAL RECONSTRUCTION

Congenital Genital Anomalies

Exstrophy and Epispadias

Exstrophy of the bladder is an uncommon condition that occurs in approximately one of every 30,000 live births, of which boys predominate in a 3:1 ratio (1,2). The defining features of exstrophy and epispadias are an open urinary tract with a protruding bladder and foreshortened epispadiac penis often combined with diastasis recti and absence of fusion of the pubic symphysis (Figure 51-1).

Although the initial postnatal diagnosis and treatment of bladder exstrophy and epispadias remain in the realm of the pediatric urologist (closure of the bladder) and pediatric orthopedic surgeon (reconstruction of the pelvic ring), it is important that the plastic surgeon be prepared, if consulted, to help reconstruction in such a child.

Different techniques have been described for penile reconstruction (3,4), and although the results of the urethral closure have drastically improved, the ideal surgical approach is still controversial. Phallic length mainly depends on antenatal development, and the majority of these patients end up with small and undeveloped penises despite the best efforts of their treating surgeons. As they pass through their postadolescent period, many of these young men will benefit from further lengthening procedures or even complete penile reconstruction. Exstrophy patients miss an umbilicus, and often they are consulting for umbilical reconstruction. Different techniques have been described with good cosmetic outcomes (5,6).

Unfortunately, in some boys, there just is not enough tissue because of underdevelopment or partial or complete loss of penile tissue after primary closure. These patients might be good candidates to undergo a phallic construction or further penile reconstruction with the use of microsurgical tissue transplantation techniques (Figure 51-2) or local pedicled perforator flaps.

Disorders of Sex Development

After standardization of the terminology, intersex conditions are now defined as disorders of sexual development (DSDs) (formerly "intersex") (7). DSD is not within the scope of this text, but the DSD classification includes conditions such as penile agenesis, extreme penoscrotal transposition with a rudimentary penis, cloacal exstrophy, micropenis, and other genital malformations with normal chromosomes and gonads. In most cases of genital ambiguity, reconstruction is done after gender assignment, which is not always obvious. Multidisciplinary teams with a lot of expertise in these pathologies are needed to guide the diagnosis and treatment in these children.

Traumatic Genital Defects

Posttraumatic genital repair is an uncommon but special chapter in surgical reconstruction. The anatomically protected position of the genitalia implies that patients who have genital injuries often have large concomitant injuries. Resuscitation and life support of the patient take precedent over any reconstruction. However, genital reconstruction is of prime relevance, and only hand, eyelid, and lip reconstructions are considered more important in the reconstructive hierarchy. Moreover, aesthetics are foremost in genital reconstruction, and the appearance of the genitalia is important to the self-esteem of a patient who is recovering from trauma. Interestingly, the genitalia appear to be a "privileged site" such that the usual postreconstructive sequelae of scarring and contracture are often absent.

Fournier's Gangrene

Classically, every necrotizing soft tissue infection in the specific region of the perineum and genitalia is termed *Fournier's gangrene*, the etiology with or without proven infection notwithstanding (8).

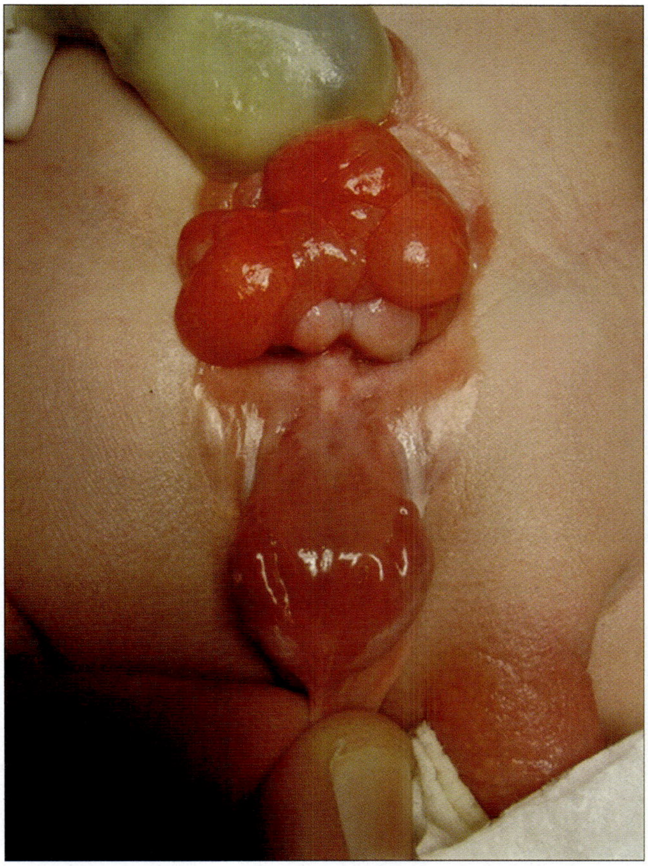

FIGURE 51-1 Exstrophy in a male patient.

Common sources of infection include various urogenital disease and local trauma but also colorectal disease (9). Several systemic conditions, including diabetes mellitus, alcoholism, heavy smoking, and acquired immunodeficiency syndrome, have been associated with Fournier's gangrene and may predispose patients to its development.

A high degree of suspicion is crucial to an early diagnosis, and the presence of marked systemic toxicity and pain out of proportion to the local findings should alert the surgeon. After the disease is identified, intravenous fluid therapy and broad-spectrum antibiotics—but most of all, immediate and aggressive surgical debridement—are critical in providing definitive treatment.

In most cases, reconstruction of the genitalia includes release of the penis and testicles from surrounding granulation tissue; release of scar contracture, and split-thickness skin grafts to the penile shaft and peripenile tissues (Figure 51-3). Flap reconstruction is seldom required.

Penile Skin Cancers

Classically, penile cancer involving the redundant preputial or penile skin can be adequately treated with circumcision or local excision. When penile cancer invades the deep structures, the excision should amount to subtotal or total penectomy. In partial- or subtotal penectomy patients, it is better to sacrifice some more superficial penile tissue, saving the remaining corporal bodies, and to accomplish a true phallic construction. The remnants of the corporal bodies can be incorporated in the base of the reconstructed penis (Figure 51-4). In patients who have had extensive superficial lymph node dissections, there are considerations with regard to recipient vessels. In these patients, angiography is performed to define the deep inferior epigastric vessels and the iliofemoral system. In most cases, surgical oncologists consult reconstructive surgeons before the ablative surgery to ensure that all considerations are recognized.

Female-to-Male Transsexualism

The reconstruction of the male genitalia in a female-to-male (FTM) transsexual individual is the most frequent indication for a phalloplasty. It is more complex than the penile reconstruction in a biologically male patient because of the added difficulties in reconstructing the fixed part of the urethra and the combination with a vaginectomy and a scrotoplasty. This specific indication will be addressed in detail further in this chapter.

METHODS OF RECONSTRUCTION

Overview of Reconstructive Options

Genital Skin Grafts

Genital skin loss occurs from burns, avulsion injuries, infections, and gangrene. As a rule, total excision of the necrotic genital tissues followed by early skin grafting produces the best results (Figure 51-5). Successful skin graft "take" is directly related to a well-vascularized wound bed, meticulous hemostasis, control of erections, infection-free environment, and adequate immobilization (10). Often a one-to-one perforated (only) split-thickness skin graft is used.

Minimally expanded meshed split-thickness skin grafts have been advocated for scrotal reconstruction (11), producing good aesthetic results in this location (see Figure 51-4). Buccal mucosa grafts can be useful in glans reconstruction.

Genital Pedicled and Local Flaps

In larger defects, there often is a need for the use of local muscle or musculocutaneous flaps, fasciocutaneous flaps, and perforator flaps in the field of male genitalia reconstruction.

Nowadays, the gracilis (purely) muscle flap is no longer considered the "workhorse of the perineum," but this muscle flap still is useful to cover and vascularize urethral anastomoses, cover exposed pelvic bones, reduce the risk of osteomyelitis, fill the perineum after exenteration, and vascularize the perineum in postirradiation injuries (12).

Formerly, more popular musculocutaneous flaps, including the vertical and transverse rectus abdominis flap (based on the deep inferior epigastric artery) (13), the gracilis musculocutaneous flap (14), the rectus femoris musculocutaneous flap (15), and the tensor fasciae lata musculocutaneous flap (16), were used occasionally in genitourinary reconstruction but have only limited use in the reconstruction of male genitalia.

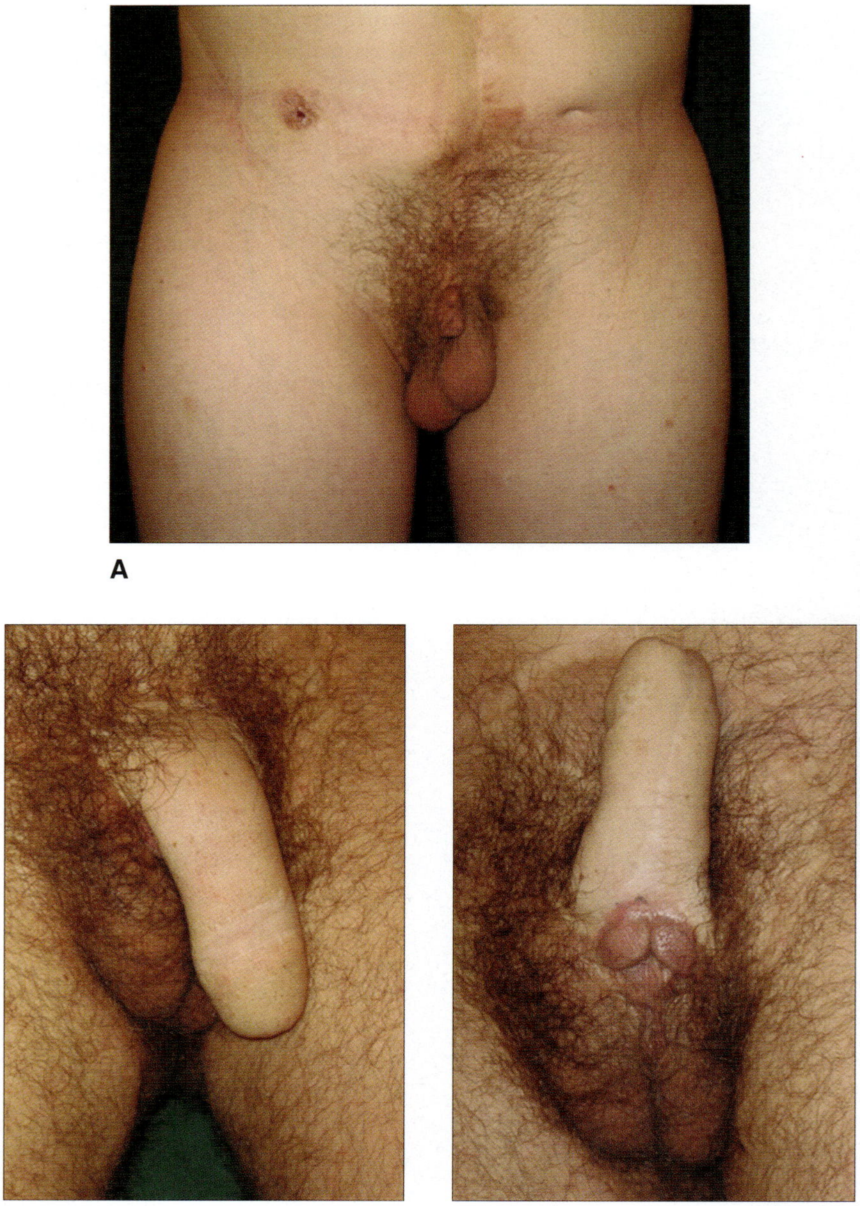

A

B C

FIGURE 51-2 (A) Bladder exstrophy in a patient with a severely underdeveloped penis who requested a complete penile reconstruction with a free radial forearm flap. (B) and (C) Postoperative result after radial forearm phalloplasty with the small glans incorporated at the base of the reconstructed penis.

Nevertheless, these reliable flaps still can be an important part of the surgeon's armamentarium in addressing genital injuries after trauma, infection, and cancer and for patients with comorbid health problems. These flaps are often the only tissues available for genital reconstruction. The trauma, cancer, infection, and comorbid disease that originally contributed to genital tissue loss may also preclude sophisticated microsurgical reconstruction. Thus, these flaps are the only hope for functional, albeit suboptimal, genital reconstruction.

Fasciocutaneous "paragenital" flaps that have been used, often with limited application, are the superficial circumflex iliac flap (17), deep circumflex iliac flap (often combined with an osseous component) (18), superficial inferior epigastric flap (19), double-pedicled composite groin flap (20), anteromedial thigh flap (21), anterolateral thigh (ALT) flap (22), gluteal–posterior thigh flap (23,24) and pudendal thigh flap (25,26). Medial thigh flaps may be based inferiorly on the perineal artery system or superiorly on the external pudendal system and branches of the profunda femoris artery. The inferiorly based flap has been called several names, including the Singapore flap (25) and the pudendal thigh flap (26). Although most descriptions of this flap have focused on vaginal reconstruction and the correction of vesicovaginal and rectovaginal fistulas, this flap has been successfully used for male genital and male urethral construction (27).

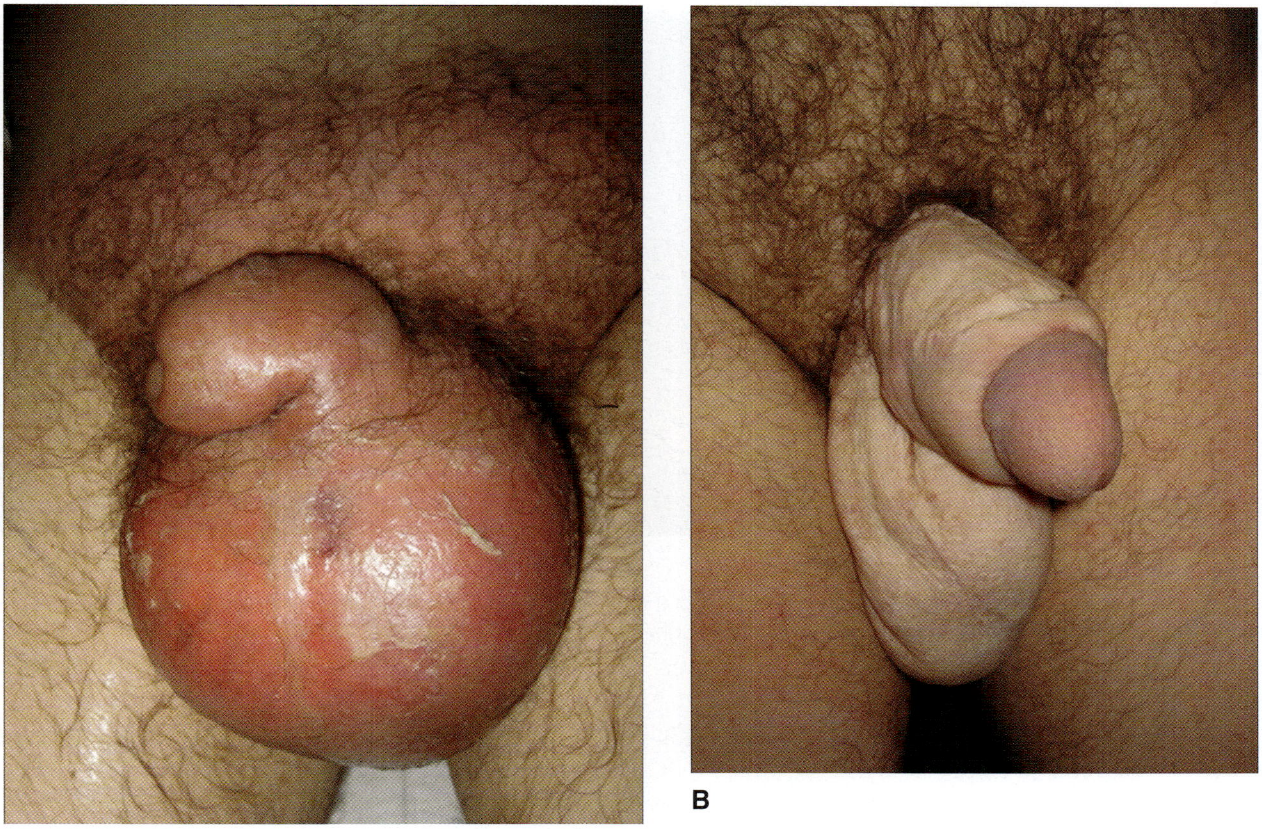

A B

FIGURE 51-3 Fournier gangrene: before debridement (**A**) and after skin grafting (**B**).

In the past decade, the musculocutaneous flaps have increasingly been replaced by their "perforator-type equivalent." Perforator flaps are considered the ultimate form of tissue transfer. Donor site morbidity is reduced to an absolute minimum, the usually large vascular pedicles provide an additional range of motion or an easier vascular anastomosis, and different tissue flaps can be combined on one single pedicle. Useful perforator flaps in the genital region include the perforator flaps originating from the inferior gluteal artery perforator (IGAP) flaps (28) and the pedicled ALT flap, which are discussed more into detail

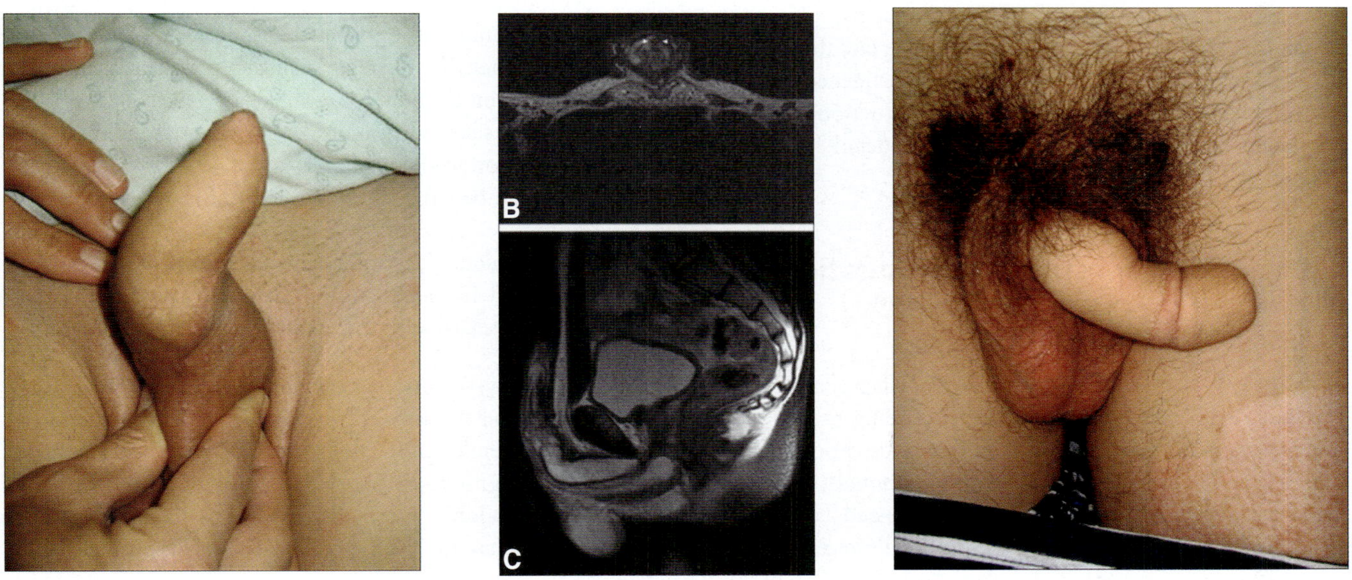

A D

FIGURE 51-4 (**A**) A hard tumor involving the whole circumference of the penis. (**B**) and (**C**) Magnetic resonance images showing disruption of both corpora cavernosa. (**D**) Postoperative result after total penile reconstruction with a free radial forearm flap.

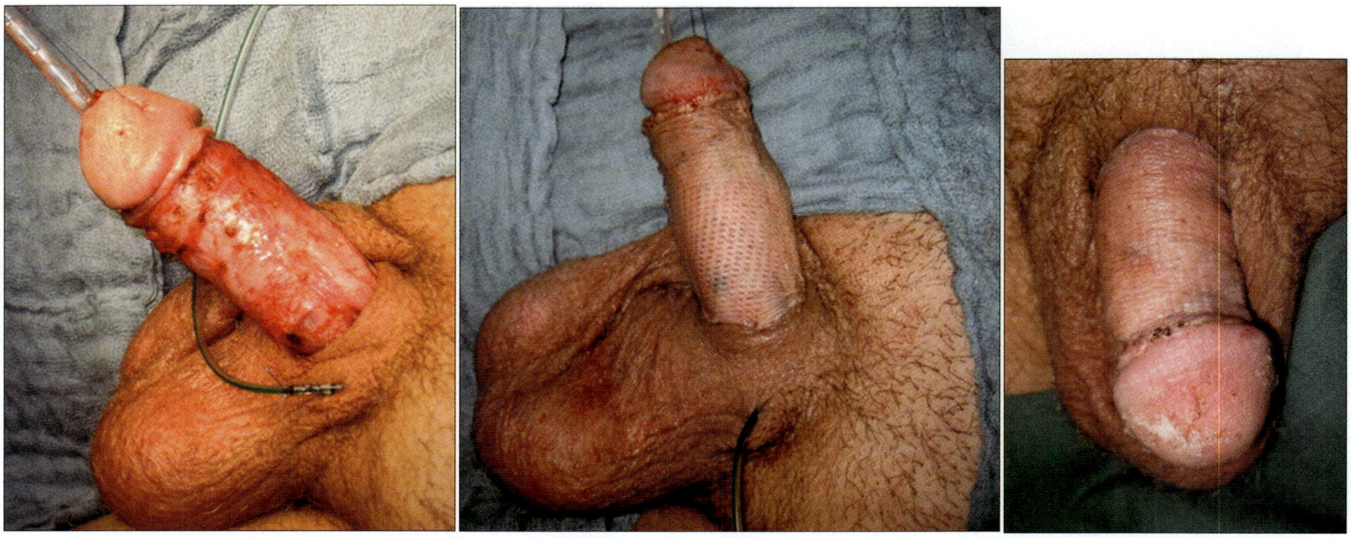

A B C

FIGURE 51-5 (A) A patient with a complete defect of the skin of the penile shaft. (B) The one-to-one perforated split-thickness skin graft is applied and sutured to the shaft. (C) A complete take of the skin graft is obtained.

under penile reconstruction. Additionally, various other pedicled perforator flaps (the so-called "lotus petal flaps") based on the external pudendal artery have also been described as possible options in the perineal area but more so in female patients (29).

Free Flaps

Microsurgical free flaps have been considered state of the art in penile reconstruction (30) because they allow for the selection of distant flaps with the transfer of free vascularized tissue and the cooptation of nerves from the donor flap to recipient nerves in the perineum. The most frequently used free flap for a phalloplasty is the radial forearm flap (RFF), or Chinese flap, which was originally described by Song et al. (31). Various other free flaps have been described, including the dorsalis pedis flap (32), deltoid flap (33), lateral arm flap (34), fibular flap (35), tensor fasciae lata flap (36), and ALT flap (37). The fact that so many techniques for penile reconstruction exist is evidence that none is considered ideal. The design and the construction of the RFF for penile reconstruction are discussed in detail later in the chapter.

Design and Construction of Specific Flaps for Penile Reconstruction

Pedicled Anterolateral Thigh Flap

In "Boys without a Penis" The ALT flap is a perforator flap based on a perforator from the descending branch of the lateral circumflex femoral artery and can be used both as a free flap (13) and as a pedicled flap (38,39). Although, overall, the free vascularized RFF (which will be discussed later) is still considered the "standard technique" in penile reconstruction, the *pedicled* ALT flap has become a new "workhorse" in perineal and male genital reconstruction, specifically in *male* patients with *congenital penile insufficiency or bladder exstrophy* (38,39). There are several reasons why in these "boys without a penis" a pedicled ALT flap can be preferred above the standard RFF (Figure 51-6):

1. A pedicled flap reconstruction avoids the technically more complex microscopic procedure and might also shorten the operation time;
2. A visible donor site scar on the forearm, often considered the signature of FTM transsexualism, is avoided and the donor site on the leg can more easily be concealed.
3. Previous reconstructive surgeries in the pelvis, groin area, and lower abdomen (e.g., in cases of bladder exstrophy) might have altered the local anatomy and vasculature, making a microsurgical anastomosis more difficult.
4. The subcutaneous fat layer is much thinner than in an FTM transsexual patient, facilitating the "(urethral)-tube-within-a-(penile)-tube" reconstruction of the penis; moreover, many exstrophy patients empty their bladders by catheterization through a continent diversion (e.g., appendicovesicostomy) and do not require an urethral reconstruction in the phalloplasty (38,39). An ejaculatory opening can be left at the ventral aspect just above the scrotum.
5. Any useful glandular, penile, and cavernosal tissue can be incorporated at the base of the newly reconstructed phallus to facilitate sexual stimulation and pleasure.

For the above-mentioned reasons, the pedicled ALT thigh flap has become the first choice for phallic reconstruction in patients with penile insufficiency, especially if no urinary reconstruction is required (13,38) such as in patients with bladder exstrophy. In addition, the shape of an ALT phalloplasty is often better than the RFF phalloplasty because of its better volume.

A recent study by Sinove et al. has clearly demonstrated that in case of penile reconstruction with a pedicled ALT flap, it is recommended to perform three-dimensional computed

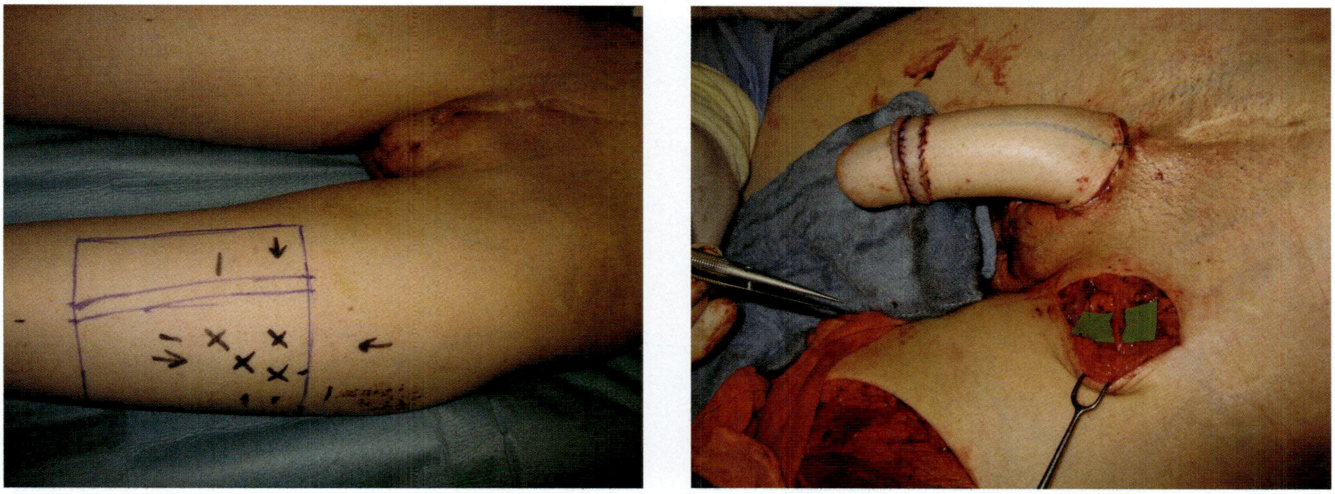

A B

FIGURE 51-6 The reconstruction of a penis with a pedicled anterolateral thigh flap. No real urethra was reconstructed (only distally to imitate a urethral meatus) here because the patient had a urostomy. (**A**) Preoperative view. (**B**) After flap inset. The ilioinguinal nerve was sutured to the lateral femoral cutaneous nerve.

tomography angiography before surgery to provide detailed information on the perforator vessel(s) and the subcutaneous tissue layer (40).

In Female-to-Male Transsexuals The fabrication of an inner tube for urethral conduit makes the ALT flap procedure more complex, especially in a biologically female transsexual patient requesting a penile reconstruction.

Theoretically, a tube-within-a-tube technique providing a good-quality inner lining of the reconstructed urethra, similar to the RFF phalloplasty, could also be performed with a pedicled ALT flap, especially in a thin individual. In most cases, however, folding the flap on itself produces a very large and bulky phallus.

An inner urethral tube can also be provided by prefabricating the ALT flap with a split-thickness skin graft. Still, the quality of the inner urethral tube when lined with skin grafts is inferior to normal skin, resulting in a higher rate of urologic complications (strictures, fistulas).

The urethral tube can also be made from another flap. Possible *pedicled* options are a groin flap (the donor area can be closed primarily), a separate perforator flap of the thigh (41), or using the remnant of a partially failed previous phalloplasty. The inner tube can also be made from a *narrow free RFF*. This flap is thin and very well vascularized (see Figure 51-10). The results of this combined (pedicled ALT + free RFF) phalloplasty procedure were similar to the results of the RFF-only phalloplasty, with regards to the urologic complication rate, and were even more pleasing from an aesthetic point of view. The resulting scar on the arm is small and located on the inner side (Figure 51-7). This scar is easily concealed and acceptable for most FTM transsexuals willing to avoid the circumferential scar. There is no reason to do a free ALT flap as described by Felici et al. because the pedicle of the ALT flap is long enough to reach the pubic area when the flap is transferred underneath the rectus femoris muscles (21,28,29,42).

Free Flap Phalloplasty

Choice of Flap Despite the multitude of free flaps that have been used and described (often as case reports), the RFF is by far the most frequently used technique (>90% of the reported cases) and universally considered the "gold standard" in penile reconstruction (13,30,43–45).

The main advantages of the RFF include the fact that the flap is thin and pliable, thus allowing the reconstruction of a well vascularized and skin-lined urethra with the so-called tube-(the urethra)-within-a-tube (the penis) technique. Moreover, the flap is easy to dissect; is predictably well vascularized; and has the greatest sensitivity of all flaps used for penile reconstruction (44) because of its multiple and easily identifiable sensory nerves, which play an important role in the extent of the recovery of tactile and erogenous sensation in the reconstructed penis.

Radial forearm Flap

Technique In a phalloplasty for an FTM individual, two surgical teams operate at the same time: the urologist in the perineal area performs the vaginectomy, the reconstruction of the fixed part of the urethra, and the scrotoplasty while the plastic surgeon dissects the free vascularized flap on the nondominant forearm (Figure 51-8). The ulnar aspect of the flap is often more hairless and therefore is usually preferred as lining for the urethra and dissected 2 cm more proximally. The medial and lateral antebrachial nerves are easily identified at the beginning of the flap elevation and dissected an additional 5 cm proximal to the skin paddle to facilitate the anastomosis to the nerves in the groin area. The forearm flap itself is dissected in a suprafascial plane, and the creation of a phallus as a tube-within-a-tube technique is performed with the flap still attached to the forearm by its vascular pedicle. A small skin flap and a skin graft are used to create a corona and simulate the (circumcised) glans of the penis.

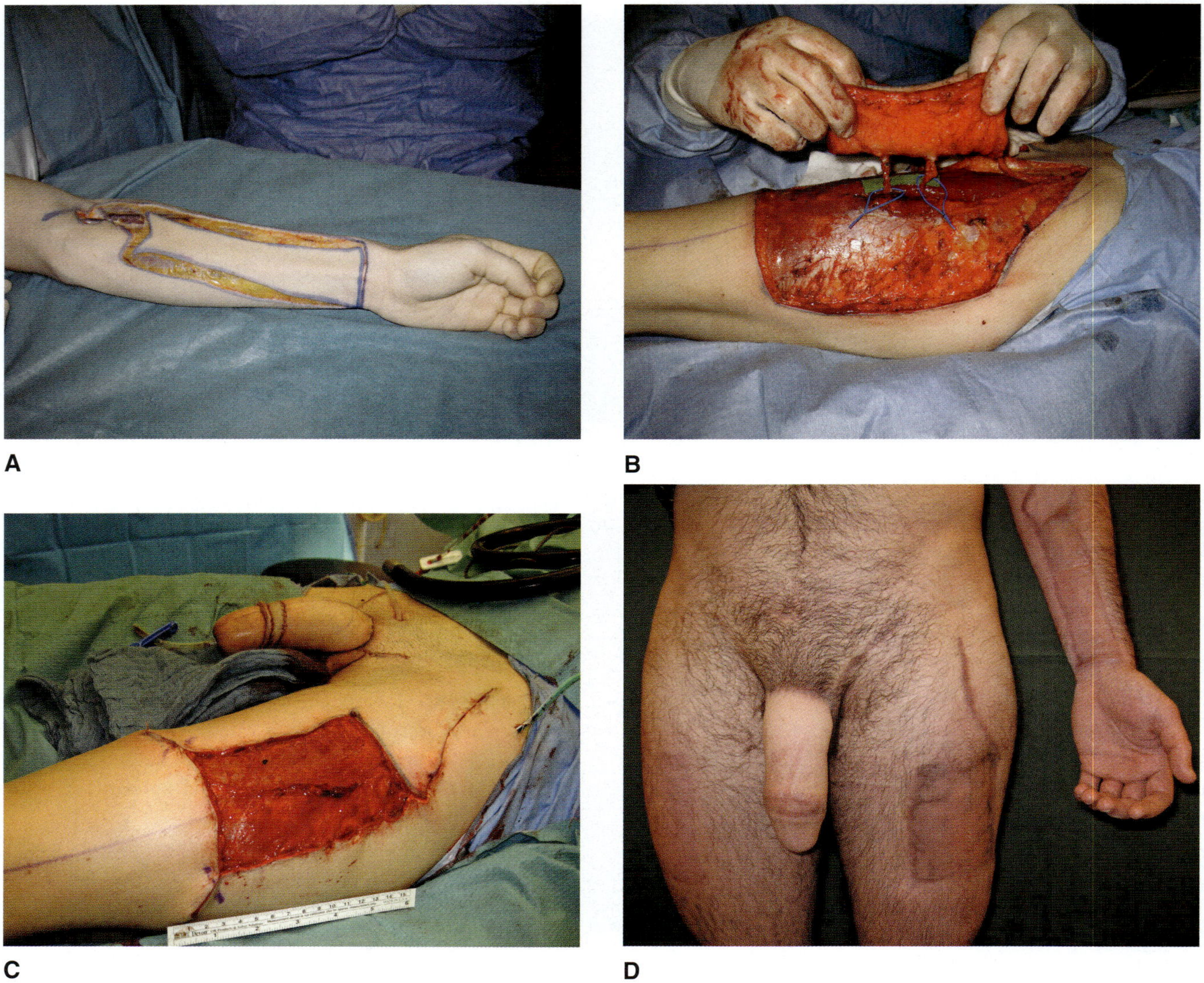

FIGURE 51-7 (**A**) Dissection of a narrow free vascularized radial forearm used for the urethra. (**B**) Dissection of the anterolateral thigh (ALT) flap will be used to wrap around the urethra. (**C**) The radial forearm flap for the urethra and ALT wrap-around put into position in the pubic area, with coronaplasty and grafting of the donor area. (**D**) Result after 9 months. The donor site on the inner aspect of the arm is inconspicuous, and the donor site on the leg can easily be covered even with shorts.

After the urethral stump is prepared and the vessels are dissected in the groin area (through a lower abdominal incision), the free flap is transferred to the pubic area (Figure 51-8E and F). First the urethral anastomosis is performed after which the radial artery is microsurgically connected to the common femoral artery in an end-to-side fashion. The venous anastomosis is performed between the cephalic vein and the greater saphenous vein. One forearm nerve is connected to the ipsilateral ilioinguinal nerve for protective sensation, and the other nerve of the arm is anastomosed to one of the dorsal penile nerves for erogenous sensation.

The defect on the forearm can be covered with full-thickness skin grafts taken from the groin area or with split-thickness skin grafts harvested from the thigh (eventually in combination with a dermal substitute). A better aesthetic aspect of the grafted donor site on the forearm might be obtained by a suprafascial dissection of the flap sparing the paratenon as well as by advancing the skin edges after harvesting of the flap and by putting extra attention to obtain a flat contour of the underlying muscle surface with careful graft placement to avoid additional wrinkling and scarring (13).

Postoperative Follow-up All patients receive a suprapubic urinary diversion after surgery. Similar to any free flap procedure, the vascularization of the penile flap is monitored after surgery, and revision of the vascular anastomosis is performed if necessary (usual in combination with the creation of an arteriovenous fistula distally to improve venous outflow).

The patients remain in bed during a 1-week postoperative period, after which the transurethral catheter is removed. At that time, the suprapubic catheter is clamped, and voiding is begun. Effective voiding may not be observed for several days. Before removal of the suprapubic catheter, a cystography with voiding urethrography is performed.

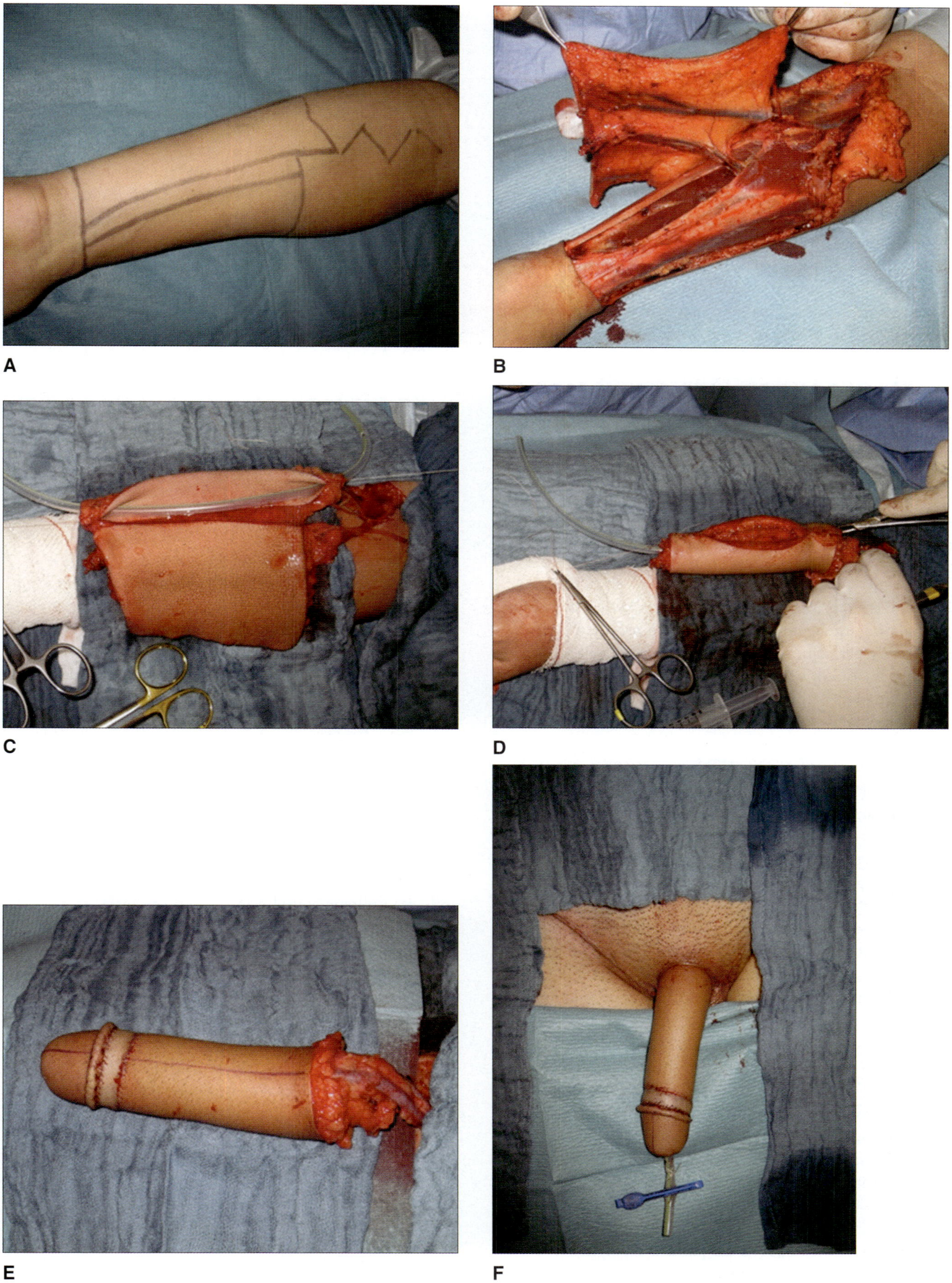

FIGURE 51-8 Standard radial forearm technique: design (A) and dissection (B) of the flap. (C) and (D) Tubing (inner tube) of the urethra and the penis itself (outer tube). (E) Creation of the glans of the penis with penis still attached to the forearm just before transfer to the pubic area. (F) Immediate postoperative result.

The average hospital stay for the phalloplasty procedure is 2.5 weeks.

Postoperative complications can include fistula or stenosis; smaller fistulas usually close by themselves, and most strictures can be resolved by simple dilatation, incision, or both. Only a smaller number of patients require a second surgical procedure (usually urethroplasty).

Tattooing of the glans can be performed after a 2- to 3-month period before sensation returns to the penis and is preferred by the majority of patients.

Implantation of the testicular prostheses can be performed after 6 months, but it is typically done in combination with the implantation of a penile erection prosthesis. Before these procedures are undertaken, sensation must have returned to the top of the penis. This usually does not occur for at least 1 year (13).

OUTCOMES AND RESULTS IN PENOSCROTAL RECONSTRUCTION

In a recent article, Monstrey et al. (13) described the largest series to date of 287 radial forearm phalloplasties performed by the same surgical team. In this large study, they investigated to what degree the radial forearm phalloplasty was able to meet the so-called ideal goals or requirements of a penile reconstruction as described by Hage et al. (46):

1. A one-stage procedure: A complete penile reconstruction, including implantation of an erection prosthesis, can never be performed in one single operation (38). In most cases, the SCM is performed as a first, often in combination with a total hysterectomy and oophorectomy (13,47) with the complete genitoperineal transformation at a later stage.
2. An aesthetic phallus: The RFF has several advantages: the flap is thin and pliable, allowing the construction of a normal sized tube-within-a-tube penis, and the flap is easy to dissect and is predictably well vascularized, making it safe to perform an (aesthetic) glansplasty at the distal end of the flap. The final cosmetic outcome of a radial forearm phalloplasty is a subjective determination, but the ability of most patients to shower with other men or to go to the sauna is the usual cosmetic barometer (Figure 51-9).

   The potential aesthetic drawbacks of the RFF are the need for a rigid prosthesis and possibly some volume loss over time.
3. Tactile and erogenous sensation: Of the various flaps used for penile reconstruction, the RFF has the greatest sensitivity (48). Usually, one antebrachial nerve is connected to the ilioinguinal nerve for protective sensation and the other forearm nerve with one dorsal clitoral nerve. The denuded clitoris was always placed directly below the phallic shaft. Later manipulation of the neophallus allows for stimulation of the still-innervated clitoris. In a long-term follow-up study on postoperative sexual and physical health, more than 80% of the patients reported improvement in sexual satisfaction and greater ease in reaching orgasm—100% in practicing postoperative FTM transsexuals (49).
4. Voiding while standing: For biological males as well as for FTM transsexuals undergoing a phalloplasty, the ability to void while standing is a high priority (50). Unfortunately, the reported incidences of urologic complications, such as urethrocutaneous fistulas, stenoses, strictures, and hairy urethras, are extremely high in all series of phalloplasties, even up to 80% (51–53). In their series of radial forearm phalloplasties, Monstrey et al. (13) still reported a urologic complication rate of 41% (119 of 287), but the majority of these early fistulas closed spontaneously, and ultimately *all* patients were able to void through the newly reconstructed penis (54).
5. Minimal morbidity: The total flap failure in the reported large series is very low (<1% or two of 287) despite a somewhat higher anastomotic revision rate (12% or 34 of 287). About 7.3% of the patients demonstrated some degree of skin slough or partial flap necrosis. This was more often the case in smokers, in those who insisted on a large-sized penis requiring a larger flap, and in patients having undergone anastomotic revision.
6. No functional loss and minimal scarring in the donor area: The major drawback of the RFF has always been the unattractive donor site scar on the forearm (Figure 51-10). Selvaggi et al. conducted a long-term follow-up study 55 of 125 radial forearm phalloplasties to assess the degree of functional loss and aesthetic impairment after harvesting such a large forearm flap and could not identify any major or long-term problem (55). With regard to the aesthetic outcome of the donor site, they found that the patients were very accepting of the donor site scar, viewing it as a worthwhile trade-off for the creation of a phallus (55).
7. Normal scrotum: For FTM patients, the goal of creating natural-appearing genitals also applies to the scrotum. In 2009, Selvaggi et al. reported on a novel scrotoplasty technique that combines a V-Y plasty with a 90-degree turning of the labial flaps, resulting in an anterior transposition of labial skin (Figure 51-11). The excellent aesthetic outcome of this male-looking (anteriorly located) scrotum, the functional advantage of fewer urologic complications, and the easier implantation of testicular prostheses make this the technique of choice (56).
8. Sexual intercourse: In a radial forearm phalloplasty, the insertion of a rigid or inflatable prosthesis is required for the patient to engage in sexual intercourse. The rigid and semirigid prostheses seem to have a high perforation rate and therefore were never used in our patients. Hoebeke et al., in the largest series to date on erection prostheses after penile reconstruction, only used the hydraulic systems available for impotent men. After 1 year, all patients had regained tactile sensitivity in their penises, which is an absolute requirement for safe insertion of an erection prosthesis (57).

A recent long-term follow-up study showed an explanation rate of 44% in 130 patients, mainly because of malpositioning, technical failure, or infection. Still, more than 80% of the patients were able to have normal sexual intercourse with penetration (49,50) (Figure 51-12).

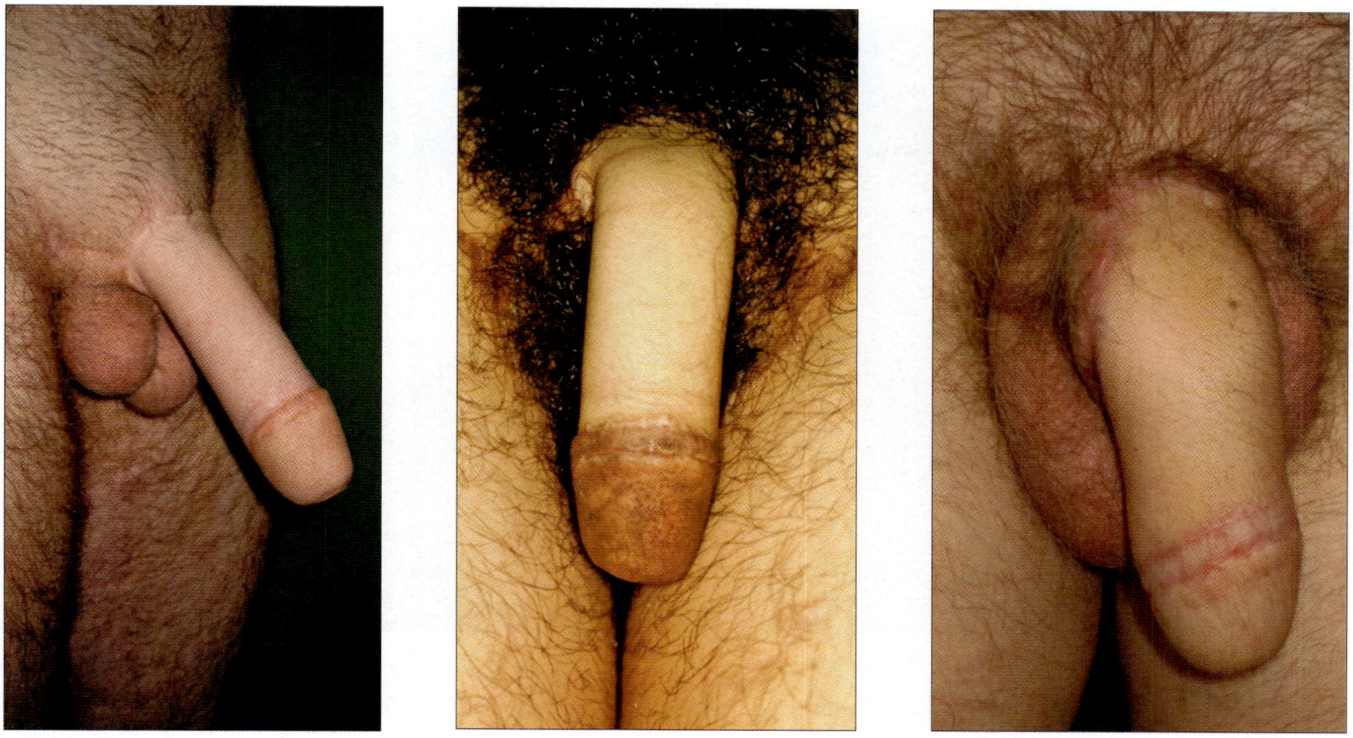

A B C

FIGURE 51-9 (A) to (C) Late postoperative results of radial forearm phalloplasties.

Fibula Flap There have been several reports on penile reconstruction with the fibular flap based on the peroneal artery and the peroneal vein (48,58,59). It consists of a piece of fibula that is vascularized by its periosteal blood supply and connected through perforating (septal) vessels to an overlying skin island at the lateral site of the lower leg. The advantage of the fibular flap is that it makes sexual intercourse possible without a penile prosthesis. The disadvantages of this technique, however, are the poor quality of the flap sensation, a pointy deformity to the distal part of the penis where the extra skin can glide around the end of fibular bone, and an impractical and inconvenient permanent erection.

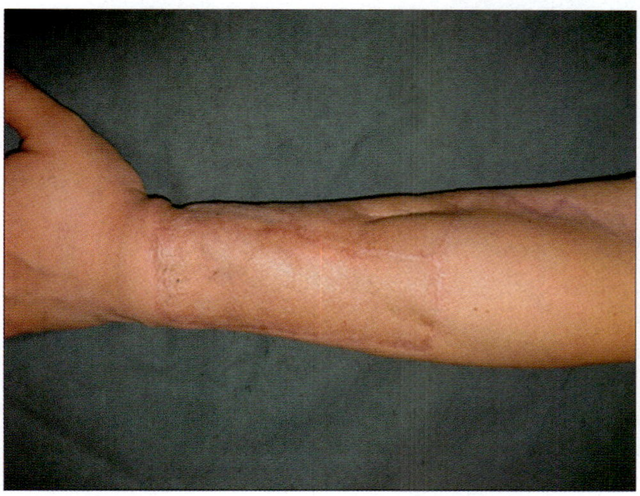

FIGURE 51-10 Late result of the donor site at the forearm.

Scrotal Reconstruction

Scrotal reconstruction adheres to the same reconstructive principles. When possible, primary closure is the procedure of choice, particularly in partial or hemilateral injuries. However, in the case of total scrotal skin loss, split-thickness skin grafts are effective if they are placed and immobilized carefully. The testicles must be fixed in an anatomically appropriate position before proceeding with graft coverage. As already mentioned, there also is a place for meshed, nonexpanded skin grafts in scrotal and perineal reconstruction because of the uneven and often biconcave contours of this region. In addition, there is an aesthetic dividend in that meshed grafts on the scrotum often emulate the scrotal rugae. The pedicled ALT can also be a valuable alternative for the reconstruction of a scrotum (Figure 51-13). In FTM transsexuals, the novel scrotoplasty provides the best results (see Figure 51-11) (56).

Metaidoioplasty

A metaidoioplasty is an operation that uses the (hypertrophied) clitoris to reconstruct the microphallus in a way comparable to the correction of chordee and lengthening of a urethra in cases of severe hypospadias. In metaidoioplasty, the clitoral hood is lifted, and the suspensory ligament of the clitoris is detached from the pubic bone, allowing the clitoris to extend out farther. An embryonic urethral plate is divided from the underside of the clitoris to permit outward extension and a visible erection (57–60). Then the urethra is advanced to the tip of the new penis. The technique is very similar to the reconstruction of the horizontal part of the urethra in a normal phalloplasty procedure. During the same procedure, a scrotal reconstruction with a transposition flap of the labia majora (as previously described) is performed combined with a vaginectomy.

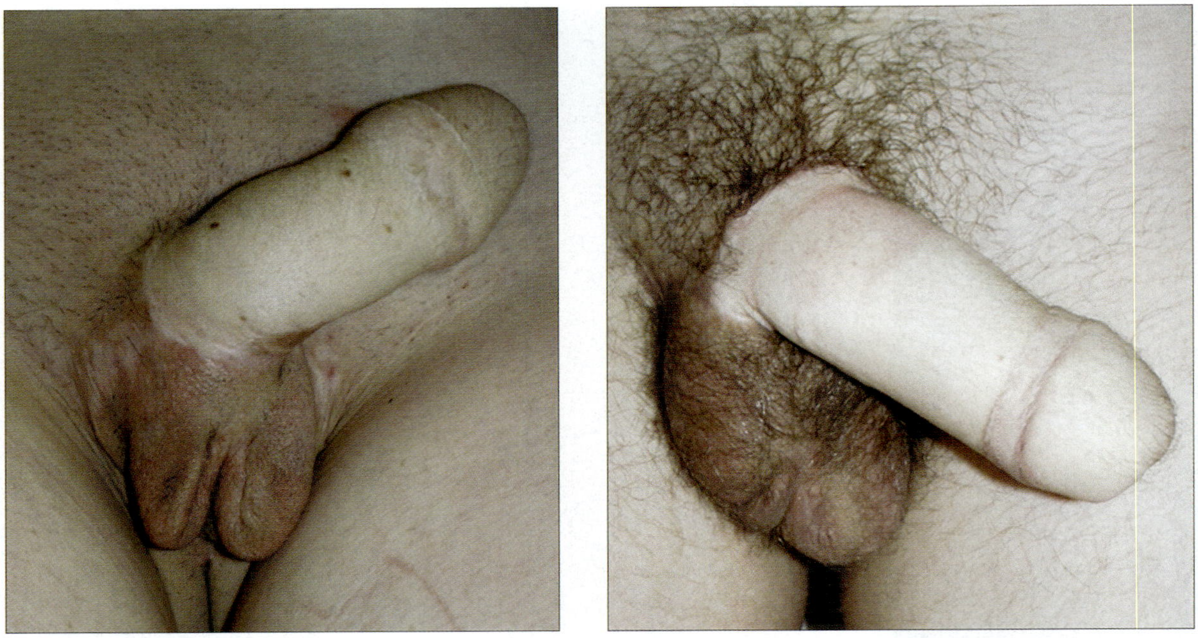

A B

FIGURE 51-11 (A) and (B) Reconstruction of a lateral-looking scrotum with two transposition flaps before and after implantation of prostheses.

Female-to-male patients interested in this procedure should be informed before surgery that voiding while standing cannot be guaranteed and that sexual intercourse will not be possible (Figure 51-14).

The major advantage of metaidoioplasty is the absence of a donor scar and the preservation of erectile function even if only in a micropenis. Another advantage is that its cost is substantially lower than that of phalloplasty. Complications of this procedure also include urethral obstruction and urethral fistula.

It is always possible to perform a regular phalloplasty (e.g., with a RFF) at a later stage and with substantially less risk of complications and operation time.

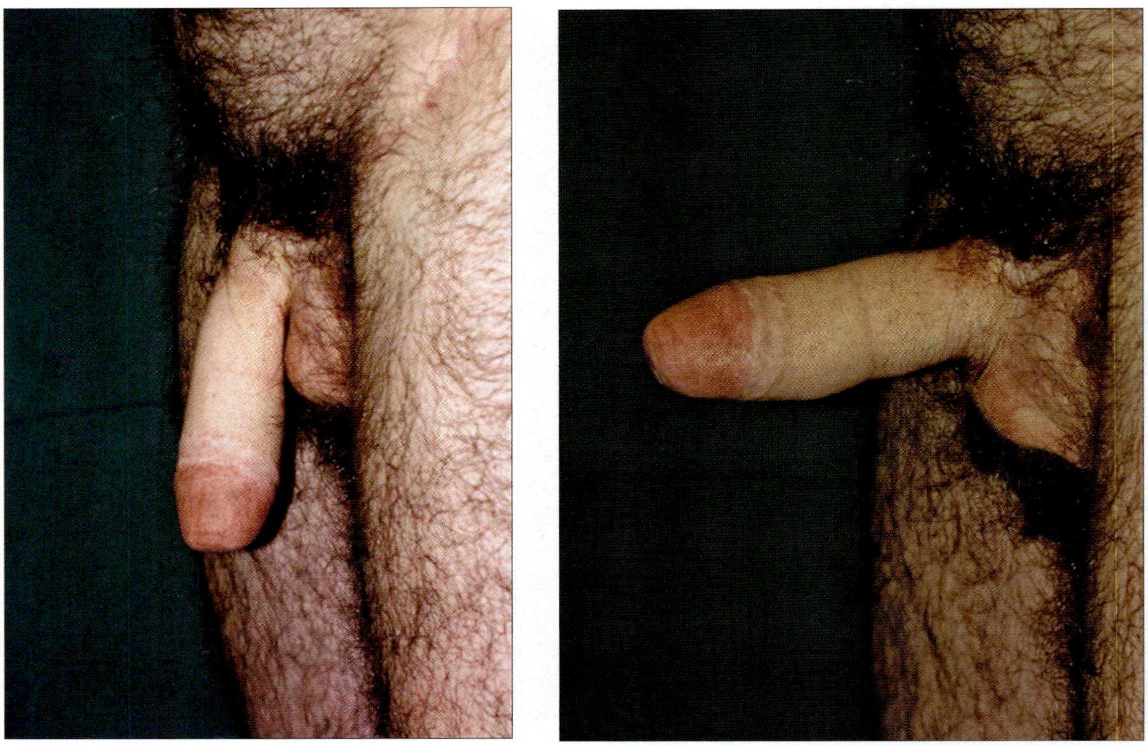

A B

FIGURE 51-12 (A) and (B) After implantation of an erection prosthesis.

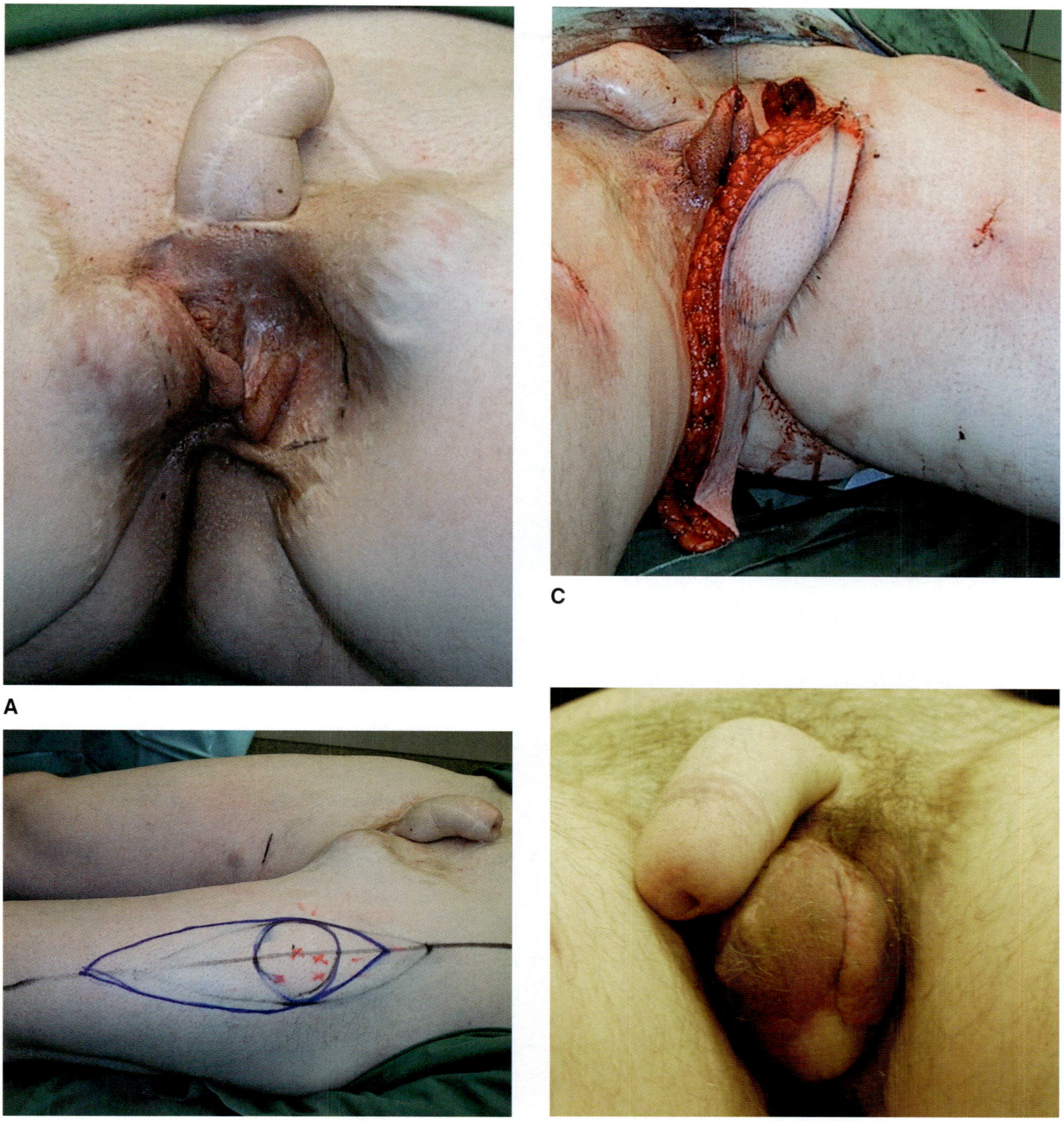

FIGURE 51-13 (A) Female-to-male transsexual patient after penile reconstruction with a lack of skin to reconstruct a scrotum. (B) Design and dissection of a pedicled anterolateral thigh (ALT) flap. (C) Transfer of the ALT flap to the pubic area. (D) Postoperative result.

PENILE IMPLANTS AFTER PENILE RECONSTRUCTION

A drawback of the RFF is the need for a rigid prosthesis. This is required for the patient to engage in sexual intercourse after surgery. Unfortunately, the limited amount of bone that can be taken from the distal radius can never function as a real rigidity device, and the risk of donor site complications is greatly increased (61,62). In addition, bone or cartilage grafts may absorb or render a pointy deformity at the distal part of the penis, where the extra skin can glide around the end of the prosthesis. Moreover, a permanently erected phallus (similar to a phalloplasty performed with a fibula osteocutaneous flap) can be an embarrassment not easily concealed.

Implantation of a penile erection prosthesis is thus the only option left, and this can be performed 126 months after the

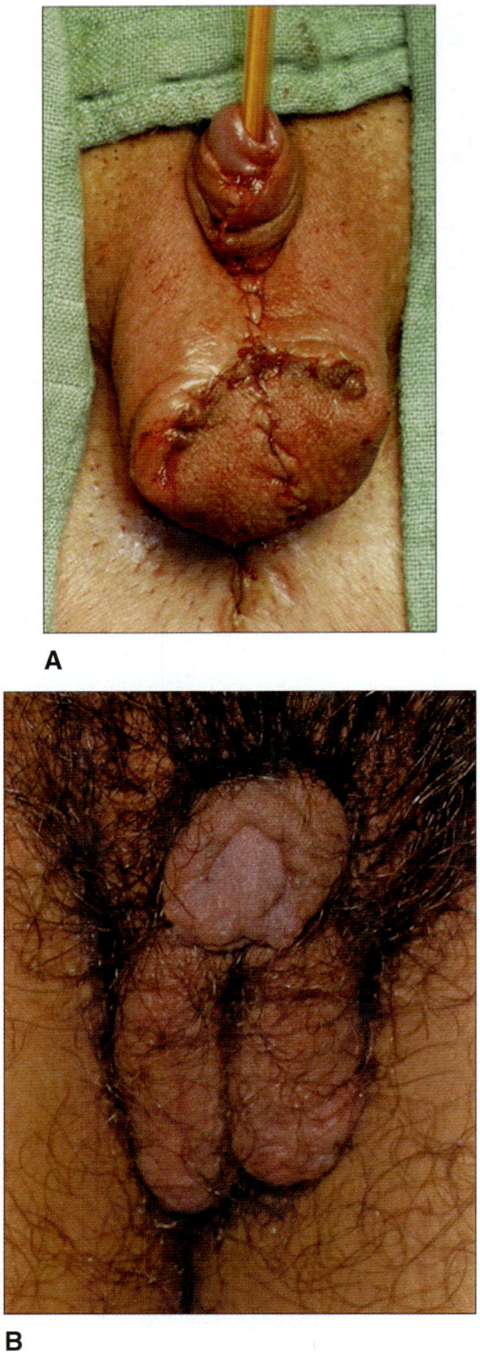

FIGURE 51-14 Metaidoioplasty: immediate (A) and late (B) postoperative results.

phalloplasty procedure because it usually takes at least 1 year before sensation has returned to the top of the penis.

Hoebeke et al. reported on the largest series to date on penile implants after a radial forearm reconstruction for FTM transsexualism (63). In their opinion, the rigid and semirigid prostheses seem to have a high perforation rate and therefore are no longer used in their patients. Instead they prefer the hydraulic systems available for impotent men, and these erection prostheses have been implanted in more than 129 patients. Initially, a one-piece hydraulic prosthesis was used (Dynaflex; AMS), usually in combination with two testicular prostheses. When this implant became unavailable, they switched to the three-piece AMS CX prosthesis. In this device, the pump replaced one testicular prosthesis. Good results were reported with the three-piece prosthesis, but they recently encountered an increase in technical failure due to leakage, probably because there was no limit to the amount of fluid that can be pumped into the cylinders as the cylinders are not placed in cavernous bodies: "overpumping" seemed to be the basis of the problem. More recently, they shifted to the two-piece device (Ambicor, AMS), a system that limits the amount of fluid available.

A long-term follow-up study indicated that in about one in four patients, a reintervention was required because of malpositioning, technical failure, or infection. A more recent long-term follow-up study showed an explanation rate of 48% in 129 patients (63). Still, more than 80% of the patients were able to have normal sexual intercourse with penetration (56). In another study, they demonstrated that patients with an erection prosthesis were more able to attain their sexual expectations than those without prostheses, although the group with prostheses more often reported pain during intercourse (49).

A major concern regarding erectile prostheses is long-term follow-up. These devices were developed for impotent men who are older and have shorter life expectancies and lower sexual drives than younger postoncologic resection patients or FTM patients who are receiving these devices.

REFERENCES

1. Jordan GH, Gilbert DA, Devine CJ Jr. *Penile reconstruction following Mohs' micrographic surgery.* Presented at American Urological Association 86th annual meeting, Toronto, Ontario, June 3, 1991.
2. Muecke EC. Exstrophy, epispadias and other anomalies of the bladder. In Harrison JH, Gittes RF, Perlmutter AD, et al (eds). *Campbell's Urology*, vol 2, 4th ed. Philadelphia: WB Saunders, 1979, pp. 1443–1468.
3. Mitchell ME, Bägli DJ. Complete penile disassembly for epispadias repair: the Mitchell technique. *J Urol* 1996;155(1):300–304.
4. Perovic S, Scepanovic D, Sremcevic D, Vukadinovic V. Epispadias surgery Belgrade experience. *Br J Urol* 1992;70:647.
5. Dewan PA. Umbilical transposition in neonates with bladder exstrophy. *Br J Urol* 1995;76(6):797–799.
6. Feyaerts A, Mure PY, Jules JA, et al. Umbilical reconstruction in patients with exstrophy: the kangaroo pouch technique. *J Urol* 2001;165(6 Pt 1): 2026–2027; discussion 2028.
7. Lee PA, Houk CP, Ahmed SF, Hughes IA. Consensus statement on management of intersex disorders. International Consensus Conference on Intersex. *Pediatrics* 2006;118(2):e488–e500.
8. Eke N. Fournier's gangrene: a review of 1726 cases. *Br J Surg* 2000;87:718.
9. Vick R, Carson C. Fournier's disease. *Urol Clin North Am* 1999;26:841.
10. Monstrey S. Personal communication, 2010.
11. McAninch JW. Management of genital skin loss. *Urol Clin North Am* 1989;16:387.
12. McCraw JB, Arnold PG, eds. *Atlas of Muscle and Musculocutaneous Flaps.* Norfolk, VA, Hampton Press, 1986, pp. 389–421.
13. Monstrey S, Hoebeke P, Selvaggi G, et al. Penile reconstruction: is the radial forearm flap really the standard technique? *Plast Reconstr Surg* 2009;124:510–518.
14. Orticochea M. A new method of total reconstruction of the penis. *Br J Plast Surg* 1972;25:347.
15. Horton CE, McCraw JB, Devine CJ, et al. Secondary reconstruction of the genital area. *Urol Clin North Am* 1977;4:133–141.
16. Santanelli F, Scuderi N. Neophalloplasty in female-to-male transsexuals with the island tensor fasciae latae flap. *Plast Reconstr Surg* 2000;105:1990.
17. McGregor IA, Jackson IT. The groin flap. *Br J Plast Surg* 1972;25:3.
18. Sun G, Huang J. One-stage reconstruction of the penis with composite iliac crest and lateral groin skin flap. *Ann Plast Surg* 1985;15:519.
19. Sun GC, Zhong AG, He W, et al. Reconstruction of the external genitals and repair of skin defects of the perineal region using three types of lateral groin Flap. *Ann Plast Surg* 1990;24:328.

20. Akoz T, Kargi E. Phalloplasty in female-to-male transsexual using a double pedicle composite groin flap. *Ann Plast Surg* 2002;48:423.
21. Ustuner TE, Mutaf M, Sensoz O. Anteromedial thigh: a source for phallic reconstruction. *Ann Plast Surg* 1994;32:426.
22. Cheng KX, Hwang WY, Eid AE, et al. Analysis of 136 cases of reconstructed penis using various methods. *Plast Reconstr Surg* 1995;95:1070.
23. Maltz M. Maltz reparative technic for the penis. In Maltz M : *Evolution of Plastic Surgery*. New York, Froben Press, 1946, pp. 278–279.
24. Gillies H, Millard DR Jr. *The Principles and Art of Plastic Surgery*, vol. 2. London, Butterworth, 1957, pp. 368–384.
25. Woods JE, Alter G, Meland B, Podratz K. Experience with vaginal reconstruction utilizing the modified "Singapore" flap. *Plast Reconstr Surg* 1992;90:270.
26. Martius H, McCall J, Bolster KA, eds. *Operative Gynecology*. Boston, Little, Brown, 1956.
27. Monstrey S, Blondeel P, VanLanduyt K, et al. The versatility of the pudendal thigh fasciocutaneous flap used as an island flap. *Plast Reconstr Surg* 2001;107:19.
28. Levine JL, Miller Q, Vasile J, et al. Simultaneous bilateral breast reconstruction with in-the-crease inferior gluteal artery perforator flaps. *Ann Plast Surg* 2009;63(3):249–254.
29. Yii NW, Niranjan NS. Lotus petal flaps in vulvo-vaginal reconstruction. *Br J Plast Surg* 1996;49(8):547–554.
30. Hage JJ, Winters HA, Van Lieshout J. Fibula free flap phalloplasty: modifications and recommendations. *Microsurgery* 1996;17:358–365.
31. Song R, Gao Y, Song Y, et al. The forearm flap. *Clin Plast Surg* 1982;9(1):21–26.
32. Cheng KX, Hwang WY, Eid AE, et al. Analysis of 136 cases of reconstructed penis using various methods. *Plast Reconstr Surg* 1995; 95(6):1070–1080.
33. Harashima T, Ionque T, Tanaka I, et al. Reconstruction of penis with free deltoid flap. *Br J Plast Surg* 1990;43:217–222.
34. Hage JJ, De Graaf FH. Addressing the ideal requirements by free flap phalloplasty: some reflections on refinements of technique. *Microsurgery* 1993;14:592–598.
35. Sadove RC, Sengezer M, McRobert JW, Wells MD. One-stage total penile reconstruction with a free sensate osteocutaneous fibula flap. *Plast Reconstr Surg* 1993;92(7):1314–1325.
36. Santanelli F, Scuderi N. Neophalloplasty in female-to-male transsexuals with the island tensor fascia lata flap. *Plast Reconstr Surg* 2000;105(6): 1990–1996.
37. Felici N, Felici A. A new phalloplasty technique: the free anterolateral thigh flap phalloplasty. *J Plast Reconstr Aesthet Surg* 2006;59:153–157.
38. Ceulemans P. *The pedicled antero-lateral thigh (ALT) perforator flap: a new technique for phallic reconstruction*. XIX Biennial Symposium of the Harry Benjamin International Gender Dysphoria (HBIGDA) Association, Bologna, Italy, April 2005.
39. Suominen S. Personal communication, 1994.
40. Sinove Y1, Kyriopoulos E, Ceulemans P, Houtmeyers P, Hoebeke P, Monstrey S. Preoperative planning of a pedicled anterolateral thigh (ALT) flap for penile reconstruction with the multidetector CT scan. *Handchir Mikrochir Plast Chir* 2013;45(4):217-222. doi: 10.1055/s-0032-1333271. Epub 2013 Mar 6.
41. Tamai S, Nakamura Y, Motomiya Y. Microsurgical replantation of a completely amputated penis and scrotum. *Plast Reconstr Surg* 1977;60:287.
42. Gilbert DA, Horton CE, Terzis JK, et al. New concept in phallic reconstruction. *Ann Plast Surg* 1987;18(2):128–136.
43. Chang TS, Hwang WY. Forearm flap in one stage reconstruction of the penis. *Plast Reconstr Surg* 1984;74(2):251–258.
44. Gilbert DA, Horton CE, Terzis JK, et al. New concept in phallic reconstruction. *Ann Plast Surg* 1987;18(2):128–136.
45. Fang RH, Kao YS, Ma S, Lin JT. Phalloplasty in female-to-male transsexuals using free radial osteocutaneous flap: a series of 22 cases. *Br J Plast Surg* 1999;52(3):217–222.
46. Hage JJ, Winters HA, Kuiper IA. The super-thin peritoneum free flap: not to be used for urethra reconstruction. *Plast Reconstr Surg* 1997;100(6): 1613–1614.
47. Weyers S, Selvaggi G, Monstrey S, et al. Two-stage versus one-stage sex reassignment surgery in female-to-male transsexual individuals. *Gynaecol Surg* 2006;3:190–194.
48. Hage JJ, Winters HA, Van Lieshout J. Fibula free flap phalloplasty: modifications and recommendations. *Microsurgery* 1996;17:358–365.
49. De Cuypere G, T'Sjoen G, Beerten R, et al. Sexual and physical health after sex reassignment surgery. *Arch Sex Behav* 2005;36:679–690.
50. Hage JJ, Bout CA, Bloem JJ, Megens JA. Phalloplasty in female-to-male transsexuals: what do our patients as for? *Ann Plast Surg* 1993;30: 323–326.
51. Walton RL, Hurwitz DJ, Bunkis J. Gluteal thigh flap for reconstruction of perineal defects. In Strauch B, Vasconez LO, Hall-Findlay EJ (eds). *Grabb's Encyclopedia of Flaps*, 2nd ed. Philadelphia, Lippincott-Raven, 1998, p. 1499.
52. Felici N, Felici A. A new phalloplasty technique: the free anterolateral thigh flap phalloplasty. *J Plast Reconstr Aesthet Surg* 2006;59:153–157.
53. Matti B, Matthews R, Davies D. Phalloplasty using the free radial forearm flap. *Br J Plast Surg* 1988;41:160–164.
54. Hoebeke P, Selvaggi G, Ceulemans P, et al. Impact of sex reassignment surgery on lower urinary tract function. *Eur Urol* 2005;47:398–402.
55. Selvaggi G, Monstrey S, Hoebeke P, et al. Donor site morbidity of the radial forearm free flap after 125 phalloplasties in gender identity disorder. *Plast Reconstr Surg* 2007;118:1171–1177.
56. Hoebeke P, De Cuypere G, Ceulemans P, Monstrey S. Obtaining rigidity in total phalloplasty: experience with 35 patients. *J Urol* 2003;169: 221–223.
57. Perovic SV, Djordjevic ML. Metaidoioplasty: a variant of phalloplasty in female transsexuals. *BJU Int* 2003;92(9):981–985.
58. Hage JJ, van Turnhout AA. Long-term outcome of metaidoioplasty in 70 female-to-male transsexuals. *Ann Plast Surg* 2006;57(3):312–316.
59. Duckett JW Jr. Transverse preputial island flap technique for repair of severe hypospadias. *Urol Clin North Am* 1980;7(2):423–430.
60. Laub DR, Eicher W, Laub DR II, Hentz VR. Penis construction in female-to-male transsexuals. In Eicher W (ed): *Plastic Surgery in the Sexually Handicapped*. Berlin, Springer, 1989, pp. 113–128.
61. Biemer E. Bedeutung und Fortschritte der chirurgischen Geslechtsum-wandlung. *Münch Med Wochenschr* 1988;130:480–482.
62. Koshima I, Tai T, Yamasaki M. One-stage reconstruction of the penis using an innervated radial forearm osteocutaneous flap. *J Reconstr. Microsurg* 1986;3:19–26.
63. Hoebeke PB, Decaestecker K, Beysens M, et al. Erectile implants in female-to-male transsexuals: our experience in 129 patients. *Eur Urol* 2009;57(2):334–340.

CHAPTER 52

Penile Replantation

James R. Sanger and Hani S. Matloub

Penile amputation is rare. Male genital amputation in adults is caused by self-mutilation, accidental masturbatory or industrial trauma, assault, and attacks by spouses in retaliation for infidelity. In Western cultures, amputation by self-mutilation is the dominant etiology. There are sporadic reports of amputation by spouses of philandering husbands. In contrast, an epidemic of penile amputations by angry wives occurred in Thailand beginning in 1973 and peaking in 1980, resulting in more than 100 amputations (1). Almost all publications regarding penile amputation and replantation consist of a single or small number of case reports with limited follow-up, resulting in anecdotal data.

Ehrich first reported, in 1929, a traumatic subtotal amputation of the distal shaft of the penis, in which the corpora cavernosa and urethra were severed, the skin was denuded, and only a small skin bridge remained. The urethra and corpora were repaired, and scrotal skin was used to cover the shaft. The penis survived; the man was able to urinate normally, and he regained erectile function (2). Subsequently Young, in 1942, reported a war injury in which the corpora cavernosa and spongiosum were transected (3). Repair resulted in incomplete erection but normal ejaculation. Dodson (4) reported survival of an amputated glans penis after suturing only the skin in 1944. Price described a patient who had severance of the corpora, retaining only a small skin bridge (5). Corporal repair resulted in survival but was complicated by urinary fistula. Erectile function recovered. Lloyd, in 1957, reported that although penile replantation was successful after repair of the corpora only, the patient was unable to experience erections (6). However, Galleher and Kaiser reported a similar case in 1961, in which erectile function, independently verified, was recovered (7).

Other authors noted significant complications with suture repair of the corpora and skin. Best et al. described a case in which a completely severed penis treated with repair of the corpora cavernosa, urethra, and skin was complicated by complete necrosis of the skin and corpus spongiosum. The corpora cavernosa survived, the urethra was subsequently reconstructed by split-thickness skin graft over a tube, and the penis and glans were buried in the scrotum. Three weeks later, the penis, with a generous portion of subcutaneous scrotal tissue, was liberated and covered with split-thickness graft. Urinary and sexual function were reported as normal, and the authors suggested that future patients be treated by denuding the skin and burying the composite autograft within the scrotum after repair of the corpora cavernosa, the urethra, and corpus spongiosum (8). Following these guidelines, McRoberts et al. successfully used this technique in two patients. Both experienced formation of an eschar of the glans penis followed by spontaneous reepithelialization but with some atrophy. The patients reported compromised erectile function (9).

Bhanganada et al. reported 18 cases of penile replantation treated by either direct repair or by repair of the corpora, urethra, removal of the shaft skin, and burying the penis in a subcutaneous position in the scrotum (1). In the later group at a second surgery, the penis was removed from the subcutaneous position, and scrotal skin was transferred to circumferentially resurface the penis. The direct repair group had poor results, with a high incidence of skin necrosis, urethral fistula, and stricture as well as impaired erections and poor sensation. Skin problems and fistulas were much less frequent in the latter group, but poor sensation and incomplete erections remained problems. The authors suggested that microvascular repair, if available, would be the ideal way to treat penile amputation (1).

In children, amputation at the time of circumcision can occur and typically involves the glans penis, including at times the very distal part of the corpora. This presents a unique problem because at this level, vessels that are adequate for microsurgical repair are frequently absent. However, at this same level, reattachment of an amputated glans as a composite graft has been successful (10,11).

Tamai et al. (12) and Cohen et al. (13) in 1977 reported the first successful microsurgical replantations of a completely amputated penis. Whereas Tamai et al. anastomosed one deep penile artery and both dorsal arteries, Cohen and colleagues repaired the dorsal arteries only. In both patients, deep dorsal and superficial dorsal veins were repaired, and microneural repairs of the dorsal nerves were done for the first time. In these patients, sensation to light touch and pinprick returned. Other reports of microsurgical penile replantation followed, with results that were clearly superior to those obtained with nonmicrosurgical techniques. Microsurgical replantation, when adequate vessels are present, is the current treatment of choice for penile amputation. Advantages include better survival rates, viability of the glans penis, return of sensation, fewer urethral strictures or fistulas, and better erection potential (14–29) (Figures 52-1 and 52-2).

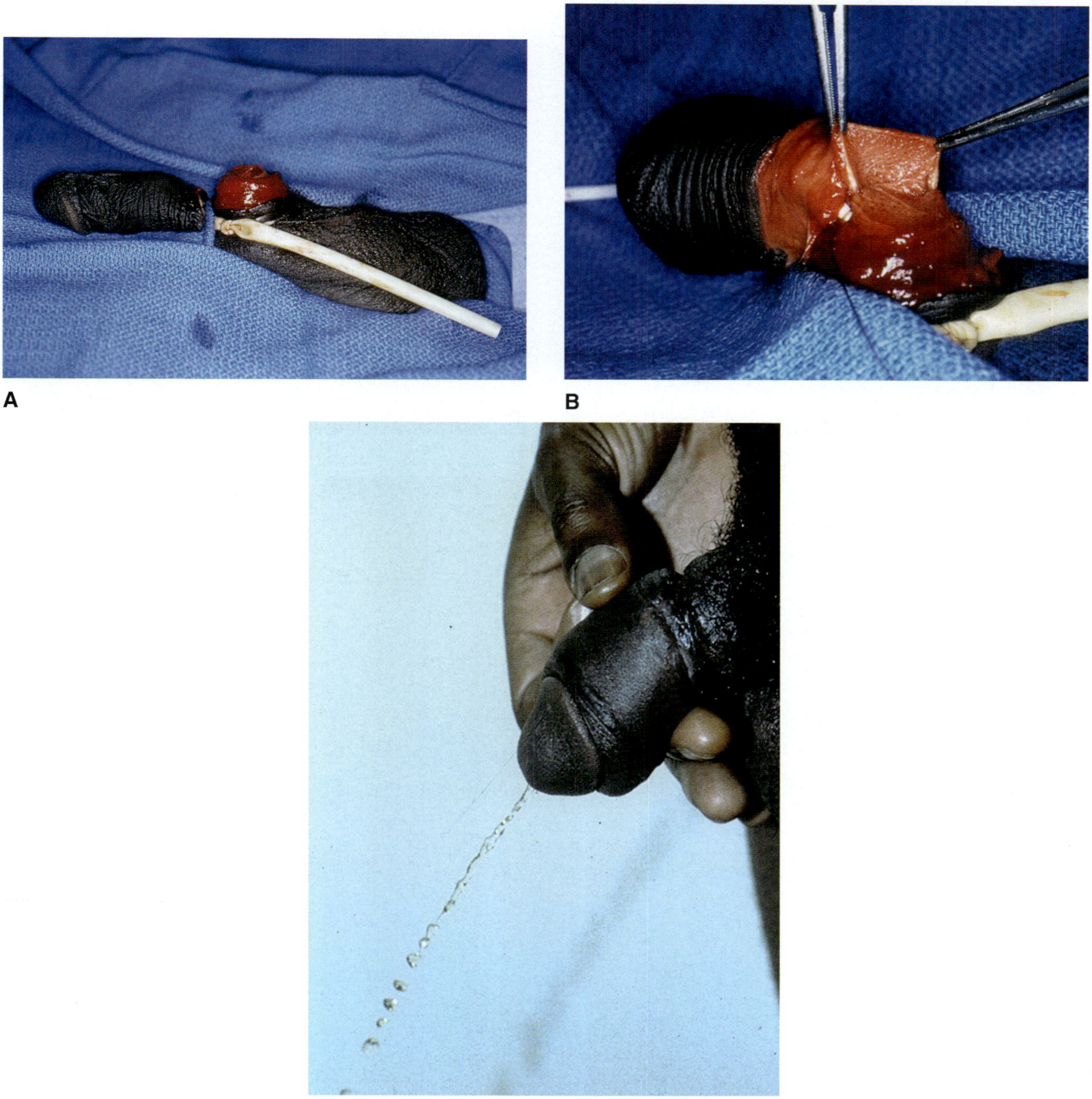

A B C

FIGURE 52-1 (A) An amputated penis in a patient who suffered acute psychosis in which "voices" demanded he "cut off" his penis. In almost all injuries, the level of amputation is at the mid to distal shaft. Adequate length is almost always present to apply a tourniquet to control hemorrhage. (B) The corpora cavernosum is repaired first and provides stability for the remaining repairs. The urinary catheter is placed through the amputated segment and across into the urethra at the base of the penile shaft but not into the bladder. (C) Postoperative result at 3 months demonstrating normal voiding. Edema in the replanted penis generally resolves after 6 months.

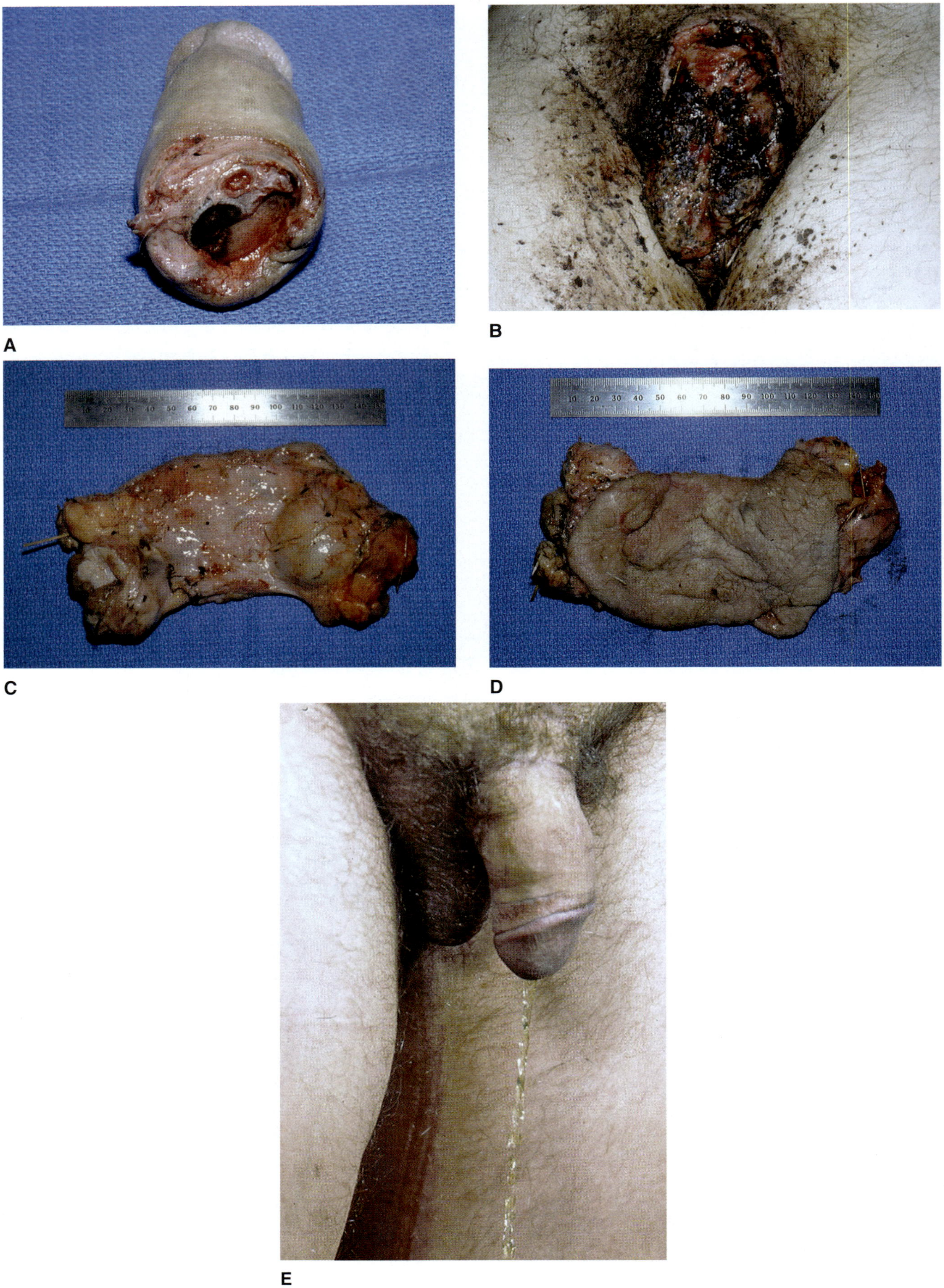

FIGURE 52-2 (A) and (B) Penile amputation in a patient with a personality disorder and alcohol intoxication. The patient first removed his penis and then amputated his scrotum and testicles. (C) and (D) The scrotum and testicles of the same patient. He had stomped on his testicles with heavy boots, and they could not be replanted. (E) One year after replantation, there is normal voiding and resolution of edema. The patient received testosterone therapy and reported normal erections.

Temporary ectopic implantation of the penis has been reported. Matloub et al. successfully implanted an amputated penis on the forearm in a patient who sustained an avulsion injury of the shaft and glans penis secondary to a riding lawnmower accident (30). Degloving of the amputated segment occurred, with the penile skin remaining anatomically attached but severely contused. There were an associated massive scrotal and perineal hematoma and extreme contamination, which precluded primary replantation. The penis was replanted at a second surgery 4 weeks later, at which time the radial artery and its venae comitantes, which had been used as the recipient vessels at the time of ectopic implantation, were harvested with the penis to provide a lengthy pedicle. The recipient vessels for replantation were the inferior epigastric artery and vein, and primary anastomosis was possible. Sural nerve grafts were coapted between the right pudendal nerve and the dorsal nerves of the penis. There was complete survival of the penis. A urethral-cutaneous fistula occurred and required a small local flap, after which urination was normal. The patient had excellent return of sensation in the glans penis but no erectile function because the proximal corpora were avulsed with the original trauma (Figure 52-3).

Successful penile replantation has been performed after prolonged ischemia times (29,31,32). Complication rates with skin loss and urethral fistula appear higher in delayed cases. With combined penile and testicular amputation, time to revascularization is more critical because the endocrine cells within the testicles are more sensitive to ischemia. In combined penis and testicle amputation, revascularization of the testicles takes precedence because irreversible damage to the testes' endocrine and reproductive cells can occur by 4 to 6 hours (28). However, the maximum warm ischemia period for testes is not known.

SURGICAL ANATOMY

A thorough understanding of the anatomy of the penis is required for successful replantation (Figures 52-4 and 52-5). The corporal bodies are unique in both their supporting structure and their neurovascular anatomy (33,34). The penis consists of three corporal bodies or cavernosa. The dorsal paired corpora cavernosum contain highly vascularized sinusoidal tissue responsible for erection. The corpora spongiosum lies ventral to the corpora cavernosa and surrounds the urethra. Layers of fascia cover these bodies. Loosely adherent skin covers the penile shaft to the level of the glans penis, or corona. At this point, the skin folds on itself to form the prepuce. The glans penis is the distal continuation of the corpora spongiosum.

Each corpus cavernosum consists of a strong layer of connective tissue or tunica albuginea, which is between 1.5 and 3.0 mm thick, and surrounds the sinusoidal tissue. Proximally at the root of the penis, the corpora cavernosum are separated from each other, and the corpora spongiosum and at that point form the crura, which attach to the pubic rami and the rami of the ischium. As the corpora approach the shaft, they unite, and the tunica albuginea fuses to form a common septum, which extends the length of the shaft. Perforations in the septum contain vascular intercommunications. Within the sinusoidal tissue is the deep penile or cavernosal artery. The tunica albuginea thins along the medial ventral surface to form a groove within which lies the corpora spongiosum.

The corpus spongiosum is also covered by a tunica albuginea, but this layer is much thinner than that of the cavernosa. Proximally, it is bulb shaped and attaches to the urogenital diaphragm. At its distal end, it forms the glans penis, which forms a cap over the ends of the corpora cavernosa. The urethra with some sinusoidal tissue fills the spongiosum.

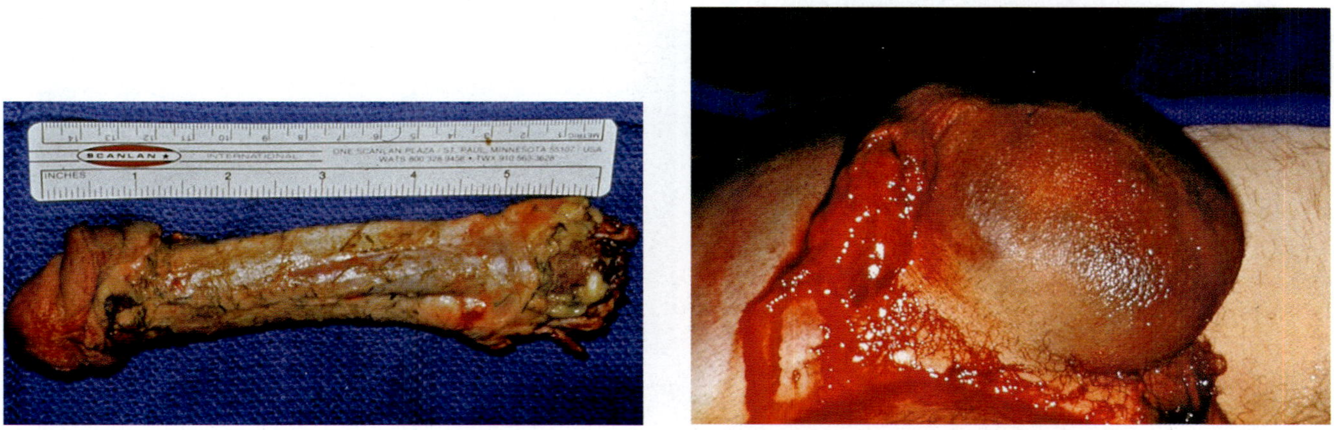

A B

FIGURE 52-3 (A) Avulsion injury with degloving of the shaft skin and preservation of the glans. Heavy contamination with grass and other foreign matter is present. (B) A massive heavily contaminated hematoma of the scrotum and perineum precludes immediate replantation. (C) One month after ectopic implantation of the penis on the right forearm using the radial artery and its venae comitantes as recipient vessels. (D) By 1 month, the severe edema has resolved, revealing that the majority of the shaft skin is preserved. (E) Elevation of the implanted penis on the radial artery and venae comitantes, which now provide long pedicle length. (F) Appearance 6 months after replantation. The patient is able to urinate normally. (Parts A, B, E, and F reproduced from Matloub, HS, Yousif NJ, Sanger JR. Case report: temporary ectopic implantation of an amputated penis. *Plast Reconstr Surg* 1994;93:408–412.)

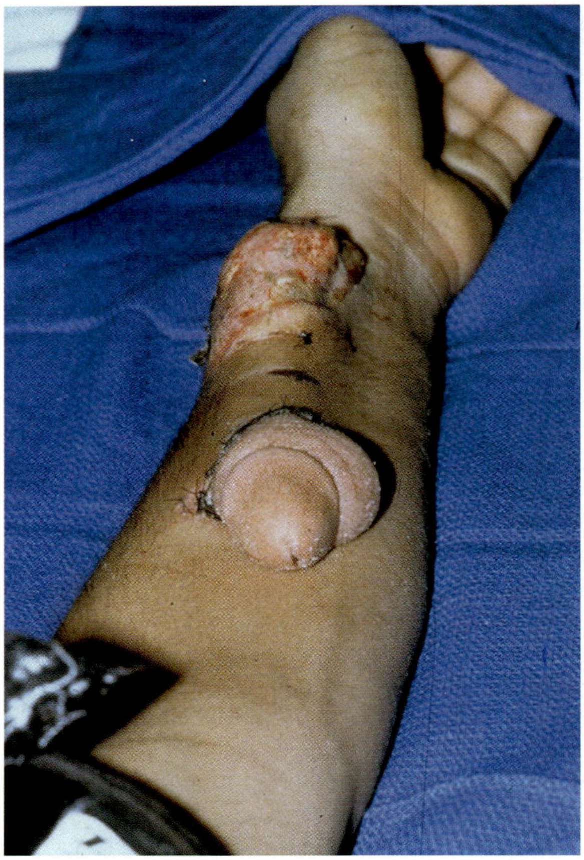

C

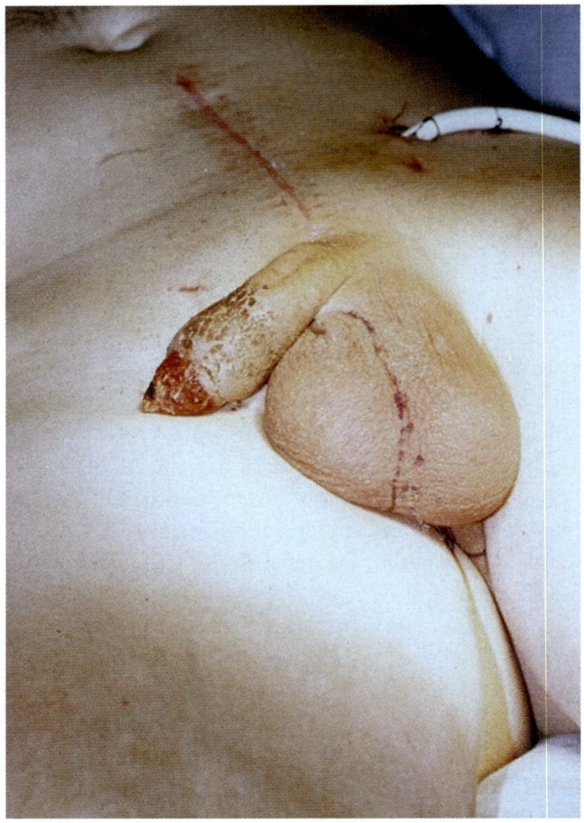

D

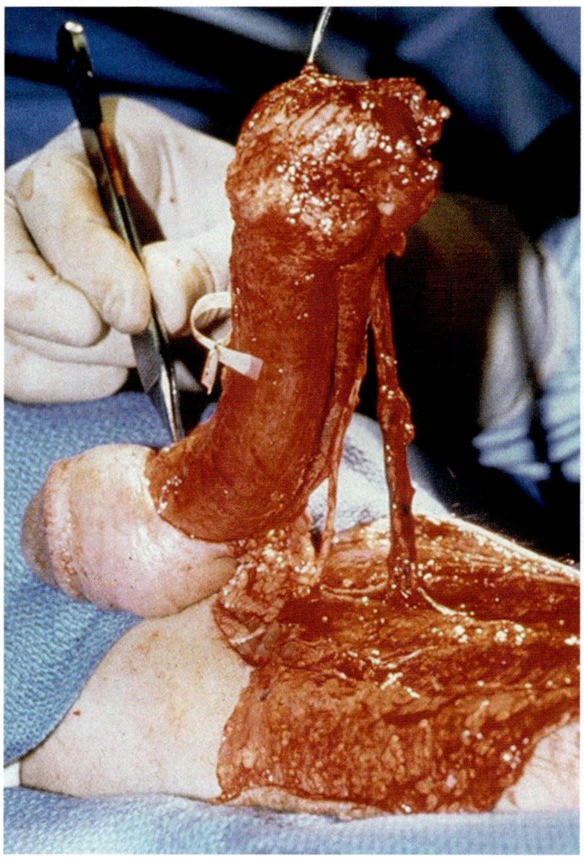

E

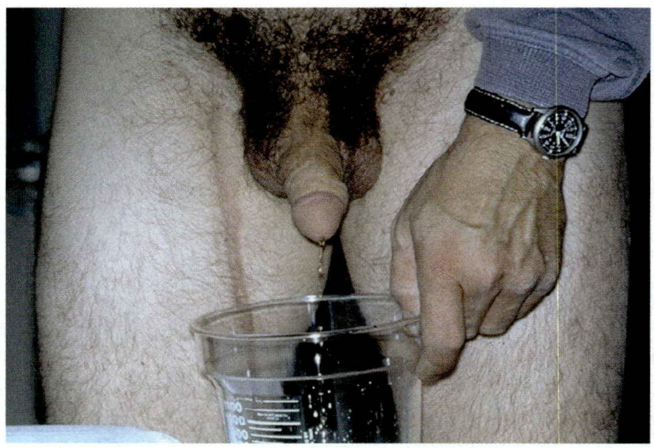

F

FIGURE 52-3 *(Continued)*

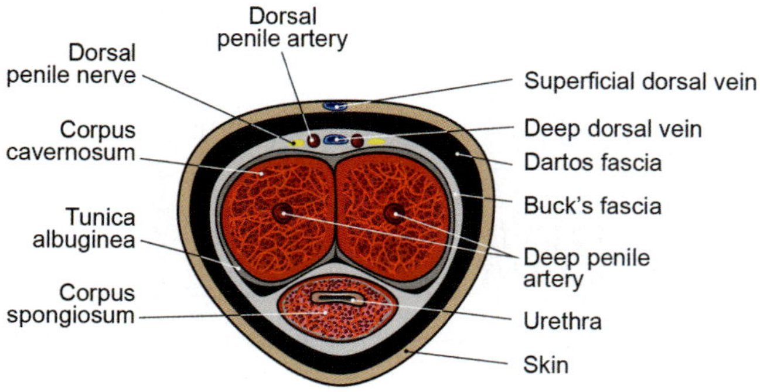

FIGURE 52-4 Cross-sectional anatomy of the penis at midshaft. The deep penile artery lies within the corpus cavernosum. The other important neurovascular structures are dorsal to the tunica albuginea and are invested by Buck's fascia.

BLOOD SUPPLY TO THE PENIS

Arterial Supply

The blood supply of the penis is derived from the internal iliac artery. Branches of both parietal and visceral vessels supply it. The visceral vessels include the superior and inferior vesical arteries, the artery of the vas deferens, and the midrectal artery. The parietal vessels are the dominant circulation and include the iliolumbar, superior and inferior gluteal, obturator, and internal pudendal arteries.

The internal pudendal artery gives off a perineal branch and continues as the penile artery. The penile artery passes through the urogenital diaphragm, traveling along the medial border of the inferior pubic ramus. At the level of the urethral bulb, it divides into the bulbourethral, cavernous, and dorsal penile arteries. The bulbourethral artery is short and can arise from the cavernous arteries, although in most cases it is the terminal branch of the penile artery. There is some variation in the origin of the cavernous branch, which is also referred to as the profunda or deep penile artery. It courses in the corpora cavernosum along the dorsal medial aspect located lateral to the cavernous vein. The cavernous artery gives off terminal branches, the helicine arteries, which supply the cavernous spaces. The cavernous arteries are the main arteries of the penis and have large numbers of helical branches that open directly into the cavernosal spaces of the corpora cavernosum during erection. The penile artery gives off the dorsal penile artery, which has a consistent course along the dorsum of the penis. The dorsal arteries are deep to Buck's fascia. The dorsal arteries give off several circumflex branches, which travel with the circumflex veins along the lateral aspect of the penis toward the ventral surface. They terminate in the glans penis and are responsible for glans engorgement during erection.

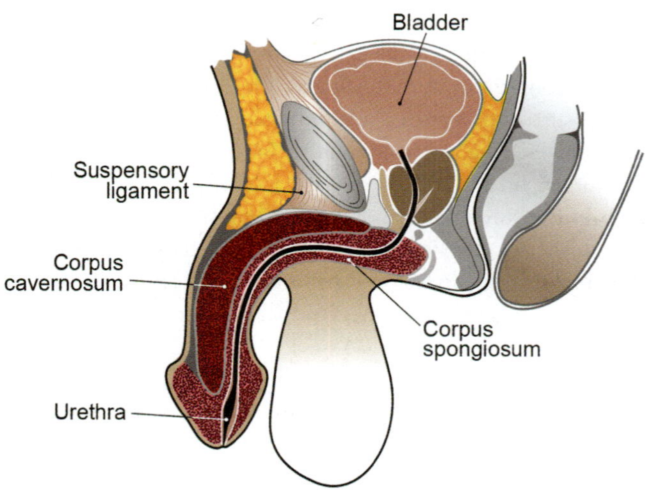

FIGURE 52-5 Sagittal view of the penis. The paired corpora cavernosum are the main erectile bodies. The corpus spongiosum contains the urethra and ends in the glans penis.

The scrotum receives its rich blood supply from vessels of the internal and external iliac artery systems. An extensive collateral circulation between the two systems exists. The femoral artery after its origin from the external iliac artery gives rise to the deep (inferior) and superficial (superior) pudendal arteries. Of these two vessels, the deep pudendal artery contributes the greatest amount to the scrotal circulation. The internal iliac artery gives rise to the internal pudendal artery. From this vessel, both direct scrotal branches and branches of the perianal artery enter the posterior aspect of the scrotum (35).

Venous Supply

The venous drainage of the penis is complex. The branches of the arteries terminate in the glans, and the first tributaries of the veins start from the glans penis. From the glans penis, small veins emerge to form the retrocoronal plexus, which then drains into the deep dorsal veins. At least one and frequently two deep dorsal veins run dorsally in the groove between the corpora cavernosa. The deep dorsal and circumflex veins drain the corpus spongiosum, including the glans penis, and the distal corpora cavernosa. The deep dorsal vein is usually an unpaired vein in the dorsal midline of the penis. These veins drain into the periprostatic plexus and then into the internal pudendal veins. In the distal two thirds of the penis, circumflex veins are present. These veins often accompany the circumflex arteries and emerge from the ventral aspect of the corpora spongiosum and course superficially to the tunica albuginea. The circumflex veins also communicate with the two lateral veins that run from the glans alongside the dorsal penile arteries. In the proximal third of the penis are several deep or cavernous veins that are located adjacent to the cavernous artery. The cavernous veins drain into the internal pudendal veins. During replantation, the deep dorsal or superficial dorsal veins are the clinically important vessels and are easily accessed for microsurgical anastomosis.

Multiple superficial veins are present on the dorsal aspect of the shaft between the Colles and Buck's fascia. Proximally, these veins frequently combine to form a single superficial vein, which usually drains into the saphenous vein.

Innervation of the Penis

The penis is innervated by autonomic (sympathetic and parasympathetic) and somatic (sensory and motor) nerves. In the pudendal canal, the dorsal nerve of the penis arises from the pudendal nerve. It enters the dorsum of the penis and travels dorsal and lateral to the dorsal penile artery. It terminates as multiple branches that innervate the glans penis. Smaller cavernous nerves can also be identified. Depending on the level of amputation, between two and four nerve repairs may be needed.

The dorsal nerve of the penis is one of the two terminal branches of the pudendal nerve; the other one reaches the scrotum. Together with the internal pudendal artery, it passes through the urogenital diaphragm and enters into the superficial perineal space, joining the penile shaft beneath the inferior pubic ligament.

Penile Fascial Layers

The subcutaneous tissue of penis (or superficial penile fascia) is continuous above with the fascia of Scarpa and below with the dartos tunic of the scrotum and the fascia of Colles. It is sometimes just called the "dartos layer." This fascia is carried forward into the prepuce.

The superficial fascia of the penis contains the superficial dorsal vein, which begins in the prepuce, anastomoses with the deep dorsal vein coming from the glans penis, and ends in the superficial inguinal veins. This loose attachment allows free movement of the skin over the deeper penile structures. Near the glans penis, the mobile penile skin becomes attached to the urethral (ventral) surface of the glans by a small skin fold called the frenulum (see Figure 52-1B). On the glans penis, the skin is firmly attached to the underlying spongy tissue.

Buck's fascia is the deep fascia of the penis. Whitish in color, it adheres to the tunica albuginea and is thick and elastic. The deep dorsal vein of the penis lies beneath the deep fascia of the penis and superficial to the tunica albuginea; it receives the blood from the glans penis and corpora cavernosa and courses backward in the midline between the dorsal arteries. Near the root of the penis, it passes between the two parts of the suspensory ligament and then through an aperture between the arcuate pubic ligament and the transverse ligament of the pelvis and divides into two branches, which enter the pudendal plexus.

The Dartos fascial layer beneath the penile and scrotal skin contains an interconnecting circulation originating from the deep and superficial external pudendal vessels and the internal pudendal vessels. Large tributaries of the deep dorsal vein encircle the penile shaft. The penile skin is vascularized by the dorsolateral and ventrolateral branches of the superficial external pudendal artery, cross-connecting with the scrotal branches of the internal pudendal artery. Because of this circulatory pattern, flaps can be harvested from the scrotal or penile skin in a transverse, circular, longitudinal, or oblique fashion and transferred to any part of the urethra, from meatus to membranous urethra, and can be used as ventral or dorsal patches.

MANAGEMENT OF THE AMPUTATED PART

Management of the amputated part is similar to that for any digital or limb amputation. During transport or while awaiting surgery, the part should be cooled. Wrapping the member in a moist saline gauze and placing it in a waterproof Ziploc bag on ice, while taking care *not* to allow freezing of the tissues, will minimize ischemic damage. Examination and cleansing of the amputated part can be initiated in the operating room, while—in addition to psychiatric and physical evaluation—stabilization of the patient is carried out in the emergency department.

PREOPERATIVE MANAGEMENT OF THE PATIENT

Penile amputation results in severe bleeding, which must be controlled initially by pressure. Application of a tourniquet using a Penrose drain may be possible if the patient is cooperative. Local anesthetic injected at the base of the shaft of the penis may facilitate application of the tourniquet. Adequate resuscitation with intravenous fluids and monitoring of vital signs are mandatory because blood loss may be massive. Blood is drawn for hematocrit and hemoglobin levels as well as for type and cross-match for possible transfusion. Preoperative antibiotics are administered. Consultation with the urology service for joint management of the patient is obtained.

Equally important to the physiologic preparation of the patient with a self-inflicted injury is psychiatric consultation. Psychotic patients are often unexpectedly docile and may appear ambivalent about amputation or replantation. They can also be severely agitated and require major sedation. Patients with personality disorders and substance abuse may be acutely intoxicated, requiring sedation and precautions for the toxicity associated with alcohol or other illicit drugs. The consulting psychiatrist determines whether sedation or antipsychotic medications need to be given preoperatively. Informed consent is at times a difficult medicolegal issue, and the psychiatric consultant facilitates obtaining it. With proper multidisciplinary care, patients with psychological impairment can safely undergo microsurgical procedures such as replantation with success rates similar to the general population and should not be denied emergency replantation (36).

PENILE REPLANTATION: SURGICAL TECHNIQUES (FIGURE 52-6)

Replantation is performed under general anesthesia because the patient is often severely agitated preoperatively, especially if the amputation was self-inflicted. Bleeding can be controlled by pressure until anesthesia is induced. Traction on the tunica albuginea of the corporal bodies facilitates placement of a tourniquet on the proximal shaft. Use of a penile tourniquet used in measurement of penile blood pressure is ideal if available. Otherwise, a Penrose drain or other elastic is sufficient. Proximal urinary diversion is recommended, and a suprapubic catheter is placed into the bladder percutaneously by the urologist.

With the tourniquet in place, adherent clots are removed and the tissue inspected. Any nonviable tissue is removed, although in most cases, the penis will have been transected sharply with minimal need for debridement. The corpora cavernosa are easily identified and are separated from each other along the fibrous penile septum (Figure 52-7). The deep penile arteries are dissected free from the surrounding

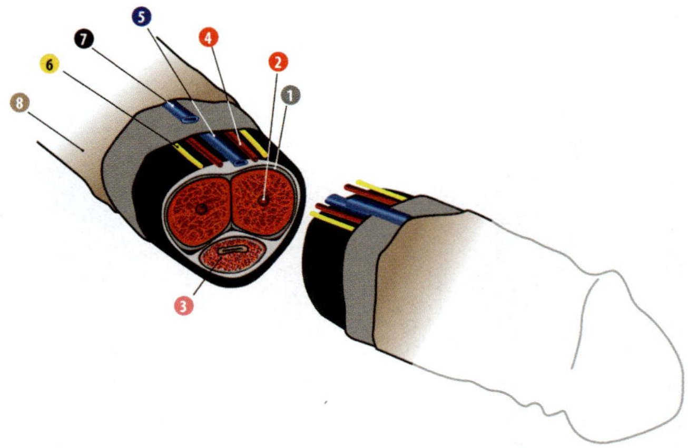

FIGURE 52-6 Replantation sequence. 1. Repair of the tunica albuginea provides stability 2. Anastomosis of the deep penile artery is done before completion of the tunica albuginea repair. 3. Repair of the urethra and tunica albuginea of the corpus spongiosum. 4 to 6. Repair of the deep dorsal vein(s), dorsal penile arteries, and dorsal penile nerves. 7. Repair of the superficial penile vein(s). 8. Skin is loosely approximated to complete the replantation.

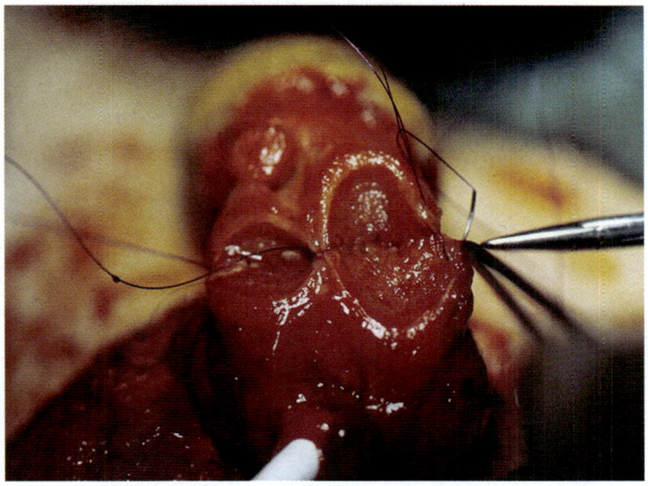

FIGURE 52-8 A running suture is used to close the corpora cavernosum, providing a watertight seal. If the deep penile artery is repaired, it is done when the tunica albuginea is about two thirds closed. Repair of the corpora cavernosum provides stability of the penis for the remaining repairs.

sinusoids and tagged with 10-0 suture. The urethra is located in the corpora spongiosum, which is ventral to the other corporal bodies. All three corpora lie within Buck's fascia, the deep investing fascia of the penis. Dorsal to the corporal bodies and beneath this fascia are the midline deep dorsal vein, the dorsal penile arteries, and the dorsal penile sensory nerves, all of which are tagged for repair. Superficial to this fascia is the superficial dorsal penile vein. After these structures are identified, the amputated member (with the corresponding structures labeled) is brought to the operating field. The ventral half of the tunica albuginea is repaired for both of the corpora cavernosum with running 4-0 locking suture (Figure 52-8). This helps stabilize the penis, which can then be supported on sterile towels.

Attention is then directed to the corpora spongiosum (Figure 52-9). A few sutures are placed in the ventral aspect of the tunica albuginea for stability. Both the proximal and distal ends of the urethra are identified. A urinary catheter is placed from the end of the penis through the urethra of the amputated part carefully across the proximal urethra. The urethra is then repaired with a 6-0 absorbable suture, usually chromic catgut, using loupe magnification. Interrupted sutures are preferred over a running suture to minimize the chance of postoperative stricture. After the urethral repair is completed, the remainder of the tunica albuginea of the spongiosum is repaired (Figure 52-10). We prefer to leave the catheter across the urethra but not in the bladder during the surgery because this provides additional stability during the vessel repairs and

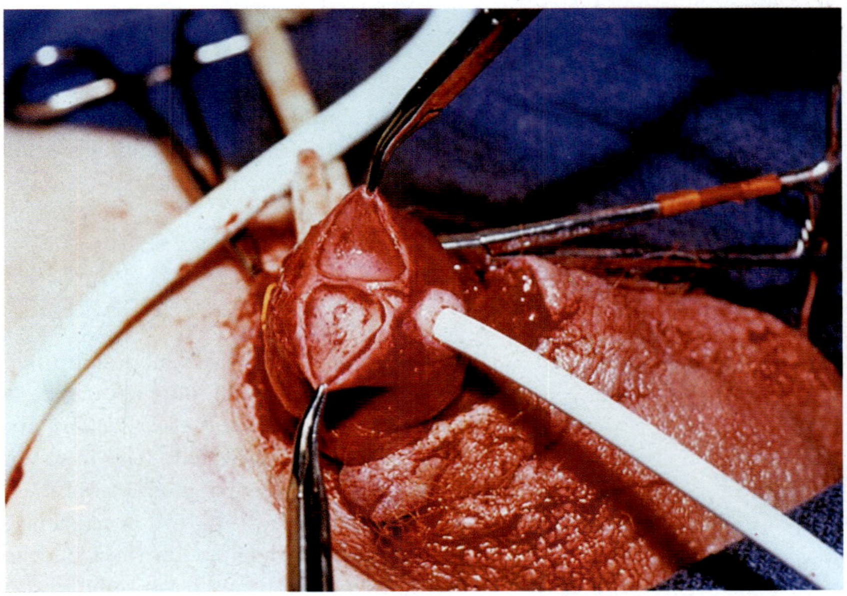

FIGURE 52-7 The proximal corpora cavernosa are prepared for suture. Note the thick tunica albuginea surrounding the corpora cavernosa.

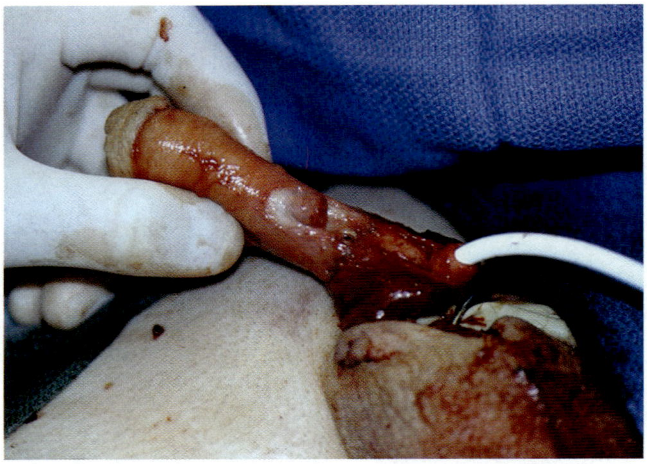

FIGURE 52-9 The repair of the corporal cavernosa is complete. The catheter will be placed into the distal urethra. The urethra is repaired with 5-0 absorbable sutures. The tunica albuginea of the corpora spongiosum is repaired with interrupted absorbable sutures.

acts as a stent to maintain the urethral diameter in the early postoperative period. It is not necessary that the catheter enter the bladder because the suprapubic tube diverts the urine.

The operating microscope is then used to prepare the deep penile arteries for repair. If possible, both arteries are repaired using 10-0 interrupted nylon sutures. Repair of the cavernous (deep penile) arteries is controversial because complete survival of the replanted penis can be achieved with successful repair of the dorsal arteries alone, but repair of the cavernous arteries may contribute to better blood flow in the corpora during erection. After repair of the deep penile arteries, the remainder of the running locking suture of the corpora cavernosa is completed. This provides a watertight closure that prevents postoperative bleeding when blood passively enters the sinusoids of the corpora cavernosum.

The dorsal penile arteries and veins are then prepared for anastomosis. Vessel size ranges between 1.0 and 2.0 mm. These vessels are easily mobilized from the surface of the underlying

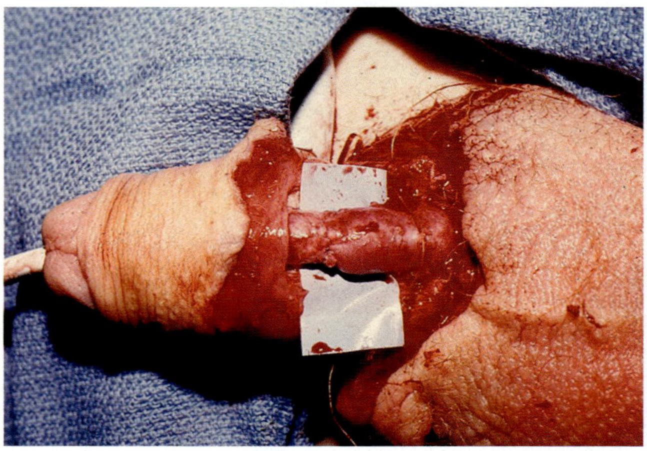

FIGURE 52-10 The urethra and corpora spongiosum have been repaired. The dorsal arteries and veins are next anastomosed followed by coaptation of the dorsal nerves.

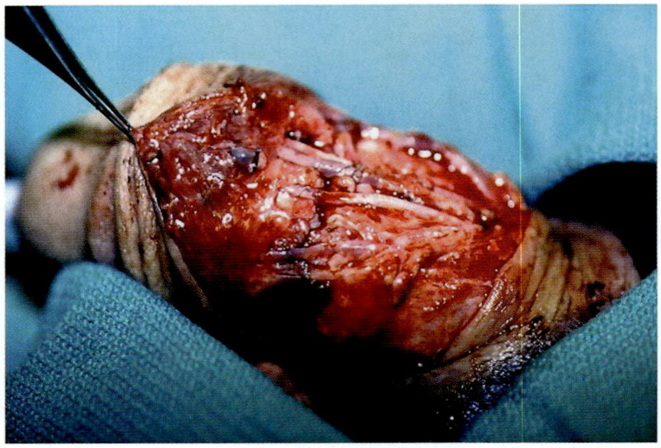

FIGURE 52-11 Completed anastomoses of dorsal arteries and veins and coaptation of dorsal sensory nerves.

tunica albuginea. Bipolar cautery is used when dividing small communicating branches. Primary repair is feasible in almost all cases. Both dorsal arteries should be repaired. The arteries are repaired with 10-0 interrupted nylon sutures. Two or more deep dorsal veins, which usually measure between 1.0 and 2.5 mm, are repaired next also with 10-0 interrupted nylon sutures. Three to four venous repairs are usually possible. In cases of more distal amputation, more vessels may be available for repair because of branching patterns (Figure 52-11).

The dorsal sensory nerves (which tend to accompany the arteries) are examined and prepared for coaptation. There are always at least two branches, but frequently several additional smaller branches are present. The right and left dorsal sensory nerves and as many branches as possible are repaired using 9-0 or 10-0 interrupted nylon sutures. This is important because recovery of sensation in the glans penis will not occur without repair of these nerves.

At this point, the tourniquet and vascular clamps are removed. Capillary fill should be apparent in the glans penis. There is often significant bleeding from the skin edges, which can easily be controlled with bipolar cautery. Buck's fascia, also known as the deep investing fascia of the penis, which surrounds the corporal bodies, can be closed at this time with absorbable sutures. The skin is then closed loosely completing the replantation. A few small sliver drains 4 to 5 mm in width, made from a rubber glove, are placed to prevent hematoma from occurring under the skin closure. These are removed after 1 or 2 days.

UNUSUAL VASCULAR REPAIRS

In almost all cases of successful penile replantation, the dorsal penile arteries and in some cases the deep or cavernous arteries have been repaired to revascularize the penis, but other vessels have been successfully used. In an unusual case in which the self-inflicted amputation level of the shaft was very distal, and the skin, which was still attached glans penis, was very proximal, a branch of the superficial pudendal artery measuring only 0.5 mm in diameter was sufficient for revascularization of the skin and glans penis (37). The posterior scrotal arteries have been successfully used to revascularize the combined avulsed penile and scrotal skin in a patient injured in an agricultural accident and in whom the shaft, although denuded of skin, maintained intact dorsal arteries and fascia (38). In combined penile and testicular amputations the testicular arteries have been repaired as well as the dorsal and deep penile arteries (28). In cases of distal amputation at or near the glans penis, in which microsurgical repair is not possible, isolation and advancement of a dorsal penile artery into the corpora spongiosum to encourage revascularization has been reported (39).

POSTOPERATIVE MANAGEMENT

Postoperative management must include close psychiatric supervision of the patient with self-inflicted amputation (26,36). Adjustment of sedation and antipsychotic medications is critical. Reamputation in the hospital has been reported (40). For this reason, patients are physically restrained in the immediate postoperative period and are under continuous observation. These measures are withdrawn when recommended by the psychiatric consultant. Long-term psychiatric care is generally needed upon discharge. A previous episode of genital mutilation or subsequent reinjury after replantation is not uncommon in this group of patients (26,40–42). In cases in which the patient has sustained accidental trauma or is a victim of violence, psychological evaluation and support are also invaluable because these patients experience posttraumatic stress syndrome and adjustment reactions.

Immediately after replantation, the patient is confined to bed rest. The replanted penis may be managed by allowing it to lie on its ventral surface with support from soft dressing. Another option that allows elevation and has been effective in reducing edema is to place a suture in the glans penis and to construct a soft foam dressing or silo to contain the penis. The suture is attached to the top of the foam, which is about 8 to 10 cm high, suspending the glans (Figures 52-12 and 52-13). This allows monitoring of the capillary fill to the glans penis and access to

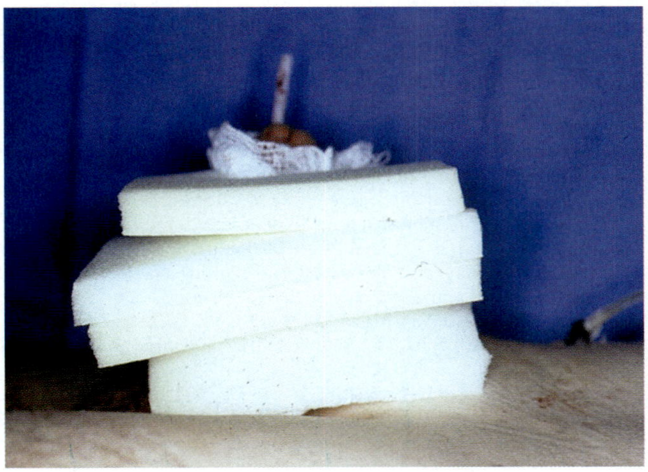

FIGURE 52-12 After loose closure of the shaft skin, a supportive dressing consisting of foam helps elevate the penis to reduce swelling. (Reproduced with permission from Sanger JR, Matloub HS, Yousif NJ, Begun FP. Penile replantation after self-inflicted amputation. *Ann Plast Surg* 1992;29:579–584.)

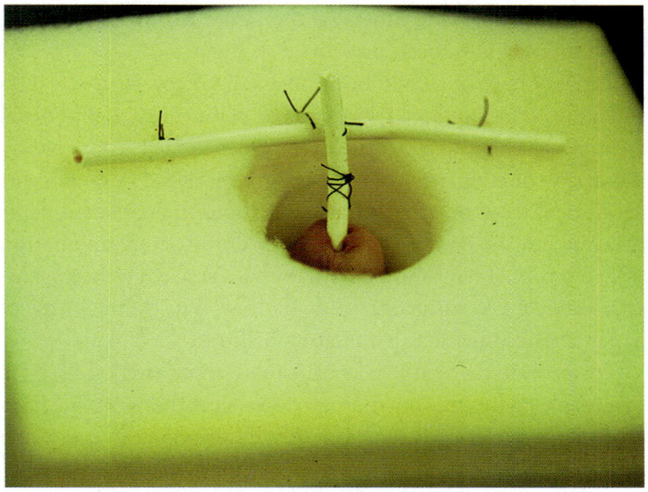

FIGURE 52-13 A suture placed through the glans or tied to the catheter helps suspend the replanted penis.

the distal dorsal shaft of the penis in the event Doppler is used to monitor the vessels. The remainder of the penis can be observed for skin problems or hematoma formation.

An alternative solution to supporting the replanted penis, which avoids external dressings or supports, incorporates a surgically created subcutaneous tunnel developed immediately cephalad to the base of the penis. The penis is covered except for the very distal shaft and glans penis, which can be observed for adequate circulation. The primary disadvantage of this technique is that a second surgical procedure is needed to remove the penis from the tunnel. Advantages include less chance of manipulation or reinjury by the patient and a normothermic environment, which should promote vasodilatation (43).

If arterial thrombosis occurs, exploration and revision of the anastomosis is the treatment of choice. For venous insufficiency, exploration and revision of the anastomosis are mandatory, but salvage of a congested penis after postoperative thrombosis of the dorsal vein by using medical leeches has been successful (37,44). Venous leeching has also been used in a nonmicrosurgical replantation using the buried penis technique in conjunction with a spongiocavernosal shunt (42). If leeching is used, careful monitoring of the hematocrit and hemoglobin level as well as intravascular volume status is important because blood flow to the penis may be quite high, especially with both intact arterial repairs and the continuous flow into the corpora cavernosa.

There is no consensus regarding the need for postoperative anticoagulation. The authors used low-molecular-weight dextran (Dextran 40) initially but currently use only 81 mg of aspirin daily. Subcutaneous heparin and intravenous heparin have also been used. Systemic anticoagulation appears unnecessary with the possible exception as an adjunct to leech therapy when no vein is available for repair.

We believe prevention of erection in the early postoperative period is valuable because engorgement of the corpora may place tension on the suture lines, which could result in bleeding. Amyl nitrate is kept at the bedside for this purpose but is rarely needed. Patients frequently lack libido because of the underlying psychiatric illness or the side effect of major sedatives that may have been prescribed to them.

Patients have generally been hospitalized for 10 to 14 days and allowed to stand after 1 week. The penis must be supported during ambulation, and traction must be avoided. Close supervision by nursing personnel during this phase is important because patients are often ambivalent about the replanted penis and may not be compliant. We allow unrestricted ambulation after 6 weeks. There should be daily assessment by the psychiatric service. On discharge from the hospital, the majority of patients enter inpatient psychiatric facilities.

Postoperative urinary leaks or fistulas occur rarely. These are best managed by continued urinary diversion and will close if no anastomotic stricture is present. Urethral stricture can usually be managed by dilatation. If there is erectile dysfunction, evaluation by the urologist is carried out. For these reasons, the patient should have a urology follow-up at least for the first year.

MANAGEMENT OF GLANS PENIS AMPUTATION

Anatomically, the glans penis is the distal continuation of the corpora spongiosum. When the amputation is on the shaft, there is adequate collateral circulation from the repaired dorsal arteries as well as corpora cavernosum vessels to assure its survival. Much of the corpora spongiosum consists of small veins; however, at the most proximal aspect of the glans, two small arteries, less than 1 mm in diameter, are present ventrally and at the lateral aspect of the urethra. The vessels get progressively smaller and move closer to the midline toward the end of the glans penis. Exploration for satisfactory vessel and microvascular repair if vessels of sufficient size are present is ideal. Successful microvascular repair has been performed in prepubertal boys who sustained amputation from circumcision trauma (10,32). However, repair of the vessels at this level may not be possible. Replantation as a composite graft is indicated in these situations and has been successful, particularly in infants injured during circumcision (39,45).

SUMMARY

Microsurgical replantation of the penis is preferred to other methods. Unlike with other techniques, direct revascularization and survival of the glans penis occurs. Furthermore, sensation is restored to the glans penis. Patients report adequate erectile function, but it is not clear whether repair of the deep penile arteries results in better erections. Penile replantation should be offered to patients even when amputation is self-inflicted because, with proper psychiatric postoperative monitoring, a successful outcome can be expected. Prior or subsequent genital mutilation is not uncommon in these individuals, however, and long-term psychiatric care is needed.

REFERENCES

1. Bhanganada K, Chayavatana T, Pongnumkul C, et al. Surgical management of an epidemic of penile amputation in Siam. *Am J Surg* 1983;146: 376–382.
2. Ehrich WS. Two unusual penile injuries. *J Urol* 1929;21:239–241.
3. Young HH. Wounds of the urogenital tract in modern warfare. *J Urol* 1942;47:59–108.
4. Dodson AI. *Urological Surgery*. St Louis, CV Mosby, 1944, p. 613.
5. Price KA. Accidental transaction of all corpora of the penis: repair with good results. *J Urol* 1952;68:620–622.
6. Lloyd FA. War injuries of the genitourinary organs: injuries of the penis. *Q Bull Northwest Univ Med School* 1957;31:378–382.
7. Galleher EP Jr, Kiser WS. Injuries of the corpus cavernosum. *J Urol* 1962;85:949–952.
8. Best JW, Angelo JJ, Milligan B. Complete traumatic amputation of the penis. *J Urol* 1962;87:134–138.
9. McRoberts JW, Chapman WC, Ansell JS. Primary anastomosis of the traumatically amputated penis: case report and summary of the literature. *J Urol* 1968;100:751–754.
10. Park JK, Min JK, Kim HJ. Reimplantation of an amputated penis in prepubertal boys *J Urol* 2001;165:586–587.
11. Aydin A, Aslan A, Tuncer S. Penile amputation due to circumcision and replantation. (Letter to Editor) *Plast Reconstr Surg* 2002;110:707–708.
12. Tamai S, Nakamura Y, Motomiya Y. Microsurgical replantation of a completely amputated penis. *Plast Reconstr Surg* 1977;60:287–291.
13. Cohen BE, May JW, Daly JSF, Young HH II. Successful clinical replantation of an amputated penis by microneurovascular repair. *Plast Reconstr Surg* 1977;59:276–280.
14. Baumeister RG, Brandl H, Chaussey C, Schilling A. Mikro-chirurgische penisreplantation nac selbstverstummenlung. *Urologe(A)* 1985;22:235–237.
15. Carroll PR, Lue TF, Schmidt RA, et al. Penile replantation: current concepts. *J Urol* 1985;133:281–285.
16. Chollet D, Rheiner P. Amputation du penis: deux methodes reconstructives. *Helv Chir Acta* 1983;50:247–252.
17. Einarsson G, Goldstein M, Laungani G. Penile replantation. *Urology* 1983;22:404–405.
18. Frey M. Successful replantation of a completely amputated penis. *Int J Microsurge* 1980;2:173–176.
19. Hamann F, Sabri W, Melchoir H. [Penis replantation following autoamputation]. *Z Urol Nephrol* 1983;76:361–367.
20. Henriksson TG, Hahne B, Hakeius L, et al. Microsurgical replantation of an amputated penis. *Scand J Urol Nephrol* 1980;14:111–114.
21. Heymann AD, Bell-Thompson J, Rathod DM, Heller LE. Successful reimplantation of the penis using microvascular techniques. *J Urol* 1977;118:879–880.
22. Strauch B, Sharzer LA, Petro J, Greenstein B. Replantation of amputated parts of the penis, nose, ear and scalp. *Clin Plast Surg* 1977;10:115–124.
23. Wei FC, McKee KH, Huerta FJ, Robinette MA. Microsurgical replantation of a completely amputated penis. *Ann Plast Surg* 1983;10: 317–320.
24. Yamano Y, Tanaka H. Replantation of a completely amputated penis by microsurgical technique: a case report. *Microsurgery* 1984;5:40–43.
25. Kitmanee M. *Penile replantation: update.* Presented at IX International Congress of Plastic and Reconstructive Surgery, New Delhi, India, March 3, 1987.
26. Sanger JR, Matloub HS, Yousif NJ, Begun FP. Penile replantation after self-inflicted amputation. *Ann Plast Surg* 1992;29:579–584.
27. Wells MD, Boyd JB, Bulbul MA. Penile replantation. *Ann Plast Surg* 1991;26:577–581.
28. Becker M, Hofner K, Lassner F, et al. Replantation of the complete external genitals. *Plast Reconstr Surg* 1997;99:1165–1168.
29. Zenn MR, Carson CC III, Patel MP. Replantation of the penis: patient report. *Ann Plast Surg* 2000;44:214–220.
30. Matloub, HS, Yousif NJ, Sanger JR. Case Report: Temporary ectopic implantation of an amputated penis. *Plast Reconstr Surg* 1994;93:408–412.
31. Ching W-C, Liao H-T, Ulusal BG, et al. Salvage of a complicated penis replantation using bipedicaled scrotal flap following a prolonged ischemia time. *J Plast Reconstr Aesthet Surg* 2010;63:e639–e643.
32. Hashem FK, Ahmed S, A-Malaq AA, AbuDaia JM. Successful replantation of penis (post-circumcision) complicated by prolonged ischemia. *Br J Plast Surg* 1999;52:308–310.
33. Breza J, Aboseif SR, Orvis BR, et al. Detailed anatomy of penile neurovascular structures: surgical significance. *J Urol* 1989;141:437–443.
34. Yachia D. Surgical anatomy of the penis and scrotum. In *Text Atlas of Penile Surgery*. London, UK, Informa Healthcare, 2007, pp. 1–9.
35. Carrera A, Gil-Vernet, Forcada P, et al. Arteries of the scrotum: a microvascular study and its application to urethral reconstruction with scrotal flaps. *BJU Int* 2008;103:820–824.
36. Lin C-H, Wei F-C, Chen C-T, et al. Microsurgical tissue transplantation or replantation in patients with psychoneurological impairment. *Plast Reconstr Surg* 2001;108:1211–1217.

37. Fan J, Eriksson M, Rosenlund AF, Nordstrom RE. An unusually avulsed penis successfully replanted by using microsurgical technique. *Plast Reconstr Surg* 1996;98:571–573.
38. Liu Y-P, Tang H-P, Yang Z-X, Pan D-D. Replantation of avulsed penoscrotal skin. *Plast Reconstr Surg* 2001;107:1800–1802.
39. Ozkan S, Gurpinar T. A serious circumcision complication: penile shaft amputation and a new reattachment technique with a successful outcome. *J Urol* 1997;158:1946–1947.
40. Silber SJ. Microsurgery of the male genitalia. In Silber SJ (ed). *Microsurgery*. Baltimore, Williams and Wilkins, 1979, p. 303.
41. Volkmer BG, Maier S. Case report: successful penile replantation following autoamputation: twice! *In J Impot Res* 2002;14:197–198.
42. Mineo M, Jolley T, Rodriguez G. Leech therapy in penile replantation: a case of recurrent penile self-amputation. *Urology* 2004;63:981–983.
43. Harris, DD, Beaghler MA, Stewart SC, et al. Use of a subcutaneous tunnel following replantation of an amputated penis. *Urology* 1996;48:628–630.
44. Pantuck AJ, Lobis MR, Ciocca R, Weiss RE. Penile replantation using the leech Hirudo Medicinalis. *Urology* 1996;48:953–956.
45. Tuerk M, Weir WH Jr. Successful replantation of a traumatically amputated glans penis. *Plast Reconstr Surg* 1971;48:499–500.

CHAPTER 53

Lymphaticovenular Anastomosis for Lymphedema

Isao Koshima, Kazuki Kikuchi, Yukio Seki, Fusa Ogata, Mitsunaga Narushima, and Makoto Mihara

Treatment for diseases of the lymphatic system, especially lymphedema of the limbs, is challenging (1–5). The true pathophysiology of lymphedema is still unknown, methods of accurate evaluation of lymphatic drainage have not been established, and treatment remains controversial. Recent *supermicrosurgical* techniques, with which vascular anastomoses smaller than 1 mm are possible, have facilitated the precise anastomosis of vessels as small as 0.3 to 0.8 mm in diameter (6–13). This technique involves a vascular anastomosis with six to eight watertight stitches using 11-0 or 12-0 nylon attached to a 50- to 30-micron needle. Using supermicrosurgery in lymphedema, the lymphatic fluid may be drained into the subdermal venular system with reasonable results.

This chapter reports our recent findings on the mechanism of development of lymphedema, the evaluation of lymphatic function, and the treatment of lymphedema, particularly using supermicrosurgical lymphaticovenular anastomosis (LVA).

MECHANISM OF LYMPHATIC FLOW

It is well known that the smooth muscle cells in the tunica media of lymphatics contract to push lymphatic fluid from the peripheral to the central portion of the body. Functioning peristalsis of the smooth muscle cells in tunica media of the lymphatics returns the lymph flow back into the venous system—specifically, the subclavicular veins—via the thoracic duct and the right lymphatic duct.

Our electron microscopic observation on biopsied lymphatics from lymphedema patients showed severe degeneration associated with minor and incomplete regeneration of the smooth muscle cells (9). As a result, diseased lymphatics lose their peristaltic function (9) (Figure 53-1). We have reported that occlusion of the lymphatics and degeneration of the smooth muscle cells might start proximally in the extremities and that the timing of the occlusion and the degeneration of the smooth muscle cells might not correspond to the duration of the edema (9).

PREOPERATIVE INDOCYANINE GREEN AND INFRARED RAY EXAMINATION TO DETECT REMAINING LYMPHATIC FUNCTION

After indocyanine green (ICG) is injected into the dermal layer of the foot, it passes proximally along the lymphatics. Using an infrared lamp, a fluorescent glow passing through the subcutaneous lymphatics can be detected as a linear streak from the distal foot to the proximal thigh. In normal legs, it usually reaches the proximal thigh within 1 hour. However, in patients with lymphedema, the linear streak does not even extend to the proximal level. Multiple spots representing dye accumulations appear near the knee joint and thigh and take a long time to do so (Figure 53-2). However, ICG injection with infrared light examination seems to be a useful new method for finding superficial lymphatics at the foot and ankle region.

DETAILED TECHNIQUE

Operative treatment is usually reserved for patients who have shown little improvement with compression therapy of at least 6 months' duration. Under local anesthesia, after making two or three 3-cm incisions on the medial aspect of the leg, the lymphatics and subdermal venules (usually 0.5 mm in diameter) are explored using loupe magnification or an operating microscope. Dissection takes place along the course of the great saphenous vein. Dye staining is not always a good indicator for

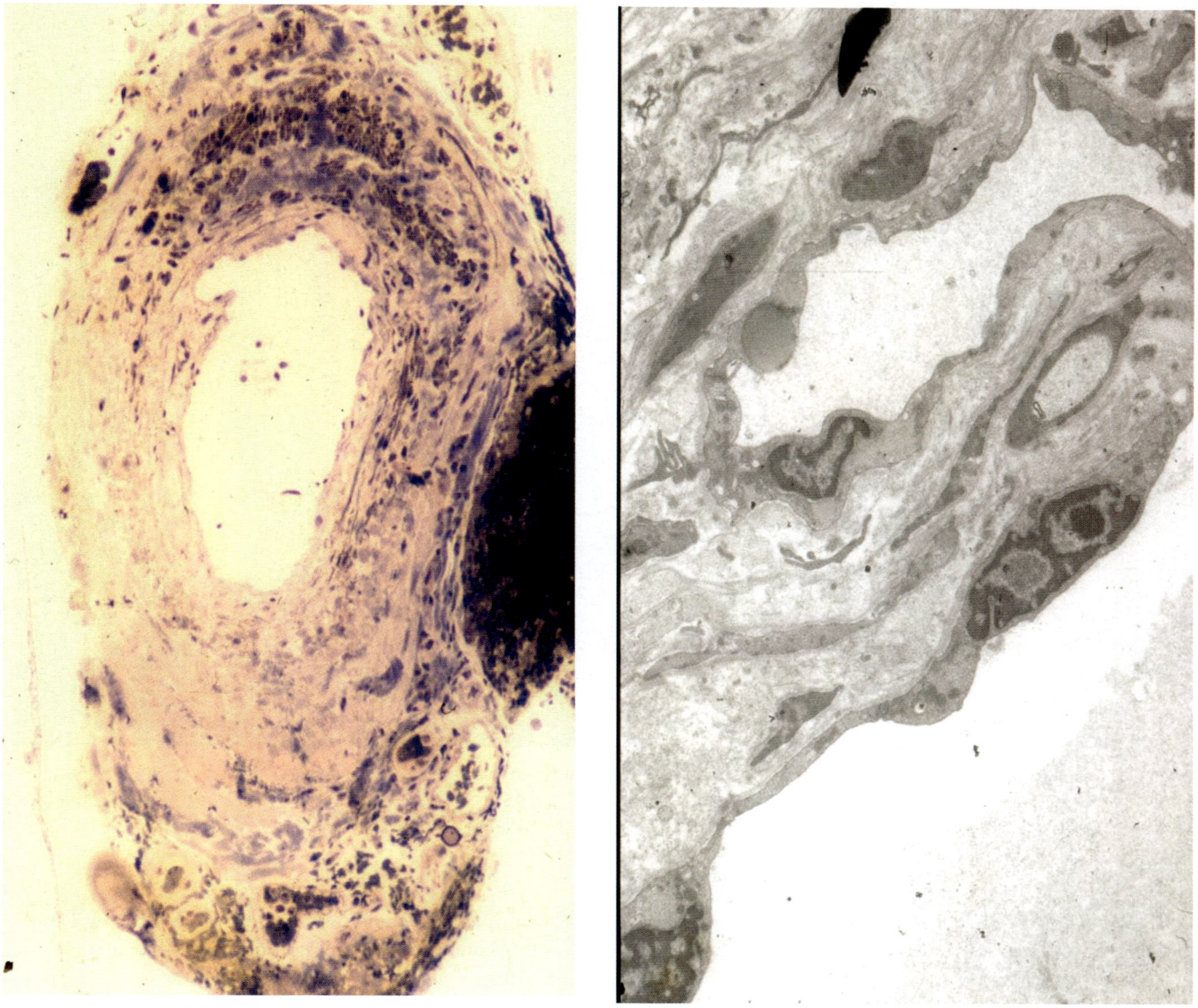

FIGURE 53-1 Biopsied specimen of a human lymphatic channel involved in lymphedema. Regenerated immature smooth muscle cells are detected under the electron microscope (left, x50; right, x3.5k). This shows smooth muscle cells within the affected lymphatics that have regenerated after their degeneration, but their drainage function is insufficient without surgical intervention such as lymphaticovenular anastomosis.

finding lymphatics because in lymphedema, their collecting function has been compromised. The subdermal venules, which exist anywhere beneath the dermis, can be usually detected adjacent to the lymphatics. Regarding the selection of these channels, lymphatics retaining some drainage function are confirmed by strong lymph backflow after they have been transected under the operating microscope. These lymphatics are selected to establish lymphaticovenous shunting. Without a vascular clamp, end-to-end LVAs between similarly sized vessels are carried out using 50- or 30-micron needles attached to 11-0 or 12-0 nylon sutures. A fine needle holder is essential, and the magnification ranges from 20 to 30 times. During anastomosis, backflow of lymphatic fluid from the end of the transected lymphatic expands both its own end and that of the recipient venule.

After the anastomosis is completed, expansion of the venule is detected as it fills up from the lymphatic flow (Figures 53-3 and 53-4). Although these operations can be completed within 2 hours, some patients with irradiated bladders require a Foley catheter. After surgery, a low-pressure bandage is applied, a vascular dilating drug (prostaglandin E1) is administered, and the patients are allowed to walk freely. About 5 or 6 hours after surgery, temporary erythema of the whole affected leg sometimes occurs because of reverse flow from the vein into the lymphatic system. These skin changes usually disappear spontaneously within 5 days. Four weeks later, the patient can wear elastic stockings on the operated limb.

TRICKS AND TIPS

- Local anesthesia is preferable to demonstrate to patients the LVA techniques. This encourages patients to perform physical treatments such as compression and massage.

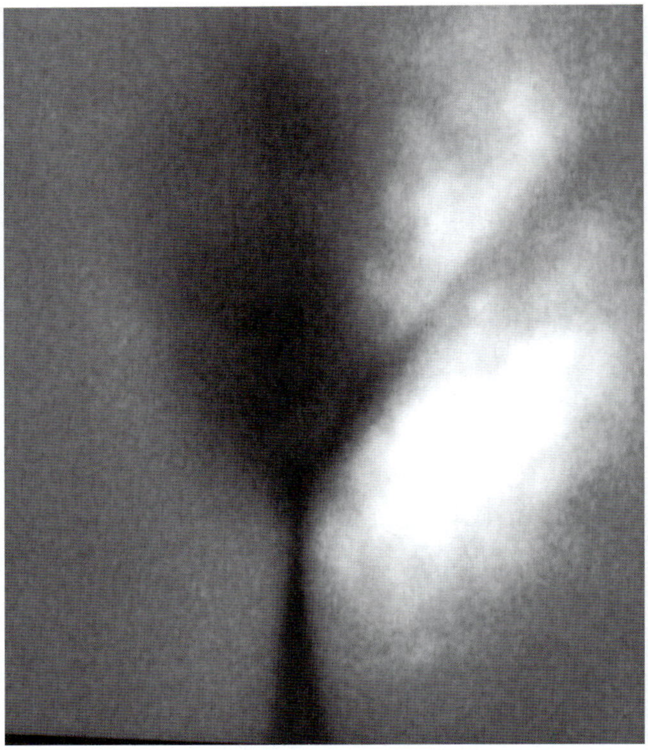

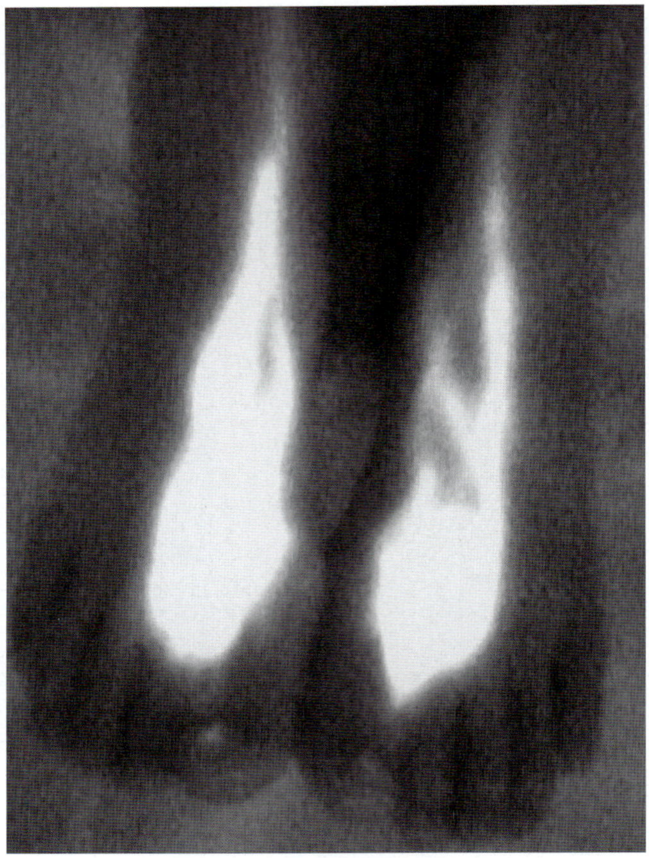

FIGURE 53-2 Indocyanine green (ICG) injection with infrared light examination in a case of lymphedema of the left leg. After injection of ICG into the skin of the bilateral first web spaces, lymphatics outlined with fluorescence are detected under infrared light. Twenty-four hours later, pooling of ICG can be detected at the area of lymphedema even in this early stage case.

- Preoperative ICG injection should be done the day *before* surgery because staining of lymphatics takes 24 hours in legs with lymphedema.
- Xylocaine E (with adrenalin) injection is preferred for the skin incision because it limits subdermal bleeding and facilitates detection of the lymphatics.
- Multiple anastomoses at the proximal level (thigh and groin) are essential to obtain better postoperative results.
- Lymph malformations with cutaneous lymphorrhea in the female genital region may be secondarily resected after primary LVA.

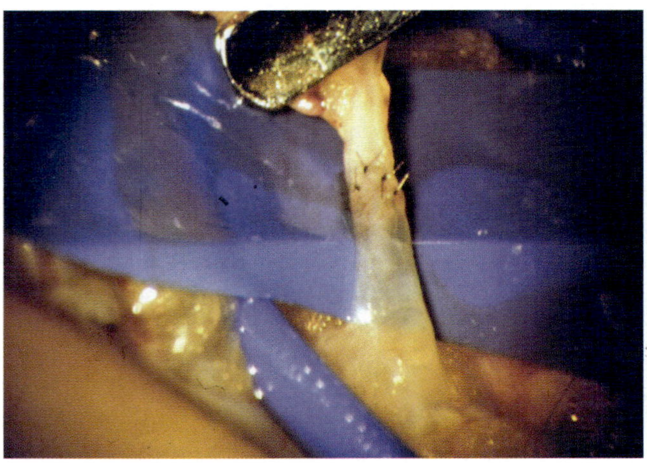

FIGURE 53-3 Supermicrosurgical lymphaticovenular anastomosis. A translucent lymphatic channel and a subdermal venule are anastomosed under the microscope.

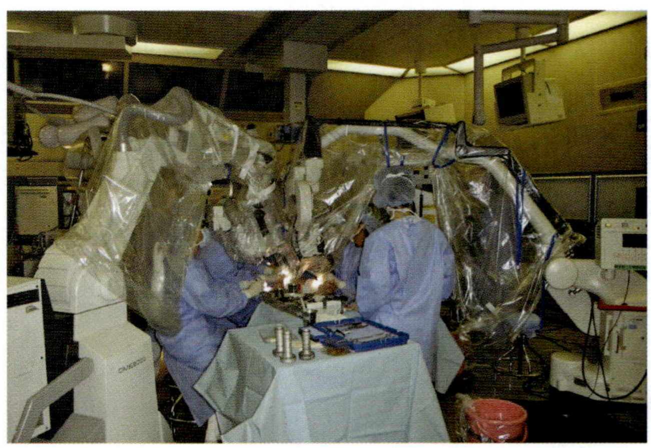

FIGURE 53-4 Under local anesthesia, four "supermicrosurgeons" start anastomoses simultaneously for bilateral lymphedema of the legs. The surgery, which includes 10 lymphaticovenular anastomoses, is usually completed in 3 hours.

COMPLICATIONS

Postoperative color changes in the skin resembling subcutaneous bleeding or erythema sometimes occur at about 5 hours after surgery. This results from reverse flow through the anastomoses (i.e., from the veins to the lymphatics). This usually clears up 1 week after surgery without the need for external compression.

Inadequate wound closure often results in lymphorrhea from the incision. Such wounds generally heal spontaneously within a few weeks.

CASE REPORTS

Case 1: Early Stage Lymphaticovenular Anastomoses Resulting in Full Recovery

A 65-year-old woman underwent left breast cancer resection 16 years earlier developed left arm edema 11 months before admission. Despite compression therapy, the left forearm was 6 cm larger than the right. Under general anesthesia, a total of six anastomoses were performed in the upper arm (two anastomoses), elbow (three anastomoses), and distal forearm (one anastomosis). After surgery, the patient maintained arm compression using a bandage. Fifteen years later, the arm remains close to normal size without the need for compression therapy (Figure 53-5).

Case 2: Congenital Leg and Scrotal Edema with Lymphorrhea

A 25-year-old man had congenital edema of right leg had scrotal lymphorrhea for 6 years. Under local anesthesia, the patient was treated with LVAs at the right ankle and scrotal area. Six months after surgery, lymphorrhea was completely absent and edema of the right leg and genital area was decreased (Figure 53-6).

Case 3: Long-Standing Facial Edema After Repeated Resection for Recurrent Pharyngeal Carcinoma

A 59-year-old man had long-standing edema of the face resulting from repeated surgery for recurrent pharyngeal cancer. Preoperative ICG injection study showed the remaining lymph drainage function through the right preauricular region. Under local anesthesia, short incisions were made through the right preauricular line and the left submandibular line. Each lymphatic channel in the right preauricular and left submandibular region was anastomosed to the superficial temporal and facial veins. After surgery, edema decreased dramatically (Figure 53-7).

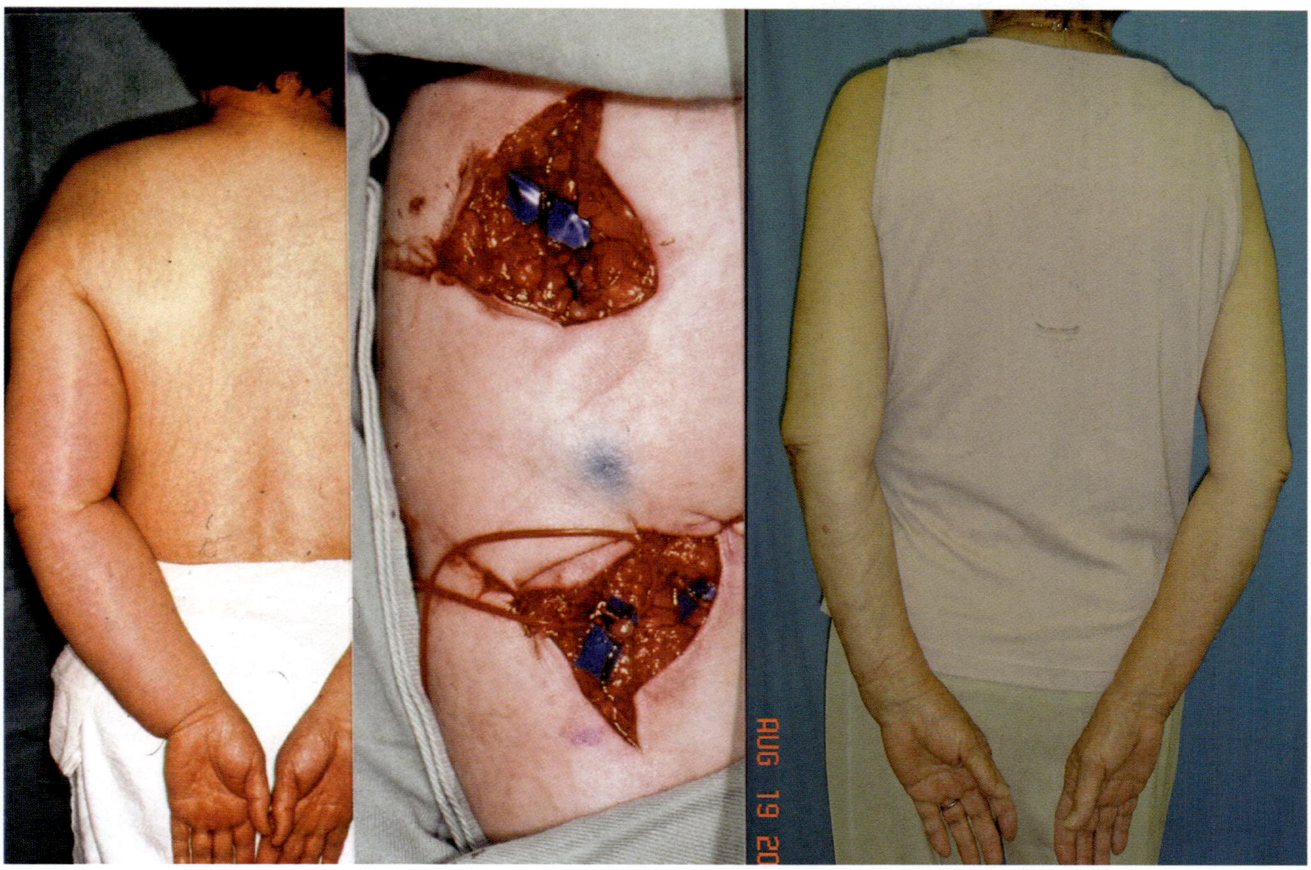

FIGURE 53-5 Case 1. (**A**) A 65-year-old woman with left arm lymphedema of 11 months' duration. (**B**) Six anastomoses were performed around the elbow. (**C**) Complete recovery shown 15 years after the operation. There was no need for postoperative compression therapy.

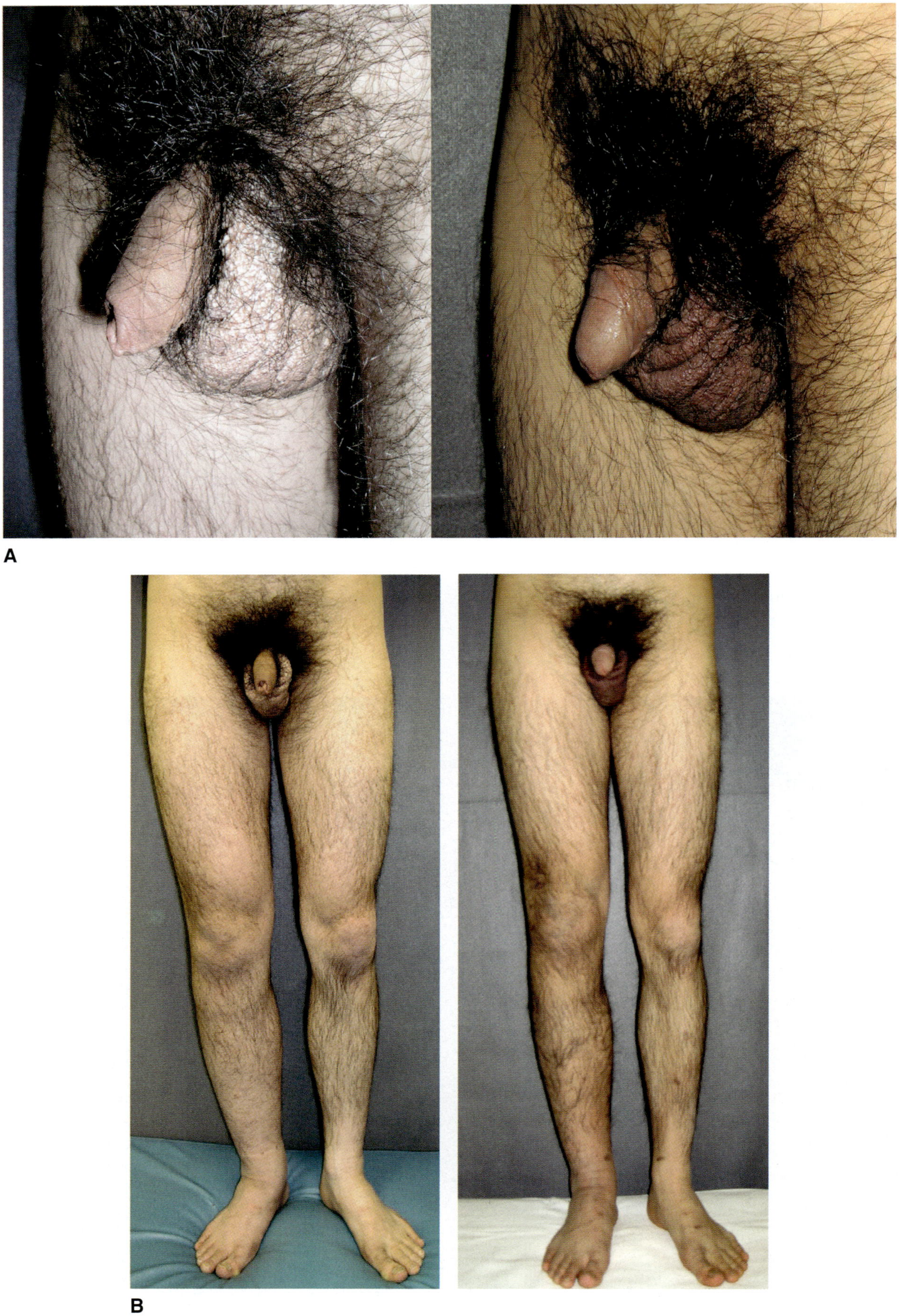

FIGURE 53-6 (**A**) Case 2. A 25-year-old man with congenital edema of the right leg and scrotal lymphorrhea for 6 years: preoperative (*left*) and improvement at 6 months after lymphaticovenular anastomosis (LVA) in the scrotum and legs (*right*). (**B**) Appearance of the legs: preoperative (*left*) and 6 months after LVA (*right*).

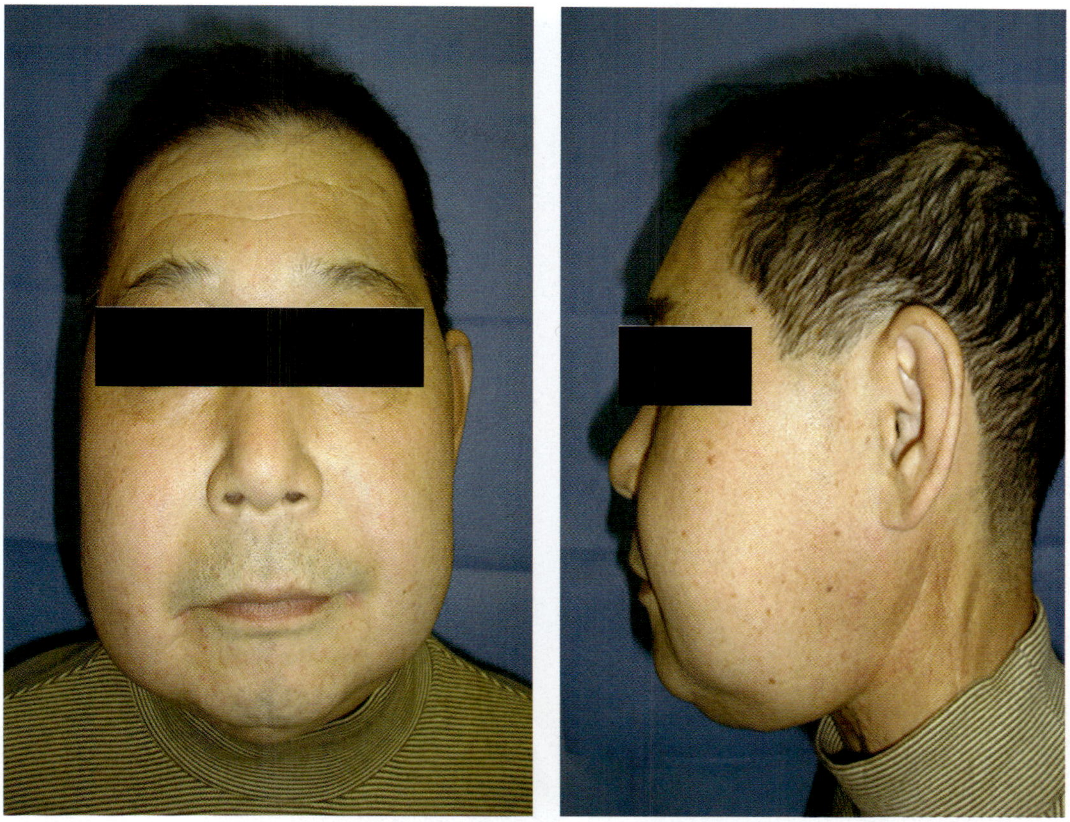

A

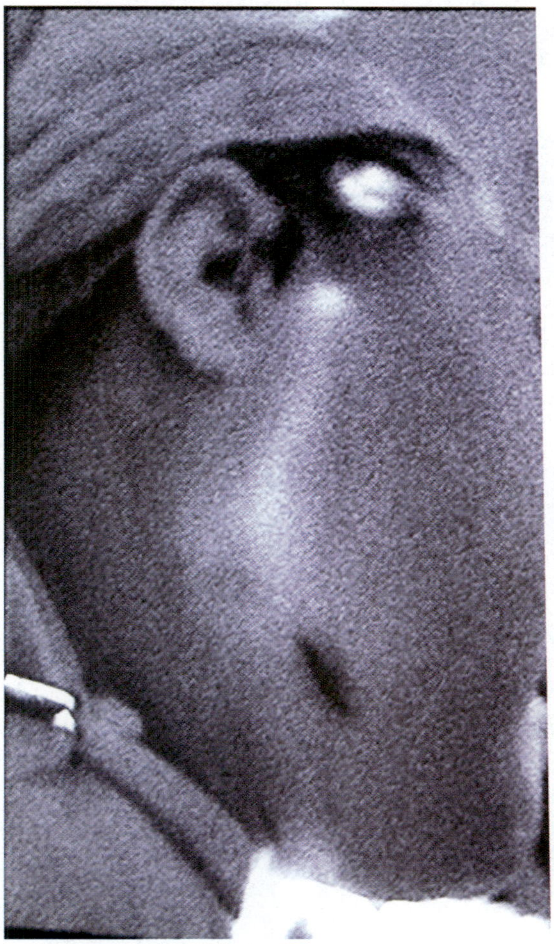

B

FIGURE 53-7 Case 3. (**A**) A 59-year-old man with long-standing edema of the face resulting from repeated surgery for recurrent pharyngeal cancer. (**B**) Indocyanine green injection study showed the remaining lymph drainage function through the right preauricular region. (**C**) With short incisions under local anesthesia, lymphaticovenular anastomosis (LVA) in the right preauricular and left submandibular regions were carried out. *Right*, LVA in the right preauricular region. (**D**) One year after LVA, edema has decreased dramatically.

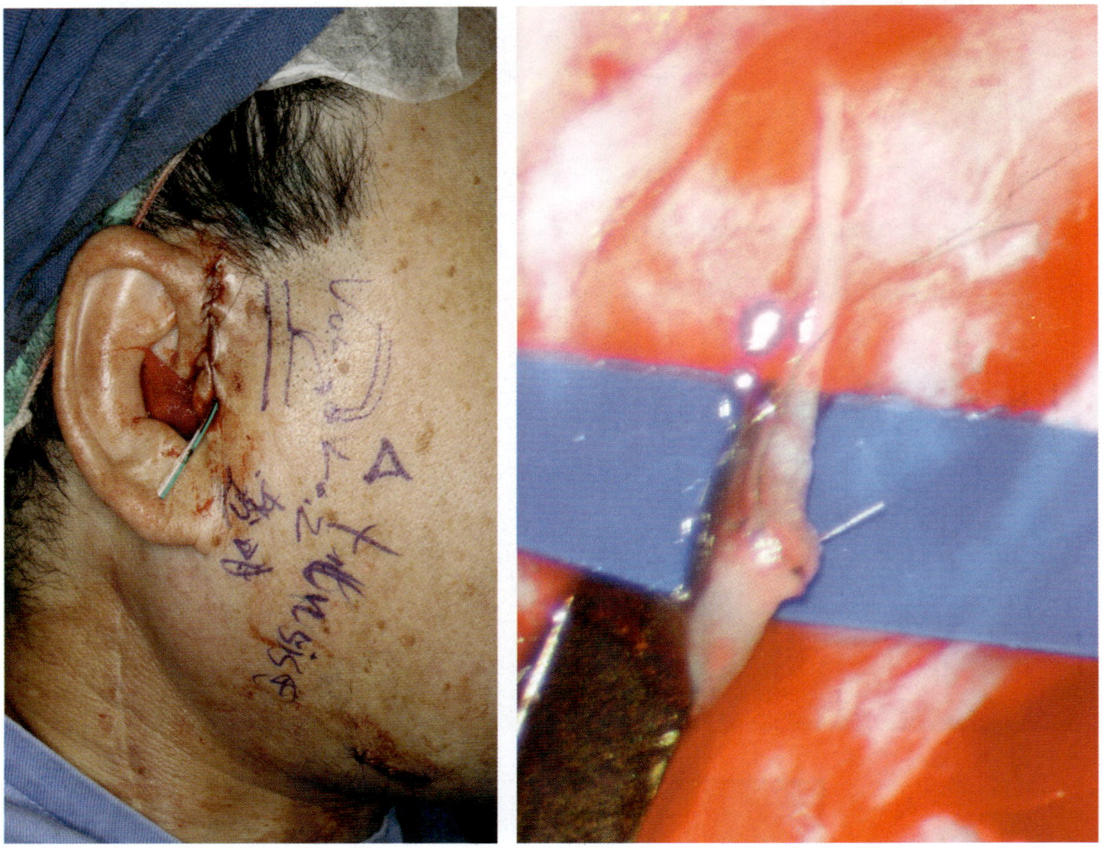

C

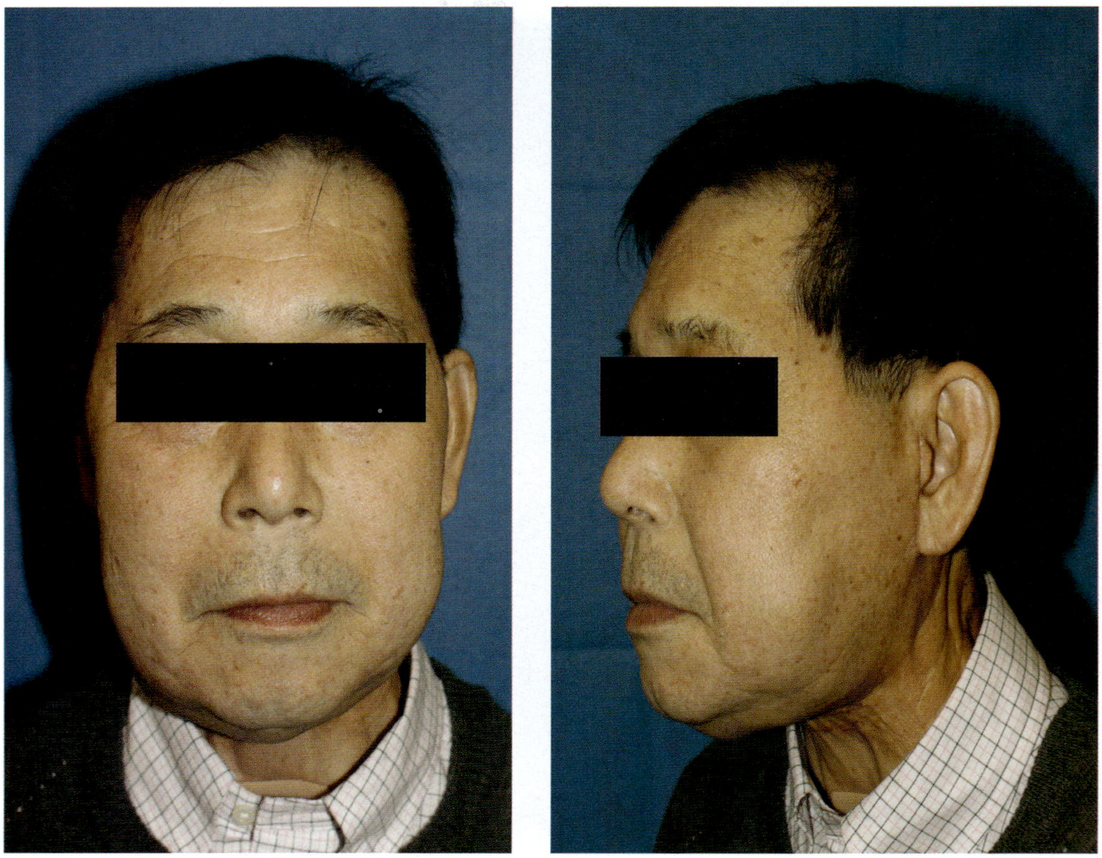

D

FIGURE 53-7 *(Continued)*

INDICATIONS FOR LYMPHATICOVENULAR ANASTOMOSIS

- Stage 0 edema: Prophylactic LVA is preferable to therapeutic LVA and has a high success rate for the prevention of lymphedema because the smooth muscle cells in the lymphatics still have normal drainage function.
- Early stage lymphedema: Complete recovery without compression may be expected with LVA because smooth muscle cells within the lymphatics are still in the predegenerate state.
- Recurrent lymphangitis: The majority of patients show a dramatic decrease in the rate of infection.
- Severe and long-standing edema in the legs: LVA should be combined with a vascularized lymphadiposal flap or vascularized lymph node transfer for best results. With LVA alone, functional recovery of the smooth muscle cells in the lymphatics cannot be expected to be adequate. Only drainage with normally functioning lymphatics and lymph nodes can be expected to help these dysfunctioning extremities. For unilateral leg edema, normal functioning lymph nodes are usually obtained from the first web space in the opposite, normal leg. The recipient site is the groin of the affected leg. For bilateral leg lymphedema, nodes are obtained from the lateral thoracic region.
- Congenital or acquired chiloabdomen: LVA in both groin regions is indicated.
- Congenital or acquired lymphorrhea of the scrotum: LVA in the scrotum and in bilateral groin regions is indicated.
- Lymphocyst formation after the resection of uterus and ovarian cancers: The cyst will disappear, and the resulting lymphedema of the leg can be prevented by LVA.
- Folliculitis with lymphorrhea in the female genital region may be resected after primary LVA.
- Severe scrotal edema caused by radiation for prostate cancer: LVA in the scrotal region is indicated.
- Long-standing facial edema after repeated resection for recurrent pharyngeal carcinoma: LVA in the preauricular and submandibular regions is effective (see Case 3).

REFERENCES

1. O'Brien BM, Chait LA, Hurwitz PJ. Microlymphatic surgery. *Orthop Clin North Am* 1977;8:405–424.
2. O'Brien BM, Sykes PJ, Threlfall GN, Browning FSC. Microlymphaticovenous anastomoses for obstructive lymphedema. *Plast Reconstr Surg* 1977;60:197–211.
3. O'Brien BM, Mellow CG, Khazanchi RK, et al. Long-term results after microlymphaticovenous anastomoses for the treatment of obstructive lymphedema. *Plast Reconstr Surg* 1990;85:562–572.
4. Huang GK, Hu RQ, Liu ZZ, et al. Microlymphaticovenous anastomosis in the treatment of lower limb obstructive lymphedema: analysis of 91 cases. *Plast Reconstr Surg* 1985;76:671–677.
5. Campisi C. Use of autologous interposition vein graft in management of lymphedema: Preliminary experimental and clinical observations. *Lymphology* 1991;24:71–76.
6. Koshima I, Soeda S, Moriguchi T, et al. The use of arteriovenous anastomosis for replantation of the distal phalanx of the fingers. *Plast Reconstr Surg* 1992;89:710–714.
7. Koshima I, Inagawa K, Urushibara K, Moriguchi T. Paraumbilical perforator flap without deep inferior epigastric vessels. *Plast Reconstr Surg* 1998;102:1052–1057.
8. Koshima I, Urushibara K, Inagawa K, et al. Free medial plantar perforator flaps for the resurfacing of plantar and foot defects. *Plast Reconstr Surg* 2001;107:1753–1757.
9. Koshima I, Kawada S, Moriguchi T, Kajiwara Y. Ultrastructural observation of lymphatic vessels in lymphedema in human extremities. *Plast Reconstr Surg* 1996;97:397–405.
10. Koshima I, Inagawa K, Urushibara K, Moriguchi T. Supermicrosurgical lymphaticovenular anastomosis for the treatment of lymphedema in the upper extremities. *Reconstr Microsurg* 2000;16:437–442.
11. Koshima I, Nanba Y, Tsutsui T, et al. Long-term follow-up after lymphaticovenular anastomosis for lymphedema in the legs. *Reconstr Microsurg* 2003;19:209–215.
12. Koshima I, Nanba Y, Tsutsui T, et al. Minimal invasive lymphaticovenular anastomosis under local anesthesia for leg lymphedema. Is it effective for stage III and IV? *Ann Plast Surg* 2004;53:1–6.
13. Campisi C, Boccardo F, Zilli A, et al. Long-term results after lymphatic-venous anastomoses for the treatment of obstructive lymphedema. *Microsurgery* 2001;21:135–139.

CHAPTER 54

Lymph Node Transfer for Lymphedema

Ming-Huei Cheng and Dung H. Nguyen

Lymphedema is a debilitating condition that is characterized by the abnormal collection of fluid and proteins within the interstitial fluid. More than 3 million patients in the United States are affected by lymphedema (1). It is often a sequela of cancer or its treatment. Postmastectomy upper extremity lymphedema (UEL) is estimated to occur in 16% to 39% of breast cancer patients and is especially prevalent in patients subjected to radiotherapy and axillary lymph node dissection (ALND) (2). Lymphedema of the lower extremities after vulva and cervical cancers affects 20% to 49% of the women postoperatively (3). It also develops in 20% of patients with melanoma after ilioinguinal lymph node dissection (3). Chronic lymphedema is associated with developmental derangements of lymphatics and hypoplasia that may be present in 55% of the affected patients. There is an increased risk of infection in these patients because of restricted protein-rich lymph flow, including dermatolymphangioadenitis, erysipelas, cellulitis, and lymphangitis. When left untreated, lymphedema can develop into a permanent, disfiguring condition that has a profound impact on the patient's functional abilities, psychosocial well-being, and overall quality of life. Early diagnosis and intervention are critical to reverse the progression of disease and to minimize its complications.

ANATOMY OF THE LYMPHATIC SYSTEM

The lymphatic fluid contains water, proteins, cells, and other macromolecules from the interstitial space. It is drained by the superficial and deep lymphatic vessels. The superficial system collects lymph from the subdermal and subcutaneous tissues through lymphatic vessels that reside in the subcutaneous tissues. The deep lymphatic system collects lymph from the tissues deep to the fascia through lymphatic channels that travel along the blood vessels. The two systems are interconnected by vessels that cross the fascia. The return pathway of lymph fluid to the intravascular circulation relies on a pressure flow gradient from the interstitium into the lymphatic capillaries and subsequently into the venous system. The right lymphatic duct drains the right torso, arm, face, and neck and empties into the right subclavian vein. The lymph from the rest of the body is drained via the thoracic duct into the left venous angle at the junction of the left internal jugular vein and the left subclavian vein. The thoracic duct is the largest of the lymphatic trunks and is responsible for emptying up to 4 L of lymph per day. When lymph drainage is disrupted anywhere along this pathway, fluid collects in the interstitial space, resulting in lymphedema.

PATHOPHYSIOLOGY OF LYMPHEDEMA

In a normal physiologic state, the lymphatic load and transport capacity are in balance. The lymphatic load is defined as the volume of lymph fluid that is present in the interstitial tissue, and the transport capacity is defined as the maximum lymph volume that is drained by the lymphatics in a given time period. When the lymphatic system becomes dysfunctional such that the transport capacity of the lymphatic system cannot keep up with the lymphatic load, lymphatic system insufficiency occurs, which leads to interstitial edema.

Lymphatic obstruction is associated with increased subcutaneous and intramuscular compartment pressures in the affected limb (4). These elevated pressures causes progressive compression of the superficial and deep lymphatic vessels, leading to diminished rates of capillary blood flow and lymphatic drainage in the lymphedematous limb (5). Hence, it is common that lymphedema coexists with varying degrees of venous insufficiency.

Lymph fluid that leaks from a severed lymphatic vessel stimulates local tissue fibrosis. This response is even more exaggerated in the presence of an infection. Progressive tissue fibrosis obstructs the residual lymphatic channels, causing further stagnation of lymph drainage, dilatation of lymphatic vessels, and eventual lymphatic valve incompetence (6). The dysfunctional lymphatic vessels are unable to absorb the excess fluid from the tissue spaces. The buildup of high osmotic pressure lymph fluid in the interstitial spaces leads to more edema and fibrosis, interfering with wound healing and predisposing the patient to infection in a vicious cycle.

Lymphedema can be classified as primary or secondary. Primary lymphedema is caused by genetic abnormalities that cause hypoplasia, hyperplasia, or aplasia of the lymphatic system components. These hereditary conditions include congenital lymphedema (Milroy's disease), lymphedema praecox, and lymphedema tarda. Secondary or acquired lymphedema is much more common and is caused by mechanical damage to the lymph vessels or lymph nodes caused by surgery, radiation, malignancy, trauma, and recurrent infections. These secondary factors cause permanent impairment of the transport capacity in the affected region and increase the likelihood of developing lymphedema in that region.

Other secondary causes of lymphedema include high altitude, chronic venous insufficiency, immobility, tourniquet effects, or the use of tamoxifen (1). In developing countries such as Southeast Asia, India, and Africa, filariasis is the most common cause of lymphedema. It is caused by chronic infection and destruction of the peripheral lymphatic system by the parasitic nematode *Wuchereria bancrofti*. Although some effective treatments are available for secondary lymphedema, there is currently no good treatment for this condition.

CANCER-ASSOCIATED LYMPHEDEMA

In developed countries, lymphedema as the result of cancer or cancer treatments is most prevalent and thus will be the focus of the remaining portion of this chapter.

Breast Cancer

In the United States, breast cancer–associated UEL is the most common cause of secondary lymphedema. It occurs as a result of tumor compression causing lymphatic vessel obstruction but more frequently from breast cancer treatment such as surgery or radiation therapy. The reported incidence of UEL after standard ALND can be as high as 56% compared with the reported 6% if sentinel lymph node biopsy (SLNB) is performed (7). UEL is more frequent with ALND because more lymph nodes are removed, and there is more disruption of dermal and subcutaneous lymphatic channels because of the more extensive dissection. In fact, many studies have shown that the severity of UEL is positively correlated with the number of lymph nodes removed and increases in a linear fashion after the removal of 10 or more lymph nodes (7,8).

Upper extremity lymphedema can be exacerbated by adjuvant radiotherapy. When both surgery and radiation therapy are performed, the frequency of UEL ranges from 6% to 48% (9). This is in contrast to an approximately 6% when a lumpectomy is performed alone (9). The incidence of UEL rises to 23% when an SLNB is combined with radiation therapy (9). Other reported predisposing risk factors include obesity, increased tumor size, tumor location in the upper outer quadrant, and postoperative wound infection. This suggests that weight reduction in obese patients, early cancer detection when tumor size is small, and prevention of postoperative infections may decrease the risk of developing postmastectomy UEL (10).

Genital Cancers

Genital carcinomas are the next most common cause of lymphedema affecting the lower extremities. In women, the incidence of lower extremity lymphedema (LEL) is highest in patients with cervical cancer (21%–49%) followed by uterine cancer (17.7%) and ovarian cancer (7.1%) (11). Although postoperative radiotherapy was found to be an independent risk factor for LEL (12), the degree of postirradiation lymphedema is strongly dependent on the type and extent of lymph node dissection performed. This is also found to be true for prostate cancer in men. The reported incidence of LEL after prostate surgery rises from 25%–50% to up to 66% when a diagnostic dissection with pelvic irradiation is converted to a therapeutic dissection with pelvic irradiation (13).

Melanoma

Melanoma-associated lymphedema is similarly related to the kind of lymph node dissection performed and whether or not postoperative radiation therapy was given. Patients who have axillary SLNB for cutaneous melanoma have a 1.7% incidence of developing UEL (14). This is in contrast to the 10% risk after a complete ALND and a stark increase to 53% after adjuvant axillary radiation therapy (15). Patients who received inguinal lymph node dissection have an approximate 30% incidence of developing LEL (16).

SYMPTOMS AND DIAGNOSIS OF LYMPHEDEMA

After cancer treatment, a patient carries a lifetime risk of developing lymphedema. The time of onset is variable and can be over weeks, months, or years (17). Lymphedema can be localized to one specific area of the limb or generalized to the entire limb. Patients typically present with complaints of feeling of heaviness in the limb; skin tightness with decreased flexibility in the hand, wrist, or ankle; and difficulty fitting into clothing in the affected area. Some patients may also develop brachial plexus radiated neuritis (18).

Untreated lymphedema lead to decrease limb function, wound healing problems, recurrent infections, and sometimes limb loss. In rare instances, lymphangiosarcoma, cancer of the diseased lymphatics, develops.

There is currently no standardized definition of lymphedema. Physical assessment includes sequential circumferential measurements at various points along the limb, volumetric measures using water displacement technique, or tissue tonometry of the affected limbs. Radiologic imaging such as computed tomography and magnetic resonance imaging might be helpful in the diagnosis by demonstrating a unique honeycomb pattern of the lymphatic channels that is specific to lymphedema and not other potential causes of edema (19).

Lymphangiography, commonly used in the past, is now replaced by lymphoscintigraphy because it caused inflammation, scarring, and atrophy of the remaining lymphatic vessels. Technetium (Tc) 99m lymphoscintigraphy is now the gold standard for evaluating the functional and morphologic changes of the lymphatic system. It is able to distinguish lymphedema from nonlymphatic causes of edema, identify pathways of lymph drainage, detect dermal backflow and number of lymph nodes, and determine the clearance times of the radiomarker (20). Its sensitivity and specificity are reported to be 73% to 97% and 100%, respectively (21).

STAGING OF LYMPHEDEMA

Lymphedema progresses from mild to severe and is categorized into three clinical stages (1):

Stage 0 (latency stage): There is a subjective complaint of feeling of heaviness or tightness in the limb with the absence of clinical symptoms of lymphedema.

Stage 1, mild lymphedema (spontaneously reversible lymphedema): The tissue is soft with pitting edema after firm pressure is applied for at least 5 seconds. Swelling is reversible and completely resolves with limb elevation.

Stage 2, moderate lymphedema (spontaneously irreversible lymphedema): The tissue now has a spongy consistency and demonstrates "nonpitting" edema caused by increased intradermal fibrosis. There is a positive Stemmer sign, which is the inability to pinch the skin of the dorsum of the fingers and toes. Clinical resolution of signs of lymphedema is not possible with limb elevation. Skin infection is also more common at this stage.

Stage 3, severe lymphedema (lymphostatic elephantiasis): Tissue swelling is irreversible because of extensive tissue fibrosis. There is increased thickness of the skin folds and significant increase in limb size, as well as skin changes such as hyperkeratosis, papillomas, cysts, and fistulas. In this state, recurrent skin and nail bacterial and fungus infections are common.

CONVENTIONAL TREATMENTS OF LYMPHEDEMA

The available treatments of lymphedema fall into three categories: rehabilitative therapies, pharmacologic agents, and surgery. The goal of therapy is to decrease the excess lymph volume as much as possible and maintain the limb at its smallest size to restore function and cosmesis to the affected limb. Effective treatment requires an interdisciplinary approach that involves multiple modalities. Patient involvement and compliance are critical to the success of the intervention.

Rehabilitative Treatment

Complex Decongestive Physiotherapy

This is the recommended treatment for lymphedema as supported by the National Lymphedema Network Medical Advisory Committee. Complex decongestive therapy (CDT) is delivered by trained therapists and uses a combination of techniques that include manual lymphatic drainage, external compression devices, exercises, and skin and nail care. The treatments act to raise the interstitial fluid pressure in the soft tissue compartments. Specifically, manual lymphatic drainage helps to break up the fibrotic tissues and stimulates lymph drainage via the functioning lymph vessels in a distal to proximal direction to push the stagnant fluid from the edematous limb. Several studies have shown volume reduction rates of more than 50% of the affected limb using CDT (22). CDT includes two phases. Phase I is the acute management phase and consists of a 4- to 6-week program in an outpatient setting with a special therapist. Phase II is the maintenance stage to be done at home by the patient or family and involves continued use of compression garments, self-massage, exercise, and proper skin and nail care. Compliance to a strict regimen can result in stabilization or modest symptomatic improvement in mild to moderate lymphedema. In severe lymphedema, the tissues are very fibrotic and require very high external compressive forces to stimulate lymphatic drainage. The effect, however, is short lived and eventually fail as a critical closing pressure is reached and all lymphatic vessels collapse and act to occlude lymph flow (23).

Compression Devices

Various compression devices are commercially available, including compression bandages, compression garments, gradient compression devices, and pneumatic compression devices. They work by providing a pressure gradient to prevent the backflow of lymphatic fluid distally. Compression devices are useful as an adjunct therapy with other rehabilitative modalities for patients with mild to moderate lymphedema. The greatest benefits are reported after 2 weeks of daily treatment (24). Garment use of at least 6 consecutive hours per day is necessary to achieve significant reduction of edema. The CDT with or without compression devices may be effective in the incomplete proximal obstructive lymphedema but is not the case with complete obstruction. Compliance is an important issue because these devices are often uncomfortable and labor intensive to put on. Proper technique must be used in applying these devices. Improper use may cause neuropathies, pain, pressure sores, and damage to the vasculature.

Pharmacologic Agents

A number of pharmacologic agents have been used for the treatment of lymphedema, including benzopyrenes, antibiotics, diuretics, and selenium. Although antibiotics are effective for the treatment of lymphedema-associated soft tissue infections, the beneficial effects of other agents have only been supported by small sample studies. Benzopyrenes, which include warfarin, have been used in Europe but are currently not approved by the US Food and Drug Administration for the treatment of lymphedema. Diuretic agents specifically have shown no benefits in the treatment of lymphedema (25).

Surgical Treatments

Debulking Procedures

The Charles procedure was the first debulking procedure (described in 1912) that involves radical excision of skin, subcutaneous tissue, and muscle fascia en bloc with primary or staged skin grafting. Since then, variations of this procedure have been reported with good results in terms of contour, improvement of function, and reduction in the incidence of secondary skin infection (26). However, there are significant drawbacks of these procedures, including wound breakdown, a 15% chance of infection, and necrosis of the skin graft (27). Liposuction as a mean of reducing the size of an involved extremity have had some success in a limited number of patients with mild to moderate lymphedema (28). Debulking procedures are performed less frequently today. It may be beneficial as an adjunct therapy to decrease the lymph load in patients with severe lymphedema after vascular lymph node transfer.

Bypass Procedures

Lymphaticovenous and lymphaticolymphatic anastomoses are microsurgical bypass procedures that are reserved for patients who have failed intensive combined medical therapy. These procedures are only effective if the venous system is competent and the regional lymphatic channels and lymph nodes are intact. Nielubowicz et al. first attempted lymphaticovenous anastomosis in the treatment of lymphedema with limited success caused by venous thrombosis at the anastomotic site (29). With refinement in the technique, direct end-to-end lymphaticovenous anastomosis can be performed with significant improvement in limb circumference, in the range of 42% to 83% in selected patients (30), as well as significant reduction in the incidence of secondary cellulitis. However, the efficacy of lymphaticovenous anastomosis and that of lymphaticolymphatic anastomosis are proportional to the number of anastomoses performed. Because of the dense fibrotic tissues in the severe edematous limb, functional distal lymphatics that are suitable for anastomosis are difficult to identify. Injection of indocyanine green (ICG) with infrared light fluorescence enhancement may facilitate the exploration of sizable lymphatics for anastomosis. The anastomosis is also technically challenging because the lymphatic vessels are tiny and thin walled. Usually, a special microscope with high magnification, ultra-fine instruments and 12-0 nylon are required for this technique. Furthermore, there are currently no reliable methods of monitoring anastomotic patency. Many lymphaticovenous or lymphaticolymphatic anastomoses that were observed to be patent in the short term eventually occluded (31–35). The persistent elevated subcutaneous or intramuscular pressures in the edematous limb may be responsible for causing obliteration of the anastomotic channels after the wound closure with 4-0 nylon (36).

Vascularized Lymph Node Transfer

A promising alternative for the management of lymphedema is microvascular transfer of groin lymph nodes to restore lymphatic drainage. Clinical and experimental studies have demonstrated that lymphatic continuity can be restored spontaneously by free tissue transfer (37). Chen et al. first described the vascularized groin lymph node transfer in the canine model in 1990 (38,39). In his studies, he found statistically significant improvement of the lymphedematous legs. Becker et al. also reported long-term significant improvement in postmastectomy lymphedema after vascularized lymph node transfer from the groin to the axilla and elbow (40). Cheng et al. transferred the vascularized groin lymph node transfer to the wrist as a recipient site with significant improvement (50% reduction rate) of postmastectomy UEL (2). Their unpublished prospective study (41) comparing vascularized groin lymph node transfer to the wrist versus the elbow in patients with postmastectomy UEL confirmed the results of the first study. Similar trend in lymphedema reduction was also observed in the elbow group, although less dramatic, at a mean follow-up period of 22 months (41). These results were supported in a prospective randomized animal study that showed similar lymphatic function in the vascularized lymph node transfer group and the sham control group and significantly better lymphatic function in the vascularized lymph node transfer group compared with the avascular lymph node transfer group (42).

MICROSURGICAL LYMPH NODE TRANSFER

Indications

Vascularized lymph node transfer is currently indicated for the treatment of lymphedema in patients who are refractory to other conventional therapies, either moderate to severe lymphedema or complete proximal obstruction revealed by Tc-99 lymphoscintigraphy. The rationale is the introduction of new lymphatic and venous channels into an involved extremity to bypass the area of lymphatic obstruction to venous drainage. Surgical candidates must have a competent venous system in the affected limb. The operative site should be free of infection and cancer recurrence.

Sources of Donor Vascularized Lymph Nodes

Anatomy of the Groin Lymph Node Flap

The groin lymph nodes are divided into the superficial and deep groups. The superficial lymph nodes, found along the superior circumflex iliac vein, primarily drain lymph from the abdominal wall (43) (Figure 54-1). Removal of these nodes therefore does not affect lymphatic drainage of the lower extremity. This makes the groin lymph nodes an attractive donor site because of the low donor site morbidity and well-concealed scar.

Cadaver studies showed that the superficial circumflex iliac artery (SCIA) arises from the common femoral artery (CFA) 2.5 cm distal to the inguinal ligament and immediately divides into superficial and deep (subfascial) branches. The superficial (but not the deep) branch supplies two or three nodes with a pedicle length of 2.5 cm (41). It arborizes within the nodal substance and continues up to the skin. The deep branch passes under the flap and at its lateral corner turns inferiorly to descend on the sartorius muscle. The descending branch sends a small vessel to the lateral corner of the flap but not to the nodes. There

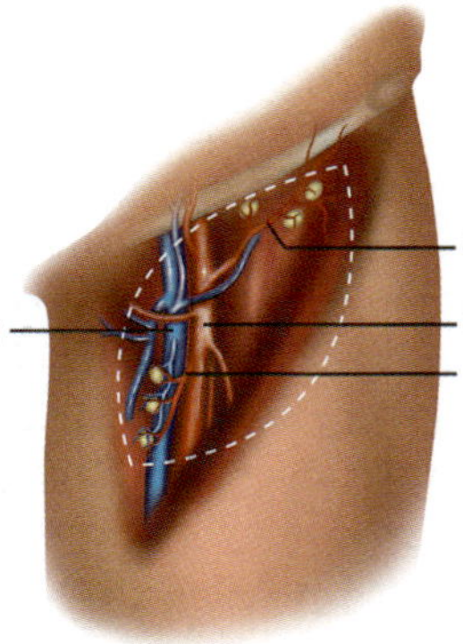

FIGURE 54-1 There are two superficial groin nodal distributions (superior row and medial column) that are located along the main branches of the common femoral artery (CFA), namely, the superficial circumflex iliac artery (SCIA) and the medial artery. Each nodal group contains two or three lymph nodes and can be harvested independently with its corresponding vascular pedicle or together at the confluence of the SCIA and medial artery at the CFA.

is also a sizable medial artery that arises from the lateral aspect of the CFA 3 cm distal to the inguinal ligament and proceeds in a superficial and lateral direction toward the skin (Figures 54-1 and 54-2). This artery supplies two or three nodes in the vicinity of the common femoral vein and the overlying skin with a pedicle length of 2.5 cm. The two nodal distributions (superior row and medial column) may not share the same primary blood supply and therefore can be theoretically harvested independently or together at the confluence of the SCIA and medial artery at the CFA (see Figure 54-1).

Anatomy of the Submental Lymph Node Flap

The submental flap was first described by Martin et al. in 1993 and has since been used widely in head and neck reconstruction (44). It is an axial pattern flap that receives one to four cutaneous perforators from the submental vessels to the skin overlying the platysma. The main perforator is typically found 3.2 cm in front of the facial artery, which pierces the platysma to give off many subdermal branches (45). A single perforator is adequate to perfuse the entire flap. Cadaver studies showed that the submental artery arises from the facial artery deep to the submandibular gland and passes medially across the mylohyoid muscle and then superficial or deep to the digastrics muscle to end on the anterior belly of the digastrics muscle posterior to the mandibular symphysis (46). The submental vein provides the venous drainage into the facial vein. There are typically two to four submental lymph nodes around the submental artery that can be included in the deep layer of the flap during flap harvest (47). The length of the submental artery is approximately 6 cm, which can be lengthened with the inclusion of the facial artery (46). The skin paddle can be up to 15 × 6 cm in most cases and still able to close the donor site primarily (48). The donor site scar is often inconspicuous. The main disadvantage to this flap is the potential injury to the marginal mandibular nerve during dissection.

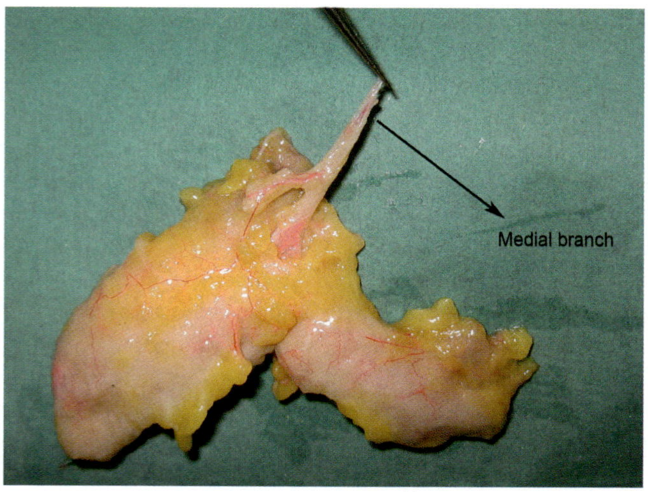

FIGURE 54-2 Cadaveric studies illustrate the medial column lymph nodes nourished by the medial artery pedicle, which comes directly off the common femoral artery.

Anatomy of the Omental Flap

There are a few case reports in the literature regarding the use of a pedicled omental flap transposition for the treatment of lymphedema that is refractory to conservative therapy. Theoretically, the omentum may be the ideal source for lymph node transfer. It provides a large surface area that harbors a large reservoir of lymph nodes and lymphatic tissues. It possesses absorptive lymph drainage capability, fights infection, has angiogenic activity, and is expendable. Through an abdominal incision, the greater omentum is harvested with either the right or left gastroepiploic vessels, depending on the location of the recipient site. The omentum is separated from the stomach carefully to preserve the gastroepiploic arcade. The omentum flap is then brought out through the abdominal incision and passed via a subcutaneous tunnel to either the axilla or inguinal region of the affected limb (49). Nakajima et al. reported marginal improvement in limb circumference after omental transposition to the axilla but marked improvement in limb function and quality of life in a patient with chronic UEL caused by breast cancer resection (49). Goldsmith and colleagues (50,51) found similar results at long-term follow-up. These authors found a marked improvement in postoperative limb range of motion and function, a significant decrease in the incidence and severity of lymphangitis, and elimination of preoperative pain in most patients. However, long and unsightly skin incisions at the recipient site are often necessary for flap inset to avoid kinking of the omentum, which can predispose to venous obstruction and thrombi formation in the smaller veins. The poor cosmetic appearance at the recipient site was thought to be unacceptable (50,51). Because of other associated serious complications with this flap, including abdominal hernia, intestinal obstruction, wound infection, dehiscence, and pulmonary embolism, omental transposition has largely fallen out of clinical practice (50).

Mechanism of Vascularized Lymph Node Transfer

The mechanism by which vascularized lymph node transfer reduces lymphedema is still under investigation. Cheng et al. (2) hypothesized that the vascularized lymph node transfer may function through an internal pump and suction mechanism

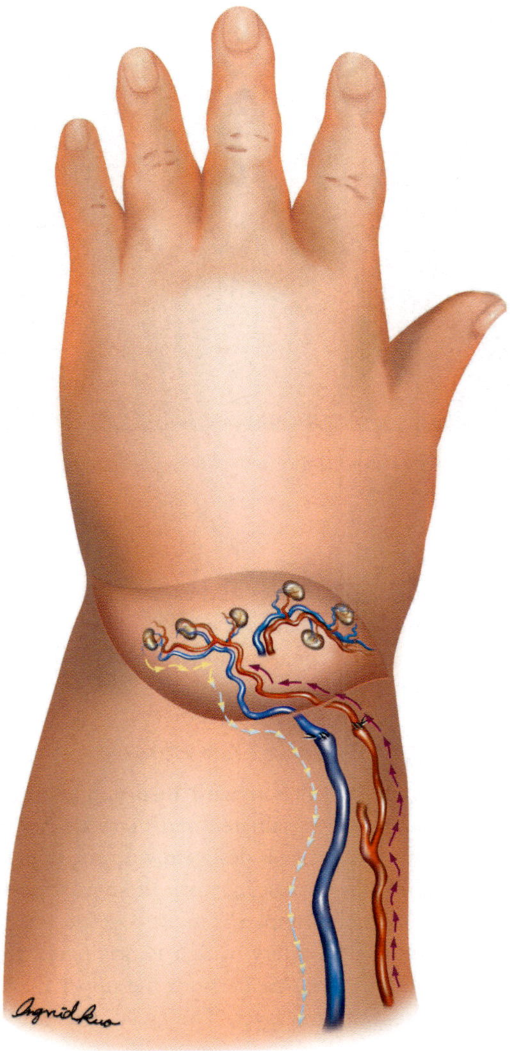

FIGURE 54-3 A vascularized groin lymph node acts by means of an internal pump and suction mechanism. The pump mechanism is driven by the high-pressure arterial flow, which provides a strong hydrostatic force within the flap. The suction is maintained by the large-caliber superficial, low-pressure cephalic vein. (Reproduced with permission from Ingrid Kuo.)

that stimulates lymphatic clearance in the lymphadematous limb (Figure 54-3). The "pump" mechanism is initiated through the high-pressure inflow across the arterial anastomosis to maintain a driving force for continuous circulation through the vascularized lymph node flap. The "suction" mechanism is continued by superficial, large-caliber, and low-pressure veins. The vascularized lymph node also provides undamaged lymphatic channels to drain the lymph from the interstitium (Figure 54-4). Lymphaticovenous connections within the flap serve as conduits for lymphatic drainage from the chronically lymphadematous tissues adjacent to the flap (see Figure 54-4). This was confirmed with intraoperative ICG fluorescence lymphogram. As the lymph is drained from the area surrounding the flap, the subcutaneous compartment pressure decreases, and more lymph is recruited from the surrounding tissue in a "catchment" effect. Over time, as the tissue compartment pressures normalize, old lymphatic channels may reopen, and lymphangiogenesis slowly recovers (52). The transferred lymph

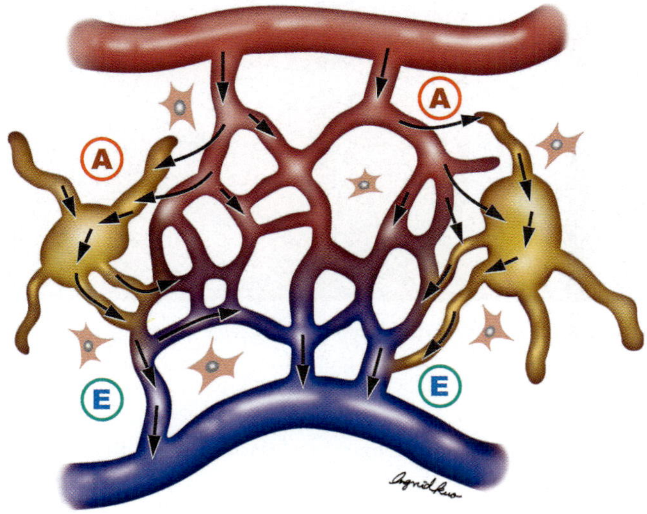

FIGURE 54-4 The lymph in the interstitial space inside the flap drains directly via afferent ducts of the transferred lymph nodes and then drains into the venous system through efferent ducts. As the lymph in the area surrounding the flap reduces, lymph fluid from nearby areas is recruited and drained through afferent ducts via a catchment effect. A, afferent ducts; E, efferent ducts. (Reproduced with permission from Ingrid Kuo.)

nodes continue to function as lymphoid organs to enhance the local immune system and may explain for the significant reduction in the incidence of postoperative cellulitis after vascularized lymph node transfer.

SURGICAL TECHNIQUE OF VASCULARIZED LYMPH NODE TRANSFER

Donor Lymph Nodes Flap Harvest

Groin Lymph Node Flap Harvest

The inguinal ligament is marked with the patient on supine position. The CFA is palpated and marked. An elliptical skin paddle 10 × 5 cm in size is designed below the inguinal ligament and medial to the CFA (Figure 54-5). The skin incision

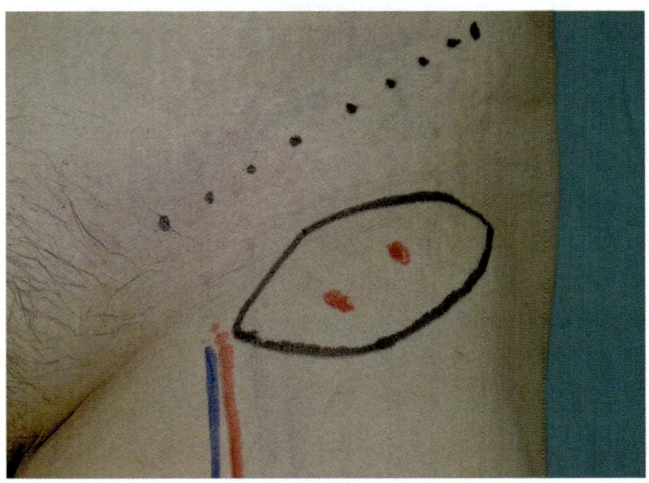

FIGURE 54-5 The design of vascularized groin lymph node flap shows an elliptical skin paddle 10 × 5 cm in size below the inguinal ligament and medial to the common femoral artery.

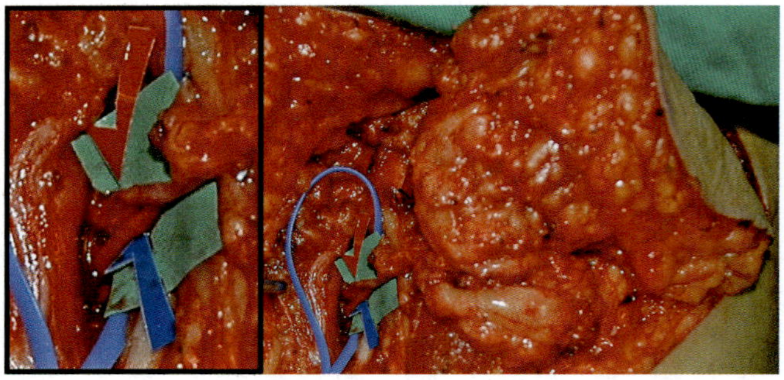

FIGURE 54-6 The medial artery (red arrow) and concomitant vein (blue arrow) are dissected and tagged with vessel loops.

is started from the upper margin of flap and deep to the fascia of sartorius. Then, the dissection may be continuously preceded to explore the CFA and its medial branch pedicle, which is small in size, 1.5 to 2 mm in diameter, and vertical to the CFA (Figure 54-6). Use of the bipolar is helpful to maintain a bloodless operative field for ease of identification of the pedicle. The medial vein 1.5 to 2.5 mm in diameter is usually not accompanied by the medial artery but travels vertically and directly drains into the common femoral vein. One may easily confuse the great saphenous vein or the superficial inferior epigastric vein. The soft tissue around the CFA should be included as much as possible during flap elevation for the inclusion of more lymph nodes, which are usually not palpable (see Figure 54-6). The perinodal soft tissue is well preserved to maintain the fine lymphatic channels and lymphatic integrity (Figure 54-7). After the medial artery and vein are identified and tagged with a vessel loop, the flap dissection can be finished from lateral to medial on the suprafascial plane. Alternatively, the superficial branch of the SCIA may be used as the pedicle. The skin paddle of this flap is important for the postoperative monitoring, tension-free wound closure without compression of the anastomoses, and better subdermal plexus lymph drainage with catchment effect. Some vessel anatomic variation may be observed.

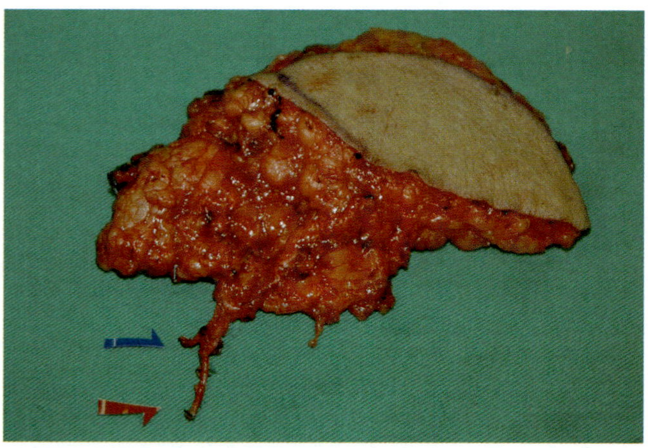

FIGURE 54-7 The vascularized groin lymph node flap is harvested with its medial artery (red arrow) and medial vein (blue arrow). The perinodal soft tissue is taken to include as many lymph nodes as possible within the flap and to preserve the fine lymphaticovenous channels.

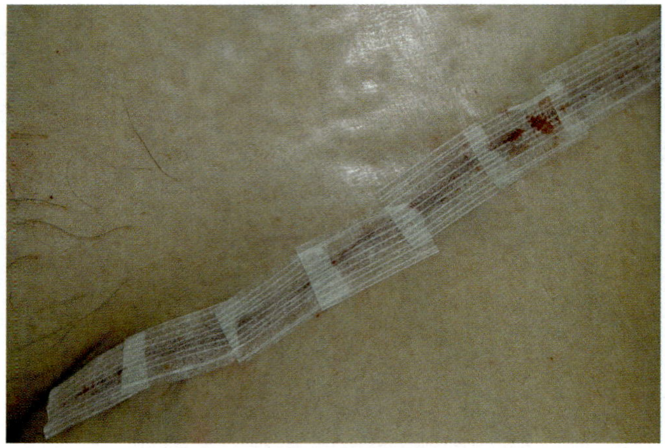

FIGURE 54-8 The groin donor site can be primarily closed with an inconspicuous scar.

However, in most clinical cases and cadaveric dissections, the medial artery and vein can always be found and dissected out. The donor site can be primarily closed with an inconspicuous scar (Figure 54-8).

Submental Lymph Node Flap Harvest

This is a newly described flap with inclusion of the lymph nodes. The facial artery is palpated and marked. An elliptical skin paddle 10 × 5 cm in size is designed with the upper border along the mandible lower margin, from the mandible angle to the symphysis. A pencil Doppler is used to detect the perforators from the submental artery, which is originated from the facial artery. The incision is made from the upper margin and deep through the platysma layer. The facial artery above the mandible bone is identified and tagged with a vessel loop at its junction with the submental artery. The dissection is continued from proximal to distal. The submental artery is dissected along its length. The marginal mandibular nerve should be tagged with a vessel loop and preserved. The facial vein with submental vein is harvested along with the submental artery. The soft tissue around the junction of submental artery and facial artery should be carefully preserved, especial surrounding the submandibular gland. The septocutaneous perforator from submental artery to the skin paddle is delicately preserved. The digastric muscle and tendon can be included to ensure the inclusion of more lymph nodes.

Recipient Site Preparation

The axilla is usually severely scarred, radiated with fibrotic skin. The recipient vessels are also hard to dissect and may need a vein graft for anastomoses. The wrist is chosen as the recipient site because the wrist is the most dependent site of the upper extremity for easy drainage of lymph fluid. After the lymph around the wrist is drained out, the lymph in the forearm area can shift down with gravity and be drained by the catchment effect. The wrist is also a healthy area for recipient vessel dissection. The elbow is an intermediate recipient site between the axilla and the wrist. With limited experience, the recipient vessels in the elbow are deep and difficult to dissect. The results of

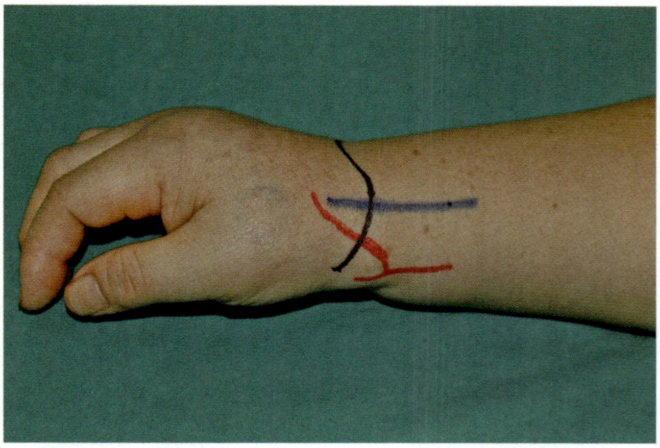

FIGURE 54-9 A curvilinear transverse incision is made on the dorsum of the recipient wrist. The superficial radial artery and the cephalic vein are used as recipient vessels.

vascularized groin lymph nodes transferred to the elbow are also not as good as to the wrist and is thus not the preferred recipient site (41).

An S-shaped incision is made on the wrist (Figure 54-9). The skin envelope is undermined to allow the groin lymph nodes flap transfer. The cephalic vein can be easily explored and tagged with a vessel loop (Figure 54-10). The radial artery's dorsal branch is located in the anatomical snuffbox, which lies beneath the extensor pollicis longus and abductor pollicis longus. It is dissected, divided, and placed on top of these extensors (see Figure 54-10). The spurt of the radial artery dorsal branch is checked before the microanastomosis because the vessel wall may be very fibrotic and may require adventitiectomy in some severe lymphedema patients. The arterial anastomosis is performed in an end-to-end fashion with 10-0 nylon. If there is a size discrepancy, the medial artery of the pedicle can be anastomosed to the radial artery in an end-to-side fashion. The double clamp can be released to check for good backflow from vein and perfusion of the entire flap. Then the venous anastomosis is completed with 10-0 nylon interrupted sutures. A size discrepancy between the venous pedicles is common but can be easily overcome using standard microvascular techniques. The wound is closed primarily over two Penrose drains. Split-thickness skin grafts may be needed on the ulnar side because the flap thickness is sometimes too large to fit for the created pocked. Care should be taken not to compress the pedicle.

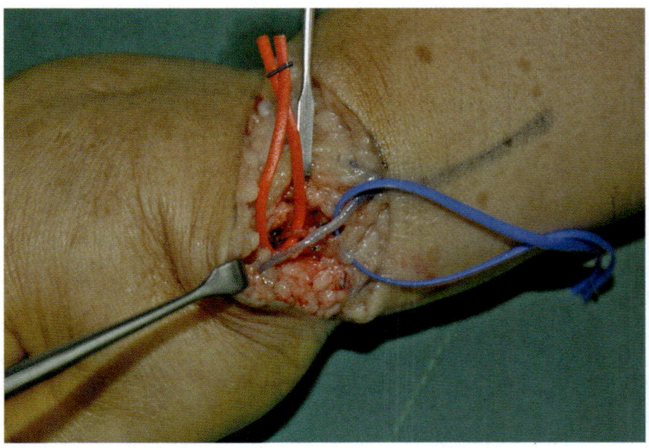

FIGURE 54-10 The recipient wrist site is prepared by exposing of the cephalic vein (blue vessel loop) and the superficial branch of the radial artery. The superficial branch of the radial artery is located beneath the extensor pollicis longus and abductor pollicis longus and is divided and placed on top of these extensors (red vessel loop).

Flap Monitoring

The patient is sent to the microsurgical intensive care unit for flap monitoring with the wrist in the neutral position. Finger flexion and extension may be started on postoperative day 3. The flap is monitored with a pencil Doppler and traditional clinical method by the experienced nursing staff every hour on postoperative day 1, every 2 hours on day 2, and every 4 hours on days 3 to 7. If the flap becomes swollen, the stitches can be removed at bedside. Heparin and low-molecular-weight Dextran are not routinely used unless there is a re-exploration and evidence of venous thrombosis. The wrist is elevated 20 to 30 degrees. No compression garment or decompression therapy is required after surgery. The patient may be discharge 7 to 10 days after surgery.

Outcomes and Results

In the clinical study by Cheng et al. (2), 13 patients were retrospectively evaluated after receiving vascularized groin lymph node transfer to the wrist for the management of postmastectomy UEL. The results showed statistically significant improvement in the lymph drainage of the lymphedematous limb, with a mean reduction rate of 50%, at a mean follow-up period of 56 months. The incidence of cellulitis was also decreased in 11 of 13 patients. Most patients reported significantly improvement of lymphedematous limb in 2 to 7 days after surgery. The patients reported that their hand and forearm became softer and the ranges of motion were also improved. The reduction of the circumference of the affected limbs was observed at 3 months after surgery. The improvement of the lymphedematous extremity is sustained because the vascularized lymph node transfer flap continues to work as a pump for lymph drainage directly to the venous system. Most of the patients are free of cellulitis after surgery. For patients with stage 3 lymphedema, the reduction rate is slowly progressive, and additional procedures such as liposuction or wedge resection of fibrotic subcutaneous tissue may be required for further decrease of the lymphatic load.

Case Studies

Case 1

A 58-year-old patient with right breast cancer underwent a modified radical mastectomy with removal of 24 lymph nodes

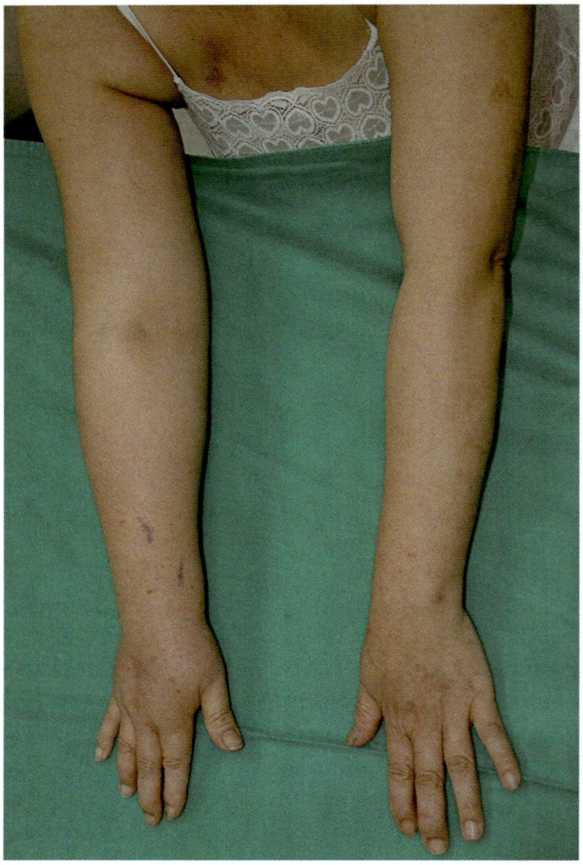

FIGURE 54-11 Preoperative photo of a 58-year-old patient with right upper extremity stage II lymphedema post modified radical mastectomy. Twenty-four axillary lymph nodes were removed during the axillary lymph node dissection. The patient also received postoperative radiation therapy. She developed two episodes of cellulitis and is refractory to conservative decongestive therapy.

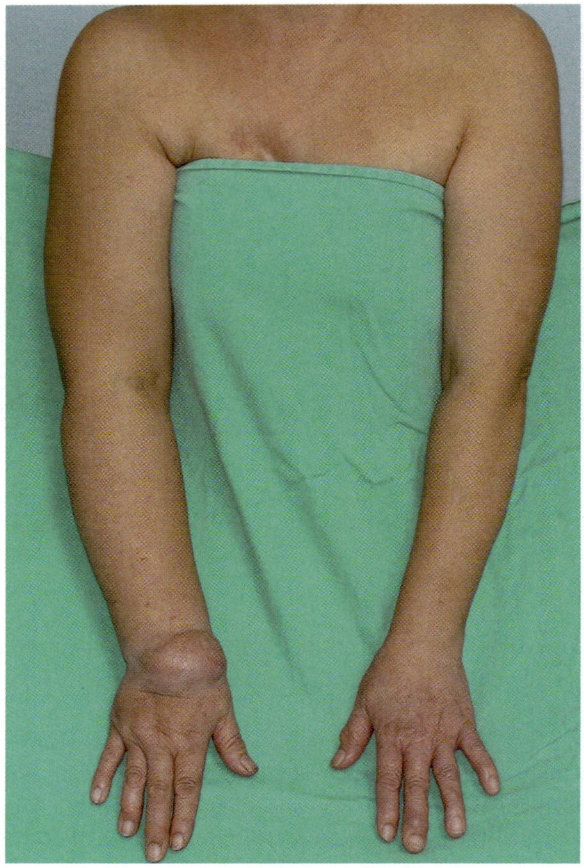

FIGURE 54-12 At a follow-up of 30 months after vascularized groin lymph node transfer to the wrist, there was a reduction rate of 52% above the elbow and 56% below the elbow in the right lymphedematous limb. The patient was satisfied with the functional outcome.

and subsequent postoperative radiation therapy. The patient developed right upper extremity stage II lymphedema for 4 years with two episodes of cellulitis, which was refractory to conservative decongestive therapy (Figure 54-11). She received vascular groin lymph node flap transfer (10 × 5 cm in size) using the wrist as a recipient site. At a follow-up period of 30 months after vascular groin lymph node transfer (VGLNT) to the wrist, there was a reduction rate of 52% above and 56% below the elbow in the right lymphedematous limb. The patient was satisfied with the functional outcome (Figure 54-12).

Case 2

A 57-year-old woman with left breast cancer patient had left UEL for 3 years after a modified radical mastectomy. She had 30 axillary lymph nodes removed and received postoperative radiation therapy. She developed three episodes of cellulitis. At 3 weeks after right vascularized groin lymph node transfer to the wrist, the patient had a reduction rate of 10% above and 4% below the elbow in left UEL (Figure 54-13). The patient received an additional wedge resection procedure of the left upper medial arm at 10 months after vascularized groin lymph node transfer. At a follow-up of 16 months, lymphoscintigraphy showed quick uptake of Tc-99 into the cephalic vein 60 seconds after subcutaneous injection of the radiolabeled tracer in the second web space. This provided the evidence for lymph drainage from surrounding tissue to the recipient cephalic vein (Figure 54-14). At a follow-up period of 24 months, the reduction rate of the left upper extremity achieved 27% above and 52% below the elbow (Figure 54-15). The patient was satisfied with the functional and cosmetic results.

Complications

The most common complication of the vascularized groin lymph node transfer is venous congestion when the flap and recipient soft tissue becomes swollen after surgery. The stitches will have to be partially released, and the flap may require a reexploration to reposition of the pedicle to relieve compression of the pedicle vein. Skin grafting may be necessary for wound coverage after suture removal. Sometimes the donor artery may be injured intraoperatively during the dissection, which may be repaired primary with 10-0 nylon.

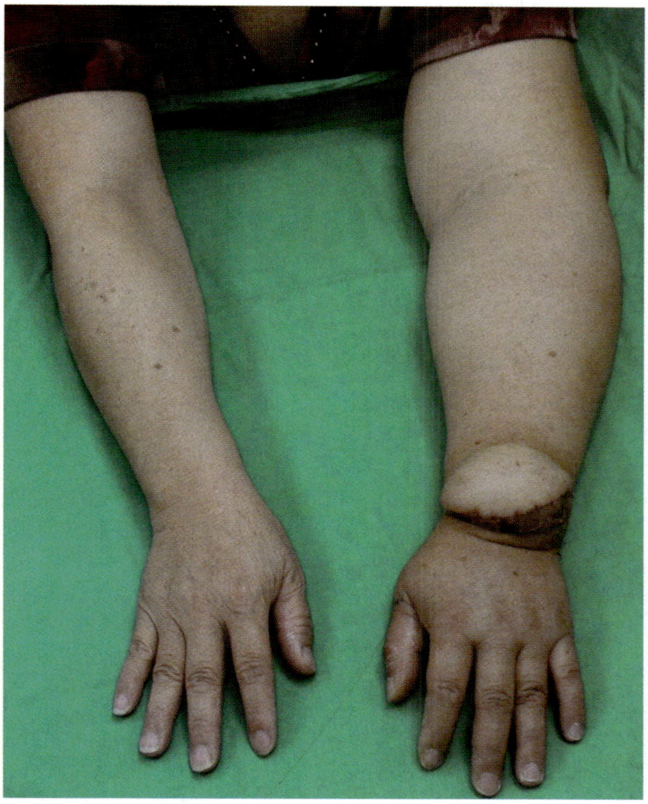

FIGURE 54-13 A 57-year-old woman with breast cancer who developed left upper extremity stage II lymphedematous after modified radical mastectomy. She had 30 axillary lymph nodes removed and received postoperative radiation therapy. She had three episodes of cellulitis before surgery. At 3 weeks after right vascularized groin lymph node transfer to the wrist, the patient had a reduction rate of 10% above the elbow and 4% below the elbow in left upper extremity.

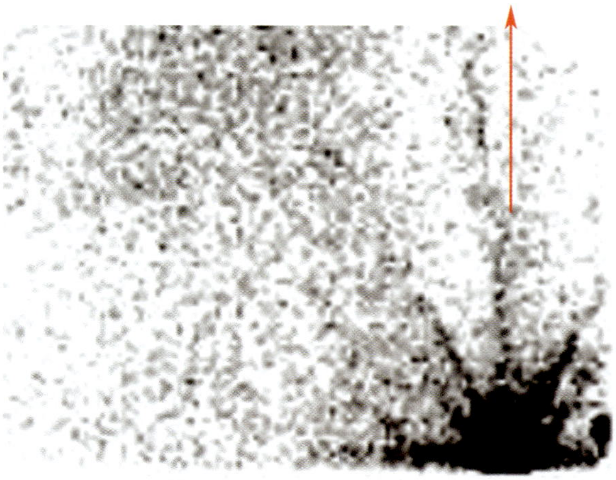

FIGURE 54-14 At a follow-up period of 16 months, the lymphoscintigraphy showed quick uptake of technetium-99 into the cephalic vein at 60 seconds after subcutaneous injection of the radiolabeled tracer in the second web space.

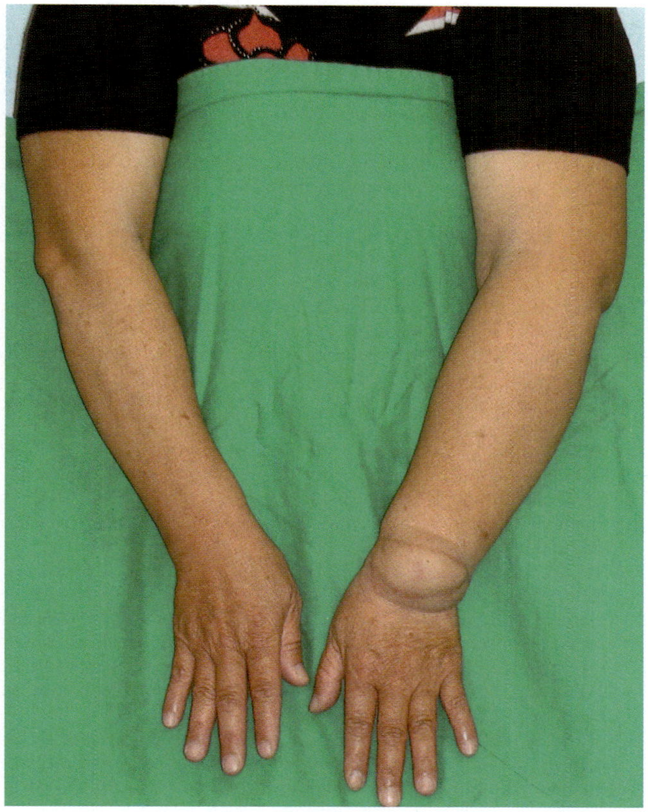

FIGURE 54-15 The patient received an additional wedge resection procedure of the left upper medial arm at 10 months after a vascularized groin lymph node transfer. At a follow-up period of 24 months, the reduction of the left upper extremity was 27% above and 52% below the elbow after vascularized groin lymph node transfer.

REFERENCES

1. Lawenda BD, Mondry TE, Johnstone PA. Lymphedema: a primer on the identification and management of a chronic condition in oncologic treatment. *CA Cancer J Clin* 2009;59(1):8–24.
2. Lin CH, Ali R, Chen SC, et al. Vascularized groin lymph node transfer using the wrist as a recipient site for management of postmastectomy upper extremity lymphedema. *Plast Reconstr Surg* 2009;123(4):1265–1275.
3. Hadamitzky C, Pabst R. Acquired lymphedema: an urgent need for adequate animal models. *Cancer Res* 2008;68(2):343–345.
4. Christenson JT, Shawa NJ, Hamad MM, Al-Hassan HK. The relationship between subcutaneous tissue pressures and intramuscular pressures in normal and edematous legs. *Microcirc Endothelium Lymphatics* 1985;2(4):367–384.
5. Qvarfordt P, Christenson JT, Eklöf B, et al. Intramuscular pressure, venous function and muscle blood flow in patients with lymphedema of the leg. *Lymphology* 1983;16(3):139–142.
6. Thompson N. The surgical treatment of chronic lymphoedema of the extremities. *Surg Clin North Am* 1967;47(2):445–503.
7. Kissin MW, Querci della Rovere G, Easton D, Westbury G. Risk of lymphoedema following the treatment of breast cancer. *Br J Surg* 1986;73(7):580–584.
8. Engel J, Kerr J, Schlesinger-Raab A, et al. Axilla surgery severely affects quality of life: results of a 5-year prospective study in breast cancer patients. *Breast Cancer Res Treat* 2003;79(1):47–57.
9. Rönkä RH, Pamilo MS, von Smitten KA, Leidenius MH. Breast lymphedema after breast conserving treatment. *Acta Oncol* 2004;43(6):551–557.
10. Meek AG. Breast radiotherapy and lymphedema. *Cancer* 1998;83(12 suppl American):2788–2797.
11. Ryan M, Stainton MC, Slaytor EK, et al. Aetiology and prevalence of lower limb lymphoedema following treatment for gynaecological cancer. *Aust N Z J Obstet Gynaecol* 2003;43(2):148–151.

12. Chatani M, Nose T, Masaki N, Inoue T. Adjuvant radiotherapy after radical hysterectomy of the cervical cancer. Prognostic factors and complications. *Strahlenther Onkol* 1998;174(10):504–509.
13. Pilepich MV, Asbell SO, Mulholland GS, Pajak T. Surgical staging in carcinoma of the prostate: the RTOG experience. Radiation Therapy Oncology Group. *Prostate* 1984;5(5):471–476.
14. Wrone DA, Tanabe KK, Cosimi AB, et al. Lymphedema after sentinel lymph node biopsy for cutaneous melanoma: a report of 5 cases. *Arch Dermato* 2000;136(4):511–514.
15. Starritt EC, Joseph D, McKinnon JG, et al. Lymphedema after complete axillary node dissection for melanoma: assessment using a new, objective definition. *Ann Surg* 2004;240(5):866–874.
16. Sabel MS, Griffith KA, Arora A, et al. Inguinal node dissection for melanoma in the era of sentinel lymph node biopsy. *Surgery* 2007;41(6):728–735.
17. Brennan MJ, Weitz J. Lymphedema 30 years after radical mastectomy. *Am J Phys Med Rehabil* 1992;71(1):12–14.
18. Gosk J, Rutowski R, Urban M, et al. Brachial plexus injuries after radiotherapy—analysis of 6 cases. *Folia Neuropathol* 2007;45(1):31–35.
19. Stanton AW, Mellor RH, Cook GJ, et al. Impairment of lymph drainage in subfascial compartment of forearm in breast cancer-related lymphedema. *Lymphat Res Biol* 2003;1(2):121–132.
20. Kramer EL. Lymphoscintigraphy: defining a clinical role. *Lymphat Res Biol* 2004;2(1):32–37.
21. Ter SE, Alavi A, Kim CK, Merli G. Lymphoscintigraphy. A reliable test for the diagnosis of lymphedema. *Clin Nucl Med* 1993;18(8):646–654.
22. Gerber L, Lampert M, Wood C, et al. Comparison of pain, motion, and edema after modified radical mastectomy vs. local excision with axillary dissection and radiation. *Breast Cancer Res Treat* 1992;21(2):139–145.
23. Miller GE, Seale J. Lymphatic clearance during compressive loading. *Lymphology* 1981;14(4):161–166.
24. McNeely ML, Magee DJ, Lees AW, et al. The addition of manual lymph drainage to compression therapy for breast cancer related lymphedema: a randomized controlled trial. *Breast Cancer Res Treat* 2004;86(2):95–106.
25. Kligman L, Wong RK, Johnston M, Laetsch NS. The treatment of lymphedema related to breast cancer: a systematic review and evidence summary. *Support Care Cancer* 2004;12(6):421–431.
26. Dumanian GA, Futrell JW. Radical excision and delayed reconstruction of a lymphedematous leg with a 15 year follow-up. *Lymphology* 1996;29(1): 20–24.
27. Karri V, Yang MC, Lee IJ, et al. Optimizing outcome of Charles procedure for chronic lower extremity lymphoedema. *Ann Plast Surg* 2010;66(4):393–402.
28. Qi F, Yang Y, Gu J, Shi Y. Long-term follow-up of the treatment of lower limb lymphedema with liposuction. *Plast Reconstr Surg* 2009;123(2): 86e–87e.
29. Nielubowicz J. Olszewski W, Sokolowski J. Surgical lympho-venous shunts. *J Cardiovasc Surg (Torino)* 1968;9(3):262–267.
30. Yamamoto Y, Horiuchi K, Sasaki S, et al. Follow-up study of upper limb lymphedema patients treated by microsurgical lymphaticovenous implantation (MLVI) combined with compression therapy. *Microsurgery* 2003;23(1):21–26.
31. Puckett CL. Microlymphatic surgery for lymphedema. *Clin Plast Surg* 1983;10(1):133–138.
32. Gilbert A, O'Brien BM, Vorrath JW, Sykes PJ. Lymphaticovenous anastomosis by microvascular technique. *Br J Plast Surg* 1976;29(4): 355–360.
33. Koshima I, Inagawa K, Urushibara K, Moriguchi T. Supermicrosurgical lymphaticovenular anastomosis for the treatment of lymphedema in the upper extremities. *J Reconstr Microsurg* 2000;16(6):437–442.
34. Koshima I, Nanba Y, Tsutsui T, et al. Long-term follow-up after lymphaticovenular anastomosis for lymphedema in the leg. *J Reconstr Microsurg* 2003;19(4):209–215.
35. Chang DW. Lymphaticovenular bypass for lymphedema management in breast cancer patients: a prospective study. *Plast Reconstr Surg* 2010; 126(3):752–758.
36. Cheng J. Discussion: lymphaticovenular bypass for lymphedema management in breast cancer patients: a prospective study. *Plast Reconstr Surg* 2010;126(3):759–761.
37. Slavin SA, Van den Abbeele AD, Losken A, et al. Return of lymphatic function after flap transfer for acute lymphedema. *Ann Surg* 1999;229(3): 421–427.
38. Chen HC, Pribaz JJ, O'Brien BM, et al. Creation of distal canine limb lymphedema. *Plast Reconstr Surg* 1989;83(6):1022–1026.
39. Chen HC, O'Brien BM, Rogers IW, et al. Lymph node transfer for the treatment of obstructive lymphoedema in the canine model. *Br J Plast Surg* 1990;43(5):578–586.
40. Becker C, Assouad J, Riquet M, Hidden G. Postmastectomy lymphedema: long-term results following microsurgical lymph node transplantation. *Ann Surg* 2006;243(3):313–315.
41. Cheng MH, Chen SC, Steven LH, Tan BK Tan, Lin CY, Huang JJ. Vascularized groin lymph node flap transfer for postmastectomy upper limb lymphedema: flap anatomy, recipient sites, and outcomes. *Plast Reconstr Surg* 2013;131(6):1286–1298.
42. Tobbia D, Semple J, Baker A, et al. Experimental assessment of autologous lymph node transplantation as treatment of postsurgical lymphedema. *Plast Reconstr Surg* 2009;124(3):777–786.
43. Becker C, Hidden G. [Transfer of free lymphatic flaps. Microsurgery and anatomical study.] *J Mal Vasc* 1988;13(2):119–122.
44. Martin D, Pascal JF, Baudet J, et al. The submental island flap: a new donor site. Anatomy and clinical applications as a free or pedicled flap. *Plast Reconstr Surg* 1993;92(5):867–873.
45. Ishihara T, Igata T, Masuguchi S, et al. Submental perforator flap: location and number of submental perforating vessels. *Scand J Plast Reconstr Surg Hand Surg* 2008;42(3):127–131.
46. Magden O, Edizer M, Tayfur V, Atabey A. Anatomic study of the vasculature of the submental artery flap. *Plast Reconstr Surg* 2004;114(7): 1719–1723.
47. Cheng MH, Huang JJ, Nguyen DH, Saint-Cyr M, Zenn MR, Tan BK, Lee CL. A novel approach to the treatment of lower extremity lymphedema by transferring a vascularized submental lymph node flap to the ankle. *Gynecol Oncol* 2012;126(1):93–98.
48. Tassinari J, Orlandino G, Fabrizio T, Calabrese L. Submental flap in facial reconstructive surgery: long-term casuistry revision. *Plast Reconstr Surg* 2010;126(3):139e–140e.
49. Nakajima E, Nakajima R, Tsukamoto S, et al. Omental transposition for lymphedema after a breast cancer resection: report of a case. *Surg Today* 2006;36(2):175–179.
50. Goldsmith HS. Long term evaluation of omental transposition for chronic lymphedema. *Ann Surg* 1974;180(6):847–849.
51. Goldsmith HS, De los Santos R, Beattie EJ Jr. Relief of chronic lymphedema by omental transposition. *Ann Surg* 1967;166(4):573–585.
52. Mellor RH, Stanton AW, Menadue L, et al. Evidence for dermal angiogenesis in breast cancer related lymphedema demonstrated using dual-site fluorescence angiography. *Microcirculation* 2002;9(3):207–219.

SECTION 4

UPPER LIMB

CHAPTER 55

Digital Replantation

Yutaka Maki

Since Jacobson and Suarez introduced microvascular surgery under the operating microscope in 1960 (1), experimental studies of microsurgery have been performed all over the world. The first successful clinical application of replantation surgery was attempted in 1962, when Malt and McKhann replanted an amputated arm (2). Chen and colleagues (3) and Inoue and colleagues (4) replanted an amputated hand in 1963. As to digital replantation surgery, Kleinert and Kasdan successfully revascularized an incompletely amputated thumb in 1962 (5). The first successful digital replantation was performed in 1965 by Komatsu and Tamai (6), who replanted a thumb amputated at the metacarpophalangeal (MCP) joint. Since then, replantation surgery has been standardized, and success rates have increased to more than 80% (7).

Surgeons who attempt replantation surgery should understand that successful replantation is not simply a matter of reattaching the amputated digit or hand but also restoring useful motion and sensation to the digits and hand. Knowledge and techniques of microvascular and peripheral nerve surgery are not enough; they also need the knowledge of basic hand surgery.

INDICATIONS FOR REPLANTATION

Indications for digital replantation have changed as surgical techniques have developed (8–12) and become standardized. In general, fingers and hands severed by guillotine-type, clean-cut amputations; trauma with crushing around the stumps; and even avulsed or degloving-type amputations can now be replanted. The presence of an artery and a vein in both stumps of the amputated part, all judged microscopically to be suitable for anastomoses, increase the chance of successful replantation. However, before surgery, the surgeon must consider (1) the predictable morbidity of the patient with an amputated digit, (2) the likelihood of viability and functional restoration of the replanted digit or hand, (3) the costs that can be reimbursed by an insurance company or worker's compensation, and (4) how long the patient will be unable to work. Most important, however, are the patient's wishes and the potential cosmetic results. The functional goals of digital replantation surgery should be to equal or better the results likely to be obtained by amputation stump closure or prosthetic replacement.

Generally accepted conditions suitable for replantation distal to the wrist are (1) thumb amputation, (2) multiple-digit amputations, (3) transmetacarpal and wrist amputations, and (4) amputation of any level of digit or hand in children (13) (Figure 55-1).

There is the extreme opinion that every amputated part should be replanted if the patient requests it and if the amputated part is suitable for replantation. However, for each individual case, the surgeon has to decide whether to replant each amputated part. If this decision cannot be made in the emergency department, it should be made after the condition of the severed vessels and nerves has been assessed under the operating microscope.

Thumb Amputation

Thumb amputations have the strongest case for replantation (14,15). A thumb–index finger pinch motion is a primary function of the hand that should be preserved if at all possible. Thumb replantation with preserved MCP joint and carpometacarpal (CMC) joint motion can provide good thumb function. Even if the interphalangeal (IP) and MCP joints are fused, a movable CMC joint makes a side or "key pinch" possible. Avulsion amputations at the MCP joint, in which flexor and extensor tendons are avulsed from the muscle belly, are candidates for replantation (Figure 55-2). If replantation is impossible, reconstruction should be considered using a wrap-around flap transfer, a second toe transfer, or pollicization, depending on the amputation level.

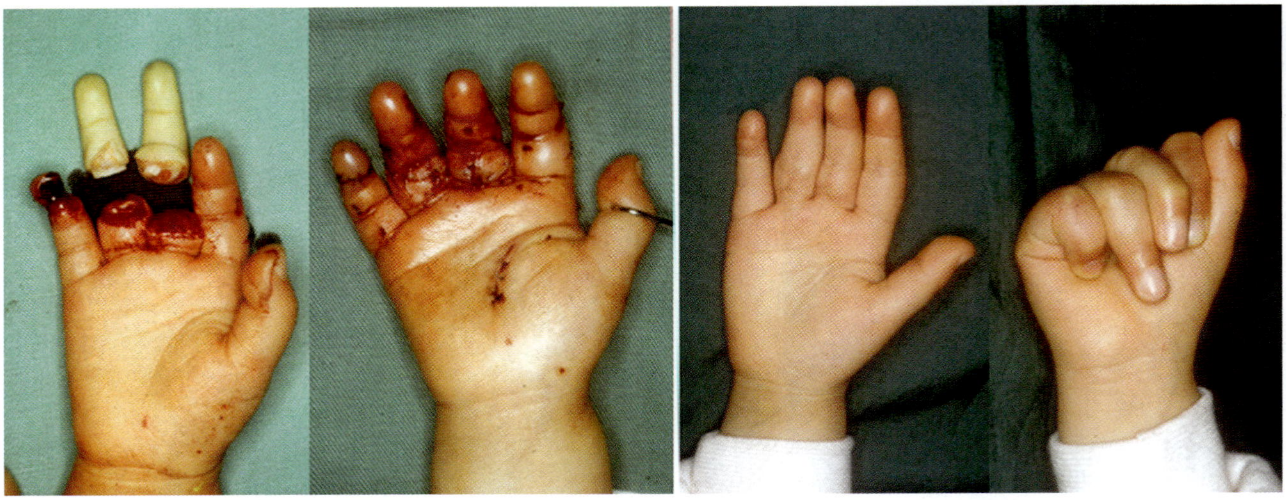

FIGURE 55-1 Multiple-digit amputation and replantation on the right hand of a 2-year-old girl. Replantation surgery started more than 12 hours after the injury. The amputation of the ring finger was at the epiphysis of the middle phalanx base. All replanted digits survived.

Multiple-Digit Amputation

In cases of multiple-digit amputations, the decision to replant all suitable amputated digits or to replant only selected digits is still controversial. Restoring pinch function is of primary importance, and restoring grip function is of secondary importance. If multiple digits are amputated in a crushing injury and are not in good condition, the amputated digit with the least damage should be replanted to the least damaged proximal stump of another digit to maintain the motion of the digit that faces the thumb to preserve pinch function, the so-called "heterotopic replantation" (Figure 55-3). If the thumb is among the amputated parts and is not suitable for replantation, another amputated digit should be transferred to the thumb ray, or the thumb should be reconstructed with a wrap-around flap transfer.

If a completely amputated digit cannot be replanted, part of the digit may be used as vascularized composite tissue to reconstruct or revascularize another amputated digit (Figure 55-4). If distal interphalangeal (DIP) and proximal interphalangeal (PIP) joint motion cannot be restored, MCP joint motion should be preserved if possible. If the MCP joint is fused, even moderate PIP and DIP motion is indispensable.

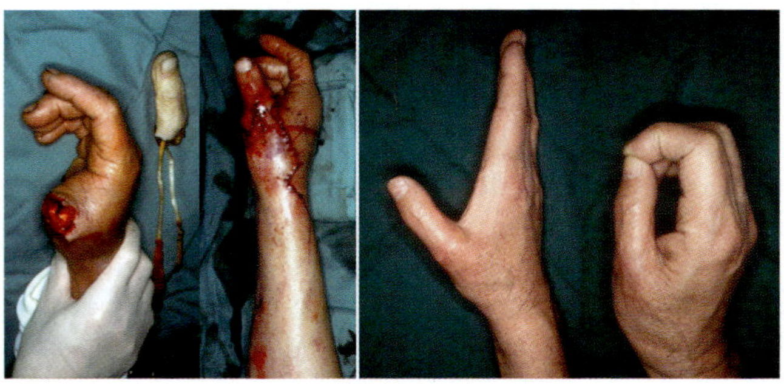

FIGURE 55-2 Complete amputation and replantation of the thumb of a 53-year-old man. The flexor and extensor tendons and the adductor pollicis were avulsed. The metacarpophalangeal joint was fused, and the tendons were not repaired. A long vein graft was placed from the interphalangeal joint to the anatomical snuffbox to reconstruct the ulnar digital artery. The ulnar digital nerve underwent secondary reconstruction with a nerve graft.

Transmetacarpal Amputation

In general, the interosseous muscles and the lateral band of the extensor mechanism are nonfunctional after replantation. Flexion of the MCP joint and extension of the PIP and DIP joint are provided by the extrinsic flexor and extensor mechanisms. To restore PIP and DIP joint extension with extrinsic extensors, a mild flexion contracture of the MCP joint is convenient; however, this type of injury gradually increases the intrinsic plus contracture and prevents finger flexion. If the first metacarpal is included in the amputation, an adduction contracture of the thumb cannot be avoided (Figure 55-5).

Wrist Amputation

In wrist amputation, the severed median and ulnar nerves can be sutured, but functional recovery of the interosseous and adductor pollicis muscles, which are innervated by the deep branch of the ulnar nerve, is poor. The situation is almost the same as that encountered in low median and ulnar nerve palsy. Successful replantation at the wrist can restore relatively good function (16).

Single-Digit Amputation

Indications for replanting a single digit are controversial. However, replanting a single digit distal to the insertion of the flexor digitorum superficialis (FDS) tendon in the middle phalanx (Tamai's zone III) can restore good function (17) (Figure 55-6). In addition, good functional results are also possible in single-digit replantations distal to the DIP joint or IP joint of the thumb (Tamai's zone I and II) (18,19). If the amputated part has not been severely crushed, sensory recovery at this level is also good even if the terminal branch of the digital nerve cannot be sutured, and amputation

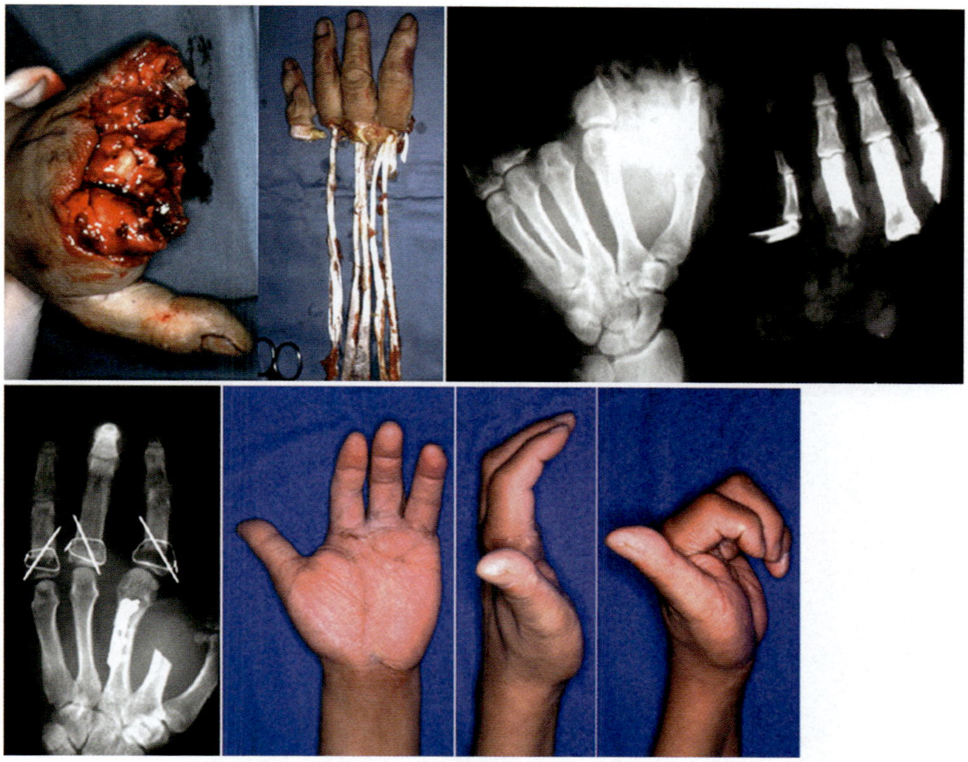

FIGURE 55-3 Complete multiple-digit amputation in a 43-year-old man. The middle finger was disarticulated at the metacarpophalangeal (MCP) joint. The flexor digitorum profundus (FDP) tendons of the index, middle, and ring fingers and the flexor digitorum superficialis (FDS) tendons of the index and middle fingers were avulsed. An arterial pedicled MCP joint of the index finger was transferred to the third ray with an intact dorsal skin flap, vein, and extensor tendons to prevent MCP joint fusion of the middle finger. The amputated index, middle, and ring fingers were replanted to the third, fourth, and fifth rays, respectively. The distal FDP tendons of the index, middle, and ring fingers were sutured to the remaining proximal FDS tendons of the ring finger and the FDP and FDS tendons of the little finger, respectively. The motion of the MCP joint on the third ray was preserved.

stump neuroma pain can be prevented. The length and cosmetic shape of the fingertip are acceptable. However, the procedure requires anastomosing vessels of less than 1 mm in diameter.

In a complete ring avulsion injury (Urbaniak's classification class III, complete degloving or complete amputation), if the amputation is distal to the insertion of the FDS tendon and the PIP joint and proximal phalanx are intact, vein and nerve grafting may restore function (20,21).

CONTRAINDICATIONS TO REPLANTATION

Replantation is not indicated when amputated parts are severely mangled or crushed or when the digit and hand are amputated at multiple levels. In these cases, sensation and range of motion are difficult to restore even if reattachment is successful. However, in children, replantation should be attempted if possible to accommodate epiphyseal growth.

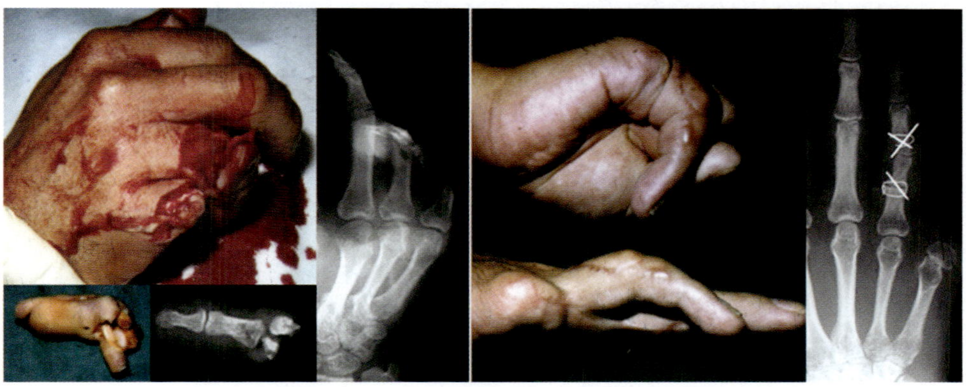

FIGURE 55-4 Complete amputation of the little finger and incomplete amputation of ring finger of a 42-year-old man. An arterialized distal interphalangeal joint with an intact dorsal skin flap and vein of the little finger were transferred as a vascularized free joint to the ring finger to restore proximal interphalangeal joint function.

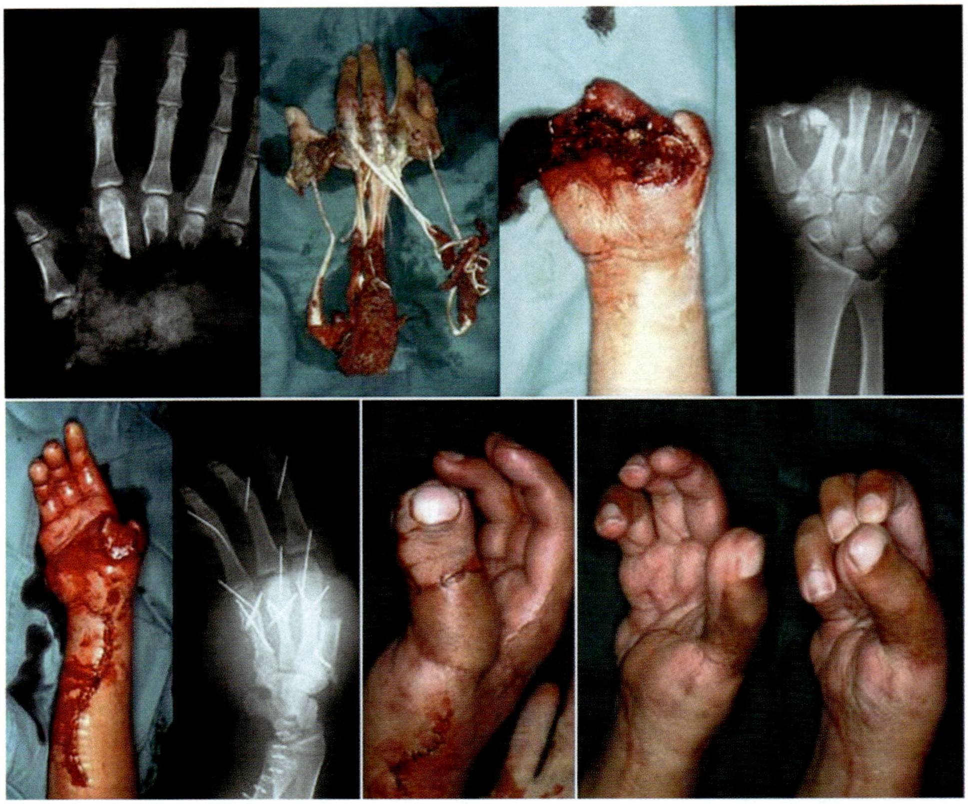

FIGURE 55-5 Complete transmetacarpal amputation, including the thumb, of an 18-year-old man. The flexor and extensor tendons of all digits were avulsed, and the second carpometacarpal joint was dislocated. He also sustained a Monteggia dislocation fracture of the same forearm. The amputated index, middle, and ring fingers were replanted to the third, fourth, and fifth rays, respectively. The flexor digitorum profundus tendons of the three digits were bundled and transferred to the flexor carpi radialis tendon, and their extensor digitorum communis tendons were bundled and transferred to the extensor carpi radialis longus tendon. One of the common digital arteries was anastomosed to the radial artery at the anatomical snuffbox, and the other was anastomosed to the ulnar artery with vein grafts. The digital nerves were sutured to the median and ulnar nerves. The thumb was reconstructed in a secondary procedure with a wrap-around flap, and its digital nerve was sutured to the radial sensory branch of the radial nerve.

Replantation is also contraindicated when the arteries to be anastomosed are severely sclerotic. Fragile or thickened intima can easily separate from the arterial wall, and atheroma degeneration can induce thrombosis and preclude patency in small arteries after anastomosis. The lumen of the vessels should be inspected before replantation is considered. In cases accompanied by other serious injuries, the general condition of the patient should be determined, and hypotension caused by blood volume loss should be corrected before replantation; treating critical injuries has a higher priority than replanting fingers and hands.

Replantations in patients with cardiac disorders, vasculitis from autoimmune diseases, uncontrolled diabetes, and so on have a high risk of failure. Patients with prolonged warm ischemic times are at risk because muscle tissue is sensitive to ischemia. If the muscle in the amputated part is to recover function, its arterial supply must be restored within 6 hours. Amputated digits have no muscle and so are less sensitive to ischemia and may therefore be replantable under warm ischemia within 12 hours of the injury. Patients with mental disorders are sometimes difficult to evaluate in brief preoperative periods. Patients who are mentally unstable may make postoperative rehabilitation difficult or impossible.

Old age is not necessarily a contraindication for replantation. In older patients with no serious disease and adequate vasculature, as established by examination under the operating microscope, replantation is not contraindicated and should be considered at the patient's request. Single-digit amputation distal to the insertion of the FDS tendon is an acceptable indication for aging patients. More proximal amputations may result in contracture of multiple joints more so than in younger adult patients.

PREPARING THE AMPUTATED PART AND THE PROXIMAL STUMP

Ideally, the amputated part should be wrapped immediately after amputation in thick dry gauze, placed in a plastic bag, stored in an ice chest, and taken to the replantation center as soon as possible. The part should not be placed directly on ice to avoid freezing the tissue.

The proximal stump should also be covered with thick gauze, and moderate compression should be applied for hemostasis. A tourniquet should not be applied on the arm during transportation because incomplete compression can induce congestion around the stump and increase the bleeding from the stump. As mentioned earlier, amputated digits have no

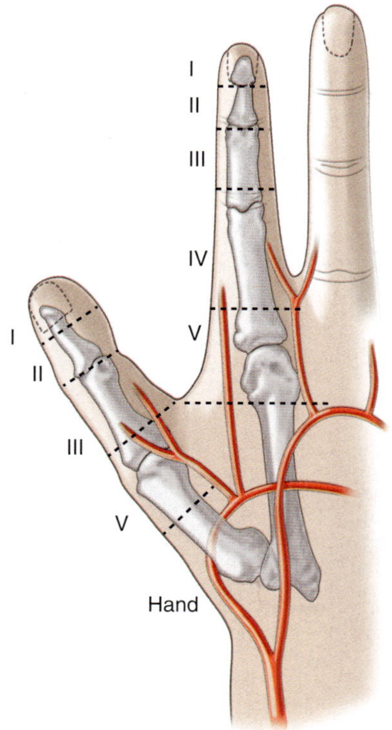

FIGURE 55-6 Tamai's zones for classifying amputation level. (Reproduced with permission from Inada Y, Fukui A, Tamai S. Digital replantation. In Tamai S (ed). *Experimental and Clinical Reconstructive Microsurgery*, p. 210.)

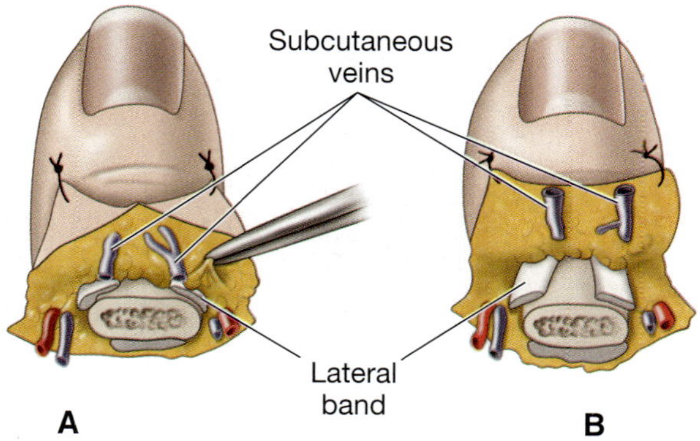

FIGURE 55-7 Approaches to finding the dorsal subcutaneous vein: along the border plane between the dermis and the subdermal fatty tissue (**A**) and along the border plane between the subdermal fatty tissue and the extensor tendon (**B**).

muscle and are less sensitive to ischemia. Cooling to 4°C up to 24 hours keeps the amputated digit replantable.

After arriving at the hospital, the amputated part is imaged radiographically and transferred to the operating room by one surgical team. It is cleaned by scrubbing and irrigation with sterile normal saline. Under surgical loupe or the operating microscope (depending on the size of the amputated part), the distal stump is debrided. The digital arteries and nerves and the dorsal subcutaneous veins are identified and marked with a thin nylon suture or with bioabsorbable dye (sterile 1% Pyoktanine blue solution) at their stumps.

Midlateral incisions are usually placed on both sides of the digit. The digital artery and nerve are exposed by dissecting Cleland ligaments longitudinally. Bone fixation and tendon suturing require dissecting both stumps at least 1.5 cm and more if necessary. The dorsal subcutaneous vein is identified by dissecting the border plane between the subdermal fatty tissue and the extensor tendon or between the dermis and subdermal fatty tissue with additional longitudinal dorsal incision if necessary (Figure 55-7). The subcutaneous vein network is in the layer of subdermal fatty tissue. If surgeons have the skill and experiences in dissecting and isolating the subcutaneous vein without bleeding from the stump before arterial anastomosis, veins can be anastomosed before arterial repair. However, if the subcutaneous vein cannot be isolated without bleeding, veins should be identified from venous bleeding from the stump after arterial anastomosis, which helps identify the small palmar subcutaneous vein at the distal phalanx level.

A second surgical team assesses the general condition of the patient with routine examination and radiographs of the injured hand and decides whether replantation is indicated. Most replantation surgeries are performed under axillary or supraclavicular regional block of the brachial plexus with the long-acting local anesthetic bupivacaine. General anesthesia is required for children, when replanting multiple digits, and for more proximal replantations. After applying a pneumatic tourniquet, the proximal stump is debrided and dissected under magnification in the same manner as was the amputated part.

The key to successful replantation is to follow this sequence: (1) meticulously isolate the vessels and nerves in both stumps, (2) assess the condition of the lumen of all vessels to ensure that they are adequate for anastomosis, (3) debride the damaged vessels and nerves in both the proximal and distal stumps, and (4) approximate the vessels and nerves without tension for anastomosis or suture. Performing the tasks in this sequence requires much experience and skill.

SEQUENCE OF REPAIRS IN FINGER AND THUMB AMPUTATION

Bone Shortening and Fixation

After preparing both stumps, resect enough bone to allow the stumps of the arteries, veins, nerves, and skin to be approximated and then anastomosed or sutured without excessive tension. How far the stump bone should be resected and which side of the stump bone should be resected more than another depends on the type of injury. If the bone stump is crushed or fragmented, resect the bone to the level where stable bone fixation can be obtained. In an avulsion injury, more bone must usually be resected until the vessel stumps can be coapted without too much tension.

In digital replantation, shortening the bone by 0.5 to 1.0 cm is common. If the amount of bone resection would be too extensive to allow coaptation of the vessels and nerves, that is, if the digit will be too short and cosmetically unacceptable after too much bone has been resected, vein and nerve grafting should be performed. If the amputation site is near a joint, such as at the base of the phalanx, the head and neck of the phalanx, metacarpus, or at the joint, the joint must be fused.

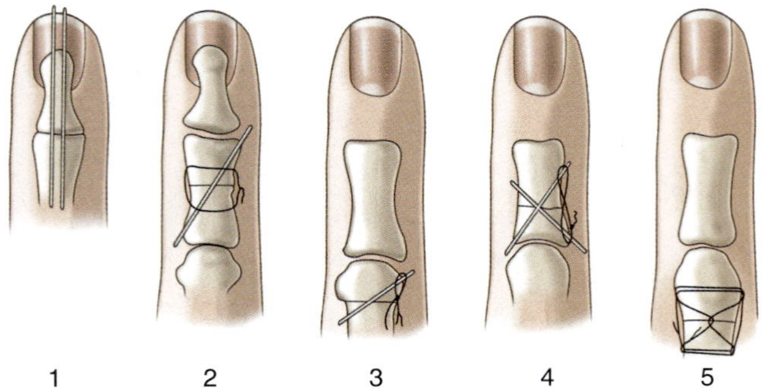

FIGURE 55-8 My preferred bone fixation techniques: (1) double-axial Kirschner wire, (2) intraosseous wiring with oblique insertion of a Kirschner wire, (3) tension band wiring, (4) crisscrossing the Kirschner wire with lateral suture wiring, and (5) double suture wiring.

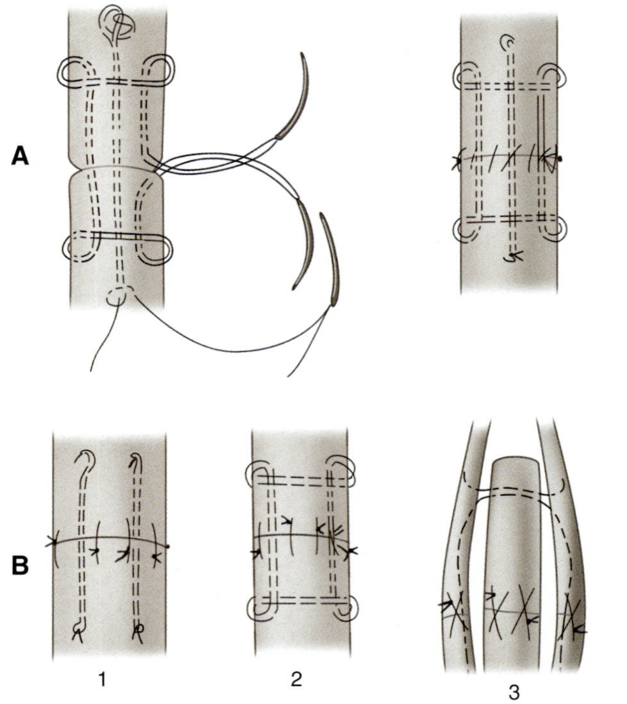

FIGURE 55-9 My preferred tendon suture technique. (**A**) To suture the flexor tendon, I use the Yoshizu type I method using double nylons with double needles and a Tsuge looped suture. (**B**) To suture the extensor tendon, I use (1) the Yoshizu type II method with a (2) a double Tsuge looped suture and (3) a figure-of-8 suture.

Bone fixation can be done in several ways. The ideal technique for replantation surgery would be simple, fast, and stable. It would allow easy correction of the rotated bone during the procedure and should not interfere with healing and tendon gliding during postoperative exercises. Insufficient or unstable bone fixation induces nonunion, which delays starting motion exercises and prolongs treatment.

The preferred bone fixation procedures are (1) single- or double-axial Kirschner wire fixation is used on the distal phalanx and DIP joint. The Kirschner wire is first inserted into the intramedullary cavity from the stump of the amputated part to the fingertip, the bone stumps are coapted, and the wire is inserted proximally. Several techniques can be used proximal to the middle phalanx, (2) intraosseous wiring with oblique insertion of a Kirschner wire (22). (3) tension band wiring, (4) crossed Kirschner wires with lateral suture wiring, and (5) double- suture wiring (Figure 55-8).

After the bone is fixed, finger alignment must be checked by flexing and extending the reattached digit to ensure that it does not cross an adjacent digit and that the index or little finger does not separate from the adjacent digit on flexion. Rotary malalignment requires revision of the fixation. If fixation is satisfactory, the periosteum of both bone stumps is sutured circumferentially, if possible, to support bony union. The periosteum is the gliding floor of the flexor and extensor tendons, and repairing it may reduce the adhesions surrounding the sutured tendon.

Extensor Tendon Repair

After bone fixation, the extensor tendon should be sutured (Figure 55-9). The extensor tendon is flat at the metacarpal level, and the extrinsic and intrinsic extensor mechanism distal to the MCP joint is thinner than at the metacarpal level. End-to-end sutures of the extensor tendon are not strong, especially distal to the MCP joint. Gaps at the suture site can create extension lag at the DIP, PIP, or MCP joints, depending on the level of amputation and the degree of extensor adhesion. I prefer to use multiple figure-of-8 sutures with 4-0 monofilament nylon distal to the MCP joint and modified Kessler sutures with 4-0 nylon and double needles on both ends (four strand, Yoshizu type II method) or with double Tsuge sutures with 4-0 looped nylon (four strand) accompanied by additional suturing proximal to the MCP joint. The central and lateral bands should be sutured separately distal to the MCP joint. In avulsion amputations, if the extensor tendon is avulsed from the muscle belly, the tendon should be transferred to an adjacent healthy extensor tendon with end-to-side interlacing sutures with maximum tension placed on the fully flexed replanted digit.

Flexor Tendon Repair

The flexor tendons should be repaired after suturing the extensor tendons and before vascular repair.

The suture should have strong tensile strength to prevent gap formation at the suture site during vascular repair, and at the same time, the replanted digit must be kept extended to maintain a good operative field. Gap formation compromises the continuity of the flexor tendon, making healing incomplete and weakening the tendon's ability to withstand tension after tenolysis. A good approach is the Yoshizu type I technique (six strand) with 4-0 double nylon and double needles and 4-0 Tsuge looped nylon with 6-0 monofilament nylon peripheral suture; its tensile strength is about 4 kg (23,24) (see Figure 55-9).

Repairing the flexor digitorum profundus (FDP) tendon is controversial when the amputation is distal to the insertion of the FDS tendon (Tamai's zone III). If the stump of the middle phalanx is close to the DIP joint or the patient is elderly and DIP joint motion cannot be expected, DIP joint tenodesis or secondary DIP joint fusion are appropriate. A sublimis finger is acceptable. However, when the patient is young and DIP joint motion can be expected, the FDP tendon should be repaired. In this case, the A4 pulley should be resected or used as the gliding floor of the repaired flexor tendon, which makes repair easy and does not disrupt DIP joint motion if parts of the C1, A3, and C2 pulleys are preserved (25).

If the amputation site is proximal to the insertion of the FDS tendon (proximal to Tamai's zone IV), only the FDP tendon is repaired except in children. The FDS tendon at this level is thin, separated distally, and cannot be sutured securely. At this level, multiple-digit amputation is common, and multiple tendons need to be repaired. Unfortunately, replanted flexor tendons are accompanied by severe scarring around the replantation site. As a result, it is difficult to restore good range of motion of the digits at this level of amputation even if both the FDP and FDS tendons are repaired.

Adhesions of the FDP and FDS tendons are unavoidable, and the tendons adhere to the surrounding sheath and gliding floor, which complicates secondary tenolysis. I recommend repairing only the FDP tendons and removing the FDS tendons. When the FDS tendons are removed from Tamai's zones IV and V, the hiatus tendinum of the distal FDS tendon stump should be opened to prevent adhesion with the FDP tendon. The FDS tendon slips along the volar plate of the PIP joint should not be removed from the volar plate to prevent bleeding from the short vinculum and to be used as the gliding floor of the FDP tendon. The proximal stump of the FDS tendon is retracted proximally and resected. If the proximal stump is to be used as a donor in a secondary tendon transfer, it should be sutured to the surrounding tissue with moderate tension to prevent myostatic contracture.

Part of the A2 or A1 pulleys should be preserved when repairing flexor tendons in Tamai's zone IV and V to prevent bowstringing of the repaired flexor tendon and to maintain effective PIP and MCP joint flexion. If the A1 and A2 pulleys cannot be preserved, the A2 pulley should be reconstructed during flexor tenolysis. In an avulsion amputation, the flexor tendon avulsed from the muscle belly is transferred to the adjacent FDP tendon with end-to-side interlacing sutures. In replantation surgery, secondary two-stage tendon grafting is not recommended. Repeated surgery under conditions of scaring and myostatic contracture with a limited source of free tendon complicates the surgery and is not time well spent. Primary tendon repair must be performed if at all possible.

Vein Repair

Whether venous repair should be done before or after arterial repair is controversial. I usually identify the subcutaneous vein at the initial dissection and repair the dorsal subcutaneous vein before arterial repair.

The most important point of venous repair is to anastomose without tension. If a tensionless anastomosis between the vein ends is impossible, a vein graft should be used to achieve it. Harvest the graft from the palmar aspect of the distal forearm, and be careful to note the direction of venous valves. If the vein is anastomosed just dorsal to the IP and MCP joints, even a gradual increase in the flexion of these joints during postoperative splinting increases the tension and compression forces on

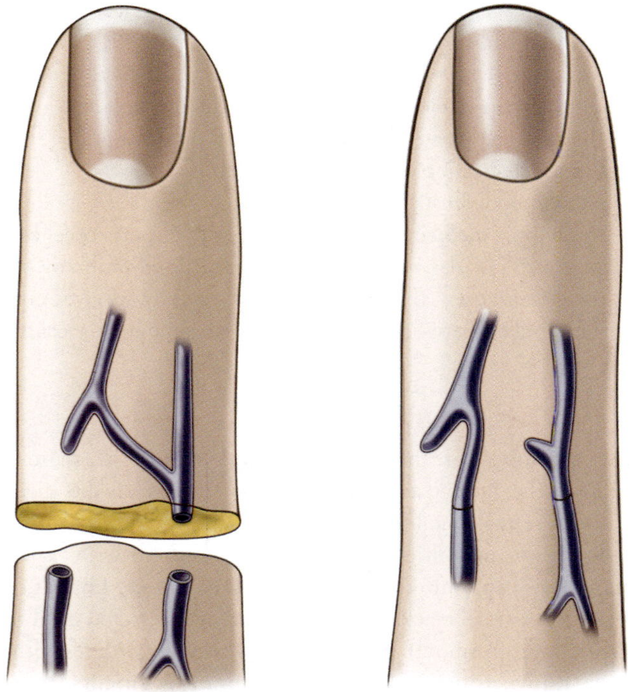

FIGURE 55-10 To increase the number of the venous anastomosis, a branch of the vein is severed and moved to another stump.

the anastomosis, possibly increasing the risk of venous occlusion. To prevent this risk, I sometimes temporarily fix the DIP and PIP joints in the extended position (for 3–4 weeks) with a Kirschner wire after the surgery.

There are two opinions on how to prevent venous congestion: repair as many subcutaneous veins as possible or repair two veins for each repaired artery. Both options are not always feasible, but both should be kept in mind (26). Venous drainage can be increased by severing the branches of the dorsal subcutaneous veins and moving their stumps to another anastomosis (Figure 55-10).

If the replantation level is in Tamai's zone II, 1-mm-caliber dorsal veins can usually be identified at the center of the dorsal aspect. If these dorsal veins are damaged, the lateral and volar aspects of the stump should be dissected to find a vein that can be anastomosed. If the replantation level is in Tamai's zone I, distal to the eponychium, the amputated part does not have a dorsal vein. In this case, the vein on the volar aspect, if it exists, can be used for the anastomosis. However, the caliber of this vein is smaller, and its wall is thinner than that of the dorsal vein, so the anastomosis requires considerable skill. In this situation, repairing the artery first helps identify the vein after it bleeds from the stump.

If the vein cannot be found, venous drainage can be maintained with any of several techniques.

1. If the backflow from one distal arterial stump is satisfactory after anastomosis of the other digital artery, this distal artery can be anastomosed to a proximal vein as a sort of arteriovenous shunt (27,28).
2. After the nail plate is removed, the nail bed can be scraped with a cotton applicator every hour to encourage bleeding.

Between scrapings, heparin-soaked gauze is placed on the raw nail bed to maintain continuous oozing (29).
3. A transverse stab incision can be made at the hyponychium and heparin-soaked gauze placed on the incision and changed if it dries to maintain oozing. A continuous heparinized saline drip on the incision is also recommended (30,31).
4. Applying a medicinal leech to the replanted part. Leeches have a risk of *Aeromonas hydrophila* infection. With any of these techniques, the replanted part hopefully survives until the capillary network reestablishes itself in about 1 week.

Arterial Repair

Any thrombus in the arterial stumps should be removed through the lumen and the damaged stumps of the digital artery trimmed. The lumen of each stump should be examined under high magnification and then washed with liberal amounts of heparinized saline. If the intima has any fibrillation, petechia, or small cracks, the artery should be resected until the surface is again smooth and normal. In sclerotic arteries with a thick intima, trimming the arterial stump by simultaneously cutting through both walls of the vessel with microscissors will tear the intima from the arterial wall. Instead, trim the stump with a spiral cut. Make a small, oblique cut at one point on the stump wall with microscissors and continue to cut the single wall of the artery around its circumference until the end comes free; do not to cut both walls at the same time (Figure 55-11).

Before coapting the arterial stumps with double clips, check the outflow from the proximal stump by releasing the tourniquet. If pulsatile arterial flow does not occur (Acland "spurt test") despite trimming the proximal stump, attempt the following procedures. (1) Dissect the artery proximally to relieve vascular tension and compression; (2) check the intima again and resect any abnormal parts of the arterial wall; (3) apply 2% Xylocaine to the external wall of the artery ; (4) warm the operating room and the patient's body; (5) irrigate the operating field with warm normal saline (procedures 3, 4, and 5 are done to relieve vasospasm); (6) increase blood pressure by infusing additional fluids; (7) correct any metabolic acidosis; and (8) if the lumen of the proximal stump is normal, anastomose the artery, close the skin, warm the area, and wait. Leaving the naked vessels exposed to the air may result in vasospasm. Some surgeons use local applications of papaverine.

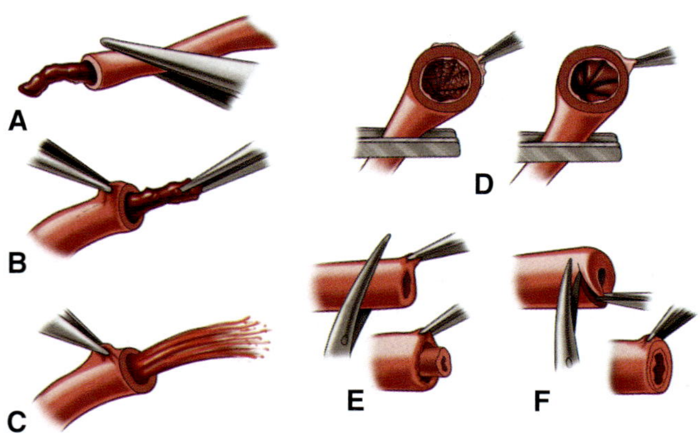

FIGURE 55-11 Techniques for trimming the stump of a vessel. (A) Squeeze the stump wall softly to remove the thrombus. (B) Pull the thrombus from the stump. (C) Confirm arterial flow from the proximal stump. (D) Check the intima for fibrillation on the surface, which can be a contraindication to anastomosis (left). A smooth surface is ideal (right). (E) Cutting both walls of the vessel at once, making a round slice, can tear the intima from the wall of the vessel. (F) Trimming the arterial wall with a spiral cut is effective for removing a sclerotic arterial wall.

If perfusion is not restored to the replanted digit soon after completing the replantation, closing the skin and keeping the digit warm for 30 minutes is the first choice. If perfusion is still not restored, determine whether the anastomosis is patent and then consider the need for reanastomosis or dissecting the distal artery to find any occlusion. Sometimes the intima far from the anastomosis in the amputated part has been damaged in a crush amputation, which occludes arterial flow.

In an avulsion amputation with a wide area of damage, subdermal bleeding along the course of the digital artery where it has separated from the surrounding tissue (the "red-line" sign) indicates the rupture of a dermal arterial branch by traction. Curling and tapering of the long arterial stump (the "ribbon sign") also indicates a traction injury. In these situations, the artery is not suitable for anastomosis and should be trimmed. If end-to-end anastomosis is not possible, a vein graft or cross-arterial anastomosis (i.e., anastomosing the radial proximal stump to the ulnar distal stump) should be considered. The vein graft must be reversed when anastomosed, and the graft should not be twisted (32). Marking a point on the surface of the vein graft with bioabsorbable dye can help indicate whether the graft has been twisted. Too much tension and too much redundancy of the anastomosis between the artery and vein graft are risk factors for occlusion. Repairing both digital arteries is preferred if possible.

In thumb replantation, positioning the thumb for anastomosing the ulnar digital artery, which has a larger caliber than the radial digital artery, is difficult. This problem can be solved by anastomosing the vein graft to the ulnar digital arterial stump of the amputated part before bone fixation (33). The proximal stump of the vein graft is routed subcutaneously along the ulnar side of the first metacarpal and anastomosed end to end or end to side to the radial artery in the anatomical snuff box after completing the other procedures that should be done before arterial anastomosis. Repeatedly inflating and deflating the pneumatic tourniquet is safe during the anastomosis and can shorten the operation and decrease blood loss.

Nerve Repairs

Nerve repair is the final procedure before closing the skin. Placing an epineurial suture with two or three stitches without tension is the basic procedure for repairing the nerve at the digital level. Both digital nerves should be repaired if possible. In finger-tip amputations (Tamai's zone I), if the tip has not been crushed severely, good sensation can be restored without suturing the nerve.

In an avulsion amputation, the digital nerve is usually avulsed from the common digital nerve, and the distal nerve stump is tapered. The nerve stump should be shortened until the normal fascicular pattern appears. A graft from the sural or medial antebrachial cutaneous nerve can bridge the gap created by the avulsion. Whether nerve grafting should be primary or secondary is controversial, especially in avulsion amputations, because judging the extent of damage is difficult.

In an avulsion amputation of the thumb, sometimes the digital nerves are avulsed from the trunk of the median nerve at the distal end of the carpal tunnel. If so and if the IP joint is fused without tendon repair, the ulnar digital nerve of the thumb can be sutured end to side to the radial digital nerve of the index finger through a perineurial window or to a sensory branch of the radial nerve on the dorsum of the first metacarpal.

Skin Coverage

Because the replanted digit and the digit or hand proximal to the replantation site become edematous after surgery, a tight skin closure may compress the anastomoses. If loose skin closure is not possible, a split-thickness skin graft without a tie-over dressing should be performed. Placing a skin graft over a vessel is safe even if it is over the anastomosis (34). If a vein graft has been used for arterial or venous repair and skin coverage is necessary at the same level, a venous flap may be indicated (35,36).

SEQUENCE OF REPAIR IN MULTIPLE-DIGIT AMPUTATIONS

When replanting multiple amputated digits, a digit-by-digit technique is not efficient. Rather, repairing the same structure in each digit at the same time before repairing the next structure can save the operating time (37).

During bone fixation, proper rotary alignment is critical; misalignment will make digits "scissor" on flexion. Ensuring bony alignment of multiple-digit replantations is more difficult than it is in single-digit replantation. After repairing the extensor tendons, only the FDP tendons are repaired proximal to the insertion of the FDS tendon. The tension of the repaired flexor tendons is checked by finger balance in the resting position and the dynamic tenodesis effect accompanied by passive wrist extension. The width of the pulley system should be preserved as much as possible during replantation.

In avulsion amputations, in which the flexor and extensor tendons are avulsed from their muscle bellies, the tendons should be transferred to new donor muscles with the same finger balance. When the amputation is proximal to Tamai's zone II, the dorsal subcutaneous vein should be repaired first if possible. Surgical time and blood loss are lower with this method than with digit-by-digit venous anastomoses guided by venous bleeding after arterial anastomosis.

SEQUENCE OF REPAIR IN TRANS-METACARPAL AMPUTATIONS

The sequence in transmetacarpal replantation is almost the same as that in multiple-digit replantation. The methods of bone fixation and tendon repair are the same, but those for vessel repair are different. At a minimum, the common digital arteries to the index and middle finger, the ring and little finger (and the princeps pollicis artery if the thumb is included), and two to three subcutaneous veins should be repaired. Sometimes a Y-shaped vein graft can be used to reconstruct the superficial palmar arterial arch and provide arterial blood flow from the proximal stump of the ulnar artery to two distal common digital arteries. Replantation at this level requires meticulous hemostasis of the distal palmar metacarpal arteries that communicate with the common digital artery to prevent retrograde bleeding into the palm after the common digital arteries are repaired (38).

For the extrinsic finger extensor mechanism to extend the PIP and DIP joints, the MCP joints of all four digits should be temporarily fixed in 30 degrees of flexion with Kirschner wires; otherwise, the finger balance assumes the intrinsic minus position and extension forces load only the MCP joints. Alternatively, maintaining the intrinsic plus position may accelerate an intrinsic plus contracture, which can be corrected by resecting the interosseous tendon. If a thumb amputated at the first metacarpal level is involved, preventing adduction contracture is important. Temporary fixation and splinting of the first intermetacarpal space with the thumb in the palmar abducted position are necessary.

SEQUENCE OF REPAIR IN WRIST AMPUTATION

If the possibility of wrist motion remains after partial carpectomy, the wrist flexor and extensor tendons and wrist capsule should be repaired. The wrist should be fixed temporarily with a Kirschner wire after the finger flexor and extensor tendons are repaired. If wrist motion is impossible, the wrist should be fused in a neutral position. The thumb abductor should be repaired in addition to the thumb extensor and finger extensors. At this level, both FDP and FDS tendons can be repaired in a relatively wide operative field. In transmetacarpal or wrist amputations, the carpal tunnel is opened to repair the flexor tendons and median nerve. In this situation, the flexor retinaculum should be reconstructed with a Z-shaped elongation to preserve the pulley function on the flexor tendons.

Dorsal fasciotomy of the interosseous muscles is needed to reduce pressure on the compartments. Both the radial and ulnar arteries and at least two to three veins should be repaired. The flexed finger MCP joints and the first intermetacarpal space with the thumb abducted away from the palm should be fixed temporarily with K wires. Edema after replantation may accelerate intrinsic minus or an ape-claw type contracture. Maintaining the intrinsic plus position of the fingers is important to prevent intrinsic minus contracture and to transmit the extrinsic extensor power to the PIP and DIP joints effectively.

DRESSING

Postoperatively, the hand should be kept in the intrinsic plus position, in which the wrist is extended and the MCP joints slightly flexed. In digital replantation, with both the flexor and extensor tendons repaired, no satisfactory position for simultaneously splinting both tendon repairs has been developed.

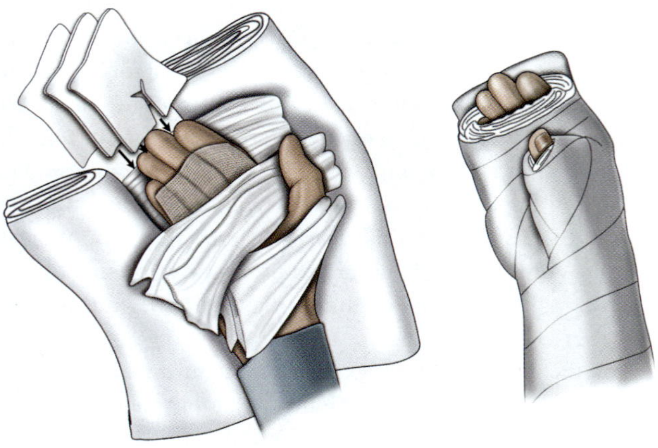

FIGURE 55-12 (A) and (B) The dressing of the hand after replantation surgery. (Reproduced with permission from Maki Y, Yoshizu T. In Tamai S (ed). *Experimental and Clinical Reconstructive Microsurgery*, p. 180.)

Wrist extension increases the tension on the repair site of the flexor tendon but decreases that on the extensor tendon, and MCP joint flexion increases on the extensor tendon but decreases that on the flexor tendon. In any case, the tensile strength of the suture should be as strong as possible to prevent elongation and rupture of the tendon.

Small squares of petrolatum gauze should be placed on the wound piece by piece so as not to constrict the replantation site circumferentially. Thin gauze is placed between the digits so as not to compress the digital artery, and thick gauze is placed on the digit and on the front and back of the hand. Unfolded gauze is placed piece by piece at the first interdigital space with the thumb abducted from the palm, and a bandage is applied with mild compression.

In digital replantation, the intrinsic plus position is maintained by a bulky dressing. In transmetacarpal or wrist replantation, mild MCP flexion and thumb palmar abduction should be temporarily fixed with Kirschner wires. A plaster splint is applied to the front or back of the hand. Fingertips should be kept out of the dressing and covered only with a removable piece of gauze so that the circulation of the replanted digit can be observed (Figure 55-12).

POSTOPERATIVE CARE AND MONITORING

After replantation surgery, the hand should be held at or slightly above the patient's heart who is nursed supine with an arm sling or pillow. The elbow and upper arm should be placed on the bed to stabilize the hand. If venous outflow is slow and congestive, the hand should be held even higher above the heart. If arterial inflow is diminished, the hand should be held below the heart. Antibiotics are given for 3 days. The patient's room should be warm, and the patient should not be allowed to smoke. Pain control and anxiety reduction are necessary to prevent vasospasm. The patient needs strict bed rest for the first 3 days, after which activity is allowed if there are no complications after the surgery.

The postoperative use of anticoagulant therapy is debated. However, in replantation surgery, damaged tissue is transferred to a damaged site, a condition completely opposite to a normal tissue transfer. I use heparin and prostaglandin E_1 (PGE_1). After the arterial anastomosis is complete, the patient receives one dose of heparin 3000 units intravenously. Then 10,000 units/day of heparin and 80 µg/day of PGE_1, diluted with 2000 mL/day drip infusion, including 500 mL of low–molecular-weight dextran, are administered for 7 days.

Patients react differently to heparin. If the bleeding from the wound and the activated partial thrombin time increase, the dose of heparin should be reduced. If the gauze dressing becomes wet and hard from bleeding around the replanted digit, the dressing should be changed, and care should be taken to prevent it from constricting the replanted site.

The most reliable monitoring method is to have a surgeon or nurse check the color, pulp turgor, capillary refill, and temperature of the digit every 1 to 2 hours for the first 3 days and then every 3 to 4 hours for the next 4 days. If the replanted digit is questionable, it should be checked more often. Continuously measuring the skin temperature of the replanted and uninjured digits with surface probes and monitoring temperature changes are useful supplementary methods for judging perfusion.

Compromised perfusion of the replanted digit may be indicated by a sudden drop in temperature of 4° to 5°C (arterial insufficiency), a temperature consistently 3°C lower than that of the normal digit (venous insufficiency), or a temperature consistently about 3°C lower than that of the normal digit with a transient 1° or 2°C decrease (transition from venous insufficiency to arterial insufficiency) (39). Temperatures below 30°C are reported to be absolute indications of anastomotic thrombosis (40). In addition, the surgeon must examine the replanted digit directly and determine whether there is a circulatory disorder by considering all of the above information. Continuous pulse oximetry has also been reported to be an effective technique of postoperative monitoring.

COMPLICATIONS AND CRITERIA FOR REEXPLORATION

When proximal arterial inflow is weak before the anastomosis and distal flow is intermittent or inconsistent despite an ideal anastomosis, postoperative intravenous heparin and PGE_1 should be continued. Continuous axillary or supraclavicular regional block of the brachial plexus with long-acting local anesthetics through a silicone catheter is recommended and should be performed before heparin is administered to prevent bleeding at the block site. However, a regional block of the brachial plexus, with a single injection of a local anesthetic that promotes vasodilatation, can also be performed in the same situation.

If a sudden change is detected, the dressing should be released or removed immediately, and tight skin stitches should be removed. In general, pale skin, loss of pulp turgor, and slow capillary refilling indicate arterial insufficiency. Skin that changes from dark red or violet to pink when the pulp is squeezed, and rapid capillary refilling, indicate venous congestion. If heparin has not been administrated continuously, one bolus of intravenous heparin (5000 units) may restore circulation (41), and a stellate ganglion block and regional block of the brachial plexus may relieve vasospasm. If perfusion does not recover rapidly after these treatments, the anastomoses should be reexplored without hesitation. Unlike the initial operation, the reexploration can be done by one surgeon and a scrub nurse.

If arterial thrombosis is diagnosed, the anastomosed artery should be resected and the thrombosis removed by squeezing the arterial wall or by removing it from the lumen. In general, an arterial thrombus elongates proximally from the anastomosis. If arterial flow appears at the proximal stump and the intimal surface looks normal after thrombectomy, reanastomosis may be successful. If the thrombus has not been removed completely and if the intimal surface of the stump shows fibrillation and the proximal stump shows no blood flow, the stumps should be resected until the intimal surface becomes normal and arterial flow is obtained. The gap between the new stumps should be bridged by a vein graft. During thrombus formation at the anastomosis site, many micro thrombi may become trapped in the distal capillaries, which will worsen distal circulation.

If venous thrombosis is diagnosed, the venous anastomosis should be resected and the thrombus removed as described earlier. Venous thrombi elongate distally from the anastomosis. If venous flow is restored to the distal stump after thrombectomy, reanastomosis may be successful. Reanastomosing the vein is almost the same as reanastomosing the artery. Late diagnosis reduces the salvage rate. In replantations in Tamai's zone I or II, if revision anastomosis of the vein is impossible, the nail plate should be removed or a stab incision should be placed in the hyponychium, as described earlier.

REHABILITATION

Whether early mobilization is possible in replantation surgery as it is in tendon surgery is still questionable. No rehabilitation technique has been established for early mobilization after simultaneous flexor and extensor tendon repair. It takes 2 weeks for proliferating endothelial cells to cover the disrupted intima (42) and 4 to 6 weeks for the media and internal elastic lamina to reconnect at the anastomosis site. During this period, flexing and extending the digit may occlude the anastomosed vessels.

Edematous joints of replanted digits are hard to move during the first few weeks after surgery. No early mobilization technique has been established for replanted digits, especially in Tamai's zones IV and V, transmetatarsal, and wrist amputations. However, incompletely amputated digits in which the flexor or extensor tendons and dorsal skin and vein remain in continuity may be suitable for early mobilization.

In general, the replanted part is immobilized for about 1 month. Mobilization of the elbow and shoulder joints of the injured extremity can begin 4 days after surgery if there are no complications. In single-digit replantation, mild passive motion of the uninjured digits can begin 8 days after surgery. Replanted digits with tendon sutures proximal to Tamai's zone III and transmetacarpal and wrist replantations can begin mobilization no earlier than 4 weeks after surgery.

Kirschner wires for temporary fixation are removed before exercises begin, and static splints to hold the fingers in the intrinsic plus position and the thumb in palmar abduction are applied after rehabilitation exercises and at night. Bone and tendon healing may progress, but the unions are still weak and may not tolerate bending or pulling. Motion exercises should be active and with assistance.

During rehabilitation, exercises that reduce extension lag but not flexion lag are the key. If both flexion and extension lag persist, flexor tenolysis and extensor tenolysis may be indicated at a later time with more than 2 months between the procedures. Because the results of extensor tenolysis are unsatisfactory in general, tenolysis should be limited to the flexor tendons. An outrigger splint is applied dorsally, and the PIP and DIP joints are kept extended with an extension block at the MCP joint. If bone union is achieved 8 weeks after surgery, passive motion exercises are added. If bone union is still questionable at this point, iliac crest bone grafting is indicated. If the range of active flexion is limited despite a full range of passive flexion 4 month after surgery, flexor tenolysis is indicated.

In wrist replantation, if the function of the abductor pollicis brevis has not recovered 6 months after surgery, opponensplasty is indicated. In general, functional recovery of the intrinsic muscles innervated by the deep branch of the ulnar nerve is poor. In transmetacarpal replantation including the thumb metacarpal and wrist replantation, hyperextension of the MCP joints of the fingers should be prevented with an extension block splint, and adduction contracture of the thumb should be prevented with a thumb abduction splint for more than 6 months to prevent an intrinsic minus posture of the fingers and an adduction contracture of the thumb (43).

The bellies of the FDP muscles (especially those of the ulnar three digits) are united; if motion in one of the three digits is limited, the motion of the other two digits will also be limited (the "quadriga" phenomenon). In this situation, suturing only the FDS tendon (sublimis finger) may be indicated from the beginning, and the FDP tendons might not be sutured.

If the patient reports dysesthesias in the replanted digit, desensitization exercises should be started. These exercises help the patient adapt to the dysesthesias by stimulating the brain through rubbing the pulp of the finger with a coarse cloth or by grasping and manipulating particulate materials with different rough surfaces (44). Stiffness of the replanted digit or hand can make it impossible for the patient to use the hand in activities of daily living and can decrease the stimulation from the hand to the brain, which can disturb sensory reeducation. Functional movement of a replanted digit is indispensable for sensory recovery.

SECONDARY OPERATIONS

Tenolysis is the most common secondary operation after replantation surgery. During rehabilitation, if extension lag can be prevented as described earlier, only flexor tenolysis is indicated. Active range of motion can be observed directly during the procedure by using a wrist block. A tourniquet should always be used despite the block if the patient can tolerate the tourniquet pain. Active flexion of the digit is evaluated 10 minutes after the tourniquet is released. Tenolysis should be continued until the active range of motion is the same as the passive range of motion. Wide dissection along the flexor tendons may be necessary.

If the A1 or A2 and the A4 pulleys were preserved during the initial surgery, there is no problem. When either the A2 or A4 pulleys were injured, pulley reconstruction is needed to prevent bowstringing of the flexor tendons and to maintain effective range of motion using a free tendon graft. After tenolysis, daily rehabilitation for at least 3 weeks is important.

An inlay-type of iliac crest bone graft is indicated for delayed union or nonunion at the site of osteosynthesis. In transmetacarpal or wrist replantation, if an intrinsic plus contracture or adduction contracture of the thumb develop and if a reverse knuckle bender or thumb web space splint is not effective, the interosseous tendon and lateral band of the extensor mechanism of the finger can be resected by Littler's procedure (45), the first web space skin can be released with a skin graft or Z-plasty. The adductor pollicis tendon can be released from the ulnar sesamoid bone at the MCP joint and the first dorsal interosseous muscle can be released from the first metacarpal. The thumb–index finger web space may need to be maintained with a temporary Kirschner wire, and a pediculed or free skin flap with adipose tissue to fill the dead space and cover the skin defect may be required. If abductor pollicis brevis function does not recover, opponensplasty of the thumb should be considered. If the thumb was not replanted, reconstructing a thumb with a wrap-around flap or distraction lengthening the remaining phalanx is indicated to restore pinch function.

RESULTS AND OUTCOMES REPORTED IN THE LITERATURE

The viability of replanted digits depend on the surgical technique, the experience of the surgeon in performing microsurgery and hand surgery, and patient selection. It is likely that an experienced surgeon can achieve a viability rate of 80% or higher (8–10,12).

Active range of motion of the replanted digit depends on the level of amputation and the extent of injured tissue. The average range of motion of the PIP joint of a digit replanted distal to the insertion of the FDS tendon is better than that of a digit replanted proximal to the FDS insertion (83 degrees vs. 35 degrees, respectively) (17).

Sensory recovery of a replanted digit depends on the level of amputation, the type of amputation, and the patient's age. Sensory recovery of digits replanted distally is better than that of those replanted proximally (46–48). Sensory recovery of a clean amputation is better than that of an avulsion or crush amputation (average static two-point discrimination for the finger, 8 mm vs. 15 mm; for the thumb, 9 mm vs. 12 mm) (49). Sensory recovery is more likely in younger patients. Recovery of motor function of the intrinsic muscles controlled by the ulnar nerve is poor. Finger-tip replantation prevents amputation stump neuroma pain. Cold intolerance occurs in most replanted digits and improves as sensation recovers up to 2 years, but it does not disappear completely (50).

REFERENCES

1. Jacobson JH, Suarez EL. Microsurgery in anastomosis of small vessels. *Surg Forum* 1960;11:243.
2. Malt RA, Mckhann C. Replantation of severed arms. *JAMA* 1964;189:716.
3. Inoue T, Toyoshima Y, Fukusumi H, et al. Factors necessary for successful replantation of upper extremities. *Ann Surg* 1967;165:225.
4. Chen ZW, Chien YC, Boa YBL. Salvage of the forearm following complete traumatic amputation; report of a case. *Chin Med J* 1963;82:632.
5. Kleinert HE, Kasdan ML. Anastomosis of digital vessels. *J Ky Med Assoc* 1965;63:106.
6. Komatsu S, Tamai S. Successful replantation of a completely cut off thumb. *Plast Reconstr Surg* 1968;42:374.
7. Tamai S. History of microsurgery-from the beginning until the end of the 1970s. *Microsurgery* 1993;14:6.
8. Kleinert HE, Jablon M, Tsai TM. An overview of replantation and result of 347 replants in 245 patients. *J Trauma* 1980;20:390.
9. Tamai S. Twenty years' experience of limb replantation: review of 293 upper extremity replants. *J Hand Surg* 1982;7:549.
10. Morrison WA, O'Brien MC, MacLeod AM. Digital replantation and revascularization. A long term review of one hundred cases. *Hand* 1978;10:125.
11. Weiland AJ, Baskin KB. Philosophy of replantation 1976–1990. *Microsurgery* 1990;11:223.
12. Fukui A, Tamai S. Present status of replantation in Japan. *Microsurgery* 1994;15:84.
13. Cheng GL, Pan DDP, Zhang NP, et al. Digital replantation in children: a long-term follow-up study. *J Hand Surg* 1998;23(suppl A):635.
14. Schlenker JD, Kleinert HE, Tsai TM. Method and result of replantation following traumatic amputation of the thumb in sixty-four patients. *J Hand Surg* 1980;5:63.
15. Arakaki A, Tsai TM. Thumb replantation: survival factors and re-exploration in 122 cases. *J Hand Surg Br* 1993;18:152.
16. Meyer VE. Hand amputations proximal but close to the wrist joint: prime candidates for reattachment (long-term functional results). *J Hand Surg* 1985;10(suppl A):989.
17. Urbaniak JR, Poth JH, Nunley JA, et al. The result of replantation after amputation of single finger. *J Bone Joint Surg* 1985;67(suppl A):611.
18. Yamano Y. Replantation of amputated distal part of the fingers. *J Hand Surg* 1985;10(suppl A):211.
19. Goldner RD, Stevanovic MV, Nunley JA. Digital replantation at the level of the distal interphalangeal joint and the distal phalanx. *J Hand Surg* 1989;14(suppl A):214.
20. Urbaniak JR, Evans JP, Bright DS. Microvascular management of ring avulsion injuries. *J Hand Surg* 1981;6:25.
21. Key S, Wernetz J, Wolff TW. Ring avulsion injury: classification and prognosis. *J Hand Surg* 1989;14(suppl A):204.
22. Lister G. Intraosseous wiring of the digital skeleton. *J Hand Surg* 1978;3:427.
23. Kusano N, Yoshizu T, Maki Y, et al. Experimental study of the new flexor tendon suture technique for postoperative early active flexion exercise. *J Hand Surg* 1999;24(suppl B):152.
24. Yoshizu T, Maki Y, Tajima T, et al. An in vitro evaluation of various new flexor repair techniques for early active motion exercise. *J Jpn Soc Surg Hand* 1997;13:1135.
25. Savage R. The mechanical effect of partial resection of the digital fibrous flexor sheath. *J Hand Surg* 1990;15(suppl B):435.
26. Matsuda M, Chikamatsu E, Shimizu Y. Correlation between number of anastomosed vessels and survival rate in finger replantation. *J Reconstr Microsurg* 1993;9:1.
27. Smith AR, Sonneveld GJ, van der Meulen JC. AV anastomosis as a solution for absent venous drainage in replantation surgery, *Plast Reconstr Surg* 1983;71:525.
28. Suzuki Y, Ishikawa K, Isshiki N, et al. Fingertip replantation with an efferent A.V. anastomosis for venous drainage: clinical report. *Br J Plast Surg* 1993;46:187.
29. Gordon L, Leitner DW, Buncke HJ, et al. Partal nail plate removal after digital replantation as an alternative method of venous drainage. *J Hand Surg* 1985;10(suppl A):360.
30. Sadahiro T. A Fish mouse incision for congestion in replantation of the amputated finger—experimental and clinical study. *J Jpn Orthop Assoc* 1979;53:411.
31. Han SK, Lee BL, Kim WK. Topical and systemic anticoagulation in treatment of absent or compromised venous out flow in replanted fingertips. *J Hand Surg* 2000;25(suppl A):659.

32. Mori K, Tajima T, Yoshizu T, et al. Influence of twist and tension of anastomosed vessels on blood flow (II. Circulation changes from lengthening of dissection and vein grafting). *J Reconstr Microsurg* 1991;7:150.
33. Shafiroff BB, Palmer AK. Simplified technique for replantation of the thumb. *J Hand Surg* 1981;6:623.
34. Yoshizu T, Katsumi M, Tajima T. Replantation of untidy amputated finger, hand, and arm: experience of 99 replantations in 66 cases. *J Trauma* 1978;18:194.
35. Honda T, Nomura S, Yamauchi S, et al. The possible applications of a composite skin and subcutaneous vein graft in the replantation of amputated digits. *Br J Plast Surg* 1984;37:607.
36. Nishi G, Shibata Y, Kumabe Y, et al. Arterialized venous skin flaps for the injured finger. *J Reconstr Microsurg* 1989;5:357.
37. Camacho FJ, Wood MB. Polydigit replantation. *Hand Clin* 1992;8:409.
38. Tonkin MA, Ames FL, Wolff TW, et al. Transmetacarpal amputation and replantation: the importance of the normal vascular anatomy. *J Hand Surg* 1988;18(suppl B):204.
39. Narisawa H, Katsumi M, Watanabe M, et al. Temperature monitoring in replantation and Vascularized free flap. *J Jpn Soc Surg Hand* 1987;4:269.
40. Stirrat CR, Seaber AV, Urbaniak JR, et al. Temperature monitoring in digital replantation. *J Hand Surg* 1978;3:343.
41. Noguchi M, Matsuzaki H, Yamamoto H. Intravenous bolus infusion of heparin for circulatory insufficiency after finger replantation. *J Reconstr Microsurg* 1999;15:245.
42. Weinstein PR, Mehdorn HM, Szabo Z. Microsurgical anastomosis: vessel injury, regeneration, and repair. In Serafin D, Buncke H (eds). *Microsurgical Composite Tissue Transplantation.* St. Louis: Mosby, 1979, p. 111.
43. Scheker LR, Chesher SP, Netscher DT, et al. Functional result of dynamic splinting after transmetacarpal, wrist, and distal forearm replantation. *J Hand Surg* 1995;20(suppl B):584.
44. Skirven TM, Callahan AD. Therapist's management of peripheral nerve injuries. In Mackin EJ, Callahan AD, Skirven TM, et al (eds). *Rehabilitation of the Hand and Upper Extremity*, 5th ed. St. Louis: Mosby, 2002, p. 599.
45. Littler JW, Cooley SGE. Restoration of the retinacular system in hyperextension of the proximal interphalangeal joint. *J Bone Joint Surg* 1965;47(suppl A):637.
46. Gelberman RH, Urbaniak JR, Bright DS, et al. Digital sensibility following replantation. *J Hand Surg* 1978;3:313.
47. Yamauchi S, Nomura S, Yoshimura M, et al. A clinical study of the order and speed of sensory after digit replantation. *J Hand Surg* 1983;8:549.
48. Murakami T, Ikuta Y, Tsuge K. Relationship between the number of digital nerves sutured and sensory recovery in replanted fingers. *J Reconstr Microsurg* 1985;1:283.
49. Glickman LT, Mackinnon SE. Sensory recovery following digital replantation. *Microsurgery* 1990;11:236.
50. Backman C, Nystrom A, Backman C. Arterial spasticity and cold intolerance in relation to time after digital replantation. *J Hand Surg* 1993;18(suppl B):551.

CHAPTER 56

Major Replantation

S. Raja Sabapathy, David Elliot, and Hari Venkatramani

Any replantation of an amputation proximal to the wrist is considered a "major replantation." These injuries cause significant functional and cosmetic impairment to an individual, also affecting body image and influencing interaction of the individual with society. When the upper limb sustains amputation distal to the wrist (minor amputation) and the part is not replanted, secondary reconstructive techniques in the form of flaps and toe transfers are available to restore useful function (1–3). After major amputation, the only alternative to replantation is a prosthesis.

Although prosthesis technology has reached a high level of sophistication in the lower limb, this is not so in the upper limb, and upper limb prostheses have still not reached a stage where they gain widespread acceptance by patients. In a study conducted in Louisville (4,5) comparing different functional levels of replanted major amputations with the best available prosthesis, the replantations outscored the prostheses. Although the study was done some time ago, the situation does not appear to have changed, despite advances in technology. Rejection of so-called "functioning" upper limb prostheses is also high: many remain in a drawer and are only taken out for clinic visits. Studies on prosthesis usage after major upper limb amputation report their abandonment in 35% to 45% of limbs, and this rate increases the more proximal the amputation (6,7).

The other option available to a hand surgeon to rehabilitate this group of patients is hand transplantation. Although transplantation is a possibility, the complexities of selection, postoperative rehabilitation, and the problems of lifelong immune suppression currently place this surgery beyond the reach of most surgical teams and their patients (8). A major breakthrough in immunology may eventually make this option of treatment more easily available in the future. However, until that time, replantation remains the mainstay of management of patients who have sustained total amputation of the upper limb proximal to the wrist and can reach microsurgeons in the very short period for which replantation is feasible.

HISTORICAL PERSPECTIVE

The first clinical replantation performed was a major replant. On May 23, 1962, a 12-year-old boy whose arm had been torn off near the shoulder in a railway accident reached the Massachusetts General Hospital in Boston within 30 minutes. Malt, a chief resident at that time, reattached and revascularized the limb. He left repair of the tendons and nerves for a second stage. A large area of skin loss near the shoulder was skin grafted on the fifth day. News of the surgery was received with both applause and scepticism as to the safety of the procedure and the possible functional outcome. By the time Malt published the case in 1964, the boy had recovered useful function, and these surgeons had done one more replant (9).

The history of major replantation surgery is only one of many in which a procedure was conceived, and often perfected, in the laboratories, and then an embarrassingly long time passed before surgeons performed the procedure clinically. Alexis Carrel, who is hailed as the father of transplantation surgery, replanted the hind leg of a dog successfully in Chicago in 1906 (10). Many centers followed this lead, and Lapchinsky in Moscow and Snyder in the University of Miami performed around 200 such replants in the 1950s. Every step that was needed to perform a replant had been practiced in many places since the beginning of the 20th century, but the jump to clinical practice was not taken for more than half a century. After the first case had been done, it was quickly repeated all over the world. Emphasis shifted from clinical possibility to the safety of the procedure and achieving a good functional result. Refinements of technique and advances in basic scientific knowledge have made major replantation a regular and safe procedure (11).

INDICATIONS FOR MAJOR REPLANTATION

Major upper limb amputation is a situation in which the surgeon has to help the patient make the decision that he or she thinks is in the best interests of the patient. It is difficult for the patient to make this decision because every patient wants every amputated part reattached and assumes that the replanted limb will be entirely normal. They are unaware of the consequences of the amputation–replantation process and the problems associated with the procedure. The enormity of the accident may also cloud the decision-making process.

The basic tenet of replantation is that the surgery must reduce the disability of the individual compared with that inherent in simple closure of the amputation stump. This must be done without putting the life of the patient at any undue risk. Because major replantation is a surgery of significant magnitude, the general condition of the patient, associated injuries, co-morbidities, and social aspects of the family have all to be taken into account in making the decision to replant. The following factors help in making the decision.

Level of Amputation and Ischemia Time

The term "major replantation" includes a wide spectrum of injuries, ranging from amputation just proximal to the wrist to amputation near the shoulder. Complications are directly related to the extent of the muscle mass in the amputated part; hence, the acceptable ischemia time is directly related to the level of injury. We have developed guidelines that are based on the level of amputation and the ischemia time at the time of the patient's arrival at the hospital (12,13) (Table 56-1). This guideline was created on the premise that the patient will have immediate access to the operating room (OR) and trained personnel will be available at the time of his, or her, arrival at the hospital. Even in institutions with this level of infrastructure, which is not common, it can take a minimum of 2 to 3 hours before the part is revascularized. A useful consideration for any unit likely to receive these patients is for near-rigid guidelines to have been set up for such cases by previous discussion with appropriate departments and administrators of the hospital, such as has been done for the management of major emergencies worldwide (14).

We have found it helpful for the first person to talk to the patient to have the guidelines available as a reminder of the protocol to be followed, both for the actual replantation procedure and to keep the ischemia time to an acceptable level. One has to be very wary of exceeding the 6-hour warm ischemia period for an above-elbow amputation because it is not possible to reduce the muscle mass in the distal part by debridement. In a below-elbow amputation, by removing all the muscle attached to the tendons in the distal part, the ischemic muscle that is the source of the reperfusion injury can be reduced, and the potential warm ischemia time can be extended.

The Nature of Injury

Guillotine amputations have a more favorable outcome than crush, avulsion, and crush–avulsion amputations. In guillotine amputations, all of the structures are cut at the same level, the need for debridement is less, and good-quality vessels and nerves are immediately available for repair. Guillotine amputations proximal to the hand have now become rare. An analysis of major replantation patients done during a 5-year period, from 1997 to 2002, in our center identified only two of 22 patients who had sustained guillotine amputations and both were just proximal to the wrist (12). Most proximal upper limb amputations are crush or crush–avulsion injuries, and if these are not considered for replantation, the number of major replantations done will be very few in any center. With technical refinements, it is now possible to replant crush, avulsion, and crush–avulsion amputations and gain useful function. Therefore, if the ischemia time is acceptable, one should take the decision to replant major amputation whatever the mechanism of injury (Figure 56-1).

Structural Integrity of the Hand

Another factor important to the decision to replant a proximal amputation is the structural integrity of the hand. If the hand of the amputated part has been severely damaged to an extent that function cannot be achieved by reconstructive surgery, then the amputated part should not be replanted (Figure 56-2). There are instances in which double-level injuries have been replanted and function has been achieved, but, here again, the hand should be structurally intact and capable of function (15,16). On rare occasions, an amputated part can be replanted and shortened to increase the length of the amputation stump to facilitate wearing of prosthesis. This mostly arises with arm amputations, in which replantation and shortening achieves a longer stump or a functioning elbow joint (Figure 56-3).

General Condition of the Patient

Because the patient must be able to tolerate a long surgical procedure, the general condition of the patient is an important determinant of whether replantation be advised. Although it is not absolutely certain how much old age and comorbidity factors, such as diabetes and hypertension, may play a role in the ultimate functional outcome, anesthetic and postoperative complications are likely to be higher in these patients and have to be considered by the surgical team and explained to the patient.

Patients with major amputations of the upper limb may have sustained concomitant injuries such as significant head, chest and abdominal injuries and multiple long bone fractures. These patients must be assessed particularly carefully in respect of the advisability of increase of risk to life by both the addition of a long operative procedure and the potential problems of reperfusion injury. Life before limb must be the watchword here.

Social Factors

Replantation after a major amputation requires commitment to rehabilitation by a patient and his or her family for a minimum period of 1 year, with the possibility of secondary procedures being necessary.

TABLE 56-1 Guidelines for Replantation According to the Level of Amputation

Level of Amputation	Time from Injury to Arrival at Hospital	Decision to Replant	Technical Considerations
A. Proximal to mid arm level	(i) ≤3 hours	Replant	Debride; fix bone; repair artery, vein, and nerve; then release the clamps ("regular sequence").
	(ii) 3–4 hours	Replant	Debride, fix bone, repair artery first, then release the arterial clamp to perfuse for 5-10 minutes with blood running out of open veins (blood replacement may be needed). Clamp the artery, repair the other structures in the regular sequence, and then release the arterial clamp only. Only release the venous clamp after a further 5 minutes.
	(iii) 4–5 hours	Replant	Use preliminary arterial shunting on arrival and then repair as in A(ii). If any delay occurs during the procedure, the arterial clamp can be released for 5 minutes once every 30 minutes.
	(iv) 5–6 hours	Grey zone for replanting	Replant only if the fingers are freely passively mobile. Otherwise, replant and do a proximal below-elbow amputation to gain length for prosthesis fitting.
	(5) >6 hours	Do not replant	Consider replanting only if the part is very well preserved and kept cool. Possible particularly in a child because the muscle mass is less. Consider preliminary arterial shunting.
B. Lower third of arm and proximal forearm	(i) ≤4 hours	Replant	Regular sequence as in A(i) above.
	(ii) 4–6 hours	Replant	Preserve the elbow by shortening on the nonjoint side.
	(iii) 6–7 hours	Replant	Arthrodese the elbow to allow more muscle debridement. After the bone fixation, repair the artery first, release the clamp for perfusion for 5-10 minutes, clamp the artery again, and then repair the other structures in the regular sequence. Then release the arterial clamp only. Only release the venous clamp after a further 5 minutes.
			Consider preliminary arterial shunting. Do replant only if the thumb is passively mobile and follow sequence as in B(ii).
	(iv) >7 hours	Do not replant	Consider replanting only if the part is very well preserved and kept cool, especially in a child because the muscle mass is less. Consider preliminary arterial shunting.
C. Midforearm to wrist level	(i) ≤6 hours	Replant	Ensure excision of muscles attached to tendons in the amputated part.
	(ii) 6–8 hours	Replant	Replant in regular sequence as in A(i).
			Debride. After the bone fixation, repair the artery first, release the clamp for perfusion for 5-10 minutes, clamp the artery again, and then repair the other structures in the regular sequence. Then release the arterial clamp only. Only release the venous clamp after a further 5 minutes.
	(iii) >8 hours	Grey zone for replanting	Replant only if the thumb is passively mobile.
			Consider preliminary arterial shunting.

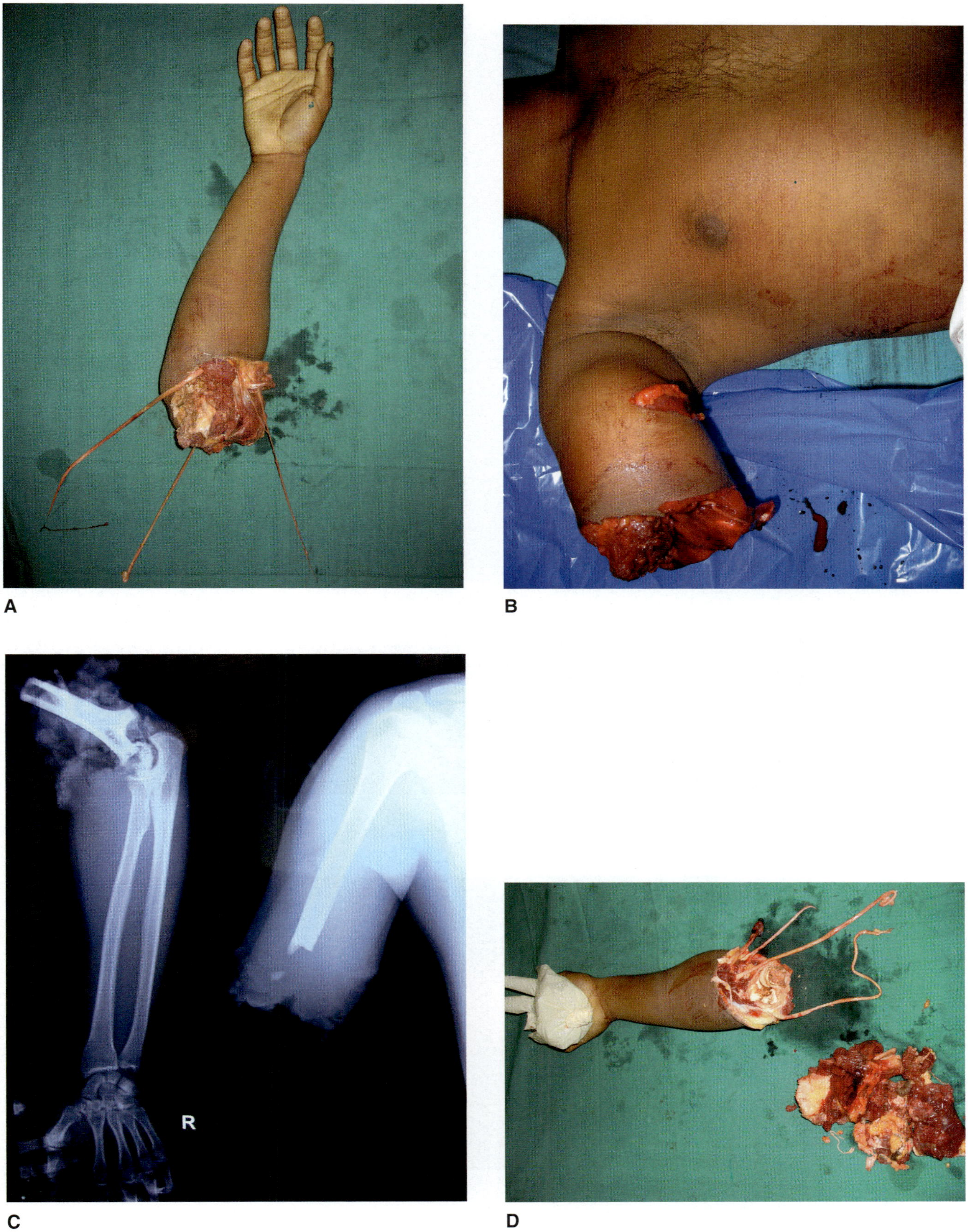

FIGURE 56-1 (A) to (C) Crush avulsion amputation of the right arm with avulsion of the nerves from a very proximal level. (D) Postdebridement photograph of the distal segment. The distal humerus had to be removed during debridement.

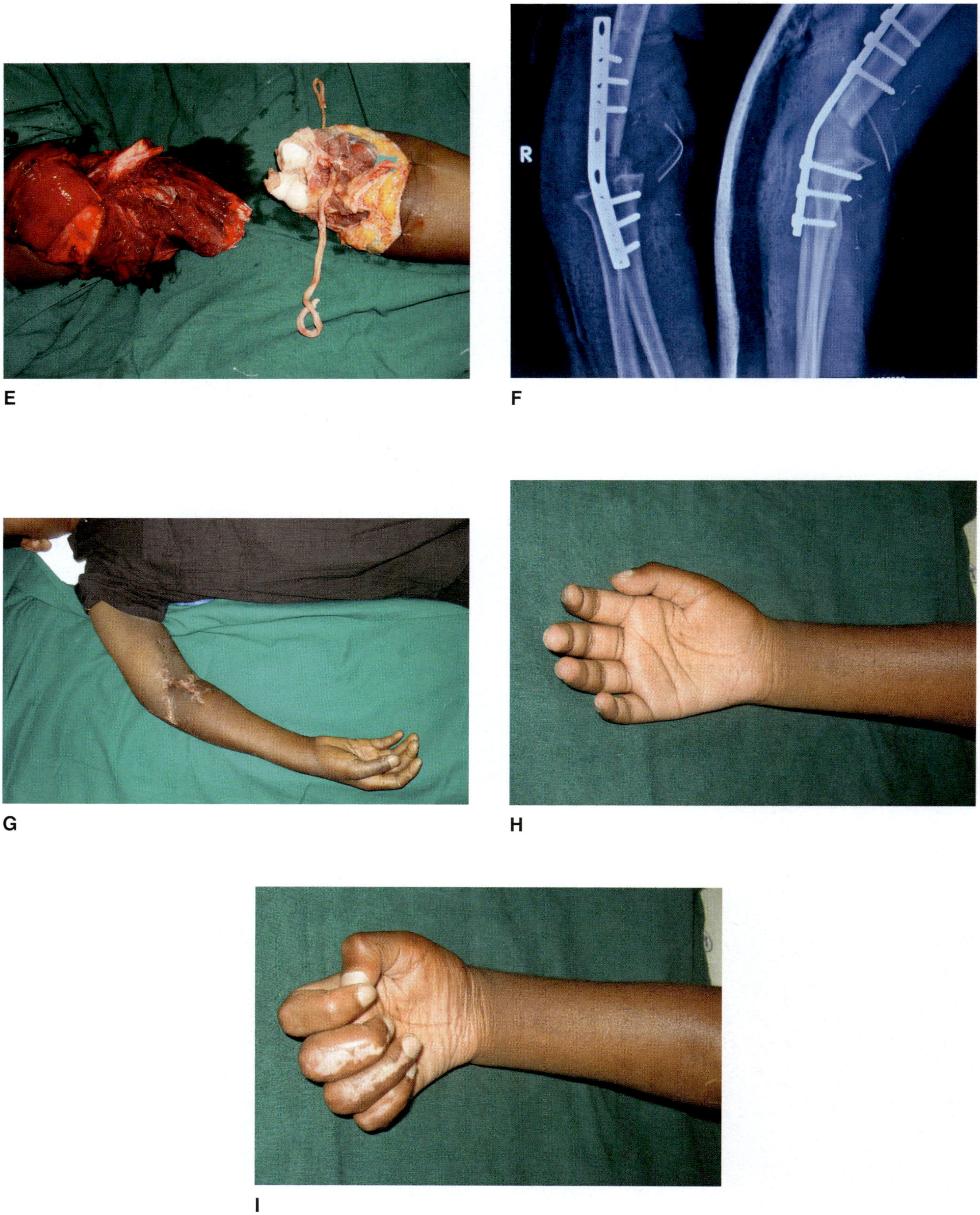

FIGURE 56-1 *(Continued)* (**E**) The prepared proximal and distal ends ready for bone fixation. (**F**) The proximal humerus fixed to the distal ulna. (**G**) Two-year follow-up. (**H**) and (**I**) The flexion and extension of the fingers achieved. The median and ulnar nerves were repaired just below the axilla.

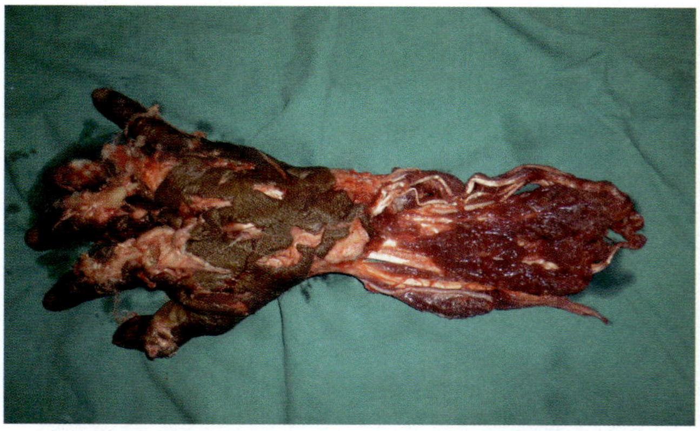

FIGURE 56-2 This crush avulsion injury is not fit for replantation because, in addition to the severe injury in the forearm, there is extensive injury to the hand with multisegment bone and soft tissue loss.

PRIMARY INDICATIONS FOR MAJOR REPLANTATION

1. The level of amputation and ischemia time are the two key determinants in deciding whether to proceed with a major replantation.
2. The hand has to be intact or reconstructable when a major replant is contemplated.
3. Scapulothoracic avulsion amputations and amputations with avulsion of the nerves from the brachial plexus are absolute contraindications to major replantation.
4. If the amputated part can be replanted without putting the life of the patient at undue risk and the above three criteria are positive, the replantation should be carried out.

TECHNICAL CONSIDERATIONS

Preparation of the Patient

Preparation starts with preparation of the patient. Success of a major replantation depends on completing the revascularization quickly. After 4 hours, the potential for damage to vital organs does not rise incrementally with time but exponentially. Time is crucial to prevent complications, so the patient must be the center of action, and all facilities must converge on the patient. In our experience of 2 decades of dealing with such cases, one factor that we have found vital to this philosophy is that these patients are admitted directly to the anteroom of the OR as soon as the patient arrives at the hospital. They bypass the emergency department and all associated delays. On reaching the OR, they can be assessed and resuscitated by senior surgeons and anesthesiologists. Radiographs, including x-ray of the amputated part, ultrasonography of the abdomen, and all routine investigations are done in the OR.

A patient with a major upper limb amputation may have associated injuries and could have sustained significant blood loss. The patient must be subjected to regular Advanced Trauma Life Support (ATLS) examination protocol and rapidly resuscitated. Resuscitation and preparation for surgery must go together. Tetanus prophylaxis and prophylactic antibiotics must also be administered. In our unit, after a preliminary ATLS survey, the patient is given a brachial block anesthesia ("on-arrival block").

We have dealt with upper limb amputations combined with head, abdominal, lower limb, and chest injuries. Of all of these, patients with chest injuries with lung damage do least well in the postoperative period. If there are associated rib fractures, the patient is carefully examined for possible lung injury. This may not be obvious on day 1. The chest radiograph may also be normal. Around the third day, opacities appear in the chest radiograph, and lung complications may occur. The services of an intensivist may be needed. We have replanted major amputations in patients with associated extradural hemorrhage and intraabdominal injuries. In these patients, it is important not to give anticoagulants in the postoperative period. Because the vessels repaired in major replants are larger diameter vessels, this is unlikely to change the outcome.

Emergency Revascularization

Warm ischemia increases the speed of muscle degradation, so every effort is taken to keep the amputated part cool during preparation for replantation. Gloves filled with ice cubes are

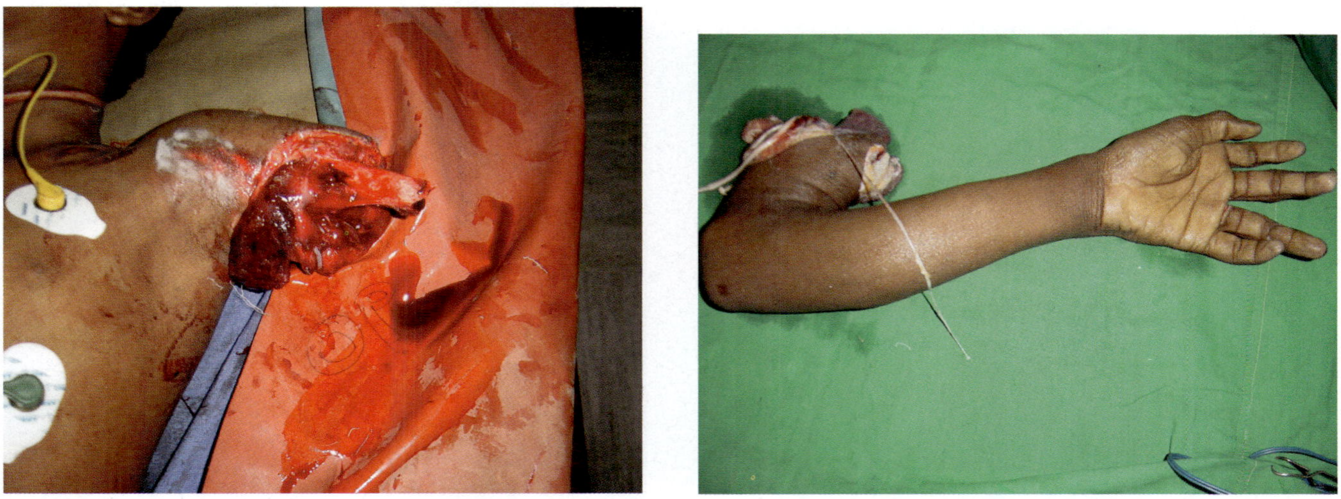

A B

FIGURE 56-3 (A) and (B) Amputation of the upper limb at the upper arm level with avulsion of the nerves from the brachial plexus and a long ischemia time. Closure of the amputation stump would need a flap.

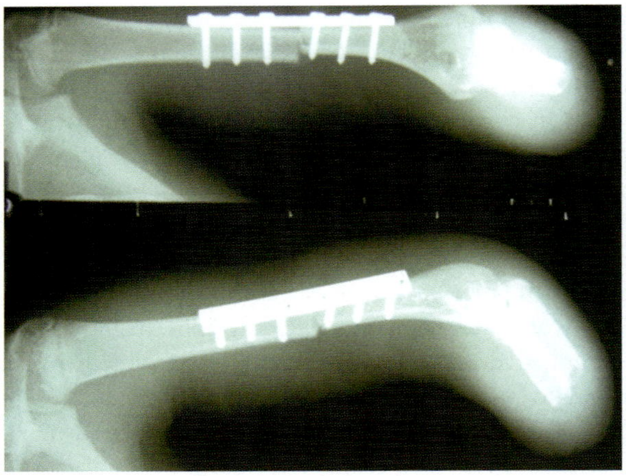

C

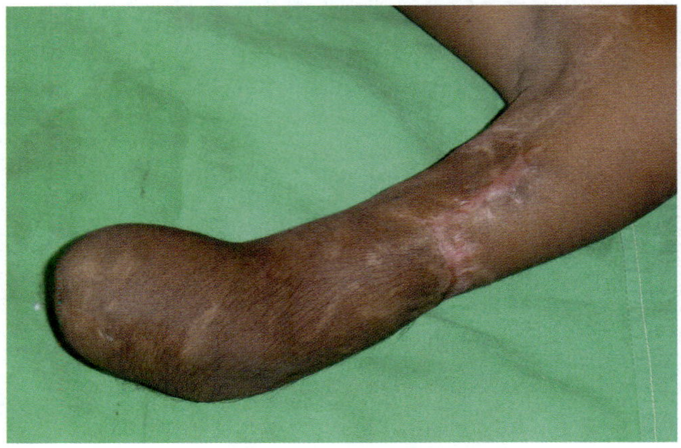

D

FIGURE 56-3 (*Continued*) (**C**) Replantation done with primary amputation at below-elbow level to increase the stump length to enable easy wearing of a prosthesis. (**D**) Long-term result of the replantation.

strapped to the part of the amputated part that is not involved in the surgical dissection (Figure 56-4). Although this does not achieve perfect core cooling, it extends the period of safe ischemia. A better, more definitive method to extend the safe period of ischemia is to perform temporary shunting of the amputated part (17). If the ischemia time is marginal, the amputated part is placed near the patient, and with the help of a vascular shunt or a plastic cannula, the distal part is revascularized (Figure 56-5). The veins are not connected, and the blood is run out of the arm and not returned to the body to avoid unwanted noxious substances getting to the kidneys. The blood is allowed to flow for about 5 minutes. Several units of blood may be lost during this reperfusion and must be available if this is done. No study has ever been done to define the exact extension of the time limit for major replantation gained by this procedure. Generally, it is thought that another hour of safe ischemic time can be gained, which is adequate to achieve full revascularization. If this cannulation is necessary, the sequence of reconnecting structures during the replantation is adjusted such that the artery is repaired soon after the skeletal fixation.

Preparation of the Amputated Part

Perfect debridement is critical and is done in a methodical manner (18). First, the skin edges are excised. Next, the vessels and nerves are identified and tagged with sutures. Then, the wound is debrided of contaminants. In badly contaminated wounds, initial tagging of the vessels and nerves prevents accidental loss of length of these structures during wound excision. Even loss of a single centimeter of length of any vessel or nerve may make the difference between direct repair and the need for a graft. The contaminants are then removed by wound excision.

The extent of the muscle mass excised depends on the type and level of injury. In guillotine amputations, the amount of muscle excised need be very little. After revascularization, the distal muscles are a combined mass and maintain their intermuscular vascular connections, so they will revascularize. However, in a crush or avulsion injury (much more common), the distal tendons are hanging free, with their muscles separated from one another. They cannot revascularize, so the muscles must be excised, leaving the tendons bare (Figure 56-6).

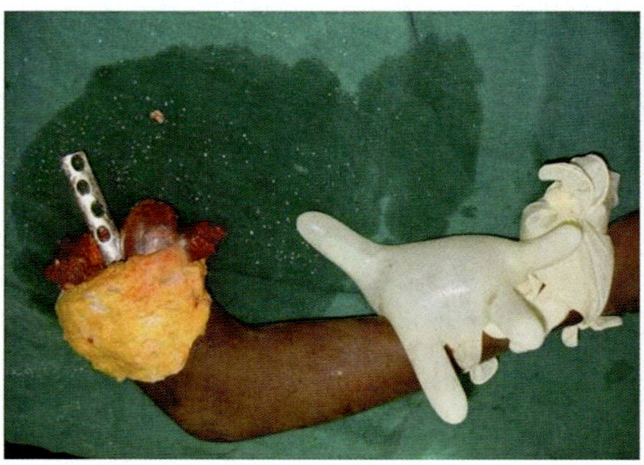

FIGURE 56-4 An arm amputation after debridement and before bone fixation. Until revascularization is done, a number of surgical gloves filled with ice similar to the ones shown are used to cover and wrap the amputated part and keep it cool.

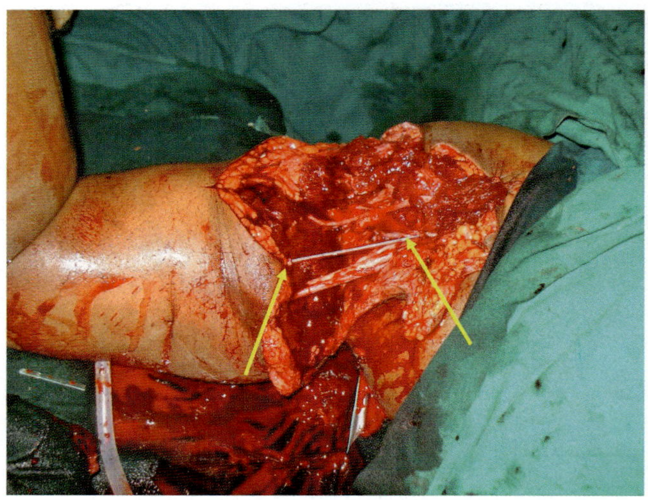

FIGURE 56-5 An above-elbow amputation with borderline ischemia time. The part is placed near the stump and perfused using a plastic shunt.

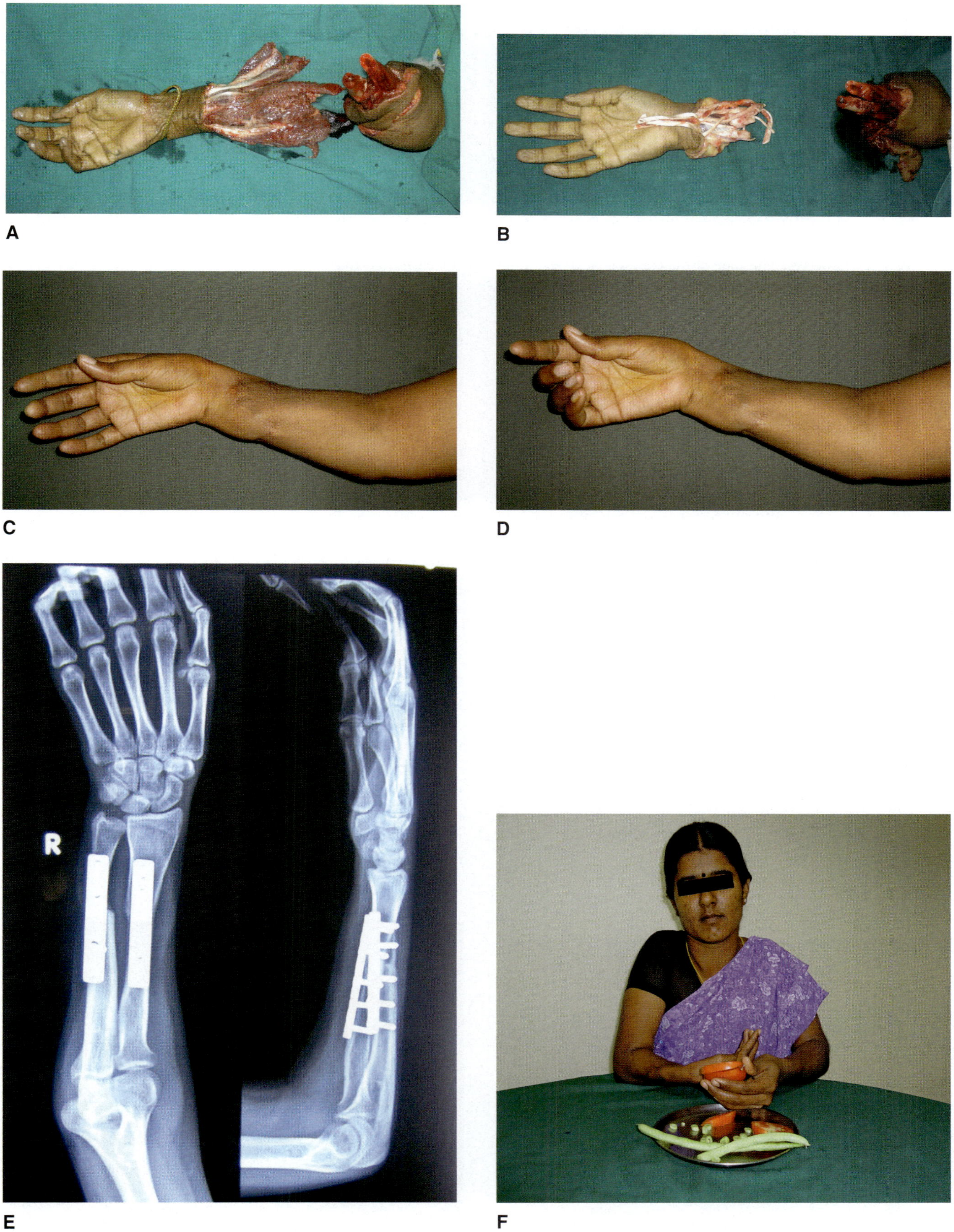

FIGURE 56-6 (A) Avulsion amputation of the forearm with muscles attached to the avulsed tendons in the distal segment. (B) All of the muscles excised during debridement, leaving the tendons bare. (C) and (D) Three years after replantation. Postoperative radiograph showing the extent of bone shortening (E) and showing the patient using the hand (F) with side-to-side thumb–index pinch to hold a knife and cut vegetables because of good recovery of the intrinsic muscles.

Retaining muscles attached to the distal tendons in a crush or avulsion injury is likely to cause infection in the replant. This is seen most obviously in a proximal forearm amputation. In an above-elbow amputation, the distal part of the biceps is usually hanging loose by its tendon and has to be excised.

Further attention is then turned to the vessels and nerves. They may be covered with contaminants. If so, it is usually possible to find a tissue plane between the adventitia and the definitive structures and strip off the contaminated tissues at this level, laying bare the vessels and nerves. We call this "skeletonization" of the vessels and nerves. The state of the vessels is next examined under the microscope, trimmed to the point of good quality, then tagged with sutures for easy identification later. This tagging is important: if they are not tagged at this stage, it is difficult to identify them in the depths of the wound after skeletal fixation.

When indicated, fasciotomies on the amputated part are done immediately after the debridement. These are always necessary unless the patient arrives within an hour of injury. After above-elbow amputation, fasciotomies of the forearm muscle compartments and the intrinsic muscles of the hand, with decompression of the median and ulnar nerves in the carpal tunnel and Guyon's canal, respectively, are required. After forearm amputations, hand fasciotomies and the same nerve decompressions only are carried out. If these are done during preparation of the amputated part, they can be done swiftly and fully. If done immediately after revascularization, there is always profuse bleeding from the wounds, and it is likely that they will be incomplete.

At all times during preparation of the amputated part, attention is given to coagulation of possible bleeding vessels. "Hemostasis" has to be achieved during dissection. This applies both to the proximal limb and the amputated part. Otherwise, after revascularization, there will be troublesome bleeding from raw areas all over the replanted distal part, increasing blood loss.

Finally, the bone ends are freshened. By this time, the patient has been anaesthetized and an examination of the proximal part has been carried out.

An impression can now be gained as to the extent of bone shortening that will be necessary to achieve primary repair of the blood vessels and nerves. Skeletal shortening of up to 10 cm is acceptable in the upper limb to make it easy to achieve bone fixation and to facilitate direct repair of the blood vessels and nerves (Figure 56-7). From long-term assessment, this shortening is acceptable to patients. In the upper limb, we usually prefer bone fixation by plating. After the degree of bone shortening and the type of fixation have been decided, the fixation can be attached to the amputated part to save time (see Figure 56-4) while work continues on the proximal part

Preparation of the Proximal Part

Debridement of the proximal part is done with the same attention to detail. The surgeon must always do this with the importance of the ischemia time in mind. Meticulous wound excision is done, as in the amputated part. Making sure of the quality of the vessels and nerves identified is the key step. There must be pulsatile flow at the end of the proximal vessel to be used for revascularization. Anything less is not acceptable. In avulsion and crush injuries, there may be another injury to the vessel proximal to the final amputation level. That, by itself, is not a contraindication to the procedure, but it must be identified and a proximal repair carried out. Replantation can only proceed if pulsatile flow is obtained at the amputation level (Figure 56-8). The nerves are trimmed to the level where they are single units covered by epineurium. In avulsion injuries, the fascicles are usually frayed and separated, and it is prudent to excise to the level where each nerve is a single unit. Too much slack on gentle pulling of the nerves can indicate avulsion at a proximal level. This has to be considered and, if suspicion arises, explored further proximally. As in the distal part, all vessels and nerves that will be repaired are identified and tagged. Failing to tag these structures with long identifiable sutures may result in an unnecessary waste of time after skeletal fixation. If the artery is repaired first, the bleeding and edema that occur may make the task even more difficult.

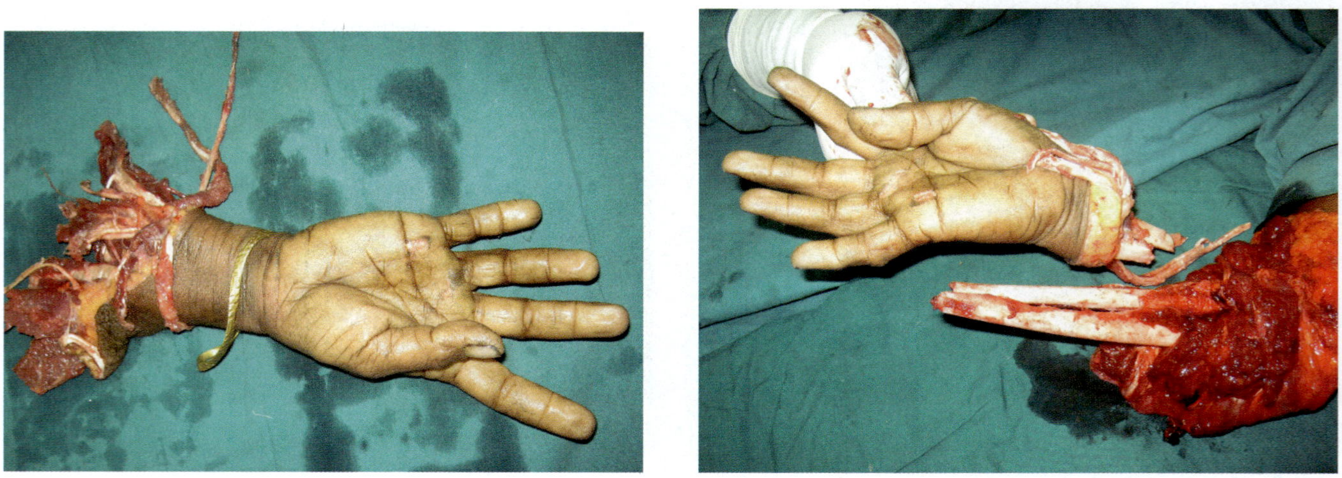

A B

FIGURE 56-7 (A) Machine injury resulting in avulsion amputation of the forearm. (B) The amputated segment placed near the proximal segment. The bare bone has to be resected.

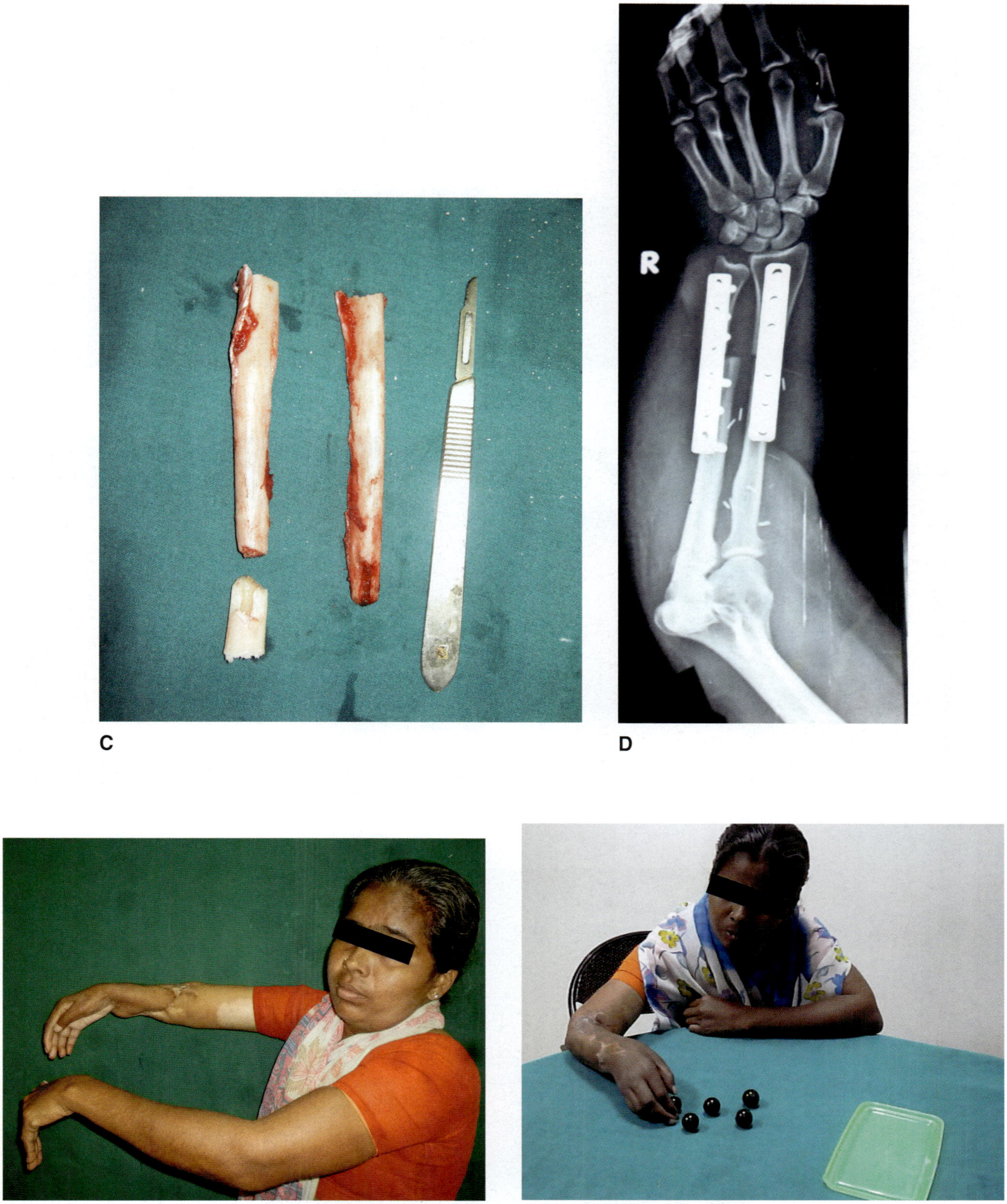

C D E F

FIGURE 56-7 (*Continued*) (**C**) Twelve cm excised segment of forearm bones. (**D**) Postoperative radiograph. (**E**) Acceptable long-term result compared with the opposite side. (**F**) When seen in isolation, the shortening is not immediately obvious.

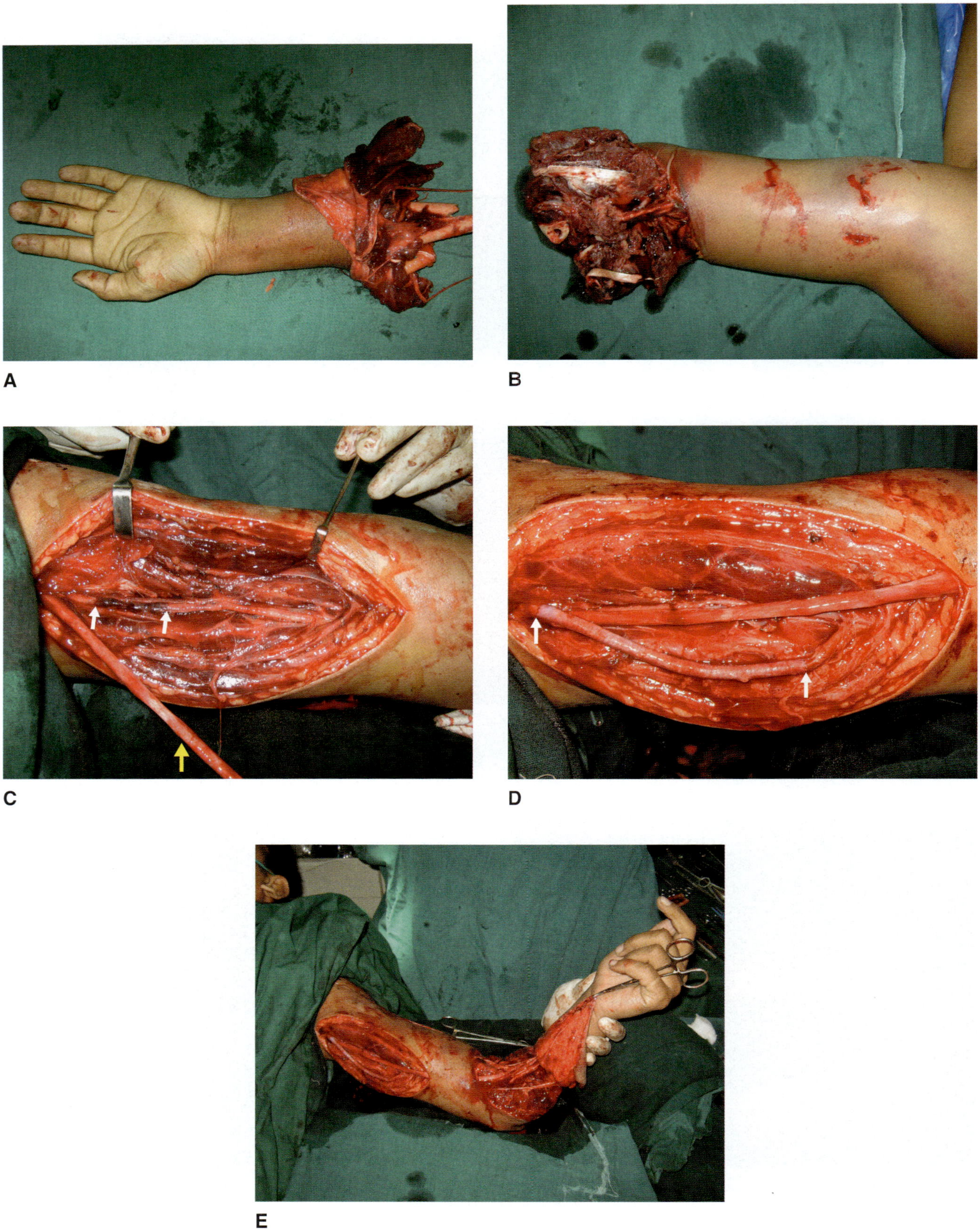

FIGURE 56-8 (A) and (B) Crush avulsion amputation of the forearm. There was no pulsation in the brachial artery in the proximal stump. (C) In-continuity segmental thrombosis in the brachial artery (between the white arrows) and the avulsed median nerve (yellow arrow). (D) The brachial artery reconstructed with a vein graft and the median nerve tunneled distally to the stump. The amputated part replanted (E) and postoperative result.

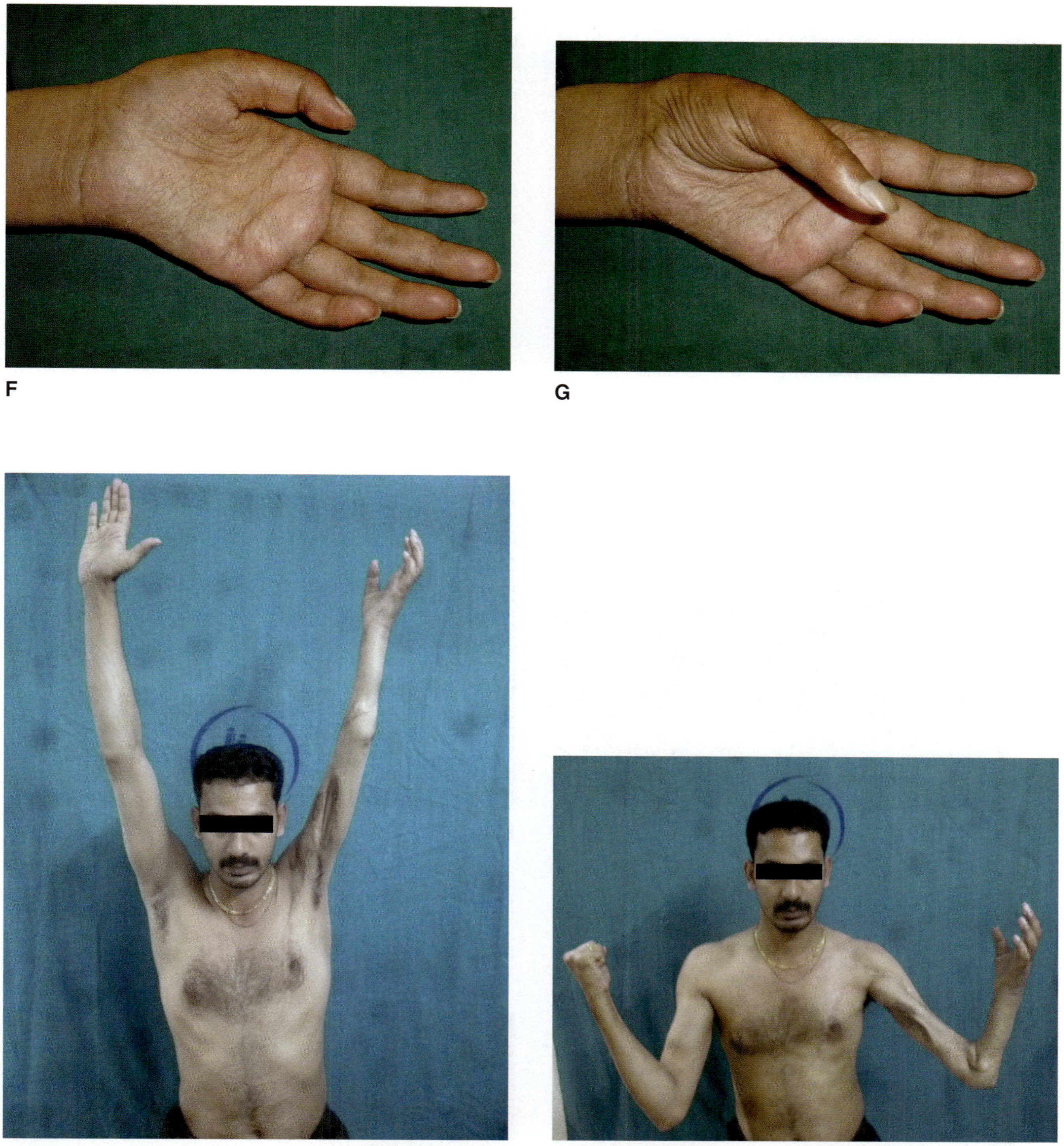

F

G

H

I

FIGURE 56-8 (*Continued*) (F to I) patient at 2 years.

Skeletal Fixation

Quick and secure skeletal fixation is an important determinant of success. Because no other step can proceed without this, it is imperative that it is done quickly. A short ischemia time is crucial for success, and time cannot be wasted in complicated techniques of skeletal fixation. Major replantations fail in many plastic surgical units because of poor orthopedic support. In our unit, senior orthopedists are involved in this step, and the procedure, in most instances, is completed in 20 minutes. Preplating of the amputated part while debridement of the proximal stump is ongoing also helps in reducing the time taken for skeletal fixation (see Figure 56-4). One cannot afford delay at this stage in a proximal replant.

Bone shortening is the single most important step in reducing bone fixation time. Ragged and oblique ends can be freshened to make clean osteotomy-like ends for fixation. In the forearm, if there is comminution, small fragments can be excised to realign the ends of the two bones easily. If the bone ends at the forearm amputation site are too comminuted, a one-bone forearm can be created. This is usually done by fixation of the proximal ulna to the distal radius, but, sometimes, it may be necessary to fix the proximal radius to the distal ulna. Under such circumstances, the two ends of the other bone are retained to stabilize the joints. In such instances, pronation and supination are retained. This is not possible when ulna-to-radius osteosynthesis is carried out (Figure 56-9).

Up to 10 cm of bone shortening is compatible with function in the upper limb. Shortening is only obvious when the two limbs are brought into close proximity. If the shortened replanted limb becomes functional, it is not obvious and, socially, the patients get along well (see Figure 56-7). Another advantage of bone shortening is that it can compensate for the segmental loss of musculotendinous units and nerves that is common in crush avulsion injuries. This allows reconnection of these structures with a single suture line and without grafts. In many instances, it may also obviate the need for flap cover, thus making the whole procedure quicker with reduction in morbidity.

Internal fixation is our favored method of skeletal fixation in major upper limb replants. Care is taken to keep the alignment correct. A fixed pronated forearm is very disabling. When forearm bones are fixed after bone shortening, the matching landmarks may not be available. In this circumstance, we keep the

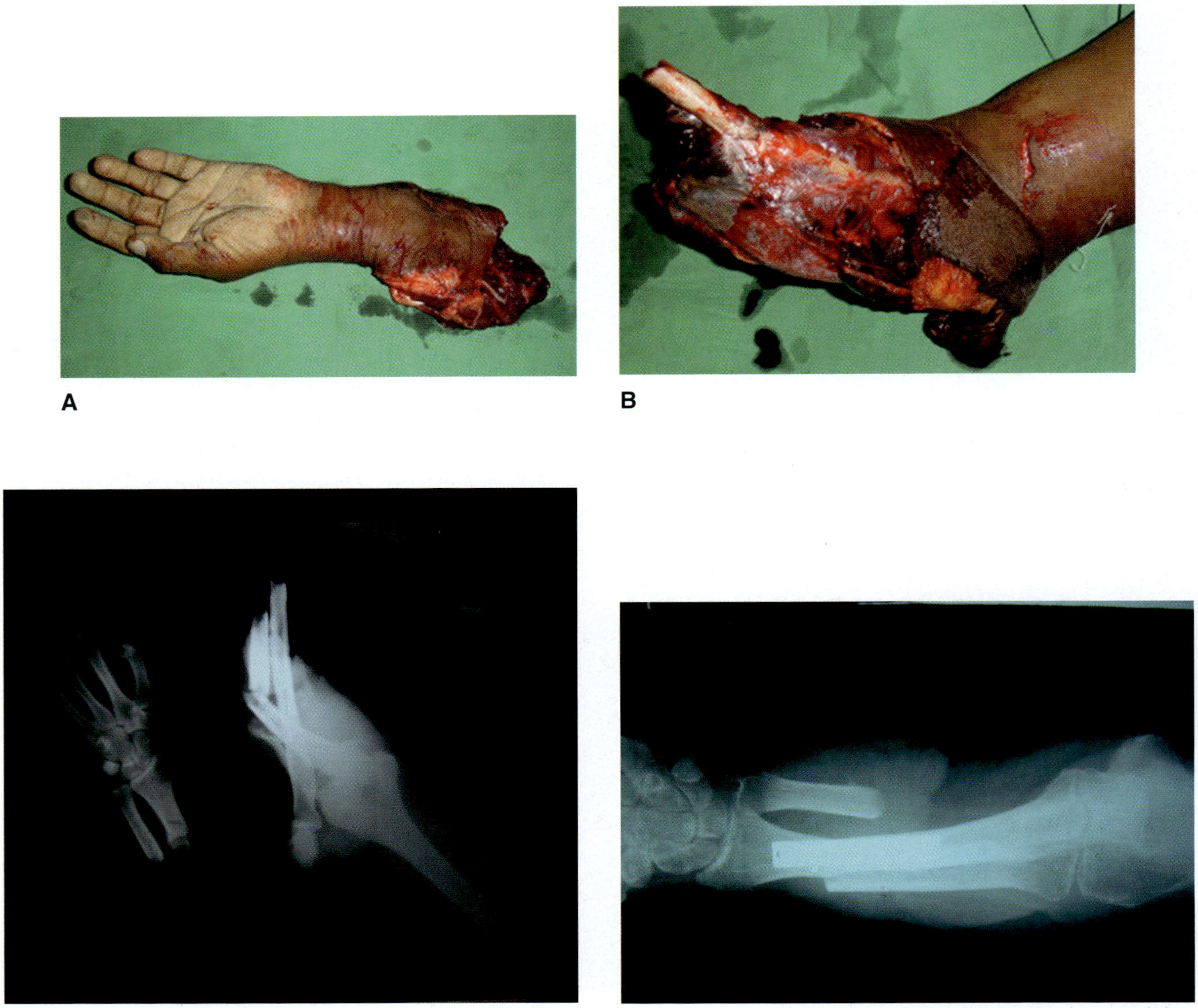

A B C D

FIGURE 56-9 (A) Avulsion amputation of the forearm. (B) The proximal segment showing extensive degloving and bone exposure. (C) Radiograph showing segmental fracture of the ulna and dislocation of the proximal radial head. (D) The free segment of ulna removed, the bone shortened, and the proximal ulna fixed to the distal radius to create a one bone forearm.

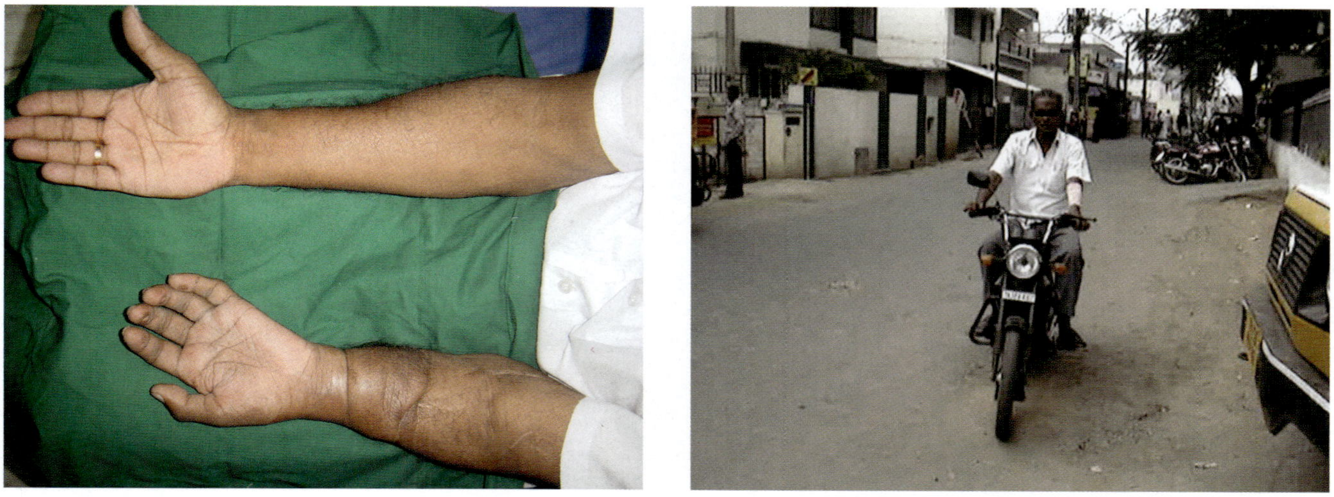

E F

FIGURE 56-9 (*Continued*) (E) and (F) Patient three-years postoperatively result with acceptable function.

proximal and distal parts in full supination and fix the forearm bones. This makes screw positioning and plate fixation easier and faster. When a one bone forearm is created, we prefer the fixation to be in the midprone position.

When the level of amputation is very near a joint, the bone resection is done on the other part of the limb to save the joint (Figure 56-10). In such instances, in addition to plating of the bones, an external fixator is used to stabilize the joint so there is no tension at the anastomosis site from movements of the joint during dressing changes.

Rarely, the limb may be avulsed through the elbow or the wrist joints. Forces required for avulsion amputation through the joints are higher than those occurring through fractures of the bones. In through-elbow amputations, we have had to arthrodese the joint by shortening of the bones proximally and distally, and this is done with 30 degrees of elbow flexion. In through-wrist amputations, movement can be retained by proximal row carpectomy. This also achieves a shortening of about 1.5 cm of length.

Some advocate use of external fixation for major upper limb replantations as a quick solution. In avulsion amputations, the bone contact obtained is critical, and, in our opinion, internal fixation achieves more reliable union. In our series of 11 arm and 42 forearm replantations (wrist level excluded), only one required secondary bone grafting to achieve bone union. This was due to a technical mistake leaving a gap at the time of primary fixation. Secondary bone grafting of nonunion in major replants has to be done with care, so one is advised to choose a procedure that gives reliable union rates and practice hard to perform this quickly. Unless bone union occurs primarily, rehabilitation of the patient cannot progress on schedule. Procedures such as secondary nerve grafting may also have to be delayed until bone union is achieved. So, even although bone fixation has to be done quickly to reduce the ischemia time, it has to be done well. The availability of surgeons with experience and shortening of the bones to viable ends are the key factors for success in achieving primary bone union.

Repair of Vessels, Nerves, and Musculotendinous Units

The sequence of repairing these structures depends on the ischemia time and the level of injury. If the amputation is proximal to the elbow, the artery must be repaired as quickly as possible. If the ischemia time is not a concern in the early stages after arrival (see Table 56-1), the veins are repaired first and then the artery. This reduces blood loss when the clamps are released. If the ischemia time is approaching the "risky" level, it is safer to do the artery first. After 4 hours, the potential for damage to vital organs rises exponentially, and it is inadvisable to take the risk of such damage. In major replants, it is always a safe practice to release the arterial clamps, keep the veins clamped for about 5 minutes, and then release the venous clamps. The blood draining from the muscles washes out accumulated and hazardous metabolites and prevents them from entering the systemic circulation. However, blood transfusion may be required if this is done.

How many vessels to repair is a common question in the mind of beginners. As many as possible is the answer! In the forearm, if possible, both arteries are repaired. Conventionally, the ulnar artery is said to perfuse the hand more than the radial artery, so it should be repaired preferentially. In our experience, we have not found a difference. Which is better probably depends more on the pattern of injury than anything else. If there is a gap in the vessels, either the radial or the ulnar artery is repaired with a graft and the circulation assessed. In the event that there is a skin defect at the level of the replant, the other artery can be used as the feeding vessel for a free flap.

The superficial veins are larger and easier to repair. However, the venae comitantes associated with the brachial, radial, and

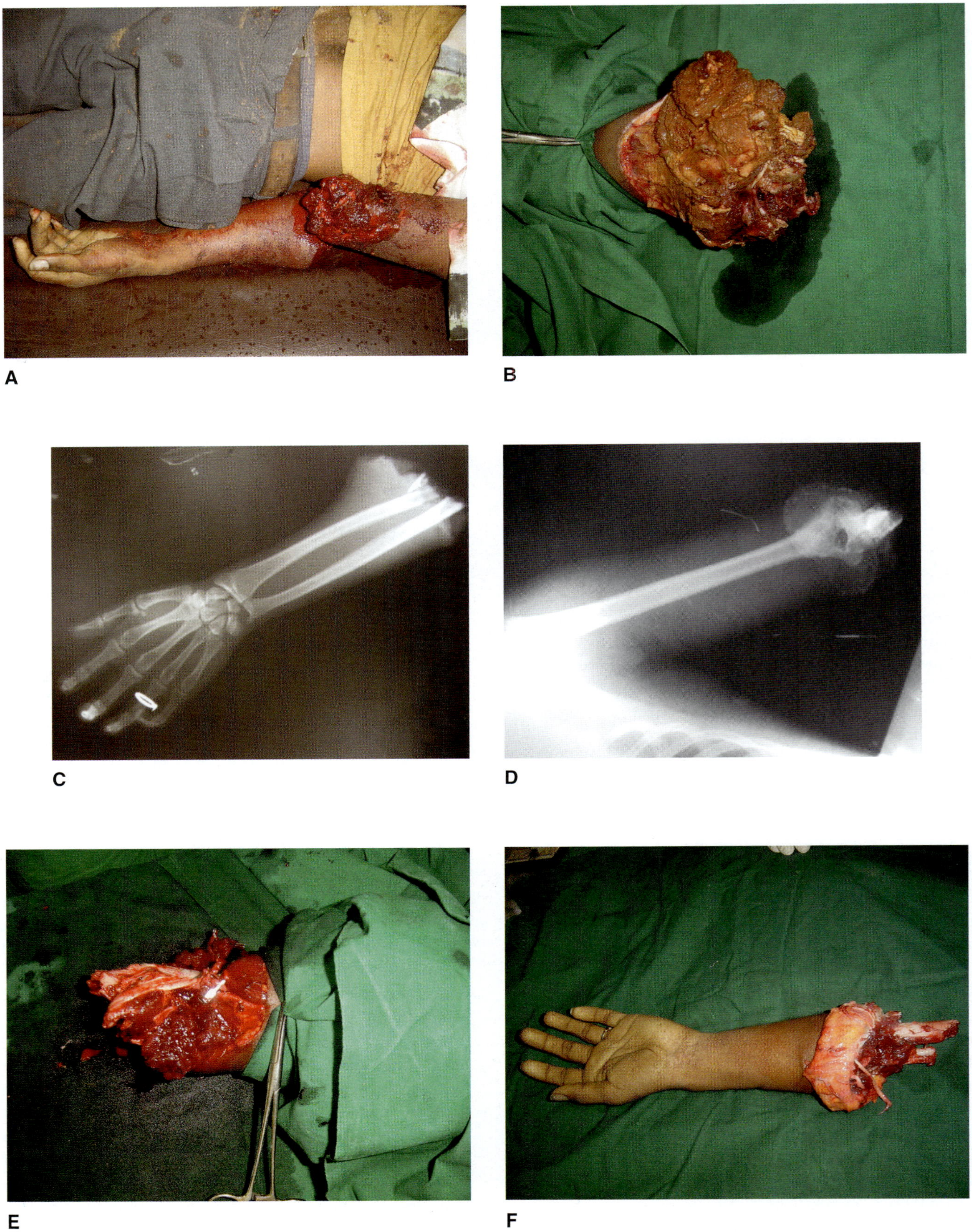

FIGURE 56-10 (A) Total crush amputation of the left elbow on arrival to the hospital. (B) Heavily contaminated proximal side before debridement. (C) and (D) Radiographs showing a short segment below the elbow joint. (E) and (F) Postdebridement photographs. The exposed bone was resected before replantation. The shortening was done predominantly in the distal segment of the bone to preserve elbow joint motion.

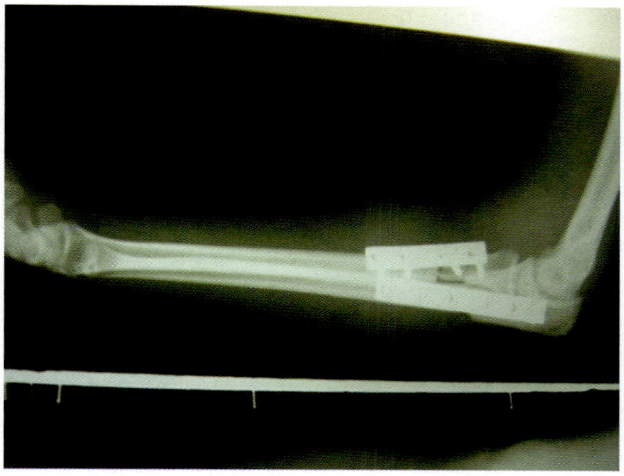

G

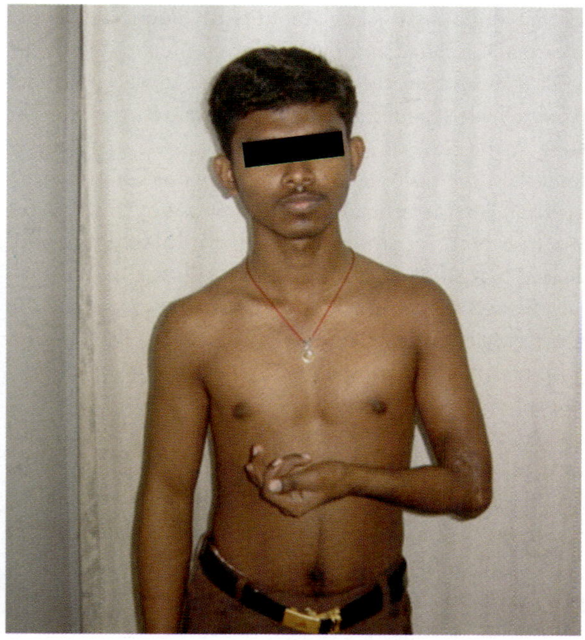

H

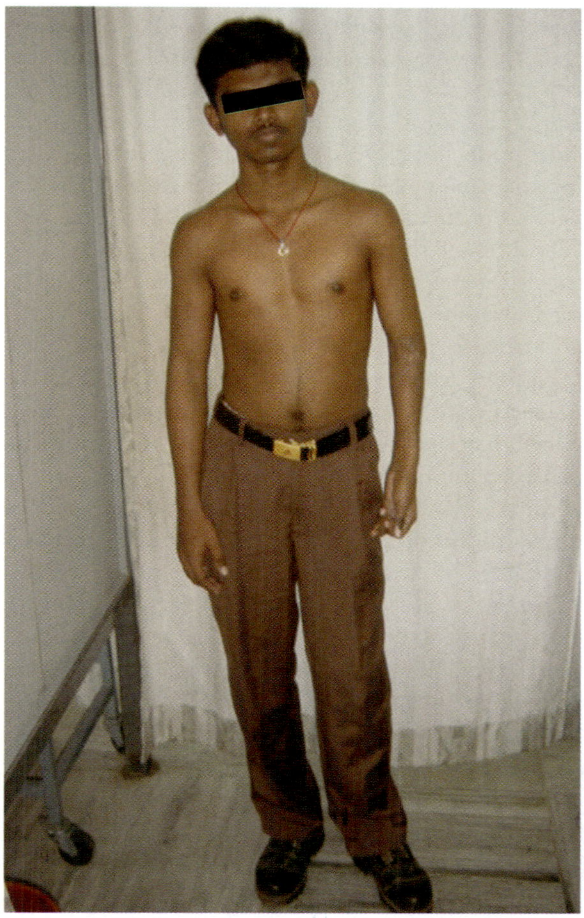

I

FIGURE 56-10 *(Continued)* (G) Postoperative radiograph showing maintenance of the elbow joint. (H) and (I) The patient achieved good elbow flexion and ultimately reached grade I functional recovery.

ulnar arteries drain significant amounts of blood. Therefore, they are carefully isolated and tagged during preparation of the amputated part and of the stump and are always repaired. Whenever we have repaired the venae comitantes, the amount of bleeding at the time of clamp release has been significantly less. Sometimes, the skin margins at the replantation site cause problems later. Any superficial vein anastomosis in such an area of skin necrosis is at risk of thrombosis. If critical to drainage of the replanted part, the replant is at risk of failure. In such situations, if the venae comitantes have also been repaired, the chances of survival of the replant are increased. If a few minutes after clamp release, there are spurting veins from the distal side, more venous repairs are necessary.

The repaired vessels must lie on a good vascular bed and must have good soft tissue cover. A gamble must never be taken on this. If a vein graft is used, this must be considered vital because the walls of a vein graft must be vascularized from their bed although the grafts carry blood. Hematoma around the anastomoses and compromised soft tissue cover are the main reasons for failure of anastomoses on the fourth or fifth day. They cause tissue death and then infection around the anastomosis, which in turn may result in thrombosis or blowout. So good care has to be taken in assessing the tissues surrounding the anastomoses, and simple nonsuction drains should be placed near the anastomoses to prevent hematoma formation.

Although the survival of the part depends on ongoing function of the vascular anastomoses, long-term function depends on the status of the nerves and the musculotendinous units, and their repairs. The key to good recovery of function is to repair good ends of the tendons and nerves. Bone shortening helps achieve good-quality nerves, muscles, and tendons for repair. If primary nerve repairs are not possible, the nerve ends are dissected, brought into the subcutaneous plane, and banked there. A mark is made on the skin over each nerve end by either leaving a suture in situ for a long period of time or by making an X scratch on the skin with a scalpel. This is particularly important on the distal side because there is no way of finding the distal end again by clinical examination or investigation. The proximal nerve end can be identified by the Tinel sign. However, this test cannot be used to detect the distal end. During secondary repair of nerves, small incisions are made, the ends are isolated, and grafts are tunneled between the repair sites. This is a very useful technique. If the nerves are left in their anatomical location, they are deep or lie close to the vessels, making dissection hazardous. A particularly useful alternative if deeper nerves cannot be brought into the subcutaneous plane is to place a Silastic tendon spacer, or several lengths of it for larger nerves, between the nerve ends and suture the distal nerve end to the Silastic rod with blue Prolene for easy vision of the suture later. This is akin to the first stage of two-stage tendon grafting. At secondary reconstruction, the nerve grafts can be passed down the tunnel created by the rod without completely opening the skin, making the second stage easier and quicker, with less risk to vital vessels, particularly if the proximal nerve end to be coapted is cut back, such that it is at a distance proximal to the vessel anastomoses.

After completion of the vessel anastomoses and revascularization of the distal part, muscle perfusion is assessed. Nonviable muscle will be obvious and must be excised. If only avulsed tendons remain in the distal part and are to be reconnected to muscle in the proximal part, the tendons are drawn through the proximal muscles with a tendon tunneler and anchored to the muscles. If tendon repairs are possible, a simple method of repair must be chosen to reduce the operating time and any good method with which the surgeon is familiar is satisfactory. At the completion of this step, only skin closure remains.

Soft Tissue Cover

The main concern at the end of the repair of the critical structures in a major replant is that the vessel and nerve repairs should not be exposed. Care must be taken to cover the repair sites with viable muscle or well-perfused skin. If there is doubt, flap cover is safer. Skin grafts have been applied over vessel repairs with success in distal replantations, but we do not recommend this practice in major replantation. If skin graft loss occurs and the vessels become exposed, emergency flap cover will be required. Exposure may also lead to infection and thrombosis of the vessels. Even if successful initially, problems may arise if a secondary procedure becomes necessary in the vicinity of the repair site(s). Subsequent flap cover is likely to be a problem because it necessitates the difficult procedure of dissecting a healed skin graft off a vessel or a nerve without damage to the vessel or nerve. For all of these reasons, skin grafts are not applied over the vessel and nerve repairs unless there is no alternative.

The need for flap cover in replantation is considerably reduced by bone shortening. Flaps are mostly required at the level of the distal third of the forearm. In more proximal replants, the vessel and nerve repair sites can usually be covered with local muscles, and flap cover is unnecessary during the emergency procedure. Because of the presence of exposed tendons in the distal third of the forearm, flap cover may be mandatory. On such occasions, we use one major forearm artery to perfuse the distal (replanted) part and the other as the inflow vessel for a free flap. The gracilis muscle flap is our choice of free flap for these cases because it wraps around the raw area well, and accurate planning of the dimensions of the flap is not necessary. This is an advantage in the acute situation. The gracilis muscle can also be stretched to cover critical areas. It can also be harvested very quickly and by a team that does not get in the way of those carrying out the upper limb procedure.

The quality of the skin suture line over the vessel repair sites has to be carefully monitored. At the first sign of any compromised vascularity of the skin, the patient should be taken to the OR, the wound debrided, and better soft tissue cover provided. In a major replant, this is important because exposure or infection around the vessel anastomoses can result in thrombosis or a blow-out. A blow-out in a major vessel is dangerous because torrential blood loss is likely in a short span of time from the partially open vessel. For this reason, if there are any doubts about the integrity of the skin cover, it is prudent to keep the patient in the hospital until the concern is allayed.

Monitoring a Major Replant

In replants distal to the wrist, monitoring is mainly concerned with the viability of the replant. In contrast, a major replant patient requires not only monitoring of the viability of the replant but also of the general condition of the patient.

Reperfusion of ischemic muscle can cause systemic disturbances, depending on the volume of the muscle mass in the distal part and the ischemic time. A delay in instituting appropriate treatment can be a disaster and even risk the life of the patient.

Major replantation is a procedure of significant magnitude that can cause massive blood loss. This may destabilize a patient who has associated comorbid factors such as diabetes, hypertension, or heart disease. Blood transfusion may also be required. The hematocrit should be maintained around 30%. Serum lactate levels are part of the routine preoperative workup. Quite often, a patient is hypovolemic on arrival, and lactate level is high. This should fall during surgery if resuscitation is being effective. Postoperatively, the serum lactate level is repeated every 6 hours until it is normal. This marker is a very reliable index of the level of tissue perfusion.

Complications associated with reperfusion injury may be dangerous. In proximal replants when the ischemia time reaches "risky" levels (see Table 56-1), certain preemptive measures are undertaken. As the surgery approaches the clamp release, the intravenous normal saline flow rate is raised to 200 mL per half hour. One mEq/kg of 8.4% sodium bicarbonate is added to the infusion 3 minutes before clamp release. Waikakul et al. (19) carried out a study correlating the potassium levels in the blood of veins draining major replants. They found that the serum potassium concentration in the amputated segment was the best objective predictor of success of major upper limb replantation. When it is higher than 6.5 mmol/L 30 minutes after reperfusion, replantation should be discontinued and amputation carried out. A high systemic venous serum potassium concentration was also found before clinical signs of reperfusion syndrome were seen.

Clinically reperfusion problems are identified by tachycardia, tachypnea, and tall tented T waves on electrocardiography (ECG). If the surgery is performed under brachial block, we have also found that the patient, who has been calm until this time, starts to sweat profusely and become restless, with tachypnoea. If the symptoms do not settle with sodium bicarbonate infusion and the serum potassium in the venous blood from the amputated part remains higher than 6.5 mmol/L, the replanted part should be amputated.

Patients undergoing major replantation have usually undergone preoperative bladder catheterization. After clamp release, the color of the urine is observed. Reddish brown or brown urine denotes frank myoglobulinuria. The presence of myoglobulinuria requires that urine output be maintained between 100 and 150 mL/hr and 100 mL of 20% mannitol (dose, 0.5 g/kg) is given over a period of 20 minutes. Sodium bicarbonate infusion is repeated. If, despite these ministrations, there are significant ECG changes and persistent severe myoglobulinuria, we seriously consider immediate removal of the replant. If the level is proximal to the elbow, the part is removed on the table. In 11 arm and 42 forearm replantations, we have experienced frank myoglobulinuria in one patient who did not respond to the above-mentioned maneuvers, and hence, the replanted part was removed on the table. We have found this to be more common in near-total amputations in which there is no opportunity for instituting cold ischemia time and debridement of the avascular muscle mass is also limited. Although myoglobulinuria may settle with high fluid input, alkalinization of the urine and use of diuretics such as mannitol, patients with proximal replants who exhibit severe renal changes have a stormy postoperative course, with subsequent lung involvement. Tachypnoea, listlessness, and failure to maintain oxygen saturation are ominous signs. If this stage is reached, it is prudent to remove the replant immediately. A stage is eventually reached when the central damage is irreversible. No life is worth a limb; this must be the non-negotiable guideline in performing major replant surgery.

A major replant patient may also have sustained other significant injuries that may manifest themselves gradually, or later. A general deterioration requires a thorough physical examination and appropriate investigations. A young boy who had an above-elbow replant became drowsy and listless around the fifth postoperative day. Although sepsis and reperfusion injury were the first things to come to mind, a computed tomography scan of the brain identified a massive extradural hemorrhage. Although we had identified and recorded a minor scalp injury on admission, he had, at no time previously, complained of headache. A major amputation is so obviously dramatic that it is possible to miss a significant head, chest, or abdominal injury. Therefore, deterioration of the patient's clinical condition at any time requires reevaluation of both the replanted part and the patient more generally.

Monitoring the replanted part itself is arguably the simplest part of the postoperative management for surgeons and requires hourly clinical examination for the first 24 hours and then once every 4 hours for the next 48 hours. Pulse oximetry is a useful aid to continuous monitoring. However, the keystone of our protocol is clinical examination. The replanted hand must look like a normal hand. If it is different in any way, either paler or more congested, the implication must be that the artery or the vein is compromised. This demands immediate attention. An abrupt loss of the pulse oximeter signal may signify arterial occlusion and decreased oxygen saturation venous compromise. However, clinical examination should override reliance on pulse oximetry alone. If the color of the fingers looks good and the blanching and capillary refill time are normal, then we wait and continue careful monitoring without recourse to exploration. However, cessation of a pulse oximeter reading that was previously normal should be taken seriously.

AVOIDING COMPLICATIONS

Most complications occur when protocols are not followed strictly. Therefore, we recommend that replantation guidelines are both written down and followed to the letter.

The effect of reperfusion from ischemic muscles is the single most important cause of serious complications. There must be a sense of urgency in the procedures performed to keep the ischemia time to a minimum. To instill this attitude into the whole team, the surgeon must lead by example. Cooling and reperfusion solutions used in solid organ transplants are not used in most major replantation centers. However, we believe that the distal part should be kept cooled by strapping ice bags to all limb parts that are not in the surgical field at all times during the procedure. Clinical signs that we have found useful in identifying severe muscle ischemia are (1) stiffness on passive movement of the fingers in above-elbow amputations and (2) increased resistance of the thumb to passive movement in below-elbow amputation. We call the latter the "stiff thumb" sign. If either of these signs is present, we do not replant. On two occasions in which we have ignored these signs and replanted, the postoperative course has been stormy and has led eventually to removal of the replant.

The other major source of complications is the wound itself. Each step of the operation has to be done as per the guidelines because this is the only way to avoid wound problems. Debridement is the key to successful outcome. Although obviously dead tissue, including any muscle attached to the proximal ends of tendons on the detached part of the limb, can be removed before revascularization, the muscles have to be debrided again after revascularization. After revascularization, ischemic muscles swell, and distal fasciotomies are essential in proximal replants. Doing this during preparation of the amputated part and before revascularization makes it easy, more complete, and less bloody.

Because revascularization can only proceed after bone fixation, this step has to be done quickly to avoid significant loss of time. Bone shortening, simple bone fixation techniques, and creation of a one bone forearm in comminuted forearm fractures are all means of reducing the time taken at this stage. Shortening of the limb also ensures that good bone, muscle/tendon, and nerve repairs are achieved. To prevent hematoma, the wound is drained with simple drains, avoiding suction drains near the vessel anastomoses.

During the postoperative period, early debridement and additional soft tissue cover are carried out without delay if the skin shows any sign of compromised vascularity. This may involve local transposition of skin flaps or a free flap. As mentioned earlier, free muscle flaps are preferred because they can be easily draped over any defect. End-to-side anastomosis proximal to the replantation anastomosis is required at the arm and elbow level. In the forearm, one of the two major vessels can be used for each purpose. One should have a very low threshold for reexploration of the wound when there are signs of tissue death, or infection, around the wound site.

REHABILITATION OF THE MAJOR REPLANTATION PATIENT

A major replantation patient is rehabilitated in the same way as a triple nerve injury patient. After replantation at the level of the distal third of the forearm and distal to the wrist, the motor units of the long flexor and extensor tendons are functional, and early motion protocols are instituted to prevent adhesion at the sites of the repairs (20). In proximal forearm and above-elbow replants, active movement of the fingers is not possible until nerve recovery occurs. In these cases, all possible proximal active movements are encouraged after 3 weeks. Distally, maintaining good passive motion at the interphalangeal and metacarpophalangeal joints and maintaining a supple first web space with the thumb in an abducted and opposition position are priorities. The forearm is positioned in supination, or in the midprone position. A fully pronated forearm is not a good position for rehabilitation because, in this position, the hand is least useful later. The splint used, and the timing of starting physiotherapy, mostly depends on the type and stability of the skeletal fixation and the tension at the vessel repair sites.

General therapy guidelines of massaging the scars and periodic follow-up for splint checks and assessing nerve recovery are routine. It is our practice to use intermittent galvanic current stimulation of motor points of the paralyzed muscle units after 6 weeks. This is continued until nerve recovery is clinically apparent. When muscle recovery starts, strengthening exercises are started. When the fingers are able to feel moving touch, sensory reeducation is started.

Depending on the level of amputation, therapy and follow-up may have to be continued for between 9 and 18 months for acceptable functional recovery to occur. It can be as much of a challenge to maintain the morale of the patient and make him, or her, comply with the therapy during this lengthy period of time as it is to do the replant itself!

SECONDARY PROCEDURES AFTER REPLANTATION

After replantation, secondary procedures are, in general, difficult to do and fraught with danger of disturbing the vessel anastomoses. For this reason, primary repair of all structures is attempted whenever possible. Major replants remain dependent on the vascular repairs for a very long time and, sometimes, permanently. Therefore, the utmost care has to be taken not to disturb the original vascular repairs at any secondary surgery. Being in possession of a good original operation note is a great help. We have found that in addition to documenting the number of arteries and veins repaired, a simple diagram of both the sites of the anastomoses and the courses of the vessels repaired and the surgeon's opinion of the critical vessel anastomoses are invaluable because the vessels and nerves may have been rerouted from their normal anatomical pathways. Transposing any nerves requiring secondary grafting into the subcutaneous tissues, or linking them with a tendon rod also makes disruption of vital anastomoses less likely.

Based on our experience, we find that secondary procedures in major replantation surgery can be grouped under three headings:

1. Procedures to promote healing or enhance function of tissues that were repaired primarily. This secondary surgery is likely to involve bony procedures for the correction of nonunions and soft tissue procedures such as tenolysis.

2. Repair of structures that were not repaired during the primary replantation procedure. This secondary surgery is likely to involve bridging gaps in tendons and nerves.
3. Procedures to enhance function. This secondary surgery is likely to involve selective arthrodesis of joints, tendon transfers, and lengthening of bones.

The timing of secondary reconstruction after major replantation does not differ from that after other major injuries and the same principles apply. The tissues must have become soft and supple. This usually occurs by 3 months.

Primary healing of the wounds is the chief determinant of the timing of secondary procedures. If there are small raw areas of skin that fail to heal primarily, these are better grafted to achieve rapid healing to allow early rehabilitation. If healing takes longer, institution of physiotherapy, scar massage, and wearing of compression garments are all delayed, and induration takes a longer time to settle. There must also be good skin cover in any area undergoing secondary surgery.

Each patient has to be individualized because the particular injury will make the requirements of each different. As a general rule, when faced later with postoperative problems, a stable skeleton has to be achieved first because soft tissue reconstruction cannot be done in the presence of a nonunion. Avoidance is key, and primary bone shortening and stable fixation reduce the incidence of nonunion. When both tendons and nerves need secondary reconstruction, it is better to do both at the same time to speed up rehabilitation. If secondary tendon procedures are performed after secondary nerve grafting, there is a risk of injuring these nerve grafts. For this reason, when we anticipate further procedures in the area, any nerve grafts are passed through extraanatomic pathways, so they will not be disturbed. Although this requires a little longer length of grafts, it is a safer option.

OUTCOMES OF MAJOR REPLANTATIONS

The outcome of major replantation is generally satisfying to the patient, particularly when compared with the alternative, but the benefit of this surgery is difficult to quantify. Any outcome assessment should stress what the patient is able to do with the replanted limb and what difference it has made to the patient's life when compared to his, or her, condition if amputation had been carried out.

Measurement of the range of motion of each joint is not as important as the patient's ability of incorporate the hand into daily activities and ability to resume normal life. The tools, which have been used in the literature, include the Chen criteria (21), the Tamai (22), the DASH (Disabilities of the Arm, Shoulder and Hand) and the Modified Carroll Scores (23). Most of these include measures to assess work capability and overall satisfaction.

Gulgonen and Ozer (24) studied the long-term results of major upper extremity replantation at a mean follow-up period of 18 years. Protective sensation was restored in all patients. According to Chen's functional recovery scale, five patients had excellent, two had good, and two had fair results. They found that grip strength, two-point discrimination, range of motion, and Chen's functional recovery scale scores did not improve after 5 years. However, Semmes-Weinstein monofilament testing and cold intolerance continued to improve for up to 10 and 12 years, respectively. They concluded that replantation of an upper extremity proximal to the wrist joint restored satisfactory upper extremity function. Sugun et al. (25) reported follow-up of 26 major replants for a mean of 11.3 years. Results according to the Chen criteria were very good, or good, in 17 patients (65.4%), moderate in three patients (11.5%), and poor in six patients (23.1%). They found correlation between the functional results and the level ($r = 0.71$) and type ($r = 0.65$) of injury, with injuries at the elbow level and avulsion injuries being associated with worse outcomes. The mean DASH score was 6.7 (range, 0–32.5), and the mean scores of Chen's grades I and II and grades III to IV patients differed significantly ($P < 0.05$). They concluded that lower DASH scores identified increased satisfaction of the patient and improved use of the replanted extremity as the "helper" arm, whereby functional deficiency is somewhat compensated. Zyluk and Walaszek (26), Patradul et al. (27) Sabapathy et al. (12), and Daoutis et al. (28) have also reported similar satisfactory outcomes in their series of replantations. Every center reporting their experience with major replantation has been very positive, reporting high levels of satisfaction among the patients.

CONCLUSION

Apart from the technical skills and infrastructure needed to perform this complex operation, a positive attitude and a sense of urgency in addressing the tasks ahead must be exhibited by the surgeon while performing major replants. There must be a patient-centric attitude with the whole team working to reduce the ischemia time, which is the single most important determinant of outcome and complications.

At the present time, replanted upper extremities perform better than the best available prosthesis. With time, patients use the replanted hand in day-to-day activities and better than the individual ranges of motion and sensory recovery of the fingers would suggest. Unlike after global brachial plexus injuries, most of the structures proximal to the level of the amputation in a replant patient are intact, and they provide for immense reconstructive possibilities in the future (Figure 56-11). Currently, replantation is also better in terms of cost, effort, and outcome than transplantation. Until there is a breakthrough in immunology, transplantation cannot become a routine procedure in most parts of the world.

The challenge is to have a good team that is willing to perform the surgery and available at the time of need, rather than a long discussion about the possible outcome.

SUMMARY

1. Functional outcome after replantation is far better than that using the best available prosthesis after major upper limb amputation.
2. The replantation surgeon must aim to get good functional outcome and not be content with mere survival of the part.

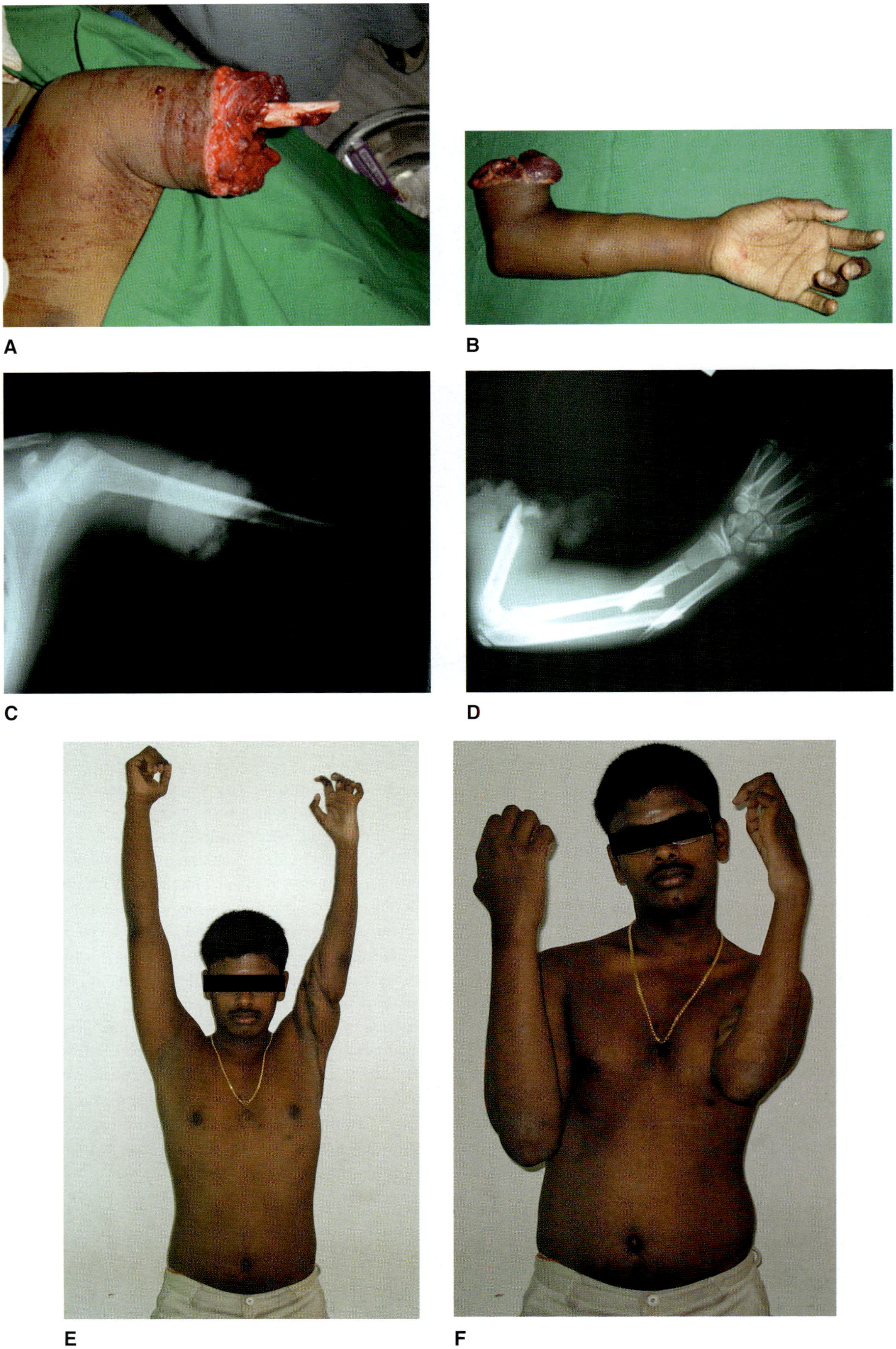

FIGURE 56-11 (A) and (B) A through-arm replant in a 12-year-old boy. (C) and (D) Radiographs showing additional fractures of both bones of the forearm. (E) and (F) Eight years later, he has full extension and flexion at the elbow and wrist and good grip strength. He underwent latissimus dorsi transfer for elbow flexion and tendon transfers for wrist extension, which helped him to achieve Chen grade 1 functional recovery.

3. In digital replants, ischemia time is not very significant; hence, the surgeon can concentrate on quality repair of structures to obtain the best possible function. For this, good microsurgical skills are essential.
4. In major replants, ischemia time is critical to avoid systemic complications, and the surgeon should concentrate on revascularizing the distal segment as quickly as possible.
5. Adequate debridement (within both the distal and proximal parts) is important in replantation surgery. Poor debridement is a common cause of late failure of the replant.
6. Bone shortening is a key step of the operative procedure. It simplifies skeletal fixation, allows primary repair of blood vessels and nerves, and may avoid the need for soft tissue cover.
7. Stable skeletal fixation is important.
8. Secondary procedures are difficult to do after major replants, and the aim is to repair all structures primarily.
9. Good operation notes, precisely detailing the structures repaired and the position of the structures not repaired prevent unnecessary, and sometimes catastrophic, exploration for secondary procedures.
10. Regular clinical examination is the best form of postoperative monitoring.

REFERENCES

1. Wei FC, el-Gammal TA, Lin CH, et al. Metacarpal hand: classification and guidelines for microsurgical reconstruction with toe transfers. *Plast Reconstr Surg* 1997;99:122–128.
2. Mardini S, Wei FC. Unilateral and bilateral metacarpal hand injuries: classification and treatment guidelines. *Plast Reconstr Surg* 2004;113: 1756–1759.
3. Kotkansalo T, Vilkki SK, Elo P. The functional results of post-traumatic metacarpal hand reconstruction with microvascular toe transfers. *J Hand Surg Eur* 2009;34:730–742.
4. Peacock K, Tsai TM. Comparison of functional results of replantation versus prosthesis in a patient with bilateral arm amputation. *Clin Orthop Relat Res* 1987;214:153–159.
5. Graham B, Adkins P, Tsai TM, et al. Major replantation versus revision amputation and prosthetic fitting in the upper extremity: a late functional outcomes study. *J Hand Surg Am* 1998;23:783–791.
6. Wright TW, Hagen AD, Wood MB. Prosthetic usage in major upper extremity amputations. *J Hand Surg Am* 1995;20:619–622.
7. Biddiss EA, Chau TT. Upper limb prosthesis use and abandonment: a survey of the last 25 years. *Prosthet Orthot Int* 2007;31:236–257.
8. Chung KC, Oda T, Saddawi-Konefka D, Shauver MJ. An economic analysis of hand transplantation in the United States. *Plast Reconstr Surg* 2010;125:589–598.
9. Malt RA, McKhann CF. Replantation of severed arms. *JAMA* 1964;189: 716–722.
10. Toledo-Pereyra LH. Classics of modern surgery: the unknown man of Alexis Carrel—father of transplantation. *J Invest Surg* 2003;16:243–246.
11. Atkins SE, Winterton RIS, Kay SP. Upper limb amputations: where, when and how to replant. *Curr Orthop* 2008;22:31–41.
12. Sabapathy SR, Venkatramani H, Bharathi RR, et al. Technical considerations and functional outcome of 22 major replantations (the BSSH Douglas Lamb Lecture, 2005). *J Hand Surg Br* 2007;32:488–501.
13. Sabapathy SR, Venkatramani H, Bharathi RR, Bhardwaj P. Replantation surgery. *J Hand Surg Am* 2011;36:1104–1110.
14. Dias JJ, Chung KC, Garcia-Elias M, et al. Recommendations for the improvement of hand injury care across the world. *Injury* 2006;37: 1078–1082.
15. Belsky MR, Ruby LK. Double level amputation: should it be replanted? *J Reconstr Microsurg* 1986;2:159–162.
16. Papanastasiou S, Sood M. Double-level replantation of the upper extremity with microvascular pulp transfer onto an intermediate macroreplant segment. *Plast Reconstr Surg* 2002;110:1294–1297.
17. Nunley JA, Koman LA, Urbaniak JR. Arterial shunting as an adjunct to major limb revascularization. *Ann Surg* 1981;193(3):271–273.
18. Gupta A, Shatford RA, Wolff TW, et al. Treatment of the severely injured upper extremity. *Instr Course Lect. Instr Course Lect* 2000;49:377–396.
19. Waikakul S, Vanadurongwan V, Unnanuntana A. Prognostic factors for major limb re-implantation at both immediate and long-term follow-up. *J Bone Joint Surg Br* 1998;80:1024–1030.
20. Scheker LR, Chesher SP, Netscher DT, et al. Functional results of dynamic splinting after transmetacarpal, wrist, and distal forearm replantation. *J Hand Surg Br* 1995;20:584–590.
21. Zhong-Wei C, Meyer VE, Kleinert HE, Beasley RW. Present indications and contraindications for replantation as reflected by long-term functional results. *Orthop Clin North Am* 1981;12:849–870.
22. Tamai S. Twenty years' experience of limb replantation-review of 293 upper extremity replants. *J Hand Surg Am* 1982;7:549–556.
23. Carroll D. A quantitative test of upper extremity function. *J Chron Dis* 1965;18:479–494.
24. Gulgonen A, Ozer K. Long-term results of major upper extremity replantations. *J Hand Surg Eur* 2012;37:225–232.
25. Sugun TS, Ozaksar K, Ada S, et al. Long-term results of major upper extremity replantations. *Acta Orthop Traumatol Turc* 2009;43:206–213.
26. Zyluk A, Walaszek I. An assessment of the results of upper limb replantation. *Chir Narzadow Ruchu Ortop Pol* 2007;72:165–173.
27. Patradul A, Ngarmukos C, Parkpian V. Major limb replantation: a Thai experience. *Ann Acad Med Singapore* 1995;24(4 suppl):82–88
28. Daoutis NK, Gerostathopoulos N, Efstathopoulos D, et al. Major amputation of the upper extremity. Functional results after replantation/ revascularization in 47 cases. *Acta Orthop Scand Suppl* 1995;264:7–8.

CHAPTER 57

Revascularization

William C. Pederson

Vascular injury to the upper extremity may be isolated but is often seen in combination with severe bony or soft tissue injury. These injuries cannot be treated in isolation, and one must be prepared to manage the soft tissue and bony injury as well as the vascular injury. Likewise, hand surgeons who manage severe injuries to the upper extremity must combine the skills of a macrovascular surgeon with those of a microneurovascular surgeon. Thus, the approach to severe vascular injuries of the hand and upper extremity must take a multimodal approach, not just addressing the vascular injury but also concomitant problems with the bone and soft tissue envelope. One must be prepared to provide bony stabilization as well as soft tissue coverage to the vascular repair when dealing with such injuries. This chapter deals with an approach to vascular injuries in the upper extremity in individuals who did not sustain a complete amputation but often require more than simple repair of the injured vessels.

VASCULAR TRAUMA IN THE UPPER EXTREMITY

Injury to the blood vessels of the upper extremity and hand is reasonably common in severe trauma, but the overall incidence compared with all trauma cases is low, generally less than 1% of all traumatic injuries (1,2). In military circumstances, most injuries to blood vessels are caused by penetrating trauma (3); however, in the civilian sector, most arterial injury is caused by blunt trauma (4). Level I trauma centers and referral centers are more likely to receive these types of injuries, especially those offering replantation services. Arterial injuries are occasionally seen with fractures but in particular with severe mangling extremity injury (5–7). Injury to the brachial artery is more frequently seen with injuries around the elbow, including supracondylar humerus fractures in children (8) and elbow dislocations (9). Gunshot wounds account for a large number of vascular injuries in the arm and hand (10,11), and severe crushing injuries caused by industrial accidents and automobile roll-overs may even cause limb amputation (12). Both proximal and more distal injuries can lead to ischemia of the hand, but because of the nature of both the collateral circulation in the upper arm and multiple arteries in the forearm, isolated injury to a single artery is not likely to cause hand ischemia.

Outcomes of arterial injury are generally more related to associated injuries (soft tissue, bone, and nerve) than with the actual arterial injury itself. Marked loss of bone or soft tissue is more likely to result in amputation than isolated injury to one of the major arteries of the limb. Some data suggest that vascular injuries in the upper arm are less likely to result in amputation than those to the forearm (13). It would also appear that (because of collateral circulation) injuries to the brachial artery are much less likely to result in severe ischemia of the hand and that thus a delay in their repair is unlikely to result in further morbidity (14,15). Unfortunately, brachial artery injuries are commonly associated with major nerve injuries to the nerves of the surrounding brachial plexus (60%–85%) (15,16). Most studies of long-term outcome note that the final functional result is more dependent on the presence or absence of major nerve injury than vascular injury (17,18). Long-term patency rates of repaired or vein grafted injured arterial segments are generally very good, and late amputation is uncommon due to ischemia.

WORKUP

In the case of a closed or penetrating injury, thorough examination of the injured extremity distal to the injury should be made. Particular attention should be paid to pulses and nerve examination. In the hand and digits, capillary refill should be evaluated, and a pencil Doppler may be helpful in evaluating flow. I do not think that a Doppler signal in one of the major distal vessels (radial or ulnar arteries) represents adequate flow in the absence of a palpable pulse. With a major crushing injury, I do not believe in repeated examinations of the wound in the emergency department. Standard radiographs should be taken of the injured limb to include the joint above and below the site of injury. If the patient is the victim of multiple traumas, there should obviously be an evaluation by the trauma team before intervention in terms of the limb. If the patient is otherwise stable and has evidence of ischemia of the distal limb, examination and management should be performed in the operating room (OR) as expeditiously as possible.

The use of arteriography remains somewhat controversial in upper extremity trauma. Traditional teaching has been that there is a 15% incidence of normal pulses distally with proximal arterial injury. As noted earlier, patients with mangling injuries or severe open fractures should probably have operative exploration to evaluate and treat potential vascular injuries. Those with closed trauma and those who have a wound in proximity to a major vessel do not necessarily require arteriography, at least in the face of a pulseless distal limb and hematoma at the site of injury. Many advocate surgical exploration in such patients without the added expense and time of performing an arteriogram (19). Most believe that a patient presenting with a proximal penetrating injury and a pulseless distal limb with evidence of a expanding hematoma provides ample indication for rapid treatment in the OR (20). If the patient has a diminished pulse on presentation compared with the other side or develops this while under observation, one should proceed with arteriography to rule out a proximal arterial injury (21). Standard arteriography may be supplanted by more modern modalities, which also precludes the necessity for an arteriographic dye load. Computed tomographic arteriography (CTA) has been shown to be able to identify arterial injury in trauma patients as well as standard dye arteriography (22). Another modality that has also shown promise is duplex ultrasonography (23). This technique uses ultrasound to evaluate the vessel, and one study showed a tremendous cost savings of using this device in the emergency setting over performing arteriography on patients with questionable vascular injury (24).

MANAGEMENT

General Principles

In the case of ischemia of the distal extremity, revascularization should be performed as expeditiously as possible. Other injuries may preclude immediate revascularization (either systemic or local), but this does not mean that the limb cannot be reperfused fairly rapidly. If there is severe bony and soft tissue injury, bony stabilization is usually undertaken before definitive revascularization. In this case, a temporary vascular shunt can be used to perfuse the distal extremity. This has been well shown to allow perfusion of the extremity, and these "temporary" shunts can be left in for several hours with a low thrombosis rate (25,26). A number of these types of shunts are available, but the Javid or Argyle 10- or 12-Fr diameter shunt is probably the most commonly used in the upper extremity (primarily in the brachial artery) (26) (Figure 57-1). Although traditionally the use of these shunts has been limited to short periods while bony fixation and soft tissue debridement have been undertaken, recent military experience with the conflict in the Middle East has shown that they can be left in for a period of many hours to 2 days with high patency rates and low rates of limb loss without requiring systemic anticoagulation (3,27,28).

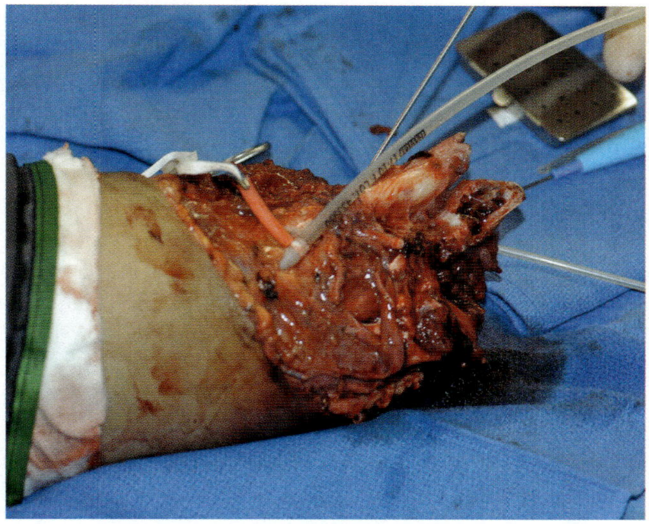

A

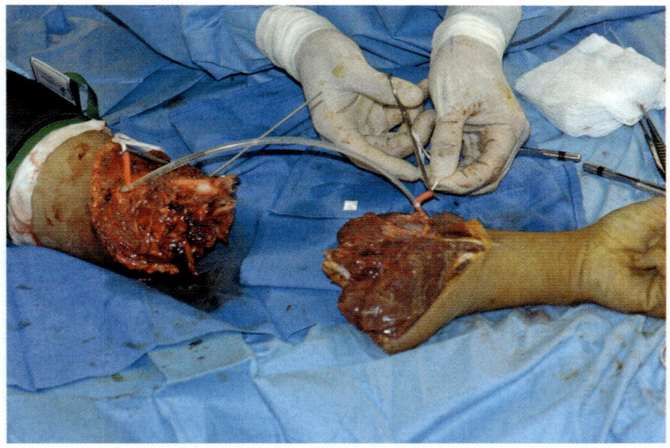

B

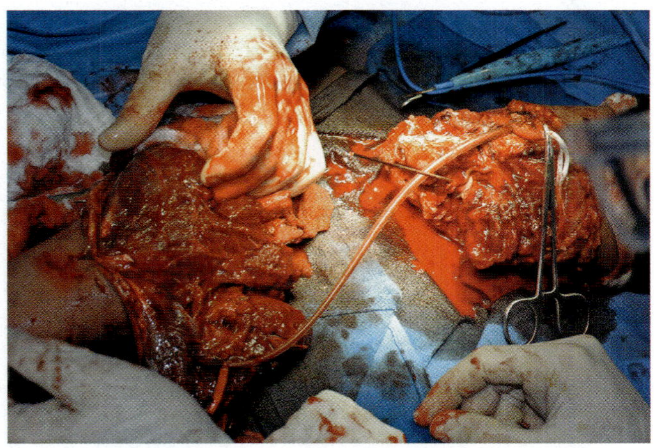

C

FIGURE 57-1 (A) View of the proximal arm on a patient after amputation at the level of the proximal forearm. A Javid shunt has been placed in the proximal brachial artery for perfusion while bony fixation is performed. Note that the shunt is held in place with an umbilical tape pulled tight around shunt with a segment of red-rubber catheter. (B) Shunt after fixation on both ends of vessel before reperfusion. (C) View after allowing perfusion via shunt. Debridement was performed and bony fixation was done with shunt in place before definitive vein grafting of defect.

Failing the use of a shunt, a vein graft of roughly the correct length can be placed between the vessel ends quickly, and then definitive orthopedic and soft tissue management can be accomplished. This approach may require revision of the length of the graft after treatment of the other injuries but is another alternative if vascular shunts are not available for some reason.

When there is adequate stable bony fixation, one can proceed with vascular repair. Initial soft tissue debridement can be performed after the tissue is perfused with a shunt, but definitive debridement is generally done after vascular repair. Depending on the status of the wound, the need for soft tissue coverage should be anticipated at the time of revascularization and debridement because vascular repairs and vein grafts should not be left exposed in the wound or simply covered with dressings. If early coverage of vessels cannot be achieved for whatever reason, one may need to consider "extraanatomic" bypass with a vein graft placed through intact soft tissues away from the site of the wound (29).

Proximal Penetrating Injury

Proximal penetrating vascular injury can be seen in gunshot wounds, stabbing-type wounds, and lacerations with glass or metal. Although not particularly common, these injuries can lead to ischemia of the forearm and hand, which may have significant sequelae. As noted earlier, however, depending on the level of injury and the presence of collateral circulation, brachial artery injuries may not immediately lead to critical ischemia downstream (14,15). They are associated, however, with a fairly high incidence of major nerve injury because the brachial artery is surrounded by the distal nerves of the brachial plexus (30,31). As noted earlier, the final functional outcome is more likely predicated on the severity of nerve injury rather than the vascular injury itself.

With an obvious penetrating vascular injury in the upper arm, surgical exploration is indicated. This is generally performed without a tourniquet because there is usually not enough room on the upper arm to allow its use. If the injury is distal enough, however, I prefer to place a tourniquet for exploration. The injury is explored via a longitudinal incision over the course of the brachial artery in the upper arm, and dissection proceeds expeditiously. These injuries will often have stopped bleeding because of vascular spasm (in the case of a transected artery) or thrombus, and dissection must proceed very carefully to prevent dislodging the clot and causing severe hemorrhage (Figure 57-2). The basis of all vascular surgery is proximal and distal control of the injured vessel, and thus the vessel should be approached first

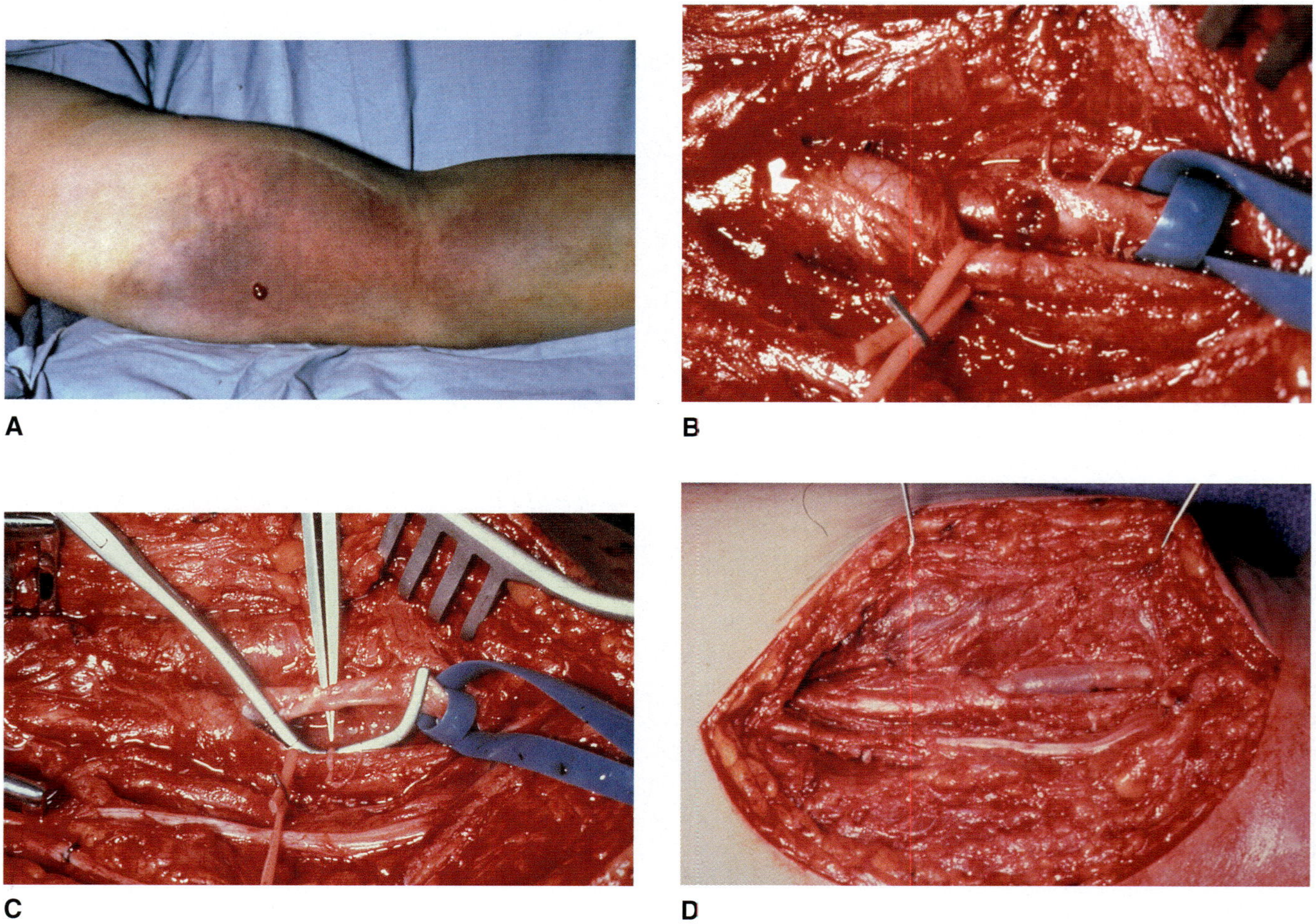

FIGURE 57-2 (A) View of a patient's proximal arm after a gunshot wound. The patient had a pulseless hand and obvious hematoma in the upper arm but good capillary refill and only mild sensory loss in a median nerve distribution. (B) View of the brachial artery behind the median nerve. Note thrombus at the site of arterial injury. (C) After control with a vascular clamp, note the through-and-through injury to the brachial artery. (D) Artery after repair with segment of reversed saphenous vein graft.

on both sides of the apparent site of injury so that control can be obtained to prevent blood loss. After the site of injury is ascertained, proximal and distal control of the artery is obtained with either vascular loops or vascular clamps. Care must be taken to avoid damage to surrounding nerves, which can happen in the face of hemorrhage from the damaged vessel and haste to gain control of the bleeding. A finger placed over the site of injury can act as an excellent method of temporary control of the bleeding while the proximal and distal vessels are carefully dissected out. If the proximal site of injury is obvious but control is difficult (because of location or surrounding nerves), control may be obtained by placing a small balloon catheter (Fogarty) into the lumen at the site of bleeding and inflating the balloon (32,33). After vascular control has been achieved, the injury must be assessed. If the injury is sharp or limited, the area of injury may be excised and the artery repaired primarily. On occasion with a partial wall injury, a vein patch graft may be used. In the majority of cases, however, a vein graft will be necessary. In these cases, most prefer to use a segment of reversed saphenous vein as the graft. This vein graft is of adequate size and tolerates arterial pressures well and is thus the graft of choice in this position. At present, the patency rates of vein graft substitutes (polytetrafluoroethylene [PTFE] or Dacron) for vessels the size of the brachial and forearm arteries remain too low to suggest these as alternatives to autologous vein (34,35).

Before performing the anastomosis, the proximal and distal vessels are irrigated with a heparinized saline solution (usually at a concentration of 100 units/cc) and the clamps or vessel loops replaced. This is a good time to evaluate proximal and distal flow in the brachial artery. There should be very brisk flow from the proximal artery and reasonably brisk flow from the distal end. If not, then catheter embolectomy should be performed with a Fogarty balloon catheter in whichever vessel flow does not appear to be appropriate. In the brachial artery, I usually repair the vessel with a 6-0 or 7-0 polypropylene vascular suture and needle using a running technique. This is generally done with loupe magnification, although the microscope can certainly be used if it will fit in the field. I prefer to perform the proximal anastomosis first and then remove the proximal vascular control and allow the graft to unwind. The graft is then clamped distally, and the appropriate length can be judged. After the graft is trimmed to the appropriate length, the distal anastomosis is performed. The clamps are removed and the arm allowed to perfuse. Distal pulses should return fairly rapidly, but this may take some time depending on the length of ischemia as well as the temperature of the limb. (Those that have been iced down may take some time to warm up and should be placed in warm lap sponges or towels.) Patients who do not have return of pulses and capillary refill may well have embolized thrombus into the radial or ulnar arteries (or both). These patients may require catheter embolectomy of the distal vessels if pulses do not return reasonably rapidly.

Fasciotomy of the forearm should be performed if there is any question as to the severity and length of ischemia. Although one can certainly wait and perform sequential measurements of the compartment pressures, it is still considered prudent to perform a fasciotomy in the face of significant warm ischemia time of the forearm muscles (4–6 hours) (36,37).

Injury with Significant Soft Tissue Loss

Wounds of the arm and forearm are frequently seen with avulsion and injury to the soft tissues with or without bony injury. These are frequent occurrences in automobile accidents (rollovers in particular) and industrial accidents involving heavy equipment. These present their own set of problems in terms of dealing with the vascular injury and concomitant soft tissue loss. Most of these patients require vein grafting of the injured segment, but thought must be given to the type and timing of soft tissue coverage of the graft. It is my experience that vascular anastomosis and particular vein grafts should not be left open or covered simply with dressings. Adequate vascularized soft tissue coverage must be available or made available to cover the anastomosis, vein graft, or both.

In most cases in the arm and hand, coverage in this type of injury requires free tissue transfer. Although a pedicle flap from the torso (i.e., a groin flap) might possibly cover the wound, this has several disadvantages. The tissue covering the graft does not import any vascularity, and in fact the hand has to be placed in a dependent position, which is detrimental in terms of controlling edema. Likewise, these types of injuries may well require a second-look procedure to perform further irrigation and debridement, and having the hand in a pedicled flap from the torso is cumbersome and inconvenient to perform such procedures later. A free flap allows for the hand and arm to be elevated to improve venous drainage of the limb and likewise brings in well-vascularized tissue. The site for anastomosis of the flap must be chosen carefully, however, because later surgery may be necessary, and vascular repairs must be in a position to allow this. Ideally, free flap anastomoses should be performed proximal to the site of vascular injury and vein bypass grafting, which provides uninjured vessels to feed the flap. At times, because of the size or nature of the wound, this may not be possible. Particularly in the case of the arterial anastomosis, hooking the free flap into the vein bypass graft provides an excellent alternative. If this is going to be necessary, a portion of the saphenous vein that includes a branch can be harvested to allow both bypass of the arterial deficit and easy end-to-end anastomosis of the free flap artery to the side branch (Figure 57-3). Regardless of the type of vein graft harvested, one should not hesitate to perform a free flap anastomosis to a vein graft in this situation because this is far better than attempting anastomosis to a damaged vessel in or near the wound.

Single-Vessel Injury in the Forearm with a Viable Hand

The necessity for repair of either the radial or ulnar artery when one is injured alone remains somewhat controversial. Early studies suggested that repair of one of the forearm vessels if the other was patent had very low patency rates (38,39). There was some thought that the quality and pressure of backflow on the divided vessel might be a predictor of patency rate, but this has not been borne out in clinical studies (40). More recent studies have shown that the results of grafting of the radial artery after radial forearm flap harvest has high patency rates, which is the opposite of what one would suspect from the studies in the 1980s (41). Interestingly, much data on the hemodynamics of the forearm vessels after harvest of the radial artery has been generated

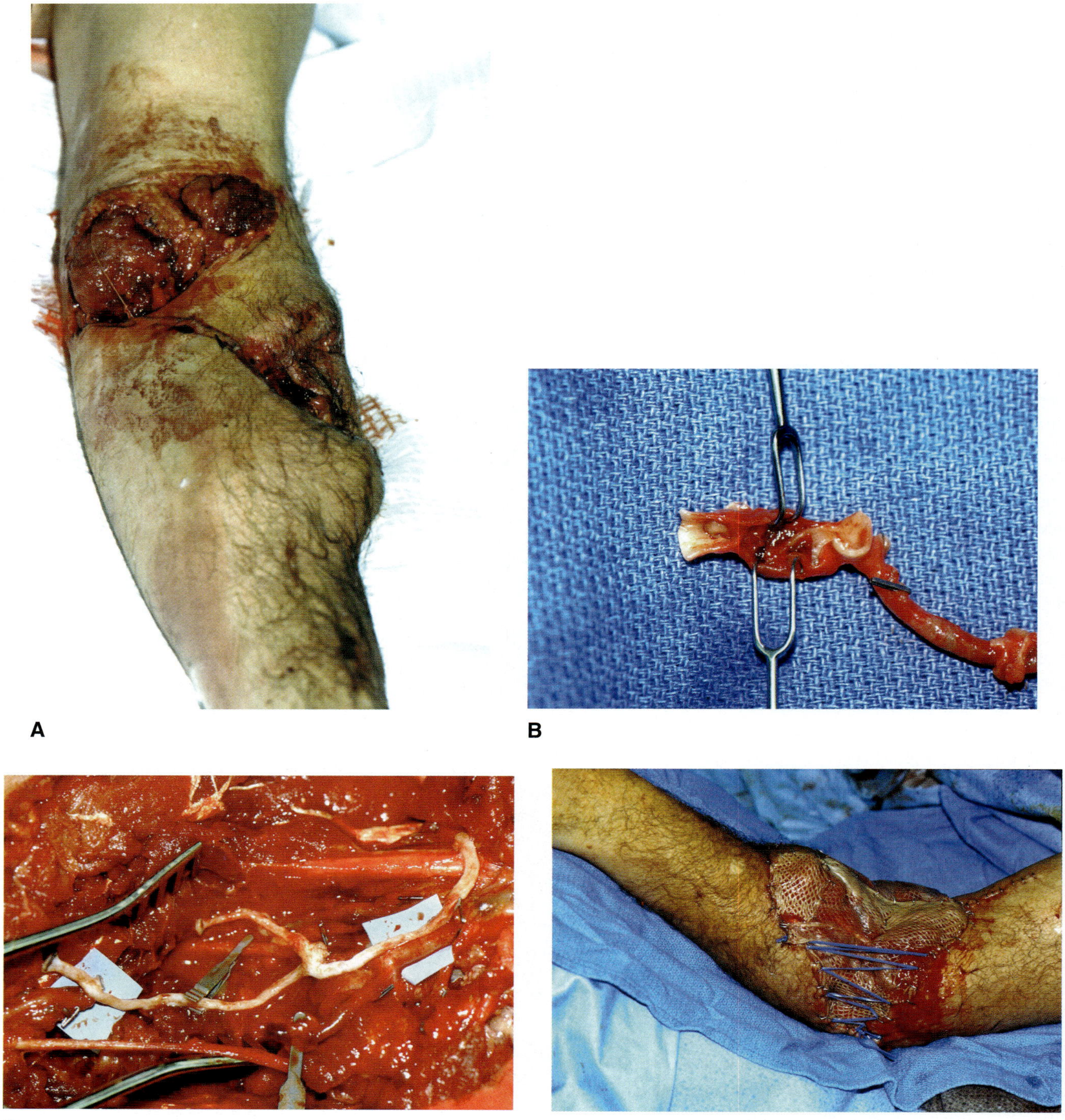

FIGURE 57-3 (A) Arm of a 46-year-old man after vehicle roll-over. The patient had a severe avulsion injury to the antecubital fossa with injury to the brachial artery and soft tissue deficit. There was no bony injury. (B) Segment of the brachial artery showing severe intimal disruption. (C) View of the saphenous vein graft in the antecubital fossa before anastomosis. Note clamps on proximal and distal brachial artery and branch for flap anastomosis coming off the superior portion of the graft. (D) The arm after completion of vascular repair, free rectus abdominis muscle, and split-thickness skin grafting. All of this was performed on the night of injury, and the patient did not require further surgery.

by cardiovascular surgeons because of their use of the radial artery for coronary artery bypass grafting. Hand ischemia after harvest of the radial artery for heart bypass is rare, but it has been reported (42). Hemodynamic studies have shown both an increase in flow in the ulnar artery after radial artery harvest (17% increase) as well as a significant increase in the diameter of the ulnar artery (15% increase) (43). Despite this, several studies have noted decreased flow in the hand, particularly to the radial-sided fingers (44). Outcome studies of patients having undergone harvest of the radial artery did not find any significant problems related to ischemia (45), but rather patients did have issues due to injury to the superficial branch of the radial nerve.

Based on personal experience and the above data, I take a case-by-case approach to single-vessel injury in the forearm. If the

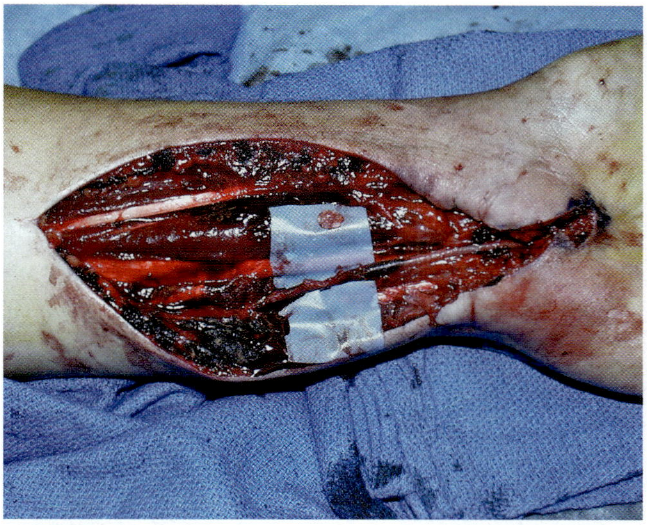

FIGURE 57-4 Forearm of a patient after a gunshot wound to the ulnar artery. The patient had apparent compartment syndrome and a large segment of damage to the vessel. The hand was well perfused with good Doppler signals in all fingertips. The artery was simply ligated proximal and distal to the site of injury.

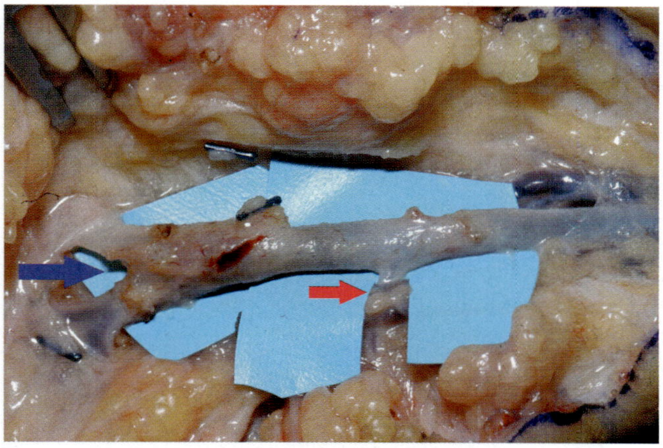

A

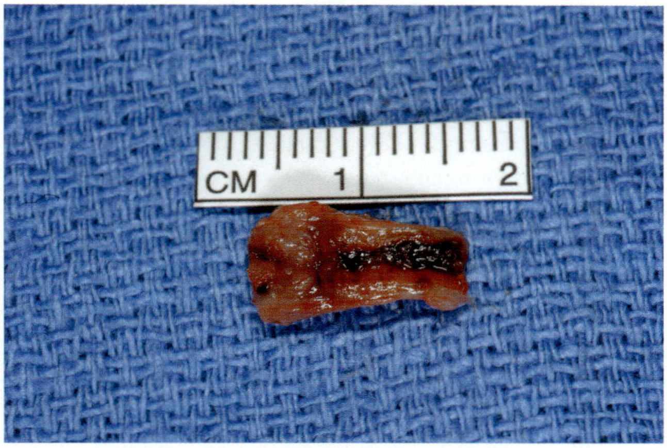

B

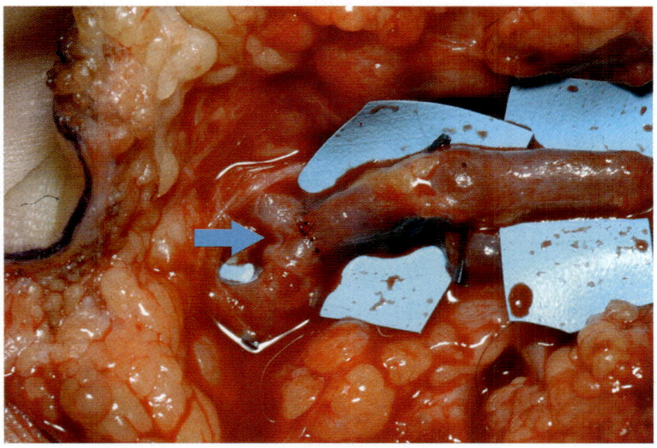

C

FIGURE 57-5 (A) Ulnar artery thrombosis in a high schoo football player who injured his hand against another player's helmet. The red arrow points to the deep branch of the ulnar artery, the blue arrow to the division at the distal end of the ulnar artery between the superficial palmar arch (above) and common digital artery to fourth webspace (below). (B) Internal view of intimal disruption at the site of injury. (C) View after reversed basilic vein graft from the forearm. Note the arrow at the site of distal anastomos s to the common lumen between the arch and digital artery to the fourth webspace.

artery can be primarily repaired after a direct sharp laceration, I often repair the vessel depending on the severity of the other injuries. If the hand is well perfused and there will be issues with soft tissue coverage of a graft or other issues which complicate a repair, I simply ligate the vessel (Figure 57-4). Patients with concomitant vascular and nerve injuries may develop apparent issues with perfusion because of hypersympathetic activity from the nerve injury in the late postoperative period. To obviate these issues, I usually repair a singly injured radial or ulnar artery in the face of a concomitant ulnar or median nerve injury.

Injuries to the Distal Circulation (Hand and Fingers)

Closed Trauma

Arterial injury and thrombosis in the hand is most commonly caused by closed trauma rather than open injury. This is manifested with ulnar artery thrombosis in the palm caused by "hypothenar hammer syndrome" and radial artery thrombosis in the anatomic snuffbox (46,47). Ulnar artery thrombosis is by far the more common problem and is usually seen in men who work with their hands who often bang the palm(s) of their hands. This leads to injury to the ulnar artery, which may be either acute (with intimal disruption and thrombosis) or chronic (with potential aneurysm formation.)

Acute injury to the ulnar artery is manifested by thrombosis and distal embolization of clot, which leads to ischemia of the digits, most commonly the ring and little fingers in my experience. The ulnar artery typically will clot at the site of injury, and clot will propagate distally to the anastomosis between the arch and the common digital artery to the fourth webspace and proximally to either the deep branch or the dorsal branch that comes off several centimeters proximal to the wrist. Most authors would agree that these individuals should be managed with surgical excision of the thrombosed segment and repair with a vein bypass graft (48,49) (Figure 57-5). This stops

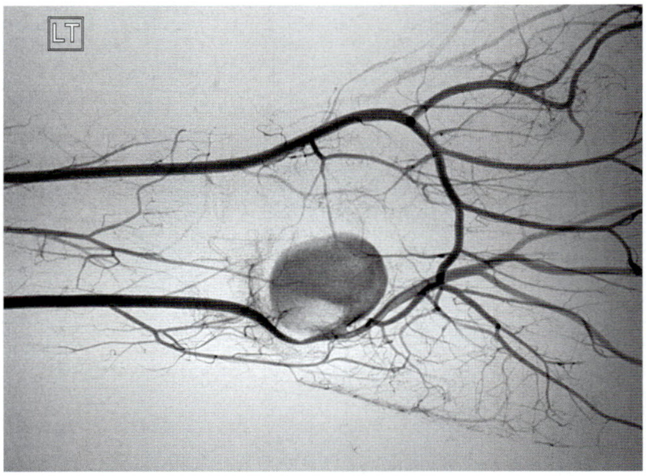

FIGURE 57-6 Arteriogram showing aneurysm of the ulnar artery after a missed injury to a vessel from a stab wound to the palm.

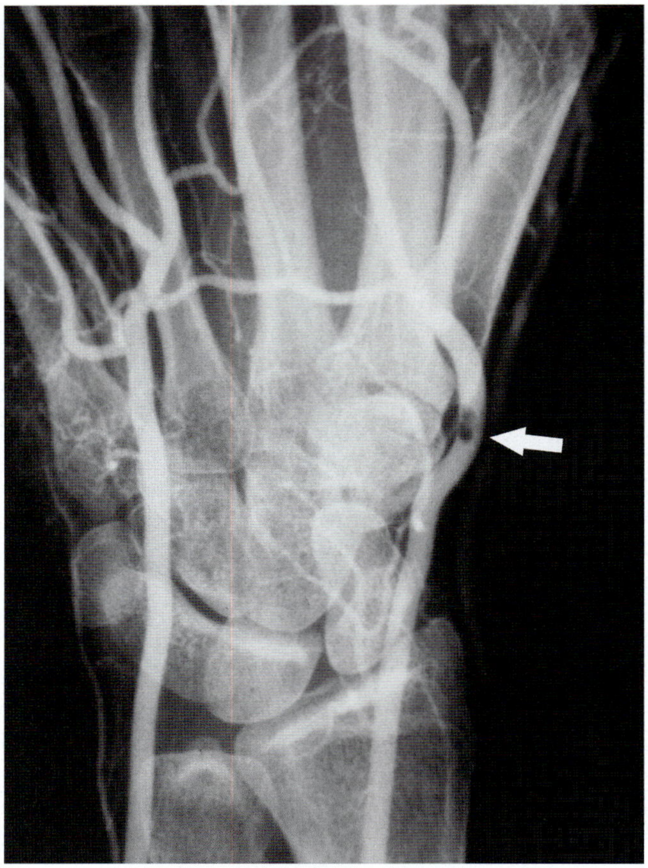

FIGURE 57-7 Arteriogram of patient presenting with ischemic index finger and thumb. Note thrombus in radial artery in snuffbox (arrow).

embolization to the fingers and restores flow via the ulnar artery. I prefer using the reversed basilic vein on the ulnar side of the forearm for ulnar artery bypass, but others use the saphenous to good effect. Midterm (2–5 year) studies on the outcomes of such grafts are generally good, with high patency rates and patient satisfaction (49). More chronic injury can lead to aneurysm formation, which also may lead to ischemic symptoms caused by distal embolization of thrombus (Figure 57-6). These patients are likewise usually managed with excision of the aneurysm and bypass grafting, although on occasion, the aneurysm can be excised and the ulnar artery brought together primarily because of redundancy in the artery.

Thrombosis of the radial artery generally occurs in the anatomic snuffbox under the extensor pollicis longus (EPL) tendon. This is in fact not really a traumatic condition but probably compression of the artery between the EPL tendon and trapezium where the artery passes between these two structures (47) (Figures 57-7 and 57-8). As with ulnar artery thrombosis in the palm, this condition leads to embolization and ischemia of the fingers, particularly the index finger and thumb. This condition should also be managed with reversed vein bypass graft, and I prefer to use the cephalic vein which is usually present in the same incision for exploration of the radial artery. Likewise, to avoid recurrence, the graft either needs to be routed over the EPL tendon or the tendon should be moved over to prevent pressure on the graft.

Open Trauma

Trauma to the arterial supply of the hand can occur with open injuries to the palm; however, to render the fingers ischemic, there must usually be severe damage to the arch. This is more likely to occur with near-amputation injuries or avulsive soft tissue damage to the palm. Simple stab wounds rarely cause ischemic problems, but missed arterial injuries may lead to aneurysm formation. These injuries should be approached individually; however, with severe injury to the palm of the hand, vein grafting may be necessary. With avulsion injuries, the patient may require reconstruction of the arch as well as the common digital vessels going into the fingers with vein grafts from the forearm or dorsal foot (Figure 57-9). Likewise, these patients may require flap coverage if the palmar skin is missing or devascularized. As with more proximal injuries, I do not believe that vascular repairs and especially vein grafts should be left without soft tissue coverage because the risk of blow-out of the artery is significant.

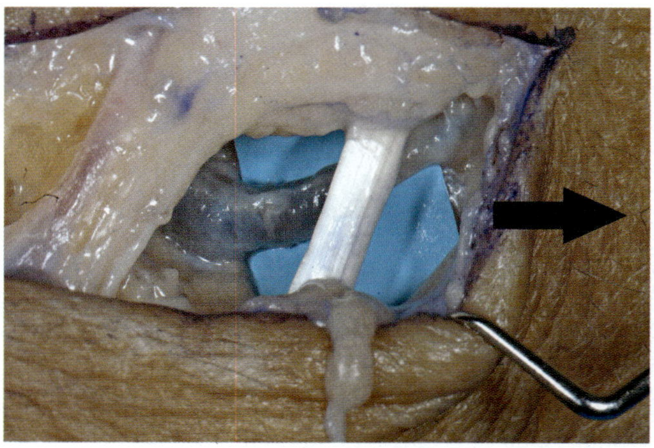

FIGURE 57-8 Thrombosis of the radial artery under the extensor pollicis longus tendon. The arrow points distally.

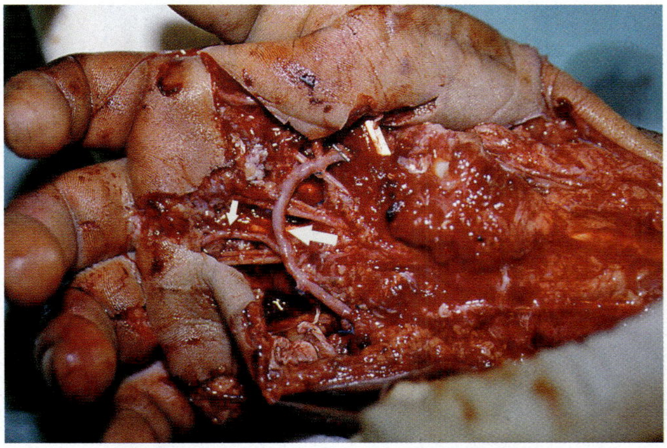

FIGURE 57-9 The palm of a patient with a severe degloving injury to the palm and avulsion of the palmar arterial arch. The arch has been reconstructed with a reversed vein graft (larger arrow), and vein grafts have been placed to two distal common digital arteries (small arrow).

Digital Artery Injury

Management of injury to the digital arteries is usually straightforward, but in most instances, unless it is an extremely sharp injury with little surrounding soft tissue injury, I believe that these should be vein grafted. Resection of the injured ends of these vessels may leave a gap in the vessel that cannot be repaired without undue tension. It is always much easier and much less time consuming to perform a vein graft to the digital artery first rather than attempting to repair a too-tight vessel. Sometimes several branches from the artery proximally and distally can be taken down to gain length, but (particularly distally) this can potentially decrease the flow into the surrounding ischemic tissues. For these reasons, I believe strongly in resecting a generous portion of the injured artery at the time of exploration and performing a vein graft if the finger is ischemic. I usually harvest small veins from the volar forearm and reverse these, and the dorsal foot can also be used for donor veins. Although the size match is not always perfect (especially in the more distal digit), these veins are of adequate size and can be anastomosed to the digital vessels without too much difficulty. If two fingers require revascularization, a bifid vein graft can be used if it is available in the forearm or dorsal foot (Figure 57-10). Many digital "revascularizations" are in essence replants, with the need for open reduction and internal fixation of the bony injury, tendon repair, and nerve and vessel repair. If the digit is hanging on by only a relative small skin bridge, it can be advantageous to simply divide this, shorten the finger, and perform a true "replant" rather than struggle around a piece of tissue that may have no value. Dorsal skin bridges often contain competent veins, however, and these should be left intact if possible.

If there is a significant wound to the finger and the digit is devascularized, provision for arterial repair and coverage should be made. Vein grafts can be covered with skin grafts, but this is far from ideal. If there are several damaged fingers and one or more are deemed nonreplantable, a "flow-through" flap may be able to be designed from one of these. A portion of the digital artery is taken with the attached skin, and the artery is used to repair another finger. This does require anastomosis of a vein as well, but usually this is not that difficult. The digital nerve can be included in the flap as well as a vascularized nerve graft (Figure 57-11).

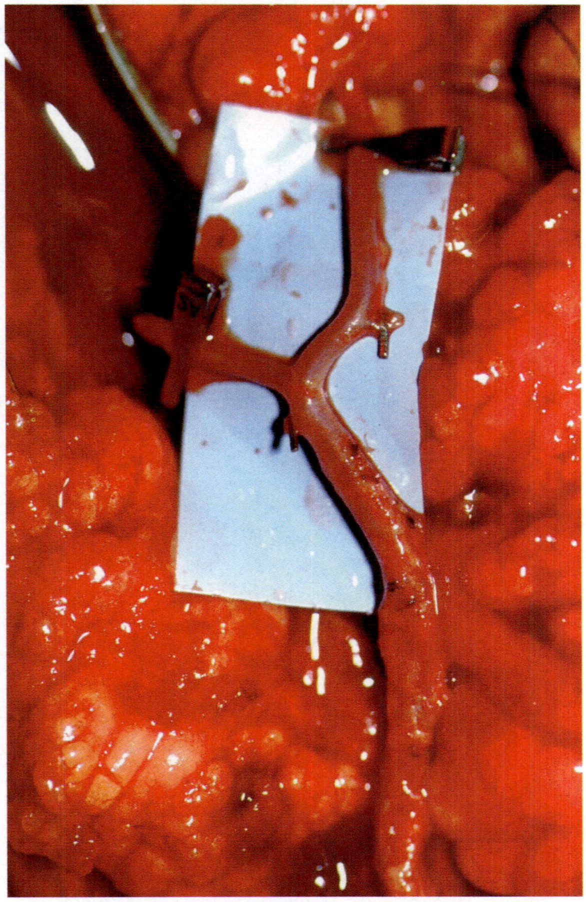

FIGURE 57-10 View of a "Y" vein graft used to repair injury to two digital vessels in the palm.

Ring Avulsions

Urbaniak and colleagues classified ring avulsion injuries into three categories (50). In class I injuries, the circulation is adequate, and standard bone and soft tissue management is appropriate. In class II injuries, the circulation is inadequate (either arterial or venous) and requires microvascular repair to restore adequate flow to the digit. In class III injuries, the finger is completely degloved or there is a complete amputation (Figure 57-12). These injuries are usually more severe than thought initially, and the emergency department physician may send a patient home with a class II avulsion injury and venous compromise without realizing the potential problems. Although some have reported decent functional results with replantation of class III injuries, I believe that these should usually not be replanted. The issues with these type of injuries involve the intervening soft tissue injury and avulsive injury to the nerves. I think that the function of a class III ring avulsion that is replanted is poor, with both

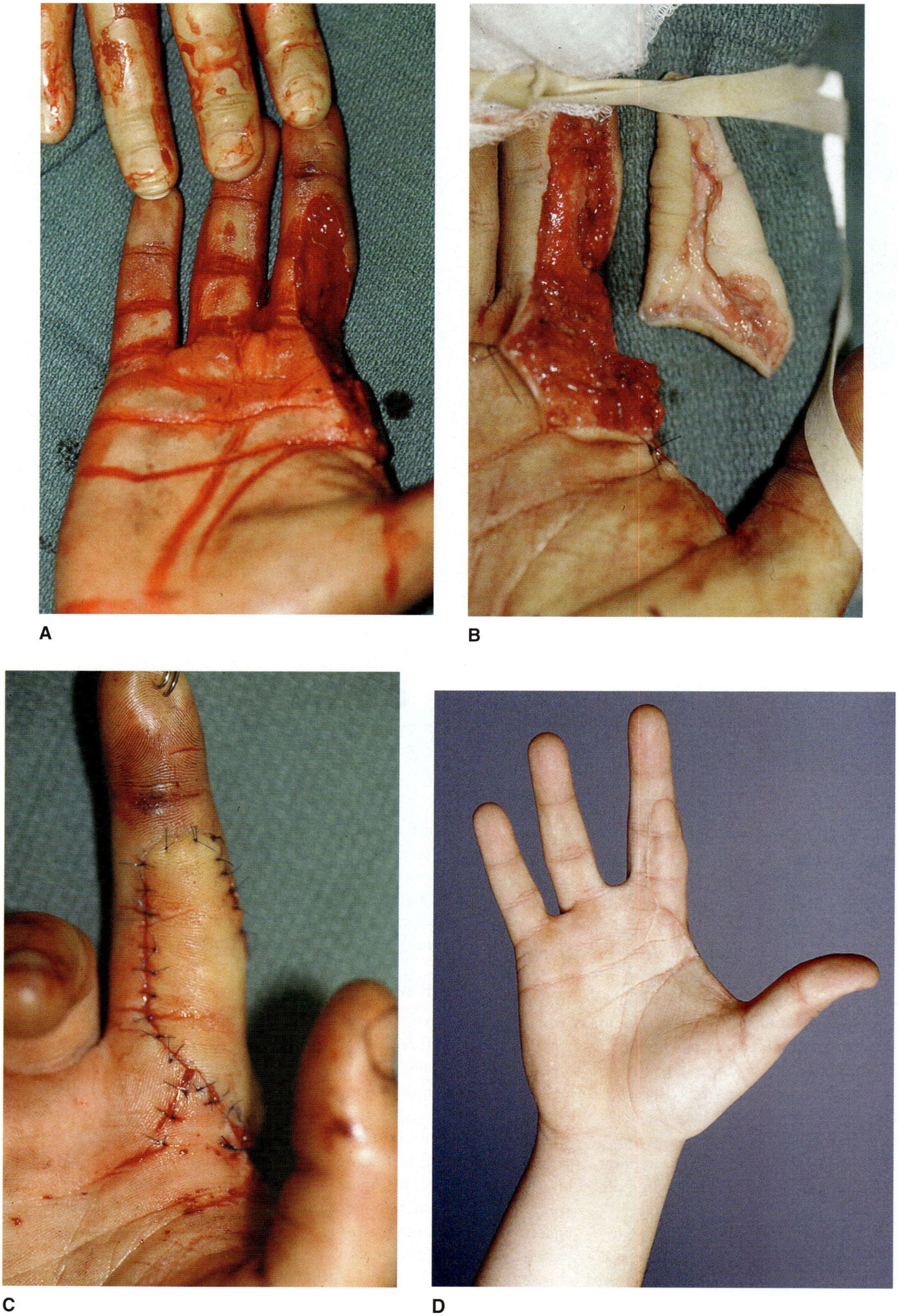

FIGURE 57-11 (A) A patient who sustained amputation of the index finger and avulsion of a portion of the base of the middle finger with loss of the digital nerve and artery. (B) A "flow-through" flap designed from the amputated index finger to repair the digital artery, nerve, and soft tissue deficit of the middle finger. (C) The flap after repair of the digital artery proximally and distally, the digital nerve, and the dorsal vein. (D) The flap 4 months after surgery.

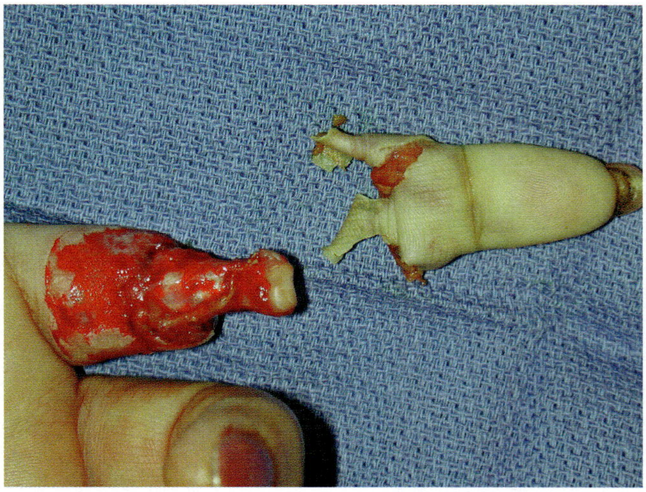

FIGURE 57-12 Class III ring avulsion. Note the significant soft tissue injury to the amputated digit and residual tissue on the finger.

poor sensation and motion. Even class II injuries may present problems with the avulsed soft tissues at the site of injury, and in these cases, one should be prepared to provide coverage of the vein graft(s) used to revascularize the digit. Small flow-through arterialized venous flaps work quite well in this situation, and the flap usually survives without difficulty and provides good cover for the included vein graft. My results with venous flow-through flaps in the venous system have not been so good, however. Nonetheless, when selecting a volar forearm vein for repair of the injured segment in a ring avulsion, the vein should be harvested with an appropriate piece of surrounding skin. This is then reversed, and arterial anastomoses are performed proximally and distally. The flap will pink up, and the skin can be trimmed as needed to provide coverage in the area of skin damage (Figure 57-13). These patients require intensive physical therapy to maximize function even if the revascularization of the digit is successful.

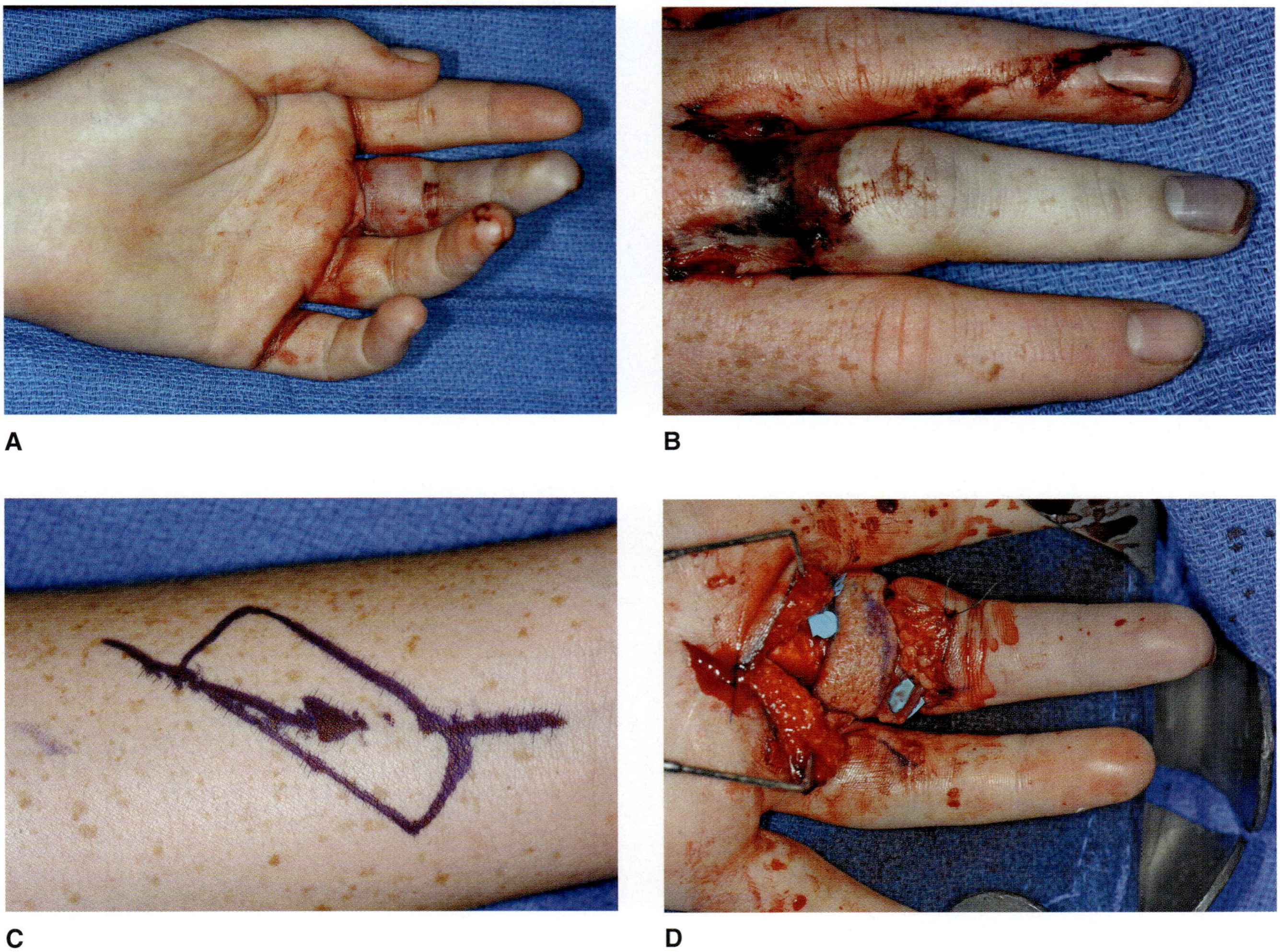

FIGURE 57-13 (A) A 20-year-old woman after a rope avulsion injury to the middle finger. (B) Dorsal view of the soft tissue injury. (C) A "flow-through" venous flap designed on the volar forearm. (D) The flap in place after the vein was anastomosed to the proximal and distal digital artery. Note the return of a pink color to the finger.

REFERENCES

1. Fitridge RA, Raptis S, Miller JH, Faris I. Upper extremity arterial injuries: experience at the Royal Adelaide Hospital, 1969 to 1991. *J Vasc Surg* 1994;20:941–946.
2. Gupta R, Rao S, Sieunarine K. An epidemiological view of vascular trauma in Western Australia: a 5-year study. *ANZ J Surg* 2001;71: 461–466.
3. Clouse WD, Rasmussen TE, Perlstein, et al. Upper extremity vascular injury: a current in-theater wartime report from Operation Iraqi Freedom. *Ann Vasc Surg* 2006;20:429–434.
4. Menakuru SR, Behera A, Jindal R, et al. Extremity vascular trauma in civilian population: a seven-year review from North India. *Injury* 2005;36:400–406.
5. Cakir O, Subasi M, Erdem K, Eren N. Treatment of vascular injuries associated with limb fractures. *Ann R Coll Surg Engl* 2005;87:348–352.
6. de Witte PB, Lozano-Calderon S, Harness N, et al. Acute vascular injury associated with fracture of the distal radius: a report of 6 cases. *J Orthop Trauma* 2008;22:611–614.
7. Schlickewei W, Kuner EH, Mullaji AB, Gotze B. Upper and lower limb fractures with concomitant arterial injury. *J Bone Joint Surg Br* 1992;74:181–188.
8. Blakey CM, Biant LC, Birch R. Ischaemia and the pink, pulseless hand complicating supracondylar fractures of the humerus in childhood: long-term follow-up. *J Bone Joint Surg Br* 2009;91:1487–1492.
9. Ayel JE, Bonnevialle N, Lafosse JM, et al. Acute elbow dislocation with arterial rupture. Analysis of nine cases. *Orthop Traumatol Surg Res* 2009;95:343–351.
10. Stein JS, Strauss E. Gunshot wounds to the upper extremity. Evaluation and management of vascular injuries. *Orthop Clin North Am* 1995;26: 29–35.
11. Trooskin SZ, Sclafani S, Winfield J, et al. The management of vascular injuries of the extremity associated with civilian firearms. *Surg Gynecol Obstet* 1993;176:350–354.
12. Ball CG, Rozycki GS, Feliciano DV. Upper extremity amputations after motor vehicle rollovers. *J Trauma* 2009;67:410–412.
13. Elsharawy MA. Arterial reconstruction after mangled extremity: injury severity scoring systems are not predictive of limb salvage. *Vascular* 2005;13:114–119.
14. Padayachy V, Robbs JV, Mulaudzi TV, et al. A retrospective review of brachial artery injuries and repairs—is it still a "training artery"? *Injury* 2010;41:843–846.
15. Zellweger R, Hess F, Nicol A, et al. An analysis of 124 surgically managed brachial artery injuries. *Am J Surg* 2004;188:240–245.
16. van der Sluis CK, Kucey DS, Brenneman FD, et al. Long-term outcomes after upper limb arterial injuries. *Can J Surg* 1997;40:265–270.
17. Shaw AD, Milne AA, Christie J, et al. Vascular trauma of the upper limb and associated nerve injuries. *Injury* 1995;26:515–518.
18. Topel I, Pfister K, Moser A, et al. Clinical outcome and quality of life after upper extremity arterial trauma. *Ann Vasc Surg* 2009;23:317–323.
19. Conrad MF, Patton JH Jr, Parikshak M, Kralovich KA. Evaluation of vascular injury in penetrating extremity trauma: angiographers stay home. *Am Surg* 2002;68:269–274.
20. Gates JD. Penetrating wounds of the extremities. Methods of identifying arterial injury. *Orthop Rev* 1994;suppl:10–12.
21. Gonzalez RP, Falimirski ME. The utility of physical examination in proximity penetrating extremity trauma. *Am Surg* 1999;65:784–789.
22. Peng PD, Spain DA, Tataria M, et al. CT angiography effectively evaluates extremity vascular trauma. *Am Surg* 2008;74:103–107.
23. Bynoe RP, Miles WS, Bell RM, et al. Noninvasive diagnosis of vascular trauma by duplex ultrasonography. *J Vasc Surg* 1991;14:346–352.
24. Ordog GJ, Balasubramanium S, Wasserberger J, et al. Extremity gunshot wounds: part one—identification and treatment of patients at high risk of vascular injury. *J Trauma* 1994;36:358–368.
25. Hancock H, Rasmussen TE, Walker AJ, Rich NM. History of temporary intravascular shunts in the management of vascular injury. *J Vasc Surg* 2010;52:1405–1409.
26. Subramanian A, Vercruysse G, Dente C, et al. A decade's experience with temporary intravascular shunts at a civilian level I trauma center. *J Trauma* 2008;65:316–324.
27. Taller J, Kamdar JP, Greene JA, et al. Temporary vascular shunts as initial treatment of proximal extremity vascular injuries during combat operations: the new standard of care at Echelon II facilities? *J Trauma* 2008;65:595–603.
28. Borut LT, Acosta CJ, Tadlock LC, et al. The use of temporary vascular shunts in military extremity wounds: a preliminary outcome analysis with 2-year follow-up. *J Trauma* 2010;69:174–178.
29. Feliciano DV. Heroic procedures in vascular injury management: the role of extra-anatomic bypasses. *Surg Clin North Am* 2002;82:115–124.
30. Diamond S, Gaspard D, Katz S. Vascular injuries to the extremities in a suburban trauma center. *Am Surg* 2003;69:848–851.
31. Manord JD, Garrard CL, Kline DG, et al. Management of severe proximal vascular and neural injury of the upper extremity. *J Vasc Surg* 1998;27:43–47.
32. Howard ER, Young AE. Control of aortic haemorrhage by balloon catheter. *Br Med J* 1971;3:161.
33. Sobeh MS, Westacott S, Blakeney C, Ham RJ. Balloon angioplasty catheters for endovascular tamponade after vascular trauma. *Injury* 1993;24:355–356.
34. Hughes K, Hamdan A, Schermerhorn M, et al. Bypass for chronic ischemia of the upper extremity: results in 20 patients. *J Vasc Surg* 2007;46:303–307.
35. Roddy SP, Darling RC III, Chang BB, et al. Brachial artery reconstruction for occlusive disease: a 12-year experience. *J Vasc Surg* 2001;33:802–805.
36. Friedrich JB, Shin AY. Management of forearm compartment syndrome. *Hand Clin* 2007;23:245–54, vii.
37. Morin RJ, Swan KG, Tan V. Acute forearm compartment syndrome secondary to local arterial injury after penetrating trauma. *J Trauma* 2009;66:989–993.
38. Gelberman RH, Nunley JA, Koman LA, et al. The results of radial and ulnar arterial repair in the forearm. Experience in three medical centers. *J Bone Joint Surg Am* 1982;64:383–387.
39. Gelberman RH, Blasingame JP, Fronek A, Dimick MP. Forearm arterial injuries. *J Hand Surg Am* 1979;4:401–408.
40. Nunley JA, Goldner RD, Koman LA, et al. Arterial stump pressure: a determinant of arterial patency? *J Hand Surg Am* 1987;12:245–249.
41. Kiehn M, Brooks D, Lee C, et al. Patency of radial arteries reconstructed after radial forearm flap harvest. *J Reconstr Microsurg* 2007;23:347–349.
42. Fox AD, Whiteley MS, Phillips-Hughes J, Roake J. Acute upper limb ischemia: a complication of coronary artery bypass grafting. *Ann Thorac Surg* 1999;67:535–536.
43. Brodman RF, Hirsh, LE, Frame R. Effect of radial artery harvest on collateral forearm blood flow and digital perfusion. *J Thorac Cardiovasc Surg* 2002;123:512–516.
44. Lee HS, Chang BC, Heo YJ. Digital blood flow after radial artery harvest for coronary artery bypass grafting. *Ann Thorac Surg* 2004;77:2071–2074.
45. Allen RH, Szabo RM, Chen JL. Outcome assessment of hand function after radial artery harvesting for coronary artery bypass. *J Hand Surg Am* 2004;29:628–637.
46. Yuen JC, Wright E, Johnson LA, Culp WC. Hypothenar hammer syndrome: an update with algorithms for diagnosis and treatment. *Ann Plast Surg* 2011;67(4):429–438.
47. McNamara MG, Butler TE, Sanders WE, Pederson WC. Ischaemia of the index finger and thumb secondary to thrombosis of the radial artery in the anatomical snuffbox. *J Hand Surg Br* 1998;23:28–32.
48. Chloros GD, Lucas RM, Li Z, et al. Post-traumatic ulnar artery thrombosis: outcome of arterial reconstruction using reverse interpositional vein grafting at 2 years minimum follow-up. *J Hand Surg Am* 2008;33:932–940.
49. Koman LA, Ruch DS, Aldridge M, et al. Arterial reconstruction in the ischemic hand and wrist: effects on microvascular physiology and health-related quality of life. *J Hand Surg Am* 1998;23:773–782.
50. Urbaniak JR, Evans JP, Bright DS. Microvascular management of ring avulsion injuries. *J Hand Surg Am* 1981;6:25–30.

CHAPTER 58

Soft Tissue Coverage of the Upper Limb

Joseph Upton

The ideal soft tissue coverage of the hand and upper limb has been and always will be in a state of evolution dependent on advances in technology, surgical technique, innovation, and the curiosity of the surgeon. When faced with a difficult wound, the surgical resident or fellow asks: "What is the best type of coverage for this problem?" The attending physician's answer should be: "It depends, and there are a lot of options." Careful analysis of any particular problem should start on the lowest rungs on the reconstructive ladder and progress through skin grafts and local and regional flaps before ascending to distant pedicle flaps and free tissue transfers. The most common mistake made by those in training is to step on the reconstructive elevator and press the button for the penthouse suite without consideration of simpler, more expeditious methods of coverage. In some clinical settings, free tissue transfer may be the best choice, but these are not common. This chapter on soft tissue coverage starts beyond those wounds covered with small skin grafts or local flaps and concentrates primarily on microvascular solutions to defects with more extensive, often composite tissue losses.

During the infancy of reconstructive microsurgery, reconstructive microsurgeons were often severely criticized by other surgical colleagues for performing radical, "unnecessary" operations for coverage of extensive wounds all over the body. At the time, we knew that what appeared to be radical operation was the most conservative approach available and in one stage achieved complete wound coverage, closed donor site, and early rehabilitation. Simultaneously, those of us who treated skeletal injuries could see the obvious advantages of early internal skeletal fixation and mobilization espoused by the A-O group in Europe. Immediate fixation and soft tissue closure followed by early rehabilitation could dismiss the common "fracture disease:" atrophy, stiffness, swelling, and pain followed by inevitable functional loss. The most important clinical imperative for us was to make sure that these free tissue transfers survived and made a significant clinical difference for the patients. It did not take long to turn most of our critics into referring physicians and often collaborators (Table 58-1). The overwhelming majority of clinical cases at that time involved coverage of the upper and lower limb.

Clinical decisions are not always easy. The majority of difficult wounds and composite tissue losses do not present in healthy patients or involve simple wounds. Most candidates for free tissue transfers have *risk factors,* which may include diabetes, smoking history, immunosuppression, obesity, radiation therapy, chemotherapy, malnutrition, peripheral vascular disease, Raynaud's phenomenon, infection, and psychiatric issues among many others. The *nature of the injury* and complexity of the wound (sharp, blunt, crush, avulsion, contaminated, clean), the presence of foreign bodies or skeletal fragments, the size of the wound, the layers of structures involved, and the patient's lifestyle are all relevant to the choice of soft tissue overage. There are no absolutes with this type of surgery, which can now be performed in every corner of the globe. Critical factors, which are often minimized, include the *surgeon's confidence* in his or her surgical ability and experience with different options, an intimate *knowledge of potential donor sites,* the facilities available, and the follow-up available to handle potential complications. Although new esoteric flaps are available and provide potentially outstanding functional outcomes, they are often not the most practical solution for the individual patient.

Although this book concentrates on operative microsurgery, *free tissue transfer,* and vascular island flaps, any discussion of upper limb coverage is incomplete without including traditional *pedicled transfer* of the same types of tissues for the same ultimate functional or aesthetic purposes. Both techniques require meticulous surgical technique, attention to detail, and a sound knowledge of both donor and recipient site anatomy.

This chapter is unusual because all the cases used for illustration of basic principles include 1- to 3-decade follow-up periods. Many of the techniques shown are not frequently used today but, interestingly, have accomplished the same goals and

TABLE 58-1 Advantages of Free Tissue Transfers

Many options to match donor and recipient tissues
Single-stage procedure
Less donor and recipient morbidity and recipient site morbidity
Possible flow-through conduits
Neurosensory potential
Quicker rehabilitation and limb elevation
Better contour
Composite tissue options

used the same principles as present-day microvascular transfers for soft tissue coverage. In retrospect, many of these transfers, including the groin and lateral arm flaps in particular, could be expeditiously used more frequently today.

INDICATIONS

Given proper debridement in an otherwise healthy patient, soft tissue coverage is needed for (1) full-thickness skin losses that cannot or should not be resurfaced with skin grafts alone, (2) wounds that are too large for local flaps, (3) defects that should not be left to granulate for weeks or months, or (4) coverage of compromised wounds with minimal healing potential. Skeletal stability should be intact with or without internal or external fixation. In the upper limb, free tissue transfers are usually indicated for larger wounds because they enable a more radical surgical debridement of nonviable or compromised tissue; can replace all of the tissue lost; and if well designed, permit vascular anastomoses outside of the zone of injury. A flap with a flow-through arterial system can be used to revascularize a devitalized digit, hand, or foot (Figure 58-1). These flaps can be very effective in small regions where specialized tissue is needed such as a thenar crease flap for the glabrous pulp surface of a fingertip or as a fascial flap to allow tendon gliding after extensor tenolyses and neurolyses in the midpalm. In contrast to the multistaged procedures required for groin or lower abdominal pedicle flaps, microsurgical transfer of similar tissue results in less scarring, concomitant tendon, nerve or skeletal reconstruction, and earlier rehabilitation (see Table 58-1)

A combination of techniques is often appropriate for coverage for a single complex defect. Skin grafts are very effective for clean wounds over muscle in the proximal forearm. Exposed hardware, nerve junctures, tendon repairs, and vascular anastomoses require full-thickness replacement. Similarly, joint contractures at all levels are reduced after full-thickness coverage of adjacent structures. Anticipated secondary reconstruction is easier beneath durable, supple soft tissue. The origin of this tissue in its new location is much less important than its ultimate function.

As reconstructive options multiply, indications change. This scenario is similar to surgical board examinations in which the questions remain the same from one decade to another while only the answers change. However, within this dynamic of change, the resilience of basic surgical principles does not and should not be altered. The conundrum of how to integrate new innovative techniques and how to change established surgical dogma is always in play and requires judicious trial and error (1–18).

The specific characteristics of each region of the upper extremity are summarized below, and examples of our preferred flaps as well as less frequently used options for coverage are presented. Toe transfers are covered in other chapters (see Chapters 26, 63, 64 and 65).

AVAILABLE FLAPS

The repertoire of flaps available to refined hand surgeons seems limitless (Tables 58-2 and 58-3). All that is really required is a composite tissue with its nutrient artery and draining vein with a lumen greater than 0.5 mm in diameter. Selection depends on matching the characteristics of the recipient tissue loss with the donor sites available as the surgeon strives to replace like tissues. All tissues within the body are potentially available. Ideally, thin skin is replaced with thin flaps, critical sensate regions with neurosensory flaps, composite tissue losses with flaps that contain the lost tissues, and areas that require tendon and joint mobility with tissue that permits gliding. The goal is to replicate normal contour and function as close as possible.

The general categories of transfers available include skin and subcutaneous tissues (*fasciocutaneous*), muscle and skin (*musculocutaneous*), bone and skin (*osteocutaneous*), fascia alone (*fascial*), and fascia and skin (*fasciocutaneous*). Within each category, smaller, more refined flaps have been isolated on smaller, perforating branches of the major axial vessels (*perforator flaps*). Tissues supplied by vessels with a diameter of 0.3 to 0.4 mm are within the capability of present-day microsurgeons; however, the margin of success is much more successful and predictable when working with vessels in the 1.5- to 2.0-mm-diameter range.

CHOICE OF FLAP

The choice of the best donor site is not always easy but should be the result of logical deductive reasoning. Most important are the patient's health and functional needs, characteristics of the tissue to be replaced, and the donor sites available. The goal should be to obtain the most functional coverage while providing proper contour, color match, and surface characteristics. The flap must be tailored to the patient. The algorithmic, reflex approach to this type of plastic surgery should be discouraged because refined soft tissue coverage often involves *more than a "cut and paste" approach*. Secondary procedures are often needed and should be part of the initial planning. It is unacceptable to transfer a bulky muscle or fasciocutaneous flap onto a thumb, hand, or forearm and discharge the patient without a long-term plan. Primary tendon, bone, and joint reconstructions should be encouraged at the time of initial coverage or soon thereafter as practical.

My personal approach with these wounds has been to first determine whether full-thickness or composite tissue replacement is more appropriate than a skin graft. One can delay for a short period of time with sequential dressing changes or temporary skin graft coverage. This solution is often appropriate when other injuries, insults, or medical conditions take a higher pri-

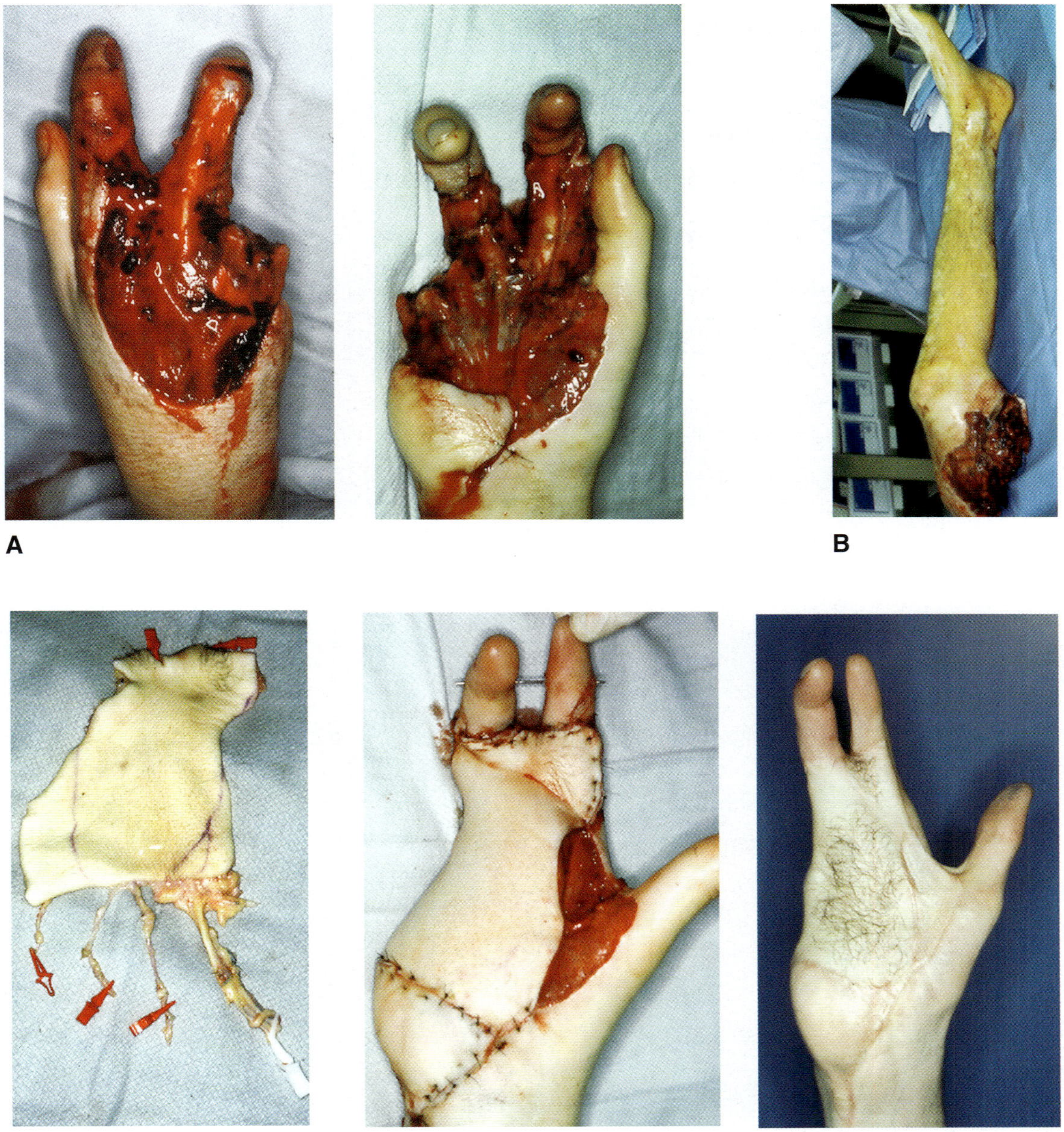

FIGURE 58-1 Dorsalis pedis flow-through revascularization. (**A**) After traction, avulsion injury to both the dorsal and palmar surfaces has been lost, the ring and small digits amputated, and the remaining long digit devascularized. (**B**) The left leg was amputated at the midfemoral level. The patient had also sustained major intracranial, liver, spleen, and cardiac injuries. (**C**) The dorsalis pedis skin was harvested as a flow-through flap from the amputated leg. (**D**) Revascularization was done 24 hours later at the bedside with loupe magnification. (**E**) Appearance 22 years later.

ority or when specialized microvascular care is not available. This option is not acceptable when there is a large amount composite soft tissue loss.

If flap coverage is most appropriate, provide it soon. We first determine the size of the defect, the characteristics of the tissue lost, and the specific anatomy of the region and then consider the ideal coverage. Often this is possible; many times it is not. A template is made, and all potential donor sites are surveyed. Comorbidities such as obesity, peripheral vascular status, associated diseases and injuries, congenital malformations, or acquired conditions become important. Does the surgeon know the donor site anatomy well? Can the transfer be performed as a pedicle or as a free tissue transfer? For example, an ipsilateral pedicle chest or groin flap may be more predictable than a free groin flap in a young child. A pedicled radial forearm fascial flap may be easier than a free temporoparietal fascia transfer to the hand. Finally, the surgeon's capability, experience, and team coupled with their success rate and the likelihood of an optimal outcome must be considered. At this stage, the *best choice* of coverage usually becomes quite evident. If indecision is affected by the patient's condition, a lack of technical support for a free tissue transfer, the confidence of the surgeon, or a lack of knowledge of the donor site, it is always best to skin graft the wound temporarily and consider the ideal coverage as a secondary option. In the trauma setting, the curious microsurgeon will feel challenged and will characteristically seek the opportunity

TABLE 58-2 Coverage Options in the Upper Limb by Region

Flaps used in digits and thumb	Local	Regional	Distant (pedicle and free transfers)
Fingertip	Advancement	Cross-finger	Toe pulp (free)
	V-to-Y palmar (Atasoy)	First dorsal metacarpal	Composite toe (free)
	V-to-Y lateral (Kutler)	Reverse cross-finger	Medial arch from foot (free)
	Palmar advance (Moberg)	Heterodigital N-V island (Littler)	Groin pedicle
	Palmar advance + FTSG (Hueston)	Local transposition	Abdominal pedicle
	Cross-finger		Thenar crease (free)
	Cross-finger fascia + FTSG		Scapular (free to pedicle)
	Homodigital ante or retrograde		
	First dorsal metacarpal flag		
	Perforator		
	Thenar		
Digit and thumb	Cross-finger	Cross-finger	Reverse radial forearm (fascia ± skin)
	Reverse cross-finger	First dorsal metacarpal (fascia ± skin)	Groin pedicle
	Homodigital-retrograde	Local advancement	Epigastric pedicle
	Local advancement	Local transposition	Spare parts (free)
	Local transposition		Distal forearm (free)
			Scapular-parascapular (free)
			Foot webspace (free)
Hand, including first webspace	Local advancement	Posterior interosseous	Groin(pedicle or free)
	Local transposition	Reverse radial forearm (fascia ± skin)	Lateral arm (free)
		Reverse dorsal ulnar forearm(Becker)	Fascia + STSG or FTSG (free)*
		first dorsal metacarpal (fascia ± skin)	Reverse radial forearm (fascia ± skin)
		Fillet from amputated part	Omentum (free)
			Muscle (free)†
			Venous skin
			Dorsalis pedis (fascia ± skin)

Fascia donor site options are parietotemporal (superficial ± deep layers), scapular, anterolateral thigh, radial forearm, lateral arm, and thoracodorsal.

†Muscle donor site options are latissimus dorsi, rectus abdominus, serratus anterior, and gracilis.

FTSG, full-thickness skin graft STSG, split-thickness skin graft.

TABLE 58-3 Specific Free Tissue Transfers for Soft Tissue Coverage of the Upper Limb

Flap	Flap Size	Artery (diameter, mm)	Nerve	Common Use as Free Transfer	Frequency (1–5)
Muscle Flaps (+STSG, +skin)					
Latissimus dorsi	Large	Thoracodorsal (2.0–3.0)	None	Arm, shoulder (pedicle); forearm, wrist	3
Rectus abdominus	Large	Deep inferior epigastric (2.0–4.0)	None	Arm, forearm	1
Gracilis	Medium	Br. med. femoral circumflex (1.2–1.8)	None	Arm, forearm (as functional muscle.)	3
Serratus anterior	Medium	Descend. branch thoracodorsal (2.0–3.0)	None	Hand, wrist	1
Fasciocutaneous					
Radial forearm	Medium	Radial (2.0–3.5)	Med. antebr. cut. nerve Forearm	Thumb, digit, hand, forearm	5
Ulnar forearm	Medium	Ulnar (2.0–4.0)	Med. antebr. cut. nerve forearm	Hand	1
Posterior interosseous	Medium	Post. interosseous (1.0–2.0)	None	Hand (dorsum)	1 (mostly pedicled)
Lateral arm	Medium	Post. rad. collat. (1.5–2.0)	Lat. cut. n. arm	Hand(first webspace)	2
Medial arm	Medium	Branches of brachial (0.8–2.0)	Med. br. cut. n. forearm	Thumb, hand	1
Deltoid	Medium	Post. hum. circum. (1.5–3.0)	Lat. br. cut. nerve	Hand, forearm, elbow	1
Scapular/parascapular	Large	Br. circumflex scapular (2.5–3.5)	None	Wrist, forearm, elbow, arm	2
Anterolateral thigh	Very large	Descend. br. lat. fem. circumflex (2.0–3.0)	Lat. fem. cut. nerve	Hand, forearm, arm	3
Groin	Medium	Superficial circum. iliac (0.8–2.0)	None	Wrist, hand, forearm	5 (mostly pedicled)
Dorsalis pedis	Small	Dorsalis pedis (0.7–1.8)	Sens. br. peroneal nerve	Digits, thumb, hand	1
Toe webspace	Small	first dorsal metatarsal (1.0–1.7)	Sens. br. peroneal nerve	Digit, thumb	1
Medial plantar	Small	Med. plantar (0.8–1.3)	Sens. br. med. plantar nerve	Thumb, digit pulp	1
first dorsal metacarpal	Small	first dorsal metacarpal (0.7–1.2)	Sens. br. rad. nerve	Thumb, digit	1
Fascial (± STSG)					
Superficial temporal	Medium	Superficial temp. (1.5–2.5)	Auriculotemporal n.	Digit, thumb, hand	3
Radial forearm	Medium	Radial (2.0–3.5)	Med. antebr. cut. n. forearm	Digit, thumb, hand	4

(continued)

TABLE 58-3 Specific Free Tissue Transfers for Soft Tissue Coverage of the Upper Limb (Continued)

Flap	Flap Size	Artery (diameter, mm)	Nerve	Common Use as Free Transfer	Frequency (1–5)
Scapular	Large	Circumflex scapular (2.5–3.5)	None	Hand, wrist	2
Anterolateral thigh	Large	Descend. br. lat. fem. circum. (2.0–3.0)	None	Wrist, forearm, hand, elbow	1
Lateral arm	Medium	Post. rad. collat. (1.3–2.0)	Lat. cut. n. arm	Hand	1
Posterior calf	Medium	Medial sural (1.2–1.4)	Sural n.	Forearm, hand	1
Others					
Omentum	Very large	Right or left gastroepiploic (2.0–4.0)	None	Arm, elbow, forearm	1
Venous	Small	Superfic. veins forearm	Med. antebr. cut. nerve	Digit, thumb, hand(dorsum)	1

to cover wounds when amputated tissues are available. Tendons, bones, arteries, nerves, skin are often available as spare parts and should not be discarded until it has been determined that they cannot be used. These are opportunities to learn and to expand one's skill set. In the patient shown in Figure 58-1, resourceful microsurgeons were able to salvage a badly compromised hand by saving a spare part in an ice bath until transfer could be performed. Despite his other critical injuries, they were not deterred by his condition and were able to both revascularize a nonviable digit and to resurface both the dorsal and palmar surfaces of the hand with a dorsalis pedis "flow-though" flap and a split-thickness skin graft harvested from an amputated lower limb. The spare part was harvested from an amputated leg, and the revascularization was performed in the intensive care unit under regional block anesthesia the next day.

Upper extremity microsurgeons should be encouraged to learn and to use newer more refined techniques such as thenar flaps for fingertip coverage, fascial flaps for dorsal hand wounds, and regional vascular island transfers for digital losses instead of relying on standard options such as muscle plus skin graft or bulky musculocutaneous flaps. During the first few decades of free tissue transfer, the primary concern was placed on the basic viability and survival of these flaps. Now a high success rate is both expected and achieved, so more emphasis should be placed upon sensation, joint mobility, tendon gliding, surface contours, and color match. The age of refinement is here, and it is no longer acceptable to resurface a palm or digit with a bulky, insensate, hirsute piece of tissue.

PREPARATION OF THE RECIPIENT SITE

Adequate debridement begins with meticulous removal of all foreign material; all devitalized tissue, including muscle; and all unusable skeletal fragments to create a healthy wound. Sequential sharp knife dissection of all nonviable and suspect tissue is best done early. We prefer an early radical initial debridement in lieu of a "wait and see" approach, which entails multiple secondary debridements. Irreversibly injured nerves should be debrided and their proximal stumps tagged while potentially viable nerves, tendons, and skin are saved. Thrombosed major vessels are resected and vein grafted in the arm and forearm. Marginal tissue is best evaluated with the tourniquet released at the end of the procedure. Lavage should be copious but not too strong to contaminate or tumese uninjured tissue planes. Repeat debridement at 24- to 48-hour intervals should be used until the entire zone of injury is ready for appropriate coverage. The suction vacuum-assisted closure (VAC) drainage system has become invaluable for temporary coverage. The major potential disadvantage is the desiccation of underlying soft tissue and bone, which should preferably be covered with local tissue. Potential recipient vessels and nerves are carefully left undisturbed outside the zone of injury. Definitive early skeletal fixation is preferred in lieu of temporary external fixation.

The preparation of both donor and recipient vascular pedicles before transfer is critical. Dissection must be preferably sharp and atraumatic. *All uninjured skeletal and soft tissue planes and structures should be respected!* In academic teaching environments, this is where the experienced attending physician should directly control the dissection because most technical mistakes occur here. Vessels with diameters of less than 1.0 mm are most vulnerable because they can be misidentified, stretched, cut, or avulsed during a quick, aggressive dissection. This is the point in the operation where an experienced surgeon slows down, eliminates all extrinsic noise and chatter, relaxes into a comfortable posture, and focuses completely on the dissection.

Flap Inset

Some caveats are involved in the inset of small free flaps within the hand distal to the wrist. Because the defects are usually small and precisely defined, a careful template must be made of the recipient site, and the flap should not exceed the template in size more than 2.0 to 3.0 mm in any dimension. Direct vertical incisions of the skin surfaces facilitate an everted skin closure. Subcuticular techniques are preferred on the dorsal surfaces. Fascial flaps and thin muscles should be advanced and secured below the adjacent recipient skin and skin grafts sutured directly and not overlapped. When long pedicles are used to larger recipient vessels such as the radial or ulnar arteries at the wrist level, the intervening tunnel must be more than capacious to avoid any kinking or twisting of the axial artery or the venae comitantes.

MONITORING

There is no ideal, flawless monitoring system, and over the past 40 years, many imaginative approaches have been used. Clinical examination of the flap and Doppler monitoring are most important. We no longer use implantable systems. Surface laser Doppler monitoring systems are a helpful adjunct to clinical appearance. Fluorescein has been used effectively. A pulse oximeter is used to monitor all toe transfers.

Full anticoagulation has many potential problems, all of which we have experienced over the past 40 years. We routinely use aspirin and low-dose heparin for hospitalized adults. More extensive anticoagulation is reserved for individual clinical circumstances such as with irradiated vessels, a known coagulopathy, vasculitis, an extensive zone of trauma, peripheral vascular disease within the upper limb, or a smoker with poor recipient vessels. Flaps to the limb have been lost when the Doppler was placed over the recipient vessel, not the vessel beneath the flap following an end-to-side anastomosis. Excessive reliance on monitoring devices is best avoided by always correlating with the clinical examination.

COMPLICATIONS

Mishaps are classified as early and late and fortunately during the past decade have become less frequent, and elective flap coverage should have a success (viability) rate well above 95%. The majority of technical problems with the dissection, vascular anastomoses, flap inset, or positioning are recognized before the operation has ended, and the vast majority of the remaining problems occur within the next 36 hours. These problems include swelling, vessel kinking, pedicle obstruction, bleeding, constrictive dressings, lack of immobilization, inappropriate medication, and mishaps during patient transport, among others.

Attention to detail makes a difference and ideally has been an integral part of the preoperative preparation. Donor sites should be closed or covered and properly immobilized. There may always be unknown clinical conditions that may contribute to flap failure. For example, we discovered homocystinuria to be the cause of thrombosis in an elective great toe transfer in a young boy and an unknown von Willebrand trait to account for repeated hematoma in a child after a large latissimus dorsi transfer to the lower extremity.

The etiology of wound dehiscence and subsequent infection can be multifactorial but will usually funnel down to lack of preparation, patient cooperation, or patient disease. Disruption of the wound invariably precedes secondary infection unless the initial wound was grossly contaminated.

Late complications such as tendon adherence, wound contracture, joint immobility, poor sensory return, and limited function are not usually related to the type or amount of flap coverage unless it has been inadequate.

THE DORSAL AND PALMAR SURFACES OF THE DIGITS AND THUMB

The normal characteristics of these skin surfaces are varied. On the dorsal surface, the ungual appendage consists of a specialized germinal and sterile nail matrix and a nail plate surrounded by nail folds and supported by a broad distal phalanx and attendant interosseous ligaments. Proximal to the nail, the dorsal skin is soft, pliable, mobile, and hirsute. It stretches easily with digital flexion and bunches like an accordion over the joint spaces with extension. In contrast, the palmar surfaces are covered with thick, glabrous skin with a notable, high-friction coefficient that limits sheer forces. The ridges of the fingertip, which comprise the "fingerprint," reinforce surface stability as do the fibrous septae, which give structure to the pulp tissue and connect the dermis to the periosteum of the distal phalanx. Additional stability of the palmar skin is provided by the dense fibrous system on either side of the neurovascular bundles (Cleland ligaments dorsal and Grayson ligaments palmar), which separate these two types of skin. The density of mechanoreceptors within the glabrous skin of the fingertip is one of the highest in the human body. It is impossible to replace these characteristics with distant or pedicled free tissue transfers. Only composite toe transfers with similar skin contain tissue with similar characteristics.

Many options for coverage of the digit and thumb are available. Some are very practical such as the skin graft, and some are quite esoteric and difficult such as the free fascial flap plus a full-thickness skin graft (Table 58-2). The major indication for free tissue transfer is usually a large defect involving multiple digits or an entire thumb. Smaller defects are usually covered with local or regional tissue. The ideal coverage situation is the traumatic injury to the hand with one or more spare parts. Here similar tissue can be placed into the recipient defect, sensation can be restored, and motion can be regained within a critical period of time. The injured carpenter shown in Figure 58-2 is a prime example. He injured or partially amputated three digits and a thumb in zone II. Border digits are normally expendable in most patients, and in this man, the index was revascularized and used several weeks later as an island transfer to reconstruct the deficient thumb. An immediate free tissue transfer was used to reconstruct a new first web space. The long-term outcome was spectacular. The most important caveats in this case were (1) to work well outside the original zone of injury for both the proximal and distal vascular anastomoses and nerve junctures and (2) to make the flap slightly larger than a precise template. The optimal vessels here were those on the injured side of the digit. Large dorsal recipient veins were present at the metacarpophalangeal (MCP) joint level. If no veins were present, we would have used a pedicled vein from an adjacent digit. The flap inset involved

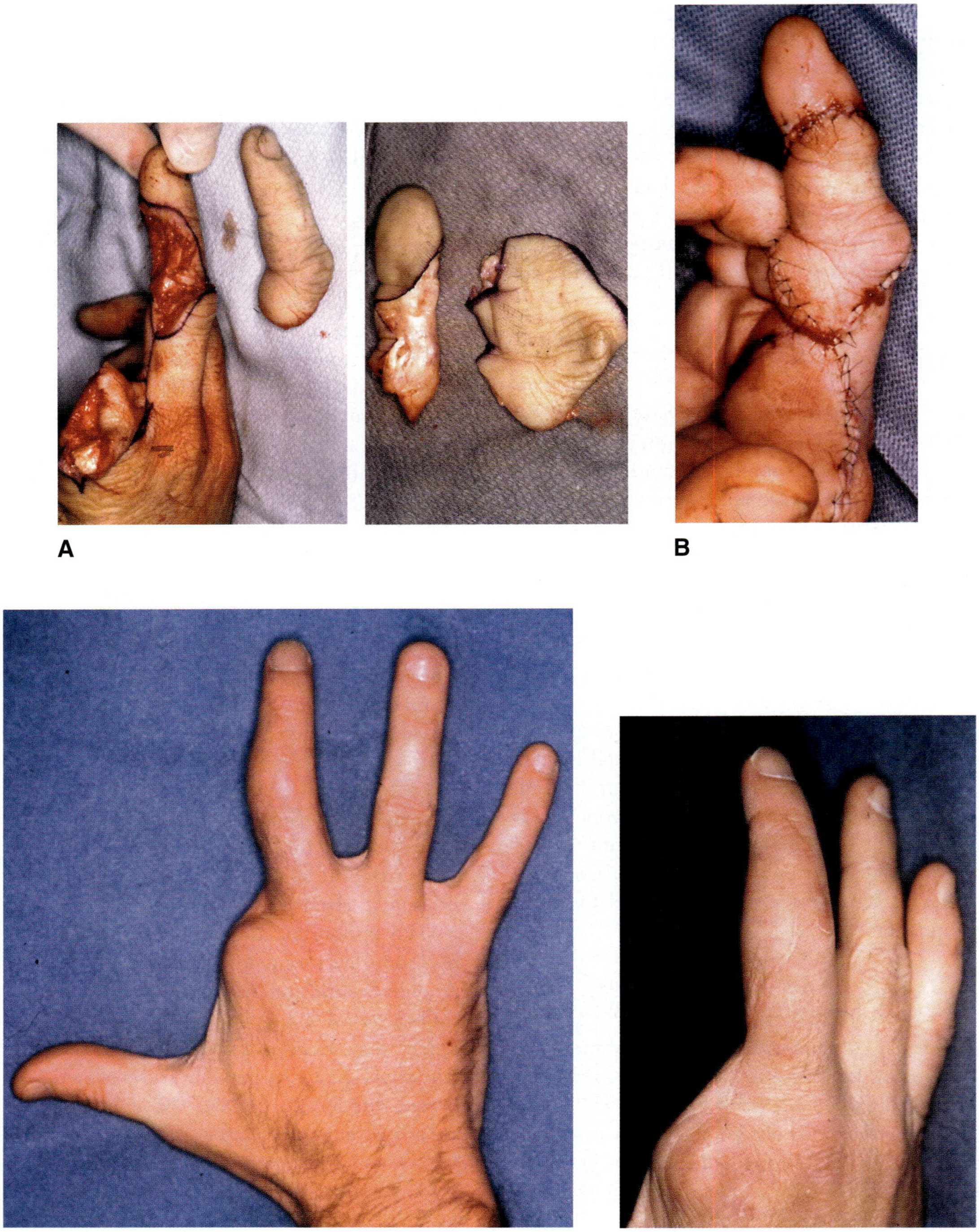

FIGURE 58-2 Amputated "spare part." (A) A skill saw injury of this carpenter resulted in amputation of the index finger and loss of all soft tissue on the radial side of the long finger. The needed composite tissue, including the neurovascular bundle, has been harvested from the amputated part. (B) Appearance after flow-through revascularization and neural junctures. (C) Appearance 17 years later. (D) Glabrous and now glabrous soft tissues have conformed well.

some cut-back incisions to avoid palmar contracture with time. Performed 30 years ago, this flap was monitored by physical examination and Doppler flow. Baby aspirin (81 mg) was given daily. The patient returned to work within 5 weeks and still works as a master carpenter. If reattached, the index finger would have been both stiff and hypersensitive in the cold climate, and the patient would have "neglected" this digit. Clinical experience has demonstrated that this assumption made 30 years ago was correct.

After severe and complicated injuries, we encourage distal digital and thumb replantation and the reattachment of composite parts such as segments of pulp or portions of nail matrices. The long-term outcome in the patient shown in Figure 58-3 with a mangled hand injury was quite predictable. The reattached fingertip, bone, tendon, and ligaments were well vascularized and functioned well in the long term. However, the joint cartilage of the fifth digit eroded, and the secondary arthritis was replaced with a silicone implant, which has broken twice because of her forceful flexion. However, the position and flexion of the slightly shortened digit has remained, and power flexion remains strong for almost 3 decades.

Homodigital and heterodigital island flaps should be used more frequently for reconstruction of glabrous pulp and dorsal skin surfaces. These regional flaps avoid the problems attendant with prolonged immobilization and joint stiffness seen with more traditional cross-finger techniques. Unfortunately, these techniques are beyond the comfort zone and skill set of most hand surgeons. The major disadvantage with island flap transfers is the venous congestion that may occur after unnecessary stripping of the neurovascular bundle. These are technically demanding dissections during which all soft tissue attached to the neurovascular bundle should remain intact and the vascular structures not skeletonized (Figure 58-4). The donor site defects will close remarkably well with dorsal skin advancement, and the need for grafts is much less than expected. In the patient shown in Figure 58-4, an extensor mechanism was reconstructed with a tendon graft and physiologic coverage was completed with a reverse radial forearm fascial flap covered with a skin graft in

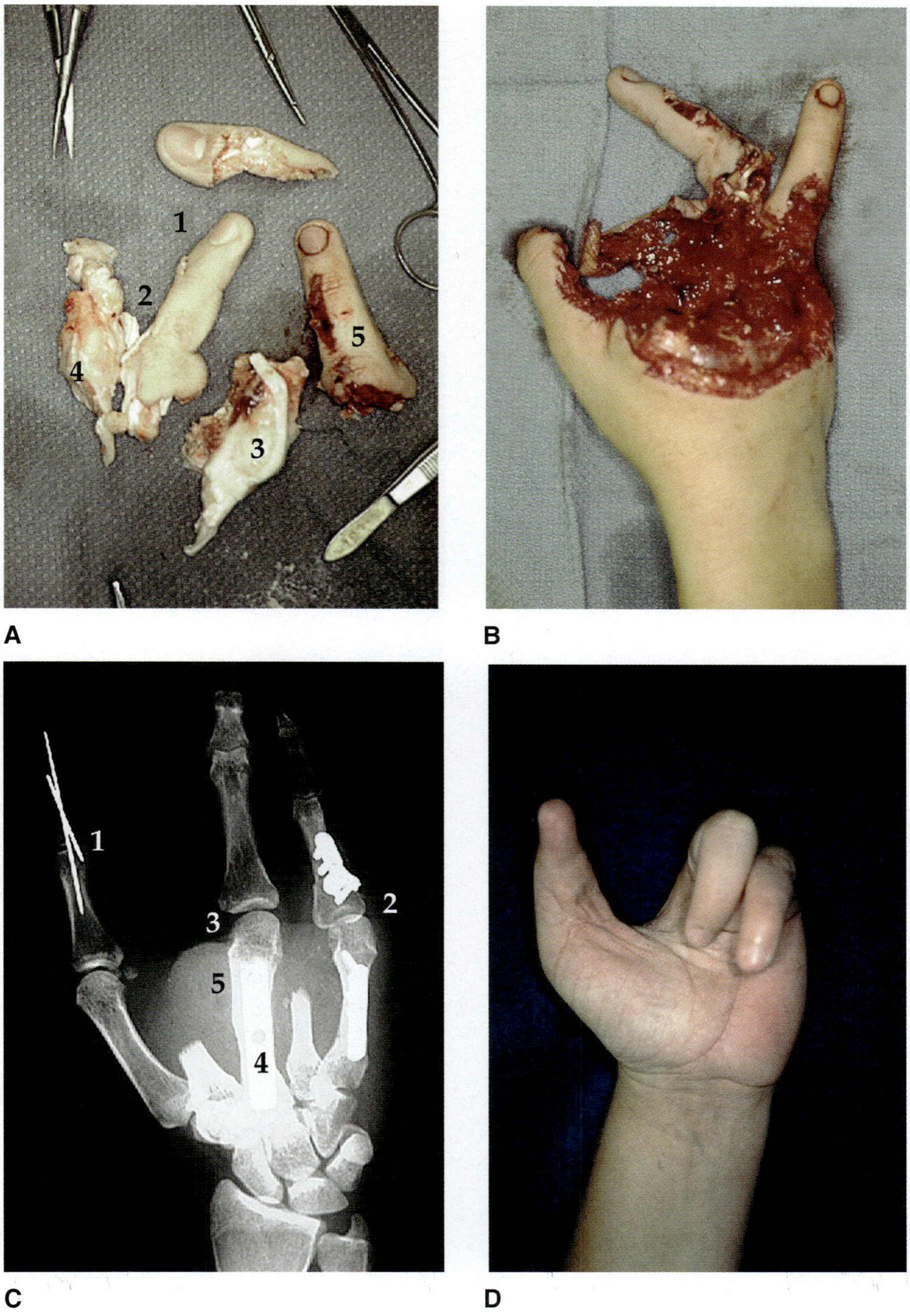

FIGURE 58-3 Vascularized and nonvascularized "spare parts." (**A**) Multiple skeletal and soft tissue pieces, including composite portions of the fingers and thumb, remain after debridement. (**B**) Appearance of the hand after a band saw accident. (**C**) Reattachment of parts included (1) replant of index tip to thumb, (2) vascularized index proximal interphalangeal joint to fifth metacarpophalangeal (MCP) joint, (3) extensor tendon for collateral ligament reconstruction, (4) intercalated bone graft for ring digit reattached onto proximal long metacarpal, and (5) replant of amputated ring finger in long position. (**D**) Flexion 5 years later.

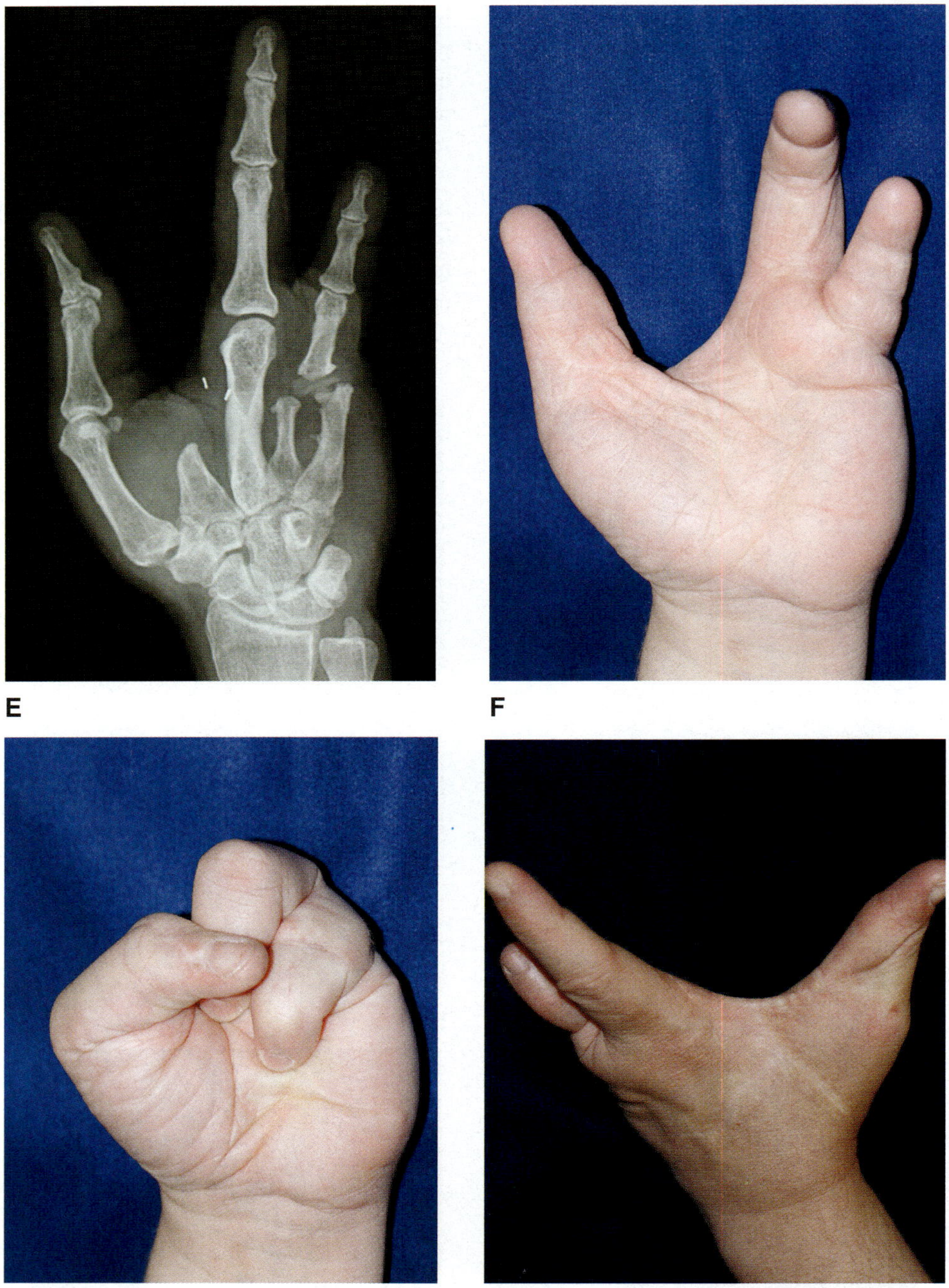

E F G H

FIGURE 58-3 (*Continued*) (E) The reattached thumb and long digits survived. The vascularized MCP joint of the fifth digit collapsed and was replaced by a silicone implant, which has broken twice but functioned well as a spacer. (F) to (H). Flexion, extension, and soft tissue contour have remained functional at 25-year follow-up. The patient recently retired after 38 years with the same machine shop.

a single stage. The portion of the neurovascular pedicle to be tunneled subcutaneously was carefully reduced in bulk.

COVERAGE OF THE DORSAL SURFACES OF THE DIGITS AND THUMB

The requirements on the dorsal surfaces are similar, but the presence of sensation is not an absolute goal. Distally, there is no substitute for a missing ungual appendage, which can only be replaced with the reattachment of an amputated part, a spare part, or a vascularized toe transfer. The germinal and sterile nail matrices and the paronychial and eponychial folds are intricate structures that are not easily reconstructed, if at all. Free matrix grafts have not gained wide acceptance as predictable procedures over the past several decades.

Skin grafts initially suffice for dorsal digit and thumb coverage, but these grafts will contract, easily adhere to underlying structures, and may fissure and ulcerate with repetitive surface torque stress. Secondary procedures are frequently required after most crush injuries, all severe avulsion injuries, and especially after difficult fractures or loss of the underlying skeleton. Full-thickness skin coverage is preferred if secondary surgery is anticipated. When the remainder of the digit or thumb is uninjured, small distal dorsal defects can be covered by homodigital

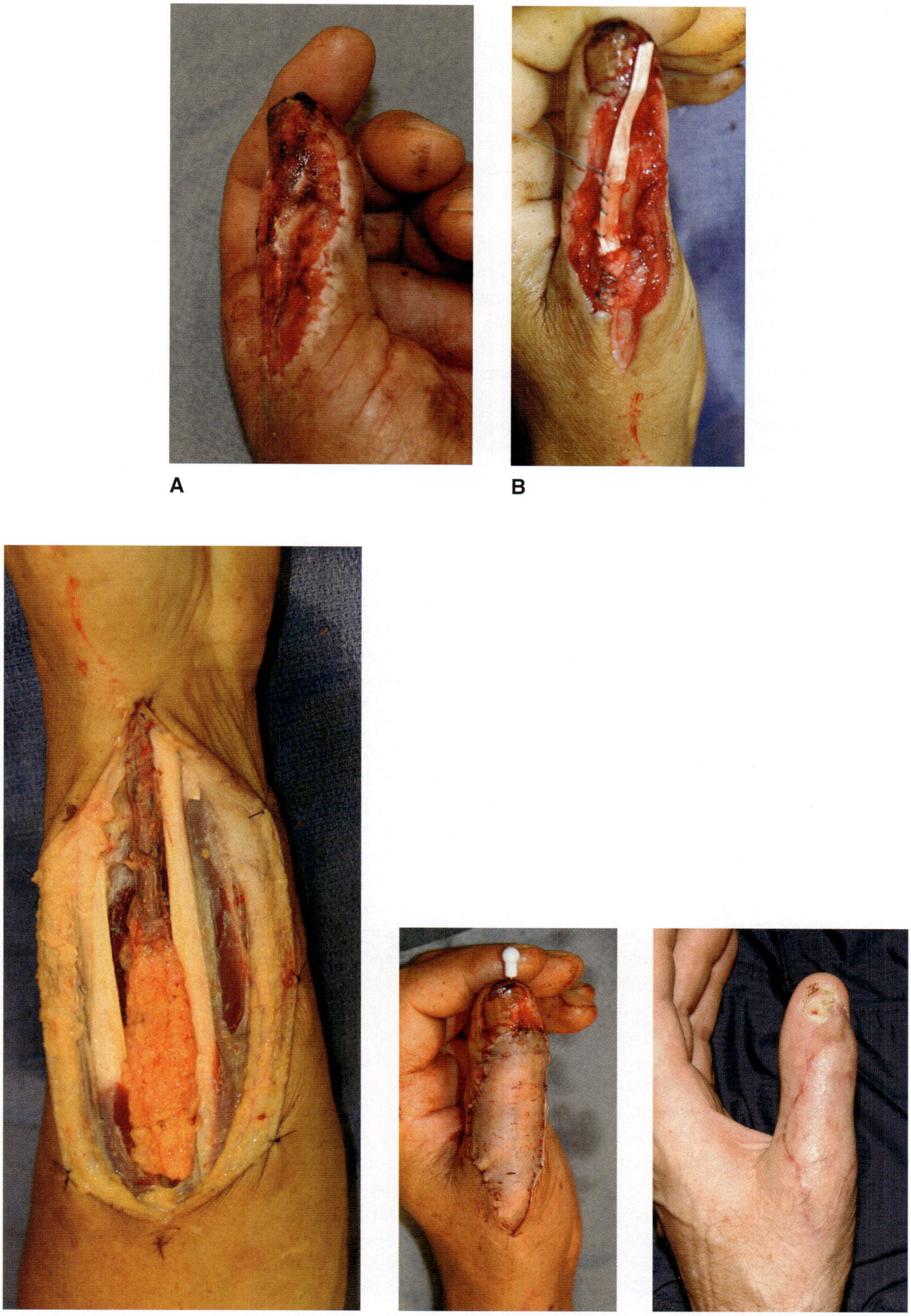

A B C D

FIGURE 58-4 Reverse radial forearm fascial flap to the thumb. (A) After an industrial roller injury, there is loss of full-thickness skin, extensor mechanism, and dorsal joint surface. (B) Primary extensor tendon graft. (C) Forearm fascia plus one layer of fat has been harvested as an island flap based distally on the radial artery. (D) Appearance after transfer, inset, and skin graft coverage at surgery and 6 weeks later.

reverse island flaps harvested from the side of the digit or with full-thickness skin grafts. For larger defects, we have used radial forearm fascial flaps with or without skin, which have been tunneled through the dorsal metacarpal space. These techniques are quick, are easy to dissect and transfer, and provide a robust blood supply to what usually is a badly injured digit or thumb. This is much less disfiguring than the local rotation of all available dorsal skin based on one side of the digit (Kutler) or thumb ("hatchet" flap).

Thin fasciocutaneous flaps or fascial flaps covered with skin grafts are ideal for these areas but may not be practical. When multiple digits or large areas are injured, transfer of a large amount of tissue with secondary digital separation and debulking is very effective and very predicable but labor intensive (see Figure 58-11). We prefer the radial forearm arterial system over the posterior interosseous arterial system because dissection is easier but have used the latter when it was not wise to compromise the radial artery. The ulnar artery is the main arterial conduit to the hand and should not be sacrificed for reverse island flap coverage in the hand. The use of its dorsal cutaneous branches has been effective for coverage at the wrist and metacarpal level.

Occasionally, a patient will present after all local options to cover an open ulcerated wound have failed (see Table 58-2). Amputation has been recommended, and the patient or family (pediatric patient) wishes to salvage the injured digit(s) or thumb. Often the MCP and proximal interphalangeal (PIP) joints are exposed; the extensor mechanism has been lost. The zone of injury often includes the metacarpal portion of the hand. In these cases, a small, thin, pliable flap with a long vascular pedicle is needed. Local and regional flap and occasionally distant pedicle options have been expended. In choosing and performing a free tissue transfer, it is important not to create additional donor or recipient site morbidity.

Free tissue transfer can be a good option when more traditional techniques fail. The patient shown in Figure 58-5 presented 1 year after a severe crush injury to his entire hand with loss of tissue on three digits. After a series of procedures, including two skin grafts, two local flaps, and a multistaged groin flap, the patient presented with no dorsal skin on the long finger and osteomyelitis. Several days before the flap transfer, a wide debridement included all infected bone, soft tissue, and pins and wires. The required portion of thin, volar forearm skin was harvested from the opposite radial forearm on a long pedicle devoid of all subcutaneous fat and areolar connective tissue. The dissection on the dorsum of the hand extended only to harvest one large dorsal vein.

The pedicle was passed through the intermetacarpal space to Guyon's canal, where recipient vessels were tortuous but uninjured. An end-to-side arterial anastomosis and two separate venous anastomoses involving two different drainage systems were performed. The major difficulty in this patient was to adequately debride his infected PIP joint and to keep it stabilized for 3 months after surgery. He regained excellent functional use because of the intact, sensate palmar skin. In this man, it was important not to redissect tissues that had taken months to heal and not to disturb his thumb, first web space, and index ray. Technical caveats included aggressive prior debridement, a wide tunnel for a thin pedicle, stable plate fixation for the PIP joint, complete inset of flap edges, and coverage with the thinnest fasciocutaneous flap available. The amount of tissue needed here was very small and the opposite radial forearm was an ideal donor site with minimal, if any morbidity.

Other free tissue transfers have been less commonly used. The most consistent, in our experience, has been the temporoparietal fascial flap (TPFF) covered with a nonglabrous thick skin graft for dorsal surfaces and a hypothenar (hand) or foot instep graft for palmar surfaces. Large pedicle groin flaps or other fasciocutaneous transfers are reserved for larger defects after electrical burns, thermal burns, major degloving injuries, and mangled wounds after farm accidents or animal maulings.

Fascial flaps, either pedicled or free, are very effectively used in the thumb and digits. They are particularly effective for resurfacing along the sides of the digits or thumb, the entire dorsal surface, and at times the palmar surfaces. These flaps are thin and mobile and can be fashioned precisely to fit the defect. They are preferably covered with thick split-skin grafts or full-thickness grafts. Glabrous skin grafts from the hypothenar region or from the instep of the foot are the best substitutes for the palmar surfaces. They are well worth the extra effort because the alternative grafts would be hyperpigmented, dry, and fissured surfaces of nonglabrous skin.

Fascial flaps as free transfers have become much less popular and expeditious for several reasons. The dissection of TPFFs is tedious and difficult and may present anomalous venous anatomy. The pedicled first or second dorsal interosseous flaps with or without dorsal skin are very effective for proximal digital and thumb defects, and the distally based radial artery forearm fascial flap easily covers all surfaces of the thumb and the proximal half of the digits (see Figure 58-4). However, the TPFFs often provide a simple solution for a small, irregular defect at the digital level. In contrast to local fascial flaps, the TPFF surface is thicker and can be used to reconstruct pulleys and the dorsal retinaculum if needed. It can be split between the frontal (anterior) and posterior (parietal) branches to cover two digits and their intradigital commissure. In the complicated reconstructive case shown in Figure 58-6, the TPFF was split and used to add bulk to both syndactylized digits, which had been lengthened and bone grafted while they were joined together. The grafts on the surface of the fascial flaps have contoured well, and the color match of the carefully selected skin is quite satisfactory. As with other free flaps a careful inset below the adjacent normal skin was performed and full-thickness grafts used for final coverage.

Radial forearm fascia as a free transfer is very effective when local tissue is not practical. The best recipient vessels are the princeps pollicis artery on the ulnar side of the thumb metacarpal, radial artery at the wrist, and occasionally common digital vessels within the palm. Fascial flaps may be more difficult to monitor, and impending problems, especially on the venous side of the circulation, may not be recognized early. There are very few outcome studies of fascial flaps. Our experience is that they are superior because they do not contract as much as grafted wounds, are thin and pliable, permit tendon gliding and joint mobility, rarely require debulking, and can be contoured

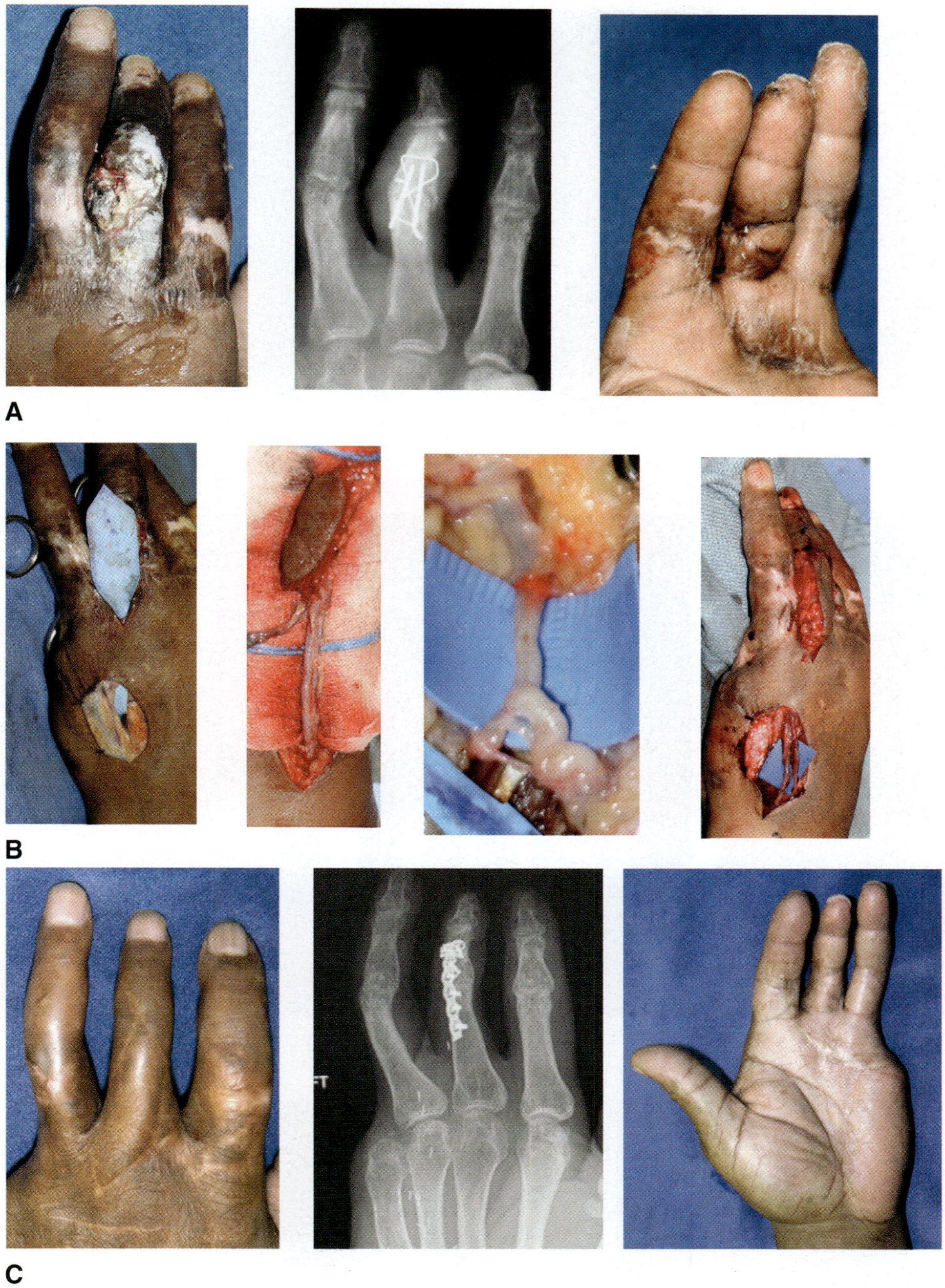

FIGURE 58-5 Radial forearm fasciocutaneous flap to digit. (**A**) Dorsal skin loss of the left long finger with secondary osteomyelitis after failed attempts for dorsal skin coverage after a severe crush injury. (**B**) The template was transferred to the contralateral forearm, where a small radial forearm flap with a long pedicle was harvested. Venous anastomosis to a large dorsal vein and end-to-side arterial anastomosis to the ulnar artery within Guyon's canal. (**C**) Twelve years later with stable dorsal coverage and a solid arthrodesis of the long finger proximal interphalangeal joint.

to create interdigital web spaces. Conversely, they require technical expertise and attention to detail.

COVERAGE OF THE PALMAR SURFACE OF THE DIGITS AND THUMB

The choices here depend on the size and location of the defect. Sensation is a key ingredient. Glabrous skin, which is only available from another digit, palmar surface, or sole of the foot, is at a premium. The quality of neural regeneration is age dependent and not always predictable. Both split- and full-thickness skin grafts taken from other regions of the body are not preferred in the long run because of hyperpigmentation, crusting, and fissuring of the nonlubricated epidermal surfaces.

Many individual local flaps are very effective for the finger and thumb pulp surfaces, provided that they are sensate, surfaced with glabrous skin, and ideally anchored to underlying bone. We prefer the use of local pulp rotational flaps (Littler), palmar V-to-Y advancement flaps (Tranquilli-Leali, Atasoy-Kleinert), and palmar advancement with glabrous skin graft (Hueston) flaps. A more extensive advancement flap (Moberg) is not used because this requires extensive dissection and often

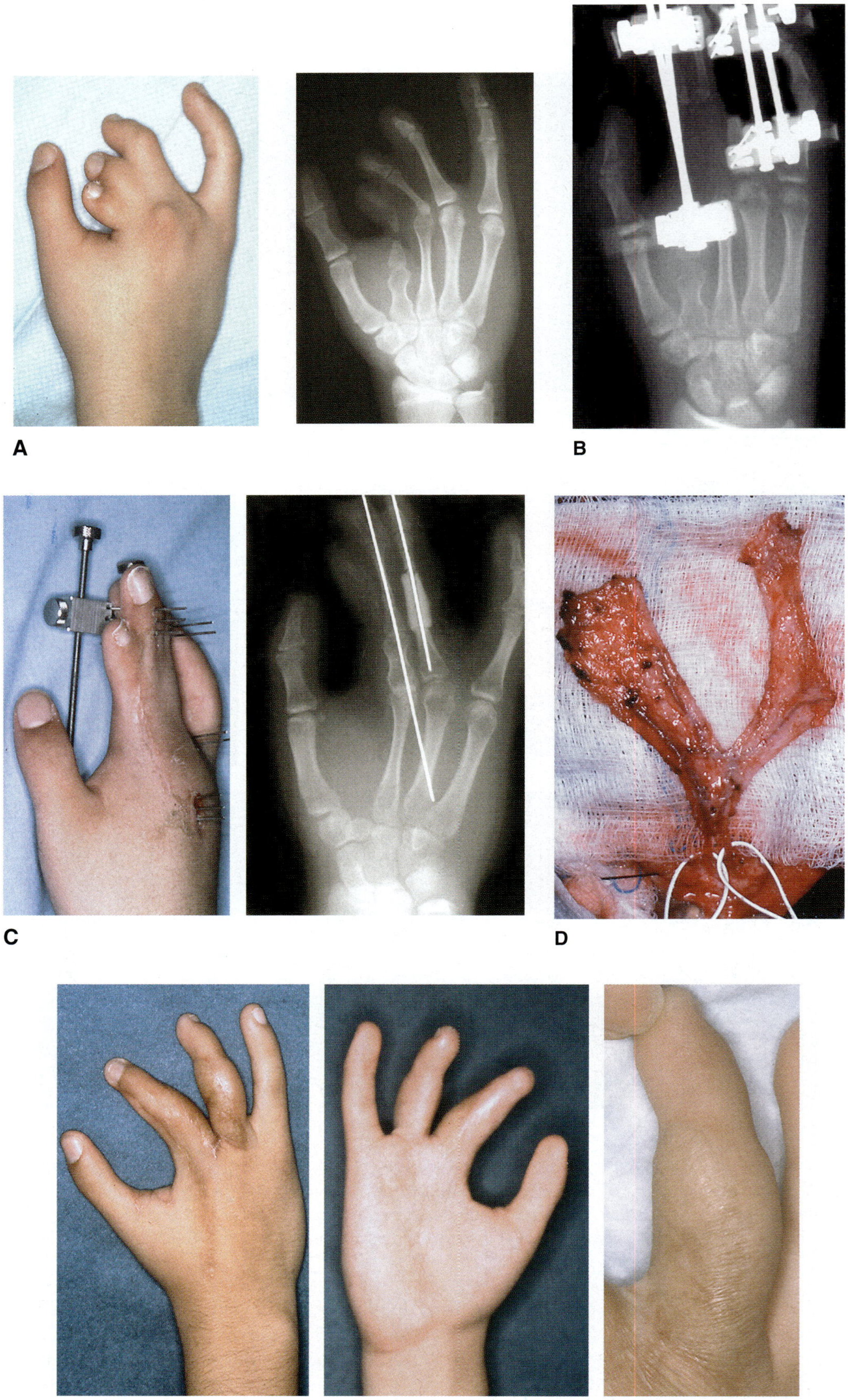

FIGURE 58-6 Split temporoparietal fascial flap (TPFF). (**A**) The clinical appearance and radiograph of the right hand symbrachydactyly in a teenage girl. The central three rays are primarily deficient. (**B**) Skeletal distraction followed disarticulation of the long digit at the metacarpophalangeal level and osteotomy of the proximal phalanx of the ring ray. (**C**) The index metacarpal and proximal phalanx is used to fill the intercalated gap on the long ray and a demineralized bone graft for the ring ray. (**D**) A split TPFF harvested on the superficial temporal vessels is wrapped around the digits at the time of syndactyly release and skin grafting. (**E**) Appearance 21 years later. The first web space was also widened with local flaps.

results in vascular compromise to the dorsal skin surface and a secondary interphalangeal joint flexion contracture.

Cross-finger pedicled transfers are very useful for smaller defects despite the potential morbidity of joint stiffness and contracture. These local flaps get tissue where it is needed. We prefer to harvest skin from the sides of adjacent digits whenever possible and use temporary pins to ensure stability of adjacent digits. Reversed homodigital flaps are very effective yet delicate procedures for pulp coverage and can be used in the emergency setting. The patient shown in Figure 58-7 sustained a sharp avulsion of this specialized palmar pulp tissue with a very limited zone of trauma. With uninjured MCP and PIP joints and intact collateral blood flow through the vincular system, he was a good candidate for this relatively new procedure. Recovery was quicker in this healthy boy than in an older adult. He returned to his job on a luxury boat within 6 weeks.

For major subtotal loss of the thumb or digit from the midportion of the metacarpal to the interphalangeal joint, toe transfer or digital transposition from another ray of the same hand are preferred. Unfortunately, these are major microvascular procedures, which are not available in all medical centers or within all hand services, which do not have plastic surgeons on the hand faculty.

The creative use of local tissue harvested from either the palmar surface or the side of adjacent digits can be quite effective for palmar coverage. The ulnar side of the thumb and fifth digit and the radial surface of the index, long, and ring digits have a much higher priority for tip-to-tip and pinching functions and

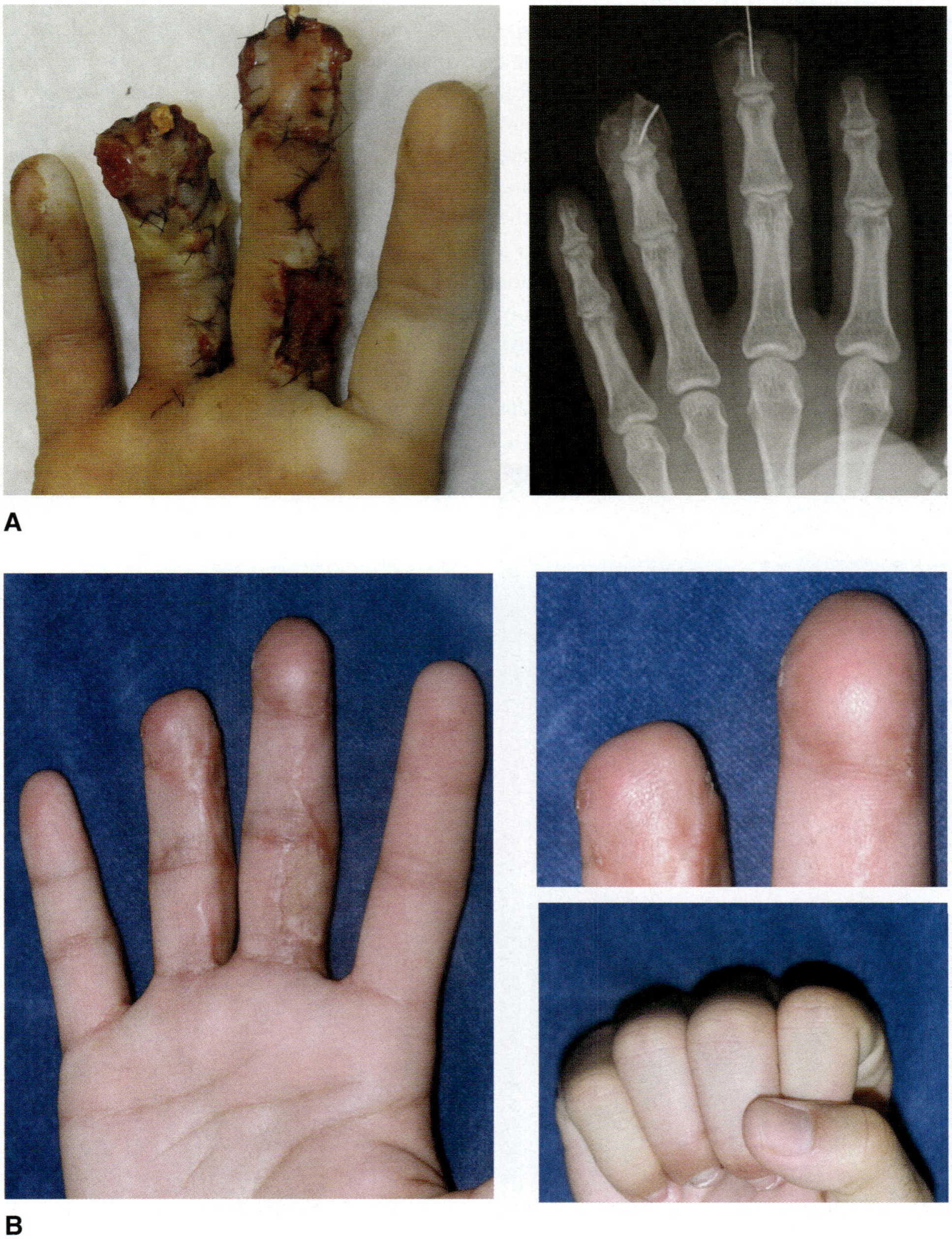

FIGURE 58-7 Homodigital island flap. (**A**) Glabrous pulp tissue on the long and ring digits was lost in a wench on a luxury sailing vessel. Only the tufts of the distal phalanges were lost. An island flap from the same digit (homodigital) was transferred from the radial side of the long digit and a local advancement for the ring within days of the injury. (**B**) Well-healed and contoured pulp surfaces within 6 weeks.

should not be used in contrast to the ulnar sides of the index, long, and ring digits. Rotation of sensate skin from one side of a fingertip to another may provide a very simple, effective solution. The major advantages are that it is easy and safe, and the disadvantage is the instability created by sectioning the fibrous septae, which anchor the pulp and skin to the distal phalanx.

A sensory nerve transfer from an intact dorsal (radial innervated) sensory nerve to a palmar digital nerve after a high median nerve injury may be all that is needed to provide protective sensation in an otherwise intact digit or thumb. The hypothenar eminence is an excellent and very underused source of glabrous skin. A large ellipse of full-thickness tissue can be harvested, and a much larger segment of split-thickness skin is available. We have used this donor site for decades in patients with Dupuytren contracture with large glabrous deficits after resection of dense fasciodermal disease (see Figure 58-10B).

There are several caveats in regard to the local transfer of tissue between digits. Hair-bearing dorsal tissue does not belong on the palmar surface of fingertips. A good alternative is a local fascial flap covered with a hypothenar graft. In multidigit (and thumb) mangled injuries, specialized glabrous skin as a "spare part" is often neglected either as a free transfer or a simple graft. Over the years, we have learned to harvest these flaps from the sides of the digits as either a regional cross-finger flap or as a neurovascular island transfer. Skin grafts coverage of these donor sites is very well tolerated (see Figure 58-7). The design of any cross-finger transposition flap for resurfacing should always respect incision placement and avoid the creation of any scar perpendicular to the flexion creases. Secondary contractures are inevitable in these hands. In children, midlateral incisions often migrate palmar with growth and eventually become the source of a flexion contracture. High midaxial incisions are preferred along the side of the digit at the juncture between the palmar, glabrous, and dorsal, hirsute skin surfaces. When local tissue transfers are being considered, potential morbidity to the donor digit is a prime consideration. The long rehabilitation and joint stiffness after a cross-finger flap in an adult may be as disabling as the original injury. However, this alternative is worth consideration if it provides the optimal functional outcome.

The transfer of more proximal portions of a digit or thumb to the fingertip level as a reverse *homodigital flap* has gained popularity but needs refinement (see Figure 58-7). As long as the vascular pedicle to the tissue being transferred is connected to the intact digital system on the opposite side of the digit, these transfers will survive. As with all vascular island flaps, venous congestion may become problematic. Incisions must be planned correctly, and plenty of room for postoperative swelling must be provided. The lateral side of the digit or thumb is the best donor region.

One of the best replacements for the palmar surface of the thumb is the *heterodigital island* transfer of glabrous skin from the ulnar side of the long digit (Figures 58-8 and 58-9). When the recipient site is large, skin should be harvested along the entire side and ulnar half of the fingertip and the donor defect closed with dorsal skin advancement and a hypothenar skin graft from the glabrous surface. The patient illustrated in Figure 58-8 was destitute because he only had one hand, in which the thumb was involved by a large, ulcerating arteriovenous malformation

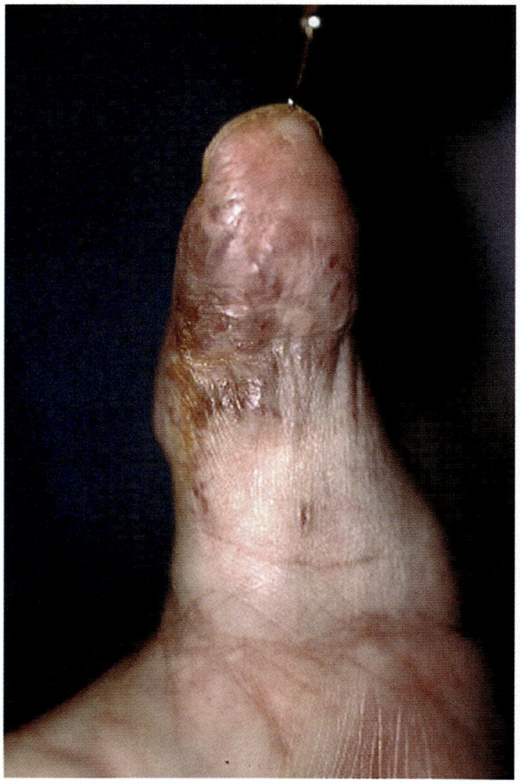

A

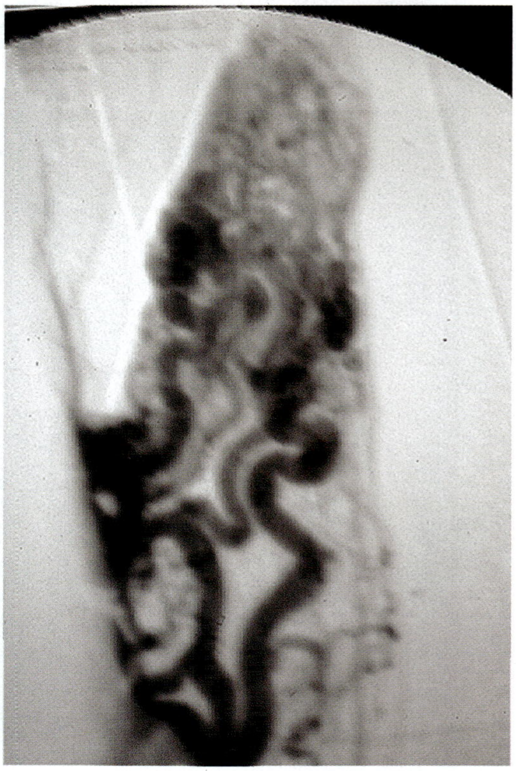

B

FIGURE 58-8 Heterodigital island transfer to thumb. (A) Since childhood, this man had an irritating, pulsatile thumb, which was the source of significant bleeding. (B) Angiogram shows an arteriovenous malformation with arteriovenous fistulas.

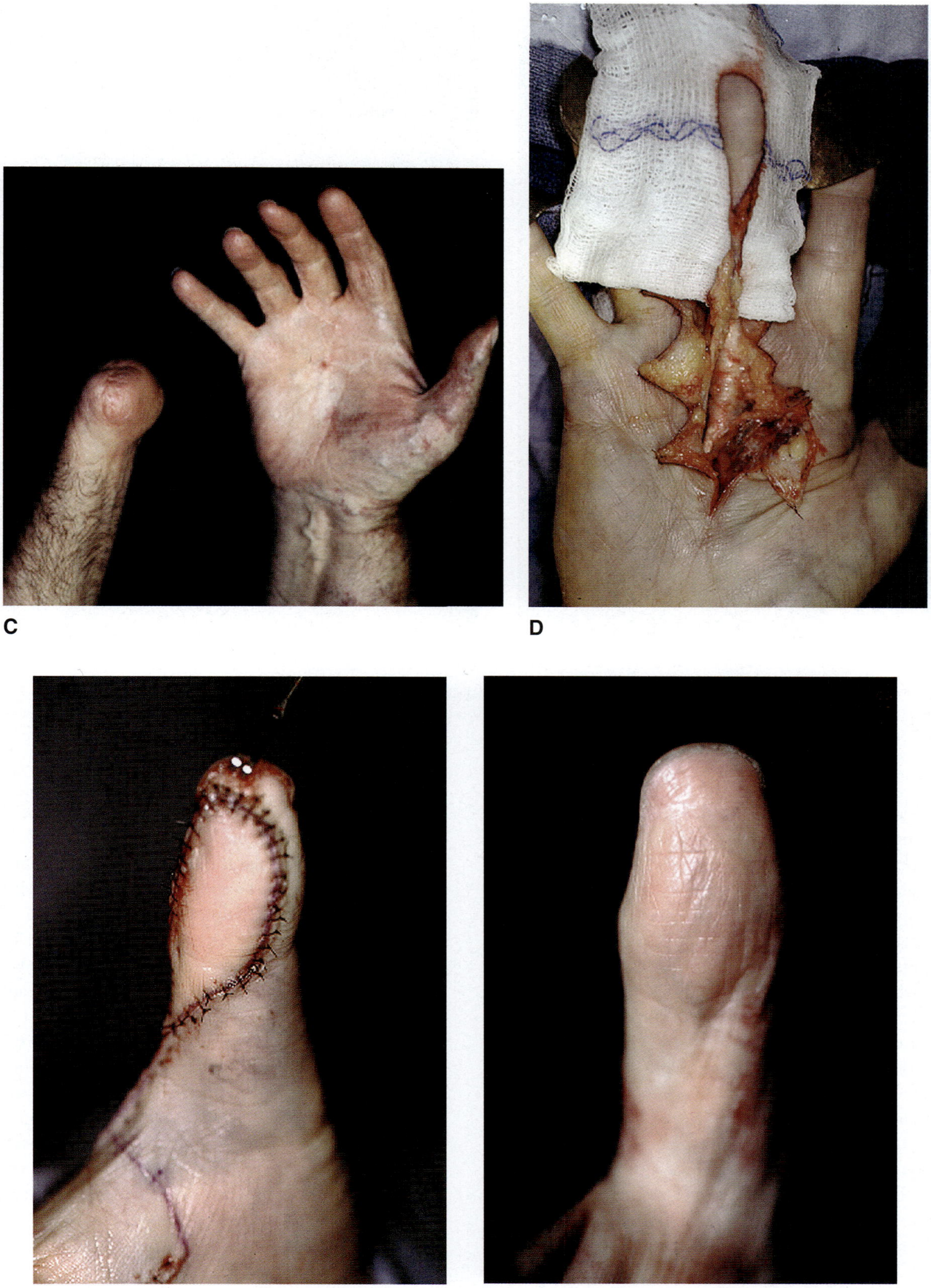

C D E F

FIGURE 58-8 (*Continued*) (**C**) There was a congenital transverse absence of the opposite hand. (**D**) Heterodigital island flap harvested from the ulnar side of the long digit. (**E**) Inset onto the entire ulnar pulp surface of the thumb. (**F**) The glabrous pulp surfaces contour well with very little scarring in contrast to nonglabrous tissue. The thumb is seen 17 years after surgery.

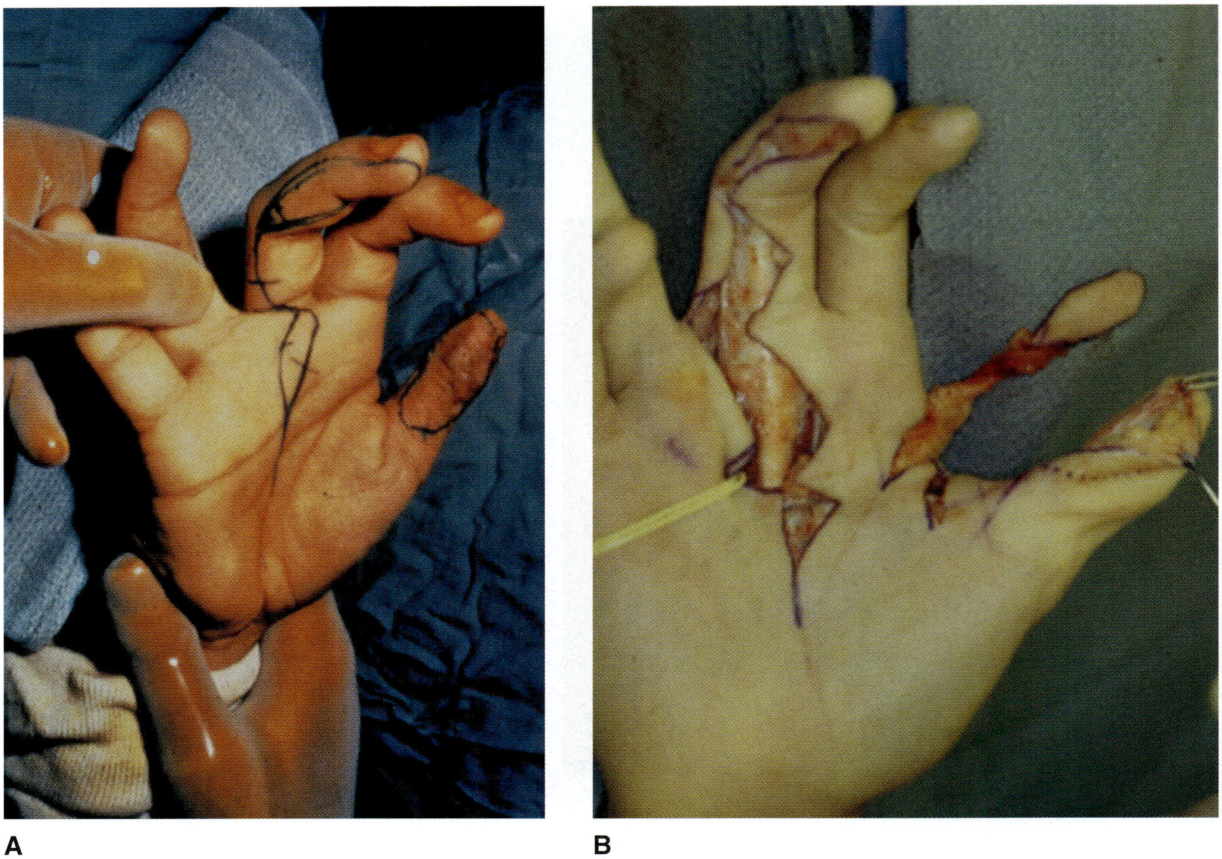

FIGURE 58-9 Island heterodigital flap transfer. (**A**) The entire ulnar surface of the digit can be used to resurface the entire pulp of the thumb. The originator of this procedure, J. William Littler, MD, wears the brown gloves here. (**B**) Pivot point of the flap is at the level of the superficial palmar arch. Kinking must be avoided.

with arteriovenous fistulas. The accumulated blood loss from his bleeding was significant. He could not tolerate ablation of his only thumb. This transfer was a simple, practical solution to a significant problem. The major technical drawback with these island transfers is venous congestion, and the primary functional problem is that the patient perceives the sensation in the donor finger instead of the thumb. This sensory "disconnect" can be obviated by coaptation of the ulnar digital nerve within the pedicle to the ulnar digital nerve of the thumb at the time of transfer or at a later date.

Another infrequently considered source of tissue is the dorsum of the hand based on the *dorsal metacarpal arterial system*. The anatomy is similar to that of the foot. Fascia with or without skin can be pedicled on the dorsal metacarpal vessels connecting to the deep palmar arches. This concept originated with the "flag" flap from the dorsal surface of the index proximal phalanx to the thumb as a pedicled transfer and has been expanded to the retrograde transfer of fascial tissue from the metacarpal level to the base of the digit or thumb. In the original "flag" operation, tissue from the dorsal surface of the index ray was transferred to the palmar surface of the thumb (Figure 58-10). The presence of a good pulse within the dorsal metacarpal interspace is imperative. The first dorsal arterial anatomy is more consistent than the second and third. When raising this tissue, it is important to include all areolar connective tissue around the pedicle with minimal surgical trauma. The flap should be transferred on a broad connective tissue pedicle and the interosseous vessels need not be skeletonized.

The free microvascular transfer of pulp tissue from the great toe, lesser toe, or the first web space of the foot provide the ideal replacement for missing pulp of the digits or thumb. However, these are esoteric alternatives not available to most hand surgeons. They are covered in other chapters. A thenar flap or cross-finger transfer of glabrous skin are the more readily available methods of coverage.

Several decades ago, there was interest in the transfer of glabrous tissue from the medial arch of the foot to the thumb. This dissection is tedious and the pedicle short but long enough for thumb pulp resurfacing. In the patient shown in Figure 58-11, the procedure was successful but the outcome unsatisfactory because of the poor sensory return, which this man needed for his precision work as a machinist. Secondary resurfacing with a heterodigital island flap provided the expected outcome. Today, alternative consideration for reconstruction would be a toe pulp flap harvested from the lateral side of the great toe, which entails a much easier dissection and longer vascular and neural pedicle length.

Venous flaps in the palmar region are much less reliable but should always be considered after mutilating injuries when spare parts are available. We have limited experience with this method and have found it to be most successful with small defects and in tissue within which an arteriovenous shunt can

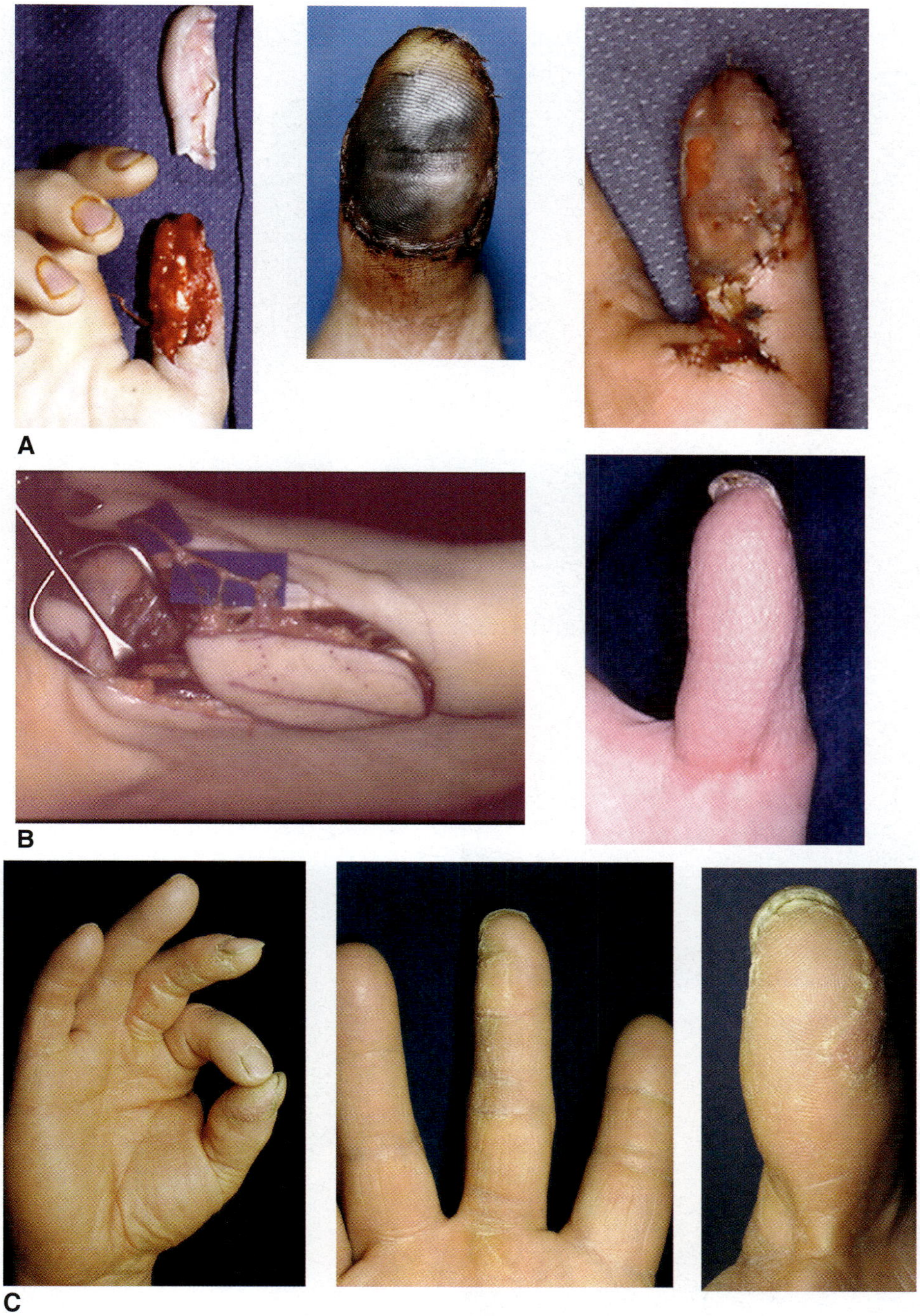

FIGURE 58-10 Medial plantar artery free flap to thumb pulp transfer. (A) The amputated part of this degloved thumb was debrided and replaced as a full-thickness graft. Typically, it did not survive. A split-thickness graft was used as temporary coverage. (B) A glabrous skin flap has been elevated based on the medial plantar artery, venae comitantes, and nerve and transferred to the thumb. Although like tissue was replaced with similar tissue, the sensation was poor, protective at best. (C) A heterodigital neurovascular transfer was then performed to restore critical sensation. The patient adapted well to the disconnected feeling of the long digit whenever he used this thumb.

be created. Preferred donor site is skin from the dorsal surface of a digit or the thin skin of the distal volar forearm. The survival rates of these flaps do not approach 90% and are plagued by congestion (see Chapter 25).

With extensive injury to multiple digits including the thumb, there is often opportunity to combine traditional pedicle flap techniques with microvascular transfers. One should not subject any patient, adult, or child to prolonged immobilization within a groin or lower abdominal flap unless absolutely necessary. A *scapular/parascapular fasciocutaneous flap* can be used creatively. As shown in Figure 58-12, the accidental detonation of a cherry bomb created significant palmar losses within this young boy's hand, including multiple digits, the entire pulp surface of the thumb, and the first web space. After debridement and syndactylization of two digits, a split scapular flap was used as a pedicle flap to resurface three separate regions. Secondary digital separation, flap debulking, and hair removal were performed within 1 year. Thirty-two years have elapsed since the surgery, and the patient has protective sensibility in all resurfaced regions, has never been injured, and has

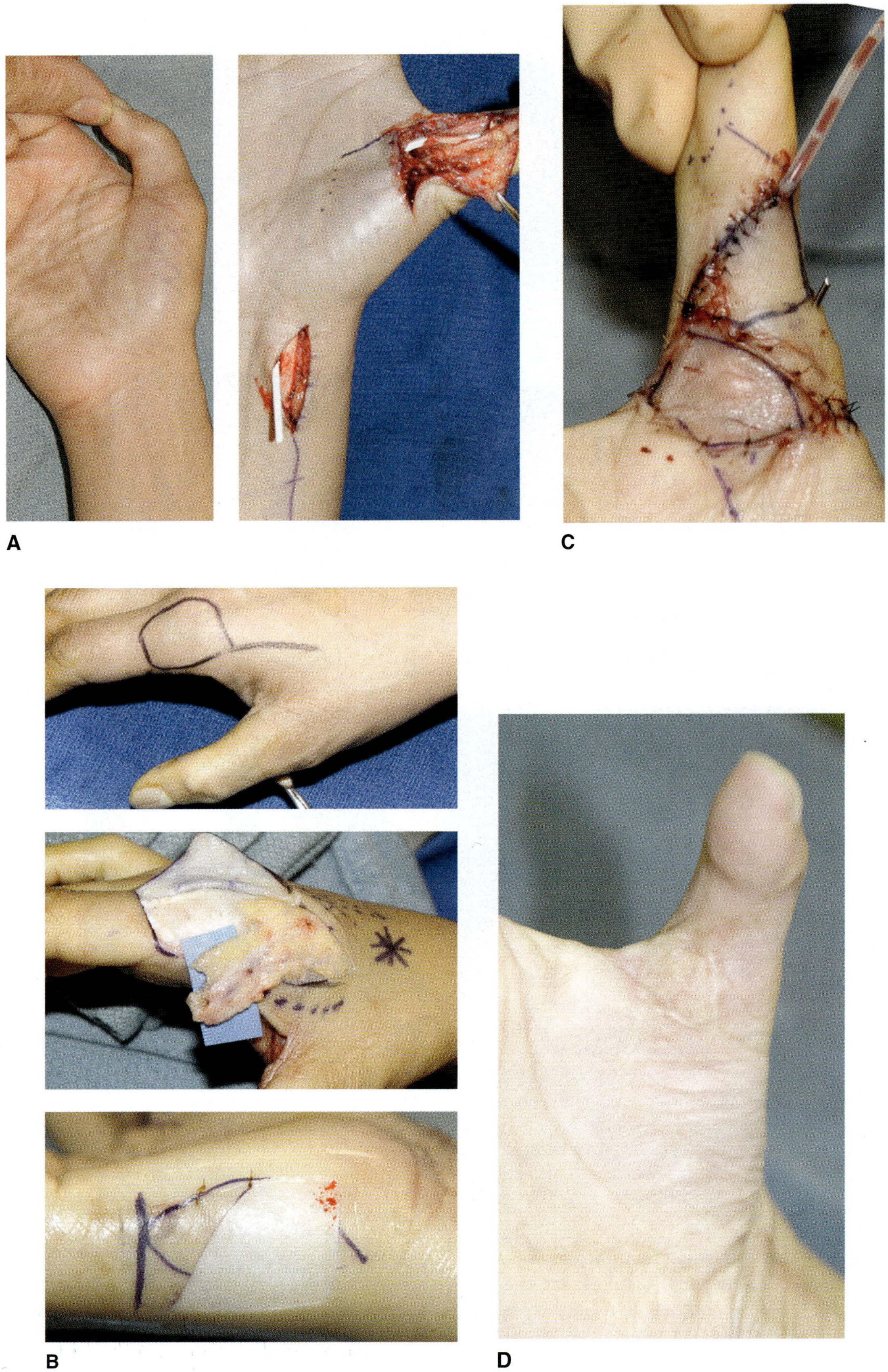

FIGURE 58-11 First dorsal metatarsal artery fascial flap. (A) The clinical appearance of a 15-year flexion contracture before and after release and insertion of a Silastic tendon spacer. (B) A fascial flap was based on the first dorsal metatarsal artery (blue star) and transposed to cover the volar thumb deficit. A thick hypothenar skin graft was taken to cover the fascial flap. (C) Vascularized coverage in a small but critical region of the hand. (D) Appearance 2 years later after the tendon graft.

completed a distinguished career in the military and claimed no disability related to his hand. These nonglabrous skin flaps on the pulp surfaces have functioned very well. This particular case highlights the use of established principles and a new technique, which at the time of this transfer was quite innovative and widely criticized as being too radical. Other fasciocutaneous flaps (see Table 58-2) can be transferred for the same purposes and can be expected to function as well. In many cases, the restoration of a true glabrous skin surface is not always possible.

There are clinical situations in which the distal pulp surface of the thumb or digit is intact and the proximal skin missing. In these hands, it is acceptable to transfer nonglabrous skin without much secondary morbidity. The thinnest, most mobile coverage would be a fascial flap covered with a thick glabrous graft harvested from the hypothenar region or instep of the foot. An all but forgotten flap would be the *dorsalis pedis fasciocutaneous* flap with sensory nerves. The case shown in Figure 58-13 illustrates the effective use of this tissue to resurface the palmar surfaces of two digits. A long or short vascular pedicle can be

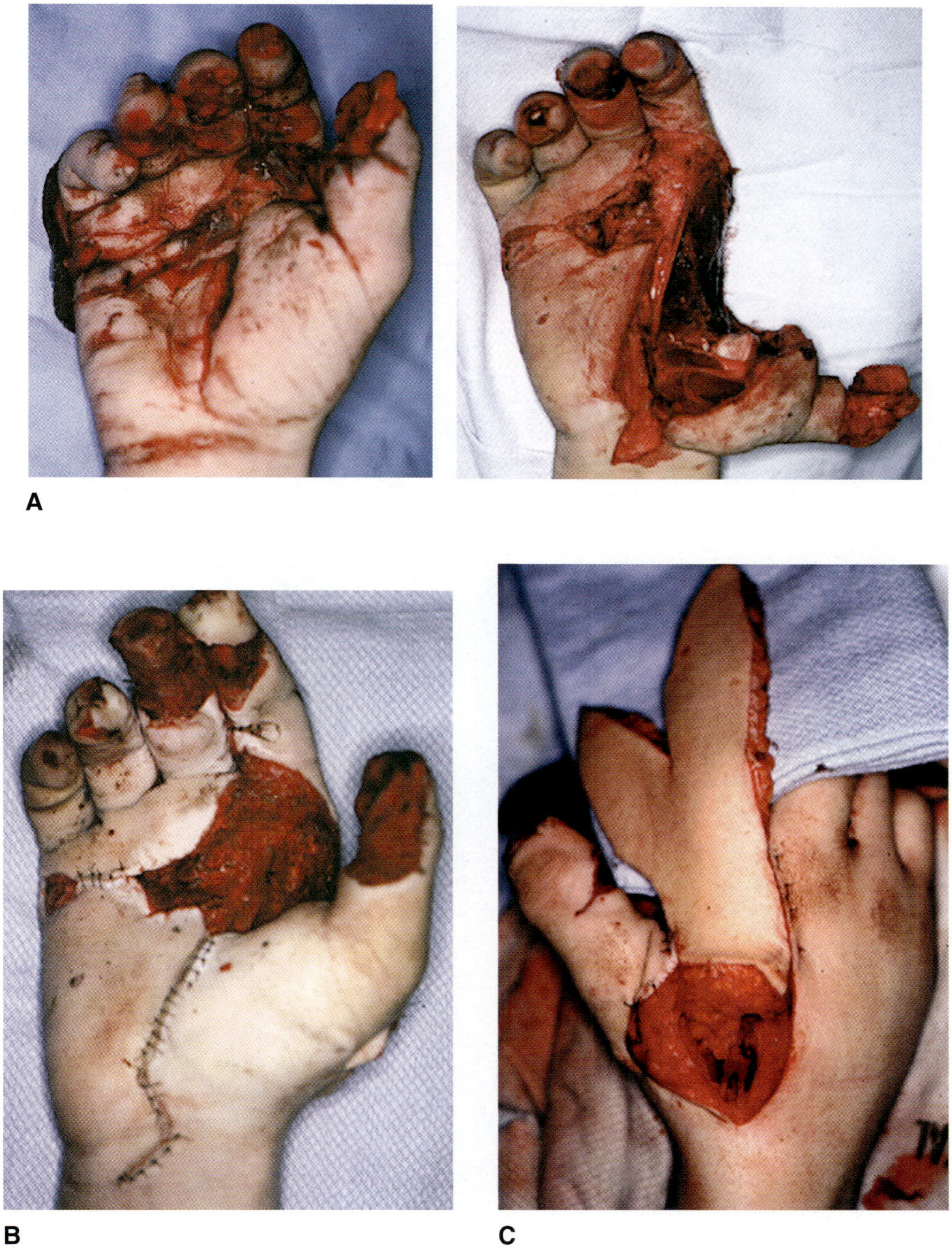

FIGURE 58-12 Split scapular flap to multiple digits and thumb. (A) Multiple fingertips and tissue within the first web space have been lost in a fourth of July fireworks explosion. The thumb is dislocated at the CMC joint, and most of the tissue within the web space has been lost. (B) After sharp debridement, three separate regions require full-thickness coverage. Local tissue has been rotated to cover the tips of three digits. (C) A scapular fasciocutaneous flap has been revascularized on the princeps pollicis arterial system.

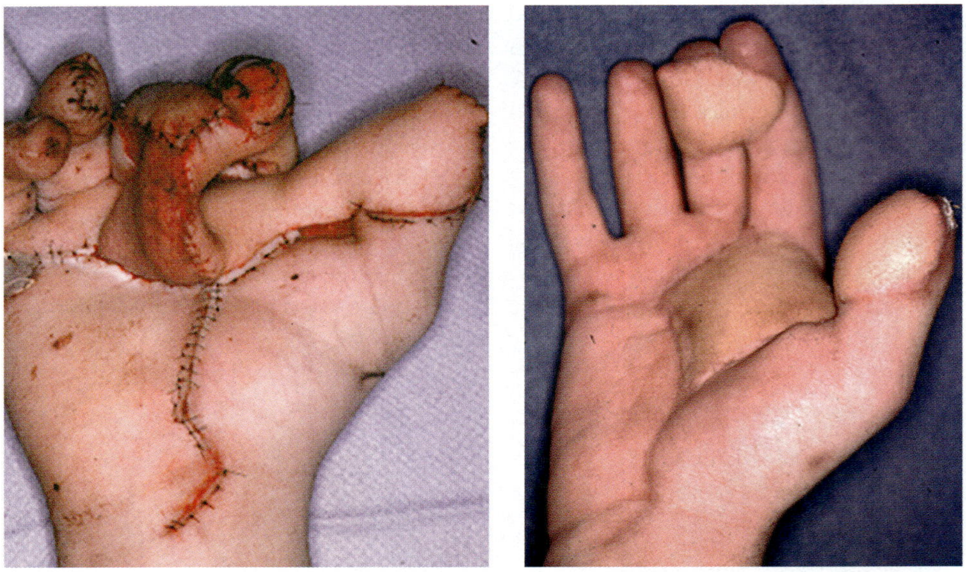

D

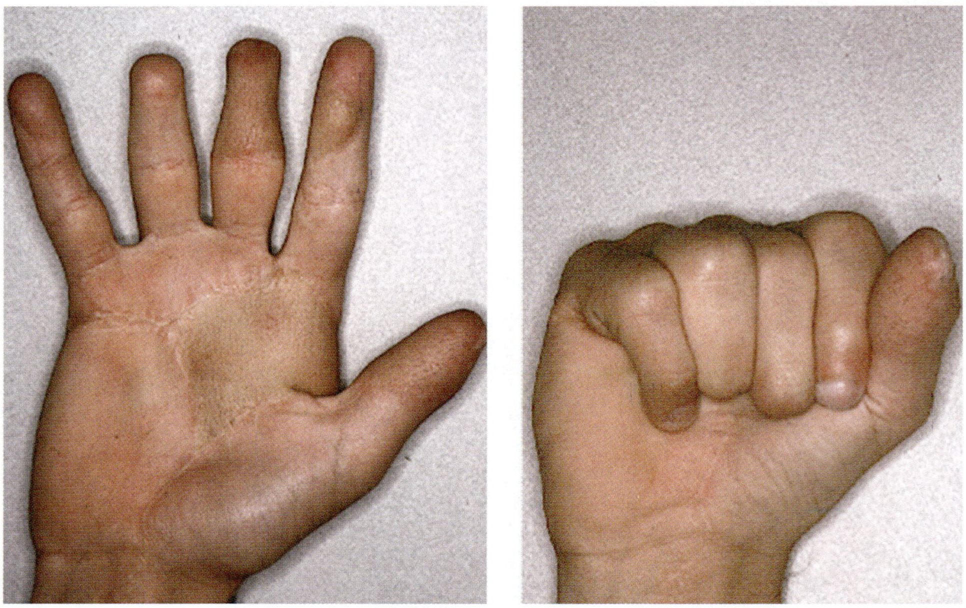

E

FIGURE 58-12 *(Continued)* (**D**) The transferred tissue is then used as a more traditional flap, which was then detached and inset in stages. (**E**) All flaps have been debulked and hail follicles removed. Protective sensation is present with a moving two-point discrimination of 8.0 mm in all distal pulp regions. Flexion of remaining joints is normal. He is seen 32 years after surgery.

harvested as needed. In this case, a localized thermal injury caused loss of full-thickness skin, both neurovascular bundles, flexor tendons, and joint exposure. After debridement, a syndactylization of the index and long digits created a larger single defect more amenable to coverage. The dorsalis pedis fasciocutaneous was raised without inclusion of the short extensor muscles and with careful identification and preservation of the direct cutaneous perforating vessels. Recipient vessels in the hand were the princeps pollicis artery and multiple dorsal veins within the first web space. The pedicle here could have been made long enough to reach the wrist if more distal vessels were not available.

The flap nerve provided a vascularized nerve graft on the radial side of the index ray. Flexor reconstruction was performed at the same time as transfer. Secondary syndactyly release and skin grafts were completed several months later. No revisions were necessary but could have been done at the second stage. The 28-year follow-up speaks for itself. Historically, the major problem with this flap has been the donor site, where meticulous surgery and immobilization is required to ensure proper healing of the skin graft. The flap is sufficiently thin in nonobese patients and usually does not require revisions. More flap than is needed should always be transferred initially.

The dorsalis pedis transfer was one of the first five free tissue transfers. The advantages were the potential long pedicle, thin tissue, and sensation. The major disadvantages are poor graft take and persistent ulceration of the donor site, a frequent complication if the skin graft is not properly applied and the foot elevated for a requisite period of time. For this reason, the similar forearm tissue is used more frequently.

When more than half of the palmar skin of a digit is missing, completion amputation is usually elected. There are extreme situations in which a patient or family may wish to salvage the digit. Free transfer of the entire first web space from the foot is a good but rarely considered donor region. The patient shown in Figure 58-14 sustained composite tissue loss at the distal phalangeal level aggravated by chronic infection and osteomyelitis. She was adamant about saving the long ray. The entire palmar surface was replaced by a first web space flap, which provided pulp with adipose tissue distally and thinner glabrous skin over the proximal and middle phalanges and flexor mechanism. In this rare case, like tissue was replaced in both glabrous and nonglabrous portions of the digit.

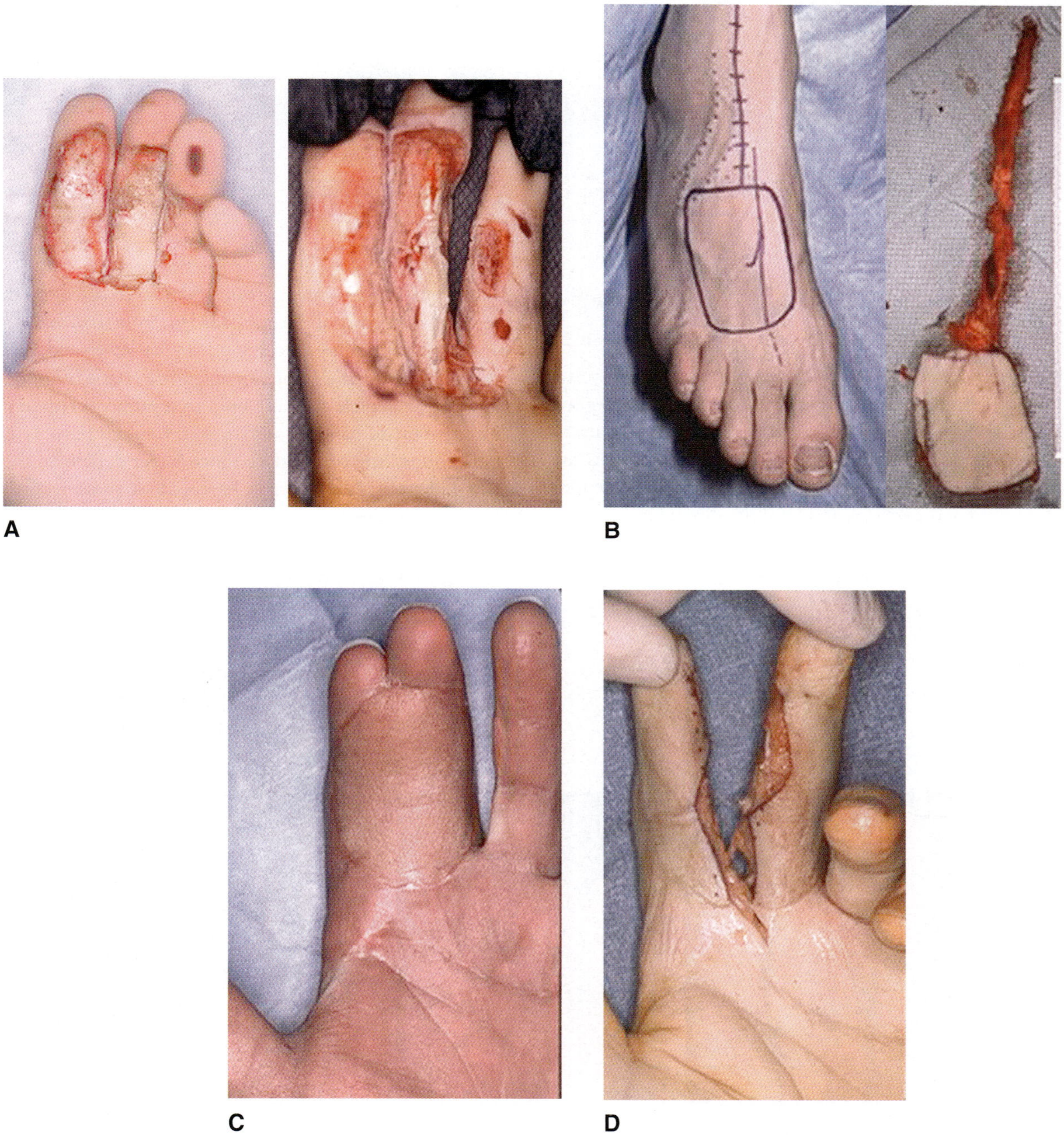

FIGURE 58-13 Dorsalis pedis flap to digits. (A) This man lost full-thickness skin and radial neurovascular bundles to index and long digits, which were compressed in a press machine. After debridement, the digits were joined together. (B) A dorsal pedis fasciocutaneous flap with long pedicle. (C) A simple, incomplete syndactyly has been created. (D) Separation was completed 3 months later and grafts placed on the sides of the digits.

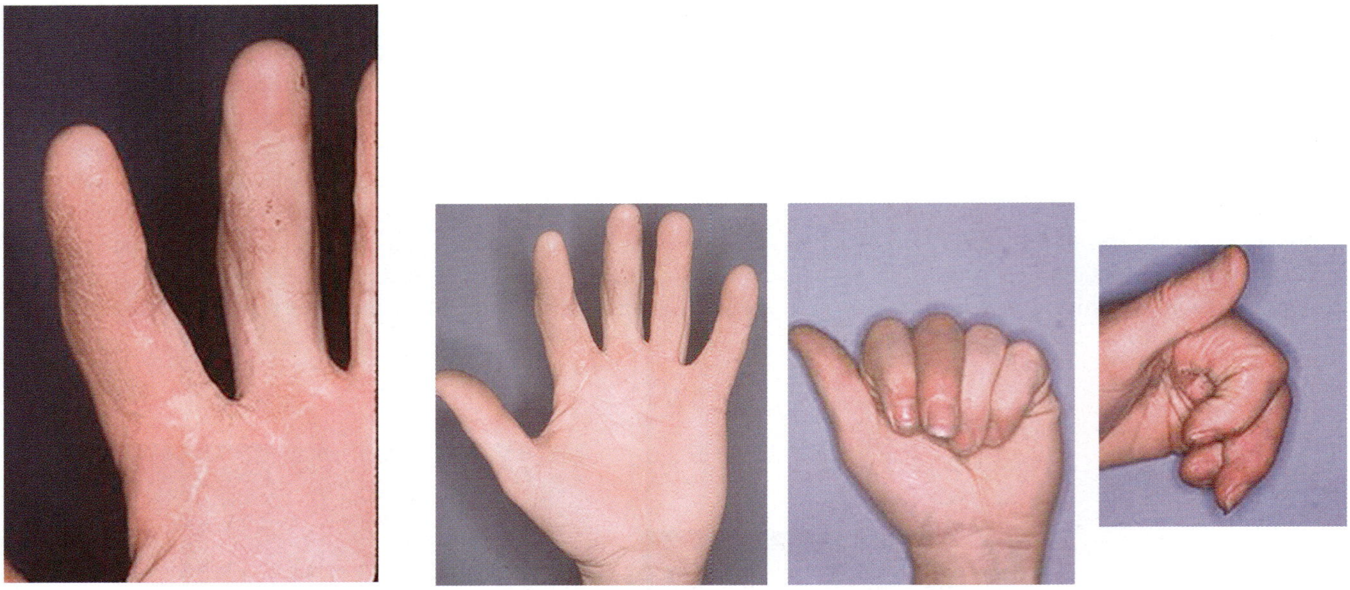

E F

FIGURE 58-13 (*Continued*) (**E**) There are no flexion contractures 6 months later. (**F**) Flexion and extension 28 years after surgery.

CIRCUMFERENTIAL COVERAGE OF THUMB OR DIGITS

The circumferential loss of both dorsal and palmar tissue on a thumb or digit is most commonly the result of a severe degloving injury, a mangling injury, or an electrical or thermal burn to the entire hand. In all cases, the soft tissue requirements are substantial for a thumb or digit. For this reason, reattachment or use of the amputated part(s) is an initial priority. Thin fasciocutaneous flaps are well suited for this purpose and are difficult to find in an obese patient. The soft tissue requirement for a circumferential loss is much greater than anticipated. In the past, we have frequently used the pedicled groin flap based on the superficial circumflex iliac system or the lower abdominal flap based on the superficial inferior epigastric vessels (Figure 58-15). Often these pedicle flaps are used to resurface a region prior to definitive toe to hand reconstruction. Enough tissue is available in this donor site to resurface much larger deficits in the upper limb. The young lady shown in Figure 58-16 presented with a ring finger she described as a "sausage" 1 year after ring avulsion injury. Reattachment was unsuccessful, and she refused amputation. The digit was covered with a multistaged groin flap. After several

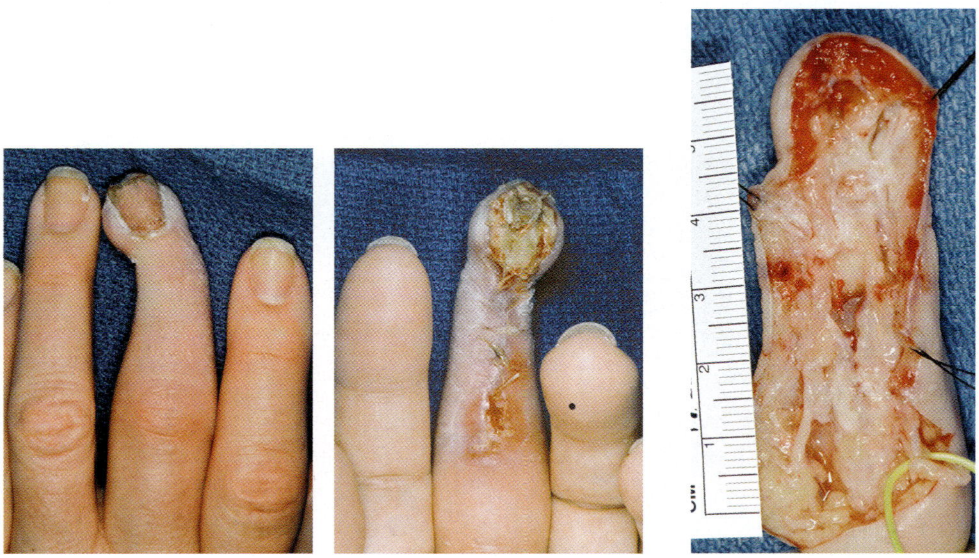

A B

FIGURE 58-14 First toe web space to the hand. (**A**) Simple skin grafts were insufficient coverage for this ring finger. Tissue has been lost and must be replaced. (**B**) After debridement, the full extent of the loss is obvious.

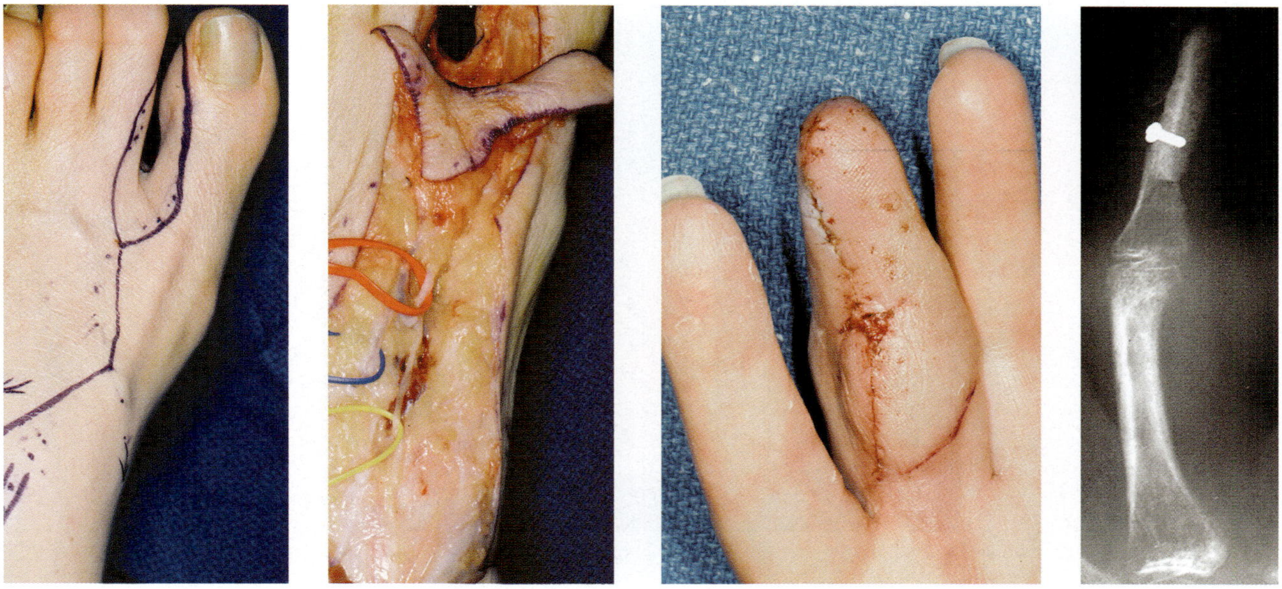

C D

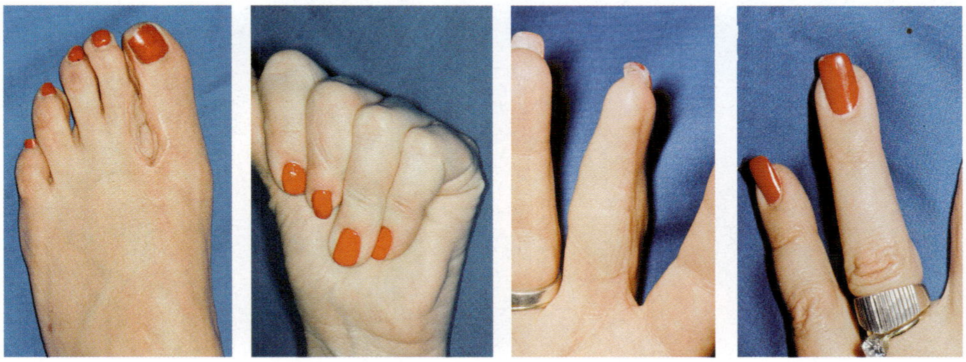

E

FIGURE 58-14 *(Continued)* (**C**) The outline and dissection of the first web space flap from the foot based on the first dorsal interosseous system draining into the dorsalis pedis artery. (**D**) Appearance after transfer, inset, and bone graft replacement of the distal phalanx. (**E**) Postoperative appearance of donor and recipient sites. Full metacarpophalangeal and proximal interphalangeal joint returned. (Used with permission from David Chiu MD.)

debulking procedures with creation of new Cleland ligaments, a second toe was transferred to the terminal phalanx. Motion at the MCP and PIP joints has been preserved. The patient was last seen 15 years after surgery and has had no additional revisions.

The thumb is the most common site for circumferential soft tissue loss from the same avulsion injuries. Because of its mobility and independence from the rest of the hand, this prime digit becomes entangled most easily. There are many special circumstances when the preservation of thumb length and mobility is only possible with a surrounding tube of soft tissue (Figure 58-17) This particular child arrived from a foreign country with her amputated thumb in a cooler 5 days after her original amputation. Although the revascularization was successful, subsequent congestion and partial soft tissue loss were predictable. Groin flap coverage enabled us to salvage length and mobility. She is now 32 years postoperative and when last seen 15 years ago demonstrated limited growth of the distal phalanx, good mobility at the MCP and interphalangeal joints, and satisfactory protective sensation with a moving two-point discrimination of 10.0 mm.

DORSAL AND PALMAR SURFACES OF THE HAND AND WRIST

Thumb Index (First) Web Space

Restoration of the first web space with supple, full-thickness skin coverage is critical for independent thumb function, which constitutes up to 50% of total hand function on most disability rating systems. Restoration of mobility to the thumb is the only reconstructive procedure given higher priority than the creation of a first web space. The area within this web space is larger than anticipated, is shaped like a tetrahedron, contains both glabrous and nonglabrous skin, and is draped over specialized intrinsic muscles. Its thin composition allows it to collapse like an accordion with adduction and to stretch with abduction and extension. Coverage requires more rather than less tissue and ideally should contain full-thickness skin.

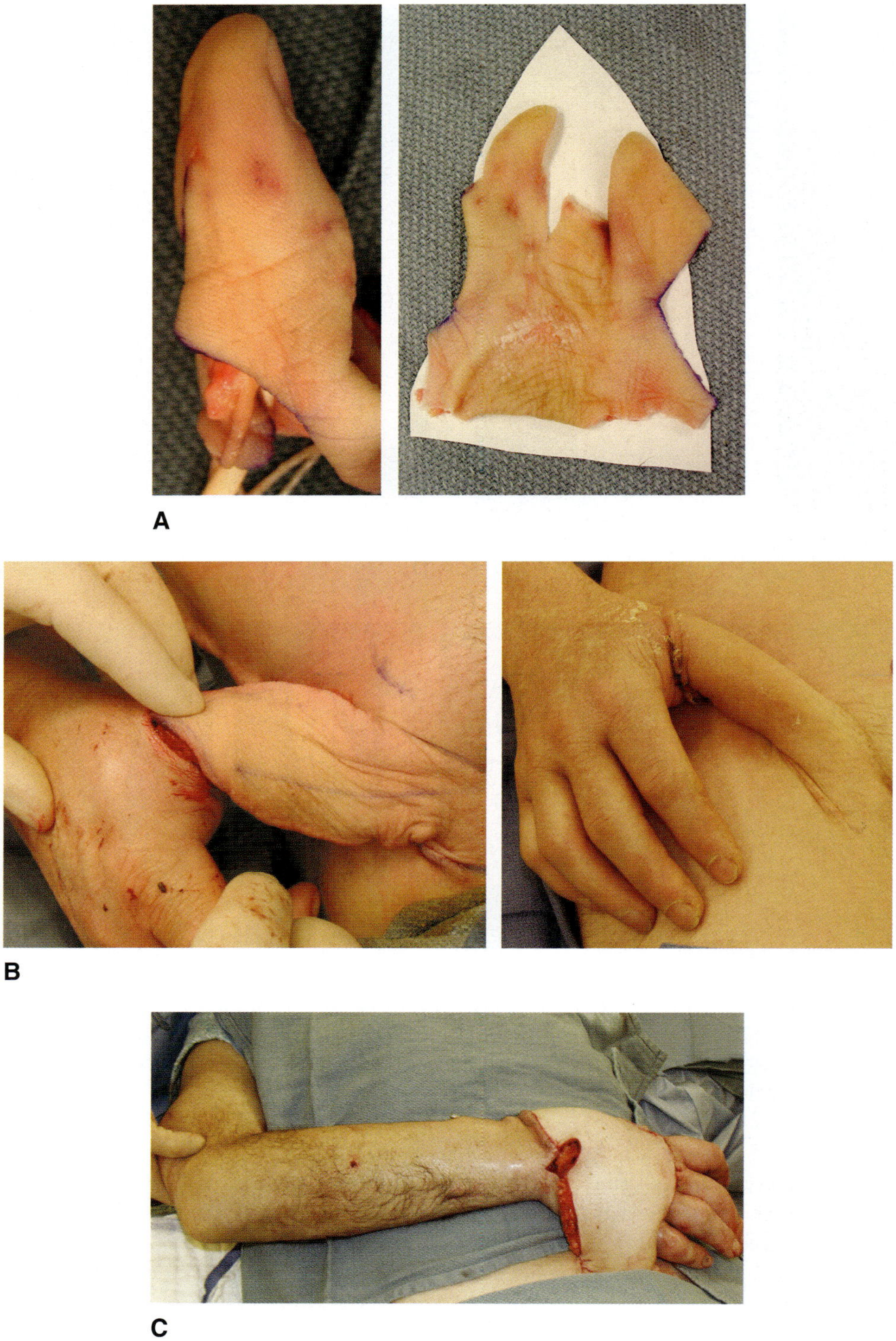

FIGURE 58-15 Abdominal pedicle flaps. (A) The Chinese "red" sign in this amputated thumb is indicative of arterial avulsion and hemorrhage very distal within the pulp tissue and is a contraindication to successful revascularization. A template has been fashioned from the filleted thumb soft tissue to calculate the precise need for tissue. (B) A groin flap has been raised and the donor site closed before inset. Several weeks later. (C) This flap for the dorsal hand and wrist has been raised on the superficial inferior epigastric arterial system. The donor region has been closed vertically.

The most common options for coverage make use of local tissues advanced, rotated, or transposed into this position. Local transposition techniques are varied and include the four-flap Z-plasty, five-flap Z-plasty, Z-plasties in series, and flaps from the dorsum of the index ray. Many direct dorsal rotation and rotation advancement techniques have been described. All are effective only if local tissue is available and the tissue deficiency is in the small or moderate range. A mini flap often produces a mini outcome. Larger deficiencies usually require additional tissue that can only be recruited from regional or distant sources.

For large deficiencies in both children and adults, there are three excellent free flap donor site options: the lateral arm, the forearm (pedicled or free), and the groin (see Table 58-3).

Transfer of a small fasciocutaneous free flap to the first web space using the princeps pollicis artery along the thumb metacarpal or radial arterial system at the wrist level is simple and elegant. This technique often avoids excessive surgical dissection within a previously injured hand. This conservative approach is often mistaken for being too bold or radical.

Free or pedicled tissue transfers into this region are reserved for severe deficiencies. It is crucial to anticipate the size of the defect after release, keep it open with a threaded K wire, make an accurate template, and plan accordingly. There is much to be gained by the formulation of a definitive reconstructive game plan during the initial treatment period. As shown in Figure 58-18, a carpenter's thumb, index, and long digits were severely injured. The thumb was subtotally amputated and all volar structure of the index and long digits were severed. Initially, the index digit was revascularized and 1 week later transferred as a vascular island to reconstruct the extensive soft tissue and skeletal losses of his thumb. A lateral arm flap was then used to construct a new web space. What appeared to be more tissue than necessary contoured well with no revision. The patient, a master carpenter, has been back at his trade for 24 years. There have been no revisions. We made a plan at the time of initial injury and stuck to it. Expeditious planning resulted in earlier healing, earlier rehabilitation, early return to work, and a maximal functional outcome.

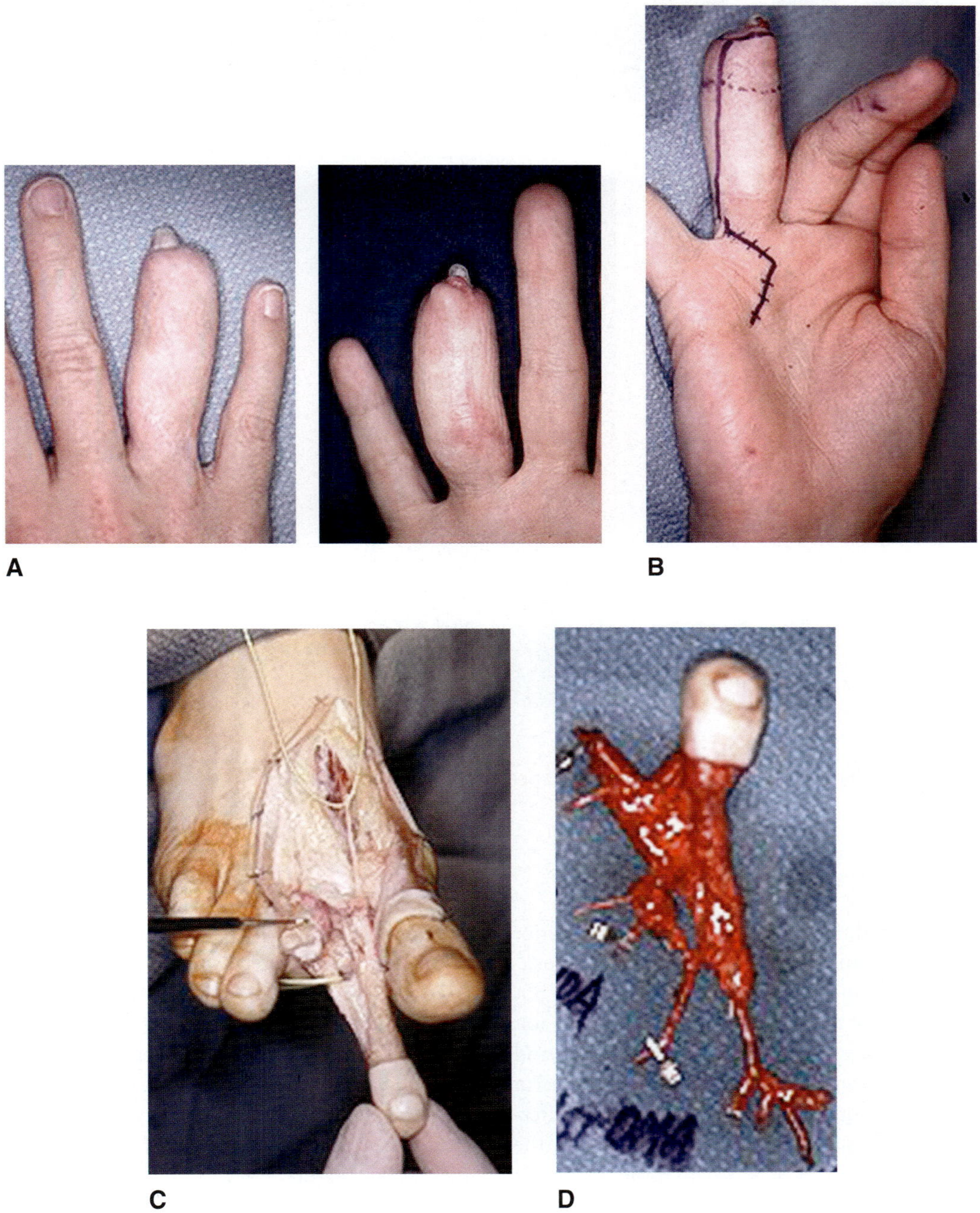

FIGURE 58-16 Groin flap for ring avulsion. (A) This ring degloving injury was initially covered with a bulky groin flap. The distal phalanx and nail are not functional. (B) Approach from a high ulnar midaxial incision. (C) A second toe has been dissected. (D) Long vascular pedicles have been isolated.

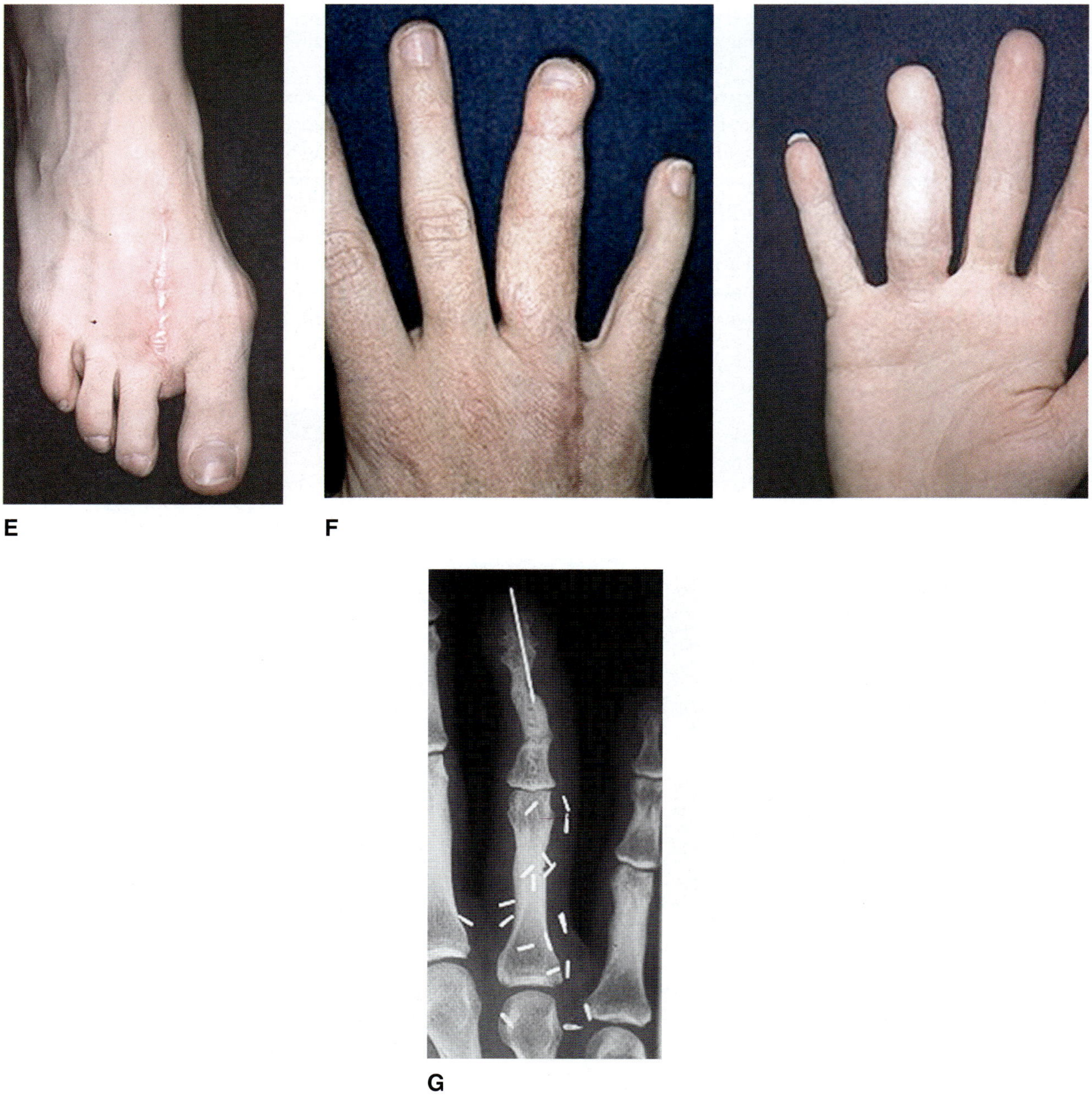

FIGURE 58-16 (*Continued*) (**E**) The donor site 1 year later. (**F**) Appearance 5 years later. (**G**) Solid arthrodesis at the distal interphalangeal joint level.

Regional vascular island flaps based on the radial, posterior interosseous, and anterior interosseous arterial systems are usually available and practical in both adults and children. Do not forget to test the patency of the palmar arch with an Allen test before raising these flaps, especially in congenital cases and particularly those with any type of radial dysplasia. The forearm is an excellent source of tissue for those with congenital differences, and these transfers can safely be completed within the first 18 months of life. Placement of adequate tissue within the first web space of the child shown in Figure 58-19 with a five-fingered hand permitted active use this digit (thumb), which had been idle in the same plane as the hand. The subcutaneous tissue plane within this flap may often be bulky in young children, but there is plenty of room within the web after the release has been completed.

The groin flap was the first free transfer to this region and is still a very good option for coverage but has been largely discarded because of the difficult dissection and variable anatomy of the superficial circumflex iliac arterial system. Another patient with radial dysplasia and a hypoplastic thumb presented with deficient circulation across the palmar arches (Figure 58-20). The Allen test result was positive. A free groin flap with its short pedicle was more than sufficient to open up this web space and allow the thumb to function in palmar abduction. The recipient vessels from the palmar arch were directly beneath the flap. Angiograms or

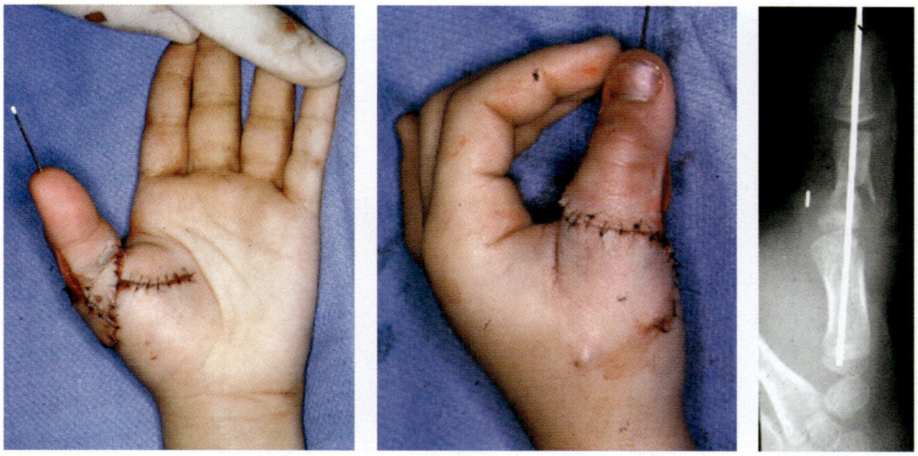

A

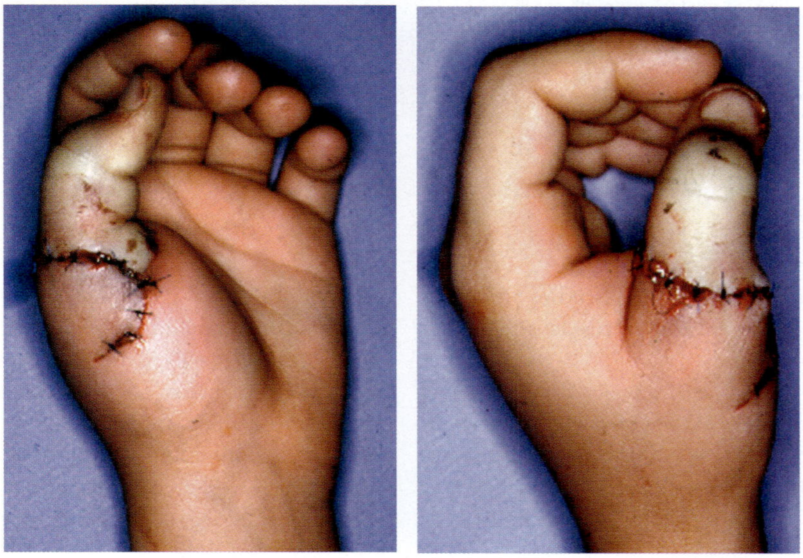

B

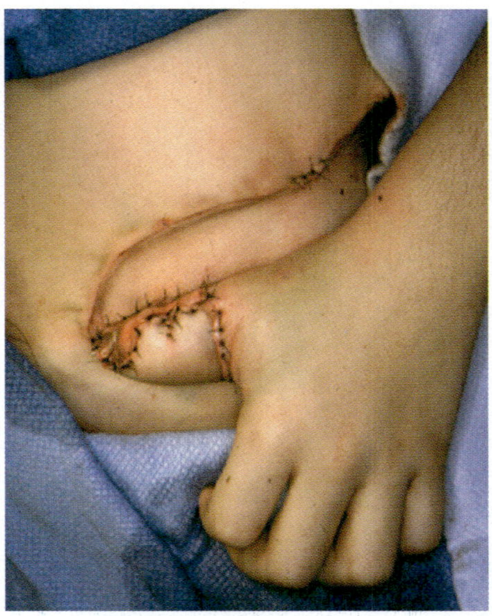

C

FIGURE 58-17 Groin flap to thumb for circumferential loss. (**A**) Appearance of revascularized thumb after 102 hours of cool ischemia. (**B**) With swelling, a portion of the volar soft tissue was lost despite anticoagulation, vasodilators, and suture removal. (**C**) Coverage with an ipsilateral groin flap and complete closure of the donor region.

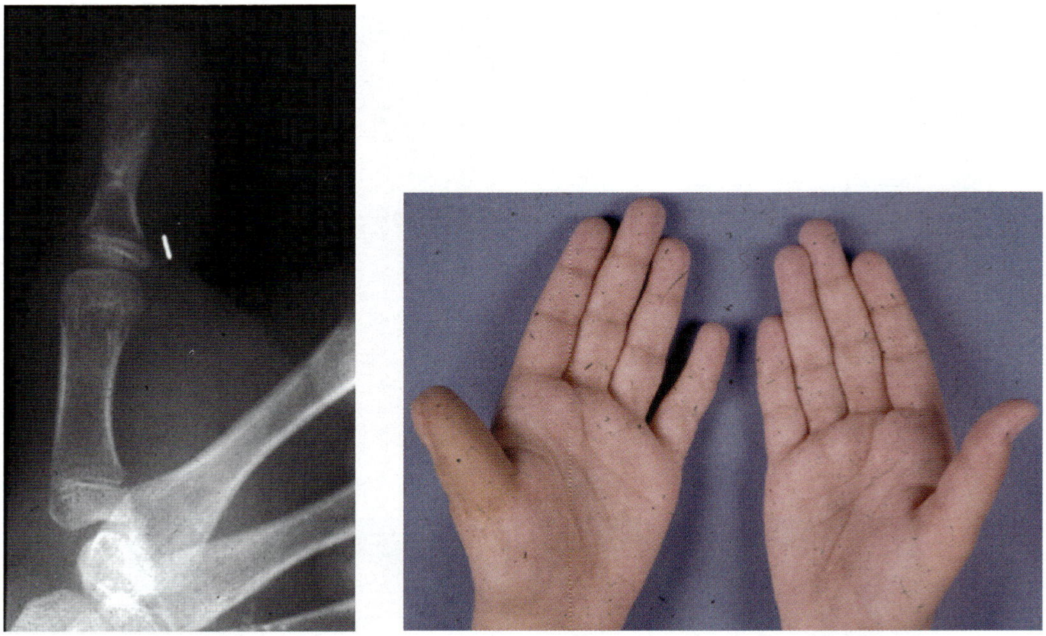

D E

FIGURE 58-17 (*Continued*) (**D**) Skeletal appearance 5 years later. (**E**) Clinical appearance 15 years later. No revisions have been done.

magnified magnetic resonance angiography studies are often necessary in children with congenital differences and radial dysplasias.

The pedicle groin flap remains as the major donor site for large- and medium-sized deficits, particularly within the first web space. The boy shown in Figure 58-21 was treated more than 30 years ago on the fourth of July after an incendiary device exploded in his left hand. The entire web space was resurfaced with full-thickness groin skin transferred as a pedicle flap. At that time, the standard technique was to identify the axial vessels before raising the flap; this maneuver was dangerous in those with an abundance of adipose tissue and was tedious because of the poorly defined anatomy. We soon learned to elevate in a retrograde fashion and identify the superficial circumflex iliac artery (SCIA) vessels directly above the fascia overlying the sartorius muscle. Secondary nerve grafting and a staged tendon

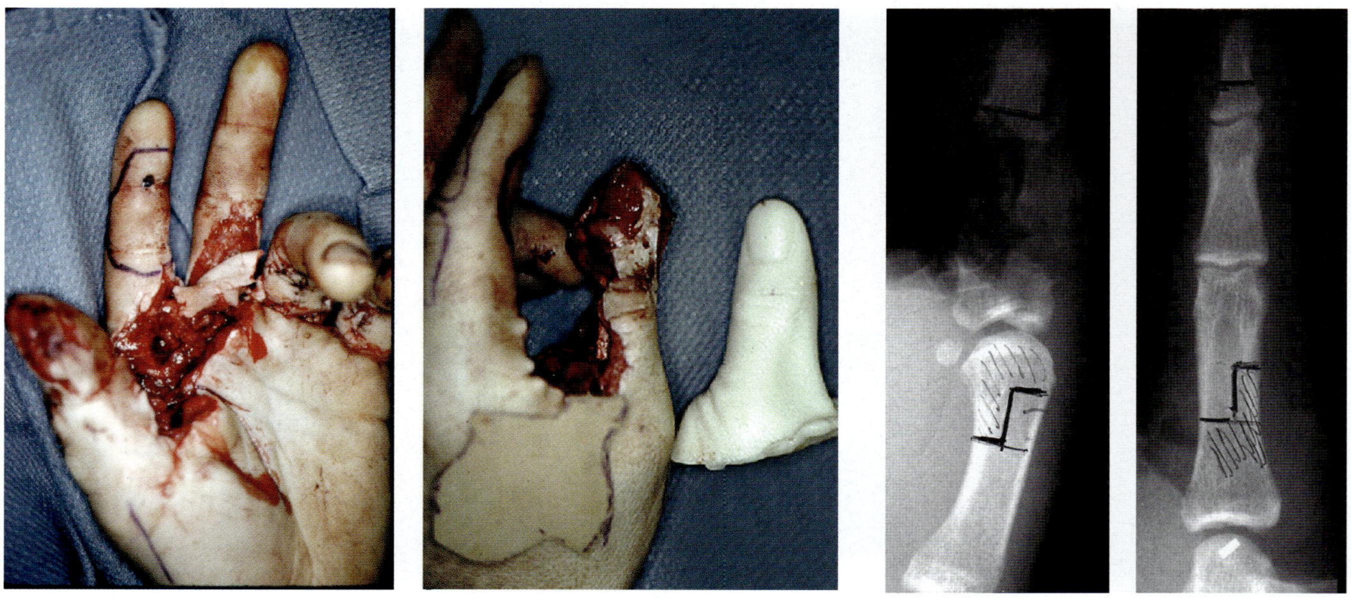

A B

FIGURE 58-18 (**A**) A table saw injury resulted in subtotal loss of the thumb and first web space. All palmar structures to the index and long fingers have been lacerated. A template has been made of the required tissue loss and a methylmethacrylate mold of the opposite thumb fabricated for accurate measurements. (**B**) The index finger (right) was used to reconstruct both the soft tissue and skeletal deficits of the thumb.

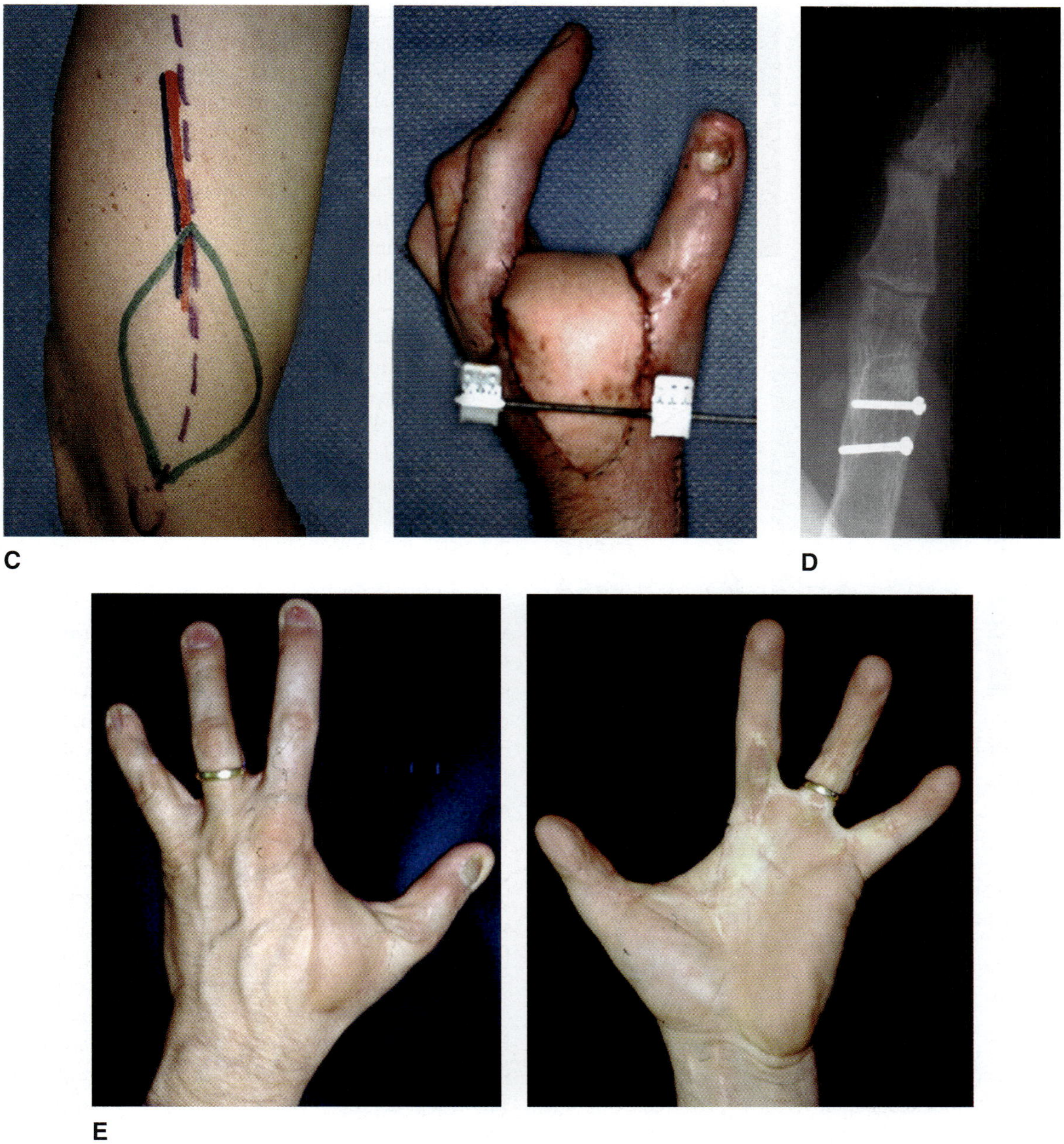

FIGURE 58-18 (*Continued*) (**C**) Distal lateral arm flap to the first web space. (**D**) Radiograph of the thumb 24 years later. (**E**) Clinical appearance of the hand. The patient was back to work in 6 months and has had no revisions.

reconstruction were easily performed. With aging, the flap has changed commensurate with weight gain and loss. It has contoured well. There have been no revisions.

As a pedicle transfer, the groin flap donor site is easy for the surgeon and burdensome for the patient and her or his family. We still use the groin and lower abdominal donor sites frequently for coverage after electrical and thermal burns in children at Shriners Hospital, where excellent nursing care is available.

Other small fasciocutaneous flaps harvested from other regions of the body will fit into this area, which does allow more bulk than the dorsal surfaces of the hand, thumb, or digit. However, a dennervated muscle covered with a skin graft is not effective because of the subsequent web space contracture, which ultimately limits thumb function.

COVERAGE OF THE DORSAL SURFACE OF THE HAND AND WRIST

The skin requirements here are the same as outlined for the digits and thumb: thin, mobile, full-thickness tissue preferably with sensation, which is preferable but not an absolute prerequisite. A simple skin graft is more than adequate for all dorsal defects, which contain well-vascularized granulation tissue, paratenon over exposed tendons, and periosteum surrounding skeletal structures. Dorsal contracture is common in this

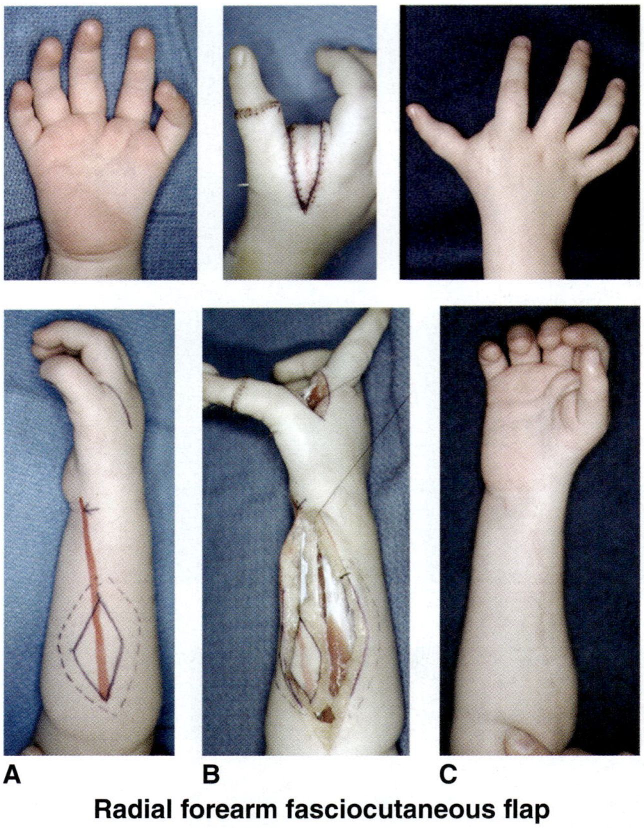

FIGURE 58-19 Radial forearm fasciocutaneous flap in a child. (**A**) Appearance of a five-fingered hand. The radial digit is triphalangeal, flexed at the proximal interphalangeal joint, and has a distal thumb metacarpal epiphysis. Outline of flap on forearm shows tetrahedral configuration. Additional fascia included with flap (dashed line). (**B**) Flap raised on the radial artery and inset into the released first web space. (**C**) Clinical appearance 2 years later. An abductor digiti quinti muscle transfer was subsequently performed to improve palmar abduction.

region, and secondary surgery is often necessary. In these patients, good full-thickness flap coverage is preferred.

For a severely mutilated hand and wrist, wound coverage is the primary goal. When simultaneous skeletal, nerve, arterial or tendon reconstruction can be completed without introducing additional morbidity to the patient, it should be encouraged. Careful planning is necessary. In fact, the staging and timing of possible secondary reconstruction should be outlined at the time of initial wound coverage. For example, placement of tendon spacers, reconstruction of the dorsal retinaculum, or repair of the extensor mechanism could easily be accomplished at the time of initial coverage. These anticipatory decisions usually influence the placement of incisions, amount of tissue to be transferred, and inset into the hand. It is a major mistake not to take the time to think and plan before any major tissue transfers. Although it is easier to adopt the "wait and see" approach, the primary surgeon is often faced with designing the secondary procedures, which could have been more easily accomplished if he or she had initially transferred enough tissue, positioned some joints differently, used a flap with sensory potential, or used a fasciocutaneous flap instead of a bulky muscle covered with a skin graft.

Our preferred option for small to moderate defects has been fascial flaps covered with full-thickness skin grafts. Either temporoparietal fascia or radial forearm fascia can cover the entire dorsal metacarpal portion of the hand (see Figure 58-4). The young girl shown in Figure 58-22 sustained significant tissue loss on the dorsum of her hand. Fractures were reduced and the extensor system repaired. In lieu of multiple VAC dressings followed by skin grafting, her wound was debrided the next day and covered immediately with a fascial flap and thick skin graft. Instead of going back to the OR for dressing changes and eventual grafting, she went straight to occupational therapy! Her function is seen 6 years later, and there have been no revisions or manipulations or tenolyses.

The original TPFF was performed at the West Roxbury VA Hospital in 1978 in an electrician shown in Figure 58-23. The previous week we had used this same tissue to cover an exposed ear reconstruction. At the time, the size of the superficial temporal vessels, the pliability of the fascial tissue, and the gliding potential for tendons and joints were obvious. The rest is history.

The pedicled groin flap based on the SCIA or a lower abdominal flap based on the superficial inferior epigastric vessels (see Figure 58-14C) are very useful here if other fasciocutaneous options are neither available nor practical. The groin flap will provide enough soft tissue to cover any portion of the dorsal hand, wrist, and forearm and is a particularly good fit for the mobile dorsal surfaces. Our use of pedicled groin flaps in severely burned children has been extensive and effective because we have access to specialized nursing required for these patients and their parents. The child shown in Figure 58-24 presented with a severe dorsal contracture after a neonatal full-thickness burn injury, which healed with hypertrophic scar formation. Skin grafts would not have been practical. A full-thickness abdominal flap covered joint releases at multiple levels, tendon reconstructions, and release of the first web space. Her anatomy and required position were more amenable to a superficial inferior epigastric flap than a standard groin flap. These flaps are the most difficult of all in young active children, and there are multiple technical caveats, including adequate sedation, parent cooperation, nursing supervision, creation of a closed system with no open wounds, provision of some mobility at the pedicle base, proper immobilization, daily dressing changes, and an amenable child. The predictable scars surrounding the flap in this Asian child were treated with intralesional steroid injections.

When extensive secondary metacarpal, wrist, or forearm skeletal reconstruction is needed, we prefer larger fasciocutaneous flaps such as the anterolateral thigh (ALT), groin, latissimus dorsi, and lateral arm donor sites usually as a staged procedure in which secondary debulking is a given necessity. Suction lipectomy for thick flaps has been a great advance. The man shown in Figure 58-25 sustained a massive crush injury with loss of all soft tissue, including all extensors on the dorsum of his hand and wrist. A series of internal pins was used instead of a cumbersome external fixation apparatus to great advantage. All fractures were reduced, tendons repaired or grafted, and the wound covered with one large ALT flap. Secondary liposuction was accomplished in one stage 1 year later.

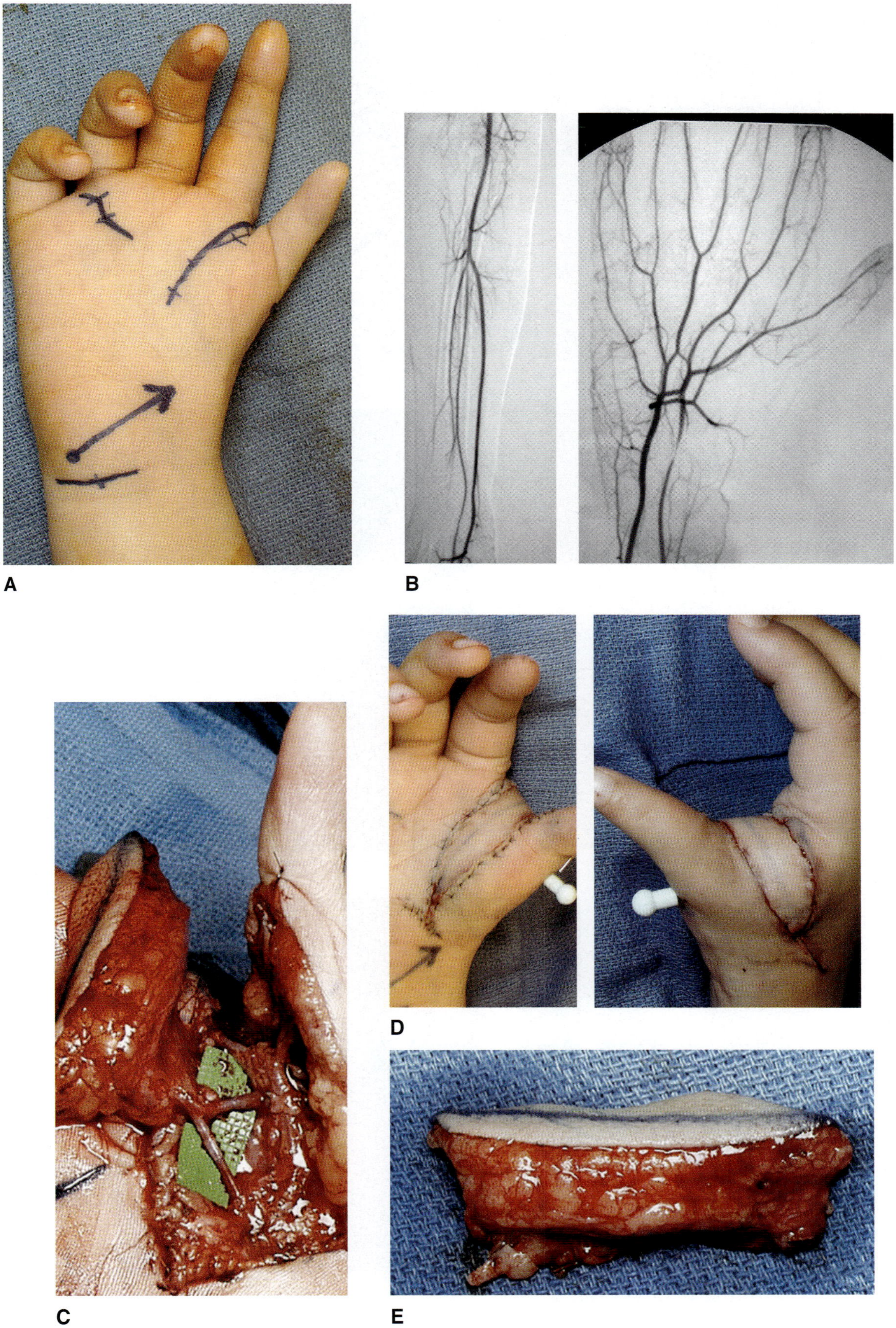

A B C D E

FIGURE 58-20 Free groin flap to first web space. (**A**) Incision marking for a type IIIA thumb hypoplasia with severe deficiency of the first web space. A ring FDS tendon transfer was also performed to improve palmar abduction of the thumb. (**B**) Angiogram shows a 2-cm-long stenosis within the radial artery. (**C**) Arterial and venous anastomoses of the free groin flap within the palm. (**D**) Inset of flap with threaded pin holding the web space in its new position. (**E**) Despite the location, these flaps are relatively thicker in young children.

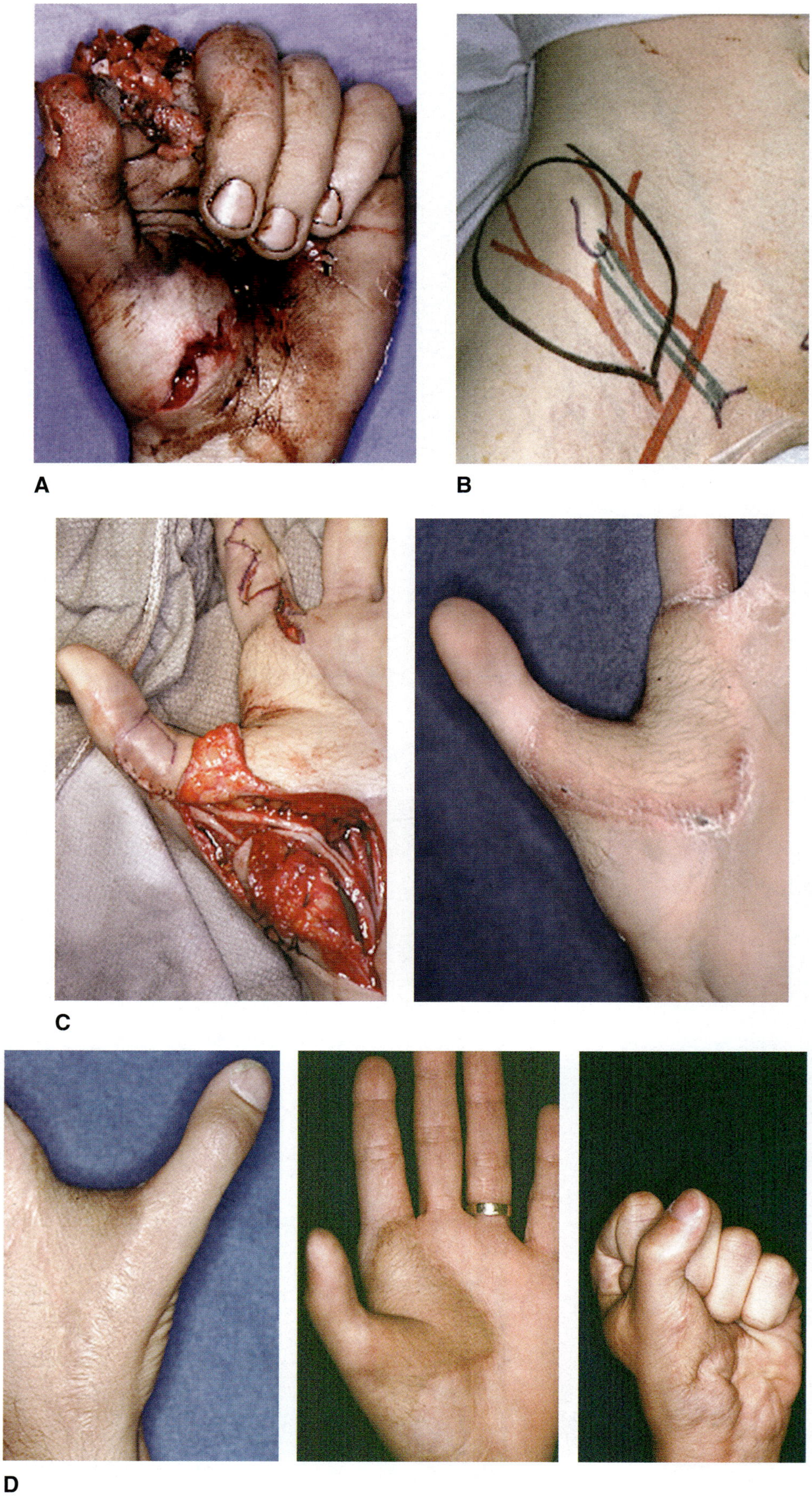

FIGURE 58-21 Pedicled groin flap to first web space. (**A**) Severe mid palmar tissue loss caused by a fireworks explosion. (**B**) Outline of the standard groin flap (black), inguinal ligament (green), deep (above), and superficial (below) circumflex iliac vessels (red). (**C**) Several months after groin flap transfer, sural nerve grafts and a tendon graft reconstruction were completed. (**D**) Function is shown 30 years later. As the patient has gained weight, the web space has enlarged commensurately.

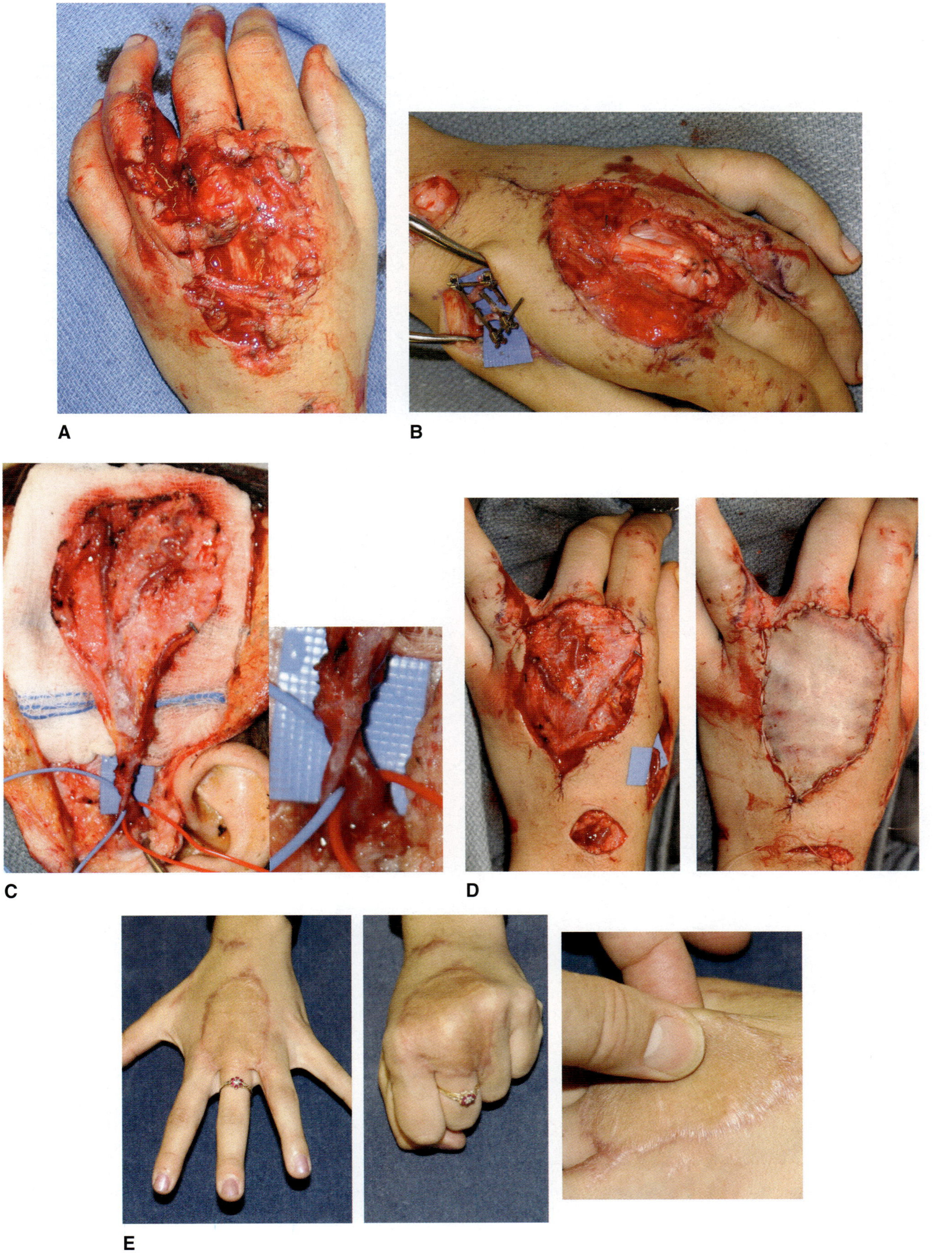

FIGURE 58-22 Temporoparietal fascial flap covered with skin graft. (A) A rollover motor vehicle accident resulted in composite loss of skin, extensor tendons, and multiple fractures. (B) Appearance of the wound after debridement, extensor tendon repairs, and preparation of recipient vessels along the princeps pollicis system. (C) Elevation of the temporoparietal fascial flap. Note the large size of the superficial temporal artery (red vessel loops) and vein (blue vessel loops) after irrigation with vasodilators. (D) The fascial flap has been revascularized, inset, and covered with a split-thickness skin graft. (E) Postoperative function with full flexion and extension and very supple mobile, thin dorsal hand coverage.

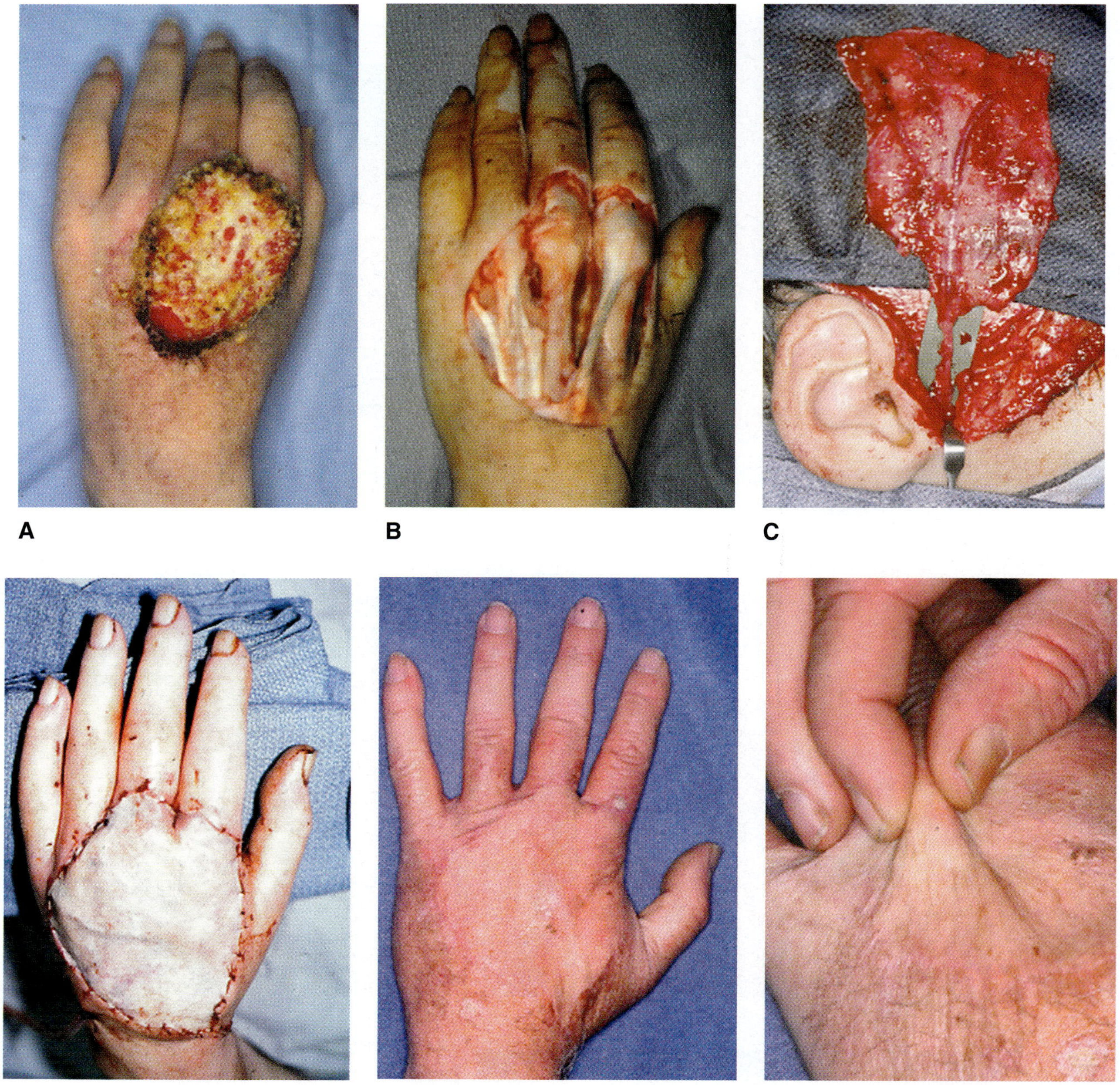

A B C D E F

FIGURE 58-23 Original temporoparietal fascial flap. (A) An invasive, exophytic squamous cell carcinoma (SCC), which had been present for many years. (B) Wide excision included full-thickness skin and several extensor tendons. (C) The temporoparietal fascia was raised very cephalad on the head with a long vascular pedicle. (D) Revascularized fascia covered with a thick split-thickness skin graft. Soft, pliable skin 15 years later. (E and F) The patient eventually died 25 years following this surgery from metastatic SCC.

COVERAGE OF THE PALMAR SURFACE OF THE WRIST OR HAND

Soft tissue requirements including sensation coupled with limited donor site availability place severe constraints on this anatomic region. Donor areas are limited because thick, durable, cornified glabrous skin is available only on the hands and feet or from a genetically identical twin. In the future, tissue engineering may help solve this very difficult problem. The uniquely designed palmar aponeurosis with its longitudinal, transverse, and deep components not only protects underlying nerves, tendons, and the arterial system but also stabilizes the overlying skin and allows passage of nutrient perforating vessels and sensory nerves. There is no flap that can replicate these features with the exception of the sole of the foot. Flaps and grafts for all regions of the body have been transferred to the palm. None is ideally successful.

The major problems with all fasciocutaneous flap transfers for large defects in this region are their bulk, the lack of sensation, hair growth, and instability. Secondary procedures are always needed. However, excellent outcomes can be achieved with persistence and correction of as many of these issues as possible. Our most durable results have been achieved with vascularized fascial flaps covered with either glabrous skin grafts

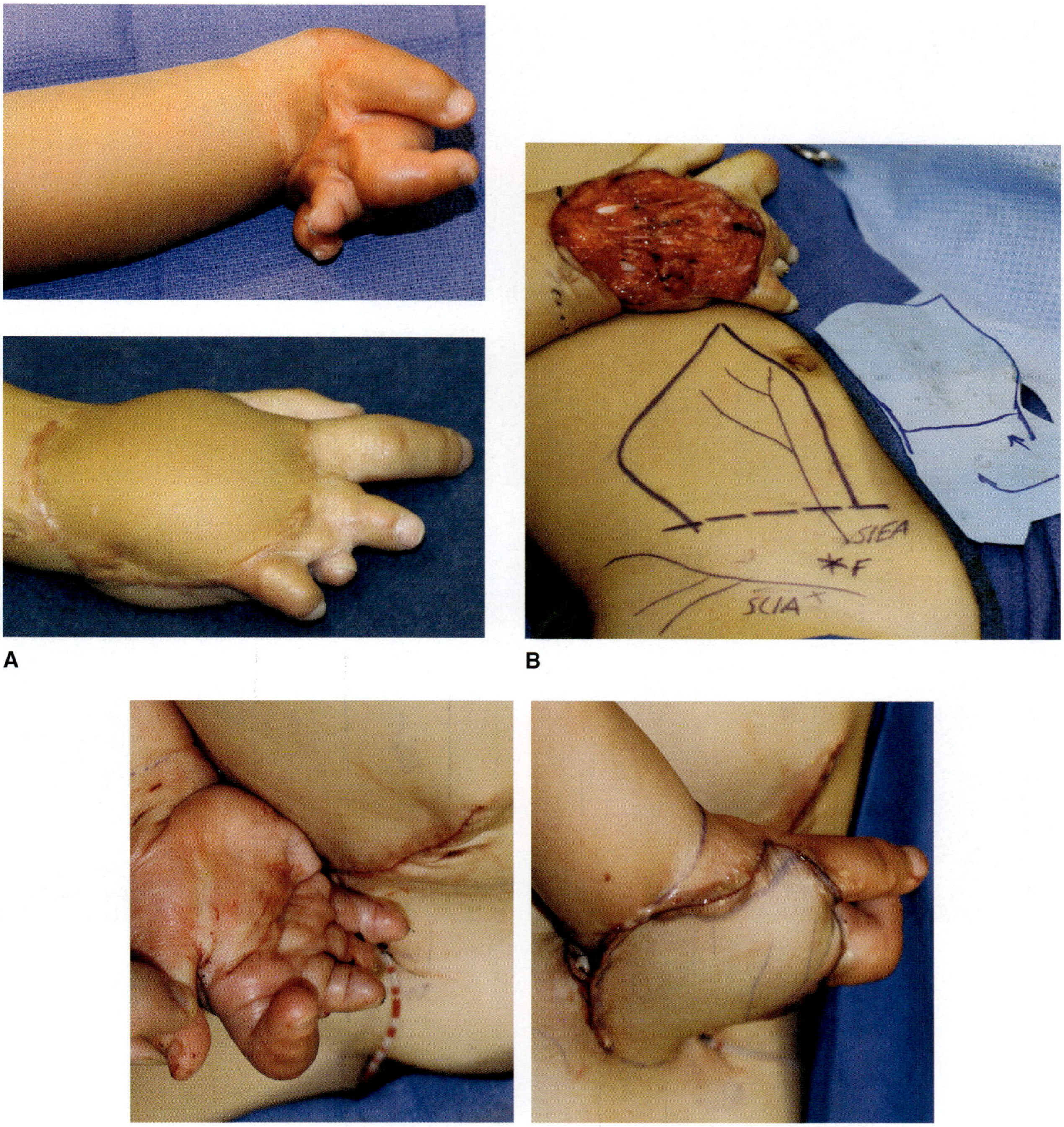

A B C

FIGURE 58-24 Lower abdominal pedicle flap to hand. (**A**) A 3-year-old child with a severe neonatal burn contracture is seen before and after release and flap transfer. (**B**) The broad inferiorly based flap contains the superficial inferior epigastric vessels. (**C**) A closed system and secure fixation and inset of the flap are necessary in mobile, active, often irritable children.

(if available) or full-thickness skin grafts. The auriculotemporal nerve on the TPFF can be coapted to the palmar cutaneous branch of the median nerve. The man shown in Figure 58-26 with a 32-year follow-up was resurfaced within 3 days of his injury; returned to work within 2 months; and has had thin, durable, sensate skin in the palm of his hand. He declined to have the grafts replaced with skin from the instep of his foot.

When a muscle covered with a skin graft is used to resurface this region, its bulk will diminish with time, but the long-term outcome will not be as satisfactory as a fascial flap covered with the same type of graft. Often small segments of the muscle may be reinnervated from underlying thenar or hypothenar intrinsic muscles and move simultaneously with contraction of these muscles. Staged flexor tendon reconstruction is difficult beneath any flap in this region, and the first stage implantation of Silastic rods should be performed during the initial procedure if at all possible. The same principle is true for large segmental nerve defects. During the past few years, we have tried to autograft dermal cells into a granulating bed before application of autogenous skin grafts but have discovered that the abundant

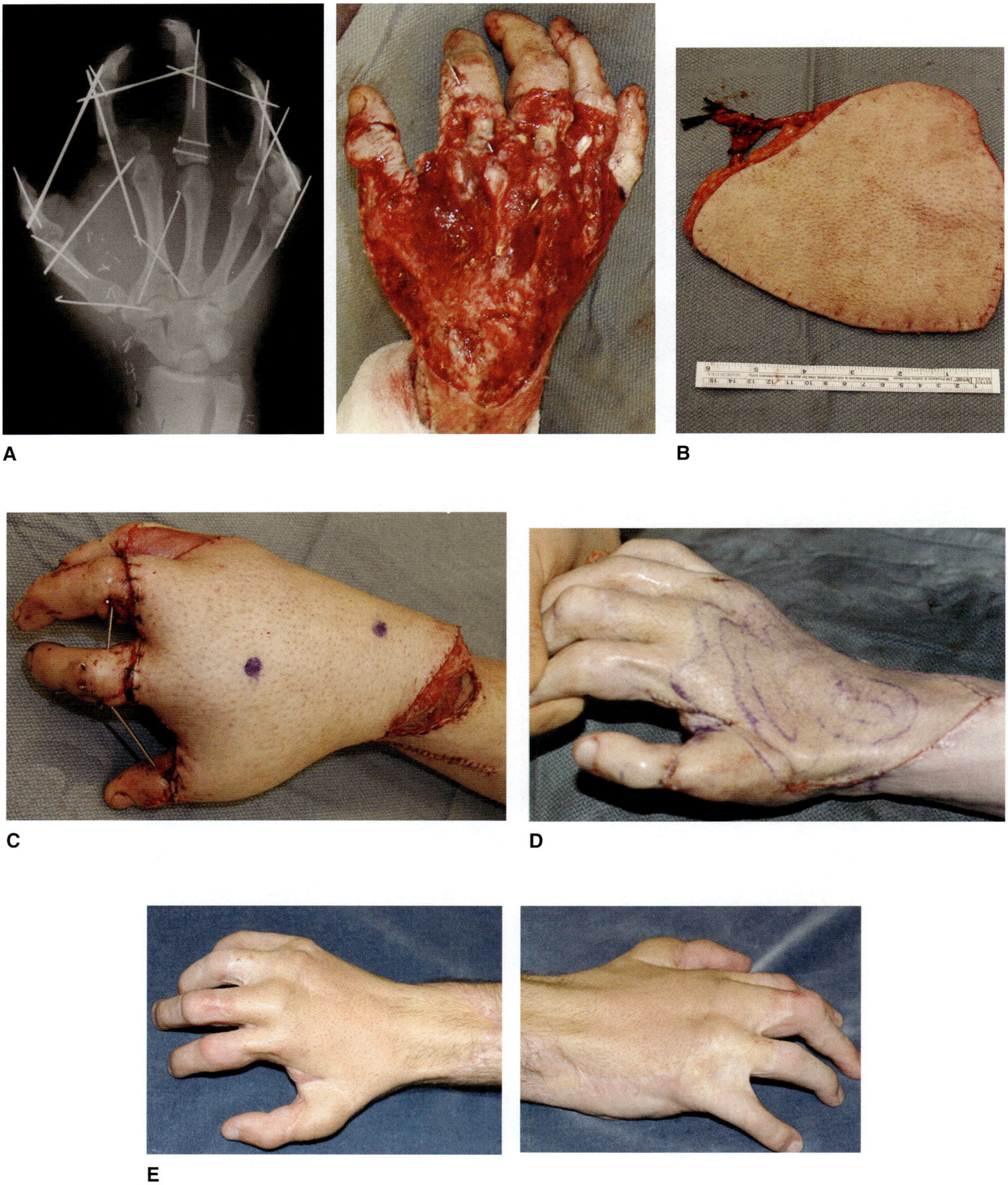

FIGURE 58-25 Anterolateral (ALT) thigh flap to hand and wrist. (**A**) Creative pin fixation after a massive crush avulsion injury to the hand allowed improved access to the dorsum of the hand devoid of soft tissue coverage. (**B**) A large ALT flap has been harvested in a large male patient. (**C**) The flap is bulky after inset and revascularization to the radial artery and cephalic vein. The thick wall of the flap proximally was skin grafted. (**D**) One year later, liposuction beneath the entire flap was completed in one stage. (**E**) Appearance 12 years later.

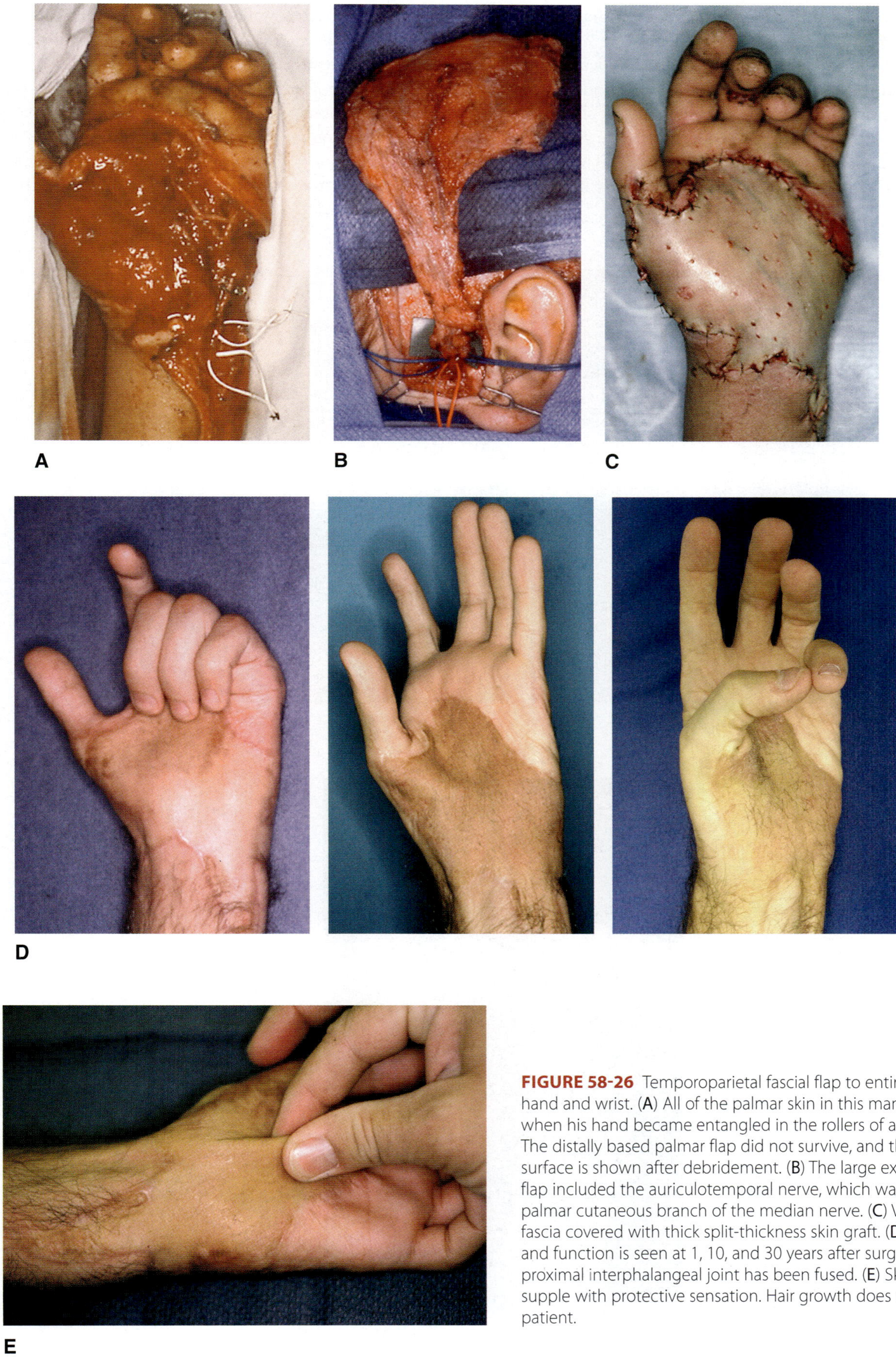

FIGURE 58-26 Temporoparietal fascial flap to entire palm of hand and wrist. (**A**) All of the palmar skin in this man was avulsed when his hand became entangled in the rollers of a printing press. The distally based palmar flap did not survive, and the palmar surface is shown after debridement. (**B**) The large extended TPF flap included the auriculotemporal nerve, which was joined to the palmar cutaneous branch of the median nerve. (**C**) Vascularized fascia covered with thick split-thickness skin graft. (**D**) Appearance and function is seen at 1, 10, and 30 years after surgery. The index proximal interphalangeal joint has been fused. (**E**) Skin is tough but supple with protective sensation. Hair growth does not bother the patient.

scar tissue resulting from this surgery is unsatisfactory for any secondary operations.

One particularly compelling indication for fasciocutaneous or musculocutaneous transfers to the wrist and hand is after mutilating degloving injuries. The 12-year-old boy shown in Figure 58-27 presented with an avulsed, ischemic hand 10 hours after a water ski towrope avulsion injury. The wrist was dislocated, all flexor tendons were avulsed, nerves were stretched but intact, and all vessels were either severed or thrombosed. Despite efforts of divers, the amputated thumb could not be retrieved. Many intrinsic muscles did not survive and were debrided within the next 10 days. A bilobed scapular flap provided sufficient coverage of the wrist and proximal palm. Flexion and sensation returned to normal parameters. He has had no flap revision or thumb lengthening. He has adapted very well but does have occasional breakdown of the scar tissue

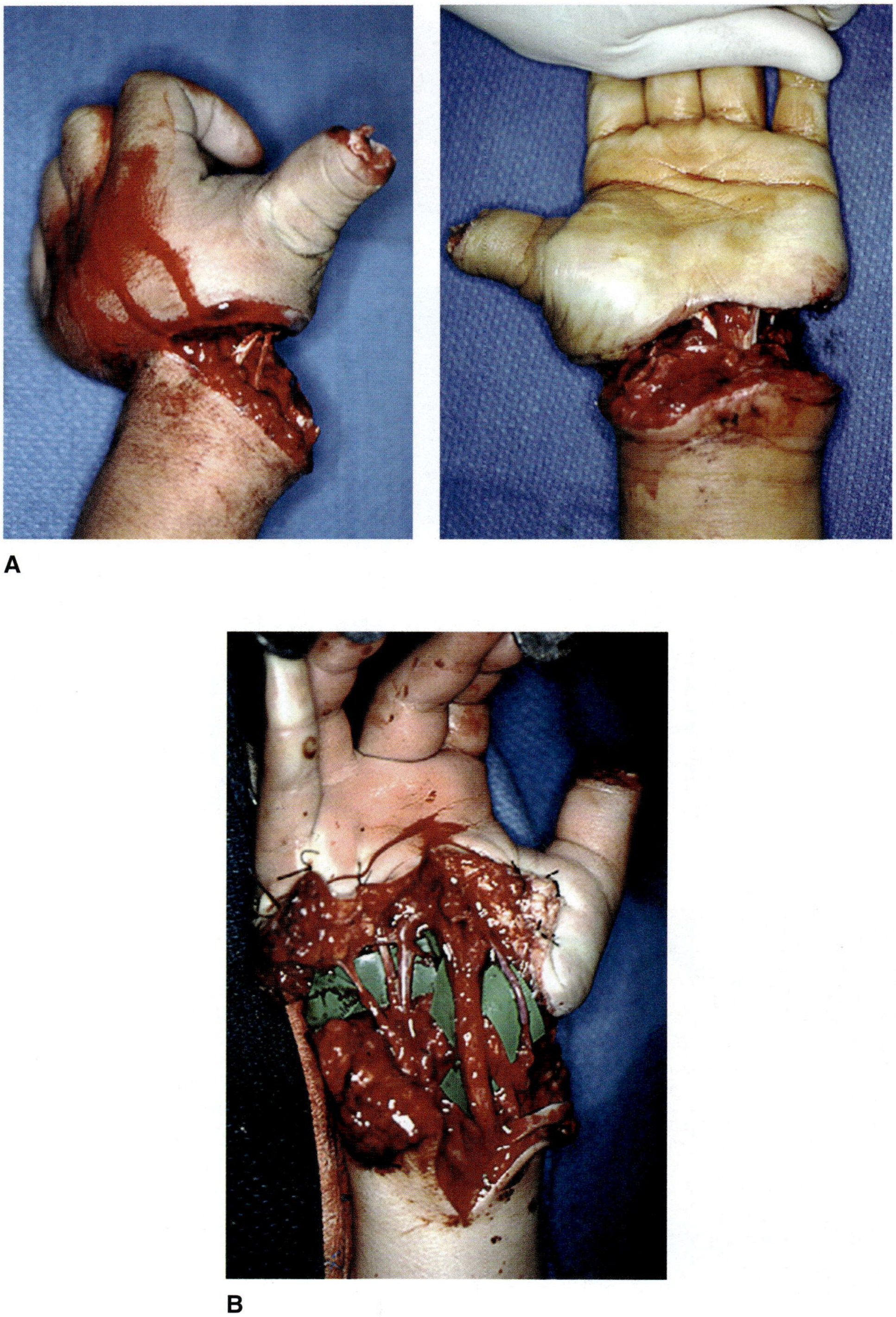

FIGURE 58-27 Split scapular flap to hand and wrist. (**A**) The thumb has been amputated at the IP joint level and the wrist completely dislocated in a water ski towrope accident. The median and ulnar nerves and radial and ulnar arteries have been transected. Many intrinsic muscles were debrided. (**B**) Appearance after primary neurovascular repairs. Flexor tendons were intact.

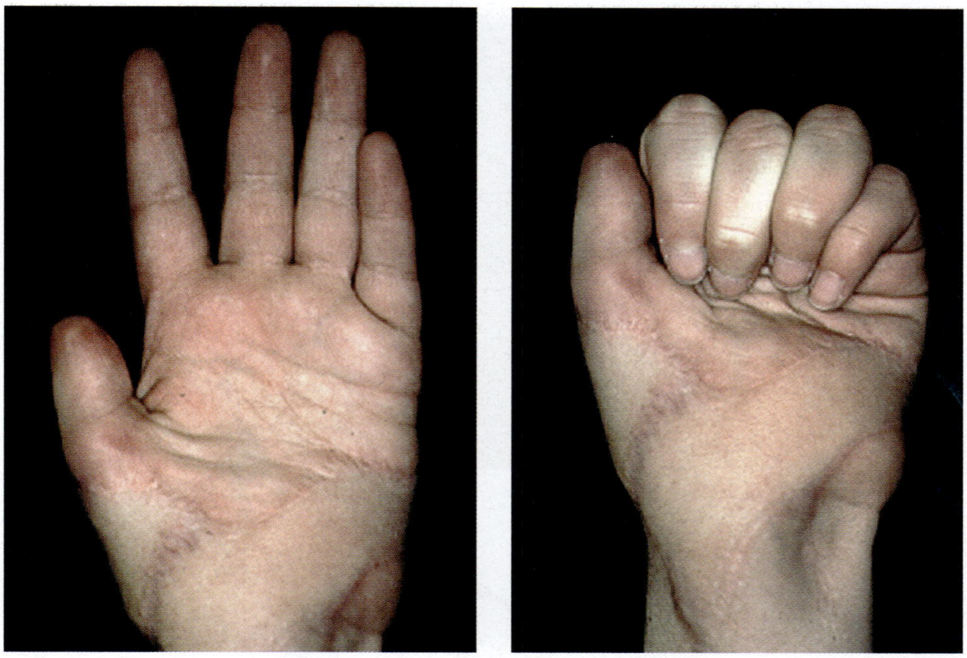

C

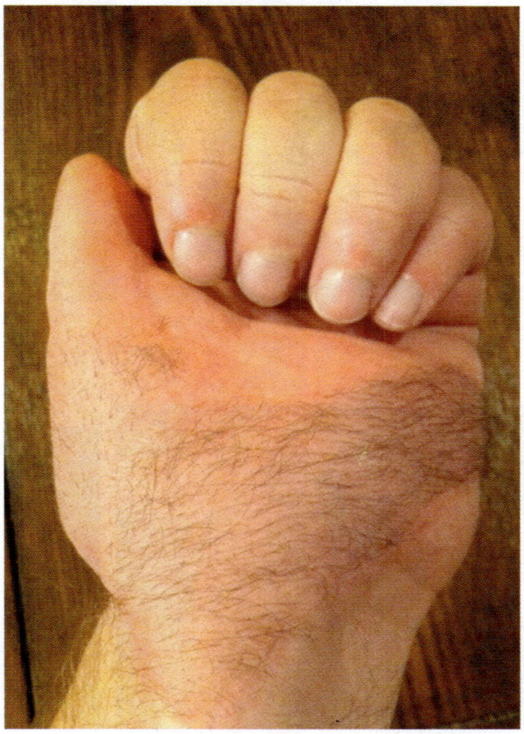

D

FIGURE 58-27 (*Continued*) (**C**) At the 5-year interval, sensation was intact, and digital flexion and extension were normal. There were no contractures. (**D**) Thirteen years after surgery, the flap bulk had increased. The patient has never noted any functional problems from the shorter thumb. He works as a sports broadcaster.

on the tip of his thumb and is not able to place his thumb in palmar abduction.

After severe mutilating farming and industrial injuries to the hand and wrist, multiple digits, the thumb, or both are missing.

These patients are candidates for toe-to-hand transfers. An excellent soft tissue bed is a prerequisite for any toe transfer. The boy shown in Figure 58-28 presented with a gangrenous stump after hand amputation at the carpal level. Debridement and graft coverage was effective only as a temporary measure. Groin flap coverage preceded a modified great toe transfer into the thumb position. More than 25 years after surgery, he uses his right hand for most activities of daily living, wears a prosthesis for executive meetings, and would not consider a hand transplant because of the morbidity of required immunosuppression.

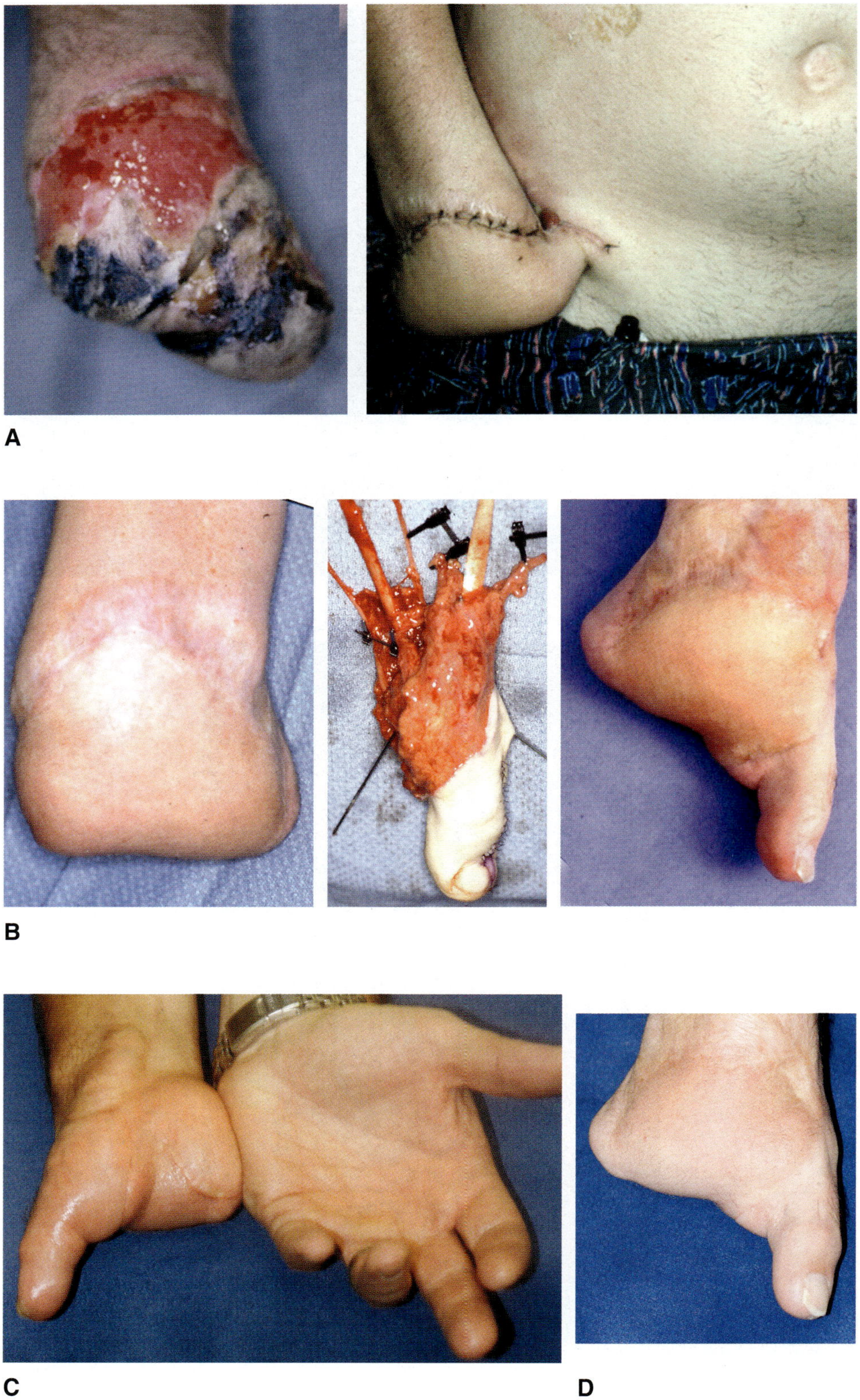

FIGURE 58-28 Groin flap to amputation stump. (A) One month after a band saw amputation of the right hand in a teenage boy working in the family business. Infection and ulceration compounded the full-thickness tissue loss. (B) Aggressive debridement and pedicled groin flap coverage effectively closed the wound and preserved length. (C) Five years later, a thumb was constructed with a modified great toe transfer. (D) The patient became a successful executive and is seen 25 years after surgery. As a right-handed golfer, he maintains a handicap index of 10 strokes.

Anterolateral thigh, latissimus dorsi, groin, scapular/parascapular, and to a lesser extent lateral arm donor sites are all effectively used in this region. Our experience with the lateral arm flap in particular has been quite encouraging because a large amount of relatively thin skin can be harvested from the arm donor site, which is then covered with a sheet graft as an entire aesthetic unit. The lateral arm donor site is also attractive because large amounts of tissue (8.0 cm × 20.0 cm) can be harvested with a primary donor site closure. In many white and most Asian patients, this skin is relatively thin. In the proximal half of the arm, it may be thick and robust, and dissection may become tedious. The lateral arm is not a good choice in obese patients.

DORSAL AND PALMAR SURFACES OF THE WRIST OR HAND

Simultaneous resurfacing of both surfaces of the wrist or hand is invariably required after severe crush, thermal, avulsion, or other industrial-related injuries. The initial consideration should be the possible use of remaining or amputated tissue as a spare part (see Figures 58-1 and 58-3). Most trauma services prefer to place a VAC and consult plastic surgery for application of a skin graft, which at best provides temporary coverage in a region that requires full-thickness flap coverage.

Prosthetic wear may be enhanced, and if toe transfer is a possibility, the extra tissue will be of great benefit. The principles and available flaps for resurfacing are similar to those previously presented.

FOREARM AND ELBOW

For smaller skin defects near the wrist or elbow, local donor tissues are available as long as they can be transposed, rotated, or advanced with intact perforating vessels. The repetitive system of arterial collaterals around the elbow joint in particular allows construction of perforator flaps from available tissue within the medial and lateral arm and volar forearm and usually obviates the need for free tissue transfers. The surgeon should always make the flap a little bit larger than the template and correct for both anticipated joint flexion and extension.

Volar or anterior wounds contract more than dorsal defects because of the lack of skeletal restraints. Full-thickness fasciocutaneous flap coverage is ideal for this region, and donor sites are usually available when simpler skin grafts are not practical. The skin in the distal third of the volar forearm is thin and mobile. A local fascial flap can be used quite effectively to cover exposed tendons and neurovascular structures, including the median nerve. Thick fasciocutaneous flaps harvested from the chest or abdomen may be cumbersome in the region when the patient has progressed through puberty and gains weight. Free fascial flaps are effective, and one forgotten application is the use of the posterior calf donor site with a vascularized sural nerve graft. The patient shown in Figure 58-29 lost volar skin and a 13-cm segment of median nerve in a grinding wheel injury. Multiple wrist flexors and superficial flexors were injured. Because the man was very hirsute, skin was not harvested with the flap. A 42-cm segment of sural nerve was divided into three cables, all of which bled with tourniquet deflation. Protective sensation returned within 18 months as well as some thenar muscle function. On his opposite forearm, a latissimus dorsi muscle was used to cover a much larger defect, but the nerve gaps could not be adequately reconstructed. A functionless intrinsic minus, claw hand deformity, has developed.

For many years, large defects on one or both surfaces of the forearm typically extending up to and sometimes including the elbow were covered with large flat muscles covered with split-thickness skin grafts. The latissimus dorsi and rectus abdominis muscles are most frequently used. Many trauma-oriented surgeons still prefer this approach. Most of these patients require

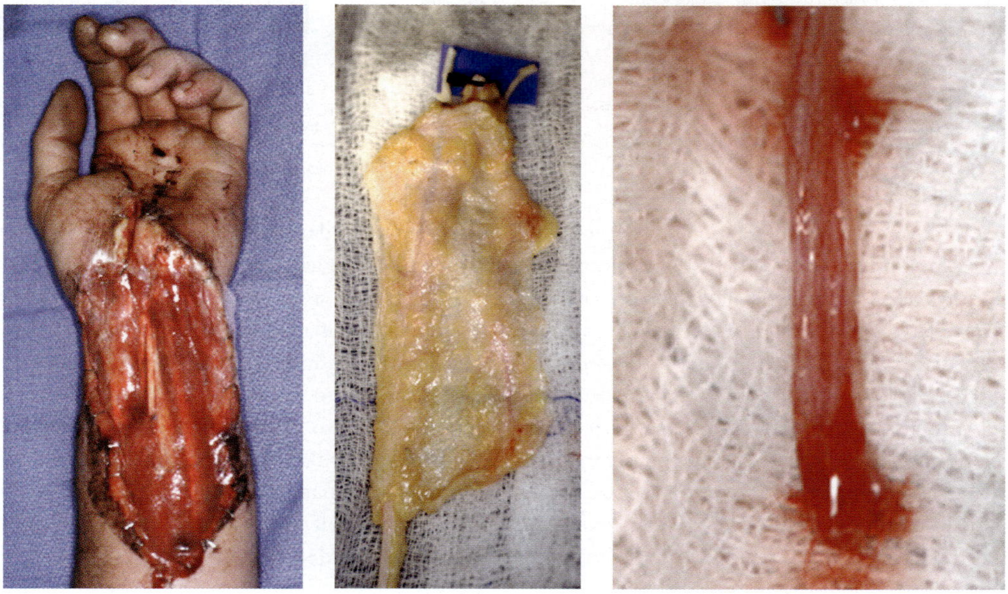

A B C

FIGURE 58-29 Posterior calf fascia and sural nerve transfer. (A) A large forearm skin defect with a 13-cm segmental defect of the median nerve. The lacerated ulnar nerve was advanced and coapted. (B) The posterior calf fascia and sural nerve have been isolated on the medial sural arterial system. (C) After revascularization, there is excellent bleeding from the most distal portion of the nerve.

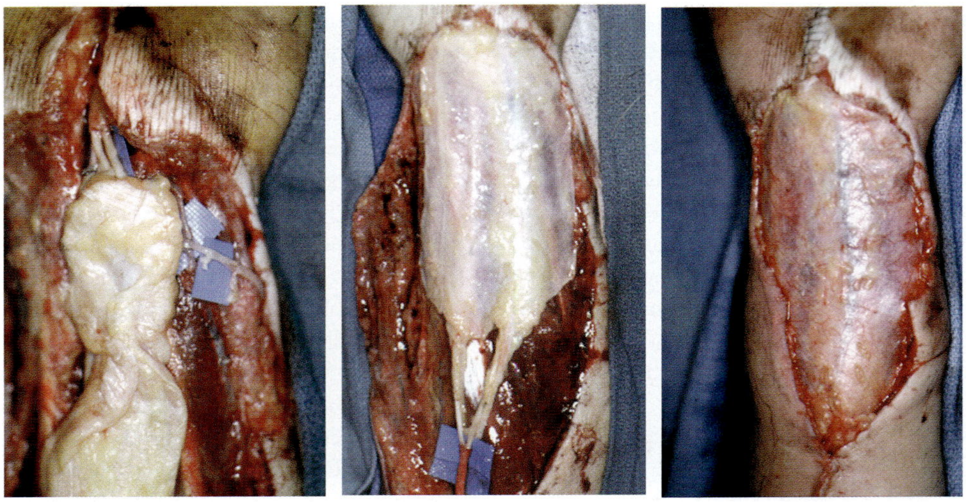

D

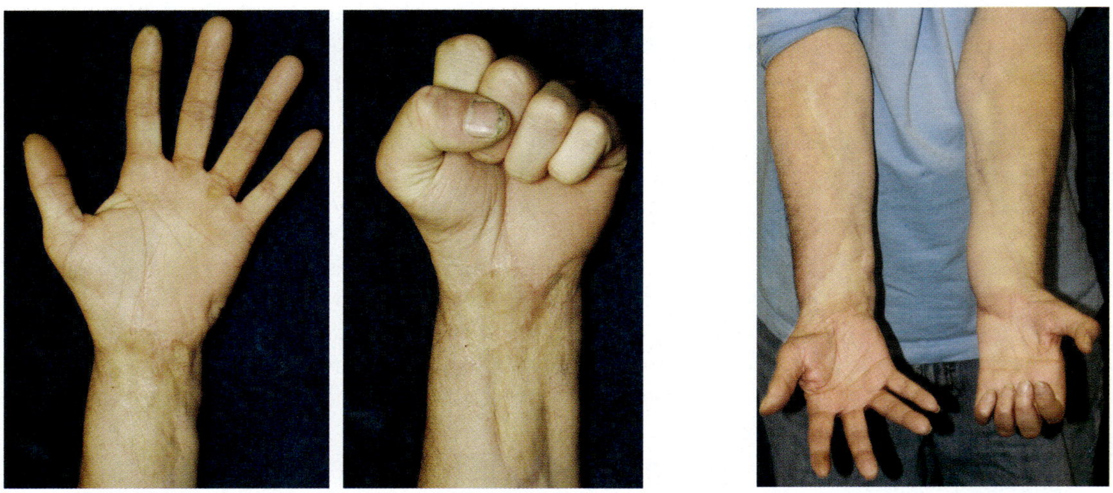

E F

FIGURE 58-29 (*Continued*) (**D**) The flap is inset and the nerve divided into three separate cables without disturbing its surrounding connective tissue. Fascia was covered with a skin graft. (**E**) Flexion and extension and good palmar abduction of the thumb are present 21 years later. (**F**) The opposite left hand which had a similar injury is clawed with minimal median or ulnar nerve function.

secondary hardware removal, nerve grafts, tenolyses, neurolyses, tendon transfers, muscle transfers, other soft tissue revisions and bone grafts. Within a few years, the muscles atrophy, and secondary contractures have created an inhospitable soft tissue environment. Secondary revisions are destined to fail. The woman shown in Figure 58-30 demonstrates the long-term inadequacy of a muscle covered with a skin graft. After a motor vehicle accident rollover avulsion injury, there was extensive circumferential loss of full-thickness tissue. Temporary wound closure was achieved with a latissimus muscle flap covered with grafts. A small island of full-thickness tissue remained on the muscle. Substance abuse and her general condition precluded more definitive resurfacing to allow secondary surgery. Within 3 years, her forearm was one solid scar. Pain and limited motion have rendered this limb useless. Transfer of her redundant lower abdominal tissues as a deep inferior epigastric artery perforator flap with secondary revision may have been a better option at the time of her original injury.

There are some other good options for these difficult wounds. If available, the latissimus dorsi, scapular, and rectus abdominis donor sites permit closure after harvest of a skin flap measuring up to 8.0 cm by 15.0 cm in most adults. One must be careful not to leave an open wound or graft over the mobile tip of the scapula, particularly in children. Larger amounts of tissue can be harvested from the thigh, where skin grafts are much better tolerated and are more of an aesthetic rather than functional burden for the patient. The versatile ALT flap has provided a welcome alternative to muscle flaps and skin grafts. After fracture reduction, tendon and nerve repairs, the wound shown in Figure 58-31 was closed completely with an anterior thigh flap, which can be harvested with minimal muscle and has large vessels and a more than adequate pedicle. Microsurgery

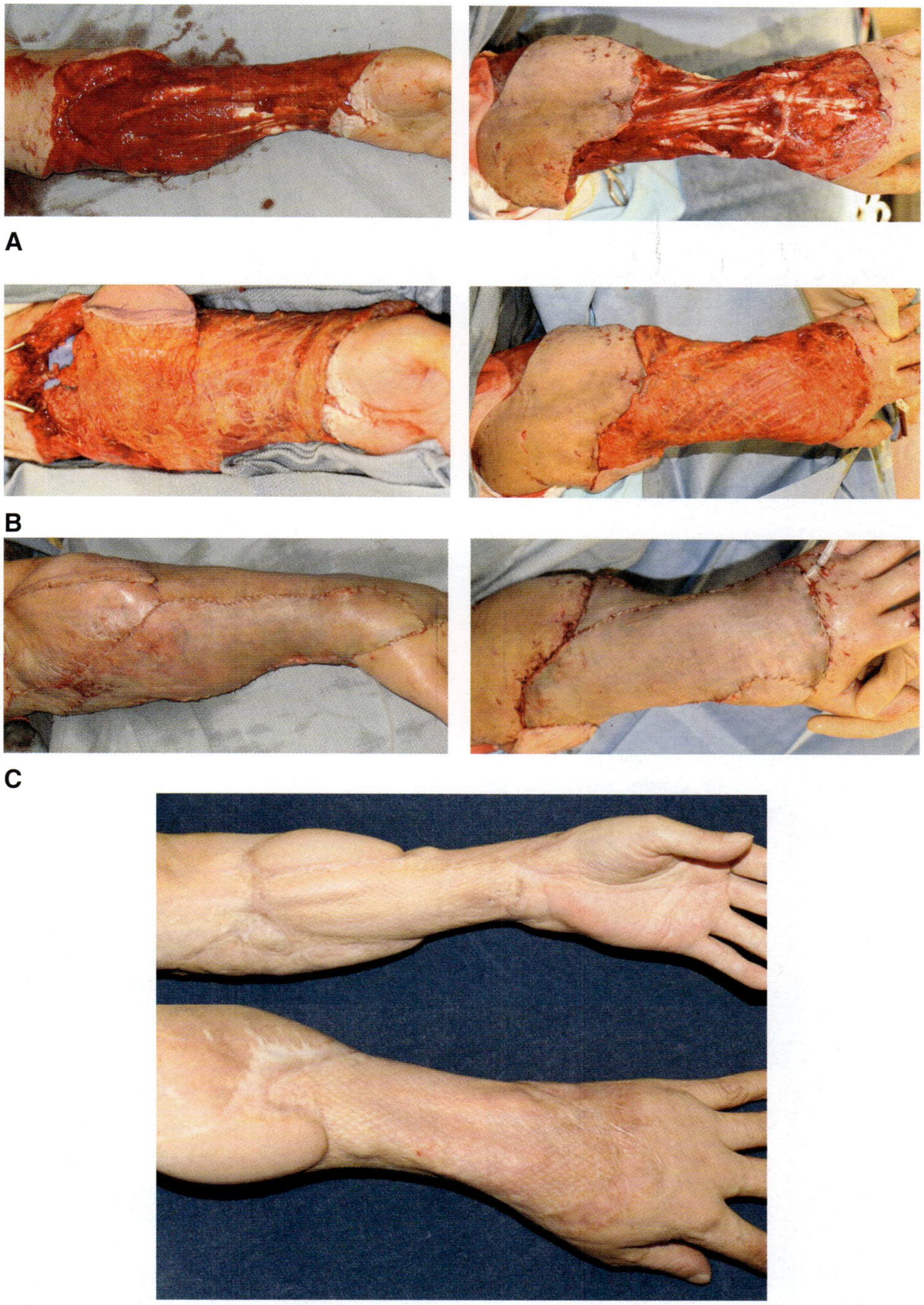

FIGURE 58-30 Latissimus dorsi muscle to forearm. (**A**) A circumferential degloving injury to the entire left forearm was associated with multiple flexor and extensor tendon lacerations and fractures of both bones. (**B**) A latissimus dorsi muscle and small skin island are wrapped around the forearm. (**C**) Muscle is covered with split-thickness skin grafts. (**D**) The same forearm 8 years later. All wounds have contracted. Tendons and muscles are contracted. The hand is functionless, and the patient has a well-established regional pain complex.

has been converted to macro surgery with this very versatile flap with large feeding vessels. Primary closure of the donor site is often possible. A small skin graft was required here.

Large defects on one or both surfaces of the forearm can be completely covered by preexpanding the groin, back, or chest before transfer as either a pedicled or free tissue transfer. The expanders should be placed beneath all fascia or muscle to be included within the flap and not within the region of the axial vessel(s) dissection. This technique is effective in children but is clearly labor intensive for the parents. Tunneling and externalizing the port in a remote area facilitate the expansion process, particularly in children. Weekly inflation can then conveniently be performed under sedation. The initial flap design, incisions, and inset should incorporate anticipated needs for secondary reconstruction. Functional muscle, vascularized bone, and neural transfers are more predictable when recipient nerves, veins, and arteries have been minimally traumatized. The child shown in Figure 58-32 fell beneath her grandfather's riding

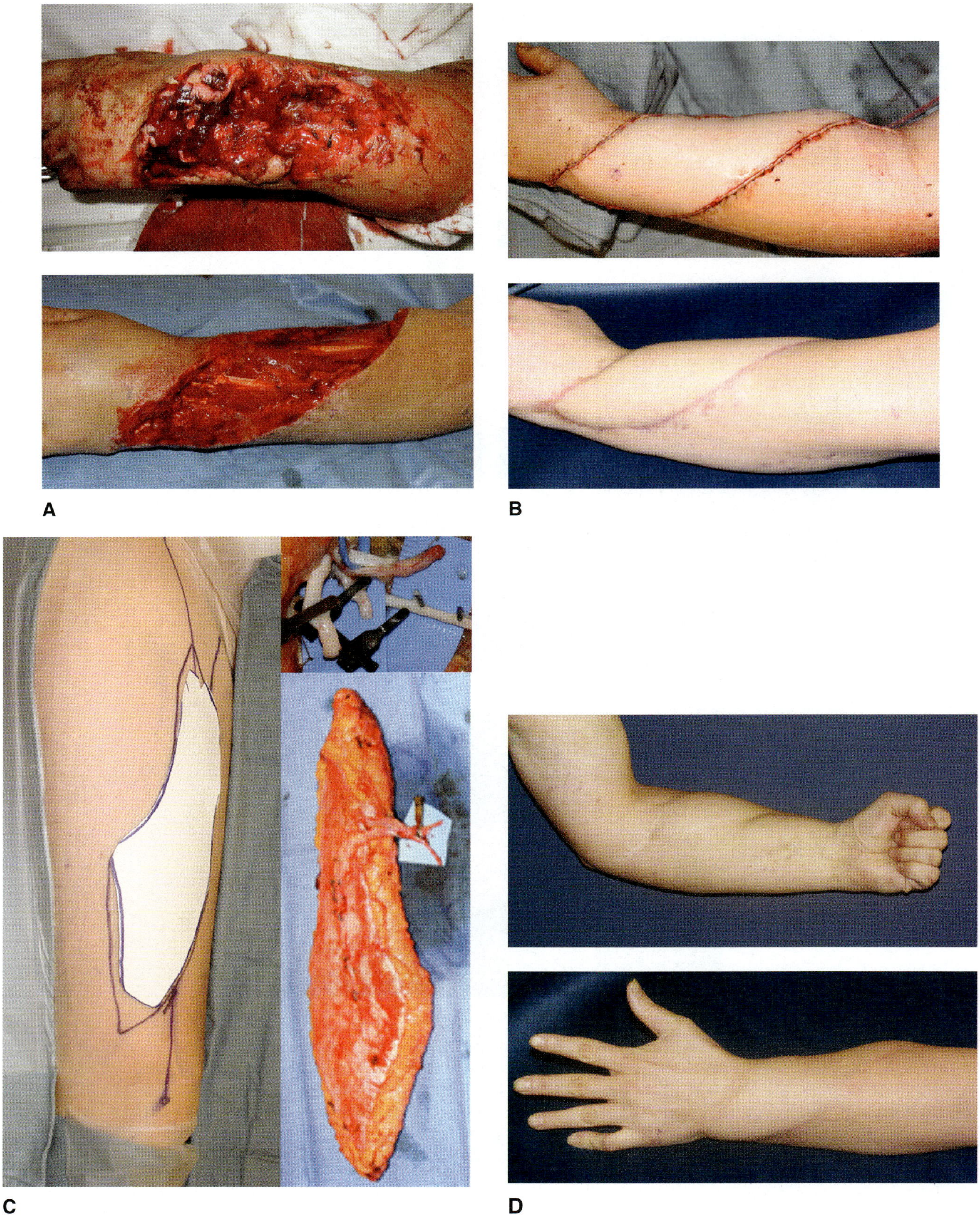

FIGURE 58-31 Anteromedial thigh fasciocutaneous flap to forearm. (A) A motor vehicle accident rollover injury resulted in extensive dorsal soft tissue loss with associated tendon, muscle, and skeletal injuries. (B) The template and harvest of this anteromedial thigh flap demonstrate the long vascular pedicle with large vessels. The inset shows conversion of microsurgery to macrosurgery. (C) Appearance after fracture reduction, tendon repair, and flap inset, all within the first 3 days after the injury. (D) Twenty-one years and no revisions later, the patient has full flexion and extension. Supination is restricted to 50 degrees. She functions very well running the engine room on an ocean fishing vessel.

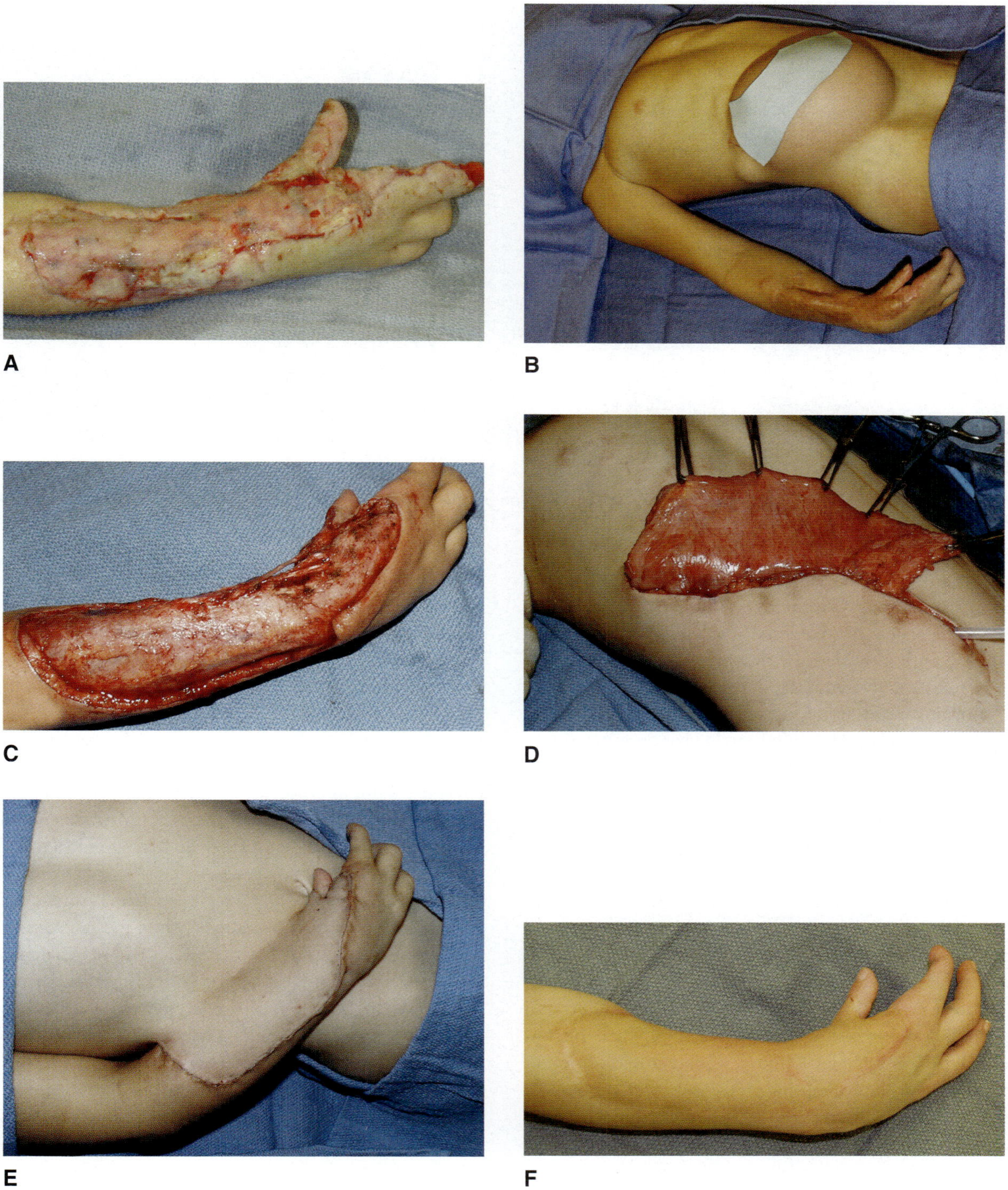

FIGURE 58-32 Expanded abdominal random flap for forearm coverage. (**A**) Temporary skin grafts have been used to cover a forearm defect after a lawnmower avulsion. (**B**) The expanded tissue in the ipsilateral abdomen will permit primary closure of the donor site. (**C**) Definitive forearm debridement. (**D**) The superiorly based abdominal flap. (**E**) Inset of the flap. (**F**) Detach and inset.

lawnmower and sustained severe damage to the radial side of the forearm and hand. Reattachment efforts succeeded in saving a portion of the thumb. Skin grafts were used as temporary wound coverage. Large expanders were placed in a position where the child would be most comfortable during limb attachment. More tissue than needed was transferred so subsequent Z-plasties could be used to lengthen the longitudinal scar on the volar forearm. Secondary procedures were easily accomplished beneath this ideal soft tissue environment. Multiple secondary procedures were performed. Skin expansion produced two things: a large flap and direct donor site closure.

There are clinical situations in which the child or adult may be too young, too active, or too sick for the procedures previously illustrated. The absolute goal is salvage of a limb, which has a reasonable degree of function. Aggressive surgery is the conservative approach when the nihilistic approach of doing nothing will fail. The child shown in Figure 58-33 presented at age 4 weeks with bilateral extensive soft tissue deficits, established contractures,

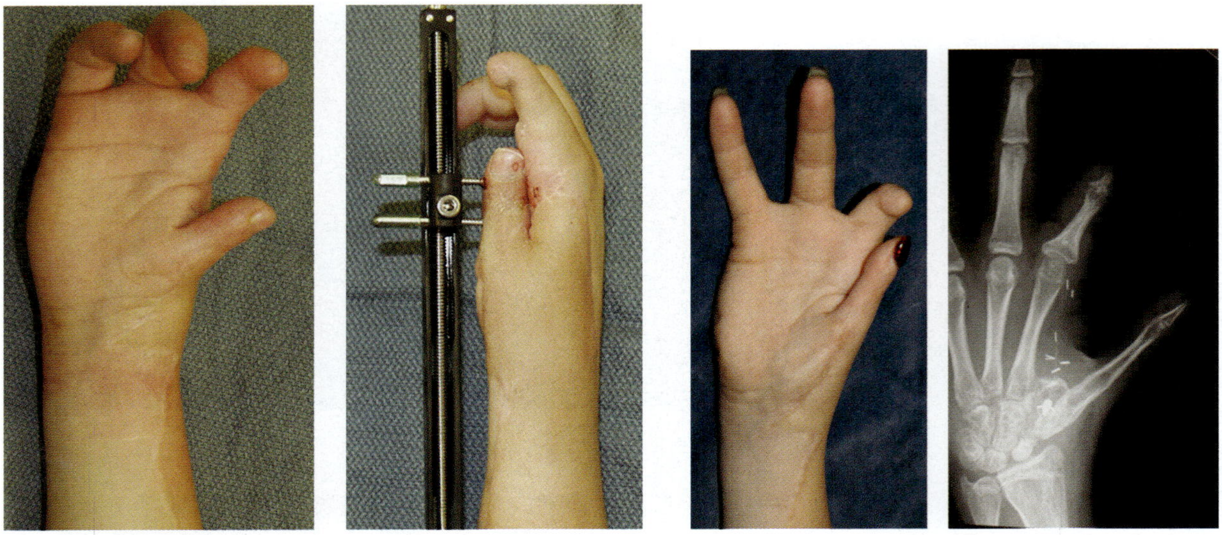

G H

FIGURE 58-32 (*Continued*) (**G**) With growth, the short thumb was lengthened to function as a radial post. (**H**) Appearance 15 years after the injury.

and osteomyelitis. Bilateral amputations were scheduled so she would not become septic. Within 3 weeks, both arms, wrists, and hands were adequately debrided and resurfaced with free flaps, which subsequently provided the proper cutaneous investment for growth, muscle and tendon transfers, neurolyses, and osteotomies. The tragic availability of her father's tissue contributed to this remarkable outcome. Her limb function has been superior to any prosthesis. This case underscores three things: the importance of soft tissue coverage, use of all available tissue, and the unexpected favorable outcome in a child.

Complex forearm wounds may be difficult to treat and involve the creative use of all available skeletal or soft tissue parts. In children, growth and function introduce problems, which cannot be precisely anticipated at the time of the original injuries. When soft tissue deficits occur early, growth and scar contracture will only accentuate the deformity. At age 2 years, the child shown in Figure 58-34 sustained an open fracture and soft tissue avulsion involving his right radius when he was dragged behind a motor vehicle. Initial wound coverage was not achieved, and the chronic, draining ulcer resulted in loss of most of the radius and a significant contracture. With time, the hand and carpus shortened and dislocated relative to the ulna. Skeletal traction was used to regain length, and his contralateral radius and forearm soft tissues were transferred from his flail opposite left upper extremity, which had been injured in the same injury. Proper wrist alignment and motion was restored. In this particular case, autogenous tissue was used in the form of a cross-forearm transfer to improve the alignment and function of his only functional hand and wrist. On the flail left side, the hand and wrist were centralized over the intact distal ulna, and a free gracilis muscle transfer was performed for elbow flexion.

ARM AND AXILLA

The characteristics of skin in this region are similar to that for the elbow and wrist: thin, mobile skin, often with a generous layer of subcutaneous adipose tissue both medial and lateral. The lateral or posterior surface is often hirsute in men. Within the axilla is a hair-bearing surface richly laden with apocrine glands. The arm consists of a large tubular bone surrounded by flexor and extensor muscle compartments, which contain large skeletal muscles. Consequently, both large and small wounds with or without exposure of nerves or bone in this region are usually well vascularized. Skin grafts are well tolerated, and the need for full-thickness coverage is not as critical for tendon motion and joint mobility. In contrast, the forearm needs a full-thickness envelope for the much smaller muscles with gliding tendons and distal retinacular structures.

In large complex wounds with exposure of these structures, free tissue may be necessary, especially if the subscapular artery and all of its potential flaps (scapular/parascapular, latissimus muscle, serratus muscle, scapular bone) from the adjacent chest wall cannot be used. All of the large flaps listed in Table 58-3 can be used and have been used effectively. Recipient vessels can be a problem. Several surgical pearls have been to use an intact, unscarred brachial system in the antecubital fossa after resurfacing of the brachial plexus and upper arm. The patient shown in Figure 58-35 demonstrates the progression of a difficult lymphatic malformation and the innovative use of microsurgery to cover a chronic, impossible wound. This patient had been followed at our Children's Hospital her entire life and had seven separate resections of a lesion that involved her entire arm and axilla. As a child and adult, she wore clothes with a special lining to hold towels, which could absorb the fluid and control the odor. Microsurgical transfers enabled us to cover the arm and brachial plexus after a massive excision. Her wound was healed and her life restored. She joined the Peace Corps and served in many developing countries as a social worker. She is now pain free, wound free, and working free for the Peace Corps at age 58 years.

Severely traumatized, burned, contracted, and scarred arms in children often need large amounts of tissue. Free tissue transfer may be difficult and donor sites limited in these small

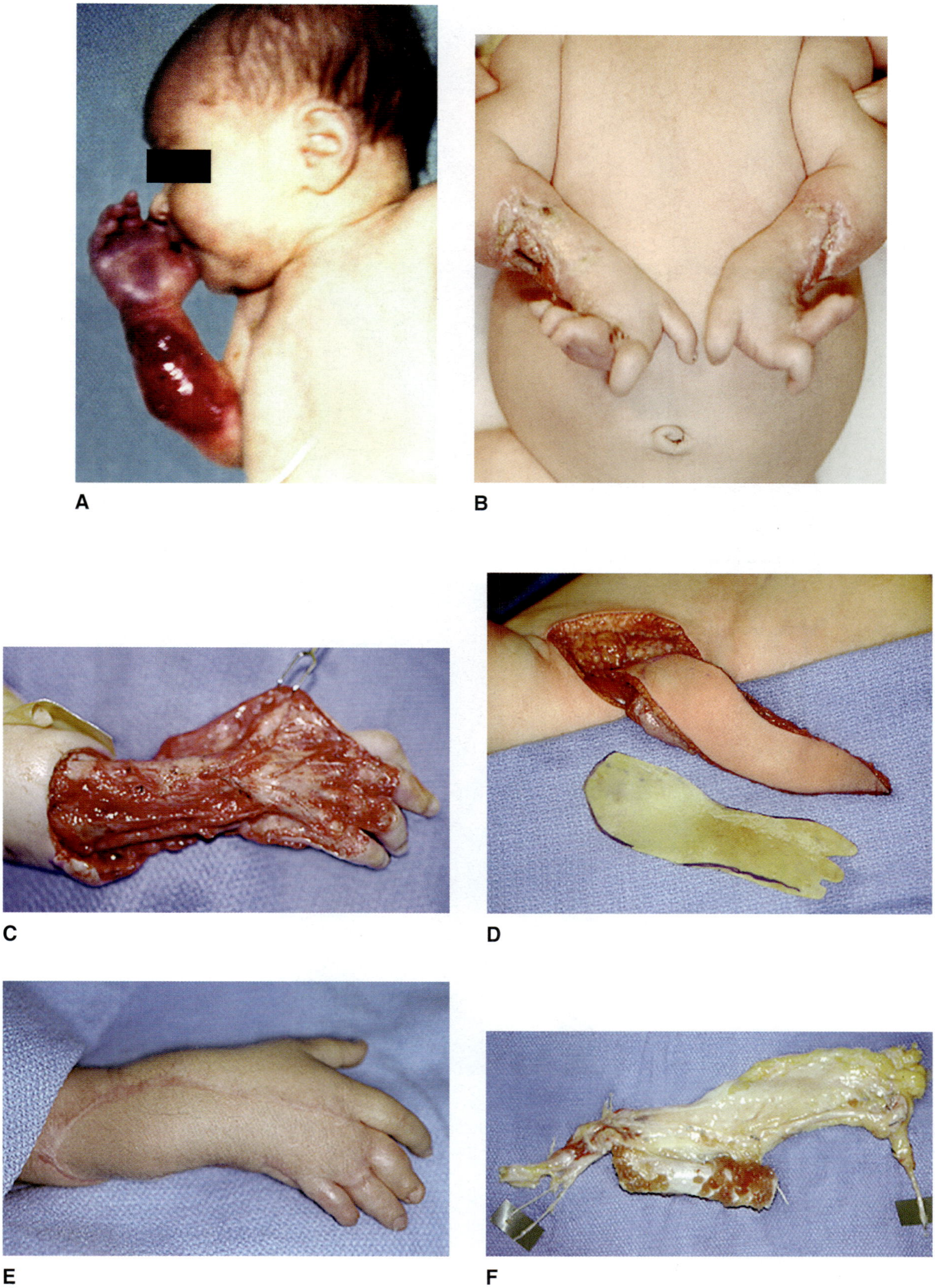

FIGURE 58-33 Bilateral latissimus dorsi musculocutaneous flaps for coverage of both forearms in an infant. (A) This dizygotic baby developed neonatal Volkmann's ischemia. Both arms are involved. She also had a unilateral cerebrovascular stroke. (B) Major contractures with infected ulnae at age 6 weeks. (C) The wound of the right forearm after release of contracture and debridement. (D) Template and latissimus dorsi musculocutaneous flap. (E) Right side 2 months after release. (F) Bone and nerve allograft harvested from the father after he had died from a ruptured aneurysm. His radius was used to reconstruct the infant's right ulna, and his radial nerves were used as grafts for both ulnar nerves.

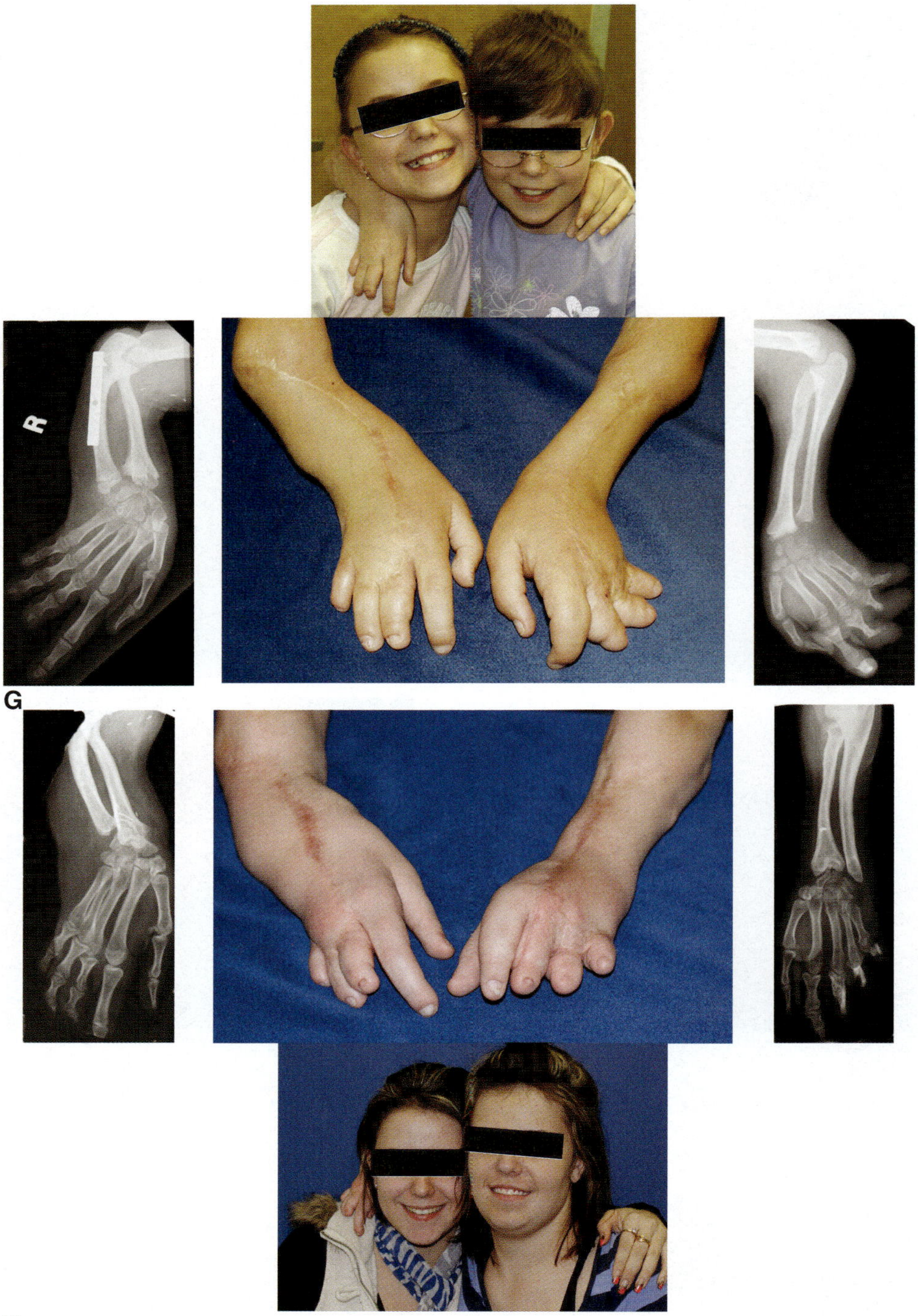

G

H

FIGURE 58-33 *(Continued)* (**G**) Twins at age 8 years. Ulnae are intact and growing, and ulnar nerve sensation is intact with 8 mm two-point discrimination. (**H**) Twins at 17 years of age. The three-ulnar digits on the left hand have been lengthened with bone grafts.

patients. Here preexpanded fasciocutaneous flaps from the ipsilateral chest wall will provide enough full-thickness tissue to wrap 270 degrees around the arm and elbow. The remaining portion along the medial arm can then be skin grafted followed by detachment of the pedicle flap and inset as the chest wall is closed primarily.

Coverage of the shoulder is a specialized problem after four-quarter amputation, traumatic amputation, problematic wounds, and brachial plexopathies. Transposition or rotation of local tissue is usually a better option than free tissue transfer. Often a filleted portion of the amputated arm or forearm can be salvaged as a pedicled island flap to provide sufficient coverage. A forgotten excellent option for coverage of extremely difficult wounds here is a free omental flap covered with a local flap or skin graft. These same tissues can be transferred, inset, and revascularized in the ipsilateral neck.

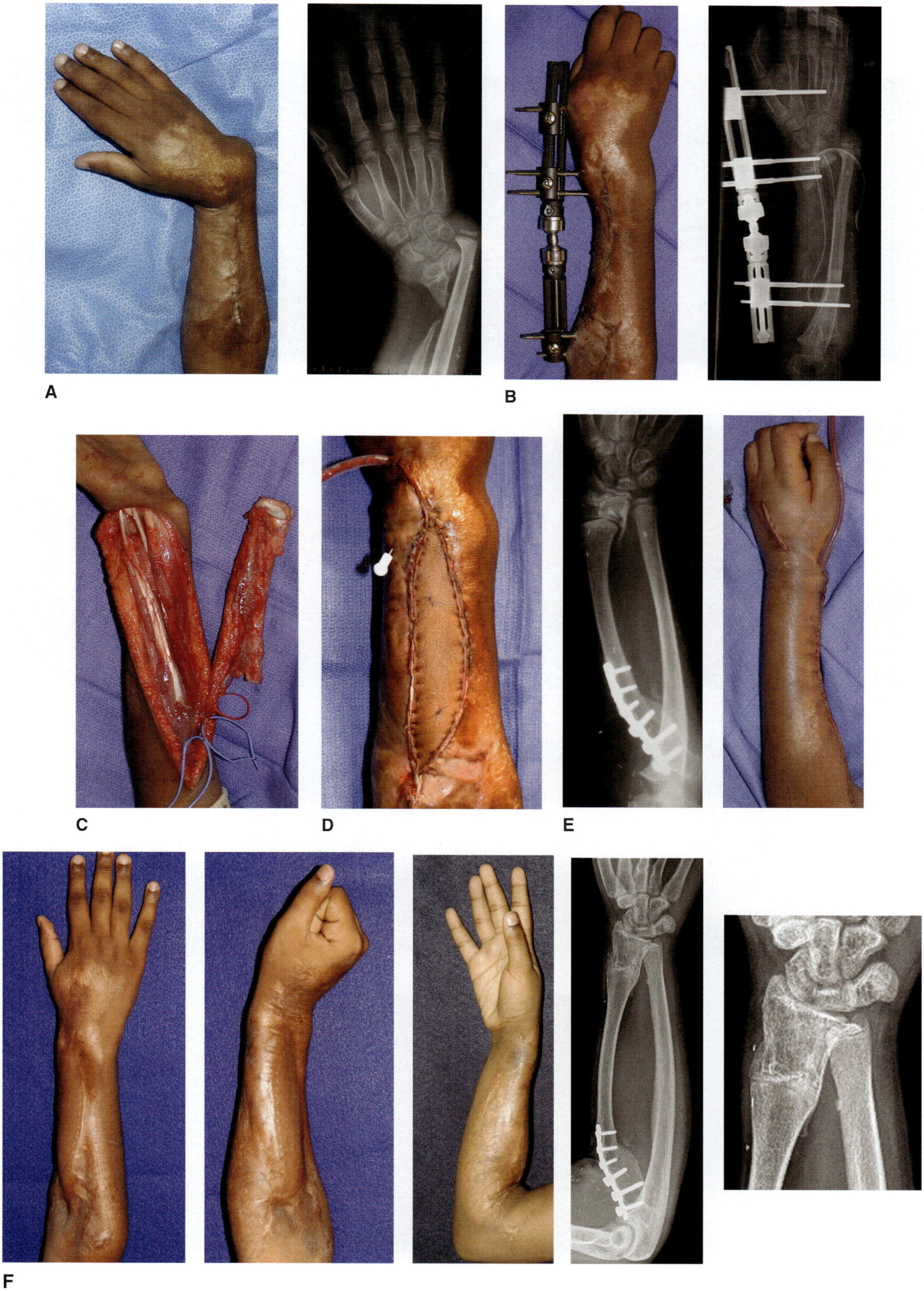

FIGURE 58-34 Radius osteocutaneous flap cross-arm transfer. (**A**) Appearance of a contracted right forearm after osteomyelitis and soft tissue loss at age 2 years. (**B**) The hand and wrist have been distracted to length. (**C**) The radius and soft tissue from the opposite flail left upper limb have been isolated as a flow-through composite tissue transfer. (**D**) After inset and revascularization. (**E**) The distal radius was placed beneath the intact distal radius of the recipient side. (**F**) There is slight radial bowing. Forearm pronation/supination and wrist flexion/extension 10 years later. Close-up radiograph shows that growth plates have closed.

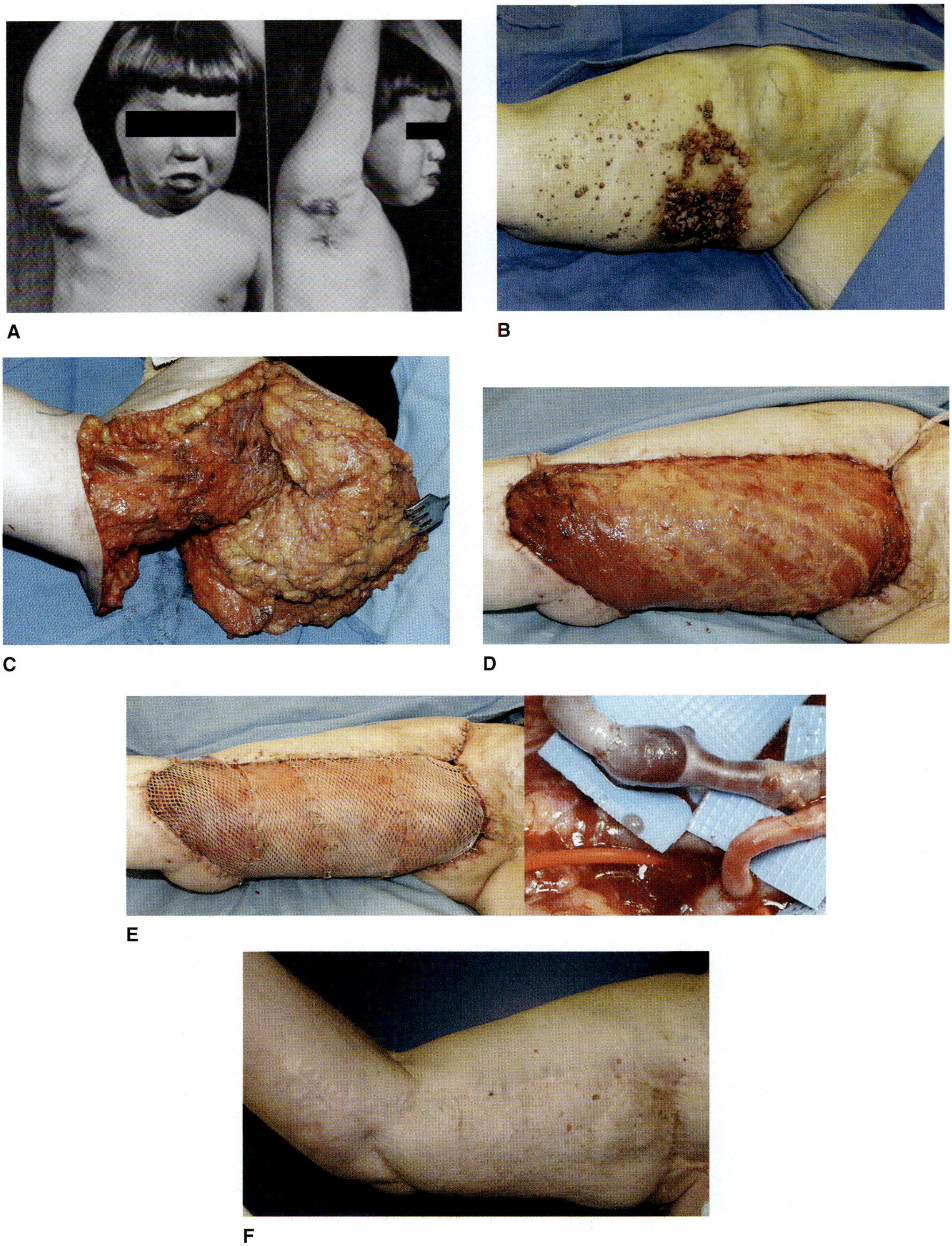

FIGURE 58-35 Latissimus dorsi muscle flap to arm and axilla. (A) Child at age 1 year with vesicular lymphatic malformation involving the arm and axilla. (B) Same patient 38 years later with chronic ulceration, maceration, and a feculent odor. (C) Resection involved complete removal of involved skin and subcutaneous planes and full dissection of the brachial plexus. (D) The contralateral latissimus dorsi muscle was transferred, revascularized, and inset. (E) Covered with a meshed spit-thickness skin graft. The inset shows macroanastomoses within antecubital fossa. (F) Follow-up at age 58 years pain free and ulcer free and with normal limb function.

REFERENCES

1. Blondeel PN, Morris SF, Hillock GG, Belgian PC (eds). *Perforator Flaps Anatomy, Technique & Clinical Applications,* vol. I. St. Louis: Quality Medical Publishing, 2006.
2. Brown DM, Upton J, Khouri RK. Free flap coverage of the hand. *Clin Plast Surg* 1997;24:57–64.
3. Brown RE, Wu TY. Use of "spare parts" in mutilated upper extremity injuries. *Hand Clin* 2003;19:73–87.
4. Chen HC, Tang YB, Mardini S, Tsai BW. Reconstruction of the hand and upper limb with free flaps based on musculocutaneous perforators. *Microsurgery* 2004;24:270–280.
5. Foucher G (ed). *Reconstructive Surgery in Hand Mutilation.* St. Louis: Mosby, Martin Dunitz, 1997.
6. Fu-Chan W, Mardini S (eds). *Flaps and Reconstructive Surgery.* St. Louis: Saunders and Elsevier, 2009.
7. Jones NF, Lister GD. Free skin and composite flaps. In *Green's Operative Hand Surgery*, 6th ed, vol. 2, pp. 1721–1756.
8. Koschnick M, Bruener S, Germann G. Free tissue transfer: an advanced strategy for post infection soft-tissue defects in the upper extremity. *Ann Plast Surg* 2003;51:147–154.
9. Levin LS, Erdmann D. Primary and secondary microvascular reconstruction of the upper extremity. *Hand Clin* 2001;17:447–455.
10. Millard DR Jr. *Principilization of Plastic Surgery.* Boston: Little, Brown and Company, 1986.
11. Moran SL, Cooney WP. Soft tissue surgery. In *Master Techniques in Orthopedic Surgery,* St. Louis: Lippincott Williams & Wilkins, 2009.
12. Neligan PC. *Plastic Surgery,* 3rd ed, vol. 6: *Hand and Upper Extremity.* Chang J (ed). St. Louis: Elsevier Saunders, 2013.
13. Netter FH. Atlas *of Human Anatomy*, 2nd ed. ICON Learning Systems, 1997.
14. Neumeister M, Hegge T, Amalfi A, Sauerbier M. The reconstruction of the mutilated hand. *Semin Plast Surg* 2010;24:77–102.
15. Pederson WC. Upper extremity microsurgery. *Plast Reconstr* Surg 2001;107:1524–1537; discussion 1538–1539, 1540–1543.
16. Strauch B, Vasconez L, Hall-Findlay EJ (eds). *Grabb's Encyclopedia of Flaps,* vol. 2: *Upper Extremities.* Boston: Little, Brown and Company, 1990.
17. Strauch B, Yu H-L, *Atlas of Microvascular Surgery.* New York: Thieme, 1993.
18. Weinzweig N, Weinzweig J. *The Mutilated Hand.* Philadelphia: Elsevier-Mosby, 2005.

CHAPTER 59

Emergency Free Flaps

Luis R. Scheker and Christiana Savvidou

The place of emergency flap coverage in reconstruction of the traumatized extremity is well established. It became popular and commonplace by the end of the 1980s, but in reality started in the latter part of the 1970s. Its development followed advances in anesthesia, pharmacology, imaging, and instrumentation and broader knowledge of the anatomy and physiology of flaps that took place from 1973 with the description of the groin flap and was aided by the formation of emergency microsurgical teams for hand and digital replantation (1).

The term "emergency free flap" was coined by Lister and Scheker in their presentation of the preliminary results to the IFSSH Post-Congress in Bloomington, Indiana, in 1983. This paper was published in 1988 reporting the success in 31 patients ranging in age from 16 to 57 years, covering defects measuring from 13 to 540 cm^2, with an average of 145 cm^2 (1). Since then multiple articles have proposed its use, and some have tried to predict the outcome depending on the location of the defect and whether it affects the upper versus the lower extremity (1–16).

Wound closure has evolved over the years with many advances developed during military conflicts from ancient times to the most recent world wars. Damage inflicted on the participants forced the treating medical team to create expedient ways to achieve wound closure and save the individuals from sepsis and death.

Closure of a clean wound has been performed immediately since the Middle Ages. Untidy wounds have been treated in different ways after the first textbook of surgery, written by Guy de Chauliac in 1363, which stated that certain wounds should be treated by delayed closure, such as ulcerated, abscessed, and contused wounds. In 1545, Ambrose Paré introduced the concept of wound cleansing, but it was Pierre Joseph Desault in the late 18th century who coined the term "debridement" (17). By the 19th century, Louis Pasteur and Robert Koch had established the concept of infection by germs. This germ theory led Joseph Lister to develop the use of carbolic acid, an antiseptic used to control infection. All of these developments led to the principle of delayed closure of contaminated wounds (multiple-stage reconstruction) (18). This concept was established even though conventional flaps were readily available and still has a place in reconstructive hand surgery, depending on the type of wound. However, several reports have shown the benefits of emergency free flap coverage of extremity injuries (1–9). These reports demonstrate that the traditionally accepted technique of delayed closure of contaminated wounds has been effectively challenged.

The most important indication for an emergency free flap is when vessels are exposed and at risk of desiccating or becoming traumatized by dressings or vacuum-assisted wound closures. After all, blood supply must be maintained or the extremity dies. Other benefits of emergency free flaps include earlier recovery, faster return to maximum range of motion, and shorter time for return to work compared with multiple-stage, delayed reconstruction.

OPTIONS FOR FREE FLAP COVERAGE

The anatomical knowledge that has accumulated following the description of pedicled flaps and the initial free groin flap has enabled the reconstructive surgeon to match "like with like" in an amazing fashion.

Today not only do we look at the functionality of the extremity but also how to minimize the morbidity of the donor site while returning the appearance of the extremity to as normal as possible in size, thickness, and color.

In selecting a free flap to reconstruct an injured extremity, we need to analyze the defect in surface area as well as depth. Every flap has a role in emergency reconstruction. Its use depends on the trauma sustained by the patient, how many extremities are involved, and what other area is affected. When the injury involves one extremity, a fasciocutaneous flap in the form of a perforator flap is now available. Depending on the size of the defect, our first choice for the injured hand is the lateral arm flap, because it has a reasonable pedicle that can be extended as shown by Acland et al. (10). It is sensate; has similar color as the hand; can be elevated under tourniquet control with a regional anesthetic block; and when using the ipsilateral lateral arm flap, the morbidity remains in the same extremity. This flap is excellent for reconstruction of the dorsum of the hand and the first web space. For females, we prefer the groin flap because the donor site can be closed primarily and the donor site is covered even with a small bathing suit. Other defects require larger flaps such as the scapular and the anterolateral thigh flap. When the defect requires bulk, the latissimus dorsi is still a good choice. For functional needs, we have used the gracilis flap even though the cutaneous part can be problematic.

For very small defects, especially for the pulp of the thumb or for segmental loss of the volar digits, when a cross-finger flap is not available, the first web space of the foot is an excellent donor site. The dorsalis pedis flap is seldom used today because its usefulness is limited by the donor site morbidity. If a large flap is elevated, the toe extensors can be exposed, and the skin grafted area frequently breaks down.

RADICAL DEBRIDEMENT

After obtaining a thorough history, examination of the injured hand is first done in the emergency department, where vascularity, sensation, active motion, soft tissue loss, and bone injury are assessed. Radiographs and laboratory studies, including wound cultures, are then obtained. Intravenous fluids and antibiotics are given. The surgeon can discuss with the patient and the family the surgical options, the realistic outcome, and the need for postoperative rehabilitation. The patient is then taken to the operating room.

The injured hand is completely evaluated under appropriate anesthesia, usually an axillary or supraclavicular block for isolated upper extremity trauma. In addition to minimizing the length of general anesthesia, the use of regional anesthesia provides postoperative vasodilation of the extremity, thus increasing blood flow to the injured areas and to the free flap. The injured hand is examined for vascularity of the digits and for injuries to the skin, tendons, bones, joints, nerves, and vessels to determine whether primary reconstruction is possible.

Adequate debridement is essential and is probably the most important factor in successful surgery. The goal of debridement is to remove all compromised or contaminated tissue. Tourniquet control is used initially during debridement to minimize bleeding and to increase visualization of anatomic structures and nonviable tissues. Debridement is completed with the tourniquet deflated to evaluate bleeding.

Debridement is begun at the periphery of the wound, where the surgeon establishes a plane of dissection between the normal and injured tissues. The idea is to excise the wound like a tumor. Fractured bone is debrided clean of small fragments that provide no structural support. Bone fragments with viable soft tissue or articular cartilage attached to them are left in place. Bone devoid of any soft tissue attachment is removed. Muscles that are severely contused and will not recover function, as well as muscles that are divided and the distal portion of which does not have any vascular supply, should also be removed. Tendons of such muscles may be woven end to side to the remaining musculotendinous units. Nonviable and even questionably viable tissue is excised back to bleeding margins. Debridement continues until only normal-appearing tissue remains. According to Godina (9), radical debridement should be a wound excision similar to that performed in cancer surgery in which the tumor is not seen by the knife; in fact, the wound "should look like the site of a surgically extirpated tumor." Certain anatomic structures, however, should be preserved. These structures include large vessels with normal flow and tendons and nerves that appear to be functional.

After the wound is considered to be clean, the tourniquet is slowly released to assess blood supply to the area; any tissue that still does not bleed and cannot be revascularized is excised. Copious irrigation of the wound by means of a bulb syringe, usually with Ringer's lactate solution, follows complete debridement. Pressure lavage should be avoided because it further damages the area involved. Cultures are taken at this point. The tourniquet is then reapplied, and further debridement is done as needed. After debridement is complete, the tourniquet is slowly released, and the wound is surveyed for significant bleeding points, which are then controlled.

If the wound appears completely healthy at this point, preparations for reconstruction are made. If the surgeon is in any doubt about the appearance of the wound, a Gram stain can be used to determine the presence of bacteria in the wound *after* debridement. Emergency reconstruction is then postponed, and antibiotic beads are placed in the wound. Free flap transfer is performed within the first 48 hours. Quantitative cultures are not useful in these cases because the results are only received after a potential flap is performed. Regular cultures and sensitivity are used to adjust antibiotic therapy to treat the appropriate bacteria after surgery. In most cases, cultures are negative after extensive debridement and profuse irrigation.

IMMEDIATE RECONSTRUCTION

The advantage of performing immediate free flap coverage is that those divided vessels can sometimes be used as recipient artery and veins. When arteries are divided and not repaired, the flow recedes to the site of the last viable branch. Also, the vascular planes are filled with fibrin-rich interstitial fluid that renders the vessels friable and difficult to manipulate, often requiring a lengthy vein graft.

If the wound is deemed appropriate for immediate free flap coverage, there is no excuse not to reconstruct bone defects with bone graft and internal fixation; this will provide the flap with a stable skeletal foundation on which to rest. Depending on the bone defect, bone can be incorporated in the flap as a fascio-osteocutaneous or an osteo-musculocutaneous flap. Sometimes there is a defect in multiple bones and it is difficult to harvest a flap with a structural geometry that corresponds to the defect. In this latter circumstance, free conventional nonvascularized bone graft should be used.

Nerve defects can be bridged using innervated flaps if there is a single nerve defect or with the use of nerve grafts either vascularized or conventional if a good tissue bed is present.

When there is a large number of flaps available for reconstruction, sculpturing the flap may not be necessary, and the defect and the donor area can be matched. However, if potential donor sites are limited because of trauma or the complexity of the patient, it may be necessary to tailor the flap by debulking or defatting the flap before inset. It is important to evert the edges of the wound for better contact between the flap and the recipient defect. If heparin is being considered, always place a drain, preferably a silicone sheath drain.

CASE PRESENTATIONS

Case presentations provide a more complete overview of the use of emergency free flaps.

A 22-year-old man had a severe extremity crush injury when his forearm was caught in a propeller. Examination showed skin loss, flexor tendon injury with a large musculotendinous defect, and neurovascular injury (Figure 59-1). After debridement of all devitalized structures, he underwent open reduction and internal fixation (ORIF) of forearm fractures, revascularization using saphenous vein grafts, nerve repair with sural nerve grafts, and a free latissimus dorsi flap for coverage of the volar forearm soft tissue defect (Figure 59-2). The patient achieved a good functional result with gradual atrophy of the latissimus muscle and a satisfactory cosmetic appearance (Figure 59-3).

A 16-year-old young man was involved in a motor vehicle accident, sustaining a crush injury of the dorsum of the left hand. Examination showed loss of skin, subcutaneous tissue, and extensor tendons and exposed metacarpal bones. The defect was more obvious after radical debridement (Figure 59-4).

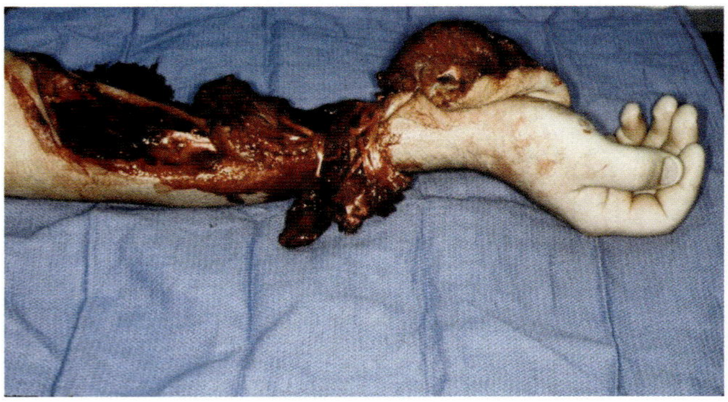

A

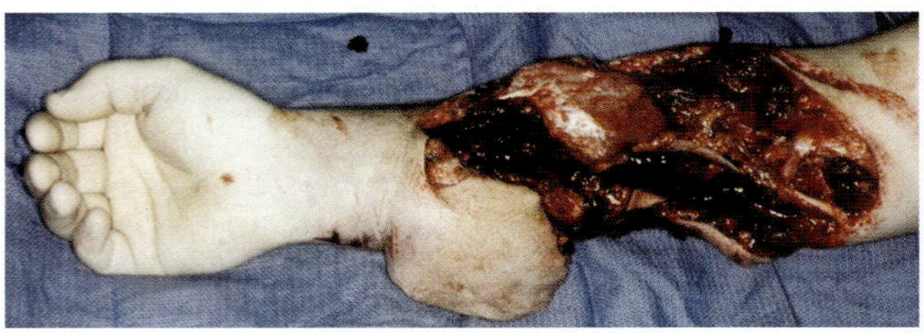

B

FIGURE 59-1 Severe crush injury of the forearm with multiple structures missing—bone, muscle, tendon, and neurovascular loss (A and B).

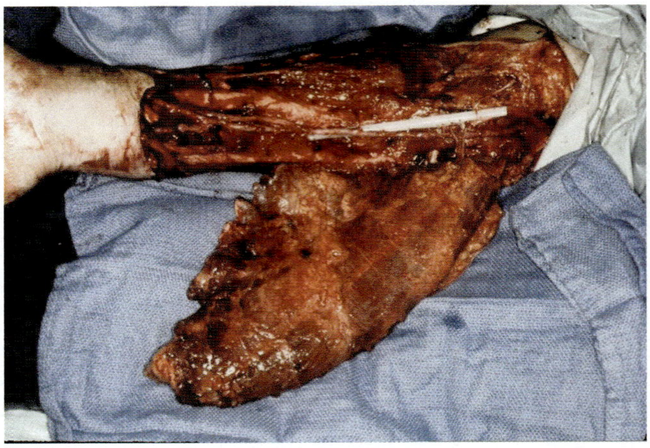

A

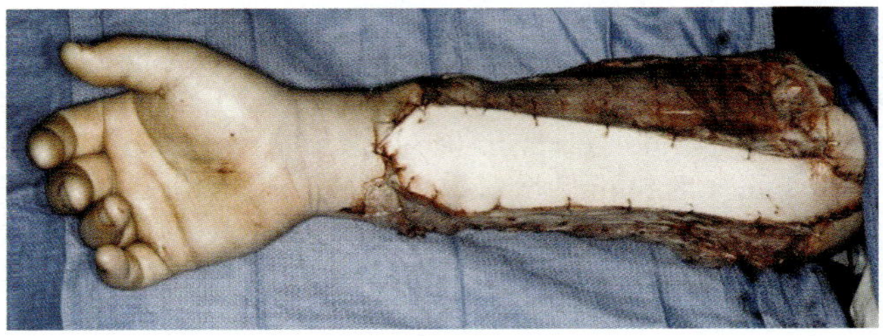

B

FIGURE 59-2 Coverage of the defect with a free latissimus dorsi musculocutaneous flap with a skin island using a saphenous vein graft and a sural nerve graft (A and B).

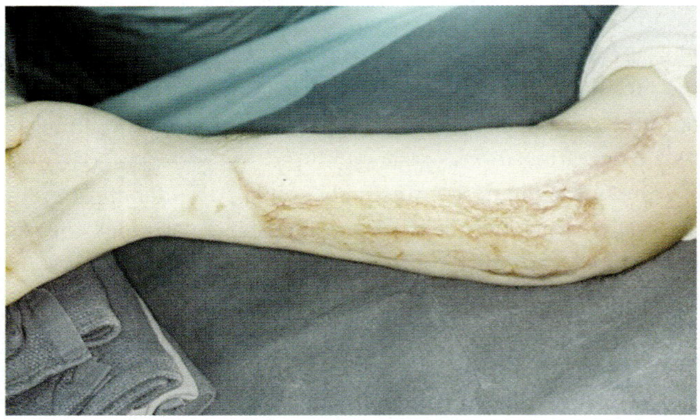

A

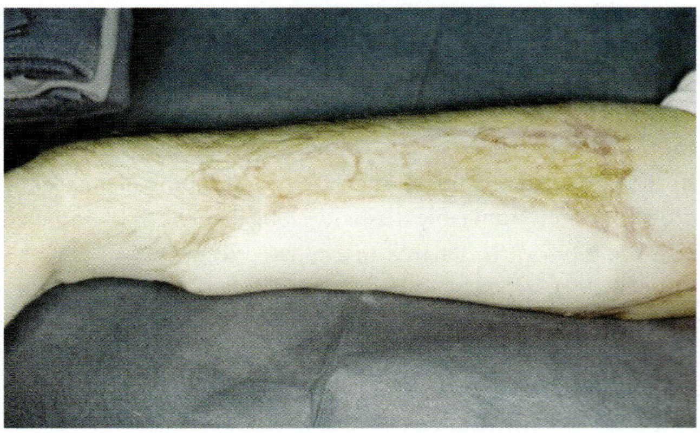

B

FIGURE 59-3 The final contour of the reconstructed forearm (A and B).

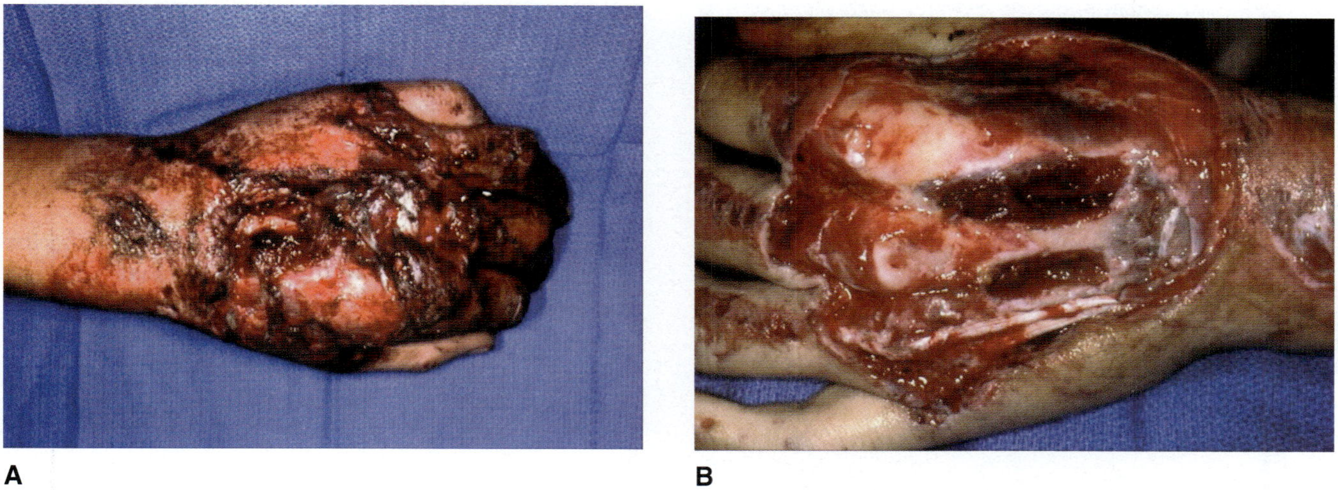

FIGURE 59-4 The injured hand before (**A**) and after (**B**) surgical debridement. The defect involves the dorsal cortices of the metacarpal bones with extensor tendon loss and a large skin defect.

Reconstruction was performed with a free lateral arm flap with tendon grafts passed through the subcutaneous fat of the flap. Extensor tendon grafts were harvested from the dorsum of the foot (Figure 59-5). The patient achieved excellent coverage and functional result (Figure 59-6).

A 19-year-old woman was involved in a motor vehicle accident rollover with a severe crush injury of the ulnar aspect of her right hand. Examination revealed a defect on the ulnar side of the dorsum of the hand with loss of exposed skin, subcutaneous tissue, extensor tendons, intrinsic muscles, and exposed

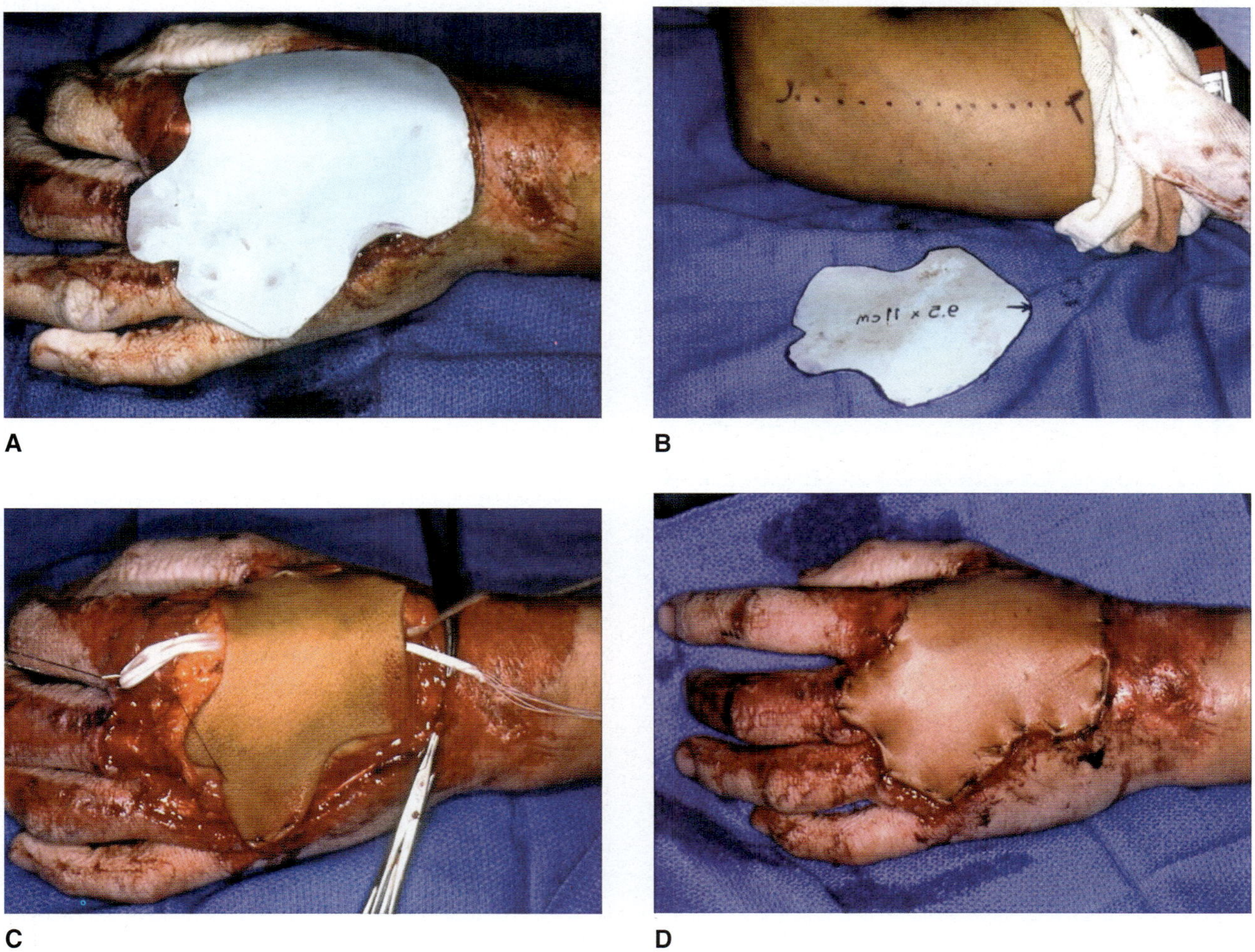

FIGURE 59-5 The flap was designed using a template of elastic bandage on the dorsum of the hand (**A**) transferred to the lateral arm donor site (**B**). Tendons from the dorsum of the foot were passed through the subcutaneous fat of the flap (**C**), and coverage of the defect was achieved (**D**).

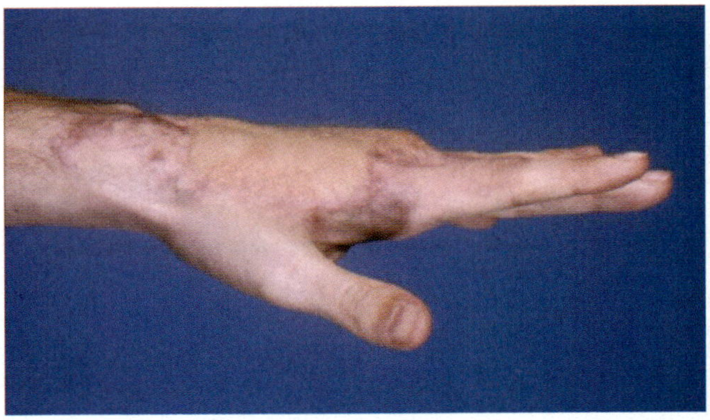

A

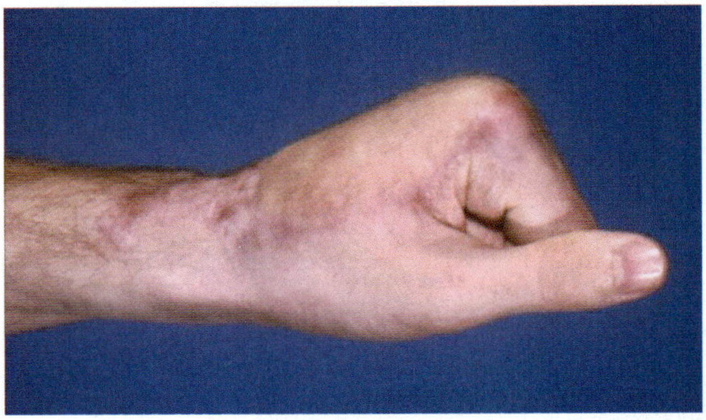

B

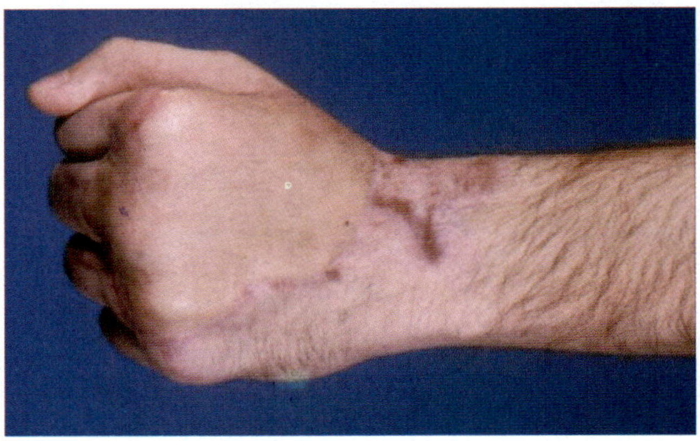

C

FIGURE 59-6 Satisfactory final result with good function and cosmetic appearance. Ability of the hand to perform extension (**A**) and flexion (**B** and **C**).

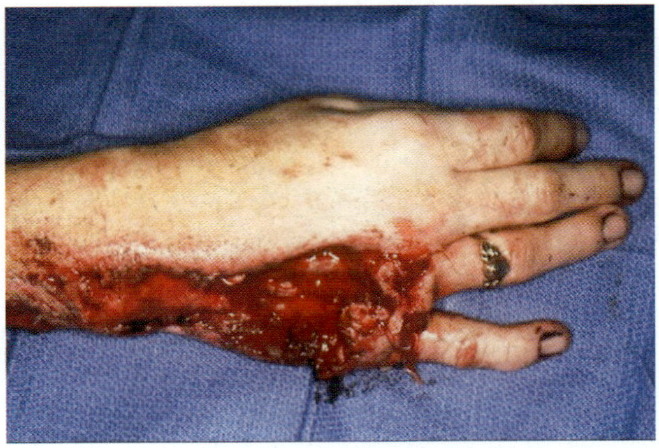

A

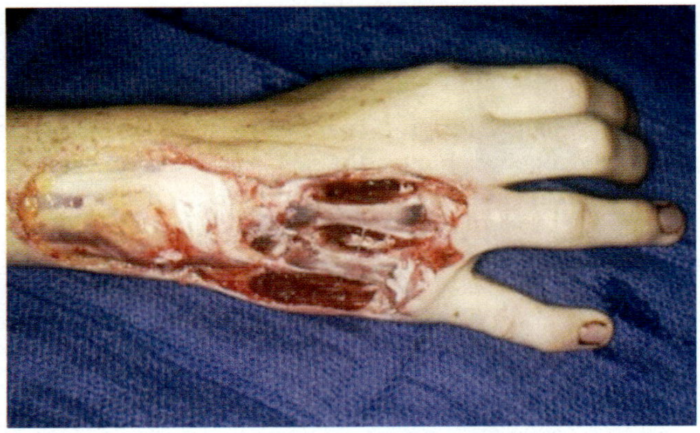

B

FIGURE 59-7 Dorsum of the hand before (**A**) and after (**B**) surgical debridement. The defect involves the fifth metacarpal head, extensor tendon loss, and a large skin defect.

metacarpal fractures with bone loss (Figure 59-7). After radical debridement, reconstruction was achieved with a free groin flap. Extensor tendons from the foot were used to reconstruct the extensor tendon defects (Figure 59-8). The patient obtained a good functional and cosmetic result (Figure 59-9).

RESULTS OF EMERGENCY FREE FLAPS

A total of 347 free flaps were performed at Christine M. Kleinert Institute from 1976 to 2001 for trauma to the upper or lower extremities and required emergency, early, or delayed coverage. Proximal limb injuries were defined as proximal to or including the knee or elbow. Distal injuries were defined as distal to and excluding the knee or elbow. When injuries crossed the elbow or knee, they were considered both a proximal and distal injury. Open or closed fracture, Gustillo grade, and fracture fixation were all evaluated to determine their impact on flap survival, infection, and overall complications. Other factors measured included timing of reconstruction, flap type, and use of vein grafts.

Total flap failure was defined as any flap loss greater than 60%. Complications were classified as minor (superficial infection, hematoma, skin graft loss) and major (flap loss, deep infection, osteomyelitis, fracture nonunion). Whereas superficial infections were defined as resolving with intravenous antibiotics, deep infections were defined as those requiring surgical intervention.

The majority of the 347 free tissue transfers were performed to the upper extremity (78.9% vs. 21.1% to the lower extremity). Most limb injuries were distal (84% vs. 13% proximal injuries vs. 3% for both). Mean age at reconstruction was 30.1 ± 15 years with injuries occurring predominantly in men (84.8%) and manual workers (73.1%). Gustillo fracture grades were 3A (2.1 %), 3B (20.5%), 3C (9.6%), and half of the patients required a fracture stabilizing procedure using either ORIF or a closed percutaneous technique. The majority (159) of the 347 flaps used were fasciocutaneous flaps (45.8%), 65 were myocutaneous flaps (18.7%), 18 were muscle only flaps (5.2%), and 105 were toe transfers

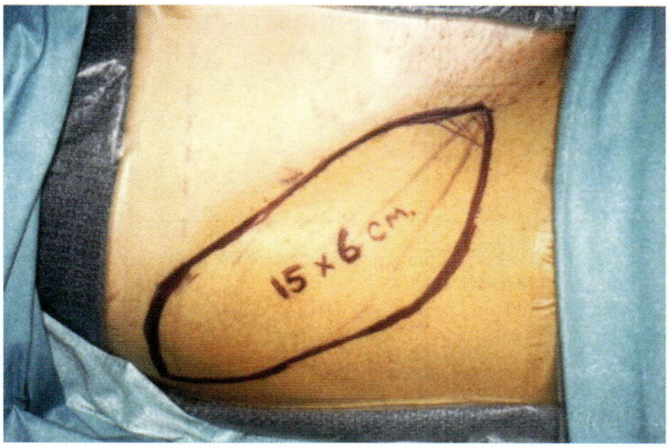

A

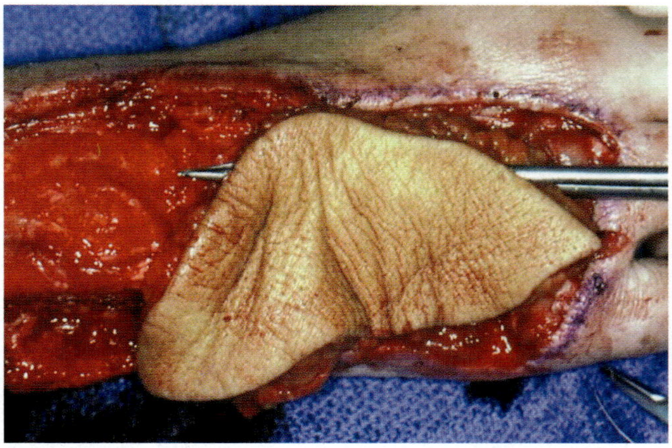

B

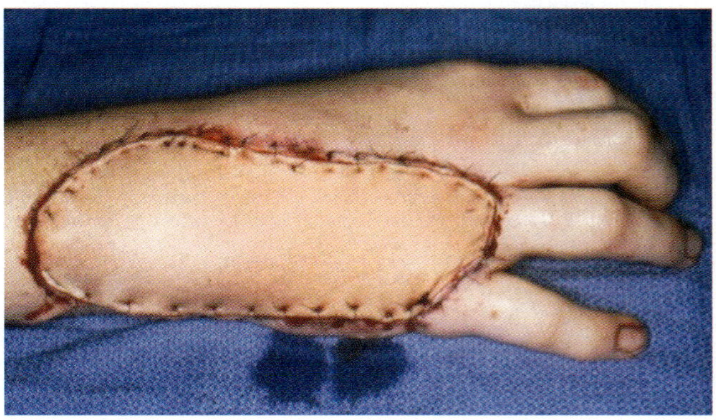

C

FIGURE 59-8 (**A**) Design of the groin flap. (**B**) Transfer of the free groin flap to the dorsal hand and preparation of the bed for the tendon grafts. (**C**) Good tissue contour and coverage.

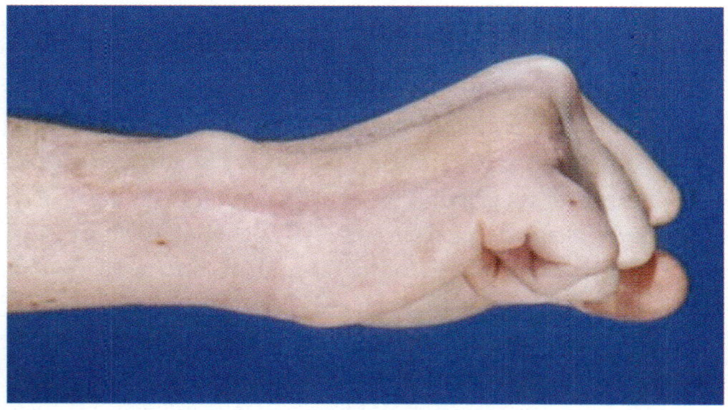

A

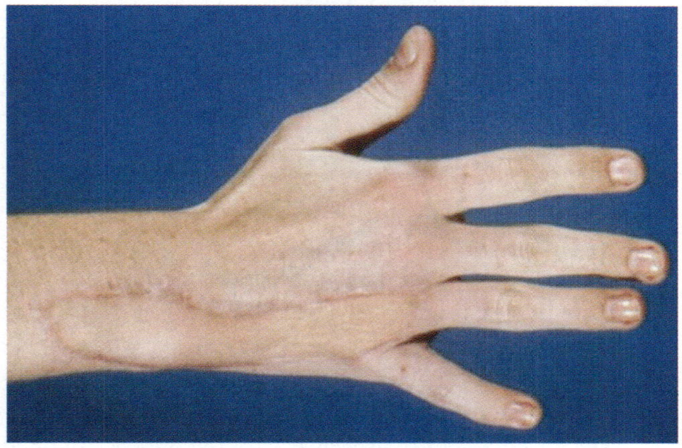

B

FIGURE 59-9 The final result after flap defatting was very good in terms of contour and cosmetic appearance. Range of motion of the hand in flexion (**A**) and extension (**B**).

(30.3%). The lateral arm flap was the most frequently used fasciocutaneous flap (74.2%) with the latissimus dorsi most often used both as a myocutaneous flap (69.2%) and a muscle flap (50%).

FLAP TYPE AND SURVIVAL

The total flap loss rate was 5.5% (19 flaps) for an overall flap survival rate of 94.5%. The failure rate for fasciocutaneous flaps was 5% (eight of 159); for myocutaneous flaps, 10.8% (seven of 65); for muscle flaps, 0%; and for toe transfers, 3% (four of 105). More than half of the fasciocutaneous flap losses occurred using the groin flap earlier in the series (failure rate, 31.3%; five of 16 groin flaps lost between 1976 and 1980). Conversely, flap survival was highest using the most common flaps such as the lateral arm flap (98.3% survival) and latissimus dorsi and rectus muscle flaps (both with 100% survival rates). Interposition vein grafts were required in 14.9% of flaps transferred.

Twenty-eight percent of free flaps were performed within 24 hours, 56% within 3 days, and 669% within 1 week. There was no significant difference in flap loss when performed within 24 hours versus after 24 hours, within 2 days versus 3 days or later, or at 6 days or less versus 1 week or more. When considering all flap losses (partial and total combined), there was no significant difference in flap loss when surgery was performed within 24 hours versus after 24 hours. The presence of a fracture, whether open (26.7%) or closed (33.6%), did not affect flap outcome. Flaps associated with a fracture fixation procedure, whether open or closed, were comparable to simple free flaps with regard to survival. Higher energy open fractures such as Gustillo grades 3A, B, and C also did not impact flap survival, nor did the use of interposition vein grafts or type of flap used for reconstruction. Revision of the venous or arterial anastomoses was associated with a 4.7 times higher risk of flap failure compared with no revision.

COMPLICATIONS

The total infection rate (osteomyelitis, 6.9%; superficial infection, 9.6%; and deep infection, 11.2%) was 16%. The total infection rate was not significantly different in emergency flaps at 24 hours or less (19.6%) versus early timing from 2 to 7 days (22.6%) or versus delayed timing after 7 days (13.1). The incidence of osteomyelitis was comparable in all three time periods, 7.2% (emergency) versus 3.8% (2–7 days) and 7.7% (after 7 days). Deep infection was not significantly correlated with timing, but the incidence of superficial infections was significantly higher in flaps performed between 2 and 7 days (17.0%) versus those performed after 7 days (7.2%). Manual workers had a 2.6 times higher risk of developing a deep infection compared with non–manual workers, but the overall total infection rate was comparable in both groups (manual workers, 17.2% versus non–manual workers, 13.1%). Smokers had a 1.8 times higher risk of deep infection compared with nonsmokers (15.0% vs. 8.3%) and twice the risk of osteomyelitis compared with nonsmokers, although the total infection rate was also comparable between both groups. Injuries to the lower extremity were three times more likely to develop an infection compared with upper extremity injuries with infection rates of 34.2% and 11.1%, respectively. Proximal injuries had a higher infection rate compared with distal injuries, 28.6% versus 13.7%, respectively.

Major complications were significantly associated with injuries to the lower extremity, as well as with the presence of open and closed fractures. Major complications were significant when a vein graft was used or the anastomoses had to be revised.

CONCLUSIONS

Increasing experience and success with elective free tissue transfers allows immediate reconstruction of severe upper and lower extremity injuries. Fewer complications, shorter hospital stays, lower cost, earlier mobilization, and increased function are some of the advantages of free flaps. Twenty-four-hour availability of a skilled microsurgical team allows the possibility of performing emergency free flaps. Radical debridement, early soft tissue coverage, and reconstruction of all missing tissue components are achieved most effectively in a single stage.

REFERENCES

1. Lister G, Scheker L. Emergency free flaps to the upper extremity. *J Hand Surg Am* 1988;13(1):22–28.
2. Del Piñal F, Pisani D, García-Bernal FJ, et al. Massive hand crush: the role of a free muscle flap to obliterate the dead space and to clear deep infection. *J Hand Surg Br* 2006;31(6):588–592.
3. Scheker LR, Ahmed O. Radical debridement, free flap coverage, and immediate reconstruction of the upper extremity. *Hand Clin* 2007;23(1):23–36.
4. Sundine M, Scheker LR. A comparison of immediate and staged reconstruction of the dorsum of the hand. *J Hand Surg Br* 1996;21(2):216–221.
5. McCabe SJ, Breidenbach WC. The role of emergency free flaps for hand trauma. *Hand Clin* 1999;15(2):275–288.
6. Scheker LR, Kleinert HE, Hanel DP. Lateral arm composite tissue transfer to ipsilateral hand defects. *J Hand Surg Am* 1987;12(5 Pt 1):665–672.
7. Levin LS, Erdmann D. Primary and secondary microvascular reconstruction of the upper extremity. *Hand Clin* 2001;17(3):447–455.
8. Del Piñal F. Severe mutilating injuries to the hand: guidelines for organizing the chaos. *J Plast Reconstr Aesthet Surg* 2007;60(7):816–827.
9. Godina M. The tailored latissimus dorsi free flap. *Plast Reconstr Surg* 1987;80(2):304–306.
10. Katsaros J, Schusterman M, Beppu M, et al. The lateral upper arm flap: anatomy and clinical applications. *Ann Plast Surg* 1984;12(6):489–500.
11. Bartlett SP, May JW, Yaremchuk M. The latissimus dorsi muscle: a fresh cadaver study of the primary neurovascular pedicle. *Plast Reconstr Surg* 1981;67:631.
12. Watson S, Craig P, Orton C. The free latissimus dorsi myocutaneous flap. *Plast Reconstr Surg* 1979;64:299.
13. Serafin D. *Atlas of Microsurgical Composite Tissue Transplantation.* Philadelphia: WB Saunders, 1996.
14. Bailey BN, Godfrey AM. Latissimus dorsi muscle free flaps. *Br J Plast Surg* 1982;35(1):47–52.
15. Henry M. Latissimus dorsi free flap salvage of recurrent chronic osteomyelitis with simultaneous elbow interposition arthroplasty. *Hand (N Y)* 2008;3(1):1–3.
16. Tobin GR, Moberg AW, DuBou RH, et al. The split latissimus dorsi myocutaneous flap. *Ann Plast Surg* 1981;7(4):272–280.
17. Drucker CB. Ambroise Paré and the birth of the gentle art of surgery. *Yale J Biol Med* 2008;81(4):199–202.
18. Huntley JS. Debridement: development of the concept. *J Perioper Pract* 2011;21(3):104–105.

CHAPTER 60

Vascularized Bone Grafts: Upper Limb

Allen T. Bishop

The use of a complex microsurgical procedure to treat bone loss or nonunion is justifiable and desirable when the use of simpler or more conventional methods will likely result in an unacceptable result. Although conventional bone grafting has been a mainstay of orthopedic reconstruction for more than a century, the use of conventional (nonvascularized) bone, whether autogenous, allogeneic, or xenogeneic, has definite limitations requiring consideration of other options. These may include prosthetic replacement, amputation, or bone transport but also may provide a good indication for a pedicled or free bone autotransplantation.

RECONSTRUCTION OF SEGMENTAL UPPER LIMB DEFECTS

Conventional Bone Grafting

Conventional bone grafting is defined as the implantation of bone without restoration of its blood supply. The graft substance may be cancellous or cortical (structural), from auto-, allo- or xenogeneic sources. In addition, a variety of inorganic or treated allogenic bone substitutes are commercially available and in frequent clinical use. Any of these materials may be used to fill voids in bone, fuse joints, span small gaps (generally <6–8 cm) caused by trauma or tumor resection, and treat nonunions.

Autograft bone remains the gold standard, providing a superior healing response compared with other sources. These grafts may be purely cancellous or corticocancellous in structure, and are most commonly obtained from the iliac crest. Other sites include the distal radius, olecranon, tibia, fibula, and distal femur and more recently from femoral reaming and aspiration (1).

Conventional bone grafting relies on the process of "creeping substitution," the gradual replacement of nonviable bone with new living bone first described by Barth (2). The process of graft incorporation requires a well-vascularized bed without shear stresses and a source of osteoblasts, most likely derived from circulating elements, because most cells within transferred conventional grafts die shortly after transfer (3). These circulating osteoprogenitor cells form osteoblasts in a metaplastic process, stimulated by the *osteoinductive* properties of the bone graft, which are strongest in cancellous bone (4). In addition, the graft provides a scaffold for vascular ingrowth and subsequent bone remodeling. This property of bone grafts is termed *osteoconduction* and may be the major role played by a conventional graft.

Conventional cortical grafts are used primarily for their ability to enhance stability across a bone or joint defect. They are slow to revascularize and are only incompletely replaced by living bone. As a result, cortical grafts become osteopenic and weaken markedly 6 to 12 months after grafting (5), at times resulting in a late stress fracture if subjected to excessive loads. This problem is more likely in longer grafts and those not adequately protected long-term with a load-sharing implant. Because of the inherent problems and limitations of conventional structural (corticocancellous) grafts, their use is generally limited to defects of less than 6 to 8 cm occurring in a bed without excessive scarring or infection and adequate soft tissue cover.

In the upper extremity, large conventional grafts are generally combined with compression plating or intramedullary rods. Autogenous conventional fibula segments have been reported to provide good results in the forearm and metacarpals (6), and intercalary structural allograft is used to reconstruct larger defects after tumor resection in the humerus, radius, ulna, carpus, and hand. Other methods may be useful at times as well, including reimplantation of the resected bone tumor after autoclaving or other sterilizing process, bone transport procedures, and prosthetic replacement.

Allograft Bone and Joint

Intercalary allograft bone must undergo the same gradual revascularization and remodeling process as conventional autograft, but the process is slower and less complete in nonautogenous bone, presumably because of local immune responses. This reaction may be modified by freezing, lyophilizing, irradiating, or decalcifying the graft or by immune modulation. One series reported 70% overall success, with relatively high complication rates, including delayed or nonunion (14%), late stress fracture (19%) (Figure 60-1), and infection (14%) (7). The use of hemi- or total joint conventional osteoarticular allografts for defects involving articular surfaces has not been as successful. In one series, proximal humerus osteoarticular grafts provided successful function in 12 of 20 patients (60%) (8). Implantation of allogeneic elbow transplants carries considerable risk of major complications, reported in as many as 70% of such cases, and resulting in implant removal in 43% of cases in one study as a result of infection, instability, bone resorption, or nonunion (9).

Prosthetic Replacement

Prosthetic replacement of long bones with fibermetal implants has been relatively seldom performed because of frequent loosening and other problems (5). Defects spanning joints in the upper extremity may be treated by resection and arthroplasty when soft tissue function provided by muscles, tendons, and neurovascular structures allows function. Hemi-, total, or constrained total shoulder arthroplasty may be possible in shoulder girdle tumor reconstruction, at times combined with an intercalary allograft. Similarly, a total elbow arthroplasty may be used in metastatic or primary bone tumors involving the distal humerus or proximal ulna. Guo and colleagues reported 78% good or excellent results in a group of 19 patients, providing both elbow function and pain relief (10). Segmental loss spanning the wrist is generally managed by arthrodesis using vascularized fibular grafting (Figure 60-8). No reports exist of the use of arthroplasty in this situation.

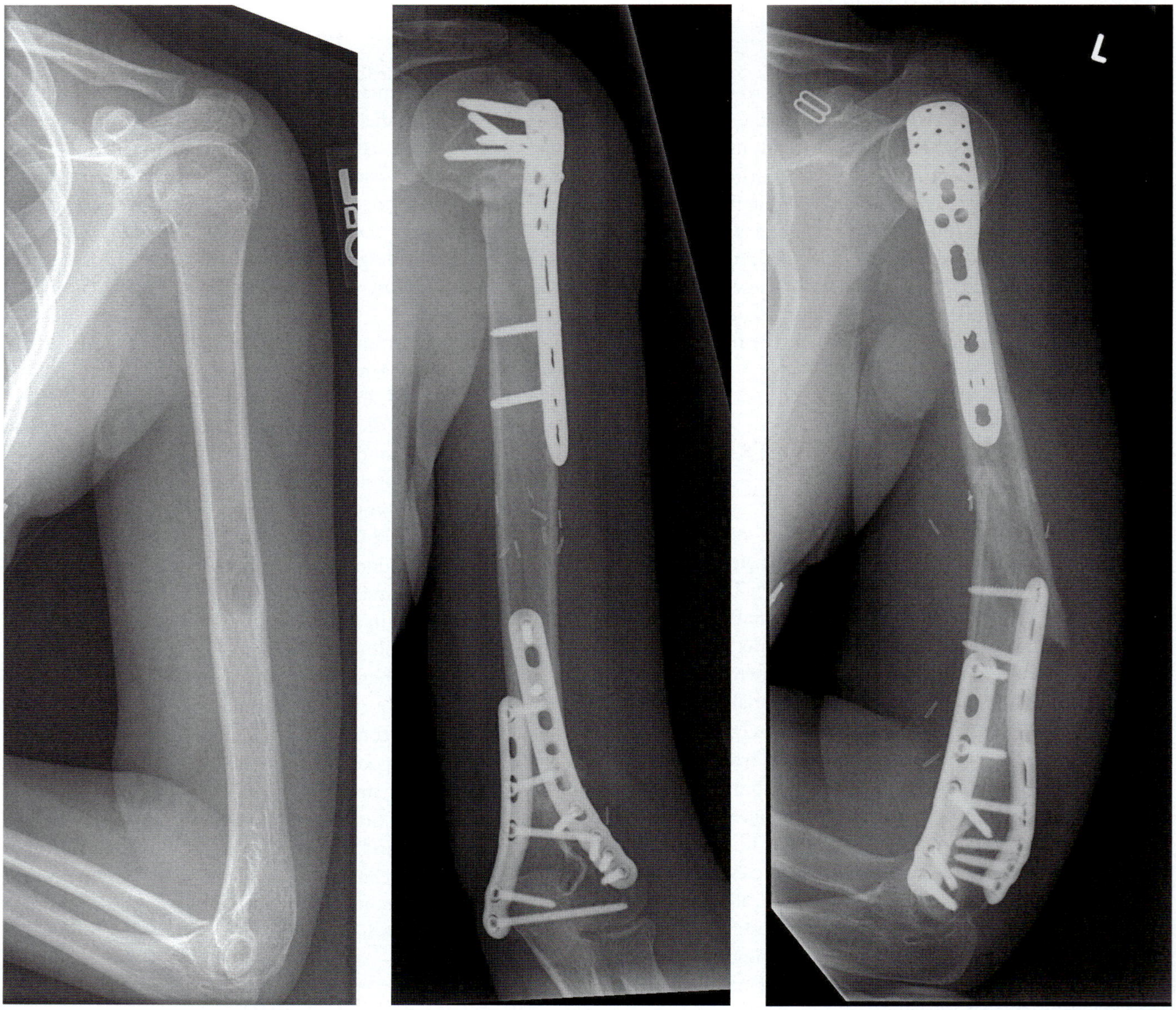

A B C

FIGURE 60-1 (A) Initial diaphyseal lesion of the left humerus. (B) Initial wide resection and intercalary allograft placement. (C) A stress fracture of the allograft occurred spontaneously 10 months later with plate failure.

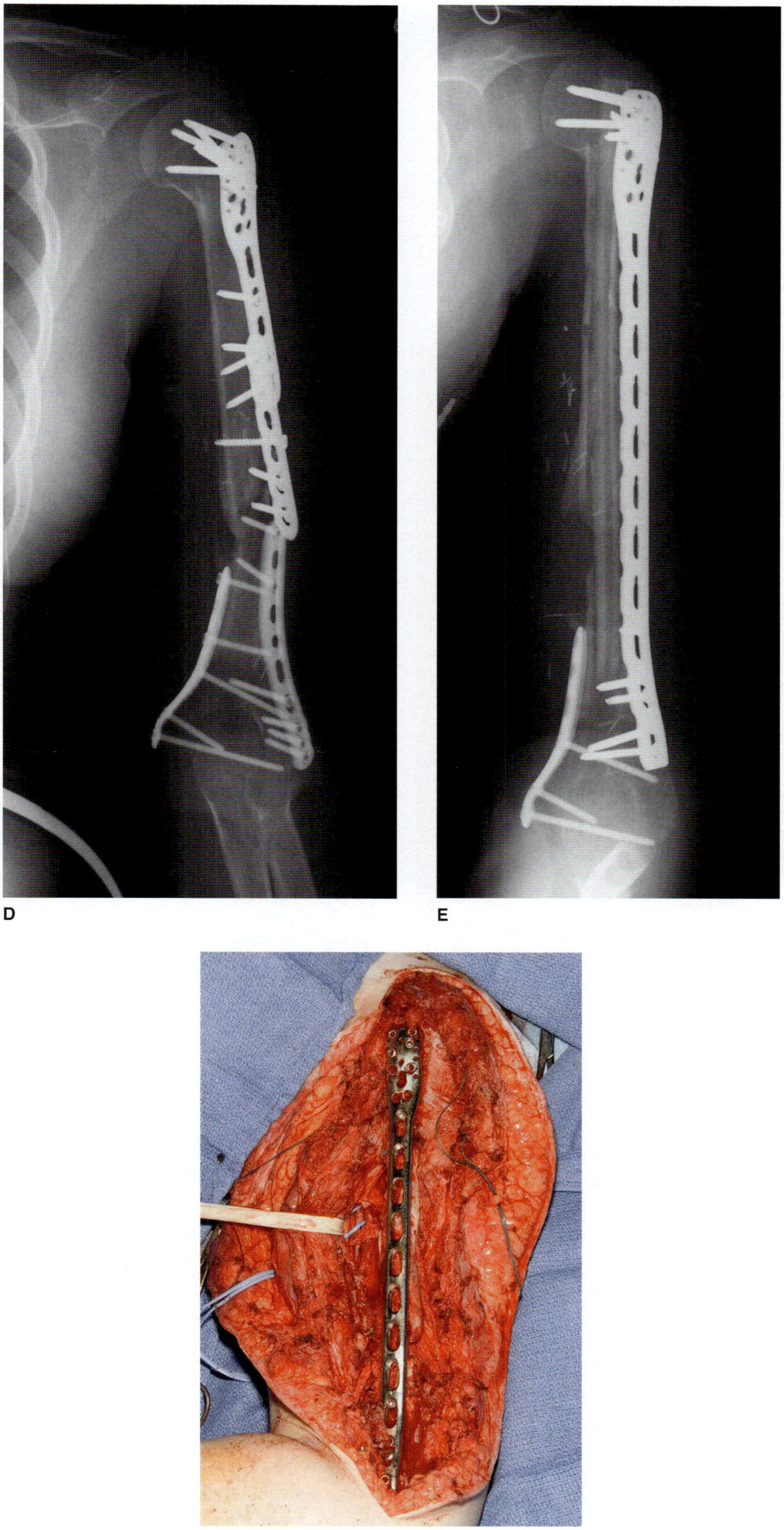

D E F

FIGURE 60-1 (*Continued*) (**D**) Subsequent iliac crest bone grafting and revision plating failed only 2 months later. (**E**) and (**F**) Reconstruction with a doweled intramedullary fibular graft and rigid internal fixation.

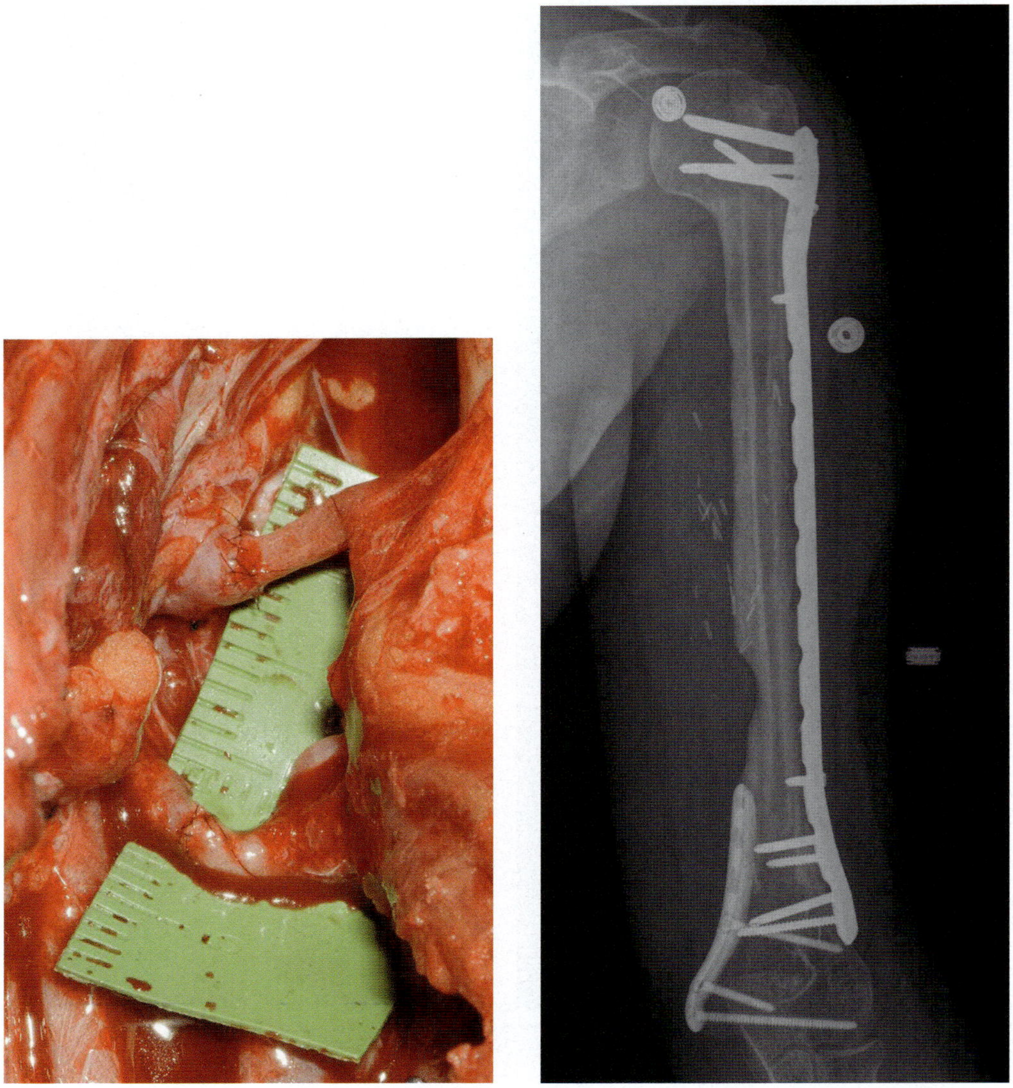

G H

FIGURE 60-1 (*Continued*) (**G**) Microvascular anastomoses were performed end to end to a local brachial artery branch and a vena comitans of the brachial artery. (**H**) Final appearance (healed at 6 months).

One-Bone Forearm

In the forearm, loss of one forearm bone may be solved, although with loss of pronation and supination, by creation of a one-bone forearm. In cases of distal radioulnar instability, this may be performed with a bone block interposition. For segmental loss, however, the distal radius is transposed to meet the proximal ulnar shaft. This procedure, when positioned in neutral or slight pronation, provides restoration of normal forearm length and stability and enables most activities of daily life. It remains a valuable salvage option in recalcitrant forearm nonunions when bone loss, soft tissue inadequacy, or joint instability at the radiocapitellar or distal radioulnar joints prevents restoration of stable, painless forearm rotation.

Bone Transport

Bone transport or distraction osteogenesis is uncommonly applied to the upper extremity, primarily in length discrepancy caused by congenital hypoplasia (11). The technique relies on bone regeneration, transporting bone into the defect after corticotomy of a long bone proximally or distally. Its use for segmental loss has been primarily applied to lower extremity trauma.

Vascularized Bone Grafting

Indications

Use of bone that retains at least a portion of its blood supply is advantageous in segmental bone defects larger than 6 to 8 cm, when soft tissue cover or local vascularity is poor, or in other special circumstances. These include cases of "biologic failure," when bone healing has failed or is unlikely to heal because of local environmental factors. Examples include failed conventional treatment; avascular or radiation-induced necrosis of bone; congenital pseudarthrosis; and local soft tissue hypovascularity or scar caused by infection, trauma, or irradiation. It is also indicated when there is need to restore longitudinal growth by epiphyseal transfer or when used as a composite or chimeric flap for composite tissue reconstruction.

Vascularized bone grafting is not a new concept. As originally described, it was limited to transfer of bone rotated on a muscle, skin, or vascular pedicle with considerable anatomic constraints. Such pedicle grafts have been performed as early as 1905, transferring the fibula to an adjacent tibial defect (12). Subsequently, many other pedicled bone flaps have been developed using rib, clavicle, iliac crest, scapula, distal radius dorsal, and palmar grafts; femoral sites, including the greater and lesser trochanters; and medial distal metaphysis or condyle, pisiform, second metacarpal, and humerus.

The same microvascular techniques that enabled development of free muscle and fasciocutaneous tissue transfers led to the experimental and clinical use of vascularized bone autotransplantation. The method was used for rib transplantation both clinically and experimentally in the 1970s (13,14), with near simultaneous development of iliac crest and fibula free tissue transfers (15–17). A variety of other potential donor free bone flap sites have been described subsequently, including (among many) use of metatarsals in association with the dorsalis pedis flap, scapula in association with scapular or parascapular flaps, radius with the radial forearm flap, segments of ulna with the ulnar artery flap, humerus with lateral arm flap, and periosteal or bone flaps from the medial femoral condyle.

Scientific Basis and Benefits of Vascularized Bone Grafting

The advantages of vascularized bone transfer over conventional grafts are many. They include more rapid union, superior osteocyte survival, improved mechanical properties, and a lower incidence of late stress fracture (18–21). Furthermore, they have the ability to hypertrophy in response to applied stress, a quality generally absent in conventional large structural auto- or allograft bone (Figure 60-2). All of these properties result from preservation of osteocyte and bone remodeling function, made possible by preservation of bone circulation.

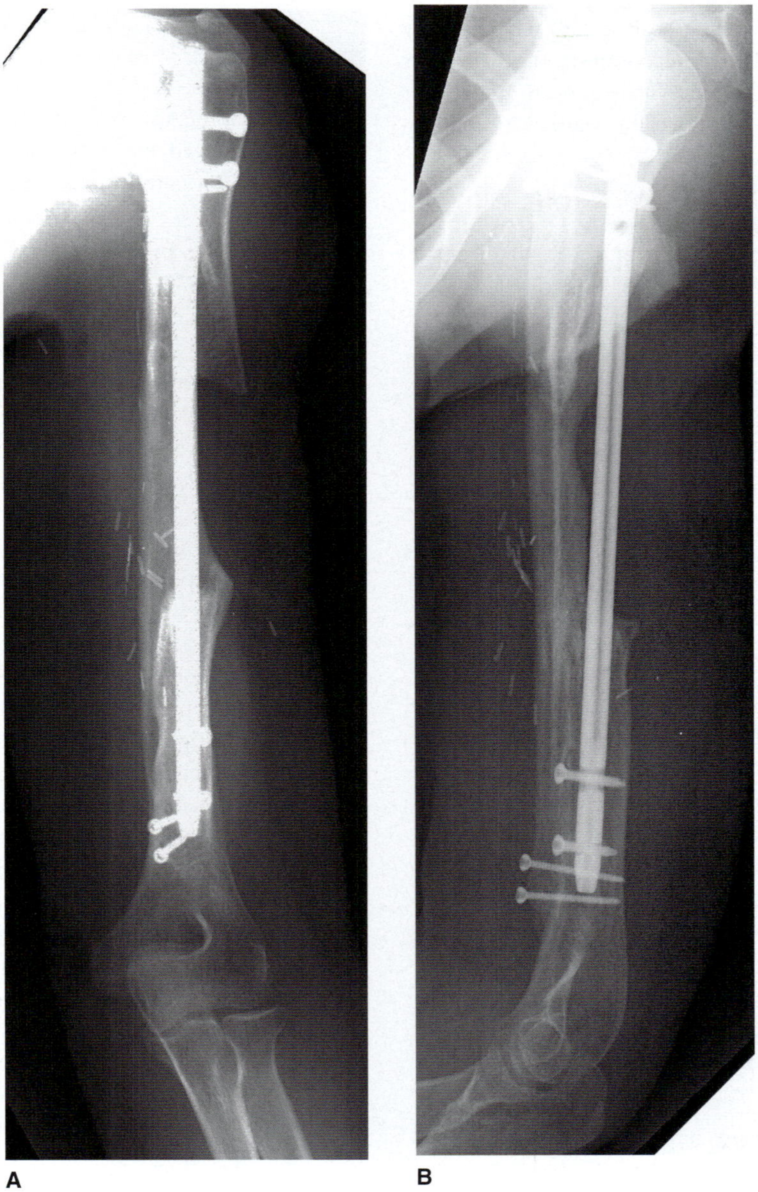

FIGURE 60-2 Visible hypertrophy of a fibular graft used to reconstruct traumatic loss of the humerus from a self-inflicted gunshot wound.

Bone blood flow has been measured at various postoperative time intervals experimentally in both canine tibia and canine distal radius models (22,23). These studies demonstrate both immediate restoration of bone blood flow resulting from preservation of bone microvascular supply, as well as a substantial hyperemic response after transplantation, with blood flow increasing fourfold over initial values with time.

The process of creeping substitution required for graft incorporation in conventional grafts does not take place in vascularized bone flaps, provided circulation is maintained. This prevents osteopenia and thus preserves normal bone material properties postoperatively. Living bone typically responds to applied stress by remodeling to meet the required loading, according to Wolff's law. Transplantation of a bone of smaller diameter or lesser strength with an adequate blood supply should therefore result in its hypertrophy over time. This is a unique property of living bone and does not occur in structural conventional auto- or allografts. Hypertrophy has been shown to result from an extraperiosteal reaction and is more likely to occur when the graft is not significantly stress shielded by extensive internal fixation or with weight bearing (20). Hypertrophy is most commonly observed in fibular transplants than other vascularized bone donors and is more likely to occur in younger individuals and in lower extremity (weight-bearing) locations.

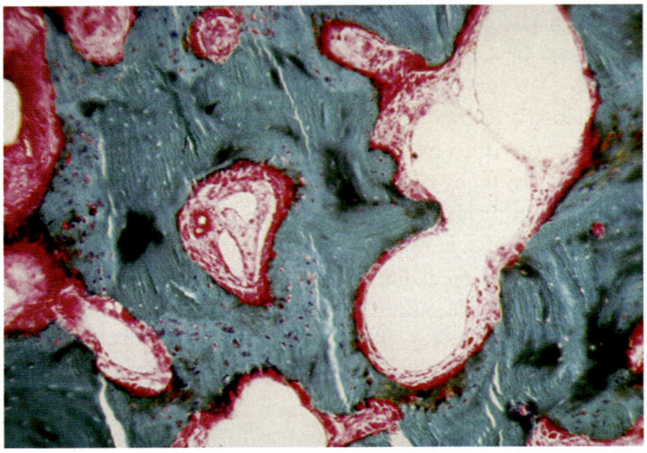

FIGURE 60-3 Histologic specimen 8 weeks after revascularization of a necrotic canine radiocarpal bone nonunion with an adjacent vascularized bone graft. Many osteoblasts rim on the surface of the trabeculae, with osteoid deposition and appositional woven bone formation and viable osteocytes which are replacing the necrotic trabecula. (Reproduced with permission from the author's laboratory, work of Dr. Toru Sunagawa [23].)

INDICATIONS FOR UPPER EXTREMITY VASCULARIZED GRAFTS

Segmental Bone Loss

Vascularized bone grafts are most often used in major defects in the axial or appendicular skeleton. They have other important uses in smaller defects, however, when avascular necrosis (AVN), irradiation, or long-standing infection require improvement in local blood flow. In the upper limb, the method has proven value in defects involving the clavicle, shoulder joint, proximal metaphysis and shaft of humerus, forearm, and radiocarpal joint and the hand. Specific applications and methods for each anatomic area are described in detail below.

Avascular Necrosis

The improved ability of vascularized dorsal radius grafts to heal carpal nonunion and revascularize adjacent necrotic bone has been shown experimentally in a canine study from our institution (23). Similarly, implantation of an arteriovenous pedicle allows identical recovery of circulation, in both cases by neovascularization (capillary proliferation and ingrowth) from the vascular tissue adjacent to the necrotic bone (24,25). New bone formation then extends into the damaged area, with ongoing evidence of remodeling histologically (Figure 60-3). The usefulness of vascularized grafts to revascularize necrotic bone has been applied to the upper extremity, including the humerus, capitellum, scaphoid, and lunate (26–31).

Other Circumstances

Other specific indications for microvascular bone transfer include poor quality of surrounding soft tissue; malignancy, where chemotherapy or irradiation may be considered postoperatively; or need for composite tissue, longitudinal growth, and failed prior conventional grafting procedures (21).

CHOICE OF FREE FLAP

Fibula

The fibula is the preferred donor bone for the majority of upper limb defects, with the exception of carpal pathology, including nonunion and AVN of the scaphoid and lunate. A length of up to 30 cm can be obtained, generally sparing the distal 7 to 8 cm to preserve ankle function. When harvested through a lateral approach, it may include an island of lateral leg skin up to 10 by 20 cm for monitoring or coverage purposes by including one or more septal perforators from the peroneal vessels, typically piercing the soleus muscle adjacent to the lateral intermuscular septum. When a skin paddle is used, skin grafting of the donor site is to be recommended. This minimizes the risk of wound breakdown and possible compartment syndrome resulting from an excessively tight closure. Osteomuscular flaps may include the flexor hallucis longus, all or a portion of the soleus or peroneal muscles using the common peroneal pedicle as well. Additionally, inclusion of the proximal fibular physis has been demonstrated to permit longitudinal growth. Inclusion of physeal vessels is required for this to occur. Current opinion favors the use of a single anterior tibial artery supplying both the physis and diaphyseal periosteum for this purpose, as described by Innocenti and colleagues (32) (see Chapter 18).

Iliac Crest

The anterior iliac crest may be used as a vascularized graft, based upon the deep circumflex iliac (DCI) vessels. The graft is a curved, membranous bone whose size and shape are not favorable for many extremity indications. Stable, rigid internal fixation is difficult to obtain in this relatively weak bone. Donor site morbidity, including incisional hernia, may occur. Graft size is limited by its shape, generally limited to no more than 10 cm. Its primary advantage is its largely cancellous nature. Reconstruction of metaphyseal defects, if not manageable by conventional grafting, may be the best indication for its use. It may be raised as a composite flap including skin based on the DCI pedicle, but loss of all or a portion of the skin flap may occur, particularly if the skin is rotated in relation to the underlying bone (33). Loss of skin paddles based on the DCI has led to a recommendation to turbocharge the flap with the superficial circumflex iliac vessels (34).

Osteocutaneous groin flaps may also be transferred as pedicle flaps to reconstruct complex wounds of the hand. The advantages frequently cited include the ability to supply vascularized bone to what is frequently a poor recipient bed for a bone graft, reconstruct both soft tissue and bony defects simultaneously, and be used in facilities without capability for microvascular surgery (35).

Scapula

Vascularized bone grafts may be obtained from the lateral border, with a scapular osteocutaneous flap, or from the medial ridge of the bone. The lateral scapular flap is based on the circumflex scapular circulation, usually taken as a composite flap. The medial flap is based on the same circulation and depends on periosteal circulation alone. Their utility as composite flaps for upper extremity reconstruction, chiefly in the hand and forearm, has been well demonstrated (36).

Rib

The rib has not been extensively used as a free tissue transfer, although it may be useful as a pedicle graft for clavicular reconstruction (37). It is not generally indicated for any other upper extremity applications because of its weak membranous bone structure, curved shape, and blood supply. It may be used with an anterior or posterior pedicle. The anterior blood supply arises from the internal mammary vessels and only supplies periosteal vessels. The posterior rib graft, which includes its nutrient artery, requires ligation of the dorsal branch of the posterior intercostal artery. Because this vessel supplies the spinal cord, the potential for causing paraplegia exists. Alternatively, ribs may be carried as part of a serratus anterior muscle flap based on the thoracodorsal vessels, again relying on periosteal blood flow.

MEDIAL FEMORAL CONDYLAR FLAP

Corticoperisoteal Flap

Because of its osteogenic capability, vascularized periosteal grafts have considerable potential for the reconstruction of bone defects. The transfer of free vascularized corticoperiosteal bone flaps seems to be ideally suited for some applications, particularly for pathologic fractures occurring after radiation, segmental bone allograft nonunions not responding to conventional bone graft, and chronic recalcitrant nonunions of long bones without substantial bone loss (38,39). The medial femoral condyle is perhaps the best source for such grafts, as described originally by Hertel and Masquelet and Doi et al. (40,41). The medial femoral condyle may also be used as a source of small, primarily cancellous structural grafts useful in the carpal bones as both bone and osteocartilaginous grafts (31,42–45).

Vascularized Bone or Osteochondral Flap

Readers are referred to Chapter 21 for details regarding medial condyle flap anatomy and harvest. It has proven utility as a corticoperiosteal flap in the upper extremity to treat radiation-induced pathologic fracture of the clavicle and forearm nonunions complicated by osteomyelitis and to revascularize the capitellum in idiopathic AVN.

It has been used in the upper limb as a vascularized bone or osteochondral free flap to reconstruct metacarpal defects and treat scaphoid nonunions with and without articular cartilage resurfacing (46–50). It is likely that the graft will find other uses as experience with this relatively new flap grows.

Pedicle Flaps

Although largely beyond the scope of a microsurgery textbook, the use of pedicled vascularized bone grafts in recent years has played an important role in carpal reconstructive problems and must be considered when planning a reconstructive surgery, along with more complex options. The use of vascularized bone grafts for carpal pathology has been described from the pisiform (51,52) metacarpal head (53), palmar and dorsal radial aspect of the radial metaphysis (54–57), or diaphysis of the ulna or radius (58). Many of these grafts require extensive dissection, need an additional surgical incision, and have limited blood supply. Palmar radius grafts in particular require dissection in proximity to important radiocarpal ligaments for elevation and implantation, have a relatively short pedicle, and have unpredictable nutrient artery locations when based on the pronator quadratus (55).

Recipient Site Factors

Clavicle

Radiation-induced pathologic fracture, segmental loss, and chronic nonunions of the clavicle have historically been demanding problems. Functional problems associated with clavicle incompetence include instability, weakness, and pain in the shoulder girdle, as well as brachial plexopathy. Because of the thin soft tissue envelope covering the bone, bulky reconstruction is desirably avoided. After failed grafting and plating or with associated osteomyelitis, conventional bone grafting is not useful. Microvascular transfer of the fibula has a high failure rate in the clavicular location in particular and is generally not a good choice for reconstruction (21,39).

We have successfully used corticoperiosteal flaps from the medial femoral condyle in these difficult circumstances, with much higher success than other reported results (39). The flap is thin and can be shaped according to the reconstructive

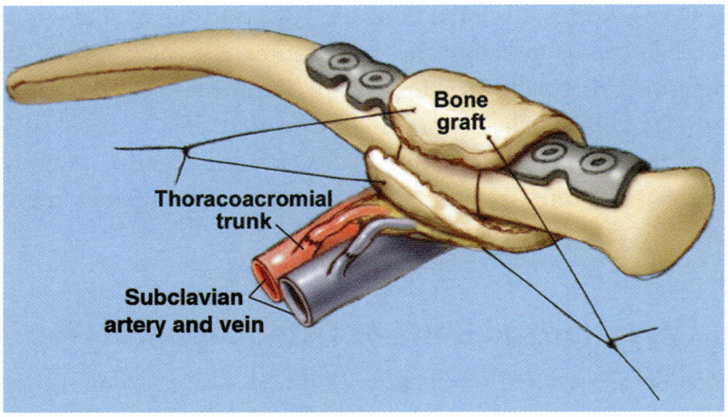

FIGURE 60-4 Use of a medial femoral condyle corticoperiosteal graft for the clavicle. The clavicle is stabilized with plate and screw fixation, filling any intercalary gaps with conventional tricortical iliac crest graft. Next, the flap is wrapped around the clavicle, enveloping the remaining exposed bone and spanning the area of reconstruction. Microvascular connections are to the thoracoacromial trunk vessels end to end. (By permission of Mayo Foundation for Medical Education and Research. All rights reserved.)

requirements without compromising its blood supply. Stabilization with a plate is generally performed using an intercalary tricortical iliac crest graft in addition when needed. The nonunion area is then enveloped with a medial femoral condyle corticoperiosteal flap, which spans the area of nonunion and nearly circumferentially enwraps the clavicle without visible bulk (Figure 60-4). It enables clavicular healing at one bone contact site, avoiding the difficulties of interposing, fixing, and healing a bridging vascularized structural graft.

Vascular connections are performed to the thoracoacromial trunk, a branch of the subclavian artery in proximity to the midclavicle. Rapid subperiosteal new bone and improved local blood flow both serve to correct the hypovascularity caused by repeated surgery, infection, or local radiation.

Case Example: Corticoperiosteal Flap

A 37-year-old woman presented with a clavicle nonunion with bone loss resulting from a prior fracture more than a decade earlier and after multiple procedures compromised by infection and nonunion. After resection of the clavicle, she presented with a chronic lower trunk brachial plexopathy causing sensory loss and intrinsic motor weakness, as well as painful shoulder girdle instability. Radiographs demonstrated a segmental midclavicle atrophic defect (Figure 60-5A). Skin and soft tissues were adequate. A corticoperiosteal flap was elevated as a free tissue transfer from the medial femoral condyle (Figure 60-5B). After clavicle stabilization with a plate and an interpositional conventional iliac crest graft, the flap was wrapped around the clavicle and secured with nonabsorbable sutures (Figure 60-5C). Thoracoacromial trunk vessels were used for vascular connections (Figure 60-5D). Healing was demonstrable several months later, with relief of the patient's neurologic symptoms (Figure 60-5E).

Shoulder

Proximal humerus defects are encountered frequently after removal of primary malignant bone tumors (giant cell tumor,

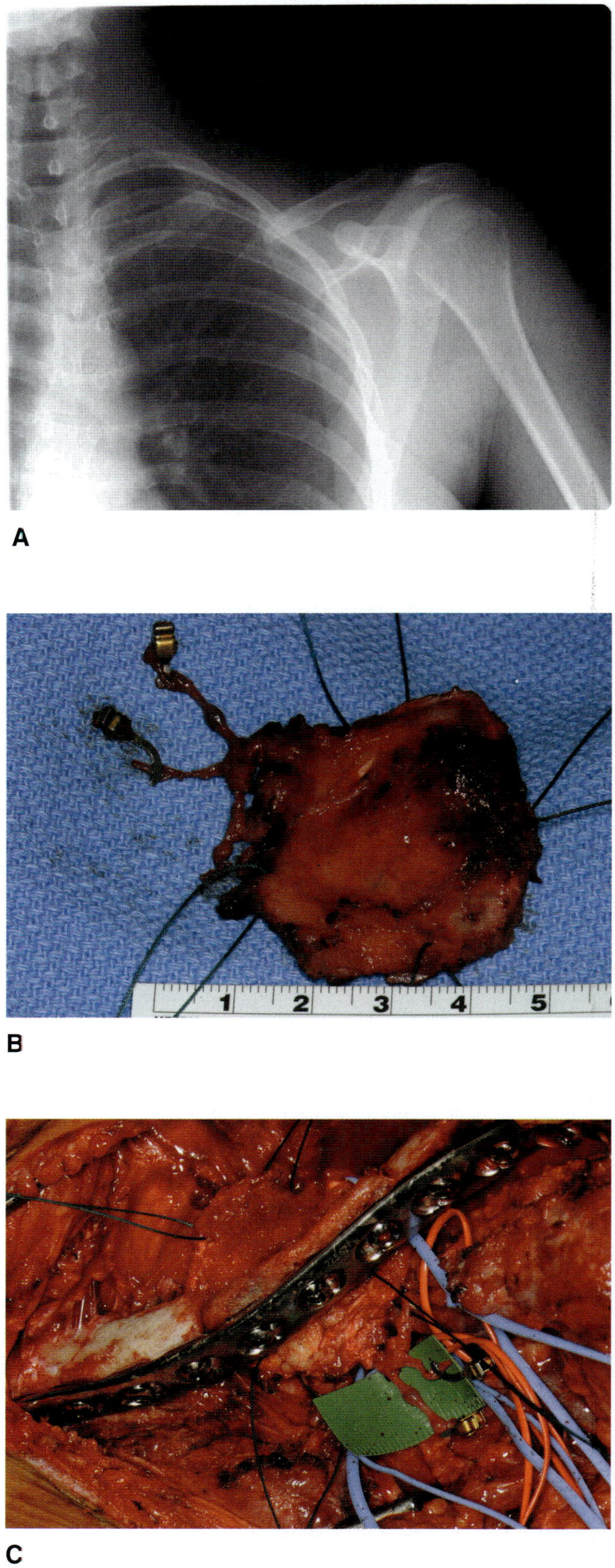

FIGURE 60-5 Clavicle nonunion with bone loss, resulting from a prior fracture and multiple procedures compromised by infection. (**A**) Segmental midclavicle atrophic defect. (**B**) Corticoperiosteal flap from the contralateral medial femoral condyle. (**C**) Clavicle stabilized with a plate and interposed iliac crest graft. The flap is positioned behind the clavicle to be wrapped and secured with nonabsorbable sutures.

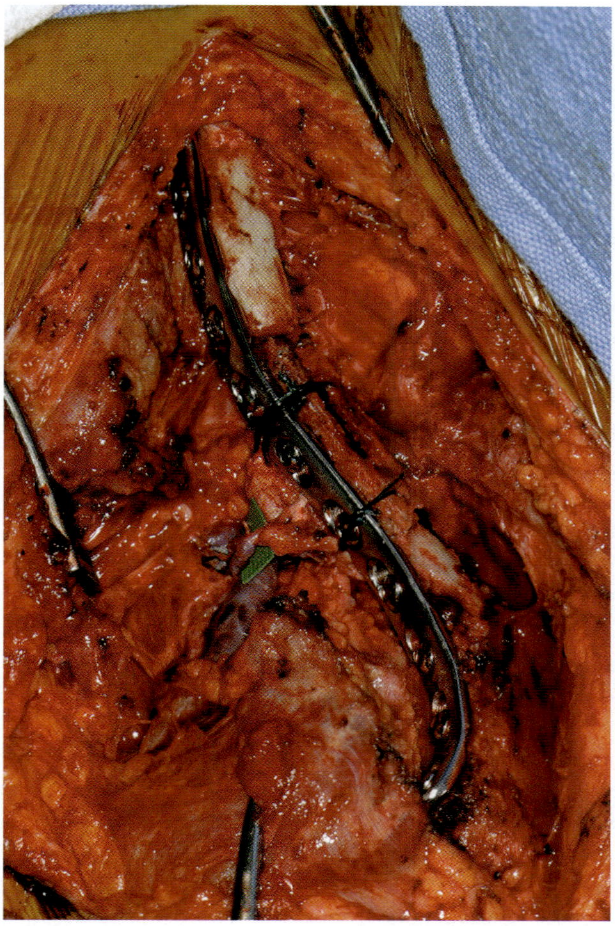

D

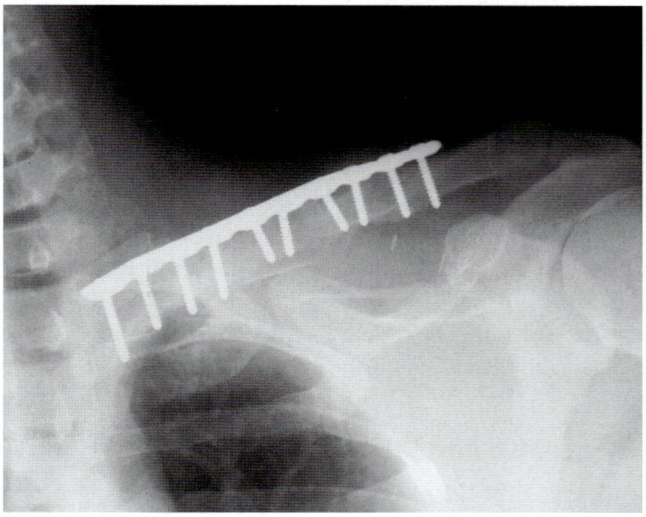

E

FIGURE 60-5 *(Continued)* (**D**) Thoracoacromial trunk vessels were used for vascular connections. The flap is in position. (**E**) Healing was demonstrable several months later, with relief of the patient's neurologic symptoms.

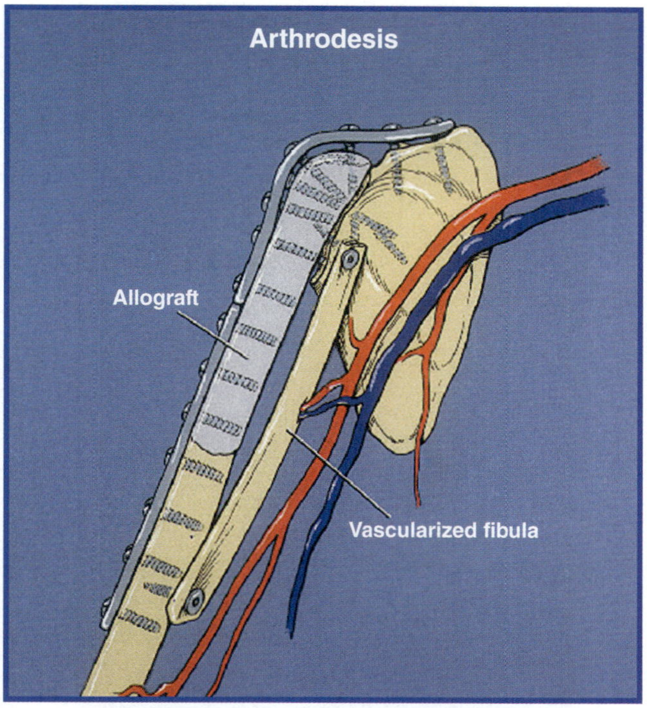

FIGURE 60-6 Shoulder arthrodesis is performed using an allograft humeral segment secured to the scapular spine for initial stability, placing a vascularized fibular strut across the construct from distal native humerus to the scapular neck. (By permission of Mayo Foundation for Medical Education and Research. All rights reserved.)

chondrosarcoma, and osteogenic sarcoma). A scapulohumeral fusion is frequently required to obtain a stable extremity permitting more distal function. This is generally obtained with a composite structural allograft secured to the distal humerus and scapula via a plate applied to the scapular spine. It is combined with a vascularized fibular strut doweled into the neck of the scapula and secured to the humerus as an onlay graft (Figure 60-6). The results of nine such arthrodeses reported by Rose et al. included seven successful fusions and two asymptomatic fibrous nonunions, all providing an effective limb-preserving reconstruction (59). An alternative is the use of a vascularized fibula to restore humerus length, suspended from the acromion with a ligamentous reconstruction as described by Linberg (60) (Figure 60-7). In a child, a fibula used for this purpose may include the fibular head, including the articular surface and physis. Appropriate microsurgical restoration of physeal blood flow using an anterior tibial artery pedicle may allow longitudinal growth to occur while also preserving some glenohumeral motion.

Humerus

Reconstruction of segmental resection of the humerus is best performed with a vascularized fibular transfer (59). When the entire diaphysis has been resected, the fibula may be positioned in an intramedullary position both proximally and distally, obtaining considerable stability from the doweled positioning. Given the diameter mismatch between fibula and humerus, with resulting substantial risk of stress fracture without load sharing, a bridging plate is recommended. Smaller diaphyseal defects require its positioning on the surface (onlay graft) because the fibula is too large to fit within the humeral diaphysis. A locked intramedullary nail or bridging plate provide needed stability in this circumstance (see Figure 60-2), at times

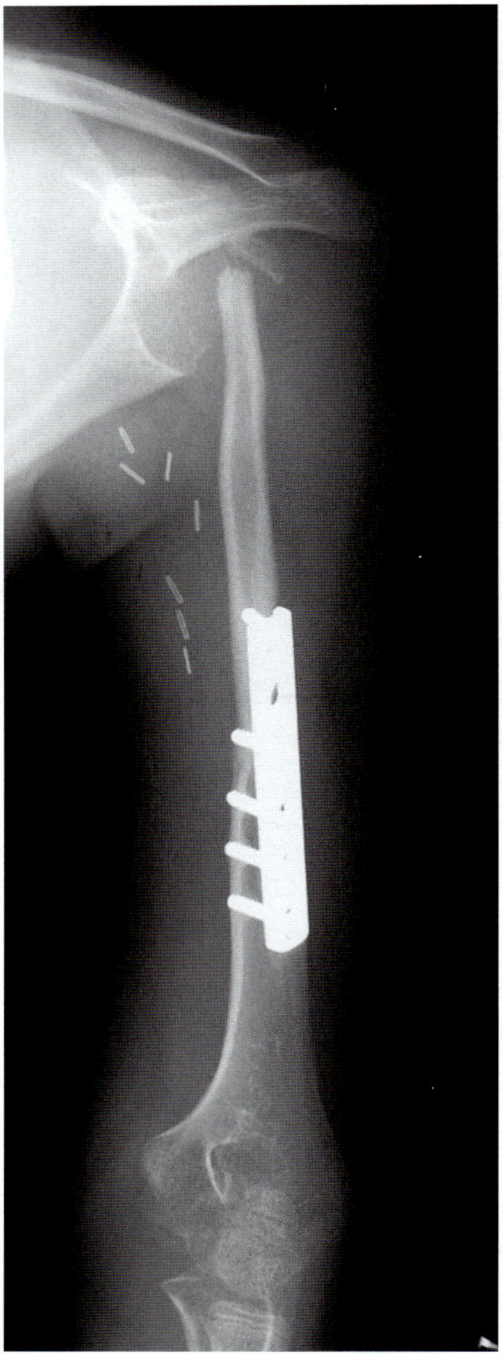

FIGURE 60-7 Osteogenic sarcoma of the proximal humerus treated by proximal humeral resection and fibular replacement of the proximal humerus with scapular suspension.

supplemented with an intercalary allograft. We generally strip the opposing periosteal surfaces (on the side opposite the peroneal pedicle of the fibula) and make a shallow depression in the cortical bone of the recipient humerus and allograft to maximize bone contact. Lag screw fixation proximally and distally is then sufficient to stabilize and compress the fibula against the humerus. Supplemental cancellous autograft bone at the allograft junction sites and along the contact area of the fibula is to be recommended. Arterial repair is generally end to side to the brachial artery, exposed as needed through a separate medial incision, with venous repairs to a vena comitans.

Rigid internal fixation of the humerus has proven to be of particular importance with fibular fracture occurring in six of 15 humeral fibular transplants in a recent series, including three of four placed into diaphyseal defects (59). As stated, either a spanning locked plate or intramedullary nail will circumvent this problem. Use of a fibula alone to span a humerus defect stabilized with either lag screws or separate proximal and distal plate fixation is the typical cause of a stress fracture. When fracture occurs, reoperation is necessary if displaced. An adequately vascularized, nondisplaced fibular fracture will often heal with nonoperative management.

Infection may also occur in these large reconstructions, requiring serial debridements, antibiotic-impregnated spacers or beads, and at times staged reconstruction. Infection was seen in 2 of 4 diaphyseal reconstructions in Rose et al.'s series (59). Despite the problems encountered, healing occurred in all four diaphyseal defects at a mean 10 months after surgery.

Case Example: Fibular Graft to Humerus

A 13-year-old female patient reported pain and swelling in the left midarm. A radiograph demonstrated a diaphyseal lesion (see Figure 60-1A). After initial treatment for suspected infection, a spontaneous pathologic fracture led to referral, magnetic resonance imaging (MRI), and a needle biopsy of a large soft tissue mass at age 16 years. The lesion proved to be Ewing sarcoma and was reconstructed with wide resection and an intercalary allograft (see Figure 60-1B). A stress fracture of the allograft occurred spontaneously 10 months later with plate failure (see Figure 60-1C). Subsequent Iliac crest bone grafting and revision plating failed only 2 months later (see Figure 60-1D). She was referred to Mayo Clinic, where a doweled intramedullary vascularized fibular graft was placed within remaining proximal and distal allograft, extending into native bone. Rigid internal fixation was provided by a 24-cm-long shoulder humeral plate (see Figures 60-1E and 60-1F). Microvascular anastomoses were performed end to end to a local brachial artery branch and a vena comitans of the brachial artery (Figure 60-1G). After surgery, a deep soft tissue wound infection responded to serial debridements, delayed wound closure, and antibiotic suppression. Complete healing occurred radiographically at 6 months (Figure 60-1H).

Forearm and Wrist

Large defects of the radius, ulna, or both lend themselves well to reconstruction by fibular transfer. The fibula is a close match in diameter to the forearm bones. Stabilization is provided by plate and screw fixation, orienting the vascular pedicle in either an orthograde or retrograde fashion as needed for optimal orientation to adjacent vessels. Care must be taken to avoid screw placement in the central third of the bone because of the proximity of the nutrient pedicle. Spanning plate fixation is generally not necessary because of the additional stability provided by a remaining forearm bone. In cases when both radius and ulna segments have been lost, a single fibula may be used for a one-bone forearm reconstruction with a spanning plate to prevent a stress fracture at plate–bone interfaces or screw holes.

Alternatively, a "double-barrel" fibular graft can be constructed to repair both radius and ulna defects with a single common vascular pedicle (61).

Lesions involving the distal radius articular surface require partial or complete wrist arthrodesis. We have generally performed a formal arthrodesis using a vascularized fibular graft for this purpose. Alternatively, conventional osteoarticular fibular grafts have been used to create a neoradiocarpal joint, or a fibula–proximal row fusion may be performed (62).

Vascular reconstruction is easily accomplished by either end to end or end to side arterial anastomosis to either radial or ulnar artery. Adequacy of collateral arterial flow through palmar arches must be confirmed preoperatively by means of an Allen's test if an end-to-end repair is to be performed. The author prefers end-to-side repairs to obviate these concerns. Venous repairs are generally end to end to cephalic or basilic veins.

Case Example: Multiply Operated Forearm and Wrist (Figure 60-8)

A 61-year-old woman presented with a painful, unstable distal ulna and ununited distal radius and wrist arthrodesis with a painful pseudarthrosis. She had a complex history that began with a closed distal both-bone fracture. An unfortunate

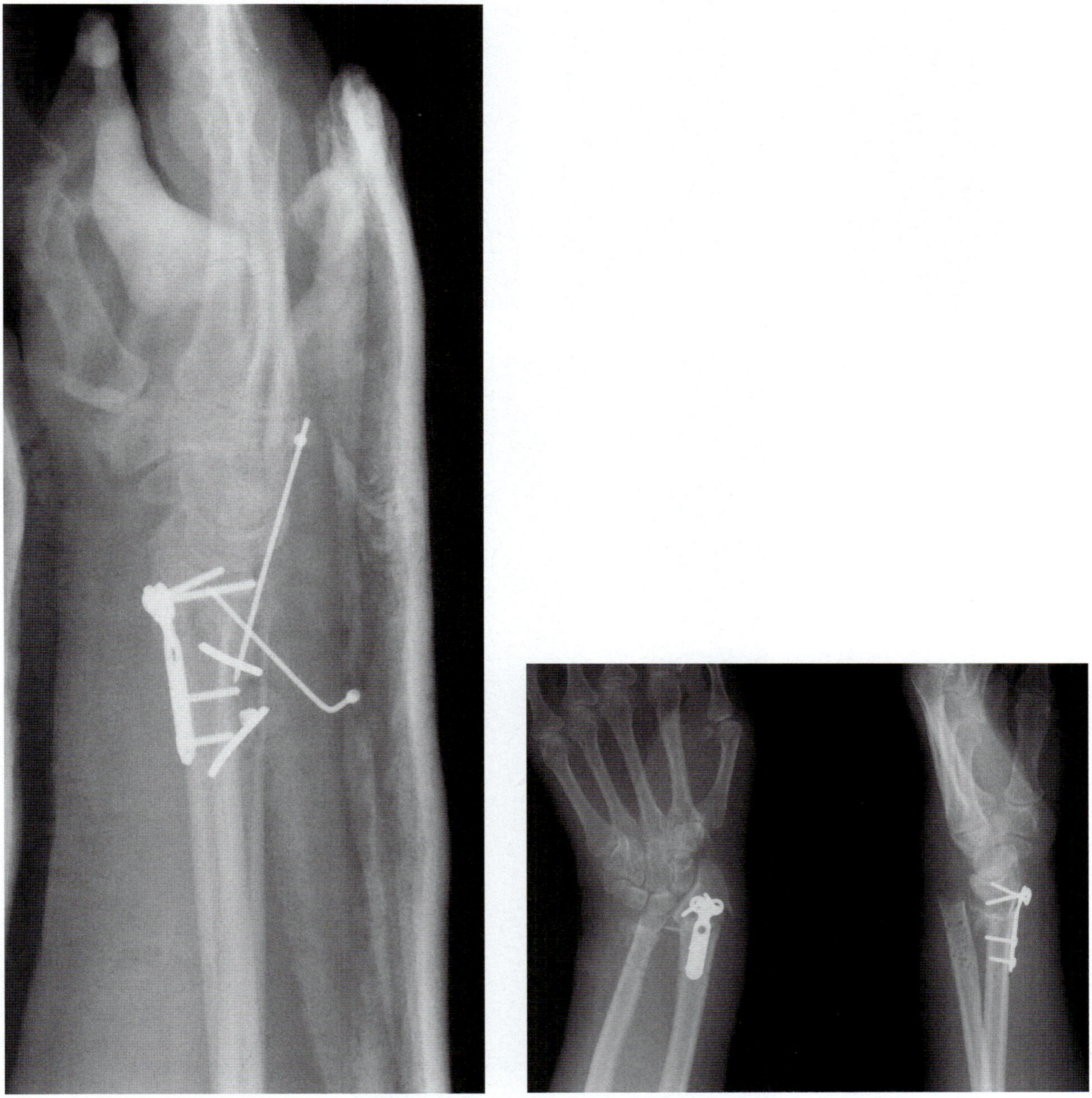

A B

FIGURE 60-8 A 61-year-old woman presented with a painful, unstable distal ulna and ununited distal radius/wrist arthrodesis with a painful pseudarthrosis. (**A**) Initial fracture fixation. (**B**) After debridement, hardware removal and ulnar head resection for infection. A resulting unstable ulna caused extensor tendon ruptures treated by tenorrhaphy of ring and small finger extensors and ulnar stump tenodesis. Continued problems led to a wrist arthrodesis with plate and screws. The third metacarpal fractured through a screw hole, requiring plate removal and metacarpal stabilization.

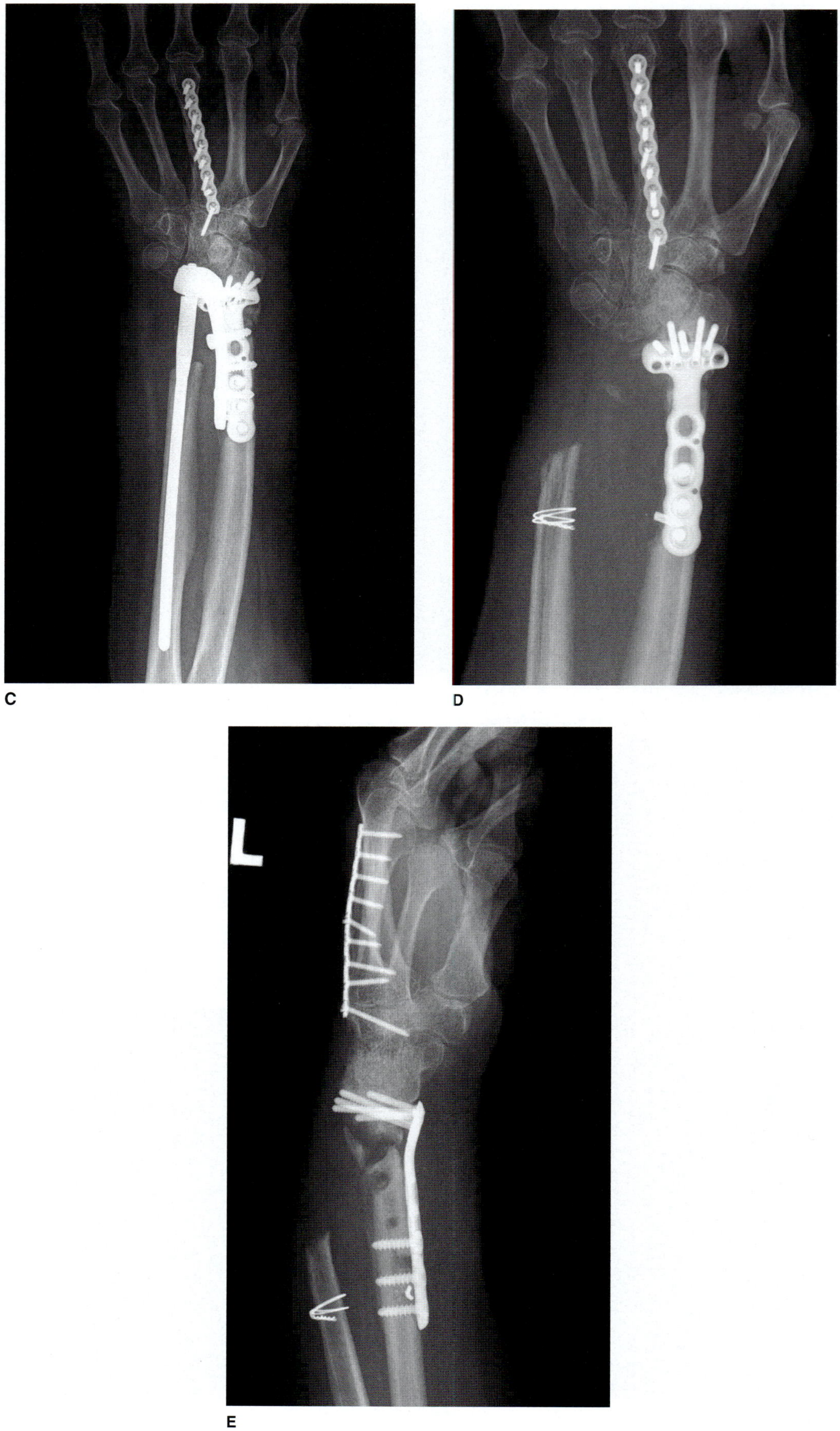

FIGURE 60-8 (*Continued*) (**C**) Distal ulnar instability was later treated with a constrained distal radioulnar prosthesis. Subsequently, the radius fractured through the implant screw holes and was fixed with a volar plate. The prosthesis later also failed because of infection with *Staphylococcus epidermidis*. (**D**) and (**E**) The hardware was removed by splitting the ulna, fixed with a cerclage wire. Intravenous antibiotics, including minocycline suppression, were used subsequently without evidence of recurrent infection.

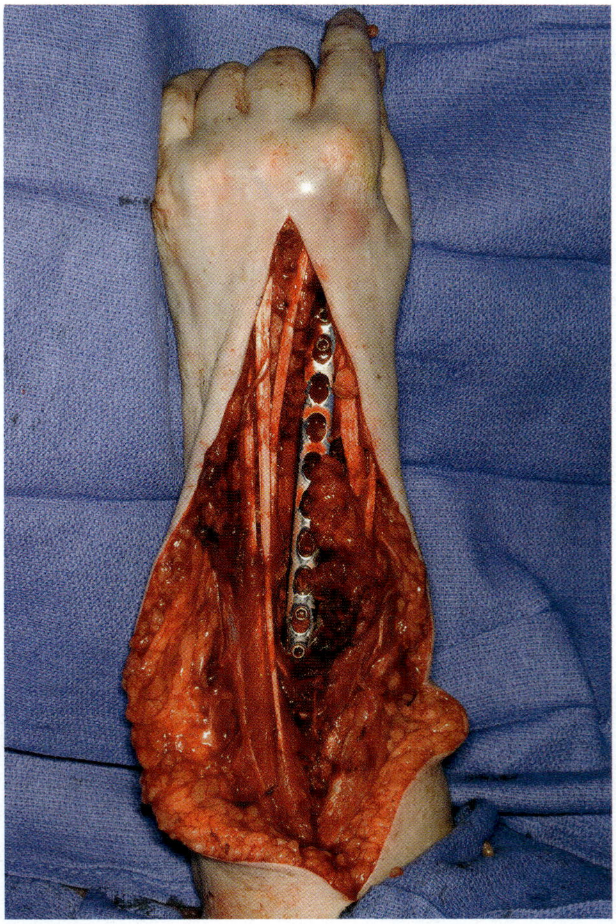

F

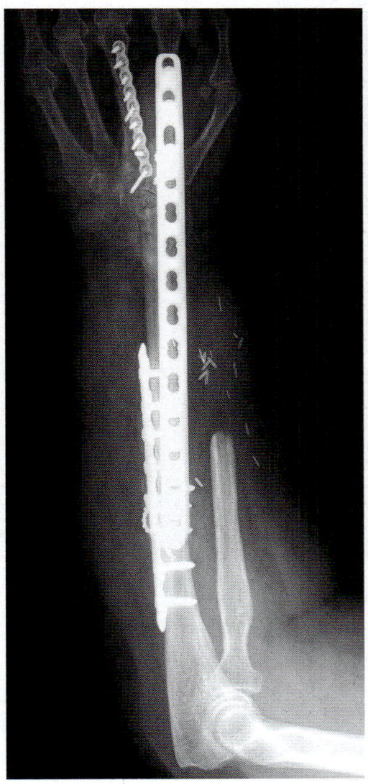

G

FIGURE 60-8 *(Continued)* (F) and (G) Stability to the wrist and distal ulna was restored with a fibular transfer creating a one-bone forearm. Radiographs suggested healing at 5 months, confirmed 1 month later by a computed tomography scan.

sequence of eight subsequent surgeries over a 5-year period followed. These included (1) initial fracture fixation and (2) debridement, hardware removal, and ulnar head resection for infection. A resulting unstable ulna caused extensor tendon ruptures treated by (3) tenorrhaphy of ring and small finger extensors, and ulnar stump tenodesis. Continued problems led to a (4) wrist arthrodesis with plate and screws. The third metacarpal fractured through a screw hole, requiring (5) plate removal and metacarpal stabilization. (6) Distal ulnar instability was later treated with a constrained distal radioulnar prosthesis. (7) Subsequently, the radius fractured through the implant screw holes and was fixed with a volar plate. (8) The prosthesis later also failed requiring removal. Stability to the wrist and distal ulna was restored with a one-bone forearm procedure using an interposed fibular graft. Radiographs suggested healing at 5 months, confirmed 1 month later by computed tomography (CT) scan.

Carpus: Scaphoid

The importance of correcting scaphoid humpback deformity and restoring blood supply in the setting of AVN has been well documented. The free vascularized medial femoral condyle graft provides both structural support to correct deformity and blood supply to promote union in the subset of patients with both scaphoid collapse and proximal pole AVN.

Indications

Scaphoid Nonunion

Numerous pedicled and free vascularized bone grafts have been described for the treatment of scaphoid nonunions, from the dorsal and palmar surfaces of the radius, iliac crest, medial femoral condyle, and metacarpal heads. The primary rationale for their use has been to improve the poor results seen in treating scaphoid nonunions associated with AVN of the proximal pole. In the presence of AVN, a meta-analysis of the literature has demonstrated conventional inlay bone grafting to have a union rate of only 47%. Vascularized grafts demonstrated a union rate of 88 percent with the same analysis (63).

Vascularized grafts may also be used in less constrained circumstances. For example, when grafting a proximal pole fracture, the adjacency of the 1,2 intercompartmental supraretinacular artery (1,2 ICSRA) pedicle to the surgical exposure provides the opportunity to use a vascularized rather than conventional graft without additional morbidity. Failed conventional grafts have been shown to heal with secondary conventional grafting (64) but may heal more quickly and reliably with a vascularized graft. In general, we have avoided using vascularized grafts in other less severe circumstances given the excellent rate of success with conventional wedge grafts for middle third fracture nonunions without associated AVN or hypovascularity (65).

1,2 Intercompartmental Supraretinacular Artery Graft

Pedicled vascularized grafts from either the dorsal or volar radius have been among the most popular such grafts. The dorsal graft,

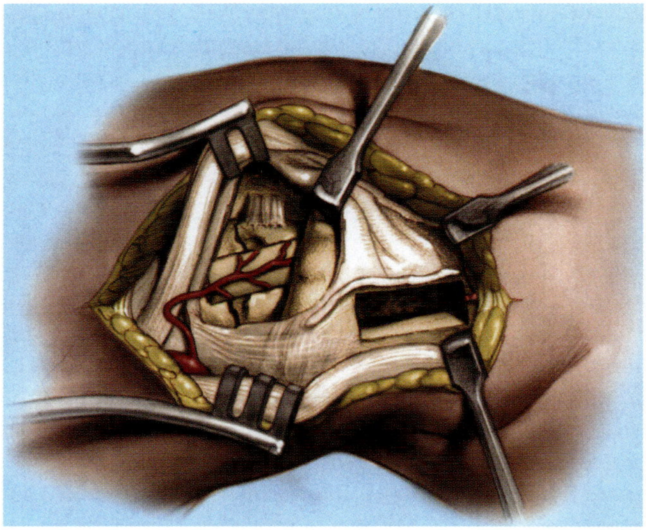

FIGURE 60-9 Pedicled grafts based upon the 1,2 intercompartmental supraretinacular artery pedicle are useful particularly for proximal pole nonunions with avascular necrosis but without carpal collapse. (By permission of Mayo Foundation for Medical Education and Research. All rights reserved.)

originally described by Zaidenberg et al. and anatomically defined by my colleagues and me, is based on the 1,2 ICSRA (55,66) (Figure 60-9). This graft is recommended for proximal nonunions without fragmentation, proximal acute fractures with comminution requiring bone grafting, and waist fracture nonunions without a humpback deformity or carpal collapse (67).

The use of a volar pedicle, originally described on a pronator quadratus pedicle, was also described by Sheetz et al. based on the palmar radiocarpal arch of vessels providing nutrient circulation to the radius (55,68). Its proximity to the important radiocarpal ligaments was thought to limit its usefulness by these authors, although it has been widely used by others for the scaphoid or lunate without significant problems (54,69). Fragmented scaphoids generally cannot be successfully treated with bone grafting and require a salvage procedure such as a four corner fusion or a proximal row carpectomy.

Medial Femoral Condyle Graft

Those presenting with both proximal pole avascularity and humpback deformity with carpal collapse represent a difficult subset of scaphoid nonunion (67). We have recently shown these to be optimally treated with the use of free medial femoral condylar wedge grafts, which both restore scaphoid length and improve local blood flow. The latter is important to promote healing to adjacent necrotic bone and to revascularize the avascular proximal pole. The free vascularized bone graft from the medial femoral condyle has several advantages. There is minimal donor site morbidity, and the bone harvested is compact cancellous bone similar in density to the scaphoid. A volar approach to the wrist may be used at the nonunion site, resulting in better visualization and access for correction of the humpback deformity with a structural autograft. Vascularized pedicled bone grafting from the distal radius typically uses a dorsal approach, limiting the placement of the graft in the scaphoid cavity and thus the correction of a humpback deformity. Additionally, the bone harvested from the distal radius, whether it is volar or dorsal, has limited structural properties. In contrast, the bone harvested from the medial femoral condyle is compact cancellous bone, and the vascular pedicle for the medial femoral condyle supplies a rich anastomotic network supplying the resected region of periosteum. The graft may be shaped into a structurally sound construct to fit the scaphoid cavity with minimal risk of devascularizing the graft. The use of a osteocartilaginous graft to resurface articular surface injury after AVN is also possible, described recently for the scaphoid but with considerable potential in other locations as well (45).

The technique of vascularized bone graft harvest from the medial femoral condyle is described in detail in Chapter 21. Placement in the scaphoid is performed through a Russe exposure using screw fixation if feasible and vascular connections to the radial artery end to side and venous anastomosis to adjacent superficial vein or vena comitans (Figure 60-10).

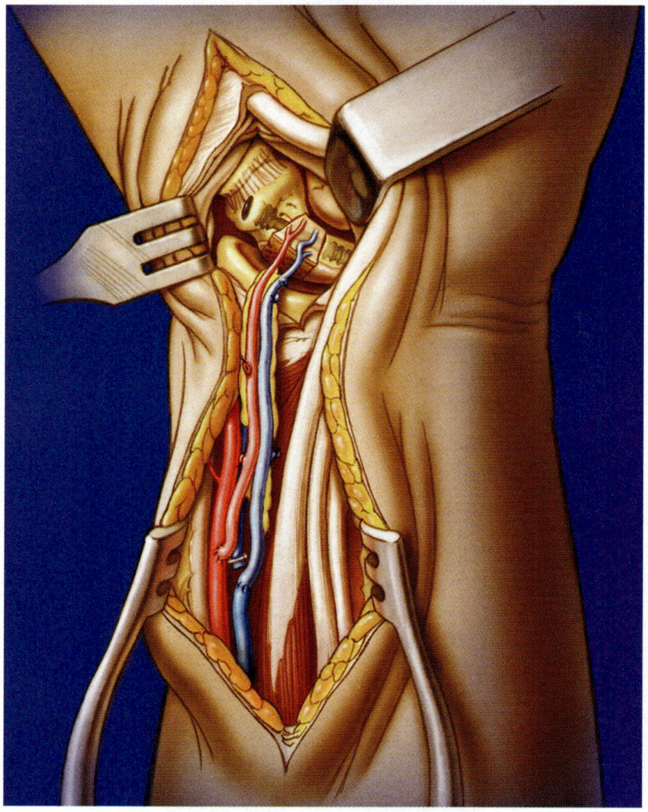

FIGURE 60-10 Placement of a free vascularized medial femoral condyle bone graft to treat a scaphoid waist nonunion with humpback deformity and avascular necrosis of the proximal portion. A Russe exposure is used for scaphoid preparation. Correction of deformity requires a volar wedge graft, often as much as 10 mm in volar proximal/distal dimension to eliminate carpal collapse deformity with an extended lunate (dorsal intercalated segmental instability). The graft is carefully shaped and positioned, and stabilized with a scaphoid screw (or Kirschner wires if a screw is not possible). Vascular connections are then made end-to-side to the radial artery and end-to-end to an adjacent vein. (By permission of Mayo Foundation for Medical Education and Research. All rights reserved.)

Case Example: Free Vascularized Graft for Scaphoid Nonunion with Avascular Necrosis and Humpback Deformity

A 14-year-old female soccer player injured her wrist in a fall on the outstretched left wrist 1 year before presentation. Symptoms resolved partially with use of a wrist brace, and no medical attention was sought for several months. She presented with an untreated scaphoid waist fracture nonunion with a humpback deformity (Figure 60-11A) and MRI evidence of avascularity (Figure 60-11B), later confirmed by absence of punctate bleeding during surgery. She was treated by correction of the dorsal intercalated segmental instability deformity and "freshening" of the nonunion site bone surface with a sagittal saw to create flat surfaces for optimal bone contact. A vascularized bone graft was harvested from the medial femoral condyle, trimmed to fit the defect, and fixed with a cannulated scaphoid screw. She was immobilized until a CT scan confirmed healing at 16 weeks after surgery.

Preiser's Disease

The rare condition termed Preiser's disease, or AVN of the scaphoid, is also amenable to treatment with vascularized bone grafts (26). This condition occurs in the absence of an acute fracture or an untreated nonunion. Case reports and clinical

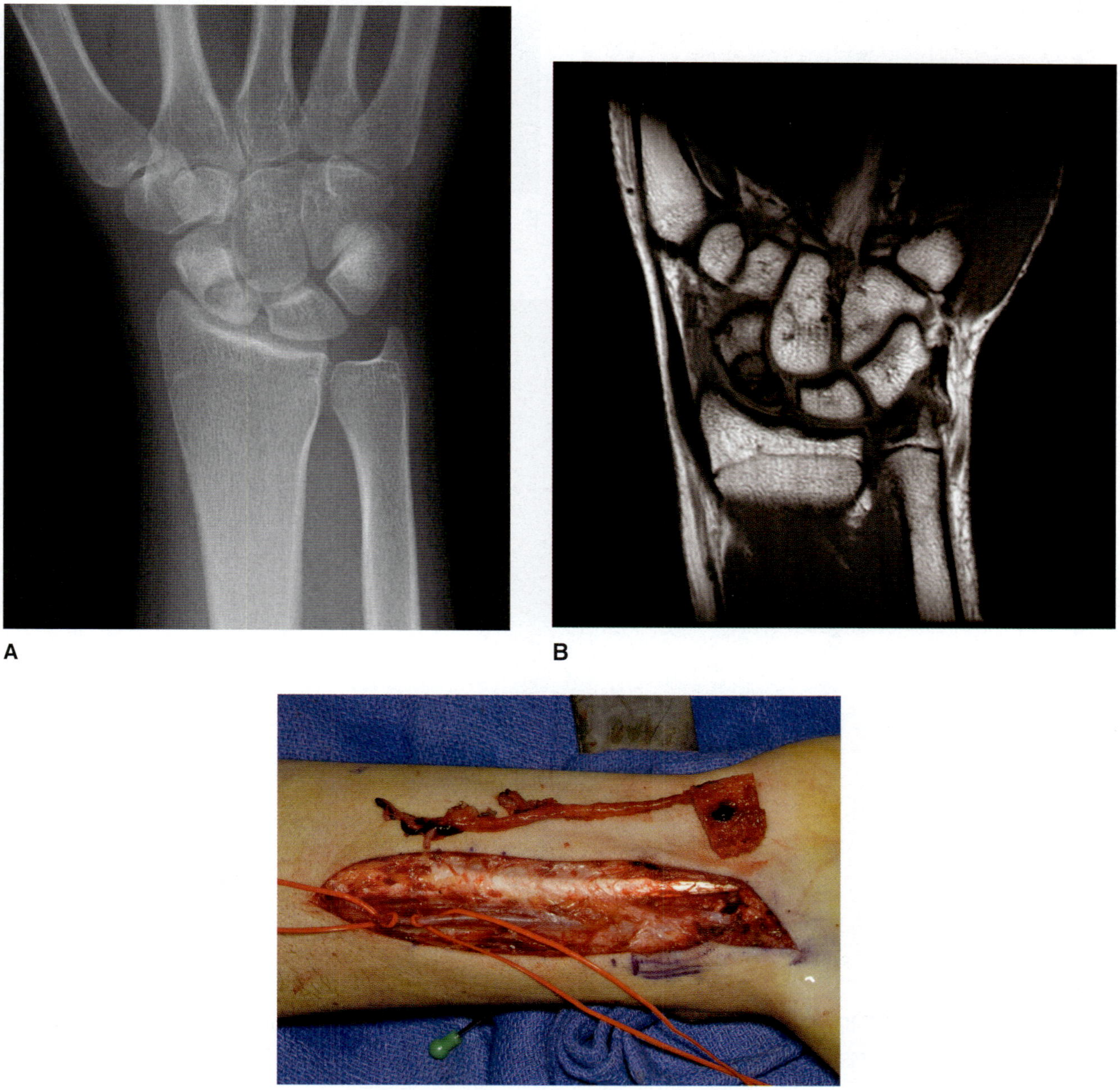

A B C

FIGURE 60-11 Scaphoid nonunion in a 14-year-old female soccer player. She presented 1 year after injury with an untreated scaphoid nonunion (B) and magnetic resonance imaging evidence of avascularity (B), later confirmed by absence of punctate bleeding at surgery. She was treated by correction of the dorsal intercalated segmental instability deformity and "freshening" of the nonunion site bone surface with a sagittal saw to create flat surfaces for optimal bone contact. (C) A vascularized bone graft was harvested from the medial femoral condyle and trimmed to fit the defect.

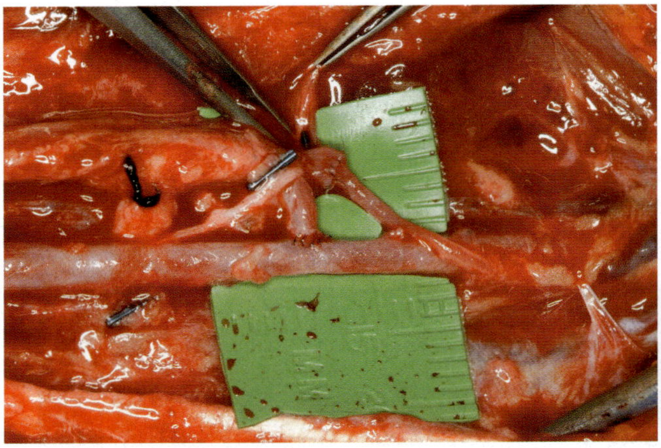

D

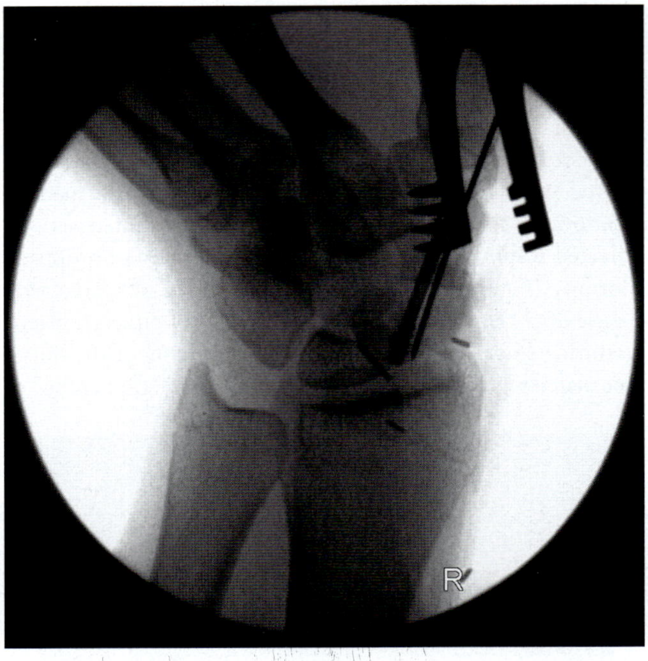

E

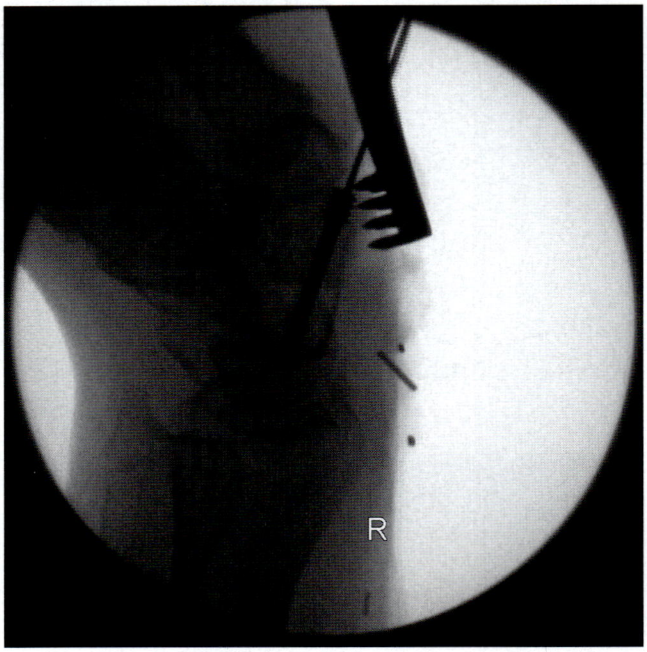

F

FIGURE 60-11 (*Continued*) (D) to (F) It was fixed with a cannulated scaphoid screw, and vascular anastomoses were performed to the radial artery end to side and a vena comitans end to end.

series have cited risk factors for disease development, including corticosteroid use, chemotherapy, systemic lupus, progressive systemic sclerosis, congenital scaphoid hypoplasia, and trauma, resulting in interruption of scaphoid blood supply. Treatment has generally been with salvage by proximal row carpectomy and four-corner fusion, with attempted salvage generally unsuccessful. A recent report of eight cases treated by 1,2 ICSRA pedicled vascularized radius grafts over a 10-year period demonstrated clinical improvement in pain, stable wrist strength, preserved wrist motion, and MRI evidence of revascularization in all cases (26). The resulting Mayo wrist score ratings were excellent in one, good in one, and fair in five. There was one poor result. It was thought that vascularized grafts were indicated in early stages of Preiser's disease before arthritic or instability changes.

Lunate

Vascularized grafts have been applied to treat osteonecrosis of the lunate (Kienböck's disease), with successful outcomes (27).

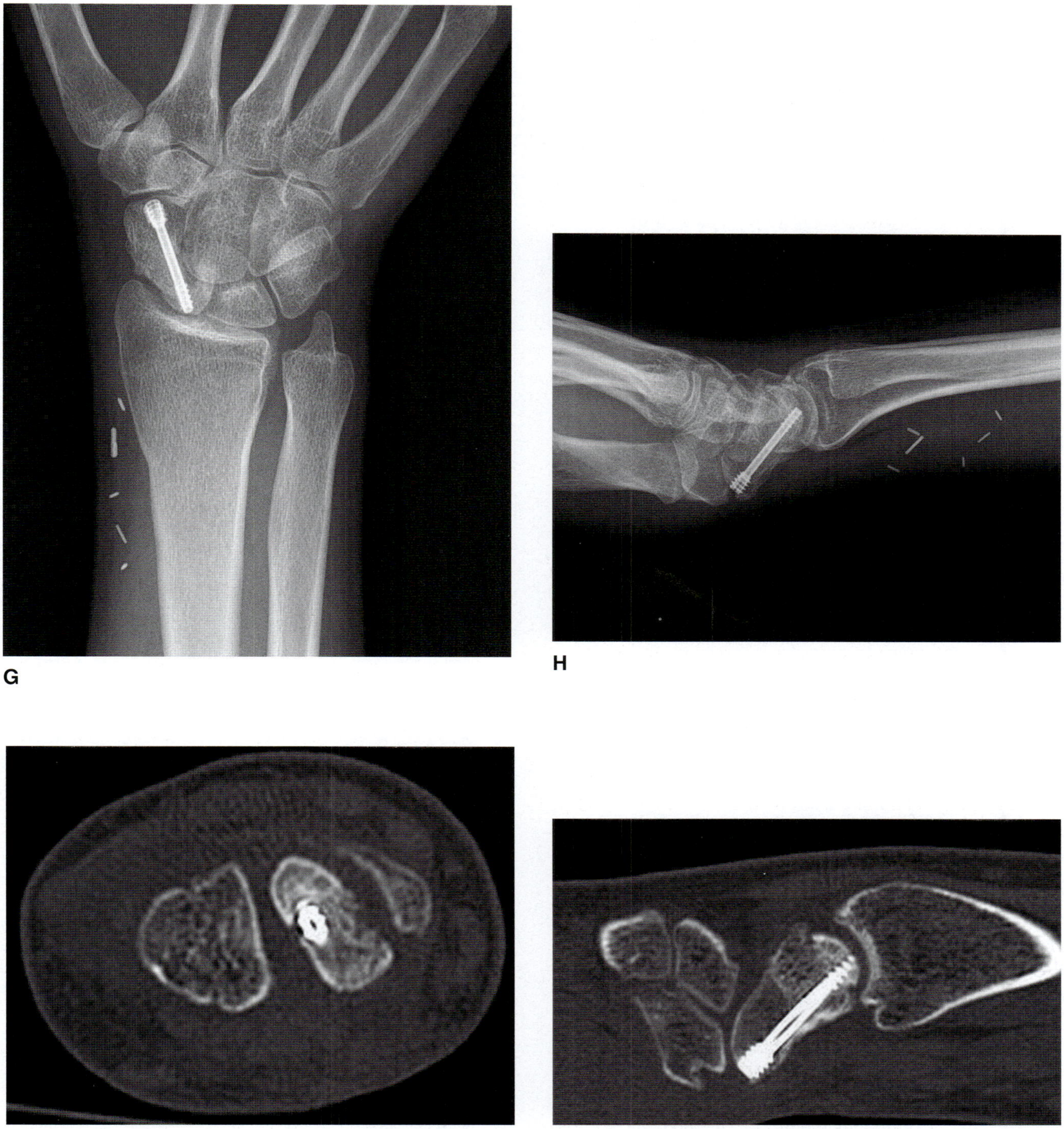

G H I J

FIGURE 60-11 (*Continued*) (G) to (J) She was immobilized until radiographs and a computed tomography scan confirmed healing at 16 weeks after surgery.

The general goal in such circumstances is to both revascularize the necrotic bone and, if collapsed, expand it to restore the normal Ståhl index (ratio of anteroposterior to proximal-distal dimension).

Lunate revascularization remains one of several options to treat this condition. Revascularization may be accomplished by vascularized bone grafting using pedicle bone grafts from the pisiform and radius or local arteriovenous bundle implantation (27,51,52,55,70). Other options commonly used may be broadly categorized as joint unloading or salvage procedures.

A consensus on a treatment algorithm for Kienböck's disease remains elusive because of our incomplete understanding of the disease's etiology; however, it has been established that AVN of the lunate leads to a predictable pattern of lunate collapse with progression to radiocarpal and midcarpal arthritis. Efforts to improve bone blood supply logically follow this understanding. The generally satisfactory results with pedicle grafting from the dorsal radius make this a reasonable option, provided the lunate is deemed salvageable (intact cartilage shell without extruded fragments).

Moran et al. reported the use of the 4 + 5 extensor compartment artery (ECA) distal radius pedicle graft for treatment of Kienböck's disease, placing the graft directly within the lunate to expand and revascularize the bone (27). Analysis of 26 such cases demonstrated 12 stage II, 10 stage IIIA, and four stage IIIB wrists. At a mean follow-up time of 31 months, motion improved from 68% to 71% of the unaffected side, grip strength improved from 50% to 89% of the unaffected side, and 92% of patients had significant improvement in their pain. Seventy-seven percent of patients showed no further collapse on postsurgical radiographs. Seventy-one percent of patients having postoperative MRI scans showed evidence of revascularization with improvement in the T2 or T1 signal. At present, microsurgical reconstruction of the lunate with free bone grafts has not been reported.

Fingers and Thumb

The small size of the long bones of the hand makes the need for vascularized bone generally less of an issue. Vascularized whole joint transfers may be performed in cases of joint destruction or loss from the hand or foot. In cases in which conventional grafts are inappropriate because of soft tissue loss, scar, or infection, vascularized grafts may be used as pedicled or free transfers. We reported one such case of osteomyelitis of the thumb metacarpal successfully reconstructed with the medial femoral condyle (71). Composite flaps from the scapular system have also been used in these circumstances, as have free lateral arm osteocutaneous and dorsalis pedis flaps.

POSTOPERATIVE MONITORING

Monitoring of vascularized bone grafts is best done in a continuous fashion if it is to be done at all, the goal being to detect arterial or venous thrombosis at a time point permitting revision of the anastomosis and preservation of bone viability. Thrombosis of the vascular pedicle in a vascularized bone graft results in conditions that are less favorable for vascular invasion and the usual process of bone graft incorporation than a conventional bone graft because of the soft tissue envelope included with the bone. Continuous monitoring methods include the use of a skin "buoy flap," thermocouple probes, and use of surface or implanted laser or ultrasound Doppler probes. Of these the buoy flap is the most feasible and easily interpreted. Direct observation of the transferred skin allows immediate return to the operating room if simpler means such as loosening the dressing, altering limb position, or trial of anticoagulation does not reverse observed changes in 1 to 2 hours.

REFERENCES

1. Kobbe P, Tarkin IS, Frink M, Pape HC. [Voluminous bone graft harvesting of the femoral marrow cavity for autologous transplantation. An indication for the "Reamer-Irrigator-Aspirator-" (RIA-) technique] [German]. *Unfallchirurg* 2008;111:469.
2. Barth H. Histologishe Untersuchungen uber Knochen Transplantation. *Beitr Pathol Anat Allg Pathol* 1895;17:65.
3. Berggren A, Weiland AJ, Dorfman A. The effect of prolonged ischemia time on osteocyte and osteoblast survival in composite bone grafts revascularized by microvascular anastomoses. *Plast Reconstr Surg* 1982;69:19.
4. Goldberg VM, Stevenson S. Natural history of autografts and allografts. *Clin Orthop* 1987;225:7.
5. Burchardt H. The biology of bone graft repair. *Clin Orthop* 1983;Apr(174):28–42.
6. Rinaldi E. Autografts in the treatment of osseous defects in the forearm and hand. *J Am Hand Surg* 1987;12:282.
7. Mankin HJ, Gebhardt MC, Tomford WW. The use of frozen cadaveric allografts in the management of patients with bone tumors of the extremities. *Orthop Clin North Am* 1987;18:275.
8. Gebhardt MC, Roth YF, Mankin HJ. Osteoarticular allografts for reconstruction in the proximal part of the humerus after excision of a musculoskeletal tumor. *J Bone Joint Surg Am* 1990;72:334.
9. Dean GS, Holliger EHT, Urbaniak JR. Elbow allograft for reconstruction of the elbow with massive bone loss. Long term results. *Clin Orthop Relat Res* 1997;341:12.
10. Guo W, Tang S, Yang RL, Ji T. [Total elbow arthroplasty after resection of tumors at the elbow] [Chinese]. *Chin J Surg* 2008;46:1734–1737.
11. Damsin JP, Ghanem I. Upper limb lengthening [review]. *Hand Clin* 2000;16:685.
12. Huntington TW. Use of a segment of fibula to supply a defect in the tibia. *Ann Surg* 1905;41:249.
13. Ostrop LT, Frederickson JM. Distant transfer of a free living bone graft by microvascular anastomoses. *Plast Reconstr Surg* 1974;54:274.
14. McKee DM. Microvascular bone transplantation. *Clin Plast Surg* 1978;5:283.
15. Taylor GI, Miller GD, Ham FJ. The free vascularized bone graft. A clinical extension of microvascular techniques. *Plast Reconstr Surg* 1975;55:533.
16. Taylor GI, Townsend P, Corlett R. Superiority of the deep circumflex iliac vessels as the supply for free groin flaps. *Plast Reconstr Surg* 1979;64:595.
17. Ueba Y, Fukikawa S. Nine years follow-up of a vascularized fibular graft in neurofibromatosis: a case report and literature review. *Orthop Trauma Surg* 1983;26:595.
18. Arata MA, Wood MB, Cooney WPD. Revascularized segmental diaphyseal bone transfers in the canine. An analysis of viability. *J Reconstr Microsurg* 1984;1:11.
19. Berggren A, Weiland AJ, Dorfman H. Free vascularized bone grafts: factors affecting their survival and ability to heal to recipient bone defects. *Plast Reconstr Surg* 1982;69:19.
20. de Boer HH, Wood MB. Bone changes in the vascularized fibular graft. *J Bone Joint Surg Br* 1989;71B:374.
21. Han CS, Wood MB, Bishop AT, Cooney WPR. Vascularized bone transfer. *J Bone Joint Surg Am* 1992;74:1441.
22. Siegert JJ, Wood MB. Blood flow evaluation of vascularized bone transfers in a canine model. *J Orthop Res* 1990;8:291.
23. Sunagawa T, Bishop AT, Muramatsu K. Role of conventional and vascularized bone grafts in scaphoid nonunion with avascular necrosis: a canine experimental study. *J Hand Surg Am* 2000;25:849.
24. Suzuki O, Bishop AT, Sunagawa T, et al. Augmented surgical angiogenesis in necrotic bone: correction of avascular necrosis with vascular endothelial growth factor (VEGF). *J Microsurg* 2002.
25. Katsube K, Bishop AT. Gene therapy for neoangiogenesis in avascular bone. *J Orthop Res* 2002.
26. Moran SL, Cooney WP, Shin AY. The use of vascularized grafts from the distal radius for the treatment of Preiser's disease. *J Hand Surg Am* 2006;31:705.
27. Moran SL, Cooney WP, Berger RA, et al. The use of the 4 + 5 extensor compartmental vascularized bone graft for the treatment of Kienbock's disease. *J Hand Surg Am* 2005;30:50.
28. Yajima H, Tamai S, Ono H, Kizaki K. Vascularized bone grafts to the upper extremities. *Plast Reconstr Surg* 1998;101:727.
29. Kakinoki R, Ikeguchi R, Nakayama K, et al. Treatment of avascular necrosis of the capitulum of the humerus using a free vascularized osteoperiosteal graft from the medial condyle of the femur: a case report. *J Shoulder Elbow Surg* 2008;17(1):e1–e4.
30. Chang CC, Greenspan A, Gershwin ME. Osteonecrosis: current perspectives on pathogenesis and treatment. [Review] [222 refs]. *Semin Arthritis Rheum* 1993;23:47.
31. Jones DB Jr, Burger H, Bishop AT, Shin AY. Treatment of scaphoid waist nonunions with an avascular proximal pole and carpal collapse. A comparison of two vascularized bone grafts. *J Bone Joint Surg Am* 2008;90:2616.

32. Innocenti M, Delcroix L, Manfrini M, et al. Vascularized proximal fibular epiphyseal transfer for distal radial reconstruction. *J Bone Joint Surg Am* 2005;1:237.
33. Bitter K, Dana T. The iliac bone or osteocutaneous transplant pedicled to the deep circumflex iliac artery. I. Anatomical and technical considerations. *J Maxillofac Surg* 1983;11:195.
34. Salibian AH, Anzel SH, Salyer WA. Transfer of vascularized grafts of iliac bone to the extremities. *J Bone Joint Surg* 1987;69(suppl A):1319.
35. Reinisch JF, Winters R, Puckett CL. The use of the osteocutaneous groin flap in gunshot wounds of the hand. *J Hand Surg Am* 1984;9(suppl A):12.
36. Hartman EH, Spauwen PH, Jansen JA. Donor-site complications in vascularized bone flap surgery. [Review] [100 refs]. *J Investig Surg* 2002;15:185.
37. Werner CM, Favre P, van Lenthe HG, Dumont CE. Pedicled vascularized rib transfer for reconstruction of clavicle nonunions with bony defects: anatomical and biomechanical considerations. *Plast Reconstr Surg* 2007;120:173.
38. Choudry UH, Bakri K, Moran SL, et al. The vascularized medial femoral condyle periosteal bone flap for the treatment of recalcitrant bony nonunions. *Ann Plast Surg* 2008;60:174.
39. Fuchs B, Steinmann SP, Bishop AT. Free vascularized corticoperiosteal bone graft for the treatment of persistent nonunion of the clavicle. *J Shoulder Elbow Surg* 2005;14:264.
40. Doi K, Sakai K. Vascularized periosteal bone graft from the supracondylar region of the femur. *Microsurgery* 1994;15:305.
41. Hertel R, Masquelet AC. The reverse flow medial knee osteoperiosteal flap for skeletal reconstruction of the leg. Description and anatomical basis. *Surg Radiol Anat* 1989;11:257.
42. Doi K, Oda T, Soo-Heong T, Nanda V. Free vascularized bone graft for nonunion of the scaphoid. *J Hand Surg Am* 2000;25:507.
43. Jones DB Jr, Burger H, Bishop AT, Shin AY. Treatment of scaphoid waist nonunions with an avascular proximal pole and carpal collapse. Surgical technique. *J Bone Joint Surg Am* 2009;2:169.
44. Larson AN, Bishop AT, Shin AY. Free medial femoral condyle bone grafting for scaphoid nonunions with humpback deformity and proximal pole avascular necrosis. *Tech Hand Up Extrem Surg* 2007;11:246.
45. Kaelicke T, Buerger H, Mueller EJ. [A new vascularized cartilage-bone-graft for scaphoid nonunion with avascular necrosis of the proximal pole. Description of a new type of surgical procedure] [German]. *Unfallchirurg* 2008;111:201.
46. Doi K, Hattori Y. The use of free vascularized corticoperiosteal grafts from the femur in the treatment of scaphoid non-union. [Review] [26 refs]. *Orthop Clin North Am* 2007;38:87.
47. Enneking WF, Gady JL, Burchardt H. Autogenous cortical bone grafts in the reconstruction of segmental skeletal defects. *J Bone Joint Surg* 1980;62(suppl A):1039.
48. Enneking WF, Mindell ER. Observations on massive retrieved human allografts. *J Bone Joint Surg Am* 1991;73:1123.
49. Eppley BL, Connolly DT, Winkelmann T, et al. Free bone graft reconstruction of irradiated facial tissue: experimental effects of basic fibroblast growth factor stimulation. *Plast Reconstr Surg* 1991;88:319.
50. Erbs G, Bohm E. [Long-term results of pisiform bone transposition in lunate necrosis] [German]. *Handchir Mikrochir Plast Chir* 1984;16:85.
51. Beck E. Die Verpflanzung des Os Pisiforme am Gafasssteil zur Behandlung der Lunatummalazie. *Handchirurgie* 1971;3:64.
52. Bochud RC, Buchler U. Kienbock's disease, early stage 3—height reconstruction and core revascularization of the lunate. *J Hand Surg Br* 1994;19:466.
53. Pierer G, Steffen J, Hoflehner H. The vascular blood supply of the second metacarpal bone: anatomic basis for a new vascularized bone graft in hand surgery. An anatomical study in cadavers. *Surg Radiol Anat* 1992;14:103.
54. Mathoulin C, Haerle M. Vascularized bone graft from the palmar carpal artery for treatment of scaphoid nonunion. *J Hand Surg Br* 1998;23:318.
55. Sheetz KK, Bishop AT, Berger RA. The arterial blood supply of the distal radius and ulna and its potential use in vascularized pedicled bone grafts. *J Hand Surg Am* 1995;20:902.
56. Shin AY, Bishop AT. Vascular anatomy of the distal radius: implications for vascularized bone grafts [review]. *Clin Orthop Relat Res* 2001;Feb(383):60–73.
57. Steinman SA, Bishop AT, Berger RA. *Vascularized Bone Grafting for Scaphoid Non-union.* Presented at American Society for Surgery of the Hand 51st Annual Meeting. Nashville, TN, 1996.
58. Guimberteau JC, Panconi B. Recalcitrant non-union of the scaphoid treated with a vascularized bone graft based on the ulnar artery. *J Bone Joint Surg Am* 1990;72:88.
59. Rose PS, Shin AY, Bishop AT, et al. Vascularized free fibula transfer for oncologic reconstruction of the humerus. *Clin Orthop Relat Res* 2005;438:80.
60. Linberg BE. Interscapulo-thoracic resection for malignant tumors of the shoulder joint region. 1928. *Clin Orthop Relat Res* 1999;358:3.
61. Jones NF, Swartz WM, Mears DC, et al. The "double barrel" free vascularized fibular bone graft. *Plast Reconstr Surg* 1988;81:378.
62. Giessler GA, Bickert B, Sauerbier M, Germann G. [Free microvascular fibula graft for skeletal reconstruction after tumor resections in the forearm—experience with five cases] [German]. *Handchir Mikrochir Plast Chir* 2004;36:301.
63. Merrell GA, Wolfe SW, Slade JF 3rd. Treatment of scaphoid nonunions: quantitative meta-analysis of the literature [see comment]. *J Hand Surg Am* 2002;27:685.
64. Carrozzella JC, Stern PJ, Murdock PA. The fate of failed bone graft surgery for scaphoid nonunions. *J Hand Surg Am* 1989;14:800.
65. Green DP. The effect of avascular necrosis on Russe bone grafting for scaphoid nonunion. *J Hand Surg Am* 1985;10:597.
66. Zaidenberg C, Siebert JW, Angrigiani C. A new vascularized bone graft for scaphoid nonunion. *J Hand Surg Am* 1991;16:474.
67. Chang MA, Bishop AT, Moran SL, Shin AY. The outcomes and complications of 1,2-intercompartmental supraretinacular artery pedicled vascularized bone grafting of scaphoid nonunions. *J Hand Surg Am* 2006;31:387.
68. Kawai H, Yamamoto K. Pronator quadratus pedicled bone graft for old scaphoid fractures. *J Bone Joint Surg Br* 1988;70:829.
69. Haerle M, Schaller HE, Mathoulin C. Vascular anatomy of the palmar surfaces of the distal radius and ulna: its relevance to pedicled bone grafts at the distal palmar forearm. *J Hand Surg Br* 2003;28:131.
70. Hori Y, Tamai S, Okuda H, et al. Blood vessel transplantation to bone. *J Hand Surg Am* 1979;4:23.
71. Sammer DM, Bishop AT, Shin AY. Vascularized medial femoral condyle graft for thumb metacarpal reconstruction: case report. *J Hand Surg Am* 2009;34:715.

CHAPTER 61

Microneurovascular Functioning Muscle Transfer: The Factors that Govern Success

Ralph T. Manktelow

Functioning muscle transfer (FMT) is a procedure that involves the microneurovascular transfer of a muscle from one location to another. FMTs are indicated when there is a major functional deficit caused by damaged, missing, or nonfunctional skeletal muscle. This procedure is indicated if a significant functional gain can be achieved with the transfer of a single functioning muscle unit. For example, in a patient with a loss of forearm flexor muscle, a muscle transfer can provide voluntary finger flexion and produce useful grip function (Figure 61-1).

Viability of a microneuromuscular muscle transfer is obtained by microvascular anastomoses between the muscle's artery and vein and a suitable artery and vein in the recipient area. Reinnervation and active muscle contraction are produced by suturing an appropriate motor nerve in the recipient area to the motor nerve of the transferred muscle.

Caution should be taken with the application of this procedure. A careful analysis of the expected outcome should be the first step in considering this procedure. If there are other extensive injuries or major anatomical deficits in the extremity, the replacement of a single motor unit may not improve the function of the extremity.

The surgical technique has been frequently discussed and described in detail (1–5). This chapter primarily focuses on the factors that govern success. Success is the provision of providing voluntary control in a viable muscle, which produces a full range of motion and power.

HISTORY

In 1970, Tamai and colleagues demonstrated the microneuromuscular transfer of functional skeletal muscle in experimental animals (6). In 1973 at the Sixth People's Hospital in Shanghai, surgeons transplanted the lateral portion of the pectoralis major muscle in a patient with Volkmann's ischemic contracture (7). This was the first clinical FMT. A good range of finger motion and substantial grip force were observed by the senior author. In 1976, Harii et al. used the gracilis to replace the muscles of facial expression in a long-standing case of Bell's palsy (8). In 1976, the authors transferred a portion of the pectoralis major to replace missing forearm musculature in a patient who had sustained forearm trauma. In the same year, they transferred the gracilis muscle for a similar indication. Both patients developed powerful voluntary grip function (9). The success of these cases stimulated additional procedures and the development of the principles of this surgery (10,11). New concepts were developed, including muscle transplantation by fascicular territory; the cutting and shaping of small segments of muscle for reconstruction of facial paralysis; the application of FMT to children's injuries, particularly for Volkman's ischemic contracture; and the use of unorthodox motor nerves for the innervation of FMT (12,13).

GENERAL PRINCIPLES

1. FMT is a complex procedure and should not be used when simpler satisfactory techniques such as a tendon transfer or tenodesis can provide an adequate result.
2. The most common pathology for which this procedure is indicated is direct muscle trauma, Volkmann's ischemic paralysis, electrical burns, postreplantation, gas gangrene, long-standing nerve injury (especially brachial plexus injury), and muscle excision for tumor (9,10,14–18).
3. The recipient extremity should have the necessary anatomical structures. These structures include an artery, vein, motor nerve, insertion site, and tendon(s) to be

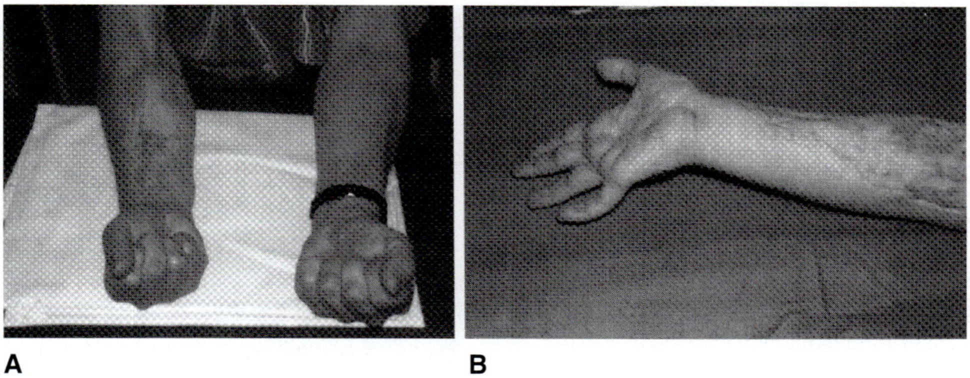

FIGURE 61-1 (A) After surgery, this patient's right forearm has a functioning gracilis muscle transfer providing all of his long finger flexor function. (B) With contraction of his intact extensors, the muscle allows full finger and wrist extension. (Reproduced with permission from Green's Operative Hand Surgery, 5th Ed. Vol 2, Ch 36.)

motored, and these key structures must be in a location that will match the same structures in the transferred muscle. Soft tissue coverage should be available to house the muscle.

4. The recipient extremity should have sufficient functional anatomy for useful limb function with the addition of the transfer and possibly other operations such as nerve repairs. This functional anatomy includes antagonistic muscles to the transferred function, intrinsic muscles to provide a balanced controlled movement, flexible joints, and sensory innervation to the distal extremity.
5. FMT has been used mostly in the upper extremity and has been used for the replacement of long flexor finger function; long extensor finger function; together with biceps, triceps, and deltoid reconstruction. Of these five applications, the most common is for long flexor finger function.
6. Although the gracilis has been the workhorse of FMT, the muscle that is the most appropriate for the recipient site requirements should be used and may be the latissimus dorsi, tensor fascia lata, serratus anterior, or others.
7. The patient must be motivated to pursue a postoperative exercise program and be willing to accept a 1- to 2-year period of improvement before maximum function is obtained.
8. FMT is a complex procedure. For a successful operation, every step must be completed correctly, from preoperative planning to late postoperative care.

FACTORS THAT GOVERN SUCCESS

Preoperative Planning

The surgeon should visualize the functional effect that a transferred muscle will likely produce. For example, for a muscle that is being used to create finger flexion in a traumatized forearm, the surgeon should consider whether useful grip be anticipated or whether a claw hand deformity will be produced because the limb lacks the critical intrinsic muscle function. Useful grip function requires other functioning structures. This will include antagonistic extensor muscles to stabilize the wrist and to extend the fingers out of the palm. The joints that will be moved by the transfer must have good passive mobility. There must be sufficient sensibility in the fingers to allow tactile functions.

In the case of a pathological tenodesis that deforms the limb or limits joint mobility such as may be seen in Volkman's ischemic contracture, it may be wise to remove the scarred muscle during a preliminary operation to allow finger and joint mobilization. Because the distal half of the muscle and the tendon of insertion of the muscle will have to glide well, there must be good soft tissue cover for this part of the transfer.

The assessment of the key recipient anatomical structures includes a site for the origin and insertion of the muscle, a donor artery and vein, motor nerve, and overlying soft tissue cover.

When the presence or condition of a suitable artery is unclear from the clinical examination, an arteriogram is useful. Arterial anastomoses in the upper extremity may be end to end or end to side. In the proximal forearm, small branches such as the ulnar recurrent and anterior interosseous arteries are available as end-to-end sources of arterial input. If the radial, ulnar, or brachial arteries are available, these vessels are excellent for end-to-side anastomoses. However, the thick wall in these vessels may make the repair more difficult than when using smaller vessels, which may be used for end-to-end anastomoses. Useful smaller arteries in the upper arm are the thoracodorsal, anterior and posterior humeral circumflex, profunda brachii, and branches of the acromiothoracic. In the lower leg, the anterior or posterior tibial are particularly useful, and end-to-side anastomoses are most reliable.

Either superficial or deep veins can be used for anastomoses. Superficial arm veins are more useful than superficial leg veins, which have a tendency to spasm. In most locations, the deep veins and venae comitantes are most suitable for anastomoses.

From the history and physical examination, it is usually possible to determine which motor nerve branches in the upper extremity are likely to be present and undamaged. Good muscle function cannot be expected without a technically sound microneural repair to an undamaged donor motor nerve. If there is significant doubt about the availability of a good motor nerve, the surgeon should explore the desired nerve and biopsy it to assess its status in a preliminary operation before the muscle transfer.

A "pure" motor nerve must be selected to provide good reinnervation. For replacement of finger long flexor musculature, the preferred motor nerves are the anterior interosseous nerve

(AIN), branches of the median nerve that had innervated the superficialis muscle, or branches of the ulnar nerve that had innervated the flexor digitorum profundus. For the dorsal (extensor) aspect of the forearm, motor branches of the posterior interosseous nerve are available. It is possible to use the motor component of a mixed nerve if the motor and sensory components of the nerve can be physically separated and identified. The motor component of the musculocutaneous nerve can be used for biceps reconstruction and the motor component of the axillary nerve for deltoid reconstruction. For triceps reconstruction, proximal branches of the radial nerve are used. For tibialis anterior reconstruction, the motor component of the tibialis anterior nerve is a good choice. A healthy, undamaged donor motor nerve should have a cross-sectional area equal or larger than that of the motor nerve of the muscle to be transferred.

If a muscle transfer to the anterior forearm is planned, an angiogram can provide valuable information about the anterior interosseous artery (AIA) and AIN. This useful recipient vessel lies beside the AIN. If the angiogram shows a normal AIA, then one can expect that the AIN, which lies adjacent to it, is also uninjured. Being deep in the forearm and protected by the radius and ulna, the AIA and AIN are frequently available as the recipient vessel and nerve for a flexor forearm transfer.

Selecting the Correct Muscle

The criteria for muscle selection are those that provide a good anatomical fit and a good physiological fit. For an anatomical fit, the location of all of the structures on the muscle and in the recipient site that are to be attached together must match like a piece of a puzzle. The physiological needs of the muscle are sufficient excursion and strength for the needs of the extremity.

The effectiveness of the transferred muscle will depend on the force and excursion of the muscle, the patient's ability to voluntarily control the muscle, and the ability of the muscle tendon unit to glide. The force of muscle contraction after transfer is related to the cross-sectional area of the contracting muscle fibers, the position of contraction on the length–tension curve, the completeness of reinnervation, and the intensity of the postoperative strengthening program. When a muscle contracts, the force of contraction depends on the number of individual muscle fibers that respond to neural stimulation. In view of the length–tension curve, it would seem reasonable to assume that a useful range of powerful muscle excursion of the gracilis is less than the maximum experimental excursion of 15+ cm but likely to be at least 8 to 10 cm (5). In our laboratory, experimental microneurovascular muscle transfer in dogs resulted in muscles that, when studied after full recovery, developed a maximum force of contraction that varied from 35% to 120% of the control muscle in the normal limb (19).

The excursion of the muscle depends on the length of the muscle fibers with most strap muscles contracting more than half of their fully extended length. During surgery, the normal excursion of the gracilis muscle can be demonstrated when its motor nerve is stimulated. After the muscle has been dissected in an adult and separated from all structures in the leg except for its vascular supply, it will shorten 15 or more cm with nerve stimulation (Figure 61-2).

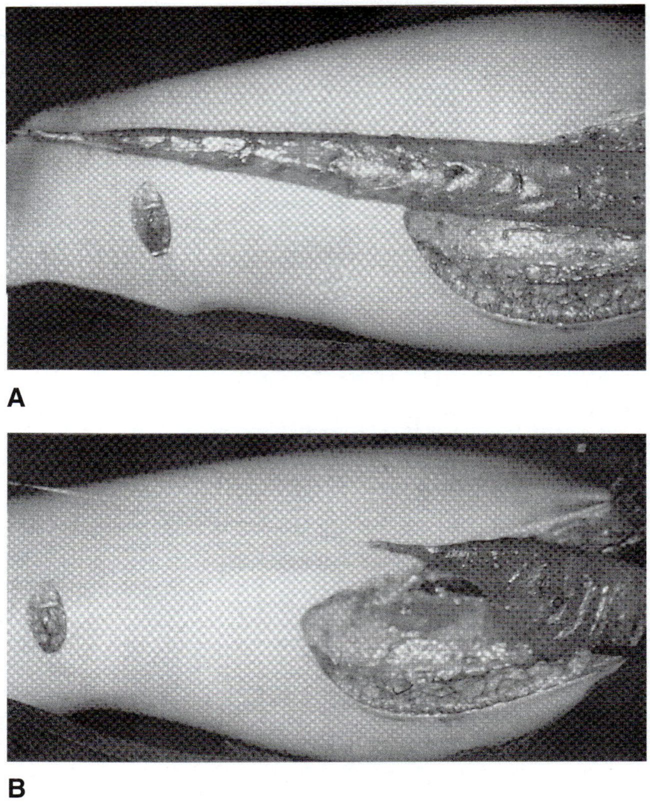

FIGURE 61-2 (A) The right gracilis muscle is separated from the surrounding structures except for the neurovascular pedicle and the attachment of its origin. (B) The motor nerve has been stimulated, and the maximum excursion of the muscle is demonstrated. The muscle has shortened 15 cm. (Reproduced with permission from Green's Operative Hand Surgery, 5th Ed. Vol 2, Ch 36.)

The gross muscle fiber arrangement of skeletal muscles are either strap or pennate. A pennate muscle has much shorter muscle fiber units than a strap muscle. These muscle fiber units insert into a central or lateral tendon. The excursion of the whole muscle is proportional to the length of these short muscle fibers rather than the overall length of the muscle itself. If a muscle fiber unit in a pennate muscle is 6 cm, the overall muscle contraction capability is slightly more than 50% of this, or just over 3 cm, and the useful range is closer to 2 cm. Although the overall muscle length may be as long as 30 cm, the entire muscle will only shorten a maximum of approximately 3 cm. If this 30-cm muscle unit were a strap muscle such as the gracilis, the contractile capability would be in excess of 15 cm with a useful range of 8 to 10 cm (Figure 61-3). However, the pennate muscle is correspondingly more powerful in its contraction inasmuch as the aggregate cross-sectional area of the pennate muscle fibers is considerably larger that those in a comparably sized strap muscle. The practical solution to muscle selection for clinical application is provided by selecting a strap muscle with a large cross-sectional area (1,19).

Available Muscles for Functional Transfer

The two muscles that have been most useful are the gracilis and the latissimus dorsi. Their anatomy and dissection technique are well described elsewhere by the authors (1,2,4). Other

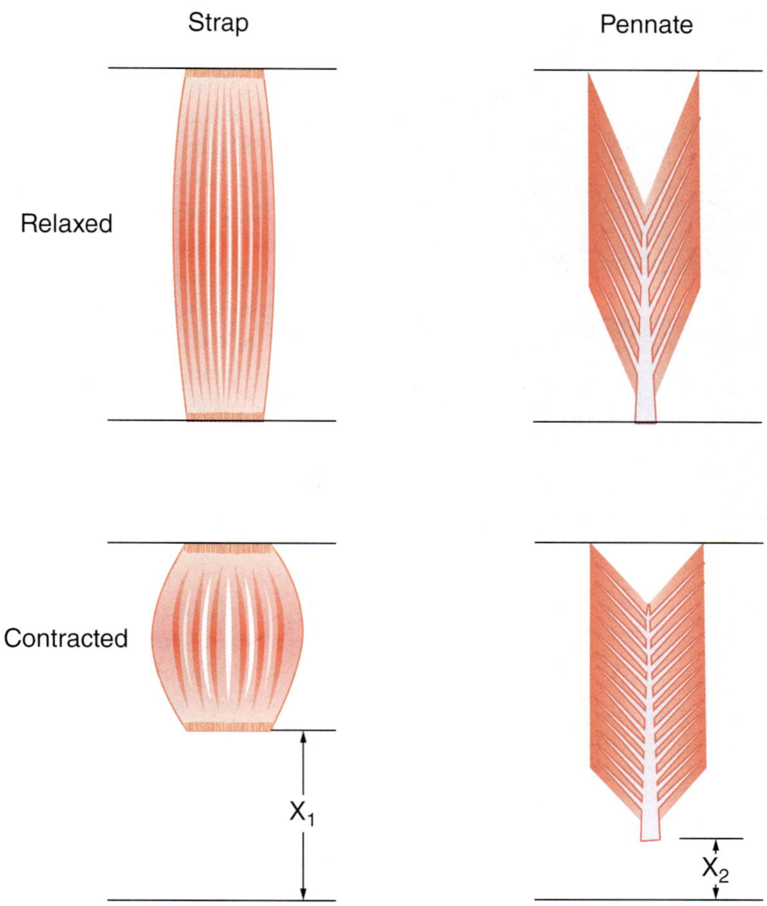

FIGURE 61-3 Schematic representation of the muscle fibers in a strap and a pennate muscle. X1 and X2 represent 50% shortening of the muscle fibers in each muscle. However, the excursions of the whole muscles are significantly different. The whole strap muscle shortens X1, which is three times the amount (X2) of the whole pennate muscle. (Reproduced with permission from Green's Operative Hand Surgery, 5th Ed. Vol 2, Ch 36.)

muscles that may be useful for FMT are the tensor fascia lata, pectoralis major, serratus anterior, pectoralis minor, and one head of the gastrocnemius.

The gracilis muscle has many advantages over other muscles. It is readily transferred by microneurovascular techniques. Muscle elevation is not difficult. The muscle's location in the inner thigh leaves an easily hidden scar, and its removal leaves no functional deficit. Furthermore, two surgical teams can usually work simultaneously, one preparing the muscle and the other preparing the recipient site. The gracilis is a good anatomical fit for most recipient locations and has a good tendon for attachment at the insertion and good fascia for attachment of the origin (Figure 61-4).

Although it can be raised as a myocutaneous flap, the cutaneous portion is only reliable over the proximal half of the muscle belly (Figure 61-5). The only consistent cutaneous perforator exits from the muscle belly at the same level as the dominant pedicle. The muscle is usually used as a muscle-only transfer because the cutaneous paddle is bulky. As long as there is good local soft tissue coverage for the distal half of the muscle and tendon, a skin graft can be applied directly to the proximal muscle belly if coverage is needed without limiting gliding distally and with good appearance. The long tendon is a major advantage because it facilitates insertion into multiple recipient tendons or into bone as for biceps, triceps, and deltoid reconstruction.

There are often multiple minor vascular pedicles supplying the gracilis, but they are not necessary for muscle perfusion except for all but the distal few centimeters of muscle. If the distal muscle does not pink up after reperfusion, it can be excised and the cut, unattached muscle fibers reattached to the tendon. Interestingly, the distal half of the muscle has a pennate type of muscle fiber architecture with fibers inserting into its tendon over the distal half of the entire muscle's length (20). This feature allows the muscle, if it is too long for the recipient area, to be shortened without dividing the tendon that lies on the posterior edge of the muscle. Because it is primarily a strap muscle, the gracilis has a long excursion that provides more than the range of motion that is required for most recipient locations. It has a moderately large cross-sectional area, which is important as the force of contraction is proportional to the cross-sectional area. However, when a large force of muscle contraction is required as in quadriceps replacement, it may be better to use a larger muscle such as the latissimus dorsi.

In cross-section, the latissimus dorsi is a much larger muscle than the gracilis and when transferred should produce a

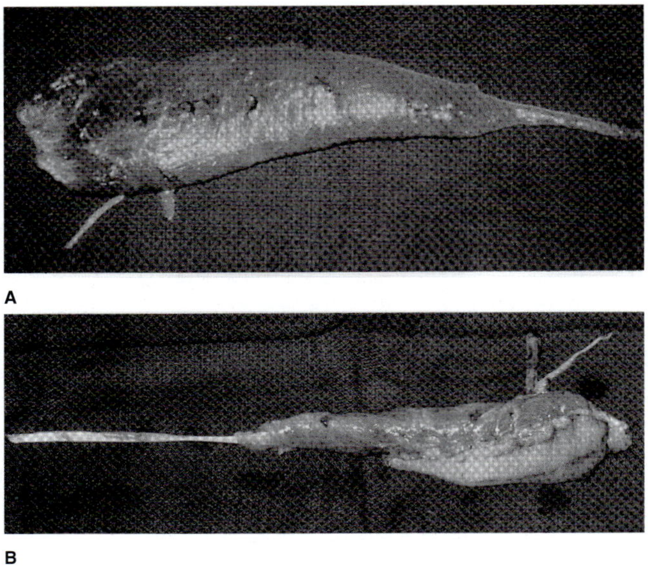

FIGURE 61-4 (A) Superficial aspect of the right gracilis muscle. The origin to the left has a short fibrous attachment to the pelvis that facilitates suture fixation in the recipient site. The motor nerve enters diagonally at the lower left, and the dominant vascular pedicle is beside it. Superficial sutures have been placed on the muscle at 5-cm intervals when the muscle was stretched to its maximum physiological length while still in the leg. The long tendon of insertion is on the right. (B) The cutaneous paddle over the proximal aspect of the muscle provides a reliable but thick skin and fat coverage. (Reproduced with permission from Green's Operative Hand Surgery, 5th Ed. Vol 2, Ch 36.)

stronger force of contraction (21). Because the latissimus dorsi is a strap muscle with long muscle fibers extending the full length of the muscle, it should provide a good excursion. However, the triangular shape of the muscle does not facilitate functional transfer of the entire muscle. There is a large discrepancy in the length of the superior muscle fibers compared with the longer inferolateral fibers. Partly for this reason, the lateral portion of the muscle is often taken for transfer while leaving the superior portion. With partial nerve sparing, some residual muscle function can be maintained. The tendon of insertion is short, and the muscle's origin has fibrous tissue to facilitate suturing on only the inferolateral half. When transferred into a linear space, the muscle is bunched up or folded upon itself. On the plus side, the thoracodorsal artery is longer and larger than the pedicle of gracilis. The two venae comitantes form a single large vein that is 3 to 6 mm in diameter, thus facilitating a reliable anastomosis to a large recipient vein and making revascularization of the latissimus dorsi quite dependable. Removal of the muscle produces only moderate weakness, which may be noticed by persons who use their shoulders vigorously in work or for sports such as tennis or cross-country skiing or sports that involve throwing.

Control of Ischemia Time

The experience in our laboratory is that muscle will survive and develop good function with up to 4 hours of ischemia time at operation room temperatures (19). A functional muscle transfer is less tolerant of a long ischemia time than a muscle that is being used only for cover. Therefore, having a reliable anastomosis is very important because you do not want to have to revise the anastomosis postoperatively. The time involved in recognizing a postoperative thrombosis, getting the patient back in the operating room, and revising the thrombosis and reestablishing perfusion can easily be longer than 4 hours. Therefore, it is important to get a perfect anastomosis in undamaged vessels and to not leave the operating room unless the muscles circulation is excellent.

Monitoring

If you are going to monitor the perfusion postoperatively, it must be done frequently and with precision. Although monitoring techniques are available, including implantable probes

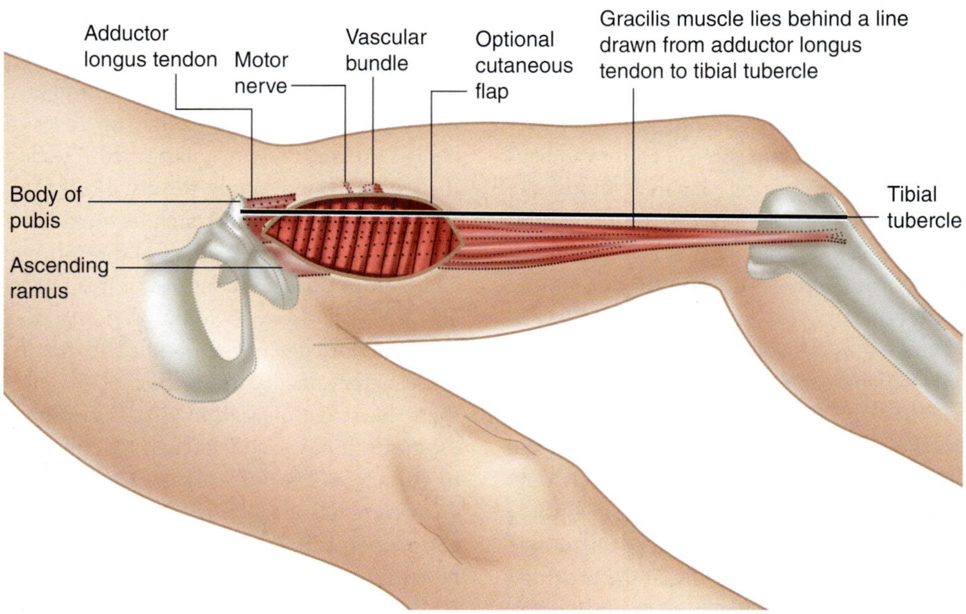

FIGURE 61-5 Skin markings identify the location of the gracilis muscle and the site of the cutaneous flap. (Reproduced with permission from Green's Operative Hand Surgery, 5th Ed. Vol 2, Ch 36.)

and oxygen monitors, visual monitoring is quite possible either through observation of the color and capillary return of the cutaneous paddle or direct observation of the muscle itself. Our preferred method is direct observation. It is done through a window created by leaving a gap in the skin closure or a window in a skin graft on the muscle. A loss of venous outflow will be quite obvious because of the dark blueness of the skin paddle or muscle belly. However, a loss of arterial flow may be more difficult to identify. With arterial obstruction, the change in a skin paddle is a loss of capillary return, and it gets paler. If the observer is unsure, a small incision into the dermis should identify the presence or absence of arterial bleeding. The change in appearance of a muscle that has developed an arterial obstruction is subtle, just a slightly granular change in the muscle's surface, which is probably related to slight dehydration. The color, however, usually remains red. The definitive test is to snip a few muscle fibers with scissors to see if there is arterial bleeding.

Setting the Muscle Tension

We developed a measuring technique that allows the muscle to be inserted at optimal tension. The technique depends on the fact that a muscle's most powerful contraction begins near the fully extended position (Figure 61-6). Choosing a muscle whose normal physiologic range of excursion is greater than that required in the recipient area ensures a full range of motion.

The technique begins after the muscle has been exposed but is still in its normal site. The muscle is stretched to its maximum physiological extended position. For example, for the gracilis, the leg is placed in full thigh abduction and knee extension. In this position, markers are placed along the surface of the muscle every 5 cm (Figure 61-7). It can then be assumed that the muscle can be safely stretched to this resting, extended length when it is transferred. After the muscle is transferred and revascularized and its origin securely attached, the muscle is stretched so that the markers are spaced 5 cm apart. The joint(s) of the extremity that are to be motored (e.g., the fingers and wrist) are then fully extended. In this position of maximum finger extension and maximum muscle stretch, the recipient tendons are placed adjacent to the tendon of the transferred muscle. Adjacent positions are marked (e.g., on the flexor tendons and on the tendon of the gracilis muscle). This marks the point at which the recipient tendon to muscle tendon repair should be done. With the joints in flexion, tendon-to-tendon fixation is accomplished without undo tension on the tendon repair. If attaching the profundus tendons of all four fingers to a transferred muscle, the tendons are woven into the transferred muscle or its tendon at the position marked. A very strong tendon weave is necessary to allow the early postoperative program of passive motion. In a muscle that does not have a tendinous portion such as the pectoralis major or some of the latissimus dorsi, the profundus tendons are inserted into the muscle. This measuring and marking procedure ensures that the muscle will allow full finger and wrist extension and provide a full range of finger flexion within the most powerful range of excursion of the muscle. This measuring principle is used in all muscle transfers to other parts of the body.

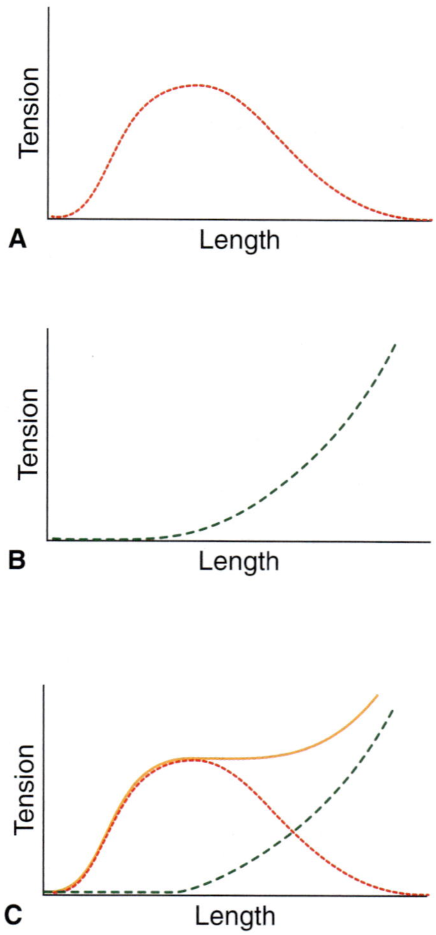

FIGURE 61-6 Graphs illustrating why the most powerful part of the muscle's excursion is from its fully extended position. As the muscle shortens toward its fully contracted length (to the left), its tension capabilities fall off markedly beginning at about 40% of the excursion. (**A**) Length–tension curve of a single muscle fiber during active contraction. (**B**) Length–tension curve of a resting whole muscle being passively stretched. Increasing tension occurs as the whole muscle is stretched because of the mechanical resistance of the muscle fibers and their connective tissue framework. (**C**) Length–tension curve (solid line) of a whole muscle under tetanic stimulation. This curve represents the sum of forces produced by active contraction and passive stretching. Note that in the muscle's stretched and extended position, the muscle's total contractile force is a combination of active muscle contraction and passive mechanical forces. (Reproduced with permission from Green's Operative Hand Surgery, 5th Ed. Vol 2, Ch 36.)

Balanced Tendon Fixation

When a single muscle is used to motor more that one tendon, care must be taken with the relative position of the each of the recipient tendons. For example, to provide finger flexion, all of the fingers should flex together to provide even contact with the object being gripped. To accomplish this, the profundus tendons are sutured in side-to-side fashion to each other in a balanced position. In the resting position, each digit will be slightly more flexed than the adjacent radial digit. A practical solution to the accurate and strong insertion of four or five tendons into one is to first interweave all of the recipient tendons together in their correct relationship side to side. The transferred tendon is

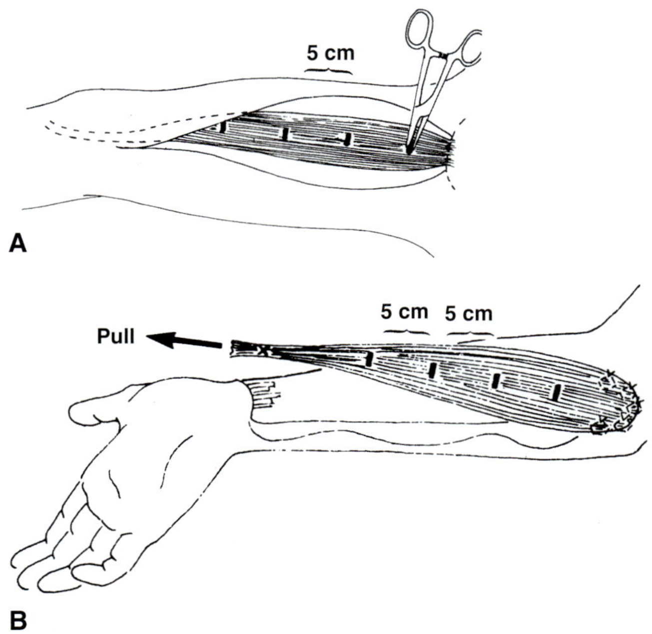

FIGURE 61-7 The technique that allows the surgeon to insert the muscle with the optimal tension for maximum muscle strength. (**A**) By abducting the thigh and extending the knee, the gracilis muscle is stretched to its maximum physiological length. Sutures or clips are placed at 5-cm intervals along the muscle while it is held stretched. (**B**) After transfer, the muscle's origin is securely fixed to the common flexor origin, and the muscle is stretched distally until the sutures are 5 cm apart. While the fingers and wrist are held in extension, marks are placed on adjacent points on the flexor digitorum profundus tendons and the gracilis tendon. This marks the location at which the gracilis tendon should be attached to the finger flexor tendons for optimum function. (Reproduced with permission from Green's Operative Hand Surgery, 5th Ed. Vol 2, Ch 36.)

then woven into this mass of joined tendons. The relative position of the recipient tendons is assessed by traction on the mass of attached tendons. Traction should produce mass flexion of the fingers in a balanced grip position. At rest, the fingers should lie in the position of function with each ulnar digit curled into the palm slightly more than the adjacent radial digit. When gripping a handle such as a tool handle, all fingers will then make secure contact and similar pressure on the handle.

When the muscle is going to produce thumb as well as finger flexion, the flexor pollicis longus should be sutured to the finger flexors in a position that has some slack so that the fingers will begin to flex before the thumb moves. In this way, the thumb, when it does flex, will come to rest on the radial side of the partially flexed index finger and provide useful key pinch rather than flex into the palm under the fingers. If the gracilis is going to be used for independent finger and thumb movements, the muscle must be split into two separate neuromuscular territories and innervated with two nerve branches that have separate function, preferably thumb and finger flexion functions (1,11,12).

One Muscle For Separate Independent Functions

It is sometimes helpful to have separately functioning parts in a single muscle. This occurs in normal anatomy, for example, in the flexor digitorum profundus, which is capable of separate finger flexion. Many muscles that are suitable for FMT can be divided into two or more separate neuromuscular functioning units. Separate longitudinal portions of the muscle can be made to contract by stimulation of a specific part of the muscle's motor nerve (1,12). Independent function is usually possible in the gracilis, pectoralis major, and latissimus dorsi. To have separately functioning parts, a muscle must be longitudinally divisible without compromising its vasculature, at least in its distal portion. This longitudinal division passes along the line dividing the separately functioning parts, which are identified by nerve stimulation.

It is desirable to have independence of long finger flexion from thumb flexion. Separate movement of the thumb allows controlled pinch and grip function. In flexor forearm reconstruction, this may be possible with the use of the AIN. As the AIN courses distally, it gives off separate ulnar branches to the profundus and separate radial branch to the flexor pollicis longus. Simply on the basis of radial and ulnar anatomical location, it is usually possible to separate the branches of the AIN into thumb and finger components. When using the gracilis, the muscle fibers are separated according to fascicular territories. A fascicular territory is a separately functioning anatomical unit that includes a portion of the motor nerve, the muscle that portion of nerve supplies, and part of the tendon of insertion. Using fascicular nerve stimulation, it is possible to split the gracilis into two musculotendinous units 90% of the time. Usually there are two to seven fascicles in the gracilis motor nerve that are visible with loupe magnification. The fascicles are gently teased apart into two groups based on their closeness to each other, and each group is labeled with a microsuture. A nerve stimulator with a microbipolar probe and a variable intensity voltage capability should be used. A tetanic stimulus will produce prolonged muscle contraction and allow the division within the muscle to be readily identified. With intraoperative stimulation of each group of fascicles, the motor territory in the muscle is identified both visually and by palpation. The division will be longitudinal along the line of the muscle fibers (Figure 61-8). By following a group of muscle fibers distally, the portion of the tendon to which these fibers is attached can be identified, and this portion can be longitudinally split from the rest of the tendon. In this way, a fascicular territory is identified and separated as an anatomical entity. By using the ulnar and the radial portions of the anterior interosseous nerve to innervate two fascicular territories of the gracilis, the muscle may be used to provide finger flexion that is separate from thumb flexion.

The nerve repairs should be done as close to the gracilis muscle as possible to minimize reinnervation time. A motor donor nerve should be undamaged and the fascicles accurately aligned under high magnification and coapted accurately without tension. After the final attachments of the muscles origin and insertion have been completed, the involved joints should be put through a full range of motion and the vascular and neural repairs observed to assess the lack of tension throughout flexion and extension.

Selecting a Suitable Motor Nerve

The donor motor nerve is critical to the success of the procedure. The nerve must be undamaged, which may create a

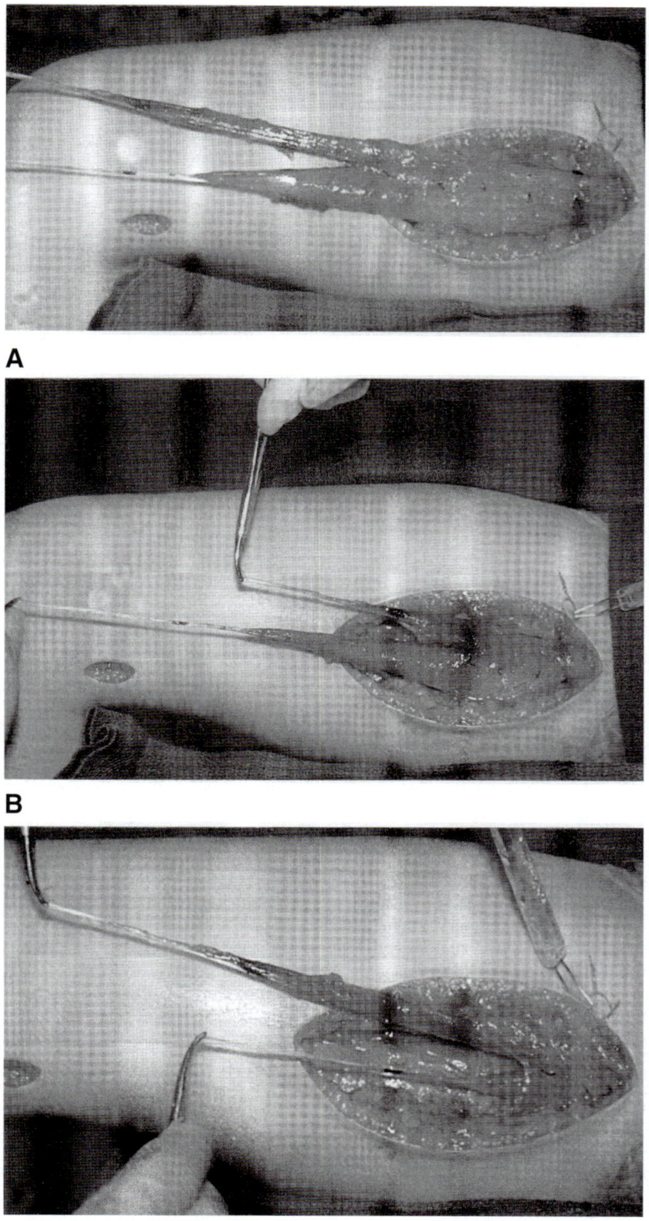

FIGURE 61-8 (A) Splitting the gracilis into two separately functioning neuromuscular units. The location of the split is identified by separating the gracilis motor nerve into two groups of fascicles and separately stimulating each group. The portions of muscle that contract are observed, and the muscle and its tendon are split along the observed functional separation. (B) Stimulation of one group of fascicles produces contraction of the upper portion of the gracilis. (C) Stimulation of the other group of fascicles produces contraction of the lower portion of the gracilis. (Reproduced with permission from Green's Operative Hand Surgery, 5th Ed. Vol 2, Ch 36.)

challenge in the trauma situation. Frequently, in an area of previous trauma, nerves will appear thickened and scarred. Usually the nerve cannot be tested by functional stimulation because the supplied muscle is missing. However, the internal appearance is most important. After cutting the nerve in cross-section, it should be examined under magnification. Our experience is that a nerve that has an intact fascicular pattern is likely to provide good reinnervation. Over the next half hour, if there is a protrusion of axoplasm from the proximal cut end of the nerve, this is further confirmation of the viability and reinnervation potential of the nerve. The other factor of importance is that the portion of the nerve that is being used is a motor portion or preferably the nerve is a pure motor nerve with no sensory function (except muscle sensory). Ideally, the motor function is the same as was present for the function being replaced or at least it had a synergistic function. However, this is not always possible as in the case of biceps reconstruction in brachial plexus injury. In this case, two to four intercostal nerves are used. The axon counts are much less in the donor nerves than in the recipient gracilis nerve, and the degree of innervation is usually less than with the much larger motor portion of the musculocutaneous nerve. Although little is known about the ability of small donor nerves to reinnervate a much larger motor nerve, it is preferred to coapt nerves of similar size and axon counts.

Identifying the Motor Portion of a Mixed Nerve

Mixed nerves with sensory and motor components such as the radial, musculocutaneous, circumflex, or tibialis anterior are useful for FMT; however, the donor nerve must be coapted to only the motor portion of the mixed nerve. A number of intraoperative methods can be used to identify each component. Often, from the gross anatomy in the extremity, it will be clear which are the sensory and the motor components simply by following the peripheral distribution of the nerve. Sometimes there will be small portions of muscle remaining that can be made to contract when the motor component is stimulated. However, if the distal portion of the nerve is absent, then another technique must be used because the cross-sectional appearance of the motor and sensory components will appear similar to the eye.

Two techniques are available. Rapid nerve staining is possible to identify motor from sensory fibers. However, this customized process with special stains usually takes at least a few hours and trained pathology personnel. However, the technique of awake nerve stimulation can be used to identify the sensory and motor components of a mixed nerve, and no staining or special personnel are required. This technique requires a microbipolar electrical probe with a nerve stimulator that has variable frequency and voltage controls, an appropriate anesthetic, and some patience. The surgical procedure involves separating the groups of fascicles in the nerve under general anesthesia. Each group of fascicles should be labeled with a fine suture so it can be identified later and held separate from the others during stimulation. The patient is awakened. An anesthetic agent should be used that can be fully reversed so that the patient rapidly becomes coherent for the stimulation. For the musculocutaneous nerve, there are usually four groups of fascicles. For the gracilis, there are two fascicles or groups of fascicles.

After anesthetic reversal with the patient now awake, each group of fascicles is stimulated with the microbipolar stimulator at different voltages. The voltage is adjusted throughout the testing procedure in keeping with the patient's response and to prevent undue discomfort. The patient is asked to identify the presence of sensation, the anatomic location of the feeling, and whether the feeling is deep or on the surface. Sensory fascicles produce a sense of discomfort, often burning, that is localized to the skin of the area in the region of the previous cutaneous innervations. The motor fascicles, when stimulated, produce an aching sensation deeper in the limb that is anatomically localized by the patient to the region of the muscle belly that the nerve used to supply.

Creating a Gliding Muscle Tendon Unit

If the transferred muscle or its tendons are stuck by adhesions, the desired movement will not occur. Although it would be ideal if the bed in which the muscle will glide is not scar tissue, there will likely be significant scar tissue in transfers after trauma or Volkman's ischemic contracture. It is more important that the overlying soft tissue envelope be healthy fatty tissue and soft flexible skin, at least over the distal half of the muscle and the site of tendon repair. This greatly facilitates gliding and allows a tenolysis if adhesions develop.

The most important factor that facilitates gliding is an early motion program (see later discussion).

Postoperative Management

It is critical in the immediate postoperative period to maintain a normal systemic circulation. A normal blood pressure in a warm patient will maintain a strong peripheral perfusion. An adequate volume of intravenous fluids is given. Urine output and core temperature are monitored. The involved extremity is slightly elevated above the heart and splinted to prevent motion. Splinting should be designed to relax the junction between the tendons and the transferred muscle. Inasmuch as the muscle is flaccid because of denervation, the amount of tension is not excessive for the tendon repairs.

Postoperative Therapy Program

There is an early and a late program. The early program consists of passive stretching of the muscle–tendon unit. This is a critical part of adhesion prevention. In the case of a forearm flexor transfer for provision of wrist and finger flexion, the program consists of active and passive extension of the fingers and wrist. This is commenced 10 to 20 days after surgery. Extension of the wrist and the fingers should be done separately and combined. The program is designed to allow full passive muscle extension and overcome any tendency to myotonic contracture. Also, and more important, passive stretching develops tissue gliding between the muscle and muscle tendon junction and the surrounding tissues. If the muscle has been inserted at the correct tension as outlined earlier, after stretching the muscle, the passive tension in the muscle will cause it to shorten and produce passive gliding, simulating the gliding motion in flexion. Thus, passive extension by the therapist or patient followed by the passive flexion induced by the mechanical tension in the muscle will develop a to-and-fro movement that will lead to a good gliding of the muscle tendon unit and healing without adhesions. When active contraction of the transfer occurs after reinnervation, active gliding of the entire unit will provide full flexion of the fingers and wrist. Full extension will also be possible. This program has resulted in a low incidence of tendon adhesions requiring subsequent tenolysis. In view of this early passive stretching program, it is obvious that the attachment of the transferred muscle and tendon to the recipient tendon(s) must be a very strong repair. Usually an interweaving tendon repair is done with multiple weaves of donor and recipient tendons and firm mattress sutures. During the period of denervation, electrical muscle stimulation to prevent atrophy is difficult to do effectively and is not believed to be necessary. In most situations, muscle movement will occur within 2 to 4 months.

The late program commences when the patient develops spontaneous contraction of the muscle. The patient must attempt active flexion frequently throughout the day. When a good range of movement develops, a program of resisted exercises is commenced and continued until maximum function is obtained. In the case of a forearm flexor transfer, this will involve resisted grip exercises and grip with wrist flexion exercises. The principles of muscle strengthening as practiced by athletes are applicable to the recovery of maximum strength of the transferred muscle with recent reinnervation. Three to five sets of 10 to 15 repetitions of each exercise are repeated daily. The amount of resistance or weight involved should be gradually increased to as much as the patient can handle and still complete the set.

Each exercise session is done to the point of fatigue. In the early stages of recovery, the exercise sessions should be done daily. A body builder would only stress a given muscle group every 48 to 72 hours to allow maximum adaptation to occur between sets. However, in this situation of muscle denervation and reinnervation, no studies are available that can be used for guidance. We believe that in the early stages of muscle recovery, daily sessions are most productive. Variation in the weights can be used to develop more muscle endurance. By using a lighter weight and more repetitions (20–60), muscle endurance can be developed. Just as an athlete would pursue an exercise program until maximum gain has been accomplished, the patient should do the same. This period of postoperative resisted exercises can take 12 to 18 months to obtain maximum strength. Concomitant with the strengthening program, there should be a functional training program to incorporate the involved extremity into normal use. This is also important for variety because repetitive exercises can be tedious. The patient is advised to use the involved extremity for activities of daily living, light sports, and manual hobbies. Incorporation of the exercise program into activities of daily living and work-stimulated activities will maintain the patient's level of interest and enthusiasm and will train the patient to incorporate the limb into his or her regular lifestyle. The patient may need to develop adaptations to normal movements, and practice will make these movements more natural and automatic.

Cortical Plasticity and Motor Relearning

The ideal nerve for reinnervation is the motor nerve that previously went to the missing muscle. However, in some cases, a different motor nerve has to be used and provide a new and different function than it had originally. Some remarkable reinnervation alternatives are available and can produce good function. When the intercostal nerves are used for biceps function, initially the patient will produce elbow flexion by taking a deep breath. However, with time, the patient will learn to contract the transferred muscle by trying to flex the elbow rather than by breathing heavily. Similarly, when an FMT is used to reconstruct the smile in a patient with facial paralysis, the motor nerve to the masseter muscle is frequently used for reinnervation of the transferred muscle. Immediately after reinnervation of the muscle, effective contraction and a smile movement are initiated by the patient trying to bite. With the passage of time, the patient learns to activate the muscle by trying to smile rather than trying to bite. Furthermore, spontaneous smiling occurs in more than half of patients (23). Something very interesting takes place in the brain, and it seems to be a cerebral cortical adaptation (24-25). It appears that the smile muscle area of the motor cortex is controlling the transferred muscle rather than the mastication area of the cortex. One of our patients had a successful biceps reconstruction by free muscle transfer innervated by the intercostal nerves. She was able to flex her elbow well and do it by thinking about doing elbow flexion. Using transcutaneous magnetic stimulation and functional magnetic resonance imaging, Chen and Anastakis showed that by 6 months, the upper limb area of the motor cortex now controlled biceps function rather than the trunk area of the motor cortex (26). These are remarkable adaptive changes in cortical representations. These changes have also been observed in association with motor skill learning and the practice of basic movements (27-29). In the future, the modulation of cortical excitability may allow us to facilitate plasticity and improve final functional outcome in patients undergoing reconstructive microsurgery.

COMPLICATIONS AND SECONDARY PROCEDURES

The most feared local complications are anastomotic thrombosis, muscle ischemia, and loss of the transfer (see earlier discussion). Infection is uncommon because the tissues have a very good blood supply.

A hematoma under the skin closure may lead to pressure on the vessels and lead to thrombosis of the anastomoses. The patient should be brought back to the operating room promptly to remove the hematoma and to stop the bleeding. Anticoagulants are not used in FMT because of the fear of bleeding.

Skin flap necrosis is a serious complication because it may limit the early postoperative exercise program and may lead to healing with excess scar tissue and result in poor tendon gliding.

Adhesions between the tendons and the tendon muscle junction limit muscle excursion and therefore limit the intended joint range of motion. A tenolysis may then be done. The timing of the tenolysis is important and should be done only after the muscle has developed good strength so gliding may be obtained immediately after the adhesions are removed. However a tenolysis is rarely required because adhesions are minimal with an early passive motion program.

In growing children, the lengthening of the transferred muscle may be less than the growth and lengthening of the rest of the extremity. To stay ahead of this potential problem, the child should be checked yearly throughout the growth period. Nighttime splinting with the muscle being placed on stretch should be adequate to deal with this issue, which is difficult to correct if it becomes established.

CLINICAL EXPERIENCE WITH FUNCTIONING MUSCLE TRANSFER

Of 62 adults and children, 31 adults were available for late postoperative follow-up of upper extremity FMT and are reported here (30). The results of surgery in children have been reported by Zuker and colleagues (13).

Adult Forearm Transfers (21)

The long flexors of the fingers alone were reconstructed in 14 patients. Long extensors and flexors of the fingers were reconstructed in four patients using two separate muscles at two separate operative procedures. Long extensors of the fingers alone were reconstructed in one patient. The etiology of muscle loss in this group included Volkmann's ischemic contracture in 11, traumatic muscle loss in six, electrical burn injury in one, and mixed motor paralysis after excision of a cervical astrocytoma in one. Seven of 19 patients required secondary procedures, including tenotomy in two, capsulotomy in one, tendon transfer in one, tenolysis in one, digital fusion in one, and metacarpophalangeal capsulodeses in four.

The follow-up revealed that the range of movement was excellent. The fingertip-to-distal palmar crease distance ranged from 0.5 to 4 cm with more than half of patients closing their fist to touch the proximal area of the palm (Figures 61-1 and 61-9). Most of the patients had full finger extension. Grip strength ranged from 14% to 81% of the opposite normal extremity, with mean grip strength 38.1%. Pinch strength ranged from 0% to 70%, with mean pinch strength 37.8% compared with the normal opposite extremity. Pinch strength was significantly weaker if thenar musculature was absent. The severity of pre transfer upper extremity injury appears to be a significant factor affecting the outcome. Two major factors that decrease the functional usefulness of the hand are the absence or weakness of intrinsic muscle function and the absence of good supination and pronation. At least protective sensation was present in all patients. If sensation was decreased, it did not appear to be a factor limiting functionality. The best grip strength was seen in male patients who pursued extensive weight training during their rehabilitation period and in patients who worked as heavy laborers. Some patients who used their upper extremity in heavy work described fatigue in the transferred muscle.

Adult Upper Arm Transfers

Of 15 adults, six had biceps, one had triceps, and eight had deltoid reconstruction. Thirteen were available for late follow-up.

Biceps Reconstruction

Loss of elbow flexion was due to musculocutaneous nerve injury in two, direct muscle loss in one, polio in one, and brachial plexus injury in two. Brachialis function was absent in all

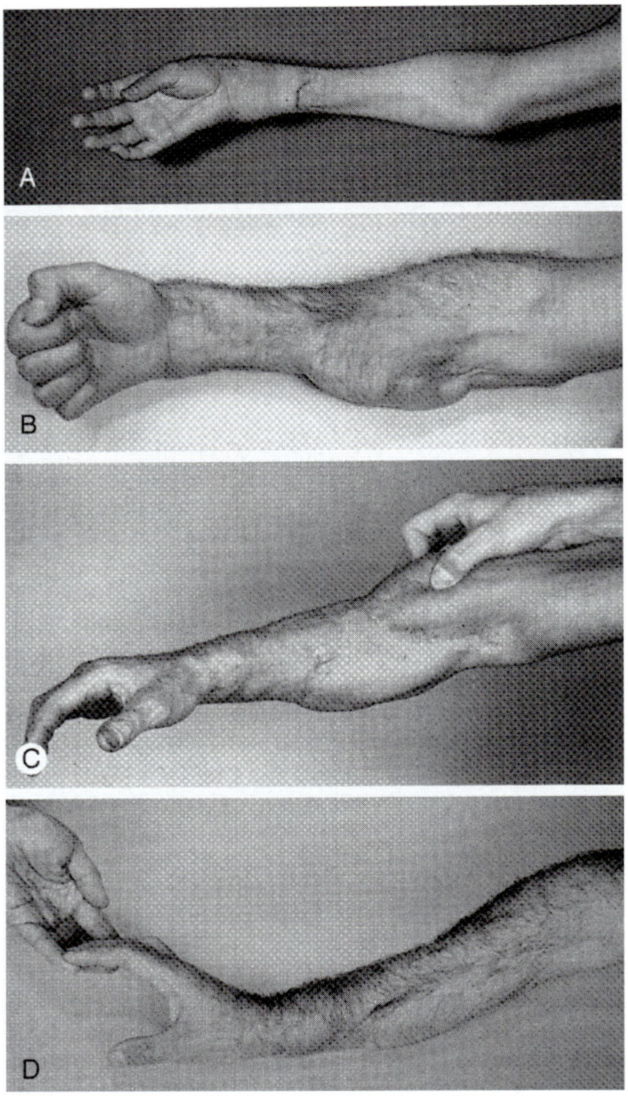

FIGURE 61-9 (**A**) Preoperative appearance of the right arm of a 22-year-old man who sustained a traumatic injury with loss of all flexor and extensor musculature except for the extensor carpi radialis longus and brachioradialis muscles. Long finger flexors were reconstructed with a pectoralis major functioning muscle transfer (FMT) and finger extension with a gracilis FMT. (**B**) Finger flexion. Note the bulging contraction of the pectoralis muscle in the proximal forearm seen along the bottom margin of the forearm. Grip strength is 24 kg measured with the Jaymar dynamometer. (**C**) Finger and thumb extension. (**D**) With relaxation of the pectoralis muscle, transfer full passive extension of the wrist is possible. (Reproduced with permission from Green's Operative Hand Surgery, 5th Ed. Vol 2, Ch 36.)

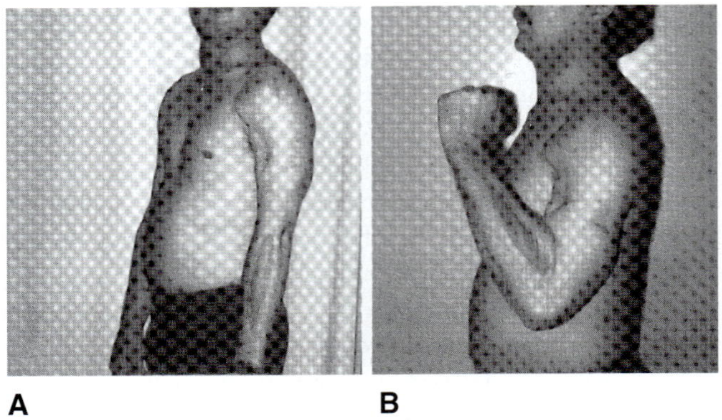

FIGURE 61-10 This patient sustained a crushing injury to his left upper arm with complete loss of the biceps and brachialis muscles. Elbow flexion was restored using the gracilis functioning muscle transfer innervated with the motor portion of the musculocutaneous nerve. (**A**) Postoperative image showing full elbow extension. (**B**) Full elbow flexion. The patient can flex his elbow to 120 degrees while holding a 7.5-kg weight in his hand. (Reproduced with permission from Green's Operative Hand Surgery, 5th Ed. Vol 2, Ch 36.)

patients. The musculocutaneus nerve was used in three patients and the intercostal nerves in three. Four biceps reconstructions were available for long term follow-up. Three patients had full active elbow flexion (M4) and were able to flex their elbows with an average weight of 5 kg held in the hand (Figure 61-10). One patient had only palpable contraction of her biceps.

Deltoid Reconstruction

The anterior deltoid was reconstructed for shoulder flexion in eight patients (Figure 61-11). The etiology of deltoid muscle loss was tumor resection in three, late recognition of axillary nerve avulsion secondary to shoulder dislocation in four, and idiopathic isolated deltoid paralysis in one. The supraspinatus muscle and secondary flexors of the shoulder were normal in each patient, but they provided only weak partial shoulder flexion. All patients in this group lacked stable shoulder flexion above the horizontal plane. Four of the eight patients had chronic subluxation of the glenohumeral joint and complained of shoulder pain before muscle transfer. In all patients, the remaining upper extremity was normal. The indication to reconstruct shoulder flexion was based on the need to flex the arm to

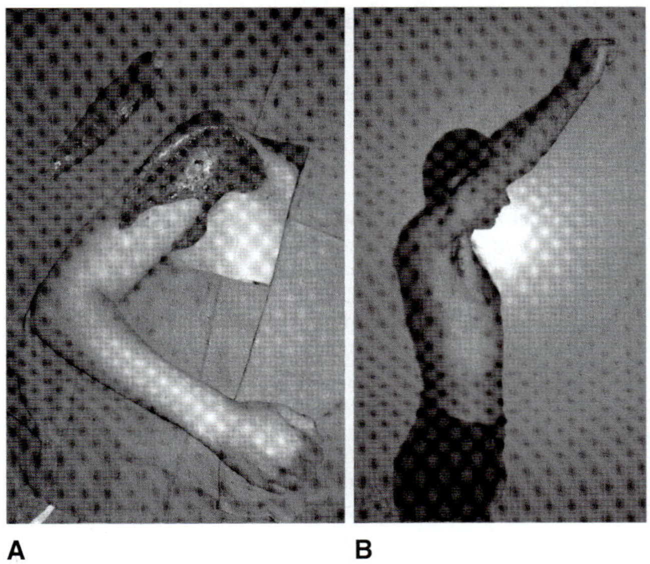

FIGURE 61-11 (**A**) Intraoperative view of the right shoulder showing the donor site and the gracilis muscle prepared for transfer. The patient has an old axillary nerve rupture caused by dislocation of his shoulder. (**B**) After transfer of muscle to the anterior shoulder, the patient can flex his shoulder to 140 degrees. (Reproduced with permission from Green's Operative Hand Surgery, 5th Ed. Vol 2, Ch 36.)

and above the horizontal plane and hold it in place. Awake nerve stimulation was used to identify the motor nerve component of the axillary nerve in seven deltoid reconstructions.

Seven patients had useful flexion of the shoulder from 60 to 170 degrees and could maintain the humerus in front of the body. One patient had no muscle contraction. All four patients with painful shoulder subluxation had a significant decrease in shoulder pain after muscle transfer. This improvement in pain was probably caused by the suspensory function of the gracilis, resulting in a decrease in traction on the glenohumeral joint capsule.

Functioning Muscle Transfer to the Leg

There has been limited experience with transfers to replace quadriceps function and to provide dorsiflexion of the foot. Our experience is in two patients with foot drop for whom we used the gracilis. Both patients developed dorsiflexion to 90 degrees and were able to discontinue using a foot-drop splint.

Functioning Muscle Transfer for Reconstruction of the Lower Face in Facial Paralysis

Facial paralysis has proven to be the largest application for FMT, and we have experience with more than 400 transfers for lower facial reconstruction. This application is covered in this book in a separate chapter by Zuker and Manktelow.

REFERENCES

1. Manktelow RT. Gracilis. Functioning muscle transplantation. In *Microvascular Reconstruction: Anatomy, Applications and Surgical Techniques*. Heidelberg, Germany: Springer-Verlag, 1986.
2. Manktelow RT. Functioning muscle transfer for reconstruction of the hand. In McCarthy JG, May JW Jr, Littler JW (eds). *Plastic Surgery*, vol. 8. Philadelphia: WB Saunders, 1990, pp. 4966–4976.
3. Manktelow RT. Functioning muscle transplantation. In Urbaniak J (ed). *Microsurgery for Major Limb Reconstruction*. St. Louis: CV Mosby, 1987.
4. Anastakis DJ. Free functioning muscle transfers. In Wolfe SW, Hotchkiss RN, Pederson WC, Kozin SH (eds) *Green's Operative Hand Surgery*. New York: Churchill-Livingstone, 2011.
5. Manktelow RT. Microsurgical muscle transfer for upper extremity motors. In Marsh J (ed). In Marsh JL. *Current Therapy in Plastic and Reconstructive Surgery*. Philadelphia: B.C. Decker, Inc., 1989.
6. Tamai S, Komatsu S, Sano S, et al. Free muscle transplants in dogs with microsurgical neurovascular anastomoses. *Plast Reconstr Surg* 1970;46: 219–225.
7. Sixth Peoples Hospital, Microvascular Service, Shanghai. Free muscle transplantation by microsurgical neurovascular anastomoses. *Clin Med J* 1976;2:47.
8. Harii K, Ohmori K, Torii S. Free gracilis muscle transplantation with microvascular anastomosis for the treatment of facial paralysis. *Plast Reconstr Surg* 1976;57:133–143.
9. Manktelow RT, McKee NH. Free muscle transplantation to provide active finger flexion. *J Hand Surg* 1978;3:416.
10. Manktelow RT, Zuker RM, McKee NH. Functioning free muscle transplantation. *J Surg Hand* 1984;9(suppl A):32.
11. Manktelow RT, Zuker RM. The principles of functioning muscle transplantation: applications to the upper arm. *Ann Plast Surg* 1989;22:275–282.
12. Manktelow RT, Zuker RM. Muscle transplantation by fascicular territory. *Plast Reconstr Surg* 1984;73:751–755.
13. Zuker RM, Egerszegi EP, Manktelow RT, et al. Volkmann's ischemic contracture in children: the results of free vascularized muscle transplantation. *Microsurgery* 1991;2(5):341–345.
14. Ikuta Y, Kubo T, Tsuge K. Free muscle transplantation by microsurgical technique to treat severe Volkmann's contracture. *Plast Reconstr Surg* 1976;58:407–411.
15. Akasaka Y, Hara T, Takahashi M. Free muscle transplantation combined with intercostal nerve crossing for reconstruction of elbow flexion and wrist extension in brachial plexus injuries. *Microsurgery* 1991;12: 346–351.
16. Chung DC, Epstein MD, Yeh MC, et al. Functional restoration of elbow flexion in brachial plexus injuries: results in 167 patients (excluding obstetric brachial plexus injury). *J Hand Surg* 1993;18(suppl A):284–291.
17. Doi K, Sakai K, Kuwata N, et al. Reconstruction of finger and elbow function after complete avulsion of the brachial plexus. *J Hand Surg* 1991;16(suppl A):796.
18. Doi K, Sakai K, Kuwata N, et al. Double free-muscle transfer to restore prehension following complete brachial plexus avulsion. *J Hand Surg* 1995;20(suppl A):408–414.
19. Tobin GR, Shusterman M, Peterson GH, et al. The intra-muscular neurovascular anatomy of the latissimus dorsi muscle: the basis for splitting the flap. *Plast Reconstr Surg* 1981;67:637–641.
20. Carlson FD, Wilkie DR. *Muscle Physiology*. Englewood Cliffs, NJ: Prentice-Hall, 1974.
21. Kuzon WM, Fish JS, Pynn BR, McKee NH. Determinants of contractile function in free muscle transfers. *Am Coll Surg Forum* 1984;35:610.
22. McKee NH, Fish JS, Manktelow RT, et al. Gracilis muscle anatomy as related to function of a free functioning muscle transplant. *Clin Anat* 1990;30:522–524.
23. Manktelow RT, Tomat LR, Zuker RM, Chang M. Smile reconstruction in adults with free muscle transfer innervated by the masseter motor nerve: effectiveness and cerebral adaptation: *Plastic Reconstr Surgery* 2006;118:885–899.
24. Donoghue JP. Plasticity of adult sensorimotor representations. *Curr Opin Neurobiol* 1995;5:749–754.
25. Karni A, Meyer G, Jezzard P, et al. Functional MRI evidence for adult motor cortex plasticity during motor skill learning. *Nature* 1995;377: 155–158.
26. Chen R, Anastakis DJ, Haywood CT, et al. Plasticity of the human motor system following muscle reconstruction: a magnetic stimulation and functional magnetic resonance imaging study. *Clin Neurophysiol* 2003; 114(12):2434–2446.
27. Karni A, Meyer G, Jezzard P, et al. Functional MRI evidence for adult motor cortex plasticity during motor skill learning. *Nature* 1995;377: 155–158.
28. Pascual-Leone A, Nguyet D, Cohen LG, et al. Modulation of muscle responses evoked by transcranial magnetic stimulation during the acquisition of new fine motor skills. *J Neurophysiol* 1995;74:1037–1045.
29. Classen J, Liepert A, Wise SP, et al. Rapid plasticity in human cortical movement representation induced by practice. *J Neurophysiol* 1998;79:1117–1123.
30. Manktelow RT, Anastakis DJ. Long term functional assessment of 32 adult microneurovascular muscle transfers for upper extremity reconstruction. *Proc Fourth International Muscle Symposium*, Zurich, Switzerland, 1995, pp. 230–233.

CHAPTER 62

Vascularized Bone Reconstruction in Children

Marco Innocenti and Carla Baldrighi

Microvascular reconstruction is widely used in the pediatric age group, but only a few articles in the literature report the results of microvascular bone reconstruction in children. The majority describe toe-to-hand transfers, which are the most frequent procedures that involve microsurgical bone reconstruction in children.

One of the reasons for the paucity of reports is related to the low incidence in childhood of major traumatic events with loss of bone that requires a vascularized bone graft. In most Western countries, severe work-related injuries, major traffic accidents, and gunshot wounds are unlikely to occur in children. In addition, the biological potential of improved healing in children accounts for a higher incidence of spontaneous bone regeneration.

However, congenital pseudoarthrosis and bone sarcomas are two conditions that occur specifically in children and adolescents. Both diseases require extensive resection of the involved segment. At present, biological reconstruction with vascularized bone graft is probably the best treatment option for these cases.

Any microsurgical procedure in very young patients is technically demanding because of the size of the anatomical structures, but it also has the advantage of the pristine condition of the vessels and the biological potential of growing individuals.

When performing microvascular bone reconstruction in children, several details concerning the anesthesia and postoperative care must be considered; room temperature, appropriate analgesia, and fluid balance need particular attention because they may compromise flap survival.

Any reconstructive plan in children must take into consideration the specific characteristics and requirements of a growing individual. In particular, skeletal reconstruction requires reliable, stable bone fixation. If the growth plate cannot be preserved or salvaged, it should be replaced whenever feasible. None of the conventional reconstructive options (prosthesis, allograft, or both) can replace the characteristics of the immature skeleton to provide a stable and durable reconstruction that maintains the growth potential of the child's bone.

Prostheses are indicated only in hip and knee reconstruction in cases of epiphyseal loss after trauma, infection, or tumor resection. Prostheses are usually custom made and not available everywhere. They can be complicated by infection and loosening of the hardware. In young individuals, because of their higher functional demands, the natural wear of the components may occur faster in the long term. The major drawback to the use of implants in children is that no growth will occur at the reconstructed joint.

Massive bone allografts have been widely used in bone reconstruction after sarcoma resection both in adults and children (1,2). They may be used either for intercalary diaphyseal reconstruction or for meta-epiphyseal reconstruction as osteo-articular grafts. The biology of allograft incorporation into host bone is a slow and incomplete process that occurs by creeping substitution (3,4) from the host bone only for a short distance beyond the host bone–allograft junction (5). This results in high rates of nonunion, fracture, and infection, which require multiple revision surgeries and sometimes amputation. In osteo-articular allografts, subchondral bone collapse with subsequent development of degenerative osteoarthritis further jeopardizes the long-term results and often requires revision surgery (5). Because of the high rate of complications, some authors believe that the use of allografts in the management of malignant bone tumors should be considered only as a temporary solution (6).

Although prostheses and allografts may be considered as an alternative to vascularized autologous bone grafts in adults, indications are very limited in the pediatric population, in which vascularized bone grafts may provide optimal reconstruction that takes advantage of the ability of the immature bone to remodel and hypertrophy.

INDICATIONS FOR VASCULARIZED BONE GRAFTS IN CHILDREN

According to the little data available in the literature, long bone reconstruction after sarcoma resection is the most frequent condition requiring a vascularized bone transfer in a child. Osteogenic sarcoma and Ewing's sarcoma are the most common bone tumors in children and adolescents (7,8). In the upper limb, they are usually located in the proximal humerus and distal radius. In the lower limb, they may have a more random distribution, although the knee region is probably most frequently involved. In terms of survival, the results of wide margin resection combined with adjuvant therapy are comparable to amputation. Therefore, limb salvage becomes the main goal in the surgical treatment of malignant bone tumors. Vascularized autologous bone grafts are probably the best available option for reconstruction of these large defects. Bone transportation techniques may be an alternative, but they take a long time, and their acceptance in small children is generally poor. Furthermore, the indication for bone lengthening in the upper limb remains controversial.

The bone defect resulting from a bone sarcoma resection may be diaphyseal, juxtaarticular, or epiphyseal. For an intercalary diaphyseal defect, a diaphyseal segment of vascularized fibula may be used, similar to adults.

Much more challenging is when the tumor is located very close to the epiphyseal plate in which effort should be used to preserve the growth plate, articular surface, or both. In both situations, only a small and sometimes a very small segment of native bone is left, and stable bone fixation with the fibula cannot be achieved biomechanically. In this situation, combing an allograft with a vascularized bone graft has been an established technique (9) and takes advantage of the structural properties of the allograft and the biological potential of the vascularized fibula.

Reconstruction of epiphyseal defects in children after resection of bone tumors presents an unique challenge to orthopedic surgeons. Issues in the pediatric population that are not present in adults include the need to maintain growth potential, the need for biological preservation of the articular surface, and the need for a long-term viable reconstruction in patients who are anticipated to survive into adulthood. For anatomical similarity, proximal fibula epiphyseal transfer is considered the best available option for reconstruction of the proximal humerus and distal radius in the upper extremity both in terms of growth and joint function (10–12).

Congenital pseudoarthrosis of long bones is the second indication for a vascularized bone transfer. This condition is characterized by segmental disturbance of periosteal bone formation followed by bowing of the affected bone, fracture, and subsequent pseudarthrosis. The disease may be related to neurofibromatosis and is more frequently located in the diaphysis of the tibia, although it may occasionally involve the forearm bones. Surgical treatment is similar to that for bone tumors and includes wide margin resection of the pathologic tissue and subsequent bone reconstruction.

This may be achieved with the Ilizarov technique or vascularized fibula transfer (13). The Ilizarov technique is a very reliable and established procedure for lower limb long bone reconstruction. The duration of the treatment, the need for meticulous and frequent care of the pin tracts, and multiple adjustments of the frame over the time period greatly limit this application in small children. In addition, the technique is difficult to apply in the upper limb, where it may be considered only to lengthen the forearm and correct the deformity as a preliminary step before definitive reconstruction with vascularized fibula (14).

Conversely, the vascularized fibular bone graft can be used in the upper limb (15,16) and is the preferred reconstructive technique for congenital pseudoarthrosis of the tibia (17–21). Weiland et al. reported 19 patients with a mean age of 5.1 years who underwent resection of the pseudoarthrosis and reconstruction with a contralateral vascularized fibula and achieved bone healing and stable reconstruction in 95% of cases (17). Kanaya et al. published a series of 10 patients in whom the tibial defect resulting from the resection was reconstructed with a vascularized fibula in eight cases and a vascularized rib in two (18). All of the vascularized fibulas except one healed in an average time of 4 months, but the two ribs failed. Similar results have been reported more recently by Sakamoto et al., Korompilias et al., and Erni et al., confirming satisfactory outcome at long-term followup (19–21).

RECONSTRUCTIVE OPTIONS

Any surgical strategy for bone reconstruction in skeletally immature patients should take into account the need to preserve the growth potential of the affected bone. In addition, a stable reconstruction is absolutely necessary in children because they are less compliant than adults in their postoperative care and rehabilitation. For these reasons, any treatment should be customized according to the age, the site, and the functional requests of the individual patient.

Among the possible donor sites for vascularized bone transfer, the fibula is the most popular choice for several reasons. It provides long, straight segments of tubular bone, which can be used in intercalary reconstruction; its blood supply is constant and reliable; its harvest straightforward; and the donor site morbidity is minimal. The diaphysis of the fibula matches the size and shape of the forearm bones and is ideal for skeletal reconstruction of this anatomical area. Furthermore, the ability of vascularized fibula to respond to the increased functional demands after the transfer by hypertrophy allows the fibula to be used to reconstruct larger diameter bones such as the humerus, femur, and tibia.

UPPER EXTREMITY

Diaphysis

Intercalary reconstruction in the upper limb in the pediatric age group is similar to reconstruction in adults.

Technical details that should be emphasized include the preparation of the junction between the graft and the recipient bone. In forearm reconstruction, there are basically two options: a transverse osteotomy and a step-cut osteotomy. The former is technically less demanding because it allows for easier control of rotation but provides only a limited contact with the recipient bone. The latter increases the bone contact surface and the stability of the implant but is also more difficult to construct (Figure 62-1). Because of the discrepancy in size in humeral reconstruction, the fibula should be inserted inside the medullary canal of the humerus. The technique may vary according to the dimensions of the two bones. In case of significant discrepancy, the medullary canal of the humerus may be reamed to allow intramedullary positioning of the fibula (Figure 62-2). For a larger cross-sectional diameter of the fibula, the graft may be placed in a groove created by a step-cut osteotomy of the humerus to increase the boney contact and facilitate bone fixation (see Figure 62-2).

The periosteum in children is particularly thick and easy to elevate. An extra flap of periosteum (Figure 62-3) should be

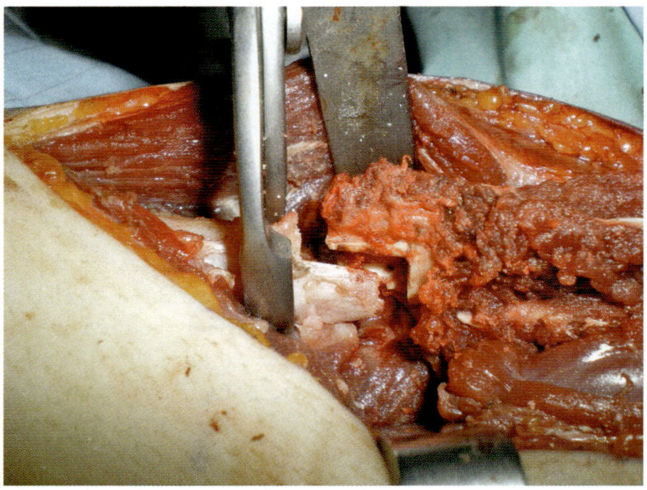

A

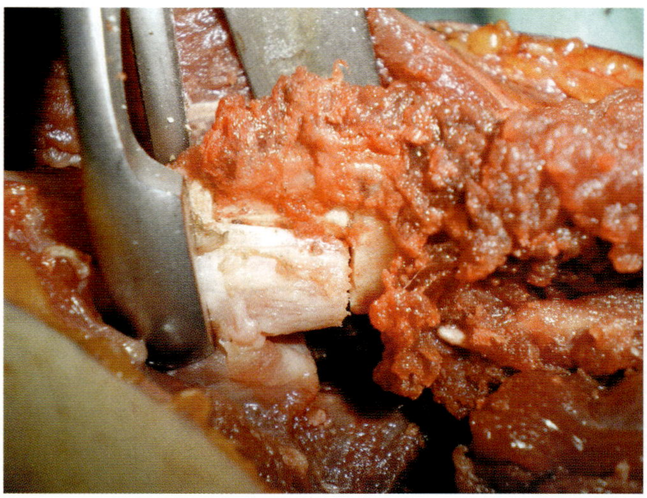

B

FIGURE 62-1 (A) and (B) Step-cut osteotomy increases the bone contact surface and the stability of an implant.

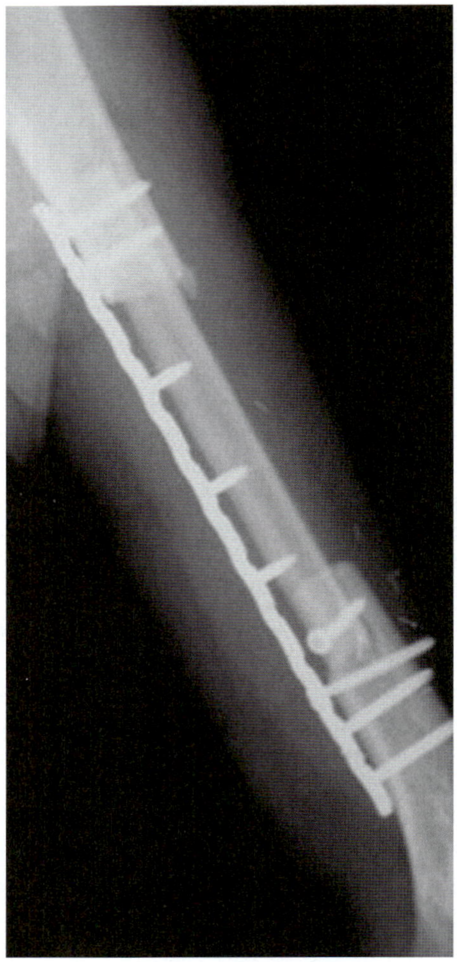

FIGURE 62-2 Intercalary reconstruction of the humerus. The proximal junction between the fibular graft and the humerus has been achieved by intramedullary positioning of the fibula; the distal junction has had a partial step-cut osteotomy. Note the minimally invasive bone fixation of the fibula by means of unicortical screws.

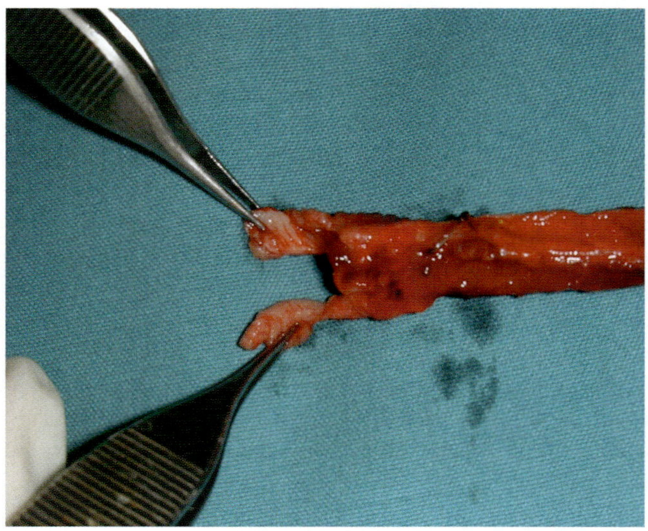

FIGURE 62-3 A flap of periosteum is harvested with the fibula to increase the potential of bony healing after being transferred to the recipient site.

harvested so it can be used to overlap the site of osteosynthesis, increasing the potential for bony healing.

For intercalary reconstruction with a vascularized bone graft in children, bone fixation should be the least invasive but as stable as possible. Titanium locking compression plates using bicortical screws in the recipient bone, and unicortical screws in the bone graft are the recommended technique for osteosynthesis. Intramedullary nailing is not applicable because of the potential harm to the endosteal blood supply, and external fixation is to be avoided, when possible, in young patients.

Epiphysis

Epiphyseal reconstruction in skeletally immature patients is much more challenging. In children, the epiphysis not only contains the articular surface but also the growth plate. Therefore, a biological reconstruction is mandatory to preserve motion and growth. Both osteoarticular allografts and prostheses are unable to provide an effective and durable reconstruction, and autologous vascularized epiphyseal transfer is the only possible option.

The first reports of nonvascularized epiphyseal transfers were published at the end of the 19th century (22–24). Failure in revascularization of the growth plate was the main reason for the discouraging results. Efforts were therefore focused on improving revascularization by reducing the thickness of the bony portion of the graft to improve revascularization from the host bone, but results did not improve significantly.

In the past 30 years, advances in microvascular surgery provided a new impetus to experimental research to investigate the feasibility of vascularized epiphyseal transfer in an animal model (25–32). Donski et al. (29) and Donski and O'Brien (30) demonstrated in skeletally immature dogs that orthotopic replantation of the distal ulna resulted in successful longitudinal growth by way of the revascularized epiphyseal plate, but growth arrest was observed in nonrevascularized growth plates. Histologic examination of the epiphyseal plates after transfer revealed that the revascularized epiphyseal plates were histologically normal, but nonrevascularized growth plates showed severe structural alteration depending on the duration of ischemia. By restoring the metaphyseal and epiphyseal blood supply, Bowen (25–28) and Nettelblad (31,32), and others demonstrated survival and growth of vascularized epiphyseal transfers.

The technique was then extrapolated to clinical practice in the 1980s when a few surgeons achieved some encouraging early results that convinced the scientific community to refine the technique and expand the indications. Several skeletal reconstructions with epiphyseal transfers have recently been described for a variety of clinical problems involving the growth plate in skeletally immature patients. In 1986, Tsai and colleagues reported eight humeral and radial reconstructions using the proximal fibula and achieved continuing axial growth in 50% of patients (33). In seven cases, a single branch of the anterior or posterior tibial artery was used, but in one case, a double vascular supply was used to supply both the epiphysis and the diaphysis. Pho et al. published their observations on three cases of epiphyseal reconstruction in children using the proximal fibula based on the peroneal artery in 1988 (34). In the same year, Zhong-Wei and Guang-Jian- reported two cases of epiphyseal transfer supplied by the peroneal artery (35). Over the past 10 years, further experience with proximal fibula epiphyseal transfer in upper limb skeletal reconstruction has been published in the literature (11,12,36). Nearly all the reports describe limited series of patients in whom the procedure has been used to reconstruct either the proximal humerus or the distal radius and ulna with increasing success because of refinement of the technique.

Our personal experience is based on 27 epiphyseal reconstructions in children ranging in age between 2 and 12 years over a period of 18 years. Nineteen patients underwent reconstruction of the proximal humerus, and eight patients underwent reconstruction of the distal radius. All children were affected by either osteosarcoma or Ewing's sarcoma. The operative technique has been gradually refined and is described in Chapter 86.

Results

Graft Survival and Growth Rate

All of the bone graft components survived and consolidated with the host bone within 3 months, indicating good blood supply and viability of the fibular diaphysis. Isotope scans showed all the grafts remained viable in the immediate postoperative period, and progressive hypertrophy was noted at long-term follow-up.

Progressive growth of the transferred bones has been evaluated by considering the tip of the physis and the growth plate as fixed landmarks and then assessing the distance between the two points over time. Evaluation of growth rate is limited to children with a follow-up period longer than 2 years. In our experience, the growth rate that can be expected after epiphyseal transfer to a heterotopic site ranges between 0.75 and 1.33 cm per year (Figure 62-4). Factors that might interfere with growth of the grafts can be summarized as follows:

- Age of the patient: Growth potential is a function of the child's age and decrease as skeletal maturity approaches.
- Recipient anatomical site: The new heterotopic location influences growth by means of mechanical and biological factors.
- Blood supply: Reliable, continuous perfusion to the graft is absolutely necessary for growth.
- Adjuvant chemotherapy: This is routinely administered preoperatively and postoperatively for bone sarcomas. Inhibition of skeletal growth is one of the reported side effects related to chemotherapy.

Although available data seem to identify the relevance of the local biological environment, longer follow-up periods and larger series are needed to confirm the role of these factors in influencing growth potential.

Functional Outcomes

Excellent results can be achieved in terms of motion and strength in reconstructions after distal radius resection. All the patients recovered nearly normal range of motion in all planes

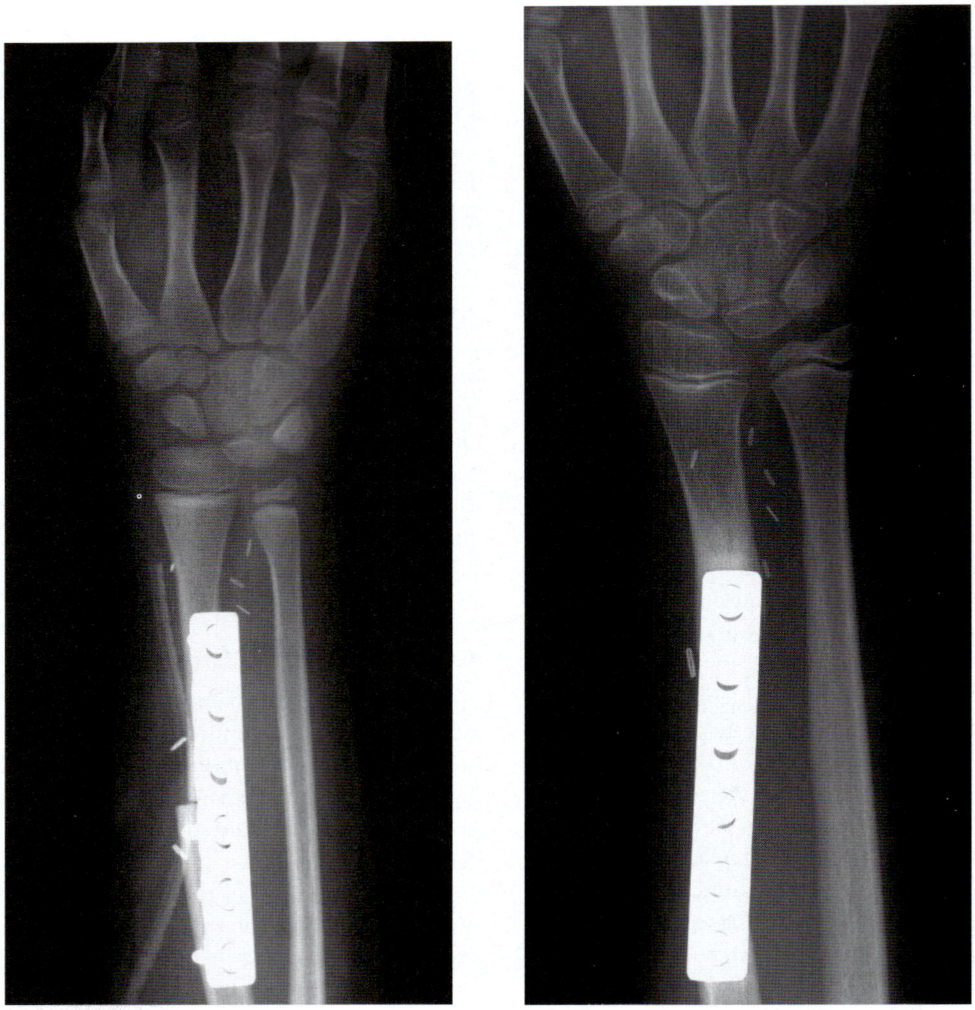

A B

FIGURE 62-4 (A) and (B) Epiphyseal transfer in distal radius reconstruction. Two years after surgery, the overall growth of the transferred fibula have been 2.4 cm. The growth rate per year has been 1.2 cm. Growth of the neoradius has matched the growth of the ulna.

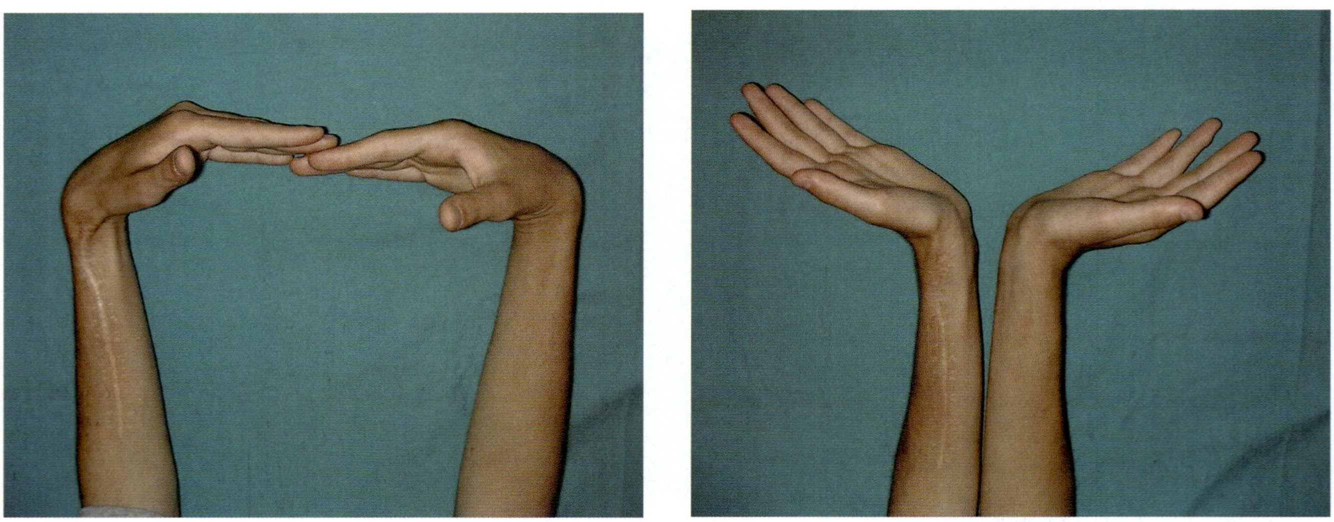

A B

FIGURE 62-5 (A) and (B) Long-term clinical follow-up. The patient has regained nearly normal range of motion of the wrist compared with the contralateral unaffected side.

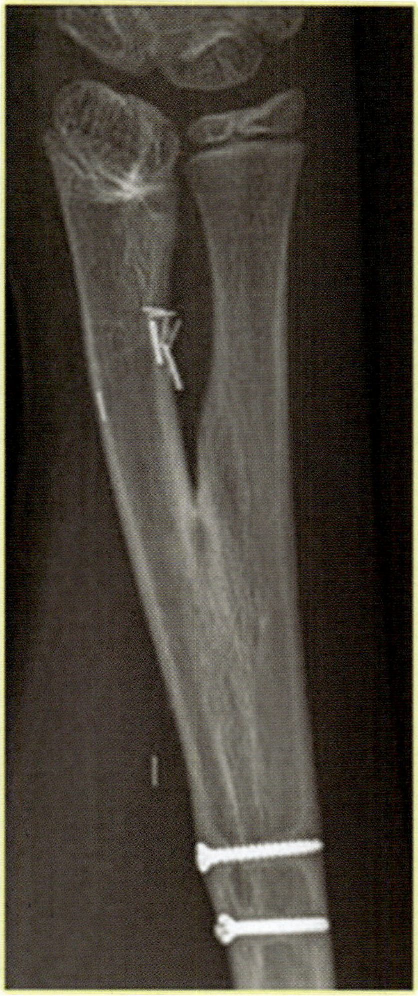

FIGURE 62-6 When the entire radius is radically resected, the fibula is fixed to the radial aspect of the ulna in a Y fashion. Loss of pronation and supination is expected in these cases, but wrist stability with a good range of motion and function is preserved.

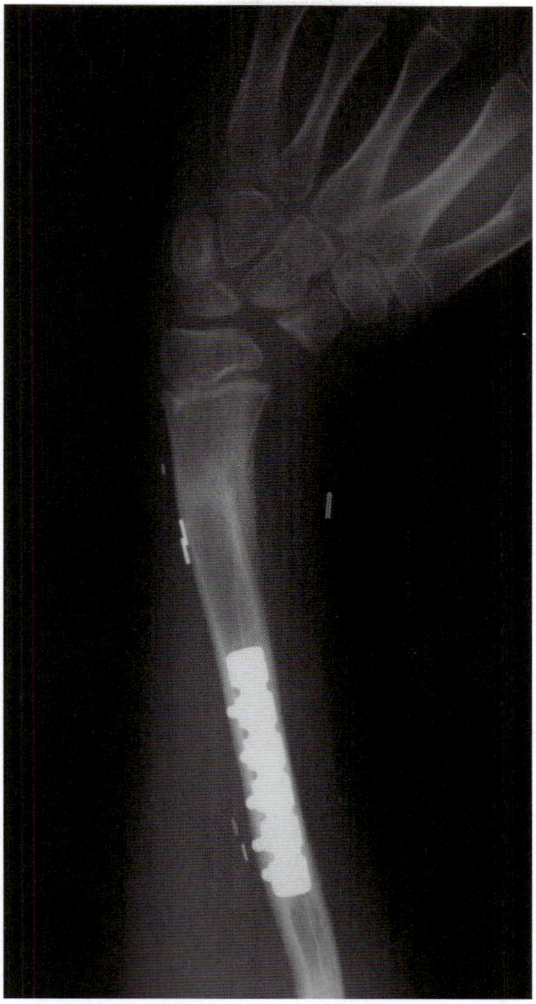

FIGURE 62-7 One-bone forearm reconstruction. When both the radius and ulna are radically resected, the surgical goal is to reconstruct a one-bone forearm. Wrist instability and late deviation are common in these cases.

(Figure 62-5). The wrists have been pain free and stable. Axial deviation and dorsal subluxation of caput ulnae have not been observed.

Loss of pronation and supination may be expected when the entire radius is involved by the tumor and a radical resection is required. In this situation, the vascularized fibula must be fixed to the radial aspect of the ulna in a Y fashion (Figure 62-6), to preserve good wrist stability and motion but prevent the ability to pronate and supinate.

The worst results in wrist reconstruction may be expected if the resection involves both the radius and the ulna. In this situation, the goal is to reconstruct a one-bone forearm, but wrist instability and late deviation are common (Figure 62-7).

Because of macroscopic anatomical mismatching, the proximal fibula is less suitable for proximal humerus replacement but still the best option (Figure 62-8). Stability of the new shoulder joint is sometimes difficult to achieve because of the difference in size and shape between the head of the humerus and the proximal fibula and because, for oncologic purposes, the en bloc excision must include the entire shoulder capsule, liga-

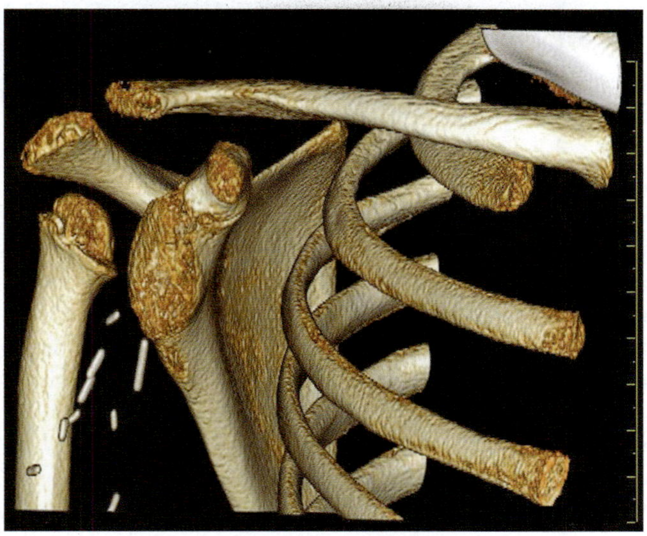

FIGURE 62-8 Proximal humerus reconstruction. Mismatching in size and shape between the proximal fibula and the proximal humerus is evident. The proximal fibula is therefore less suitable for proximal humerus reconstruction but is still the best option.

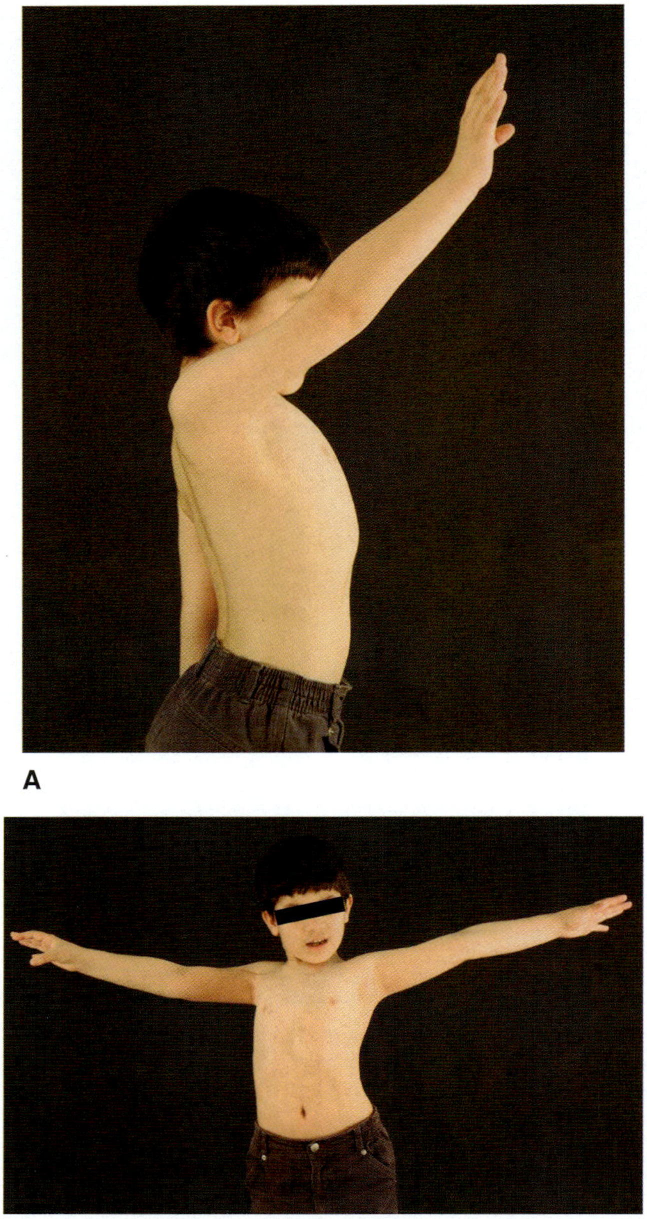

A

B

FIGURE 62-9 (**A**) and (**B**) Functional outcome in a case of proximal humerus reconstruction. Lack of abduction is the major functional impairment that occurs in proximal humeral reconstruction.

ments, and muscles. This results in a relatively high incidence of subacromial displacement of the fibular head. However, the functional outcome of proximal humerus reconstructions is usually more than acceptable for the daily activity of patients, and the majority of them are able to swim and practice other sports involving the use of the upper limb (Figure 62-9). Lack of abduction, which ranges between 50 and 90 degrees in our series, is the major functional impairment that can be expected in proximal humeral reconstruction.

Remodeling

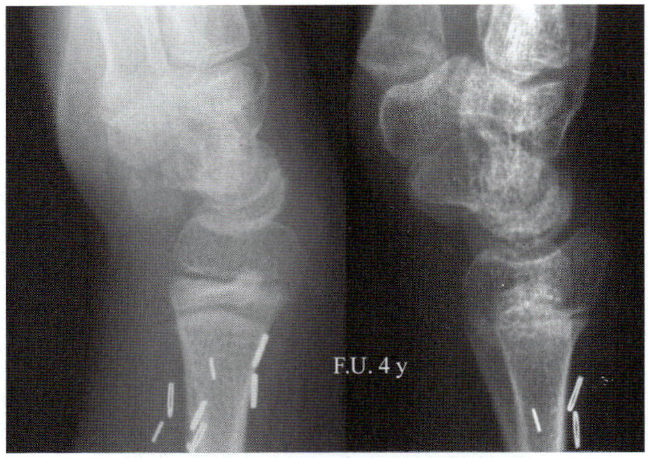

FIGURE 62-10 Long-term radiographic follow-up. At 4 years of follow-up, the transferred fibula epiphysis has remodeled, developing a concave surface to meet the functional demands of the reconstructed wrist joint.

The proximal fibular physis shows remarkable plasticity when transferred to a heterotopic location. Such adaptive modification is much more evident in wrist reconstruction because the loading stress in the radiocarpal joint is definitely more significant than that in a suspended joint such as the glenohumeral joint. After surgery, the load stress at the distal articular surface of the new wrist joint leads to progressive development of a concave surface, which improves contact with the proximal carpal row (Figure 62-10).

Complications

Instability of the knee joint may be one of the donor site complications. However, in our series, stable fixation of the lateral collateral ligament augmented with a residual strip of biceps femoris tendon to the lateral aspect of the tibia prevented instability in all cases. In contrast, injury to the motor branches of the peroneal nerve is very difficult to avoid. Direct neurotization and immediate neurorrhaphy are recommended to reduce the incidence of permanent palsies, which have been observed in two patients in our series.

Fractures are more likely to occur in humeral reconstructions because of excessive mechanical stress. In our experience, the use of more elastic implants has significantly reduced the incidence of fractures of the transferred fibula.

Subacromial displacement of the fibular physis is a relatively common complication. Although this condition does not significantly interfere with the final functional outcome, it should be prevented by improving the quality of soft tissue reconstruction.

Failure to achieve longitudinal growth is a major complication that has been observed in five patients in our series. In two of these growth failures, the proximal fibula epiphyseal transfer was based on the peroneal artery alone as the vascular pedicle. Premature growth plate arrest was observed in both patients a few months after surgery. In the remaining three patients, the transfer was based on the anterior tibial artery and failure was probably attributable to damage to the recurrent epiphyseal branch during transfer into the recipient site.

LOWER EXTREMITY

Hypertrophy of the transferred fibular bone segment is observed in almost all patients, especially in the weight-bearing segment, although this phenomenon takes time to occur.

Single-barrel fibula reconstruction in the lower limb is often complicated by stress fractures, and secondary procedures, either conservative or surgical, may be necessary. Double-barrel fibula reconstruction (37) may be used for short defects, which are rare in oncologic patients because of the extent of the resection. To achieve a more reliable reconstruction in long defects, it has been suggested to combine a massive allograft with a vascularized fibula by assembling the two components in various ways (9). The massive allograft provides initial stability, and the vascularized fibula provides the biological potential to prevent the consequences of mechanical failure of the allograft over the medium and long term. As the allograft undergoes resorption or stress fractures, the loading stress is gradually shifted to the vascularized fibula, which responds by hypertrophy. In addition, the stability of the allograft allows a small epiphyseal bone fragment to be preserved in resections close to a joint and provides a foundation for reinsertion of tendons and ligaments to allow restoration of joint stability.

Assembly of the fibula and the allograft may vary according to the size of the recipient bone and the level of resection. In diaphyseal reconstruction of the femur, the vascularized fibula may be positioned either medial to the allograft or within the medullary canal of the allograft. In both constructs, direct contact of the vascularized fibula with both the proximal and distal stumps of the recipient femur is important. In a side-by-side construct, the fibula is positioned along the axis of maximal load (medially) to produce a rapid hypertrophic response.

Intramedullary concentric location of the fibula is the most frequent type of construct in the lower limb. In this construct, the fibula is more protected from loading and hypertrophy is slow but consistent (Figure 62-11). In a series of 36 patients, these allograft-vascularized fibula combinations showed three possible types of behavior (38). In 13 patients, the allograft maintained its architecture without resorption or fractures. Nevertheless, the inlaid fibula underwent slow but progressive hypertrophy, which led to gradual integration with the allograft. A dense line on the allograft endosteum was the first sign of bony bridging heralding fusion of the two grafts. In eight patients, fracture or nonunion of the allograft occurred. The fibula responded promptly with rapid hypertrophy, which again induced bony bridging with the allograft. In three patients, no change in size or density of the fibula was followed by fracture with no callus formation. This was interpreted as a failure to restore adequate blood supply to the transferred fibula.

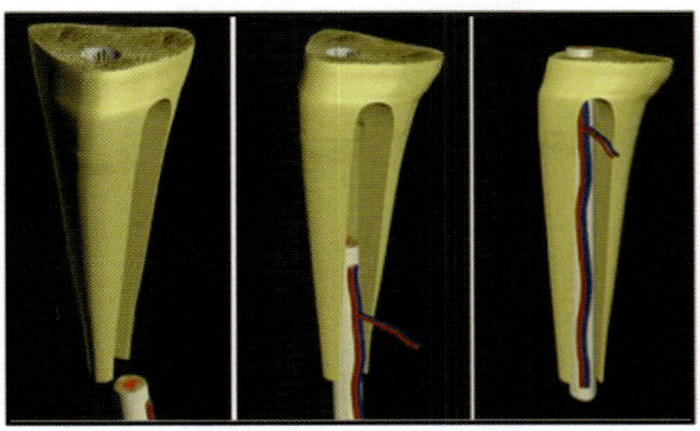

FIGURE 62-11 Diagrammatic representation of intramedullary positioning of a vascularized fibula into the allograft in a concentric fashion. The fibula extends beyond the allograft proximally and distally to contact the recipient bone.

Operative Technique

- A massive, frozen allograft of the appropriate size is defrosted in an aseptic environment in the operating room. The choice of the allograft is planned preoperatively according to the location and extent of the segment to be reconstructed.
- The allograft is placed in a vise and cut at the desired length using an oscillating saw. The medullary canal is reamed to allow an intramedullary positioning of the autologous fibula (Figure 62-12). If the transverse diameter of the fibula is compatible with the allograft medullary canal, only a window for the vascular pedicle needs to be drilled in the allograft cortex at the level of the selected recipient vessels (Figure 62-13). Alternatively, when the fibula has a larger diameter than the medullary canal of the allograft, a longitudinal strip of allograft cortex should be resected and the fibula press fit into the slot (Figure 62-14).
- Two key points are necessary to guarantee the success of the procedure: (1) a perfect contact between the allograft and the recipient bone and (2) an extra length of fibula, which should exceed the length of the allograft by 2 cm proximally and distally. In this way, the vascularized fibula has adequate contact with the recipient bone, allowing a certain amount of load to pass directly through the fibula and promote hypertrophy.

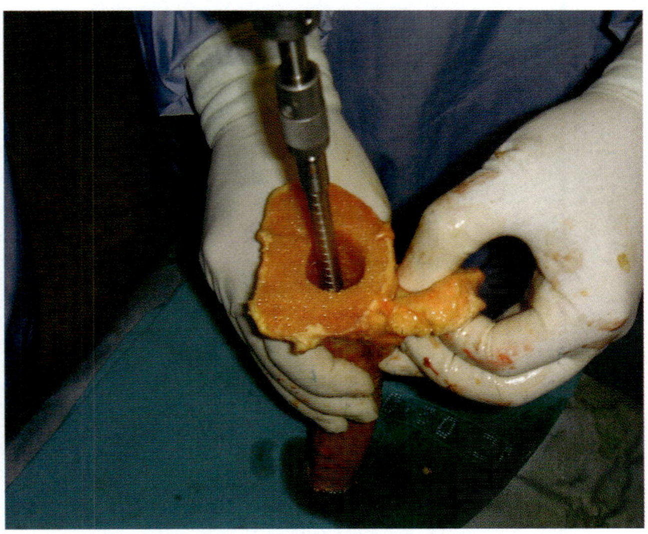

FIGURE 62-12 Reaming the allograft medullary canal to accommodate the autologous fibula.

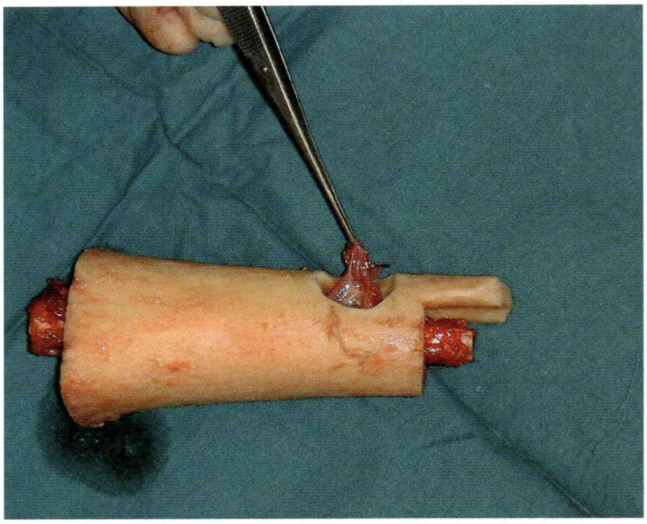

FIGURE 62-13 The transverse diameter of the fibula is compatible with the allograft medullary canal. A window for the fibula vascular pedicle is made in the allograft cortex to allow anastomoses with the recipient vessels.

- Bone fixation is of paramount importance and varies according to the type of reconstruction. If the resection is very close to the epiphyseal plateau, only screw fixation can be used, but a plate is preferred at the diaphyseal level (Figure 62-15). For intercalary reconstruction of the middiaphysis, either two compression plates (Figure 62-16) or only one long bridging plate (Figure 62-17) may be used. Double-plate fixation has the advantage of producing better compression at the osteosynthesis sites, but a single bridging plate has the advantage of avoiding a weak point between the two plates.
- The recipient vessels must be dissected for an adequate length to allow the anastomoses to be performed without tension or kinking

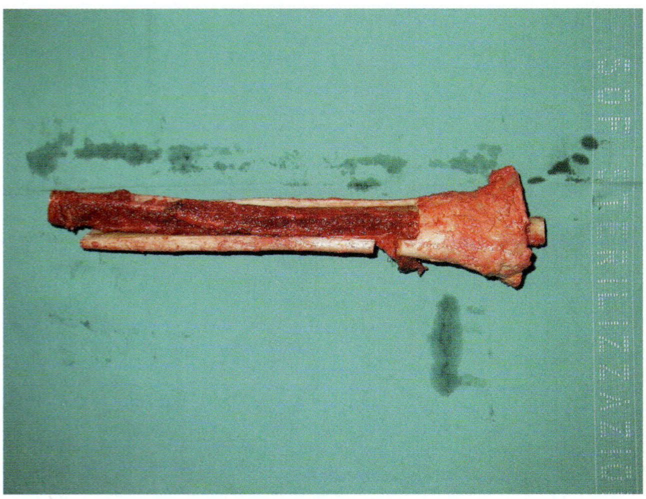

FIGURE 62-14 The fibula is larger than the medullary canal of the allograft. A longitudinal strip of allograft cortex is resected, and the fibula is lodged in press-fit fashion into the slot.

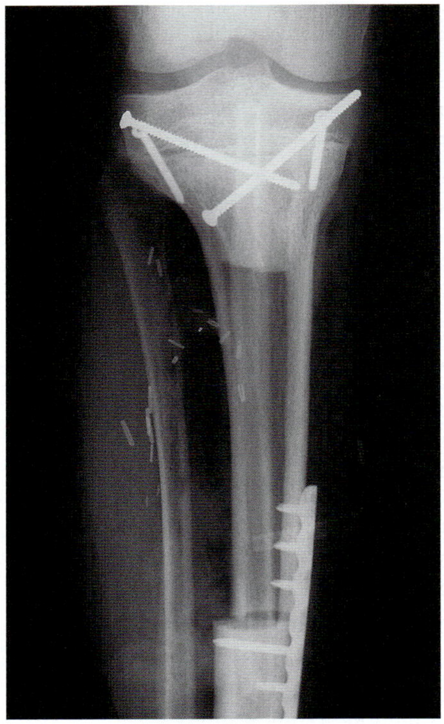

FIGURE 62-15 A small portion of the epiphyseal plateau is left after resection. Screw fixation is recommended at this site. A plate is used at diaphyseal level between the allograft and recipient tibia.

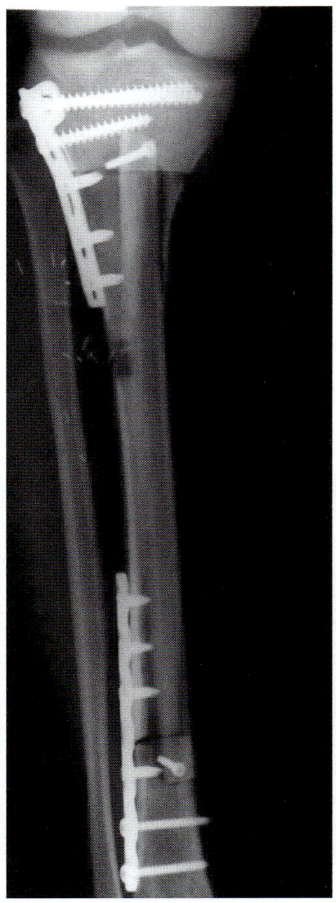

FIGURE 62-16 Intercalary reconstruction of the tibia. Two compression plates are used for bone fixation between the tibia and the allograft.

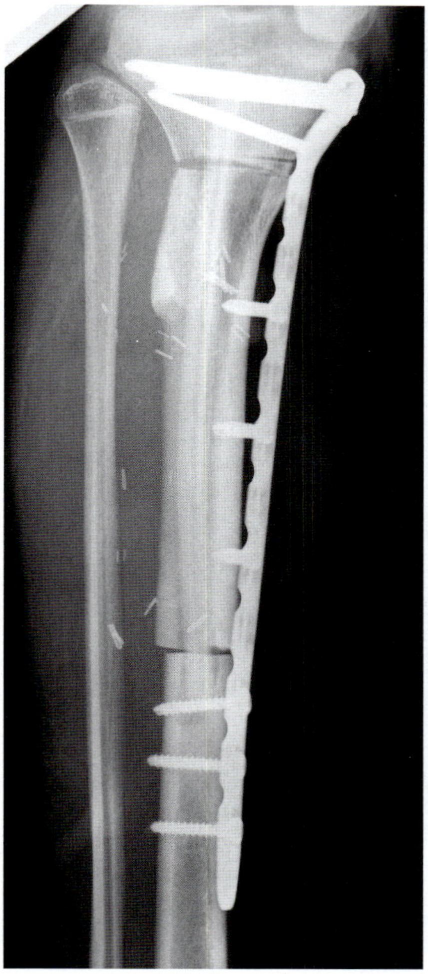

FIGURE 62-17 Intercalary reconstruction of the tibia. A long bridging plate is used for bone fixation between the tibia and the allograft.

Results

A series of 90 patients has recently been evaluated (39,40). Thirty-three cases involved intercalary reconstruction of the femur and the remaining 57 involved the tibia. The average follow-up period has been 9 years (range 3–17 years), and the average length of the bony defect was 16 cm (range, 7–26 cm).

A high percentage of patients (73%) healed in one operation and did not require any further surgery. According to the Musculo-Skeletal Tumor Society (MSTS) functional scoring system, six patients who had a failed reconstruction because of infection and seven patients who underwent amputation because of local recurrence of the tumor were excluded. Of the remaining 77 patients, 72% achieved an excellent result, 20% a good result, 5% a fair result, and 3% a poor result.

In our experience, the combination of a massive allograft and a vascularized fibula has proved to be an optimal and durable reconstruction for large bony defects in the lower extremity. This procedure is based on taking advantage of the properties of the two components: the allograft provides initial stability and protects the vascularized fibula from excessive mechanical stress, and the biological potential of the vascularized fibula guarantees a good long-term result in case of fracture or resorption of the allograft. However, allograft resorption has not been the most frequent finding in our series. More often, slow hypertrophy of the fibula led to progressive fusion to the inner surface of the allograft, and with subsequent bony remodeling, the eventual creation of a unique bone resulting from the fusion of the two grafts (Figure 62-18). The technique has

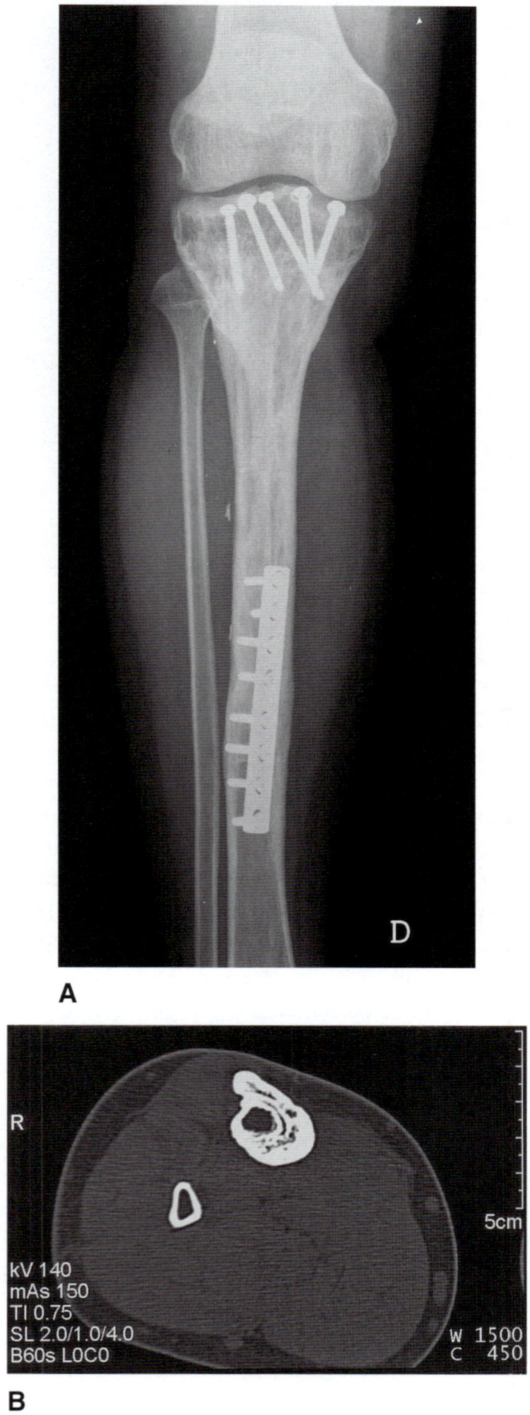

FIGURE 62-18 (A) Long-term radiographic follow-up. Over time, the vascularized fibula shows progressive hypertrophy and fuses with the inner surface of the allograft, forming one solid unit. (B) Computed tomography imaging shows the process of progressive fusion between the hypertrophied fibula and the inner surface of the allograft.

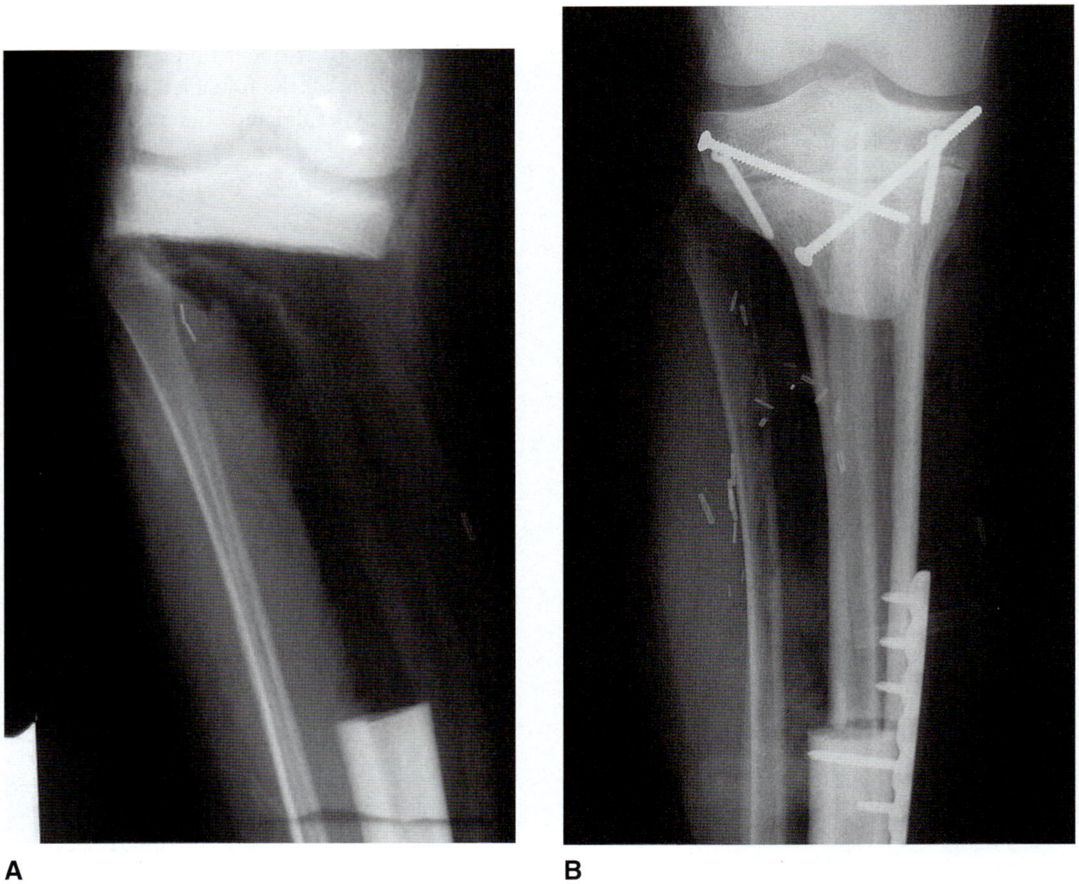

FIGURE 62-19 Concentric vascularized fibula and allograft assembly. This technique is especially advantageous in cases of intraepiphyseal resection when only a thin layer of epiphyseal plateau remains (A). Proximal bone fixation is achieved with only four screws, taking advantage of both the stability of the allograft and the biological potential of the vascularized fibula (B).

proven to be particularly useful in intraepiphyseal resections in which only a thin layer of epiphyseal plateau can be preserved (Figure 62-19). In these situations, a vascularized fibula alone would require a transarticular external fixator for at least 3 months with possible residual stiffness of the joint. Alternatively, an allograft alone would require very stable bone fixation that cannot be achieved when only a thin portion of the epiphysis remains after the resection.

In summary, the technique described is particularly indicated for lower limb skeletal reconstruction in children. It provides a durable reconstruction for very long resections and salvage of the epiphysis and improves the functional results. The vascularity of the fibula is the cornerstone for both success of the reconstruction and successful management of complications. The stability of the osteosynthesis of the allograft is essential to achieve early union and avoid complications.

REFERENCES

1. Ogilvie CM, Crawford EA, Hosalkar HS, et al. Long-term results for limb salvage with osteoarticular allograft reconstruction. *Clin Orthop Relat Res* 2009;467(10):2685–2690.
2. Raskin KA, Hornicek F. Allograft reconstruction in malignant bone tumors: indications and limits. *Recent Results Cancer Res* 2009;179:51–58.
3. Aro HT, Aho AJ. Clinical use of bone allografts. *Ann Med* 1993;25(4):403–412.
4. Delloye C, de Nayer P, Allington N, et al. Massive bone allografts in large skeletal defects after tumor surgery: a clinical and microradiographic evaluation. *Arch Orthop Trauma Surg* 1988;107(1):31–41.
5. Enneking WF, Campanacci DA. Retrieved human allografts: a clinicopathologic study. *J Bone Joint Surg Am* 2001;8(7):971–986.
6. Rödl RW, Ozaki T, Hoffmann C, et al. Osteoarticular allograft in surgery for high-grade malignant tumours of bone. *J Bone Joint Surg Br* 2000;82B:1006–1010.
7. Gloeckler Ries LA, Reichman ME, Riedel Lewis D, et al. Cancer survival and incidence from the Surveillance, Epidemiology, and End Results (SEER) program. *Oncologist* 2003;8:541–552.
8. Abed R, Grimer R. Surgical modalities in the treatment of bone sarcoma in children" *Cancer Treat Rev* 2010;36:342–347.
9. Capanna R, Bufalini C, Campanacci M. A new technique for reconstructions of large metadiaphyseal bone defects: a combined graft (allograft shell plus vascularized fibula). *Orthop Traumatol* 1993;159–177.
10. Innocenti M, Ceruso M, Manfrini M, et al. Free vascularised growth plate transfer after bone tumor resection in children. *J Reconstr Microsurgery* 1998;14(2):137–143.
11. Innocenti M, Delcroix L, Manfrini M, et al. Vascularized proximal fibular epiphyseal transfer for distal radial reconstruction, *J Bone Joint Surg Am* 2004;86A(7):1504–1511.
12. Innocenti M, Delcroix L, Balatri A. Vascularized growth plate transfer for distal radius reconstruction. *Semin Plast Surg* 2008;22(3):186–194.
13. Ohnishi I, Sato W, Matsuyama J, et al. Treatment of congenital pseudarthrosis of the tibia: a multicenter study in Japan. *J Pediatr Orthop* 2005;25(2):219–224.
14. Mateev M, Imanaliev A. Two-stage reconstruction in congenital pseudarthrosis of the forearm using the Ilizarov technique and vascularized osteoseptocutaneous fibula. *J Reconstr Microsurg* 2006;22(3):143–148.
15. Charles YP, Diméglio A, Chammas M. Congenital pseudarthrosis of the forearm. Report of two cases and review of the literature. *Chir Main* 2009;28(1):26–32.

16. Bae DS, Waters PM, Sampson CE. Use of free vascularized fibular graft for congenital ulnar pseudarthrosis: surgical decision making in the growing child. *J Pediatr Orthop* 2005;25(6):755–762.
17. Weiland AJ, Weiss AP, Moore JR, Tolo VT. Vascularized fibular grafts in the treatment of congenital pseudarthrosis of the tibia. *J Bone Joint Surg Am* 1990;72(5):654–662.
18. Kanaya F, Tsai TM, Harkess J. Vascularized bone grafts for congenital pseudarthrosis of the tibia. *Microsurgery* 1996;17(8):459–469.
19. Sakamoto A, Yoshida T, Uchida Y, et al. Long-term follow-up on the use of vascularized fibular graft for the treatment of congenital pseudarthrosis of the tibia. *J Orthop Surg Res* 2008;3:13.
20. Korompilias AV, Lykissas MG, Soucacos PN, et al. Vascularized free fibular bone graft in the management of congenital tibial pseudarthrosis. *Microsurgery* 2009;29(5):346–352.
21. Erni D, De Kerviler S, Hertel R, Slongo T. Vascularised fibula grafts for early tibia reconstruction in infants with congenital pseudarthrosis. *J Plast Reconstr Aesthet Surg* 2010;63(10):1699–1704.
22. Wenger HL. Transplantation of epiphyseal cartilage. *Arch Surg* 1954;50:148–151.
23. Wilson JN. Epiphyseal transplantation. A clinical study. *J Bone Joint Surg* 1966;48A:245–256.
24. Graham WC. Transplantation of joints to replace diseased or damaged articulations in hand. *Am J Surgery* 1954;88:136–141.
25. Bowen CVA, O'Brien BM. Experimental study of the microsurgical transfer of growth plates. *Can J Surg* 1984;27:446.
26. Bowen CVA. Experimental free vascularized epiphyseal transplants. *Orthopaedics* 1986;9:893–898.
27. Bowen CVA, Ethridge CP, O'Brien BMcC, et al. Experimental microvascular growth plate transfers. Part 1—investigation of vascularity. *J Bone Joint Surg Br* 1988;70B:305–310.
28. Bowen CVA, O'Brien BMcC, Gumley GJ. Experimental microvascular growth plate transfers. Part 2—investigation of feasibility. *J Bone Joint Surg Br* 1988;70B:311–314.
29. Donski PK, Carwell GR, Sharzer LA. Growth in revascularized bone grafts in young puppies. *Plast Reconstr Surg* 1979;64:239–243.
30. Donski PK, O'Brien B. Free microvascular epiphyseal transplantation: an experimental study in dogs. *Br J Plast Surg* 1980;33:169–178.
31. Nettelblad H, Randolph MA, Weiland AJ. Physiologic isolation of the canine proximal fibular epiphysis on a vascular pedicle. *Microsurgery* 1984;5:98–101.
32. Nettelblad H, Randolph MA, Weiland AJ. Free microvascular epiphyseal plate transplantation. An experimental study in dogs. *J Bone Joint Surg Am* 1984;66:1421–1430.
33. Tsai TM, Ludwig L, Tonkin M. Vascularized fibular epiphyseal transfer: a clinical study. *Clin Orthop* 1986;210:228–234.
34. Pho RW, Patterson MH, Kour AK, Kumar VR. Free vascularized epiphyseal transplantation in upper extremity reconstruction. *J Hand Surg Am* 1988;13:440–447.
35. Zhong-Wei C, Guang-Jian Z. Epiphyseal transplantation. In Pho RW, (ed). *Microsurgical Technique in Orthopaedics*. London: Butterworths, 1988, pp. 121–127.
36. Ghert M, Colterjohn N, Manfrini M. The use of free vascularized fibular grafts in skeletal reconstruction for bone tumors in children. *J Am Acad Orthop Surg* 2007;15(10):577–587.
37. Jones NF, Swartz WM, Mears DC, et al. The "double-barrel" free vascularized fibular bone graft. *Plast Reconstr Surg* 1988;81:378–385.
38. Manfrini M, Vanel D, De Paolis M, et al. Imaging of vascularized fibula autograft placed inside a massive allograft in reconstruction of lower limb bone tumors. *AJR Am J Roentgenol* 2004;182(4):963–970.
39. Capanna R, Campanacci D, Belot N, et al. A new reconstructive technique for intercalary defects of long bones: the association of massive allograft with vascularized fibular autograft. Long-term results and comparison with alternative techniques. *Orthop Clin North Am* 2007;38(1):51–60, vi.
40. Innocenti M, Abed Y, Beltrami G, et al. Biological reconstruction after resection of bone tumors of the proximal tibia using allograft shell and intra-medullary free vascularized fibular graft: long term results. *Microsurgery* 2009;29(5):361–372.

CHAPTER 63

Toe Transfer for Traumatic Thumb Amputations

Wayne A. Morrison

Along humans' evolutionary path from the primordial slime to sedentary slob, when survival skills changed from fleet of foot to sleight of hand and communication skills from foot stomping to thumb texting SMS, the relative roles of the hallux and the thumb have seen a progressive reversal in functional importance. Commensurate with their changing roles, the disability profiles have shifted from stubbed toes to overuse of the flexor pollicis longus appropriately dubbed "nintendinitis." Losing a thumb today has serious consequences for work and lifestyle.

The toe contains all of the unique physical and aesthetic qualities that constitute a thumb: glabrous, innervated skin nonshear adherent and padded pulp, a nail to stabilize the skin sleeve, a skeleton, joints, and appropriate tendons. These qualities were recognized at the end of the 19th century by Nicoladoni (1–3), who transferred both the second and great toes for thumb replacement in a staged pedicled manner but without nerve repair. In the more leisured times of the first half of the 20th century, patients were regularly committed to periods of prolonged hospitalization, and they deferred totally to the wisdom and whim of the daring, bold, or courageous surgeon. Pedicled transfers including toes in various forms were intermittently reported, notably by Lambret, Clarkson and Gillies (4), and Freeman. However, they remained a rarity because of trophic ulceration and poor function most likely from poor vascularization, lack of sensation, and skeletal instability.

From the era of the first microvascular repair and digital replantation, it was obvious to many that a toe could theoretically be transferred by microvascular means to create a thumb. Free hallux transfer was first realized in monkeys by Buncke and colleagues (5), and in 1968, Cobbett (6) performed the first human big toe transfer. This was soon followed by Buncke and colleagues (7) and independently by Yang (8), who in 1977 reported a series of 40 cases of second toe transfer in the Chinese literature. O'Brien and colleagues (9) in Australia closely followed, and subsequently Chung and Wei (10) assumed the mantle of dogen of toe transfer after accumulating an extraordinary experience of traumatic reconstructions consequent to Taiwan's rapid industrialization program.

Microvascular toe transfer, first perfected more than 40 years ago, remains a rarely performed procedure in most major hand surgical units, yet from functional, aesthetic, and technical viewpoints, it is one of hand surgery's most sophisticated and satisfying operations. Its rarity relates no doubt to patients' concerns about adding insult to injury and a heightened concern for taking care of what they have left. As Lady Bracknell quipped in Oscar Wilde's play, *The Importance of Being Earnest,* "To lose one parent may be regarded as misfortune, to lose both looks like carelessness." Cultural and aesthetic issues and concerns with walking are other legitimate reservations that also account for its infrequent performance. Surgeons are no longer seen by the better educated "Me" generation as the super heroes of yesteryear but more as businessmen marketing a product. From the surgeon's point of view, inexperience and the anxiety that the procedure is an all-or-nothing outcome deter many. Sadly, as a result, many surgeons commit patients to alternative procedures that are multistaged and doomed from the outset to be at best compromises and in many cases futile.

OPTIONS

Thumb reconstruction has been described using whole toes, either the hallux or second toe, and as a modified hallux using either the "wrap-around" (11–13) or "trimmed toe" (14) techniques.

INDICATIONS

Who needs a toe transfer, and who in their right mind would submit to one? Toe transfers can be considered for partial and complete thumb loss. The challenge is to convince the individual of the wisdom and indeed the sanity of your recommendations. As with all surgical procedures, the indications are based on a balance of benefit versus risk or morbidity. The benefits of toe transfer are not difficult to see given that the toes are essentially the same structure functionally and aesthetically apart from size as the missing part. Rarely in reconstructive surgery there is an option to find a potentially dispensable donor that is a replica of the missing part. Balancing this are the risk of technical failure and the morbidity of an absent toe. Microvascular transfers always carry a failure risk, and toes are technically more demanding than most, and for posttraumatic reconstructions, recipient vessels may also be suboptimal. Realistically, in most mortals' hands, this risk of failure is of the order of 5%.

Most studies evaluating the foot after hallux and second toe transfers at or distal to the metatarsophalangeal joint have reported minimal functional morbidity (12,15–19). Neuromas have been reported (20). Partial toe transfers with grafted secondary defects risk higher morbidity from ulceration and pain. Aesthetic morbidity, however, is real, especially for women with open footwear, and this can only be quantified through the eyes of the beholder.

Alternative options for thumb reconstruction are pollicization or osteoplastic procedures. The former is classically indicated when the index tip is also damaged or amputated. Otherwise, the sacrifice of a normal index finger in the context of an already damaged thumb, except for congenital four-fingered hands in which thenar muscle reconstruction is possible from the transferred intrinsics, seems unjustified. Osteoplastic reconstructions are typically multistaged; complex; prone to complications; and in the end, suboptimal.

Eventually, the indication for a particular surgical procedure is that which the patient directs you to do. Given that toe transfer remains rare, it would suggest that the patients "vote with their feet" and despite any eloquent entreaties based on evolutionary logistics, it is generally difficult to convince them of the benefits of trading a toe to make a thumb. Sadly, many patients are so daunted by the prospects of toe transfer or of the alternatives that they elect to do nothing and accept permanent disability.

Reconstruction of the thumb demands an understanding of its key functional and aesthetic components, what is missing in this particular case, and what reconstructive options are available to replace them. Key functional elements of the thumb are length, sensation, a well-padded nonshearing pulp, skeletal stability, and mobility. Whereas sensation is largely a property of the distal thumb, mobility is a proximal property. In their discussions about thumb reconstructions, many patients are motivated as much by appearance as function, so aesthetic elements should not be underestimated.

For amputations distal to the interphalangeal (IP) joint, it is not loss of length per se that diminishes function but the loss of unique soft tissue. The soft tissue cover of the remaining proximal thumb is a poor compromise for the lost distal skin sleeve that houses much of the thumb's critical function. Fingerprinted skin, a dense plexus of sensory nerve endings; stable, nonswivel, padded pulp; and nail, which stabilizes the pulp and magnifies sensation, are all components of the distal phalanx. Thumb mobility depends on an intact trapeziometacarpal joint and functioning thenar muscles. Ideally, the basal joint and one other are necessary to permit positioning of the thumb tip for useful opposition to the digits and to avoid excessive rigidity of the thumb skeletal column. Loss or stiffness of one of the more distal joints can be readily compensated for.

TOE SELECTION

Toe selection takes into account function and aesthetics. For amputations distal to the metacarpophalangeal (MCP) joint—and these are by far the commonest injury—no added joint or motors are needed, and the deficits are length, sensation, and aesthetics. The ideal toe selection would be a reduced hallux, or augmented second toe. Hallux modifications include the "wrap-around" flap and "trimmed-toe" procedures. The former degloves the toe skin and requires an iliac crest bone graft but preserves the toe on the foot. The trimmed toe reduces toe skeleton size directly and includes the reconstituted IP joint but totally sacrifices the toe. The second toe can be expanded by the simultaneous insetting of the adjacent lateral hemi pulp of the hallux as an island flap on the same common vascular pedicle (21). This procedure preserves most of the big toe but sacrifices the second. For thumb amputations at or proximal to the metatarsophalangeal joint, a second joint is required, and in proximal amputations, added skeleton is required, so that the toe selection needs to be a whole toe either the hallux or second toe. Both are obviously mismatches, but the hallux is aesthetically preferable and, although bulky, can be secondarily reduced. Its large size compensates for its lack of precision pinch. Osteotomy can be taken obliquely through the head of the first metatarsal to include the essential elements of the joint, articular surface of the head, collateral ligaments, and volar plate but preserve the plantar weight-bearing components. It also includes a dorsal sliver of metatarsal bone shaft up to 2 cm in length for use as skeletal lengthening for the thumb. This design maintains the medial weight-bearing platform width of the foot and facilitates direct dorsal skin closure.

Alternatively, the second toe can be selected, including its metatarsophalangeal joint. This has the advantage of a lesser secondary defect, but it contains an extra joint and is aesthetically unattractive at the thumb site being obviously a toe. The incorporation of the big toe adjacent hemipulp into the volar part of the second toe combined with bulbous tip reduction can significantly improve the appearance (21).

When the thumb amputation includes the trapeziometacarpal joint and thenar muscles, then the second toe with its metatarsal and associated extrinsic and intrinsic tendons is the only realistic toe reconstructive option. Basal joint mobility can be restored using a Swanson silicone MCP joint prosthesis stemmed into the metatarsal shaft distally and the carpal remnant proximally. The alternative is a nontoe option pollicizing the adjacent index finger. This level of amputation as with transmetacarpal amputations requires preliminary or simultaneous skin flap cover for critical components of the transferred toe.

TECHNIQUE

Ipsilateral big and contralateral second toes are chosen so that the vascular pedicle will drape through the dorsal aspect of the first web in the hand. Racquet-shaped toe incisions are designed in the metatarsophalangeal crease on the plantar surface and extend around dorsally to include a small V-flap. From this point, the incision extends proximally to access the dorsal venous and arterial systems (Figure 63-1).

The common vascular anatomy of all whole or partial toes is based on the dorsalis pedis and first dorsal-metatarsal artery systems; this was originally best described by Gilbert and colleagues (22) (Figure 63-2). Where the dorsal vasculature is deficient, the plantar system is reciprocally large but short and may necessitate vein grafting. In the skin incision design for big toe transfers, under no circumstances should skin be removed proximal to the level of the metatarsophalangeal joint to ensure adequate primary closure over the vulnerable dorsal aspect of the remaining metatarsal head. A separate, more proximal skin island can be incorporated on the same dorsalis pedis vascular pedicle, and this flap can be oriented variably to cover critical toe tendon and vascular tissue at the new thumb site (23) (Figure 63-3). Here skin grafts will readily take on paratenon and capsular tissues of the toe transfers so that total flap cover is often unnecessary.

Hallux osteotomy is obliquely through the metatarsal head as mentioned to preserve the weight-bearing plantar aspect of the metatarsal and avoid long-term morbidity. Functional

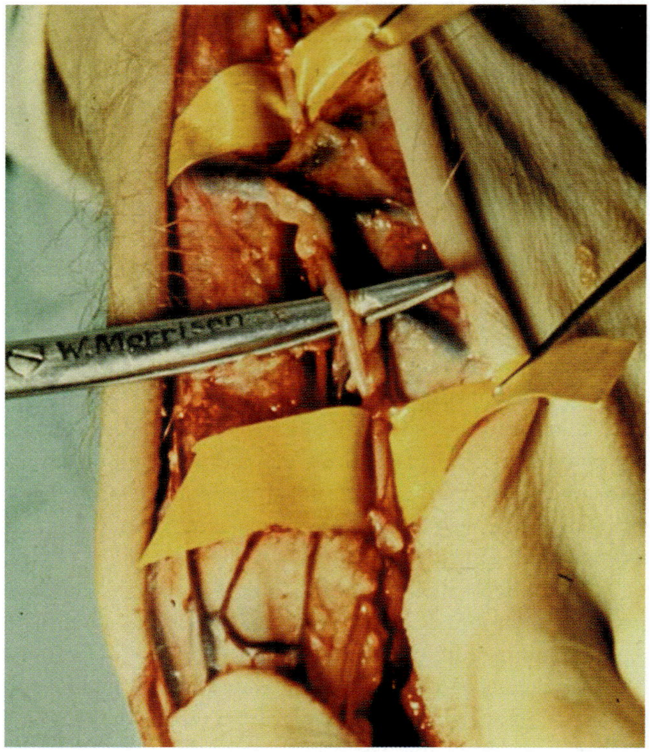

FIGURE 63-2 Common vascular anatomy.

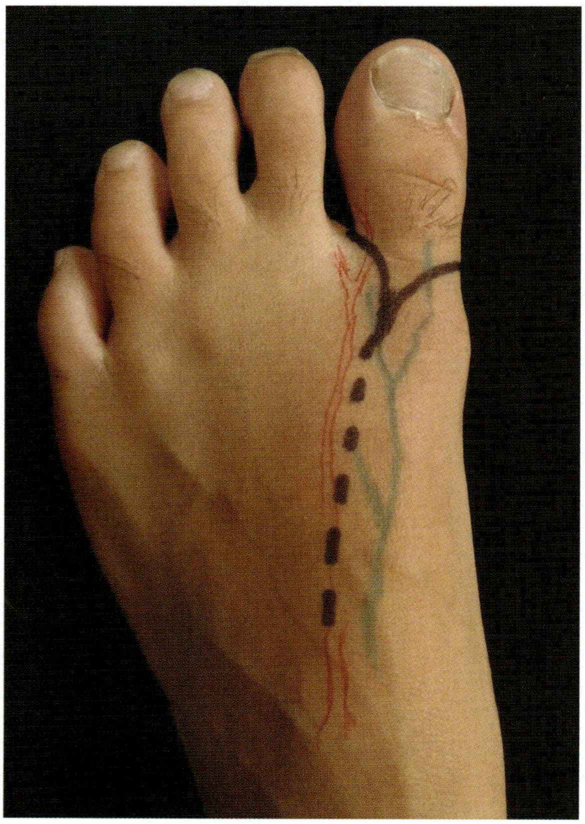

FIGURE 63-1 Big toe transfer incisions.

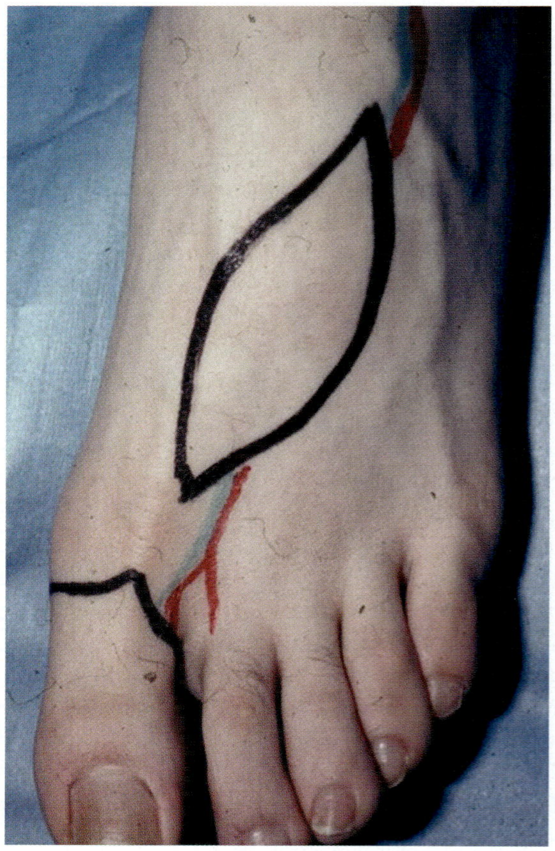

FIGURE 63-3 Dorsalis pedis flap in continuity.

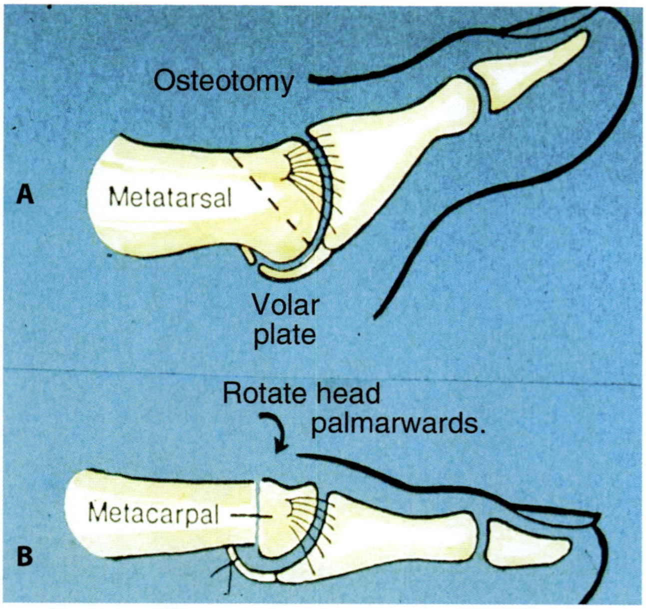

FIGURE 63-4 Oblique osteotomy through the metatarsal head with the metatarsophalangeal joint.

components of the metatarsophalangeal joints are incorporated with the transfer (Figure 63-4). Even when the toe joint is not required, it is preferable to remove the dorsal knuckle of the metatarsal head to facilitate skin flap closure.

Both long and short extensors and the flexor hallucis as well as intrinsic tendon stumps are taken sufficiently proximal for direct repair to their thumb compartments. The flexor is usually tethered to adjacent tendons in the sole, and long lengths cannot be harvested simply by tenotomy at the level of the medial malleolus.

The two digital nerves are included with the toe.

Spasm is common after pedicle dissection, and it is important after completion of the toe dissection to release the tourniquet before dividing the pedicle to confirm adequate vascularization of the toe. Failure to perfuse after tourniquet release may be due to spasm or direct vessel damage, and it is important that this is recognized before transfer to the hand. Spasm usually recovers with time. Vasodilators, warm packs, and gravity by hanging the foot over the operating table may resolve the problem. If these are unsuccessful, vessel damage should be excluded by dissecting the vessel distally and teasing away the periadventitia to observe pulsations. As a last resort, the artery may be divided at its proximal limit and infused with 2 to 3 mL of fresh blood in a pulsatile manner. This will immediately overcome spasm, and the pink flush confirms patency. Otherwise, it will identify the site of any leaks or physical obstruction.

Wrap-around (11–24) and trimmed-toe (14) dissections are more complex. In the wrap-around technique (Figure 63-5) the toe is degloved except for a medial skin bridge that extends around the tip (Figure 63-5A). The width of this bridge is the difference in circumference of the toe and the opposite thumb (Figure 63-5B). The dorsal toe skin flap is elevated from the extensor tendon and immediately at the level of the tendon's insertion into the base of the proximal phalanx the germinal matrix is elevated subperiosteally with the flap distally to the level of the eponychial fold. The distal half of the distal phalanx at the level of the eponychial fold is osteotomized and is included with the nail complex in the transfer (Figure 63-6), and the remaining intact toe stump is resurfaced by folding the medial flap around the remaining bevelled distal phalanx. A cross-toe flap from the dorsum of the adjacent second toe resurfaces the plantar defect of the hallux, and a thick skin graft is used to cover the dorsal aspects of the big and second toes. The cross-toe flap is divided after 4 weeks. The wrap-around technique as originally published (11) was soon modified to incorporate the distal half of the distal phalanx in the transfer because this stabilizes the nail bed and is otherwise discarded to facilitate closure of the toe stump. The volume of the bone graft is deliberately greater than the original thumb skeleton to compensate for the absent tendon volume, and the second toe cross-toe flap is now used to resurface the plantar aspect of the hallux rather than the dorsum to improve the padding on the plantar surface (12). The wrap-around for thumb amputations through the proximal phalanx requires an iliac crest bone graft interposed between the residual base of the proximal phalanx and the distal phalanx component of the toe (see Figure 63-5A). The length of this graft should rarely exceed 2 cm because the thumb without a distal joint can afford to be shorter than normal to avoid problems with rigidity. It is also important to realize as mentioned earlier that the circumferential bulk of the bone graft must be sufficient to fill the toe skin sleeve. This not only replaces the volume of the original thumb skeleton but also those of the flexor and extensor tendons and joint capsule. Bone grafts of these short lengths, when interposed between proximal and distal segments of vascularized bone, readily survive and do not atrophy. In young children, there is a theoretical risk of bone atrophy and poor growth, and the procedure is contraindicated. The toe sleeve is then folded around the graft and loosely sutured (see Figure 63-5B).

The trimmed-toe procedure (14) also retains the medial skin bridge on the foot, which facilitates foot closure and involves a primary skeletal reduction along its medial aspect to match thumb dimensions. The IP joint is included but requires reconstruction of the medial collateral ligament, which is elevated in the skeletal reduction. The toe is disarticulated through the metatarsophalangeal joint. Compared with the wrap-around procedure, this reduces complications from foot scar but necessarily sacrifices the whole toe. To patients, the option of retaining the big toe is often the critical issue in deciding whether they will consider toe transfer as a realistic option for thumb reconstruction.

THUMB STUMP DISSECTION

Because of the racquet incision design for toe amputation at the metatarsophalangeal crease to preserve plantar skin on the foot, the volar skin cover of the toe is usually deficient relative to the dorsal skin. With healed thumb stumps, it is possible to accommodate to this by designing a U-shaped access incision based palmarward so that when opened, it will afford flap cover to the plantar aspect of the toe. As previously mentioned, in some cases of more proximal amputation, preliminary or simultaneous flap cover from a separate source will need to be anticipated to ensure coverage of nongraftable toe components.

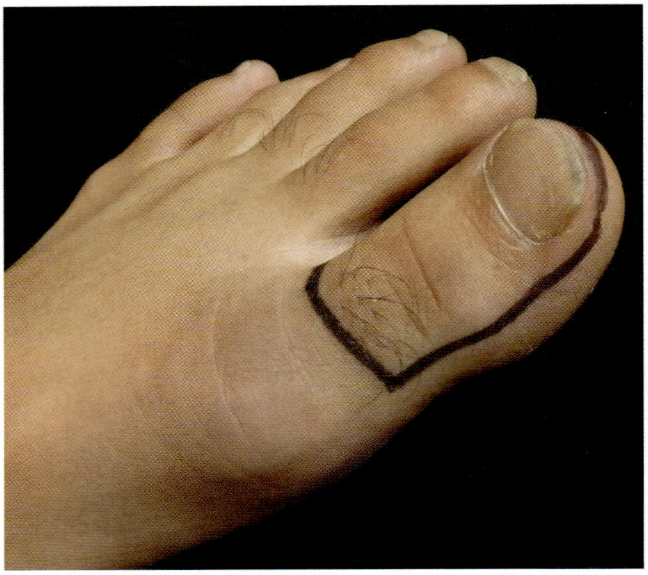

A

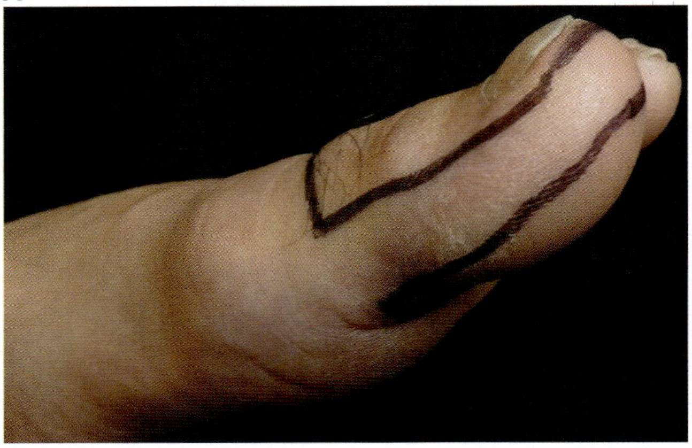

B

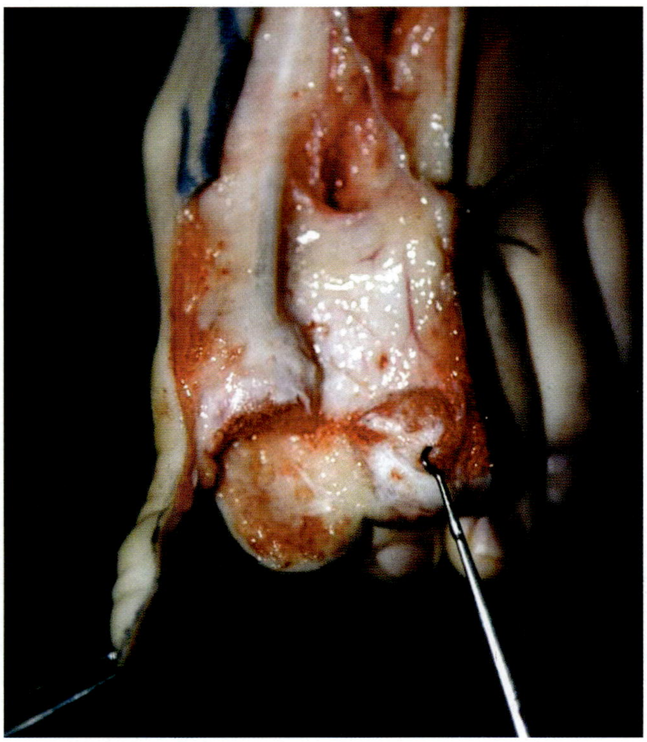

C

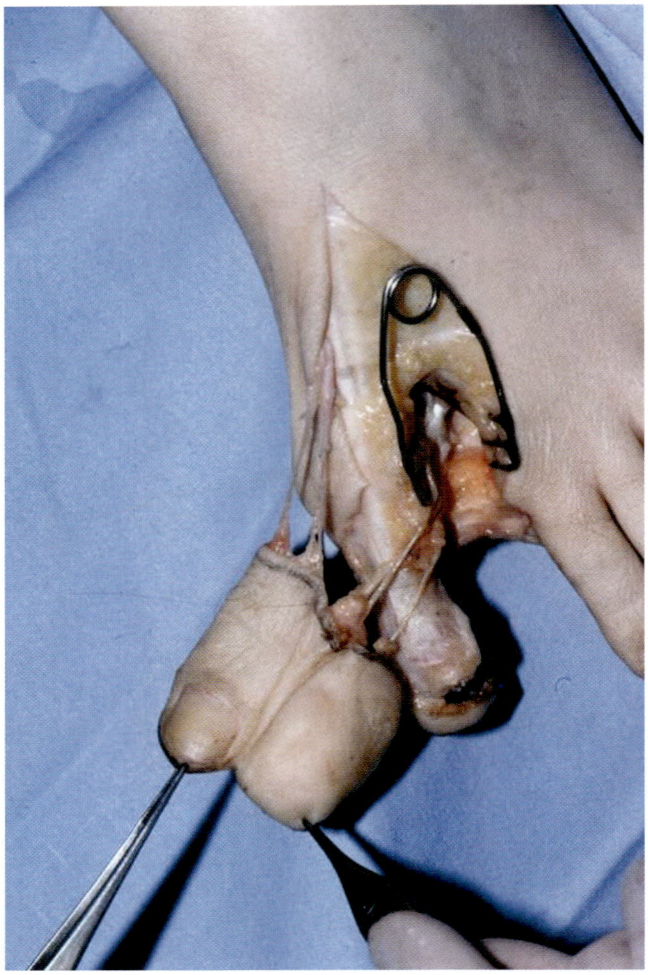

D

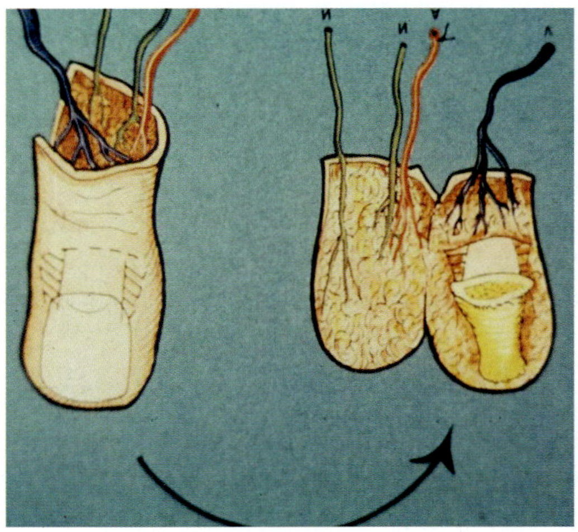

E

FIGURE 63-5 Wrap-around markings. (A) Dorsal. (B) Medial. (C) Osteotomy of the distal phalanx. (D) Flap elevated in the vascular pedicle. (E) Germinal matrix with a toe flap.

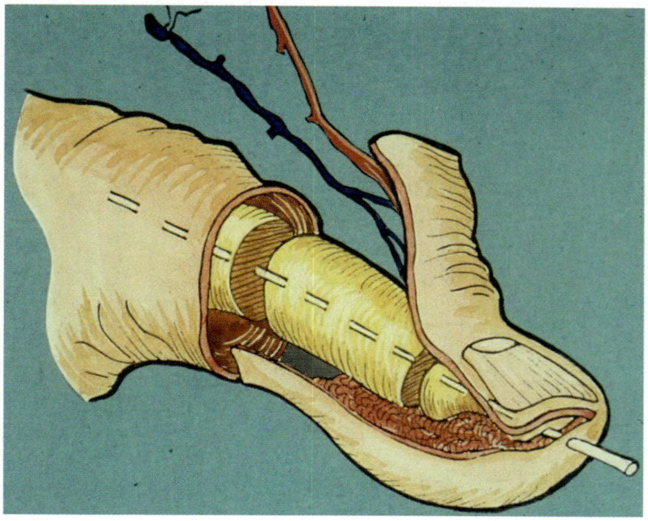

F

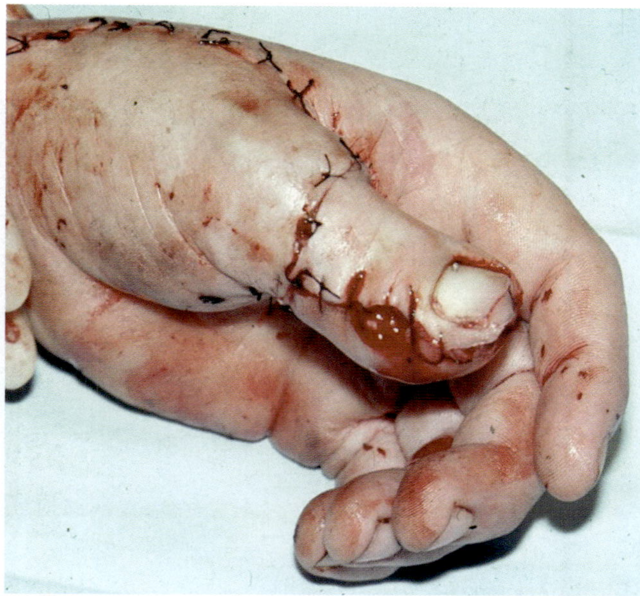

G

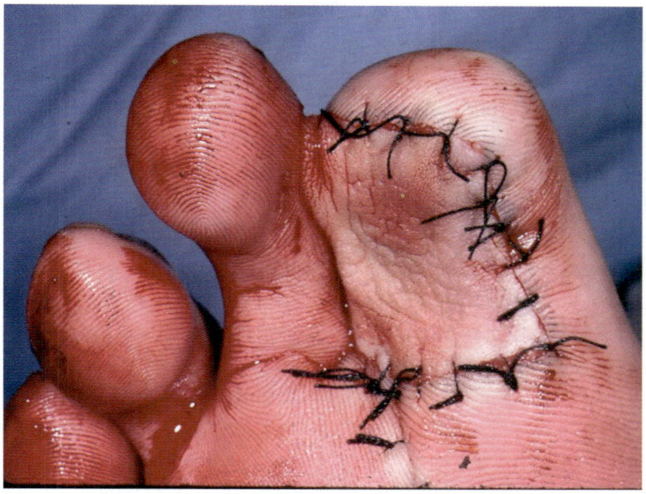

H

FIGURE 63-5 *(Continued)* (**F**) Iliac bone graft interposed. (**G**) Flap wrapped around iliac crest bone grafts. (**H**) Cross-toe flap.

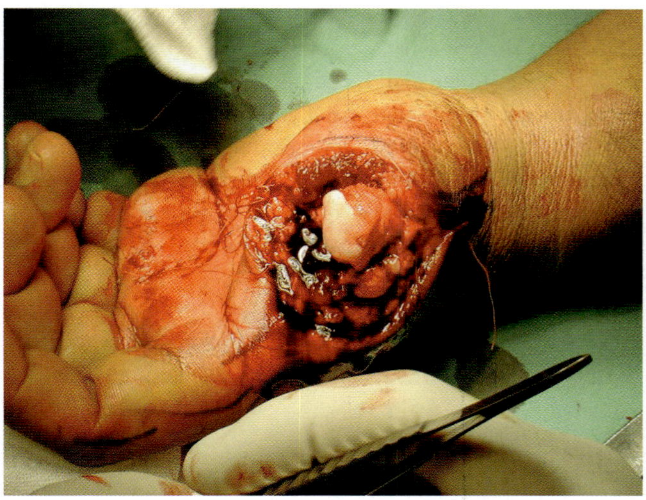

A

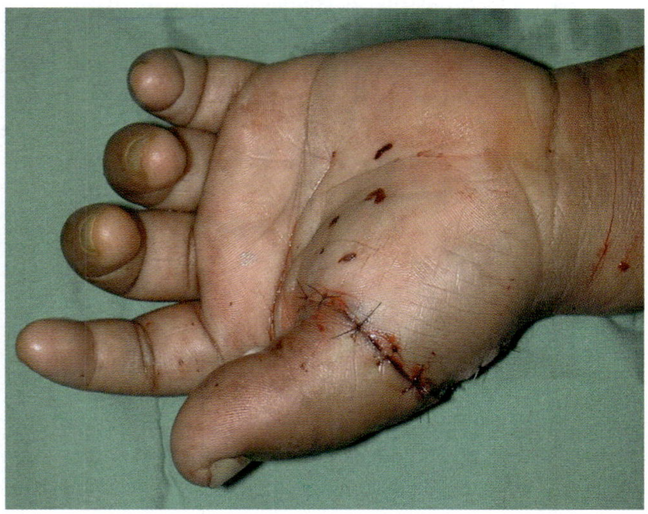

B

FIGURE 63-6 Case 1. (**A**) Amputated thumb through the metacarpophalangeal joint. (**B**) Hallux transfer.

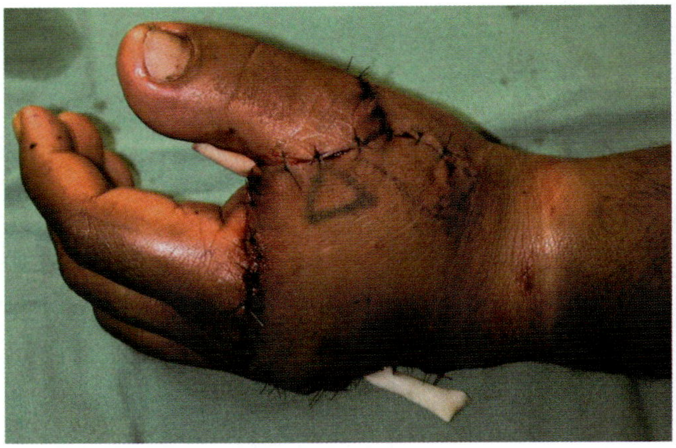

C

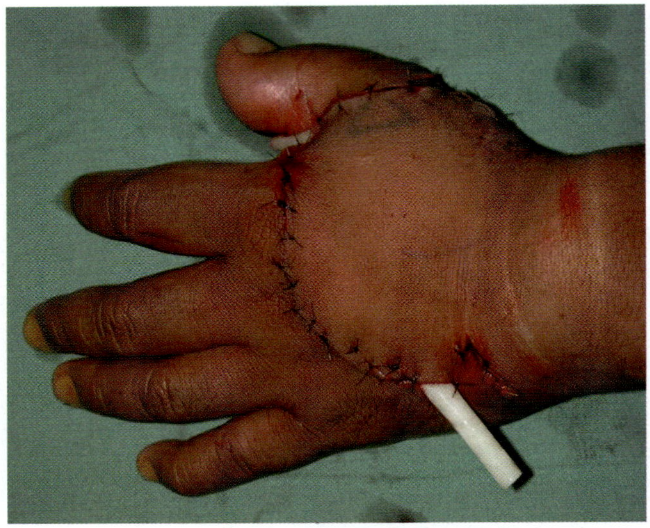

D

FIGURE 63-6 (*Continued*) (C) and (D) Dorsal hand rotation flap to facilitate closure.

Except for segmental toe flap transfers in which vessels may be taken distally in the foot, whole and modified toes will depend on the dorsal vasculature, and it is generally safer to harvest the vessels proximally at the dorsalis pedis level for anastomosis to the cephalic and radial artery systems.

In the hand, the dorsal branch of the radial artery and cephalic vein in the snuff box region are usually available for anastomosis. A wide tunnel should be created for the vessel pedicle over the first web and the dorsum of the first metacarpal to the proximal snuff box incision. It is unwise to use an incision to link the two sites because postoperative swelling may necessitate release of sutures and risk pedicle exposure.

BONE FIXATION

Bony fixation needs to be oriented such that when the toe is in opposition and abduction, it opposes to the pulps of the radial aspects of the index and middle fingers to form a tripod pinch. Exaggerated radial abduction can be used to compensate for mild first-web contracture. It is preferable for the new thumb to be on the short side because of its inevitable reduced flexibility. Initial axial Kirchner wire fixation through the joint allows rotation to be corrected, and it is then maintained with two crossed Kirschner wires, ideally leaving joints free so that the longitudinal pin can then be removed. Plating may be preferable for more proximal metacarpal osteosynthesis.

TENDON REPAIR

Whole and trimmed-toe transfers, which include joints unlike the wrap-around procedure, require tendon reconstruction. The hallux is bulky and stiff and masks any intrinsic tendon deficiency. This contrasts with the second toe, which has an extra joint and is intrinsically unstable. Here whereas the arc of rotation of the IP joint is predominantly in flexion, the metatarsophalangeal joint naturally extends. To counter this, the metatarsal fixation to the metacarpal should be angled volarward combined with dorsal capsulotomy of the metatarsophalangeal joint. A Kirschner wire is inserted longitudinally across the IP joints in full extension, and both flexor and extensor tendons are repaired under maximum tension. The wire is retained for 2 to 3 months if possible.

After avulsion injuries, the extensor pollicis brevis (EPB) and extensor pollicis longus (EPL) tendons may not be available in which case the extensor indicis proprius can be transferred for EPL reconstruction. The extensor hallucis brevis tendon resides on the ulnar side of the new thumb's extensor tendon when the ipsilateral toe is chosen and may be transferred beneath the extensor hallucis longus for repair of the EPB or discarded. Repair of the extensor brevis tendon of the second toe to the thumb EPB helps to tension the IP joints in extension. Repair of the short muscles of the thumb, when available, to the intrinsic tendons of the toes will stabilize and potentially afford some activation of extension of the toe IP joints.

VESSELS

The vascular pedicle should be tunneled over the dorsum of first metacarpal and delivered through a separate snuff box incision where the dorsal branch of the radial artery and cephalic veins have been prepared. End-to-end anastomoses here should be technically simple. For distal amputations in the region of the IP joint, wrap-around and trimmed-toe pedicles may be anastomosed to the dominant ulnar digital artery at the MCP joint crease level. Access to this vessel is difficult, and intimal damage may persist from the original injury.

NERVES

Both digital nerves are repaired to their toe counterparts.

SKIN CLOSURE

Thumb skin closure at the base of the toe is often difficult because of limited skin. Tight closure combined with postoperative swelling risks vascular compression, causing spasm and

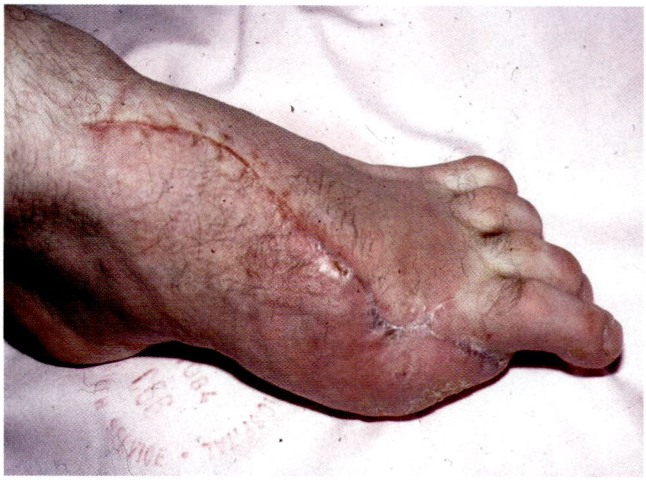

FIGURE 63-7 Hallux transfer foot closure.

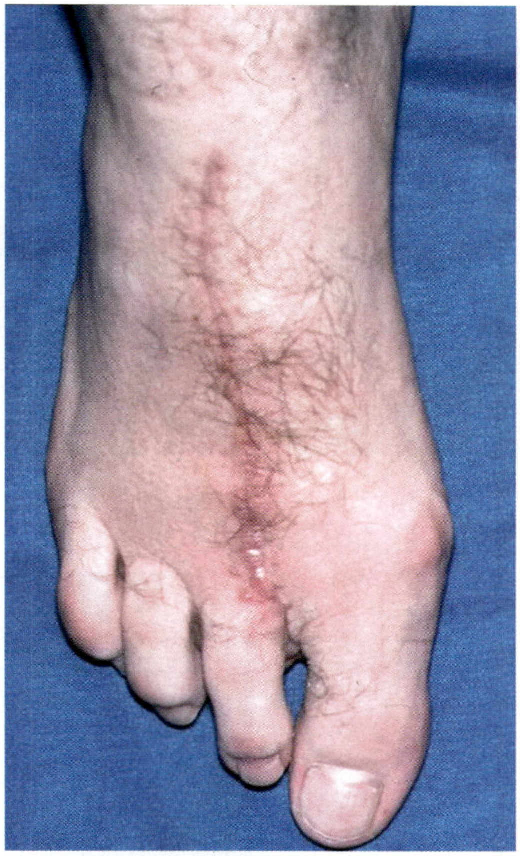

FIGURE 63-8 Second toe transfer foot closure.

thrombosis, and small skin grafts are preferable to tight closure even if they require secondary removal. Access incisions in the hand should avoid the direct path of the vascular pedicle so that even if they cannot be totally closed, skin grafts will not lie directly over exposed vessels.

In the foot, skin incisions for the big and second toes must be designed to permit direct closure of the toe stumps.

CASES

Case 1

This case demonstrates an amputation for tumor through the MCP joint with skin taken more proximally. Reconstruction was achieved using a hallux transfer taken at the MTP joint. The new MCP joint consisted of proximal thumb and distal toe joint surfaces. Skin shortage was closed with a rotation flap from the dorsum of the hand (see Figure 63-6).

Representative foot closure defects include the hallux transfer (Figure 63-7) and second toe transfer (Figure 63-8).

Case 2

A thumb amputation at the midmetacarpal level has been treated with the hallux transfer, including the dorsal metatarsal head and neck and collateral ligamentous system. Skin shortage was closed with an island dorsalis–pedis flap in continuity (Figure 63-9).

Case 3

A degloving amputation of the thumb through the proximal phalanx has been repaired with a wrap-around flap (Figure 63-10).

POSTOPERATIVE MONITORING

Bandaging should be loose, not circumferential, and allow as much visualization of the toe as possible. Monitoring is the same as for any free flap according to the conventions of the particular surgical team. Because of the tendency to spasm, the hand level should not be higher than the level of the heart.

COMPLICATIONS

Hand

The main anxiety is anastomotic thrombosis and meticulous discipline to the principles of microvascular surgery, especially ensuring normal recipient vessels, is paramount to success. Wide tunnels and loose skin closure to prevent vessel kinking and compression have been mentioned.

Foot

Wound breakdown from flap edge necrosis is best avoided by planning access incisions that conserve skin on the foot and minimize undermining. Longitudinal incisions directly over the vascular pedicle are preferable to curvilinear or especially Z-shaped designs that have no logic.

SECONDARY SURGERY

Secondary surgery is unusual after toe transfers and is especially hazardous to blood vessels and nerves. Stiff but stable thumbs are preferable to mobile, unstable ones, and although tendon adhesions are common, the benefits of tenolysis are limited because there is a real risk of damage to neurovascular structures. Debulking procedures for the hallux may be considered, and a midline

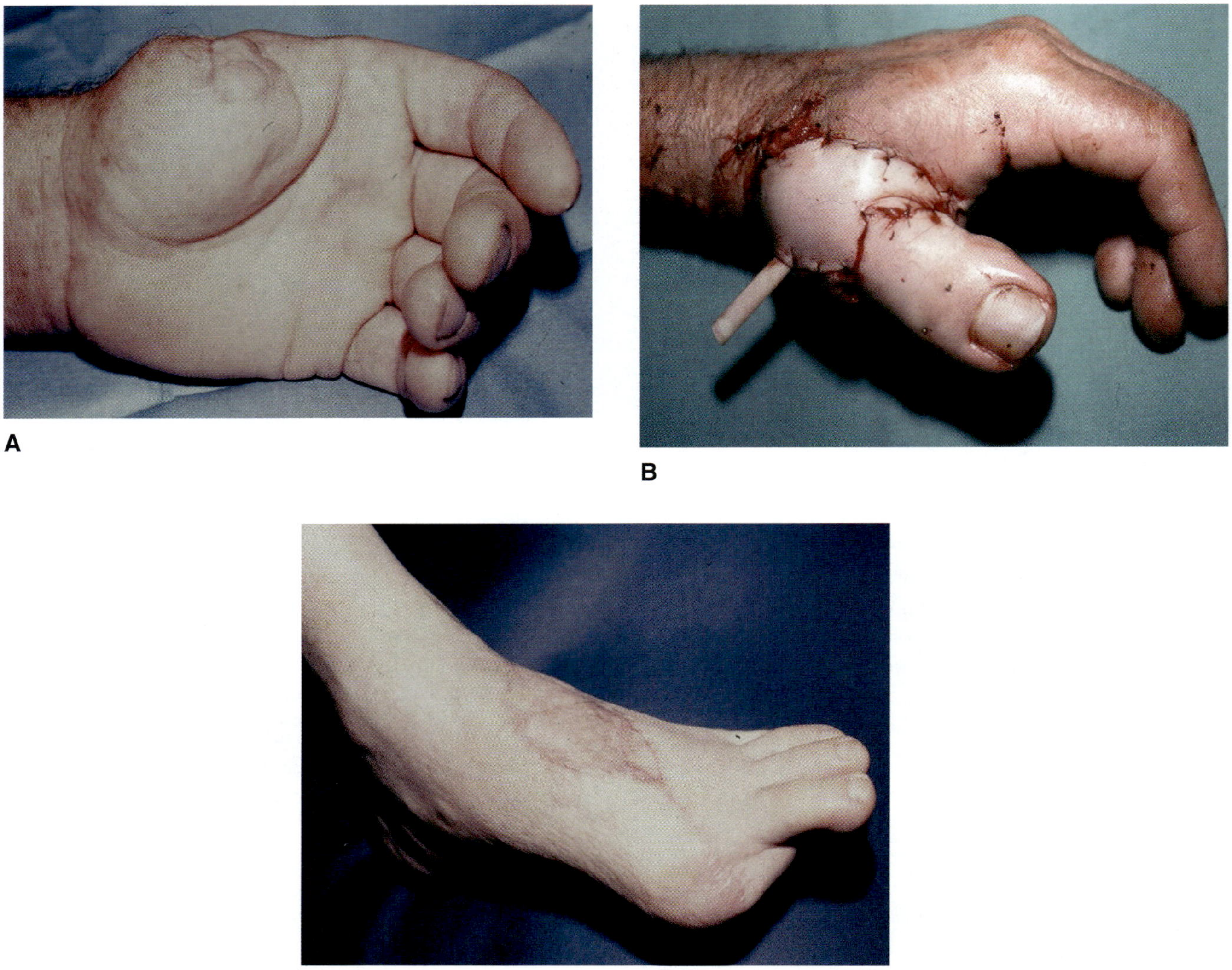

A B C

FIGURE 63-9 Case 2. (**A**) Amputated thumb through the metacarpal. (**B**) Closure with a dorsalis pedis island flap in continuity with the big toe transfer. (**C**) Foot closure, skin graft to proximal foot.

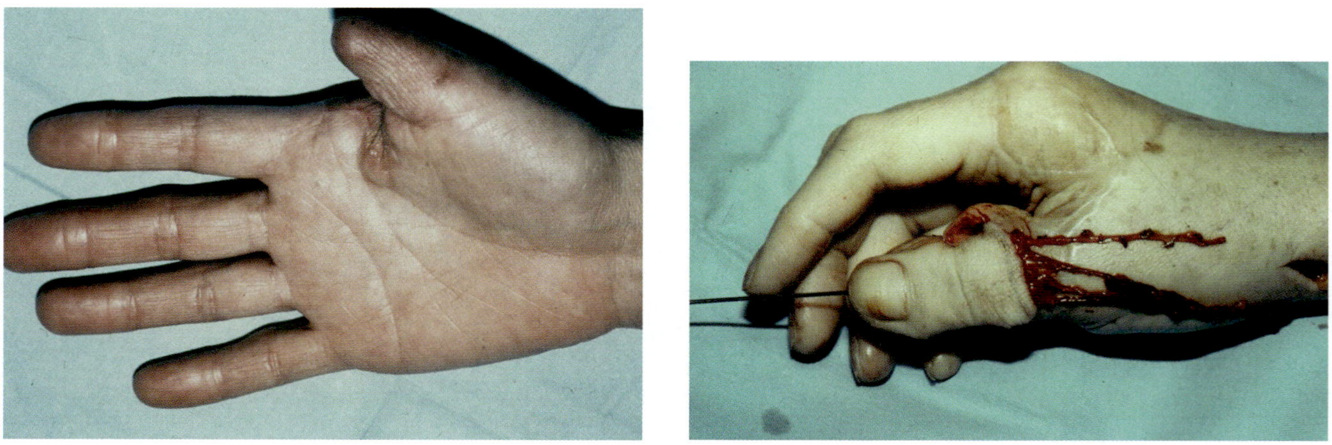

A B

FIGURE 63-10 Case 3. (**A**) Amputation through the proximal phalanx associated with degloving. (**B**) Wrap-around flap: intraoperative view.

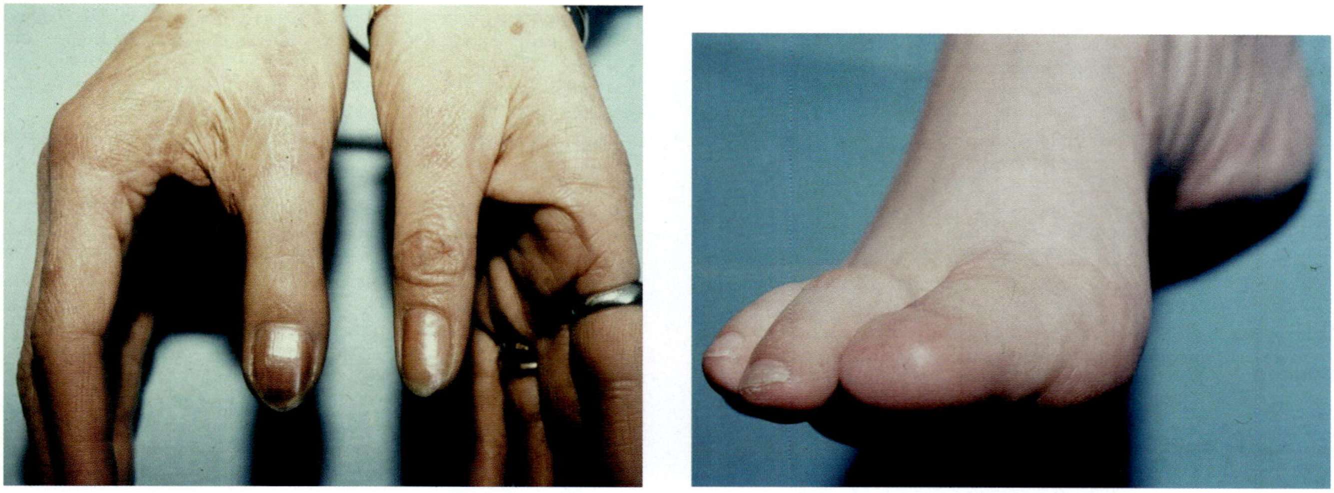

C D

FIGURE 63-10 *(Continued)* (**C**) Result at 2 years. (**D**) Foot defect.

longitudinal elliptical pulp excision can improve appearance considerably in both whole and partial toe transfers (24,25). However, the shape and size of the toes are determined by their skeletons, and unless bony reduction is done such as with the trimmed-toe procedure, then the obvious bulky characteristics of the hallux will remain.

RESULTS

In plastic surgery, it is said that "nothing ruins a good result like a long term follow up" (26). Toe transfers by contrast improve with time and their functional results are generally very good, especially for subtotal amputations (12,15–19). Toes naturally contain all of the characteristics of a thumb apart from cosmetic size match. The range of movement of the IP joint is limited, but it is stable, and pinch is strong because this is largely determined by adductor function, which in most cases remains preserved. Sensory return depends on the honesty of the examiner, the level and nature of the original nerve injury, and the age of the patient. Two-point discrimination is variably reported as optimistically matching the normal thumb to considerably more conservative and more realistic estimates. Aesthetically, the reconstruction that most closely matches the normal thumb is the wrap-around technique, but this is only applicable in amputations distal to the MCP joint.

Foot

Scars, skin grafts, and neuromas on the foot are a potential source of chronic discomfort and ulceration, leading to problems with footwear. This particularly applies to grafts over the distal portion of the toe stump where excessive skin has been removed.

FUTURE

Happily for those who would find it difficult to accept the concept of a toe transfer as a trade-off for a new thumb, they are less likely to have to face the decision because of increased workplace safety and a steady decline in traumatic accidents.

As continuing evolutionary pressures force the thumb to expand and toes to shrink, nature might eventually provide the perfect match with a donor bred for transfer, and patients will again give the "thumbs up" to toe transfers. Alternatively, our tissue engineers might be able to regenerate a thumb from "pixie dust" (27). Until then the plastic surgeon's urge to express his or her artistic bent and inventive flare with one of our few remaining "show and tell" operations needs to be tempered by the reality that the owners of the toes have the last say. No longer are patients in the thrall of the eminent and daring surgeon, and they are reluctant to entrust their toes on a voyage to unknown or uncertain destinations.

For the moment, toe transfer remains a niche operation for limited application by select surgeons. In the right place, on the right patient, and using the right toe choice, it can be a truly spectacular and elegant procedure that restores immediate and unrivalled function to the thumb and with appropriate planning and care minimal morbidity.

REFERENCES

1. Nicoladoni C. Daumenplasfik und Organischer Ersatz der Fingerspitze. *Arch Clin Chri* 1900;61:606.
2. Nicoladoni C. Wien Klin Wochenschr. *Daumenplasfik* 1897;10:663.
3. Huemer GM. Carl Nicoladoni and the concept of toe-to-hand transfer at the turn of the nineteenth century. *Plast Reconstr Surg* 2005;115(5): 1432–1433.
4. Clarkson P, Furlong R. Thumb reconstruction by transfer of big toe. *Br Med J* 1949;2(4640):1332.
5. Buncke HJ Jr, Buncke CM, Schulz WP. Immediate Nicoladoni procedure in the Rhesus monkey or hallux-to-hand transplantation, utilising microminiature vascular anastomoses. *Br J Plast Surg* 1966;19(4): 332–337.
6. Cobbett JR. Free digital transfer. Report of a case of transfer of a great toe to replace an amputated thumb. *J Bone Joint Surg Br* 1969;51(4): 677–679.
7. Buncke HJ Jr, McLean DH, George PT, et al. Thumb replacement: great toe transplantation by microvascular anastomosis. *Br J Plast Surg* 1973;26(3):194–201.
8. Yang DY. Thumb reconstruction by free second toe transplantation. Report of 40 cases. [Chinese]. *Clin J Surg* 1977;15:13.
9. O'Brien BM, MacLeod AM, et al. Hallux-to-hand transfer. *Hand* 1975;7(2):128–133.

10. Chung KC, Wei FC. An outcome study of thumb reconstruction using microvascular toe transfer. *J Hand Surg Am* 2000;25(4):651–658.
11. Morrison WA, O'Brien BM, MacLeod AM. Thumb reconstruction with a free neurovascular wrap-around flap from the big toe. *J Hand Surg Am* 1980;5(6):575–583.
12. Morrison WA, O'Brien BM, MacLeod AM. Experience with thumb reconstruction. *J Hand Surg* 1984;9(3):223–233.
13. Doi K, Kuwata N, Kawai S. Reconstruction of the thumb with a free wrap-around flap from the big toe and an iliac-bone graft. *J Bone Joint Surg Am* 1985;67(3):439–445.
14. Wei FC, Chen HC, Chuang CC, Noordhoff MS. Reconstruction of the thumb with a trimmed-toe transfer technique. *Plast Reconstr Surg* 1988;82(3):506–515.
15. Poppen NK, Norris TR, Buncke HJ Jr. Evaluation of sensibility and function with microsurgical free tissue transfer of the great toe to the hand for thumb reconstruction. *J Hand Surg Am* 1983;8(5 Pt 1):516–531.
16. Frykman GK, O'Brien BM, Morrison WA, et al. Functional evaluation of the hand and foot after one-stage toe-to-hand transfer. *J Hand Surg Am* 1986;11(1):9–17.
17. Gulgonen A, Gudemez E. Toe-to-hand transfers: more than 20 years follow-up of five post-traumatic cases. *J Hand Surg Br* 2006;31(1):2–8.
18. Buncke GM, Buncke HJ, Lee CK. Great toe-to-thumb microvascular transplant after traumatic amputation. *Hand Clin* 2007;23(1):105–115.
19. Kotkansalo T, Vilkki SK, Elo P, Luukkaala T. Long term functional results of microvascular toe-to-thumb reconstruction. *J Hand Surg Eur* 2011; 36(3):194–204.
20. Maloney CT, DeJesus R, Dellon AL. Painful foot neuromas after toe-to-thumb transfer. *J Hand Surg Am* 2005;30(1):105–110.
21. Zhao J., Tien HY, Abdullah S, Zhang Z, Aesthetic refinements in second toe-to-thumb transfer surgery. *Plast Reconstr Surg* 2010;126(6): 2052–2059.
22. Gilbert A, Daniller A, Strauch B (eds). Composite tissue transfer from the foot: anatomic basis and surgical technique. In Daniller A, Strauch B, (eds). *Symposium on Microsurgery*, vol. 15. St. Louis: CV Mosby, 1976.
23. Willemart G, Kane A, Morrison WA. Island dorsalis pedis skin flap in combination with toe or toe segment transfer based on the same vascular pedicle. *Plast Reconstr Surg* 1999;104(5):1424–1429.
24. O'Brien B, Morrison WA. *Reconstructive Microsurgery*. St. Louis: Churchill Livingstone 1987; 294–308, 359–369.
25. May JW Jr. Aesthetic and functional thumb reconstruction: great toe to hand transfer. *Clin Plast Surg* 1981;8(2):357–362.
26. Krisek T. Personal communication, 1999.
27. Badylak. Pixie dust. 2010.

CHAPTER 64

Toe-to-Hand Transfers for Finger Reconstruction

Wee-Leon Lam and Fu-Chan Wei

BRIEF HISTORY OF CONVENTIONAL OPTIONS

In the history of hand surgery, reconstruction of fingers has probably played a less dominant role than the thumb when dealing with the severely injured hand. In general, if the major prehensions of key pinch, lateral pinch, and power grasp are grossly preserved, then finger reconstruction was not seen as a worthwhile venture.

Increasing demands from modern-day employment, hobbies, and psychological concerns have probably led to new indications for finger reconstruction. Before the advent of microsurgery, various conventional "nonmicrosurgical" methods have been attempted to improve the function of either single finger loss or to treat the metacarpal hand, including phalangization with first web space deepening (1), distraction lengthening (2), and the use of nonvascularized bone blocks with pedicled flaps for finger reconstruction (3). Most of these methods were either ineffective in restoring a satisfactory prehensile pattern or require a lengthy rehabilitation period with multiple procedures. Without effective restoration of length and sensibility, hand function continues to be compromised, and the search continued for a more optimum method of finger reconstruction.

The introduction of toe-to-hand transfers has allowed the possibility of replacing missing fingers and missing components of fingers with almost identical composite tissues through a single-stage surgery with minimal donor morbidity. With technical refinements and increased experience, there is now a wealth of literature that bears testament to the acceptance of toe-to-hand transfer as the "gold standard" in replacing missing fingers and its established superiority over other nonmicrosurgical and conventional methods (4,5). This chapter highlights some of the important principles and recent advances using toe-to-hand transfer techniques for finger reconstruction. Readers are referred to other chapters for some of the surgical aspects, including toe harvest and anatomical considerations as well as toe-to-finger transfer for congenital anomalies, with the focus in this chapter mainly on the initial assessment, decision making, flap inset, and outcomes in traumatic finger amputation reconstruction.

INDICATIONS FOR THE SPECIFIC TOE TRANSFER

Despite the initial hesitations in the use of toes for finger or finger component reconstruction, there are now various established options. Certain guidelines can be drawn from examination of the injured hand that facilitates subsequent decision-making for choosing the right type of toe flap, with three main considerations: the level of amputation, which finger(s) is (are) involved and whether the amputation is single or multiple.

Proximal or Distal Finger Reconstruction

Proximal or distal amputation is defined by its relation to the insertion of the flexor digitorum superficialis (FDS) tendon (6), generally considered to be the base of the middle phalanx. Distal to this level, the fingertip is considered the end organ of touch (7), with the volar pulp and its accompanying glabrous skin that prevents excessive gliding and shearing and a nonslippery surface for grasping, with the highest innervation density compared with anywhere else on the body surface. On the dorsal surface, the nail plays an important functional role in facilitating sensibility of tip pinch, as well as an aesthetic role.

In our experience, successful toe-to-hand transfers for distal finger amputation can universally produce satisfying outcomes, as achieved by a wide variety of options, including the use of vascularized nail grafts (8,9), pulp flaps (10), wrap-around flaps (11), and the partial second or third toe (12) depending on what tissues are missing. These operations are rewarding because of the rapid and one-stage restoration of function and cosmesis without significant donor site morbidity (Figure 64-1).

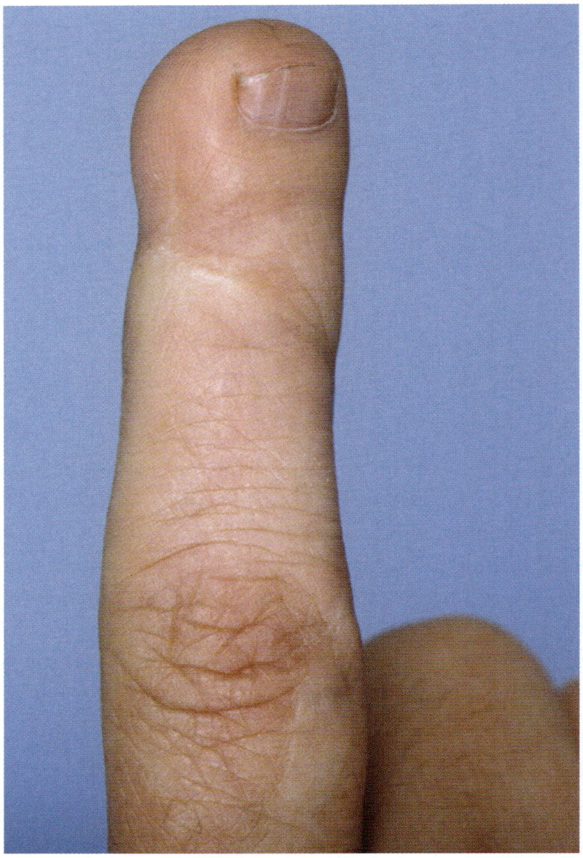

A

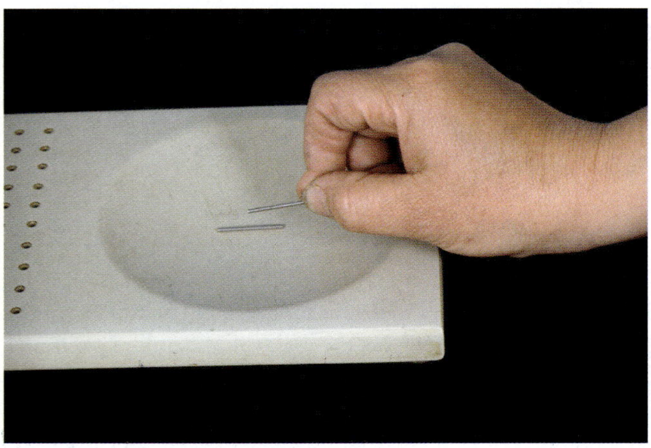

B

FIGURE 64-1 (**A**) and (**B**) Second toe-to-hand transfer for distal finger reconstruction. Note the satisfactory length and appearance achieved. Finger function is usually excellent because of preservation of the proximal interphalangeal joint.

In contrast to distal finger amputations, free toe transfers or even replantation of single proximal finger amputations has often been considered as unnecessary or even contraindicated. Both replantation as well as toe-to-hand transfer for fingers amputated at this level has been the subject of debate for many years (13). A reconstructed finger that is unable to flex at the proximal interphalangeal joint is considered more of a liability than an asset to the patient. Another concern relates to the length of the reconstructed finger. In distal finger amputation, the second toe transfer is always able to restore its original length to produce a more desirable aesthetic appearance. However, a toe reconstruction to replace a proximal finger amputation will typically result in a shorter finger and consequently a more unnatural looking hand. Therefore, a toe transfer for a single proximal finger amputation should only be offered to selected patients who are very clear about their goals and who are willing to accept the limitations of a proximal toe transfer. Furthermore, single proximal finger toe-to-hand transfer should only be considered for index and middle finger amputation because of the limited total active movement (TAM) that can be expected and should not be carried out for the ring and little fingers if the objective is to achieve a better power grip.

Multiple Finger Reconstruction

Decision making for patients with multiple finger amputations are largely guided by the specific occupational and cosmetic needs of the patient. In general, two adjacent fingers should be reconstructed wherever possible to allow a stable, tripod pinch or hook grip (14,15), lateral stability, a stronger hook grip, and a wider span for grasping larger objects compared with single pulp-to-pulp pinch (16) (Figure 64-2). In our experience, patients who received single toe transfer for pulp-to-pulp pinch often complained of opposing fingers slipping off each other while trying to make a firm pinch. There is also a tendency of the isolated reconstructed finger to go into ulnar deviation without the stabilizing effect of the intermetacarpal ligaments (Figure 64-3). The reconstruction of a tripod pinch seems to prevent this from happening by providing a counter force on the ulnar side of the finger. The reconstruction of two adjacent fingers can be accomplished either by bilateral toe transfers (either the second or third toe) or a combined second and third or third and fourth toe transfers depending on the integrity of the web space. If the amputations are distal to the web space, bilateral lesser toes are preferred to prevent a syndactylous appearance. If the amputations are proximal to the web space, then a combined two-toe unit is recommended to replace the missing fingers as well as reconstruct the web space in one setting (17). Another guiding factor is the length of the remaining finger; which should not be longer than that of a normal little finger when considering combined second and third toe transfers to ensure a smooth finger arcade during cylinder-grasp prehension. We have previously recommended the preferential reconstruction of the radial two fingers for patients who require fine pinch and the ulnar two fingers for manual workers who require a strong grip (17). However, we have found that in the latter

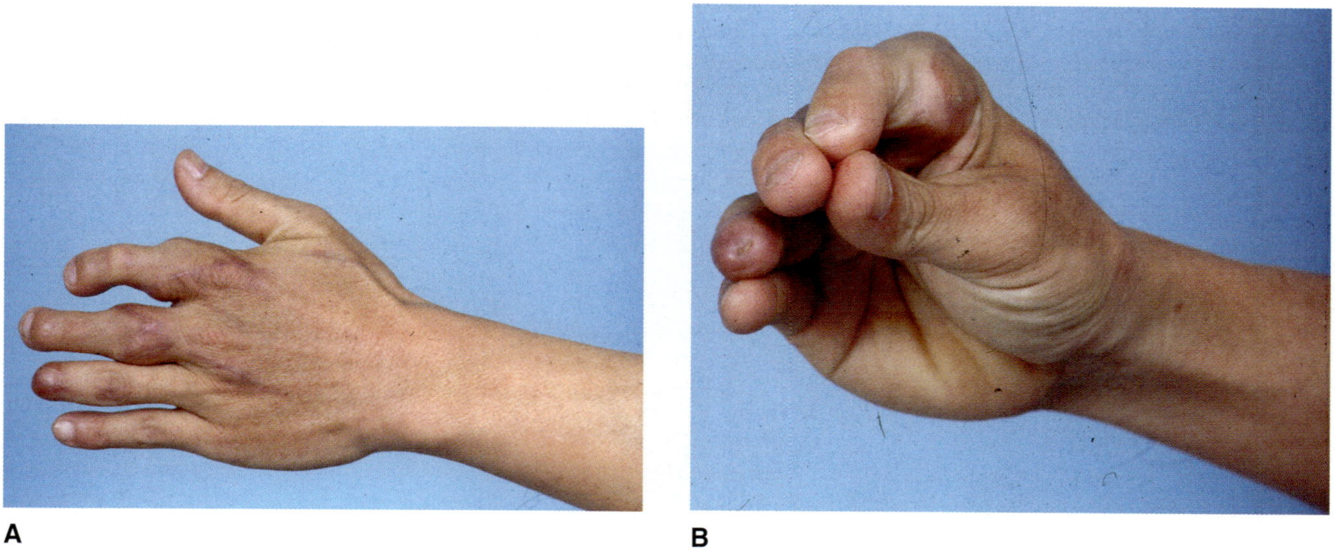

FIGURE 64-2 (**A**) and **B**) Reconstruction of a tripod pinch allowing increased lateral stability, a stronger hook grip, and a wider span.

group, a central reconstruction (middle and ring) often produces a better outcome because even the most perfect ulnar construct may not be able to fulfill its goal in recreating the power grasp because of the limited range of motion. The different toe flaps and their commoner indications are as listed in Table 64-1.

Metacarpal Hand Reconstruction

A classification system based on reconstructive options and different stages of injury has been proposed for the metacarpal hand from our department (15,18) that takes into account the level of finger amputations and involvement of the thumb (Tables 64-2 and 64-3). This classification system grades the severity of injury and provides guidelines for different reconstructive strategies. Type I refers to an injury with four-finger proximal amputations without the thumb or only distal thumb involvement that still preserves its functional length (distal to the interphalangeal [IP] joint). In type IA injuries in which the finger amputation level is distal to the metacarpophalangeal (MCP) joint, the choice is between bilateral lesser toes or a combined toe unit for the reconstruction of adjacent digits, depending on the integrity of the web space. In type IB injuries, in which the amputation level is through the joints with intact articular surfaces, combined second and third toes can be transferred as composite joint transfers. More proximal injuries (type IC) in which the finger amputation level is proximal to the MCP joints usually require the harvest of combined second and third toes as transmetatarsal transfers (Figure 64-4).

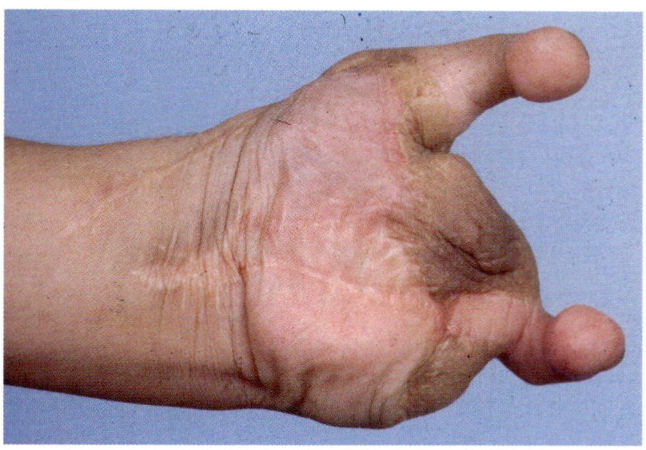

FIGURE 64-3 Single pulp-to-pulp toe reconstruction showing the tendency of the reconstructed toe to go into ulnar deviation.

Type II metacarpal hand injuries describe four-finger proximal amputations but with thumb amputation proximal to its functional length. The reconstruction of fingers follow a similar decision-making process as for type I defects, but reconstruction of the thumb is determined by the presence or absence of a functional thenar musculature. If the thenar muscle is intact or possesses adequate function (types IIa and IIb), a one-stage procedure to reconstruct the thumb and two adjacent fingers is recommended. If the thenar muscle is inadequate (IIC), the thumb reconstruction should be delayed until after the finger reconstruction, with the thumb position and length first determined by the aid of a prosthesis while the reconstructed fingers assume their final positions (Figure 64-5). Reconstruction of thumb defects in type II metacarpal hand obviously has implications for donor site morbidity. When the left great toe (our preferred option) has been used for thumb reconstruction, then the donor site for finger transfers has to be shifted to the third toe on the ipsilateral foot for a single toe harvest or the other foot for a combined second and third toe.

Decision making in bilateral metacarpal hand injuries can be incredibly complex and requires a careful discussion with the patient regarding a balance between the reconstructive goals and an acceptable level of donor morbidity. Bilateral type II injuries may require up to but not exceed five donor toes to achieve a functional level of prehension (19) without causing excessive gait disturbance. In general, a great toe is usually harvested from the left foot for the dominant thumb

TABLE 64-1 Indications for Various Toe Transfers or Toe Components for Finger Reconstruction

Types of Toe Flaps	Indications
	Distal Finger
Vascularized nail graft	• Traumatic dorsal fingertip amputations • Nail reconstruction after tumor excision • Painful or aesthetically unacceptable nails (e.g., posttraumatic nail hook deformity)
Pulp and hemi-pulp flap	• Small volar pulp defects for dominant sides of fingers where sensation is critical • Resurfacing of unstable or painful scar (e.g., previous failed or unsatisfactory skin grafts or local flaps)
Lesser toe wrap around flap	• Reconstruction of circumferential or dorsal hemi-circumferential loss of skin and nail (distal to the proximal portion of the middle phalanx) • Partial distal thumb degloving injury
Partial toe flap (second or third) (complete unit harvested distal to the proximal interphalangeal joint)	• Distal finger reconstruction (distal to the insertion of the flexor digitorum superficialis or an intact proximal interphalangeal joint)
	Proximal Finger
Total second toe flap (harvested at proximal phalangeal level as a composite joint or transmetatarsal level)	• Reconstruction of isolated proximal finger amputation (in carefully selected patients only; see text) • Preferred choice for congenital hand reconstruction • Thumb reconstruction for nondominant hand in the metacarpal hand • As bilateral second toes for reconstruction of tripod pinch in amputations distal to the web space (multiple finger amputations and metacarpal hand; see Tables 64-2 and 64-3)
Third toe flap	Similar indications to the second toe but for use when: • The second toe is not available or not suitable for transfer as a result of previous injury, surgery, or deformity • The second toe has been reserved or used for thumb reconstruction • The second toe is located in the same foot where the great toe has been removed (usually for thumb reconstruction in bilateral metacarpal hands). • The third toe provides a better size match for finger reconstruction than the second toe
	Multiple Fingers
Combined second and third toe flap	• Reconstruction of tripod pinch in amputations proximal to the web space for multiple finger amputations (the remaining finger must not be shorter than the little finger) • Reconstruction of tripod pinch in amputations proximal to the web space for the metacarpal hand (see Tables 64-2 and 64-3)
Combined third and fourth toe flap	Similar to the combined second and third toe flap but for use when: • The second toe is needed for gait preservation • The second toe has been planned for thumb or other finger reconstruction (as in bilateral type II metacarpal hand) • The second toe is unavailable

TABLE 64-2 Type I Metacarpal Hand Classification and Recommended Toe Transfer Reconstruction

Classification	Level of Finger Amputation	Finger Reconstruction
IA	Amputation distal to MCP joint	Combined second and third toe or third and fourth toe transfers with osteosynthesis at proximal phalanxes
IB	Amputation through MCP joint with intact joint articular surface	Combined second and third toe or third and fourth toe transfers with composite joint repair for stabilization
IC	Amputation proximal to MCP joint	Combined second and third toe or third and fourth toe transfers with osteosynthesis at metacarpus

MCP, metacarpophalangeal.

TABLE 64-3 Type II Metacarpal Hand Classification and Recommended Toe Transfer Reconstruction

Classification	Level of Thumb Amputation	Finger Reconstruction	Thumb Reconstruction	Stage
IIA	Distal to the metacarpal neck	Combined second and third toe or third and fourth toe	Whole or trimmed great toe	Simultaneous fingers and thumb reconstruction
IIB	Proximal to the metacarpal neck with adequate thenar muscle function	Combined second and third toe or third and fourth toe	Whole or trimmed great toe after metacarpal lengthening or bone augmentation Transmetatarsal second toe	Simultaneous fingers and thumb reconstruction
IIC	Any level with inadequate thenar musculature	Combined second and third toe or third and fourth toe	Same as in IIA or IIB Tendon transfer to restore opposition may be needed	Staged with fingers reconstruction first
IID	Any level with damaged carpometacarpal joint	Combined second and third toe or third and fourth toe	Same as in IIA or IIB Immobile thumb post	Staged with fingers reconstruction first

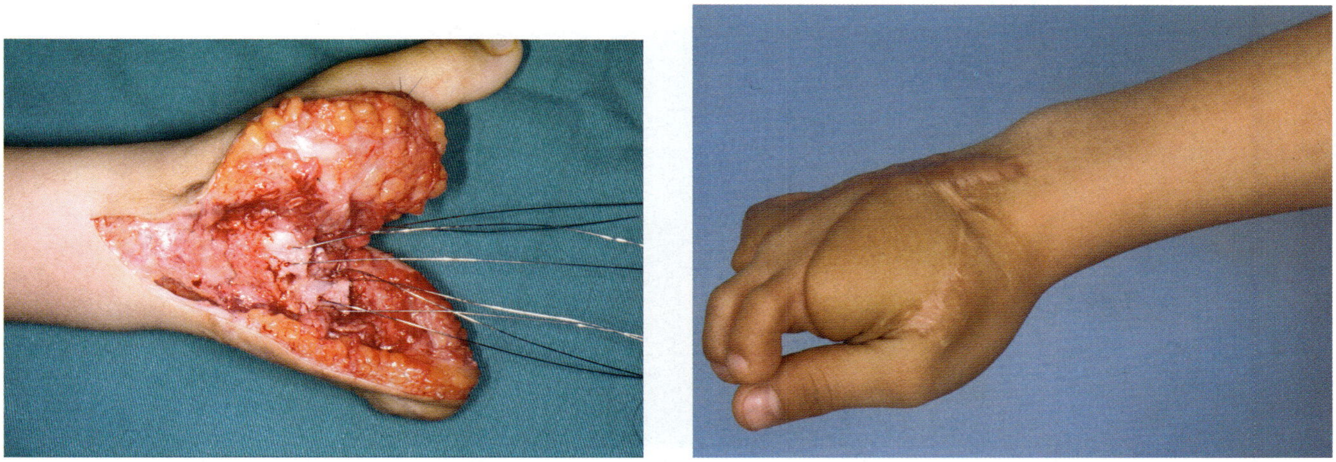

A **B**

FIGURE 64-4 (**A**) and (**B**) Reconstruction of a metacarpal hand defect that is proximal to the web space with combined second and third toe transfers.

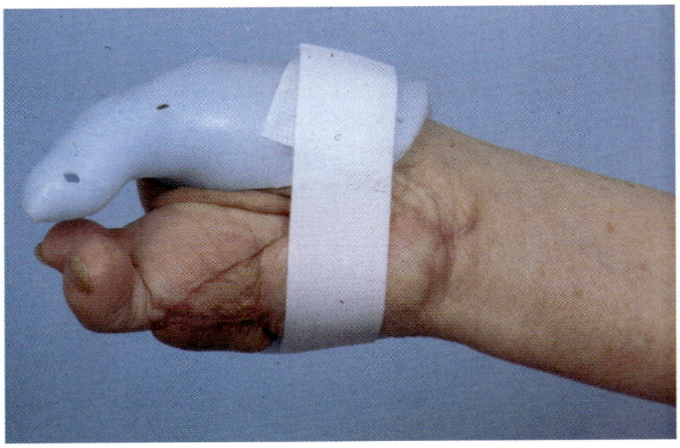

FIGURE 64-5 The use of a temporary prosthesis for type IIC metacarpal hand to predetermine the length and position of the future thumb.

reconstruction together with a combined two-toe reconstruction from the opposite foot to achieve a tripod pinch. In the nondominant hand, single finger pulp-to-pulp pinch is considered adequate with the use of a lesser toe for both thumb and one-finger reconstruction (19) (Figure 64-6).

PREPARATION OF RECIPIENT SITE

Preparation of the Recipient Site During Initial Debridement

Preparation of the recipient site starts with initial management of the injured hand. If toe-to-hand transfers are planned, all viable lengths of bone, tendons, and neurovascular bundles should be carefully preserved to facilitate the future toe transfer. By maximal preservation of all relevant anatomical structures, extensive dissection of the toe and the need for nerve, tendon, and vein grafts during toe transfer becomes less necessary. Excessive shortening of the digital skeleton to achieve primary closure of the wound should also be avoided. Bone stumps as short as 5.0 mm in length can be used for effective osteosynthesis with intraosseous wiring in toe-to-hand transfers (20). An intact MCP joint cartilage surface should be preserved for composite joint repair during toe transfer. Preservation of the extensor mechanism in the finger is important for maintaining a balanced function between the intrinsic and extrinsic systems to achieve good extensor function and to avoid a boutonniere deformity. Conservative debridement of the flexor tendons

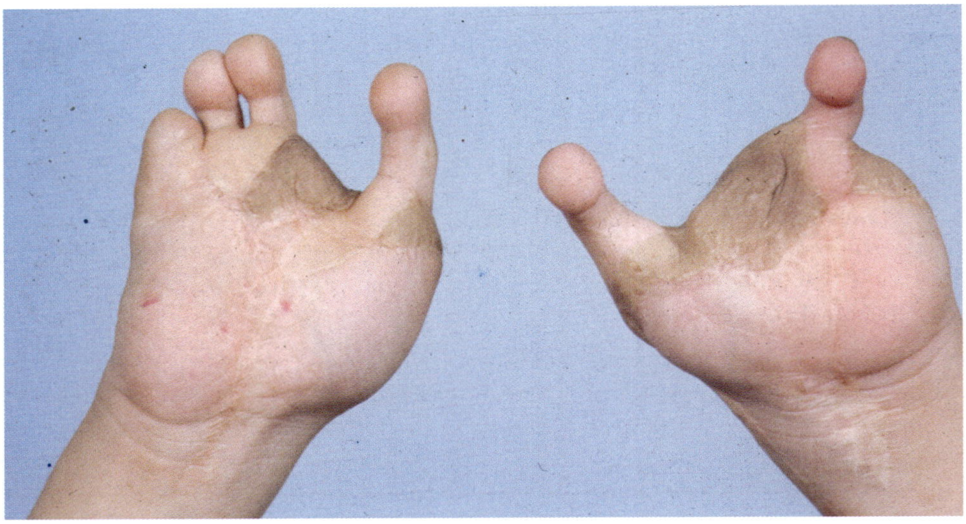

A

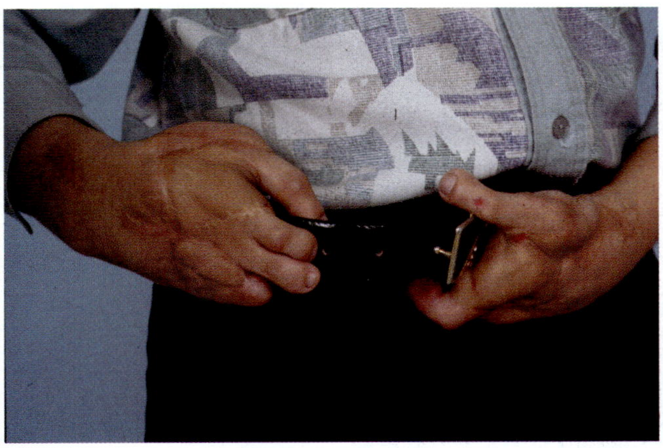

B

FIGURE 64-6 (**A**) and (**B**) Reconstruction of bilateral metacarpal hands with a total of five toes to provide a tripod pinch on the right dominant hand and a single pulp-to-pulp pinch on the nondominant hand.

should be performed for the same reasons. The traditional "pull-and-cut" method of digital nerves to prevent neuroma formation should be prohibited. For coverage of skin defects, the use of local flaps must be avoided because they may increase scarring and sacrifice a potential recipient vessel for future toe transfer. If additional soft tissue and skin cover is needed, a better option is offered by a distant pedicled groin flap, which can also be used for the creation of an adequate web space. Furthermore, excess skin on the recipient hand subsequently allows less dorsal foot skin to be harvested with the transferred toe, affording direct closure of the donor site and overall better cosmesis (21).

Primary versus Secondary Toe-to-Hand Transfers

The optimal timing for performing toe-to-hand transfers depends on the severity of the injury, the condition of the wound, the patient's ability to comprehend information, surgeon's training and background, and hospital facilities. Primary transfer is defined as performing the toe transfer when the wound is still open, which can be acute, subacute, or chronic. A primary toe-to-hand transfer can be safely performed provided the debridement and washout can convert the wound into a clean bed, with success and complication rates similar to that of secondary reconstruction (22). In contrast to primary transfer, a secondary transfer is performed only after the wound is completely healed, achieved either by a pedicled groin flap or direct closure. The timing for secondary transfer is usually months after the original injury. In properly selected patients, a primary reconstruction is recommended to facilitate a one-stage procedure, earlier rehabilitation, and return to work.

Preparation of Recipient Site During Toe-to-Hand Transfer

Whether primary or secondary toe-to-hand transfer is being performed, appropriate initial management of the injured hand allows a smooth transition between the initial debridement and the subsequent inset of the toe transfer. Because the actual procedure of toe harvest is discussed in detail in other chapters, only the salient points as they relate to flap inset will be mentioned here.

Two-Team Approach

A two-team approach is advocated in which one team harvests the toe(s) and the other prepares the recipient site and allows for less operative and anesthetic time, as well as for less surgeon fatigue and stress. To avoid unnecessary dissection in the foot, the two teams should have constant communication regarding the required lengths of tendons, nerves, and vessels.

Incisions

Cruciate incisions are always used in the stump (23,24); the objective is to create four equal triangular skin flaps that will interdigitate with the V-shaped flaps of the transplanted toe (25). The skin flaps are adequately undermined to remove all scar and redundant subcutaneous tissues at the amputated stumps and to permit adequate mobility and a telescoping effect, which can prevent an unappealing, bulbous "cobra"-shaped deformity at the toe–finger stump junction.

Vessels (Artery and Vein) Preparation

After adequate exposure, care is taken to identify suitable recipient vessels for anastomoses. By definition, a good recipient artery is one that should spurt spontaneously and forcefully, and this should be dissected proximally until a healthy stump is found. After it is located, it should be meticulously dissected for an adequate distance with careful stripping of the adventitia layer to reduce the risk of vasospasm.

For distal finger reconstruction, a separate incision at the ulnar side (index, middle, and ring fingers) or radial side (little finger) of the proximal phalanx or distal palm can be made to identify the proper digital or common digital artery for anastomosis. A tunnel can then be made between the proximal recipient artery and the amputation stump. Skeletonizing of the neurovascular bundles is useful to permit smooth tunneling. For more proximal amputations, the common digital arteries or the superficial palmar arch are all possible options. Although more commonly used for the thumb than fingers, another useful recipient vessel is the radial artery in the anatomical snuff box. A separate incision in the snuff box is usually required to access this vessel, with additional benefits being the simultaneous identification of the terminal branches of the cephalic vein for venous anastomosis. If two separate incisions are used, the subcutaneous tunnel must be wide enough to allow passing of the donor vessel without compression.

Although the vein:artery anastomosis ratio has been recommended to be 2:1 by some authors, in our experience, usually one venous anastomosis is sufficient. Usually veins on the dorsal aspect of the finger or hand are dissected and used as the recipient vessel. In judging the suitability of the vein, good backflow indicates adequate drainage because the external appearance alone is not reliable.

Bone and Joint Preparation

With the use of intraosseous wires as a stable form of osteosynthesis, only a bone length of 0.5 cm is necessary to allow the periosteal dissection to be kept to a minimum to maximize the blood supply to the bone ends. Further trimming of the bone edges with either a burr or oscillating saw to produce a smooth bony stump surface facilitates good contact and promotes osteosynthesis with the transferred toe. If composite joint repair is planned, the joint capsule and ligaments should be carefully dissected and properly preserved while the cartilage surface is exposed.

Tendon Preparation

As mentioned, the extensor tendon and its various intrinsic attachments should be preserved as much as possible during the initial management as well as at the time of the recipient preparation for toe transfer. In more proximal reconstructions, it may be worthwhile to dissect out the lumbricus and interosseous muscles for repair to the corresponding structures from the toe harvest. Location of the flexor tendons may be difficult at times because of proximal retraction. Proximal incisions may be necessary; if so, these should observe the basic principles of hand incisions such as avoiding the crossing of joint creases. If the carpal tunnel is opened for tendon retrieval, then it should be decompressed fully. Flexor tendon repair at the wrist level is seldom required. When located proximally, either the flexor digitorum profundus (FDP) or sublimis tendons can be used for repair to the transferred flexor digitorum longus tendon of the toe. When there is great difficulty in locating enough recipient tendons (e.g., in multiple digit amputations), the flexor tendons of two transplanted toes can be sutured to one proximal tendon. Primary transfer of the sublimis flexor tendon from the adjacent finger can also be performed if no flexor tendon is found in the amputated finger. Any tendon adhesions should be freed to ensure smooth gliding of the repaired tendon at the end of the procedure.

Nerve Preparation

Preoperative identification of the approximate positions of the recipient nerves may be performed by percussion for Tinel's sign in the stump. After skin flap elevation in the amputation stump, neuromas of the digital or common digital nerves can usually be identified close to the wound edges. The nerves used for neurorrhaphy should be dissected to a point where they have a normal or close to normal fascicular appearance in cross-section as determined by loupe or operating microscope magnification. When no suitable digital nerves can be found, then other proximal nerves in the palm such as the palmar cutaneous branch of the median nerve or dorsal branches of the ulnar nerve may be selected as recipient nerves. If necessary, end-to-side neurorrhaphy to the adjacent or any available nerve can also be an alternative option.

BONY FIXATION INSET AND SCULPTING OF THE TOE TRANSFER

The suggested sequence of a toe transfer is as follows: (1) skeletal fixation, (2) extensor tendon repair, (3) flexor tendon repair, (4) skin tailoring and temporary closure, (5) nerve repair, (6) arterial anastomosis, (7) venous anastomosis, and (8) final skin closure.

Skeletal Fixation

As mentioned, bony fixation can be achieved with the use of parallel or sagittal intraosseous wiring. We have previously reported a nonunion rate of 1.5% in 68 toe-to-hand transfers after an average 30 months of follow-up (20). The advantages of using this bony fixation technique include the following:

1. It is a simple and reliable method, applicable to stumps as short as 5.0 mm.
2. It provides stable yet semirigid fixation, which allows earlier postoperative rehabilitation as well as correction of any slight angulation and malrotation in the early postoperative period.
3. It causes minimal disruption to the overlying tendon during periosteal dissection, which may reduce the need for secondary tenolysis.

Two parallel 1.0-mm holes are made through both cortices in the distal part of the phalanx of the transferred toe and the amputated stump of the finger in a dorsal-volar direction. About 2.0 mm of healthy bone between the holes and the bony edge in the skeletal stump is sufficient for bone healing. After placing the toe in its proper position in the hand, the angle and rotation of the fingers are determined. Two stainless steel wires (28 gauge) are then introduced through the corresponding holes and twisted carefully while the position of the toe is adjusted. To avoid tethering of soft tissues, the wire ends must be placed in the extensor side and away from the site of osteosynthesis.

For composite joint repair, the volar plate and collateral ligaments of the toe are sutured to the corresponding structures in the hand under proper tension to prevent postoperative instability of the repaired joint. This technique has been used mostly with combined second and third toe transfer at the MCP joint. Long-term results with composite MCP joint reconstruction have shown an active range of motion of 52 degrees on average (26,27).

Tendon Repair

The extensor digitorum longus tendon is sutured to the corresponding recipient extensor tendon of the finger with the IP and MCP joints in full extension to minimize postoperative extensor lag. If available, the extensor digitorum brevis can be sutured to the dorsal (extensor) expansion to enhance IP joint extension, although the result of this reconstruction is not predictable. The hand is then turned over for repair of the flexor tendon. Against the tension of the extended toe, the flexor repair is adjusted until the natural cascade of the hand is reached. In distal finger amputation with an intact FDS insertion, the FDP is repaired mainly to provide stability in power pinch. If the proximal FDP stump is not available, the flexor tendon of the toe can be sutured to the distal portion of the FDS insertion or an annular or cruciate pulley. For proximal finger toe-to-hand transfers, only the FDP tendon is repaired. Tenorrhaphies are performed usually in zone III to avoid entrapment of the repair site by the remaining pulleys during tendon excursion. However, in distal toe transfer, the flexor digitorum longus tendon is usually repaired in zone II. To further prevent the transferred lesser toe from clawing, a single K-pin is then inserted through the IP joints to maintain the finger in full extension. Other modalities include the use of night splints with the finger in hyperextension, at least during the first year (23,28).

Skin Tailoring and Temporary Closure

After the bone and tendons have been repaired, the artery and vein of the toe transfer are brought to the corresponding recipient sites, and when their reach is confirmed, the skin is temporarily closed. Adjustments are made to the skin flaps at this point. It is important to ensure a tensionless closure but at the same time prevent a bulky appearance by trimming off any excess skin. After confirmation that a tension-free closure can be achieved, a minimal number of sutures are then removed to permit enough access only for the microsurgical anastomoses. This technique allows minimal handling of the entire hand construct without disturbing the anastomoses once they are completed. It also ensures that that no excessively tight closure or wound closures lie directly over the anastomoses.

NERVE REPAIRS

Coaptation of the nerves is performed in an end-to-end fashion with 10-0 nylon sutures, bringing the epineurium of the two nerve ends together in a tensionless repair. Usually, only the proper or common digital nerves are repaired. However, both the deep and superficial peroneal nerves included in the transferred toe can also be repaired to the proper or common digital nerves or any sensory nerve available to maximize the toe innervation. If only one suitable recipient nerve is present proximally, then multiple donor nerves can be coapted to this nerve.

VESSEL ANASTOMOSES

The arterial anastomosis is performed first. After it is completed, capillary refill in the skin and venous backflow are observed for at least 5 minutes. If the blood outflow is sluggish or inadequate, the arterial anastomosis and the entire course of the artery need to be rechecked with further adventitiectomy performed if necessary. If perfusion of the toe remains dubious and a second artery is available in both the transferred toe and recipient site, an additional arterial anastomosis can be considered, for example, in combined second and third toe transfers. An additional guide in combined second and third toe transfers as to whether a second set of anastomosis is required can be from observation of the third toe upon release of tourniquet and before detachment; if the toes pink up simultaneously or in quick succession, then it is unlikely that a second anastomosis would be needed (29). After the arterial anastomosis is performed, the overlying wound is then closed while proceeding to the venous anastomosis. After these are performed, all of the remaining wounds are then closed. If there is some observed tension after skin closure, partial closure and skin grafting of the partially opened surface is advisable. However, this is uncommon if adequate preoperative planning has been performed. Small Silastic drains are used to prevent hematoma formation. It is important to ensure that the placement of these drains avoids any possible contact with the vessels or the vascular anastomosis.

POSTOPERATIVE MONITORING

Immediate Postoperative Period

After the procedure, patients are transferred to a microsurgical intensive care unit (MICU) for close monitoring of the transferred toe and kept for a minimum of 3 to 5 days. This immediate postoperative care is critical to ensure the success of the microsurgical procedure. If an intensive care facility is not available, patients should nursed by experienced staff who are trained in the routine monitoring of free flaps. Besides flap monitoring, each patient is carefully monitored to ensure they are warm, well hydrated, and pain free. The patient's hand is kept slightly elevated above the level of the heart, with the proximal palm and wrist gently wrapped and the finger tips exposed for continuous observation of perfusion. Despite the increasing use of objective monitoring technologies, clinical observation still remains our method of choice for early detection of vascular compromise. In assessing the adequacy of perfusion to the transferred finger or thumb tip, capillary refill, temperature, swelling, and flap color are used as parameters that are checked every hour within the first 48 hours and then every 3 to 4 hours for the next 3 days while the patient is in the MICU. Another convenient method of monitoring toe-to-hand transfers is the pulse oximeter, which can detect early loss of the arterial pulse as well as provide a continuous display of oxygen saturation (30).

Dressings

Bulky dressings are not recommended for the following reasons: (1) blood clots retained around the wound could induce vasospasm and compress the anastomosis, (2) a theoretical higher risk of infection may result, (3) early postoperative rehabilitation is prevented, and (4) observation and correction of any malrotation are difficult because it should be carried out early enough before bone healing.

An initial bolus of 100 cc of Dextran 40 (low-molecular-weight heparin) is rapidly administered intravenously 10 minutes before completion of the arterial anastomosis followed by continuous infusion (25 mL/hr) during the next 4 to 5 days. Oral aspirin (81 mg/day) is also administered for the first 2 weeks to reduce the risk of platelet aggregation. Prophylactic antibiotics are used both in elective cases and in primary toe transfers. The donor foot is gently covered with nonadherent gauze over the wound sites and supplemented by a light fluff dressing. No splints are used in the donor foot or the recipient hand. Two days later, the foot is uncovered without further dressings.

POTENTIAL COMPLICATIONS

Other than general complications that may relate to a lengthy anesthetic, the most common complication in the immediate postoperative period is vascular compromise caused by vasospasm or thrombosis. Emergency reexploration of the anastomoses is required after failed bedside measures such as release of sutures, topical application of lidocaine, and fluid optimization. Revision of an anastomosis using another arterial pedicle may be required in certain cases, such as in combined toe transfers. Venous compromise is less common and is usually correctable. Other complications including skin flap necrosis or wound healing problems with resultant exposed structures must be remedied as soon as possible to prevent desiccation of tendons or neurovascular bundles, which can result in poor function and aesthetic result.

Longer term complications may be directly related to the original injury or indirectly as a result of suboptimal reconstruction which are often correctable by secondary procedures (see next section).

SECONDARY SURGERY

The rate of secondary procedures is around 14% to 20% after toe-to-hand transfers (31,32). Revision procedures for functional improvement such as tenolysis, arthrodesis, and web space deepening usually yield good results (31). Flexor tenolysis is the commonest secondary procedures described for most series but occur in a smaller percentage of cases in our series

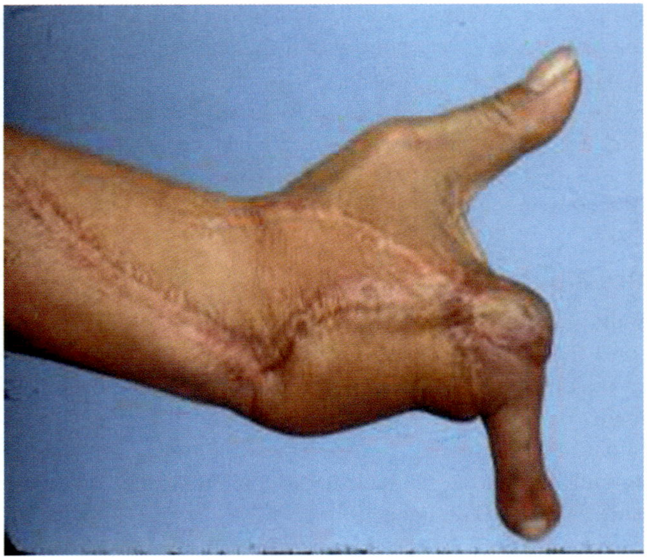

FIGURE 64-7 Subluxation in a reconstructed composite joint caused by inadequate repair of the collateral ligaments.

compared with others, probably because of the method of bony fixation and also the implementation of a comprehensive rehabilitation program with an emphasis on earlier active and passive movement (33). Other secondary surgeries may be required for bone and joint revisions. An unstable joint may result, for example, from a loose repair during composite joint transfer (Figure 64-7). In addition, a malrotated finger may require rotational osteotomy to permit better opposition to the thumb.

Revision procedures for esthetic improvement are usually minor, and aim to increase the resemblance of the toe to the finger or thumb (25,34). The commonest procedure is a pulp plasty carried out under local anesthesia to reduce the bulbous appearance of the toe, although other procedures, including scar revision and flap thinning, may be required.

OUTCOMES OF TOE-TO-FINGER TRANSFERS

Success of microsurgical toe-to-hand transfer compares favorably with that of other free tissue transfers, with failure rates generally not exceeding 5% in most series in adult and pediatric populations (35–37). In our series of 2005 procedures in 1779 patients carried out over a 20-year period (1985–2010) at Chang Gung University in Taoyuan, Taiwan, a success rate of 97% was achieved. In terms of range of motion, an average total range of motion of 50 to 60 degrees is usually achievable for the proximal and distal IP joints (27,28). If a metatarsophalangeal joint has been transferred to reconstruct the MCP joint, the expected range of movement should average 50 degrees or 52 degrees if a composite joint reconstruction has been carried out via a metatarsophalangeal joint disarticulation during harvest (15).

In general, both grip and pinch strength after thumb reconstruction average 75% to 80% of the opposite thumb (23,39). Independent strength assessment in finger reconstructions is more difficult to measure and is often dependent on an intact thumb function to produce a stable tripod or pulp-to-pulp pinch. Furthermore, restoring the prehensile patterns of the hand may be a much more valid measure of outcome and has been achieved in most series, especially after reconstructions for multiple finger amputations and the metacarpal hand deformity (6,40,41).

Appearance and Sensory Outcomes

A major advantage of toe-to-hand transfer is the replacement of tissue that bears a near-normal resemblance of what was lost. Our series of toe transfers for isolated finger amputations has found that restoration of the digital arcade and storage function of the hand to be useful both functionally and psychologically (42). With improved sensory recovery comes an enhanced appreciation of the reconstructed digits and a better overall integration into the body. These improvements largely depend on a comprehensive sensory reeducation program as described. Performing the toe-to-hand transfer surgery within 1 month of the injury has also been shown to lead to better sensory results (43). Overall, the average recovery of two-point discrimination should not be expected to exceed approximately 7 to 8 mm (44,45).

Donor Site Outcome Evaluation

Foot morbidity is completely acceptable after isolated harvest of the second toe (11,46) (see Figure 64-6). In contrast, foot deformity appears to be more evident after great toe or combined second and third toe harvest. Although we have previously advocated the use of nonvascularized bone blocks to replace harvested metatarsals after combined second and third toe transfer at the transmetatarsal level, this is no longer routine in our practice because we have found that the great toe and the heel provide adequate compensation for avoidance of any problems with walking or take-off. Regardless of the number of toes harvested, the potential donor defect should always be discussed in detail with the patient, with the needs individualized to lifestyle, hobbies, and concerns over appearance.

REFERENCES

1. Huguier P. Replacement du pouce par son metacarpien, par l'aggrandissement du premier espace interosseox. *Arch Gen Med* 1874;23:78–82.
2. Matev IB. The bone-lengthening method in hand reconstruction: twenty years' experience. *J Hand Surg Am* 1989;14:376–378.
3. Foucher G, Van Genechten F, Merle M, Michon J. Single stage thumb reconstruction by a composite forearm island flap. *J Hand Surg Br* 1984;9:245–248.
4. Tsai TM. 2nd & 3rd toe transplantation to a transmetacarpal amputated hand. *Ann Acad Med Singapore* 1979;8:413–418.
5. O'Brien BM, Brennen MD, MacLeod AM. Simultaneous double toe transfer for severely disabled hands. *Hand* 1978;10:232–240.
6. Wei FC, Epstein MD, Chen HC, Chuang CC, Chen HT. Microsurgical reconstruction of distal digits following mutilating hand injuries: results in 121 patients. *Br J Plast Surg* 1993;46:181–186.
7. Dellon AL. Sensory re-education after fingertip injury and reconstruction. In Foucher G (ed). *Fingertip and Nailbed Injuries.* New York: Churchill Livingstone, 1991.
8. Koshima I, Soeda S, Takase T, Yamasaki M. Free vascularized nail grafts. *J Hand Surg Am* 1988;13:29–32.
9. Cheng G, Fang G, Hou S, et al. Aesthetic reconstruction of thumb or finger partial defect with trimmed toe-flap transfer. *Microsurgery* 2007;27:74–83.
10. Logan A, Elliot D, Foucher G. Free toe pulp transfer to restore traumatic digital pulp loss. *Br J Plast Surg* 1985;38:497–500.

11. Wei FC, Chen HC, Chuang DC, Chen S, Noordhoff MS. Second toe wrap-around flap. *Plast Reconstr Surg* 1991;88:837–843.
12. Woo SH, Lee GJ, Kim KC, Ha SH, Kim JS. Cosmetic reconstruction of distal finger absence with partial second toe transfer. *J Plast Reconstr Aesthet Surg* 2006;59:317–324.
13. Boeckx W, Jacobs W, Guelinckx P, Van de Kerckhove E. Late results in replanted digits. Is replantation of a single digit worthwhile? *Acta Chir Belg* 1992;92:204–208.
14. Wei FC, Colony LH. Microsurgical reconstruction of opposable digits in mutilating hand injuries. *Clin Plast Surg* 1989;16:491–504.
15. Wei FC, el-Gammal TA, Lin CH, Chuang CC, Chen HC, Chen SH. Metacarpal hand: classification and guidelines for microsurgical reconstruction with toe transfers. *Plast Reconstr Surg* 1997;99:122–128.
16. Tsai TM, Jupiter JB, Wolff TW, Atasoy E. Reconstruction of severe transmetacarpal mutilating hand injuries by combined second and third toe transfer. *J Hand Surg Am* 1981;6:319–328.
17. Wei FC, Chen HC, Chuang CC, Noordhoff MS. Simultaneous multiple toe transfers in hand reconstruction. *Plast Reconstr Surg* 1988;81:366–377.
18. Mardini S, Wei FC. Unilateral and bilateral metacarpal hand injuries: classification and treatment guidelines. *Plast Reconstr Surg* 2004;113: 1756–1759.
19. Wei FC, Lutz BS, Cheng SL, Chuang DC. Reconstruction of bilateral metacarpal hands with multiple-toe transplantations. *Plast Reconstr Surg* 1999;104:1698–1704.
20. Yim KK, Wei FC. Intraosseous wiring in toe-to-hand transplantation. *Ann Plast Surg* 1995;35:66–69.
21. el-Gammal TA, Wei FC. Microvascular reconstruction of the distal digits by partial toe transfer. *Clin Plast Surg* 1997;24:49–55.
22. Yim KK, Wei FC, Lin CH. A comparison between primary and secondary toe-to-hand transplantation. *Plast Reconstr Surg* 2004;114:107–112.
23. Wei FC, el-Gammal TA. Toe-to-hand transfer. Current concepts, techniques, and research. *Clin Plast Surg* 1996;23:103–116.
24. Woo SH, Kim JS, Seul JH. Immediate toe-to-hand transfer in acute hand injuries: overall results, compared with results for elective cases. *Plast Reconstr Surg* 2004;113:882–892.
25. Wei FC, Chen HC, Chuang DC, et al. Aesthetic refinements in toe-to-hand transfer surgery. *Plast Reconstr Surg* 1996;98:485–490.
26. Wilson CS, Buncke HJ, Alpert BS, Gordon L. Composite metacarpophalangeal joint reconstruction in great toe-to-hand free tissue transfers. *J Hand Surg Am* 1984;9:645–649.
27. Strauch RJ, Wei FC, Chen SH. Composite finger metacarpophalangeal joint reconstruction in combined second and third free toe-to-hand transfers. *J Hand Surg Am* 1993;18:972–977.
28. Gilbert A. Discussion in: The second toe flap. In Serafin D (ed). *Atlas of Microsurgical Composite Tissue Transplantation.* Philadelphia: Saunders, 1996, pp. 616–618.
29. Cheng MH, Wei FC, Santamaria E, et al. Single versus double arterial anastomoses in combined second- and third-toe transplantation. *Plast Reconstr Surg* 1998;102:2408–2412; discussion 2413.
30. Jones NF. Gupta R. Postoperative monitoring of pediatric toe-to-hand transfers with differential pulse oximetry. Reconstruction of severe transmetacarpal mutilating hand injuries by combined second and third toe transfer. *J Hand Surg Am* 2001;3:525-529.
31. Yim KK, Wei FC. Secondary procedures to improve function after toe-to-hand transfers. *Br J Plast Surg* 1995;48:487–491.
32. Carlsen B, Jones NF. Radical resection of a massive venous malformation of the thumb and immediate reconstruction with a microsurgical toe transfer. *J Hand Surg Am* 2007;32:1587–1591.
33. Wei F-C. Toe to Hand Transplantations. In D Green RH, W Pederson, S Wolfe (ed). *Green's Operative Hand Surgery.* St. Louis: Churchill Livingstone, 2005, pp. 1835–1863.
34. Wei FC, Yim KK. Pulp plasty after toe-to-hand transplantation. *Plast Reconstr Surg* 1995;96:661–666.
35. Foucher G, Medina J, Navarro R. Microsurgical reconstruction of the hypoplastic thumb, type IIIB. *J Reconstr Microsurg* 2001;17:9–15.
36. Poppen NK, Norris TR, Buncke HJ Jr. Evaluation of sensibility and function with microsurgical free tissue transfer of the great toe to the hand for thumb reconstruction. *J Hand Surg Am* 1983;8:516–531.
37. Gu YD, Zhang GM, Cheng DS, et al. Free toe transfer for thumb and finger reconstruction in 300 cases. *Plast Reconstr Surg* 1993;91:693–700; discussion 1–2.
38. Wei FC, Yim KK. Single third-toe transfer in hand reconstruction. *J Hand Surg Am* 1995;20:388–394; discussion 95–96.
39. Chung KC, Wei FC. An outcome study of thumb reconstruction using microvascular toe transfer. *J Hand Surg Am* 2000;25:651–658.
40. Fumiaki S, Wei FC, Sassu P, et al. Multiple toe transplantations to reconstruct three amputated neighbouring distal fingers by heat press injury—a case report. *J Plast Reconstr Aesthet Surg* 2009;62:e309–e313.
41. Wei FC, Coessens B, Ganos D. Multiple microsurgical toe-to-hand transfer in the reconstruction of the severely mutilated hand. A series of fifty-nine cases. *Ann Chir Main Memb Super* 1992;11:177–187.
42. Demirkan F, Wei FC, Jeng SF, et al. Toe transplantation for isolated index finger amputations distal to the proximal interphalangeal joint. *Plast Reconstr Surg* 1999;103:499–507.
43. Chu NS, Wei FC. Recovery of sensation and somatosensory evoked potentials following toe-to-digit transplantation in man. *Muscle Nerve* 1995;18:859–866.
44. Whitworth IH, Pickford MA. The first toe-to-hand transfer: a thirty-year follow-up. *J Hand Surg Br* 2000;25:608–610.
45. Morrison WA, O'Brien BM, MacLeod AM. Experience with thumb reconstruction. *J Hand Surg Br* 1984;9:223–233.
46. Buncke G (ed). *Lengthening by Toe Transfer.* London: Martin Dunitz, 1997.

CHAPTER 65

Toe-to-Hand Transfers for Congenital Anomalies of the Hand

Neil F. Jones

Buncke first performed an experimental microsurgical toe-to-hand transfer in a monkey in 1964 (1). This was followed by the first microsurgical second toe transfer to the hand in a human by Yang in 1966 followed by the first great toe–to–thumb transfer based on the plantar arterial system by Cobbett (2) and a great toe–to–thumb transfer based on the first dorsal metatarsal artery (FDMA) by Buncke (3). Many surgeons are now capable of performing successful transfers of the great toe and second toe as well as simultaneous double toe transfers and combined second and third toe transfers for posttraumatic reconstruction of amputations of the thumb and multiple digits; this is described in Chapters 63 and 64. Great toe transfers have further evolved to minimize the harvest of tissues from the foot and customize the appearance of the great toe similar to a thumb with the techniques of the Morrison (4) "wrap-around" flap, the Wei (5) "trimmed toe" transfer and the Upton (6) modified great toe transfer. Similar toe transfers have also been used for posttraumatic reconstruction of children's hands with success rates comparable to those in adults (7).

Conventional nonmicrosurgical treatment of congenital anomalies of the hand in children usually involves pollicization of the index finger for children with hypoplastic or absent thumbs (8) and nonvascularized toe phalangeal bone grafting and distraction lengthening of hypoplastic digits caused by symbrachydactyly, cleft hand, and congenital constriction ring syndrome (9). The first microsurgical toe-to-thumb transfers to reconstruct congenital anomalies of the hand were performed in 1976 by O'Brien et al. (10) in two children with thumb hypoplasia. Nyarady et al. (11) reported a second toe-to-thumb transfer for thumb hypoplasia in 1983. Following these early case reports and small series (12–14), several surgeons around the world have developed increasing expertise performing larger series of microsurgical toe-to-hand transfers to reconstruct various congenital anomalies of the hand (15–31). Children born with symbrachydactyly (32), transverse deficiencies, cleft hand (33), and congenital constriction ring syndrome can be considered for reconstruction with toe-to-hand transfers. Even though toe-to-thumb transfers have been described for the treatment of isolated hypoplasia or absent thumb (34,35), the gold standard remains pollicization of the index finger (8,25,36). However, if the thumb is involved in congenital constriction ring syndrome and the carpometacarpal joint and thumb metacarpal are present along with the thenar muscles, these children are excellent candidates for toe-to-thumb transfers. Similarly children with more severe radial longitudinal deficiencies with sequential absence of the thumb, index, middle, and ring fingers, microsurgical toe-to-thumb transfer becomes the preferred technique for reconstruction (36).

INDICATIONS FOR TOE-TO-HAND TRANSFERS FOR CONGENITAL ANOMALIES OF THE THUMB (21)

1. Congenital constriction ring syndrome affecting the thumb but with preservation of the carpometacarpal joint, metacarpal, and thenar muscles (Figures 65-1 to 65-6)
2. Severe radial longitudinal deficiencies with an absent thumb and radial digits but with one or two ulnar border digits
3. Severe monodactylous form of cleft hand with absent thumb, index, middle, and ring fingers but with preservation of the small finger
4. Severe arteriovenous malformation affecting the thumb and radial side of the hand

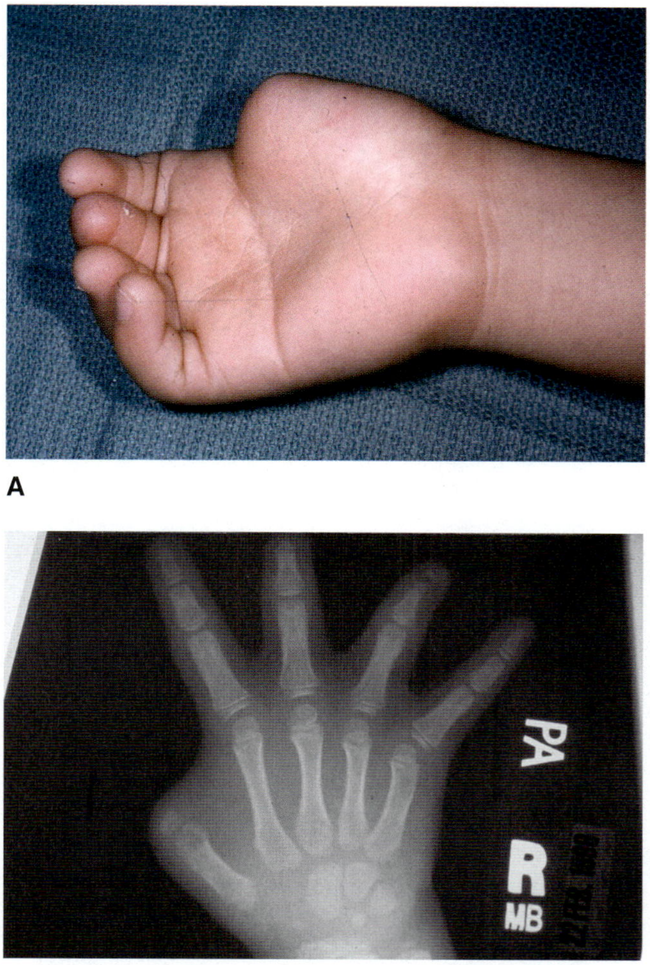

A

B

FIGURE 65-1 Preoperative photograph (**A**) and radiograph (**B**) of a 2-year-old girl with congenital constriction ring syndrome affecting her right thumb and index and middle fingers.

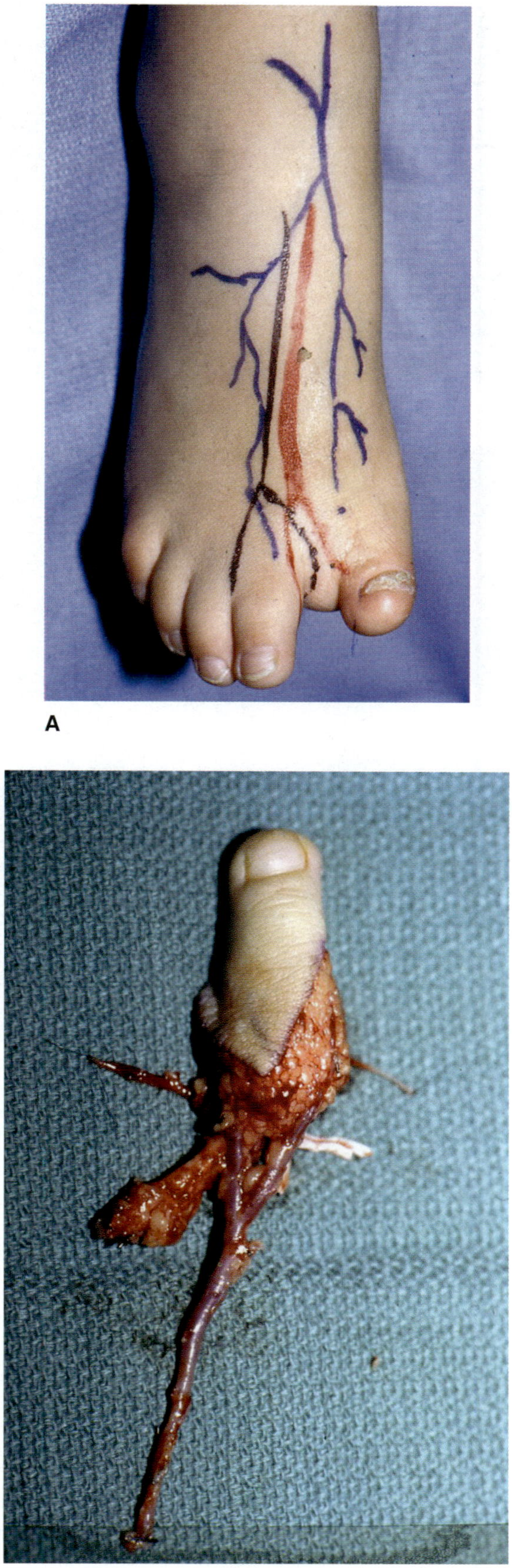

A

B

FIGURE 65-2 Congenital constriction ring syndrome also caused an above-knee amputation of the left lower extremity and an abnormality of the right great toe, so a right second toe transfer was selected (**A**) and (**B**).

INDICATIONS FOR TOE-TO-HAND TRANSFERS FOR CONGENITAL ANOMALIES OF THE FINGERS (21)

1. Severe transverse deficiencies or ulnar longitudinal deficiencies with absence of all four fingers but with preservation of the thumb
2. Monodactylous form of symbrachydactyly with absence of all four fingers but with preservation of the thumb (Figures 65-7 and 65-8)
3. Complete absence of all five digits distal to the metacarpals (Figures 65-9 to 65-12)

PREOPERATIVE ASSESSMENT

During the initial consultation with the parents of a child born with a congenital anomaly of the hand, the surgeon should allow the parents to express their hopes and expectations for treatment because the parental response to their child being born with a congenital anomaly is similar to the bereavement response. The parents must not only deal with their own sense

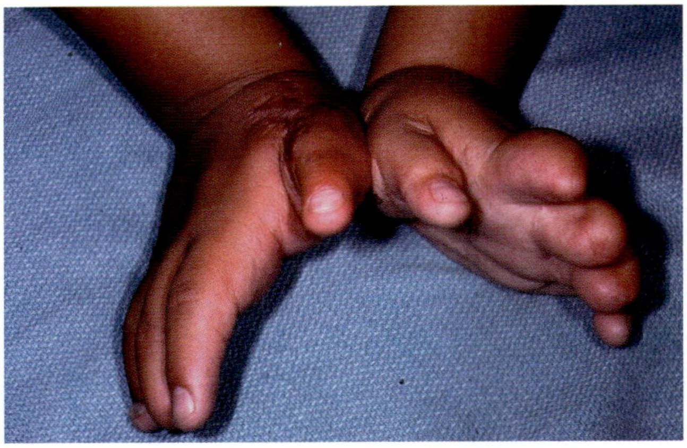

A

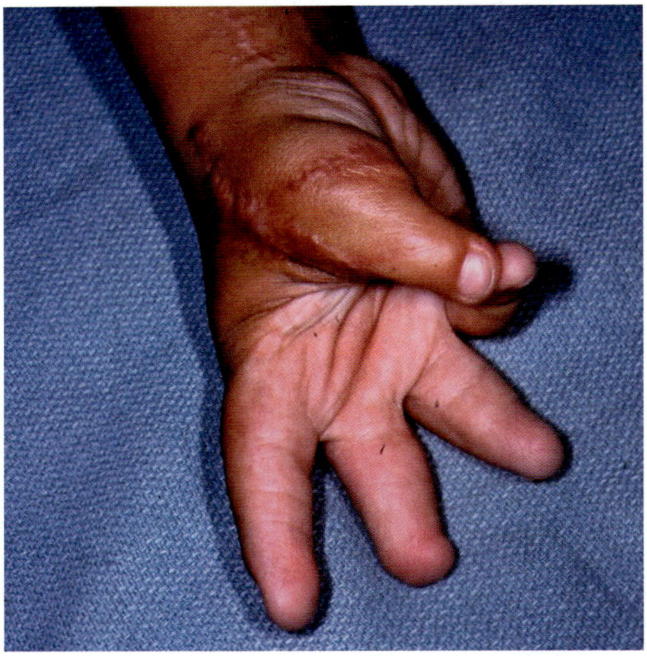

B

FIGURE 65-3 Three years after surgery, the right second toe to right thumb transfer has comparable appearance to the normal left thumb (**A**) and excellent opposition to the small finger (**B**).

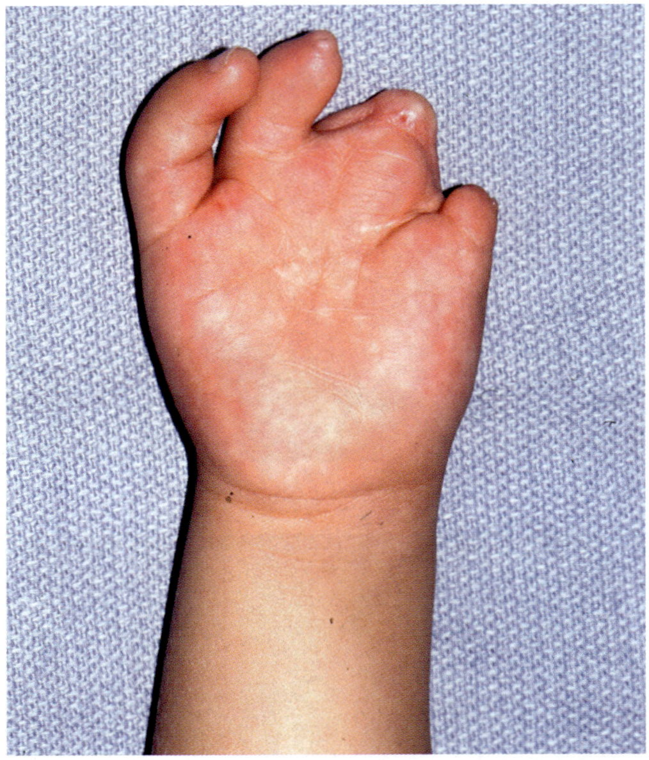

A

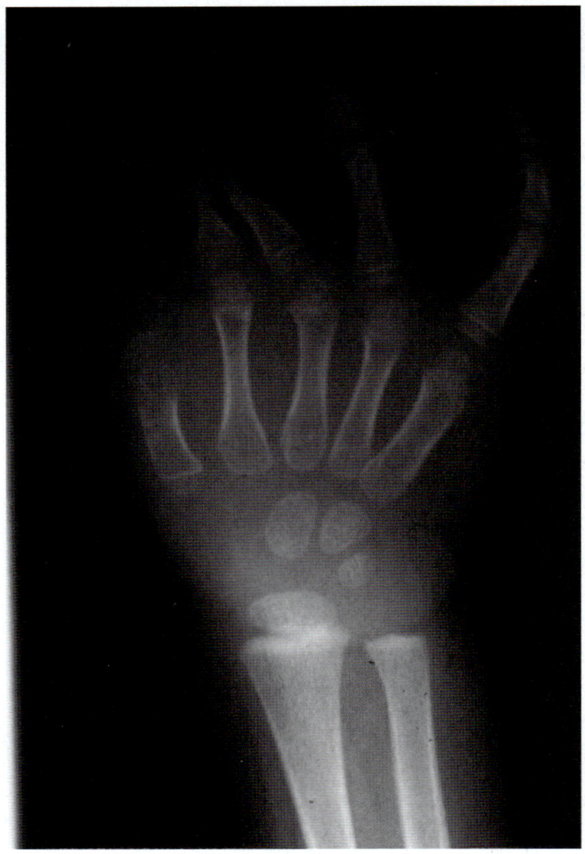

B

FIGURE 65-4 Preoperative photograph (**A**) and radiograph (**B**) of a 2-year-old girl with severe congenital constriction ring syndrome affecting the right thumb and index, middle, and ring fingers.

of loss but also have the obligation to make decisions on the treatment of their child. Some surgeons have recommended that the parents and child meet with a clinical psychologist because it has been shown that psychological counseling may be important in decision making in pediatric hand surgery (37–39).

Other surgeons show photographs and videos of children with similar anomalies before and after reconstruction with toe transfers or simulate the size and shape and position of a toe transfer using models fabricated from fast-setting dental compound. We have found the best form of counseling is to have the parents meet with parents of children who have previously undergone microsurgical toe transfers and even arrange to meet and see a child who has undergone a toe transfer. Now that some of these children who have had a toe transfer are in their late teens or early 20s, they themselves become the ideal

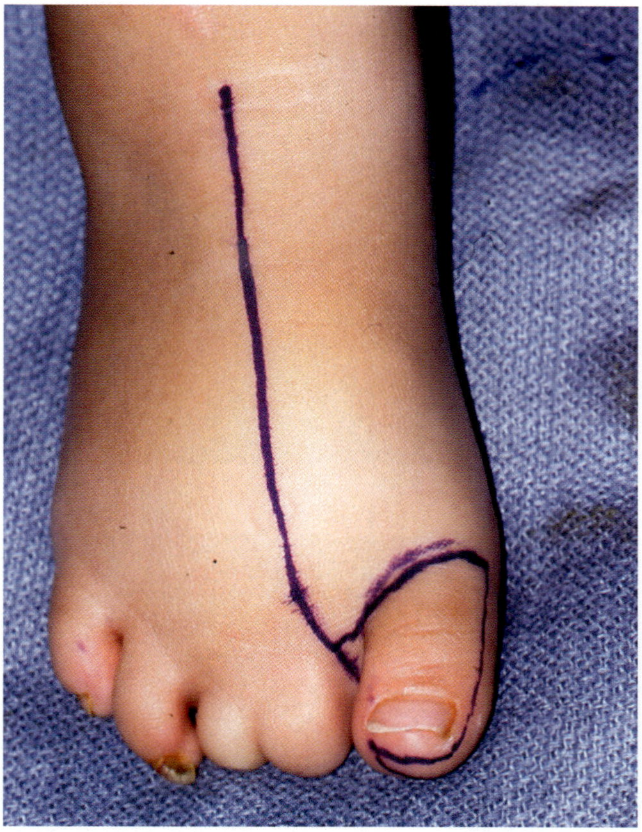

A

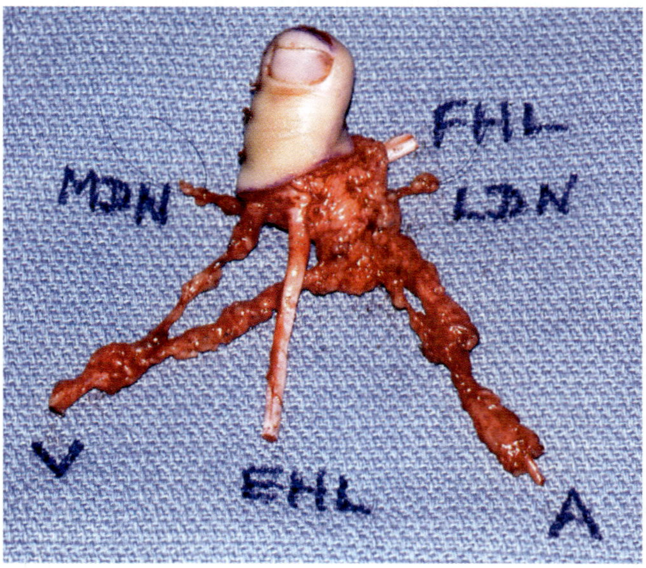

B

FIGURE 65-5 Because the second and third toes in both feet were affected by congenital constriction ring syndrome, a trimmed right great toe transfer was designed (**A**) for transfer to the hand (**B**).

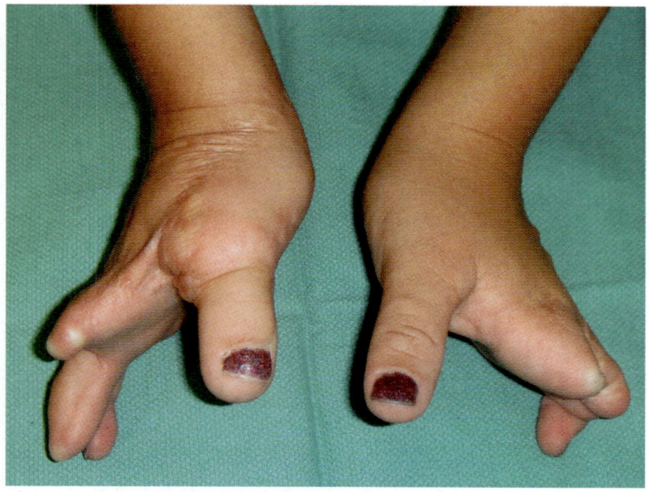

A

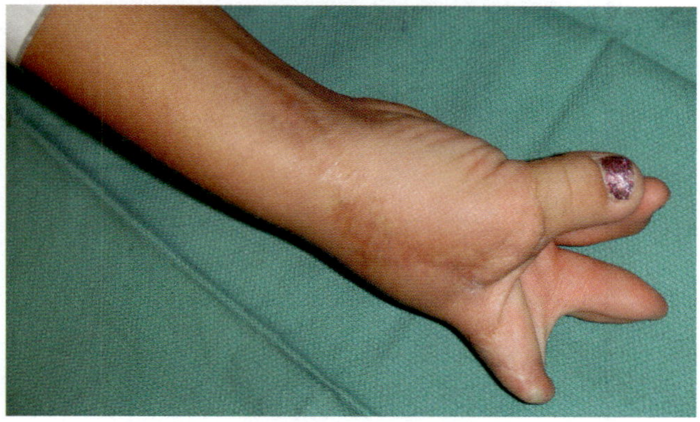

B

FIGURE 65-6 Two years after surgery, the trimmed right great toe–to–right thumb transfer has comparable appearance to the normal left thumb and excellent opposition to the only normal small finger.

advocates for counseling parents of children with congenital anomalies.

A detailed examination of the child's upper extremity should be performed except for a very young child when the movements of the extremity should be observed while the child is playing. The spine, chest, and shoulder should be examined for abnormalities such as Poland's syndrome. The presence or absence of the radiocarpal joint as well as the number and size of the metacarpal bones should be recorded as well as the presence or absence of the thumb and the presence or absence of a thumb carpometacarpal joint. Dimpling of the skin over the ends of the metacarpals may indicate the presence of flexor tendons.

The child's feet should be examined because some congenital differences of the upper extremity may be associated with congenital differences of the lower extremity (33). The child's foot can be positioned close to the hand so the parents and the child can visualize what the transferred toe might look like. Plain radiographs of both hands and wrists and both feet should be obtained to determine the presence of metacarpals and, most important, whether the thumb carpometacarpal joint is present. The need for preoperative angiography of either the upper or lower extremity is debatable. Greenberg and May (40) suggested a lateral angiogram of the foot was helpful in identifying the location and size of the FDMA. However, most surgeons agree that a preoperative angiogram is not necessary, and information regarding the presence and depth of the FDMA can be obtained from examination of the foot with a pencil Doppler probe.

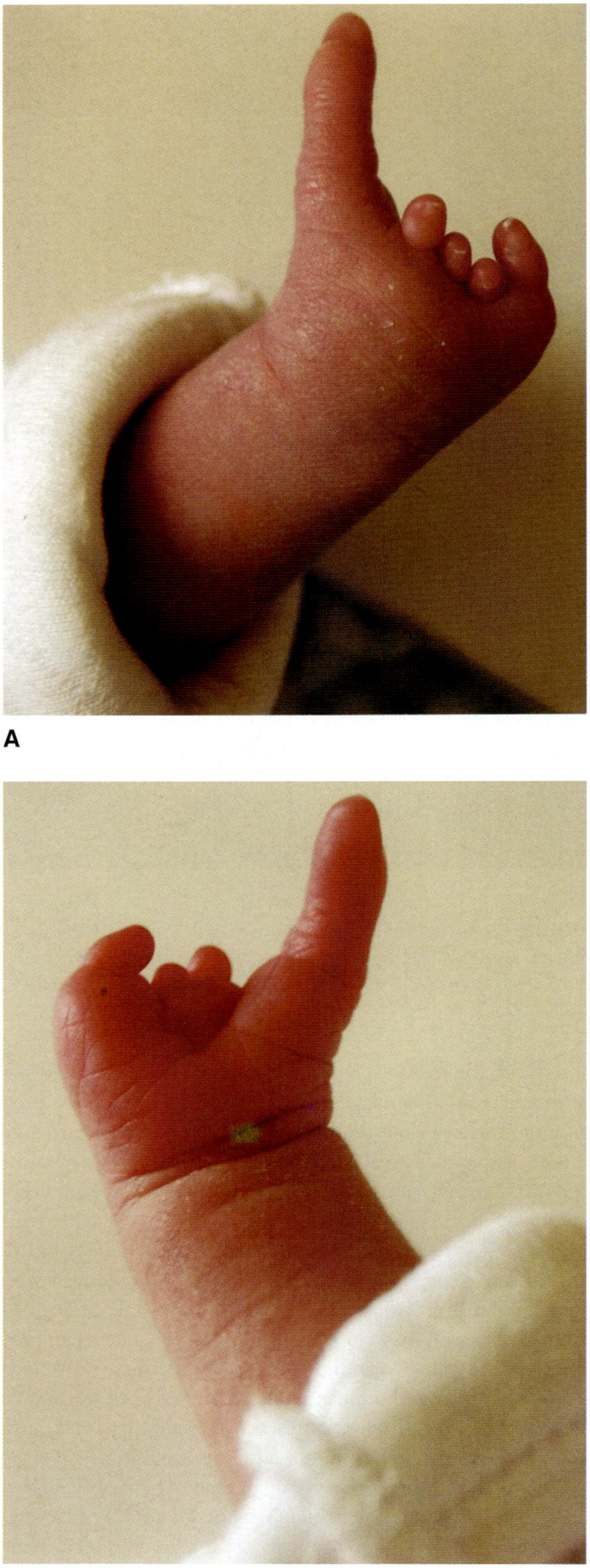

A

B

FIGURE 65-7 Dorsal (**A**) and palmar (**B**) photographs of a 6-month-old girl with symbrachydactyly of her right hand with a normal thumb but absence of all four fingers, represented just by nubbins.

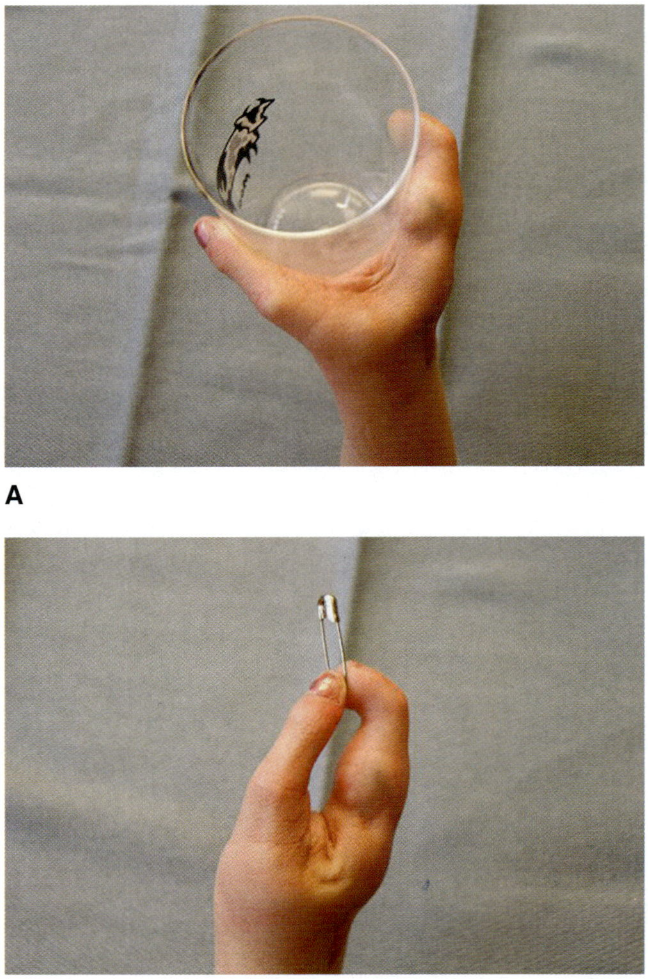

A

B

FIGURE 65-8 Five years after a right second toe–to–small finger transfer, the child has excellent grasp between the thumb and second toe transfer into the small finger position (**A**) and very precise fine pinch between the thumb and toe transfer (**B**).

Preoperative evaluation by the child's pediatrician should always be performed to exclude any associated abnormalities of the cardiopulmonary, hematopoietic, gastrointestinal, and genitourinary systems as well as to exclude any syndromes.

Alternative nonmicrosurgical reconstructive options such as distraction lengthening and nonvascularized toe phalangeal bone grafting should be discussed with the parents. An older child with a unilateral defect or with a near normal thumb may be considered for a prosthetic hand or fingers.

The choice of using a great toe or second toe transfer must be explained to the parents. Although a great toe transfer, especially the trimmed toe technique, may produce the best cosmetic result for thumb reconstruction (see Figures 65-4 to 65-6) and resemble a thumb (5,6), most parents have difficulty with a decision to "mutilate" a normal foot even if it means providing improved function to the hand, and therefore they tend to choose the second toe because of the more inconspicuous donor site in the foot. Also in cultures where sandals are worn, a second toe transfer is preferred for thumb reconstruction so that the thong remains in position between the great toe and third toe. The Morrison "wrap-around" flap cannot be

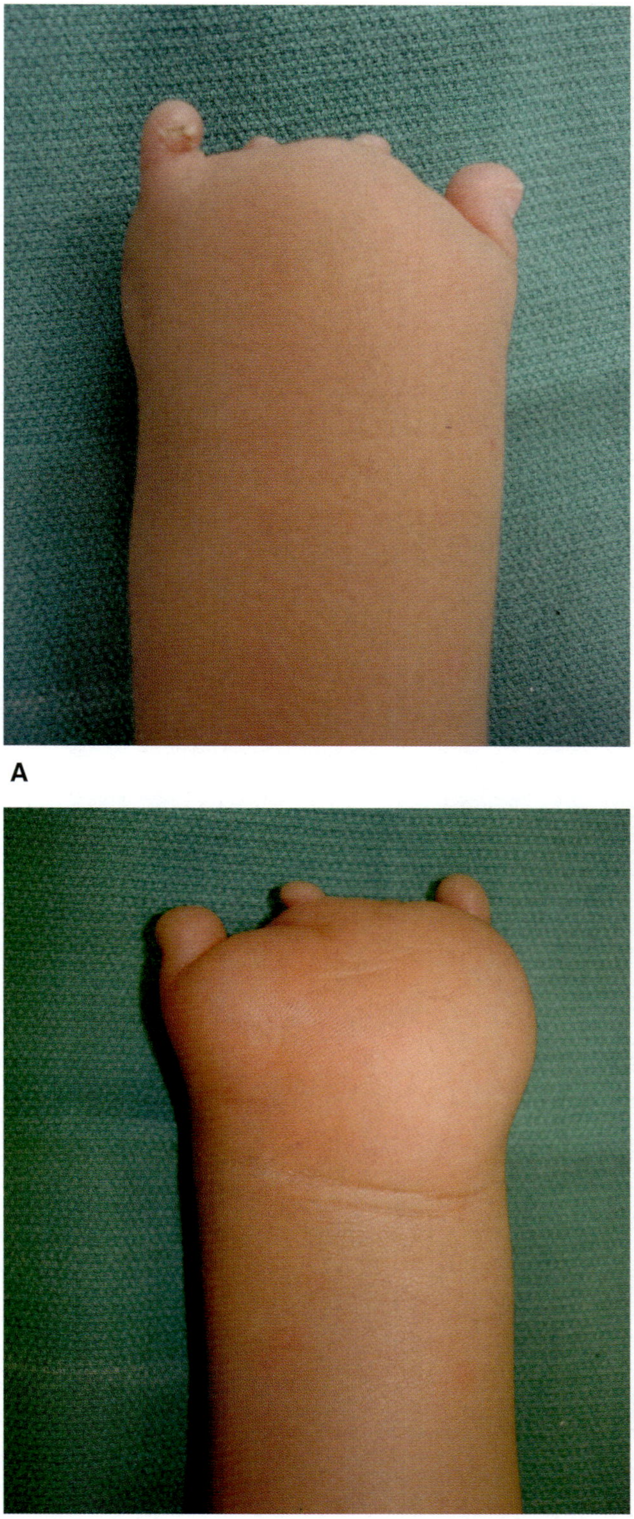

A

B

FIGURE 65-9 Dorsal (A) and palmar (B) photographs of a 2-year-old boy with symbrachydactyly affecting all five digits of his left hand.

used in small children because it does not provide the possibility of further growth (4). The parents can be reassured that sporting activities are not significantly affected by a second toe transfer, but some impairment in push-off and running speed and difficulties walking on uneven or sloped surfaces have been documented by gait analysis after great toe transfer (41).

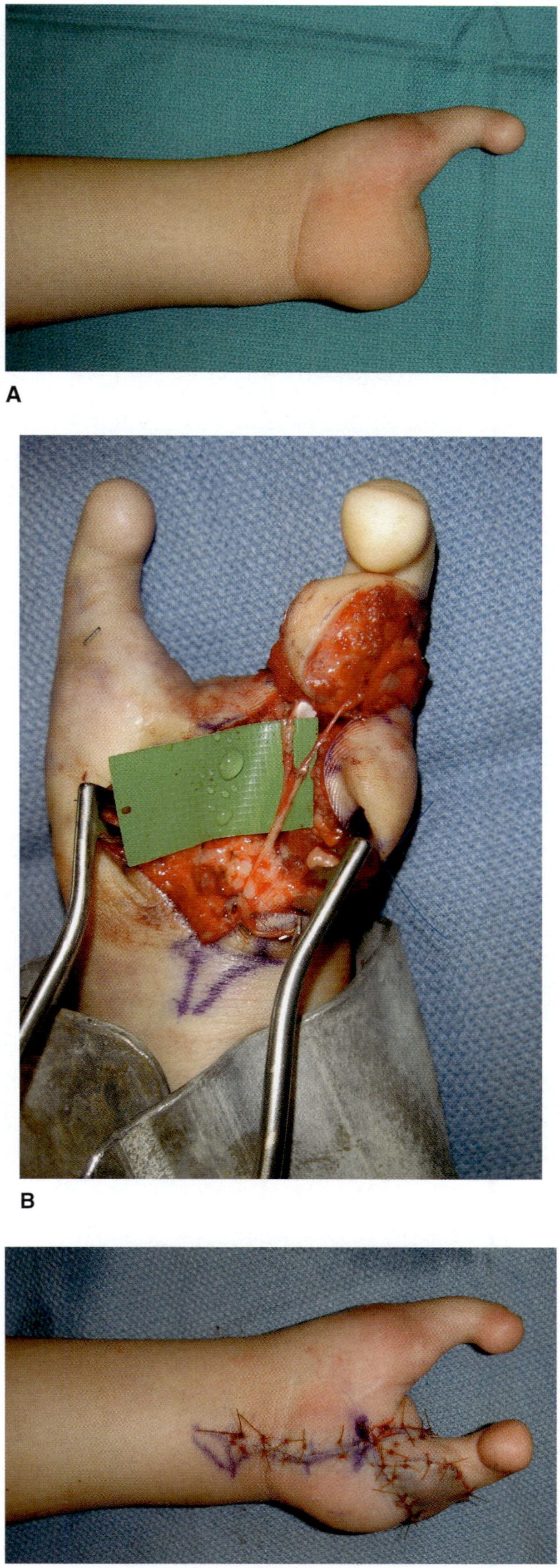

A

B

C

FIGURE 65-10 The child underwent staged second toe transfers, first into the thumb position (A) and 6 months later into the small finger position (B and C).

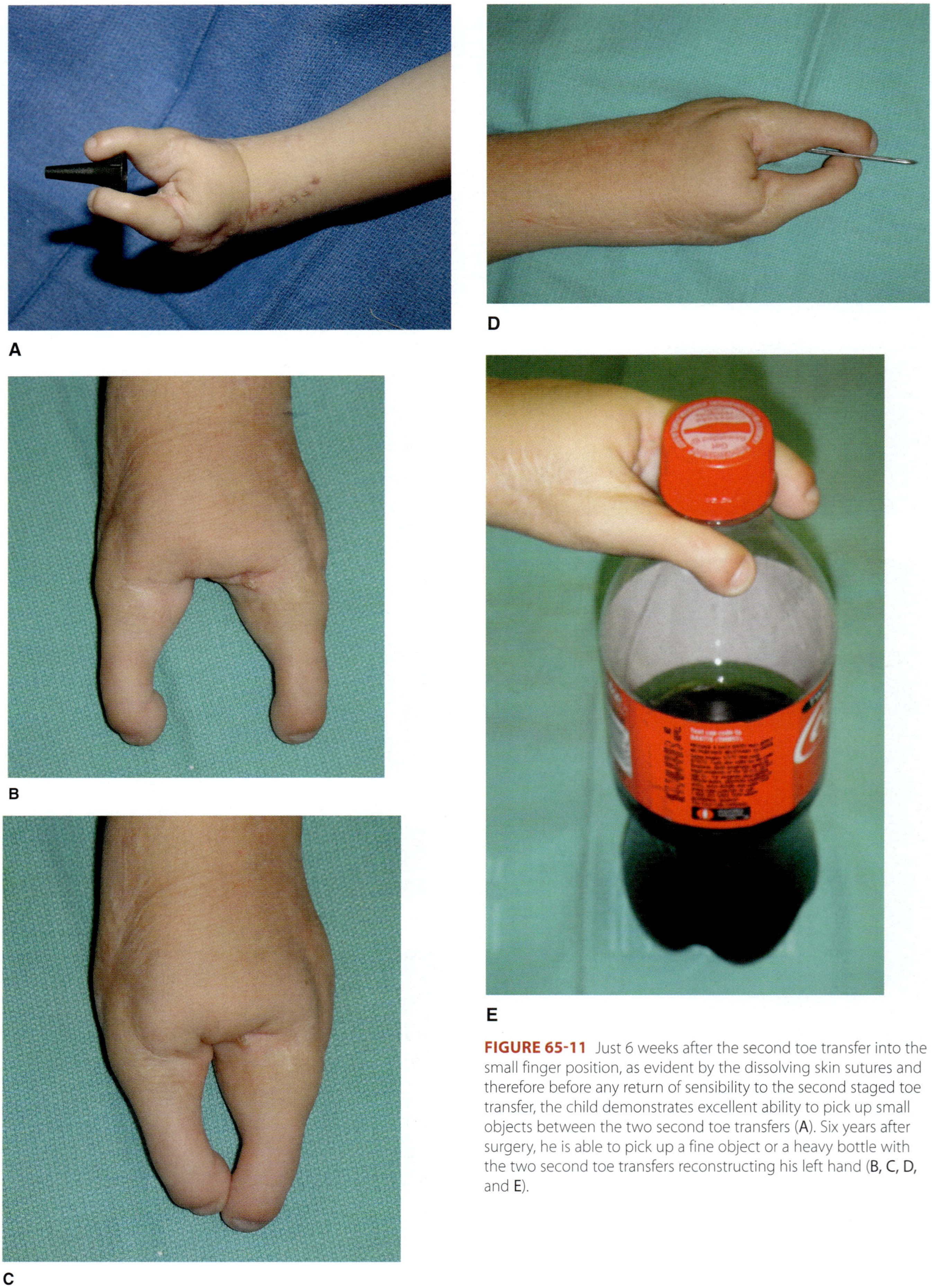

FIGURE 65-11 Just 6 weeks after the second toe transfer into the small finger position, as evident by the dissolving skin sutures and therefore before any return of sensibility to the second staged toe transfer, the child demonstrates excellent ability to pick up small objects between the two second toe transfers (**A**). Six years after surgery, he is able to pick up a fine object or a heavy bottle with the two second toe transfers reconstructing his left hand (**B**, **C**, **D**, and **E**).

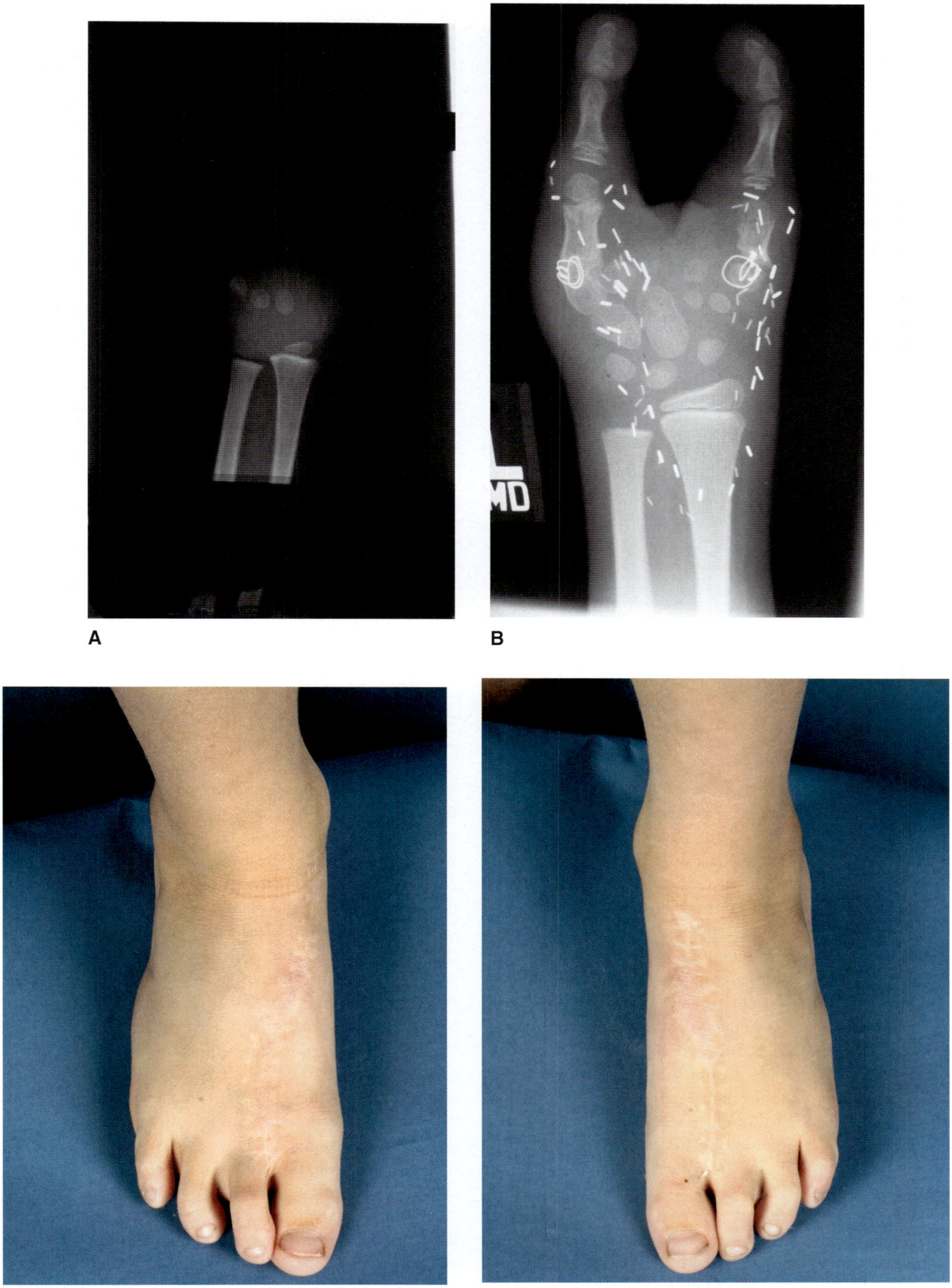

FIGURE 65-12 Preoperative (A) and 2 years after surgery (B) radiographs showing reconstruction of his left hand with staged sequential second toe transfers into the thumb and small finger positions. Appearance of the donor feet 2 years after surgery, right (C) and left (D).

For finger reconstruction, the second toe is always used. A single second toe transfer can be placed in the ring or small finger position to allow both pinch and grasp (see Figures 65-7 and 65-8). For absence of all four fingers, bilateral toe transfers can be considered, one into the small finger position and one into the middle finger position to allow three-point pinch. Bilateral second toe transfers can be performed either in two stages or simultaneously (21,30). Very occasionally, a combined second and third toe transfer can be considered. A child with one normal hand but a contralateral aplastic hand or a contralateral hand with a single digit, either the thumb or small finger, should still be considered for a toe transfer. For the aplastic hand, one toe should be transferred into the thumb position and one toe into the middle, ring or small finger position to allow both pinch and grasp (see Figures 65-9 to 65-12) (21,24,31).

TIMING

Although it is technically possible to perform a toe transfer before the patient is 1 year of age, most surgeons now recommend waiting until 18 months of age when the digital vessels are larger (19) and the anesthetic risk lower (42). In addition, waiting longer allows the family more time to make an informed decision about the necessity for reconstructive surgery. Successful toe transfers have been reported in children older than 10 years of age (43), but generally cortical integration may be better if the toe transfer is performed by the age of 3 years.

CONTRAINDICATIONS

The most obvious contraindications to toe transfers for congenital anomalies of the hand are absence or significant deformity of the toes, a transverse deficiency of the hand proximal to the carpus, and psychosocial factors in the parents or child. However, even in children with severe cleft foot deformities, the abnormal great toe can be transferred to the hand, and then the new thumb can be straightened by arthrodesis or correctional osteotomies at a second stage (33). Even transverse deficiencies proximal to the carpus have been reconstructed by Vilkki by splicing the second toe metatarsal into the distal radius (31,44). Absent digital nerves or median or ulnar nerves are not a contraindication because a nerve transfer can be performed using the uniformly present superficial branch of the radial nerve transferred to the digital nerves of the toe transfer. Similarly, inadequate radial or ulnar arteries at the level of the wrist are not a contraindication because arterial inflow can be provided by a long vein graft from the brachial artery at the elbow.

The family must be realistic and be able to accept the fact that a toe transfer may require emergency revision of the microsurgical anastomoses and can potentially fail, leaving the child with the same deficit in the hand and now a new deformity in the foot. If the parents are unable to accept this potential risk of failure, a toe transfer should not be considered.

POSITIONING AND MARKING

Toe transfer surgery is performed under general anesthesia, occasionally supplemented with an axillary block or continuous brachial plexus infusion to increase the peripheral circulation to the hand and for postoperative pain relief (42). A Foley catheter is used to monitor the child's urine output and overall fluid status, but central venous catheters are not used routinely. A sterile tourniquet is applied to the thigh because a skin graft may need to be harvested from the thigh or groin, but only a regular tourniquet is applied to the upper arm of the involved extremity. An 8-mHz pencil Doppler probe is used to mark out the location of the dorsalis pedis artery and posterior tibial artery in the donor foot. The dorsalis pedis artery is traced distally into the FDMA lying between the great toe and second toe metatarsals. The presence and potential depth of the FDMA can be assessed from the presence or absence and the intensity of the Doppler signal. The thigh tourniquet can be elevated temporarily to 150 mm Hg and potential dorsal veins marked.

SURGICAL TECHNIQUE

If only one surgical team is available, dissection usually commences with the hand to confirm that recipient tendons and nerves are available to repair to the tendons and nerves of the toe transfer. If two teams are available, dissection of the hand and foot can be performed simultaneously.

Dissection of the Donor Foot

Dissection of the foot is performed under tourniquet control after exsanguination with an Esmarch bandage or just by elevating the lower extremity to leave some blood within the venous system. A racquet-shaped incision is used to harvest the great toe or a V-shaped incision is used to harvest the second toe. For a second toe harvest, the midpoint of the webspace between the great toe and second toe and the midpoint of the webspace between the second toe and third toe is marked, and dorsal and plantar triangular flaps are designed from these two points proximally to their apex at the level of the MTP joint. The dorsal incision is extended proximally in either a longitudinal fashion or a lazy S shape to the level of the extensor retinaculum. Usually a dominant dorsal vein can be identified and dissected distally to the level of the dorsal V-shaped flap and proximally to its origin from the greater saphenous vein at the level of the extensor retinaculum. The extensor hallucis longus (EHL) is dissected proximally and divided if transferring the great toe. Alternatively, the extensor digitorum communis (EDC) is dissected and divided proximally when transferring the second toe. The extensor tendon should be harvested as long as possible to provide enough length in cases in which the proximal motor units are short or deficient. The deep peroneal nerve is identified proximally and traced in a proximal-to-distal direction to the proximal margin of the V-shaped dorsal flap. The fascicles of the deep peroneal nerve supplying the toe to be transferred, either the great toe or the second toe, are divided from the main trunk

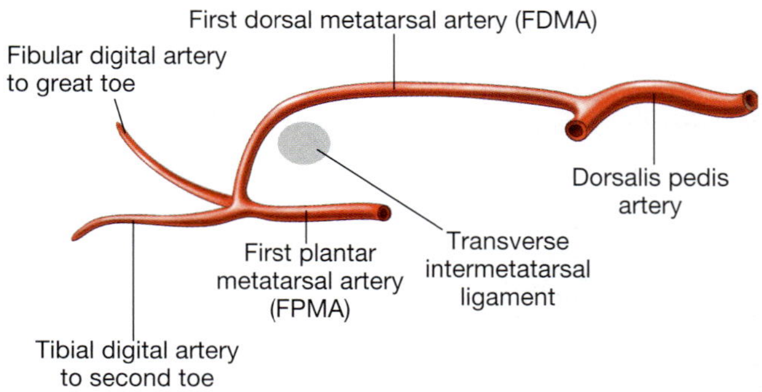

FIGURE 65-13 Anatomy of the first dorsal metatarsal artery and the first plantar metatarsal artery, the vascular supply of both a great toe or second toe transfer.

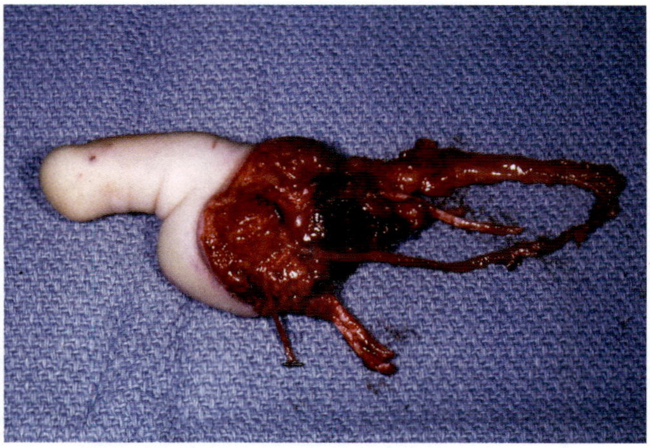

FIGURE 65-14 Creation of an AV loop on a back table by anastomosis of the first plantar metatarsal artery (FPMA) to the saphenous vein, which serves to elongate the FPMA with the saphenous vein itself acting as the interposition vein graft.

of the deep peroneal nerve for later repair to the superficial branch of the radial nerve in the hand.

The FDMA is initially identified distally in the webspace between the great toe and second toe (45). The FDMA may lie in a dorsal, intramuscular, or plantar position in relation to the interosseous muscles. After the FDMA has been identified, the communicating branch between the FDMA and the first plantar metatarsal artery (FPMA) is visualized passing over and distal to the intermetatarsal ligament (Figure 65-13). The ligament is divided and the FPMA dissected farther proximally through the plantar incision. A decision can then be made as to whether the dorsal or plantar arterial system is dominant. If the FDMA is considered to be large enough and in a superficial position, the FDMA can be dissected in a distal-to-proximal direction to its origin from the dorsalis pedis artery. At the junction of the FDMA and dorsalis pedis artery, a communicating branch passes deep to anastomose with the plantar arch and is ligated. The dorsalis pedis artery can be dissected further proximally to the level of the extensor retinaculum by dividing the extensor hallucis brevis tendon. If the FDMA is very small caliber or lies in a deep intramuscular or plantar position, the FPMA can be chosen as the dominant arterial system. The FPMA is obviously shorter than the dorsalis pedis–FDMA arterial system, and therefore the FPMA has to be extended with an interposition vein graft anastomosed on a back table. Occasionally, the FPMA can be anastomosed to the saphenous vein to create an AV loop on a back table. This serves to elongate the FPMA with the saphenous vein itself acting as the interposition vein graft (Figure 65-14). If the second toe is being transferred, the fibular digital artery to the great toe is ligated and divided. Similarly, if the great toe is being transferred, the tibial digital artery to the second toe is ligated and divided.

Alternatively, the dorsalis pedis artery can be dissected in a proximal-to-distal direction into the FDMA. Occasionally, if the great toe is being transferred, it may be transferred on the medial plantar arterial system (46). If the great toe is being transferred in a child with a congenital cleft foot, it can be transferred on the posterior tibial arterial pedicle (33).

The flexor hallucis longus tendon to the great toe or the flexor digitorum longus and flexor digitorum brevis tendons to the second toe are identified through the plantar incision and are divided as far proximally as possible. The medial and lateral plantar digital nerves are identified on either side of the flexor tendon sheath and traced proximally to their bifurcation from the common digital nerves (Figure 65-15). Usually, extra length is necessary, and the bifurcation from the common digital nerve can be split more proximally using microforceps and microscissors. Before finally transecting each digital nerve, the digital nerves are tagged with a small microclip to facilitate their identification after the toe is transferred to the hand.

If the second toe is being transferred, an osteotomy of the second toe metatarsal is performed at the metaphyseal flare. If the great toe is being harvested, the osteotomy is usually performed at the level of the metatarsophalangeal (MTP) joint because a more proximal osteotomy through the great toe metatarsal may interfere with gait. After the osteotomy has been performed, final dissection of the chosen arterial and venous pedicles may be performed to increase their length. The tourniquet is then deflated to allow reperfusion of the toe, and the vascular pedicle can be irrigated with 1:20 papaverine solution or 2% plain Xylocaine solution to relieve any vasospasm. The toe is wrapped in a laparotomy pad bathed with warm irrigating solution. Before transfer to the hand, the toe should appear pink with excellent capillary refill and should have an excellent Doppler pulse.

Dissection of the Hand

If two teams are available, dissection of the hand and foot may be performed simultaneously; otherwise, the hand should be dissected before the foot to ensure that adequate recipient tendons and nerves are present in the hand. The tendon and nerve anatomy is usually very anomalous in symbrachydactyly, but in congenital constriction ring syndrome, the flexor and extensor tendons and digital nerves are present out to the level of the amputation.

The dorsum of the hand is explored first before the palmar aspect to expose the extensor tendons, the superficial radial nerve, a recipient vein, and the dorsal branch of the radial artery in the anatomical snuff box through either a transverse incision at the level of the wrist or a longitudinal incision from

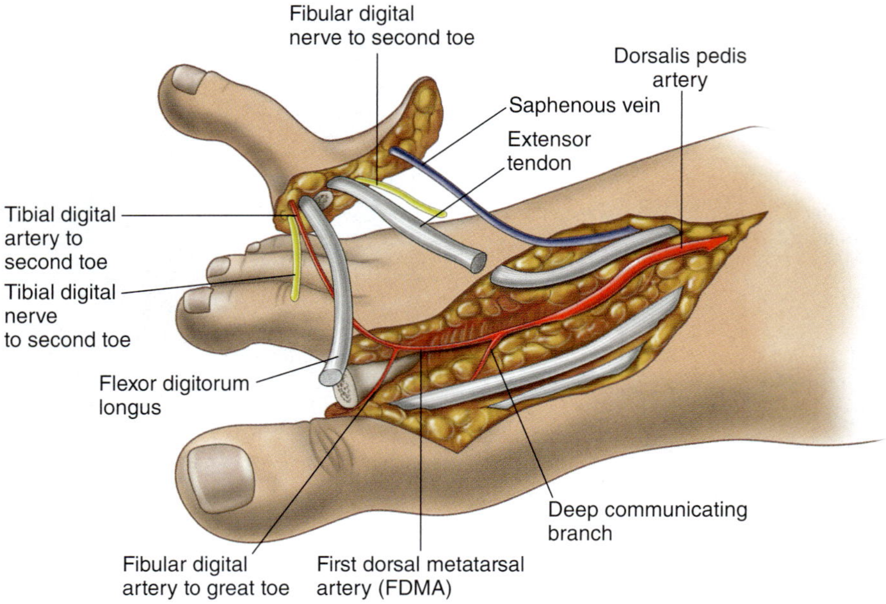

FIGURE 65-15 Anatomy of the dorsal venous drainage of the foot and the superficial and deep peroneal nerve distribution to either the great toe or second toe.

the selected metacarpal, so that the V-shaped dorsal skin flap of the toe transfer will interdigitate. The extensor tendons are usually normal, unlike the flexor tendons, and one extensor tendon is selected that has good gliding and amplitude. A dorsal vein is identified and tagged for the later venous anastomosis. For a toe-to-thumb transfer, the dorsal branch of the radial artery passing through the anatomical snuff box is dissected for the arterial anastomosis.

The palmar surface of the hand is explored through a Bruner zig-zag incision. The median and ulnar nerves may need to be identified at the level of the wrist and dissected distally to identify common digital nerves or proper digital nerves for later repair to the plantar digital nerves. The flexor tendons are dissected either proximal or distal to the transverse carpal ligament, but a portion of the transverse carpal ligament should always be left intact to prevent bowstringing. The flexor tendons are commonly fused together in symbrachydactyly. One of the tendons should be selected and released from the fusion mass, sometimes if necessary all the way proximally into the midforearm to the musculotendinous junction. Finally, the stump of the metacarpal is cleared of periosteum, and dorsal-palmar and radial-ulnar drill holes are made with a 0.035-in K-wire for the subsequent osteosynthesis of the toe metatarsal to the metacarpal using 90-90 intraosseous wiring. Twenty-eight-gauge dental wire may be provisionally passed through the drill holes. The incisions in the hand are closed with staples to prevent excessive swelling, and the tourniquet on the upper arm is deflated.

Transfer of the Toe to the Hand

After the toe transfer has been allowed to reperfuse for at least 20 minutes and all the structures in the hand have been identified and tagged, the tourniquet on the leg is reinflated. The arterial and venous pedicles are ligated with 3-0 or 4-0 silk ties and reinforced with small microclips. If the second toe has been transferred, the gap between the great toe and the third toe is closed by repairing the intermetatarsal ligament using 2-0 or 3-0 Ethibond suture. Meticulous hemostasis is performed, but if there is persistent drainage, a small Jackson-Pratt drain is placed. The skin is closed with interrupted 4-0 chromic catgut mattress sutures. Obviously, closure of the foot defect after harvesting a great toe does not require reconstruction of the intermetatarsal ligament.

The upper arm tourniquet is reinflated to 250 mm Hg to provide a bloodless field to allow bony osteosynthesis, repair of the extensor and flexor tendons, and nerve repairs. The rotation and length of the toe transfer are then determined by placing the base of the toe metatarsal at the proposed site of osteosynthesis of the metacarpal and checking the relationship of the toe transfer to the remaining digits or to the proposed location of a future toe transfer. The exact rotation of the toe transfer and length of the toe metatarsal are marked on the corresponding surfaces of the toe metatarsal and metacarpal. Excess length of the toe metatarsal is removed with an oscillating saw. Osteosynthesis is accomplished using 90-90 intraosseous wiring between the toe metatarsal and the recipient metacarpal. Dorsal-palmar and radial-ulnar drill holes are made in the toe metatarsal using a 0.035-in K-wire, and the previously placed 26-gauge stainless steel dental wires are then passed through these holes and twisted clockwise while at the same time pulling perpendicular to the site of osteosynthesis. As the wire reaches its maximal tension, the surface of the stainless steel dental wire changes from a glistening, shiny appearance to a dull gray. Some surgeons use crossed K-wires or longitudinal K-wires, arguing that they are quicker to insert, do not damage the growth plate, and are stable enough to allow bony union. If the toe transfer has been harvested through the MTP joint, the base of the proximal phalanx of the toe transfer can be fixed to the metacarpal in the hand either with intraosseous wires or crossed K-wires. This arrangement only allows flexion of the toe transfer at the proximal interphalangeal (PIP) and distal interphalangeal (DIP) joints. In some toe-to-thumb transfers, there is absence of a carpometacarpal joint; in such circumstances, the toe metatarsal can be fixed directly to the scaphoid or even spliced into the radial aspect of the radial styloid as described by Vilkki (31,44).

After osteosynthesis has been achieved, any propensity for hyperextension at the MTP joint of the toe transfer is prevented by suturing the volar plate to soft tissues more proximally or to the metatarsal to limit extension to a neutral 0 degrees. The EHL to the great toe or the EDC to the second toe is then repaired to the selected extensor tendon in the hand with the toe transfer in full extension at the metacarpophalangeal, PIP, and DIP joints and the selected recipient tendon at its resting tension. The extensor tendon repair is performed with multiple 4-0 nylon horizontal mattress sutures and a running locked suture to allow early motion. Tethering of the extensor tendon repair to an adjacent extensor tendon may produce a quadriga effect; therefore, adjacent extensor tendons are released. Usually, only one flexor tendon, the flexor hallucis longus in a great toe transfer or the flexor digitorum profundus tendon in a second toe transfer is repaired to a recipient flexor tendon in the hand or at the wrist level. Occasionally, a flexor tendon graft may be necessary to make up the discrepancy in length between the flexor tendon in the toe transfer and a flexor tendon with suitable excursion at the wrist, or alternatively, a primary tendon transfer may be required. The flexor tendon repair is again accomplished using several mattress sutures supplemented with a running locked suture. Any adjacent flexor tendons that might tether the newly reconstructed flexor tendon to the toe transfer are divided to prevent a potential quadriga effect.

Neurorrhaphy of the medial and lateral digital nerves of the toe transfer are then performed to the stump of the proper or common digital nerves in the hand in an end-to-end epineurial fashion under the operating microscope using 10-0 nylon sutures. If there is a gap between the digital nerves of the toe transfer and recipient nerves in the hand, interposition nerve grafts may be necessary using either the superficial or deep peroneal nerves in the foot. Occasionally, the digital nerves of the toe transfer may need to be extended with nerve grafts and then repaired end to side to the median or ulnar nerves at the wrist. Alternatively, a nerve transfer can be performed using the superficial branch of the radial nerve transferred from the dorsal aspect of the first webspace and repaired to one or both of the digital nerves of the toe transfer in the palmar incision.

The microsurgical anastomoses are performed after the second period of tourniquet inflation. The venous anastomosis is usually performed before the arterial anastomosis. The proximal end of the vein to the toe transfer is anastomosed end to end to the selected vein over the dorsal aspect of the wrist under the operating microscope using standard microsurgical techniques using 10-0 nylon sutures. After the venous anastomosis has been completed, the recipient vein is occluded just proximal to the anastomosis with a small microvascular clamp. The site of the arterial anastomosis depends on whether the dorsal or plantar arterial system of the toe transfer was harvested and the location of the recipient radial or ulnar artery. End-to-end or end-to-side anastomosis to the ulnar artery or the dorsal branch of the radial artery in the anatomical stuff box can be performed if there is a long dorsalis pedis–FDMA or posterior tibial artery pedicle. If the FPMA arterial pedicle has been harvested, it is usually too short to reach the radial artery or ulnar artery at the wrist. Occasionally, it can be anastomosed to the superficial palmar arch or to a common digital artery, but it is usually better to elongate the FPMA with an interposition vein graft anastomosed on a back table before performing the osteosynthesis and tendon and nerve repairs. The interposition vein graft can then be anastomosed end to end to the radial artery in the anatomical snuff box or the ulnar artery at the wrist. Occasionally, the FPMA can be anastomosed to the saphenous vein to create an AV loop on a back table. This serves to elongate the FPMA with the saphenous vein itself acting as the interposition vein graft (see Figure 65-14).

The tourniquet is then deflated, leaving a single microvascular clamp on the proximal side of the venous anastomosis to create a high-pressure column of blood flowing through the toe transfer to expand any collapsed vessels caused by vasospasm. The anastomoses are irrigated with 1:20 papaverine, and the hand is bathed with warm irrigating solution. The toe transfer should turn pink and have excellent capillary refill. The patency of the arterial and venous anastomoses can be confirmed by the Acland "milking test," and the vascular clamp can be removed from the proximal side of the venous anastomosis.

The incisions are loosely closed with interrupted 4-0 chromic catgut sutures, and if there is any tension on the closure, split-thickness or full-thickness skin grafts should be liberally used. Any skin graft can be excised at a later date to improve the appearance of the hand. A sterile pulse oximeter probe is applied to the nail plate of the toe transfer before the dressings are applied for continuous postoperative monitoring of the patency of the arterial and venous anastomoses (47). A loose sugar-tong splint is applied to the upper extremity, and the foot is immobilized in a posterior plaster of Paris splint with the foot in neutral position.

POSTOPERATIVE CARE

The child is monitored in a pediatric intensive care unit for 1 to 2 days after surgery. The hand and foot are elevated, and the hand is kept warm with a heating blanket. The toe transfer can be observed hourly for color and capillary refill, but differential pulse oximetry is a simple technique for continuous and noninvasive monitoring of toe transfers and is superior to temperature monitoring (47). One pulse oximeter is placed on the toe transfer in the operating room, and a second pulse oximeter is placed on the contralateral index finger. The pulse rate on the toe transfer corresponds to the patency of the arterial anastomosis, and any loss of the pulse rate compared with the contralateral pulse oximeter may be an indication that the arterial anastomosis has thrombosis. The oxygen saturation (SaO_2) corresponds to the patency of the venous anastomosis, and any persistent drop in the SaO_2 when compared with the contralateral SaO_2 may indicate thrombosis of the venous anastomosis. If the color, capillary refill, or pulse oximeter indicates compromised perfusion to the toe transfer, the child should be immediately returned to the operating room for reexploration and possible revision of the microsurgical anastomoses.

Anticoagulation with Dextran 40 (0.36 mL/kg/hr) is continued for 5 days, and 81 mg of aspirin is started on postoperative day 1 and continued for 4 weeks. The Dextran infusion is reduced to half on postoperative day 6 and discontinued on day 7. A first-generation cephalosporin is administered intravenously for 48 hours after surgery, and intravenous fluids are maintained until the child tolerates a normal diet. The dressings on the hand and foot are changed on postoperative days 5 to 7. If there is any concern with perfusion to the toe transfer, the cast and dressings should be immediately released or completely removed because occasionally the plaster splint and dried blood can combine to form a constrictive "cast," producing external compression on the microsurgical anastomoses. The child can begin to ambulate as soon as he or she feels comfortable with the foot. The plaster hand and foot splints are removed at the first postoperative visit at 2 weeks, and "take" of any skin grafts is assessed. The foot incision may occasionally require local wound care for minor dehiscence or oral antibiotics for localized cellulitis. A removable thermoplast splint is fabricated to protect the toe transfer, and the parents are instructed to begin passive and active range of motion exercises of the toe transfer. A hand therapist may assist with therapy if the family is apprehensive. If K-wires have been inserted for bony fixation, they are usually removed 4 to 6 weeks after surgery.

RESULTS AND OUTCOMES

The first microsurgical toe transfer for reconstruction of a congenital hand anomaly in a child was reported by O'Brien et al. (10), who successfully transferred the great toe to reconstruct thumb hypoplasia in two children. May et al. (13) reported a 9-year-old boy with aplasia of the thumb and index and middle fingers of both hands treated by bilateral great toe–to–thumb transfers. Nyarady et al. (11) performed the first second toe–to–thumb transfer for thumb hypoplasia. The first series of pediatric toe-to-thumb transfers was reported by Yoshimura (12), who successfully performed 12 toe transfers, of which one child had an absent thumb and index and middle fingers and another child had congenital constriction ring syndrome. Larger series have subsequently reported success rates greater than 96%.

Gilbert (19) reported 21 second toe transfers in 17 children with congenital hand differences to reconstruct four thumbs and 17 fingers in children between the ages of 18 months and 3 years. There was one reexploration for venous thrombosis but no failures. Gilbert found that the results were better in children with congenital constriction ring syndrome than those with congenital aplasia because structures were more normal proximally. Restoration of motion was minimal at the PIP and DIP joints of the toe transfers with mean active combined motion of 40 degrees. The majority of the children were unable to discriminate any difference in sensation between the toe transfer and normal fingers. Growth of the toe transfers was similar to that of the contralateral second toe, and no deficits in gait were observed.

Lister (26) reported 12 children who underwent a second toe transfer to reconstruct the thumb for congenital constriction ring syndrome, symbrachydactyly, and transverse arrest. Tu et al. (35) described 11 children between the ages of 18 months and 6 years who underwent toe transfers to reconstruct a hypoplastic thumb as an alternative to pollicization. One child required immediate reexploration for venous occlusion, and one child failed for a success rate of 91%. Mean total active range of motion was 60 degrees, and sensation was regained in all toe transfers with an average two-point discrimination of 4.2 mm.

Shvedovchenko (29) reported 103 successful toe transfers in 66 children between 3 and 14 years of age, some with congenital differences of the hand. Vilkki (31) performed 18 toe transfers in children between 2 and 12 years of age for congenital adactyly with one failure caused by anesthesia complications and five reexplorations. Kay (22–24) successfully transferred 66 toes in 40 children for congenital anomalies, traumatic loss, or infection, of which five toe transfers required reexploration. Total active range of motion was less than expected with an average of 60 degrees, and tenolysis was performed secondarily in 15 children and tendon transfers in seven children. All of the children achieved protective sensibility, and in children in whom two-point discrimination could be measured, the median was 5 mm. A total of 76% of the parents were very satisfied with the results of the toe transfer surgery (48), and most parents and children thought that the surgery had positively affected the child's psychosocial well-being (39). Foucher et al. (17,18) reported 65 toe transfers in 58 children who achieved a mean total active range of motion of 38 degrees but a mean extension lag of 25 degrees and mean two-point discrimination of 5 mm. There were no failures if two arteries were anastomosed, but there were two failures when only one artery was anastomosed. Van Holder et al. (30) reconstructed 14 children with congenital constriction ring syndrome, symbrachydactyly, and transverse failure with staged double second toe transfers. Mean total active flexion achieved was 80 degrees with a mean extension lag of 20 degrees. All of the toe transfers regained sensibility and provided improved function and appearance; however, all 14 children required at least one secondary procedure. Richardson et al. (28) performed 18 toe transfers in 13 children with symbrachydactyly. A total of 85% of parents were happy with the appearance and function of their child's reconstructed hand. Jones et al. (21) reported 100 toe transfers in 79 children with congenital anomalies of the hand. Eight toe transfers (8%) required reexploration of the microsurgical anastomoses; two toe transfers (2%) failed. All children regained protective sensation. Toe transfers have also been performed for reconstruction of congenital differences in older children. Spokevicius (43) successfully transferred four toes in three children with congenital differences between 11 and 17 years of age.

The range of motion of the transferred toe is unpredictable and is the most common indication for secondary revision. Passive range of motion exceeds active range of motion, but despite this, tenolysis is rarely useful (24). Most motion occurs at the MTP joint, and there is usually minimal active motion at the DIP joint and an extension lag at the proximal interphalangeal joint, so that a flexion deformity of the toe transfer is a frequent outcome (15,26). Consequently, a toe transfer performed for finger reconstruction functions largely as a post to assist in grasp. Vilkki (31) reported that ability to pinch was restored in 14 of 17 children with congenital adactyly. Jones et al. (21) reported that 66 of 68 children regained pinch and grasp function after toe transfers.

Growth of a toe transfer is related to the surgical technique of osteosynthesis, ischemia time, venous stasis, innervation, and infection. Gilbert (20) reported that 10 of 85 epiphyseal plates developed premature closure. Vilkki (31) reported normal or near-normal growth of 11 toe transfers with a mean follow-up period of 4 years. Kay and Wiberg (23) reported that growth of a toe transfer ranged between 70% and 104% of the contralateral toe. Chang and Jones (49) performed a radiographic analysis of growth after 23 toe transfers for congenital anomalies and demonstrated that 96% of the epiphyseal plates remained open on postoperative radiographs, there was increasing serial growth of the transferred toe compared with preoperative radiographs, and growth of the toe transfer was exactly the same as the growth of the contralateral toe. The second toe is approximately 5 cm long in a 2-year-old child and provides an immediate and much greater increase in length compared with nonvascularized toe phalangeal bone grafting or distraction lengthening and a more guaranteed potential for serial growth.

Virtually every large series of toe transfers has documented that all the children regain protective sensibility, and many recover two-point discrimination of 4 to 6 mm (18,19,21,23,24, 26,28,30,35).

All of the large series of toe transfers report minimal or no morbidity in the donor foot.

CONCLUSION

Microsurgical toe-to-hand transfer has become an accepted and most rewarding technique in the armamentarium of the pediatric hand surgeon for reconstruction of congenital differences of the hand in children, although it remains a technically challenging undertaking requiring a high level of microsurgical skill on the part of the surgeon and the trust and patience of the child's parents. Preoperative counseling of the parents with the opportunity to meet or speak with other children and families who have undergone toe transfers is very helpful. The appropriate age for toe transfer is probably between 2 and 3 years, although the procedure can still be successful in older children. Differential pulse oximetry simplifies postoperative monitoring. Toe transfers provide sensation and some limited range of motion, but parents should be made aware that sensation will take 3 to 6 months to return and that motion of the transferred toe may continue to improve over a 1- to 2-year period. Most of these children will require secondary tenolyses, tendon transfers, bone grafting, arthrodeses, osteotomy, or scar revision to achieve their optimal functional and aesthetic outcome. A child who is able to write his or her name for the first time or who can now ride a bicycle or who can participate in sports provides the surgeon with far more feedback than the most sophisticated outcome instruments.

REFERENCES

1. Buncke HJ, Buncke CM, Schultz WP. Immediate Nicoladoni procedure in the Rhesus monkey, or hallux-to-hand transplantation, utilizing microminiature vascular anastomoses. *Br J Plast Surg* 1966;19:332–337.
2. Cobbett JR. Free digital transfer: report of a case of transfer of a great toe to replace an amputated thumb. *J Bone Joint Surg* 1969;51B:677–679.
3. Buncke HJ, McLean DH, Geroge PT, et al. Thumb replacement: great toe transplantation by microvascular anastomosis. *Br J Plast Surg* 1973;26: 194–201.
4. Morrison WA, O'Brien BM, MacLeod AM. Thumb reconstruction with a free neurovascular wrap-around flap from the big toe. *J Hand Surg* 1980;5:575–583.
5. Wei FC, Chen HC, Chuang CC, Noordhoff MS. Reconstruction of the thumb with a trimmed-toe transfer technique. *Plast Reconstr Surg* 1988; 82:506–515.
6. Upton J, Mutimer KL. A modification of the great toe transfer for thumb reconstruction. *Plast Reconstr Surg* 1988;82:535–538.
7. Wei FC, Mardini S. Reevaluation of the technique of toe-to-hand transfer for traumatic digital amputations in children and adolescents. *Plast Reconstr Surg* 2003;112:1870–1874.
8. Buck-Gramcko D. Pollicization of the index finger: method and results in aplasia and hypoplasia of the thumb. *J Bone Joint Surg* 1971;53A:1605–1617.
9. Miyawaki T, Masuzawa G, Hirakawa M, Kurihara K. Bone-lengthening for symbrachydactyly of the hand with the technique of callus distraction. *J Bone Joint Surg* 2002;84A:986–991.
10. O'Brien BM, Black MJ, Morrison WA, Macleod AM. Microvascular great toe transfer for congenital absence of the thumb. *Hand* 1978;10:113–124.
11. Nyarady JP, Szekeres, Vilmos Z. Toe-to-thumb transfer in congenital grade III thumb hypoplasia. *J Hand Surg* 1983;8:898–901.
12. Yoshimura M. Toe-to-hand transfer. *Plast Reconstr Surg* 1980;66:74–83.
13. May J, Smith RJ, Peimer C. Toe-to-hand free tissue transfer for thumb construction with multiple digit aplasia. *Plast Reconstr Surg* 1981;67: 205–213.
14. Meals RA, Lesavoy MA. Hallux-to-hand transfer during ankle disarticulation for multiple limb anomalies. *JAMA* 1983;249:72–73.
15. Eaton CJ, Lister GD. Toe transfer for congenital hand defects. *Microsurgery* 1991;12:186–195.
16. Foo IT, Malata CM, Kay SP. Free tissue transfers to the upper limb. *J Hand Surg* 1993;18B:279–284.
17. Foucher G. Le transfert d'orteil dans les malformations congenitales de la main. *Bull Acad Natl Med* 1997;181:1737–1744; discussion 1744–1745.
18. Foucher G, Medina J, Navarro R, Nagel D. Toe transfer in congenital hand malformations. *J Reconstr Microsurg* 2001;17:1–7.
19. Gilbert A. Toe transfers for congenital hand defects. *J Hand Surg* 1982;7A:118–124.
20. Gilbert A. Reconstruction of congenital hand defects with microvascular toe transfers. *Hand Clin* 1985;1:351–360.
21. Jones NF, Kaplan J. Indications for microsurgical reconstruction of congenital hand anomalies by toe-to-hand transfers. *Hand* 2013;8:367–374.
22. Kay SP, Wiberg M. Toe to hand transfer in children. Part 1: technical aspects. *J Hand Surg* 1996;21B:723–734.
23. Kay SP, Wiberg M, Bellew M, Webb F. Toe to hand transfer in children. Part 2: functional and psychological aspects. *J Hand Surg* 1996;21B: 735–745.
24. Kay S, McGuiness C. Microsurgical reconstruction in abnormalities of children's hands. *Hand Clin* 1999;15:563–583.
25. Lister G. Reconstruction of the hypoplastic thumb. *Clin Orthop Rel Res* 1985;195:52–65.
26. Lister G. Microsurgical transfer of the second toe for congenital deficiency of the thumb. *Plast Reconstr Surg* 1988;82:658–665.
27. Lister G. Toes to the hand. In Flatt A (ed). *Pediatric Hand Surgery.* 1991, p. 180–192.
28. Richardson PWF, Johnstone BR, Coombs CJ. Toe-to-hand transfer in symbrachydactyly. *Hand Surg* 2004;9:11–18.
29. Shvedovchenko IV. Toe-to-hand transfers in children. *Ann Plast Surg* 1993;31:251–254.
30. Van Holder C, Giele H, Gilbert A. Double second toe transfer in congenital hand anomalies. *J Hand Surg* 1999;24B:471–475.
31. Vilkki SK. Advances in microsurgical reconstruction of the congenitally adactylous hand. *Clin Orthop Rel Res* 1995;314:45–58.
32. Foucher G, et al. La symbrachydactylie, classification et traitement. A propos d'une serie de 117 cas. *Chirurgie de la Main* 2000;19:161–168.

33. Chang J, Jones NF. Simultaneous Toe-to-hand transfer and lower extremity amputations for severe upper and lower limb defects: the use of spare parts. *J Hand Surg* 2002;27B:219–223.
34. Harashina T, Inoue T, Fujino T, et al. Reconstruction of a floating thumb with an excess big toe. *J Reconstr Microsurg* 1994;10:11–15.
35. Tu YK, Yeh WL, Sananpanich K, et al. Microsurgical second toe-metatarsal bone transfer for reconstructing congenital radial deficiency with hypoplastic thumb. *J Reconstr Microsurg* 2004;20:215–225.
36. Michon J, Merle M, Bouchon Y, Foucher G. Functional comparison between pollicization and toe-to-hand transfer for thumb reconstruction. *J Reconstr Microsurg* 1984;1:103–112.
37. Bradbury ET, Kay SP, Tighe C, Hewison J. Decision-making by parents and children in paediatric hand surgery. *Br J Plast Surg* 1994;47:324–330.
38. Bradbury ET, Kay SPJ, Hewison J, The psychological impact of microvascular free toe transfer for children and their parents. *J Hand Surg* 1994;19B:689–695.
39. Bellew M, Kay SP. Psychological aspects of toe-to-hand transfer in children: comparison of views of children and their parents. *J Hand Surg* 1999;24B:712–718.
40. Greenberg B, May J. Great toe-to-hand transfer: role of the preoperative lateral angiogram of foot. *J Hand Surg* 1988;13A:411–414.
41. Frykman GK, O'Brien BM, Morrison WA, MacLeod AM. Functional evaluation of the hand and foot after one-stage toe-to-hand transfer. *J Hand Surg* 1986;11A:9–17.
42. Inberg P, Kassila M, Vilkki S, et al. Anaesthesia for microvascular surgery in children: a combination of general anaesthesia and axillary plexus block. *Acta Anaesthesiol Scand* 1995;39:518–522.
43. Spokevicius S, Radzevicius D. Late toe-to-hand transfer for the reconstruction of congenital defects of the long fingers. *Scand J Plast Reconstr Surg Hand Surg* 1997;31:345–350.
44. Foucher G. The "stub" operation—modification of the Furnas and Vilkki technique in traumatic and congenital carpal hand reconstruction. *Ann Acad Med Singapore* 1995;24:73–76.
45. Wei FC, Silverman RT, Hsu WM. Retrograde dissection of the vascular pedicle in toe harvest. *Plast Reconstr Surg* 1995;96:1211–1214.
46. Koman LA, Weiland A, Moore JR. Toe-to-hand transfer based on the medial plantar artery. *J Hand Surg* 1985;10A:561–566.
47. Jones NF, Gupta R. Postoperative monitoring of pediatric toe-to-hand transfers with differential pulse oximetry. *J Hand Surg* 2001;26A: 525–529.
48. Schenker M, Wiberg M, Kay SP, Johansson RS. Precision grip function after free toe transfer in children with hypoplastic digits. *J Plast Reconstr Aesthet Surg* 2007;60:13–23.
49. Chang J, Jones NF. Radiographic analysis of growth in pediatric microsurgical toe-to-hand transfers. *Plast Reconstr Surg* 2002;109: 576–582.

CHAPTER 66

Free Joint Transfers

Vaughan Bowen

Small joints in the hand may be damaged by congenital abnormalities, trauma, or disease. Table 66-1 lists numerous surgical techniques that have been developed for managing patients with joint damage in the hand. Each technique has advantages and disadvantages. Many factors need to be considered when choosing the best technique for a specific patient's problem. The most important consideration, however, should be hand function, including dexterity in the radial digits, and grip in the ulna fingers. Good-functioning joints are critical to hand activity. In an adult's hand, they need to be mobile, pain free, and stable. In a child's hand, they also need the potential for growth and development.

HISTORICAL BACKGROUND

Synthetic and Biological Joint Reconstructions

Synthetic reconstructions have been very successful for managing clinical problems in large joints such as the hip, knee, and shoulder. Vascularized joint transfers have been almost exclusively used for the reconstruction of damaged hands, although, even there, Silastic interposition, pyrocarbon, metal–polyethylene, and biological joint replacements have been widely used and produce satisfactory results in the majority of cases.

In 1986, Foucher et al. (1) compared the results of a number of different kinds of joint reconstruction. At the metacarpophalangeal (MCP) joints, they found that the range of motion in vascular joint transfers was similar to that obtained with Swanson Silastic implants. The advantages of vascularized joint transfers, however, were that they were applicable to the most severe problems with compound tissue loss, especially if it involved the extensor tendon, skin, and volar plate. Vascularized joint transfers could also be structured to contain functional epiphyseal plates, which gave them an advantage in the management of complex problems in children.

No studies have compared the results of vascularized joint transfers with pyrocarbon or metal–polyethylene joint replacements.

Experimental Nonvascularized and Vascularized Joint Transfers

Summaries of the work done with nonvascularized joint transfers and other studies leading to the first vascularized joint transfers have been published (2–10). Although there are some reports of reasonably successful isolated cases, the results of nonvascularized joint transfers were generally disappointing. They underwent tissue necrosis, and although their bone could be replaced and remodeled, the hyaline cartilage was replaced with fibrocartilage. The joints became dysfunctional. If epiphyseal plates were included, growth was unpredictable and usually retarded or nonexistent.

In 1967, Buncke et al. (2) described the short- and long-term clinical, radiographic, histologic, and fluorescent microscopy features of joints in successful experimental microsurgical replantations in rat knee and monkey toe and finger models. They concluded that whereas nonvascularized transplants undergo extensive degenerative change, vascularized transplants survive completely and maintained their normal cellular architecture and function.

Other researchers published similar results in their experiments on vascularized joint transfer studies (6,9). Hurwitz (6) showed that experimental vascularized whole-joint transfers were indistinguishable macroscopically and microscopically from normal joints, and they only had a slight restriction in movement.

The possibility of using vascularized partial joint transfers has been investigated experimentally (6) and clinically (11). They proved to be inferior, and the movement achieved was much less than in vascularized whole-joint transfers. There are only a few clinical indications for their use. They may be a useful option for:

TABLE 66-1 Surgical Techniques for the Management of Damaged Joints in the Hand

Osteotomy
Extraarticular
Intraarticular
Arthroplasty
Synthetic
Spacers
Implants
Metal
Polyethylene
Pyrocarbon
Biologic, autogenous
Soft tissue interposition arthroplasties
Nonvascularized whole joint transfers
Vascularized partial joint transfers
Vascularized whole joint transfers
Biologic, allogeneic
Vascularized allograft joint transplants
Arthrodesis
Other options
Denervation
Amputation
Tissue engineering

1. Reconstructing the thumb after a transarticular amputation at the MCP joint in a patient in whom some MCP joint movement is required.
2. Reconstructing a proximal phalanx with lost or damaged articular surfaces at each end.
3. Reconstructing an articular surface in joints outside the hand in usual clinical situations. For instance, the proximal fibula has been used to reconstruct the distal radius (12) and the elbow (13) for cases in which there has been massive bone loss or resection.

Recognizing the limited choice of donor tissue and hoping to avoid donor site morbidity, some investigators have studied the possible use of allografts (14,15). If adequate systemic immunosuppression is given, the functional results are very similar to those with autografts. Without immunosuppression, vascular rejection limited survival and was associated with articular cartilage destruction and loss of function within 6 to 8 months (5).

Development of Technique for Clinical Cases

The foot has been thought of as a good source of donor tissue since the early days of reconstructive microvascular surgery (16,17). Tsai et al. (9) did a primate study in which the surgical technique was readied for clinical application.

Clinical Vascularized Joint Transfers

Vascularized joint transfers are mostly done for reconstruction of small joints in the fingers and thumb. The early medical literature (2,8,9,17–22) demonstrated that vascularized joint transfers could be satisfactorily used to solve difficult clinical problems that did not lend themselves to synthetic joint replacements. Case reports (17,18,22) and small clinical series (8,19–21) documented microsurgical and functional success. Subsequently bigger series (1,7,11,23–27) and review papers have been published (3,5,10,28) detailing indications, technique, results, and complications.

FREE TISSUE TRANSFERS AVAILABLE FOR JOINT RECONSTRUCTION

Nowadays, by far the most frequently used donor site for vascularized joint transfers is the second toe. Because it is possible to remove the whole second ray from the foot on its microvascular pedicle, surgeons have numerous choices of donor tissue. Greater or lesser portions of the ray can be harvested as needed for the specific reconstruction being done. It is also possible to remove part or all of the adjacent big toe or third toe, either as isolated sources of donor tissue or combined with components from the second toe.

Another source of donor tissue has been other finger joints. These can be harvested as homodigit (4,5,29) or heterodigit transfers (5,25). They can be moved as free transfers or as islands (4,5,25). Their use has been restricted to relatively uncommon, specialized circumstances when it is anticipated that the potential donor site morbidity from their loss will be low.

Table 66-2 lists the donor sites that have been used as free tissue transfer. The table includes the numerous types of variation that have been used in structure and application.

THE SECOND TOE DONOR SITE

Second Toe Advantages and Disadvantages

The second toe is a source of well-vascularized autogenous tissue with a well-understood, long, and reasonably predictable vascular pedicle. The vessels are large enough for reliable microvascular anastomosis. The rich vascularity is a useful quality for posttraumatic recipient sites that are poorly vascularized. Second toe joints are well matched in size and shape to the small joints in the hand. Vascularized transfers can be harvested as composite grafts with a thin, flexible overlying skin flap, which can be used for postoperative monitoring or soft tissue cover. They can also be harvested with tendon, usually on the extensor side. The cut surfaces of the distal metacarpal and phalanges are very satisfactory for osteosynthesis. The bone is of good quality for internal fixation and provides an excellent surface for bone healing. Epiphyseal plates are similar in location to those in the hand, although growth potential is less. The foot donor site is easily accessible and distant to the hand, so that a separate team of surgeons can work at the donor site at the same time as the recipient site is being prepared.

TABLE 66-2 Free Tissue Transfers for Joint Reconstruction

1. Second toe MTP joint
    - Joint alone
    - Joint with overlying tendon
    - Joint with skin flap with or without skin flap
    - Immature donor tissue with two epiphyseal plates
2. Second toe PIP joint
    - Joint alone
    - Joint with overlying tendon
    - Joint with skin flap with or without skin flap
    - Immature donor tissue with single epiphyseal plate
3. Variations in donor tissue site
    - Autograft whole joint or partial joint
        - From the second toe
        - From another toe
        - From another part of the hand
            - Homodigital joint transfer
            - Heterodigit joint transfers (free or as an island)
            - "Digit bank" joints
        - Proximal fibula as a partial joint transfer
    - Allograft whole joint or partial joint
4. Variations in application
    - Standard whole toe joint transfer
    - Inverted whole toe joint transfer
    - Flow-through flap
    - Twisted two toe

MTP, metatarsophalangeal; PIP, proximal interphalangeal.

There are some disadvantages in using the second toe as a donor site. Sometimes the anatomical dissection to raise the donor tissue can be difficult, especially if there are vascular anomalies. The phalanges are smaller than those in the hand, which means that there may be less bone for reconstruction and for positioning internal fixation. The anatomical structure of the metatarsophalangeal (MTP) joint is different to the hand. Specifically, the joint functions in hyperextension rather than in flexion, which is required for MCP joint reconstruction. A number of techniques have been developed to manage this difficulty (see later subsection on osteotomy configuration). Primary healing in the foot has been a problem, although advances in surgical technique have reduced difficulties. It is, however, important to ask patients about their work and leisure activity patterns to make sure there are no contraindications for using the foot as a donor site.

Skeletal Structure of the Foot Second Ray

An adult second metatarsal is a miniature long bone 6 to 7 cm in length. The shaft is made of hard cortical bone. It is 1 cm in diameter. The head is made of cancellous bone with a thin outer cortex. It is 1.5 to 2 cm in diameter.

The MTP joint differs from an MCP joint in that it lies in hyperextension and tends to function into hyperextension. Unlike the MTP joint, the interphalangeal (IP) joints in the toes function in flexion in a manner similar to those in the hand.

The second toe MTP joint transplant differs from the proximal interphalangeal (PIP) joint transplant in that it has greater growth potential. The MTP joint transplant has two epiphyseal plates, one at the distal end of the metatarsal and one at the proximal end of the proximal phalanx. There is no epiphyseal plate at the distal end of the proximal phalanx, so the PIP joint transplant only has one epiphyseal plate at the proximal end of the middle phalanx.

The toe phalanges and IP joints are smaller than those in fingers but otherwise are relatively similar.

Arterial Supply to the Second Toe and Its Joints

The blood supply to the foot, specifically, the blood supply to the dorsalis pedis system and free tissue transfers developed from the toes, was extensively studied using cadaver dissections, latex injection studies (18), and radiographic studies. Wei et al. (30) summarized the literature and focused on the variations that had previously been classified. Although it is important to recognize that anatomical variations occur, a clear understanding of the typical vascular anatomy is the foundation for surgical success.

Many different types of free tissue transfer can be elevated from the vascular pedicle. These include dorsalis pedis free flaps, second metatarsal vascularized bone grafts, vascularized joint transfers, microvascular free toe transfers, and other customized complex composite tissue free tissue transfers.

Manktelow (31) published a very clear and detailed description of the microsurgically relevant anatomy of the blood supply to the second toe and its components. The anterior tibial artery changes its name to the dorsalis pedis artery as it crosses the ankle to enter the foot. The dorsalis pedis artery is 2 to 3 mm in diameter. It passes deep to the extensor retinaculum and runs lateral to the extensor hallucis longus tendon. In the hindfoot, it stays deep, lying on the surface of the talus, navicular, and second cuneiform bones and their associated ligaments, giving off tarsal branches to supply them and the soft tissues in the region. It then runs along the groove between the first cuneiform and the base of the second metatarsal, where it is crossed by the extensor hallucis brevis muscle. In this location, it runs alongside the deep peroneal nerve on its medial side and may give off the arcuate artery, the origin of the second, third, and fourth dorsal metatarsal arteries, on its lateral side. The dorsalis pedis artery terminates at the proximal end of the interspace between the first and second metacarpals. A communicating branch descends close to the surface of metatarsal bone bases to join the plantar arterial system.

More distally, the second metatarsal and second toe received their blood supply from the first dorsal metatarsal artery and the first plantar metatarsal artery.

Typically, the first dorsal metatarsal artery arises as a terminal branch of the dorsalis pedis artery at the interspace at the proximal ends of the first and second metacarpals, where the communicating branch descends to the planter arterial system. This, however, is not always the case. Variations are common. Vessels may vary in size and position from this typical anatomical description. Manktelow (31) reviewed the original literature describing these variations (32) and warned about confusing variations in the origin of the first dorsal metatarsal artery. In particular, he emphasized the possibility that the first dorsal metatarsal artery may arise from plantar vessels. There is no dorsalis pedis artery in 3% to 12% of feet. In 3% to 7%, it is a continuation of the peroneal artery. When there is a dorsalis pedis artery, the first dorsal metatarsal artery may still arise from the plantar system. Although it most commonly lies dorsally, in as many as 34% of dissections, its origin and course was deep to or within the interosseous muscles. Distally, however, it always ended up dorsal to the deep transverse intermetatarsal ligament.

The second metatarsal blood supply comes from branches of the first dorsal metatarsal artery, which first perforate the first dorsal interosseous muscles, and then supply periosteal vessels. One or two branches of the periosteal vessels supply the intramedullary circulation by penetrating the cortex through one or two nutrient foramena at each end.

In the region of the transverse intermetatarsal ligament between the first and second MTP joints, the distal ends of the first dorsal and first plantar metatarsal arteries are linked by communicating arteries. Digital arteries branch off at this location and run distally as the lateral digital artery of the big toe and medial digital artery of the second toe.

Venous Drainage of the Second Toe and Its Joints

Venous blood drains through two different pathways, the venae comitantes and the superficial dorsal veins. Both systems are useful for draining free tissue transfers from the second toe.

A small superficial dorsal vein originates on each side of each toe in the subcutaneous tissues. These run proximately as the dorsal metatarsal veins. At the proximal end of the metatarsals, they form dorsal arches, which drain medially into the long saphenous vein and laterally into the short saphenous vein. The long saphenous vein runs proximally anterior to the medial malleolus. The short saphenous vein runs posterior to the lateral malleolus.

Venae comitantes accompany all of the arteries in the foot. They drain all the deep structures: bones, joints, and deep muscles. There is extensive linking and communication. The venae comitantes of the planter and dorsal systems are linked. The venae comitantes also communicate with the superficial dorsal veins.

Associated Skin Flaps

A number of options are used to harvest skin with donor joints from toe donor sites (3,5,7,10,23,24,27). These can be used for soft tissue reconstruction or for postoperative monitoring. Branches of the main vascular pedicle enable the surgeon to harvest a dorsalis pedis flap, localized skin from the second toe, or skin from the adjacent big toe with a donor joint from the second toe.

INDICATIONS

Table 66-3 summarizes the factors to be considered when planning a vascularized joint transfer.

Overall Considerations

Although vascularized joint transfers come close to providing the ideal arthroplasty goals (24) of pain-free motion, stability, durability, and the potential for growth in children, they are complex and demanding surgical procedures, with the disadvantage of a donor site with its own potential complications. Indications for their use are similar to the simpler synthetic or biological arthroplasties, which are perfectly satisfactory most of the time. The indications for vascularized joint transfers are

TABLE 66-3 Factors to Be Considered When Planning a Vascularized Joint Transfer

1. Overall considerations
    - Joint to be reconstructed
    - Nature of the joint pathology
    - Degree and extent of tissue damage
    - Goals
    - Surgical complexity
    - Resources available
    - Advantages and disadvantages compared with simpler techniques
2. Patient-related considerations
    - Age
    - Heath status
    - Hand dominance
    - Occupation
    - Donor site considerations
    - Expectations
3. Functional considerations in the hand
    - Need for stability
    - Need for mobility
    - Structure and function in the digit to be reconstructed
        - Skeletal structures
        - Flexor tendon function
        - Extensor tendon function
        - Soft tissue cover
        - Neurovascular status
    - Structure and function in the undamaged part of the hand

TABLE 66-4 Unique Features of Vascularized Joint Transfers That Make Them a Good Choice for Solving Certain Specific Complex Problems

1. They preserve joint architecture and articular cartilage.
2. They can fill segmental defects with composite tissue (bone, cartilage, ligaments, extensor tendon, skin) in a single-stage reconstruction.
3. They have inherent stability with intact collateral ligaments and volar plate.
4. They can provide growth potential in children.
5. They probably have good longevity and durability.

limited and restricted to relatively rare or unusual situations when they can provide solutions to difficult problems that cannot be solved by simpler procedures.

Almost all vascularized joint transfers are used for hand reconstruction. Many factors need to be analyzed in forming specific treatment plans for individual patients (10). Vascularized joint transfers, however, have a number of unique features that make them the best choice for solving specific problems that tend to be complex in nature. These are listed in Table 66-4.

In considering whether a vascularized joint transfer is indicated for an individual patient, patient related factors and hand function should be carefully evaluation.

Patient-Related Considerations

Patient-related factors such as age, health status, hand dominance, occupation, and expectations need to be considered. Older patients tend to be poor candidates. Tsai et al. (10) noted that the best results were obtained in patients younger than 40 years of age. Patients also need to be highly motivated (10) to make the transfer function well. It is also important to ask patients if they are involved in any recreational or work activities that may put high demands on their feet. These might be a contraindication for a foot donor site. Surgeons should be especially cautious about using the foot for harvesting donor tissue in young, physically active people.

Functional Considerations in the Hand

It is important to consider overall hand function when planning the reconstruction. In some, joint stability may be more important than mobility, but in others, movement is the most important factor. When stability is more important than movement, arthrodesis may be the best option. If mobility is important and the quality of bones and soft tissues is good, synthetic or biological joint replacements are often the best choice. If mobility is important and the quality of bones and soft tissues is not good, a vascularized joint transfer may be a good option. Do not fail to take into consideration the importance of good postoperative management after a vascularized joint transfer. This is vital to maximize the functional result as well as for maintenance of function in the rest of the reconstructed hand.

INDICATIONS

General Indications for Vascularized Small Joint Transfers in the Hand

General indications for vascularized joint transfer have been published (7,24). These are listed in Table 66-5.

Specific Indications for Vascularized Toe Joint Transfers to the Hand

Typical posttraumatic joint reconstructions that have been done with vascularized joint transfers have been:

1. Thumb MCP joint or IP joint injury with epiphyseal plate damage
2. Finger MCP joint or PIP joint injury with epiphyseal plate damage
3. Injury involving both PIP and distal interphalangeal (DIP) joints. One option is to consider DIP joint fusion and PIP joint reconstruction.
4. Children with an unstable injured thumb MCP joint associated with IP joint injury in the same digit
5. Thumb carpometacarpal (CMC) joint reconstruction using second toe MTP joint donor

Joint damage in children with complex tissue loss and epiphyseal plate damage is probably the main indication for vascularized toe joint transfers to the hand (8).

Free joint transfers have been used to reconstruct congenital hand deformities, but the results are not as good as in those used to reconstruct traumatic defects (24). Symphalangism is the main indication. Some investigators have indicated that the technique should not be used in cases of Poland's syndrome (7,24). Foucher et al. (23) described reconstructing the thumb CMC joint in rare cases of Blauth III thumb hypoplasia, noting that the reconstruction provided an acceptable cosmetic result, satisfactory stability, mobility (which could be improved with muscle–tendon transfer), and the potential for growth.

Young adults with local causes of digital joint destruction are also a strong indication for free joint transfers because the surgical results tend to be good in this group. Chen et al. listed specific indications in young adults (26):

TABLE 66-5 General Indications for Vascularized Small Joint Transfers in the Hand

1. Painful posttraumatic arthritis
2. Posttraumatic joint instability or joint destruction
3. Posttraumatic deformity
4. Joint reconstructions when other replacement options cannot be used or may not be the best option
5. Complex trauma involving joint and other adjacent tissues
6. Multiple PIP joint injuries
7. Congenital deformities

PIP, proximal interphalangeal.

SECTION 4

TABLE 66-6 Prerequisites for Good Results from Vascularized Joint Transfers (24)

1. Functioning flexor tendons in the involved digit
2. Functioning extensor tendons in the involved digit
3. Age younger than 40 years
4. Good neurovascular status to the digit
5. Strong patient motivation
6. Good rehabilitation facilities

(Reproduced with permission from Ellis PR, Hanna D, Tsai TM: Vascularized single toe joint transfer to the hand. J Hand Surg 16-A:160, 1991.)

1. Use should be restricted to young adults younger than the age of 40 years
2. Cases of complex tissue loss but with normal flexor tendon function
3. MCP joint reconstruction in the second and third rays
4. PIP joint reconstruction
5. Cases with multiple PIP joint involvement
6. Joints in which arthrodesis was contraindicated, such as an MCP joint when both the PIPJ and DIPJ were stiff

PREREQUISITES

If a free joint transfer is being considered, a number of prerequisites need to be fulfilled. These are listed in Table 66-6. Ennis (7,10,24) particularly emphasized how important it is to have functioning musculotendinous units, especially good flexor tendons, to move transferred joints. Poor results and even ankylosis will result if musculotendinous unit function is unsatisfactory or absent.

The presence of good neurovascular status in the digit is also a necessary prerequisite. Patent digital arteries are particularly important for island transfers.

RECONSTRUCTIVE VARIATIONS AND THEIR INDICATIONS

Vascularized toe transfers can be used in many different ways to reconstruct problems in the hand. Table 66-7 lists a variety of different ways the procedure can be used for hand reconstruction (11).

In their 1990 review (23) of free vascularized toe joint transfers to the hand, Foucher et al. included three cases of double transfer and six cases of twisted two toes MTP joint transfer. The double transfers consisted of:

1. PIP and DIP joints from the same toe to reconstruct one finger
2. MTP and PIP joints from the same toe to reconstruct two separate fingers
3. PIP joints from the second and third toes to two separate finger sites

The twisted two toes MTP joint transfers were custom-made reconstructions for thumbs amputated at the base. Nail, skin, and bone, harvested from the big toe on a first web vascular pedicle, was combined with a vascularized second toe joint (with or without its own skin flap) to make a new thumb.

TABLE 66-7 Ways Vascularized Joint Transfers from the Second Toe Can Be Used to Reconstruct the Hand (11)

1. Vascularized PIP joint transfer to reconstruct the finger PIP joint
2. Vascularized MTP joint transfer to reconstruct the finger MTP joint
3. Combined vascularized MTP joint and PIP joint transfer to reconstruct two adjacent MCP joints
4. Combined vascularized transplants consisting of two MTP joints to reconstruct two adjacent MCP joints
5. Combined vascularized transplant of the PIP joint of the second and third toe to reconstruct two adjacent PIP joints
6. Vascularized MTP joints transfer to reconstruct the sum CMC joint

CMC, carpometacarpal; MTP, metatarsophalangeal; PIP, proximal interphalangeal.
(Reproduced with permission from Hierner R, Berger AK: Long-term results after vascularized joint transfer for finger joint reconstruction. J Plast Reconstr Aesthet Surg 61:1338, 2008.)

Foucher et al. also described the use of donor joints from the hand either as homodigital or heterodigital transfers (4,5,25,29) and as free tissue transfers or as islands (4,5,25). In 1990, Foucher et al. described an unusual case (29) of the successful transfer of a DIP joint as an island to reconstruct the PIP joint in the same digit. They called this a homodigital joint transfer. The joint achieved rapid bone healing, 15 of 80 degrees of motion, lateral stability, and long-term preservation of articular cartilage. They later published the results of a small series (25). Foucher et al. described the concept of a "digit bank," pointing out that amputated and nonreplantable digits could provide joints, with intact vascular pedicles, that could be used for reconstructing other parts of a mutilating hand injury (4). Foucher et al. published the results of these heterotopic joint transfers (25), comparing the results of a series of island joint transfers (seven homodigital islands and seven heterodigital islands) with free toe joint transfers to the hand.

Cavadas et al. (33) used another island variation, the on-top plasty, in multidigit amputations.

Koshima et al. (34) described a variation in which a flow-through vascularized toe joint transfer was used to reconstruct a digit with segmental loss of tissue. They listed numerous benefits and advocated using the technique for segmental loss problems.

VASCULARIZED JOINT TRANSFERS OUTSIDE THE HAND

In 1995, Vilkki and Salonen (35) described their research into the possibility of using vascularized joint transfers for acromioclavicular joint reconstruction using skeletal and cadaver models. In 2002, Vilkki et al. (36) described a clinical case in which they reconstructed a temporomandibular joint (TMJ) with an ipsilateral second toe MTP joint in a 4-year-old girl. Others

(3,26) have also described using toe joints for TMJ reconstruction. In 1998, Vikki (37,38) described a technique for using vascularized joint transfers to reconstruct the wrist in radial club hands. Chen et al. (3) described toe joint transfers to the elbow.

RECIPIENT SITE PREPARATION

Preoperative Planning

The recipient site circulation should be carefully evaluated preoperatively. Clinical examination, which should include an Allen test, can be augmented with Doppler ultrasonography. Hekali et al. (39) used recipient site arteriography, believing it was important to determine which arteries could be used. Foucher et al. (25) regarded preoperative recipient site arteriography as mandatory. Plain radiographs should also be obtained to obtain skeletal measurements for preoperative planning of the osteotomy and osteosynthesis sites.

Recipient Site Dissection

The operation is best done with two surgical teams and simultaneous recipient site and donor site dissections. If there is only one surgical team, the recipient site should be prepared first. The finger joint to be replaced is exposed. This is usually done dorsally, leaving the neurovascular structures and flexor tendons on the volar side undamaged. If cutaneous scarring is present, it should be excised and replaced with flap skin harvested with the donor tissue. Similarly, the extensor mechanism should also be explored, and if it needs to be replaced, tendon should also be harvested with the donor tissue. The damaged joint is then excised with osteotomies in the bones on each side of it. All damaged bone should be removed leaving viable healthy bone for the proximal and distal osteosyntheses. The shape of the osteotomies should be carefully considered during preoperative planning. Transverse osteotomies, oblique osteotomies, and step-cut osteotomies all have advantages and disadvantages. The recipient site vessels should be prepared next. Two options for recipient vessels are an interdigital artery or the radial artery in the anatomical snuff box. Foucher et al. (23) called these the "short" or "long" transfers. Tsai et al. (10) advocated going to the anatomical snuff box even if it means using vein grafts. This is an easy and accessible site for anastomosis. The dorsal branch of the radial artery and a tributary the cephalic vein in this location are large and often out of the zone of previous trauma and its subsequent scarring.

DONOR SITE PREPARATION

Preoperative Planning

The circulation to the foot should be checked preoperatively. In particular, it is important to establish that there is a dorsalis pedis system to use as a donor site pedicle and that there is a posterior tibial system to supply the foot after the donor tissue has been taken. Clinical examination can be done by compressing either the posterior or the anterior tibial vessels at the ankle and feeling for a pulse in the other. Doppler ultrasonography is also useful (24). Arteriography (39) can also be used if there is any doubt. Plain radiographs of the donor joint should also be obtained to make sure there is no preexisting arthritis and to obtain small bone measurements for preoperative planning of the osteotomy of the donor sites.

The Second Toe Donor Site Dissection: Proximal Interphalangeal and Metacarpophalangeal Joints

The second toe PIP joint is the most commonly used free joint transfer. After the harvest of this donor tissue is understood, variations can be planned with ease because they follow the same general pattern. Harvesting the MCP joint is very similar to PIP joint preparation except that the skeletal divisions are made at more proximal levels.

Dissection can be from proximal to distal or in a retrograde manner from distal to proximal, a technique preferred by Wei et al. (30), arguing that it eliminates confusion arising from description of the vascular anatomy and its variations in the first web.

To harvest the PIP joint, a curved skin incision is made on the dorsum of the foot and extending into the second toe. The first dorsal metatarsal artery is identified. It is only necessary to identify the dorsalis pedis if a longer pedicle is required. If this is necessary, the dissection should be continued proximally. A planter incision is also needed to identify the first plantar metatarsal artery. Care should be taken to look for anatomic variations so that the vessels are not damaged. The medial digital artery of the second toe is ligated distally at the level of the DIP joint, carefully preserving the fine branches that vascularize the PIP joint. The lateral digital artery to the second toe is carefully left intact to supply the distal part of the toe after the PIP joint has been harvested. The dorsal veins; dorsal venous arch; and, if necessary, saphenous vein are prepared at the same time as the arteries. The skeleton is divided with a disarticulation through the DIP joint and an osteotomy through the proximal phalanx at a site determined during preoperative planning (the skeletal divisions are through the PIP joint and metacarpal for MCP joint harvest). The joint and its associated bones are then mobilized from the remaining tissues in the toe, with care taken to leave the lateral neurovascular bundle and the medial nerve intact. The extensor tendon and a dorsal skin island can also be included if needed (24). When the donor tissue has been raised as an island flap, the tourniquet should be released and blood allowed to flow for 20 to 30 minutes.

Donor Site Variations

Multiple variations for donor site dissection have been described. The donor site can be dissected in many different ways to customize the transfer to the specific needs of an individual patient. As long as the surgeon understands the anatomy and its variations of the various foot donor sites and is careful to preserve foot function, a huge number of donor site variations are possible. The more common choices, listed earlier, include which toe, which toe joint, single or multiple toe joints, length of bone to be harvested, inclusion or exclusion of extensor tendon, inclusion or exclusion and location of associated skin flap, length of vascular pedicle, and which veins to be used for outflow.

Repair of the Donor Site Defect

A number of different techniques have been described to repair the foot to minimize donor site problems.

The skeletal resection is usually managed by either leaving the donor toe as a resection arthroplasty or by making a bony fusion across a defect using iliac crest graft or bone resected from the hand. Reconstructions have been internally fixed with K wires or compression screws. Soft tissue closure needs to be durable. Options for skin closure have consisted of skin grafts, syndactylization, local flaps or cross-toe flaps, and toe fillet flaps.

Singer et al. (40) argued that second toe preservation was not essential and that amputation might be preferable to a problematic toe reconstruction, although they pointed out the problem with flip-flop use in people without a second toe.

INSETTING, SKELETAL FIXATION, AND PREPARATION FOR MICROVASCULAR ANASTOMOSIS

The length of bone taken with the joint is estimated at the time of preoperative planning. The actual length harvested is determined by intraoperative measurement of the size of the recipient site defect after the damaged joint and any associated poor quality bone has been removed.

Table 66-8 lists a number of factors that need to be considered when fitting the transferred joint into its recipient site.

Skeletal Length

Foucher et al. (1,23) emphasized that the skeletal length of the transferred joint should be slightly shorter than the available space so that it does not have to be forced to flex. Chen et al. (26) also said that the fit is better short than long but warned not to make the extensor too lax or lag will occur.

Volar Plate

Foucher et al. (1) advocated removing residual volar plates during recipient site preparation to debulk the digits. This allows the flexor tendons to come closer to the transferred joint. This reduced their leverage and improved tendon balance in the reconstructed digit.

TABLE 66-8 Factors to Be Considered When Fitting the Transferred Joint Into Its Recipient Site

1. Skeletal length
2. Volar plate
3. Flexor tendon pulleys
4. Osteotomy configuration
5. Neurovascular structures
6. Internal fixation
7. Extensor tendon reconstruction
8. Skin cover

Flexor Tendon Pulleys

Pulley damage should be appraised at the time of recipient site preparation (1). This is particularly important in PIP joint injuries in which the distal end of the A2 pulley and the A3 pulley are often damaged. The flexor tendons can be evaluated and tenolysis done if needed through the space created when the damaged joint is removed (10). When the transferred PIP joint reconstruction is inset, the best results can be obtained when the flexor tendon pulley system is intact to the rim of the transfer.

Osteotomy Configuration

The shape of the osteotomies and cut ends of both the donor and recipient bones can vary according to need. Transverse osteotomies are technically straightforward but have the smallest surface area for bone healing and may not be as good as other configurations for internal fixation. Ellis et al. (24) described the use of transverse osteotomies in earlier cases but in later cases, when a functioning extensor tendon was present, they used a step-cut osteotomy. Oblique osteotomy cuts (18) help reduce hyperextension when MTP joints are used as donors. Ellis et al. (24) described using a dorsal step-cut osteotomy to preserve the insertion of the extensor tendon central slip. It is important to have as big a surface contact area between donor and recipient as possible. It is best if this can be cancellous bone because this will provide the best condition for rapid healing at the osteosynthesis site.

Neurovascular Structures

After both recipient and donor sites have been prepared, the free tissue transfer can be made. The donor site vascular pedicle is ligated, the vessels divided, and the joint transferred to the hand. If the microvascular anastomoses will be done in the anatomical snuff box, the vascular pedicle may either be tunneled under the skin on the dorsum of the hand, or the dorsal skin may be opened and the vessels positioned under direct vision.

Internal Fixation

Internal fixation is a technical challenge because of the small size of the transplanted tissue and often because of the small size of the recipient bones. When the operation is being done in children, the difficulties are even greater because of the need to avoid damage to the epiphyseal plates. Internal fixation is usually achieved with a combination of interosseous wire loops and K-wires because the osteosynthesis sites are almost always too small for satisfactory screw or plate fixation. Internal fixation can be difficult and should be done with care. The free joint transfer should be positioned as accurately as possible, avoiding angulatory or rotatory malalignment, a difficult task with tissues that are small and often not ideally matched. Every effort should be made to achieve good bone contact to minimize the risk of delayed bone healing or nonunion. When the operation is being done in children, epiphyseal plate damage from either surgical dissection or internal fixation should be avoided to minimize the risk of growth arrest or retardation. Epiphyseal plates will continue to grow in small transplants, but care should be taken to preserve as much of the periosteum as possible to maintain best possible blood supply to the epiphyseal plates. Reduction in blood supply to them will result in growth retardation.

Interosseous wire loop fixation has been used (9,26). It works but is not very stable. After initially using this technique, Tsai et al. subsequently modified their technique to include longitudinal K-wire fixation (20) because of problems with boutonniere deformities. Kuo et al. (21) used K-wire fixation. Smith and Jones (22) used a combination of interosseous wire loops and K-wire fixation. Foucher et al. (25,29) used longitudinal pins for their homodigital transfers. They also described (23) the use of K-wires buried in bone and cemented intramedullary fixation "corkscrews."

Plate and screw fixation would theoretically be best, but the bones are too small. Additionally, fixation should not cross epiphyseal plates. The most common fixation currently being done is a combination of interosseous wire loops and K-wires.

Tsai et al. (10) recommended pinning the DIP joint in full extension and leaving the K-wire in place for 4 weeks postoperatively to enhance PIP exercises.

Extensor Tendon Reconstruction

The best situation is if the extensor tendon can be preserved. For PIP joint replacement, a distal step-cut osteotomy (24) is a good way to preserve the central slip insertion. If the extensor mechanism is absent or in poor condition, it should be reconstructed using donor extensor tendon taken from the toe with the joint transfer. It is important to avoid extensor tendon lag. Tsai et al. (10) recommended pinning the toe in full extension with a longitudinal K-wire to reduce the risk of lag. It should be noted that the extensor tendon of an MTP joint transfer cannot be used as a graft if the joint is inverted.

Skin Cover

It is frequently necessary to take a skin flap with the transfer. This is often essential for wound closure. It also has the advantage of being a convenient monitor of vascularity. The original technique of harvesting a dorsomedial skin island over the PIP joint necessitated preservation of the poorly developed second toe extensor tendon and resection of the finger extensor tendon. This was not ideal, especially if the finger extensor tendon was intact. Tsai et al. (10,24) modified the technique to preserve the finger extensor tendon, harvesting the skin flap either from the lateral side of the second toe or from the great toe, carefully preserving it on its own vascular pedicle.

If a large area of resurfacing is necessary in the hand, a dorsalis pedis flap can be harvested with the joint (22). Preoperative planning is important. The skeletal fixation determines the orientation and position of the transfer and needs to be considered carefully when planning the design of the skin flap harvest. Smith and Jones (22) described a technique for maintaining the overlying skin flap when an MTP joint transfer is inverted. An alternative technique for preserving the skin flap is to use the oblique osteotomy cuts described by Mathes et al. (18).

MICROVASCULAR ANASTOMOSIS

After the transfer has been inset and internally fixed, the tendons repaired, and the skin flap sutured into place, the microvascular anastomoses are done. At least two veins should be anastomosed for venous drainage (10). Anastomoses can be done in the hand close to the free joint transfer or in the anatomical snuff box, with or without vein grafts, as described earlier. Wounds are then closed and dressings applied.

POSTOPERATIVE MANAGEMENT

General Management of the Patient

The general management of the patient who has had a toe joint transferred to the hand should be the same as for any other free tissue transfer operation. Patients should be given adequate analgesics. Fluid volume should be sufficient to give ample circulation through the transfer. Antibiotics, anticoagulants, and plasma expanders may be used according to patient needs and surgeon preference. Patients should be nursed in a warm, draft-free environment. They should not be given caffeine or exposed to cigarette smoke.

Donor Site Management

It is important to be concerned about donor site morbidity. Efforts should be taken to minimize problems in the foot and to obtain good quality primary healing.

Recommendations for the management of the foot donor site vary among authors, but there is general agreement that patients should have 10 days of complete bed rest postoperatively, and then start gradual ambulation. A walking cast should be used for 4 weeks. Patients should not use a crutch with the operated hand. It takes a number of months before patients are able to walk normally.

Recipient Site Management

At the end of the toe joint to hand operation, a bulky soft dressing is applied and reinforced with a plaster of Paris or fiberglass splint. Care should be taken to leave the skin island exposed for monitoring. The operated hand should be elevated in the postoperative period. Various forms of monitoring devices have been used (10), but none is perfect. Clinical observation of vascularity in the skin island by experienced nurses is still the best way to monitor viability of the transfer. Color, temperature, and capillary refill should be charted at frequent intervals. Postoperative dressings should be changed to light dressings when rehabilitation of movement is started. The timing of this varied in different series (7,10,21,25,26), but the general principle has been to start motion as early as possible. If the extensor mechanism was preserved, gentle active range of motion can be started as early as the second postoperative day using a protective dorsal splint. It is not necessary to wait for bony union before starting movement, provided that the skeletal fixation is satisfactory. If the extensor mechanism had to be reconstructed, range of motion exercises should be delayed until the surgeon believe it is safe to start, which should be no later than 4 weeks after the operation. Percutaneous K-wires should be removed at 4 weeks. If the DIP joint was pinned in extension, its splint should also be removed at 4 weeks and then DIP joint motion started. Reconstructed fingers should have extension splints at night for 4 months. Dynamic flexion splinting can be used, if necessary, in the later stages of rehabilitation.

POTENTIAL COMPLICATIONS

Potential complications after vascularized joint transfer operations are listed in Table 66-9.

Generalized Complications

The potential for anesthetic and generalized surgical complications is similar to that of any other microsurgical free tissue transfer case.

Donor Site Complications

Donor site problems in the foot have been a problem in some cases. The literature does not document a lot of detail about these. Some patients complained of difficulty with footwear. In particular, difficulty wearing flip flops has been described. Other patients have complained about postoperative gait disturbance and foot pain. Sometimes this is related to neuroma formation at the site of digital nerve transaction; at other times, it may be skeletal in nature. The aesthetic appearance of the donor site has been a concern to some patients. In general, however, improved hand function has been good enough to overshadow concerns about most of the donor site problems, which, with careful attention to detail during harvest, have tended to be relatively mild.

As written in the section on preoperative planning, many donor site concerns can be avoided by asking patients about their functional activities and expectations during the stage of preoperative planning. In particular, it is important to know if patients are involved in sports, dancing, or work that has high demands on the feet. There may be contraindications for using the foot as a donor site.

TABLE 66-9 Potential Complications After Vascularized Joint Transfers Operations

1. Generalized complications
Similar to any other surgical operation
Similar to any other microvascular procedure
2. Donor site complications
Altered function in the foot
Difficulty wearing footwear
Foot pain
Neuroma
Musculoskeletal
CRPS
Poor aesthetics appearance
3. Recipient site complications
Microvascular failure
Infection
Pain
Joint pain
CRPS
Stiffness
In the transferred joint
In the rest of the hand
Skeletal deformity
Contractures
Poor aesthetic appearance
Malrotation
Skin loss

CRPS, complex regional pain syndrome.

Recipient Site Complications

The most devastating complication from a vascular joint transfer is complete loss of the donor tissue from microvascular failure. This is not very common. It has been reported as occurring in 7% of cases (11). Reoperation is worthwhile and has resulted in salvage in many, but not all, cases (8,23,24). Microsurgical failure has been more frequent in primary and emergency transfers than in cases done for secondary reconstruction (1).

Infection has been reported as occurring in 7% cases (11). Both wound infections and pin tract infections have been described.

The most common cause for disappointing results has been functional failure from pain and stiffness, which has been reported in 20% of cases (11). This may just be localized to the vascularized joint transfer, but it can also affect the adjacent joints or even involve the whole hand. During rehabilitation, care must be taken to rehabilitate not just the transferred joint but also to maintain motion in the rest of the hand.

Flexion deformity in PIP joints has been a big problem. It may be the result of multiple factors (1). Attention to technical details, better internal fixation (20), and extension splinting have been used to manage the problem. Other skeletal complications encountered include malrotation, which has required reoperation in some cases, and growth retardation or acceleration in children.

Poor aesthetic appearance has been a problem for some patients (40). Cold intolerance has been reported as 61% in the hand and 31% in the donor foot (23). Other complications have included skin loss, scar contracture, and complex regional pain syndrome (CRPS) at both the donor and recipient sites.

Foucher et al. (23) found that even patients with successful reconstructions had difficulty returning to work, attributing this to the severity of the cases. The average time to return to work was 274 days (range, 30–1050 days). A total of 57% change their jobs, and only 10.5% returned to their previous employment.

Secondary Surgery

Secondary surgery has been necessary in more than 50% of cases (11,23). Extensor tenolysis and capsulotomy have been the most common procedures. They have been worthwhile for improving range of motion. Correction of skeletal malalignment, when it has occurred, has also been a useful operation.

Chen et al. (41) described a two-stage reconstruction with two periods of rehabilitation. His results showed that the technique improved the results of free joint transfer.

OUTCOME

The medical literature contains numerous papers describing the outcome of vascularized joint transfers. Some researchers reported relatively large series (1,3,4,7,10,11,23–26). All the studies are retrospective. Some of the cases described had unusual, unique clinical problems. Most of the rest had difficult clinical conditions, such as many of the congenital cases, or difficult versions of more common problems, such as the posttraumatic cases. The very nature of these problems was the indication for vascularized joint transfers, but their heterogeneity was such that scientifically well-designed, high-quality comparative studies could not be done. The published studies, however, contain valuable information documenting innovative thinking about methods to reconstruct difficult problems, useful technical ideas, and clear and detailed descriptions of the type of outcomes that can be expected. Table 66-10 summarizes the most important outcomes.

O'Brien et al. published results from Melbourne in 1984 (8). The group contained four children and three adults who had finger and thumb joints reconstructed with joints harvested from a foot (six cases) or a functionless finger (one case). Six were successful, resulting in retention of joint space; stability; painless functional range of motion; and, in children, continued growth. A long-term follow-up of the four children was published in 1988 (40). The best results were in the MTP joint to MCP joint transfers. These had a stable, painless, functional range of motion with near normal growth. The results of toe PIP joint to finger PIP joint were disappointing. The transfers did not achieve good active extension and had limited growth potential.

TABLE 66-10 Summary of Outcomes

1. Loss of graft: Uncommon. Usually results from microvascular failure and infection. Reoperation is worthwhile and salvages some.
2. Range of motion: The most important outcome parameter. Final ranges of motion vary and depend on a number of factors, including the specific donor joint used, technical factors, the patient's age, the nature of the problem being treated, recipient site factors, and other patient factors (including rehabilitation).
3. Growth: Growth is important outcome when the operation is for a congenital anomaly or posttraumatic joint destruction in a child. Growth continues after transplantation. It is better with MTP joint transfers because they contain two epiphyseal plates compared with PIP joint transfers, which only contain one. The rate of growth is difficult to assess but is probably close to normal. Growth retardation will occur if the epiphyseal plates have reduced circulation, but growth acceleration is also possible.
4. Aesthetic appearance: Aesthetic result is both personal and technical. It tends to be better in children than in adults.

MTP, metatarsophalangeal; PIP, proximal interphalangeal.

Results of transfers done in Louisville have been published (7,10,24). In a combined series (24) of adult and pediatric patients 31 single-joint free tissue transfers were harvested from toes and used to reconstruct finger MCP or PIP joints in 26 patients. Twenty-six transfers were done to reconstruct posttraumatic joints and five for congenital anomalies. The average follow-up period was 22.6 months. In posttraumatic reconstructions, the average range of motion was in an arc of 30 degrees, positioned between 18 and 48 degrees. In the congenital anomalies, the average range of motion was in an arc of 13 degrees, positioned between 14 and 27 degrees. There was a high rate of complications. Overall, 50% of the patients experienced complications, but most were described as being minor. Local complications were listed as malrotation, skin loss, boutonniere deformity, infection, and vascular insufficiency (four cases). General complications, not involving the transferred joint, were listed as donor site hematoma, donor site CRPS 1, osteonecrosis of graft, donor sites scar contracture, anemia, and recipient site CRPS 1. Fifteen of the joint transfers required tenolysis. The authors noted that all tenolysis operations were done for posttraumatic problems. Results of 19 joint transfers done in children with joint and epiphyseal plate destruction were published separately (7). In two transfers, the epiphyseal plates closed prematurely. In all, the rest growth was almost normal. MCP joint reconstructions with either an MTP joint or an MCP joint achieved 39 to 75 degrees of range of motion, MCP joint reconstructions with a PIP joint achieved 38 to 51 degrees of range of motion, and PIP joint reconstructions with a PIP joint achieved 22 to 39 degrees of range of motion.

Results of transfers done in Taipei have been published (3,26). A review of 51 toe joint transfers (3) showed that all were done for posttraumatic problems except for two used to manage congenital deformities. Fifteen MTP joints were used to reconstruct MCP joints. Nine toe PIP joints were used to reconstruct MCP joints. Twenty-two toe PIP joints were used to reconstruct hand PIP joints. There were three postoperative vascular problems, two of which were salvaged by reoperation. Functionally, MTP joint transfers to MCP joints achieved a mean range of motion of 27 degrees. Toe PIP joint transfers to MCP joints achieved a mean range of motion of 34 degrees. Toe PIP joint transfers to hand PIP joints achieved a mean range of motion of 23.5 degrees. Nineteen required secondary surgical procedures.

In 2001, Kimori et al. (27) published the results of 12 finger joint reconstructions in Hiroshima. Second toe PIP joints were transferred in patients ages 7 to 47 years. Follow-up periods ranged from 9 to 48 months. There were no microvascular failures. Bone union occurred in all cases. Preoperative joint pain deformity and instability were resolved in all cases. The average range of motion was 59 degrees for PIP joint reconstructions and 54 degrees for MCP joint reconstructions. None of the patients complained of pain or functional deficits in the donor foot.

Hierner and Berger (11) published long-term (3–15 years) results after vascularized joint transfer for finger joint reconstruction in Germany. Their retrospective clinical study described the results of 16 vascularized joint transfers in patients ages 2 to 42 years. The risk of failure (ischemia, tendon adhesions, joint stiffness) was 10%. The amount of active motion obtained depended on etiology, age, donor site, and recipient site. Transfers done for trauma had a greater active range of motion than those done for congenital defects. Transfers in children had better active range of motion than those done in adults. The authors recommended amputating the whole second ready after harvesting the graft from the second toe. Motion in the transplanted joints was intermediate in range and better for whole-joint transfers than partial transfers. Arthritic changes occurred in 75% of the partial vascularized joint transfers compared with 0% of the complete joint transfers even after 15 years of follow-up. Growth continued normally in immature transfers. Technical complications (usually tendon adhesion or skeletal mal alignment) were common and seen in 50% of transfers. They recommended the extensor tenolysis should be done earlier than 6 months after transplantation.

Foucher et al. have published extensively on the subject of vascularize joint transfers. Results of their transfers done in Strasbourg have been published (1,4,23,25). They also published an extensive review (5) of their large experience. They described the rationale, development, indications, and results for the many options and variation of vascularized joint transfers procedures that can be done. They have clearly illustrated technical details and listed critical points.

REFERENCES

1. Foucher G, Hoang P, Citron N, et al. Joint reconstruction following trauma: comparison of microsurgical transfer and conventional methods. A report of 61 cases. *J Hand Surg* 1986;11-B:388.
2. Buncke HJ, Daniller AI, Schultz WP, et al. The fate of autogenous whole joints transplanted by microvascular anastomoses. *Plast Reconstr Surg* 1967;39:333.
3. Chen SHT, Wei FC, Chen HC. Vascularized toe joint transplantation. *Hand Clin* 1999;15:613.
4. Foucher G, Citron N, Sammut D. Compound vascularized island joint transfer in hand surgery. *French J Orthop Surg* 1991;5:32.
5. Foucher G. Vascularized joint transfers. In Green DP, Hotchkiss RN, Pederson WC, Wolffe SW. *Green's Operative Hand Surgery*, 5th ed. Philadelphia: Elsevier Churchill Livingstone, 2005, p. 1813.
6. Hurwitz PJ. Experimental transplantation of small joints by microvascular anastomoses. *Plast Reconstr Surg* 1979;64:221.
7. Ishida O, Tsai TM. Free vascularized whole joint transfer in children. *Microsurgery* 1991;12:196.
8. O'Brien B, Gould JS, Morrison WA, et al. Free vascularized small joint transfer to the hand. *J Hand Surg* 1984;9(5):634–641.
9. Tsai TM, Ogden L, Jaeger SH, et al. Experimental vascularized total joint autografts—a primate study. *J Hand Surg* 1982;7:140.
10. Tsai TM, Wang WZ. Vascularized joint transfers: indications and results. *Hand Clin* 1992;8:525.
11. Hierner R, Berger AK. Long-term results after vascularized joint transfer for finger joint reconstruction. *J Plast Reconstr Aesthet Surg* 2008;61:1338.
12. Pho RW. Malignant giant-cell tumor of the distal end of the radius treated by a free vascularized fibular transplant. *J Bone Joint Surg* 1981;63:877.
13. Cavadas PC, Landin L, Thione A, et al. Reconstruction of massive bone losses of the elbow with vascularized bone transfers. *Plast Reconstr Surg* 2010;126:964.
14. Yaremchuk MJ, Sedacca T, Schiller AL, et al. Vascular knee allograft transplantation in a rabbit model. *Plast Reconstr Surg* 1983;71:461.
15. Muramatsu K, Doi K, Akino T, et al. Results of vascularized joint allograft under immunosuppression with cyclosporine. *Microsurgery* 1993;14:527.
16. Morrison WA, O'Brien BM, MacLeod AM. The foot as a donor site in reconstructive microsurgery. *World J Surg* 1079;3:43.
17. Rose EH. Reconstruction of central metacarpal ray defects of the hand with a free vascularized double metatarsal and metacarpophalangeal joint transfer. *J Hand Surg* 1984;9A(1):28–23.
18. Mathes SJ, Buchmann R, Weeks PM. Microvascular joint transplantation with epiphyseal growth. *J Hand Surg* 1980;5:586.
19. Wray RC, Mathes SM, Young VL, et al. Free vascularized whole-joint transplants with ununited epiphyses. *Plast Reconstr Surg* 1981;67:519.
20. Tsai TM, Jupiter JB, Kutz JE, et al. Vascularized autogenous whole joint transfer in the hand—a clinical study. *J Hand Surg* 1982;7:335.
21. Kuo ET, Zhao YC, Zhang ML. Reconstruction of metacarpophalangeal joint by free vascularized autogenous metatarsophalangeal joint transplant. *J Reconstr Microsurg* 1984;1:65.
22. Smith PJ, Jones BM. Free vascularized transfer of the metatarsophalangeal joint to the hand. A technical modification. *J Hand Surg* 1985;10B:109.
23. Foucher G, Sammut D, Citron N. Free vascularized toe-joint transfer in hand reconstruction: a series of 25 patients. *J Reconstr Microsurg* 1990;6:201.
24. Ellis PR, Hanna D, Tsai TM. Vascularized single toe joint transfer to the hand. *J Hand Surg* 1991;16A:160.
25. Foucher G, Lenoble E, Smith D. Free and island vascularized joint transfer for proximal interphalangeal reconstruction: a series of 27 cases. *J Hand Surg* 1994;19A:8.
26. Chen SHT, Wei FC, Chen HC et al. Vascularized toe joint transfer to the hand. *Plast Reconstr Surg* 1996;98:1275.
27. Kimori K, Ikuta Y, Ishida O, et al. Free vascularized toe joint transfer to the hand. A technique for simultaneous reconstruction of the soft tissue. *J Hand Surg* 2001;26B:314.
28. Foucher G, Nagle DJ. Microsurgical reconstruction of fingers and fingertips. *Hand Clin* 1999;15:597.
29. Foucher G, Lenoble E, Sammut D. Transfer of a composite island homodigital distal interphalangeal joint to replace the proximal interphalangeal joint. *Ann Chir Main* 1990;9:369.
30. Wei FC, Silverman RT, Hsu WM. Retrograde dissection of the vascular pedicle in toe harvest. *Plast Reconstr Surg* 1995;96:1211.
31. Manktelow RT. *Microvascular Reconstruction. Anatomy, Applications and Surgical Technique*. Berlin: Springer-Verlag, 1986.
32. May JW Jr, Chait LA, Cohen BE, et al. Free neurovascular flap from the first web of the foot in hand reconstruction. *J Hand Surg* 1977;2:387.
33. Cavadas PC. Microvascular free on-top plasty in multidigital amputations. *J Plast Reconstr Aesthet Surg* 2007;60:720.
34. Koshima I, Inagawa K, Sahara K, et al. Flow-through vascularized toe-joint transfer for reconstruction of segmental loss of an amputated finger. *J Reconstr Microsurg* 1998;14:453.
35. Vilkki SK, Salonen EJ. Experimental models for microsurgical joint reconstruction in the upper extremity. *Ann Acad Med Singapore* 1995;24(suppl):58S.
36. Vilkki SK, Hukki J, Nietosvaara Y, et al. Microvascular temporomandibular joint and mandibular ramus reconstruction in hemifacial microsomia. *J Craniofacial Surg* 2002;13:809.
37. Vilkki SK. Distraction and microvascular epiphysis transfer for radial for radial club hand. *J Hand Surg* 1998;23B:445.
38. Vilkki SK. Vascularized joint transfer for radial club hand. *Tech Hand Up Extrem Surg* 1998;2:126.
39. Hekali P, Vilkki S, Solonen K. Arteriography before toe to hand free tissue transfer operation. *Eur J Radiol* 1981;1:285.
40. Singer DI, O'Brien BM, McLeod AM, et al. Long-term follow-up of free vascularized joint transfers to the hand in children. *J Hand Surg* 1988;13A:776.
41. Chen HC, Tang YB, Chen S, et al. Improving the result of vascularized joint transfer in hand joints: two-stage reconstruction with two periods of rehabilitation. *Tech Hand Up Extrem Surg* 1998;2:262.

CHAPTER 67

Nerve Repair in the Upper Extremity

Rolfe Birch

THE MEDIAN AND ULNAR NERVES

After a nerve is divided, the sooner the distal segment is connected to the cell body and proximal segment, the better the result will be. The quality of treatment of the wound at first operation and the timing of repair of the nerves are factors within the control of clinicians. The past 20 years has seen extensive laboratory work that confirms clinical evidence that the central nervous system suffers after interruption of a peripheral nerve. The rapidity and the severity of that response to violent proximal nerve injury is the overarching biological imperative that must guide action (1).

History

Bland Sutton (2) relates that in the 1870s, JW Hulke, then surgeon to the Middlesex Hospital in Mortimer Street, London, repaired the cut median and ulnar nerves of a woman. Bland Sutton continues: "This was the first instance of a successful secondary suture of a divided nerve in London. Surgeons had been afraid to stitch a cut nerves in this way for fear of tetanus." At the London Hospital, Horsley (3) and Sherren (4), who reported 50 cases, practiced primary suture. Sherren's account of the success of a median nerve graft performed by Dean in 1896 is probably the earliest adequately studied such case. The principles governing the repair of war nerve injuries were established in World War I. They include resection of scar until a healthy bed is secured, excision of damaged nerve until healthy stumps are reached, and tension-free suture by adequate mobilization and flexion of adjacent joints or grafting. Of grafting, Tinel (5) wrote: "When the distance between the segments of the nerve trunk is too great to permit direct suture *the only legitimate operation is nerve grafting*." The proper treatment of war wounds was implemented by Robert Jones in that same war (6); the wound should be treated by debridement, excision, and delayed closure. He instituted hospitals dedicated to rehabilitation; from these came the definition of the requirements for successful operations of reconstruction. The Second World War saw the rapid reinstitution of rehabilitation units, and the work of the five special hospitals designated for nerve injuries was analyzed in the Medical Research Council Special Report No. 282 (7). Young (8) summarized some of this work. Nerve grafting in all its forms was studied. The first evidence of axonal transport was revealed. The rate of nerve regeneration, effects of disuse, regeneration of proprioceptors, maturation of regenerated fibers, and significance of retrograde influence were among the fields of enquiry. Collectively, this work marked a most important stage in improving understanding of regeneration and of applying those lessons to clinical practice: here was an example of what has become known, in fashionable circles, as "translational research."

Results of repairs were graded by strict, even stringent, criteria. About 50% of 1441 sutures made a useful recovery; a similar outcome is seen in the 67 cases of grafts. Primary and secondary sutures were compared to the detriment of the former: "Formal nerve suture should be undertaken at the earliest moment when it is possible to recognize the extent of damage to the nerve, excise the injured segment, and bring together the mobilized nerve ends without the prospect of undue postoperative tension." These are painful but important findings: the lesson is that the results of operating on peripheral nerves depend to an extent hardly matched in any other branch of surgery on the skill of the surgeon and the quality of the technique. Woodhall and Beebe (9) brought together the experience of the military surgeons of the United States. On the basis of 3148 nerve sutures in war wounds, they said that "delay in suture involves a loss of, on average, about 1% of maximal performance for every six days of delay." From the Vietnam War, Omer and his colleagues (10,11) emphasized the harmfulness of delay and found that grafts were disappointing. Pedicle nerve grafting gave better results. A review of publications (12) describing 13,000 nerve injuries from conflicts suggests that the first operation to the wound is most important; arterial injuries must be repaired and sepsis prevented. Unfavorable factors include delay before repair; extensive damage to the nerve, adjacent soft tissues, and skeleton; the presence of arterial injury;

TABLE 67-1 Median and Ulnar Nerves: Lesions and Repairs, 1977 to 2004

	Median		Ulnar	
	Lesions (*n*)	Repairs (*n*)	Lesions (*n*)	Repairs (*n*)
Closed infraclavicular traction lesion (see Table 67-4)	58	30	63	25
Penetrating missile wounds	98	43	113	53
Glenohumeral dislocation	50	3	51	4
Fracture dislocation at the elbow, children	83	18	109	22
Fracture dislocation at the elbow, adults	30	4	31	4
Volkmann's ischemic contracture in supracondylar fractures, children	24	0	19	2
High repairs (see Table 67-5)	117	117	99	99
Low repairs (see Table 67-6)	134	134	130	130
Totals	594	349	615	339

and the level of lesion. The material on which this chapter is based is set out in Table 67-1.

Nerve Anatomy

The median nerve contains fibers passing through the spinal nerves C6, C7, C8, and T1, and its severance effectively ruins hand function. The ulnar nerve conveys fibers from C7, C8, and T1, and its severance reduces power grip to 50% and, if untreated, to severe deformity within the hand. Although such variations as a Martin Grűber anastomosis are significant, those in the distribution of the spinal nerves forming the brachial plexus are more important. At least one third of patients with complete lesions of C5, C6, and C7 retain powerful extension of their digits, and this is seen in some patients in whom only the first thoracic nerve has survived.

The formation and relations of the three *cords* are variable, and indeed their designations are somewhat misleading. Immediately inferior to the clavicle, the posterior cord lies *lateral* to the axillary artery, the medial cord *behind* and the lateral cord *in front*. The cords assume their appropriate relations about the axillary artery deep to pectoralis minor. The axillary artery may pass anterior to the three cords and the median nerve. The nerves and cords are tethered by the pectoralis minor, and here is the most common site of rupture in violent traction injuries to the infraclavicular brachial plexus.

Not infrequently, the ulnar nerve arises as two or three branches from the medial cord. The greatest variation in formation of trunk nerves is found within the lateral cord. The lateral root of the median nerve may arise as two or three branches, and in some cases it appears as a branch of the musculocutaneous nerve. It is useful to be aware of these variations of the formation of the plexus and of its relation to the great vessels because they can cause difficulties during urgent exploration.

The neurovascular bundle is found in its sheath in the lower part of the axilla: most medial is the axillary and brachial vein; the nerves are grouped around the lower part of the axillary and the brachial arteries (Figure 67-1). The axillary artery is

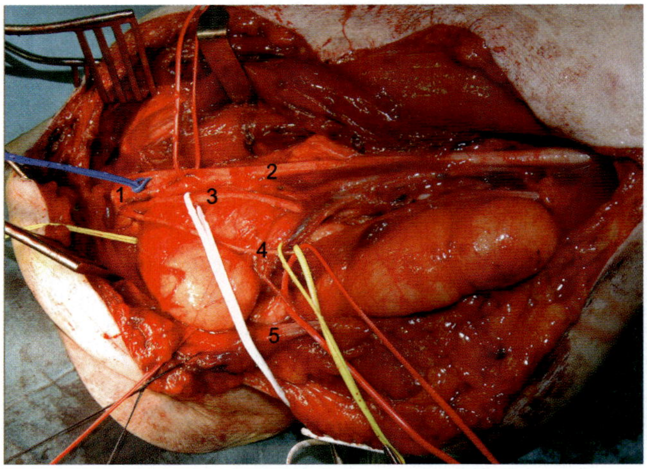

A

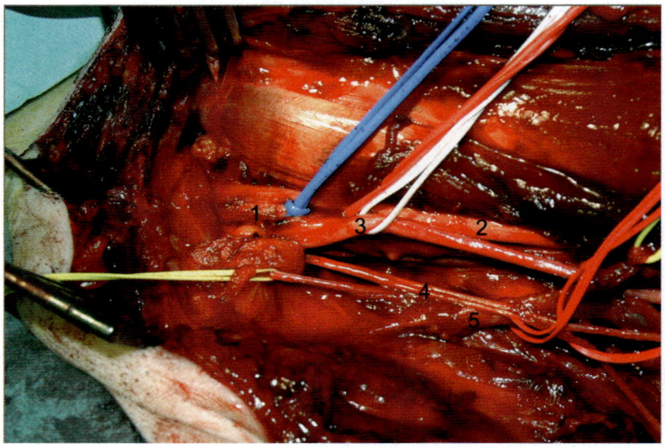

B

FIGURE 67-1 The infraclavicular brachial plexus splayed over a massive lipoma. The axillary artery (1) is marked by the blue sling, the median nerve (2) by a red sling, and the ulnar nerve (3) by a white sling. The medial cutaneous nerve of the forearm (4) is seen, and the radial nerve (5) lies deep to the tumor. The appearances before (**A**) and after (**B**) removal of the tumor. (© Copyright 2011 Rolfe Birch.)

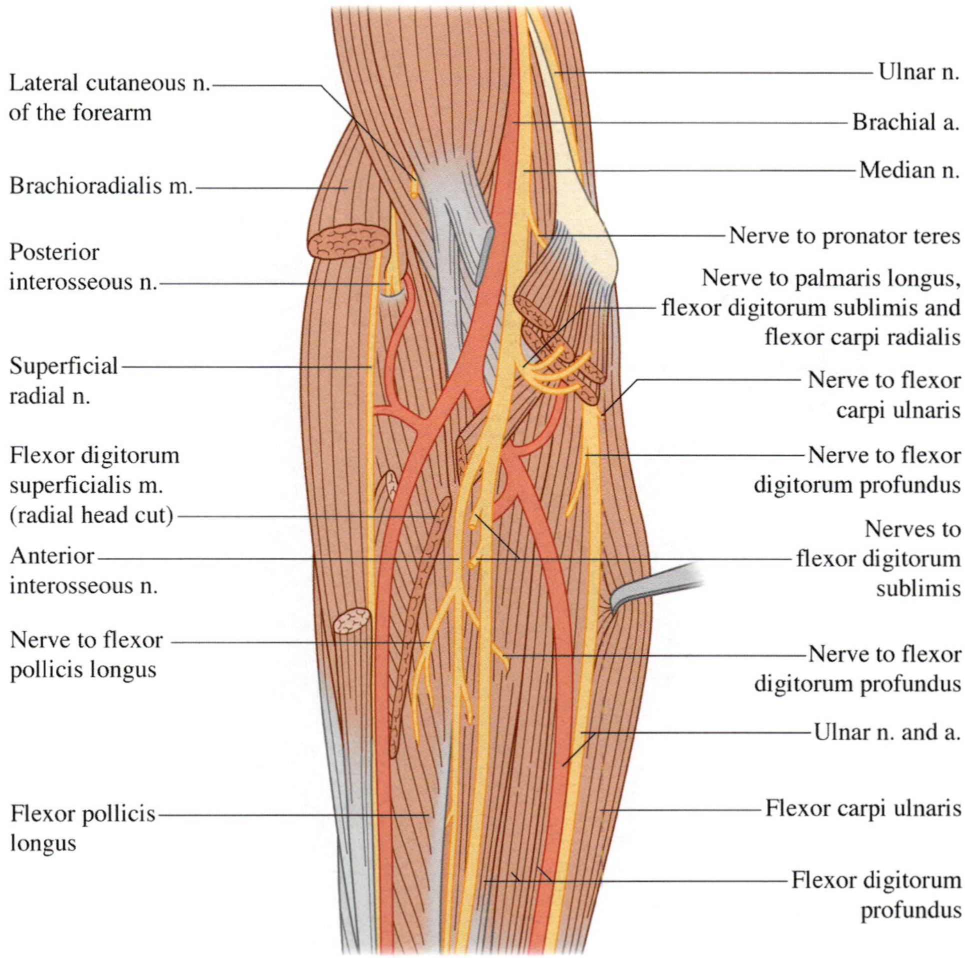

FIGURE 67-2 The anterior aspect of the right elbow. m, muscle; n, nerve. (© Copyright 2011 Rolfe Birch.)

embraced by the two roots of the median nerve, which starts on its lateral side and crosses it in the arm. The ulnar nerve and the medial cutaneous nerve of the forearm are on the medial side of the artery. The former passes posteriorly about halfway down the arm to pierce the medial intermuscular septum and to lie between it and the medial part of the triceps muscle, to which it usually gives a branch. The median nerve is easily displayed at and just below the elbow and in the lower part of the forearm through a sinuous incision winding down from the elbow (Figure 67-2). At elbow level, it is found medial to the brachial artery. It then descends between the superficial and deep heads of the pronator teres and can to some extent be mobilized by division of the deep (ulnar) head of the pronator teres. The nerve runs down the forearm between the deep and superficial flexor muscles, loosely attached by areolar tissue to the deep surface of the flexor digitorum superficialis. It can be exposed in this part of its course by separating the flexor superficialis from its radial origin and retracting the muscle. The anterior interosseous nerve is now displayed. The anterior interosseous nerve and its accompanying artery may be damaged by compression because of swelling in the deepest part of the flexor compartment of the forearm. The nerve enters the hand just deep to and between the tendons of the palmaris longus and flexor carpi radialis.

The "bottleneck" (13) of the carpal tunnel is formed posteriorly and laterally by the concavity of the carpus. It is roofed by the flexor retinaculum and anchored medially to the pisiform and hamate bones and laterally to the scaphoid and the trapezium (Figure 67-3). The width of the retinaculum is about 2.5 cm; its length is about the same. Proximally, it blends with the antebrachial fascia and distally with the palmar aponeurosis. The tendon of the palmaris longus is attached to it anteriorly. A deep lamina on the radial side is attached to the medial lip of a groove on the trapezium. Between this layer and the more superficial part lies the tendon of the flexor carpi radialis muscle in its synovial sheath. On the ulnar side, a localized thickening of the antebrachial fascia extends laterally from the pisiform bone as a superficial part of the retinaculum, passing superficial to the ulnar nerve and vessels to blend with the retinaculum lateral to them. Lanz (13) illustrates 12 variants of the main nerve and its motor branch. In most cases, the motor branch arises from the radial side of the nerve in the carpal tunnel and runs laterally, soon branching to supply the opponens and abductor pollicis brevis, and often part of the flexor pollicis brevis. A particular hazard for the surgeon is produced by an origin from the ulnar side of the nerve and a course across it, either deep or superficial, to the retinaculum. The palmar cutaneous branch arises from the median nerve about 7 cm above

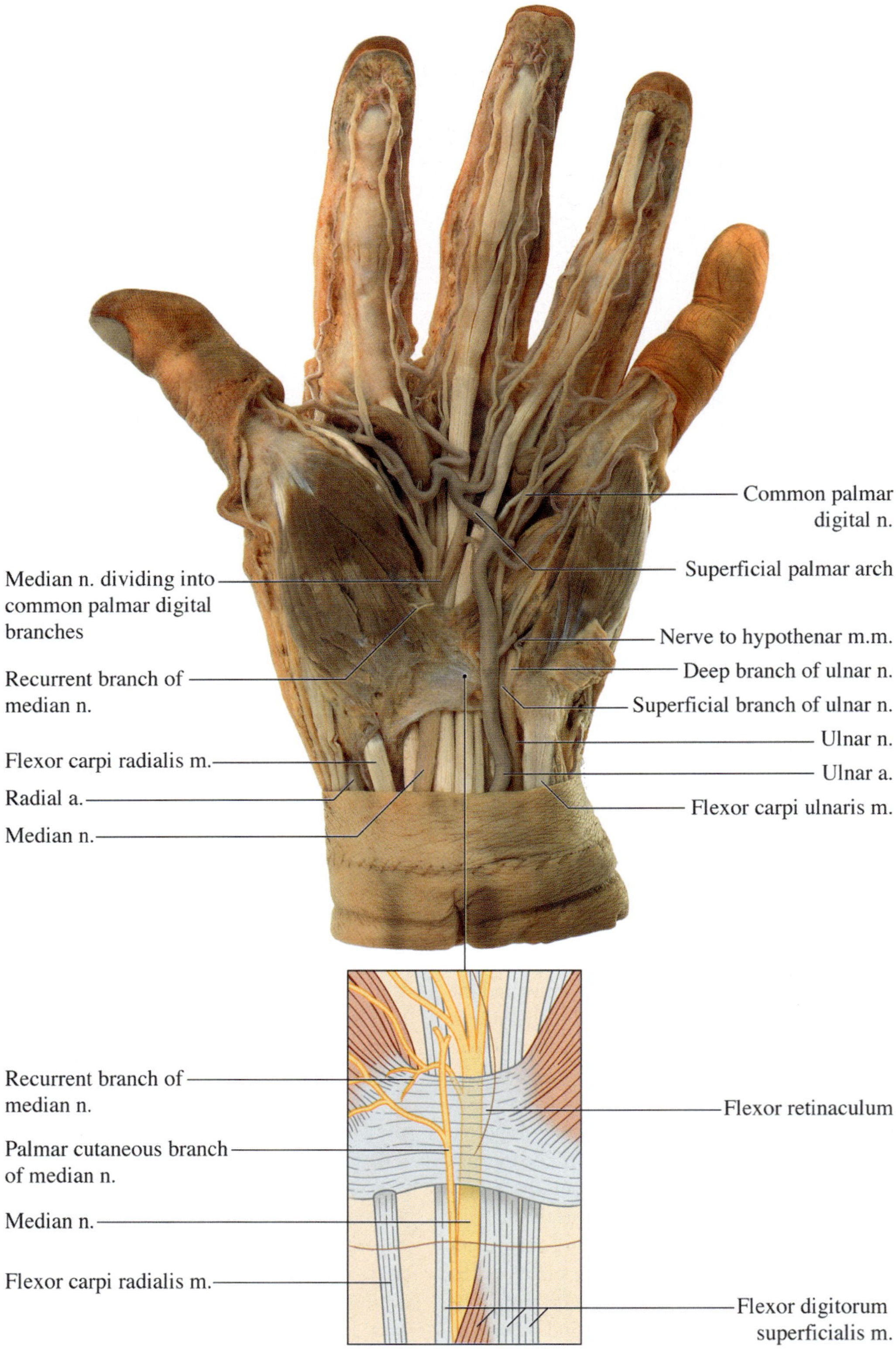

FIGURE 67-3 The median and ulnar nerves in the left hand. The inset shows the normal course of the median nerve at the wrist and the palmar cutaneous nerve. m, muscle; n, nerve. (© Copyright 2011 Rolfe Birch.)

the wrist crease and runs distally, medial to the tendon of the flexor carpi radialis to innervate the skin over the thenar eminence and the radial side of the proximal part of the palm. Damage to this can cause a profound, persistent painful state.

As the ulnar nerve approaches the elbow, it runs behind the medial intermuscular septum and then passes subcutaneously behind the medial epicondyle of the humerus in the retrocondylar groove. Schroeder and Scheker (14) define the "arcade of Struthers" thus: "the arcade was better described as a fibrous canal with an average length of 5.7 cm, its openings, at either end, were 3.9 and 9.6 cm proximal to the medial epicondyle." The components of the arcade include not only the tough medial intermuscular septum of the arm but also the sheath of the medial head of triceps, which can be seen enveloping the nerve, as well as the internal brachial ligament. The ulnar nerve then passes superficial to the medial capsule of the elbow joint and deep to the arcade, joining the two origins of the flexor carpi ulnaris muscle (the arcuate ligament). This is the "cubital tunnel." The nerve then runs between the flexor carpi ulnaris and flexor digitorum profundus muscles, joining the ulnar artery in its course down the forearm. The muscular branches arise just below the elbow. The nerve is vulnerable to external pressure. It may be compressed between the arcuate ligament and the medial capsule, and with relaxation of this ligament, it may become hypermobile, dislocating forward when the elbow is flexed. Because of the excursion required of it during movement of the elbow, it may be stretched during flexion if its movement is restricted by changes caused by damage by external pressure. The ulnar nerve and artery pass down the forearm within a well-defined sheath that is found deep to the anterior margin of flexor carpi ulnaris. The nerve and artery may become tightly compressed by swollen anoxic muscle and later by postischemic fibrosis. Arterial bleeding from a wound on the ulnar aspect of the forearm indicates damage to the ulnar nerve. The dorsal branch of the ulnar nerve is at risk during operations about the distal third of ulna and the dorsum of the wrist (see Figure 67-13).

The ulnar nerve divides into its superficial (sensory) and deep (motor) components at about wrist level. Both components run into Guyon's space (Figure 67-4). The superficial branch passes superficially to supply the palmaris brevis and the skin of the medial two digits; the deep branch runs between the abductor and the flexor of the little finger to pierce the opponens and then runs across the deep palmar space with the deep palmar arch, ending by supplying the adductor and flexor brevis of the thumb and the first palmar interosseous muscle. Deep as it is, the deep branch is vulnerable to wounds from glass or knives. The nerve is best followed by an incision beginning above the wrist, entering the ulnar side of the palm and curving across the distal palm in a crease. It is isolated in the upper part of the incision lateral to the tendon of flexor carpi ulnaris and medial to the ulnar artery and followed to its bifurcation. Then the deep branch is followed between the hypothenar muscles. Its deep course has to be revealed by mobilization of the deep and superficial flexor tendons. The multitude of the motor branches of this nerve, to most of the intrinsic muscles of the hand, has to be borne in mind during this exposure, although it is impossible to avoid some of these in a scarred field.

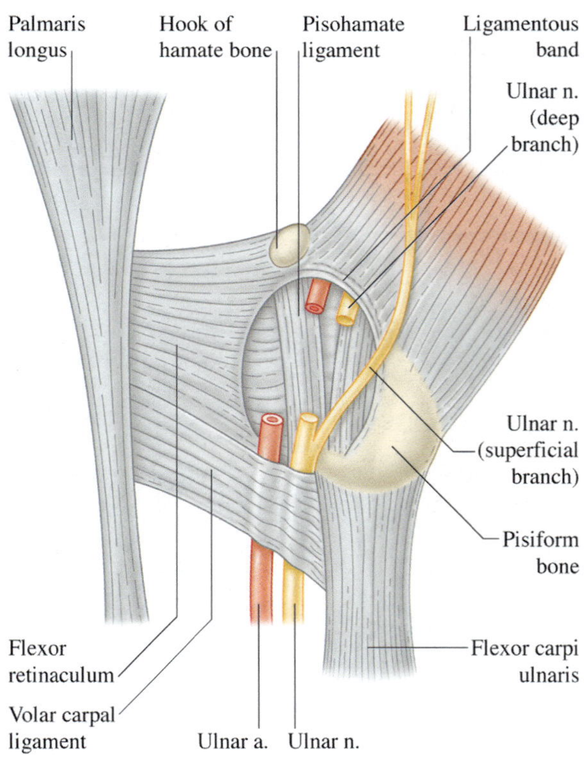

FIGURE 67-4 Guyon's space. Note the possibilities for entrapment at and distal to the volar carpal ligament. a, artery; n, nerve. (© Copyright 2011 Rolfe Birch.)

Vascular Injuries

Axilla Wilbourn (15) has described the medial brachial fascial compartment, which extends from the axilla to the elbow and is bounded by the tough medial intramuscular septum and the axillary sheath, and suggests that bleeding into this compartment is responsible for the majority of infraclavicular plexopathies after regional block. Wilbourn's comment bears repeating: "Distal pulses are normal as they are with most compartment syndromes because the elevated pressure, although sufficient to collapse the vasae nervori, is far below mean arterial pressure. Ultrasound, MR (magnetic resonance imaging) and CT (computed tomography) may reveal the vascular lesion, but, considering the very brief time available for surgical decompression before irreversible nerve damage occurs, obtaining these is rarely justified." The 16 patients described by Stenning et al. (16) probably fall into the syndrome described by Wilbourn. There was, in all of these cases, an injury to the axillary artery or one of its offsets caused by dislocation of the shoulder or fracture of the proximal humerus. The diagnosis of continuing bleeding into the axillary sheath was made by the delayed onset of nerve palsy or the deepening of the lesion while under observation. There were 87 nerve palsies. A favorable outcome was seen in all cases in which urgent repair of the artery and decompression of the axillary sheath were performed. The outcome for function within the hand in another patient in whom the diagnosis was delayed by 8 weeks is shown in Figure 67-5.

Elbow The collateral circulation at the elbow rests on alternative pathways that accompany the radial nerve (the radial collateral artery), the ulnar nerve (the superior ulnar collateral artery), and sometimes the median nerve. This network may maintain perfusion of the forearm and hand in cases in which the brachial artery has been divided *when there is no associated fracture or dislocation,* but the situation is very much worse if nerves are entrapped within the fracture or compressed by hematoma. Wajcberg et al. (17) used high-resolution ultrasonography to measure the rate of flow through the brachial artery in adults and in children. Flow was calculated by multiplying the velocity-time interval of the Doppler flow

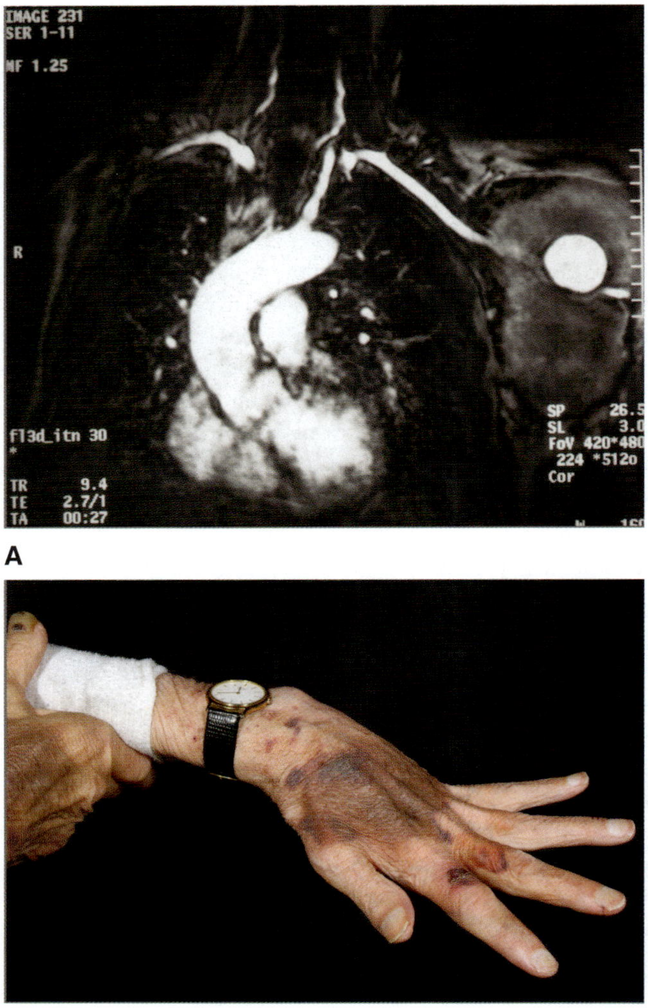

A

B

FIGURE 67-5 A fracture of the left proximal humerus was complicated by an expanding hematoma in a 63-year-old man. Two attempts to occlude the torn posterior circumflex artery by interventional radiology failed. He was seen at 8 weeks by which time he was in right heart failure and in great pain, and he had a complete infraclavicular plexopathy on the left side. A total of 6 L of altered blood was removed from the axilla. His pain was relieved. Recovery was particularly poor in the radial and median nerves. (**A**) Magnetic resonance angiogram before surgery. (**B**) The left hand 4 years after surgery. (© Copyright 2011 Rolfe Birch.)

signal by the heart rate and the cross-sectional area of the vessel according to Laplace equation: BF (blood flow) = $[\pi \times (D/2)]^2 \times$ FV (flow velocity). The mean diameter of the brachial artery in children between 4 and 5 years of age is 2.7 mm, which provides a resting flow of *about 200 mL/min*. The reader will at once note the significance of the diameter of the vessel from the equation of Laplace, and this factor is emphasized by Poiseuille's law, which states that flow through a tube is affected by three variables: the radius (to the power 4), the total tension in the wall, and the pressure gradient. The diameter of the superior ulnar collateral artery at the elbow in children is no more than 1 mm. This caliber provides flow of *about 20 mL/min*, assuming that the pressure gradient is the same as that in the brachial artery itself and that the collateral pathways are intact.

Depth of Lesion

It is helpful to the clinician to bear in mind two facts: (1) a nerve that has been transected or ruptured cannot recover until it is repaired, and (2) a lesion of a peripheral nerve that remains in continuity but that continues to be subjected to the cause of that lesion will deepen until the cause is removed. The speed of that deepening is related to the cause. A nerve crushed by a plate or by an encircling suture may recover if that cause is removed within a minute or two. It is unlikely to recover if it is not relieved for more than 2 or 3 hours. A nerve subjected to continuing traction and ischemia from an expanding hematoma or to compression and ischemia within a swollen ischemic limb will recover if the situation is corrected within 4 to 6 hours. A nerve trapped within a fracture or joint will probably survive for a number of days unless internal fixation has been done (Figure 67-6). It may be years before the situation becomes irretrievable for a nerve subjected to radiotherapy or exposed to continuing traction from a malunited fracture. The cardinal symptom of the persistence of a noxious agent is pain.

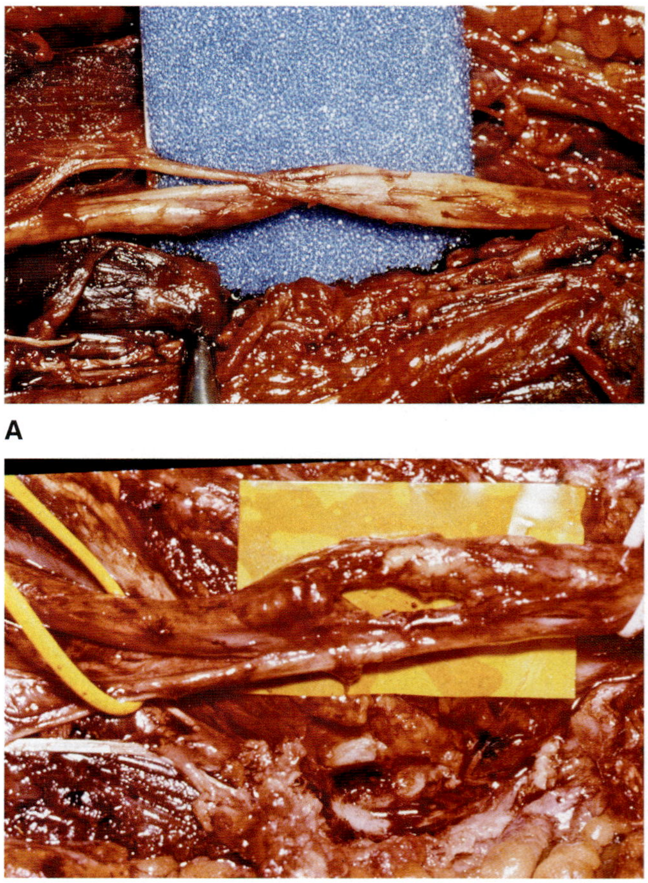

A

B

FIGURE 67-6 Deepening of the lesion. (**A**) The median nerve extricated from the supracondylar fracture in a 9-year-old girl at 3 days from injury. There was complete recovery. (**B**) The median nerve extricated from the supracondylar fracture in a 13-year-old girl 8 weeks after injury. There was no recovery. (© Copyright 2011 Rolfe Birch.)

Neurapraxia-Conduction Block

Transient Ischaemic Block Large myelinated fibers are first affected; C fibers and autonomic fibers escape. Recovery of all modalities occurs within a few minutes of return of perfusion. The effect of temporary ischemia is well illustrated by the behavior of the main nerves during emergency repair of a main artery. Conduction persists for about 1 hour while the artery is being controlled and repaired. Then conduction diminishes before altogether ceasing. Conduction returns within a few minutes after removal of clamps and restoration of flow. A similar process is seen in nerves exposed distal to a suprasystolic cuff.

With severe and prolonged pressure, there is local demyelination and more prolonged conduction block (PCB) (18). The myelin is squeezed proximally and distally from underneath the tourniquet so as to invaginate into the proximal and distal sheaths of the nodes of Ranvier. A PCB that may last for weeks or months results. If the cause of the local demyelination persists in the form of, for example, a bony projection causing pressure and distortion or of external pressure by hematoma, the block persists. In these, removal of the external pressure is rapidly followed by recovery in lesions that had persisted for several years (1). The autonomic fibers are usually spared but not necessarily so. Seddon (19) observed the characteristic features of conduction block caused by bullets: paralysis exceeds loss of sensation, the nerves responsible for proprioception are more deeply affected than those conveying light touch sensation, and vasomotor and sudomotor function is least affected. It is likely that this lesion is provoked by a momentary displacement or stretching of the nerve trunks. This explanation cannot account for the PCB of blast injuries in which the patient is exposed, at close range, to the shock wave of an explosion without any wound or fracture and with no signs of significant injury to the soft tissues.

It is unwise to make a diagnosis of neurapraxia when there is (1) persisting pain, (2) a strong Tinel's sign at the level of lesion, or (3) a pulseless limb. Conduction block may prove to be only the first step toward something much worse. Ischemia affects first the large fibers; discriminative sensibility and vibration sense are first affected (20). It is not easy to test these modalities when ischemia is developing because of damage to a main vessel associated with a fracture of a long bone, but if action is not taken until superficial sensibility is lost, it will come too late.

Degenerative Lesions: Axonotmesis and Neurotmesis

The situation is wholly different when the lesion is serious enough to cause interruption of the axon. Then follows Wallerian degeneration, which affects the axon, the cell body, and the Schwann cell ensheathment and its myelin sheath. There are changes in the endoneurial cells and, over longer periods of time, in the motor and sensory end organs. Distal to the site of injury, the axon degenerates, and there is a granular disintegration of the cytoskeleton and axoplasm, which are converted over succeeding days into amorphous debris. Motor conduction in the distal segment ceases about 3 days after injury. The essential difference between neurapraxia and the different types of degenerative lesion is the persistence of conduction in the distal segment of the nerve in the former and its disappearance in the latter. Conduction disappears within 1 hour of an ischemic lesion but persists for hours or even days after transection or rupture. The early disappearance of conduction is the hallmark of impending or actual "critical" ischemia.

The continuity of the Schwann cell basal laminae from proximal to distal segment maintains the original pathways for regrowth of axons. Gutmann and Sanders (21) and Seddon (19), in extensive studies of mammalian and human nerves, showed that crushing, or "firm squeezing," was followed by reconstitution of the nerve. It is the difference between preservation and destruction of continuity that underlies the division of degenerative lesions between those with the potential for spontaneous recovery (axonotmesis) and those that will not recover (neurotmesis) unless action is taken. We (1,22) prefer a further simplification of the classification as "degenerative" and "nondegenerative." The first question to be asked is, "Is this lesion degenerative (i.e., axonotmesis or neurotmesis) or nondegenerative (i.e., neurapraxia or conduction block)?"

Diagnosis

The object of the clinician must be to recognize an injury as soon as possible and then to determine the nerve or nerves affected, the level or levels of injury, and the extent and depth of the lesion or lesions.

The history is important: high-velocity injury; compound fracture and wounding; accidental, criminal, surgical, or all three are likely to mean that there has been a serious lesion. The use of a knife, often enough in the hand of a surgeon, is an indication that a nerve is likely to have been partly or completely severed. Advice from witnesses or emergency paramedical staff is always valuable. The subclavian artery is ruptured in as many as 30% of cases of violent traction injury of the infraclavicular portion of the brachial plexus. Arterial injury is frequent in fracture dislocations of the shoulder and elbow. It is important always to search for other injuries before embarking on treatment of the nerve lesion. The site and nature of the wound or wounds must be observed. In closed injuries, the presence of swelling and bruising may give some indication of severity.

The early *symptoms* of acute nerve injury are abnormal sensations, alteration or loss of sensibility, weakness, motor paralysis, impairment of function, and sometimes pain. Sometimes the patient is aware of warming and dryness of all or part of an extremity (Figure 67-7).

Neuropathic pain is never easy to recognize in an injured patient who is probably confused, distressed, and in pain. It can be distinguished from the pain of fracture or dislocation by loss of sensation; by painful, spontaneous sensory symptoms (dysesthesias) expressed throughout the territory of the nerve; and by lancinating or shooting pain irradiating into the distribution of the nerve. A constant crushing, bursting, or burning pain in the otherwise undamaged hand indicates serious and continuing injury to major nerves. Progression of sensory loss with a deep bursting or crushing pain within the muscles of the limb, often accompanied by allodynia, indicates impending critical ischemia until proven otherwise.

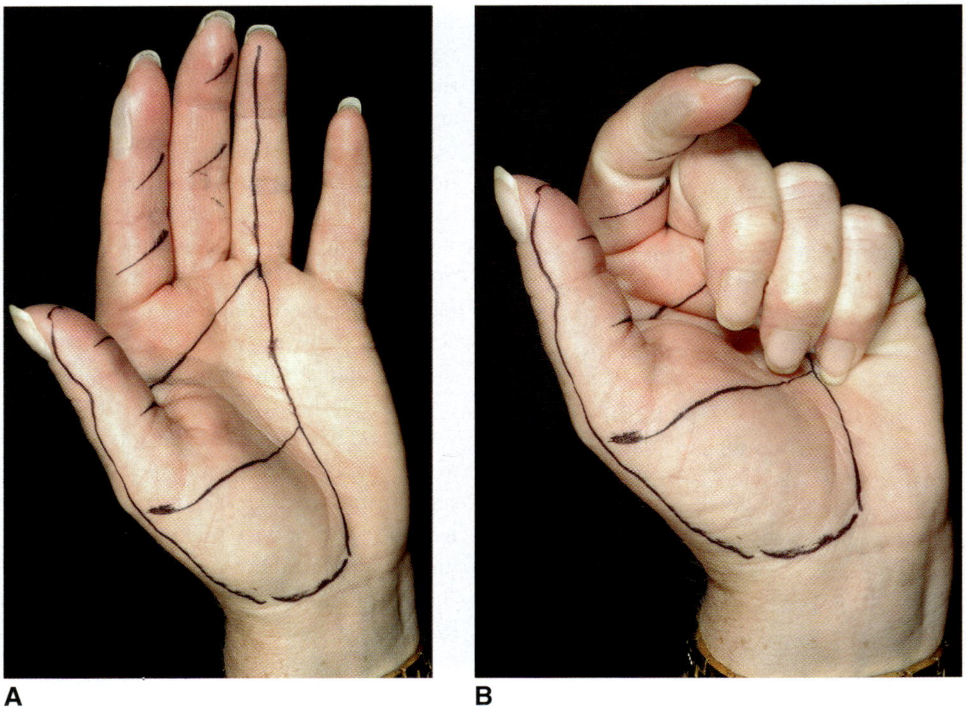

FIGURE 67-7 (A) and (B) Sympathetic paralysis seen within a few days of transection of the median nerve at the elbow. (© Copyright 2011 Rolfe Birch.)

Examination should enable the clinician to extend the knowledge afforded by the history and the narrative of symptoms to permit accurate diagnosis to be made. All findings should be recorded in such a manner that the record will be intelligible later not only to the examiner but also to others. Unfortunately, the signs of acute nerve injury have to be sought at a time when the patient may be the least able to cooperate in an examination—soon after wounding, when there is likely to be distress and when the general condition may be affected by loss of blood and other injuries. The examination often has to be done in the often unfavorable surroundings of an accident and emergency department. After operation, the patient's response is likely to be distorted by postoperative pain, the effects of recent general anesthesia, or sedative or analgesic drugs. These are no conditions for a quiet and comprehensive "neurologic examination," yet this is the time when the fact of nerve injury must at least be recognized if the best result is to be obtained from treatment. *The examiner should at all times bear in mind that if there is a wound over the line of a main nerve and if there is any suggestion of loss of sensibility or impairment of motor function in the distribution of that nerve, it must be regarded as having been cut until and unless it is proved otherwise* (Figure 67-8).

In the absence of wounding, clinicians should be able to arrive at an accurate diagnosis of the *level* and *depth* of a lesion by clinical examination. A sound grasp of the level of the branches of the trunk nerves and of the contribution to those nerves coming from individual spinal nerves is a prerequisite. "*Aids to Examination of the Peripheral Nervous System*" (23) is essential reading.

Sympathetic paralysis is one almost infallible sign of deep lesion. It is always present in the first 48 hours after injury to the median and ulnar nerves or their cutaneous branches. *A strong Tinel's sign* at the level of a closed lesion indicates that axons are ruptured. Other early signs that indicate a deep injury to a nerve include changes in texture of the skin, rather like "goose pimples"; development of a skin rash; and hypersensitivity surrounding the area of anesthesia. In a small child, there may be an abnormal posture of the denervated digits. The immersion test is useful in small infants: the injured hand is placed in warm water for a few minutes; the skin of a denervated digit fails to wrinkle.

Two weeks after a complete degenerative lesion, sensory loss is well defined, and wasting begins. Anhidrosis is still present, but with the degeneration of peripheral fibers, the warm isothermia of the skin gives way to poikilothermia and later to cold isothermia. As time goes by, the changes of disuse appear and include thinning of the skin, even ulceration from accidental injury, loss of substance in the tips of the digits, loss of skin markings, constant coldness and cyanosis, stiffness of joints, contractures, and unmistakable wasting. Nails become brittle and discolored and are prone to infection. Hair growth is disturbed, and hairs are often coarse. These changes occur rapidly in the ischemic limb; they are far less in PCB.

The very real difficulty of recognition of rupture of a nerve trunk in a closed fracture may be overcome by the use of high-resolution ultrasonography (24).

Techniques

The object of nerve repair is the accurate coaptation of healthy conducting elements without tension. In practical terms, this means accurate coaptation of the bundles. This is done after skeletal injuries have been stabilized and vessels repaired and after muscles, tendons, the joint capsule, and the synovium have been drawn together, restoring gliding planes. Cover by healthy full-thickness skin is essential. In delayed repair, the

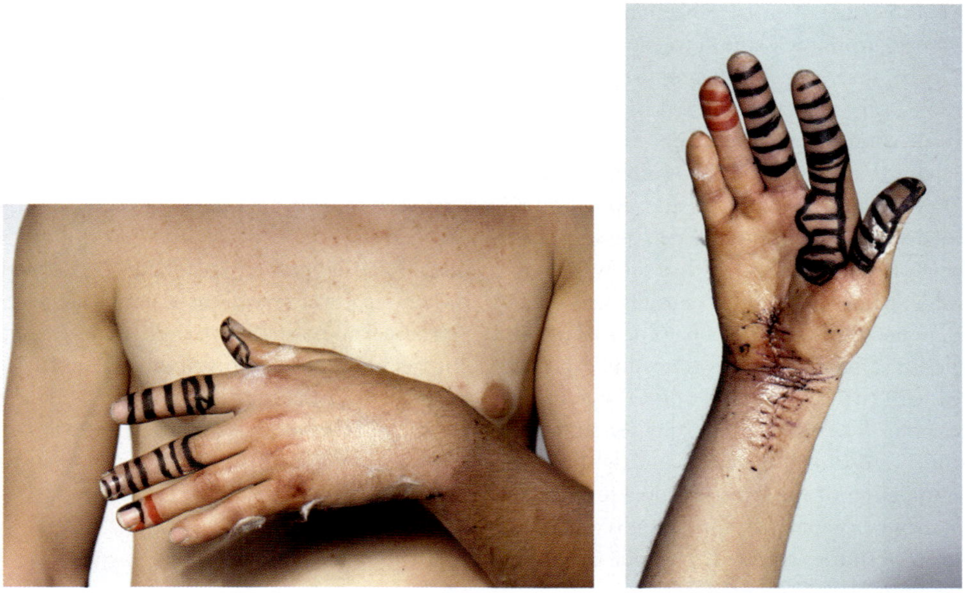

A B

FIGURE 67-8 (A) Typical area of loss of sensibility after division of the median nerve at the wrist, sparing the palmar cutaneous branch. (B) The area of sensory loss and "clawing" of the little and ring fingers after division of the ulnar nerve in the forearm. (© Copyright 2011 Rolfe Birch.)

incision is planned so that a skin flap is raised over the nerve, and the nerve ends are cut back progressively until healthy pouting bundles show in the cut surfaces. Resection is less in urgent repairs. No more than 1 to 2 mm of nerve is removed in tidy wounds. Finding the right level of section in the closed traction rupture or in an untidy wound is much easier in urgent repairs when there is still conduction in the distal trunk. In high ruptures, a nerve the stimulator is moved slowly from the stumps toward healthy tissue until a somatosensory evoked potential becomes detectable (proximal stump) or until muscular activity returns (distal stump). This usually coincides with a healthy-looking nerve face; the amount of tissue resected is usually between 5 and 10 mm. More nerve must be resected in late cases; when there has been sepsis, as much as 4 cm of the proximal and distal stumps are irretrievably fibrosed. Palpation of the nerve detects the difference between soft, healthy tissue from the firm or hard, scarred segment.

Then the ends must be united, preferably by end-to-end suture. As long as the gap after resection is small, little mobilization of the nerve is needed to close it, and the repaired nerve lies without tension, without excessive flexion of adjacent joints. One simple test as to the advisability of direct suture of a nerve trunk at the wrist or in the forearm involves passing an epineurial suture of 6-0 nylon, with the wrist flexed to no more than 30 degrees. If this suture will draw the stumps together without tearing the epineurium and without causing blanching of the epineurial vessels, then primary suture is reasonable. Failing that, grafting is necessary. It will be seen that in many circumstances, it is better to bridge a gap with a graft than to force direct suture; it is better to resect to healthy bundles and create a wide gap than to resect too little to facilitate direct suture. Anterior transposition of the ulnar may provide at most 3 cm. No gaps in the median nerve in the forearm can be closed by end-to-end suture.

It is often easy to match bundle to bundle simply by looking at the nerve end under the microscope or with loupes, although the changing architecture of the nerve along its length makes this difficult when a long gap has to be bridged. Accurate matching is assisted by the orientation of epineurial vessels and by making a sketch of the prepared nerve ends indicating the size and the disposition of different bundles. When the operation is done soon after injury, it is easy to effect an "electrophysiological orientation" (25). The possibilities of histochemical identification of nerve fibers are reviewed by Brushart (26).

Suture Techniques

Orgell (27) described a modified fascicular suture, "group fascicular suture," and he concluded that because there was little difference between the results of epineurial and perineurial suture, epineural suture was "the technique of choice for most acute nerve lacerations." Spinner (28) thinks that a "fascicular" suture is useful in distal median and ulnar repairs and emphasizes that the most important cause of failure is "inadequate resection of injured nerve back to healthy tissue." During an urgent or emergency operation, the surgeon should indeed proceed to a neat epineurial suture using 6-0 or 7-0 sutures or to immediate grafting if circumstances permit. Many excellent results follow this approach in severe cases of injury or when the nerve has been inadvertently divided during an operation.

I prefer bundle (fascicular) suture combined with epineurial suture for most main nerves. In the early days after division of a nerve, bundles are mobile within the epineurium, and epineurial suture risks malalignment. Dissection within the nerve is avoided because this surely leads to fibrosis. The needle is passed through the condensed inner epineurium and the perineurium to secure accurate coaptation of larger bundles. The repair is completed by epineurial suture. In delayed repair, fibrosis within the epineurium stabilizes the bundles so that they cannot rotate within the epineurium. In these, epineurial suture may be adequate. The atrophy of the distal stump and the extent of fibrosis in both increase the difficulties in neglected cases.

In both primary and secondary sutures, the areolar adventitial tissue is dissected back from each stump to expose the true epineurium. In fascicular suture, matched bundles, identified by size and by position in the nerve, are united by perineurial sutures of 9-0 or 10-0 nylon. After these "key" bundles have been united, the coaptation is completed by passing sutures of 8-0 or 9-0 nylon through the perineurium and epineurium. The nerve can be rotated on a saline-soaked dental swab, first from one side and then from the other, so that the whole circumference is accessible. Between 18 and 25 sutures are used to repair the adult median nerve at wrist level. In epineurial repair, orientation of bundles is achieved as well as is possible, and the epineurium is united with two lateral sutures of 8-0 nylon, the ends of which are left long. The repair of the anterior surface is completed with sutures of 8-0 or 9-0 nylon, and the nerve is then rotated by manipulation of the lateral sutures so that the posterior epineurium can be coapted. If fibrin glue is available, this reduces the number of sutures required. The glue is applied after key sutures have been placed (Figure 67-9).

Grafting

When possible the medial cutaneous nerve of the forearm (MCNF) from the damaged limb is used. The superficial radial nerve (SRN) and the lateral cutaneous nerve of the forearm (LCNF) provide valuable innervation to the skin of the hand, and *neither should be used unless the parent nerve is irretrievably damaged.*

No graft should be harvested until the injured nerves have been exposed and the extent of lesion defined and the gap between the prepared nerve ends measured. This is a good time for the surgeon to pause for a few minutes of reflection so the repair can be properly planned. This is particularly important when repairs of several main nerves are necessary. A map of the proximal and distal nerve ends is prepared outlining the pattern of the bundles in each stump and measuring the length of the gap between the prepared stumps. Then a calculation is made of the number of grafts required for each nerve and the disposition and length of the grafts that are cut to about 15% more than the measured gap.

Harvest and Preparation of the Graft The MCNF is harvested from the arm through a straight incision. One anterior branch will be seen in the middle of the arm, lower down the nerve divides into two branches that straddle the main brachial vein. The terminal 4 cm of the posterior interosseous nerve (PIN) provides useful material for grafting

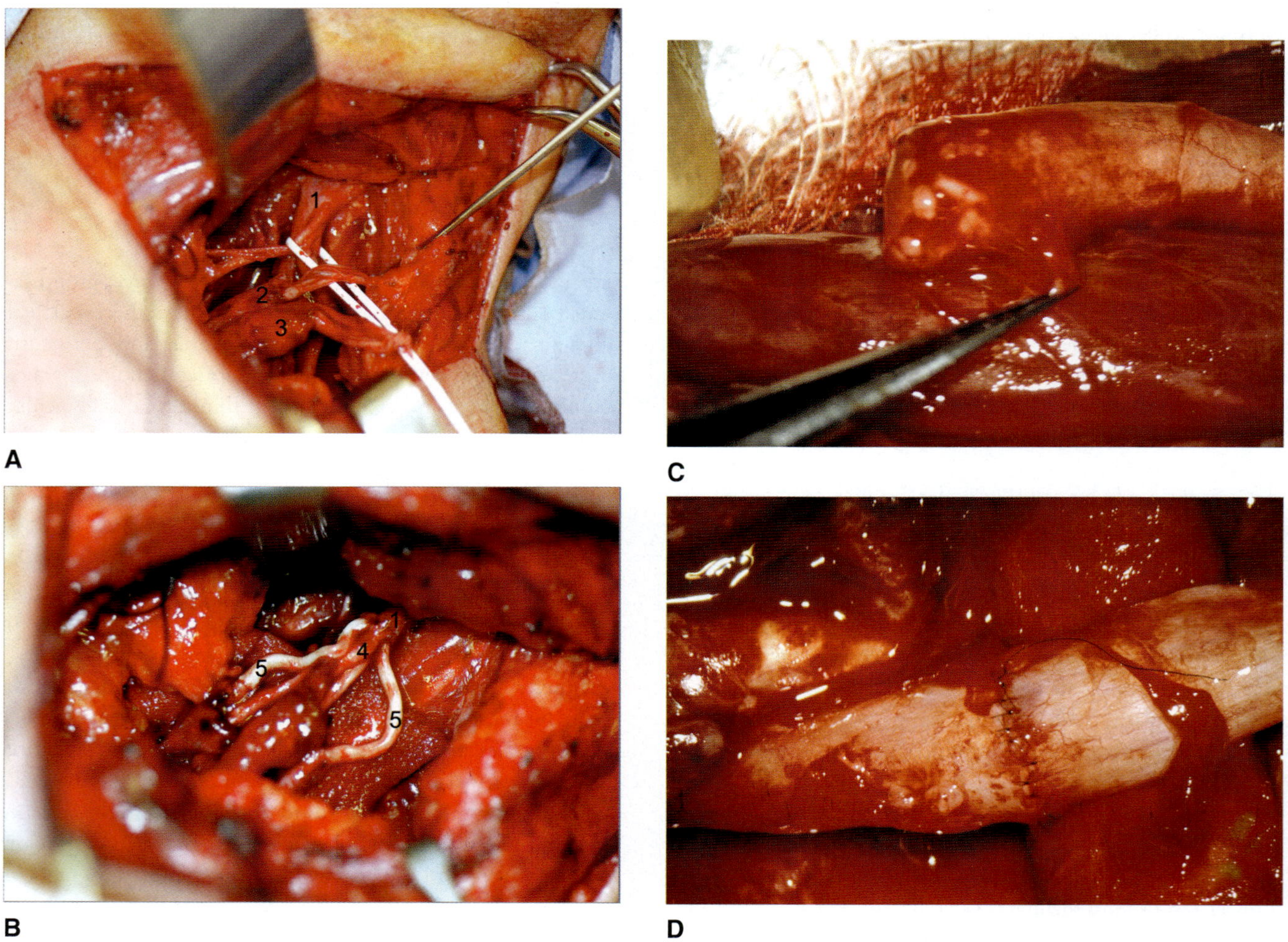

FIGURE 67-9 Primary suture of the median nerve at the wrist. (A) The meso neurium adventitia is cleared. (B) The pattern of the bundles is examined. (C) The first sutures pass through the perineurium of the larger bundles followed by epiperineurial sutures. (D) The nerve is rolled on a swab for access to the posterior aspect. The completed repair is seen next. (© Copyright 2011 Rolfe Birch.)

palmar digital nerves instead of the sural nerve. The sural nerve will be needed if two or more nerves require grafting. In the supine position, the lower limb(s) is elevated by a stoical assistant or the knee is flexed to about 70 degrees with the foot resting on the table. The nerve is exposed through a long midline incision beginning laterally in the distal third of the leg to a point midway between the posterior aspect of the lateral malleolus and the lateral margin of the Achilles tendon. The incision may be extended into the popliteal fossa as a Z. Up to 50 cm of graft is available. The grafts, tenderly handled, are laid between saline-soaked swabs and cut to appropriate length with a new scalpel blade or with vascular scissors. The nerve ends are prepared so that the fascicles protrude and are laid in the prepared bed, which must be healthy and unscarred. Fixation is usually by fibrin glue, but the grafts can be sutured initially with two lateral sutures of 9-0 nylon. Because the individual strands of the grafts are likely to be around the same size as the individual bundles, the suture unites epineurium of the graft to perineurium of the bundle (Figure 67-10).

It is better to graft the proximal stump of the nerve first, leaving the distal ends of the grafts laid out across the bed before proceeding to the distal stump, matching as far as is possible, fascicle to fascicle. It is very important, after both ends have been coapted, to carefully inspect the grafts and the suture lines to make certain that during the union of one end the union of the other end has not been disturbed.

It is better to bridge the gap with grafts if intact fascicles have been separated from the lesion. All nerve repairs must be isolated secluded from bare bone, tendon, or lacerated muscle by healthy tissue. Grafts are stabilized by closing healthy synovium, fat, or muscle over them. It is necessary to restate that repairs of nerves and vessels must be covered by healthy, full-thickness skin. Split-thickness skin grafts induce severe fibrosis, which strangulates.

The limitations to conventional nerve grafting include the limited amount of cutaneous nerve available, the different architecture between cutaneous nerves and main nerves, the disproportion in the volumes of conducting nerve tissue and connective tissue and in the caliber of nerve fibers, and the specificity of Schwann cells either to motor or to sensory axons. We have seen a high rate of failure among more than 4000 grafts of trunk nerves carried out since 1965. Wide retraction of the stumps in closed traction lesions is usual, and it is a simple matter to draw the nerves back to their normal position during an operation performed within the first 1 or 2 days. It is always easy to be wise after the event, but it now seems that suture would have been the better way forward in some of our cases, particularly for nerves injured at the elbow, knee, and wrist. In an earlier study of repair of the median and ulnar nerves at the wrist and forearm (29), there was no detectable difference in the results between the 25 repairs and the 35 grafts. The gap after resection of the neuroma was measured with the elbow extended and the wrist at 20 degrees dorsiflexion. The average gap was 2.5 cm in the repairs and 5.5 cm in the grafts. Trumble (30) provides sound advice about reasonable methods of diminishing the gap between nerve stumps by careful mobilization and by positioning of adjacent joints and he emphasizes that the gap is always longer in delayed repairs. Whenever possible, the stumps of transected or ruptured nerves should be approximated at the first operation when circumstances prevent primary repair. Clinicians must never forget that nerve grafts obtain their blood supply from the bed in which they lie. The lessons of the First World War were restated by Seddon (31): "Since the wounds of nerves that call for repair by grafting are usually extensive the need for the replacement of skin scars by healthy tissue arises with corresponding frequency. Nothing less than a full thickness flap or tube pedicle graft will suffice

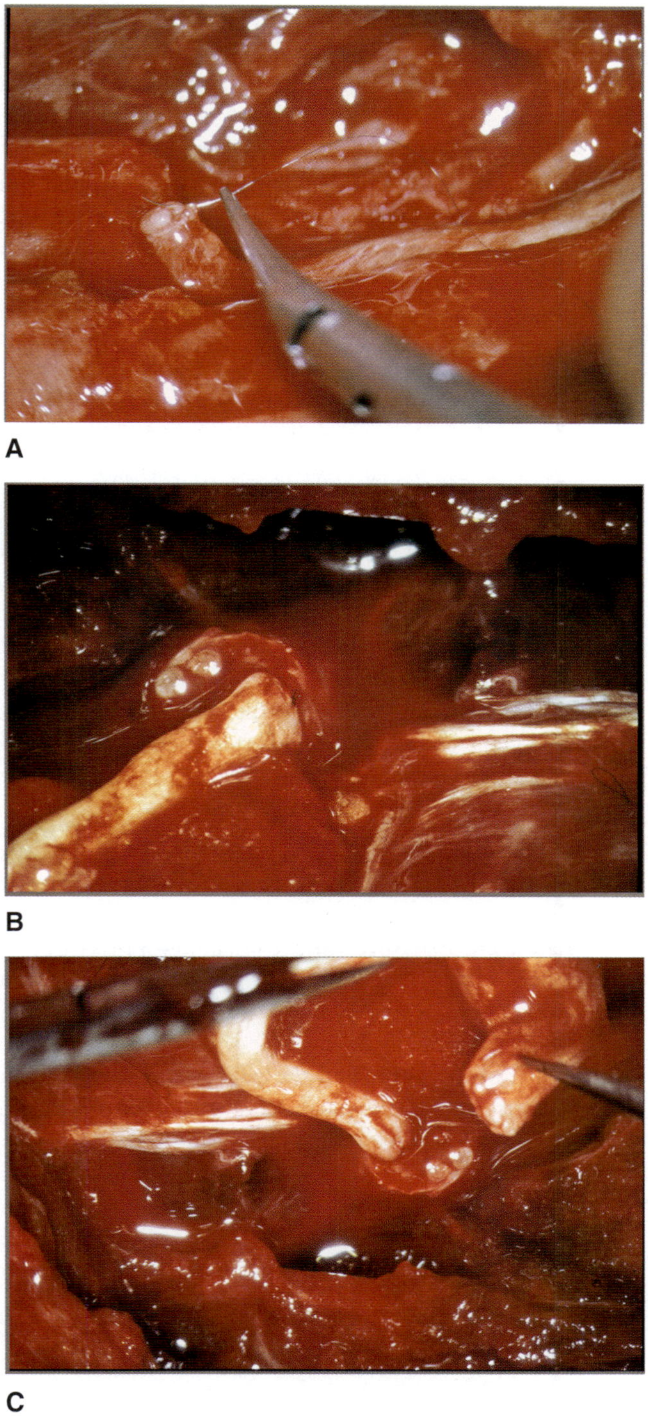

FIGURE 67-10 In nerve grafting, the suture coapts epineurium of the graft to perineurium of the bundle. (© Copyright 2011 Rolfe Birch.)

since it is important the graft should lie, so far as is possible, in healthy well vascularized tissue." Leaving a nerve graft within scarred muscle or underneath a split-thickness skin graft just will not do.

Entubulation In 1997, Lundborg et al. (32) published a significant paper describing a prospective randomized trial comparing silicone entubulation and suture of median and ulnar nerves in the forearms of 18 patients. Recovery was studied most thoroughly, and no significant difference in outcome between the two groups was noticed.

Nerve Transfers in Infants Anand and Birch (33) studied 24 patients with severe birth lesions of the brachial plexus; the plexus had been repaired in 20 of the patients. The recovery of sensation was far better than that of skeletal muscle motor recovery and sympathetic function. Sensation was normal in all dermatomes for at least one modality in 16 examined hands, and there was accurate localization in the dermatomes of avulsed spinal nerves that had been reinnervated by intercostal nerves transferred from remote spinal segments. The poor recovery of muscle function in these children may reflect the greater vulnerability of the immature nervous system to avulsion or proximal axonotomy.

Nerve Transfers in Adults Őzkan (34) treated 20 cases of irreparable lesions of ulnar or median nerves by transfer of the digital nerve from the inner to the outer side of the appropriate digit. Extensive sensory retraining was used in all patients, and accurate localization was restored in 18. Battiston and Blanzetta (35) reported useful recovery in six of seven cases of high ulnar lesions by transfer of the distal part of the anterior interosseous nerve and the palmar cutaneous branch of the median nerve to the ulnar nerve at the wrist. We have transferred the dorsal branch of the ulnar nerve or the MCNF to the median nerve with modest success. Although transfer of the intercostal nerves to the lateral or medial cords often improves the trophic state of the skin of the hand in adults with severe injuries to the brachial plexus, it is usual to find that stimulation of the reinnervated skin is referred to the chest wall (36).

The lesion in continuity presents a most difficult problem. If bundles can be seen traversing the lesion and if there is conduction across it, I leave things be. But if the lesion is not recovering or if it is causing severe pain and if there is no obvious local cause external to the nerve for that pain, then resection and repair must be considered. External neurolysis (i.e., decompression of the nerve working outside the epineurium) is reasonable, but there should be no undue delay before reverting to resection and nerve grafting if there is no progress to recovery. If the chief problem is pain and the pain seems to be arising from the nerve lesion, it is my practice to place an indwelling catheter close to the proximal trunk and infuse local anesthetic for 2 to 3 days. Resection is performed if—and only if—the block abolishes pain (37,38). The traction lesion in continuity is a common finding during exploration, and it is very difficult. The nerve, which is usually in the axilla or at the knee, is exposed after a severe closed traction injury and is found elongated by one third or more. The epineurial blood vessels are torn, but the perineurium and individual bundles appear intact. The damaged segment may exceed 25 cm in length, and resection and repair of such extensive lesions is scarcely feasible. Useful recovery occurs naturally in one third to half of these injuries. It seems that the damaged segment acts as an imperfect graft because the perineurium is in continuity and at least some of the Schwann cells survive (38).

Postoperative Care

Repairs need protection during at least the first 3 weeks after repair and longer than this in many secondary sutures. The method used in the postoperative care of severe wounds at the wrist is as follows (Figure 67-11). The splint holds the elbow at 90 degrees of flexion, the wrist at between 30 and 40 degrees of flexion, the metacarpophalangeal (MCP) joints at about 70 degrees of flexion, and the proximal interphalangeal (PIP) joints at no more than 30 degrees of flexion. The dorsal splint extends to the tips of the fingers and the palmar splint to the PIP joints only. The splints are bandaged so that there is restriction but not rigid immobilization. Gentle, active flexion of the fingers and the thumb is encouraged from the outset. The arm is supported in a sling, but there should be encouragement of gentle active lateral rotation and of elevation of the shoulder to 90 degrees from the first postoperative day. At 3 weeks, the splints and the skin sutures are removed. The next splint does not restrict the elbow. The wrist is splinted to prevent extension beyond 20 degrees. The dorsal hood, which again extends to the tips of the fingers, blocks the MCP joints to 30 degrees short of extension and the PIP joints to 30 degrees short of extension. Increasingly, vigorous active flexion of the fingers and the thumb is now permitted, and gentle active flexion at the wrist is also encouraged within the confines of the splint, bandaged as it is to the forearm and hand. In direct sutures of nerves in the elbow region, the first splint is replaced by a hinged splint at 2 weeks after the operation. This permits active flexion but blocks extension. The range of permitted movement is increased at weekly intervals by adjusting the hinge. By 6 weeks, splints are discarded, and vigorous active flexion against resistance is introduced. Now, gentle passive extension stretching can be introduced for the fingers and the thumb. Early gentle active movements within the confines of the splint and the bandages are encouraged.

It is, of course, very important during the period of recovery to maintain the mobility of the joints some or all of whose governing muscles are paralyzed and to warn the patients of the danger, especially in cold weather, of accidental damage to the anesthetic skin. Most of the work on passive movements of the joints can be done by the patient or by his or her parents, but weekly supervision by a therapist is useful in keeping the mind concentrated on the work during the long march toward recovery. In the case of the MCP joints of the fingers and the carpometacarpal joint of the thumb, dynamic splints are useful, but the problem of the stiff MCP joint in the paralyzed hand persists.

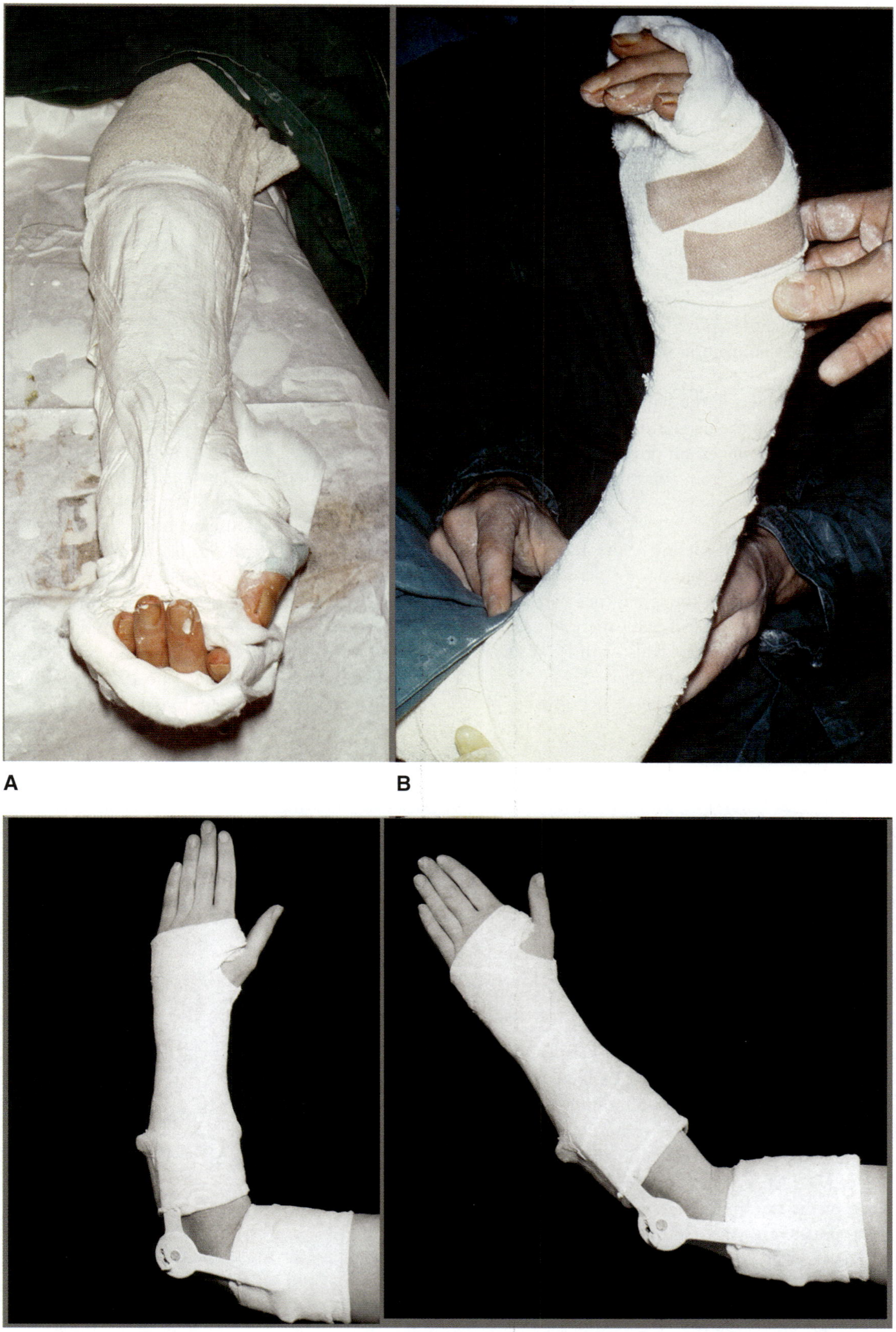

A B C D

FIGURE 67-11 Protection after nerve repair. (A) and (B) Plaster splint after repair of both nerves and flexor tendons at the wrist. (C) and (D) Hinged plaster splint with adjustable block. (© Copyright 2011 Rolfe Birch.)

Neuropathic Pain

Injury to a nerve may lead to a number of events that underlie neuropathic pain (37):

1. Spontaneous firing in nociceptor and other neurons and abnormally increased firing in response to noxious stimulation
2. Sensitization of the axons, with their cell bodies in the dorsal root ganglion and the dorsal horn of the spinal cord, so that pain and sensory disturbance is increasingly experienced in new areas outside the distribution of the injured nerve
3. Sensitization of mechanoreceptive neurons or a change in their behavior, so that nonpainful stimuli are perceived as pain
4. Afferent and efferent fibers in the sympathetic system, which are conveyed with the nerve trunks, are involved in the injury, and may to some extent provoke or maintain symptoms and signs arising from abnormalities of the level of lesion or more

The spread of pain beyond the lesion of the injured nerve is a common example of central sensitization. Increased somatic C-fiber and A-delta fiber input in the spinal cord may account for the enhanced biceps reflex seen in one patient with neurostenalgia from a median nerve injury. This, with his pain, was abolished by revision repair and resurfacing.

Important principles in the treatment of neuropathic pain include (39):

1. Removal of the cause
2. Promotion of healing or regeneration
3. Correction of the microenvironment of the nerve
4. Restoration of afferent pathways
5. Modulation of the central inhibitory pathways
6. Reduction of sympathetic overactivity
7. Changing pain thresholds by modification of emotional or behavioral components of pain interpretation. Operation is necessary in the first four of these and may be needed to reduce sympathetic activity.

The median and ulnar nerves are notoriously susceptible to one of three pain syndromes, which are classified as follows (37,40). A strong, painful Tinel's sign is almost always present at the level of such a lesion in all three syndromes.

Causalgia is the most severe of the neuropathic pain states. It is usually caused by a high partial injury to the median, ulnar, and tibial nerves or the trunks of origin with associated arterial injury. Pain is spontaneous, persistent, often burning; extends throughout the limb; and is worsened by physical and emotional stimuli. The patient has excessive sweating and vasomotor disturbance. Allodynia and hyperpathia are intense. Forty-eight patients with causalgia have undergone surgery since 1975. The median and ulnar nerves or their nerves of origin were involved in 28 of these. Penetrating missile wound was the cause in 21 patients; there was false aneurysm or arteriovenous fistula in 11. Operation was done to correct the cause, repair the arterial lesion, and repair the damaged nerve; an indwelling proximal catheter was used for the infusion of local anesthetic for at least 72 hours. Sympathectomy was performed in the first six patients. Sympathectomy can be extremely effective in the relief of causalgia (41). In Kline and Hudson's case (42), causalgia after a gunshot wound to the infraclavicular part of the brachial plexus was relieved only temporarily by repair of a false aneurysm of the axillary artery and neurolysis of the lateral cord; only sympathectomy later cured the pain. However, I have not used sympathectomy since 1998 (37).

Neurostenalgia is caused by persisting tethering, compression, distortion, or ischemia of an intact or repaired nerve. Pain is confined to the distribution of the nerve, and sympathetic overactivity is rare. These patients, together with those who have true causalgia, are the most rewarding to treat by operation. In most cases, the nerve trunk is intact, and the lesion is neurapraxia (PCB) or at worst axonotmesis. The nerve is in some way irritated, tethered, compressed, or ischemic, and treatment of the cause relieves the pain. Tethering or entrapment of the nerve induces sharp, lancinating pain (Figure 67-12). In ischemia, the pain is constant, deep seated, and rather poorly localized and is usually described as burning, crushing, or bursting. A hematoma, which falls short of causing ischemia of a limb, will result in scar, which can be a potent cause of tethering of the nerve and neurostenalgia.

In *posttraumatic neuralgia* (PTN), pain is initially confined to the territory of the nerve without florid sympathetic overactivity. Dysesthesia and lancinating pain are usual in nerves with a cutaneous component, but pain is deep, boring, and poorly localized in nerves passing to muscle. The subsequent extension of pain into adjacent areas indicates central sensitization. Many of the worst cases of PTN followed damage to a terminal branch where it lies in the superficial fascia. The only method of treatment with any hope of lasting success is the restoration of a normal input of nonpainful impulses; this normally

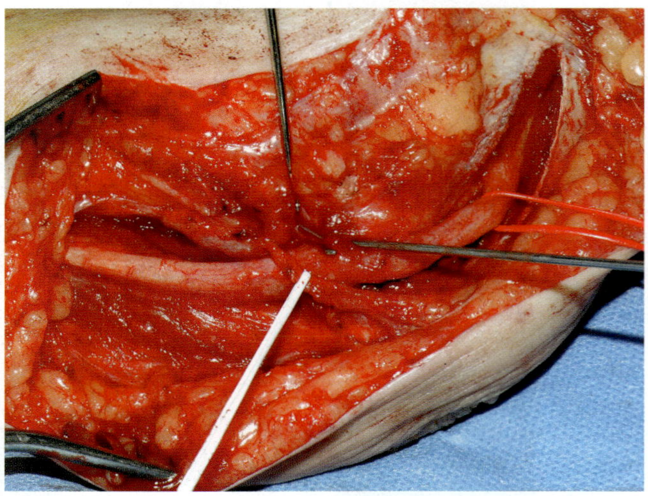

FIGURE 67-12 A 38-year-old woman experienced intense pain and a partial lesion of the ulnar nerve after arthroscopic repair of the capsule of the elbow joint. Her pain was worsened by attempted extension at the elbow. The nerve was exposed 4 days later; it had been caught by a clip. The clip was removed, and her pain was relieved. There was considerable recovery in the ulnar nerve, but she did not recover vasomotor and sudomotor control, and there was persistent weakness of the intrinsic muscles. (© Copyright 2011 Rolfe Birch.)

involves successful repair of the affected nerve or nerves. These cases produce the most difficulty in treatment, and it is a salutary reflection that many of these injuries were caused by surgeons and doctors in the course of treatment. The propensity of the pain caused by injury to cutaneous nerves to evolve so that it spreads to adjacent skin with extension of the area of allodynia and the development of excessive sweating and of vasomotor instability often leads to diagnosis of *complex regional pain syndrome*," an error that consigned several hundreds of patients whom we have seen to fruitless and even to harmful treatment by infusions, blocks, and powerful drugs and even to a suggestion that the patient has some form of psychological disturbance (Figure 67-13).

Nerve Injuries in Fractures or Dislocations

Seddon (43), in speaking about nerves injured in the arm and at the elbow, thought that recovery could be awaited if two conditions were met. "The first is: reasonable apposition of the bony fragments and the other *complete certainty that there is no threat of ischaemia of the forearm muscles*". The extensive review from Siegel and Gelberman (44) found that 85% of nerve palsies recovered spontaneously from closed fractures and 65% to 70% after open fractures. Ninety percent of the nerves that went on to recovery had done so by 4 months; in these, the predominant lesion must have been conduction block. Their indications for exploring the nerve included (1) the fracture needs internal fixation, (2) associated vascular injury, (3) wound exploration of an open fracture is necessary, and (4) irreducible fracture or dislocation irreducible. There are two more: (1) the lesion deepens while under observation, and (2) the lesion occurred during surgery for internal fixation.

I follow the following principles in the approach to nerves injured by skeletal injury:

1. Clinical examination usually permits the distinction between conduction block and degenerative lesions.
2. A diagnosis of neurapraxia should not be made in the presence of significant neuropathic pain. This suggests that the noxious agent is still at work on the nerve.
3. Deepening of the lesion while under observation indicates bleeding until proven otherwise.
4. The diagnosis of neurapraxia cannot be regarded as secure until the persistence of conduction in the distal segment of the nerve is demonstrated after about 8 days after the injury.
5. Tinel's sign at the level of closed lesion shows that at least axons have been ruptured. An advancing sign distinguishes between (axonotmesis) and (neurotmesis). This investigation should enable the clinician to come to a view about the likelihood of recovery at no later than 6 weeks from the injury (45).
6. If a surgeon elects to convert a closed fracture to an open one by whatever technique, then the lesion of the nerve should be exposed. The nerve, indeed the nerve with the adjacent artery, may be in the fracture or in the joint. Both will certainly be displaced from their normal positions.
7. A complete lesion of the nerve strengthens the case for open treatment.

The Elbow

The elbow is a notorious area of difficulty in treating nerve injuries, especially in children. The close proximity of all

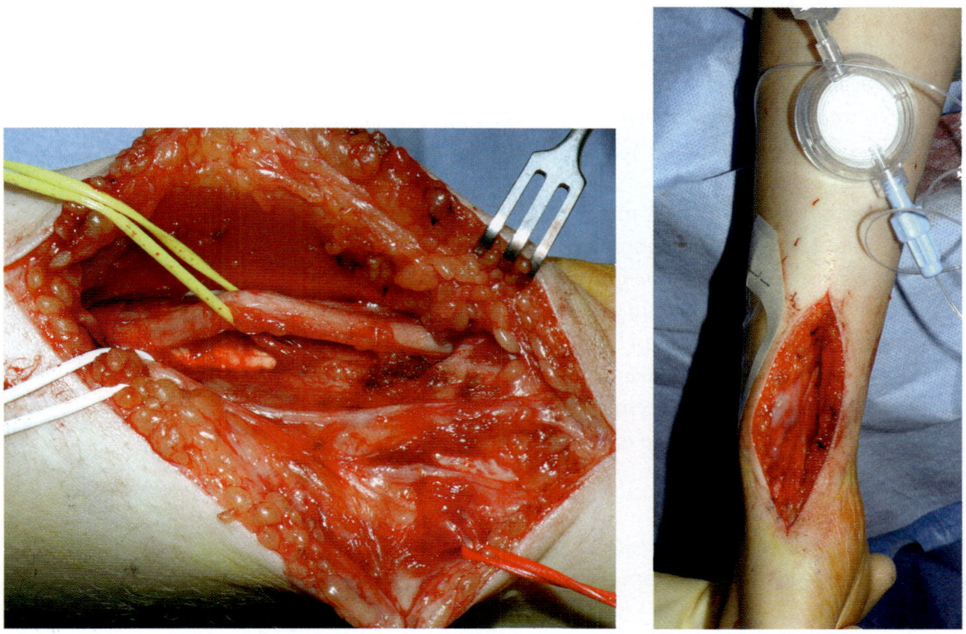

A B

FIGURE 67-13 Posttraumatic neuralgia misdiagnosed as complex regional pain syndrome type I in a 12-year-old girl. (**A**) A branch of the dorsal division of the ulnar nerve has been partially transected by the arthroscope. (**B**) The nerves were bathed in fibrin glue after neurolysis; a catheter has been inserted for prolonged nerve block. This child had been given fruitless treatment for 12 weeks. The referral was prompted by an educational psychologist's concern about her mental deterioration. Pain was relieved with surgery. (© Copyright 2011 Rolfe Birch.)

trunks to bone makes them vulnerable to displacement into the fracture or joint, often accompanied by the brachial artery. Since 1975, 239 nerve lesions (202 median and ulnar) after fracture or dislocation of the elbow in children have been explored. A total of 114 lesions (56.4%) were incurred during first operation. The nerves were found to be entrapped within the fracture, impaled on a bone spike, compressed by swelling or fibrosis, or tethered or transfixed by pins, and 27 nerves required repair. Most of these injuries could have been prevented by exposing the nerve during open reduction and internal fixation.

Volkmann's Contracture and the Supracondylar Fracture Seddon (43) described 38 cases and observed that: "paralysis was by far the most frequent manifestation of ischemia with depression of sensibility (a certain indication of nerve involvement) and a reduction or loss of voluntary power." A more recent study examined 26 children who presented to the first hospital with a "pink pulseless hand" after supracondylar fracture (46). The brachial artery had been explored, as an emergency, in five children in whom recovery was good. Twenty-one fractures were treated by internal fixation at the first operation. The brachial artery and the affected nerves were subsequently explored in 21 children. The artery was constricted by dense scar tissue deep to the bicipital aponeurosis (12 cases) or trapped within the fracture (9 cases). In all cases, pulsatile flow returned after decompression of the vessel. The flexor compartment was worst affected (21 cases). The intrinsic muscles were affected in nine hands. The extensor compartment was least affected; the five patients were successfully treated by serial stretching and splinting. Fifty-six main nerves were injured. Ischemia of the nerve that was compounded by compression from swollen or infarcted muscle caused the lesion in 41 nerves. Thirteen nerves were trapped in the fracture. Two nerves had been divided by a Kirschner wire during internal fixation. Preservation or recovery of modalities of cutaneous sensibility and of vaso- and sudomotor function was noted at the first examination in 14 of the median and ulnar nerves.

Recovery of cutaneous sensibility and of small muscle function in the hand was generally good after decompression but recovery into the flexor and extensor muscles of the forearm was determined by the extent of post ischemic fibrosis. In general, the nerves recovered far better than the flexor muscles of the forearm after decompression. The extent of growth disturbance was evident only in a long-term review. Children with seemingly good early results after corrective surgery had recurrence of deformity with significant defects at skeletal maturity (Figure 67-14).

Iatrogenic Injuries in Adults The risks to the PIN and of ischemic injury to the ulnar nerve during operations for fractures or dislocations at the elbow are well known. New methods bring new risks. Five nerves were transected during arthroscopic procedures at the elbow, and six more were ruptured by the drill during operations of "closed" reduction or during the application of an external frame. Thirty-four other nerve lesions incurred during "minimal access surgery" required exploration.

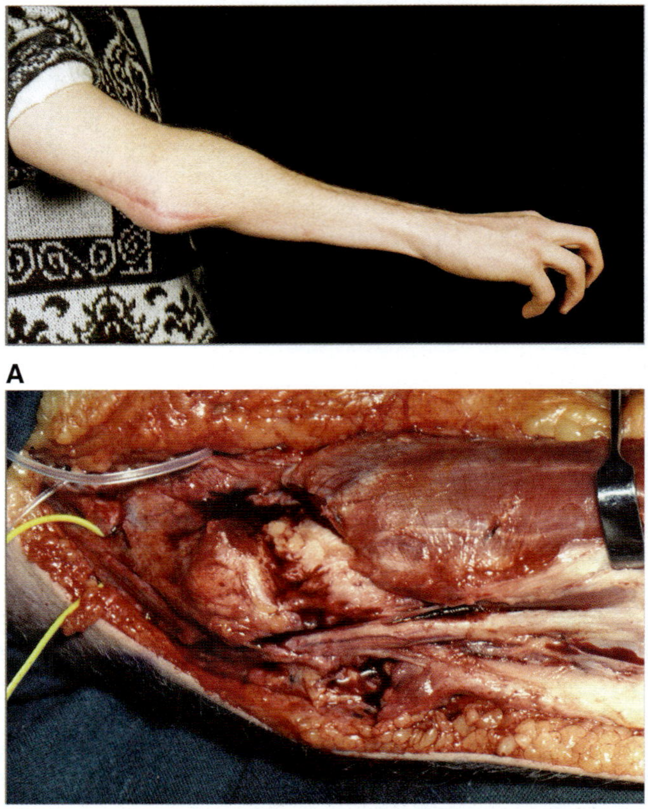

FIGURE 67-14 Volkmann's ischemic contracture. (**A**) The ulnar nerve exposed during flexor muscle slide 8 weeks after supracondylar fracture. The epineurial vessels and the ulnar recurrent collateral vessels are occluded, and the nerve is compressed by the swollen, infarcted muscle. (**B**) There is some recurrence of deformity, and the forearm and hand are shorter than on the uninjured side. ()

CONCLUSIONS

1. Circulation must be restored. Rupture of a brachial artery from a supracondylar fracture in a child is rare. The artery is usually compressed by the bicipital aponeurosis or becomes entangled within the fracture. Ischemia is inevitable if the brachial artery is occluded and if a main nerve or nerves, with attendant vessels, are trapped in the fracture.
2. Neuropathic pain or severe pain persisting after reduction of a fracture or deepening of a nerve lesion indicates impending ischemia until proven otherwise.
3. If the skeletal injury is complicated by a nerve palsy and if the surgeon thinks it necessary to expose the fracture, then it is wise to identify and trace the affected nerve. Entrapment or other distortion of the nerve is more likely than rupture.
4. A deep lesion of a nerve that becomes evident after an operation strongly suggests that the nerve has been cut or entrapped.
5. In adults, the ulnar nerve requires careful handling. The collateral vessels are better taken with the nerve during anterior transposition.
6. No case of isolated anterior interosseous palsy has been encountered among the 295 children's nerves injured by

fractures or dislocations involving the distal humerus seen since 1975. It may be that the fibers in the median nerve destined for the anterior interosseous nerve are selectively vulnerable to injury at the elbow; it is more likely that a partial lesion of the whole median nerve was not detected at initial presentation. The anterior interosseous nerve is particularly susceptible to ischemic anoxia because of its location in the depths of flexor compartment, and it is likely that some reported cases are examples of anoxic conduction block.

War Wounds

A War Nerve Injury Clinic was established at the Defence Medical Rehabilitation Unit at Headley Court, Surrey 7 years ago. Three hundred servicemen and -women who had sustained more than 850 injuries to the peripheral nerves have been seen. Most modern war wounds are caused by explosive devices; they are multiple and complex (Figure 67-15). Avulsion, laceration, blast, and crush combine to tear and shred tissues of all compartments. Heavy contamination with dirt and debris is usual, and meticulous debridement is the essential first step in time-limited resuscitative surgery. The field hospital policy of emergency restoration of arterial flow and extensive decompression led to a remarkably low incidence of ischemic fibrosis; the sole case occurred in a patient in whom the brachial artery was ligated. Many of the wounded have sustained severe injuries or even amputations of lower limbs, so it is important to restore the highest level of function possible in the upper limbs and hands. Some of the findings in the first 100 consecutive patients (261 nerves) are presented here.

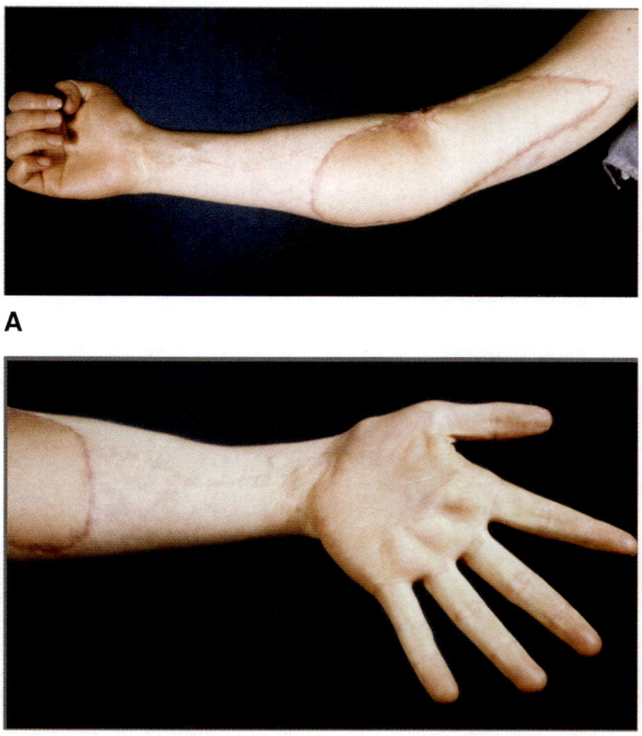

A

B

FIGURE 67-15 An example of reconstruction from an earlier conflict. (A) and (B) A 28-year-old ambulance driver sustained a missile wound to the elbow, which destroyed the brachial artery and median nerve during a terrorist attack in Northern Ireland in 1980. The artery and the nerve were repaired primarily and the skin defect replaced by split skin graft. The artery thrombosis about 3 days later, the nerve repair failed, and she developed severe pain. Six month later, both the artery and nerve were repaired again, scar tissue was excised, and skin cover was provided by a free latissimus dorsi myocutaneous flap. Fasciocutaneous flaps are preferred for the wounds of current conflict. (© Copyright 2011 Rolfe Birch.)

The Wound The severity of damage at the level of the nerve lesion is probably unparalleled; fracture in 50%, arterial injury in 32%, moderate or severe muscle loss in 28%, and moderate or severe skin loss in 50%. Two or more nerves were injured in 70% of patients. Nerve lesions were more common (54%) in the lower limbs. The two definitive studies (7,9) of peripheral nerve injury in World War II found that 62% were in the upper limb and that a single nerve was involved in more than 65% of cases. Gousheh (47) found arterial injury in 20% of 369 war wounds of the brachial plexus. The studies from Roganovic and his colleagues (48,49) noted arterial injury in 13.4% of 2239 peripheral nerve injuries from the Balkan wars; 702 injuries to the common peroneal nerve were complicated by fracture in 45.9%, injury to main artery in 24.4%, and severe soft tissue loss in 24.8%.

Prolonged Conduction Block The median time to onset of recovery was 4.17 months in the 116 nerves with PCB. It was 3.8 months in the penetrating missile wound group (45 nerves) compared with 4.7 months in the explosion group (71 nerves) ($P = 0.0001$).

Nerve Repairs Forty-six nerves were repaired, 36 at a median interval of 6 days and 11 at a mean interval of 90 days. There were 10 primary sutures and 25 primary grafts. Seven free fasciocutaneous flaps were used in the early repairs. Revision repairs were later done in three of the repairs and five of the grafts, and nine neurolyses were performed. Ten free fasciocutaneous flaps were required in the revision operations. The overall results in the 46 repairs were 15 good (32.6%), 19 fair (41.2%), and 12 poor (26.1%).

Pain Secondary operations were necessary in 36 patients with persisting neuropathic pain. Thirty of them experienced such relief after operation that analgesic medication was considerably reduced or abandoned. Relief was dramatic for some patients, who experienced it when they awoke from the anesthetic. The operations included six revision repairs, 11 neurolyses of nerves that had been repaired, and neurolysis in 19 patients. The causes of persisting pain included displaced bone fragments; heterotopic bone; the proximity of implants; retained metallic fragments or suture material; and most commonly, scar tissue, which enveloped and constricted the nerve. Resurfacing with free fasciocutaneous flaps was used in 15 patients.

Grading of Outcome: Factors Affecting Recovery

Three grades are used (36):

1. Good, which means that recovery of function is substantial, that it enables the patient to use the limb and

to lead a normal life without difficulty and that they are not troubled by pain or over reaction.

2. Fair, which implies recovery of function that is useful but that falls far short of normal. The patient is sufficiently aware of the hand or the foot that he or she does not damage it. Muscle power of Medical Research Council grade 2 or 3 restores some balance across a joint, and it may be possible to supplement this with the appropriate muscle transfer to enhance, for example, flexion of the elbow or extension of the wrist.
3. Poor, which means no or insignificant recovery. This grade is used in all cases with persisting spontaneous neuropathic pain, hypersensitivity, or overreaction. Some patients with cold sensitivity were unable to continue in their previous occupations (Tables 67-2 and 67-3).

All systems of measurement have their defects, and it seems the more closely one looks at the result of a nerve repair, the more defects are revealed. The grade "excellent" was given to a few distal repairs (29,42). The outcome is set out according to the cause of injury: the "tidy" wound from a knife, glass, or scalpel; the "untidy" wound from an axe, saw, penetrating missile, open fracture or dislocations, or burn; and the closed traction lesion (Tables 67-4 to 67-7).

Two factors outweigh all others: delay before repair and the violence of the injury. In some patients, the failure to repair the subclavian or axillary arteries led to such a poor limb that repair of nerves was either abandoned or not even attempted. The infraclavicular closed traction lesion, so often associated with rupture of the axillary artery, fared particularly badly. The difference between urgent and delayed repair is striking.

Age The recovery of cutaneous sensation in a child is usually remarkably good. An earlier study of primary repair of 30 adult

TABLE 67-2 Grading of Results in Median and Ulnar Nerves Repaired in the Infraclavicular Region, the Axilla, and the Arm (High Lesions)

Median	
Good	Long flexor muscles, MRC ≥4 Localization to digit without hypersensitivity Return of sweating
Fair	Long flexor muscles, MRC ≥3 Protective sensation; moderate or no hypersensitivity Sweating diminished or absent
Poor	Long flexor muscles, MRC ≤2 Protective sensation but severe hypersensitivity or no sensation
Ulnar	
Good	FCU and FDP little and ring, MRC ≥4 Intrinsic muscles MRC ≥2 Localization to little and ring fingers; no hypersensitivity Return of sweating
Fair	FCU and FDP little and ring fingers, MRC ≥3 No intrinsic muscle function Protective sensation little and ring fingers No or moderate hypersensitivity Little or no sweating
Poor	FCU and FDP little and ring fingers; MRC, 2 No intrinsic muscle function Protective sensation with severe hypersensitivity or no sensation No sweating

FCU, flexor carpi ulnaris; FDP, flexor digitorum profundus; MRC, medical research council.

TABLE 67-3 Methods of Grading of Results of Median and Ulnar Nerves Injured Below the Elbow (Low Lesions)

Grade	Motor	Sensory	Equivalent on Seddon's Grading
Excellent	Power MRC, 5 No wasting or deformity No trophic changes	Function indistinguishable from normal hand; good stereognosis, no hypersensitivity; 2PD equivalent to uninjured digits	Good M5, S4
Good	Power MRC, 4–5 Abolition of paralytic deformity Minimal pulp wasting	Accurate speedy localization; can recognize texture or objects; minor cold sensitivity and hypersensitivity; 2PD <8 mm at tips of fingers	Good M5, S3+
Fair	MRC ≥3 Pulp wasted	Some accurate localization to digit; no sweating; stereognosis; 2PD >8 mm; significant cold sensitivity and hypersensitivity	Fair M3, S3
Poor	MRC ≤3 Trophic changes	No sweating; sensation or severe cold sensitivity and hypersensitivity	Bad M0, 1, S0, 1 or 2

MRC, medical research council; 2PD, two-point discrimination.

TABLE 67-4 Results of Repair of 55 Median and Ulnar Nerves in Closed Infraclavicular Traction Lesions*

	Early: Within 14 days (33 Nerves)	Late: After 15 days; Mean, 22 weeks (22 Nerves)
Good	14	2
Fair	13	7
Poor	6	13

*These nerves were ruptured in 42 of the 89 patients. The axillary artery was ruptured in 31 cases.

digital nerves (50) found that only 27% of the patients rated their result as excellent, and 40% complained of persistent hyperesthesia at 2 years. It seems that sensory recovery after a well-executed primary repair of the median nerve at the wrist is regularly better than that seen after digital nerve repair. However, many patients report striking improvement in sensation with quite sudden loss of cold sensitivity and hypersensitivity some years after repair. Repair of high lesions in patients older than 65 years of age was often followed by the relief of pain and with it improvement in the patient's mental well-being. Older patients may be more likely to develop severe pain after injury to a nerve (37).

Level of Injury The recovery of the small hand muscles after repair of the distal motor branches is scarcely ever matched by that seen after high repairs, and in some patients, it may be better to proceed to tendon transfer after it is clear that the high repair is progressing.

Anatomy of the Radial Nerve

The radial nerve, the terminal branch of the posterior cord, is the largest of the main nerves within the upper limb and contains fibres passing through the spinal nerves from C6 to T1. The lateral head of triceps and brachioradialis (BR) are consistently innervated by C6: the long head of triceps, the radial wrist extensors (extensor carpi radialis longus [ECRL] and extensor carpi radialis brevis [ECRB]), and the extensor digitorum communis (EDC) by C7 and the extensor muscles to the thumb by C8 and sometimes by T1. The nerve passes down the limb like a double spiral starting in the axilla, it is anterior to the axis of the limb, but it curves posteriorly around the upper humerus before reemerging into the anterior compartment after piercing the intermuscular septum. At the elbow, the SRN and PIN migrate into the posterior aspect of the forearm. Between its origin and its entrance into the spinal groove, the nerve receives fewer arteries than elsewhere along its course. The first 8 to 10 cm of the nerve may not have a nutrient artery, so this segment is only supplied by descending intraneural channels and will be relatively avascular if transected at its origin. The profunda brachii artery accompanies the nerve in the spiral groove. Bleeding from it compresses the nerve. The nerve lies closest to the humerus, where it pierces the lateral intermuscular septum as it passes through a short tunnel bounded by bone and unyielding fascia. Here, the nerve is tethered, which is a common level of rupture, entrapment, or compression.

Some generalizations regarding the radial nerve:

1. For many patients, elbow extension is a good deal more important than elbow flexion, particularly for those who use walking aids or have a spinal cord injury. Wrist

TABLE 67-6 Repair of 264 Median and Ulnar Nerves in Tidy Wounds Injured Between the Distal Wrist Crease and Elbow in Adults Age 16 to 65 Years, 1979 to 2004

	Repair Type (*n*)			
Outcome	Primary Repair	Delayed repair	Graft	Total
Excellent	13	2	2	**17**
Good	52	15	34	**101**
Fair	25	30	52	**107**
Poor	2	16	21	**39**
Total	**92**	**63**	**109**	**264**

TABLE 67-5 216 High Repairs of Median and Ulnar Nerves in Adults and Children, 1975 to 2000*

	Median (*n* =117)					Ulnar (*n* =99)			
Outcome	Tidy wounds	Untidy wounds	Closed traction	Total	Outcome	Tidy wounds	Untidy wounds	Closed traction	Total
Good	8 (36.4)	6 (16.2)	3 (5.2)	**17 (14.5)**	Good	5 (33.3)	5 (14.3)	0 (0)	**10 (10.1)**
Fair	10 (45.4)	16 (43.3)	22 (37.9)	**48 (41)**	Fair	7 (46.7)	16 (45.7)	24 (49)	**47 (47.5)**
Poor	4 (18.2)	15 (40.5)	33 (56.9)	**52 (44.5)**	Poor	3 (20)	14 (40)	25 (51)	**42 (42.4)**
Total	**22**	**37**	**58**	**117**	**Total**	**15**	**35**	**49**	**99**

*There were 125 arterial injuries (58%). Twenty of the 27 good results followed repair within 48 hours of injury. Seven of these results were in children. Results of repair at 3 months or more after the untidy wound or closed traction lesion were uniformly bad. Operation was not considered or attempted repair was abandoned in 31 patients presenting with a delay of 3 weeks or more because of ischemic fibrosis or sepsis.

TABLE 67-7 Recovery of Sensation After Repair of 129 Digital Nerves*

	Adults		Children (Age 15 Years or Younger)	
Grade	Repair within 48 hr of injury	Repair 2 wk or more after injury	Repair at varying intervals after injury	
Excellent	1	0	17	**18**
Good	33	9	8	**50**
Fair	24	11	2	**37**
Poor	16	8	0	**24**
Total	**74**	**28**	**27**	**129**

*Seventeen digital arteries and 20 flexor tendons were repaired in the primary operation.

extension is the cornerstone of hand function; extension and abduction of the thumb open out the web space, the basis of prehensile function (Figure 67-16). Many patients with median nerve palsy are able to use the sensate skin on the sides of the thumb and index finger to great effect.

2. The level of lesion has perhaps a greater effect on the recovery of distal muscles than in any other peripheral nerve. It is very unusual to see restoration of extension of the digits even after a well-executed primary repair of a wound in the axilla. Conversely, repair of the PIN is usually gratifying (Figure 67-17).
3. Most lesions of the radial nerve are compound; there is injury to the skeleton, the main vessels, and the soft tissues at the level of lesion. The effect of this on regeneration is often profound.
5. Exposure of the nerve is not easy, and this may account for some injuries incurred during operation but cannot explain their increase (Table 67-8).

We are chiefly concerned with aspects of diagnosis, exposure, and the prevention of iatrogenic injury.

Pain

Causalgia arising from lesions of the radial nerve is uncommon, accounting for two of our 48 operated cases. *Neurostenalgia* is much more common (51). Persistent pain within the distribution of the radial nerve after skeletal injury or beginning after operation for such an injury is a sure indication that the nerve continues to be damaged by bone, entrapment, or suture or implant. Most common is the problem of PTN from injuries to the cutaneous branches of the nerve, particularly to the SRN (Figure 67-18).

Diagnosis and Level of Lesion

In high lesions, it is important to examine muscles innervated by branches from the posterior cord, which is easy enough for the teres major (lower subscapular nerve) and latissimus dorsi (thoracodorsal nerve). Early diagnosis of rupture of the circumflex nerve remains one of the most difficult conundrums in the

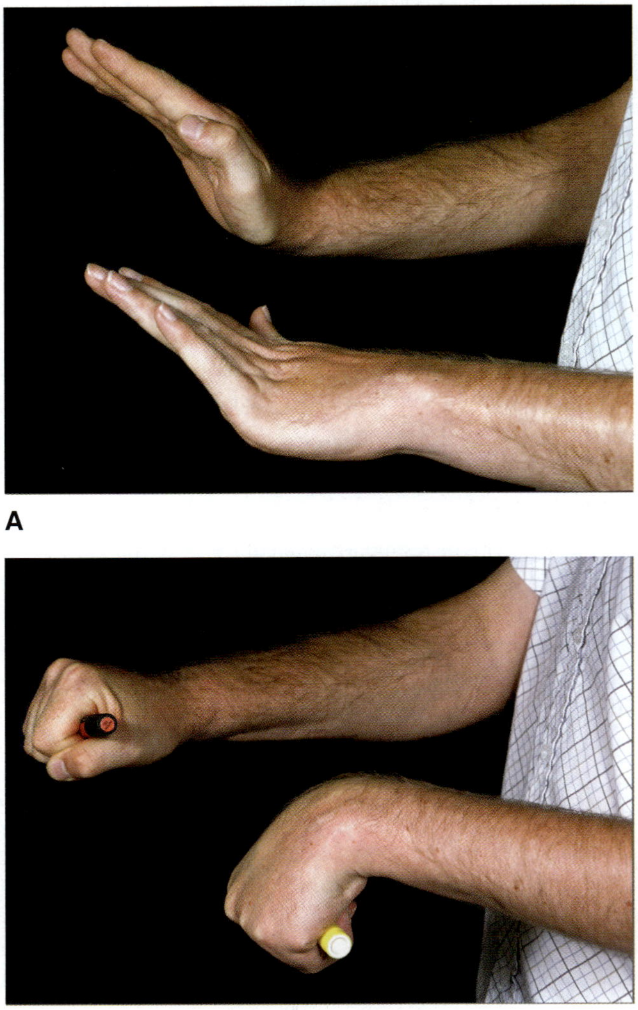

A

B

FIGURE 67-16 The importance of wrist extension. (A) and (B) This 31-year-old graphic designer sustained bilateral lesions of the brachial plexus. Avulsion of C7 on the right was treated by flexor to extensor transfer, achieving a power grip at 50% of estimated normal. On the left, C6, C7, and C8 were avulsed, and only one flexor digitorum superficialis muscle was available for transfer to the extensor digitorum communis and extensor pollicis longus. Power grip was negligible. (© Copyright 2011 Rolfe Birch.)

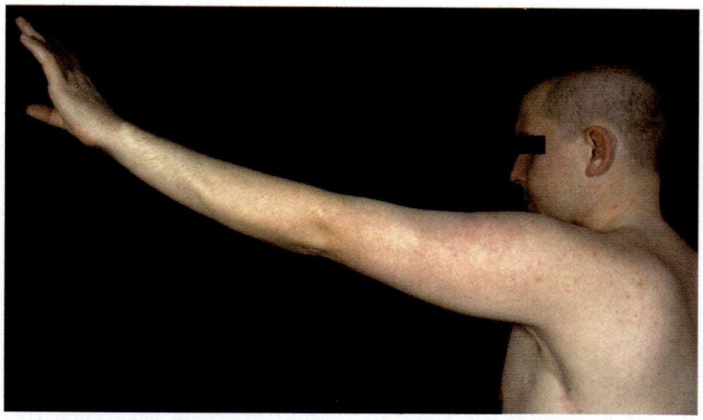

FIGURE 67-17 The outcome 2 years after repair, on the day of injury, of a stab wound of the circumflex, musculocutaneous, and radial nerves and of the axillary artery. Elbow and wrist extension recovered, but muscle transfer was needed for extension of the digits. (© Copyright 2011 Rolfe Birch.)

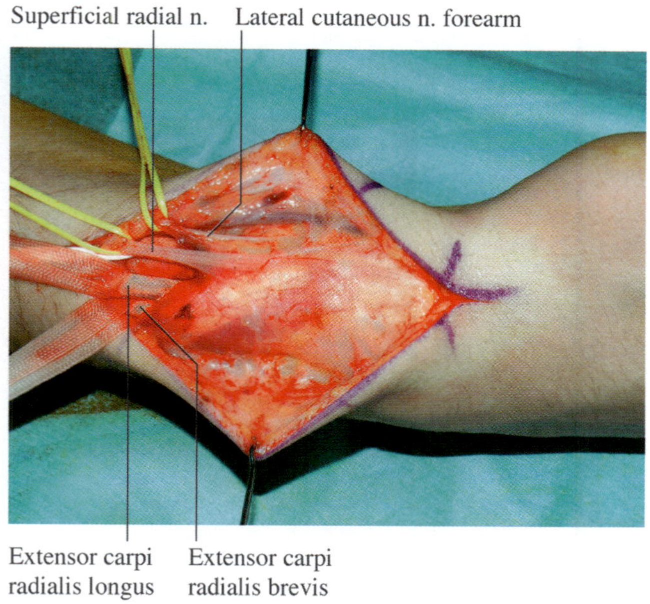

FIGURE 67-18 The terminal branches of the superficial radial and lateral cutaneous nerves of the forearm seen during operation at the right wrist. n, nerve. (© Copyright 2011 Rolfe Birch.)

examination of the peripheral nerves. The nerve is deeply seated and Tinel's sign is rarely detectable. The patient is in pain, and voluntary movement is affected by that pain as well as by the restraint of any sling. The extent of loss of cutaneous sensation is variable; there may not be complete anaesthesia. Patients with an intact suprascapular nerve and an intact rotator cuff are able to initiate abduction, and many can fully elevate the arm. One reliable test is to examine the posterior third of the deltoid with the fingers and ask the patient to thrust the arm back. It should be possible to detect activity in the muscle even when the arm is supported in a sling. The triceps is paralyzed in high axillary lesions. The lateral head of triceps is paralyzed when the nerve is damaged posterior to the humerus. If the lateral head of triceps is active but the BR and ECRL are paralyzed, then the lesion lies between the lateral intermuscular septum and about 5 cm above the lateral epicondyle. The sensory loss in high lesions extends to the lateral aspect of the elbow and proximal forearm (Figure 67-19).

Depth of Lesion

The preservation of some modalities of sensation is, of course, one of the important features of conduction block. Many patients volunteer that the skin within the distribution of the affected nerve is not numb; rather, it "feels different." It is possible to detect dryness of the skin by moving the fingertip from normal to affected skin, but vasomotor paralysis is much more difficult to detect.

Tinel's sign is particularly helpful in the analysis of closed lesions of the radial nerve. The examiner's finger percusses along the course of the nerve from *distal* to *proximal* starting well below the presumed level of the lesion. The patient is asked to say when the advancing finger elicits a wave or a surge of "pins and needles" or abnormal sensations, which may be painful, into the distribution of the nerve, which must be clearly indicated by the examiner. The sign can be regularly elicited on the day of injury in a conscious patient. The level of the sign should be measured from a fixed point such as the lateral epicondyle or styloid process of the radius and the distance entered into the records. A strongly positive Tinel's sign indicates that axons are ruptured at that level. Subsequent centrifugal progression indicates regeneration (52). The behavior of the Tinel's sign was studied in 134 cases from the 227 compound lesions seen between 2000 and 2007 (45). Some of these were closed

TABLE 67-8 Radial Nerve Injuries

Nerves (*n*)	Arterial Injury or Compartment Syndrome	Repairs	Neurolysis or Decompression	Good Spontaneous Recovery, Often After Decompression
1965 to 1998				
738	92 (12.5%)	330	N/A	301 (40.8%)
2000 to 2007				
227	30 (15.3%)	72 (31.7%)	53 (23.2%)	103 (45.4 %)

*Excluding nerves injured by shoulder dislocation.
†Excluding nerves injured by fracture dislocation at the elbow in children younger than 15 years of age.
‡The incidence of iatrogenic injury was about 5% in the early series but 23.8% in the later series.
N/A, not applicable.

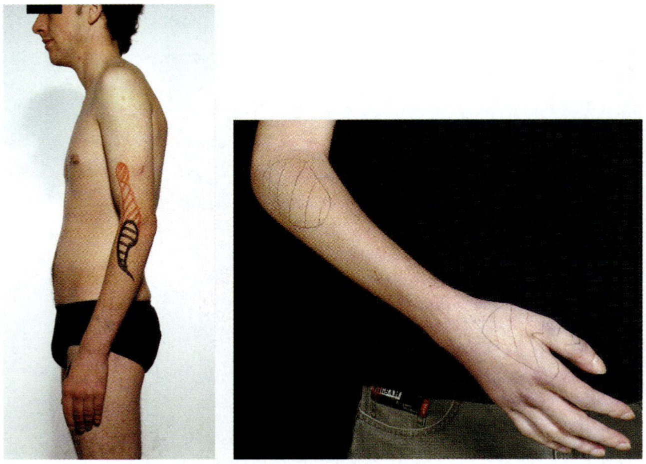

A B

FIGURE 67-19 (**A**) Sensory loss in high lesion of the radial nerve. (**B**) There is early recovery into the wrist extensors after repair. (© Copyright 2011 Rolfe Birch.)

lesions; in others, the initial wound had healed. A strong static Tinel's sign indicated rupture or entrapment in 72 nerves. In 41 of these, the static sign was converted into a progressing one after extricating the nerve from the fracture or other cause of distortion. The remaining 31 nerves were repaired. A strongly progressing Tinel's sign was followed by spontaneous recovery in 103 cases, including the 41 nerves that progressed after neurolysis. There were five misleading progressing Tinel's signs. In two of these, the nerve was explored because the anticipated recovery into the muscles had not occurred; part of the nerve was caught within the fracture. In the other three cases, the extensor muscles of the forearm were damaged by ischemia or by direct injury (Figure 67-20).

Confirmation that a closed lesion has a favorable prognosis is demonstrated by finding activity in the first relevant muscle by four weeks in about one third of cases and by eight weeks in more than 60% (12,53–56).

Radial Nerve Injury with Fractures of the Humerus

Ekholm et al. (57) analyzed 401 fractures (98% closed) from a population of 1.8 million treated over 2 years. The incidence of radial palsy was 8%, which is close to the figure supplied to Seddon (43) by Böhler. Ekholm et al. confirmed the important observation made by Holstein and Lewis (58): "For only a short distance near the lateral supracondylar ridge is the nerve in direct contact with the humerus, and it is in this area that the nerve pierces the lateral intermuscular septum before passing onto the surface of the brachialis muscle. From our anatomical dissections, the nerve has least mobility at this point, and, in our opinion, it is this lack of mobility that is a prime factor contributing to the nerve injury." The likelihood of spontaneous recovery for the radial palsy caused by a closed diaphyseal injury has been recorded as 80% or better (59–61). The vulnerability of the nerve in fractures of the distal third of the humerus is emphasized by, among others, Livani et al. (62), who described six cases of such fractures associated with radial nerve palsy in which the nerve was interposed or compressed or

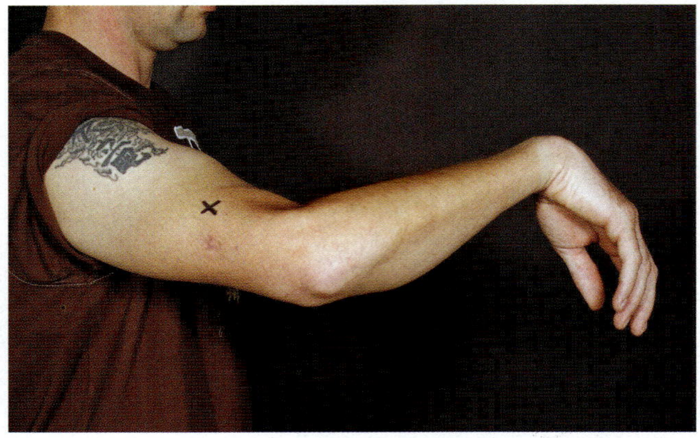

A

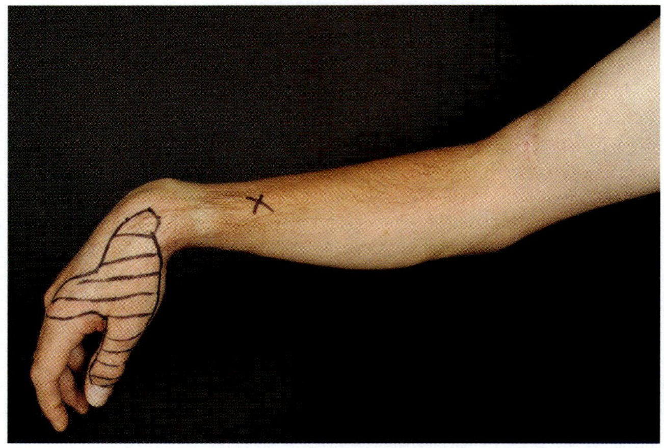

B

FIGURE 67-20 (**A**) Ten weeks after primary suture of the radial nerve, the strong Tinel's sign was static. A further repair by graft was performed, which was successful. (**B**) A progressing Tinel's sign proved misleading in this case of radial palsy. Three quarters of the nerve was trapped within the fracture site. (© Copyright 2011 Rolfe Birch.)

deviated to such an extent that spontaneous recovery was "impossible, improbable or unpredictable."

There is general agreement that open humeral shaft fractures with radial nerve palsy require exploration of the nerve at the same time as debridement of the wound (43,44,54,56,63–66).

Thirty percent of the cases sent to Seddon (43) did not recover; the lesions were unfavorable in about 50% of our own, but it is important to emphasize that most cases were referred by orthopaedic surgeons because they were unfavorable. These figures should not generally be applied.

Surgical Exposure of the Radial Nerve (38)

1. The forequarter of the limb should be prepared and toweled in such a way that the upper limb can be freely moved about and that it can be placed across the patient's chest or can be moved onto a side table. This facilitates combined anterior with posterior incisions.
2. Incisions must be adequate and extensile so that the lesion of the nerve can be exposed adequately and the arteries safely controlled.
3. Difficulties of dissection in a scarred field may be improved by identifying structures in healthy tissue proximal and distal to the level of injury.

The Infraclavicular Lesion

The Exposure of Fiolle and Delmas (67) This affords full display of the supra-, retro-, and infraclavicular plexus; of the second part of the subclavian to the terminal axillary artery; and of the subclavian and axillary veins deep to the clavicle. It is the exposure of choice in the closed infraclavicular rupture of vessels and nerves. The incision is T-shaped, the vertical limb running in the deltopectoral groove, retracting the cephalic vein medially, and then curving into the apex of the axilla underneath the fold of pectoralis major (Figure 67-21). In urgent cases, a Gigli saw is used to divide the clavicle at the lateral edge of the sternocleidomastoid muscle; otherwise, a hole is drilled and prepared for a compression screw, inclined at 45 degrees to the long axis of the clavicle. Subsequent fixation is made easier by contouring a plate to the bone and drilling and preparing one hole in the lateral fragment. The clavicle is cut at 90 degrees to the axis of the hole for the compression screw. It is possible, in some cases, to avoid cutting the clavicle. The bone can be drawn upward or downward by a nylon tape.

The fascia at the root of the axilla is divided, and the finger develops a plane between the pectoralis major and minor in front and the axillary bundle behind. The pectoralis major is detached from the humerus. The pectoralis minor is reflected with care taken to protect the musculocutaneous nerve. The limb is rolled into lateral rotation so that the trunks, divisions, and cords of the brachial plexus are displayed with their accompanying vessels.

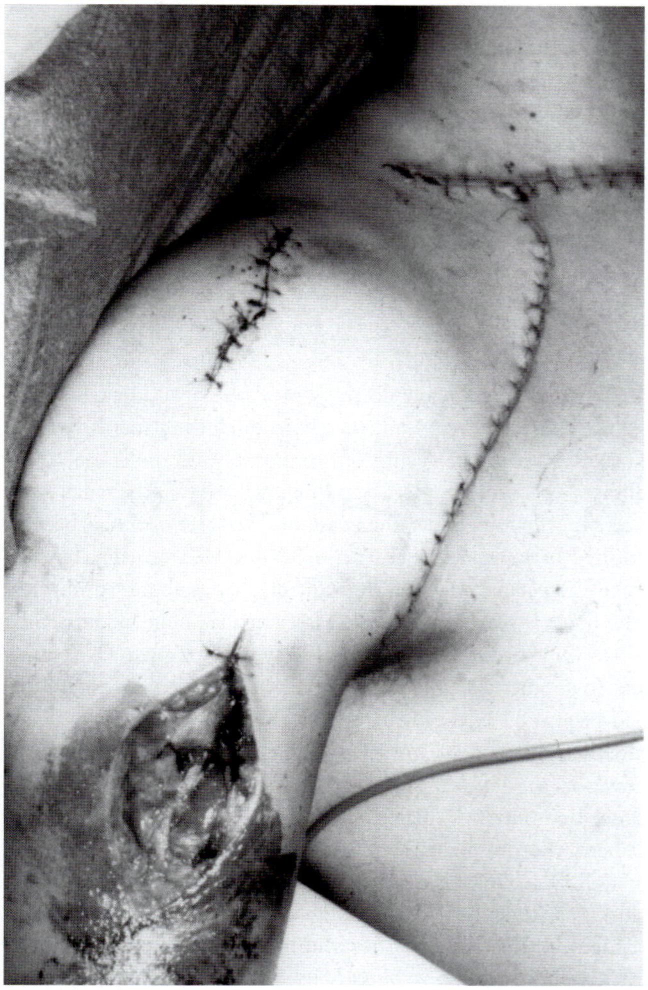

FIGURE 67-21 The Fiolle and Delmas exposure. The incision at the shoulder was made for the purpose of inserting an intramedullary nail. The wound, caused by the fracture, has been left open. (© Copyright 2011 Rolfe Birch.)

The High Lesion The proximal part of the nerve is fairly easily displayed in the upper part of an axillobrachial incision, but I do not hesitate to reflect part or whole of the pectoralis major and minor from their insertions in difficult situations in which bleeding may prove difficult to control.

The Arm Finding the middle part of the radial nerve, the part most likely to be in trouble, is rather more difficult. It is identified through a posterior incision and by separation of the superficial part of the triceps (the long and lateral heads) from its deep head (the medial head). The V-shaped interval between the upper parts of the long and lateral heads, the "seam of the half-sleeve" (68), is defined and opened from above down toward the olecranon (Figure 67-22).

Further exposure of the radial nerve is anterior to the lateral head of the triceps muscle by entering the interval between the biceps and brachialis anteriorly and BR and ECRL posteriorly. The incision continues across the anterolateral aspect of the elbow into the forearm, where the nerve and its branches are found in the valley between the brachialis and BR. There are important branches from this segment of the nerve. The nerve to brachialis, passing anteromedially, is often seen about 5 finger breadths above the lateral epicondyle. The nerve to BR passes posterolaterally about 2 cm more distal, and more distally still is the branch to ECRL. After that, usually two branches to ECRB, the origin of the SRN, and the first part of the PIN before it dives down behind the supinator, can be seen (Figure 67-23).

This display is not easy in a scarred field bleeding from branches of the profunda brachii artery is a nuisance. Following the anteromedial side of the nerve protects the nerves to the BR and ECRL, but it is important to be on the lookout for the nerve to brachialis and for cutaneous nerves passing to the arm and forearm. Although it is often possible to palpate the nerve with the tip of the finger, I do not hesitate to extend the incision distally to assist in finding the nerve where the valley opens out.

The Posterior Interosseous Nerve In the Henry (68) approach, the incision is made on the posterolateral aspect of the upper forearm between the mobile mass of BR, ECRL and ECRB, and EDC. The interval between the ECRB and the EDC is then opened and the supinator muscle exposed. The PIN passes between the superficial and deep parts of this muscle to emerge at the lower margin of the superficial part and to run for about 4 to 5 cm before breaking up into its terminal (motor) branches. The point of emergence can quite easily be found and the nerve then followed proximally by division of the superficial part of the muscle along its line (Figure 67-24).

Iatrogenic Injuries of the Radial Nerve

The continuing increase in the number of these injuries to the radial nerve is deeply disturbing (69). Even worse is the apparent trend toward doing nothing after the event is recognized, sitting tight "waiting and seeing" rather than intervening.

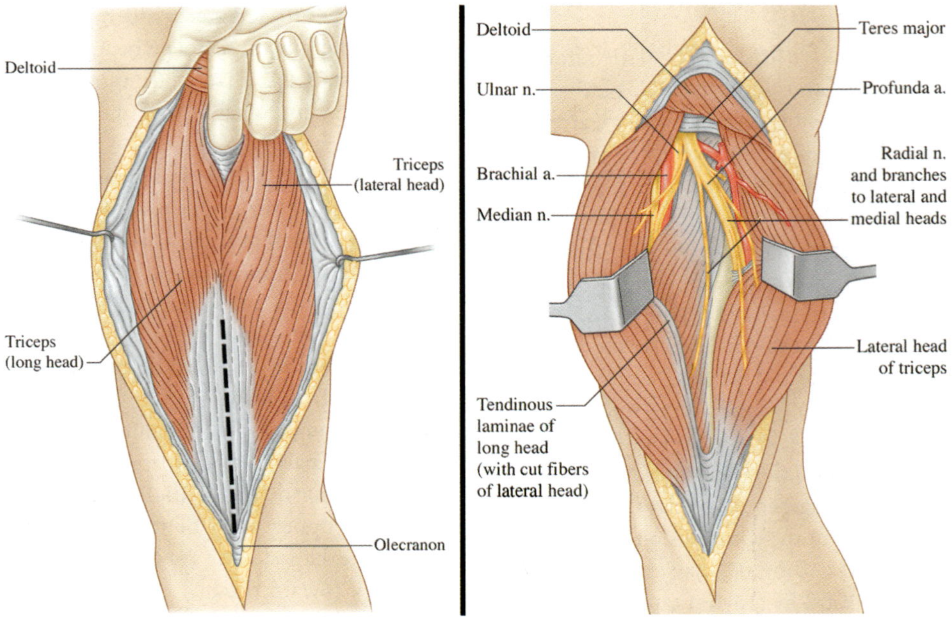

FIGURE 67-22 Exposure of the radial nerve in the arm. The "seam of triceps" (68). The finger is introduced between the long and lateral heads and separated. The opening of the "seam" reveals the radial nerve from the start of its course on the back of the humerus to the piercing of the lateral intermuscular septum. a, artery; n, nerve. (© Copyright 2011 Rolfe Birch.)

1. It must be reemphasized that the surgeon who deems it necessary to perform internal or external fixation in the presence of a radial nerve palsy should always explore that nerve. A surgeon who does not do this is asking for trouble.
2. In the unfortunate event that a radial nerve palsy is detected after closed manipulation and reduction, then the possibility that the nerve has become trapped in the fracture will be revealed by inspection of a radiograph. If the fragments are gapped apart, then it is likely that the nerve and adjacent soft tissues are preventing reduction.

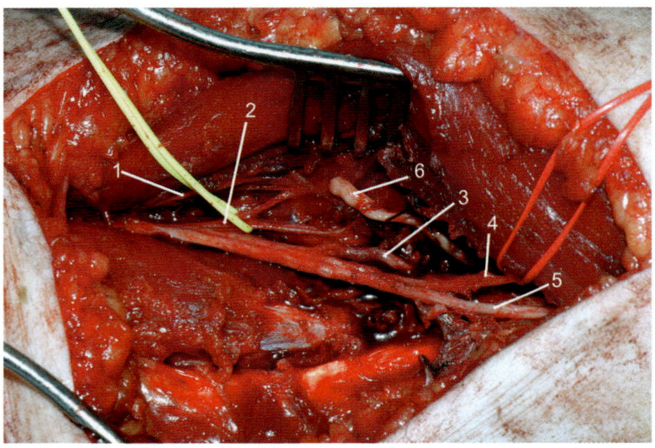

FIGURE 67-23 The radial nerve at the elbow exposed during repair of the posterior interosseous nerve cut during operation for a fracture of the radial head. The nerve is seen in the valley between brachioradialis and biceps lying on fibers of brachialis. The nerves to the brachioradialis (1), to the extensor carpi radialis longus and brevis (2), the proximal part of the posterior interosseous nerve, (3) a further branch to the extensor carpi radialis brevis (4), and the superficial radial nerve (5) are shown. A segment of the lateral cutaneous nerve of the forearm (6) has been prepared as a graft. (© Copyright 2011 Rolfe Birch.)

3. For a radial nerve palsy occurring after an operation, it is reasonable to await recovery *if and only if* the surgeon noted that the nerve was intact and had not become displaced into the fracture or damaged by an implant at the time of wound closure.
4. The most common level of injury was the junction of the upper two thirds and lower third of the arm. "Blind" drilling is especially dangerous; in three cases, more than 10 cm of nerve was avulsed.

We have seen a number of cases in which the operating surgeon acted with commendable alacrity. Three cases of accidental transection of the nerve were immediately sutured; the patients went on to excellent recovery. A surgeon, coming toward the end of a very difficult operation of internal fixation, realized that the radial nerve had slipped from under the assistant's retractor and had become crushed between the plate and the bone. He immediately extricated the nerve; the duration of the crush was about 10 minutes. The nerve was explored 6 weeks later, at that surgeon's insistence; it had fully reconstituted, and recovery was complete (axonotmesis). In another case, the radial nerve was damaged by cement that had been used in the treatment of a pathological fracture in the proximal third of the humerus. The first surgeon reexplored the nerve on the following day and found that the nerve was lying close, but not immediately adjacent, to extruded cement. The cement was trimmed away. The nerve recovered. In a case of intramedullary nailing of a humeral shaft fracture, a complete radial palsy was noted on the evening of operation. The nerve was exposed, it was found crushed within the fracture site, and it was extricated. The duration of compression was about 12 hours, and recovery was complete (axonotmesis). Operating on a closed fracture converts it into an open fracture no matter how small the incision used. Operating through small incisions or by means of the arthroscope compels the surgeon to work blind in cases in

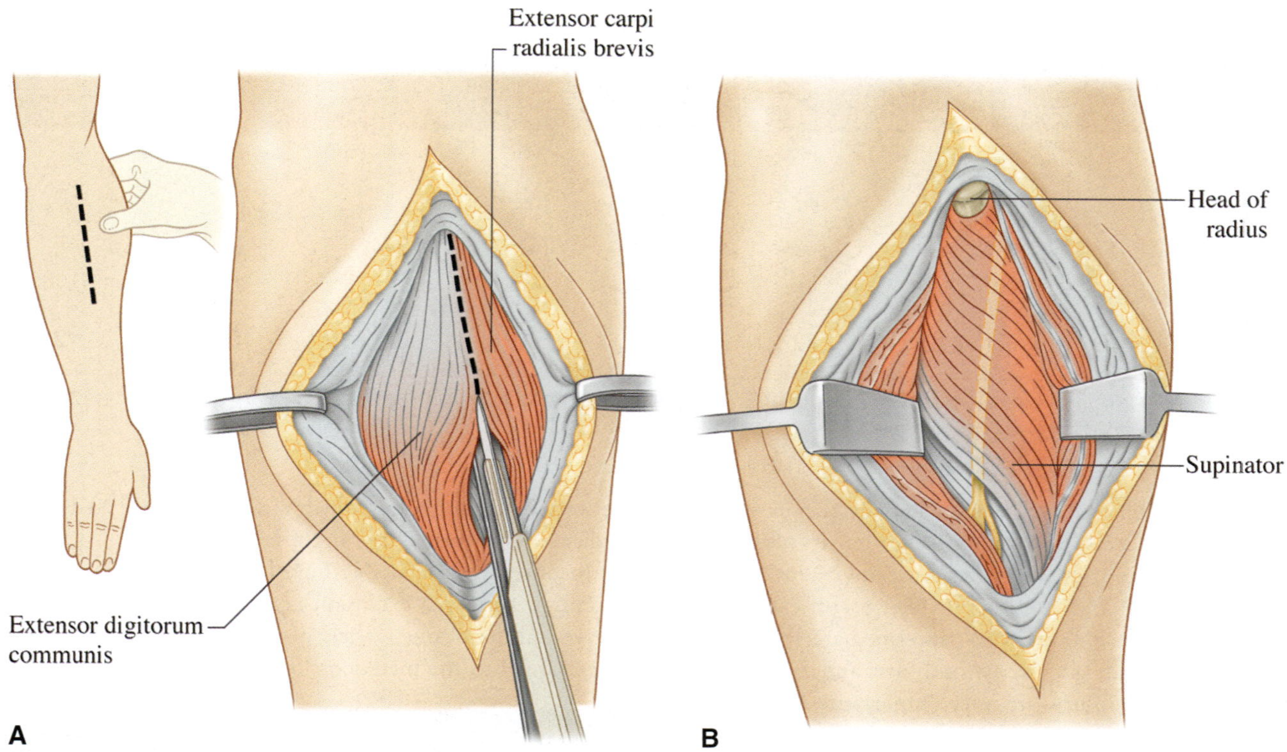

FIGURE 67-24 Exposure of the posterior interosseous nerve (after Henry [68]). (**A**) The incision and the separation of the extensor carpi radialis brevis from the extensor communis. (**B**). The posterior interosseous nerve and supinator exposed. (© Copyright 2011 Rolfe Birch.)

which normal topographic anatomy has been distorted by the injury (Figures 67-25 and 67-26).

Results of Repair of the Radial Nerve

Zachary (70) found that 90% of the 114 radial nerve repairs, treated at one of the five special hospitals in World War 2, and followed for a minimum of five years regained extension of the wrist and 61% regained some extension of the digits. Independent extension of the thumb and the index finger was restored in 36%. These are remarkably good results considering that these were war injuries and that some loss of the nerve trunk was inevitable. Shergill et al. (71) reported 260 radial nerve repairs. Sixteen of 18 PIN repairs were successful. The 242 main radial nerve repairs were classed into four groups:

1. Open tidy wounds from glass, a knife, or scissors
2. Open untidy wounds from penetrating missile injury, open fracture, or contaminated wounds (52)
3. Closed traction injuries, usually associated with fractures of the humerus (62)
4. Associated rupture of the axillary or brachial artery (55)

The results were graded by the extent of recovery of proximal and distal muscles. A "good" result for a high lesion

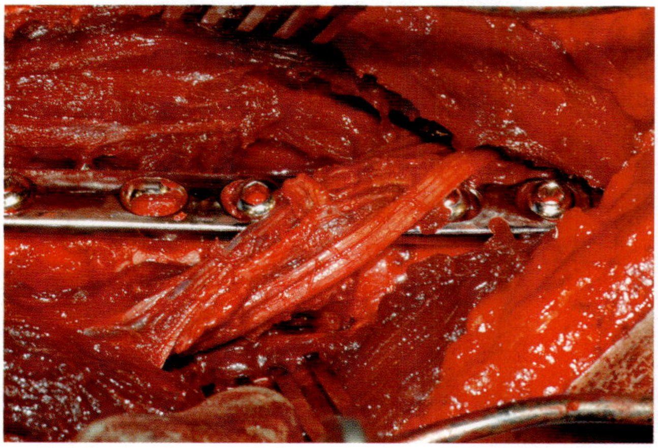

FIGURE 67-25 The appearance of a radial nerve after extrication from beneath a compression plate 48 hours after the first operation. Pain was relieved, but there was only incomplete recovery, so later flexor to extensor transfer was necessary. (© Copyright 2011 Rolfe Birch.)

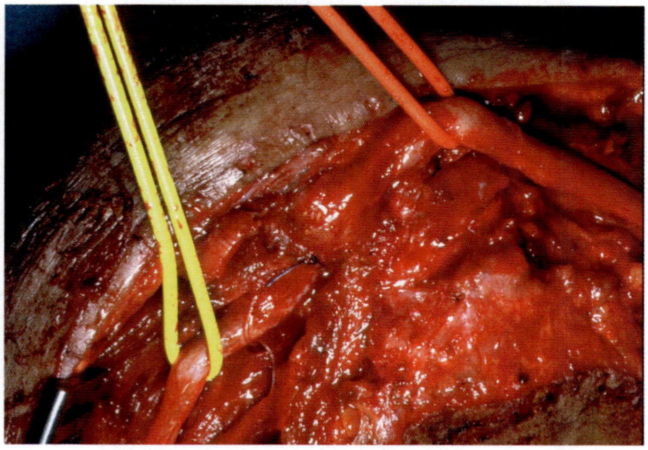

FIGURE 67-26 Rupture of the radial nerve in a closed fracture of the humerus. The stumps are embedded within the fracture, which had been nailed. (© Copyright 2011 Rolfe Birch.)

TABLE 67-9 Results of 242 Radial Nerves Repairs

		Good		Fair		Poor	
Wound	**Nerves (*n*)**	*n*	%	*n*	%	*n*	%
Open "tidy"	73	28	38	30	41	15	21
Open untidy	52	13	25	13	25	26	50
Closed traction	62	19	31	17	27	26	42
Associated arterial injury	55	12	22	8	14	35	64
Total	**242**	**72**	**30**	**68**	**28**	**102**	**42**

Adapted from Shergill G, Birch R, Bonney G, Munshi P. The radial and posterior interosseous nerves: results of 260 repairs. *J Bone Joint Surg* 2001;83B:646–649.

required powerful elbow extension and extension of wrist against gravity, whereas a "good" result for repairs of the nerve below the nerves to triceps requires powerful extension of the wrist and digits. A "fair" result provided useful extension at the elbow (high lesion) or wrist (intermediate lesion). The nature of the wound; the severity of injury; and, in particular, associated arterial injury are very important. Results were poor in 15 (21%) of the open tidy group but in 35 (64%) of the arterial injury group (55). There was some degree of ischemic damage to the muscles of the forearm in all cases in which there was a delay of more than 8 hours before restoration of arterial flow (Table 67-9). Of the 77 nerves repaired within 14 days of injury, 49% achieved a good result. Only 28% of the 169 late repairs achieved this grade; the mean delay was 27 weeks. There were no good results from repairs when the interval exceeded 12 months. A later study of 227 radial nerve lesions excluded the "tidy" wounds, so this study group is similar to Shergill's groups 2, 3, and 4 (Table 67-10).

Thirty-six of the 72 repairs (50%) were graded good, an improvement over 30% good results in the earlier series, The method of repair has not changed, and it would seem that the two groups are broadly comparable. The one difference is the interval between injury and repair, which was, on average, 190 days in the earlier series; it was 58 days in the later series.

In otherwise irreparable high lesions, restoration of elbow extension and wrist extension is a great boon for the patient. Nerve transfer of one fascicle of the ulnar nerve in the arm to the nerve(s) to the medial or long head of triceps and of one

TABLE 67-10 227 compound lesions of the radial nerve, 2000 to 2007

Level of Lesion		**Depth of Lesion**	
High (above lateral head of triceps)	64	Conduction block	27
Intermediate	129	Axonotmesis	97
Low	34	Neurotmesis	103

*Excluding nerves injured by shoulder dislocation.
†Excluding nerves injured by fracture dislocation at the elbow in children younger than 15 years of age.
‡The *total* number of iatrogenic injuries was 54 (23.8%).
§The total number of nerves repaired was 72 (31.7%).
||The total number of nerves extricated or decompressed ("neurolysis") was 53 (23.2%).

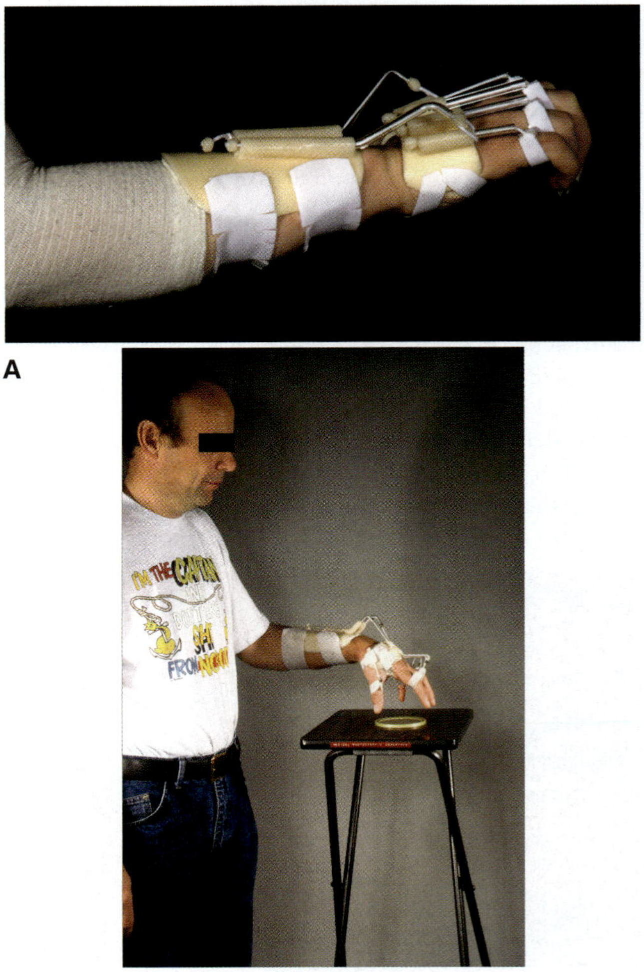

A

B

FIGURE 67-27 (A) A very elaborate splint for radial nerve palsy. (B) Active extension for the wrist, fingers, and thumb is provided. The appearance of impracticability is belied by the fact that the patient found this splint extremely useful, so useful that he declined operation. (© Copyright 2011 Rolfe Birch.)

fascicle from the median nerve at the elbow (usually a fascicle passing to the superficial flexor origin) to the nerve to ECRB has been reliably effective.

Rehabilitation after Radial Nerve Injury

Radial nerve palsy is, for many patients, far worse than median or ulnar nerve lesions. These patients require close and careful supervision by the surgeon to mitigate that disability and to prevent progression to a fixed deformity. The surgeon should not pass the responsibility to therapists or "rehabilitation services." Well-made dynamic splints are valuable. In some patients, they make the difference between holding on to their job or losing it or maintaining their independence or losing it (Figure 67-27).

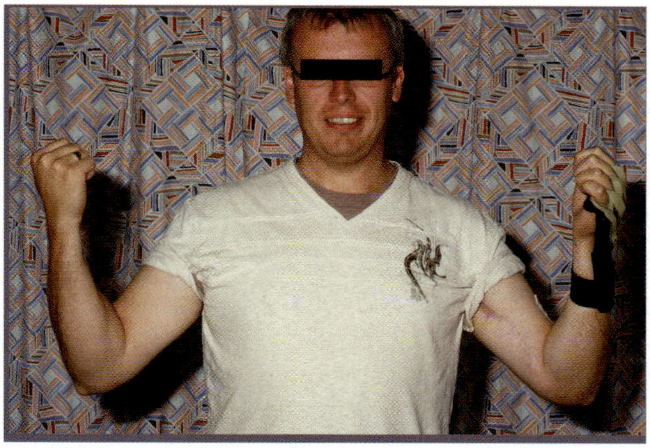

A

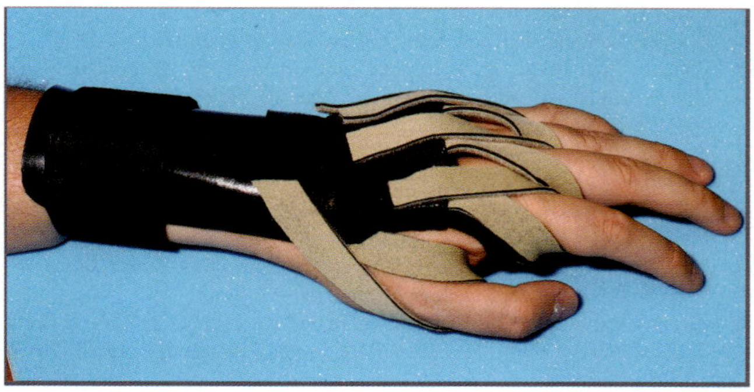

B

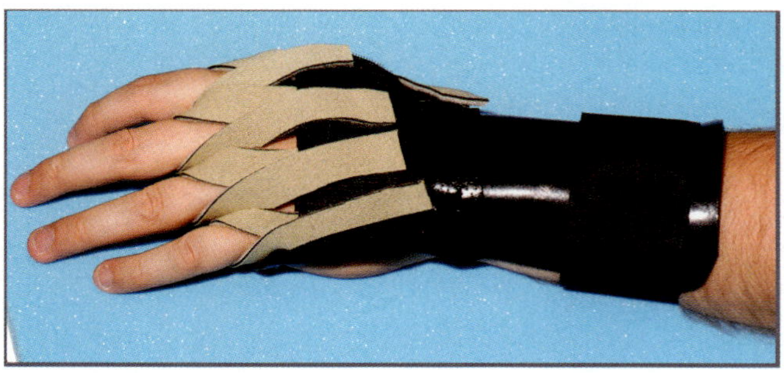

C

FIGURE 67-28 (A) Emergency repair of the brachial artery and musculocutaneous nerve was successful in this 34-year-old man. The graft for the radial nerve restored extension of the elbow. (B) and (C) A low-profile splint has been fitted as a prelude to flexor to extensor tendon transfers. (© Copyright 2011 Rolfe Birch.)

Flexor–to–extensor tendon transfers are an integral part of the process of rehabilitation and should be undertaken when it is clear that the nerve is not recovering and the condition of the limb and the patient permits. I do not favor combining radial nerve repair with a tendon transfer for wrist extension at the same time because it is always important to ensure that the skeleton is stable, the wounds have healed, the joints are mobile, and the proposed motors are of adequate power (Figure 67-28).

ACKNOWLEDGMENTS

The figures are reproduced with permission from Birch R. *Surgical Disorders of the Peripheral Nerves*, 2nd ed. UK: Springer, 2011.

REFERENCES

1. Birch R. Reactions to injury. In *Surgical Disorders of the Peripheral Nerves*, 2nd ed. UK: Springer, 2011, pp. 77–114.
2. Bland-Sutton J. Injuries of the peripheral nerves. In *The Story of a Surgeon*. Methuen, 1930, pp. 34–37.
3. Horsley V. On injuries to peripheral nerves. In *The Practitioner*, vol. 10. 1899, pp. 131–144.
4. Sherren J. *Injuries of Nerves and their Treatment*. London: James Nisbet and Co., 1908.
5. Tinel J. *Nerve Wounds*. Revised and edited by Joll CA. London: Ballière Tindall and Cox, 1917.
6. Jones R. *Orthopaedic Surgery of Injuries*. London: Oxford University Press, 1921.
7. Seddon HJ (ed). *Peripheral Nerve Injuries*, Medical Research Council Special Report Series No. 282. HMSO, 1954.
8. Young JZ. First evidence of axonal transport. In Dyck PJ, Thomas PK, Griffin JW, et al. (eds). *Peripheral Neuropathy*, 3rd ed.
9. Woodhall B, Beebe GW (eds). *Peripheral Nerve Regeneration*. VA Medical Monograph. Washington, DC: US Government Printing Office, 1956.
10. Omer GE, Eversmann WW. Peripheral nerve problems. In Burkhalter WE. (ed). *Orthopaedic Surgery in Vietnam*. Washington, DC: Office of the US Army Surgeon General and Center of Military History, 1994.
11. Omer GE. Peripheral nerve injuries and gunshot wounds. In Omer GE, Spinner M, Van Beek AL (eds). *Peripheral Nerve Problems*, 2nd ed. Philadelphia: WB Saunders, 1998, pp. 398–405.
12. Birch R. Compound nerve injuries. In *Surgical Disorders of the Peripheral Nerves*, 2nd ed. UK: Springer, 2011, pp. 303–374.
13. Lanz U. The carpal tunnel syndrome. In Tubiana R (ed). *The Hand Volume IV*. St. Louis: WB Saunders, 1993, pp 463–486.
14. Schroeder HP, Scheker LR. Redefining the "arcade of Struthers." *J Hand Surg* 2003;28A:1018–1021.
15. Wilbourn AJ. Brachial plexus injuries. In Dyck PJ, Thomas PK (eds). *Peripheral Neuropathy*, 4th ed. Philadelphia: Elsevier Saunders, 2005, pp. 1339–1373.
16. Stenning M, Drew S, Birch R. Low energy arterial injury at the shoulder with progressive or delayed nerve palsy. *J Bone Joint Surg* 2005;87B: 1102–1106.
17. Wajcberg E, Thoppil N, Patel S, et al. Comprehensive assessment of post ischaemic vascular reactivity in Hispanic children and adults with and without diabetes mellitus. *Paediatr Diabetes* 2006;7:329–335.
18. Fowler TJ, Danta G, Gilliatt RW. Recovery of nerve conduction after a pneumatic tourniquet: observations in the hind limb of a baboon. *J Neurol Neurosurg Psychiatry* 1972;35:638–647.
19. Seddon HJ. Three types of nerve injury. *Brain* 1943;66:237–288.
20. Mackinnon SE, Dellon AL. Ischaemia of nerve: loss of vibration sensibility. In *Surgery of the Peripheral Nerve*. New York: Thieme, 1988, p. 57.
21. Gutmann E, Sanders FK. Recovery of fiber numbers and diameters in the regeneration of peripheral nerves. *J Physiol* 1943;101:489–518.
22. Birch R, Bonney G, Wynn Parry CB. Reactions to injury. In *Surgical Disorders of the Peripheral Nerves*, 1st ed. London: Churchill Livingstone, 1998, p. 37–56.
23. O'Brian M (ed). *Aids to the Examination of the Peripheral Nervous System*, 4th ed. London: Elsevier, 2000.

24. Cokluk C, Aydin K. Ultrasound examination in the surgical treatment for upper extremity peripheral nerve injuries: part I. *Turk Neurosurg* 2007;17(4):277–282.
25. Kato H, Minami A, Kobayashi M, et al. Functional results of low median and ulnar nerve repair with intraneural fascicular dissection and electrical fascicular orientation. *J Hand Surg* 1998 23A:471–482.
26. Brushart TM. Nerve repair and grafting: histochemical identification. In Green EP (ed). *Operative Hand Surgery*, 4th ed. New York: Churchill Livingstone, 1999, pp. 1388–1389.
27. Orgell MG. Epineurial versus perineurial repair of peripheral nerves. In Tertzis JK (ed). *Microreconstruction of Nerve Injuries*. London: WB Saunders, 1987, pp. 97–100.
28. Spinner RJ. Operative care and technique. In Kim DH, Midha R, Murovic JA, Spinner RJ. (eds). *Kline and Hudson's Nerve Injuries*, 2nd ed. Philadelphia: Saunders Elsevier, 2008, pp. 87–106.
29. Birch R, Raji ARM. Repair of median and ulnar nerves. *J Bone Joint Surg* 1991;73B:154–157.
30. Trumble TE. Overcoming defects in peripheral nerves. In Gelberman RH (ed). *Operative Nerve Repair and Reconstruction*. Philadelphia: JB Lippincott, 1991, pp. 507–524.
31. Seddon HJ. The use of autogenous grafts for the repair of large gaps in peripheral nerves. *Br J Surg* 1947;35:151–167.
32. Lundborg G, Dahlin L, Dohi D, et al. A new type of "bioartificial" nerve graft for bridging extended defects in nerves. *J Hand Surg* 1997;22B:299–203.
33. Anand P, Birch R. Restoration of sensory function and lack of long-term chronic pain syndromes after brachial plexus injury in human neonates. *Brain* 2002;125:113–122.
34. Őzkan T, Őzer K, GülgŐnen A. Restoration of sensibility in irreparable ulnar and median nerve lesions with use of sensory nerve transfer: long-term follow up of 20 cases. *J Hand Surg* 2001;26A:44–51.
35. Battiston B, Blanzetta M. Repair of proximal ulnar by distal transfer-reconstruction of high nerve lesions by distal double median to ulnar nerve transfer. *J Hand Surg* 1999;24(A):1185–1191.
36. Birch R. Regeneration and recovery. In *Surgical Disorders of the Peripheral Nerves*, 2nd ed. UK: Springer, 2011, pp. 115–144.
37. Birch R. Pain. In *Surgical Disorders of the Peripheral Nerves*, 2nd ed. UK: Springer, 2011, pp. 527–562.
38. Birch R. Operating on nerves. In *Surgical Disorders of the Peripheral Nerves*, 2nd ed. UK: Springer, 2011, pp. 231–302.
39. Willner C, Low PA. Pharmacologic approaches to neuropathic pain. In Dyck PJ, Thomas PK, Griffin JW, et al (eds). 1993.
40. Birch R, Bonney G, Wynn Parry CB. Pain. In *Surgical Disorders of the Peripheral Nerves*, 1st ed. London: Churchill Livingstone, 1998, pp. 373–404.
41. Jebara VA, Bechir S. Causalgia: a war time experience—report of 20 treated cases. *J Trauma* 1987;27:519–523.
42. Kline DG, Hudson AR. *Nerve Injuries*. Philadelphia: WB Saunders, 1995.
43. Seddon HJ. Common causes of nerve injury In *Surgical Disorders of Peripheral Nerves*, 2nd ed. New York: Churchill Livingstone, 1975, pp. 67–88.
44. Siegel DB, Gelberman RG. Peripheral nerve injuries associated with fractures and dislocations. In Gelberman RH (ed). *Operative Nerve Repair and Reconstruction*. Philadelphia: JB Lippincott, 1991, pp. 619–633.
45. Birch R. Clinical aspects of nerve injury. In *Surgical Disorders of the Peripheral Nerves*, 2nd ed. UK: Springer, 2011, pp. 145–190.
46. Blakey CM, Biant LC, Birch R. Ischaemia and the pink, pulseless hand complicating supracondylar fractures of the humerus in children. *J Bone Joint Surg* 2009;91B:1487–1498.
47. Gousheh J. The treatment of war injuries in the brachial plexus. *J Hand Surg* 1995;20A:S68–S76.
48. Roganovic Z. Missile caused complete lesions of the peroneal nerve and peroneal division of the sciatic nerve: results of 157 repairs. *Neurosurgery* 2005;57:1201–1212.
49. Roganovic Z, Mesovic S, Kronja G, Savic M. Peripheral nerve lesions associated with missile induced pseudo aneurysms. *J Neurosurg* 2007;107:765–775.
50. Goldie BS, Coates CJ, Birch R. The long term results of digital nerve repair in no man's land. *J Hand Surg* 1992b;12B:75–77.
51. Denmark A. An example of symptoms resembling tic douloureux produced by a wound in the radial nerve. *Med Chir Trans* 1813;4:48.
52. Kato N, Birch R. Peripheral nerve palsies associated with closed fractures and dislocations. *Injury* 2006;37:507–512.
53. Bowden REM, Scholl DH. Recovery of nerves. In Seddon HJ (ed). *Peripheral Nerve Injuries*, Special report series, No. 282. Medical Research Council, 1954, pp. 16–24.
54. Shah JJ, Bhatti NA. Radial nerve paralysis associated with fractures of the humerus. *Clin Orthop Rel Res* 1983;172:171–176.
55. Shaw JL. Sakellarides H. Radial nerve paralysis. *J Bone Joint Surg* 1967;49A:899–902.
56. Ring D, Chin K, Jupiter JB, Boston MA. Radial nerve palsy associated with high-energy humeral shaft fractures. *J Hand Surg* 2004;29A:144–147.
57. Ekholm R, Adami J, Tidermark J, et al. Fractures of the shaft of the humerus. *J Bone Joint Surg* 2006;88B:1469–1473.
58. Holstein A, Lewis GR. Fractures of the humerus with radial nerve paralysis. *J Bone Joint Surg* 1963;45A:1382–1388.
59. Sonneveld GJ, Patka P, van Mourik JC, Broere G. Treatment of fractures of the shaft of the humerus accompanied by paralysis of the radial nerve. *Injury* 1987;18:404–406.
60. Pollock FH, Drake D, Bovill EG, et al. Treatment of radial neuropathy associated with fractures of the humerus. *J Bone Joint Surg* 1981;63A: 239–243.
61. Larsen LB, Barfred T. Radial nerve palsy after simple fracture of the humerus. *Scand J Plast Reconstr Surg Hand Surg* 2000;34:363–366.
62. Livani B, Belangero WD, Castro de Medeiros R. Fractures of the distal third of humerus with palsy of the radial nerve. *J Bone Joint Surg* 2006;88B:1625–1628.
63. Venouziou A, Gougoulias N, Dailiana Z, et al. Surgical treatment of radial nerve lesions associated with fractures of the humeral shaft. *J Hand Surg* 2007;32E:43–44.
64. Vichard P, Tropet Y, Landecy G, Briot JF. Parlaysies radiales contemporaines des fractures de la diaphyse humérale. *Chirurgie* 1982;108:791–795.
65. Foster RJ, Swiontkowski MF, Bach AW, Sack JT. Radial nerve palsy caused by open humeral shaft fractures. *J Hand Surg* 1993;18A:220–222.
66. Pollock RC, Birch R. Complete transposition of the radial nerve complicating an open fracture of the shaft of humerus. *Injury* 1999;30:623–625.
67. Fiolle J, Delmas J. In Cumston CG. (trans ed). *The Surgical Exposure of the Deep Seated Blood Vessels*. London: Heinemann, 1921, pp. 61–67.
68. Henry AK. Extensile exposure. *Upper Limb*, 4th ed. Edinburgh: Churchill Livingstone, 1975.
69. Birch R. Iatrogenous injuries. In *Surgical Disorders of the Peripheral Nerves*, 2nd ed. UK: Springer, 2011, pp. 483–526.
70. Zachary RB. Results of nerve sutures. In Seddon HJ (ed). *Peripheral Nerve Injuries*. Special report series No. 282. Medical Research Council, 1954, pp. 354–387.
71. Shergill G, Birch R, Bonney G, Munshi P. The radial and posterior interosseous nerves: results of 260 repairs *J Bone Joint Surg* 2001;83B: 646–649.

CHAPTER 68

Nerve Repair and Nerve Grafting in the Upper Extremity

Minoru Shibata

HISTORY OF NERVE REPAIR

The greatest contribution to understanding peripheral nerve injury was made by Augustus Waller during the 19th century (1). His detailed description of the histologic changes that occur in the distal axon after disconnection from the nerve body has subsequently been referred to as Wallerian degeneration. There were an enormous number of peripheral nerve injuries in World War I, and analysis of the results of treatment among the registered casualties provided an opportunity to compare several different methods of nerve repair. Elsberg recognized the detrimental effect of traction on nerve regeneration and recommended perineurial and epineurial apposition of the nerve ends with matching of the fasciculi (2). He also recognized the importance of the coaptation of the nerve ends without tension. The first description of nerve grafting was reported by Philipeaux and Vulpian in 1870, but there was no real scientific interest before World War I (2). Huber evaluated nerve autografts, allografts, and xenografts in experimental models and achieved the most favorable results from nerve autografts. Nerve grafting including allografting was performed on many war casualties, but the results of nerve grafting were mostly unsatisfactory. Nerve grafting was only performed occasionally after World War I.

Remarkable work with regards to the natural history of nerve injury and nerve repair was reported in 1918 by Tinel (3), who demonstrated that regenerating axons are very reactive to stimulation, and the advancing regenerating axons can be followed by tapping over the nerve. This observation is now well known as Tinel's sign.

By the start of World War II, the techniques of direct nerve repair had not changed significantly. Highet and Holms demonstrated histologically massive fibrosis of failed nerve repairs associated with postoperative stretching after direct nerve repair (4). They confirmed this clinical observation with a well-designed canine experiment to investigate the effect of stretching after nerve repair. Because of the unfavorable results of stretching, nerve grafting was reevaluated to reconstruct significant nerve gaps. In the early years of World War II, the convincing efficacy of nerve grafting was confirmed experimentally, but the clinical results of nerve grafting remained poor except for Bunnell's successful results with digital nerves.

Sir Herbert Seddon reintroduced autogenous nerve grafting in 1947 as an effective reconstructive procedure for nerve injuries with a segmental defect and achieved 51.9% partial to good recovery (5). He recommended using a graft about 15% longer than the defect and developed a classification of nerve injuries with three categories, neurapraxia, axonotmesis, and neurotmesis, based on his experience with a considerable number of peripheral nerve injuries. Sunderland subsequently devised a more detailed classification with five categories (6).

After World War II, the first major development was the introduction of microsurgical nerve repair by Smith in 1964 (7). This advance was followed by the reintroduction of nerve grafting and intraoperative nerve monitoring. Millesi demonstrated the superiority of nerve grafting compared with end-to-end nerve repair under excessive tension and changed the practice of clinical nerve repair (8). In his technique, nerve grafts were interposed between the fascicles under the operating microscope, which was different from Seddon's technique of cable grafting.

The management of neuroma in continuity, categorized as a Sunderland sixth-degree lesion, has remained controversial. Kline et al. introduced the technique of recording evoked nerve action potentials from the distal nerve stump (9) and applied this clinically as well as reporting an algorithm for the management of the neuroma in continuity.

More recently, two older techniques of nerve transfer and end-to-side nerve repair have been reintroduced and recognized as useful alternatives in the armamentarium for nerve repair.

Oberlin et al. described the transfer of fasciculi from the ulnar nerve to the musculocutaneous nerve and demonstrated its superiority over other methods of neurotization in restoring elbow flexion in patients with C5-C6 or C5-C6-C7 brachial plexus palsy (10) (Figure 68-1). This technique has become the procedure of choice for restoration of elbow flexion. Other nerve transfers have been devised and offer superior alternatives to address the unique difficulties associated with both isolated proximal and devastating multiple nerve injuries (see Chapter 71).

End-to-side nerve coaptation is indicated when the proximal end of a divided motor, sensory, or mixed nerve is not available for repair. In 1899, Kennedy first described end-to-side nerve coaptation of the divided distal end of the facial nerve to the side of the intact hypoglossal nerve (11). In this case, he performed an epineurial window and deliberately divided axons of the hypoglossal nerve to induce axonal sprouting. This was the first report of the successful use of end-to-side nerve coaptation to provide functional recovery in situations when traditional nerve repairs were not applicable. May et al. reintroduced this end-to-side nerve coaptation with deliberate axonotomy, and this procedure became an acceptable surgical procedure for reconstruction of facial nerve injuries (12). End-to-side nerve repair was reintroduced experimentally by Viterbo et al. (13), who demonstrated reinnervation of the rat tibialis anterior muscle by an end-to-side coaptation between the distal end of the divided peroneal nerve and the side of the intact tibial nerve. In the original studies, an epineurial window was created at the end-to-side coaptation with no intentional deliberate axonotomy, but more recent studies have shown that end-to-side coaptation when a perineurial window is created but without a deliberate axonotomy is more effective for both motor and sensory reinnervation (14) (see Chapter 69).

WALLERIAN DEGENERATION AND NERVE REGENERATION

Since the landmark paper by Augustus Waller in 1850 (1), nerve degeneration and regeneration have been studied extensively and have provided a better understanding of peripheral nerve physiology. According to Gaudet et al. (15) and Rotshenker (16), the inflammatory response associated with cellular and molecular events is initiated by axonal disintegration in the distal nerve stump. This response activates nearby Schwann cells

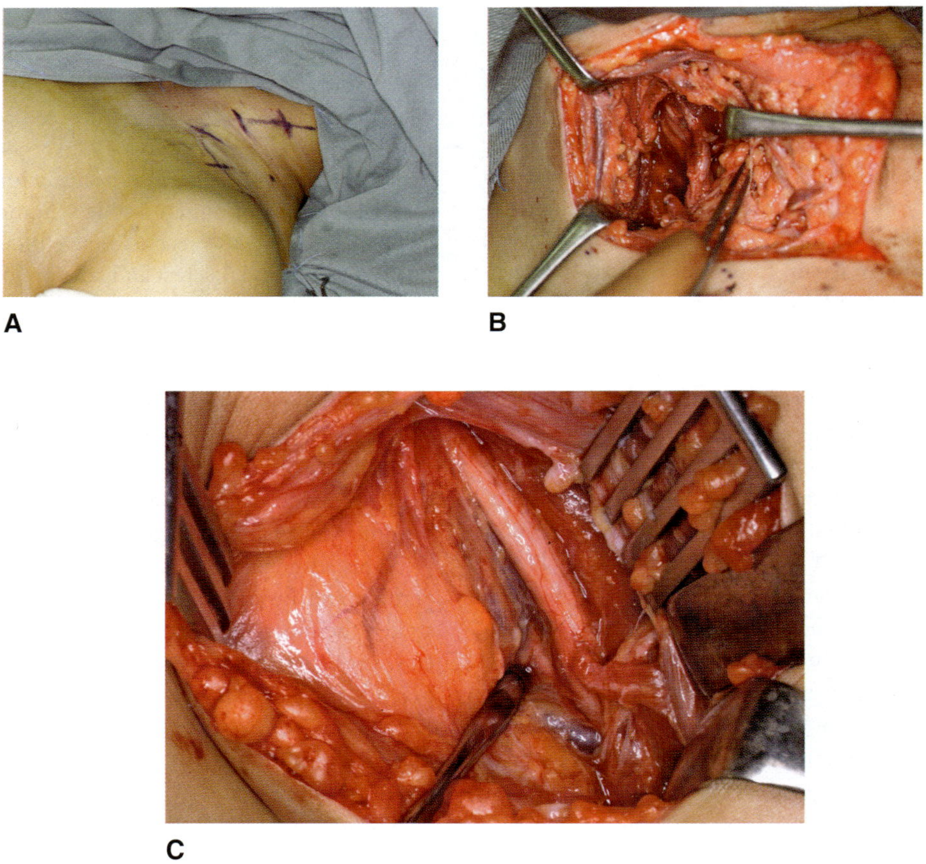

FIGURE 68-1 (A) and (B) A 21-year-old girl with a left C5, 6 root avulsion in a motor vehicle accident. Nerve transfers were performed for reconstruction of shoulder and elbow motion. Exploration of the left brachial plexus 2 weeks after injury identified pooling of cerebrospinal fluid and redundant C5 and C6 nerve roots. (C) Median nerve transfer (donor) to the motor branch of the musculocutaneous nerve (recipient) using end-to-side nerve coaptation with an epineurial window. The spinal accessory nerve was transferred to the suprascapular nerve.

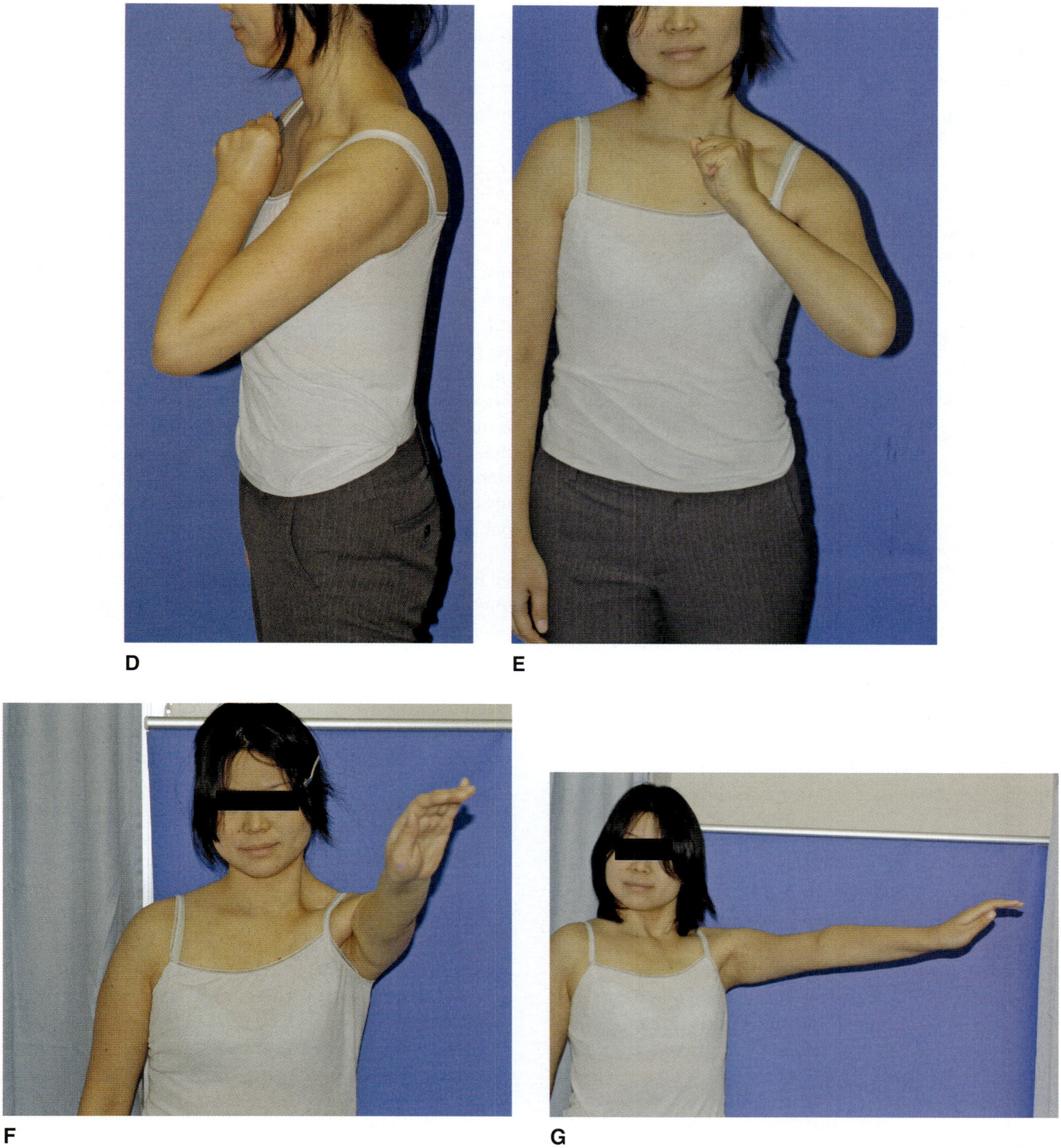

FIGURE 68-1 *(Continued)* (D) and (E) Seven years after surgery, elbow flexion recovered to M5. Gripping of the ipsilateral hand facilitates elbow flexion. (F) and (G) Seven years after surgery, anterior and lateral elevation of the left shoulder has been regained after the spinal accessory nerve to suprascapular nerve transfer.

and resident macrophages via receptors sensitive to tissue damage. Denervated Schwann cells respond to injury by shedding myelin, proliferating, phagocytosing debris, and releasing cytokines that recruit bloodborne monocytes and macrophages. Macrophages take over the bulk of phagocytosis within days of peripheral nerve injury before leaving the nerve after remyelination has occurred. The inflammatory response associated with the peripheral nervous system is far more efficient compared with that of the central nervous system. Wallerian degeneration serves as a prelude for successful nerve repair when these requirements are met. In contrast, functional recovery is poor when the injury fails to produce an efficient innate immune response of Wallerian degeneration. Figure 68-2 shows progression of Wallerian degeneration and axon regeneration after peripheral nerve injury. A single axon with associated myelinating Schwann cells is shown. Although myelin phagocytosis and degeneration occurs within the basal lamina (purple), the basal lamina is shown only in panel 1 for clarity. The process is as follows:

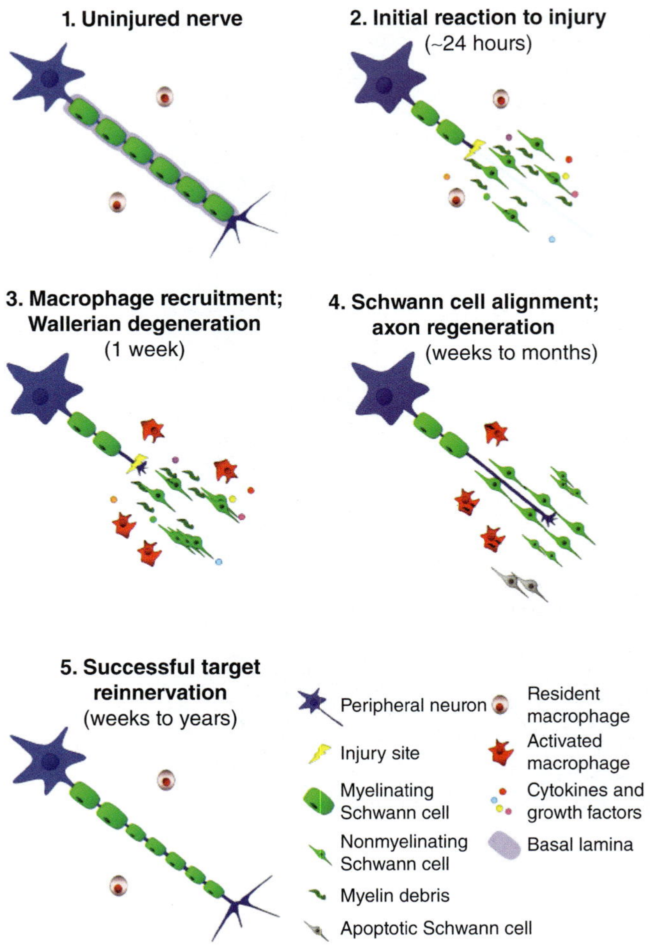

FIGURE 68-2 Schematic representation of Wallerian degeneration. (Reproduced with permission from Gaudet AD, Popovich PG, Ramer MS. Wallerian degeneration: gaining perspective on inflammatory events after peripheral nerve injury. *J Neuroinflammation* 2011;8:110–123.)

(1) The endoneurium of an uninjured nerve consists of axons; associated Schwann cells (myelinating and nonmyelinating); and resident, inactivated macrophages. (2) Soon after peripheral nerve injury, denervated myelinating Schwann cells release their myelin. These Schwann cells then proliferate within their basal lamina tubes, produce cytokines and trophic factors, and phagocytose detached debris. In addition, the reaction within the neuron cell body begins; this is characterized by cell soma hypertrophy, displacement of the nucleus to an eccentric position, and dissolution of Nissl bodies. (3) Wallerian degeneration is well underway within 1 week of injury. Soluble factors produced by Schwann cells and injured axons activate resident macrophages and lead to recruitment of hematogenous macrophages. The activated macrophages clear myelin and axon debris efficiently and produce factors that facilitate Schwann cell migration and axon regeneration. (4) After a lag period, injured axons form a growth cone and begin to regenerate along bands of Bugner formed by Schwann cells. These tubes provide a permissive growth environment and guide extending axons toward potential peripheral targets. Schwann cells that have been chronically denervated (e.g., for a few months) are less supportive of regrowth and are more likely to undergo apoptosis. (5) If the axon is able to traverse the injury site, and its environment supports its growth along the entire distal stump, then the axon can connect with peripheral targets. Although myelinating Schwann cells do remyelinate the regenerated portion of an axon, the myelin is thinner, and the nodal length is shorter than in the uninjured portion of an axon.

TIMING OF NERVE REPAIR

During World War II, nerve repair surgery was delayed for 2 to 3 weeks because of wound contamination, and it was believed that a 3-week delay was optimal to facilitate the best regeneration potential. However, no clinical data supported the view that delayed primary repair would be advantageous over an immediate primary repair. Because of advances in the understanding of nerve physiology, surgeons can now understand how peripheral nerves react to trauma, as well as the alterations that occur both in the peripheral and central nervous systems. With increasing time after injury, the results of nerve repair become progressively worse as a result of fibrosis in the distal nerve segment, atrophy of Schwann cells, and advanced loss of neurons. The surgeon can only influence a few factors that affect the functional outcome. The timing of nerve repair and reconstruction is one of the most influential factors on the results after nerve injury (17). Recent understanding of intracellular signaling pathways that are rapidly initiated in neurons and in nonneuronal cells to promote nerve regeneration has made the timing of nerve repair and reconstruction more important. Experimental and clinical data clearly confirm the advantage of early nerve repair and reconstruction after injury. An injured nerve needs to be swiftly repaired or reconstructed together with an early appropriate rehabilitation program for both motor and sensory recovery. Nerve transfers can be considered to shorten the time for muscle reinnervation.

Time from Injury

The appropriate timing for exploration of a closed nerve lesion, such as an incomplete brachial plexus injury or birth palsy, may be a difficult decision. Designation of the optimal time for surgery has been dogmatic because it parallels our understanding that time-dependent, irreversible changes occur in the motor end plates. Therefore, in a proximal nerve lesion, the longer the target muscle is denervated, the lower the likelihood of successful reinnervation. In general, the optimal time for surgical intervention of a closed nerve injury has been believed to be before 6 months. Despite these general recommendations, several innovative surgeons have challenged this dogma and have performed early surgical exploration and reconstruction. However, early surgery might not allow sufficient time for spontaneous reinnervation, but waiting too long can lead to irreversible failure of the motor end plates, resulting in complete failure of reinnervation. Early exploration and reconstruction 3 to 6 weeks after injury may be indicated if there is a severe pre- or postganglionic brachial plexus injury. Early surgical exploration before the development of scar and neuroma formation allows easier exploration and more accurate identification of injured structures. However, because of the severity of concomitant injuries associated with brachial plexus injuries, early exploration is often not possible. In the past, routine exploration has been performed 3 to 6 months after injury in patients

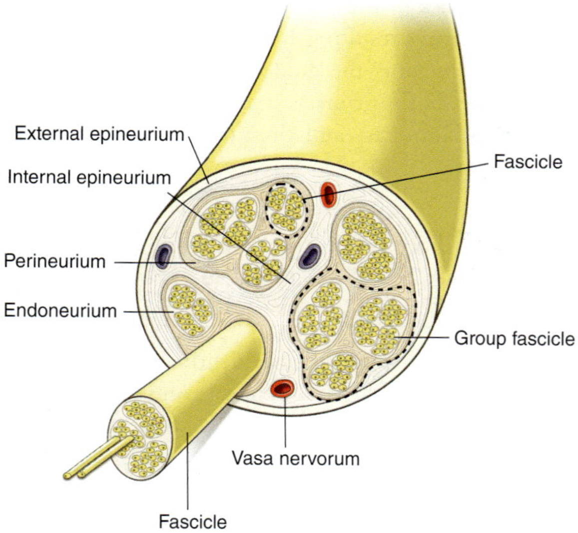

FIGURE 68-3 Cross-sectional anatomy of a peripheral nerve.

who have not demonstrated adequate reinnervation over time. The results of delayed (9–12 months) or late (>12 months) surgery are known to be poor because the time for the nerve to regenerate to the target muscles is greater than the survival time of the motor end plates after denervation. In these delayed situations, irreversible changes occur in the muscle cells and useful functional motor recovery cannot be achieved. For these cases, microvascular transfer of a normal muscle innervated by an uninjured motor nerve transfer may be indicated.

ANATOMY OF THE PERIPHERAL NERVE (FIGURE 68-3)

Sunderland investigated the intraneural fascicular anatomy of the peripheral nerves and described an intermingling of the fascicles (18). However, Jabaley et al. reported a more constant plexiform fascicular anatomy, with individual group fasciculi maintaining their position in the same quadrantic relationship over significant distances (19); similar arrangements have been described by several other investigators (20). There are theoretical advantages for group fascicular repair compared with epineurial repair. However, this has not been conclusively proven either experimentally or clinically. The fascicular pattern of the median and ulnar nerves is relatively constant at the level of the distal forearm and wrist over distances of several centimeters. The fascicular anatomy in this area allows either group fascicular repair or epineurial repair. Electrical stimulation of group fascicles in the distal and proximal ends of the nerve may provide additional information as to which are motor group fascicles and which are sensory group fascicles. The author believes that epineurial or epineurial–perineurial repair, taking care to match the fascicular pattern in each of the two nerve ends or matching the position of blood vessels on the surface of the epineurium, is as good as group fascicular repair.

EPINEURIAL NERVE REPAIR

In preparation for a nerve repair, the nerve ends may be wrapped circumferentially with a membranous material and cut with a razor blade or scalpel. Alternatively, the nerve ends are cut on a firm surface such as a tongue depressor. Excessive fascicular protrusion ("oozing" of the nerve fibers) can be controlled to some extent using a pair of microscissors. Preparation of a fresh, sharply cut nerve can be achieved with minimal debridement under loupe magnification or under a microscope. For a delayed primary or secondary nerve repair, the nerve ends should be trimmed back far enough to excise fascicles involved by heavy scarring. Each nerve stump—the neuroma and glioma—should be serially sectioned until a normal-appearing fascicular cross-section becomes visible instead of dense amorphous scar tissue.

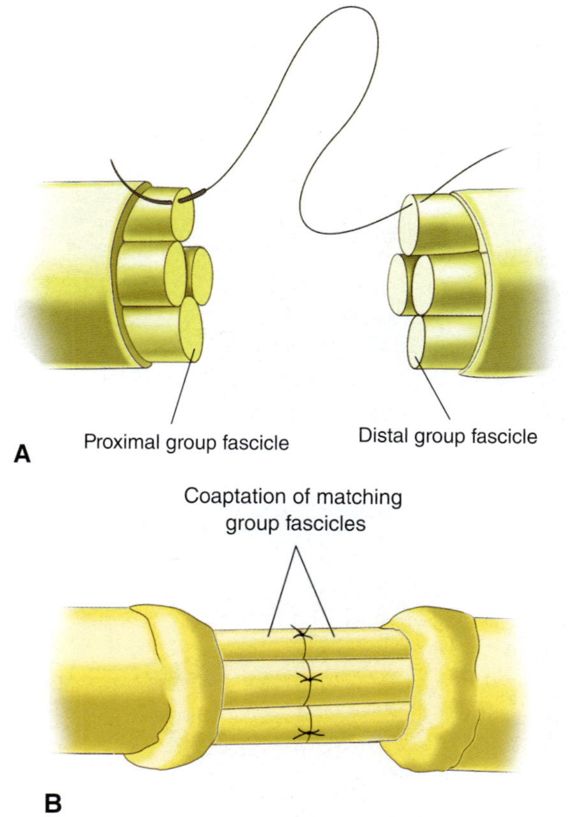

FIGURE 68-4 (A) and (B) Schematic representation of epineurial nerve repair.

In an epineurial repair, sutures are placed in the external epineurium around the circumference of the nerve (Figure 68-4). Mirror images of the cross-sectional arrangement of fascicles in the proximal and distal nerve stumps are aligned rotationally. Alternatively, surface landmarks such as the longitudinal epineurial vessels pattern are aligned by placing key sutures (Figure 68-5). Additional sutures are placed to secure coaptation. Coaptation with minimal tension is preferable; too much tension may result in strangulation of the ends or result in excess scar formation. If one or two 8-0 nylon sutures are unable to maintain approximation of the two nerve ends, nerve grafting is indicated. This test is also true for digital nerve repair using 10-0 nylon sutures. A nerve conduit may be considered if the gap distance is short (preferably <1 cm) to allow regeneration directed by neurotropism (21,22). An epineurial repair does not achieve absolutely correct matching of the fascicles in the proximal and distal nerve stumps and may result in malalignment and displacement of fascicles. Theoretically, fascicular repair may be more

SECTION 4

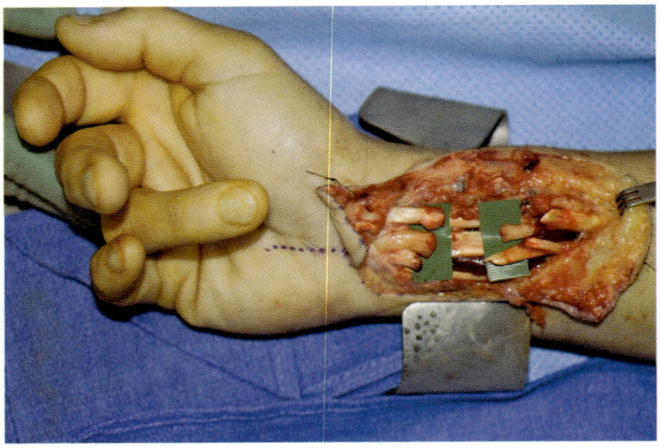

A

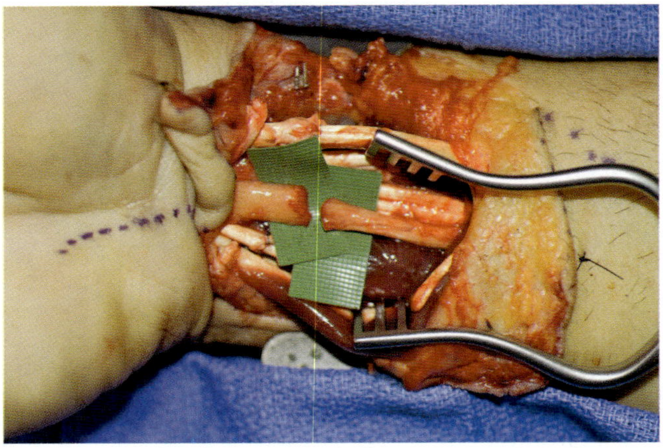

B

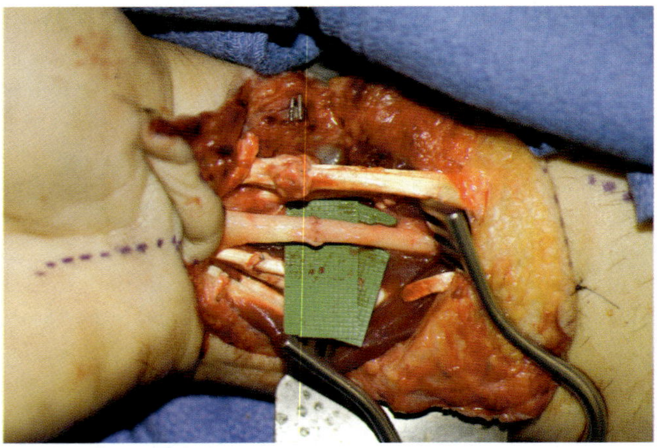

C

FIGURE 68-5 (A) and (B) "Spaghetti" right wrist with laceration of flexor tendons and median nerve. (C) Epineurial repair of the median nerve. (Used with permission from Dr. Neil F. Jones, MD.)

advantageous for perfect fascicular matching compared with epineurial repair. There have not been stringent enough experimental and clinical comparisons of the results of these two nerve repair techniques. No study has been able to provide conclusive evidence to document that one technique is superior to the other. Because of the difficulty in identifying matching fascicles in the proximal and distal nerve ends; as well as the scarring resulting from fascicular dissection, epineurial repair remains the gold standard nerve repair technique for the both primary and secondary nerve repair because of its simplicity and the minimal scarring resulting from dissection.

INTERNAL TOPOGRAPHY OF THE MEDIAN AND ULNAR NERVES AND GROUP FASCICULAR NERVE REPAIR

The median and ulnar nerves have identifiable group fascicular patterns at the wrist, which is the most common site of injury for these nerves. At this level, anatomical dissection allows the identification and matched coaptation of group fascicles (Figure 68-6). The motor branch of the median nerve travels in the palmar and radial aspect of the median nerve over about a 7-cm distance from 3 cm proximal to the wrist crease to the distal edge of the transverse carpal ligament and is identifiable both visually and by dissection (Figure 68-7). The motor branch of the ulnar nerve bifurcates within Guyon's canal and is separately identifiable in the dorsal and ulnar aspect of the ulnar nerve for approximately 8 cm proximally (20) (Figure 68-8). Group fascicular repair theoretically allows the repair of motor-to-motor and sensory-to-sensory group fascicles and therefore reduces the potential for fascicular mismatching. Group fascicular repair is a more clinically useful technique compared with fascicular repair; however, the theoretical superiority of this procedure has not been proven either experimentally or clinically.

SUTURES VERSUS NERVE GLUE

Fibrin glue was introduced more than 30 years ago and has been studied experimentally and clinically and compared with microsurgical suture repair. Sameem et al. reviewed the use of fibrin glue for peripheral nerve repair and identified 181 potential studies and finally analyzed 16 studies, of which 14 were animal studies, one was a cadaveric study, and one was a human study (23). They concluded that even though the majority of these studies used animal models, most indicated that the performance of fibrin glue was equal, if not superior, to microsutures for peripheral nerve repair. Most histopathologic studies revealed equivalent or improved results when using fibrin glue compared with microsutures. The main criticism of fibrin glue relates to its ability to consistently hold the nerve ends together and maintain the tensile strength of the repair. Critics cite gapping and complete failure of the repair as the main disadvantages when fibrin glue is used alone without sutures. However, two studies have reported positive biomechanical data. In the first study, the fibrin glue group had significantly greater resistance to gapping than the no-glue group, with no differences in peak load (24). In the second study, although the fibrin glue repair was significantly less resistant than suture repair immediately after the repair and on postoperative day 7, mechanical resistance became equal on postoperative days 14 and 28. Interestingly, the fibrin glue group had a final mechanical resistance that was greater than conventional suture repair (25).

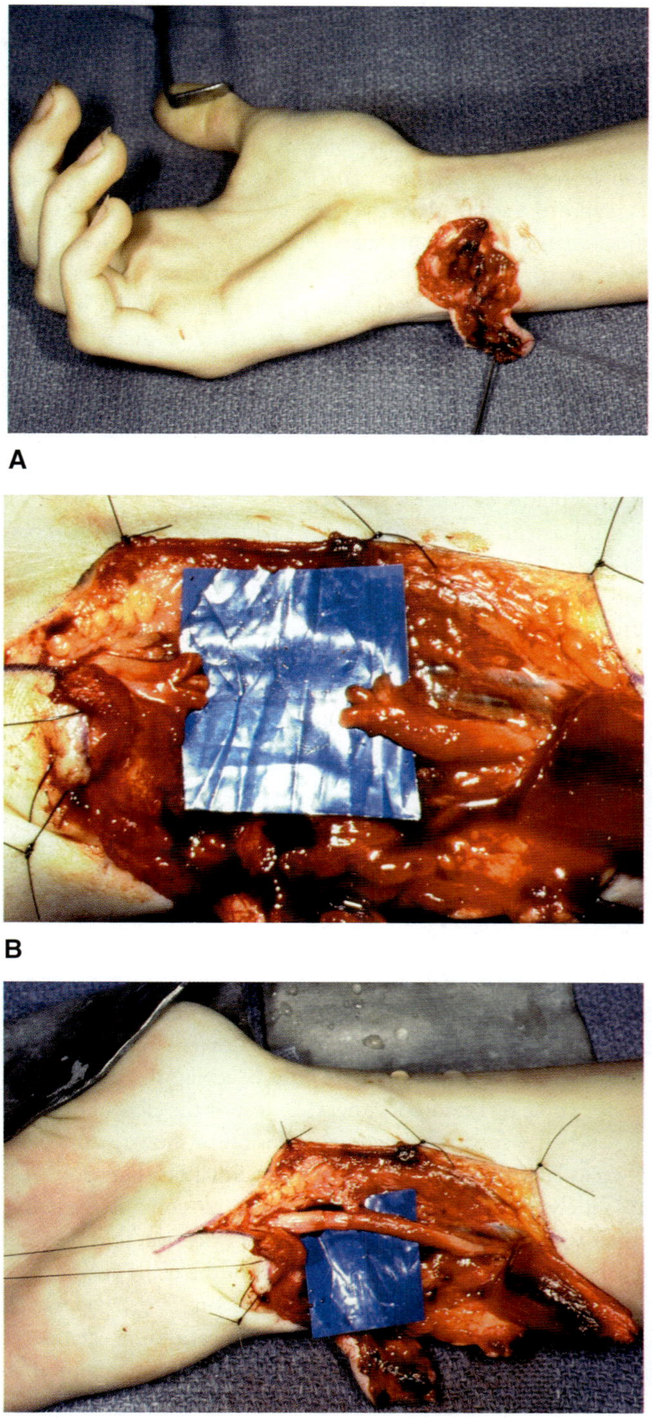

FIGURE 68-6 (A) and (B) Laceration of the right ulnar nerve at the wrist. The proximal and distal nerve stumps were separated into three group fascicles using "awake electrical stimulation." (C). Group fascicular repair of the ulnar nerve. (Used with permission from Dr. Neil F. Jones, MD.)

Overall, many authors have reported that fibrin glue is a quicker and easier modality to use than microsuture repair. However, there is not one well-controlled human trial assessing the efficacy of fibrin glue compared with microsutures.

Fibrin glue is extremely useful in facilitating the handling of sural nerve grafts. Multiple sural nerve grafts can be initially glued together at their ends and the construct trimmed using a razor blade. This construct of glued sural nerve grafts is then placed in the nerve defect with reversed polarity and temporarily glued to the proximal and distal nerve ends before placing microsutures.

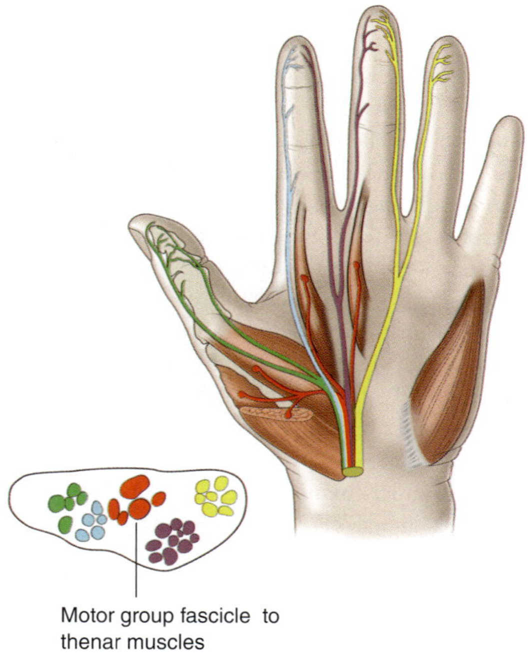

FIGURE 68-7 Internal topography of the median nerve at the wrist.

DIGITAL NERVE REPAIR

The digital nerves to the radial three and a half digits are terminal branches of the median nerve, and the digital nerves to the ulnar one and a half digits are terminal branches of the ulnar nerve. The common digital nerves are deep to the superficial palmar arch, but the digital nerves are superficial to the digital arteries. The digital neurovascular bundles are located on either side of each digit just dorsal to Grayson's ligament

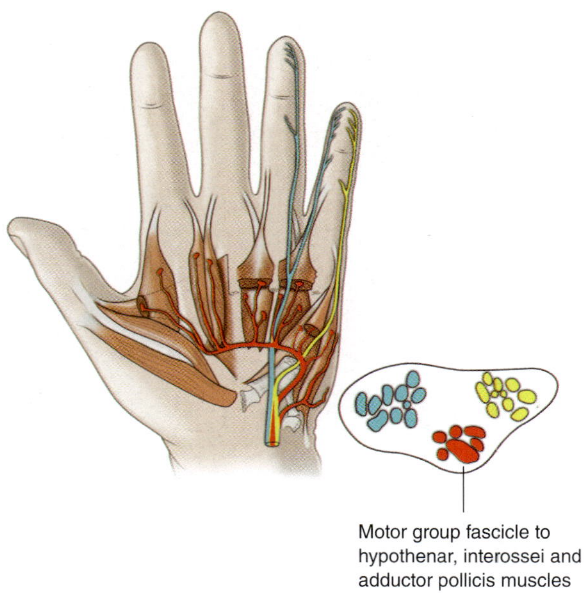

FIGURE 68-8 Internal topography of the ulnar nerve at the wrist.

and palmar to Cleland's ligament. The radial neurovascular bundle of the thumb and index finger and the ulnar neurovascular bundle of the little finger are located slightly closer to the midline of the digit. Each digital nerve bifurcates into at least three and occasionally more branches at the distal interphalangeal joint. A Bruner's incision is used for dissection of the digital nerves. A digital nerve laceration is prepared for repair by trimming the nerve ends with microscissors under loupe magnification or under the operating microscope. Epineurial coaptation using two to four 9-0 or 10-0 nylon sutures is adequate for end-to-end digital nerve repairs, with the metacarpophalangeal (MCP) and IP joints positioned in full extension (Figure 68-9). If the defect is longer than 5 mm, 9-0 or 10-0 nylon sutures may fail to maintain the approximation; in such a situation, nerve grafting is indicated. The sural nerve or medial antebrachial cutaneous nerves (MABCNs) are options for grafting a digital nerve defect. A similar graft could be harvested from the lateral antebrachial cutaneous nerve. However, this nerve receives contributions from branches of the superficial radial nerve. The terminal branch of the posterior interosseous nerve running on the interosseous membrane in the distal forearm can either be used as a conventional nonvascularized graft for digital nerve reconstruction or as a vascularized nerve graft based on the dorsal branch of the anterior interosseous artery (26). Vein conduits and synthetic conduits, such as polyglycolic acid (PGA) or bovine collagen tubes, may provide similar results for digital nerve repair as autogenous nerve grafting (see Chapter 70).

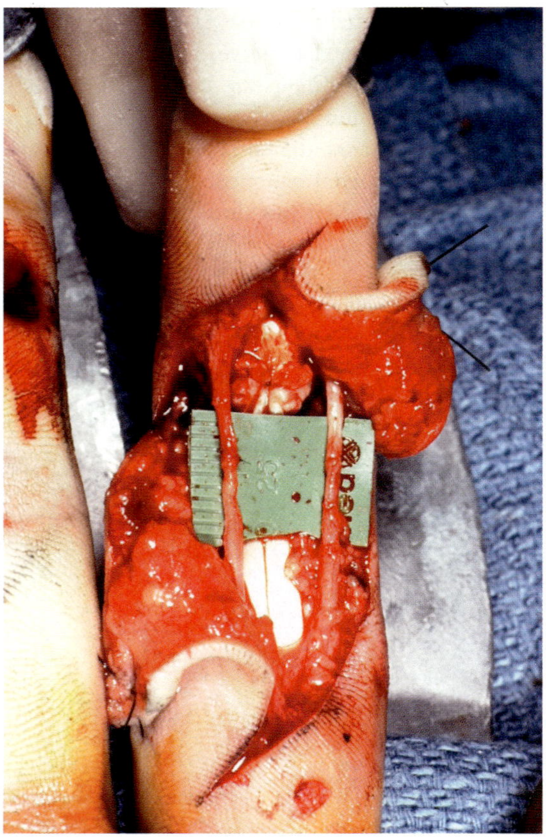

FIGURE 68-9 Epineurial repair of both digital nerves. (Used with permission from Dr. Neil F. Jones, MD.)

RESULTS OF DIGITAL NERVE REPAIRS

Digital nerves consist of pure sensory nerve fibers. Therefore, the results of direct repair or nerve grafting of digital nerves can be evaluated more precisely compared with other mixed motor and sensory peripheral nerves.

Paprottka et al. recently reported a systematic review and meta-analysis of the outcomes of sensory recovery after digital nerve repair (27). A total of 2997 common or proper digital nerve repairs from 182 clinical papers provided the basis for their analysis. End-to-end coaptation or nerve grafts achieved slightly more precise two-point-discrimination and more S4 results by the Highet classification than end-to-side coaptations. Within the Highet S3+ outcomes, there was a higher incidence of end-to-side coaptations compared with end-to-end coaptations or nerve grafting.

End-to-end nerve repairs from 1980 to the present had better sensory recovery outcomes than nerve repairs between 1965 and 1979. This was interpreted to reflect the improved results after the introduction of the operating microscope. Sensory recovery after digital replantation was significantly better in younger patients than older patients. There was no statistical significant difference in the timing of nerve repair and sensory recovery. There was also no difference in sensory recovery with differing gap lengths up to 4 cm after reconstruction with synthetic conduits or vein conduits.

HOW TO GAUGE TENSION ON THE NERVE COAPTATION SITE

The most detrimental effect on nerve regeneration is too much tension at the repair site. The position of the joints proximal and distal to the repair site obviously affects the tension on the nerve repair. Surgeons may be deluded into believing that tension can be overcome by flexion of either the wrist or the elbow both during and after surgery. However, extension of the wrist or elbow 3 weeks later ruins the recovering nerve function. Therefore, it is absolutely mandatory to determine the tension on the nerve repair with the wrist and elbow joints in extension that provides maximal tension on the approximation of the nerve ends.

It is difficult to precisely gauge tension at the coaptation site during surgery. It can be determined by holding each nerve end in jeweler's forceps and gauging the tension required to bring the two ends together under the operating microscope (Figure 68-10). Alternatively, a suture can be placed through the epineurium of the proximal and distal nerve ends and the surgeon can decide whether this suture will hold the two ends together. Nerve grafting should be considered if an 8-0 nylon suture cannot hold the ends of the median, ulnar, or radial nerves together or a 10-0 nylon suture for a digital nerve. If these approximating sutures fail to hold the two nerve ends together, nerve grafting is indicated.

HISTORY OF NERVE GRAFTING

The first nerve graft was performed by Philipeaux and Vulapian in 1863 in dogs. The first human nerve graft was performed by Albert in 1876 (2). Bielschowsky and Unger reported better

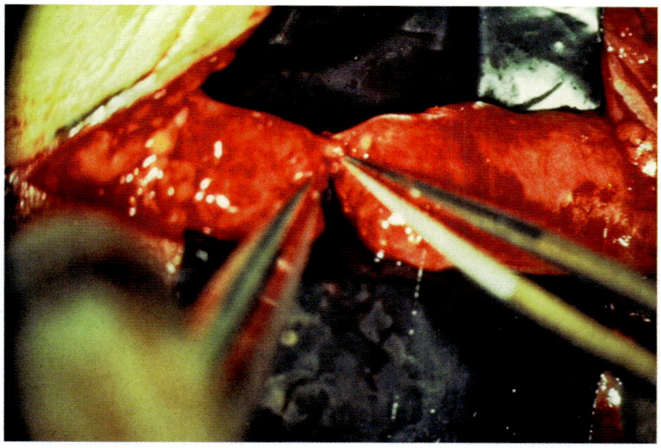

FIGURE 68-10 Use of two jeweler's forceps to gauge tension on a digital nerve repair under the operating microscope. (Used with permission from Dr. Neil F. Jones, MD.)

survival of cutaneous nerve grafts compared with nerve trunk grafts. Seddon established the technique of cable nerve grafting in 1947 (5). St. Clair Strange introduced the pedicled nerve graft technique by connecting two parallel nerves such as the median and ulnar nerves in the forearm to reconstruct one of these nerves (28). The early results of nerve grafting were pessimistic and only used as a salvage procedure when the defect was too large to be approximated. Direct nerve repair achieved by flexion of the adjacent joints was preferred. However, a high failure rate of these nerve repairs under tension resulted. The most recent advance in nerve grafting was the introduction of microneural surgery in 1964 by Smith (7). Millesi demonstrated both experimentally and clinically that nerve grafting by avoiding tension produced better results than direct nerve repair under tension (29). Millesi et al. reported that interfascicular nerve grafting achieved better results compared with simple cable nerve grafting; however, significant differences between these two techniques has not yet been well documented (8,30). In 1976, Taylor and Ham introduced the concept of vascularized nerve grafting similar to a free tissue transfer (31).

INDICATIONS FOR NERVE GRAFTING RATHER THAN NERVE REPAIR UNDER TENSION

Defining the critical length of a nerve defect or the amount of tension that can be tolerated in an end-to-end nerve repair remains undetermined. The results of experimental studies comparing direct nerve repair with nerve grafting to bridge defects up to 2 cm in length are conflicting. Practically, a decision for direct repair of the median, ulnar, and radial nerves in the arm or forearm can be made if an 8-0 nylon suture will hold the nerve ends together with the elbow in extension and the wrist in about 20 degrees of extension or if a 10-0 nylon suture will approximate the ends of a digital nerve with the MCP and IP joints in extension. If these approximating sutures are unable to hold the nerve ends together, nerve grafting should be performed. The length of graft should be sufficient to avoid any tension with the adjacent joints in extension. There is a tendency for a nonvascularized nerve graft to shrink, and about 10% extra graft length should be harvested. More important, the joints must be kept in the extended position for a few weeks after the surgery.

DONOR NERVES FOR NERVE GRAFTING

Selection of which donor nerve graft to harvest depends on several factors. The diameter of the nerve graft influences revascularization. If a nerve with a diameter greater than 3 mm, such as the common peroneal or ulnar nerve, is used as a nonvascularized nerve graft, central necrosis of the nerve graft will occur. Smaller diameter nerves are therefore selected as single or multiple strands for cable grafting (Figure 68-11). Sensory nerves are chosen because donor site morbidity is minimal, and revascularization is less of a problem. The length of graft required also influences the donor nerve selection.

The sural nerve is the most frequently used donor nerve and typically consists of a medial component arising from the tibial nerve and a lateral component arising from the lateral sural cutaneous nerve or common peroneal nerve (32).

The ipsilateral donor site of the MABCN may be beneficial. The scar along the medial aspect of the upper arm and the proximal medial aspect of the forearm is relatively invisible. The MABCN arises from the medial cord of the brachial plexus, and its fibers are derived from the C8 and T1 spinal nerves. The nerve courses down the ulnar aspect of the arm medial to the brachial artery, pierces the deep fascia with the basilic vein at about the middle of the arm, and divides into volar and ulnar branches. If the proximal portion of the nerve is harvested, sensation will be lost over the anteromedial aspect of the upper arm and the ulnar half of the forearm. Birch suggests that it is a useful ipsilateral graft donor site, and about 25 cm of length of nerve graft can be harvested (33). The proximal portion of this nerve can be divided into several 4-cm-long cable grafts for defects in the median, ulnar, or radial nerves. For longer nerve defects, cables harvested from one or both sural nerves can be used to reconstruct the defect. The sural nerve remains the first choice for cable grafts for the median, ulnar, and radial nerves.

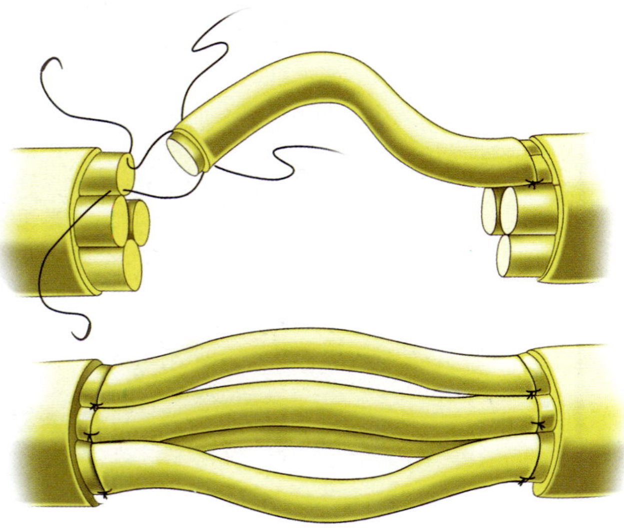

FIGURE 68-11 Schematic representation of cable nerve grafting.

One of the branches of the MABCN harvested from the proximal forearm is a useful donor for digital nerve defects. If the proximal portion of the MABCN has to be harvested, a painful neuroma may occur.

The lateral antebrachial cutaneous nerve is the sensory branch of the musculocutaneous nerve and passes below the cephalic vein and divides at the elbow joint into volar and dorsal branches. The lateral antebrachial cutaneous nerve is also potentially an ipsilateral donor nerve. However, because this nerve has significant anatomical communication with the superficial radial nerve, harvesting this nerve as a graft may result in neuroma problems or irritable sensory changes over the distal radial forearm and dorsal wrist.

SURGICAL TECHNIQUE OF NERVE GRAFTING

Autogenous sural nerve is the most frequently used cable graft for bridging a defect in the median, ulnar, or radial nerves (Figure 68-12) and sural nerve, MABCN, or terminal branch of the posterior interosseous nerve for digital nerve defects (Figure 68-13).

After harvesting the nerve graft, the direction of polarity is marked. The graft is divided into several segments, each measuring about 10% longer than the defect to compensate for postoperative ischemic shortening plus a few millimeters for stump debridement. The nerve segments are laid side by side with the same direction of reverse polarity to minimize axonal dispersion from the side branches. The ends of each cable graft are glued together using fibrin glue. The cables between the nerve ends should be left unglued to allow for better revascularization of each graft, especially the central cables. Both ends are wrapped with a strip of rubber band to construct one large cable, and both ends are then trimmed with a razor blade to obtain a uniform transverse surface to allow end-to-end coaptation to the proximal and distal nerve stumps.

The joints proximal and distal to the nerve defect should be positioned in extension. The prepared graft is then placed into the nerve defect, and there should be no tension at either coaptation site. Coaptation is begun by placing two sutures 180 degrees opposite to each other. Coaptation is then completed by placing additional sutures between the nerve ends and the nerve graft around the circumference or by using fibrin glue.

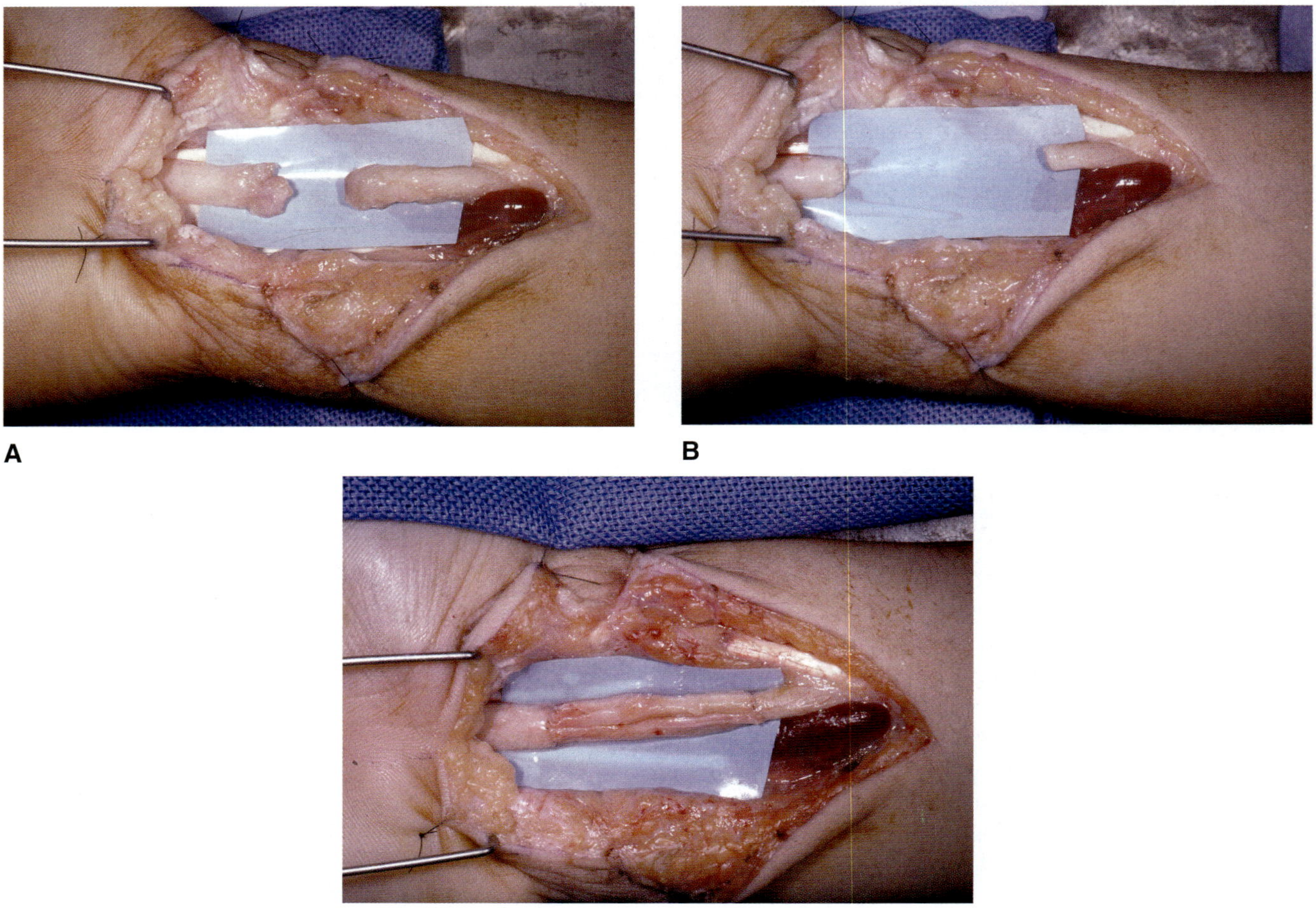

A B C

FIGURE 68-12 (A) and (B) Missed right median nerve laceration. The proximal and distal nerve ends were serially sectioned back to a normal-appearing fascicular pattern (C). Four sural nerve cable grafts in reverse polarity were used to reconstruct this 4-cm defect. (Used with permission from Dr. Neil F. Jones, MD.)

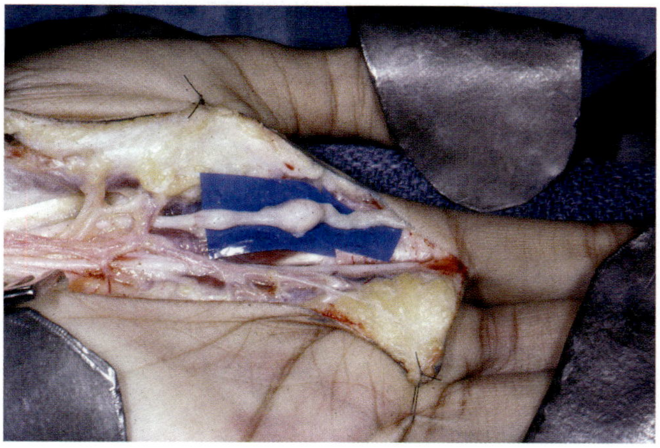

A

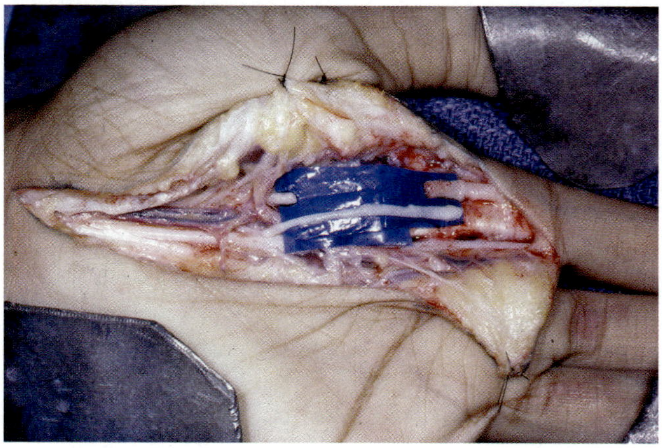

B

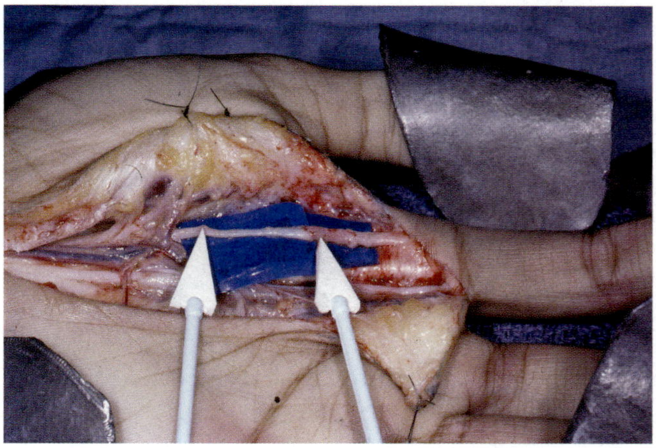

C

FIGURE 68-13 (A) Neuroma of the radial digital nerve to the left index finger. (B) After resection, there was a 2.5-cm nerve gap. (C) A nerve graft was harvested from the distal portion of the posterior interosseous nerve. (Used with permission from Dr. Neil F. Jones, MD.)

There is no evidence that wrapping the two coaptation sites of a nerve graft with either a short segment of vein graft or a synthetic conduit or nerve wrap will prevent axonal dispersion. It is important to maintain the joints in an extended position for 14 days after surgery. If the adjacent joints are held in flexion after surgery, adhesions will form around the graft and prevent elongation of the graft.

INDICATIONS FOR VASCULARIZED NERVE GRAFTS:

The nature of the recipient bed, the anatomical location of the nerve defect and the size of the affected nerve are the important factors in any decision to use a vascularized nerve graft. A vascularized nerve graft may be more indicated in a severely scarred recipient bed than in a less scarred bed. There are theoretical advantages for considering a vascularized nerve graft in a more proximal anatomical location and for long nerve defects.

ANATOMY OF POTENTIAL DONOR SITES FOR VASCULARIZED NERVE GRAFTS

To minimize any donor site morbidity, only two nerves are potential candidates for vascularized nerve grafting, the sural and ulnar nerves. The vascularized sural nerve may be considered for any nerve reconstruction in a poorly vascularized bed and the ulnar nerve pedicled on the superior ulnar collateral artery as a vascularized trunk nerve graft only in patients with irreparable C8 and T1 root avulsions.

The sural nerve is the most useful donor nerve, not only for conventional nerve grafting but also for vascularized nerve grafting. The sural nerve was originally described as a vascularized nerve graft by arterializing the reversed lesser saphenous vein that accompanies the sural nerve (Figure 68-14). Leclere et al. described the blood supply of the sural nerve from the superficial sural artery (SSA) (34). The medial sural nerve can be elevated based on the SSA system as a vascularized nerve graft (Figure 68-15). Septocutaneous perforators of the SSA extend laterally to also supply the lateral cutaneous branch of the sural nerve. The vascular pedicle of the SSA continues to its popliteal origin with the nerves. The average length of the vascular pedicle from the popliteal crease to the distal aspect of the lateral gastrocnemius muscle, where the nerve is enveloped by well-vascularized fascia is 18 cm on average (range, 15–25 cm). The mean length of the pedicle before the artery joins the medial sural nerve is 4.5 ± 1.9 cm (range, 2.0–7.9 cm). The average diameter of the SSA is 1.4 ± 0.4 mm (range, 0.5–2.0 mm). The accompanying vena comitans has an average diameter of 2.0 ± 0.8 mm (range, 1.0–3.9 mm), but a separate subcutaneous vein may occasionally need to be dissected with an average diameter of 3.5 ± 0.4 mm (range, 3.0–4.0 mm).

An alternative blood supply to vascularize the sural nerve is the peroneal artery system, which supplies the fascia through the posterolateral crural septum (Figure 68-16). If the peroneal artery system is used, a chimeric flap containing fibula bone and the sural nerve can be harvested.

ST. CLAIR STRANGE ULNAR NERVE-TO-MEDIAN NERVE PEDICLED VASCULARIZED NERVE GRAFT

Survival of a nerve graft depends on its revascularization. Central necrosis of a nonvascularized trunk nerve graft with a diameter greater than the common peroneal nerve was well documented in the middle of the 20th century. In 1946, St Clair Strange described an interesting two-stage operative

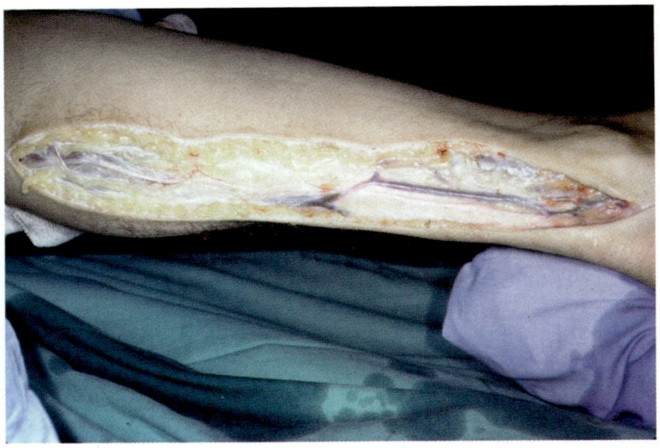

A

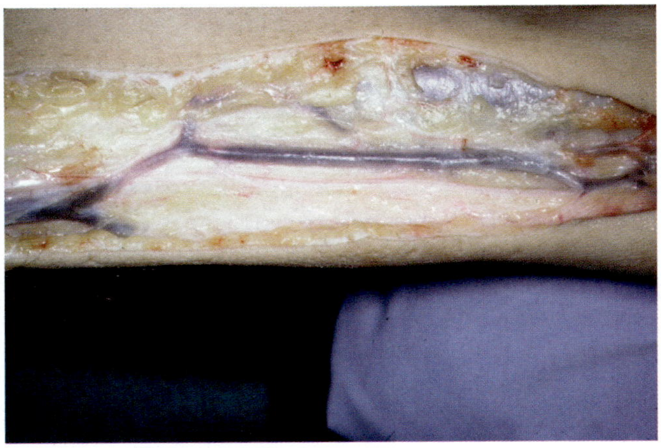

B

FIGURE 68-14 (A) and (B) Anatomy of the right sural nerve with the lesser saphenous vein anteriorly. This allows the sural nerve to be used as a vascularized nerve graft by arterializing the reversed lesser saphenous vein. (Used with permission from Dr. Neil F. Jones, MD.)

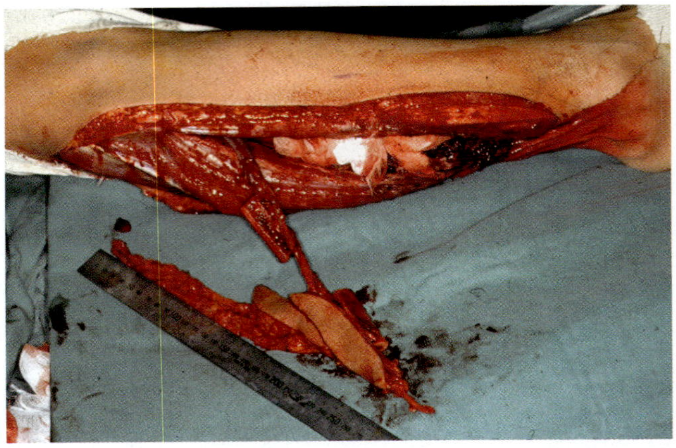

A

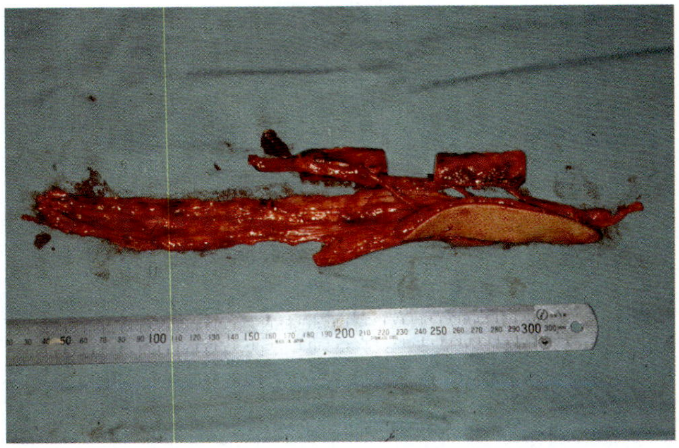

B

FIGURE 68-16 (A) and (B) A vascularized sural nerve graft within the peroneal fascia based on the peroneal artery.

procedure using a pedicled major trunk nerve graft (28). A patient who had sustained a shell injury had complete destruction of the median and ulnar nerves over a distance of 12 cm, from 6 cm below the elbow to 6 cm above the wrist. A pedicled vascularized nerve graft was devised using the ulnar nerve to repair the defect in the median nerve. At the first stage, the neuromas of the median and ulnar nerves were resected so that there was good fascicular anatomy at the proximal ends of both nerves. The prepared proximal stumps of the median and ulnar nerves were coapted in a U-shaped fashion. The ulnar nerve was then transected 13.5 cm proximal to its stump, but the epineurium and extrinsic blood supply was kept intact. At a second stage 32 days later, the transection site of the proximal ulnar nerve was identified and

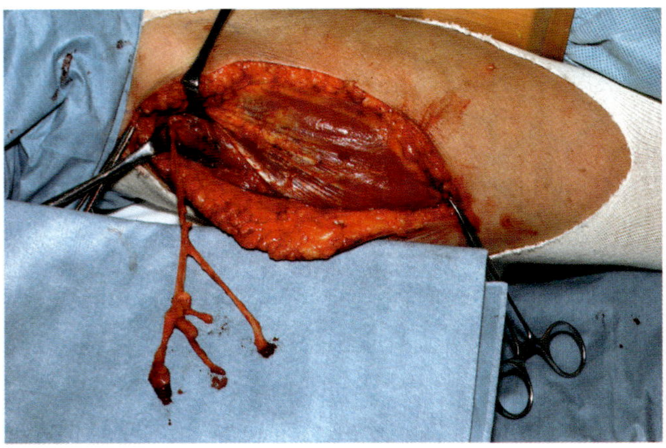

A

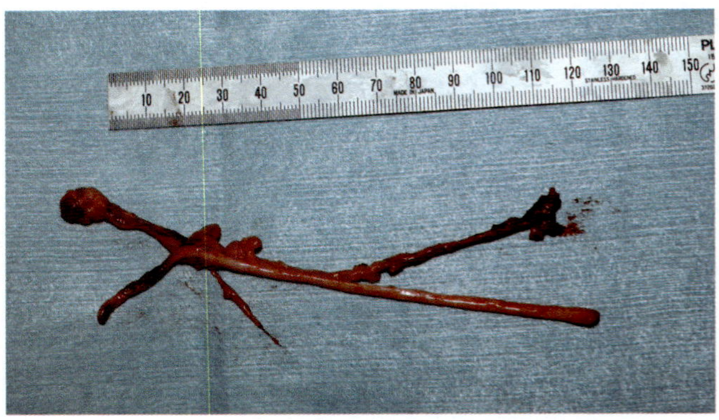

B

FIGURE 68-15 (A) and (B) A vascularized sural nerve graft based on the superficial sural artery.

completely divided and transposed down through a subcutaneous tunnel so the proximal ulnar nerve could be coapted to the distal median nerve stump. There was brisk bleeding from the proximal ulnar nerve stump, confirming this two-stage procedure as the first example of nerve reconstruction using a vascularized major trunk nerve graft.

Greenberg et al. reported five cases of St. Clair Strange pedicled vascularized nerve grafting with a mean follow-up period of 10 years (35). Protective sensation was achieved in the median nerve distribution, and all patients had active use of their hands, but none had meaningful two-point discrimination.

SURGICAL TECHNIQUE OF VASCULARIZED NERVE GRAFTING:

The sural nerve and lesser saphenous vein are harvested together with the intervening fascia between them. The distal end of the lesser saphenous vein is then anastomosed to a recipient artery to allow arterial blood to flow through the lesser saphenous vein and into the sural nerve. There is no venous anastomosis (see Figure 68-14).

The technique for transferring the sural nerve as a vascularized cable graft is to fold the sural nerve graft like a "concertina" but only transect the nerve into segments. Each nerve segment receives a blood supply from the extrinsic vessel (lesser saphenous vein or SSA) running alongside the nerve. A nerve segment with no accompanying extrinsic artery can still remain perfused if the nerve is elevated as the component of a neurofascial flap, based on the SSA system or the peroneal artery system.

In patients with a C8 and T1 preganglionic root avulsion brachial plexus injury, the ulnar nerve can be used as a vascularized trunk nerve graft. The ulnar nerve is supplied primarily by the superior ulnar collateral artery and occasionally by the inferior ulnar collateral artery. A long vascularized nerve graft can be elevated on either the superior or inferior ulnar collateral artery vascular pedicle and used to bridge the distance from the contralateral C7 root to the median nerve in the injured upper arm. The ulnar nerve is divided at the wrist and dissected in a suprafascial plane to the level of the medial intermuscular septum. The medial intermuscular septum is excised, and the ulnar nerve is released from the cubital tunnel. At the level of the mid-upper arm, the superior ulnar collateral artery with one or two venae comitantes is identified as it joins the ulnar nerve on its lateral aspect. The pedicle is carefully protected, and the ulnar nerve is then dissected proximally. The median nerve is also identified at this level. The tourniquet is deflated, and satisfactory perfusion to the ulnar nerve is confirmed. The median and ulnar nerves are then divided at this level, and the proximal ulnar nerve stump is coapted to the distal median nerve stump. The distal end of the ulnar nerve is then passed subcutaneously across the chest and neck to the contralateral C7 nerve root.

The ulnar nerve supplied by the superior ulnar collateral artery has become well accepted as either a free or pedicled vascularized nerve graft for reconstruction of patients with irreversible nerve injuries such as C8 and T1 root avulsions (36). Terzis et al. reported 151 reconstructions using a vascularized ulnar nerve graft for traumatic brachial plexus palsy. They concluded that vascularized ulnar nerve grafting is an appropriate solution for brachial plexus injuries with C8 and T1 root avulsion, with outcomes that are superior to those achieved with conventional nerve grafting (37).

COMPARISON OF RESULTS OF VASCULARIZED NERVE GRAFTS AND CONVENTIONAL NERVE GRAFTS

Several experimental studies have compared the results of vascularized nerve grafts with nonvascularized nerve grafts. Vascularized nerve grafts have been postulated to be superior to conventional nerve grafts, especially in scarred recipient beds with a poor vascular supply. However, the results still remain controversial. Some studies have not found any difference between the results of vascularized and conventional nerve grafting (38,39). On the other hand, some experimental studies have concluded that the results of vascularized nerve grafting are superior to conventional nerve grafting even in normal recipient beds (40,41).

Only two clinical studies have compared the results of vascularized and conventional nerve grafting, and one is a case report. Doi et al. compared the speed of recovery and the long-term outcomes of 27 vascularized and 22 conventional sural nerve grafts in upper extremity injuries. They concluded that vascularized nerve grafting is indicated when the defect is longer than 6 cm, is associated with an extensive skin defect, or nerve grafting is performed after replantation. In all other situations, conventional nerve grafting achieved equally good results (42).

Mackinnon and Kelly reported one patient who underwent simultaneous vascularized and nonvascularized nerve grafting in the same forearm (43). Two branches of the MABCN were identified proximal to the elbow and traced distally. A single sural nerve (as a conventional nonvascularized nerve graft) was used to graft from one branch of the MABCN to the ulnar side of the median nerve at the wrist. The superficial radial nerve (as a vascularized nerve graft) was used to graft from the other branch of the MABCN to the radial aspect of the median nerve. In this unique situation, histologic and clinical evaluations were better for the vascularized nerve graft 2 years after surgery.

Further clinical studies will be necessary to compare the results of vascularized and nonvascularized nerve grafting using small-diameter nerve grafts in a normal recipient bed to confirm the clinical efficacy of vascularized nerve grafting.

TREATMENT OF NEUROMAS

Partial or total transection or traction or chronic compression of a peripheral nerve containing sensory nerve fibers can result in a painful neuroma. The basic principle of treatment of a severed nerve is to coapt the nerve ends with or without an interposition nerve graft to prevent the development of a painful neuroma and to restore function. Although there may be some degree of neuroma formation at the coaptation site, a significant number of nerve fibers will regenerate beyond the repair site to their distal targets if an adequate nerve repair is performed.

Between 10% and 25% of all patients with an amputation injury have chronic stump pain caused by the development of a postamputation neuroma (44). Pain, paresthesias, and a positive Tinel's sign are the common symptoms and signs of a painful postamputation neuroma. A multitude of techniques have been described to solve this difficult problem, suggesting that there is no single definitive treatment method. Watson et al. summarized the current concepts of treatment of neuromas of the hand and upper extremity (45).

If there is an appropriate distal nerve stump and sensory receptors are available, nerve grafting can provide the direction for the regenerating axons from the proximal nerve stump. There may still be some irritation from the local neuroma that forms at the coaptation sites, especially for sensitive sensory nerves such as the superficial radial nerve. Wrapping the nerve coaptation sites with a nerve tube may confine the suture site neuroma to a minimum. If the nerve gap is short (<2 cm), a vein conduit or synthetic nerve tube can be used to bridge the defect. If the nerve gap is longer, an interposition nerve graft may be used to diminish pain and achieve some degree of sensory recovery. Nerve wrapping can be used at the graft coaptation sites to avoid painful suture neuromas. If the distal nerve is not available and sensory recovery is critical, a free neurosensory flap, such as the first web space from the foot, may allow nerve regeneration from the injured proximal sensory nerve into the sensory nerve of the skin flap.

If multiple previous operations have failed to control the pain, the proximal nerve stump is managed in one of four ways, translocation without excision of the neuroma; translocation of the nerve into either bone or muscle, or coverage of the neuroma with a soft tissue flap.

Translocation of the Nerve without Excision of the Neuroma

Herndon et al. described the translocation of an amputation neuroma to an unscarred site where the neuroma would not be irritated when the hand was used and reported excellent results in 82% of patients (46). They carefully isolated the neuroma with its fibrous capsule and its proximal nerve from surrounding scar tissue and translocated it away from local pressure or trauma deep into a muscle or a web space or between the shafts of the metacarpals without any tension on the nerve. A dorsal location is preferable to a palmar location to avoid pressure on the neuroma with normal activity of the hand. A fine absorbable suture is placed through the fibrous capsule (not the neuroma itself) and tied. Another knot is tied 3 to 4 mm away from the neuroma. The free ends of the suture are then tunneled subcutaneously and passed out through the skin with a straight needle proximal to the new location selected for the neuroma. The second knot remains deep to the dermis, ensuring that the neuroma is at least 3 to 4 mm below the surface of the skin. The proximal nerve trunk is carefully examined to make certain that there is no tension or twisting along its new course.

Translocation of the Nerve Into Bone

Translocating a neuroma into the medullary cavity of bone is one of the oldest techniques (47,48). The logic underlying this procedure is to contain the nerve stump within a hard compartment, to restrict the size of the neuroma, and to protect it from external irritation. Specific details include adequate mobilization of the proximal nerve, avoiding tension on the transposed nerve, avoiding implantation just distal to a joint, and securing the translocated neuroma at its entrance into the bone. The author believes that this technique is one of the most reliable procedures to treat painful neuromas.

Translocation of the Nerve Into Muscle

Prevention of neuroma formation after excision of a painful neuroma by implantation into muscle was reported in a rabbit model by Teneff in 1949 (49), but Moszkowicz had already reported the first clinical case treated in this way in 1918 (50). Dellon and Mackinnon implanted the superficial radial nerve into the undersurface of the brachioradialis muscle after first resecting the neuroma and then dissecting the nerve proximally enough to avoid any tension on the transferred nerve (51). They reported good to excellent pain relief in 82% of patients. The pronator quadratus muscle can be used similarly for implantation of a neuroma of the palmar cutaneous branch of the median nerve. This technique is one of the most widely used surgical procedures to treat painful neuromas.

Coverage of the Neuroma with a Vascularized Soft Tissue Flap

Coverage of painful neuromas or neuromas in continuity with vascularized flaps, such as the hypothenar fat flap, reverse pedicled Becker flap, or reverse radial forearm fascial flap or even free flaps, have been reported to be effective for pain relief of difficult problems such as recalcitrant carpal tunnel syndrome, which presents with a painful neuroma in continuity–like condition (52). Coverage of a painful neuroma of the palmar cutaneous branch of the median nerve with a pedicled pronator quadratus muscle flap may be similar, although the effect may be due more to implantation of the neuroma into muscle.

REFERENCES

1. Waller A. Experiments on the section of the glossopharyngeal and hypoglossal nerves of the frog, and observations of the alterations produced thereby in the structure of their primitive fibres. *Philos Trans R Soc London* 1850;140:423–429.
2. Naff NJ, Ecklund JM. History of peripheral nerve surgery techniques. *Neurosurg Clin North Am* 2001;12:197–209.
3. Tinel J. *Nerve Wounds*. New York: W Wood & Co., 1918, p. 317.
4. Highet WB, Holmes W. Traction injuries to the lateral popliteal nerve and traction injuries to peripheral nerves after future. *Br J Surg* 1943;30:212.
5. Seddon HJ. The use of autogenous grafts for the repair of large gaps in peripheral nerves. *Br J Surg* 1947;35:151.
6. Sunderland S. A classification of peripheral nerve injuries producing loss of function. *Brain* 1951;74(4):491–516.
7. Smith JW. Microsurgery of peripheral nerves. *Plast Reconstr Surg* 1964;33:317.
8. Millesi H, Meissl G, Berger A. The interfascicular nerve-grafting of the median and ulnar nerves. *J Bone Joint Surg Am* 1972;54(4):727–750.
9. Kline DG, Hackett ER, May PR. Evaluation of nerve injuries by evoked potentials and electromyography. *J Neurosurg* 1969;31:128.
10. Oberlin C, Beal D, Leechavengvongs S, et al. Nerve transfer to biceps muscle using a part of ulnar nerve for C5–C6 avulsion of the brachial plexus: anatomical study and report of four cases. *J Hand Surg Am* 1994;19:232–237.
11. Kennedy R. On the restoration of coordinated movement after nerve crossing with interchange of function of the cerebral cortical centers. *Phil Trans R Soc Lond (Biol)* 1901;194:127–162.

12. May M, Sobol SM, Mester SJ. Hypoglossal-facial nerve interpositional-jump graft for facial reanimation without tongue atrophy. *Otolaryngol Head Neck Surg* 1991;104:818–825.
13. Viterbo F, Trindade JC, Hoshino K, Mazzoni Neto A. Latero-terminal neurorrhaphy without removal of the epineurial sheath: experimental study in rats. *Rev Paul Med* 1992;110:267–275.
14. Oyamatsu H, Koga D, Igarashi M, et al. Morphological assessment of early axonal regeneration in end-to-side nerve coaptation models. *J Plast Surg Hand Surg* 2012;46(5):299–307.
15. Gaudet AD, Popovich PG, Ramer MS. Wallerian degeneration: gaining perspective on inflammatory events after peripheral nerve injury. *J Neuroinflammation* 2011;8:110–123.
16. Rotshenker S. Wallerian degeneration: the innate-immune response to traumatic nerve injury. *J Neuroinflammation* 2011;8:109–113.
17. Dahlin LB. The role of timing in nerve reconstruction. *Int Rev Neurobiol* 2013;109:151–164.
18. Sunderland S. The intraneural topography of the radial, median and ulnar nerves. *Brain* 1945;68:243–298.
19. Jabaley ME, Wallace WH, Heckler FR. Internal topography of major nerves of the forearm and hand: a current view. *J Hand Surg* 1980;5:1–18.
20. Chow JA, Van Beek AL, Bilos ZJ, et al. Anatomical basis for repair of ulnar and median nerves in the distal part of the forearm by group fascicle suture and nerve-grafting. *J Bone Joint Surg Am* 1986;68:273–280.
21. Hasegawa J, Shibata M, Takahashi H. Nerve coaptation studies with and without a gap in rabbits. *J Hand Surg Am* 1996;24(2):259–265.
22. Lundborg G, Rosén B, Dahlin L, et al. Tubular repair of the median or ulnar nerve in the human forearm: a 5-year follow-up. *J Hand Surg Br* 2004;29:100–107.
23. Sameem M, Wood TJ, Bain JR. A systematic review on the use of fibrin glue for peripheral nerve repair. *Plast Reconstr Surg* 2011;127:2381–2390.
24. Isaacs JE, McDaniel CO, Owen JR, Wayne JS. Comparative analysis of biomechanical performance of available "nerve glues." *J Hand Surg Am* 2008;33:893–899.
25. Nishimura MT, Mazzer N, Barbieri CH, Moro CA. Mechanical resistance of peripheral nerve repair with biological glue and with conventional suture at different postoperative times. *J Reconstr Microsurg* 2008;24: 327–332.
26. Shibata M, Ogishyo N. Free flaps based on the anterior interosseous artery. *Plast Reconstr Surg* 1996;97(4):746–755.
27. Paprottka FJ, Wolf P, Harder Y, et al. Sensory recovery outcome after digital nerve repair in relation to different reconstructive techniques: meta-analysis and systematic review. *Plast Surg Int* 2013;2013:704589.
28. Strange FG. An operation for nerve pedicle grafting: preliminary communication. *Br J Surg* 1947;34:423–425.
29. Millesi H. Nerve transplantation for reconstruction of peripheral nerves injured by the use of the microsurgical technic. *Minerva Chir* 1967;15:22(17):950–951.
30. Millesi H, Milessi G, Berger A. Further experience with interfascicular grafting of the median, ulnar and radial nerves. *J Bone Joint Surg Am* 1976;58:209.
31. Taylor GI, Ham FJ. The free vascularized nerve graft. A further experimental and clinical application of microvascular techniques. *Plast Reconstr Surg* 1976;57:413–426.
32. Riedl O, Frey M. Anatomy of the sural nerve: cadaver study and literature review. *Plast Reconstr Surg* 2013;131(4):802–810.
33. Birch R. *Green's Operative Hand Surgery*, 6th ed. Wolfe SW, Pederson WC, Hotchkiss RN, Kozin SH (eds). St. Louis: Elsevier, 2011, p. 1052.
34. Leclère FM, Eggli S, Mathys L, Vögelin E. Anatomic study of the superficial sural artery and its implication in the neurocutaneous vascularized sural nerve free flap. *Clin Anat* 2012 Mar 29. doi: 10.1002/ca.22054. [Epub ahead of print].
35. Greenberg BM, Cuadros CL, Panda M, May JW. St. Clair Strange procedure: indications, technique, and long-term evaluation. *J Hand Surg Am* 1988;13A:928–935.
36. Birch R, Dunkerton M, Bonney G, Jamieson AM. Experience with the free vascularized ulnar nerve graft in repair of supraclavicular lesions of the brachial plexus. *Clin Orthop Relat Res* 1988;237:96–104.
37. Terzis JK, Kostopoulos VK. Vascularized ulnar nerve graft: 151 reconstructions for posttraumatic brachial plexus palsy. *Plast Reconstr Surg* 2009;123(4):1276–1291.
38. Settergren CR, Wood MB. Comparison of blood flow in free vascularized versus nonvascularized nerve grafts. *J Reconstr Microsurg* 1984;1:95–101.
39. Iwai M, Tamai S, Yajima H, et al. Experimental study of vascularized nerve graft: evaluation of nerve regeneration using choline acetyltransferase activity. *Microsurgery* 2001;21:43–51.
40. Shibata M, Tsai TM, Firrell J, et al. Experimental comparison of vascularized and nonvascularized nerve grafting. *J Hand Surg Am* 1988;13:358–365.
41. Koshima I, Harii K. Experimental study of vascularized nerve grafts: morphometric study of axonal regeneration of nerves transplanted into silicone tubes. *Ann Plast Surg* 1985;14:235–243.
42. Doi K, Tamaur K, Sakai K, et al. A comparison of vascularized and conventional sural nerve grafts. *J Hand Surg* 1992;17A:670–676.
43. Mackinnon S, Kelly L, Hunter DA. Comparison of regeneration across a vascularized versus conventional nerve graft: case report. *Microsurgery* 1983;9:226–233.
44. Ducic I, Mesbahi AN, Attinger CE, Graw K. The role of peripheral nerve surgery in the treatment of chronic pain associated with amputation stumps. *Plast Reconstr Surg* 2008;121:908.
45. Watson J, Gonzalez M, Romero A, Kerns J. Neuromas of the hand and upper extremity. *J Hand Surg* 2010;35A:499–510.
46. Herndon JH, Eaton RG, Littler JW. Management of painful neuromas in the hand. *J Bone Joint Surg* 1976;58A:369–373.
47. Mass DP, Ciano MC, Tortosa R, et al. Treatment of painful hand neuromas by their transfer into bone. *Plast Reconstr Surg* 1984;74:182–185.
48. Goldstein SA, Sturim HS. Intraosseous nerve transposition for treatment of painful neuromas. *J Hand Surg Am* 1985;10(2):270–274.
49. Teneff S. Prevention of amputation neuroma. *J Int Coll Surg* 1949;12(1):16–20.
50. Moszkowicz L. Zur Behandlung der schmerzhaften neuroma. *Zentralbl. Chir* 1918;45:547.
51. Dellon AL, Mackinnon SE. Treatment of the painful neuroma by neuroma resection and muscle implantation. *Plast Reconstr Surg* 1986;77:427–438.
52. Becker C, Gilbert A. The ulnar flap. *Handchir Mikrochir Plast Chir* 1988;20(4):180–183.

CHAPTER 69

End-to-Side Nerve Repair

Fausto Viterbo

End-to-end neurorrhaphy describes the coaptation of a proximal nerve stump to the distal nerve stump using sutures or fibrin glue. This type of repair can only be performed if the proximal and distal nerve stumps are close to each other. Otherwise, nerve grafts are necessary when there is a segmental defect between the proximal and distal nerve stumps. Occasionally, the proximal nerve stump is not available, so a nerve transfer is performed. A branch of an adjacent nerve is divided and sutured end-to-end to the distal nerve stump. The nerve to be sacrificed is always chosen so that the muscles or sensory distribution it innervates are less important than the muscles or sensory distribution that requires reinnervation. An example is the "hypoglossal–facial" nerve transfer for the treatment of facial palsy, in which the hypoglossal nerve is divided and the proximal hypoglossal nerve is sutured to the distal facial nerve stump. Facial tone is improved, but part of the tongue atrophies. If the proximal nerve stump is not available or the necessary nerve graft would be too long, another recent option is an end-to-side neurorrhaphy without dividing the donor nerve. This neurorrhaphy can either be end-to-side or side-to-end.

Ballance et al. (1) performed the first side-to-end nerve repair in 1895 for a patient with facial nerve palsy. The distal stump of the facial nerve was sutured into an incision made on the lateral aspect of the spinal accessory nerve. Facial movements returned but were associated with synkinetic shoulder movements. Balance et al. (1) and Harris and Low (2) also described this side-to-end neurorrhaphy not only for facial palsy but also for upper brachial plexus avulsions. Sherren (3) described using the hypoglossal nerve for this end-to-side neurorrhaphy; however, the inconvenience of associated synkinetic movements remained in this case between the tongue and the face. Sherren also recommended making a longitudinal or transverse incision in the donor nerve so that the axons of this healthy nerve would be sectioned, allowing contact between the axons of both nerves. Invariably, all of these techniques caused functional impairment in the muscles innervated by the spinal accessory or hypoglossal nerves. Thereafter, except for the publication of Gatta (4), there is a "gap" in the literature, with no reports on this subject until 1989 when Krivolutskaia et al. (5) treated facial palsy by end-to-side neurorrhaphy with scarification of the lateral aspect of the donor nerve using a needle tip and reported complete functional rehabilitation in four of seven patients. May et al. (6) interposed a nerve graft connecting the distal stump of the injured facial nerve to the hypoglossal nerve after producing a partial incision but avoiding complete transection of the hypoglossal nerve, but this still resulted in complete atrophy of the hemitongue.

All of these techniques involved a lateral incision in the donor nerve before suture of the recipient nerve (Figure 69-1). These incisions (1,3,6), or scarification (5) in the lateral aspect of the donor nerve, allowed the divided axons to sprout inside the recipient nerve, producing an ETS connection between the endoneurial tubes of both nerves (Figure 69-2). However, the muscles or sensory distribution innervated by the donor nerve may be compromised.

Viterbo et al. (7) introduced the end-to-side technique without any incision in the donor nerve, thereby avoiding impairment to this donor nerve. In experimental studies in rats, they divided the peroneal nerve and sutured the distal stump to the lateral aspect of the intact tibial nerve without removing any epineurium (Figures 69-3 to 69-5). For the first time, they achieved muscle reinnervation without impairment to the donor nerve. Therefore, they identified a new phenomenon, the growth of axons from an intact donor nerve into the distal stump of a recipient nerve. This research resulted in controversial discussions about whether an intact axon can induce lateral sprouting across a barrier of epineurium, perineurium, and endoneurium. A subsequent repercussion of this research was that any nerve could potentially be used as a donor nerve, introducing exciting new surgical possibilities.

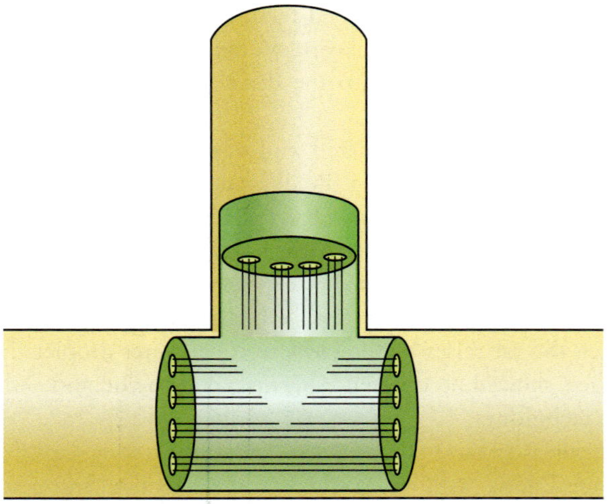

FIGURE 69-1 Balance's end-to-side neurorrhaphy. An incision is made in the donor nerve itself, not just an epineurial window.

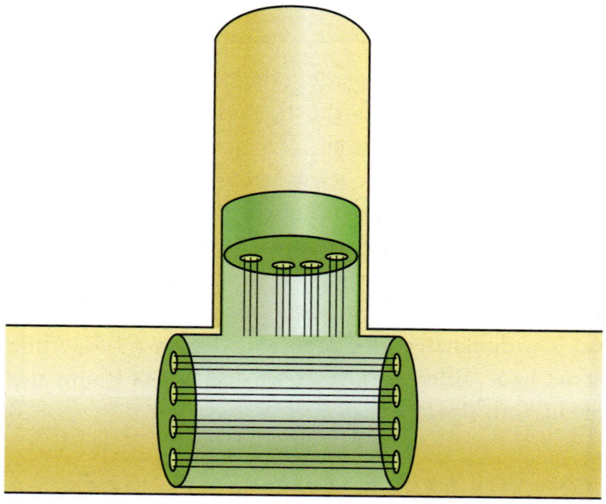

FIGURE 69-4 Viterbo's end-to-side neurorrhaphy. In thicker nerves, an epineurial–perineurial window is made.

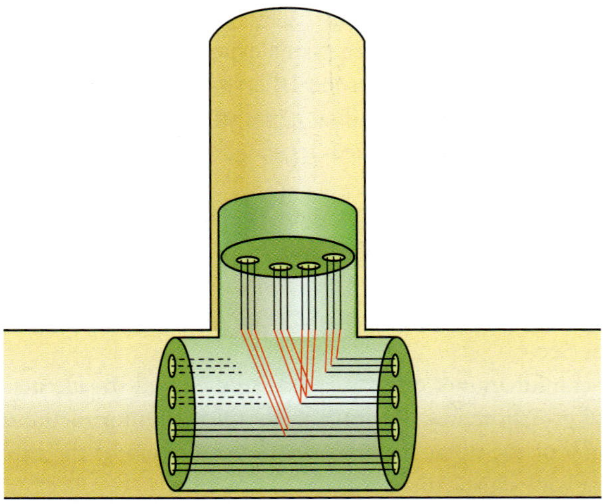

FIGURE 69-2 Balance's end-to-side neurorrhaphy may allow end-to-end interface between donor and recipient endoneurial tubes.

In 1994, Viterbo et al. (8,9) described the same experimental model but used an epineurial–perineurial window and two ETS neurorrhaphies of a nerve graft to connect the tibial nerve and the distal stump of the peroneal nerve. According to Viterbo et al. (7,8), end-to-side neurorrhaphy allows axons from the donor nerve to sprout inside the distal stump of the recipient nerve, reinnervating previously denervated muscles but without harming muscles innervated by the donor nerve. Axonal sprouting after end-to-side neurorrhaphy, with or without removing an epineurial window, has been confirmed by several authors (10–17) and several studies have demonstrated the effectiveness of end-to-side neurorrhaphy in reinnervating previously paralyzed muscles controlled by the recipient nerve. However, little is known about deficits that can occur in the donor nerve, as well as to the muscles innervated by the donor nerve.

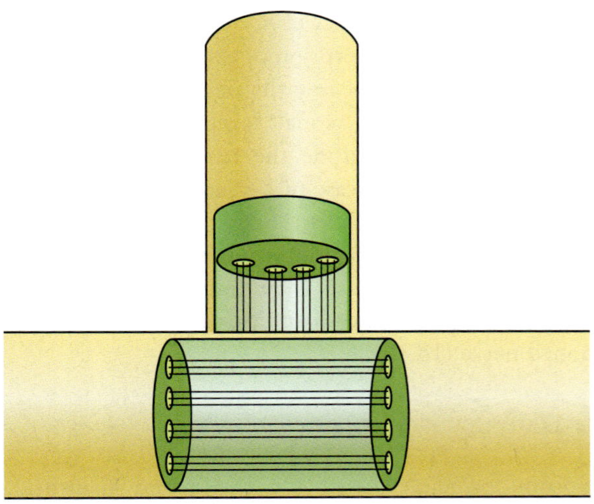

FIGURE 69-3 Viterbo's end-to-side neurorrhaphy. In thin nerves, the epineurium and perineurium are not removed, and no epineurial window or incision is made into the donor nerve.

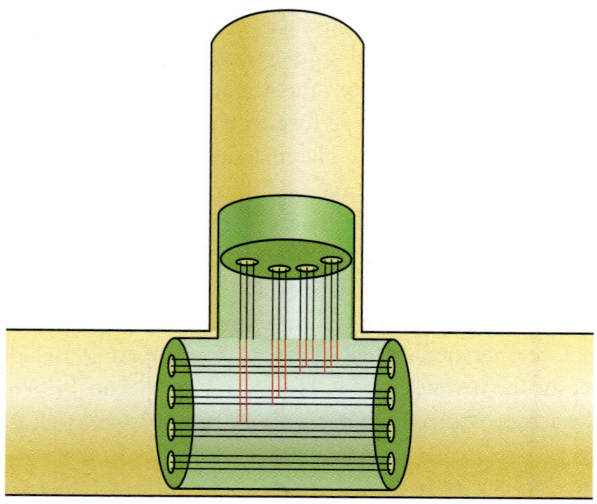

FIGURE 69-5 In Viterbo's end-to-side neurorrhaphy, axons sprout laterally from the donor nerve to reach the recipient nerve. There is no injury to the axons in the donor nerve.

NOMENCLATURE

There are controversies regarding the nomenclature in the end-to-side or side-to-end in the literature. Ballance et al. (1) described the technique as an ETS anastomosis. Viterbo et al. (8–10) have used both the terms latero-terminal neurorrhaphy (side-to-end) and ETS according to the donor and recipient nerves. If the donor nerve is sutured to the lateral aspect of the recipient nerve, the term *end-to-side* is used (Figure 69-4). If the recipient nerve is sutured to the lateral aspect of the donor nerve, it is designated as side-to-end (Figure 69-5). Although there are basic differences, the term *end-to-side* is now used to represent both situations.

SELECTIVE EXPERIMENTAL STUDIES

Viterbo et al. (7) introduced the experimental model of "tibial–peroneal nerve and tibial cranial muscle" in rats. The peroneal nerve was divided and its distal nerve stump sutured to the lateral aspect of the intact tibial nerve without performing an epineurial window in the donor tibial nerve. The tibial cranial muscle is innervated exclusively by the peroneal nerve and is palpable, enabling clinical monitoring of the end-to-side neurorrhaphy. A possible explanation of the end-to-side phenomenon without a deliberate epineurial window in the donor nerve is the possibility of axonal sprouting from the proximal stump of the peroneal nerve to the distal stump of the peroneal nerve, the phenomenon of "motor contamination." To prevent the possibility of motor contamination of the distal peroneal nerve as a result of axonal sprouting from the proximal peroneal nerve stump, Viterbo et al. (7) buried the proximal stump of the peroneal nerve in the adjacent muscle. The same authors published a similar study in 1994 (8) but with an epineurial–perineurial window in the donor tibial nerve and without injuring the endoneurial tubes within the tibial nerve.

Lundborg et al. (10) divided the peroneal nerve, and after a 7-day period of predegeneration, the distal stump of this nerve was sutured end-to-side to the tibial nerve. After 90 days, electrophysiologic stimulation of the tibial nerve proximal to the end-to-side neurorrhaphy produced contraction of the gastrocnemius and cranial tibial muscles, suggesting lateral axonal sprouting had occurred from the donor to the recipient nerve.

Matsumoto et al. (11) performed end-to-side neurorrhaphy in a Y-shaped silicone tube. The intact tibial nerve was placed in the proximal silicone tube and exited from one of the two distal bifurcations. The distal stump of the peroneal nerve was inserted in the other distal bifurcation, leaving a 1-mm gap between the distal stump of the peroneal nerve and the tibial nerve. Twenty-one days after surgery, 66% of the animals demonstrated sensory axonal regeneration across the gap, reinnervating the distal stump of the peroneal nerve. However, motor axonal regeneration was not observed in any animal even 12 weeks after the surgery.

In a similar study, Akeda et al. (12) performed ETS coaptation using a T-shaped silicone tube. The tibial nerve was inserted into the transverse limb of the T, and the distal stump of the divided peroneal nerve was inserted into the vertical stem of the tube and positioned end-to-side to the tibial nerve without sutures or an epineurial window. Six weeks after the surgery, axons had regenerated into the distal stump of the peroneal nerve.

Liao et al. (13) evaluated end-to-end versus end-to-side neurorrhaphy in rats using the ulnar nerve as the donor nerve and the musculocutaneous nerve as the recipient nerve. The end-to-end technique resulted in faster and better restoration of muscle strength and better electrophysiologic results. However, the "grooming test," which is a functional test in which the rat raises its forepaws to clean water droplets from its face, showed no difference between end-to-end and end-to-side techniques.

Lykissas et al. (14) repaired 6- and 12-mm-long gaps in the peroneal nerve with a nerve graft and two end-to-end neurorrhaphies and compared this technique with a "bypass" nerve graft with two end-to-side neurorrhaphies above and below the defect. After 5 months, walking track analysis and axon counts showed no difference between these two techniques. They suggested that this bypass graft with two end-to-side neurorrhaphies could be considered in patients with long nerve gaps.

Jaberi et al. (15) used the same experimental design in rabbits by sectioning the peroneal nerve and suturing its distal stump end-to-side to the tibial nerve after removing an epineurial window and confirmed regenerating axons in the distal peroneal nerve.

Mennen (16) investigated end-to-side neurorrhaphy in primates by dividing the ulnar nerve and suturing its distal stump end-to-side to the intact median nerve and observed lateral sprouting from the median nerve to the distal stump of the ulnar nerve.

Schmidhammer et al. (17) also studied end-to-side neurorrhaphy in primates by suturing the distal stump of the deep branch of the ulnar nerve to the motor branch of the median nerve with satisfactory results.

These initial findings have been confirmed in rats, rabbits, and primates with ongoing investigation of the mechanism of axonal sprouting, including whether there is selective sensory or motor sprouting, whether an epineurial–perineurial window is necessary and whether there is downgrading of the donor nerve and the influence of nerve growth factors (10–17). It is now known that absorption of the epineurium and perineurium occurs after some months and then axonal sprouting starts laterally (14,18). Axonal sprouting from inside the intact donor nerve to inside the recipient nerve probably occurs because of the release of nerve growth factors. Direct contact between the recipient nerve stump and the intact donor nerve allows interaction between the Schwann cells of both nerves, which increases the production of nerve growth factors, which induce and direct axonal sprouting inside the sectioned nerve (18,19).

TECHNICAL CONSIDERATIONS

The same principles used for end-to-end neurorrhaphy should be strictly applied to end-to-side neurorrhaphy. Magnification, microsurgical instruments, and gentle handling are mandatory. Epineurial coaptation is performed with

8-0 to 10-0 microsutures depending on the size of the nerves. Important technical points to be considered specific to end-to-side neurorrhaphy are:

1. The recipient nerve should be coapted perpendicular to the donor nerve. Any obliquity in the relationship is indicative of tension (Figure 69-6A).
2. The surgeon must ensure proper contact of the recipient nerve to the donor nerve (Figures 69-6B and 69-6C).
3. The needle should be passed carefully to include only the epineurium.
4. The number of microsutures depends on perfect coaptation and ranges from two to four microsutures.
5. If there is a discrepancy in the diameter of the donor and recipient nerves (e.g., a small donor with larger recipient), instead of placing sutures in the donor epineurium, sutures can be placed in the soft tissues surrounding the donor nerve in order not to injure the axons of the donor nerve.
6. Whether to perform an epineurial–perineurial window or not depends mainly on the size of the nerve. We recommend performing an epineurial window only in nerves with a diameter greater than 1.5 to 2 mm. For example, it is not necessary to make a window in branches of the facial nerve, but a window is necessary in the brachial plexus trunks or nerves.
7. In some situations, the donor nerve lies deeply, which makes an end-to-side neurorrhaphy difficult. We recommend using a single "embracing" suture. The needle is first passed through the epineurium of the recipient nerve followed by passing the needle completely around the perimeter of the donor nerve. The needle is then passed back through the epineurium of the recipient nerve 180 degrees opposite to

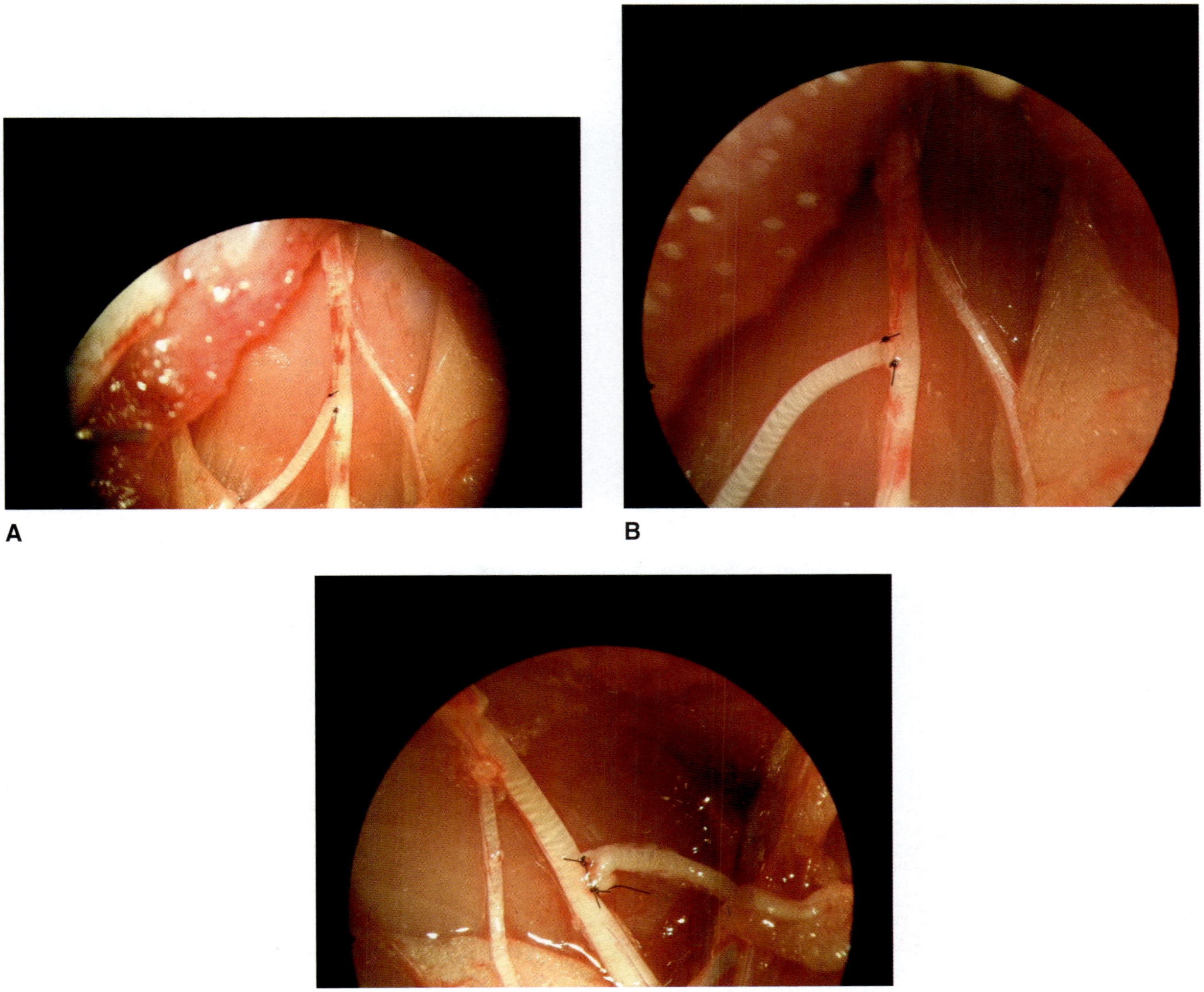

A B C

FIGURE 69-6 (A) End-to-side neurorrhaphy with an unfavorable oblique angle between the recipient nerve and the donor nerve, indicative of tension at the site of repair despite good coaptation. (B) Properly coapted end-to-side neurorrhaphy, in which the recipient nerve is oriented perpendicular to the donor nerve without tension and with good contact between them. (C) Unfavorable end-to-side neurorrhaphy with improper coaptation and inadequate contact of the recipient nerve to the donor nerve.

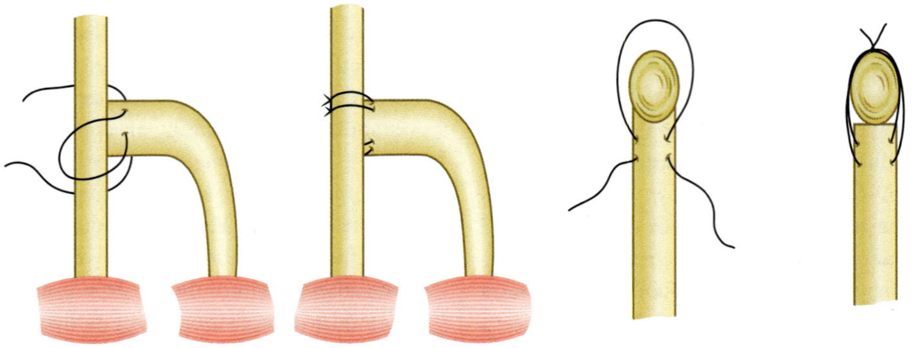

FIGURE 69-7 End-to-side neurorrhaphy with one "embracing" nylon suture.

the previous suture pass before the two suture ends are tied around the outside of the donor nerve, not too tightly and not too loosely, just to coapt the recipient nerve against the side of the donor nerve (Figure 69-7).

8. Although fibrin glue is used in end-to-end neurorrhaphy, we do not recommend its use in end-to-side neurorrhaphy.

CLINICAL APPLICATIONS

End-to-side neurorrhaphy has been used for many clinical applications with satisfactory results (19–33), but some authors have reported poor results (14,34–37).

Facial Nerve Palsy

Traditional cross-face nerve grafting is usually performed using two end-to-end neurorrhaphies (38). A disadvantage is that a branch of the facial nerve on the healthy side has to be divided to act as the donor nerve. If too many branches are divided, the patient will develop bilateral facial palsy (Figure 69-8).

Viterbo (39,40) proposed a cross-face nerve graft with two end-to-side neurorrhaphies for the treatment of facial palsy. In this technique, the right and left facial nerve trunks are identified through bilateral preauricular incisions. The buccal or zygomatic branches (or both) can be bridged to each other using sural nerve grafts coapted by end-to-side neurorrhaphies (Figure 69-9).

Samii et al. (21) performed end-to-side sural nerve grafts after resection of a schwannoma of the facial nerve, with satisfactory function 18 months later.

Frey et al. (41) treated seven patients with facial nerve palsy using a cross-face nerve graft end-to-end into a healthy zygomatic nerve branch and end-to-side into the corresponding branch on the side with incomplete facial nerve palsy. Three of seven patients achieved functional improvement as well as static and dynamic symmetry.

Yamamoto et al. (25) reported nine patients with facial nerve palsy reinnervated from the opposite hypoglossal and facial nerves with improvement in House-Brackmann scores. Postoperative electromyography showed dual innervation of the

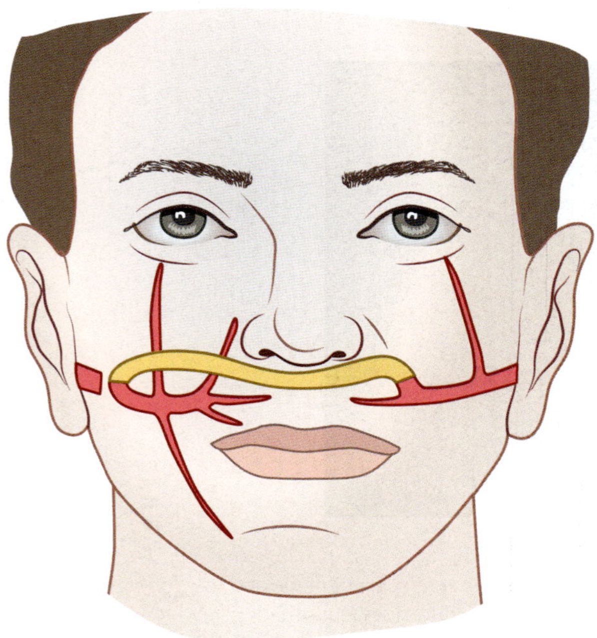

FIGURE 69-8 Scaramella's end-to-end cross-face nerve graft.

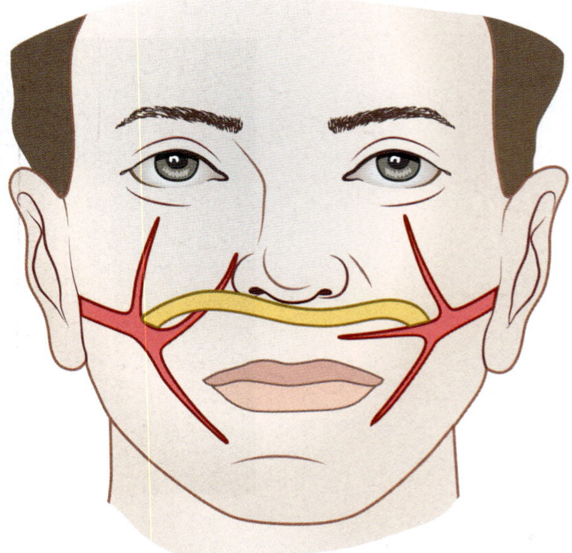

FIGURE 69-9 Viterbo's end-to-side cross-face nerve graft. Theoretically, a larger number of nerve fibers can be transferred across the face, and the procedure can be performed early.

paralyzed face from the opposite facial nerve or hypoglossal nerve. No patients developed hemitongue atrophy or synkinesis associated with tongue movement.

Labbé (42) described neurotization of a temporalis muscle elongation by end-to-side sural nerve grafts in an attempt to achieve a spontaneous smile. The sural nerve graft was sutured end-to-side to the buccal branch of the normal facial nerve, and the distal end of the sural nerve graft was sutured end-to-end to the distal stump of one of the three branches that innervates the temporalis muscle.

Viterbo (43) has combined cross-face end-to-side sural nerve grafts with an ipsilateral temporalis muscle flap, in which the cross face nerve graft neurotized the temporalis muscle with good results (Figures 69-10 and 11).

Upper Extremity

Viterbo et al. (44) published a clinical case report of a patient with a complete upper root brachial plexus avulsion for 6 years treated by end-to-side nerve grafts bridging the phrenic nerve to the C5 to C6 nerve roots. One year after surgery, electrophysiologic studies demonstrated reinnervation in the triceps, pectoralis major, and infraspinatus but no return of muscle contraction.

Franciosi et al. (45) treated five patients with brachial plexus avulsions of the C5, C6, and C7 roots by end-to-side neurorrhaphy between the proximal ulnar nerve and the musculocutaneous nerve, resulting in return of biceps muscle contraction within 6 months in all patients.

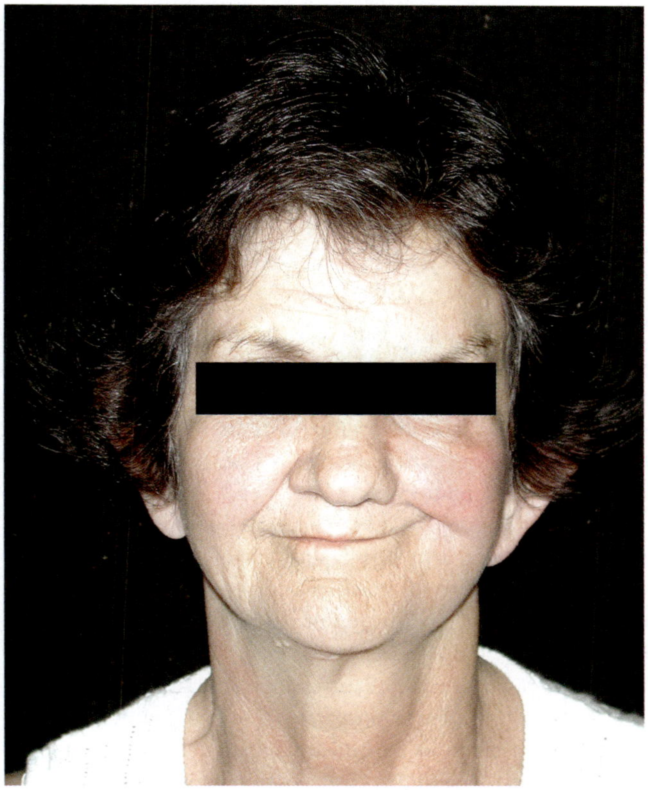

FIGURE 69-11 Postoperative result.

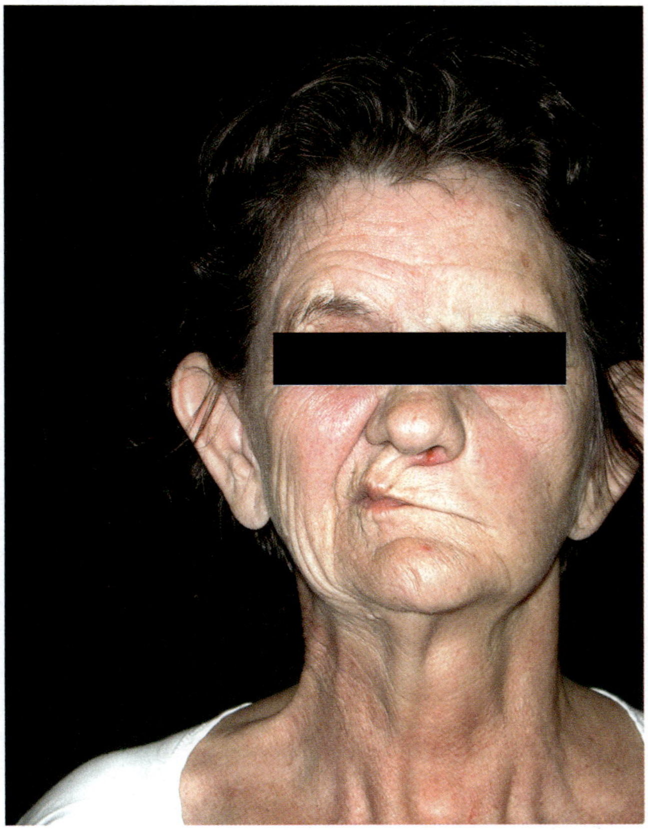

FIGURE 69-10 Facial palsy in a 59-year-old woman 8 months after resection of an acoustic neuroma. She underwent a buccal–buccal end-to-side cross-face sural nerve graft and an ipsilateral temporalis muscle transfer elongated with fascia lata.

Mennen (46) used end-to-side neurorrhaphy for reconstruction of brachial plexus injuries and concluded that the technique was simple, produced satisfactory results, and was preferable to nerve grafts in most cases.

However, Bertelli and Ghizoni (35) failed to achieve any motor recovery in C5 to C6 root avulsions after performing an end-to-side neurorrhaphy with an epineurial window to the radial nerve.

Amr et al. (28) treated five patients with brachial plexus injuries, one C5 and C6 rupture; one C7, C8, and T1 avulsion; and three complete C5, C6, C7, C8, and T1 avulsions. The ruptures were treated by nerve grafts and the avulsions had their roots implanted end-to-side into the spinal cord. After 2 years, two patients achieved M4 shoulder abduction and flexion and elbow flexion and improved pain.

Ray et al. (29) described a C5 to C6 avulsion treated by end-to-side innervation of the suprascapular nerve by the spinal accessory nerve and reported excellent functional recovery of shoulder abduction and flexion and elbow flexion.

For axillary nerve lesions, Viterbo (47) has performed nerve grafts end-to-side to the radial nerve to provide direct muscle neurotization of the deltoid with good results.

Voche and Quattara (48) treated nerve injuries in the palm or digits by end-to-side neurorrhaphy with an epineurial window and claimed that the results of end-to-side neurorrhaphy are comparable to nerve grafts or vein conduits.

Magdi Sherif and Amr (33) reported four median and ulnar nerve lacerations at the wrist level treated by end-to-side nerve grafts between the motor fascicles of the ulnar and median nerves. After 4 months, three of the four patients started to recover movement of the affected hand muscles and electrophysiologic studies confirmed nerve conduction through the nerve grafts.

Battiston et al. (22) performed end-to-side nerve repairs using vein grafts filled with muscle and achieved good results in sensory nerve reconstruction, especially digital nerves.

Restoration of Sensation in the Lower Extremity

To restore sensibility after harvest of the sural nerve, Viterbo et al. (49) repaired the distal stump of the sural nerve end-to-side to the superficial peroneal nerve. Two patients were unable to discriminate any anesthetic area in their foot, demonstrating that this technique prevents the loss of sensation caused by harvesting the sural nerve.

Kalbermatten et al. (26) randomly divided 30 patients undergoing lateral arm free flap coverage of the lower leg into two groups. The lateral brachial cutaneous nerve was sutured end-to-side to the lateral aspect of the tibial nerve in one group, but patients in the second control group did not undergo any nerve repair. One year after surgery, pain, temperature sensibility, two-point discrimination, and Semmes-Weinstein testing findings were better in the end-to-side group.

Viterbo and Ripari (50) treated two patients with paraplegia by bridging the intercostal nerves above the spinal cord injury and the sciatic nerve below with two sural nerve grafts repaired end-to-side. Both patients showed improved sensation and did not develop pressure ulcers (Figure 69-12).

Restoration of Sensation in the Breast

Slezac et al. (51) attempted to restore sensibility to the reconstructed breast by reinnervating a transverse rectus abdominis myocutaneous (TRAM) flap using an end-to-end nerve repair between the 11th and 12th intercostal nerves and the lateral cutaneous intercostal nerves.

Doncatto et al. (52) attempted reinnervation of the reconstructed breast by end-to-side neurorrhaphy of one or both 11th intercostal nerves to the lateral surface of the fourth, fifth, sixth, or seventh intercostal nerves. A total of 81.5% of the end-to-side patients achieved superficial touch, but only 11.5% of the noninnervated patients regained this degree of sensibility.

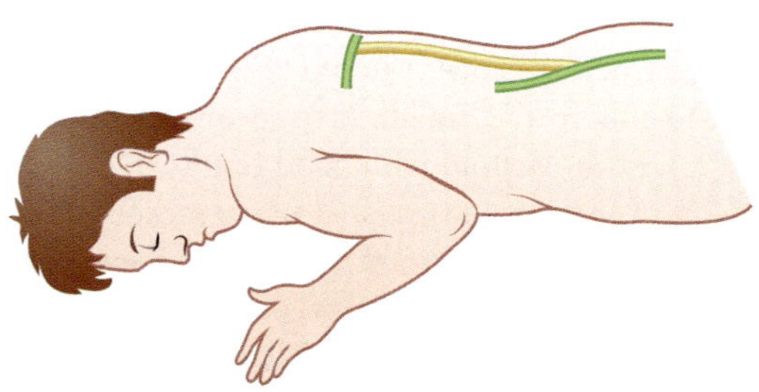

FIGURE 69-12 Pressure ulcers in a paraplegic could potentially be prevented by two end-to-side sural nerve grafts between the intercostal nerves above the spinal cord injury and the sciatic nerve.

THE FUTURE

End-to-side neurorrhaphy has an enormous potential to be applied to a variety of nerve injuries and conditions. The absence of any damage to the donor nerve means that any nerve can be considered as a potential donor nerve and allows early surgery to be performed to prevent muscle atrophy. Future research will provide a better understanding of the role of nerve growth factors and enzymes in end-to-side nerve repair.

REFERENCES

1. Ballance CA, Ballance HA, Stewart P. Remarks on the operative treatment of chronic facial palsy of peripheral origin. *Br Med J* 1903;2:1009–1013.
2. Harris W, Low VW. On the importance of accurate muscular analysis in lesions of the brachial plexus and the treatment of Erb's palsy and infantile paralysis of the upper extremity by cross-union of the nerve roots. *Br Med J* 1903;24:1035–1038.
3. Sherren J. Some points in the surgery of the peripheral nerves. *Edinb Med J* 1906;20:297–332.
4. Gatta R. Sulla anastomosi latero-terminale dei tronchi nervosi. *Arch Ita Chir* 1938;48:155–171.
5. Krivolutskaia EG, Chumasov EI, Matina VN, et al. End-to-side type of plastic repair of the facial nerve branches. *Stomatologiia (Mosk)* 1989;68(6):35–38.
6. May M, Sobol SM, Mester SJ. Hypoglossal-facial nerve interpositional-jump graft for facial reanimation without tongue atrophy. *Otolaryngol Head Neck Surg* 1991;104(6):818–825.
7. Viterbo F, Trindade JC, Hoshino K, Mazzoni A. Latero-terminal neurorrhaphy without removal of the epineural sheath: experimental study in rats. *São Paulo Med J* 1992;110:267–275.
8. Viterbo F, Trindade JC, Hoshimo K, Netto AM. End-to side neurorrhaphy with removal of epineural sheath; an experimental study in rats. *Plast Reconstr Surg* 1994;94(7):1038–1047.
9. Viterbo F, Trindade JC, Hoshino K, Neto AM. Two end-to-side neurorhaphies and nerve graft whit removal of the epineural sheath: experimental study in rats. *Br J Plast Surg* 1994;47:75–80.
10. Lundborg G, Zhao Q, Kanje M, et al. Can sensory and motor collateral sprouting be induced from intact peripheral nerve by end-to-side anastomosis? *J Hand Surg Br* 1994;19(3):277–282.
11. Matsumoto M, Hirata H, Nishiyama M, et al. Schawnn cells can induce collateral sprouting from intact axons: a experimental study of end-to-side neurorrhaphy using a Y-chamber model. *J Reconstr Microsurg* 1999;15: 281–286.
12. Akeda K, Hirata H, Matsumoto M, et al. Regenerating axons emerge far proximal to the coaptation site in end-to-side nerve coaptation without a perineurial window using a T-sharped chamber. *Plast Reconstr Surg* 2006;117(4):1194–1203.
13. Liao WC, Chen JR, Wang YJ, Tseng GF. The efficacy of end-to-end and end-to-side nerve repair (neurorrhaphy) in the rat brachial plexus. *J Anat* 2009;215(5):506–521.
14. Beris A, Lykissas M, Korompilias A, Mitsionis G. End-to-side nerve repair in peripheral nerve injury. *J Neurotrauma* 2007;24(5):909–916.
15. Jaberi FM, Abbas BP, Nezhad ST, Tanideh N. End-to-side neurorrhaphy: an experimental study in rabbits. *Microsurgery* 2003;23:359–362.
16. Mennen U. End-to-side nerve suture in primate (Chacma Baboon). *Hand Surg* 1998;21:1.
17. Schmidhammer R, Redl H, Hopf R, et al. Synergistic terminal motor end-to-side nerve graft repair: investigation in a non-human primate model. *Acta Neurochir Suppl* 2007;100:97–101.
18. Brenner MJ, Dvali L, Hunter DA, et al. Motor neuron regeneration through end-to-side repairs is a function of donor nerve axotomy. *Plast Reconstr Surg* 2007;120(1):215–223.
19. Hayashi A, Yana A, Komuro Y, et al. Collateral sprouting occurs following end-to-side neurorrhaphy. *Plast Reconstr Surg* 2004;114:129–137.
20. Pardini AG Jr, Freitas AD, Plentz EG. Avaliação da sensibilidade após neurorrafia término-lateral de nervos digitais: nota prévia. *Rev Bras Ortop* 2005;40(9):543–554.
21. Geuna S, Papalia I, Tos P. End-to-side (terminolateral) nerve regeneration: a challenge for neuroscientists coming from an intriguing nerve repair concept. *Brain Res Rev* 2006;52(2):381–388.
22. Samii M, Koerbel A, Safavi-Abbasi S, et al. Using an end-to-side interposed sural nerve graft for facial nerve reinforcement after vestibular schwannoma resection. Technical note. *J Neurosurg* 2006;105(6):920–923.

23. Battiston B, Tos P, Conforti LG, Geuna S. Alternative techniques for peripheral nerve repair: conduits and end-to-side neurorrhaphy. *Acta Neurochir Suppl* 2007;100:43–50.
24. Millesi H, Schmidhammer R. Nerve fiber transfer by end-to-side coaptation. *Hand Clin* 2008;24(4):461–483.
25. Papalia I, Cardaci A, D'alcontre FS, et al. Selection of donor nerve for end-to-side neurorrhaphy. *J Neurosurg* 2007;107:378–382.
26. Yamamoto Y, Sekido M, Furukawa H, et al. Surgical rehabilitation of reversible facial palsy: facial—hypoglossal network system based on neural signal augmentation/neural supercharge concept. *J Plast Reconstr Aesthet Surg* 2007;60(3):223–231.
27. Kalbermatten DF, Wettstein R, von Kanel O, et al. Sensate lateral arm flap for defects of the lower leg. *Ann Plast Surg* 2008;61(1):40–46.
28. Pondaag W, Gilbert A. Results of end-to-side nerve coaptation in severe obstetric brachial plexus lesion. *Neurosurgery* 2008;62(3):656–663.
29. Amr SM, Essam AM, Abdel-Meguid AM, et al. Direct cord implantation in brachial plexus avulsions: revised technique using a single stage combined anterior (first) posterior (second) approach and end-to-side side-to-side grafting neurorrhaphy. *J Brachial Plex Peripher Nerve Inj* 2009;19:4–8.
30. Ray WZ, Kasukurthi R, Yee A, Mackinnon SE. Functional recovery following an end to side neurorrhaphy of the accessory nerve to the suprascapular nerve: case report. *Hand (N Y)* 2009;5(3):313–317.
31. Tos P, Artiaco S, Papalia I, et al. End-to-side nerve regeneration: from the laboratory bench to clinical applications. *Int Rev Neurobiol* 2009;87: 281–294.
32. Viterbo F, Amr AH, Stipp EJ, Reis FJ. End-to-side neurorrhaphy: past, present, and future. *Plast Reconstr Surg* 2009;124(6):351e–358e.
33. Frey M, Michaelidou M, Tzou CH, et al. Proven and innovative operative techniques for reanimation of the paralyzed face. *Handchir Mikrochir Plast Chir* 2010;42(2):81–89.
34. Sherif Magdi M, Amr AH. Intrinsic hand muscle reinnervation by median-ulnar end-to-side bridge nerve graft: case report. *J Hand Surg Am* 2010;35(3):446–450.
35. Kayikçioğlu A, Karamürsel S, Ağaoğlu G, et al. End-to-side neurorrhaphies of the ulnar and median nerves at the wrist: report of two cases without sensory or motor improvement. *Ann Plast Surg* 2000;45:641–643.
36. Bertelli JA, Ghizoni MF, Nerve repair by end-to-side coaptation or fascicular transfer: a clinical study. *J Reconstr Microsurg* 2003;19:313–318.
37. Pannucci C, Myckatyn TM, Mackinnon SE, Hayashi A. End-to-side nerve repair: review of the literature. *Restor Neurol Neurosci* 2007;25(1): 45–63.
38. Landwehrs GM, Brüser P. Clinical results of terminolateral neurorrhaphy in digital nerves. *Handchir Mikrochir Plast Chir* 2008;40(5):318–321.
39. Scaramella L. L'anastomosi tra i due nervi facciali. *Arch Otolaryngol* 1971;82:209.
40. Viterbo F. Cross-face termino-lateral neurorrhaphy: a new method for treatment of facial palsy. *Plastic Surg Forum* 1992;15:356–358.
41. Viterbo F. A new method for treatment of facial palsy: the cross-face nerve transplantation with end-to-side neurorrhaphy. *Revista da Sociedade Brasileira de Cirurgia Plástica Estética e Reconstrutiva* 1993;8(1,2,3):29–38.
42. Frey M, Giovanoli P, Michaelidou M. Functional upgrading of partially recovered facial palsy by cross-face nerve grafting with distal end-to-side neurorrhaphy. *Plast Reconstr Surg* 2006;117(2):597–608.
43. Labbé D. *Lengthening of temporalis myoplasty and spontaneous smile.* 10th International Microsurgical Symposium. Botucatu, Brazil, September 19–20, 2008.
44. Viterbo F. *Orthodromic temporal flap in facial palsy.* 10th International Microsurgical Symposium. Botucatu, Brazil, September 2008.
45. Viterbo F, Franciosi LF, Palhares A. Nerve grafting and end-to-side neurorrhaphies connecting the phrenic nerve to the brachial plexus. *Plast Reconstruct Surg* 1995;96(2):494–495.
46. Franciosi LF, Modestti C, Mueller SF. Neurotization of the biceps muscle by end-to-side neurorrhaphy between ulnar and musculocutaneous nerves. A series of five cases. *Analles Chir Main (Ann Hand Surg)* 1998; 17(4):362–367.
47. Mennen U. End-to-side nerve suture in clinical practice. *Hand Surg* 2003;8(1):33–42.
48. Viterbo F. *Deltoid neurotization with ETS.* 10th International Microsurgical Symposium. Botucatu, Brazil, September 19–20, 2008.
49. Voche P, Ouattara D. End-to-side neurorrhaphy for defects of palmar sensory digital nerves. *Br J Plast Surg* 2005;58:239–244.
50. Viterbo F. Restoration of sensitivity after removal of the sural nerve—a new application of lateral-terminal neurorrhaphy (case report). Revista da Sociedade Brasileira de Cirurgia Plástica Estética e Reconstrutiva 1993;8(1,2,3):85–89.
51. Viterbo F, Ripari, WT. Nerve grafts prevent paraplegic pressure ulcers. *J Reconstruct Microsurg* 2008;24(4):251–253.
52. Slezac S, Mcgibbon B, Dellon AL. The sensational transverse rectus abdominis musculocutaneous flap (TRAM): return of sensibility after TRAM breast reconstruction. *Ann Plast Surg* 1992;28:210.
53. Doncatto L, Hochberg J, Caleffi M. O retalho TRAM com reinervação sensitiva para reconstrução mamária. *Revista Brasileira de Mastologia* 1995;5(3):20–23.

CHAPTER 70

Nerve Conduits

David T. W. Chiu and Paul S. Cederna

Peripheral nerve defects occur as a result of nerve injury related to trauma or surgical resection of nerve lesions. The surgeon is called upon to repair the nerve defect and to provide the best motor and sensory functional outcome for the patient. Ideally, the nerve is repaired by direct coaptation through either nerve stump mobilization or nerve rerouting and transposition (1). When these maneuvers are inadequate to provide a tensionless repair, other techniques must be used. Much work has been conducted on developing an alternative to traditional nerve repair using either nerve autografts or nerve conduits, including vein grafting, basal lamina scaffolds, nonabsorbable or absorbable conduits, and tissue-engineered constructs. The purpose of this chapter is to give an overview of the current concepts in nerve grafts and alternative peripheral nerve conduits used in clinical applications and in scientific investigation.

HISTORY

The history of nerve repair has its beginnings in 300 AD, when Galen differentiated nerves from tendons (2). Despite periodic efforts at nerve repair, amputation was the primary procedure for patients who sustained severe peripheral nerve injuries (2). In 1870, Philipeaux and Vulpian performed an experiment in which they used a segment of the lingual nerve to reconstruct the damaged hypoglossal nerve (3). In 1880, Gluck used decalcified bone grafts as a bridge graft for reconstruction of nerve gaps (4). In 1891, Bungner described the use of the brachial artery to repair a nerve defect as a form of biologic nerve conduit (5). In 1904, Foramitti (6), and in 1915, Nageotte (7) observed initial nerve regeneration in an arterial and vein graft followed by subsequent graft disintegration. In 1927, Bunnell reported on successful autogenous nerve grafting, and in 1947, Seddon reported the cable graft technique for repair of nerve gaps (8). In 1972, Millesi et al. (9) and Berger and Millesi (10) demonstrated that tensionless nerve grafting yielded better results than primary nerve coaptation under tension. In 1980, Chiu et al. (11–13) demonstrated, first in an animal model and then in humans, successful histologic and clinical evidence of nerve regeneration across a nerve gap reconstructed with autogenous vein graft. For further review, many comprehensive historical reviews are available in the literature (8,14–22).

ANATOMY

The neuron is the basic anatomical unit of the nervous system. It consists of the cell body, or perikaryon; dendrites and a single axon, which extends far beyond the spinal cord, reaching into the periphery. The axon hillock, where the axon takes off from the cell body, is also the site at which the action potential of the neuronal cell is generated. The axon has numerous microtubules and neurofilaments bounded by axolemma. Protein is generally synthesized in the perikaryon and transported down the axon via the microtubule system in an antegrade fashion. Axons are surrounded by glial cells, known as Schwann cells, in the peripheral nervous system. The Schwann cells form a myelin sheath and insulate a segment of the axon. In the peripheral nervous system, a single axon may be myelinated by as many as 500 Schwann cells. The area between two successive areas of myelination is known as a node of Ranvier.

Peripheral nerves are cable-like structures consisting of axons and supporting collagen and connective tissue. The endoneurium, which consists of delicate strands of collagen circumscribing an individual myelinated axon or a group of nonmyelinated axons, defines the outer border of a nerve fiber and provides nourishment and mechanical support. Aggregation of several nerve fibers constitutes a fascicle, which is surrounded by the perineurium. This is a layer of connective sheaths consisting of collagen and perineurial cells that provides tensile strength to the nerve and contributes to the blood–nerve barrier. Multiple fascicles are organized into group fascicles surrounded by connective tissue known as interfascicular epineurium. The anatomical boundary of the peripheral nerve is delineated by a layer of well-defined connective tissue known as the extrafascicular epineurium. This is the layer that carries blood vessels and neurons to the nerve trunk. When the epineurium is injured, it responds by producing collagen and therefore scar tissue (3,23).

NERVE REPAIR

Primary nerve repair takes place within the first 1 or 2 weeks after injury and is preferred over secondary or delayed repair if the following four conditions are met: (1) a sharply divided nerve without crush, (2) a well-perfused wound bed without contamination, (3) a lack of associated musculoskeletal injuries, and (4) a patient who is free from associated systemic injury and stable enough to undergo surgery. Successful repair of a peripheral nerve injury has two critical requirements: (1) tension-free repair and (2) maintenance of the longitudinal excursion of the peripheral nerves. Nerve repair methods include epineurial repair, group fascicular repair, fascicular repair, and a mixture of these techniques (2,3,18).

NERVE GRAFTS

The pioneering work of Seddon (24) and then Millesi et al. (9,25) forms the fundamental basis for the reconstruction of the peripheral nerve. There are three types of available nerve grafts, xenografts, allografts, and autografts. Xenografts have not been successful because of the inability to overcome acute and chronic rejection. Peripheral nerve allografts have not achieved broad acceptance because of the need for long-term, systemic, nonspecific immunosuppression to prevent rejection. However, peripheral nerve allografts are currently being studied extensively and are coming closer to clinical application (26,27) Autografts provide both a conduit with a basal lamina structure and maintain the Schwann cells that provide an excellent scaffold for nerve regeneration (Figure 70-1) (3). The technique of nerve grafting has evolved from the trunk graft, cable graft, and pedicled nerve graft into the interfascicular nerve graft. The free vascularized nerve graft further extends the domain of nerve grafting when the wound bed is unfavorable or the nerve gap is excessively long.

COMMONLY USED AUTOGRAFTS

Trunk Graft

The trunk graft uses the whole segment of a nerve interposed between the cut ends of a damaged nerve. This type of graft has had limited success because the center of the graft may become necrotic and fibrotic before penetration of neovasculature. This phenomenon can be attributed to the thickness of the graft and the compromised blood supply to the central portion of the graft (3).

Cable Graft

The cable graft is formed by uniting the strands of nerve graft segments into a single unit and then using this whole unit as a graft to reconstruct a nerve gap; these nerve constructs closely resemble a natural nerve trunk (8). The nerve segments that are placed in the central position become vulnerable to ischemia because revascularizations, which occurs first at the periphery, may not reach the central graft segments before central necrosis.

Interfascicular Graft

The interfascicular nerve graft was initially described by Millesi et al. in 1972 (9). In this technique, the strands of the grafted nerves are interposed between carefully dissected groups of fascicles in the damaged nerve. This has the advantage of allowing each nerve graft to have optimal contact with the surrounding tissue, permitting better vascularization of the graft (8).

Vascularized Graft

Finally, there are limited reports in the literature of free vascularized nerve grafts, a technique pioneered by Taylor and Ham (28). A distinct advantage of this approach is the inherent blood supply to the donor nerve. Birch et al. (29) reported their experiences reconstructing the brachial plexus with the ulnar nerve vascularized by the ulnar artery or ulnar collateral artery. They believe that the recovery is better than with traditional nerve grafting because of the improved blood supply to each fascicle. It has been proposed that the vascularized graft should be used when there are extensive nerve gaps, skin defects, and poorly vascularized wound beds.

Sources of Nerve Grafts

There are certain criteria that one must keep in mind when choosing a nerve graft: (1) the nerve graft must be expendable and not cause an undesirable donor site deficit, (2) the ratio between the nerve fibers and the fibrous content must be favorable, and (3) the nerve graft must be thin enough to survive free grafting. There are many sources for cutaneous nerve grafts, but the most popular is the sural nerve. The sural nerve can be harvested to a length of 30 to 40 cm with minimal functional deficit to the patient (8). There are many additional sources of peripheral nerve grafts that fulfill all of the criteria above, including the medial antebrachial cutaneous nerve, the lateral antebrachial cutaneous nerve, the dorsal antebrachial nerve, and the lateral femoral cutaneous nerve. The superficial branch of the radial nerve is a potential source for autogenous nerve grafts; it has densely packed fascicles and a small amount of epineurial tissue but is associated with a significant sensory deficit in the hand. It is recommended that this nerve never be taken with a concomitant median nerve injury. The dorsal branch of the ulnar nerve can similarly be obtained but should also not be used with a concomitant median nerve injury (3). The posterior interosseous nerve is a good choice for digital nerve repair in terms of size and lack of residual sensory deficit after harvesting because it is an articular branch; however, the nerve tissue–to–fibrous tissue ratio is poor (30). The choice of graft depends on the surgeon's preference and the nature and location of the injury. The patient must also fully understand the deficit that will result after nerve harvest. A preoperative nerve block will help the patient appreciate the resulting deficit after the nerve is harvested. Nerve grafts must be placed in a

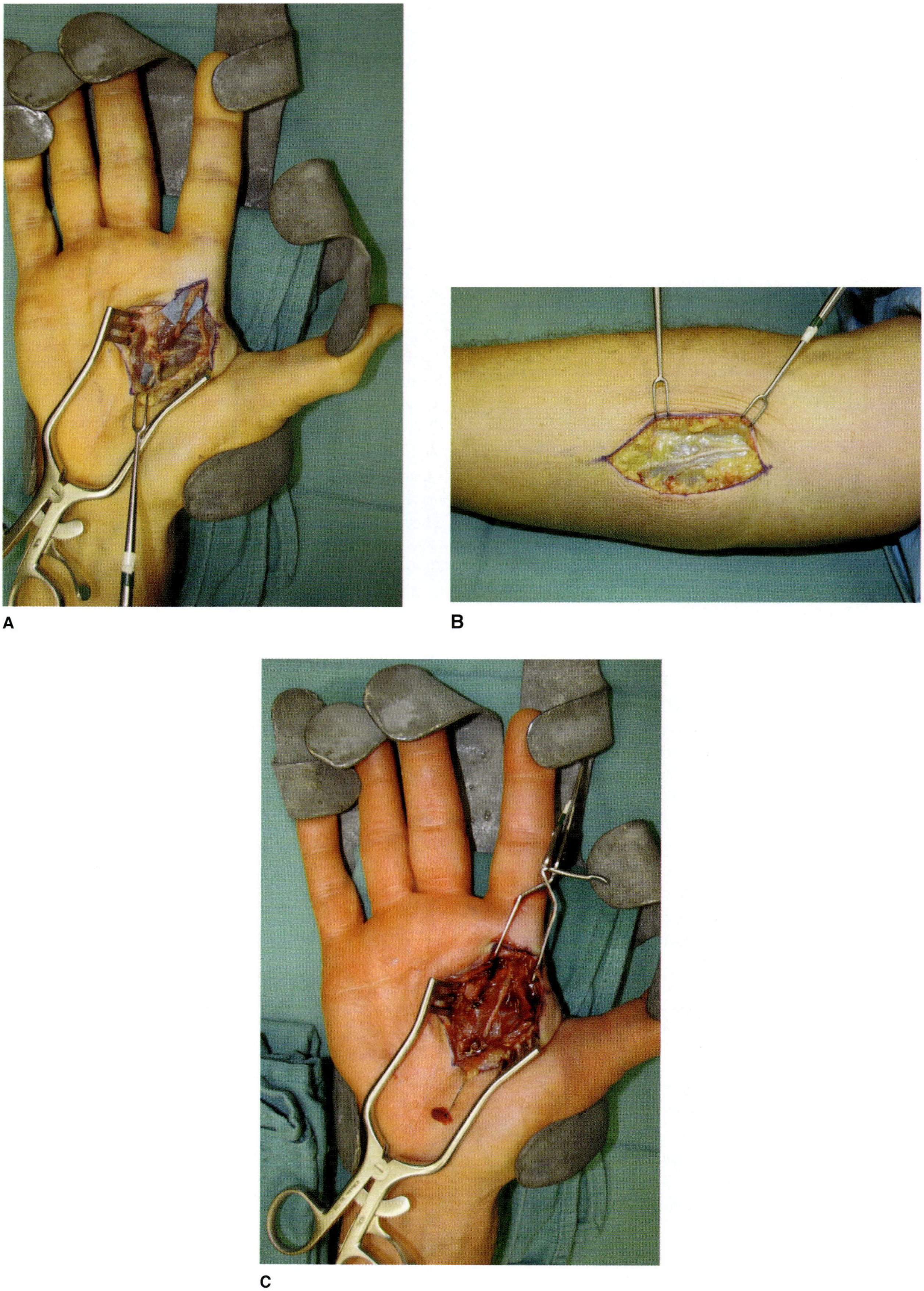

FIGURE 70-1 Right hand digital nerve repair with autogenous nerve graft. (A) A 3-cm defect in the radial digital nerve to index finger after penetrating trauma. (B) Right medial antebrachial cutaneous nerve graft. (C) A 3-cm autogenous nerve graft reconstruction of the digital nerve gap.

suitable bed, and the length of the graft should not be too long to be redundant or too short to cause tension at the nerve coaptation site.

NERVE CONDUIT

The natural configuration of peripheral nerve contributed to its being confused with tendon in time of antiquity. Historically, many different types of conduits were used to reconstruct gaps in peripheral nerves, including bone tubes, magnesium tubes, and vascular conduits. The early effort known as "tubulization" was "an unqualified failure," a conclusion drawn by Sir Sydney Sunderland as late as 1978. However, Chiu et al. recognized that the foundation of success in peripheral nerve reconstruction is an intrinsic capacity of axons to regenerate (11). A bridge graft should work if it provides "the regenerating nerve fibers with a passage that is protected from the surrounding scar tissue by a resilient barrier—a barrier that also allows regenerating nerve fibers the metabolically active environment favorable for growth and maturation"; this is the concept of a conduit. Veins were chosen because they are readily available and are biologically resilient and because veins are substantial enough to act as a barrier against scarring but permeable enough to support a favorable internal milieu for nerve regeneration. The early success of using vein conduits to reconstruct nerve gaps marked the evolution from tubulization to nerve conduit and brought about a new era of nerve reconstruction. Since that revolutionary work, a number of peripheral nerve conduits have been developed experimentally and used clinically, including autogenous biologic conduits, nonautogenous biologic conduits, and nonbiologic conduits.

Autogenous Biologic Conduits

The most widely recognized and commonly used biologic conduits for bridging peripheral nerve defects are vein and skeletal muscle conduits.

Vein

The most popular autogenous biologic nerve conduit is the autogenous venous nerve conduit (AVNC), introduced by Chiu in 1980. He demonstrated successful nerve regeneration through an AVNC in a 1-cm defect in a rat sciatic nerve (11–13,31–33). These findings were corroborated by Suematsu et al. in 1988 (34). The successful clinical application of AVNCs was validated by Chiu and Strauch in 1990 (12). In a single blinded, controlled prospective clinical study, they reported a series of 15 nerves repaired with AVNCs after resection of symptomatic neuromas in the hand and forearm. There was successful return of two-point discrimination. Chiu and Strauch (12,32) found that nerve gaps of 3 cm or less could be repaired successfully and demonstrated the efficacy of AVNCs in both acute and delayed nerve repairs of digital nerves. Strauch et al. (35), using the rabbit model, confirmed their excellent growth and return of function of peripheral nerves repaired with AVNCs up to 3 cm in length. The technique of repair is a telescoping venoneurorrhaphy in which the nerve stumps are telescoped into the lumen of the vein conduit and anchored by 9-0 or 10-0 nylon suture. A potential drawback with vein grafting is that the vein wall may collapse. However, Tseng et al. (13) have demonstrated in rats that hematoma and thrombin within the vein keep the conduit patent. A limitation of AVNC is that its success has only been demonstrated in peripheral sensory nerves with small defects (<3 cm). Yet the lack of complications, consistent clinical success, and cost effectiveness continue to sustain its clinical applicability (Figure 70-2).

Muscle and Nerve

The use of muscle and nerve conduits has been recorded by multiple authors. The premise is that the longitudinally oriented basal lamina in skeletal muscle and the extracellular matrix are effective in directing nerve regeneration. This hypothesis was based on similarities between the basal lamina of muscle and the endoneurial tubes of degenerating nerves (36–38). Studies in animals and humans have demonstrated that both fresh and denatured muscle conduits can lead to successful regeneration and even lead to superior results compared with end-to-end suture (39–42). The disadvantages of muscle are the risk of nerve fibers regenerating in an extraendoneurial environment, resulting in a decrease of the number of axons reaching the end organ. Another disadvantage is the added donor site defect necessary for muscle harvest (37). For a more detailed review of the use of muscle for peripheral nerve repair, the reader is referred to Meek et al (37). Acellularized peripheral nerve constructs have been investigated experimentally and used clinically for the repair of peripheral nerve gaps while at the same time minimizing or eliminating allogenicity (Figure 70-3) (43–47).

Nonautogenous Biologic Conduits

Collagen

Collagen is a major component of the extracellular matrix. Collagen constructs have been designed to guide peripheral nerve regeneration and are currently being studied in animal models and human trials, with promising results (48–52). In a study by Archibald et al. (49), a collagen-based nerve guide was used for the repair of nerves at the wrist in primates and showed functional recovery similar to nerve autografts. Keilhoff et al. (51) demonstrated in rats that collagen type I/III tubes were well integrated and revascularized and allowed nerve regeneration. A number of collagen-based peripheral nerve conduits have been approved for use in humans (Figure 70-4).

Synthetic Conduits

The search for an "off-the-shelf," nonimmunogenic material that supports axonal sprouting and elongation across long nerve gaps has prompted research into constructs derived from synthetic materials. The benefits of synthetic materials are that they are readily available, there is an unlimited supply, and they do not lead to any donor site deficit in the same way as harvesting an autogenous nerve graft will lead to an area of numbness and possible paresthesia or dysesthesia. The synthetic constructs provide a physical conduit for guiding axonal regeneration across nerve gaps. The synthetic conduits fall into two large

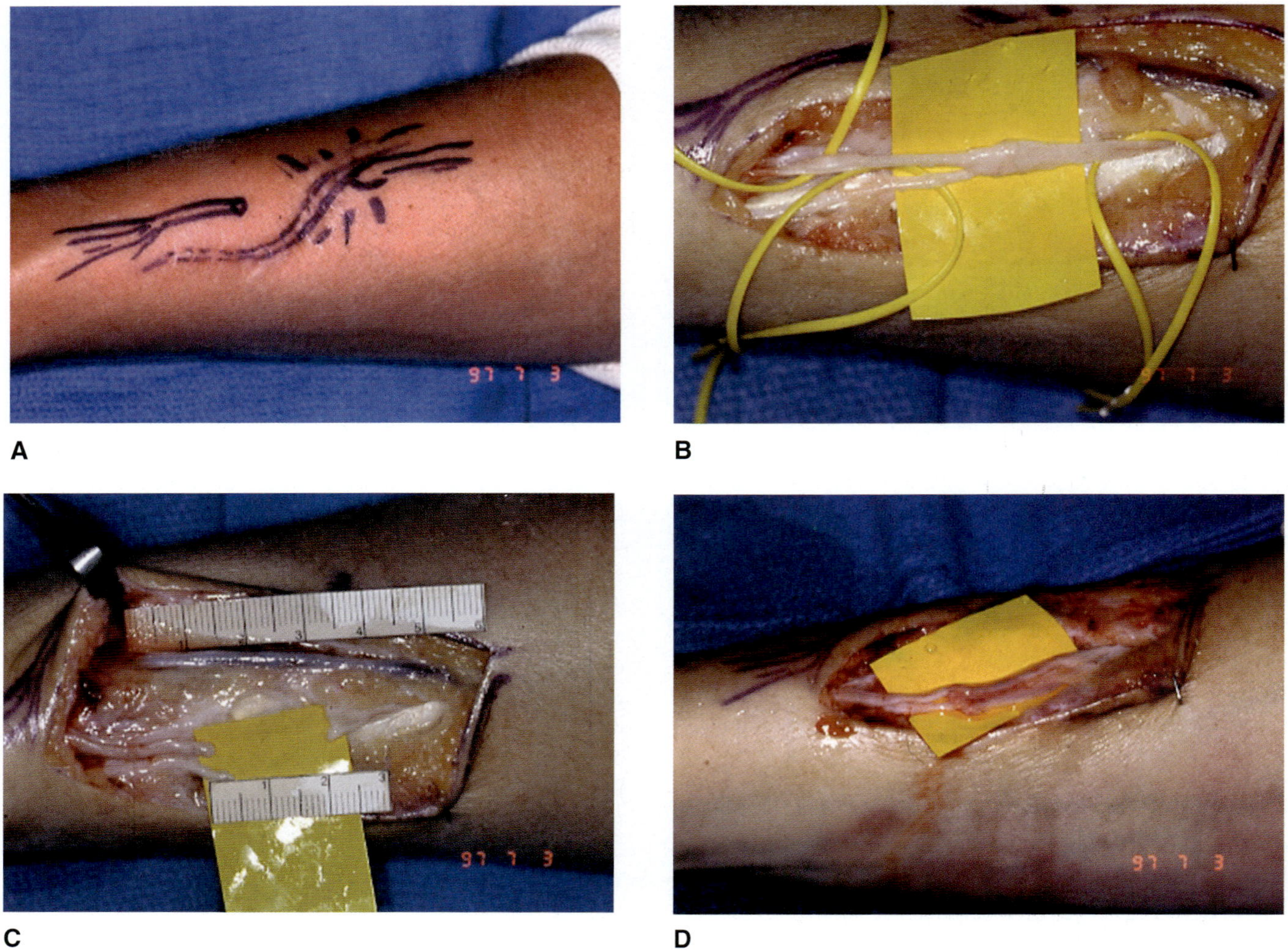

FIGURE 70-2 (A) Exquisitely tender with a positive Tinel's sign at a laceration scar on the radial aspect of the right forearm of a 34-year-old cleaning lady. (B) Exploration revealed a neuroma in continuity of the superficial radial nerve. (C) After resection of the neuroma in continuity of the superficial radial nerve, there left a nerve gap of the two fascicules of 1.7-2 cm, respectively. The ruler was placed behind the adjacent superficial cephalic vein. (D) The fascicular defect of the radial nerve was bridged with a segment of reversed cephalic vein as nerve conduit. AVNC, autogenous venous nerve conduit.

categories, nonabsorbable and absorbable conduits. Numerous conduits have been used in the past or are currently available. Outlined here are the most commonly used absorbable and nonabsorbable synthetic conduits.

Nonabsorbable Conduits

Silicone Tube Silicone tubes were some of the first synthetic conduits to be used in vivo for the reconstruction of nerve gaps. Silicone tubes are nonpermeable and have the potential benefit of retaining all of the secreted neurotrophic substances near the ends of the divided nerve. In 1991, Lundborg et al. reported successful neural regeneration across 5-mm nerve gaps using a silicone tube (53,54). The success of this technique was so profound that Lundborg began to use silicone tubes as an alternative to direct suture repair for peripheral nerve injuries that did not have a peripheral nerve gap. Long-term follow-up of patients treated for median and ulnar nerve deficits demonstrated that the use of a silicone tube was at least as good as direct suture repair (55). A significant improvement in the perception of touch 3 months after surgery in patients who underwent reconstruction with silicone tubes was reported. However, a subpopulation of patients in these studies did require surgical removal of the silicone tube because of irritation and a foreign body reaction. In these cases, excellent neural regeneration was noted within the silicone tube with the location of the original nerve injury being virtually impossible to identify. In 1999, Braga-Silva described the use of silicone tubes for the late repair (the mean length of time between the injury and repair was 101 days) of median and ulnar nerves in the forearm, with gaps of up to 3 cm (56). However, as was noted by Lundborg, the silicone tubes did create irritation of the nerve and required removal in seven of the 26 implanted tubes. Indeed, this is one of the major problems faced through use of nonabsorbable conduits.

Hydrogel Conduits Hydrogels are a class of biomaterials that are cross-linked, water-soluble polymers. There has been a great interest in these polymers for tissue regeneration purposes because they are biocompatible, hydrophilic, stable, and compliant. The biostable hydrogels contain water content

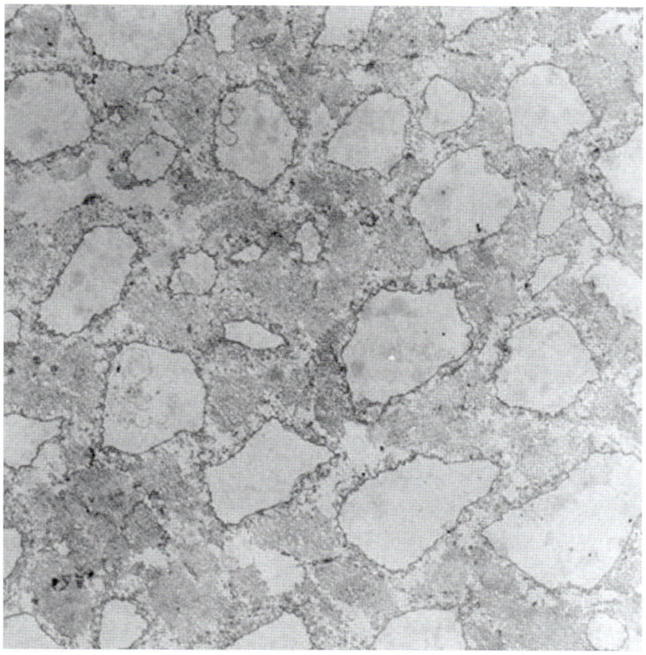

FIGURE 70-3 Scanning electron micrograph of acellular peroneal nerve. Note the patent endoneurial conduits.

similar to human tissues, making them soft and compliant, leading to low sheer stresses on tissues. This is particularly valuable in nerve applications in which any stress placed directly on the nerve can lead to axonal pruning, axonal disruption, pain, and motor and sensory deficits. As early as 1982, cultured neurons were noted to become attached to hydrogel substrates and to experience nerve fiber growth on the same substrate (57). Since that time, hydrogels have been used for reconstruction of nerve gaps in animal studies and in clinical trials. Despite substantial theoretical benefit of the hydrogel constructs, this has not translated into the successful reconstruction of longer nerve gaps (>2 cm). However, these constructs have been used as a scaffold for the creation of more bioactive nerve grafts with cellular elements and growth factors. In 1992, Aebischer and colleagues examined the efficacy of hydrogel tubes seeded with syngeneic Schwann cells for reconstruction of 8 mm rat sciatic nerve gaps. In this study, they demonstrated extensive peripheral nerve regeneration through the semipermeable, synthetic hydrogel guidance channel seeded with Schwann cells (58). In 2003, Midha and colleagues reported the use of synthetic hydrogel tubes for reconstruction of 10 mm rat sciatic nerve gaps. They not only demonstrated reasonable axonal regeneration across these gaps but also noted that when additional growth factors and collagen gel were added to the lumen of these tubes, axonal regeneration was enhanced further (59). These studies and many others provided evidence that the biostable hydrogel nerve constructs were an ideal scaffold for creation of more complex nerve grafts. Currently, these polymer hydrogels come in many different formulations and configurations, including cross-linked poly-hydroxyethyl-methacrylate (pHEMA) and poly-*N*-(2-hydroxypropyl)-methacrylamide (pHPMA). These constructs serve as the scaffold for many different bioactive nerve guidance channels. However, as a "stand-alone" nerve

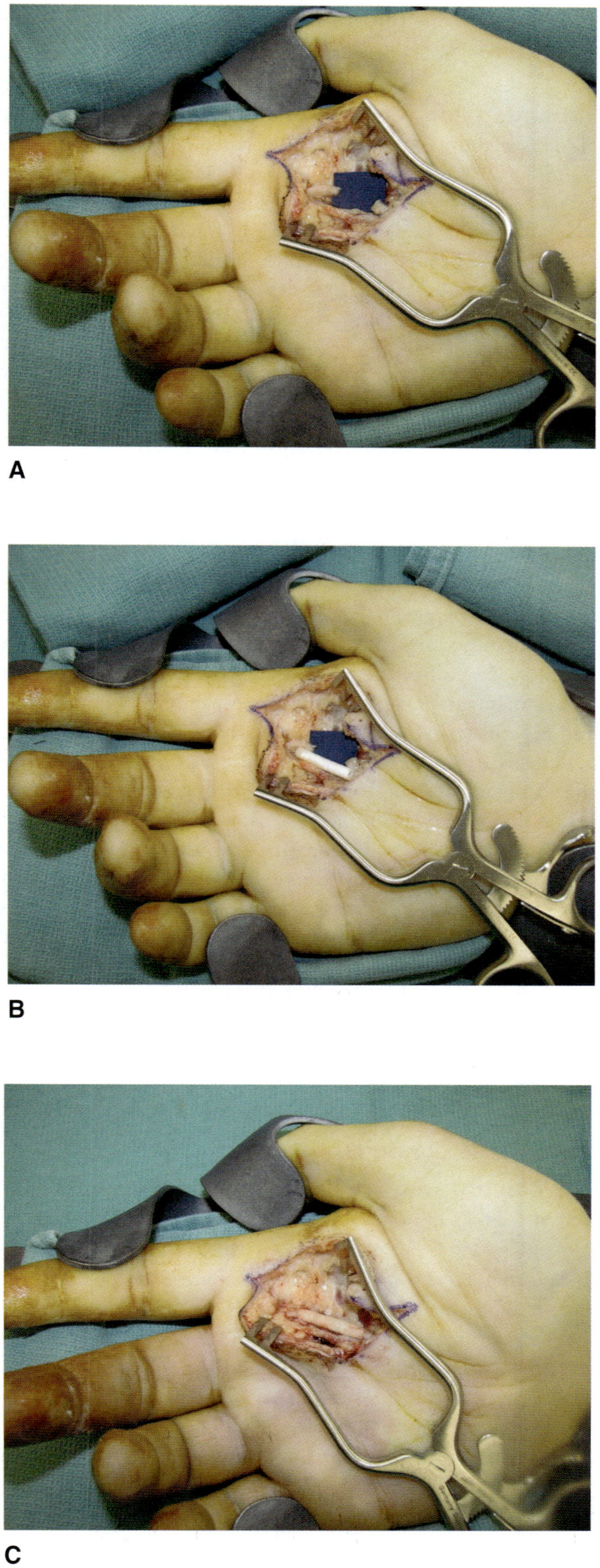

FIGURE 70-4 Right hand digital nerve repair with nerve conduit. (**A**) A 1.5-cm defect in the ulnar digital nerve to index finger after resection of neuroma. (**B**) A 2.0-cm Integra NeuraGen nerve guide. (**C**) A 2.0-cm nerve conduit reconstruction of 1.5-cm digital nerve gap.

guidance channel, hydrogel conduits allow axonal regeneration across only short nerve gaps (<2 cm).

Expanded Polytetrafluoroethylene In 1985, Rice et al. described use of a polytetrafluorinated ethylene compound (Gore-Tex; WL Gore and Associates, Flagstaff, AZ) tubing in the repair of rat sciatic nerve gaps. They demonstrated that using thin-walled (0.36-mm) polytetrafluoroethylene (PTFE) tubing to reconstruct short sciatic nerve gaps provided functional results comparable to the results achieved with nerve grafts or vein interposition grafts (60). In 1989, Aesbischer and colleagues published the use of the PTFE tubes as nerve guidance channels for the reconstruction of 4-mm gaps in the sciatic nerve in mice. In addition, they added electrically charged particles on to the surface of the PTFE for the purposes of enhancing neural regeneration. Four weeks after surgery, they were able to demonstrate enhanced neural regeneration when electrically charged nerve guidance channels, PTFE in this case, were used for nerve gap reconstruction (61). In 1998, Stanec and Stanec described their use of expanded polytetrafluoroethylene (Gore-Tex) tubes in two manuscripts. The first manuscript was a case report in which a 22-year-old woman underwent reconstruction of a 2.9-cm ulnar nerve gap with an expanded PTFE conduit and experienced sensory and motor recovery. The PTFE tube had to be removed after surgery because of irritation, but the exploration demonstrated macroscopically normal nerve inside the conduit (62). In the second study, 43 patients had median and ulnar nerves reconstructed with PTFE tubes. They concluded that nerve gaps up to 40 mm allowed functional recovery in 79% of patients; however, in gaps larger than 40 mm, only 13% had functional recovery. Only one patient needed to have the tube removed (63). Since that time, numerous basic science and clinical studies have supported the use of PTFE grafts for bridging small nerve defects (<3 cm). The wealth of information will support the use of this conduit for 2-cm gaps or smaller.

Absorbable Conduits

Polyglactin and Polyglycolic Acid Conduits The first use of an absorbable nerve conduit was described by Molander and colleagues in 1982 when they reconstructed 7- to 9-mm nerve gaps in a rabbit tibial nerve with polyglactin 910, a resorbable synthetic material (64). After absorption of the mesh, the authors noted numerous regenerating axons and organized fascicles within the nerve sheath. One year later, the same authors reported their results comparing neural regeneration through a polyglactin conduit and conventional nerve grafting in the short rabbit tibial nerve gap model. They found very little difference in nerve healing between the two groups when morphometric observations and electromyographic recordings were performed (65). Indeed, this was the first step toward a dramatic increase in materials science and engineering to produce a better biodegradable nerve conduit.

The polyglycolic acid (PGA) conduit was the first biodegradable nerve conduit approved for human use in the United States and Europe. It is a synthetic polymer that begins to degrade by hydrolysis 3 months after surgery and is typically resorbed by 6 to 8 months. The product of degradation is glycolic acid, which is nontoxic to the nerve and to the patient. In 1990, Mackinnon and Dellon demonstrated the clinical use of absorbable PGA tubes to bridge digital nerve gaps (0.5–3.0 cm). In this prospective study of secondary digital nerve repairs with a mean gap of 1.7 cm, they demonstrated comparable functional results when nerve gaps were repaired with either PGA conduits or autogenous nerve grafting (66). In 2000, Weber et al. described a prospective, randomized, multicenter study of the use of PGA tubes versus standard repair. They studied 136 nerve transections occurring in the hand in 96 patients and found that repair with PGA conduit produced superior results for short gaps of less than 4 mm compared with end-to-end repair. For longer defects, they demonstrated superior results when compared with nerve autografts (67). Very few studies have demonstrated a superior functional outcome from using of any biologic or synthetic conduit for peripheral nerve gap repair compared with an autogenous nerve graft. However, it is clear that for shorter nerve gaps, use of synthetic conduits can provide very good results.

Poly(DL-Lactic-Co-Glycolic Acid) and Poly(L-Lactic Acid) Conduits

Recently, there have been increasing efforts toward developing more complex biodegradable, synthetic conduits for reconstruction of nerve gaps. Through the precise manufacturing of conduits with varying sizes, configurations, internal scaffolding, internal channels, and variable permeability, scientists and engineers have hoped to increase the length of the nerve gap that can be successfully bridged. In 1998, Widmer et al. described the manufacturing of porous, biodegradable tubular conduits for guided tissue regeneration. The biomechanical properties of the poly(DL-lactic-co-glycolic acid) (PLGA) and poly(L-lactic acid) (PLLA) constructs were studied before and after 8 weeks of degradation. The potential for seeding the constructs with cellular elements and bioactive substances was also investigated. Both of the PLGA and PLLA constructs were shown to have great promise for the regeneration of tissues with a tubular structure such as long bones, blood vessels, or peripheral nerves (68). One year later, Evans and colleagues reported on the use of PLLA constructs for reconstruction of 1-cm sciatic nerve defects in rat hindlimbs. Sixteen weeks after surgery, they noted that nerve fiber density in the distal sciatic nerve for the PLLA constructs was similar to that of the isogenic nerve grafts (69). Over the next few years, both the PLLA and PLGA constructs were intensely scrutinized to optimize the structural characteristics of the conduits to enhance the potential for neural regeneration across long nerve gaps (70). In 2003, Vacanti and colleagues described the precise fabrication of PLGA conduits that were porous, and biodegradable; had longitudinal channels; and had "dimensionally tolerance" to enhance neural regeneration across nerve gaps (71). Since that time, numerous PLGA nerve conduits have been created for the reconstruction of nerve gaps. Most recently, the PLGA and PLLA conduits have been loaded with various growth factors and cellular elements to enhance neural regeneration across longer nerve gaps.

Tissue-Engineered Conduits

Along with the effort of precise fabrication of synthetic constructs with the optimal microarchitecture to promote, enhance, and guide peripheral nerve regeneration across a longer nerve gap, biologic scaffolds have similarly been the focus of intense research through modification of the external and internal structure to promote axonal regeneration over longer distances. However, with all of the advances that have been made in tissue engineering and material science, the longest nerve gap that can be successfully reconstructed with either a biologic or synthetic construct is less than 3 cm. Of course, there are scattered reports of constructs that can bridge slightly longer gaps, but to date, there has been no consistent series of reports identifying a single type of biologic or synthetic construct for successful reconstruction of longer gaps. The major issues that have prevented this success is the lack of trophic support and cellular elements that can provide the appropriate series of biologic signals necessary to promote axonal elongation across longer gaps.

Two main concepts guide the development of new technologies to enhance peripheral nerve regeneration across longer nerve gaps: (1) create a conduit that mimics the important biologic features of the normal peripheral nerve, including the scaffold and the trophic support, and (2) modify or enrich the synthetic or biologic constructs with the appropriate cellular elements that promote regeneration.

The creation of a bioactive peripheral nerve construct to enhance peripheral nerve regeneration across long nerve gaps has been attempted for decades. The concept is that the appropriate trophic support provided within a peripheral nerve construct will enhance axonal sprouting, guide elongation, and lead to more successful end organ reinnervation. Most neurotrophic factors belong to one of three families: (1) neurotrophins, (2) glial cell-line derived neurotrophic factor family ligands, and (3) neuropoietic cytokines (72). Neurotrophins are released by target tissues and act to prevent apoptosis of neurons and induce progenitor cells to produce neurons. The neurotrophic factors most commonly studied to enhance peripheral nerve regeneration within a nerve conduit are nerve growth factor (NGF), brain-derived neurotrophic factor (BDNF), neurotrophin-3 (NT-3), and neurotrophin-4 (NT-4). NGF was the first neurotrophin identified and has been the subject of more than 11,000 publications since 1964. The addition of NGF to peripheral nerve constructs has been shown to dramatically enhance axonal regeneration across peripheral nerve defects (73). However, this enhanced axonal regeneration has not translated into dramatic improvements in the distance over which peripheral nerve conduits will support regeneration. BDNF is one of the most active substances to stimulate peripheral nerve regeneration and as a result has been the subject of intense scrutiny. Similar to NGF, the addition of BDNF has been shown to increase axonal regeneration but has not been shown to significantly increase the distance over which the axons regenerate. Glial growth factor has been identified as a potent stimulator of neural regeneration and has been shown to increase the number of Schwann cells and axonal regeneration when added to conduits for reconstruction of 2- to 4-cm rabbit common peroneal nerve gap (74). Ciliary neurotrophic factor has also been used as a luminal filler in silicone conduits to reconstruct 10-mm defects in rat sciatic nerve gaps and has produced an increase in motor axonal regeneration and enhanced myelination (75).

Hundreds of additional studies have investigated the various neurotrophic factors in biologic and synthetic constructs to help provide neuroregeneration across longer nerve gaps (76). The search for a single growth factor to enhance peripheral nerve regeneration across long gaps has been relatively unsuccessful, and as a result, scientists have increased the complexity of their trophic signaling by combining synergistically acting growth factors from different neurotrophic families to enhance peripheral nerve regeneration. This has been successfully accomplished by Madduri et al., who combined glial cell-derived neurotrophic factor (GDNF) with NGF to produce a dramatic enhancement in early axonal regeneration in a 10-mm rat sciatic nerve gap (77). However, the successful reconstruction of long nerve gaps remains unsolved with either the addition of growth factors to a conduit or providing constitutively expressed growth factors within a conduit.

The second strategy that has been used to enhance neuroregeneration across long nerve gaps has been to modify or enrich the synthetic or biologic constructs with the appropriate cellular elements that promote neuroregeneration. This has been accomplished in a number of different ways with either the addition of Schwann cells, one of the critical cellular elements required for axonal elongation, or the addition of stem cells to provide the trophic support and guidance to enhance peripheral nerve regeneration across longer nerve gaps. One of the original strategies to provide the appropriate trophic support through incorporation of cellular elements within the construct was to fill an autogenous vein graft with pieces of nerve graft. This bioengineered nerve graft was successfully used in human and animal studies with satisfactory results for gaps larger than 3 cm (78,79). This approach is very effective because it delivers Schwann cells into the nerve gap to enhance neural regeneration across longer nerve gaps. However, this approach also adds fibroblasts to the conduit, which may compromise neural regeneration across the nerve gap. As a result, investigators have chosen to simply add Schwann cells, the critical element for axonal elongation and remyelination, to the constructs. In 2003, Haase and colleagues demonstrated successful axonal sprouting, elongation, and muscle reinnervation when a chemically acellularized peripheral nerve graft was used to reconstruct a 2-cm nerve gap in the rat peroneal nerve model; however, the nerve graft did not support axonal regeneration across a 4-cm gap (44). When isogenic Schwann cells were added to the construct, there were successful axonal regeneration and muscle reinnervation across a 4-cm nerve gap. It has been consistently demonstrated in a number of investigations that the addition of Schwann cells to any type of peripheral nerve conduit can enhance the distance over which successful axonal regeneration will occur. In the instance of vein conduits filled with Schwann cells, nerve gaps up to 6 cm have been successfully bridged in the rabbit model (80). Through the addition of Schwann cells to the constructs, we have been able to successfully enhance the length over which successful axonal regeneration can occur. This has been the major focus of research in the area of peripheral nerve conduits over the past 15 years and will continue to be an important focus in the coming years.

Most recently, scientists have begun to investigate the possibility of using stem cells as a source of trophic support for regenerating axons. The theoretical advantage of using mesenchymal stem cells (MSCs) or adipose-derived stem cells (ASCs) is that they can be a source of Schwann cells without having to harvest an autogenous nerve graft as a source of Schwann cells. Attempts to isolate, purify, and amplify Schwann cells from the peripheral nerve of an adult animal has proven to be extremely challenging and as a result may not be the best strategy for providing Schwann cells to peripheral nerve conduits for reconstruction of nerve gaps. On the other hand, MSCs and ASCs are a readily available source of cells that are easily isolated and can be induced down a neural cell lineage to have a Schwann cell–like phenotype (81,82). Most recently, ASCs have not only been induced down a neural cell lineage but have also been shown to produce myelin, enhance neurite outgrowth in vitro, and increase neural regeneration within a conduit in vivo (83,84). It is quite possible that in the years to come, ASCs or MSCs will become a readily available source of Schwann cells for incorporation into bioactive nerve grafts for the reconstruction of long nerve gaps.

CONCLUSIONS

The ideal nerve reconstruction would provide a tensionless repair, with no additional scarring, no increase in operative time, no nerve entrapment, and enhanced neural regeneration. Bioengineered conduits represent an alternative to autogenous nerve grafting in selected patients for peripheral nerve repair. Clinical studies have demonstrated that vein, muscle, silicone tubing, PGA tubes, and combinations of these conduits hold promise as successful alternates. Molecular modulation of the internal structure of the conduit could hold the promise of an ideal nerve conduit and form the future of peripheral nerve surgery. Future clinical studies will provide information comparing different techniques to provide surgeons with more reconstructive options for reconstruction of patients with peripheral nerve injuries.

REFERENCES

1. Trumble TE, McCallister WV. Repair of peripheral nerve defects in the upper extremity. *Hand Clin* 2000;16:37–52.
2. Diao E, Vannuyen T. Techniques for primary nerve repair. *Hand Clin* 2000;16:53–66.
3. Wilgis EFS. Nerve repair and grafting. In Green DP (ed). *Operative Hand Surgery*. 2nd ed. Vol 2. New York: Churchill Livingstone, 1988, pp. 1373–1404.
4. Gluck T. Uber neuroplastik auf dem wege der transplantation. *Arch Klin Chir* 1880;25:606–616.
5. Bungner O. Uber die degenerations und regenerations—Vorgange am nerven nach verletzungen. *Beitr Pathol Anal* 1891;10:321.
6. Foramitti C. Zur technic der nervennaht. *Arch Klin Chir* 1904;73: 643–648.
7. Nageotte J. Le processus de la cicatrisation des nerfs. *CR Soc Biol (Paris)* 1915;78:249.
8. Millesi H. Techniques for nerve grafting. *Hand Clin* 2000;16:73–91.
9. Millesi H, Meissl G, Berger A. The interfascicular nerve-grafting of the median and ulnar nerves. *J Bone Joint Surg Am* 1972;54:727–750.
10. Berger A, Millesi H. Nerve grafting. *Clin Orthop Relat Res* 1978;133: 49–55.
11. Chiu DT, Janecki I, Krizek TJ, et al. Autogenous vein graft used as a conduit for nerve regeneration. *Surgery* 1982;91:226–233.
12. Chiu DT, Strauch B. A prospective clinical evaluation of autogenous vein grafts used as a nerve conduit for distal sensory nerve defects of 3 cm or less. *Plast Reconstr Surg* 1990;86:928–934.
13. Tseng CY, Hu G, Ambron RT, Chiu DT. Histologic analysis of Schwann cell migration and peripheral nerve regeneration in the autogenous venous conduit (AVNC). *J Reconstr Microsurg* 2003;19:331–340.
14. Seddon H. *Surgical Disorders of the Peripheral Nerves*. Baltimore: Williams & Wilkins, 1972.
15. Mackinnon S, Dellon AL. *Surgery of the Peripheral Nerve*. New York: Thieme, 1988.
16. Sunderland S. *Nerve Injuries and Their Repair: A Critical Appraisal*. New York: Churchill Livingstone, 1991.
17. Terzis JK, Sun DD, Thanos PK. Historical and basic science review: past, present, and future of nerve repair. *J Reconstr Microsurg* 1997;13: 215–225.
18. Lundborg G. A 25-year perspective of peripheral nerve surgery: evolving neuroscientific concepts and clinical significance. *J Hand Surg Am* 2000;25:391–414.
19. Hall S. Nerve repair: a neurobiologist's view. *J Hand Surg Br* 2001;26: 129–136.
20. Naff NJ, Ecklund JM. History of peripheral nerve surgery techniques. *Neurosurg Clin North Am* 2001;12:197–209.
21. Dvali L, Mackinnon S. Nerve repair, grafting, and nerve transfers. *Clin Plast Surg* 2003;30:203–221.
22. Lundborg G. *Nerve Injury and Repair*. Edinburgh: Churchill Livingstone, 1988.
23. Choi M, Chiu DTW. Nerve physiology and repair. In Trumble TE, Budoff JE, Cornwall R (eds). *Hand, Elbow & Shoulder: Core Knowledge in Orthopaedics*. Philadelphia: Mosby Elsevier, 2006, pp. 222–223.
24. Seddon HJ. Nerve grafting. *J Bone Joint Surg Br* 1963;45:447–461.
25. Millesi H, Meissl G, Berger A. Further experience with interfascicular grafting of the median, ulnar, and radial nerves. *J Bone Joint Surg Am* 1976;58:209–218.
26. Evans PJ, Midha R, Mackinnon SE. The peripheral nerve allograft: a comprehensive review of regeneration and neuroimmunology. *Prog Neurobiol* 1994;43:187–233.
27. Mackinnon SE, Hudson AR, Bain JR, et al. The peripheral nerve allograft: an assessment of regeneration in the immunosuppressed host. *Plast Reconstr Surg* 1987;79:436–446.
28. Taylor GI, Ham FJ. The free vascularized nerve graft: a further experimental and clinical application of microvascular techniques. *Plast Reconstr Surg* 1976;57:413–426.
29. Birch R, Dunkerton M, Bonney G, et al. Experience with the free vascularized ulnar nerve graft in repair of supraclavicular lesions of the brachial plexus. *Clin Orthop Relat Res* 1988;237:96–104.
30. Dellon AL, Seif SS. Anatomic dissections relating the posterior interosseous nerve to the carpus, and the etiology of dorsal wrist ganglion pain. *J Hand Surg Am* 1978;3:326–332.
31. Chiu DT, Smahel J, Chen L, Meyer V. Neurotropism revisited. *Neurol Res* 2004;26:381–387.
32. Chiu DT. Autogenous venous nerve conduits: a review. *Hand Clin* 1999;15:667–671.
33. Chiu DTW. Autogenous vein graft as a conduit for nerve regeneration. *Surg Forum* 1980;31:550.
34. Suematsu N, Atsuta Y, Hirayama T. Vein graft for repair of peripheral nerve gap. *J Reconstr Microsurg* 1988;4:313–318.
35. Strauch B, Ferder M, Lovelle-Allen S, et al. Determining the maximal length of a vein conduit used as an interposition graft for nerve regeneration. *J Reconstr Microsurg* 1996;12:521–527.
36. Strauch B. Use of nerve conduits in peripheral nerve repair. *Hand Clin* 2000;16:123–130.
37. Meek MF, Varejao AS, Geuna S. Use of skeletal muscle tissue in peripheral nerve repair: review of the literature. *Tissue Eng* 2004;10:1027–1036.
38. Meek MF, Coert JH. Clinical use of nerve conduits in peripheral nerve repair: review of the literature. *J Reconstr Microsurg* 2002;18:97–109.
39. Glasby MA, Gschmeissner SE, Huang CL, De Souza BA. Degenerated muscle grafts used for peripheral nerve repair in primates. *J Hand Surg Br* 1986;11:347–351.

40. Norris RW, Glasby MA, Gattuso JM, Bowden RE. Peripheral nerve repair in humans using muscle autografts: a new technique. *J Bone Joint Surg Br* 1988;70:530–533.
41. Pereira JH, Bowden RE, Gattuso JM, Norris RW. Comparison of results of repair of digital nerves by denatured muscle grafts and end-to-end sutures. *J Bone Joint Surg Br* 1991;16:519–523.
42. Pereira JH, Palande DD, Subramanian A, et al. Denatured autologous muscle graft in leprosy. *Lancet* 1991;338:1239–1240.
43. Haase SC, Cederna PS, Dennis RG, Kuzon WM. Peripheral nerve reconstruction using acellular nerve grafts. *Surg Forum* 2000;51:607–609.
44. Haase SC, Rovak JM, Dennis RG, et al. Recovery of muscle contractile function following peripheral nerve gap repair with an acellularized peripheral nerve graft. *J Reconstruct Microsurg* 2003;19:241–248.
45. Mungara AK, Cederna PS: The CD40/CD40L Co-stimulatory pathway in nerve allograft rejection. *J Am Coll Surg* 2003(suppl);197:S60.
46. Rovak JM, Bishop DK, Boxer LK, et al. Peripheral nerve transplantation: the role of chemical acellularization in eliminating allograft antigenicity. *J Reconstruct Microsurg* 2005;21:207–213.
47. Brown DL, Bishop DK, Wood SY, Cederna PS. Short-term anti-CD40L co-stimulatory blockade induces tolerance to peripheral nerve allografts, resulting in improved skeletal muscle function. *Plast Reconstruct Surg* 2006;117:2250–2259.
48. Li ST, Archibald SJ, Krarup C, Madison RD. Peripheral nerve repair with collagen conduits. *Clin Mater* 1992;9:195–200.
49. Archibald SJ, Shefner J, Krarup C, Madison RD. Monkey median nerve repaired by nerve graft or collagen nerve guide tube. *J Neurosci* 1995;15:4109–4123.
50. Chamberlain LJ, Yannas IV, Hsu HP, et al. Collagen-GAG substrate enhances the quality of nerve regeneration through collagen tubes up to level of autograft. *Exp Neurol* 1998;54:315–329.
51. Keilhoff G, Stang F, Wolf G, Fansa H. Bio-compatibility of type I/III collagen matrix for peripheral nerve reconstruction. *Biomaterials* 2003;24:2779–2787.
52. Harley BA, Spilker MH, Wu JW, et al. Optimal degradation rate for collagen chambers used for regeneration of peripheral nerves over long gaps. *Cells Tissues Organs* 2004;176:153–165.
53. Lundborg G, Dahlin LB, Danielsen N. Ulnar nerve repair by the silicone chamber technique. Case report. *Scand J Plast Reconstr Surg Hand Surg* 1991;25:79–82.
54. Lundborg G, Rosen B, Abrahamson SO, et al. Tubular repair of the median nerve in the human forearm. Preliminary findings. *J Hand Surg Br* 1994;19:273–276.
55. Lundborg G, Rosén B, Dahlin L, et al. Tubular versus conventional repair of median and ulnar nerves in the human forearm: early results from a prospective, randomized, clinical study. *J Hand Surg Am* 1997;22:99–106.
56. Braga-Silva J. The use of silicone tubing in the late repair of the median and ulnar nerves in the forearm. *J Hand Surg Br* 1999;24:703–706.
57. Carbonetto ST, Gruver MM, Turner DC. Nerve fiber growth on defined hydrogel substrates. *Science* 1982;216:897.
58. Valentini RF, Vargo TG, Gardella JA Jr, Aebischer P. Electrically charged polymeric substrates enhance nerve fibre outgrowth in vitro. *Biomaterials* 1992;13:183.
59. Midha R, Munro CA, Dalton PD, et al. Growth factor enhancement of peripheral nerve regeneration through a novel synthetic hydrogel tube. *J Neurosurg* 2003;99:555.
60. Rice DH, Burstein FD, Newman A. Use of polytetrafluorinated ethylene compound in peripheral nerve grafting. An experimental study. *Arch Otolaryngol* 1985;111:259.
61. Valentini RF, Sabatini AM, Dario P, Aebischer P. Polymer electrical guidance channels enhance peripheral nerve regeneration in mice. *Brain Res* 1989;480:300.
62. Stanec S, Stanec Z. Ulnar nerve reconstruction with an expanded polytetrafluoroethylene conduit. *Br J Plast Surg* 1998;51:639.
63. Stanec S, Stanec Z. Reconstruction of upper-extremity peripheral-nerve injuries with ePTFE conduits. *J Reconstr Microsurg* 1998;14:227.
64. Molander H, Olsson Y, Engkvist O, et al. Regeneration of peripheral nerve through a polyglactin tube. *Muscle Nerve* 1982;5:54.
65. Molander H, Engkvist O, Hagglund J, et al. Nerve repair using a polyglactin tube and nerve graft: an experimental study in the rabbit. *Biomaterials* 1983;4:276.
66. Mackinnon SE, Dellon AL. Clinical nerve reconstruction with a bioabsorbable polyglycolic acid tube. *Plast Reconstr Surg* 1990;85:419.
67. Weber RA, Breidenbach WC, Brown RE, et al. A randomized prospective study of polyglycolic acid conduits for digital nerve reconstruction in humans. *Plast Reconstr Surg* 2000;106:1036.
68. Widmer MS, Gupta PK, Lu L, et al. Manufacture of porous biodegradable polymer conduits by an extrusion process for guided tissue regeneration. *Biomaterials* 1998;19:1945.
69. Evans GR, Brandt K, Widmer MS, et al. In vivo evaluation of poly (L-lactic acid) porous conduits for peripheral nerve regeneration. *Biomaterials* 1999;20:1109.
70. Li J, Shi R. Fabrication of patterned multi-walled poly-l-lactic acid conduits for nerve regeneration. *J Neurosci Methods* 2007;165:257.
71. Sundback C, Hadlock T, Cheney M, Vacanti J. Manufacture of porous polymer nerve conduits by a novel low-pressure injection molding process. *Biomaterials* 2003;24:819.
72. Deister C, Schmidt CE. Optimizing neurotrophic factor combinations for neurite outgrowth. *J Neural Eng* 2006;3:172.
73. Lee AC, Yu VM, Lowe JB 3rd, et al. Controlled release of nerve growth factor enhances sciatic nerve regeneration. *Exp Neurol* 2003;184:295.
74. Mohanna PN, Terenghi G, Wiberg M. Composite PHB-GGF conduit for long nerve gap repair: a long-term evaluation. *Scand J Plast Reconstr Surg Hand Surg* 2005;39:129.
75. Han J, Zhang J, Zhang Y. A functional evaluation on peripheral nerve regeneration enhanced by targeted muscular injection of ciliary neurotrophic factor. *Zhongguo Xiu Fu Chong Jian Wai Ke Za Zhi* 2000;14:87–89.
76. Wood MD, MacEwan MR, French AR, et al. Fibrin matrices with affinity-based delivery systems and neurotrophic factors promote functional nerve regeneration. *Biotech Bioeng* 2010;106:970.
77. Madduri S, di Summa P, Papaloizos M, et al. Effect of controlled co-delivery of synergistic neurotrophic factors on early nerve regeneration in rats. *Biomaterials* 2010;31:8402.
78. Tang JB. Group fascicular vein grafts with interposition of nerve slices for long ulnar nerve defects: report of three cases. *Microsurgery* 1993;14:404.
79. Tang JB. Vein conduits with interposition of nerve tissue for peripheral nerve defects. *J Reconstr Microsurg* 1995;11:21.
80. Strauch B, Rodriguez DM, Diaz J, et al. Autologous Schwann cells drive regeneration through a 6-cm autogenous venous nerve conduit. *J Reconstr Microsurg* 2001;17:589.
81. Safford KM, Hicok KC, Safford SD, et al. Neurogenic differentiation of murine and human adipose-derived stromal cells. *Biochem Biophys Re Commun* 2002;294:371.
82. Kingham PJ, Kalbermatten DF, Mahay D, et al. Adipose derived stem cells differentiate into a Schwann cell phenotype and promote neurite outgrowth in vitro. *Exp Neurol* 2007;207:267.
83. Xu Y, Liu L, Li Y, et al. Myelin-forming ability of Schwann cell-like cells induced from rat adipose-derived stem cells in vitro. *Brain Res* 2008;1239:49.
84. Di Summa PG, Kingham PJ, Raffoul W, et al. Adipose derived stem cells enhance peripheral nerve regeneration. *J Plast Reconstr Aesthet Surg* 2010;63:1544.

CHAPTER 71

Nerve Transfers

Christophe Oberlin

Since the introduction of nerve transfers for reconstruction of traumatic brachial plexus injuries, they have been applied more recently to obstetric brachial plexus palsy (1–3). Nerve transfers represent an alternative to anatomical reconstruction by means of nerve grafting and increase the reconstructive options to improve the final results. The surgeon has to decide: which function is to be restored by nerve grafting and which function by nerve transfer? Which is the more reliable procedure? Does the age of the patient, the delay after injury, or the type of trauma influence this choice?

CONCEPT OF NERVE TRANSFERS

Definitions

A nerve transfer involves partially or totally cutting a healthy normal nerve and suturing it to the distal stump of a paralyzed nerve. This implies that sacrifice of the "donor nerve" is likely to have minimal or no consequences for the patient. There are two different nerve transfers, terminal nerve transfers and proximal fascicular nerve transfers.

Terminal Nerve Transfers (Figure 71-1)

In some cases, a donor nerve is cut completely with potential sacrifice of the end organ, a muscle, or sensory receptors. It should be clearly established what, if any, are the permanent sequelae resulting for the patient. Any such sequelae should be less important than the overall improvement resulting from the nerve transfer. This therefore implies that a nerve transfer has to be successful or the sequelae close to zero. These transfers are termed *terminal nerve transfers* because there is complete division of the terminal branch of a donor nerve.

Proximal Fascicular Nerve Transfers (Figure 71-2)

In some cases, isolated fascicles of a nerve are used as the donor nerve fibers, preserving the major part of the donor nerve and maintaining complete sensory and motor function of this nerve (4). Minimal donor site morbidity has been widely confirmed in the literature (5–11). The mechanism remains unclear, probably partly central by brain plasticity and partly distally in which the relative denervation is compensated by distal collateral sprouting. This type of transfer is termed *proximal fascicular nerve transfer*, proximal because the dissection is performed at a proximal level of a nerve and fascicular because technically only a single group fascicle from the donor nerve is sutured to a distal nerve stump.

Historical Aspects

Historical review (12) reveals that what we call "proximal fascicular nerve transfer" today corresponds to "nerve anastomosis, technique C" published by Sherren in London in 1906 (Figure 71-3). True "end-to-side suture" is a completely different technique and consists of excising an epineurial "window" on the donor nerve and then suturing the distal stump of a recipient nerve to the "epineurial window" (Figure 71-4) (13). True "end-to-side" nerve sutures seems to provide lesser functional results than proximal fascicular nerve transfers; the end-to-side nerve suture technique is described in Chapter 69.

DISCUSSION

When a surgeon has to choose between an anatomical nerve reconstruction by means of conventional nerve grafting or nerve transfer, why use a nerve transfer? One of the most important parameters influencing the result is the quality of the axons in the proximal nerve stump. We know that this is difficult to assess intraoperatively, especially in stretch injuries, even with the help of histologic techniques. Conversely, we know precisely the number of myelinated axons in each potential nerve transfer from published anatomical studies. We also know the proportion of sensory and motor axons in each potential nerve transfer,

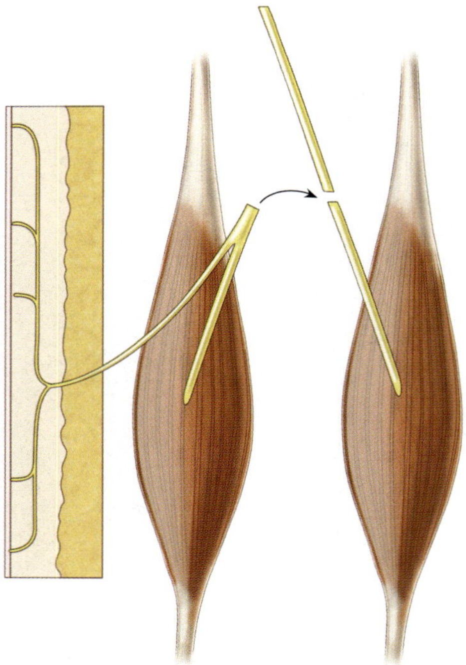

FIGURE 71-1 Terminal nerve transfer. The donor nerve is completely transected with sacrifice of the motor or sensory end organ and transferred to the recipient nerve.

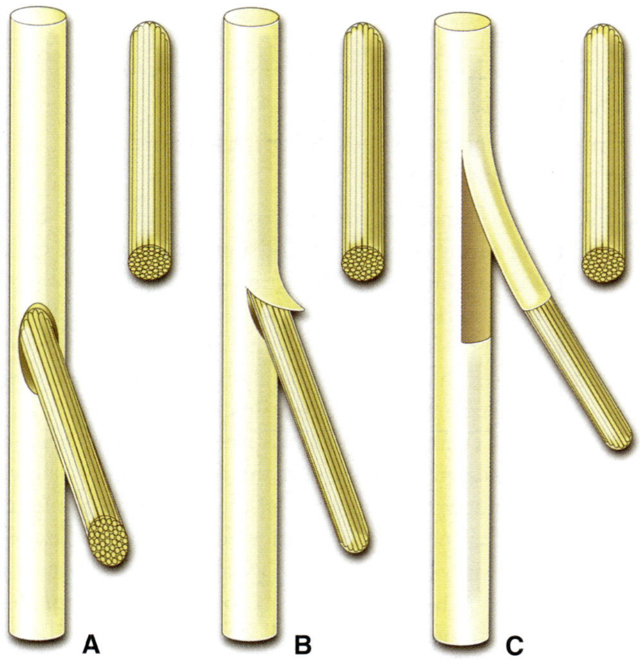

FIGURE 71-3 Different types of nerve transfers according to Sherren 1906, quoted in Papalia (2009). Type A seems to correspond to the "true end-to-side technique" by Viterbo, and type C corresponds to fascicular nerve transfer.

allowing us a choice when trying to restore either sensation or motor function. Anatomic dissections have allowed the identification of potential donor nerves very close to the motor nerves of target denervated muscles that could potentially be used for reconstruction of motor function. The length and duration of axonal regrowth is therefore shortened, which is a major factor in influencing outcomes (14). This fact is of such crucial importance that even in some sharply transected nerve injuries, some nerve transfers have proved to provide better results than classical nerve repairs or grafting!

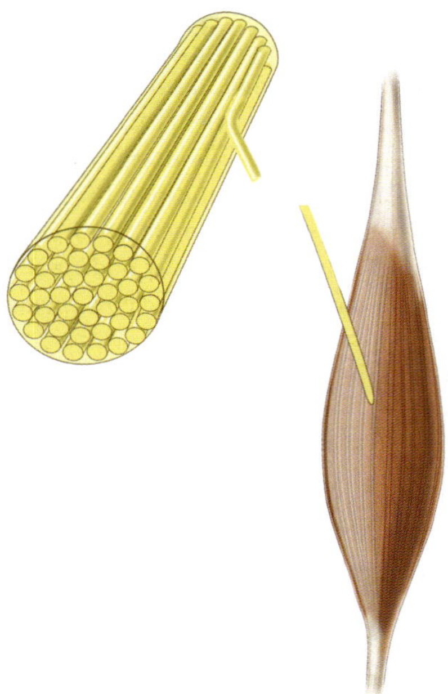

FIGURE 71-2 Fascicular nerve transfer. One fascicle is separated from the main nerve and used as donor fibers, preserving the main part of the nerve trunk, maintaining complete sensory and motor function of this nerve.

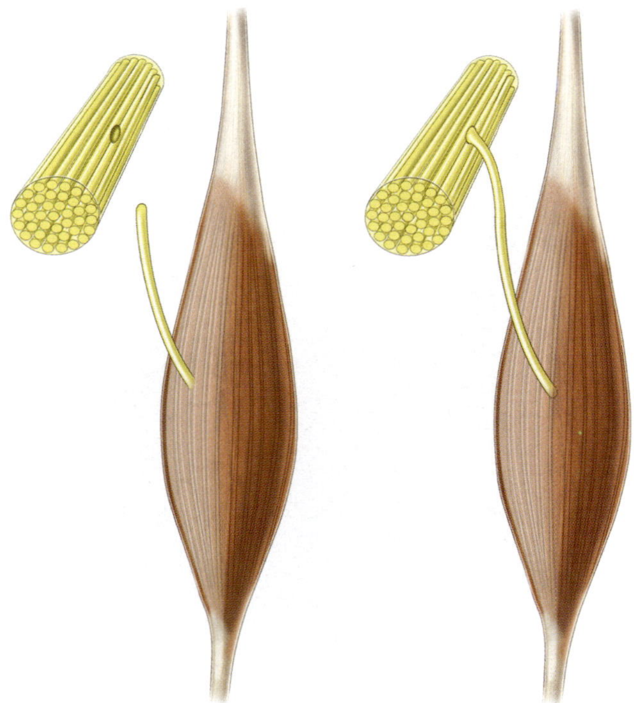

FIGURE 71-4 "True end-to-side" nerve transfer. This technique consists of excising a small epineurial "window" on the main donor nerve and then suturing the distal stump of the recipient nerve to the epineurial window.

POSSIBLE NERVE TRANSFERS IN THE UPPER EXTREMITY

Shoulder

Spinal Accessory Nerve to Suprascapular Nerve (Figure 71-5)

Thousands of spinal accessory nerves have probably been divided to be transferred to either the suprascapular nerve or to the musculocutaneous nerve. Dissection of the spinal accessory nerve on the anterior surface of the trapezius muscle allows preservation of the innervation to the upper portion of the muscle. However, this results in a paralysis of the mid and lower trapezius of a terminal nerve transfer. In cases of partial brachial plexus palsy, if reinnervation of the rotator cuff and deltoid muscles is successful, harvesting of the spinal accessory nerve produces a characteristic deformity of the shoulder. An important question that needs to be considered regarding the use of the spinal accessory nerve is: is it logical to paralyze a major muscle of the scapula–thoracic articulation to improve shoulder motion? Furthermore, in cases of failed reinnervation and persistent paralysis of the shoulder, the prognosis of a shoulder fusion is clearly worse if the spinal accessory nerve has been previously harvested (41 degrees of elevation against 68 degrees in our series of shoulder fusions) (15).

Radial Nerve to Axillary Nerve (Figure 71-6)

The idea to use a branch of the radial nerve to reinnervate the axillary nerve was first suggested in the 1940s (16), but Somsak Leechavengvongs published an anatomical study and detailed operative technique to provide reliable results (17). Somsak showed that the nerve to the long head of the triceps is long enough to be cut and turned upward to be sutured without tension to the motor component of the axillary nerve. In our experience, evaluation of the reduction in strength of elbow extension can be performed using a conventional scale placed on a table in front of the patient. The elbow is flexed 90 degrees, and the patient is asked to actively extend the joint (Figure 71-7). Elbow extension on the normal side is routinely 8 to 14 kg. The Somsak transfer is a "terminal" type of transfer and results in approximately a 30% reduction in strength of elbow extension (18).

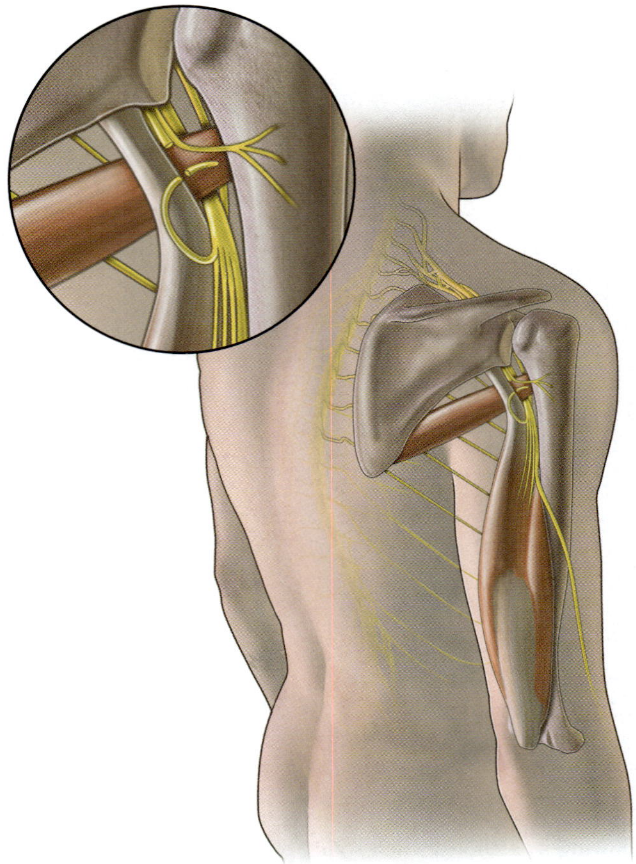

FIGURE 71-6 Radial nerve to axillary nerve transfer. A branch of the radial nerve is used to reinnervate the axillary nerve. The nerve branch to the long head of the triceps is long enough to be cut and turned back and sutured without tension to the motor component of the axillary nerve.

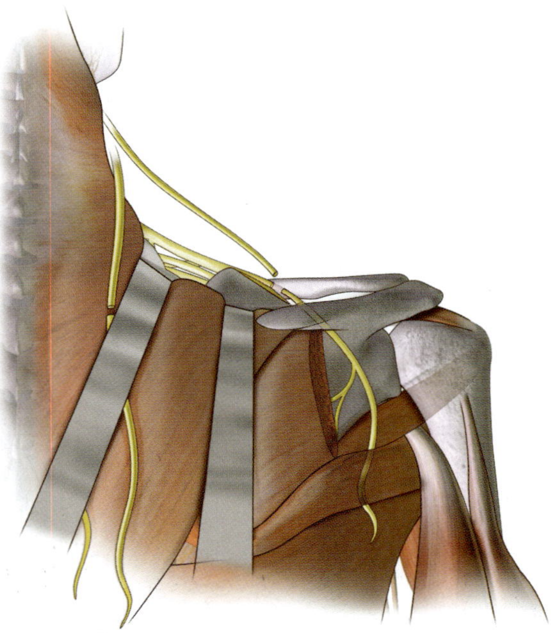

FIGURE 71-5 Spinal accessory nerve to suprascapular nerve transfer. Dissection of the nerve on the anterior aspect of the trapezius muscle preserves the innervation to the upper part of the muscle.

Brachial Plexus to Spinal Accessory Nerve (Figure 71-8)

Most spinal accessory nerve injuries are caused by surgeons during lymph node biopsy. In these cases, secondary repair is relatively easy. The nerve repair is close to the trapezius muscle, and results are reported to be satisfactory. But in rare situations such as resection of large tumors or irradiation, the proximal stump of the spinal accessory nerve is unavailable or of poor quality. In these cases, a nerve transfer from the brachial plexus itself is a simple procedure. A fascicle is harvested from the posterior aspect of the upper cord and coapted directly to the distal spinal accessory nerve at its entry into the trapezius muscle so that an agnostic contraction of the trapezius will be produced by

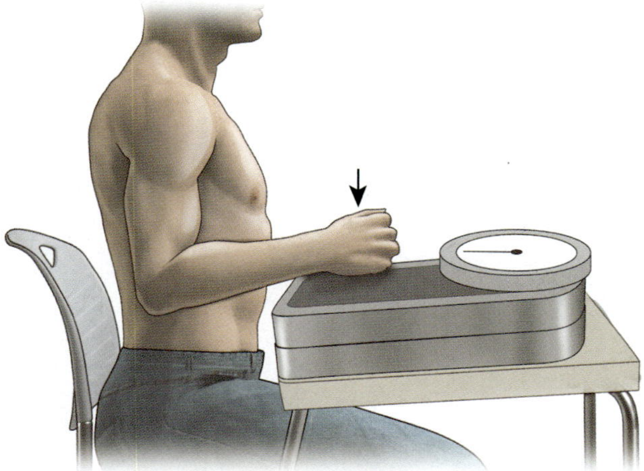

FIGURE 71-7 Assessment of strength of elbow extension. A conventional scale is put on a table in front of the patient. The elbow is flexed 90 degrees, and the patient is asked to actively extend the elbow.

abducting the shoulder and extending the elbow. Electrical stimulation will guide the choice of which motor fascicle to select by producing a contraction of the deltoid muscle or triceps. This technique is likely to become a routine procedure after resection of some extensive carcinomas of the neck.

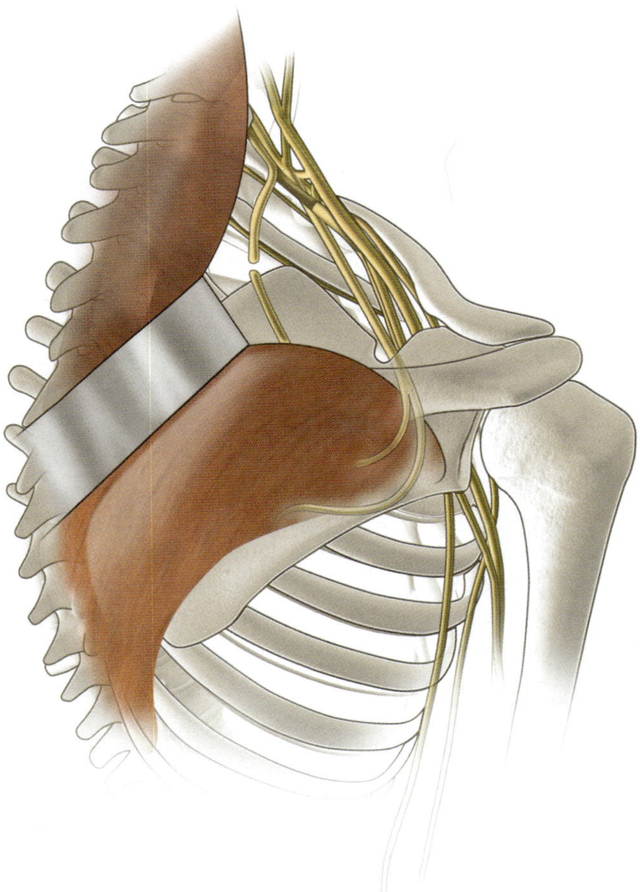

FIGURE 71-8 Plexus to spinal accessory nerve transfer. A fascicle is harvested from the posterior aspect of the brachial plexus and directly coapted to the distal spinal accessory nerve at its entry into the trapezius muscle.

Elbow

Double Ulnar and Median Nerve to Biceps and Brachialis (Figure 71-9)

I performed my first fascicular nerve transfer from the ulnar nerve in 1992, published 2 years later (4). The patient had a concomitant traumatic paraplegia and a C5 and C6 avulsion. The routine procedure at that time was either (1) a Steindler procedure, or transfer of the pectoralis minor to the biceps, or (2) transfer of the triceps to the biceps. This last option was almost always successful, but lack of elbow extension was a major problem because this particular patient with paraplegia absolutely needed to maintain elbow extension. Before undertaking the surgery, I asked myself: "What is the closest normal nerve to the biceps muscle that I want to restore?" The ulnar nerve was the obvious candidate because I knew from clinical "tardy ulnar palsy" that compression of a large part of the ulnar nerve is possible while still retaining normal function. I presumed, however, that fascicles were likely to contain both motor and sensory axons. The operation was a success without any observable morbidity. However, I had made two wrong assumptions: The sensory and motor fascicles were not spread randomly inside the ulnar nerve: after using electrical stimulation intraoperatively, I observed that one can easily distinguish motor and sensory fascicles. A large motor fascicle is frequently found in the anteromedial quadrant of the nerve with an ideal size to match the biceps nerve. The second mistake was that the absence of donor nerve morbidity does not correlate with the mechanism of preservation of function in the chronic denervation of tardy ulnar palsy. In the latter situation, muscle strength does not decrease for a long time because there is distal collateral sprouting from the remaining nerve fibers, resulting in "giant motor units," which have been repeatedly observed in electrophysiologic studies. There is no published electromyography study looking at nerve transfers, but the fact that there is no immediate deficit in the distal ulnar nerve suggests an immediate compensation mechanism that may be central in origin rather than peripheral.

The first series using this technique (5,9) showed approximately 85% good results but with some failures, particularly in elderly patients; those with long preoperative delay; and those with C5, C6, C7 palsies. Interestingly, I observed some cases presenting clinically as a C5, C6, C7 palsy but revealing C5, C6, C7, and C8 avulsions on myelography, and intraoperatively, the ulnar nerve failed to react to direct electrical stimulation. All of the active forearm muscles were innervated by the median nerve. In these situations, I was forced to use some median nerve fascicles to reinnervate the biceps. Mackinnon and colleagues (10) reported reinnervating both elbow flexor muscles, the biceps with an ulnar nerve fascicle, and the brachialis with the pectoral nerve (7). It was advantageous to combine the two nerve transfers, the median nerve being closer to the nerve to the brachialis, thus preserving the pectoralis nerve function because it is a terminal nerve (10,11). We have observed that the double transfer to biceps and brachialis provides better results than one single transfer to biceps (19).

At the beginning of our experience with the median nerve fascicle transfer, two complications of anterior interosseous nerve palsy occurred (20). In these cases, we harvested too large a

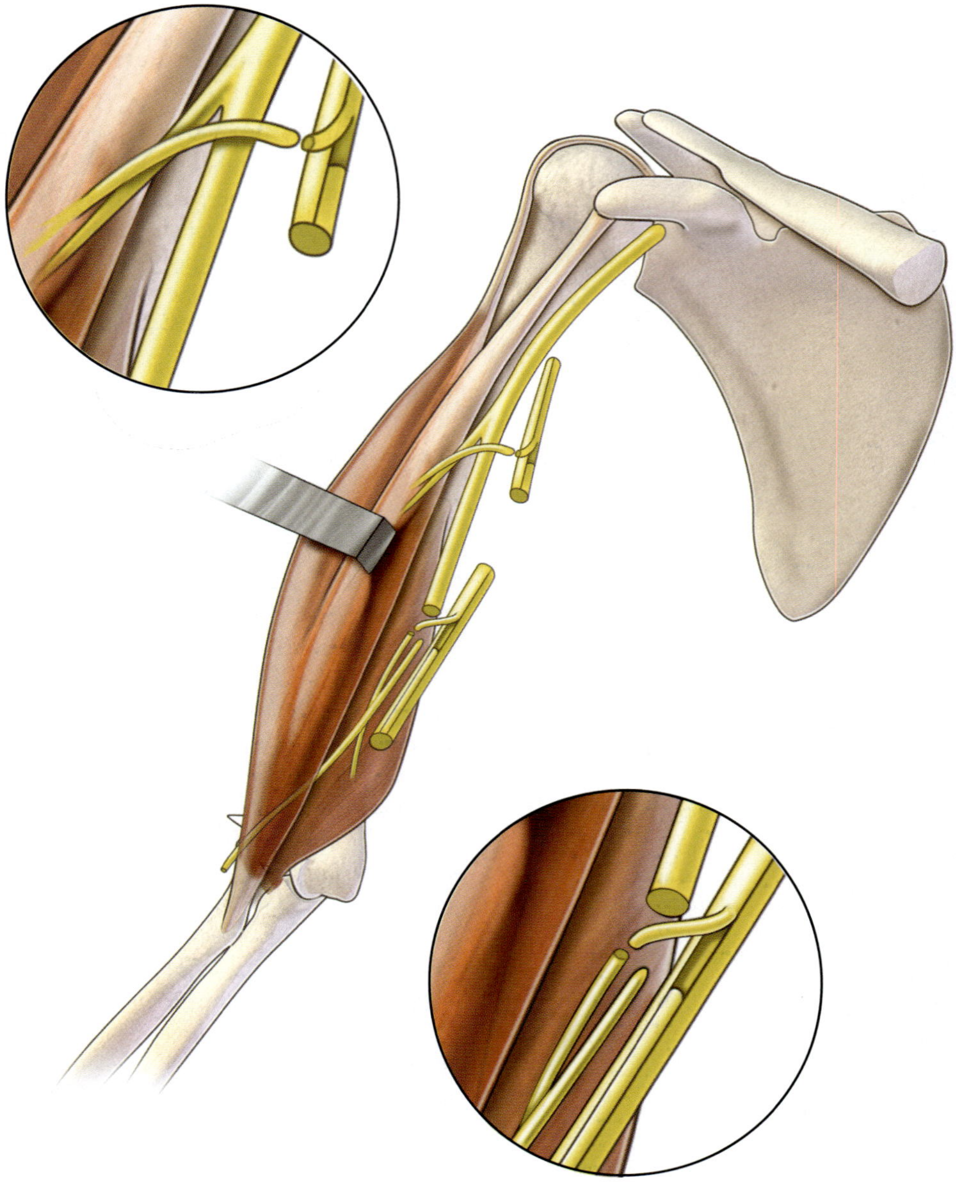

FIGURE 71-9 Double ulnar and median to biceps and brachialis nerve transfers. A fascicle from the ulnar nerve is transferred to the motor nerve to the biceps and a fascicle from the median nerve is transferred to the motor nerve to the brachialis muscle.

fascicle from the median nerve at a level where the anterior interosseous nerve forms inside the main nerve trunk. This fascicle is actually too large to coapt to the nerve to the brachialis and must be preserved at least partially; otherwise, the nerve transfer becomes a "terminal" type and will result in a definite morbidity.

Ulnar Nerve to Triceps Nerve (Figure 71-10)

The transfer of a fascicle from the ulnar nerve to reinnervate the branch of the radial nerve to triceps is also useful in cases of posterior cord palsy. A traction injury of the posterior cord results in an extensive neuroma deep in the axilla and retroclavicular area. Anatomical nerve grafting is not easy and may require an osteotomy of the clavicle. Intraoperative evaluation of the quality of the cross-sections of the nerve stumps after excising the neuroma is not simple, and the size of the cord may lead to a shortage of sural nerve grafts. Therefore, the results are frequently poor, with some contraction of the deltoid muscle or some marginal recovery in the triceps. My current technique consists of transferring an ulnar nerve fascicle onto the motor nerve to the long head of the triceps, intercostal nerve to the axillary nerve, and tendon transfers for the palsy of the wrist and finger extensors.

Forearm and Hand

Motor Nerve Transfers

There are only a few reports of motor nerve transfers at the forearm level. Such nerve transfers are only possible if some healthy muscles in the forearm are deliberately denervated in an attempt to reinnervate some other muscles. Practically, this involves denervating muscles that are normally used for tendon transfers. This presupposes that the results of such nerve transfers should always be better than the functional results of the classical tendon transfers. This has to be confirmed with

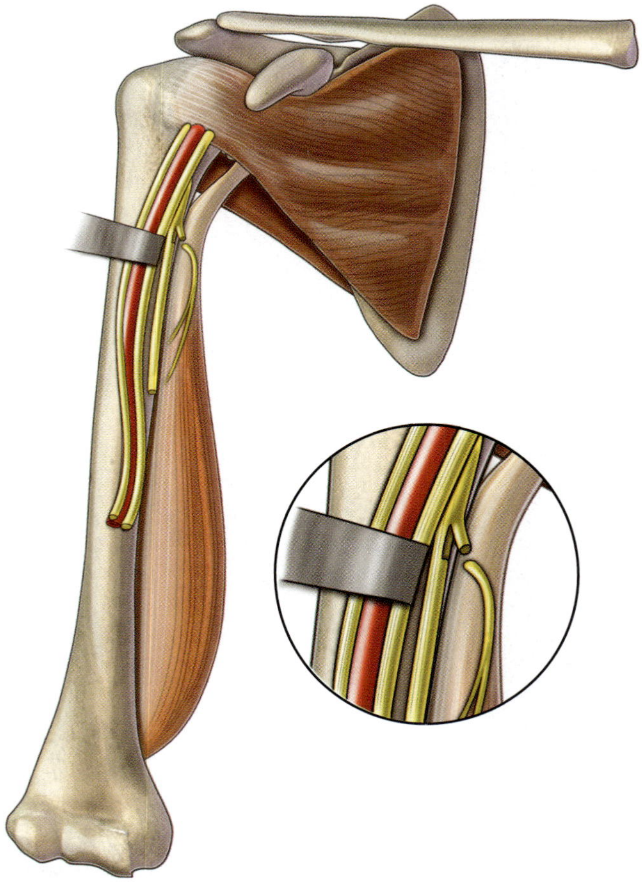

FIGURE 71-10 Ulnar to triceps transfer. A fascicle from the ulnar nerve is transferred to a branch of the radial nerve to the triceps in cases of posterior cord palsy.

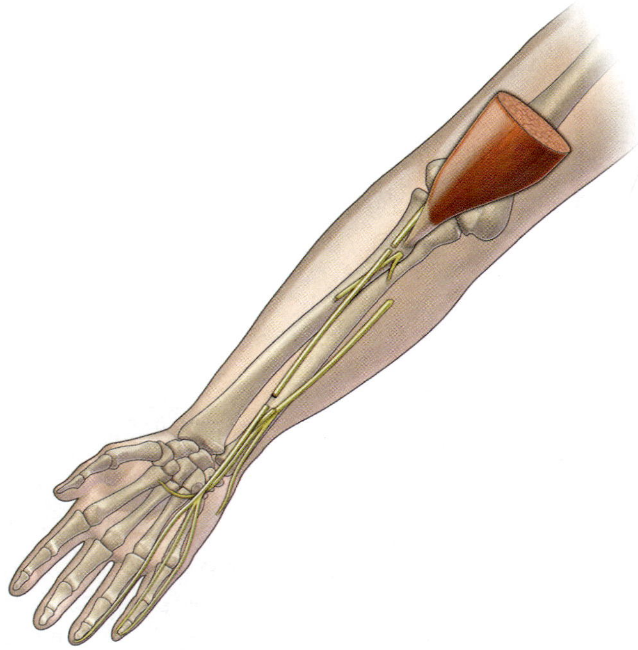

FIGURE 71-11 Sensory nerve transfer from the lateral antebrachial cutaneous nerve of the forearm to the ulnar nerve. The lateral antebrachial cutaneous nerve of the forearm is cut at the elbow crease, elongated with a sural nerve graft, and the distal end of the graft is sutured to the sensory component of the ulnar nerve (split proximally from the motor component).

detailed and sophisticated data (21), including strength measurements and overall active motion of the digits.

Brown et al. recently proposed that radial nerve palsy be treated by means of nerve transfers from the volar aspect of the forearm rather than tendon transfers (22). The results, especially thumb extension, look interesting.

Another nerve transfer has been proposed by Bertelli and Ghizoni (23) for cases of midlevel tetraplegia. In these patients, wrist extension is strong, indicating that the supinator muscle remains innervated. Sacrifice of the nerve to the supinator is probably without functional consequence because supination can be provided by the biceps. Therefore, the nerve to supinator could be used to reinnervate the finger extensor or flexor muscles.

Sacrifice of the terminal branch of the anterior interosseous nerve to the pronator quadratus muscle has been proposed to reinnervate the deep motor branch of the ulnar nerve in devastating injuries to the ulnar nerve (24–26).

Sensory Nerve Transfers

Sensory Nerve Transfer from the Lateral Cutaneous Nerve of the Forearm (Figure 71-11)

Complete loss of sensation in the hand may result in severe burn injuries or pressure sores, leading sometimes to finger amputations. In most cases, protective sensation can be restored by conventional median or ulnar nerve repairs. In some cases, it is not possible, for example, in C8 to T1 brachial plexus palsies. We described the transfer of the lateral antebrachial cutaneous nerve of the forearm to the sensory component of the ulnar nerve for these patients using 10- to 15-cm-long interposition sural nerve grafts (27).

Radial Nerve to Median Nerve

Sensory reconstruction of the palm by nerve transfers from a normal radial nerve has been proposed for cases of median or median-ulnar nerve palsy. Gousheh reported a series from the Iran–Iraq War (28). However, reconstruction of the median or ulnar nerves by nerve grafting provides a high percentage of satisfactory sensory recovery. We still do not know how long after a nerve injury grafting is not likely to provide return of sensation. Even after a long delay, can an anatomical nerve reconstruction be proposed for complete lack of sensation? One can imagine that multiple nerve grafting procedures have been necessary in some patients, exhausting all the possible nerve graft donor sites. Patients with a normal radial nerve have very good sensation on the dorsum of the thumb, index finger, and first web space. The question is: is it logical to partially destroy that normal sensation to provide lesser sensation in the median or ulnar nerve territory?

Intercostal Nerve Transfers (Figure 71-12)

My experience concerns the use of the third to sixth intercostal nerves. Harvesting the second intercostal nerve is not recommended because it provides a large sensory contribution to the

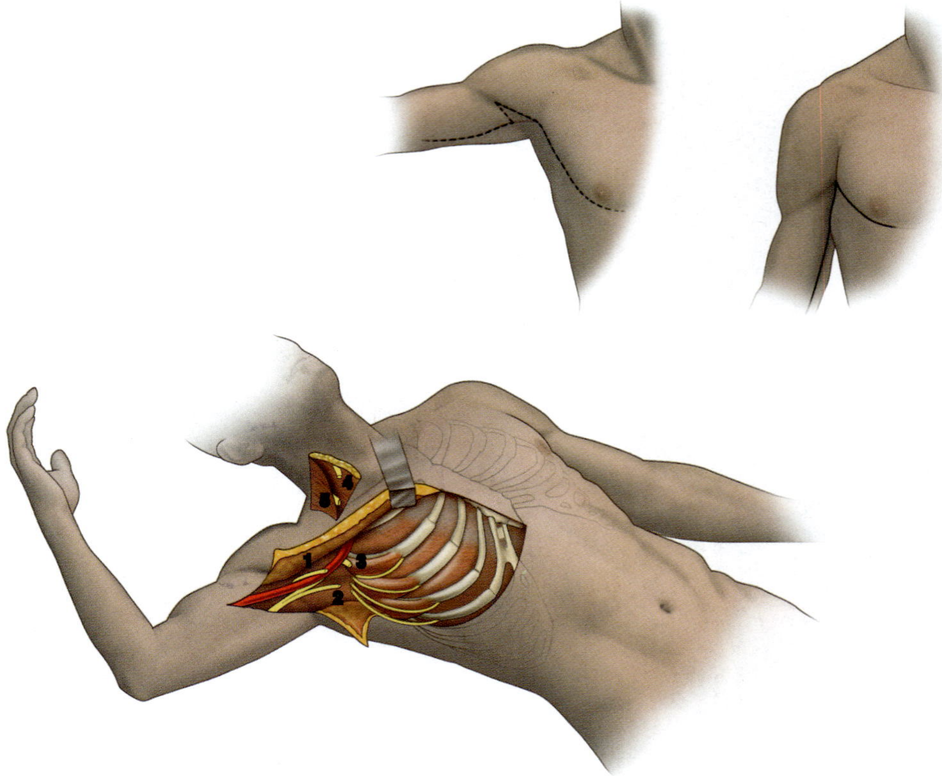

FIGURE 71-12 Intercostal nerve transfer. Four intercostal nerves are harvested through a long brachiothoracic incision following the distal border of the pectoralis major muscle. Intercostal nerves can be transferred to the musculocutaneous nerve (1), the triceps (2), or the axillary nerve (3). This long subpectoral approach is our first choice technique even in cases of sub- and retroclavicular brachial plexus injury. Nerve reconstructions from a graftable C5 root (4) or from the spinal accessory nerve (5) are performed through a separate cervical approach.

medial cutaneous nerve of the arm and preserving this sensation is crucial. Another reason not to use the second nerve is its relatively short length because of the narrower size of the upper thorax, making it difficult to reach the recipient nerve. The current technique consists of dissecting the intercostal nerves as far medially as possible, to the costochondral junction, to allow direct suture to the recipient nerve. A cadaveric study (29) showed that the mean length of intercostal nerves varied from 11 to 12 cm. Of course, by dissecting the intercostal nerve completely along the intercostal space, all of the motors fibers to the intercostal muscles are also severed. Measurement of the cross-sectional area of the nerve fascicles at different points of the same intercostal nerve demonstrated a 33% loss of the cross-sectional area, from the anterior axillary line to the level of the cartilaginous part of the rib. This same study also reported a mean cross-sectional area of 2.64 mm^2 for the cross-sectional area of the musculocutaneous nerve compared with 0.23 mm^2 for one intercostal nerve at the parasternal level, suggesting a minimum of four intercostal nerves are required to neurotize the musculocutaneous nerve. I have never observed any respiratory problems after intercostal nerve transfers and use them even in cases of phrenic nerve palsy (relatively common in brachial plexus trauma). In my experience, I have only observed two cases of respiratory insufficiency after plexus injury, necessitating a phrenic plicature. Of course, the intercostals were preserved in these two patients.

Cross-C7 Nerve Transfer (Figure 71-13)

We have performed 42 cases of cross-C7 transfer (19), most of them according to Terzis' technique: only one part of the root is transected and lengthened using two to four sural nerve grafts. Initially, I used the posterior component of C7, supposed to contain more motor axons than the anterior component as recommended by Xu et al (30). I quickly found, using intraoperative nerve stimulation, that the anterior component also contains motor fascicles for the pectoral muscles and triceps. Because the harvesting is easier from the volar component, this became our routine technique. We have used the pedicled ulnar nerve as a graft only when sural nerves are not available, typically in patients with associated lower limb amputations.

POSSIBLE NERVE TRANSFERS IN THE LOWER EXTREMITY

Thigh

Femoral Nerve Palsy

Femoral nerve palsy caused by trauma, surgery, or tumor resection results in a severe functional incapacity. In our experience, nerve grafting has been possible in all cases. Transfer of the obturator nerve to the femoral nerve has been reported by Campbell and colleagues (31) with a satisfactory result. We are

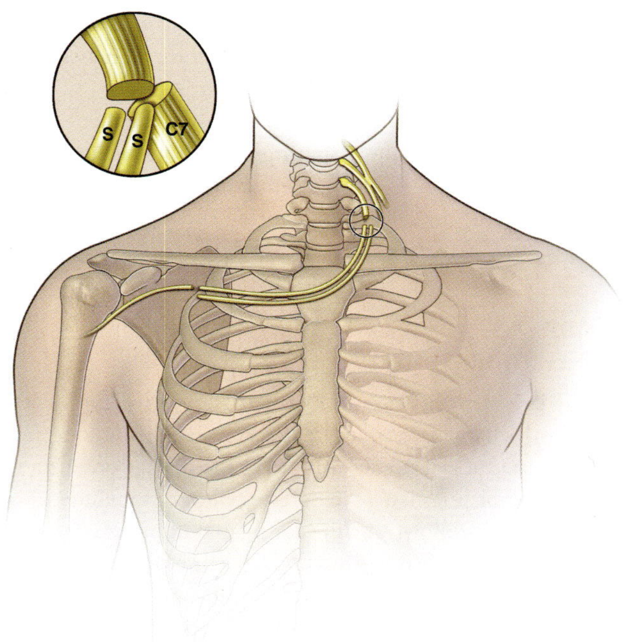

FIGURE 71-13 Cross-C7 transfer. Fascicles from the motor part of C7 are cut and elongated with two sural nerve grafts (or a pedicled vascularized ulnar nerve graft). The distal coaptation is variable (musculocutaneous, median nerve, and so on).

not convinced that such a procedure will become routine because the obturator nerve is small compared with the size of the femoral nerve. In addition, in a high femoral nerve palsy, including paralysis of the psoas muscle, sacrificing the obturator nerve will produce complete palsy of hip flexion because the adductor muscles participate in hip flexion, leading to severe instability of the hip. In low femoral nerve palsy with quadriceps paralysis, we have been able to find and graft the proximal stump of the femoral nerve in all cases.

Leg and Foot

Peroneal Nerve Palsy

Peroneal nerve rupture associated with a knee dislocation may cause a stretch elongation of the nerve, which results in a long nerve gap (sometimes >15 cm) after debridement. Conventional treatment is a tendon transfer to restore dorsiflexion of the ankle. Patients complain of an inability to extend the toes and the great toe. We have developed a transfer of the nerves to the flexor of the great toe and the flexor of the toes to the nerve to the extensors of the great toe and the nerve to the toes.

Through the same long medial incision used to harvest the tibialis posterior tendon, the motor nerves to the flexors of the great toe and toes are identified by electrical stimulation. The common origin of these two nerves is separated from the posterior tibial nerve to produce a 10- to 12-cm-long nerve transfer. The interosseous membrane is widely excised, and the tibialis posterior tendon is transferred to the dorsum of the foot. A second incision is made on the anterior aspect of the middle third of the leg and the interval between tibialis anterior and the toe extensor muscles identified. The sensory branch of the anterior tibial nerve is identified distally and separated proximally from the rest of the nerve (the branches to the extensors). The recipient motor nerves to the toe extensors are therefore identified and cut proximally, allowing direct suture to the donor motor nerve transferred anteriorly through the interosseous membrane. The results of our series are currently being evaluated.

We have no experience of other nerve transfers for peroneal nerve palsy, such as using the nerve to the lateral head of gastrocnemius (32,33).

SURGICAL TECHNIQUES OF COMMON NERVE TRANSFERS

Communication with the anesthesiologist is mandatory before any motor nerve transfer to ensure that only short-acting paralytic agents are used during induction of anesthesia to allow intraoperative nerve stimulation.

Somsak Leechavengvongs Procedure

The patient is positioned supine with the upper extremity retracted across to the opposite chest. After the incision along the posterior border of the deltoid muscle, Leechavengvongs perfectly described the complicated anatomy and dissection of the axillary nerve in the quadrilateral space. The nerve gives off a branch to teres minor and then a sensory branch and usually two motor branches: one to the posterior deltoid and one to the mid and anterior deltoid. By identifying the sensory branch during the dissection, the surgeon can then focus on the remaining motor branches. The deeper and most volar branch is probably the anterior motor branch, which is selected for the nerve transfer. The radial nerve is then identified, and one of its branches to the triceps is selected by electrical stimulation. Currently, any one of these branches can be used. It is rerouted superiorly and coapted to the anterior branch of the axillary nerve.

Double Nerve Transfer for Elbow Flexion

The surgical incision on the medial aspect of the arm lies between the midpoint of the axilla and the medial epicondyle and is facilitated by placing the shoulder in external rotation (34). The incision starts approximately three finger breadths from the axilla (at the level of the distal edge of the insertion of the pectoralis major into the humerus) and extends to approximately three finger breadths proximal to the medial epicondyle corresponding with the bicipital groove.

The skin and subcutaneous tissues are incised down to the brachial fascia, which is incised along the posterior edge of the biceps. The ulnar and median nerves are easily identified just deep to the brachial fascia. The medial brachial and medial antebrachial nerves lie within the surgical field and should be protected. The biceps muscle is retracted laterally away from the humerus, gently lifting and rotating the muscle to visualize the deep surface along its medial border. The musculocutaneous nerve lies on the deep surface of the medial border of the biceps and is often covered by a thin layer of fascia and fatty tissue. Dissection of the musculocutaneous nerve is carefully performed from proximal to distal until the first motor branch to the biceps is identified. This branch usually enters the middle third of the biceps proximally with respect to the dominant vascular pedicle to the biceps from the brachial artery. The vascular pedicle travels more transversely than the nerve and should be preserved. More distal dissection of the musculocutaneous nerve is done to evaluate the pattern of innervation to the biceps. The majority of patients (62%) have a single branch from the musculocutaneous nerve (MCN) that bifurcates to supply the short and long heads of the biceps muscle separately (type I pattern). However, a substantial percentage of patients have two, and less commonly, three separate branches from the musculocutaneous nerve. After identifying all of the branches, proximal intrafascicular dissection of the nerve should be done, separating out the fascicles to the biceps as far proximally as possible. When there is more than one branch to the biceps, it is sometimes possible through proximal intrafascicular dissection of the MCN nerve to identify a single motor group fascicle, which can be used for neurorrhaphy. Proximal intrafascicular dissection of the musculocutaneous nerve is carried out under the operating microscope as far proximally as the limits of intrafascicular bridging allow, usually this is 2 to 4 cm. The fascicles are divided from the main trunk of the musculocutaneous nerve as far proximally as possible, and then they are rotated toward the ulnar nerve.

We prefer to perform the intrafascicular dissection of the ulnar nerve under the operating microscope using microsurgical dilating forceps to spread between the fascicles to help protect intrafascicular connections. Dissection of the ulnar nerve is started distal to the level of the motor branch to the biceps from the musculocutaneous nerves so that the harvested fascicle(s) will have sufficient length to reach the musculocutaneous nerve branch to the biceps muscle without tension. The donor fascicle(s) are divided as far distally as possible to allow these donor fascicles to be rotated toward the recipient motor branch.

If reinnervation of the brachialis muscle is planned and there is adequate distal function of the median nerve innervated muscles, then the branch of the musculocutaneous nerve to the brachialis is identified and dissected. In most cases, the musculocutaneous nerve branch to the brachialis is a single branch, around 4.5 cm distal to the branch to the biceps, arising from the posteromedial side of the musculocutaneous nerve, and slightly thinner than the terminal sensory branch (the lateral antebrachial cutaneous nerve). The brachialis motor branch is mobilized from the main trunk of the musculocutaneous nerve and rotated toward the median nerve. Distal intrafascicular dissection of the median nerve is performed as described earlier for the ulnar nerve dissection.

A nerve stimulator is used to identify the donor fascicles of the median and ulnar nerves. A nerve stimulator with precise variable settings used by anesthesiologists for placement of nerve blocks is ideal for such identification. Placing the grounding needle close to the neurolyzed segment of the donor nerve provides more precise localization of the dominant function innervated by the selected fascicle. We have not found it necessary to have an exact cross-sectional match of the donor and recipient nerves and prefer to have a smaller rather than larger donor fascicle. When there is more than one motor branch to biceps, we recommend reinnervation of both branches using two separate donor fascicles from the ulnar nerve.

Neurorrhaphy of the donor fascicles to the recipient motor branches is done under the operating microscope using 11-0 or 10-0 nylon suture on a 70- to 75-micron needle, placing two sutures at 180 degrees, and augmenting the repair with fibrin glue.

Intercostal Nerve Transfer to Musculocutaneous Nerve

The good results obtained from intercostal nerve transfers to restore both elbow flexion and extension justify the long incision from the medial upper arm along the distal border of the pectoralis major muscle to the parasternal line. In women, this thoracic incision follows the inferior mammary crease, resulting in a very acceptable scar. Clinically, dissection of the intercostal nerves is a demanding technique, necessitating hypotension to prevent excessive bleeding. The use of cautery is forbidden until the nerve has been completely elevated. After the nerve has been cut distally (medially), it is reflected laterally. To improve the distal rotation of the nerve, the proximal portion must be dissected further, necessitating division of the large first sensory perforating branch. In some women, this has resulted in a loss of sensation over the breast, which suggests that peeling off the perforating branch rather than sacrificing it might be better.

RESULTS AND OUTCOMES OF NERVE TRANSFERS FROM THE LITERATURE

Spinal Accessory to Suprascapular Nerve

The results of spinal accessory to suprascapular nerve transfers are controversial in the literature. Merrell, in a prominent meta-analysis (35), reported 98% M3 or M4 shoulder abduction. What is strange is that only a very few cases of M4 were obtained (three of 50). This suggests that what was classified as M3 by many authors was probably exaggerated. We agree with other authors that the spinal to suprascapular nerve transfer is fraught with technical difficulties and gives only 25% good results (8,17,36). Malessy and colleagues reported a detailed evaluation of his own series (37) with only 25% to 30% M3 to M4 results. My experience is the same. Grafts from C5 to the suprascapular nerve provide even poorer results. In summary, the suprascapular does not seem to be a very good recipient nerve in adult complete brachial plexus injury. For this reason, we increasingly perform a shoulder fusion, although it is necessary to preserve the spinal accessory nerve in this event.

Double Nerve Transfers for Elbow Flexion

Transfer of fascicles from the ulnar and the median nerve to the two motor branches of the musculocutaneous nerve has now proven to be the best nerve reconstruction to restore elbow flexion. Unfortunately, some patients are still referred very late after a brachial plexus injury. Because of the proximity of the donor axons to the target, this technique can even be used in some late presentations. In my experience, the longest delay in presentation that resulted in good biceps function was 18 months after a C5, 6, 7 lesion. The alternative in late cases is a free muscle transfer reinnervated from ulnar fascicles. The results of the double transfers seem to be better than a single transfer. I compared the results of 34 single transfers with the results of the first 34 consecutive double transfers, which revealed an obvious improvement: less M2 to M3 results and better strength of the M4 (e.g., 9 kg in a C5, 6, 7 clinical and radiologic palsy) (Figure 71-14) (9).

In the literature, an M4 recovery can encompass a very broad range of clinical outcomes. Therefore, some studies have suggested an additional parameter of being able to hold a weight with the elbow at 90 degrees of flexion, and several studies have defined functional success as the ability to support a minimum

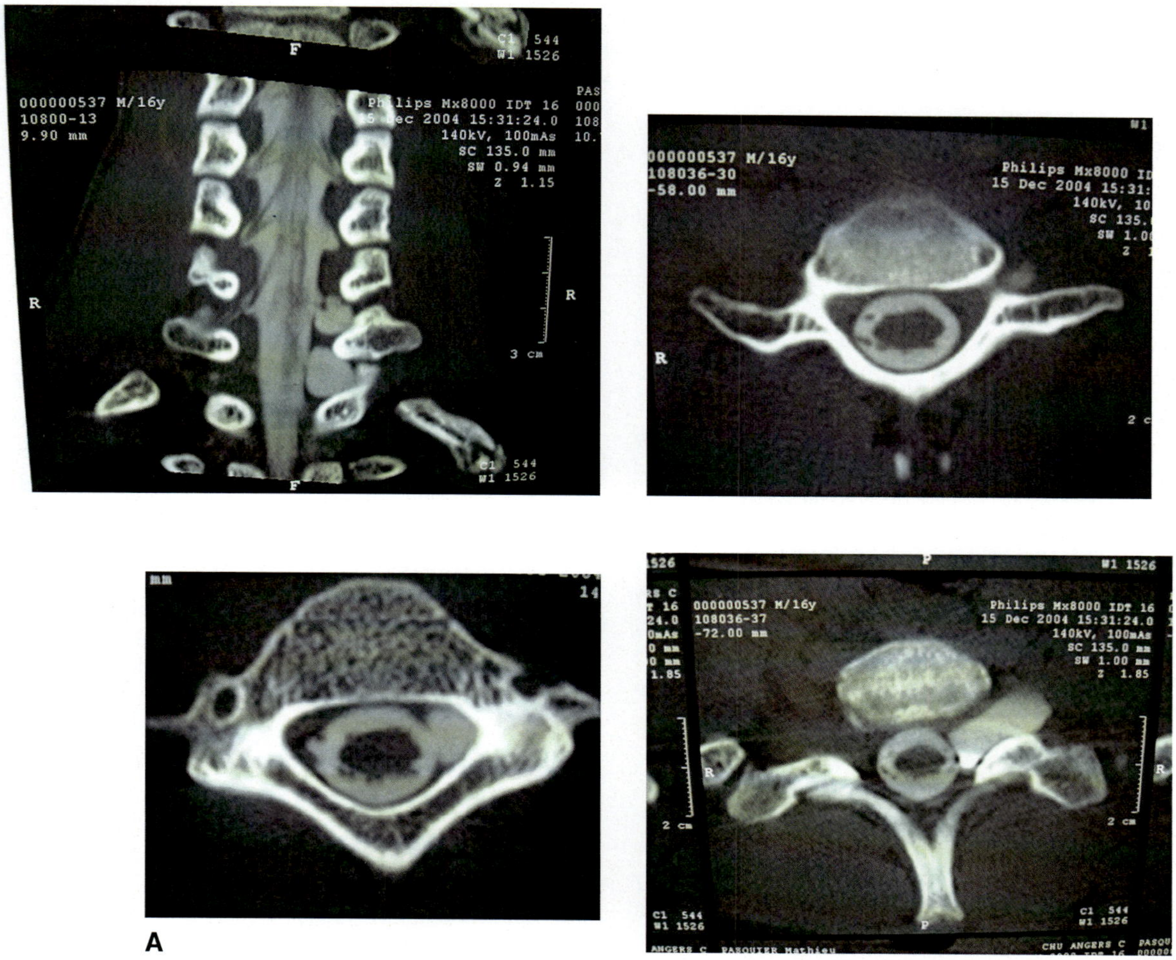

A

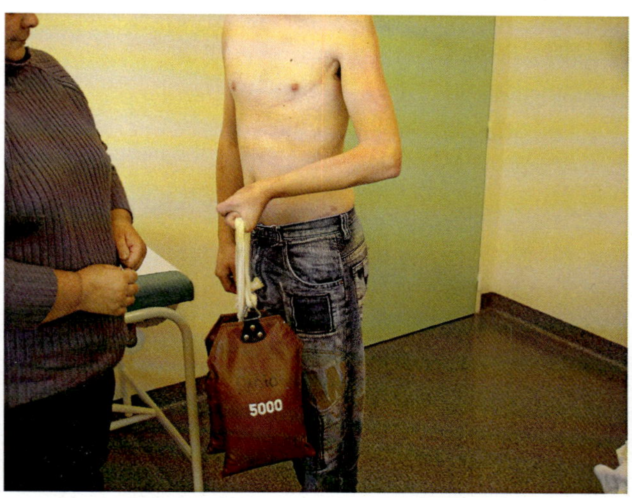

B

FIGURE 71-14 Results of a double nerve transfer for restoring elbow flexion in a case of C5 to C7 root avulsion from the medulla. (A) Myelogram showing avulsion at three levels. (B) The patient can flex the elbow with 9 kg in his hand. The shoulder has been fused, the triceps reinnervated by intercostal nerve, and wrist and finger extension reconstructed by tendon transfers.

of a 0.5-kg weight. No long-term deficits have been reported in the literature from the ulnar to biceps nerve transfer either by clinical examination in some studies or by clinical examination in conjunction with formal testing of pinch, grip, and two-point discrimination in other studies. Mild temporary deficits were reported in two studies. Twelve transient paresthesias affecting the small and ring fingers resolved within a few weeks of surgery. Sungpet and colleagues (38) tested wrist flexion, grip strength, pinch, and two-point discrimination on postoperative day one and found no change in grip strength, pinch, or two-point discrimination but five of 36 had lost one MRC grade strength of wrist flexion. This recovered fully at final follow-up. Paradoxically, most authors report improvement in grip and pinch strength at final follow-up, probably because of the increased use of the arm facilitated by functional recovery of the biceps.

Stevanovic (20), identified a total of 100 cases in three large series with outcomes for elbow flexion using fascicles from either the median or ulnar nerve for reinnervation of the biceps. Eighty percent of patients recovered M4 or more motor strength for elbow flexion, 9% recovered M3 function, and 11% had less than M3 recovery. There was a higher failure rate in the series reported by Teboul (9), in part because of the longer preoperative delay to surgery (>2 years in three cases). Clinical evidence of biceps reinnervation was seen at an average of 3 months, with a range from 2 to 7 months. Recovery of M3 function ranged between 4 and 13 months. For patients who recovered M4 function, elbow flexion strength ranged between 0.5 and 7 kg.

Factors that affected outcome included the length of delay to surgery as well as the severity of brachial plexus injury. A low preoperative grip strength suggests a more extensive degree of plexus injury, despite intact function, and may help predict outcome. When C5-C6 lesions were analyzed separately from C5, 6, 7 injuries, outcomes were better in the C5-C6 group. Even though a delay to surgery seems to be correlated with a worse prognosis, the series by Teboul et al. (9) reported two patients operated on at 12 months after injury, both of whom recovered M4 biceps recovery. Age was not correlated with poorer outcomes; however, brachial plexus injuries generally occur in a younger age group, and there were fewer patients in the older than 40-year age group. In reporting outcomes of intercostal nerve transfers for elbow flexion, Nagano et al. found that no patient older than 40 years recovered M4 motor function. Interestingly, in the two series in which specific patient data is provided, there were eight patients age 40 years or older (range, 40–66 years) of which five patients recovered M4 function, with the oldest patient in the series achieving the best elbow flexion strength.

We have reported two anterior interosseous nerve palsies (19), which did not recover. We had difficulty identifying a donor fascicle from the median nerve, which was just size matched to the branch of the musculocutaneous nerve to the brachialis muscle rather than performing intrafascicular dissection. We elected to use this "large" fascicle from the median nerve, with the resultant distal deficit.

In conclusion, double nerve transfers for restoring elbow flexion provide such good results that they are our first choice even in cases of isolated musculocutaneous nerve rupture (Figure 71-15).

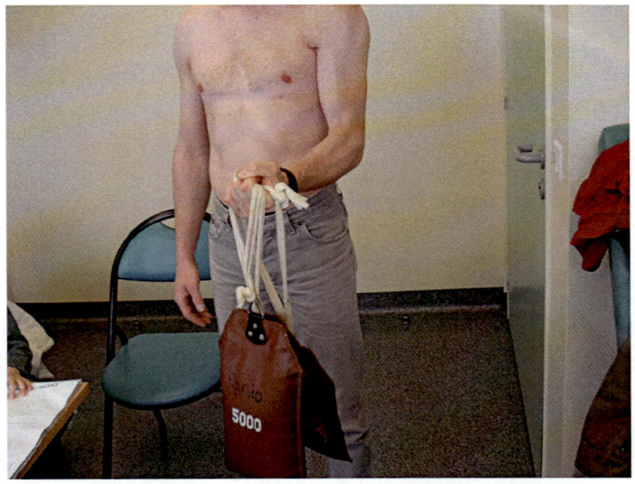

FIGURE 71-15 Results of a double nerve transfer for restoring elbow flexion in a case of isolated musculocutaneous nerve rupture.

Somsak Leechavengvongs Procedure

We reviewed 40 Somsak procedures performed between 2004 and 2009 for deltoid palsy, including 26 upper plexus palsies, 14 axillary palsies, and three cases of associated suprascapular palsy. The age range was from 16 to 68 years, and the average delay before surgery was 8 months (3–27 months). The strength of shoulder abduction and elbow extension was evaluated at a mean follow-up of 17 months (12–38 months).

In the upper plexus group (n = 26), 10 patients recovered M4 deltoid strength (average of 142 degrees of shoulder abduction), 11 patients were M3 (average of 68 degrees of shoulder abduction), three patients were M2 (average of 23 degrees of shoulder abduction), and two patients were M0. The average gain of shoulder abduction for this group was 55 degrees.

In the isolated axillary nerve group (n = 11), nine patients recovered M4 (average of 147 degrees of shoulder abduction), one was M3, and one was M2. In the three axillary nerve lesions associated with suprascapular palsy, two patients were M4 (average of 14 degrees of shoulder abduction), and one was M2. The average gain of abduction for the axillary nerve group was also 55 degrees.

Eight patients had a long delay between the injury and surgery (11–27 months), but six of them had M4 deltoid strength (Figure 71-16), and two were M3. There was no difference in outcome between the patients operated within 6 months and those operated after a 12-month delay.

Similarly, of the 12 patients older than 40 years old (oldest 68 years), seven had M4 deltoid strength, four patients were M3, and one was a failure.

The postoperative strength of elbow extension was compared with the normal side in 25 patients. The mean loss of triceps strength after a Somsak procedure was 28%.

Intercostal Nerve Transfers

Our series of 51 intercostal transfers to the nerve of the long head of triceps (19), performed between 1999 and 2004, resulted in 19 M4 triceps recovery, 16 M3, seven M2, and only four complete failures (78% fair or good results). These good

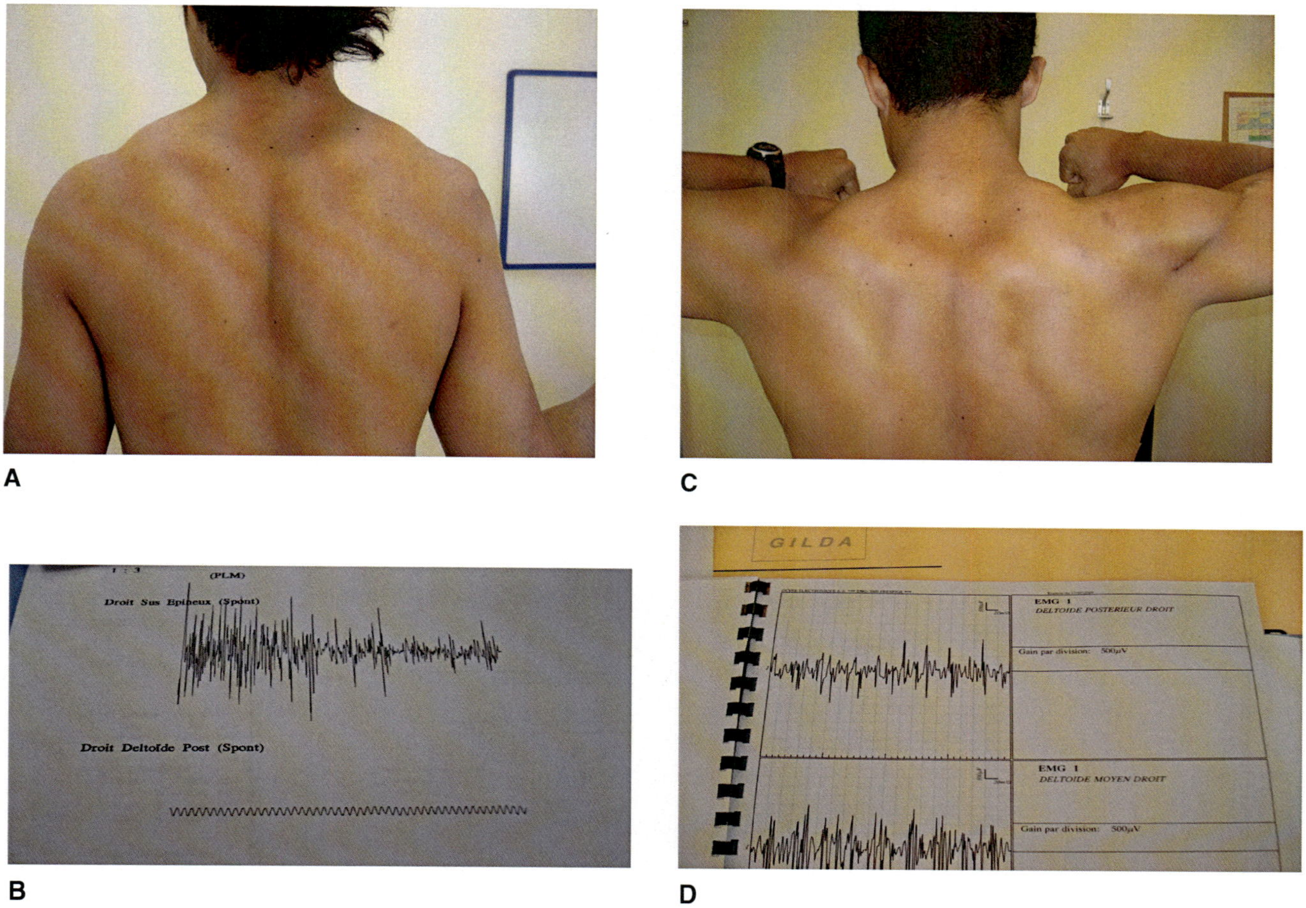

FIGURE 71-16 Isolated right axillary nerve palsy operated 23 months after an iatrogenic injury in a professional rugby player. (A) Preoperative status. Deltoid atrophy is obvious. (B) EMG of the posterior deltoid muscle postoperatively. (C) Deltoid muscle 18 months postoperatively. (D) EMG postoperatively.

results have encouraged us to consider intercostal nerve transfers as the first choice for elbow flexion reconstruction in complete brachial plexus palsy (Figure 71-17). Poor results are specifically due to a delay of more than 6 months after injury. Another interesting point is the comparison between the results of complete palsies (n = 25) and partial palsies (n = 26). Four good and 15 fair results were achieved in complete palsies and 15 good and six fair results in partial palsies. The better results in partial palsies are likely to be due to some spontaneous recovery of the triceps muscle in some C5, 6, 7 palsies.

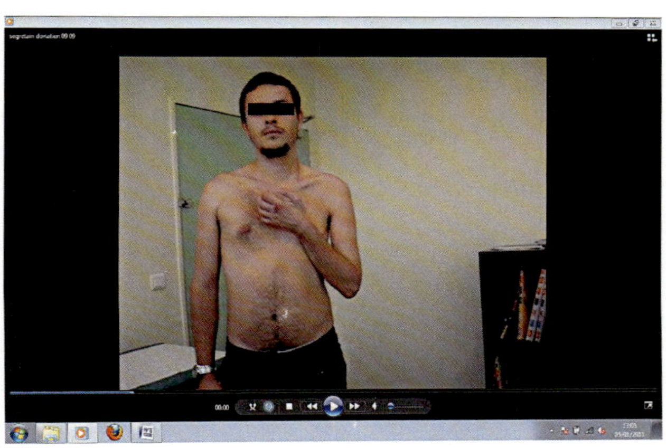

FIGURE 71-17 Result of the transfer of four intercostal nerves to the musculocutaneous nerve to restore elbow flexion. The shoulder and wrist have been fused secondarily.

A literature review (39–41), especially the meta-analysis by Merrell (35), reveals similar results for intercostal nerve transfers to the musculocutaneous nerve for elbow flexion: 72% good results from 27 different series.

Cross-C7 Transfers

We have published 42 cases of cross-C7 transfers, with a follow-up period of 4 years (19). In half of the cases, the distal target was the musculocutaneous nerve and the rest different trunks or nerves. We obtained some very good results, especially for elbow flexion (Figure 71-18), but the complete study revealed only 30% M3 to M4 muscle target reinnervation Specifically, the results for hand and forearm function were very poor. Another difficulty has been the initiation of contraction of the recipient muscles (e.g., the biceps) and simultaneous contraction of some muscles on the donor side (e.g., the triceps or the pectoralis muscle). In almost all cases, this co-contraction persists, even after a mean follow-up period of 4 years.

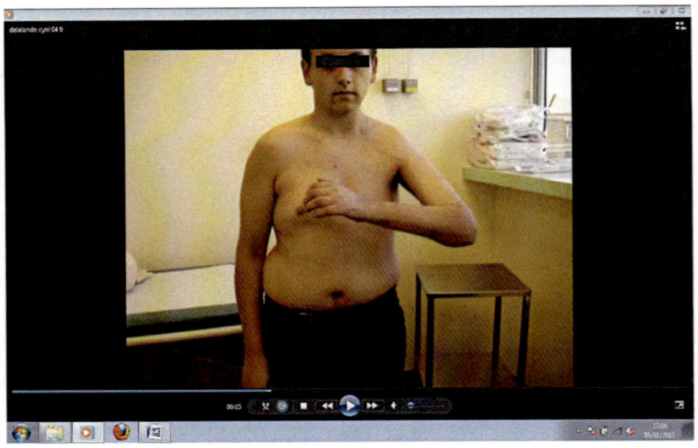

FIGURE 71-18 Result of a cross-C7 transfer to the musculocutaneous nerve in a complete avulsion injury. The shoulder and wrist have been fused. Contralateral contraction of the right pectoral muscle is necessary to produce flexion of the left elbow.

Analysis of the literature regarding the cross-C7 technique is confusing. Some authors report minimal or no morbidity on the donor side. However, we have observed patients who describe transient numbness of the third finger, but all cases resolved spontaneously. McGuiness and Kay (42) described the prespinal route for a C7 transfer, the graft being tunneled between the spine and the esophagus to shorten the distance between C7 and the recipient nerve. The largest series of results of 21 cross-C7 transfers to the median nerve with a follow-up period of 3 years (43) revealed only 29% M3 to M4 muscle recovery. Our conclusion is that the cross-C7 technique produces no morbidity, but is, in our hands, an unreliable procedure in adults. Furthermore, brain plasticity is unable to allow completely independent movement in most of the cases.

CONCLUSIONS

In severe extensive nerve injuries, such as brachial plexus injuries, nerve transfers are now a definitive part of the armamentarium of nerve reconstruction alongside nerve grafting. Some terminal nerve transfers are used routinely such as intercostal nerve transfers. Proximal fascicular nerve transfers have only recently become routine procedures both in adults and children. The results seem so favorable that these techniques can be considered even for some isolated single nerve injuries. The advantages and disadvantages of some terminal nerve transfers, such as the use of the spinal accessory nerve and the nerve to the long head of triceps, are still debated. Some nerve transfers have been abandoned, such as the hypoglossal nerve (44). However, the concept of nerve transfers will surely continue to evolve in both the upper and lower extremities.

REFERENCES

1. Al-Qattan MM. Oberlin's ulnar nerve transfer to the biceps nerve in Erb's birth palsy. *Plast Reconstr Surg* 2002;109(1):405–407.
2. Shigematsu K, Yajima H, Kobata Y, et al. Oberlin partial ulnar nerve transfer for restoration in obstetric brachial plexus palsy of a newborn: case report. *J Brachial Plex Peripher Nerve Inj* 2006;29;1:3.
3. Kawano K, Nagano A, Ochiai N, et al. Restoration of elbow function by intercostal nerve transfer for obstetrical paralysis with co-contraction of the biceps and the triceps. *J Hand Surg Eur Vol* 2007;32(4):421–426.
4. Oberlin C, Beal D, Leechavengvongs S, et al. Nerve transfer to muscle using a part of ulnar nerve for C5-C6 avulsion of the brachial plexus: anatomical study and report of 4 cases. *J Hand Surg* 1994;19A:32–237.
5. Loy S, Bhatia A, Asfazadourian H, Oberlin C. Ulnar nerve fascicle transfer onto to the biceps muscle nerve in C5-C6 or C5-C6-C7 avulsions of the brachial plexus. Eighteen cases. *Ann Chir Main Memb Super* 1997;16(4):275–284.
6. Leechavengvongs S, Witoonchart K, Uerpairojkit C, et al. Nerve transfer to biceps muscle using a part of the ulnar nerve in brachial plexus injury (upper arm type): a report of 32 cases. *J Hand Surg Am* 1998;23(4): 711–716.
7. Tung TH, Novak CB, Mackinnon SE. Nerve transfers to the biceps and brachialis branches to improve elbow flexion strength after brachial plexus injuries. *J Neurosurg* 2003;98(2):307–312.
8. Bertelli JA, Ghizoni MF. Reconstruction of C5 and C6 brachial plexus avulsion injury by multiple nerve transfers: spinal accessory to suprascapular, ulnar fascicles to biceps branch, and triceps long or lateral head branch to axillary nerve. *J Hand Surg* 2004;29A:131–139.
9. Teboul F, Kakkar R, Ameur N, et al. Transfer of fascicle(s) from the ulnar nerve to the biceps in the treatment of upper brachial plexus palsy, *J Bone Joint Surg Am* 2004;7:485–490.
10. Mackinnon SE, Novak CB, Myckatyn TM, Tung TH. Results of reinnervation of the biceps and brachialis muscles with a double fascicular transfer for elbow flexion. *J Hand Surg Am* 2005;30(5):978–985.
11. Liverneaux P, Diaz LC, Beaulieu JY, et al. Preliminary results of double nerve transfer to restore elbow flexion in upper type brachial plexus palsies. *Plast Reconstr Surg* 2006;117(3):915–919.
12. Papalia I, Geuna S, D'Alcontres FS, Tos P. Origin and history of end-to-side neurorrhaphy. *Microsurgery* 2007;27(1):56–61.
13. Viterbo F, Trindade JC, Hoshino K, Mazzoni Neto A. End-to-side neurorrhaphy with removal of the epineurial sheath: an experimental study in rats. *Plast Reconstr Surg* 1994;94(7):1038–1047.
14. Samii A, Carvalho GA, Samii M. Brachial plexus injury: factors affecting functional outcome in spinal accessory nerve transfer for the restoration of elbow flexion. *J Neurosurg* 2003;98(2):307–312.
15. Atlan F, Durand S, Fox M, et al. Functional outcome of glenohumeral fusion in brachial plexus palsy. A report of 54 cases. *J Hand Surg Am* 2012;37(4):683–688.
16. Lurje A. Concerning surgical treatment of traumatic injury of the upper division of the brachial plexus (Erb's-type). *Ann Surg* 1948;127: 317–326.
17. Leechavengvongs S, Witoonchart K, Uerpairojkit C, et al: Nerve transfer to deltoid muscle using the nerve to the long head of the triceps. Report of 7 cases. *J Hand Surg* 2003;28(4):633–638.
18. Belkheyar Z, Michau H, Diverrez J-P, Oberlin C. Transfer of a part of the triceps nerve to the axillary nerve in case of deltoid palsy: Somsak procedure. Review of 40 cases with more than one year follow-up. *J Hand Surg Eur Vol* submitted.
19. Oberlin C, Durand S, Belheyar Z, et al. Nerve transfers in brachial plexus palsies. *Chir Main* 2009;28(1):1–9.
20. Stevanovic M. Nerve transfer for restoration of elbow flexion: the modified Oberlin procedure. In Slutsky D (ed). *Upper Extremity Nerve Repair—Tips and Techniques: A Master Skills Publication.* Chicago: American Society for Surgery of the Hand, 2009, pp. 193–205.
21. Talby Y. Submitted.
22. Brown JM, Tung TH, Mackinnon SE. Median to radial nerve transfer to restore wrist and finger extension: technical nuances. *Neurosurgery* 2010;66(3 suppl):75–83; discussion 83.
23. Bertelli JA, Ghizoni MF. Transfer of supinator motor branches to the posterior interosseous nerve in C7-T1 brachial plexus palsy. *J Neurosurg* 2010;113(1):129–132.
24. Battiston B, Lanzetta M. Reconstruction of high ulnar nerve lesions by distal double median to ulnar nerve transfer. *J Hand Surg Am* 1999;24(6):1185–1191.
25. Ustün ME, Oğün TC, Büyükmumcu M, Salbacak A. Selective restoration of motor function in the ulnar nerve by transfer of the anterior interosseous nerve. An anatomical feasibility study. *J Bone Joint Surg Am* 2001;83A(4):549–552.
26. Novak CB, Mackinnon SE. Distal anterior interosseous nerve transfer to the deep motor branch of the ulnar nerve for reconstruction of high ulnar nerve injuries. *J Reconstr Microsurg* 2002;18(6):459–464.
27. Oberlin C, Teboul F, Severin S, Beaulieu JY. Transfer of the lateral cutaneous nerve of the forearm to the dorsal branch of the ulnar nerve, for providing sensation on the ulnar aspect of the hand. *Plast Reconstr Surg* 2003;112(5):1498–1500.
28. Gousheh J. The treatment of war injuries of the brachial plexus. *J Hand Surg Am* 1995;20(3 Pt 2):S68–S76.

29. Asfazadourian H, Tramond B, Dauge MC, Oberlin C. Morphometric study of the upper intercostals nerves: practical application for neurotizations in traumatic brachial plexus palsies. *Ann Chir Main* 1999;18:243–253.
30. Xu JG, Gu YD, Wang H, et al. Comparative experimental study on treatment outcome of nerve transfer, using selective C7 nerve root vs. phrenic nerve. *Microsurgery* 2004;24(2):143–146.
31. Campbell AA, Eckhauser FE, Belzberg A, Campbell JN. Obturator nerve transfer as an option for femoral nerve repair: case report. *Neurosurgery* 2010;66 (6 suppl Operative);discussion 375.
32. Flores LP. Proximal motor branches from the tibial nerve as direct donors to restore function of the deep fibular nerve for treatment of high sciatic nerve injuries: a cadaveric feasibility study. *Neurosurgery* 2009;65 (6 suppl):218–224; discussion 224–225.
33. Pirela-Cruz MA, Hansen U, Terreros DA, et al. Interosseous nerve transfers for tibialis anterior muscle paralysis (foot drop): a human cadaver-based feasibility study. *J Reconstr Microsurg* 2009;25(3):203–211.
34. Oberlin C, Ameur NE, Teboul F, et al. Restoration of elbow flexion in brachial plexus injury by transfer of ulnar nerve fascicles to the nerve to the biceps. *Tech Hand Up Extrem Surg* 2002;6(2):86–90.
35. Merrell GA, Barrie KA, Katz DL, Wolfe SW. Results of nerve transfer: techniques for restoration of shoulder and elbow function in the context of a meta-analysis of the English literature. *J Hand Surg* 2001;26A(2): 303–314.
36. Thomeer RT, Malessy MJ. Surgical repair of brachial plexus injury. *Clin Neurol Neurosurg* 1993;95(suppl):65–72.
37. Malessy MJ, de Ruiter GC, de Boer KS, Thomeer RT. Evaluation of suprascapular nerve neurotization after nerve graft or transfer in the treatment of brachial plexus traction lesions. *J Neurosurg* 2004;101(3):377–389.
38. Sungpet A, Suphachatwong C, Kawinwonggowit V. One-fascicle median nerve transfer to biceps muscle in C5 and C6 root avulsions of brachial plexus injury. *Microsurgery* 2003;23(1):10–13.
39. Nagano A, Tsuyama N, Ochiai N, et al. Direct nerve crossing with the intercostal nerve to treat avulsion injuries of the brachial plexus. *J Hand Surg Am* 1989;14(6):980–985.
40. Samardzic M, Grujicic D, Antunovic V. Nerve transfer in brachial plexus traction injuries. *J Neurosurg* 1992;76:191–197.
41. Samardzic M, Rasulic L, Grujicic D, Milicic B. Results of nerve transfers to the musculocutaneous and axillary nerves. *Neurosurgery* 2000;46: 93–101; discussion 101–103.
42. McGuiness CN, Kay SP. The prespinal route in contralateral C7 nerve root transfer for brachial plexus avulsion injuries. *J Hand Surg Br* 2002;27(2):159–160.
43. Songcharoen P, Wongtrakul S, Mahaisavariya B, Spinner RJ. Hemi-contralateral C7 transfer to median nerve in the treatment of root avulsion brachial plexus injury. *J Hand Surg Am* 2001;26(6):1058–1064.
44. Vacher C, Dauge MC, Bhatia A, et al. Is the hypoglossal nerve a reliable donor nerve for transfer in brachial plexus injuries? *Plast Reconstr Surg* 2003;112(2):708–710.

CHAPTER 72

Obstetric Brachial Plexus Palsy

Isaac Harvey and Howard M. Clarke

The brachial plexus is the network of nerves that connects the brain and spinal cord with the upper limb. It transmits both sensation from and motor function to the upper limb. Injuries can occur to the brachial plexus during the birth process as a result of traction on the brachial plexus. Injuries most commonly occur in standard vertex presentation delivery but can also occur in breech delivery and cesarean section. Injuries to the plexus at the time of birth regardless of cause are referred to as obstetric brachial plexus palsies (OBPPs). Similar to other closed peripheral nerve injuries, the forces applied to the plexus frequently result in lesions with a mixed spectrum of severity. The injury may be complete in which all nerves of the brachial plexus are affected or incomplete in which only part of the plexus is affected. The degree of damage to a given nerve root ranges from no injury to neurapraxia to neurotmesis. The prognosis for the affected limb and therefore the indications for surgery vary markedly depending on the severity of the injury to this complex network of nerves. The challenge of predicting severity and therefore outcome in this complex network of nerves is central to the management of these difficult patients and is a source of controversy amongst experts in this area. The majority of infants with OBPPs fall into the category of incomplete palsy that will recover or improve spontaneously to a level as good or better than could be expected from surgical intervention. It has been estimated that between 8% and 25% fall into the severely affected range that would reasonably be expected to achieve improved, although not perfect, outcomes from surgery (1–3). The key to the initial management of these injuries is the differentiation of infants who are likely to benefit from surgical intervention from those who will recover equally well spontaneously. The indications, timing, and techniques for surgery in OBPP are not uniform among major centers involved in brachial plexus, and several varied systems for reporting outcomes have been reported. This has led to difficulty comparing treatment and outcomes across varying treatment indications and regimens. This chapter discusses the history of obstetric brachial plexus surgery, natural history, initial approach to patients, brachial plexus anatomy, and indications and timing of surgery, as well as surgical technique, outcomes, and complications.

History

The first description of obstetric brachial plexus injury in the medical literature was in 1768 by Smellie (4), who described bilateral upper limb palsies in an infant he had delivered by applying traction to the head with forceps. In 1872, Duchenne gave the first anatomical description of the muscles involved in OBPP (5). Two years later in 1874, Erb performed electrical stimulation studies that localized the lesion that he identified to the upper roots, hence the nomenclature of upper root injuries as "Erb's palsy" (6). Subsequently in 1885, Klumpke delineated a further subset of brachial plexus palsy in which the lower roots are affected (7); this has become known as "Klumpke's palsy."

Since these original descriptions in the late 19th century, the treatment of OBPP has advanced in sometimes halting steps along two paths. The first path directed attention at restoration of the neural anatomy aiming to achieve reinnervation of the denervated muscles. In 1903, Kennedy first described resection and primary repair of the lesion (8), at this early stage recognizing the importance of complete resection of neuroma to normal fascicular anatomy and repair of the nerves without tension (although he achieved this by immobilizing the affected shoulder and neck together). Throughout the early part of the 20th century, several authors continued to report favorable outcomes of primary nerve surgery (9–11) advocating early neurosurgical intervention in affected children. In 1925, Sever (12) reported on 1100 cases, and in 1930, Jeppson (13) reported on the treatment of obstetric palsy with disappointing outcomes. In 1947, Seddon (14) attempted repair of an upper root palsy using sural nerve grafts, with similarly disappointing results. This led him to advocate against primary nerve repair. The combined effect of these experiences led to a near halt in primary nerve surgery for brachial plexus surgery for almost 50 years. As such, the second path of treatment of OBPP dominated between the 1930s and 1980. This path focused surgical efforts away from primary nerve surgery to rebalancing of the remaining soft tissues in the form of muscle transfers and releases.

As early as 1913, Fairbanks (15) focused attention on the internal rotation contracture that occurs in OBPP and described an operation to release the capsule of the shoulder joint and the subscapularis and supraspinatus tendons and partially that of infraspinatus. This concept of rebalancing muscular and ligamentous forces around the shoulder was further expanded by several authors (16) who developed tendon transfers to complement the release of contracted structures about the shoulder and add power to the weakened motion, particularly of external rotation.

In 1967 with the advent of modern microsurgical techniques, Milessi and colleagues (17) were able to demonstrate in laboratory animals that better recovery with less scar was possible by using proper microsurgical technique and appropriately delicate instruments for nerve repair. They correlated this with clinical reports in humans of improved outcome from microsurgical repair of peripheral nerves both motor and sensory. This led to a resurgence of interest in nerve surgery for OBPP. In 1980, Gilbert and colleagues (18) began to report favorable outcomes for microsurgical reconstruction using sural nerve grafts to anatomically reconstruct the injured plexus. In cases in which insufficient proximal elements of the plexus were available for this type of reconstruction, several authors introduced nerve transfers to neurotize the plexus from extra plexal sources such as the accessory and intercostal nerves. Other authors have demonstrated the utility of the contralateral C7 and phrenic nerves as donors for neurotization in specific plexus palsies. Taylor and Ham (19), Ikuta and colleagues (20), and others further added to the microsurgical armamentarium to treat OBPP with the introduction of free muscle transfers and vascularized ulnar nerve grafts. Since then, multiple reports in the literature with large numbers with long-term follow-up demonstrate the efficacy of primary microsurgical and secondary reconstruction in combination to increase the function of the upper limb in OBPP.

Epidemiology

Obstetric brachial plexus palsy occurs in 0.38 to 2.6 per thousand term births (3,21–27). Risk factors that have been identified relate to increased fetal size and difficulties during delivery. They include gestational diabetes (odds ratio [OR], 1.9), forceps delivery (OR, 3.4), vacuum extraction (OR, 2.7), and shoulder dystocia (OR, 76.1) (28). Breech delivery, multiparity, and history of a previous child with a brachial plexus injury have all been reported as independent risk factors for injury (24,26,29–32). Although shoulder dystocia is very common in births resulting in OBPP, it is by no means a prerequisite. It has been reported that 25% of OBPPs occur in the absence of shoulder dystocia (33). A fetal birth weight 500 to 1000 g greater than average is the most consistent associated factor in many reports. This is becoming increasingly important because the average birth weight in many developed countries is rising as are average maternal body mass index and rates of maternal diabetes (all associated risk factors). It could be assumed that despite ongoing advances in perinatal care, these increasing trends will likely lead to an increase, rather than a decrease, in the number of infants presenting with OBPP in the future.

Anatomy

Critical to the understanding of the obstetric brachial plexus palsy is an understanding of the anatomy of the brachial plexus. The neurons subserving motor function in the upper limb have their cell bodies present in the anterior horn of the grey matter of the spinal cord (Figure 72-1). The axons of these anterior

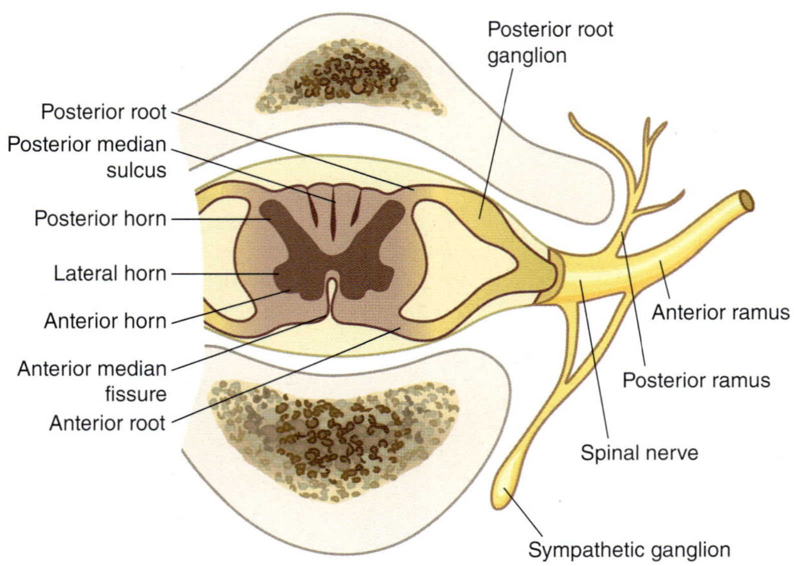

FIGURE 72-1 Cross-section of the spinal cord demonstrating the anterior and posterior rootlets and the location of the dorsal root ganglion.

horn cells project from the spinal cord via the anterior rootlets and emerge through the intervertebral foramina. Before exiting the intervertebral foramina, they are joined by the sensory neurons from the upper limb. These sensory cells have their cell bodies in the dorsal root ganglia; their axons extend along the dorsal roots to join the motor fibers before passing through the intervertebral foramina as the mixed spinal nerve. The brachial plexus most commonly originates from spinal levels C5 to T1. If C4 gives a significant contribution to the upper trunk, then the plexus is described as being prefixed. If T2 gives a significant contribution to the lower trunk then the plexus is described as being postfixed. Approximately 22% of plexuses are prefixed, but only 1% are found to be postfixed (34). Cases in which the plexus appears to be prefixed or postfixed by less than a complete spinal level are also seen. The brachial plexus can be divided in a proximal to distal direction using the terminology of roots, trunks, divisions, cords, and branches (Figure 72-2).

In dissection of the plexus, roots are found between the scalenus anterior and medius muscles, trunks in the posterior triangle, divisions behind the clavicle, cords around the second part of the subclavian artery, and branches in the axilla. In the standard description of the brachial plexus, the C5 and C6 roots join to form the upper trunk, the C7 root continues as the middle trunk, and the C8 and T1 roots join to form the lower trunk. Each trunk then splits into anterior and posterior divisions. The posterior divisions all join to form the posterior cord. The anterior divisions of the upper and middle trunks join as the lateral cord and the anterior division of the lower trunk continues as the medial cord. All of the muscles in the upper limb are innervated by the brachial plexus. The major nerves of the upper limb are the terminal branches of the brachial plexus. The musculocutaneous nerve originates from the lateral cord, the ulnar nerve from the medial cord, the radial and axillary nerves from the posterior cord, and the median nerve from a contribution from both the medial and lateral cords. Other branches arise from the plexus roots, trunks, and cords. Specifically, the dorsal scapular nerve (to rhomboids) arises from the C5 root along with a contribution to (or not infrequently from) the phrenic nerve. The suprascapular nerve arises from the posterior division of the upper trunk, and the long thoracic nerve arises from the posterior aspects of the C5 to C7 roots. The lateral pectoral nerve originates from the anterior division of the upper trunk, and the medial pectoral nerve originates from the medial cord. The thoracodorsal and upper and lower subscapular nerves arise from the posterior cord.

Pathogenesis

During delivery, lateral cervical flexion and distraction of the cervical spinal column away from the shoulder may lead to traction being applied to the nerves of the brachial plexus. At each root level within the plexus, this can result in varying degrees of injury from neurapraxia (chemical disruption of the nerve with intact structure) to rupture (in which the connection of the root with the spinal cord is still intact but damage occurs more distally along the course of the nerve) to avulsion (in which the rootlets are torn from the spinal cord). In a vertex presentation, lateral cervical flexion at delivery and distraction of the cervical spine from the shoulder create a gradient of increasing traction from the upper to the lower cervical roots

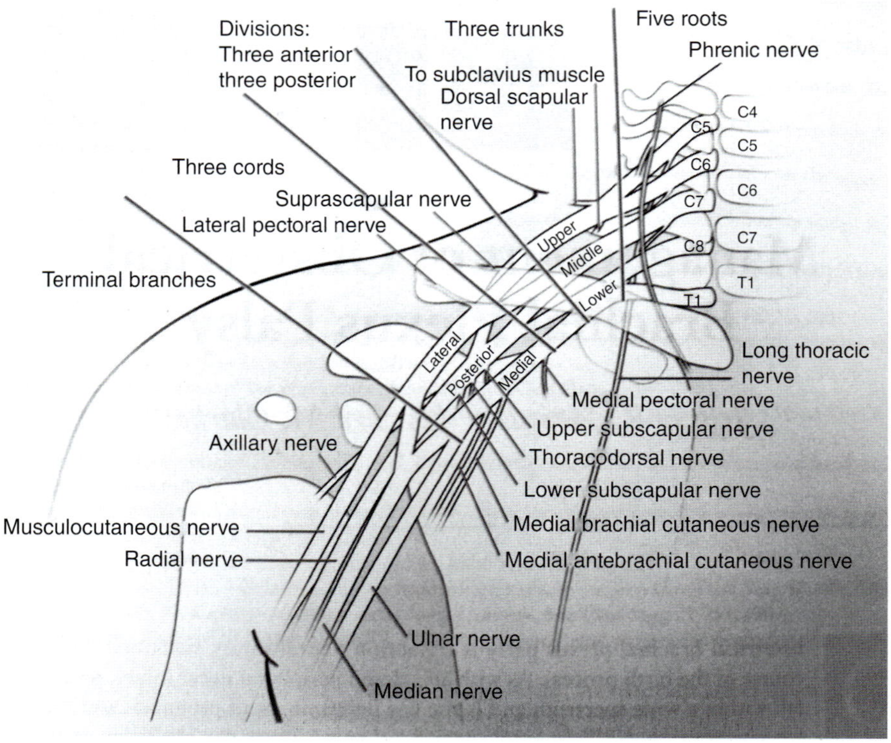

FIGURE 72-2 Anatomy of the brachial plexus. (Republished with permission of Taylor & Francis Group LLC, from Management of obstetric brachial plexus palsy by Marcus JR and Clarke HM in *Practice of Pediatric Plastic Surgery.* 2008, pp. 1427-1453; permission conveyed through Copyright Clearance Center, Inc.)

(10,35). This was elegantly demonstrated by Metaizeau et al. (36,37), who studied the effects of traction on the brachial plexus in stillborn infants. By immobilizing the shoulder and applying lateral traction to the head, force requirements and pattern of injury were determined. They were able to determine that 20 to 40 kg of force was required to produce injury, the upper roots are more likely to rupture (88%) than avulse, and the lower roots are four times more likely than upper roots to avulse. This is because the roots of C5 and C6 are anchored to the transverse process of their corresponding cervical vertebrae by a dense fibrous sheath, giving them some protection against avulsion. The lower roots do not have this attachment. Also, the upper roots exit the spinal cord in a transverse manner and then take an abrupt turn inferiorly after exiting the spinal foramina. The lower roots take a more transverse course. The weakest point (elastic limit) in the lower roots is the point at which they leave the spinal cord, hence the increased chance of avulsion. The exception to this general rule of upper root rupture and lower root avulsion was noted by Gilbert in breech deliveries (38). In this situation, there is a much higher incidence of upper root avulsion.

The differentiation of root rupture from avulsion is an important but difficult issue. A ruptured root leaves an intact connection with the spinal cord that will provide a potential source of sprouting axons with which to reinnervate the arm. An avulsed root torn from the spinal cord does not. An avulsed root is therefore not useful in neurosurgical reconstruction of the plexus at present. It is worthy of note that no preoperative method currently available has 100% accuracy at differentiating root rupture and avulsion. The only definitive way of differentiating rupture and avulsion within the spinal canal would be by laminectomy and direct inspection of the rootlets. Laminectomy is not considered safe in infants, so we are left with some uncertainty as to the state of the roots of the plexus even after operative exploration. The various methods used to help differentiate these lesions are discussed later in this chapter.

Diagnosis

An infant with OBPP presents with failure to move the arm or abnormal posturing of the affected arm. The initial presentation varies from the commonly described Erb's palsy posture in which the shoulder is internally rotated and adducted, the elbow extended, the forearm pronated, and the wrist flexed, to the completely flaccid arm of a total palsy. In fact, the Erb's palsy presentation may be seen in more extensive lesions than the typically described upper trunk lesion and a lone T1 root in continuity can be sufficient to produce this appearance (39). Rarely, a lower trunk palsy (Klumpke's paralysis) is seen (34).

The key to diagnosis is an accurate history and examination. The history should record the maternal history, the antenatal period, details of the birth, and the postnatal course. We use a check sheet to ensure complete histories are obtained from each patient (Figure 72-3). Attention is directed toward both child and maternal factors and particular note taken of factors known to predispose to brachial plexus injury. Of particular importance are the position of the limb shortly after birth and the time course of the development of any movement in the affected arm since birth.

Several important mimics of OBPP must be looked for. These include a "pseudo paralysis" from fracture of the clavicle or humerus. In this situation, the infant avoids using the arm because of pain from the fracture. Some believe that concurrent fracture of the humerus or clavicle is an indication of the amount of force applied to the plexus, although the literature does not support an association between humerus or clavicle fracture and prognosis. Other congenital limb anomalies must be looked for. Other causes of upper limb spasticity must be sought, including brain injury or infarction and placental embolism in which clot from the placenta passes through a patent foramen ovale and then to the limb, causing ischemic injury. After these causes are excluded, examination of the infant's plexus injury may proceed.

Comprehensive examination of a newborn's brachial plexus is often thought to be difficult because of size and the patient's lack of ability to follow commands. Because of this, the involvement of an experienced physical or occupational therapist can be very helpful in assessing motor function in these small infants. The infant is placed on a clean sheet on a padded floor or large low bench in the examination room. In this manner, the brachial plexus team can examine the infant efficiently and critically in a safe environment. Older, cooperative children may stand for the examination. The child is undressed down to the diaper. The position of the head and neck is assessed and note made of the presence or absence of torticollis. When present, this should be treated with physiotherapy or rarely in persistent cases with surgery. This will help avoid persistent neck and resultant skull deformities. Whether true torticollis is present or not, children with OBPP tend to look away from the side of the lesion.

The position of the arm is noted as previously mentioned. Preserved elbow flexion in the absence of elbow extension suggests a conducting neuroma of the upper trunk accompanied by C7 avulsion. Abdominal and thoracic symmetry with respiration are assessed to detect phrenic nerve injury. The shoulder is assessed for evidence of subluxation or, rarely, frank dislocation. Horner's syndrome (ptosis, miosis, anhydrosis, and enophthalmos) indicates injury to the T1 root level proximal to the level where the sympathetic fibers separate from the motor fibers. These arise from the T1 nerve root level just after the nerve leaves the intervertebral foramen.

In an attempt to simplify the continuum of plexus injuries, Narakas and Slooff categorize OBPP into four groups. These groups warrant mention because they figure prominently in the literature, although they are perhaps too gross to guide management. Narakas correlates prognosis with these four groups. The mildest clinical group (I) is represented by the classic upper trunk C5 to C6 (Erb's) palsy, with initial absence of shoulder abduction and external rotation, elbow flexion, and forearm supination. Wrist and digital flexion and extension are intact. Successful spontaneous recovery is believed to occur in as many as 90% of infants in this group (40). Group II represents an extended upper trunk lesion and includes additional involvement of C7, adding absent wrist and digital motion to the deficits listed in category 1. These infants have the classic "waiter's tip" posture of their hand and wrist. Group III consists

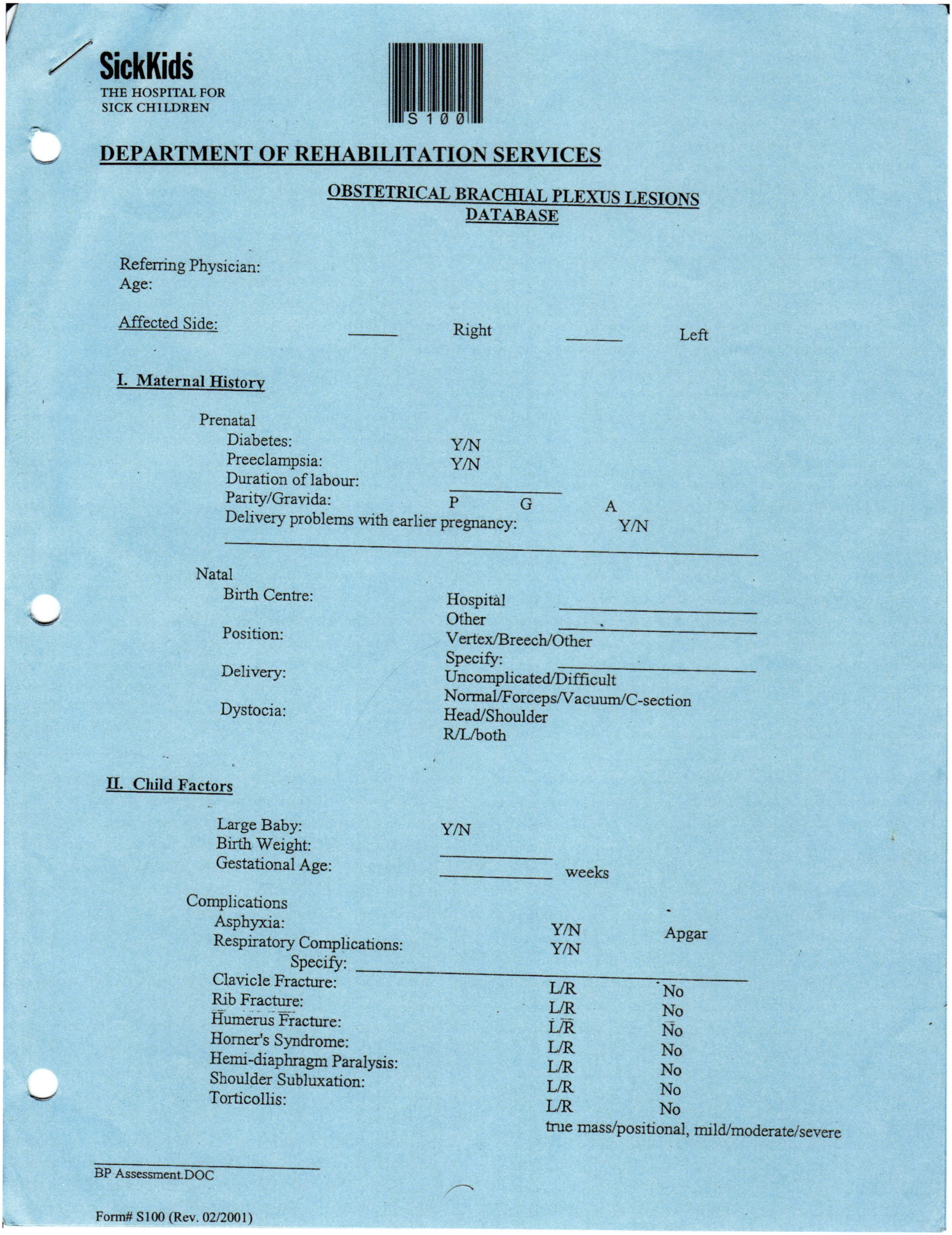

SickKids
THE HOSPITAL FOR SICK CHILDREN

S100

DEPARTMENT OF REHABILITATION SERVICES

OBSTETRICAL BRACHIAL PLEXUS LESIONS DATABASE

Referring Physician:
Age:

Affected Side: _____ Right _____ Left

I. Maternal History

Prenatal
- Diabetes: Y/N
- Preeclampsia: Y/N
- Duration of labour: __________
- Parity/Gravida: P G A
- Delivery problems with earlier pregnancy: Y/N

____

Natal
- Birth Centre: Hospital __________ Other __________
- Position: Vertex/Breech/Other Specify: __________
- Delivery: Uncomplicated/Difficult Normal/Forceps/Vacuum/C-section
- Dystocia: Head/Shoulder R/L/both

II. Child Factors

- Large Baby: Y/N
- Birth Weight: __________
- Gestational Age: __________ weeks

Complications

Asphyxia:	Y/N	Apgar
Respiratory Complications:	Y/N	
Specify: ______________________		
Clavicle Fracture:	L/R	No
Rib Fracture:	L/R	No
Humerus Fracture:	L/R	No
Horner's Syndrome:	L/R	No
Hemi-diaphragm Paralysis:	L/R	No
Shoulder Subluxation:	L/R	No
Torticollis:	L/R	No
	true mass/positional, mild/moderate/severe	

BP Assessment.DOC

Form# S100 (Rev. 02/2001)

FIGURE 72-3 Data sheet for recording information on patients with obstetric brachial plexus palsy.

III. Arm Resting Posture

LEGEND: B = birth; P = presently

Flail arm ______ No ______ Yes (If yes, go to Part IV)

______ Internal Rotation
______ External Rotation
______ Adduction
______ Normal
______ Flaccid

Elbow
______ Flexion
______ Extension
______ Normal
______ Flaccid

Forearm
______ Pronation
______ Supination
______ Normal
______ Flaccid

Wrist
______ Flexion ______ Radial Deviation
______ Extension ______ Ulnar Deviation
______ Normal ______ Flaccid

Digits
______ Fisted Hand
______ Intrinsic Minus
______ Normal
______ Flaccid

IV. Other Changes

Temperature
______ Normal
______ Increased
______ Decreased

Colour Change
______ Normal
______ Pale/Mottled
______ Other: ______________

V. Motor Development

____
____
____
____
____
____

BP Assessment.DOC

FIGURE 72-3 *(Continued)*

SickKids
THE HOSPITAL FOR SICK CHILDREN

S100

DEPARTMENT OF REHABILITATION SERVICES

VI. Active Movement

LEGEND:

0 = no muscle tone or contraction
1 = muscle contraction, no motion
2 = joint motion 1/2 range
3 = joint motion > 1/2 range
4 = full joint motion

gravity eliminated

5 = joint motion 1/2 range
6 = joint motion > 1/2 range
7 = full range

against gravity

Involved side: R/L ______________________________

____

Shoulder Abduction ______________________________

Shoulder Adduction ______________________________

Shoulder Flexion ______________________________

Shoulder Ext. Rot. ______________________________

Shoulder Int. Rot. ______________________________

Elbow Flexion ______________________________

Elbow Extension ______________________________

Forearm Pronation ______________________________

Forearm Supination ______________________________

Wrist Flexion ______________________________

Wrist Extension ______________________________

Finger Flexion ______________________________

Finger Extension ______________________________

Thumb Flexion ______________________________

Thumb Extension ______________________________

BP Assessment.DOC

Form# S100 (Rev. 02/2001)

FIGURE 72-3 *(Continued)*

VII. Passive ROM

Shoulder	Flexion	=	______
	External Rotation	=	______
	Internal Rotation	=	______
Elbow	Flexion	=	______
	Extension	=	______
	Supination	=	______
	Pronation	=	______
Wrist	Extension	=	______
	Flexion	=	______
	Ulnar Deviation	=	______
	Radial Deviation	=	______
Hand	Long Flexor Tightness		Present/Absent
	Long Extensor Tightness		Present/Absent
	Thumb Long Flexor Tightness		Present/Absent
	Thumb Long Extensor Tightness		Present/Absent

Analysis

Plan

Positioning:

Range of Motion:

Stimulation:

Follow up: ____

BP Assessment.DOC

FIGURE 72-3 *(Continued)*

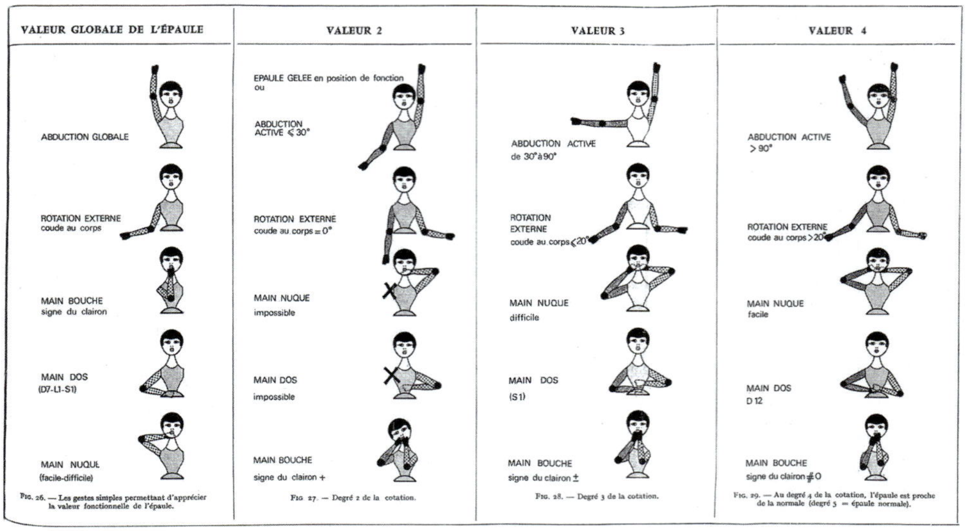

FIGURE 72-4 Mallet classification for upper limb function in obstetric brachial plexus palsy. (Reproduced with permission from Mallet J. Paralysie obstétricale du plexus brachial. Traitement des séquelles. Primauté du traitement de l'épaule.—Méthode d'expression des résultats. *Rev Chir Orthop Reparatrice Appar Mot* 1972;58(suppl 1):166–168.)

of a flail extremity but no Horner's sign. The most severe involvement (group IV) is manifested as a flail extremity and Horner's sign. These infants may have an associated phrenic nerve palsy with an elevated hemidiaphragm. These infants have limited spontaneous recovery.

The motor examination is central to prognosticating the need for surgery. In adults, the Medical Research Council (MRC) muscle grading system is widely used to quantify muscle strength for individual muscles. This familiar scale divides muscle function into grades 0 through to 5 with 0 being no contraction and 5 being normal power. In brachial plexus injury, Mallet (41) introduced a scoring system to assess specific limb movements that together give an assessment of overall limb function (Figure 72-4). This classification system assesses active shoulder abduction, external rotation, hand to nape of neck, hand behind the back, and hand to mouth. Patients are graded on their ability to perform these movements and the presence or absence of maladaptive patterns that may be used to achieve these movements. Unfortunately, both of these scoring systems require participation by the patient and the ability to follow commands. For this reason, they are impossible to use in the infant with OBPP. Gilbert and Tassin introduced a 4-point grading scale that assesses movement both with gravity eliminated and against gravity (Table 72-1). This system does not require the ability of the patient to follow commands and so is applicable to infants. It grades muscle function into 4 grades. M0 is no contraction, M1 is contraction with movement, M2 is slight or complete movement with gravity eliminated, and M3 is complete movement against the weight of the corresponding segment of the extremity. This scale is simple and easy to apply and is widely recognized. However, because it must cover a wide range of ability within the four available muscle grades, it may not be possible to discern more minor variations in muscle ability.

We use the Active Movement Scale (AMS) as developed at the Hospital for Sick Children by Clarke and Curtis (Table 72-2). This assesses 15 motions of the upper limb and assigns a grade of 0 to 7. The assigned grade is based on the active range of movement with gravity eliminated and against gravity. Grades 0 to 4 are assessed with gravity eliminated. A patient must achieve grade 4 (full motion with gravity eliminated) before being allowed to score 5, 6, or 7. The scale assesses movement within the available passive range of the potentially affected joints. The motions assessed are shoulder flexion, abduction, and external and internal rotation; elbow flexion and extension and pronation and supination; and wrist, finger, and thumb flexion and extension. A score of 0 is no contraction, 1 is contraction with no motion, 2 is motion less than or equal to half the available range, 3 is motion greater than half the available range, and 4 is full range of motion with gravity eliminated. Five is motion less than or equal to half the available range against gravity, 6 is greater than half the available range of motion against gravity, and 7 is full motion against gravity. The AMS provides a subtle and sensitive instrument with which to document both initial muscle function and subsequent muscle recovery.

TABLE 72-1 Gilbert and Tassin Classification of Upper Limb Function in Obstetric Brachial Plexus Palsy

Observation	Muscle Grade
No contraction	M0
Contraction with movement	M1
Slight or complete movement with weight eliminated	M2
Complete movement against the weight of the corresponding segment of the extremity	M3

Reproduced with permission from Gilbert A, Tassin TL. Réparation chirurgicale du plexus brachial dans la paralysie obstétricale. *Chirurgie* 1984;110(1):70–75.)

TABLE 72-2 The Active Movement Scale

Observation	Muscle Grade
Gravity Eliminated	
No contraction	0
Contraction; no motion	1
Motion ≤1/2 range	2
Motion >1/2 range	3
Full motion	4
Against Gravity	
Motion ≤1/2 range	5
Motion >1/2 range	6
Full motion	7

Reproduced with permission from Clarke HM, Curtis CG. An approach to obstetric brachial plexus injuries. *Hand Clin* 1995;11(4):563–580; discussion 580–581.)

The scale has been validated in clinical studies showing high inter- and intrarater reliability among both experienced and inexperienced physiotherapists (42).

It is important that the motor examination is precise, reliable, and reproducible but also that the examination is applicable across the full range of the child's development, including both before and after surgery. This allows comparison of pre- and postoperative measures as well as comparative studies among patients.

Prognosis, Natural History, And Indications For Surgery

An understanding of the natural history of OBPP is critical to any management decision regarding these cases. The majority of children with OBPP will recover spontaneously. A smaller proportion of patients will not show good recovery and would experience a better outcome from surgery than from natural recovery. The prognosis of a given plexus lesion depends on the severity of injury (Sunderland grade of injury) to each nerve root. Those with Sunderland grade 1 injuries (neurapraxia) would be expected to show near complete recovery within the first few months of life, but higher grades of injury require axonal regrowth, so they take a correspondingly longer time period to recovery, if that recovery occurs at all. The degree of recovery depends on the number of axons that cross the damaged site and successfully reach their target muscle motor end plate. Because there is no reliable imaging test to differentiate the degree of nerve injury or to quantify axonal regrowth, repeated accurate clinical assessment is mandatory. Much effort has been devoted to determining patients who will progress to adequate spontaneous recovery versus who that require surgery to achieve the maximum possible outcome.

Most authors agree that when surgical intervention is required, it should be performed as early as possible to maximize the benefit to the patient. In experiments in which neurons were selectively prevented from regenerating for periods of up to 1 year (chronic axotomy) or denervation of the distal nerve stump was prolonged for long periods (more than 1 year), it has been demonstrated that (1) chronic axotomy, in of itself, reduces regenerative capacity to about 33% of normal when regenerating axons do not make target connections within 3 to 4 months, and (2) motor neurons progressively fail to regenerate their axons into distal nerve stumps containing atrophic Schwann cells; as few as 5% are successful in regenerating their axons if denervated nerve stumps are not reinnervated. The progressive decay in regenerative capacity after chronic axotomy and chronic denervation followed exponential time courses so that immediate nerve repair is key to regenerative success (43). It must also be borne in mind that over long distances, this limited time window of regenerative success will impact on the capacity of the nerves to regenerate their axons. Hence, even immediate nerve repair may have limited return of function after very proximal injuries.

In reading the literature, many authors use the term "recovery" in an unspecified sense regarding prognostication of recovery from OBPP. It is often unclear if recovery means "any recovery," which would include MRC and AMS grade 1, or full recovery (MRC grade 5 and AMS grade 7). In these studies, interpretation of the reported results is difficult.

There are two circumstances in which the indication for nonoperative management or surgery is quite clear from early on. The first is when there is evidence of return of some neurologic function within 1 month in all affected muscle groups. These patients can almost universally be expected to recover normal neurologic function without the need for surgery (3,44–46). Indeed, an undefined but probably large number of these patients are never seen in a specialized clinic and are absent from published series. The second circumstance is that of the severe presentation of a flail limb with Horner's syndrome that fails to improve over the first 3 months. These patients can expect a poor functional outcome if surgery is not undertaken (23,47,48). In the series reported by Waters (3), 12% fell into the first group with recovery by 1 month, and 5% fell into the Horner's syndrome group. This leaves more than 80% of referrals between these two extremes, where indications for operative or nonoperative management are not as clearly defined.

Surgery is indicated if the outcome from that surgery is expected to be better than the predicted spontaneous recovery. Many authors have assessed the natural history of unoperated OBPP and have attempted to use criteria based on the physical assessment to help determine which patients are likely to achieve satisfactory spontaneous recovery and which patients will derive benefit from surgical intervention. The landmark study by Tassin and Gilbert (46) documented the results of spontaneous recovery over 10 years in 44 children who had not undergone surgical reconstruction. They found that complete recovery was possible if the deltoid and biceps had MRC muscle grade 1 by the second month, that results were good but recovery incomplete if biceps and deltoid recovered by 3 to 3.5 months, and that results were highly unsatisfactory if biceps was not MRC grade 3 by 5 months. Because of perceived difficulties in the assessment of deltoid function in infants, they used the criteria of biceps function alone. They concluded that the absence of any biceps function at 3 months of age is an indication for surgery. This recommendation is perhaps the most widely adopted indication for surgery. In a detailed analysis of the natural history of OBPP, Michelow et al. (27) reported on the changes in active movement in 66 infants over a 12-month period. They demonstrated that 92% of all patients recover spontaneously from OBPP to a level equivalent to or better than that expected from surgery, but 8% would achieve better outcomes from surgical reconstruction. In this detailed analysis, it was found that absence of elbow flexion alone at 3 months incorrectly predicted a poor recovery of function 12.3% of the time. On analysis of the recorded movements in these patients, they found that when elbow flexion; elbow extension; and wrist, finger, and thumb extension were combined into a "test score," poor recovery was incorrectly predicted 5.2% of the time. Therefore, an additional 7.1% of children could be spared surgery and still be expected to achieve a good recovery when this more comprehensive score was used (Table 72-3). A test score of less than 3.5 at 3 months of age is strongly predictive of a poor outcome and is an indication for operative intervention . Waters (3) followed 66 patients monthly for a minimum of 2 years, recording outcomes on the Mallet scale. He compared outcomes of nonoperative treatment and surgical reconstruction based on the month that biceps function was seen to return. He found that patients who recovered biceps function between 3 and 6 months of age did not proceed to normal global function. Additionally, those who were operated on at 6 months of age because of failure of recovery of the biceps had better outcomes than those who recovered function at 5 months of age but did not have surgery. He concluded that if the biceps had not returned by 5 months, then any recovery would likely be inferior to surgical reconstruction and recommended operating on patients with failure of biceps recovery by 5 months. This lends further weight to the notion that the specific timing of recovery is an important factor in prognosis and that surgical outcome can surpass natural recovery in carefully selected patients.

TABLE 72-3 The Hospital for Sick Children Active Movement Scale Conversion for Use in Calculating Test Score

Muscle Grade	Converted Score
0	0
1	0.3
2	0.3
3	0.6
4	0.6
5	0.6
6	1.3
7	2.0

Reproduced with permission from Michelow BJ, Clarke HM, Curtis CG, et al. The natural history of obstetric brachial plexus palsy. *Plast Reconstr Surg* 1994;93(4):675–680.

Strömbeck (49) studied 247 patients, dividing patients into groups based on the number of injured roots and comparing those who had surgical intervention with those managed nonoperatively. A total of 54% of their studied patients recovered biceps function by 3 months and progressed to satisfactory function. Unchanging total plexus palsy at 3 months was seen in 13%, and all were recommended for surgery. A total of 33% were observed for late recovery defined as recovery of biceps function by 6 or 9 months. Those who did not regain function at these later times were recommended for surgery. They found that late recovery did occur and that there was no significant difference in the group that underwent surgery and the group that did not, except for improved shoulder movement in upper plexus lesions undergoing surgery. This led the authors to reject the 3-month hypothesis altogether, instead waiting for a "late recovery." Although there are certainly some patients who do not achieve biceps function by 3 months and do go on to functional recovery, at least half do not. The use of the test score reduces the number of incorrect prediction over the use of biceps recovery alone. If used in the Strömbeck study, it may have led to offering surgery to some patients at an earlier stage.

On careful analysis of the natural history of OBPP, Michelow et al. (45) identified a subset of patients who have evidence of biceps function and pass the test score at 3 months of age but who do not progress to adequate function. At repeated examination between 3 and 6 months of age, if the patient fails to demonstrate any improvement in active movement scores, it is believed that he or she is not likely to show further improvement and will fall into this category of early partial recovery with an early plateau and limited long-term biceps and shoulder function. Surgery is offered for these patients at 6 months of age in our institution.

Of patients who show spontaneous recovery, the majority of this recovery is complete by the age of 9 months. If a patient is unable to bring the hand to the mouth using biceps antigravity movement at this age, then it is unlikely he or she will ever achieve this. To this end, Clarke et al. use the "cookie test" at 9 months of age. In this test, the child is given a small plain cookie in the affected hand. The arm is held at the patient's side to prevent abduction of the shoulder. If the patient is able to bring the cookie to his or her mouth with less than 45 degrees of cervical flexion, the patient passes the test. If the patient is unable to bring the cookie to the mouth, he or she fails the test, and surgery is offered.

In our approach to assessment of patients with OBPP, infants are evaluated regularly during the first year. Patients with documented Horner's syndrome or clinical evidence of T1 avulsion are offered early surgery at about 8 weeks of age to allow for possible recovery of neurapraxia of the T1 root and appropriate preoperative testing. At the 3-month evaluation, AMS scores are converted using a standard formula to obtain a test score ranging from 0 to 10. A test score of less than 3.5 of 10 is an indication for surgery at that age. In a small number of selected patients, surgery may be recommended at 6 months of age for those children that have passed the test score at 3 months of age but have failed to show improvement in their AMS scores. A final decision for surgery, based on physical examination findings and degree of recovery, is made at

9 months of age. At that time, we recommend surgery for patients who may have passed the 3-month test but sufficient further improvement has not been observed by 9 months of age, as measured by the "cookie test." We only rarely rely on only one piece of data at one time to make a final decision regarding surgery. Brachial plexus injuries are complex lesions, and the patterns of reinnervation are neither completely understood nor completely predictable. Because of this, repeated examination by experienced examiners over a number of visits is essential.

Imaging And Electrodiagnostic Studies

The place of imaging in assessment of patients with OBPP remains controversial and varies from center to center. This is largely because sensitivity and specificity rates for determining whether an individual root is intact, ruptured, or avulsed still fall short of the desired 100%. Because of this, all imaging and electrodiagnostic results must be taken in the clinical context of the particular child and his or her injury and recovery status.

Plain radiographs may be used in the initial assessment, and a chest radiograph may demonstrate clavicular or rib fractures (which can affect intercostals as a potential source for neurotization) or the position of the diaphragm (elevated, suggesting a potential phrenic nerve lesion). Radiographs of the humerus may be ordered to document a suspected humeral fracture.

Ultrasonography may be used in the preoperative assessment to visualize the diaphragm during inspiration and expiration to assess phrenic nerve function. It may be used later in children with a persistent, passively tight internal rotation contracture of the shoulder to rule out a posterior glenohumeral subluxation.

Computed tomography (CT), CT myelography, and magnetic resonance imaging (MRI) have all been used to differentiate avulsion from rupture in an effort to aid surgical planning. The accuracy and predictability of these tests are not the same for all roots, and avulsed roots can exist despite a normal myelogram. Chow et al. (50) examined the CT myelogram findings of 261 roots and compared them with the surgical findings. They found that when a pseudomeningocele was seen, the sensitivity was 0.63, specificity was 0.85, and positive predictive value was 0.4 for root avulsion. If a pseudomeningocele is identified but no rootlets could be identified traversing the sac, sensitivity was 0.37, specificity was 0.98, and positive predictive value was 0.74. The presence of pseudomeningoceles with or without rootlets was not a sensitive indicator of root avulsions. Root avulsions were better predicted by identifying the absence of rootlets in a pseudomeningocele. If myelography is to be performed, it is better to perform the myelography at least 1 month after the injury to allow for the pseudomeningocele to be sealed and to prevent the dye from flowing freely to the surrounding spaces.

Magnetic resonance imaging has been used in many centers for preoperative evaluation because it has the added advantage of good visualization of the brachial plexus beyond the spinal foramina. Visualization of the intradural portion of the rootlets is difficult with this method because of the insufficient contrast between the subarachnoid space and the neural structures, a problem caused mainly by cerebrospinal fluid pulsatility. The reliability of MRI for detecting root avulsion injury differs for each involved root. Tsai et al. (51) compared the findings of MRI in adults with surgical findings in operations in which C4 to T1 hemilaminectomies were performed and direct inspection of the cord and rootlets undertaken. They found that C6, C7, and C8 yielded high agreement values between MRI and surgical findings, ranging from 86% to 94%. C5 manifested the lowest agreement values: 54% on ventral root assessment.

Electrodiagnostic studies are used by some centers to help determine the status of the plexus. Electromyography (EMG) of specific muscle groups is thought to help distinguish both the level of plexus injury and the recovery status of the affected muscles and is used widely in adults. The results are highly operator dependent and can be falsely optimistic concerning the chances of recovery from a plexus lesion. Most surgeons believe that clinical examination is a better prognostic indicator than EMG. With regard to intraoperative electrophysiologic testing, Dupree et al. (52) demonstrated that there was no correlation between the findings on intraoperative somatosensory evoked potentials by an expert neurophysiologist and operative findings.

At our institution, the decision to operate is based entirely on the clinical findings as described previously. After the decision has been made that a patient is a suitable candidate for surgery, imaging is performed that will aid in planning the operative management. Ultrasonography of the diaphragm is obtained to assess phrenic nerve function because a preexisting phrenic nerve palsy cannot be expected to improve after surgery, but a traction injury of a previously functioning phrenic nerve can be expected to recover postoperatively over time. A CT myelogram is obtained to aid in assessment of root avulsion.

Operative Intervention

The patient is intubated with a nasotracheal tube, and the tube is secured to the membranous septum with a 2-0 or 3-0 silk suture to minimize the possibility of intraoperative extubation. The operation begins with the child in the prone position in preparation for bilateral sural nerve harvest. The infant is placed on an abdominal support to facilitate positioning. Both lower extremities are prepared, sterile tourniquets are applied, and the sural nerves are harvested through three transverse incisions measuring 2 cm in length (one posterior to the lateral malleolus; one at the popliteal fossa; and one at the distal belly of the gastrocnemius muscle belly, anticipating the point at which the nerve becomes subfascial). The use of a 0-degree, 4-mm, 18-cm endoscope facilitates identification of the peroneal branch and other potentially useful branches when placed in the distal most incision. Usually, approximately 13 to 15 cm of sural nerve can be harvested from each leg in a 10-kg infant. The nerves are marked with ink to preserve orientation and then placed in a damp sterile container in a refrigerator. The incisions are then closed with absorbable sutures (Figure 72-5).

The child is then turned supine and placed at the extreme head of the table as close to the side of the table as possible. All pressure points are meticulously padded. "Egg crate" type padding,

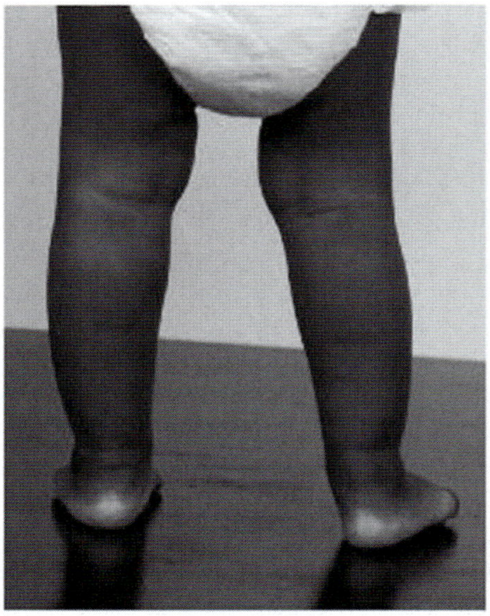

FIGURE 72-5 Incisions used for endoscopic sural nerve harvest seen 6 months after surgery. (Reproduced with permission from Capek L, Clarke H. Endoscopically assisted sural nerve harvest in infants. *Semin Plast Surg* 2008;22(1):25–28.)

without an additional ring for the head, works well. A small beanbag is placed under the padding beneath the scapulae to provide moderate neck extension. Intraoperative fluids are limited to maintenance fluids only to prevent pulmonary edema. Urine output, measured by a Foley catheter, is anticipated to be low. The ipsilateral hand, arm, chest, neck, and head are prepped into the field. The head is turned away from the side with the lesion. A clear drape is used to facilitate the anesthesia team's visualization of the head and endotracheal tube and a clear adherent plastic is used to cover the ear. The hand is secured in a sterile towel clipped to the drapes to allow easy visualization of the hand during intraoperative nerve stimulation (Figure 72-6).

A number of incisions are available to approach the brachial plexus. We favor marking an incision posterior to the sternocleidomastoid muscle, curving gently at the insertion on the clavicle

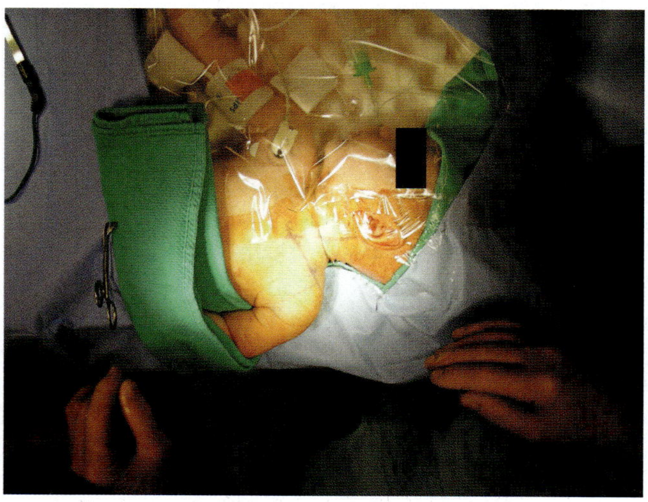

FIGURE 72-6 Draping with a clear plastic drape to allow visualization of the nasotracheal tube throughout surgery and support of the arm with a sterile towel and clip.

and continuing laterally toward the deltopectoral groove. An extensile exposure is marked for use if necessary along the deltopectoral groove, but this is usually not needed. The V-shaped incision is sufficient for exposure of the contents of the posterior triangle without the need for self-retaining retractors and heals quite well. A supraclavicular exposure is used. An incision is made through the skin and the extremely thin platysma in a single layer. The triangular flap of skin and platysma is retracted laterally. Supraclavicular nerve branches are seen crossing the inferior, transverse limb of the incision and are divided as they cross the clavicle. Following them proximally will lead to the fourth cervical root of the cervical plexus, which marks the superior limit of the dissection and serves as a landmark when identifying the C5 root. Other branches of the cervical plexus, including the great auricular nerve and lesser occipital nerves, are preserved. The C4 contribution to the cervical plexus can be used as graft material if needed. The sternocleidomastoid muscle is identified, and dissection is undertaken just lateral to it. The clavicular head of the sternocleidomastoid muscle is partially divided to facilitate exposure. The external jugular vein lies over the sternocleidomastoid muscle at its lateral border, and it may or may not be necessary to divide this vein. The omohyoid muscle is located and dissected, stay sutures are placed in the tendinous condensation found in the middle of the muscle, and it is divided here. Deep to the omohyoid muscle lies the fat pad of Brown, an adipolymphatic layer that is dissected and retracted laterally to expose the neuroma. The transverse cervical artery and vein are located centrally in the field, dissected, and divided to facilitate exposure followed by division of the suprascapular artery and vein located at the superior margin of the clavicle or just deep to the bone itself. A lateral sweeping motion with a gauze sponge draped over the index finger is very effective in separating this fat pad from the underlying clavicle. The neuroma is usually quite prominent and firm. The phrenic nerve, the only nerve that courses from lateral to medial as it descends the neck, is usually draped across the external surface of the neuroma at this level. The phrenic nerve can be seen coursing from C4 distally. It often gives contributions to C5, as evidenced by the nerve being thicker proximal to C5 and thinner distally, indicating that it has given axons to C5 before entering the thorax. The phrenic nerve is stimulated with a bipolar nerve stimulator, and the twitch of the diaphragm can be palpated and visualized. The phrenic nerve must be dissected carefully from the neuroma and, in most cases, from the C5 root to allow access to a healthy C5 stump. The neuroma is then dissected. The anterior scalene muscle, which lies anterior to the brachial plexus, may be adherent to the neuroma. The middle scalene, lying posterior to the plexus, may also be scarred. The long thoracic nerve of Bell lies posterior to the plexus within the middle scalene muscle. It can be preserved during the dissection if possible but may require division to provide adequate proximal access to healthy roots. The C4 root serves as a landmark for locating the C5 root, which is dissected up into its foramen. After C5 is dissected, C6 and C7 are located and dissected. Proceeding inferiorly in the neck, each foramen progressively appears closer than the previous one (i.e., the distance between C5 and C6 appears greater than the distance between C6 and C7). The more inferior the foramen, the more posteriorly it is located. In the case of an empty foramen, the root has likely been avulsed. The injured plexus can be distorted by progressive contraction of the neuroma along its length. Avulsions and ruptures also distort the remaining plexus. In the case of very long lesions, the dissection can be carried inferior to the clavicle by separating the fibers of the pectoralis major muscle from the lower border of the clavicle and, if necessary, detaching the origin of the pectoralis minor muscle from the coracoid process. The upper trunk should be visible at this point. The suprascapular nerve lies along the lateral border of the plexus. The middle trunk may be adherent to the upper trunk, depending on the level of the lesion. The subclavian artery is located overlying the lower trunk. It should be safely dissected away from the plexus to allow inspection of the C8 and T1 roots and their foramina. The dorsal scapular artery is found either between the upper and middle trunks or between the middle and lower trunks and should be divided to facilitate exposure. The C8 and T1 roots lie deep in the operative field but, with retraction of the clavicle, can be readily visualized without dividing the clavicle or extending the incision into the deltopectoral groove. The T1 root lies immediately superficial to the parietal pleura. If the pleura is violated, as demonstrated by air bubbles in a saline-flooded field, it may be possible to seal the leak with fibrin glue (Tisseel; Baxter International, Deerfield, IL) or rarely it may become necessary to insert a chest tube. After the T1 and C8 roots are identified, they are traced proximally. Dissection continues distal to the neuroma to define where the nerve appears undamaged. The roots are then stimulated directly with a nerve stimulator, and the responses in the extremity are noted. A root that has been avulsed will not conduct distally even though the nerve may appear normal in the case of an intraforaminal avulsion.

The neuroma is then transected at its midportion. The structures distal to the neuroma are separated. The lesion can vary significantly both in level and in overall length. The nerves are transected with a fresh #15 blade at levels where they feel supple and appear fascicular and healthy. It is helpful to cut against a tongue blade or an empty scalpel handle to obtain a clean cut. The cut must be made proximal to any scar to allow axonal regeneration from healthy axons to occur. The cut section of the stumps are inked for orientation and sent for toluidine blue frozen section staining. It is often helpful to tag the epineurium of the distal stump of the suprascapular nerve with a 6-0 polypropylene suture to facilitate subsequent retrieval. The proximal level of transection is then determined. Sometimes a root avulsion is clear. For example, if there is an empty foramen, then there is no proximal stump available for grafting. Also, if the dorsal root ganglion is visible, then that root is clearly avulsed and not usable. The presence of the dorsal root ganglion can be verified on intraoperative histology, in which ganglion cells can be readily visualized. For lesions in continuity, dissection is carried out to what appears to be healthy tissue, and the nerve is transected. Sometimes this can mean removing portions of the anterior and middle scalene muscles purely to improve visualization to the level of the foramen. The nerves are transected proximally and stained for orientation, and the stumps are sent to the neuropathology department for histologic evaluation along with the distal stumps. Essentially, all of the neuroma must be cleared from the potential nerve coaptation site, or scarring will prevent axonal regeneration. If the distal nerve stump appears appropriate histologically, it is suitable to receive axons by means of grafts or transfers.

Histologic examination of the nerve stumps is imperative because it has been shown that visual inspection of the nerve stumps alone is insufficient to determine the intraneural architecture. When intraoperative frozen section of the nerve stumps is used, this leads to re-resection of at least one nerve stump in 25% of patients. When the stumps are re-resected, there is a clear demonstrable improvement in the histologic grade of the stumps (53).

Determining the suitability of the proximal stumps as potential donors is more problematic. Even if the proximal stump appears suitable on histologic examination (very little scarring, good fascicular pattern, and no ganglion cells), an intraforaminal avulsion cannot be ruled out. Multiple factors must be considered in making the diagnosis of an intraforaminal avulsion, including the clinical examination, CT myelography, intraoperative direct nerve stimulation, histology, and the "feel" of the nerve at transection.

When surgery is indicated by the clinical examination, neurolysis alone, without neuroma excision and grafting, is inappropriate. Lin et al. have demonstrated that although the early results of neurolysis in Erb's palsy are encouraging, they are not sustained over the longer term (54). They found that patients undergoing neurolysis for Erb's palsy or total plexus palsy were no better off 4 years after surgery than those undergoing spontaneous recovery, but patients who underwent sural nerve grafting showed measurable improvement in seven movements on the AMS.

In summary, all of the elements of the brachial plexus that do not demonstrate normal fascicular appearance or those that do not produce appropriate muscle movements on direct nerve stimulation are resected and reconstructed.

RECONSTRUCTION OF THE BRACHIAL PLEXUS

After the proximal and distal targets are adequately prepared, nerve reconstruction is begun. Reconstruction is performed using nerve grafts and nerve transfers. In contrast to the priorities in adult brachial plexus surgery, priority must be given to reinnervation of the hand first followed by restoration of elbow flexion and finally shoulder stability. Because of the short distances for regrowth and the infant's neural plasticity, good outcomes for reinnervation of the hand can be expected that would not be seen in adults with a similar injury. The distances from the available proximal stumps to the distal stumps are measured, and the distribution of the available grafts is planned. Because the distances between the proximal and distal stumps are typically 3 to 4.5 cm and one can usually obtain approximately 25 to 30 cm of graft material, six to 10 sural nerve grafts are typically feasible. Grafts from the cervical plexus are used where additional graft material is needed. Usually 2.5 to 3 cm of graft is obtainable from this source. Grafts are preferentially directed from the original root to the originally intended target (anatomical grafting). When the proximal stump is not available to innervate the intended distal nerve, other sources of

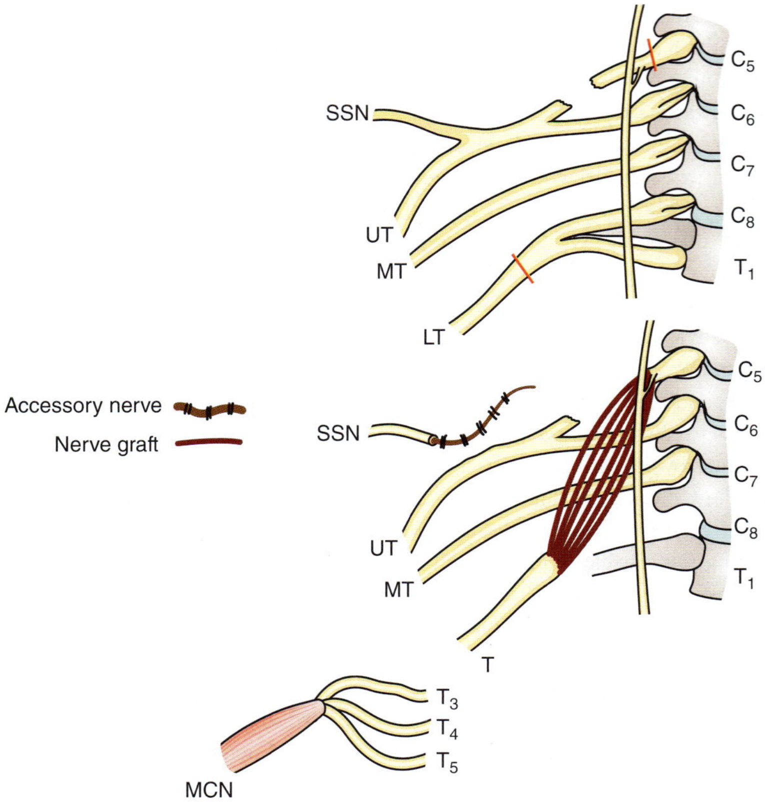

FIGURE 72-7 Schematic of accessory nerve to suprascapular nerve transfer, grafting from C5 to the lower trunk, and transfer of three intercostals to the musculocutaneous nerve.

axons must be used, either from within the plexus (intraplexus neurotization) or from outside the plexus (extraplexus neurotization). Sural nerve grafts are reversed to minimize axonal drop off from side branches. Grafts placed using anatomical grafting are arranged to take advantage of the gross internal topography of the proximal stumps. Therefore, in a situation suitable for anatomical grafting, the most cephalad portion of the C5 root would be coapted to the suprascapular nerve, the posterior aspect to the posterior division of the upper trunk, and the anterior aspect to the anterior division of the upper trunk. Grafts are arranged in the desired location beginning in the depths of the wound, and fibrin glue (Tisseel) is used for nerve coaptations. No sutures are necessary for the nerve graft coaptations. The use of fibrin glue allows sectioning of the proximal stump deep within the intervertebral foramen, where suturing would be difficult if not impossible. Fibrin glue also allows the grafts to be distributed easily and selectively over the cut face of the appropriate stump. Sameem et al. (55) reviewed the use of fibrin glue in peripheral nerve repair and found that the results of most studies indicated fibrin glue to be equal or superior to microsutures.

Nerve transfers are indicated in cases in which multiple root avulsions have occurred, resulting in a paucity of donor axons from the proximal stumps. Transfer of the distal part of the spinal accessory nerve to the suprascapular nerve is the most commonly performed nerve transfer. This transfer is usually performed through the existing supraclavicular exposure. The nerve is located on the deep surface of the trapezius muscle and traced distally into the upper back beyond the proximal branches serving the upper and middle trapezius to prevent shoulder droop. It is divided as far distally as possible to provide sufficient length for direct coaptation to the suprascapular nerve. As an alternative, one may approach the spinal accessory–to–suprascapular nerve transfer through a separate posterior incision with the patient prone. The advantage of the posterior approach is that it allows one to obtain a more distal coaptation between the spinal accessory to the suprascapular nerve, thus reducing the distance from the coaptation to the motor end plates. The disadvantage is that it requires a separate exposure. Intercostal nerve transfers can also be used where insufficient donor axons are available, particularly in cases with only one viable proximal root. In that situation, three intercostal nerves can be used to reconstruct the musculocutaneous nerves, the spinal accessory nerve is transferred to the suprascapular nerve, and the available proximal root is grafted to the lower trunk (Figure 72-7). Contralateral C7 transfer has been reported in obstetric brachial plexus reconstruction, but this transfer is not widely practiced. Our indication for contralateral C7 transfer would be the rare case with five root avulsions.

POSTOPERATIVE CARE

At the completion of the procedure when the incision is closed, the patient is fitted with a Velpeau sling made from a single length of cotton stockinette (Figure 72-8). This sling is maintained continuously for 3 weeks. When applied, this maintains the shoulder in a position of adduction and internal rotation and the elbow in a position of 90 degrees of flexion. We have used this inexpensive sling in 350 cases of primary plexus reconstruction and have found it to be very well

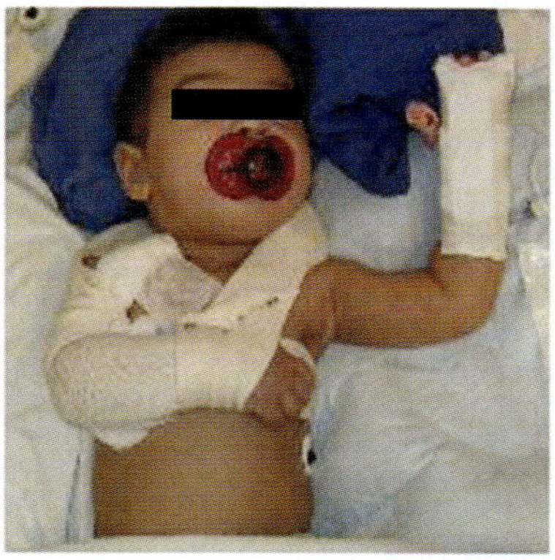

FIGURE 72-8 At the end of the operation the upper limb is secured in a Velpeau sling made from cotton stockinette for a period of three weeks. (Reproduced with permission from Gilbert, A., J.L. Tassin. Réparation chirurgicale du plexus brachial dans la paralysie obstétricale. Chirurgie 1984:110(1):70-75.)

tolerated by infants and easy to maintain and adjust by parents or caregivers.

COMPLICATIONS

Complications arising from primary surgery have been documented in a retrospective series (56). The overall complication rate was 33.5%, with no deaths. Accidental extubation occurred in 2.9% of patients; all of these occurred in the first half of the study. This problem was addressed by suturing the endotracheal tube to the membranous septum and by using transparent drapes for visualization of the tube. After this, no accidental extubations occurred. Postoperative fluid overload occurred in 14 patients (8.1%), three (1.7%) of whom developed pulmonary edema. Intensive care unit admission was required in two of those patients. Diuretic treatment was required in seven patients. No patient receiving less than or equal to 4 mL/kg/hr developed fluid overload, but 50% of the patients receiving greater than or equal to 10 mL/kg/hr did. Currently, the authors strictly limit total intravenous fluids to 4 mL/kg/hr or less. Other complications include wound infection (2.3%), seroma (1.2%) and respiratory complications along with hemidiaphragm paralysis (6.4%), atelectasis (2.9%), pleural effusion (1.7%) pneumothorax (1.7%), and chylothorax (0.6%).

CONCLUSION

Microneurosurgical reconstruction of the brachial plexus in OBPP is a relatively new area of expertise. The potential for significantly improving the function of an affected infant's limb is high in carefully selected cases. Identification of these cases continues to be one of the major challenges in OBPP surgery. Refinements in the criteria for selection of patients likely to benefit from surgery continue to be made because of rigorous scientific recording of pre- and postoperative status using reliable and validated instruments. We can expect that as the field continues to evolve, these criteria will be further refined and other questions answered by the application of scientific methods.

REFERENCES

1. Greenwald AG, Schute PC, Shiveley JL. Brachial plexus birth palsy: a 10-year report on the incidence and prognosis. *J Pediatr Orthop* 1984;4(6):689–692.
2. Sherburn EW, Kaplan SS, Kaufman BA, et al. Outcome of surgically treated birth-related brachial plexus injuries in twenty cases. *Pediatr Neurosurg* 1997;27(1):19–27.
3. Waters PM. Comparison of the natural history, the outcome of microsurgical repair, and the outcome of operative reconstruction in brachial plexus birth palsy. *J Bone Joint Surg Am* 1999;81(5):649–659.
4. Smellie W. *A Collection of Cases and Observations in Midwifery. To Illustrate His former Treatise, or First Volume, on that Subject*, 4th ed, vol. II. London: D. Wilson, G. Nicol, 1768:446–448.
5. Duchenne GBA. *De l;Électrisation localisée et de son application à la pathologie et à la thérapeutique par courants induits et par courants galvaniques interrompus et continus*, 3rd ed. Paris: Librairie J. B. Baillière et fils, 1872, p. 1120.
6. Erb W. Ueber eine eigenthümliche Localisation von Lähmungen im Plexus brachialis. *Verhandlungen. Heidelberg: Naturhistorisch-medizinischer Verein*; 1874, pp. 2:130–136.
7. Klumpke A. Contribution à l'étude des paralysies radiculaires du plexus brachial. *Rev Med* 1885;5:591–616.
8. Kennedy R. Suture of the brachial plexus in birth paralysis of the upper extremity. *Br Med J* 1903;I:298–301.
9. Sharpe W. The operative treatment of brachial plexus paralysis. *JAMA* 1916;66:876–881.
10. Taylor AS. Brachial birth palsy and injuries of similar type in adults. *Surg Gynecol Obstet* 1920;30:494–502.
11. Taylor AS. Results from the surgical treatment of brachial birth palsy. *JAMA* 1907;48(2):96–104.
12. Sever JW. Obstetric paralysis. Report of eleven hundred cases. *JAMA* 1925;85(24):1862–1865.
13. Jepson PN. Obstetrical paralysis. *Ann Surg* 1930;91:724–730.
14. Seddon HJ. The use of autogenous grafts for the repair of large gaps in peripheral nerves. *Br J Surg* 1947;35:151.
15. Fairbank HAT. A lecture on birth palsy: Subluxation of the shoulder-joint in infants and young children. *Lancet* 1913;I:1218–1223.
16. L'Episcopo JB. Tendon transplantation in obstetrical paralysis. *Am J Surg* 1934;25(1):122–125.
17. Millesi H, Ganglberger J, Berger A. Erfahrungen mit der Mikrochirurgie peripherer Nerven. *Chir Plast Reconstruct* 1967;3:47–55.
18. Gilbert A, Khouri N, Carlioz H. Exploration chirurgicale du plexus brachial dans la paralysie obstétricale. Constatations anatomiques chez 21 malades opérés. *Rev Chir Orthop Reparatrice Appar Mot* 1980;66:33–42.
19. Taylor GI, Ham FJ. The free vascularized nerve graft: a further experimental and clinical application of microvascular techniques. *Plast Reconstr Surg Radiol Anat* 1976;57:413.
20. Ikuta Y, Yoshioka K, Tsuge K. Free muscle transfer. *Aust N Z J Surg* 1980;50(4):401–405.
21. Sjoberg I, Erichs K, Bjerre I. Cause and effect of obstetric (neonatal) brachial plexus palsy. *Acta Paediatr Scand* 1988;77(3):357–364.
22. Clarke HM, Al-Qattan MM, Curtis CG, Zuker RM. Obstetrical brachial plexus palsy: results following neurolysis of conducting neuromas-in-continuity. *Plast Reconstr Surg* 1996;97(5):974–982; discussion 983–984.
23. Clarke HM, Curtis CG. An approach to obstetrical brachial plexus injuries. *Hand Clin* 1995;11(4):563–580; discussion 580–581.
24. Eng GD, Koch B, Smokvina MD. Brachial plexus palsy in neonates and children. *Arch Phys Med Rehabil* 1978;59(10):458–464.
25. Hardy AE. Birth injuries of the brachial plexus: incidence and prognosis. *J Bone Joint Surg Br* 1981;63-B(1):98–101.
26. Levine MG, Holroyde J, Woods JR Jr, et al. Birth trauma: incidence and predisposing factors. *Obstet Gynecol* 1984;63(6):792–795.
27. Michelow BJ, Clarke HM, Curtis CG, et al. The natural history of obstetrical brachial plexus palsy. *Plast Reconstr Surg* 1994;93(4):675–680; discussion 681.
28. Gilbert WM, Nesbitt TS, Danielsen B. Associated factors in 1611 cases of brachial plexus injury. *Obstet Gynecol* 1999;93(4):536–540.
29. Al-Qattan MM, Clarke HM, Curtis CG. The prognostic value of concurrent phrenic nerve palsy in newborn children with Erb's palsy. *J Hand Surg Br* 1998;23(2):225.
30. Jennett RJ, Tarby TJ. Brachial plexus palsy: an old problem revisited again. II. Cases in point. *Am J Obstet Gynecol* 1997;176(6):1354–1356; discussion 1356–1357.
31. Jennett RJ, Tarby TJ, Kreinick CJ. Brachial plexus palsy: an old problem revisited. *Am J Obstet Gynecol* 1992;166(6 Pt 1):1673–1676; discussion 1676–1677.

32. Specht EE. Brachial plexus palsy in the newborn. Incidence and prognosis. *Clin Orthop Relat Res* 1975(110):32–34.
33. Perlow JH, Wigton T, Hart J, et al. Birth trauma. A five-year review of incidence and associated perinatal factors. *J Reprod Med* 1996;41(10): 754–760.
34. al-Qattan MM, Clarke HM, Curtis CG. Klumpke's birth palsy. Does it really exist? *J Hand Surg Br* 1995;20(1):19–23.
35. Sever JW. Obstetric paralysis: its etiology, pathology, clinical aspects and treatment, with a report of four hundred and seventy cases. *Am J Dis Child* 1916;12(6):541–578.
36. Métaizeau JP, Gayet C, Plenat F. Les lésions obstétricales du plexus brachial. *Chir Pediatr* 1979;20(3):159–163.
37. Métaizeau JP, Prévôt J, Ligier JN. Les paralysies obstétricales (Etude expérimentale, déductions pronostiques et indications thérapeutiques). *Méd Hyg* 1982;40:617–624.
38. Gilbert A. Long-term evaluation of brachial plexus surgery in obstetrical palsy. *Hand Clin* 1995;11(4):583–94; discussion 594–595.
39. Fattah A, Curtis CG, Agur AM, Clarke HM. Functional contribution of T1 to the brachial plexus in infants. *J Hand Surg Eur Vol* 2012;37(3): 237–243.
40. Slooff ACJ. Obstetric brachial plexus lesions and their neurosurgical treatment. *Clin Neurol Neurosurg* 1993;95(suppl):S73–S77.
41. Mallet J. Paralysie obstétricale du plexus brachial. Traitement des séquelles. Primauté du traitement de l'épaule.—Méthode d'expression des résultats. *Rev Chir Orthop Reparatrice Appar Mot* 1972;58(suppl 1): 166–168.
42. Curtis C, Stephens D, Clarke HM, Andrews D. The active movement scale: an evaluative tool for infants with obstetrical brachial plexus palsy. *J Hand Surg Am* 2002;27(3):470–478.
43. Fu SY, Gordon T. The cellular and molecular basis of peripheral nerve regeneration. *Mol Neurobiol* 1997;14(1-2):67–116.
44. Eng GD, Binder H, Getson P, O'Donnell R. Obstetrical brachial plexus palsy (OBPP) outcome with conservative management. *Muscle Nerve* 1996;19:884–891.
45. Michelow BJ, Clarke HM, Curtis CG, et al. The natural history of obstetrical brachial plexus palsy. *Plast Reconstr Surg* 1994;93(4):675–680.
46. Gilbert A, Tassin JL. Obstetrical palsy: a clinical, pathologic, and surgical review. In Terzis JK (ed). *Microreconstruction of Nerve Injuries*. Philadelphia: WB Saunders, 1987, pp. 529–553.
47. Gilbert A. Indication and strategies. In Gilbert A (ed). *Brachial Plexus Injuries*. London: Martin Dunitz, 2001, pp. 205–210.
48. Al-Qattan MM Clarke HM, Curtis CG. The prognostic value of concurrent Horner's syndrome in total obstetric brachial plexus injury. *J Hand Surg Br* 2000;25(2):166–167.
49. Strömbeck C, Krumlinde-Sundholm L, Forssberg H. Functional outcome at 5 years in children with obstetrical brachial plexus palsy with and without microsurgical reconstruction. *Dev Med Child Neurol* 2000;42(3):148–157.
50. Chow BCL, Blaser S, Clarke HM. Predictive value of computed tomographic myelography in obstetrical brachial plexus palsy. *Plast Reconstr Surg* 2000;106(5):971–977.
51. Tsai PY, Chuang TY, Cheng H, et al. Concordance and discrepancy between electrodiagnosis and magnetic resonance imaging in cervical root avulsion injuries. *J Neurotrauma* 2006;23(8):1274–1281.
52. Dupere M, Vajsar J, Moncada M. *The use of intraoperative somatosensory evoked potentials in the diagnosis of nerve root avulsion in obstetrical brachial plexus palsy*. Eighth Congress of the International Federation of Societies for Surgery of the Hand, Istanbul, Turkey, 2001.
53. Murji A, Redett RJ, Hawkins CE, Clarke HM. The role of intraoperative frozen section histology in obstetrical brachial plexus reconstruction. *J Reconstr Microsurg* 2008;4(3):203–209.
54. Lin JC, Schwentker-Colizza A, Curtis CG, Clarke HM. Final results of grafting versus neurolysis in obstetrical brachial plexus palsy. *Plast Reconstr Surg* 2009;123(3):939–948.
55. Sameem M, Wood T, Bain J. A systematic review on the use of fibrin glue for peripheral nerve repair. *Plast Reconstr Surg* 2001;127(6):2381–2390.
56. La Scala GC, Rice SB, Clarke HM. Complications of microsurgical reconstruction of obstetrical brachial plexus palsy. *Plast Reconstr Surg* 2003;111(4):1383–1388.

CHAPTER 73

Traumatic Brachial Plexus Reconstruction

David Chwei-Chin Chuang

Traumatic brachial plexus injuries (BPIs) can cause devastating deficits in the upper extremity with often lifelong functional, occupational, and social sequelae. Before the era of microsurgery, surgical treatment was highly unpredictable and disappointing. Because of advances in reconstructive microsurgery and more understanding of the effects of nerve transfers and functioning free muscle transfers (FFMTs), significant improvement in the functional outcome of the brachial plexus reconstruction can be achieved consistently. Timely referral to a center with expertise in brachial plexus reconstruction is essential to achieve optimal outcomes.

The complexity of the brachial plexus and rigor of brachial plexus reconstruction places high demands on both the treatment team as well as the injured patient. A skilled treatment team and an informed patient, who is motivated and committed to the surgery and even more important to the demanding rehabilitation, have the best chances to obtain a favorable outcome.

The aim of this chapter is to give a comprehensive overview of our experience of the anatomy, level of injury with numbered description, timing of surgical intervention, preoperative evaluation, surgical management, postoperative rehabilitation, management of sequelae, and results and outcomes of brachial plexus reconstruction.

ANATOMY

The brachial plexus is formed by the anterior rami of the lower cervical (C5–C8) and the first thoracic (T1) spinal nerves. It gives motor innervation to muscles of the shoulder, including all anterior and posterior chest muscles related to glenohumeral joint movement and muscles of the entire upper limb (extrinsic and intrinsic). It supplies sensory innervation to the entire upper limb except the skin over part of the medial aspect of the upper arm. In the *prefixed brachial plexus,* C4 provides a significant contribution to C5. In the *postfixed brachial plexus,* T2 has significant contributions to T1. Clinically, the prefixed type is more commonly seen than the postfixed.

Each spinal nerve is formed by the union of the ventral root (motor fibers) and the dorsal root (sensory fibers). Each root is in turn formed by a number of rootlets. The cell bodies (neurons) of the motor fibers are located in the anterior horn of the spinal cord, and the cell bodies of the sensory fibers reside in the dorsal root ganglion located within the intervertebral foramen, immediately outside the dura mater of the spinal cord. The dorsal and ventral roots unite distal to the ganglion to form a mixed spinal nerve, which passes through the interscalene space between the scalene anterior and middle muscles. Just distal to the scalene muscles, the five postganglionic spinal nerves unite to form the three trunks: upper (formed by C5 and C6), middle (C7 itself), and lower trunk (formed by the C8 and T1 spinal nerves). Each trunk divides into anterior and posterior divisions just proximal to or directly under the clavicle. Through these divisions, the nerves exchange fibers and rearrange to unite a second time, just distal to the clavicle to form the cords. Lateral and medial cords are anterior compartment nerves, passing anterior to the subclavian artery. The posterior cord is a posterior compartment nerve, passing posterior to the subclavian artery. The cords run in front of the subscapularis muscle and behind the pectoralis minor muscle. Each cord has two or more terminal branches to the peripheral nerves. However, numerous anatomical variations of the brachial plexus do exist and should always be kept in mind (1,2).

MICROANATOMY

The microanatomy or fascicular topography of the brachial plexus has been extensively studied and described (3,4). Marked changes in fascicular topography occur every 10 mm. This is especially true at the level of the upper trunk, where interfascicular crossovers are so extensive that direct repair or repair with short nerve grafts will frequently lead to co-contractions because

SECTION 4

TABLE 73-1 Different Classifications by Different Surgeons for Level of Brachial Plexus Injury (6)

Leffert	Two levels	Supraclavicular injury (supraganglionic, infraganglionic, and sub- or retroclavicular) and infraclavicular injury
Wood	Two levels	Supraclavicular (roots, trunks, and divisions), infraclavicular (cords and branches)
Terzis	Three levels	Root, supraclavicular postganglionic, infraclavicular
Millesi	Four levels	Supraganglionic root, infraganglionic root, trunk, and cord
Alnot	Four levels	Preganglionic root, postganglionic root, supra- and retroclavicular, and infraclavicular
Chuang	Four levels	Preganglionic root, postganglionic spinal nerve, pre- and retroclavicular, and infraclavicular
Narakas	Five levels	Supraganglionic root, infraganglionic spinal nerve, infraganglionic trunk, retroclavicular and terminal branches
Mackinnon	Six levels	
Boome	Eight levels	

of aberrant reinnervation of muscles. This aberrant reinnervation is mainly found in patients with obstetric brachial plexus palsy patients (5) but rarely in adult BPI due to its long nerve gap. Throughout the plexus, connective tissue is more abundant than neural tissue. All of these factors contribute to why the results of brachial plexus nerve surgery are so unpredictable. Knowledge of the internal topography of the plexus can be helpful in connection of corresponding nerve fibers with bridging nerve grafts.

DISPUTED ANATOMY

Various classifications of the level of BPI have been proposed: two levels, three levels, four levels, five levels, six levels, and eight levels of injuries by different experts (Table 73-1). These numerous classifications have made the understanding of the anatomy of the brachial plexus complex and confusing. The most confusing part is the term *postganglionic roots*. Some anatomists use the term *root* for the nerves in the interscalene space before formation of the trunks (1). However, some call this part the *spinal nerve* (6-9). In fact, after the dorsal root ganglion, both ventral and dorsal roots continue for only a few millimeters (5 mm) in distance and unite to become a mixed nerve, where it is no longer a root (Figure 73-1). Therefore, the components of the brachial plexus are roots (spinal cord + rootlets + roots), spinal nerves, trunks, divisions, cords, and terminal branches.

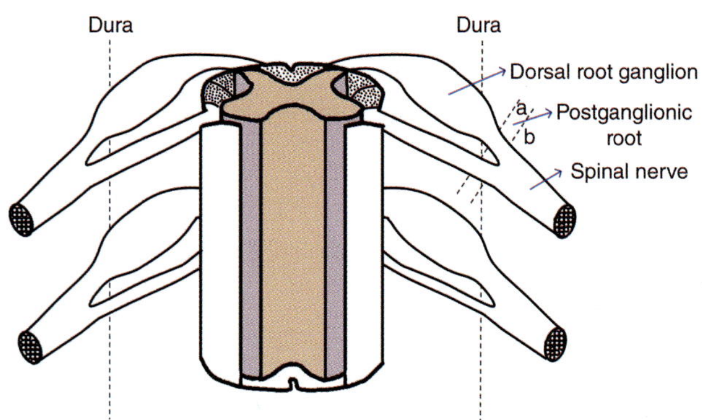

FIGURE 73-1 Schematic showing the relationship of the cord, roots, dorsal root ganglion, and spinal nerve. (Reproduced with permission from David Chwei-Chin Chuang and Lee-Min Lee.)

LEVEL OF INJURY

To avoid confusion of the anatomical terminology, we have described a clearer classification of brachial plexus lesions by simply using numbers for the levels of injury (Figure 73-2).

- Level 1 injury, a lesion inside the (vertebral) bone, is a preganglionic root injury involving the spinal cord, rootlets or roots, or dorsal root ganglion at or close to the dura mater. The incidence here is the highest, around 70%.
- Level 2 injury, a lesion inside the muscles (interscalene space, proximal to the origin of the suprascapular nerve), is a postganglionic spinal nerve injury. The incidence of pure level 2 injury is about 8%.

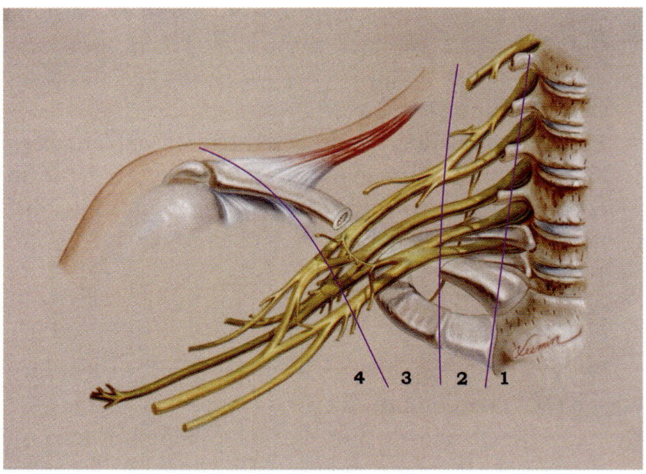

FIGURE 73-2 Anatomy and numbered levels of brachial plexus injury. Level 1 injury is preganglionic root injury, level 2 injury is postganglionic spinal nerve injury, level 3 injury is pre- and retroclavicular injury (trunk and divisions injury), and level 4 injury is intraclavicular injury (cords and terminal branches injury). (Reproduced with permission from David Chwei-Chin Chuang and Lee-Min Lee.)

- Level 3 injury is a lesion located in the pre- and retroclavicular space, including trunks and divisions. The incidence of pure level 3 injury is low, about 5%.
- Level 4 injury is an infraclavicular injury, including cords and terminal branches in and proximal to the axillary fossa. The incidence of pure level 4 injury is the second highest, about 17%.

The same nerve may have extensive injury from level 1 down to level 2 or continuously down to level 3. Such extended level injury is seen quite frequently. In addition, different nerves may have different levels of injury. For instance, C5 and C6 level 2 (rupture) injury is quite often accompanied with C7-T1 three roots level 1 injury or C5 level 2 injury with a C6-T1 level 1 injury. However, skip-level lesions are rare: for instance, C5 and C7 level 1 injury but with C6 intact or C5 injury involving levels 1 and 3 but with level 2 intact. The term *supraclavicular BPI* will cover a large zone lesion, including level 1, level 2, or level 3 injuries. In the following pages, we will detail our management of adult BPI using the numbered level classification.

Two types of lesions are seen in BPI, avulsion and rupture. Both are traction injuries but with different characteristics. Root avulsion is a very frequent BPI because of its weak supporting structures. Attempts in performing spinal cord implantation with or without nerve graft have shown unsatisfactory clinical result. This implies that in an avulsion injury, only the distal end is available, but the proximal stump is absent or unsuitable for repair. *Root injury* is an obscure term that may mean avulsion from the cord (true avulsion) or rupture or stretch at the rootlets or roots. Root avulsion in BPI is usually accompanied by dural tearing and a cerebrospinal fluid leak with cyst formation, termed a *pseudomeningocele* (Figure 73-3). However, in some cases, the root can be avulsed at its origin with an intact dural cone and no cyst formation, called *avulsion in situ*. The nerve root may remain inside the spinal canal or at the dural orifice, showing a grossly normal appearance or loosening with curvature of the spinal nerve at the time of surgical intervention despite established paralysis. Most often, however, the entire avulsed roots, including ventral roots, dorsal roots, and ganglia, retract and migrate downward to the interscalene or preclavicular region.

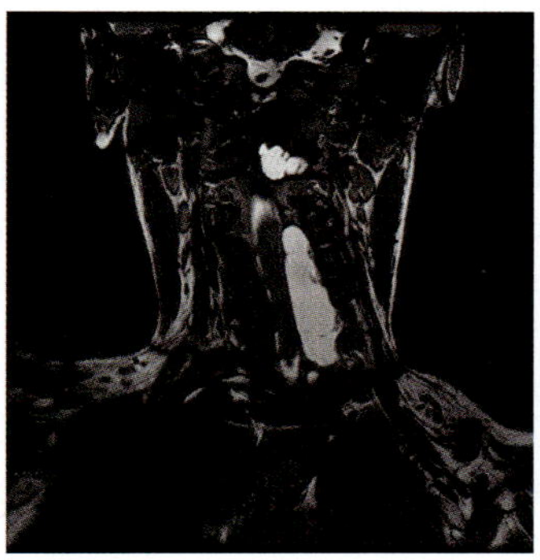

FIGURE 73-3 One cut of the three-dimensional magnetic resonance image showing C3 and C5-C8 pseudomeningoceles.

PATHOPHYSIOLOGY AND DEGREE OF NERVE INJURY: TIMING OF NERVE EXPLORATION

The timing of nerve exploration depends on the degree of nerve injury. The degree of peripheral nerve injury can be classified into neurapraxia, axonotmesis, and neurotmesis (Seddon classification [10]) or grade 1 to 5 injury (Sunderland classification [11]). Seddon's axonotmesis or Sunderland's second-degree injury start to show Wallerian degeneration at the proximal and distal stumps. Seddon's neurotmesis or Sunderland's third- to fifth-degree injury has the potential for aberrant reinnervation after nerve regeneration. In Sunderland's fourth or fifth-degree injuries, only nerve repair can succeed in restoring continuity. In the first-, second-, and third-degree injuries, spontaneous recovery may occur. In cases of penetrating injury by sharp objects, there is always no argument for immediate exploration or within a few days after the accident for direct nerve repair. Some surgeons advocate exploration of a closed BPI as early as possible (12,13) because of the advantages of easy diagnosis of root avulsion and avoidance of the problem of scar dissection. However, most brachial plexus surgeons recommend exploration within 5 months, and more are favoring between the third and fourth months after injury (6,14–16). In cases of closed BPI, the degree and extent of the injury are usually difficult to judge soon after injury. However, there is only one chance for nerve repair or reconstruction. The benefits of waiting outweigh the advantages of too early surgery.

MANAGEMENT OF ADULT BRACHIAL PLEXUS INJURIES

More than 1700 adult patients with brachial plexus palsy have been treated by the author between 1985 and 2010. Most adult BPIs are closed injuries. Accurate assessment of the extent and severity of the brachial plexus damage in closed BPI is important. The preoperative evaluation and diagnosis should include the following information: mechanism of injury; present condition and past history; clinical evaluation of motor, sensory, and Tinel's sign; pain character, Horner's syndrome; vascular lesions; mobility of diaphragm; ancillary investigations such as plain chest and cervical spine radiographs; advanced imaging studies (three-dimensional magnetic resonance imaging [MRI] and magnetic resonance angiography [MRA]); and electrodiagnostic studies (needle electromyography [EMG] and nerve conduction velocity [NCV]).

ETIOLOGY OF ADULT BRACHIAL PLEXUS INJURIES

Brachial plexus injuries may be caused by trauma such as motorcycle accidents (the most common, ~80%) or traction injury by rolling machine or conveyor belt, high-speed falls, compression injury by heavy objects or shoulder dislocation, penetrating injury by sharp objects or gunshot wounds, or iatrogenic injury by surgeons for tumor resection (e.g., brachial plexus schwannoma). Other causes are tumors (primary or secondary), infections (e.g., enterovirus, polio infection), inflammation (e.g., irradiation neuritis), and toxins (e.g., injection injury).

PATIENT HISTORY

The patient's history helps to classify the degree and extent of injury and to determine the need and strategy for surgical intervention. Whereas a history of shoulder dislocation or glenoid fracture may have a high incidence of level 4 injury, a history of cervical spine injury or a vertebral fracture level 1 root injury is more likely. Arterial injury and repair implies the site of nerve injury. For instance, traction on the arm by a rolling machine or conveyor belt often causes an open wound in the axilla and extensive ecchymosis around the shoulder and chest and rupture of the axillary vessels, and level 4 BPI should be highly suspected. Segmental thrombosis of the subclavian artery is usually associated with a C8-T1 Level 1 root injury. A history of rib fractures and chest intubation prohibits the use of intercostal nerve transfers because of a higher failure rate (17). Limping caused by a femur fracture with osteomyelitis or nonunion will also affect intercostal nerve transfers because of poor exercise tolerance for rehabilitation. Extreme causalgia, often seen in cases with root avulsion, is also a major predictive factor for poor results caused by poor rehabilitation. In addition, a partial Brown-Séquard syndrome (hemitransection of the spinal cord with ipsilateral upper motor neuron lesion below the level of the lesion and contralateral abnormal sensation to pain and temperature that may not be at the same level) (18) is also seen in level 1 injury.

CLINICAL EVALUATION

Clinical evaluation is the essential and most important step in establishing the diagnosis of site and degree of injury which determines the treatment and prognosis. This evaluation is usually performed at 2 months after injury.

Motor Examination

Motor examination should be completed muscle by muscle in a distal-to-proximal direction and recorded using the British Medical Research Council scale (M0–M5) (19) for different muscle strengths.

Sensory Examination

Performing complete sensory tests, such as pain and temperature appreciation, static and moving two-point discrimination, constant touch, and vibration, in BPI is both unnecessary and illogical. However, sensory evaluation should include the pinprick pain test and Tinel's sign. Differentiation of the pinprick test from areas of normal to abnormal sensation to map out the area of sensory disturbance is enough for most BPI patients. Sensory grading is based on the British MRC scale (S0–S4), modified by adding a grade for sensory overreaction (S2+) (19). Such sensory evaluations can give some clues about the level and degree of BPI. Hoffman-Tinel's sign is an important clinical sign to determine the location of a neuroma or to judge the regeneration of the injured nerves. Palpation or percussion in the neck, at the supraclavicular Erb's point (clavicular insertion of the sternocleidomastoid muscle), at the infraclavicular coracoid process of the scapula, and along the routes of different peripheral nerves may induce an electrical current sensation (like "pins and needles") running down from the shoulder to the hand, and constitutes a positive Tinel's sign. Tinel's sign should be localized to the point where maximal pain is elicited. If the Tinel's sign remains at a fixed point, implying retardation of nerve growth, surgical exploration is warranted. If the Tinel's sign advances from supraclavicular to infraclavicular and further down the arm or forearm at successive examinations, a "wait-and-see" approach is recommended because it might indicate a Sunderland first- to third-degree lesion. A weak or absent Tinel's sign in the neck region usually indicates a total root avulsion. Evaluating the location by Tinel's sign may provide useful information. Horner's syndrome (miosis, ptosis, enophthalmos, and anhidrosis) is a sign of sympathetic nervous system disturbance. It indirectly implies avulsion of T1 and C8 roots because the sympathetic fibers from the T1 to T2 sympathetic ganglion are quite close to the preganglionic fibers of T1 and C8. This syndrome may regress with time. It is a more reliable sign in adult BPI but less accurate in obstetric BPI.

Vascular Injury Examination

Absence or weakness of pulsation of the radial artery at the wrist indicates vascular injury of the axillary or subclavian artery. Whereas subclavian artery occlusion might indicate a level 1 lesion, axillary artery occlusion might be associated with a level 4 lesion. Vascular injury should be taken into account when considering the use of a vascularized ulnar nerve graft for reconstruction because the ulnar artery needs to be ligated, harvested, and transferred together with the ulnar nerve. In addition, care must be taken if an FFMT is performed for elbow flexion reconstruction when there is absence of radial artery pulsation. Splint immobilization to keep the elbow flexed more than 90 degrees will easily compromise the digital peripheral circulation and potentially cause digital gangrene if the radial artery pulsation is absent.

Root Injury Pain

Brachial plexus root injury pain is a characteristic symptom in the BPI. It is somehow like a scar pain inside the spinal cord or roots. Typically, root pain has no precise distribution and is described as an electric shooting pain occurring for a short duration (seconds) that resolves spontaneously but recurs. The pain can be induced by cold temperatures and sometimes be relieved by a distraction mechanism by concentrating on other tasks such as working, exercising, doing garden care, or in some cases by changing posture or by massage. This characteristic pain is called *deafferentation pain*. The *root shooting pain* or *root scar pain* is usually intolerable and may persist forever but often occurs less frequently 6 months after the accident. The pain is more intolerable in elderly patients, usually causing poorer results after reconstruction. But it can be better tolerated and accepted over time by younger patients. This pain is rarely seen in children or in obstetric palsy patients.

Imaging Studies: Plain Radiography, Magnetic Resonance Imaging, and Magnetic Resonance Angiography

Plain radiographs of the chest and cervical spine are required. Chest radiographs should include inspiration and expiration views to exclude diaphragmatic palsy. Cervical spine radiographs are evaluated for any fracture of the transverse or spinous process as well as vertebral bodies. Cervical scoliosis and neck rigidity are possible sequelae of neurologic injury.

In recent years, the invasive imaging studies (e.g., cervical myelography) have gradually been replaced by noninvasive MRI (20). MRI imaging with various investigative techniques is very helpful in the diagnosis of level 1, level 2, or even level 3 injuries. The MRI cervical spine myelogram (Figure 73-4) offers a brief image for the level 1 lesion. The technique of the MRI three-dimensional (3D) FIESTA (Fast Imaging Employing Steady-state Acquisition) offers continuous slices (240 images) of the anteroposterior plane similar to a movie, and the outline of different cyst formations, even including the direction of leak of a fistula, can be seen (Figure 73-5). Different 3D source data from coronal, axial, and oblique views; side-by-side comparison of normal and injured nerve rootlets (Figure 73-6); and different planes of ventral and dorsal rootlets using the curve planar reformat (CPR) technique (Figure 73-7) are all reconstructed to demonstrate the respective rootlets in better perspective. 3D MRI diffusion weighted imaging (DWI) techniques can also offer views of the level 2 or even the level 3 nerve structures. The valuable and accurate data provided by the various MRI techniques allow surgeons to make more confident judgments on the level of injury of BPI. This is especially true of level 1 lesions. MRA offers additional information about any associated injury to the subclavian artery.

Electrodiagnostic Studies

Electrodiagnostic studies, mainly consisting of NCV and needle EMG, can be used to localize the lesion and to assess its severity. Abnormal low amplitude of the sensory action potential (SNAP) indicates a ganglionic or postganglionic lesion. Conversely, the pick-up sensory action potentials taken from a paralytic limb is evidence of a preganglionic root lesion. The presence of fibrillation potentials on needle EMG may suggest that the lesion is at least an axonotmesis. Reduction in the amplitude of the compound muscle action potentials during motor nerve conduction studies indicates an axonal loss rather than a neurapraxia lesion.

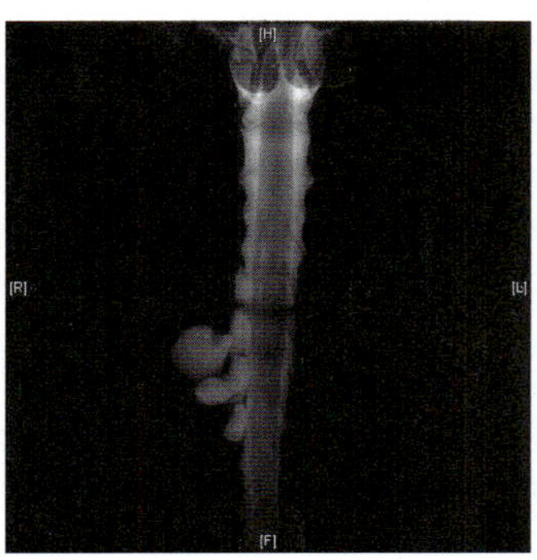

FIGURE 73-4 C5-T1 total root avulsion shown by three-dimensional magnetic resonance imaging myelogram.

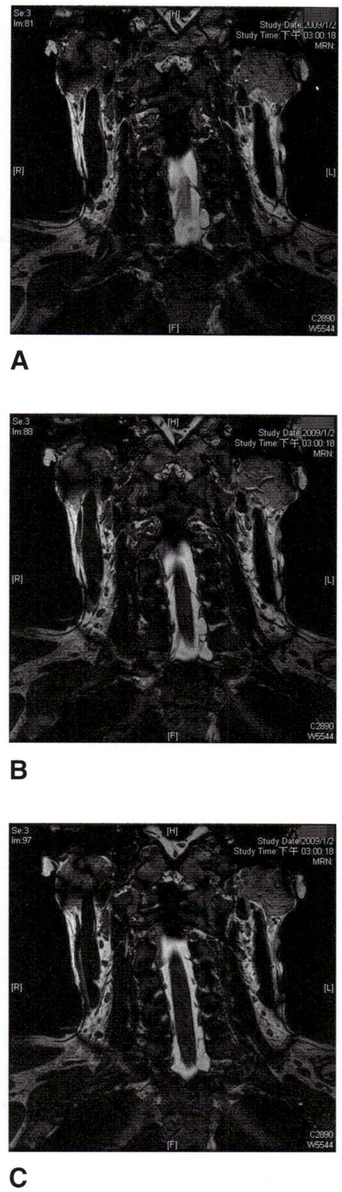

FIGURE 73-5 (A) to (C) C6, C7, C8 cysts on images 81, 88, and 97 done with the three-dimensional magnetic resonance image FIESTA technique.

SURGICAL TREATMENT

Surgery is the treatment of choice for adult BPI in both closed and open injuries.

In an open injury in the neck caused by a knife or other sharp object, significant motor and sensory deficits are very suspicious for division of the brachial plexus. Exploration and nerve repair is indicated immediately or within a few days after the trauma. Direct end-to-end neurorrhaphy with 6-0 to 9-0 nylon is very

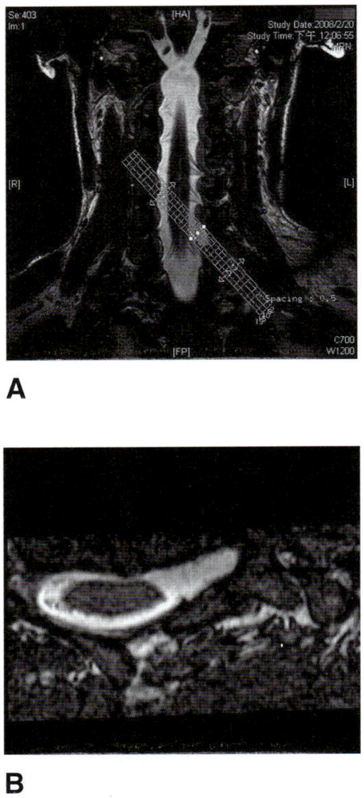

FIGURE 73-6 (A) and (B) Oblique cuts with side-by-side comparison of normal and injured nerve rootlets (left C7 pseudomeningocele).

possible, and excellent results can be expected. The golden time for primary end-to-end repair is within 1 week for supraclavicular and within 2 weeks for infraclavicular penetrating lesions (8). After the golden time, nerve grafts are usually required after resection of the neuroma.

However, for closed BPI, the main reason for the delayed exploration is to establish the diagnosis of the site and degree of the lesion. Management of these patients can be considered in the following six stages:

- Stage 1: Stabilization stage (first month); includes stabilization of vital signs, bone fractures, or joint dislocations
- Stage 2: Diagnostic stage (second month); includes clinical examination and ancillary investigations to establish the diagnosis of the lesion; start physiotherapy to prevent soft tissue swelling and joint stiffness, delay muscle atrophy by electric stimulation; and psychologic education before surgery
- Stage 3: Surgery (third to fifth months). If the patient fails to show any return of function by 5 months, surgical intervention is indicated. Nerve reconstruction at 5 months shows no difference with surgery at the third month in our series. However, the results of muscle strength grading after nerve reconstruction more than 6 months after injury are usually significantly weaker compared with a denervation time less than 6 months. Therefore, it is unwise to just perform brachial plexus reconstruction more than 6 months after injury. Local muscle transfer or FFMT to enhance the results is often necessary.
- Stage 4: Postoperative care (3–4 weeks postoperatively) and rehabilitation (3–4 years)
- Stage 5: Late reconstruction for deformities or deficits (during the third or fourth year after surgery)
- Stage 6: Salvage stage (fifth or sixth year after surgery), including amputation and treatment of intolerable pain

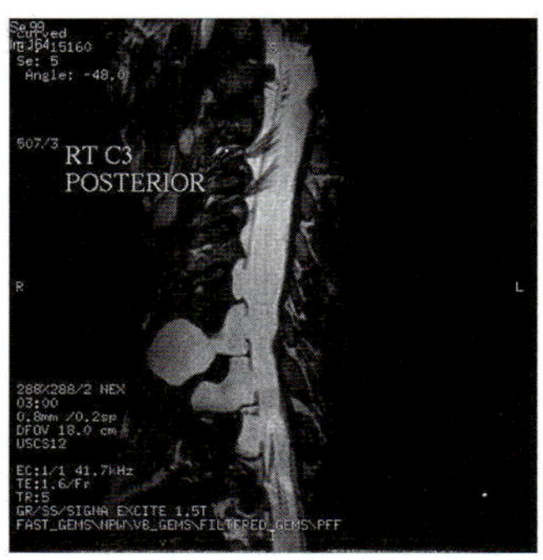

FIGURE 73-7 Different planes of ventral and dorsal rootlets using the curve planar reformat technique (C5-T1 total root avulsion).

In late nerve repairs for chronic cases (1 year after injury), the muscles have undergone a long period of denervation and atrophy, which is replaced by connective tissue and fat. Late nerve repair in such circumstances is useless and usually leads to poor results. Effective physical therapy and constant electric stimulation can only postpone the onset of muscle atrophy but cannot prevent the muscle from eventually undergoing atrophy. FFMTs or banked nerve grafts from ipsilateral or contralateral nerve transfers followed by secondary FFMTs are the option for such chronic cases.

Surgical Technique of Exploration of the Supraclavicular Brachial Plexus

A C-curved incision, starting from the midpoint of the posterior border of the sternocleidomastoid muscle and curving laterally parallel to and above the clavicle, is a popular incision for a supraclavicular approach. A platysma musculocutaneous flap is elevated along the C-curved incision. Dissection beneath the sternocleidomastoid muscle is made to the internal jugular vein, a landmark for the uppermost medial dissection. The supraclavicular sensory nerves are the landmarks for the uppermost cranial dissection. The omohyoid muscle transverses just behind the sternocleidomastoid muscle and is looped and spared if possible; this is an important landmark for possible secondary exploration. Below the omohyoid muscle, there is abundant adipofascial tissue containing rich lymphatic ducts, lymph nodes, and the transverse cervical vessels. A similar C-shaped incision along the internal jugular vein medially and the subclavian vein inferiorly is made and a superiorly-based adipofascial flap is elevated. The lymphatic tissues, including the ducts coming from the deep plane of the internal jugular vein, should be coagulated or ligated before division to avoid postoperative lymph leakage and chylus formation. The transverse cervical artery and vein in the deeper plane of the adipofascial tissue are preserved if possible and potentially may be used as the recipient vessels for a vascularized ulnar nerve graft. The phrenic nerve and scalene anterior muscle are seen following elevation of the adipofascial flap elevation. The subclavian artery lies just beneath the scalene anterior muscle and should be carefully protected. The dominant transverse process of C5 above the supraclavicular sensory nerves is palpable. If necessary, the fibrotic scalene anterior muscle attached to the C5 transverse process can be detached and segmentally excised to expose the C5 and C6 spinal nerves: the spinal nerve above the C5 transverse process is C5, and the spinal nerve below is the C6 spinal nerve. The C7 spinal nerve is usually located a little farther away from the C6 spinal nerve. The C8 and T1 spinal nerves and lower trunk are then identified deeper underneath the subclavian artery. Sometimes the C8 is quite close or adherent to the C7 spinal nerve.

Technique of Exploration of the Infraclavicular Brachial Plexus

For the infraclavicular approach, an incision is made just along the deltopectoral groove and extended upward to meet the supraclavicular incision or downward to the medial sulcus of the biceps. Chuang's triangle (8) is a triangle bordered by the main branch of the cephalic vein medially, the clavicle laterally, and the edge of the deltoid muscle inferiorly. Some of the deltoid and clavicular portion of the pectoralis major muscle can be detached to increase exposure of the triangle area. Under the clavicle, the subclavius muscle is noted. Under the subclavius muscle, the lateral and posterior cords as well as the suprascapular nerve can be seen. From here, the suprascapular and infrascapular fossae are connected through an avascular plane without the need to osteotomize the clavicle. The clavicle and the subclavius muscle are lifted together by passing a rolling gauze. The "white line" is an intermuscular septum between the clavicular and sternal parts of the pectoralis major muscle. Splitting the septal white line, the underlying pectoralis minor muscle and infraclavicular brachial plexus can now be seen. The first and most anterior cord encountered beneath the upmost part of the pectoralis minor muscle is the lateral cord. The Y-shaped limbs from the lateral and medial cords will become the median nerve. The subclavian artery can easily be found between the Y-shaped limbs. The posterior cord lies posterior to the subclavian artery and has two terminal branches: the larger one is the radial nerve, and the smaller one is the axillary nerve. In the upper arm, the musculocutaneous nerve penetrates the coracobrachialis muscles and can be found between the biceps and coracobrachialis muscles. Sometimes it is an anatomical variation and arises from the median nerve. The axillary nerve in the axilla can be found at the humeral neck, above the tendinous portion of teres major, accompanied by the lateral circumflex humeral artery.

Other ancillary incisions may be required for additional sources of donor nerve transfers:

- Neck: Upwardly extend the incision for the spinal accessory nerve.
- Chest: A semicircular incision for the intercostal nerves
- Inframental incision for the hypoglossal nerve
- Medial arm incision for the biceps and brachialis motor nerve branches
- Contralateral neck: Similar C-curved incision for the contralateral C7 spinal nerve

SURGICAL TREATMENT AND TECHNIQUES

The surgical options for brachial plexus reconstruction are neurolysis (mostly external neurolysis), direct nerve repair (indicated for a penetrating injury), nerve grafts (free nerve grafts or vascularized ulnar nerve grafts), nerve transfers, and FFMTs. Decision making for these surgical options depends on the level of injury.

Level 1 Injury (Preganglionic Root Injury)

Nerve transfers, pedicled muscle transfer, and FFMT provide the only possibilities for functional restoration.

Nerve Transfer

A nerve transfer is a technique in which a physiologically functioning nerve is intentionally divided (with low donor nerve morbidity) and transfer to a distal more important but irreparable motor nerve or a paralyzed muscle. The procedure is optimally performed within a golden time period, within 5 months of the injury, to reinnervate the paralyzed muscle(s) (aiming for restoration of M4 muscle strength). Nerve transfers can be broadly classified into three categories: extraplexus, intraplexus, and close-target (or distal) nerve transfers.

Extraplexus Nerve Transfer

Extraplexus nerve transfer involves the transfer of a neighboring nerve from outside the brachial plexus from either the ipsilateral or the contralateral neck to the avulsed brachial plexus to neurotize a paralytic nerve. The commonly used donor nerves are mostly aimed at motor reinnervation. These include the phrenic nerve, the spinal accessory (XI) nerve (accessed by an anterior neck approach), deep motor branches of the cervical plexus (cervical motor branches [CMBs]), the hypoglossal nerve (XII), and the contralateral C7 spinal nerve (CC7). (Figure 73-8).

Intraplexus Nerve Transfer

Intraplexus nerve transfer is an option in cases of nonglobal root avulsion when at least one spinal nerve is ruptured and still available for transfer, not to its original pathway but to other more important nerves of the brachial plexus. For example, in a C5 and C6 level 2 rupture injury in which the C5 stump is healthier than the C6 stump, the C5 fibers are intentionally transferred to C6 (or the anterior division of the upper trunk) to restore elbow flexion. The distal C5 (or the posterior division of the upper trunk and suprascapular nerve) are then innervated by the partially injured C6 (Figure 73-9). This strategy acknowledges that elbow flexion has priority over shoulder function.

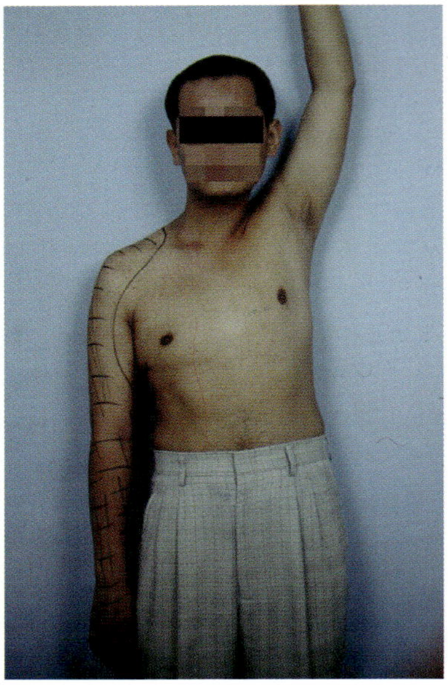

A

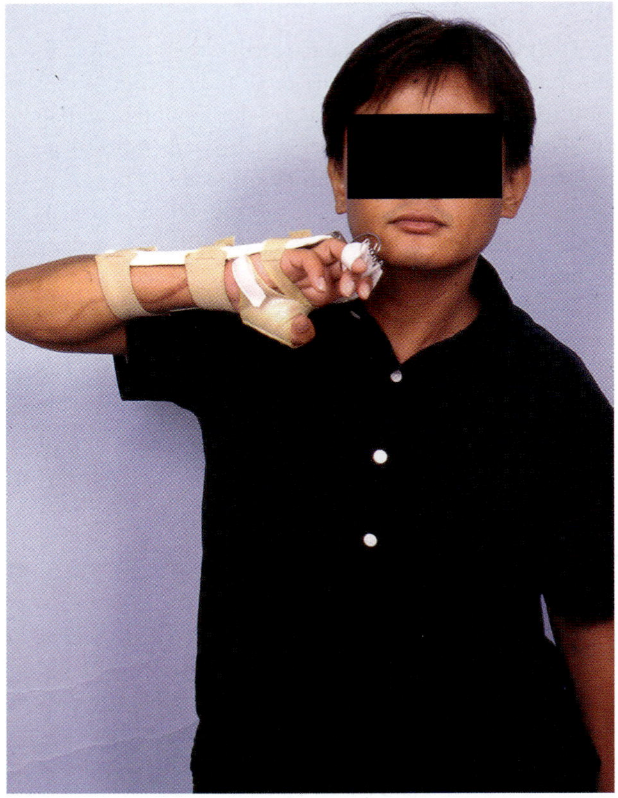

B

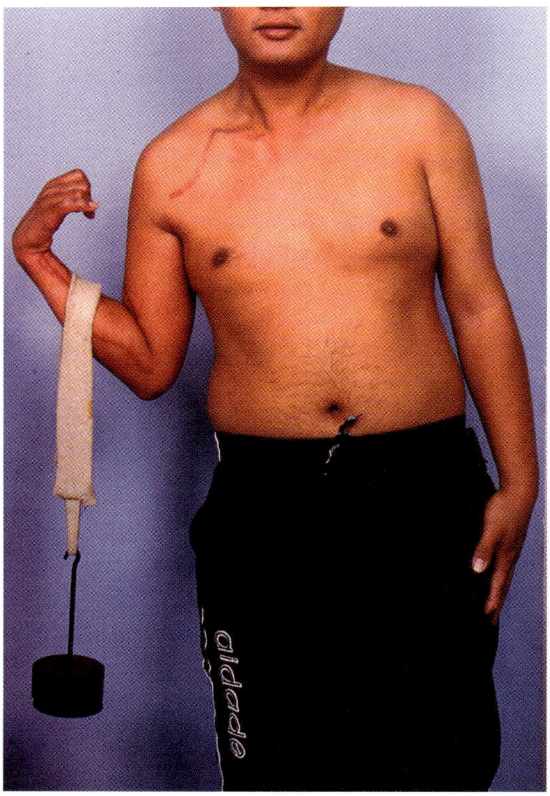

C

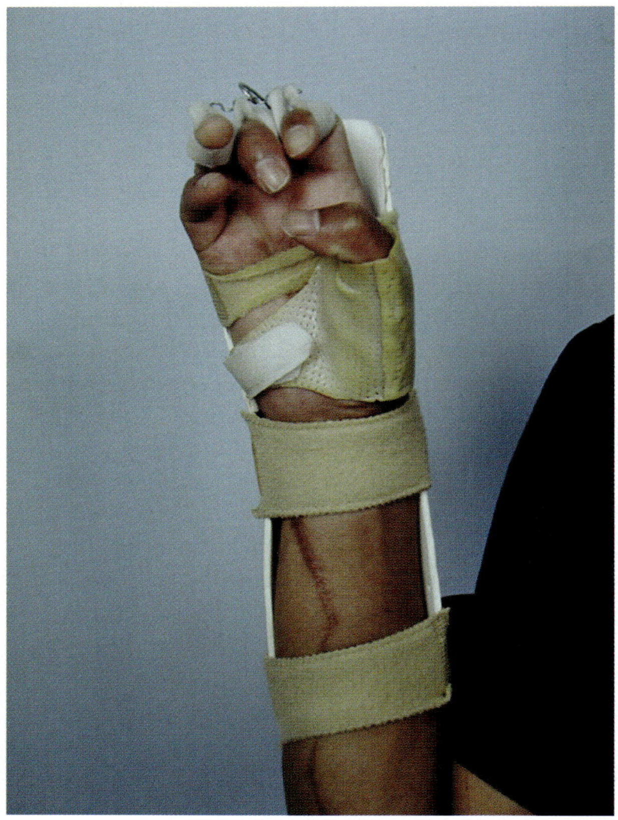

D

FIGURE 73-8 (A) A 29-year-old man with a right brachial plexus injury, C5-T1 total root avulsion, underwent a XI transfer to the suprascapular nerve and left contralateral C7 transfer to the musculocutaneous and median nerves with a vascularized ulnar nerve graft 2.5 months after a motorcycle accident. (B) to (D) Results 3 years later show 90-degree shoulder elevation, M4 elbow flexion, and M3 finger flexion.

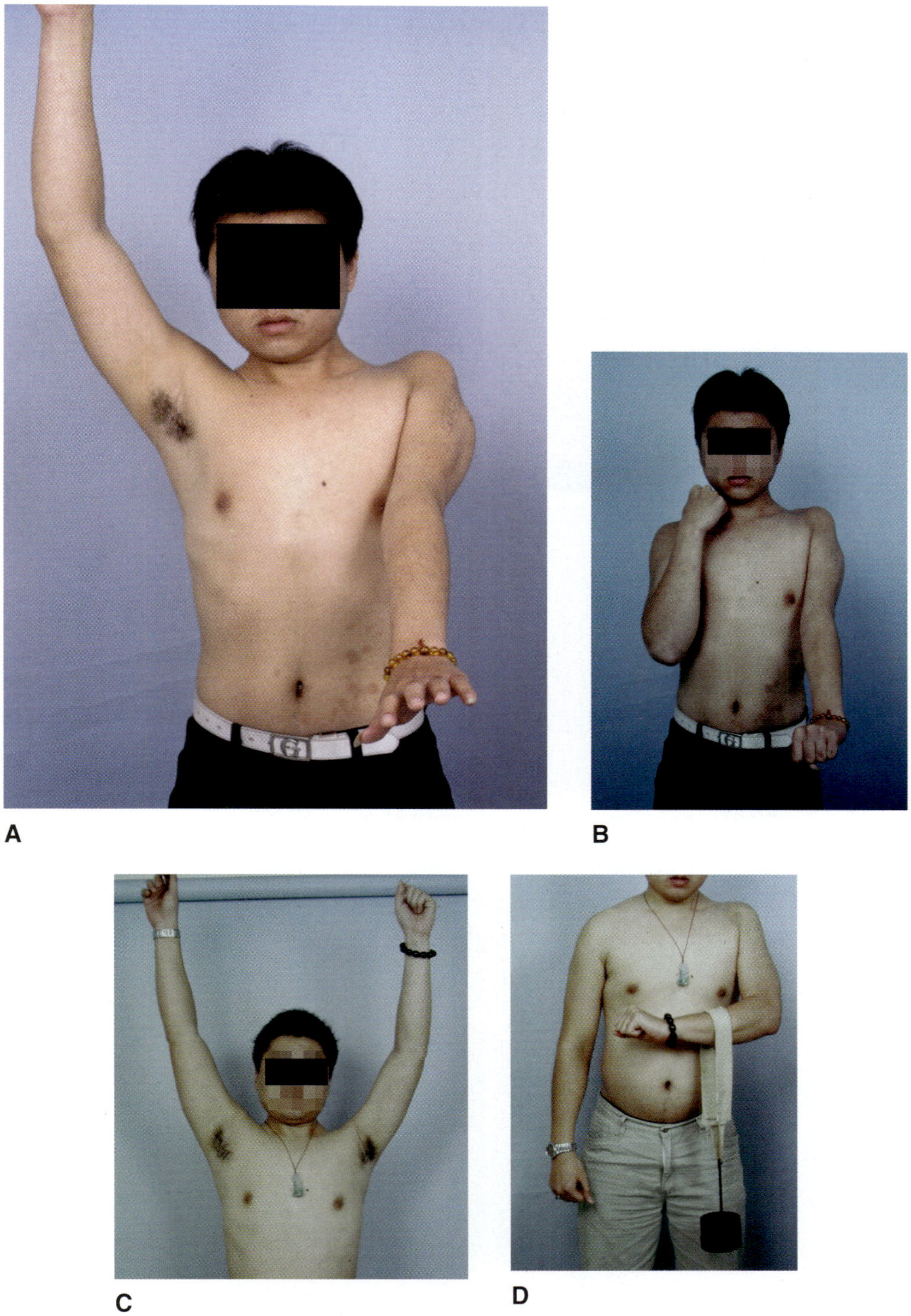

FIGURE 73-9 (A) to (D) A 25-year-old man with a left brachial plexus injury with rupture injury of C5-C6 at level 2, with a healthier C5 stump than C6 stump, underwent C5 nerve grafting to the anterior division and C6 nerve grafting to the posterior division of the upper trunk plus phrenic nerve transfer to the suprascapular nerve. (C) and (D) Results show good shoulder and elbow function 3 years after surgery.

Extraplexus and intraplexus nerve transfers are both considered as proximal nerve neurotizations (Figure 73-10).

Close-Target Nerve Transfer (or Distal Nerve Transfer)

Close-target nerve transfer is a procedure that provides direct coaptation at a more distal site closer to the neuromuscular junction, thus achieving faster recovery of motor outcomes. Close-target nerve transfer is defined as a procedure outside of the supra- and infraclavicular fossae. Examples include:

1. Spinal accessory nerve (XI) transfer to the suprascapular nerve via a posterior approach
2. Partial ulnar nerve transfer to the motor branch to the biceps
3. Partial median nerve transfer to the motor branch to the brachialis (Figure 73-11)

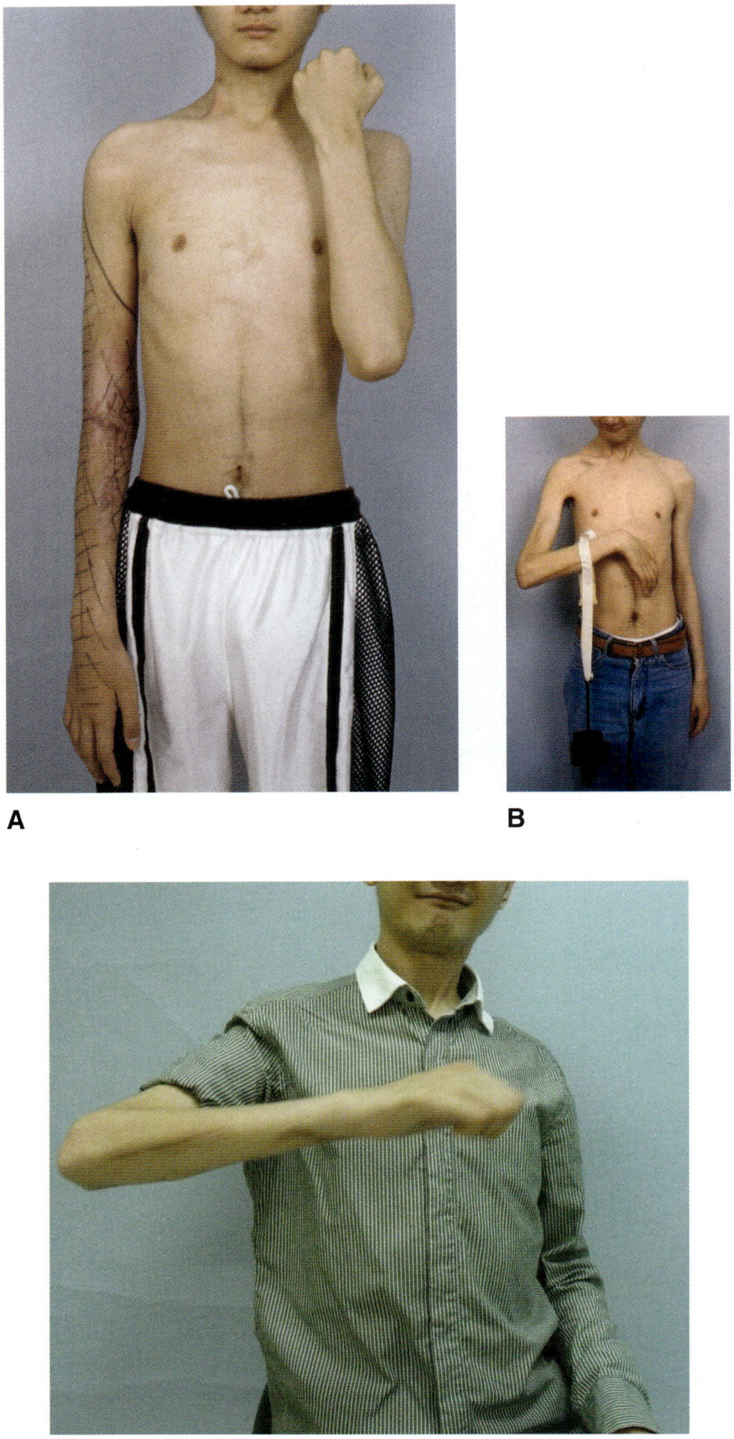

A B

C

FIGURE 73-10 (A) A 21-year-old male with a right brachial plexus injury with rupture C5 and root avulsions at C6-T1 underwent a phrenic nerve transfer to the posterior cord with a nerve graft, XI nerve transfer to the suprascapular nerve directly, and C5 transfer to the musculocutaneous and median nerves together with a vascularized nerve graft. (B) and (C) Results 5 years after surgery show nearly 90-degree shoulder abduction, M4 elbow flexion, M2 elbow extension, and M3 finger flexion after wrist and thumb arthrodeses.

4. Long head of triceps branch transfer to the axillary nerve
5. Intercostal nerve (IC) transfers to the motor branch to the biceps or the entire musculocutaneous nerve or the nerve to the long head of the triceps
6. Anterior interosseus nerve transfer to the radial or posterior interosseus nerve
7. Terminal branch of the anterior interosseus nerve transfer to the deep motor branch of the ulnar nerve at the wrist

Close-target nerve transfer is considered a distal nerve transfer. Selecting proximal or distal nerve transfers as a reconstructive strategy is now the subject of much debate. Proximal nerve transfer is traditionally still the main reconstructive procedure.

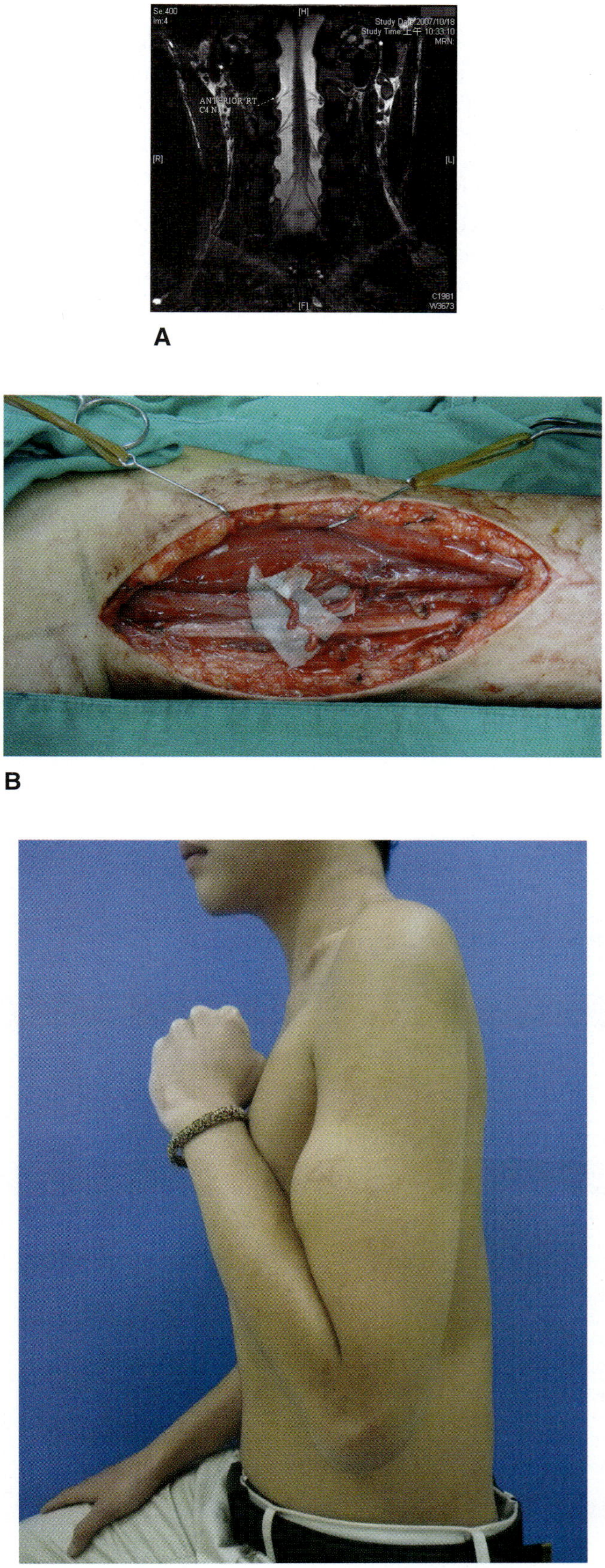

A

B

C

FIGURE 73-11 (**A**) A 20-year-old man with a left brachial plexus injury with C5-C6 root avulsions. (**B**) Transfer of a branch of the ulnar nerve to the biceps motor nerve and transfer of a branch of the median nerve to the brachialis nerve. (**C**) Result 1 year, 9 months after surgery showing M4 elbow flexion.

End-to-side neurorrhaphy (terminolateral neurorrhaphy) is a technique that transfers the distal end of a paralytic and irreparable nerve to the side of an intact nerve through an epineurotomy window for both motor and sensory reconstruction (21). It may be used in either proximal or distal nerve transfers. However, most brachial plexus surgeons are reluctant to use this technique or only use this technique as an adjuvant technique.

RECONSTRUCTIVE STRATEGIES WITH NERVE TRANSFERS FOR DIFFERENT FUNCTIONS

Reconstructive strategies with nerve transfers for different functions are quite individualized and depend on the intraoperative findings, the surgeon's philosophy, the patient's condition, and the patient's functional requirements. Different numbers of root injury or availability have different reconstructive strategies (23–25).

For the Shoulder

Reconstruction for shoulder abduction in a level 1 lesion should take priority over shoulder adduction. If the supraspinatus, infraspinatus, and deltoid muscles are innervated simultaneously, results are predictably better. The phrenic, XI, and XII nerves; the CMB; part of C5 or C6; the long thoracic nerve; the branch to the long head of the triceps; the medial pectoral nerve; the IC nerves; and CC7 have all been reported as donor nerves for shoulder abduction, but the phrenic and XI nerves are the most commonly used donor nerves for shoulder abduction. The recipient nerves for shoulder abduction in order of priority are the distal C5 (combined suprascapular nerve and posterior division of the upper trunk), the suprascapular nerve, the dorsal division of the upper trunk, and then the axillary nerve (26). A study of the author's series of patients demonstrated that triple nerve transfers produced the best and consistently reliable results for shoulder elevation: an average of 160 degrees of shoulder abduction was achieved after triple nerve transfers, 85 degrees after double nerve transfers, and 65 degrees after single nerve transfer (27).

For the Elbow

In a level 1 injury, reconstruction of elbow flexion is always the first priority. Donor nerves for elbow flexion include the IC nerves, XI nerve with or without a nerve graft, the phrenic nerve with or without a nerve graft, partial ulnar nerve, partial median nerve, the pectoral nerve, the thoracodorsal nerve, and CC7. The recipient nerve is the musculocutaneous nerve (mixed nerve), the motor branch to biceps, or the motor branch to brachialis.

Elbow extension is a lesser priority for reconstruction. Phrenic nerve transfer to the distal C5, to the posterior division of the upper trunk, or to the radial nerve with a nerve graft can often provide elbow extension. Some authors have described transferring two or three IC nerves to the branch to the long head of the triceps to achieve elbow extension.

For the Fingers

In global (C5-T1) level 1 injuries, the priority for reconstruction of finger function depends on the procedure used: nerve transfer or FFMT. Traditionally, reconstruction of finger flexion is preferable to finger extension, which can sometimes be helped with a dynamic extension splint. In a C5 rupture with four root avulsions, C6-T1 transfer of C5 to the median nerve (see Figure 73-10) or in a total root avulsion (C5-T1), transfer of the CC7 to the median nerve (see Figure 73-8) can be performed to achieve finger and wrist flexion as well as finger sensation. Both procedures require a vascularized ulnar nerve graft. In total root avulsions or four-root avulsion with a C5 rupture, nerve reconstruction first or FFMT first is a subject of much debate. Whereas nerve reconstruction first is a strategy of proximal-to-distal reconstructive priority; FFMT first is a strategy of distal-to-proximal reconstructive priority. Nerve reconstruction first by multiple nerve transfers aims to achieve a complete one-stage reconstruction for shoulder, elbow, and hand functions (23); FFMT is used predominantly as an additional reconstruction to enhance results at a later stage. However, FFMT first is an alternative approach (28). In the first stage, a long free muscle transfer (usually gracilis muscle) is positioned from the clavicle down to the extensor digitorum communis muscle and innervated by the XI nerve. In the second stage, a second long free muscle transfer is placed from the second rib down to the flexor digitorum profundus muscle and innervated by IC nerves. With this strategy, nerve reconstruction using C5, contralateral C7, or IC nerve transfers becomes an adjuvant procedure for restoring shoulder or elbow function. Comparison between the proximal-to-distal reconstructive strategy (nerve reconstruction first, free muscle transfer later), and the distal-to-proximal strategy (free muscle transfer first, then nerve reconstruction) in total root avulsions (level 1) is illustrated in Table 73-2.

Pedicle Muscle Transfer

Pedicled muscle transfer is indicated in nonglobal BPI such as a C5-C6 level 1 injury with intact C7-T1. Local latissimus dorsi muscle transfer for elbow flexion or finger flexion or even for shoulder abduction, local pectoralis major muscle transfer or local pectoralis minor muscle transfer for elbow flexion, part deltoid transfer for elbow extension, forearm flexors transfer for wrist or finger extension, and forearm muscle transfers for intrinsic muscle palsy are all examples of pedicled muscle transfers. The issue of using a reinnervated muscle transfer as a pedicled muscle transfer is also contentious. Preoperative muscle strength examination is very important but difficult. In a pedicled muscle transfer, it should be at least M4 muscle strength; otherwise, many of these transfers are useless and wasted. For example, using a local latissimus dorsi muscle transfer for elbow flexion in a C5 and C6 ± C7 avulsion injury usually results in M3 but not M4 muscle strength compared with a latissimus dorsi muscle transfer for traumatic loss of biceps and brachialis, which always results in M4 muscle strength. The reason for this difference in outcome is the condition of the thoracodorsal nerve, which originates from

TABLE 73-2 Comparison of "Proximal to Distal" and "Distal to Proximal" Reconstructive Priorities for Total Root Avulsion

	Proximal to Distal	Distal to Proximal
Philosophy	Traditional strategy	New strategy
Reconstructive priority	Shoulder and elbow first, then finger	Finger and elbow first, then shoulder
Brachial plexus exploration	Yes	Maybe not
Nerve Reconstruction		
For shoulder	Yes	May or may not be needed
For elbow	Yes	Need FFMT
For finger	Yes	Need FFMT
Stages	One stage Complete reconstruction	Multiple stages
Rehabilitation period	At least 4 yr	2 yr
Patient selection	Highly motivated, intelligent patient	Less intelligent and impatient patient
Predicted Outcomes		
Shoulder elevation	Better (≥60 degrees)	Shoulder fusion (10–30 degrees), M3-M4
Elbow flexion	Usually better M4	
Finger flexion	M2-M4	M3
Finger extension (EDC)	M0	M2-M3

EDC, extensor digitorum communis; FFMT, functioning free muscle transfer.

C6-C8. In the first example of an upper plexus injury, the thoracodorsal nerve is actually an injured nerve; in the second example of traumatic muscle loss, the thoracodorsal nerve is normal.

Functioning Free Muscle Transfers

Functioning free muscle transfer describes the transfer of a muscle using microvascular anastomoses for revascularization and microneural coaptation to a recipient motor nerve for reinnervation. The use of FFMT in brachial plexus reconstruction is one example of the application of nerve transfer (29). It has been shown to be effective and has become increasingly popular. The gracilis myocutaneous FFMT is most commonly used and best choice of donor muscle in brachial plexus reconstruction. Commonly used donor nerves include the XI, the IC, the phrenic nerve, the CC7 nerve, part of the ulnar nerve, and part of the median nerve and more proximally from the infra- or supraclavicular nerves, which requires elongation with a nerve graft and followed by an FFMT in a two-stage procedure. The results of FFMT are better than those achieved with a local muscle transfer. FFMT is especially useful for restoration of elbow and hand function in a global plexopathy. Indications for FFMT in BPI include acute or chronic root avulsion, root injury with failed nerve transfer (muscle strength less than M3), or BPI with associated Volkmann's contracture of the forearm.

Level 2 Injury

Disruption at the level of the spinal nerve with neuroma formation and dense scar tissue involving the scalene muscles are the main findings in this type of injury. Nerve rupture may occur in one or multiple spinal nerves. The clinical differential diagnosis between level 1 and 2 injury is of great importance with regard to the surgical approach and prognosis. Reconstruction for this level of injury includes neurolysis, nerve repair, nerve grafts, C-loop vascularized ulnar nerve graft, nerve transfer (if associated with a level 1 lesion in other spinal nerves), and palliative reconstruction.

Level 3 Injury

Level 3 injury involves the trunks and divisions. Nerve rupture with neuroma formation and dense scar tissue are the usual findings. Bypass nerve grafting is required to reestablish the connection between the supra- and infraclavicular brachial plexus. Osteotomy of the clavicle is often required for exposure, especially for injuries involving the lower trunk, to allow nerve grafting or direct neurolysis. Multiple nerve grafts are required. A C-loop vascularized ulnar nerve graft is sometimes helpful to reduce the number of nerve grafts needed, especially in cases of extensive injury.

Level 4 Injury

Level 4 injury involves the cords and their terminal branches. Level 4 injuries are usually limited to this zone only and rarely have more proximal level involvement. Level 4 injuries are usually caused by nerve ruptures and only rarely avulsion of the distal nerve. Avulsion can occur at the bone margin such as the suprascapular nerve at the scapular notch, the axillary nerve at the humeral neck, or the radial nerve at the spinal canal inlet or can occur at the muscle attachment such as the musculocutaneous nerve from the biceps surface. In closed level 4 injuries, the nerve damage is variable, ranging from simple isolated nerve injuries (axillary, musculocutaneous, or radial nerve) to lesions of all cords or all terminal branches. Level 4 injuries have particular characteristics that present specific difficulties in surgical dissection and repair because of dense scar tissue. There is a high incidence of vascular injury, rupture, or segmental occlusion of the subclavian or axillary arteries. Detachment of the insertion of the sternal portion of pectoralis major muscle by Z-lengthening is often required. For penetrating injuries, vascular and nerve repairs are usually performed simultaneously. Traction injuries at level 4 are usually associated with fractures of the proximal humerus or glenoid scapula. The nerve damage is extensive. Long nerve grafts are usually required to bridge the nerve gap, usually more than 8 cm in length. Sometimes a C-loop vascularized ulnar nerve graft is harvested from the paralyzed forearm and used for median and radial nerve reconstruction. The results are usually good with less aberrant reinnervation and better prognosis. In nerve avulsion from the muscle, nerve grafting of the proximal nerve stump and direct implantation into the muscle (nerve-to-muscle neurotization) yield fair results around M3. FFMT is another option to consider for reconstruction of these particular cases.

POSTOPERATIVE MANAGEMENT AND REHABILITATION

Immediate postoperative splinting for 3 weeks is required after nerve grafts or nerve transfers. Thereafter, retraining and rehabilitation should start, including physiotherapy (to avoid joint stiffness), muscle stimulation (to delay muscle atrophy), biofeedback, and occupational therapy. Patients should be followed periodically every 3 to 4 months with the surgeon and twice a month with a physical therapist. Patients are encouraged to have electric muscle stimulation at home (twice a day) regularly. For intercostal nerve transfers, passive shoulder elevation should be restricted to less than 90 degrees for 6 months. Regular follow-up in the rehabilitation center and outpatient clinics is tremendously important and should be explained to the patient before and emphasized again after surgery.

"Induction exercises" (or motivation exercises) are important muscle exercises for patients with nerve transfers. The original function of the donor nerve must be practiced to induce movement in the target muscles newly innervated by the nerve transfer. For example, patients who have undergone phrenic or intercostal nerve transfers must increase their deep breathing rate by running or long walks to induce movement in their target muscles. Similarly, tongue to palate push-up exercises in hypoglossal nerve transfers, shoulder adduction, or grasp exercises of the contralateral normal limb in contralateral C7 transfers all have the same effect. Various nerve transfers have different induction exercises. Induction exercises are started when movement of the innervated muscles becomes palpable (M1). The action of induction exercises is comparable to an internal electrical stimulator.

PALLIATIVE RECONSTRUCTION FOR SEQUELAE DEFORMITIES

Palliative reconstruction can be considered when deformities persist after maximal recovery, either after spontaneous incomplete recovery or after nerve reconstruction. Palliative reconstructive procedures include tendon or muscle transfers, FFMTs, tenodeses, and arthrodeses. Alternatively, orthotics and prostheses can be used for assistance. Patients at this stage should be encouraged to recognize their disabilities and attempt to use their incompletely recovered limb. In a completely failed reconstruction or if the patient perceives the injured limb to be a useless dead weight, amputation may need to be considered.

RESULTS AND OUTCOMES

Restoration of Shoulder Abduction: Comparison of Nerve Transfers versus Nerve Grafts

The author retrospectively studied 62 reconstructions of shoulder abduction with at least 2 years of follow-up, separated into three groups: C5 nerve grafts (seven patients), C5 nerve grafts plus XI nerve transfer or phrenic nerve transfer (eight patients), and only phrenic or spinal accessory nerve transfer (42 patients). The recipient nerves selected for shoulder abduction were distal C5, posterior division of the upper trunk, suprascapular nerve, or axillary nerve. Results showed shoulder abduction of 108.57 ± 54.29 degrees in the group of C5 nerve grafts, 107.50 ± 60.42 degrees in the group of combined C5 nerve grafts and nerve transfers, and 84.05 ± 44.01 degrees in the group of extraplexus nerve transfers. Successful shoulder abduction of 90 degrees or more was 57.1% in the C5 nerve grafts, 62.5% in the combined C5 nerve grafts and nerve transfers, and 54.8% in the nerve transfers. The conclusion from this study was "do not neglect the C5 stump for reconstruction." C5 nerve grafts combined with nerve transfers produced better results than nerve transfers alone for shoulder abduction.

Restoration of Elbow Flexion by Nerve Transfer: Comparison of Proximal versus Distal Nerve Transfers

A total of 188 patients who underwent musculocutaneous nerve neurotization to restore elbow flexion were evaluated. Musculocutaneous nerve neurotization from C5, the medial cord, C8, contralateral C7, the spinal accessory nerve, or the phrenic nerve comprised the group of proximal nerve transfers. Musculocutaneous nerve neurotization from partial ulnar nerve or partial median nerve comprised the distal nerve transfers. Intercostal nerve transfers to the musculocutaneous nerve were classified in a separate group. There was no significant difference in the successful recovery of elbow flexion (M >3) between proximal and distal nerve transfers. Even though the speed of recovery was faster in distal nerve transfers, 19 months versus 23.9 months, the difference was also not significant. The only statistically significant difference was the speed of recovery between partial ulnar nerve with or without partial median nerve fascicles and intercostal nerve transfers ($P = 0.046$). However, a number of patients with distal nerve transfers had persistent grip strength deficits resulting from the donor nerve transfers.

Results of Adult Brachial Plexus Reconstruction with the Level of Injury

It is difficult and impractical to provide patients and their families with expectations about the results of treatment. However, after successful nerve grafting of level 4 injuries, M4 with 180 degrees of shoulder elevation, M4 or M4+ elbow flexion or extension, M3 to M3 + forearm finger flexion or extension, and M2 or less of intrinsic hand muscles can usually be expected. After successful multiple nerve transfers for total root avulsions, 60 degrees or more shoulder abduction, M4 elbow flexion, and M2-M3 finger flexion can be achieved. In addition, M2-M3 wrist and finger extension can be obtained after FFMT in late reconstructions.

CONCLUSION

Closed traction injuries of the brachial plexus are always disabling. "For somebody who has nothing, a little is a lot." The healing process, surgeon, patient, and rehabilitation program are the main factors influencing the outcome of the treatment. The healing process is influenced by the patient's age; the degree, extent, and location of injury; and the time interval between the injury and surgery. The surgeon can directly influence the overall outcome, but assurance of functional restoration is unpredictable. A thorough knowledge of the gross and internal anatomy of the brachial plexus, an understanding of nerve pathophysiology, meticulous microneurovascular skills, and familiarity with conventional hand reconstruction are all basic requirements for brachial plexus reconstructive surgeons. The patient's desire and cooperation is also an important determining factor, especially for patients who undergo nerve transfer. A rigorous rehabilitation program should include intensive physiotherapy, pain management, and direction in using the disabled limb to return to normal life and work or retraining for another occupation. However, the outcome for patients undergoing surgical reconstruction for a BPI is now more optimistic than ever before.

REFERENCES

1. Gray H, Goss CM. *Gray's Anatomy*, 26th ed. Philadelphia, Lea & Febiger, 1955, pp. 1038–1058.
2. Leffert RD. *Brachial Plexus Injuries*. New York, Churchill Livingstone, 1985, pp. 1–38.
3. Slingluff CL, Terzis JK, Edgerton MT. The quantitative microanatomy of the brachial plexus in man. Reconstructive relevance. In Terzis JK (ed). *Microreconstruction of Nerve Injuries*. Philadelphia: WB Saunders, 1987, pp. 285–324.
4. Narakas A. Surgical treatment of traction injuries of the brachial plexus. *Clin Orthop* 1978;133:71–90.
5. Chuang DC, Ma HS, Wei FC. A new evaluation system to predict the sequelae of late obstetric brachial plexus palsy. *Plast Reconstr Surg* 1998;101:673–685.

6. Chuang DC. Adult brachial plexus injuries. In Neligan P (ed). *Plastic Surgery*, 3rd ed, vol. VI. Philadelphia: Saunders Elsevier, 2011.
7. Sunderland S. Brachial plexus injuries. *Clin Neurol Neurosurg* 1993;95 (suppl):S1–S2.
8. Chuang DC. Adult brachial plexus injuries. In Mathes SJ, Hentz VR (eds). *Plastic Surgery*, 2nd ed, vol. 7. Philadelphia: Saunders Elsevier, 2006, pp. 515–538.
9. Chuang DC. Adult brachial plexus reconstruction with the level of injury: review and personal experience. *Plast Reconstr Surg* 2009;124(suppl): 359e–369e.
10. Seddon HJ. Three types of nerve injury. *Brain* 1943;66:238–288.
11. Sunderland S. A classification of peripheral nerve injuries producing loss of function. *Brain* 1951;74:491–516.
12. Boome RS. General discussion on the brachial plexus. In Boome RS (eds). *The Brachial Plexus*. New York: Churchill Livingstone, 1997, pp. 1–17.
13. Narakas A. Surgical treatment of traction injuries of the brachial plexus. *Clin Orthop* 1978;133:71–90.
14. Alnot JY. Traumatic paralysis of the brachial plexus: preoperative problems and therapeutic indications. In Terzis JK (eds). *Microreconstruction of Nerve Injuries*. Philadelphia: WB Saunders, 1987, pp. 325–345.
15. Millesi H. Brachial plexus lesions: classification and operative technique. In Tubiana R (ed). *The Hand*. Philadelphia: WB Saunders, 1988, pp. 645–655.
16. Terzis JK, Verkris MD, Soucacos P. Outcomes of brachial plexus reconstruction in 204 patients with devastating paralysis. *Plast Reconstr Surg* 1999;104:1221–1240.
17. Chuang DC, Yeh MC, Wei FC. Intercostal nerve transfer of the musculocutaneous nerve in avulsed brachial plexus injuries—evaluation of 66 patients. *J Hand Surg* 1992;17A:822–828.
18. Nordin L, Sinisi M. Brachial plexus-avulsion causing Brown-Séquard syndrome. *J Bone Joint Surg Br* 2009;91:88–90.
19. Lister G. *The Hand*, 3rd ed. Edinburgh: Churchill Livingstone; 1993, pp. 233–236.
20. Yoshikawa T, Hayashi N, Yamamoto S, et al. Brachial plexus injury: clinical manifestation, conventional imaging findings, and the latest imaging techniques. *Radiographics* 2006;26:S133–S134.
21. Chuang DC. Nerve transfers in adult brachial plexus injuries: my methods. *Hand Clin* 2005;21:71–82.
22. Viterbo F, Trindade JC, Hoshino K, Mazzoni AL. End-to-side neurorrhaphy with removal of the epineurial sheath: an experimental study in rats. *Plast Reconstr Surg* 1994;94:1038–1047.
23. Narakas AO. Neurotization or nerve transfer in traumatic brachial plexus lesions. In Tubiana R (ed). *The Hand*. Philadelphia: WB Saunders, 1987, pp. 656–683.
24. Oberlin C. Nerve transfer to biceps muscle using a part of ulnar nerve for C5-6 avulsion of the brachial plexus—anatomical studies and report of four cases. *J Hand Surg* 1994;19A:232–237.
25. Mackinnon SE, Novak CB, Myckatyn TM, Tung TH. Results of reinnervation of the biceps and brachialis muscles with a double fascicular transfer for elbow flexion. *J Hand Surg* 2005;30A:978–985.
26. Chuang DC, Wei FC. Restoration of shoulder abduction by nerve transfer in avulsed brachial plexus injuries—evaluation of 99 patients with various nerve transfers. *Plast Reconstr Surg* 1995;96:122–128.
27. Cardenas-Mejia A, O'Boyle, CP, Chen KT, Chuang DC. Evaluation of single-, double-, and triple-nerve transfers for shoulder abduction in 90 patients with supraclavicular brachial plexus injury. *Plast Reconstr Surg* 2008;122:1470–1478.
28. Doi K, Sakai K, Kuwata N, et al. Double-muscle technique for reconstruction of prehension after complete avulsion of brachial plexus. *J Hand Surg* 1995;20A:408–414.
29. Chuang DC. Nerve transfer with functioning free muscle transplantation. *Hand Clin* 2008;24:377–388.

CHAPTER 74

Double Free Muscle Transfers

Kazuteru Doi

Several surgical approaches (1–4), including implantation of nerve roots into the spinal cord and nerve transfers with or without free muscle transfers, have been developed to restore prehension for total paralysis of the brachial plexus. Most of these procedures, other than the double free muscle transfer (DFMT) technique (5–9), have not provided functional improvements for patients in their daily activities.

The DFMT technique achieved a dramatic revolution in the treatment of total paralysis of the brachial plexus by providing universal prehensile function, although several requirements, including successful free muscle transfers, stability of the proximal joints, and prolonged postoperative rehabilitation, are absolutely necessary for the success of this procedure.

Several authors have followed our procedures (10–13), but their functional outcomes (13) are less satisfactory than ours because their patients did not complete the postoperative rehabilitation program, which usually needs at least 1 year after surgery, and they did not understand the basic biomechanics of DFMT (14).

OUTLINE OF DOUBLE FREE MUSCLE TRANSFER

The double free gracilis muscle transfer technique consists of five established, but modified, reconstructive procedures (8):

1. Exploration of the brachial plexus and repair of the ruptured motor nerves, if possible
2. The first free muscle transfer, neurotized by the spinal accessory nerve, for elbow flexion and finger extension
3. The second free muscle transfer, neurotized by the fifth and sixth intercostal nerves, for finger flexion
4. A cross-nerve procedure using the third and fourth intercostal nerves to neurotize the motor branch of the triceps muscle for elbow extension, performed simultaneously with the second muscle transfer
5. The intercostal sensory rami coapted to the medial cord of the brachial plexus to restore sensibility to the hand

DONOR MUSCLE SELECTION

The gracilis is the best choice for the donor muscle. The latissimus dorsi, gracilis, and rectus femoris muscles were all used as donor muscles in the initial period of reconstruction by this technique. Long-term results showed that the latissimus dorsi did not provide satisfactory finger function because of adhesion of the muscle to the fabricated pulley system and rupture of its tendon caused by ischemic necrosis of the portion distal to the pulley. The rectus femoris is a bipennate muscle and has less excursion, resulting in poor finger function.

INDICATIONS

Not all patients with a total paralysis of the brachial plexus are candidates for DFMT. Suitable patients should be younger than 40 years old and have sustained the injury within the preceding 6 months. They should not have sustained any injury to the subclavian or axillary arteries nor had any injury or history of surgery to the donor motor nerve (the spinal accessory or the intercostal nerves). They should be motivated and have financial and emotional support to participate in a prolonged postoperative rehabilitation program (6).

Although all of our patients older than 40 years of age showed normal reinnervation of the transferred muscles, the ultimate muscle power achieved in these older patients was too weak to perform prehensile function despite satisfactory elbow flexion. In DFMT, supplemental procedures, such as cross-nerve transfer for shoulder function and elbow extension, are indispensable to achieving useful prehension (7,15). These procedures should be conducted within 6 months of injury before atrophy of the denervated muscles becomes irreversible. Patients who sustained brachial plexus injury more than

6 months previously can be assessed as possible candidates for surgery according to their shoulder and elbow function after spontaneous recovery of the upper C5 or C6 roots or after preceding surgical procedures. Patients who have sustained major injuries of the subclavian or axillary arteries, which have been repaired with artificial or autogenous vein graft, may potentially be candidates for DFMT, provided the two donor vessels are proven to be patent by preoperative angiogram, although occlusion of donor vessels is not unusual.

However, they are not good candidates because of the risk of vascular compromise of the vascular anastomoses. The recovering spinal accessory nerve should be avoided for use as the donor motor nerve. Displaced rib fractures are usually accompanied by intercostal nerve injury, and these patients should not be enrolled as candidates for DFMT. Causalgia is not a contraindication for DFMT, and severe pain always subsides after the procedure. Patients tolerate pain without medication during the periods of reconstructive surgery and postoperative rehabilitation.

PREOPERATIVE EVALUATION

Even when total palsy exists, fewer than 20% of patients demonstrate avulsions of all five roots of the plexus (9). In particular, the C5 nerve root is usually spared from avulsion, and this nerve root is a key root for functional improvement of the DFMT by shoulder reconstruction. There are many methods of evaluating the level of nerve root injury and hence the need for nerve root repairs in brachial plexus injury. They include preoperative clinical examination, electrophysiological studies, radiologic studies, intraoperative macroscopic and microscopic evaluation, intraoperative electrical stimulation, histopathologic studies, somatosensory evoked potentials, evoked spinal cord potentials (ESCPs), and choline acetyltransferase (CAT) activity measurements (16). ESCP and CAT activities were found to be the most reliable techniques for evaluating the possibility of requiring nerve root repairs, but both techniques are not universally available.

We have tried to assess the possibility of requiring nerve root repair of the C5 nerve root using preoperative clinical evaluation without using these two techniques and found that Tinel's sign, sensation in the C5 area, and electromyographic (EMG) study of the infraspinatus muscle are not helpful in assessing the possible need for nerve root repair of the C5 nerve root. However, we found a highly significant correlation between a combination of the radiologic findings, macro- and microscopic examination of the nerve root during surgical exploration, and direct electrical stimulation, with the possibility of requiring nerve root repair of the C5 nerve root. Among the radiologic parameters, a coronal view in a computed tomography myelogram is the most simple and reliable indicator (17). However, we now prefer coronal views of 1.5-T magnetic resonance imaging, which provide clear images of the injured cervical nerve roots without any invasive technique.

OPERATIVE TECHNIQUE

Timing

The timing of the various reconstructive procedures is important and is guided by several criteria. Procedures 1 and 2 were performed simultaneously at the first operation, but recently, we have performed these procedures in two stages because of the prolonged duration of the combined surgery. Procedures 3, 4, and 5 are performed at a third stage, usually 2 or 3 months after the first free muscle transfer. Sometimes the order of procedures 2 and procedures 3 to 5 is reversed, when more than 6 months has elapsed, because procedure 2 only consists of a free muscle transfer, but procedures 3, 4, and 5 include a motor nerve repair. If the motor nerve of the triceps muscle was repaired in procedure 1, then the motor branch of the biceps muscle is repaired in procedure 4 to strengthen elbow flexion, or it can be used as a supplementary donor muscle for secondary reconstruction of failed or weak finger flexion or elbow extension.

Procedure 1

The two upper cervical roots, C5 and C6, are explored through a transverse cervical skin incision. When the C5 or C6 nerve root is available as a donor, neurotization of the suprascapular nerve and posterior division of the upper trunk is performed with a sural nerve or vascularized ulnar nerve graft (Figure 74-1) (18).

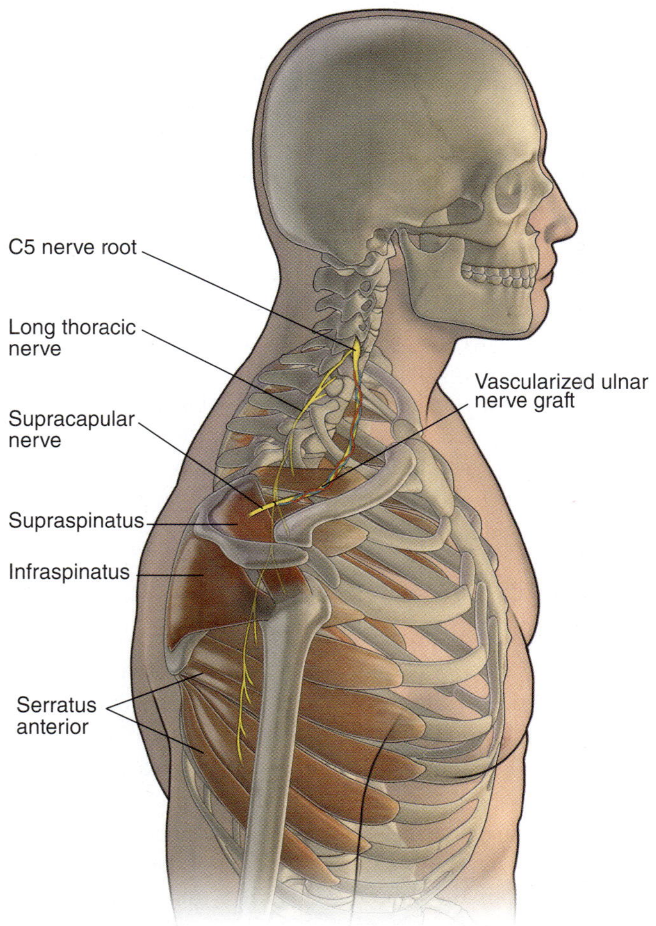

FIGURE 74-1 Procedure 1. The C5 nerve root is connected to the suprascapular nerve by a vascularized ulnar nerve graft based on the superior ulnar collateral artery and vein to restore shoulder function. The serratus anterior muscle is partially functioning from the spared proximal C5 nerve root. n, nerve. (Redrawn with permission from Doi K. Management of total paralysis of the brachial plexus by the double free-muscle transfer technique. *J Hand Surg* 2008;33E:240.)

If the C5 or C6 nerve root is not available, then the contralateral C7 nerve root is chosen as the donor motor nerve and is transferred to the suprascapular nerve, the long thoracic nerve, and the posterior division of the upper trunk using a vascularized ulnar nerve graft (7).

Procedure 2

Simultaneous elbow flexion and finger extension are reconstructed with a free muscle transfer using the spinal accessory nerve as the motor nerve (Figure 74-2).

Preparation of the Spinal Accessory Nerve as Donor Nerve (19)

A 10-cm transverse incision is made along the clavicle from its midportion to the acromioclavicular joint (see Figure 74-1). The upper part of trapezius, which inserts on the clavicle and the acromioclavicular joint, is divided with a monopolar coagulator. The divided upper part of the trapezius is retracted posteriorly. The spinal accessory nerve can be found on the anterior surface of the trapezius; however, identification of the nerve at this site is difficult because it is embedded in adipose tissue. The landmark for detection of the spinal accessory nerve at this site is the transverse cervical artery and vein. These vessels enter the muscle at the base of the neck and then descend vertically midway between the vertebral column and the medial border of the scapula, accompanied by the spinal accessory nerve. After identification of the vessels, a nerve stimulator is used to probe around the vessels to identify the distal part of the spinal accessory nerve. Small branches from the cervical plexus are frequently found around the vessels, but these branches are comparatively small, and the response of the trapezius to electrical stimulation is weak. The spinal accessory nerve is always found in the adipose tissue on the anterior surface of the trapezius. A small branch to the upper part of the trapezius should be preserved. The terminal division of the nerve is dissected distally as far as possible, divided, and transferred to the supraclavicular fossa for coaptation. Transecting the nerve at the level of the scapular spine usually provides enough length to reach the supraclavicular fossa.

Preparation of the Recipient Vessels

By incorporating a the deltopectoral skin incision, beginning proximally at the clavicle and extending distally over the coracoid to the axillary crease, the deltopectoral interval is developed, exposing the cephalic vein, which is isolated and traced proximally. The cephalic vein is clamped at its distal end and cut at a suitable length to be the recipient vein.

The thoracoacromial artery and venae comitans are isolated on the pectoralis minor muscle, and traced deeper to their bifurcation from the subclavicular artery and vein after the tendinous origin of the pectoralis minor muscle is detached from the coracoid process.

Attachment of the Gracilis Muscle and Preparation of the Tunnel for Passing the Motor Nerve

A tunnel for passing the motor nerve of the gracilis muscle from the infraclavicular fossa to the supraclavicular fossa is made underneath the clavicle by blunt dissection using a mosquito clamp, and a Penrose drain is passed through this tunnel. Several anchoring sutures are passed through the lateral clavicle and anterior acromion for reattachment of the detached trapezius muscle and for the attachment of the gracilis muscle.

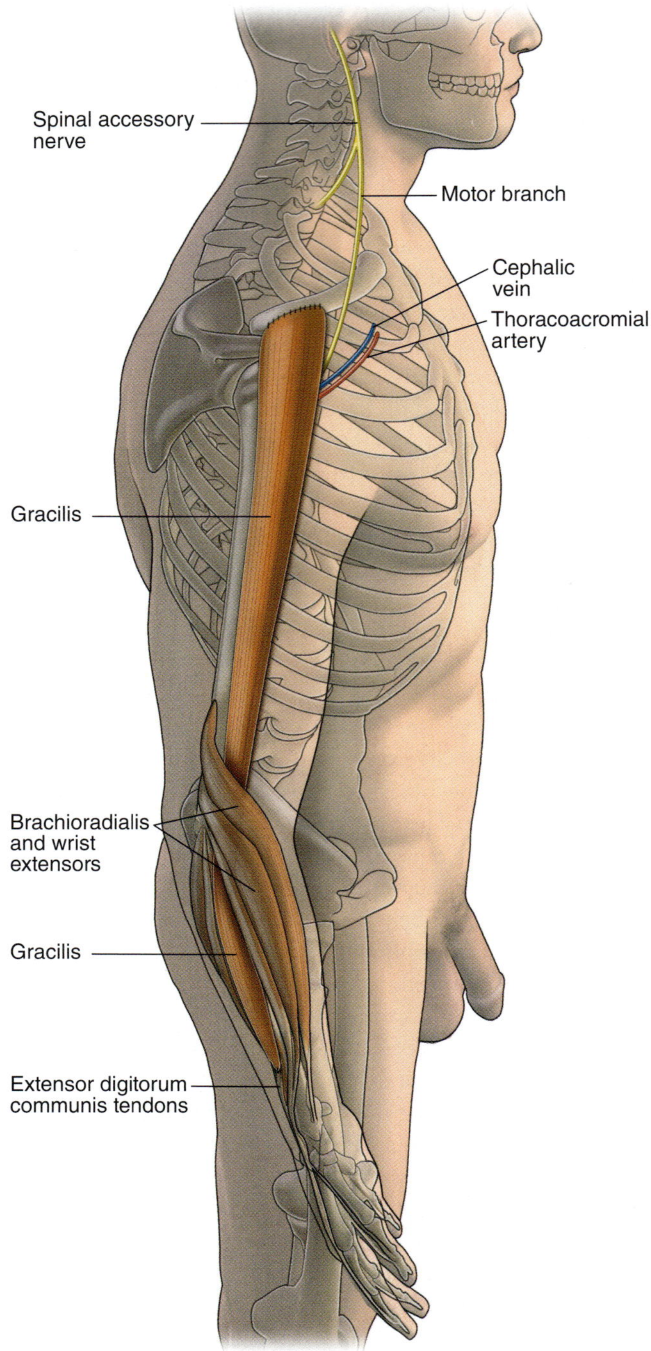

FIGURE 74-2 Procedure 2. The first free muscle transfer is attached to the clavicle proximally and the extensor digitorum communis tendons distally for simultaneous reconstruction of elbow flexion and finger extension. The gracilis is vascularized by the thoracoacromial artery and cephalic vein and innervated by the spinal accessory nerve. a, artery; n, nerve; v, vein. (Redrawn with permission from Doi K. Management of total paralysis of the brachial plexus by the double free-muscle transfer technique. *J Hand Surg* 2008;33E:240.)

Preparation of the Recipient Bed for the Gracilis Muscle

Longitudinal skin incisions are made on the lateral aspect of the elbow and the dorsal aspect of the forearm. A subcutaneous tunnel is prepared between the deltopectoral and elbow incisions for passage of the gracilis muscle. Through the elbow incision, the pulley to prevent bowstringing of the gracilis muscle is made beneath the brachioradialis and wrist extensor muscles, and a Penrose drain is placed. Through the dorsal forearm incision, the extensor digitorum communis tendons are divided at their musculotendinous junctions.

Harvesting of the Gracilis Muscle (20)

The gracilis muscle from the contralateral thigh is selected because the orientation and location of its neurovascular bundle match the site of the recipient vessels. The length of the gracilis muscle should be sufficiently long to span the distance between the acromion and midforearm without tension. This is verified by measuring the length of the gracilis muscle from its pubic origin to tibial insertion.

We harvest the gracilis muscle with an accompanying skin flap through three small skin incisions assisted by endoscopy (21,22). The gracilis muscle has a type 2 vascular pedicle, with a dominant vascular pedicle originating from the profunda femoris vessels and a single motor nerve originating from the obturator nerve. During harvest, it is important to include the entire fascia around the muscle to ensure vascularity of the skin paddle and enhance muscle gliding in its new bed. Mobilization of the adductor longus muscle allows the pedicle to be dissected to its origin from the profunda femoris vessels, achieving maximal length of the available pedicle. Lengthening the gracilis tendon with a periosteal strip provides a gracilis muscle long enough to span the distance from the clavicle to the distal forearm. The main complications are related to the donor site and include delayed healing, infection, and scar-related problems. The functional deficit is negligible after harvest of a gracilis muscle.

The First Gracilis Muscle Transfer

The gracilis muscle is placed on the anterior aspect of the shoulder, and the proximal origin of the muscle is fixed to the lateral half of the clavicle using the previously placed anchoring sutures.

The motor nerve of the gracilis muscle is passed through the tunnel underneath the clavicle guided by the Penrose drain and coapted to the middle and distal branches of the spinal accessory nerve in the supraclavicular fossa.

Microvascular anastomoses are then performed between the medial circumflex femoral artery and vein of the gracilis muscle and the thoracoacromial artery and vein or the cephalic vein in the infraclavicular fossa.

A straight, direct route for the free muscle transfer is created from its origin to its final insertion to maximize its force of contraction. It is placed subcutaneously on the lateral aspect of the upper arm and the dorsal surface of the forearm, deep to the brachioradialis and radial wrist extensor muscles, just distal to the elbow, to prevent bowstringing. This position is optimal for elbow flexion and finger extension, although grip may weaken when the elbow is flexed. The distal tendon of the transferred gracilis muscle is sutured to the extensor digitorum communis tendons. It is essential that the correct muscle tension is reproduced in the upper limb before final suturing of the muscle to the finger extensors.

Proper muscle tension is critical for good postoperative function. We previously described (5,6,8,9) that the original muscle length should be restored by stretching the muscle until the distance between the markers, which were previously placed on the surface of the muscle before harvesting at 5-cm intervals, as described by Manktelow et al. (23) again become 5-cm intervals. However, we no longer use this technique because we harvest the gracilis muscle with the overlying fascia, which does not contract equally with the muscle, and therefore markers on the fascia are not indicative of the resting muscle tension.

The correct muscle tension is adjusted with the shoulder in 60 degrees of abduction and 15 degrees of anterior flexion, the elbow in 150 degrees of flexion, and the wrist in neutral with the fingers in full extension. With maximal distal traction on the muscle, the position of coaptation is marked on the extensor digitorum communis tendons and the gracilis muscle tendon. The elbow is then flexed to 90 degrees, and with the wrist in neutral and the fingers fully flexed, the donor gracilis muscle tendon and extensor digitorum communis tendons are sutured. The correct tension of the transfer is then evaluated by using the tenodesis principle.

Procedures 3 to 5

Finger flexion is reconstructed using a second free muscle transfer (Figure 74-3) performed 2 to 3 months after the first operation after improvement in postoperative contracture of the elbow and finger joints. The fifth and sixth intercostal nerves are used as donor motor nerves and the thoracoacromial artery and venae comitans as the recipient vessels for the second gracilis muscle transfer. The third and fourth intercostal nerves are simultaneously coapted to the motor branch to the triceps muscle to restore elbow extension (Figure 74-4), and the sensory rami of the second intercostal nerve are sutured to the median nerve to restore hand sensibility, all during the second operation (see Figure 74-4).

Preparation of the Recipient Site

A longitudinal medial upper arm and axillary incision extends along the lower border of the pectoralis major muscle from the anterior axillary fold toward the sternum, curving slightly medially toward the xiphoid process. In women, the incision is placed in the inframammary fold for better cosmesis. Flaps are developed on either side of the incision, with care taken not to injure the intercostobrachial nerve, which usually appears in the axillary subcutaneous fat and is used as the donor sensory nerve. The intercostobrachial nerve is isolated and traced to its bifurcation from the second intercostal nerve. The lateral division of the median nerve and the motor branch to the triceps muscle are identified and divided from their bifurcation from the lateral and posterior cord in the axilla. The thoracodorsal artery and venae comitans are also isolated and prepared as recipient vessels for the second free muscle transfer.

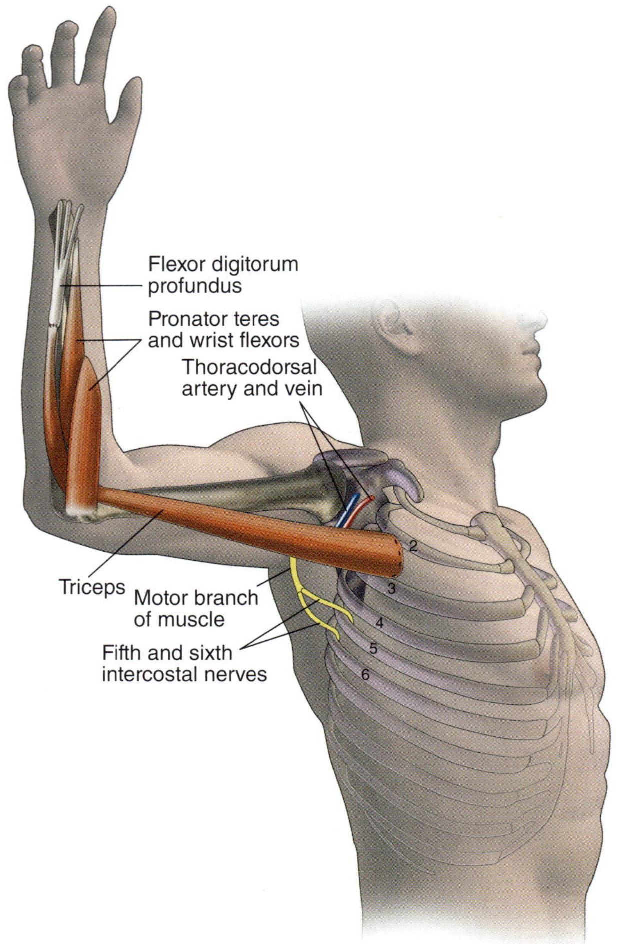

FIGURE 74-3 Procedure 3. The second free muscle transfer is attached to the second and third ribs proximally and the flexor digitorum profundus tendons distally for restoration of finger flexion. The gracilis is vascularized by the thoracodorsal artery and vein and innervated by the fifth and sixth intercostal nerves. a, artery; v, vein. (Redrawn with permission from Doi K. Management of total paralysis of the brachial plexus by the double free-muscle transfer technique. *J Hand Surg* 2008;33E:240.)

The third to the sixth intercostal spaces are exposed by blunt dissection underneath the pectoralis major and minor muscles (24). The clavicle and first rib can easily be palpated and the number of the ribs identified. The periosteum is incised with a Bovie over the midline of the anterior surface of the rib, from the midaxillary line to the costochondral junction, with care taken not to injure the serratus anterior muscles. The periosteum of each rib is then carefully elevated with a periosteal elevator. The denuded rib is elevated with a Farabeuf retractor and the free edge of the periosteum is retracted with Kocher forceps to expose the intercostal nerves. The intercostal nerve runs with the intercostal artery and vein along the inferoposterior edge of the rib. A longitudinal incision is then made along the deep surface of the periosteum, medial to the midclavicular line, with a #15 scalpel. At this level, the intercostal muscles are thin, and the nerve is easier to identify. If the intercostal nerve is not visualized, looking for a bleeding point on the periosteum and the lateral sensory rami of the intercostal nerve will identify the intercostal nerve.

Depending on the length of intercostal nerve required to reach the recipient nerve, the dissection may be extended medially to the costochondral junction. Laterally, the dissection is extended to the deep surface of the serratus anterior muscle slips. We prefer and advocate preserving the serratus insertion if it is not completely paralytic or has been reinnervated by surgery. For the intercostal nerve transfer to reach the recipient nerve is facilitated by passing the nerves through a tunnel created in the muscle.

The gracilis muscle is attached to the second and third ribs by anchoring sutures passed through drill holes in the ribs.

Before the gracilis muscle transfer is positioned, the intercostobrachial nerve is coapted to the median nerve, and the motor branch to the triceps muscle is coapted to the third and fourth intercostal nerves using 10-0 monofilament nylon sutures.

The Second Gracilis Muscle Transfer

The second gracilis muscle is harvested from the ipsilateral thigh and placed in the axillary incision. The proximal attachment of the muscle is sutured to the second and third ribs, making sure the monitoring skin flap is positioned superficially.

The medial circumflex femoral artery and vein of the gracilis muscle are anastomosed to the thoracodorsal artery and vein.

To activate finger flexion, the gracilis muscle is placed along the medial aspect of the upper arm and forearm, so as not to become a secondary elbow flexor. The muscle is passed under the pronator teres and wrist flexors just distal to the elbow. The distal portion of the gracilis muscle is thin and tendinous and can easily be passed through a small hiatus deep to the forearm flexor muscles. The distal tendinous portion of the gracilis is sutured to the flexor digitorum profundus tendons. To determine the correct tension, the shoulder, elbow, and wrist are in the same position as described earlier and the fingers are placed in full flexion. The medial circumflex femoral vessels of the gracilis muscle are anastomosed to the thoracodorsal artery and vein. The fifth and sixth intercostal nerves are coapted without tension to the motor nerve of the obturator nerve to the second gracilis muscle transplant.

POSTOPERATIVE VASCULAR MONITORING

Postoperative perfusion of the innervated free muscle transfer has only been monitored by conventional skin flap parameters. However, we have experienced three clinical cases, in which conventional monitoring of the skin flap did not reflect the vascularity of the underlying innervated free muscle transfer. After revision of the compromised microsurgical anastomoses, even though the skin flap survived, the gracilis muscle did not survive completely or recover functionally because the response to ischemia of skin and muscle varies. From an experimental study of compound muscle action potentials (CMAPs) for monitoring innervated free muscle transfers in rabbits, we have applied CMAP monitoring in clinical cases. After the completion of the neurovascular anastomoses, epidural electrode are inserted into the subfascial plane of the gracilis muscle. The waveform of the potentials and amplitude and latency are monitored continuously every 60 minutes. Amplitude and latency of the potentials were calculated as a percentage of their baseline value. Clinical examination of the

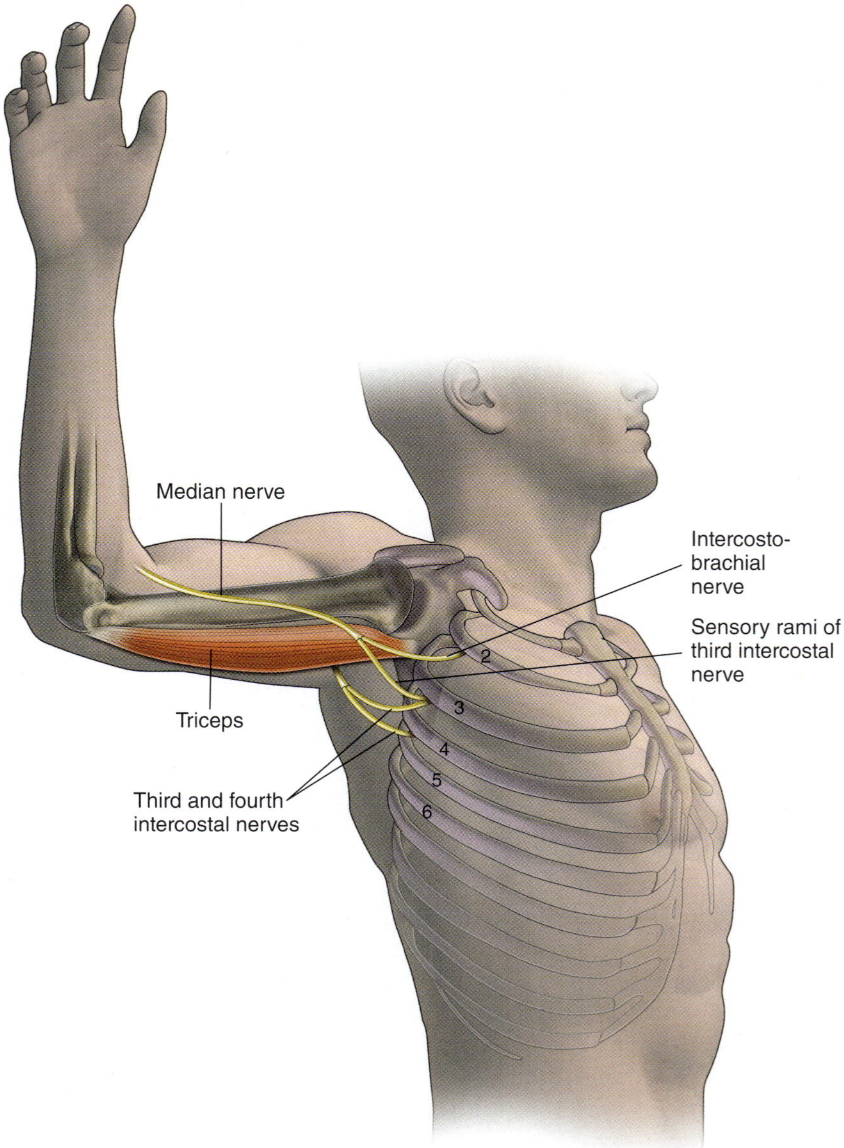

FIGURE 74-4 Procedures 4 and 5. During the same operation as the second free muscle transfer, the third and fourth intercostal nerves are transferred to the motor branch of the triceps to stabilize the elbow against the antagonist flexor, when the posterior division of the upper trunk has not been repaired previously. In the same operation, sensory reconstruction is performed by transfer of the intercostobrachial nerve and sensory rami of the third intercostal nerve to the medial root of the median nerve. n, nerve. (Redrawn with permission from Doi K. Management of total paralysis of the brachial plexus by the double free-muscle transfer technique. *J Hand Surg* 2008;33E:240.)

monitoring skin flap was carried out simultaneously. Whenever the amplitude of the CMAP decreased acutely more than 50% from the previous one without any signs of vascular compromise of the skin flap, immediate reexploration and revision of the anastomoses resulted in complete survival of the muscle transfer and good functional recovery.

POSTOPERATIVE IMMOBILIZATION

After each muscle transfer, the upper limb is immobilized with the shoulder in 30 degrees of abduction and flexion and 60 degrees of internal rotation; the elbow in 100 degrees of flexion; the wrist in neutral position; and the fingers in full flexion or extension, depending on the function to be restored using an arm brace and cast for 8 weeks and subsequently by a sling to prevent subluxation of the glenohumeral joint until recovery of the shoulder girdle muscles.

POSTOPERATIVE REHABILITATION

Low-frequency electrical stimulation of the denervated gracilis muscle transfer, which is not strong enough to move the fingers, is used until EMG reinnervation is seen. Through all of the phases of rehabilitation, a static plastic splint is used to maintain the wrist in a neutral position and all three finger joints in the intrinsic-plus position to prevent an intrinsic-minus deformity developing during rehabilitation.

Before 1999, our routine postoperative protocol did not allow any passive mobilization during the first 6 weeks after surgery.

Then gentle passive exercises of the shoulder, elbow, and all finger joints (but not the wrist) were started.

After EMG documentation of reinnervation of the transferred muscle, usually performed between 3 and 8 months after surgery, EMG feedback techniques using small portable myotrainers with surface electrodes, MYO ANALYZER and MA-230 (MINATO, Osaka, Japan), are started to train the transferred muscle to move the elbow and fingers because the patients usually have difficulty contracting each muscle effectively. Surface electrodes are placed on the monitoring skin flap of each muscle transfer. The myotrainer or myomonitor allows the patient or therapist to see what the muscle is doing and thereby learn better control. Initially, the first free muscle transfer for elbow flexion and finger extension is reinnervated from the terminal branch of the spinal accessory nerve and is activated by movement of the scapula. The second free muscle transfer for finger flexion is reinnervated from the fifth and sixth intercostal nerves and is activated by maximal inspiration or expiration. EMG feedback has been very helpful in the early stages to allow the patient to visualize and hear activity. After gaining more appropriate feedback, patients can work on strengthening their own muscles and can achieve contraction of the transferred gracilis muscle without having to simulate the original muscle action, such as adducting the scapula or respiration.

After recovery of active elbow and finger motion, EMG feedback to train for independent finger flexion and extension is started. Simultaneous flexion of the elbow should be prevented by the antagonistic action of the triceps muscle, which depends on reinnervation from the third and fourth intercostal nerves. The patients are taught a home exercise program to activate the individual gracilis transfers and triceps muscle.

The patients usually stay for 2 months after the second free muscle transfer and then attend a nearby rehabilitation center two or three times a week and visit our clinic every 1 to 3 months for another $1^1/_2$ to 2 years.

Finally, most patients with satisfactory recovery of active finger motion develop an intrinsic-minus finger deformity but can use their hand for hook grip. To increase the strength of the hook grip and arm–trunk prehension, progressive resistance exercises, consisting of strengthening finger flexion, elbow flexion, and shoulder adduction with pulleys and weights, are recommended. The patients are then started on skilled activities, such as lifting, holding, carrying, and pinching.

Early Mobilization Technique

After 1999, early passive mobilization was introduced (25), although other rehabilitation protocols, such as the postoperative brace and sling and electrical muscle stimulation, were continued, as described earlier. One week after free muscle transfer, all patients were referred to the rehabilitation center for early passive mobilization therapy consisting of tendon compression and tenodesis exercises.

The tendon compression technique is performed by compressing the tendinous portion of the transferred gracilis muscles at the elbow to move the fingers into extension or flexion, depending on the type of reconstruction. At the same time, the therapist holds the patient's wrist in the neutral position with the fingers in flexion or extension to resist the therapist's compression with the elbow in the extended position to make the gracilis tendon taut (16).

The previous technique included tendon compression at the elbow, but more recently, this has been abandoned. Free movement of the fingers by passive flexion and extension of the wrist and passive-assisted movement at the metacarpophalangeal (MCP) joints with the wrist in a reciprocal position to reduce tension is now performed.

This combined maneuver is included in the postoperative program after double free gracilis muscle transfers and is continued until active movement of the fingers occurs.

After successful reinnervation of the muscle, subsequent management is the same as the conventional program.

POTENTIAL COMPLICATIONS

Vascular Compromise

In our initial series of 146 free muscle transfers, when postoperative viability was assessed by a conventional skin monitoring flap, 143 transfers had no postoperative vascular compromise and achieved satisfactory motor function. However, three patients, despite successful revision of postoperative thrombosis of the arterial anastomoses, developed partial or complete necrosis of the muscle even though the accompanying skin flap survived and did not achieve any functional recovery.

Conventional monitoring of a skin flap does not promptly reflect compromised perfusion to an innervated free muscle transfer because ischemia affects skin and muscle differently. Earlier more rapid detection of vascular compromise by CMAP monitoring is imperative to provide functional muscle recovery after revision of the anastomoses.

After postoperative monitoring of CMAPS, 34 of 35 free muscle transfers survived without any signs of vascular compromise of the monitoring skin flap. In one free muscle transfer, the CMAP amplitude decreased acutely, although clinical evaluation of the monitoring skin flap did not indicate vascular compromise. Reexploration revealed occlusion of the venous anastomosis, and successful revision of the anastomosis resulted in good functional recovery of the muscle transfer.

Some authors do not recommend revision of thrombosed anastomoses because there is no chance of salvage (10,12,13,23). However, we disagree and recommend CMAP monitoring to allow potential salvage of a compromised muscle transfer. Our recent survival rate of free muscle transfers with CMAP monitoring is 100%.

Tendon Adhesions

Despite the powerful contraction and the high amplitude of the compound action potential of the transferred muscle, poor range of finger motion indicates adherence of the tendons. The compression test of the tendon at the elbow does not produce further movement of the finger joints. These patients will benefit from tenolysis of the transferred muscle and the recipient tendons. Tendon adhesions mostly occur underneath the pulley at the elbow and around the tenorrhaphy site.

Causalgia

Half of our patients complained of causalgia before surgery, and although we never treated their pain problems, other than by administration of conventional analgesics, they did not complain of too much pain during follow-up.

SECONDARY RECONSTRUCTION

Wrist Arthrodesis

In some of our patients, the wrist remained unstable after wrist splinting; these patients required wrist arthrodesis to stabilize this joint. Our technique of wrist arthrodesis is modified from the standard technique of compression plate fixation in order to cater for the specific requirements of double free gracilis muscle transfers (26). A titanium low-contact, dynamic compression (LCDC) wrist fusion plate is applied to the index finger metacarpal and to the dorsoradial surface of the distal radius after the extensor carpi radialis longus and brevis tendons are removed. The wrist is fused in neutral position or slight extension with slight ulnar deviation.

Control of Claw Finger Deformity

Claw finger deformity frequently develops after satisfactory recovery of finger flexion and extension and should be prevented by a static volar splint, but most patients need secondary procedures, including Zancolli's MCP joint capsulodeses or temporary interphalangeal joint fixation with K-wires, depending on the patient's choice after a preoperative simulation with a splint (27).

RESULTS AND OUTCOMES

Over a period of 14 years between March 1992 and September 2005, 67 patients have undergone the DFMT procedure for prehensile reconstruction after complete paralysis of the brachial plexus. Sixteen patients with a free muscle transfer using the latissimus dorsi or the rectus femoris muscle and two patients in whom a partially recovered spinal accessory nerve was used as the donor nerve were excluded. Of the remaining 49 patients who have undergone double gracilis muscle transfers, three patients did not return for rehabilitation after surgery, and one patient has had less than 24 months of postoperative follow-up. One patient had successful revision of a postoperative anastomotic thrombosis, but she developed partial ischemic necrosis of the gracilis muscle. The remaining 44 patients with a mean follow-up period of 40 months (range, 24–164 months) after the second free muscle transfer were analyzed to assess the long-term results.

Mean active shoulder abduction and flexion was 26 degrees (range, 0–70 degrees). The mean arc of shoulder rotation was 57 degrees (range, 0–150 degrees). Mean active elbow flexion was 114 degrees (range 70–145 degrees).

The mean total active range of motion (TAM) of the fingers was 45 degrees (range, 0–110 degrees). Forty patients (97%) obtained more than 20 degrees of TAM (Figure 74-5).

The power of lifting with a hook grip was examined using a specially designed machine (Digital Hanging Scale; Kansai Scale Co., Osaka, Japan) in 25 patients. The mean power of hook grip lifting was 4.1 kg (range, 0–14 kg) (Figure 74-6).

Sensory recovery was also satisfactory, with most patients achieving protective sensation in the hand (28,29).

RECENT MODIFICATIONS

The contralateral C7 to the suprascapular and long thoracic nerve transfers did not provide useful functional recovery of the shoulder. We now prefer the phrenic nerve to suprascapular nerve transfer and the third and fourth intercostal nerve transfers to the long thoracic nerve for shoulder reconstruction. Stabilization of the elbow joint when moving the fingers by the triceps muscle has been abandoned. Outcomes of the recent modifications of the DFMT will be reported soon.

ACKNOWLEDGMENT

Most figures in this paper have been published in 2008, The British Society for Surgery of the Hand, vol 33, no. 3, 2008, ©Sage Publications Ltd. All rights reserved.

REFERENCES

1. Carlstedt T. *Central Nerve Plexus Injury*. London: Imperial College Press, 2007, p. 139.
2. Chuang DCC, Ma HS, Borud LJ, et al. Surgical strategy for improving forearm and hand function in late obstetric brachial plexus palsy. *Plast Reconstr Surg* 2002;109:1934.
3. Liang C, Yu-Dong G, Shao-Nan Hm et al. Brachial plexus root avulsions in children—a report of 12 cases. *J Hand Surg* 2007;32A:96.
4. Songcharoen P, Wongtrakul S, Mahaisavariya B, et al. Hemi-contralateral C7 transfer to median nerve in the treatment of root avulsion brachial plexus injury. *J Hand Surg* 2001;26A:1058.
5. Doi K, Sakai K, Kuwata N, et al. Double free muscle transfer to restore prehension following complete brachial plexus avulsion. *J Hand Surg* 1995;20A:408.
6. Doi K, Muramatsu K, Hattori Y, et al. Restoration of prehension with the double free muscle technique following complete avulsion of the brachial plexus. Indications and long-term results. *J Bone Joint Surg* 2000;82A:622.
7. Doi K, Hattori Y, Ikeda K, et al. Significance of shoulder function in the reconstruction of prehension with double free muscle transfer after complete paralysis of the brachial plexus. *Plast Reconstr Surg* 2003;112:1596.
8. Doi K. Management of total paralysis of the brachial plexus by the double free muscle transfer technique. *J Hand Surg* 2008;33E:240.
9. Hentz VR, Doi K. Traumatic brachial plexus injury. In Green DP, Hotchikiss RN, Pederson RX, Wolfe SW (eds). *Green's Operative Hand Surgery*, 5th ed. Philadelphia: Elsevier, 2005, p. 1351.
10. Bishop AT. Functioning free muscle transfer for brachial plexus injury. *Hand Clin* 2005;21:91.
11. Gu LQ. Current advances in treatment of brachial plexus injury in China. *J Jpn Soc Reconstr Microsurg* 2005;18:87.
12. Shin AY, Spinner RJ, Steinmann SP, et al. Adult traumatic brachial plexus injuries. *J Am Acad Orthop Surg* 2005;13:382.
13. Adams JE, Kircher MF, Spinner RJ, et al. Complications and outcomes of functional free gracilis transfer in brachial plexus palsy. *Acta Orthop Belg* 2009;75:8.
14. Doi K, Hattori Y, Tan SH, et al. Basic science behind functioning free muscle transplantation. *Clin Plast Surg* 2002;29:483.
15. Doi K, Shigetomi M, Kaneko K, et al. Significance of elbow extension in reconstruction of prehension with reinnervated free muscle transfer following complete brachial plexus avulsion. *Plast Reconstr Surg* 1997;100:364.
16. Hattori Y, Doi K, Dhawan V, et al. Choline acetyltransferase activity and evoked spinal cord potentials for diagnosis of brachial plexus injury. *J Bone Joint Surg* 2004;86B:70.

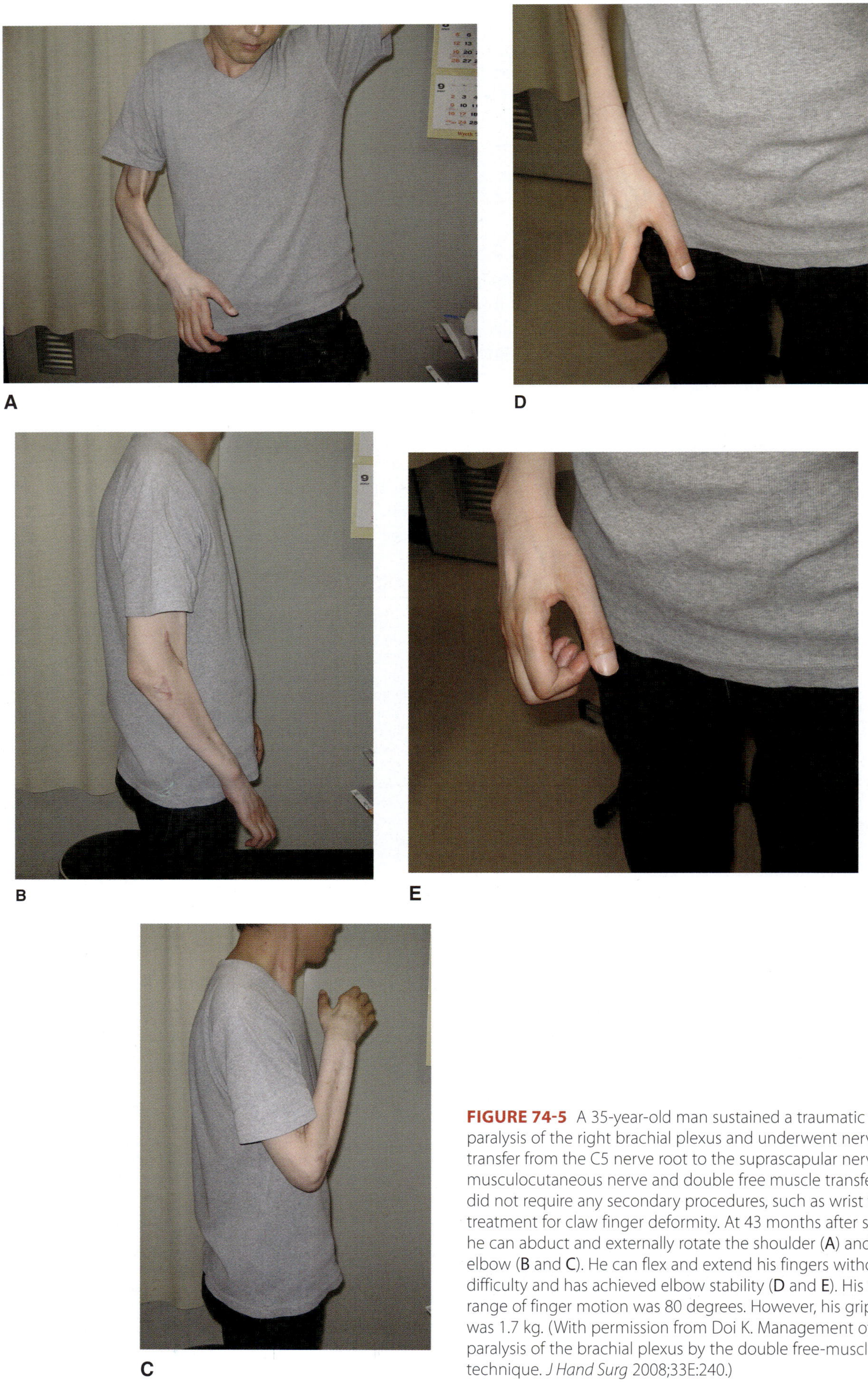

FIGURE 74-5 A 35-year-old man sustained a traumatic total paralysis of the right brachial plexus and underwent nerve transfer from the C5 nerve root to the suprascapular nerve and musculocutaneous nerve and double free muscle transfers. He did not require any secondary procedures, such as wrist fusion or treatment for claw finger deformity. At 43 months after surgery, he can abduct and externally rotate the shoulder (**A**) and flex the elbow (**B** and **C**). He can flex and extend his fingers without any difficulty and has achieved elbow stability (**D** and **E**). His total active range of finger motion was 80 degrees. However, his grip strength was 1.7 kg. (With permission from Doi K. Management of total paralysis of the brachial plexus by the double free-muscle transfer technique. *J Hand Surg* 2008;33E:240.)

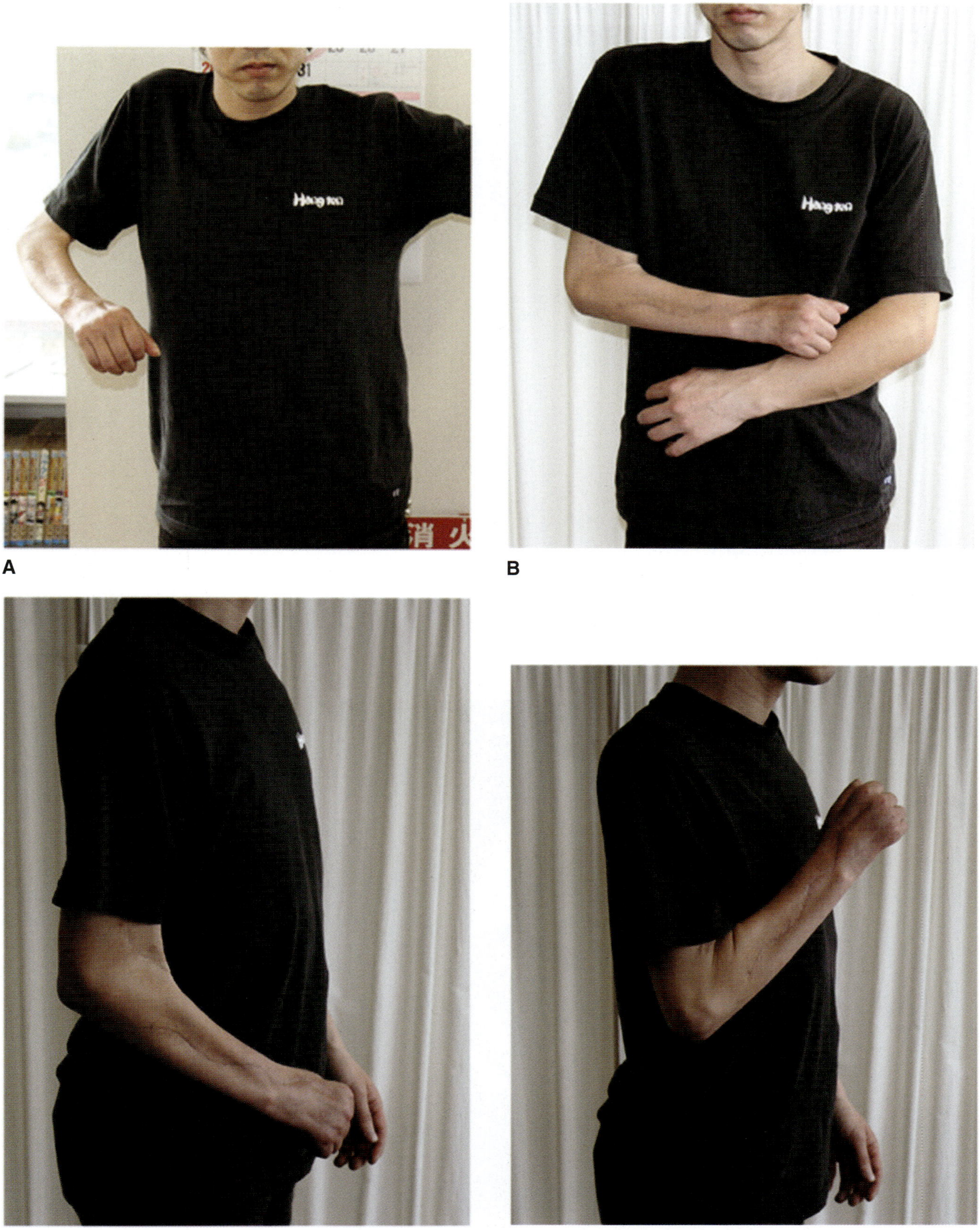

A B

C D

FIGURE 74-6 A 23-year-old man sustained a traumatic complete paralysis of the right brachial plexus with postganglionic injury of the C5 and C6 roots and preganglionic injury of the C7, C8, and T1 roots. He underwent nerve grafting between the C5 and C6 nerve roots and the anterior and posterior divisions of the upper trunk. Double free muscle transfers were performed. Secondarily, he underwent arthrodesis of the wrist and Zancolli's capsulodeses of the metacarpophalangeal joints. Three years after surgery, he has satisfactory functional recovery of the shoulder, including (**A**) shoulder abduction and internal rotation; (**B**) shoulder adduction and internal rotation of the elbow (**C** and **D**), elbow flexion and extension, and fingers. Total active range of finger motion is 80 degrees.

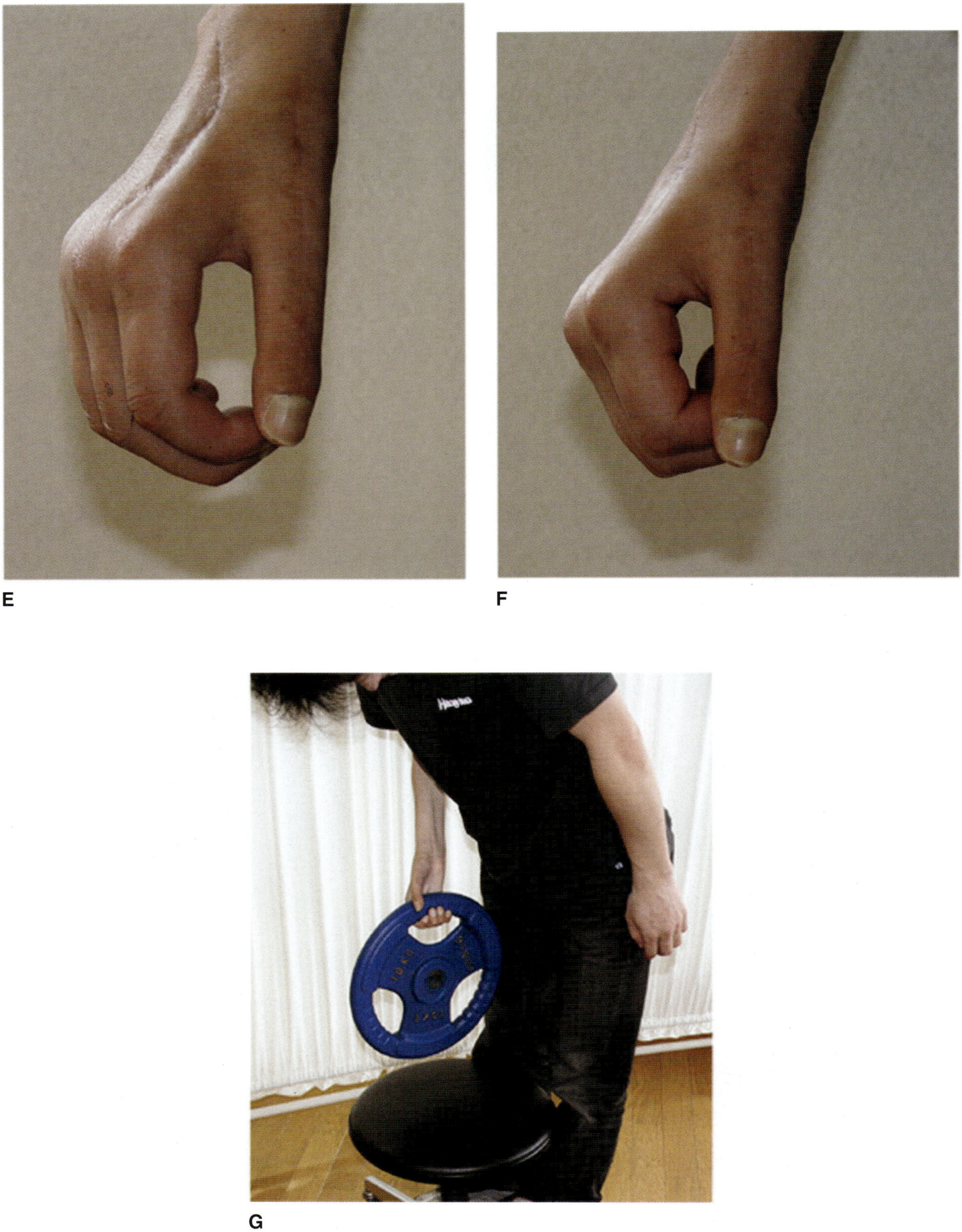

FIGURE 74-6 (*Continued*) (**E**) Finger extension; (**F**) finger flexion; and he can lift a 10-kg barbell (**G**). (With permission from Doi K. Management of total paralysis of the brachial plexus by the double free-muscle transfer technique. *J Hand Surg* 2008;33E:240.)

17. Yamazaki H, Doi K, Hattori Y, et al. Computerized tomography myelography with coronal and oblique coronal view for diagnosis of nerve root avulsion in brachial plexus injury. *J Brachial Plex Peripher Nerve Inj* 2007;2:16.
18. Hattori Y, Doi K. Vascularized ulnar nerve graft. *Tech Hand Up Extrem Surg* 2006;10:103.
19. Hattori Y, Doi K, Toh S, et al. Surgical approach to the spinal accessory nerve for brachial plexus reconstruction. *J Hand Surg* 2001;26A:1073.
20. Addosooki AI, Doi K, Hattori Y, et al. Technique of harvesting the gracilis for free functioning muscle transplantation. *Tech Hand Up Extrem Surg* 2006;10:245.
21. Doi K, Hattori Y, Tan SH, et al. Endoscopic harvesting of the gracilis muscle transfer for reinnervated free muscle transfer. *Plastic Reconstr Surg* 1997;100:1817.
22. Addosooki AI, Doi K, Hattori Y. Technique of harvesting the gracilis for free functioning muscle transplantation. *Tech Hand Up Extrem Surg* 2006;10:245.
23. Manktelow RT, Zuker RM, McKee NH. Functioning free muscle transplantation. *J Hand Surg* 1984;9A:32.
24. Wahegaonkar AL, Doi K, Hattori Y, et al. Technique of intercostal nerve harvest and transfer for various neurotization procedures in brachial plexus injuries. *Tech Hand Up Extrem Surg* 2007;11:184.
25. Doi K, Hattori Y, Yamazaki H, et al. Importance of Early passive mobilization following double free gracilis muscle transfer. *Plastic Reconstr Surg* 2008;121:2037.
26. Addosooki A, Doi K, Hattori Y, et al. Wrist arthrodesis after double free muscle transfer in traumatic total brachial plexus palsy. *Tech Hand Up Extrem Surg* 2007;11:29.
27. Takka S, Doi K, Hattori Y, et al. Selection of grip function in double free gracilis transfer procedures after complete paralysis of the brachial plexus. *Ann Plast Surg* 2005;54:610.
28. Ihara K, Doi K, Sakai K, et al. Restoration of sensibility in the hand after complete brachial plexus injury. *J Hand Surg* 1996;21A:381.
29. Hattori Y, Doi K, Sakamoto S, et al. Sensory recovery of the hand with intercostal nerve transfer following complete avulsion of the brachial plexus. *Plast Reconstr Surg* 2009;123:276.

CHAPTER 75

Neurolysis, Neuroma in Continuity, and Recurrent Nerve Compression Syndromes

David E. Sieber, Carrie Black, and Allen L. Van Beek

This chapter will focus on indications and techniques for neurolysis, treatment of neuromas in continuity, and recurrent nerve compression syndromes in the upper extremity.

The definition and classification of peripheral nerve injuries has been well described by Seddon (1) and Sunderland (2), which range from nerve bruising to complete transection. The healing process that occurs can include cicatricial scar tissue to nonfunctional segments in continuity to complete transection with a nerve gap. The indications and operative techniques for each of these situations will be discussed.

NEUROLYSIS

Neurolysis, or the technique of freeing a nerve from surrounding scar tissue, is a component of most reconstructive procedures involving peripheral nerves. Because of the delicate characteristics of a nerve, including reactivity and vascularity, it is essential to start the dissection in healthy tissue away from the site of injury. Tracking the nerve distally and proximally toward the site of injury minimizes the potential of causing further damage to the nerve (Figure 75-1).

There are three possible levels of dissection when manipulating the nerve's supportive connective tissue. *Epineurotomy* is the term used when the circumferential epineurium is opened on its surface. When looking at a damaged nerve in the operating room (OR), this layer is usually already opened. *External neurolysis* refers to freeing the external epineurium and fibrosis that surrounds the nerve making the fascicles readily visible but not separated into individual groups or single fascicles. To preserve segmental circulation, it is prudent to leave a small area of intact epineurium along one edge of the nerve. *Internal neurolysis* refers to the manipulation of the nerve's internal epineurium as well as the external epineurium and results in the skeletonization of fascicles or groups of fascicles. There is a greater risk for compromising the vascularity of the nerve with this technique. The perineurium should not be opened during neurolysis except for when the internal contents of the fascicle are being prepared for end-to-side nerve repairs. Many authors have described techniques and indications for external and internal neurolysis in certain clinical settings (3–9).

Freeing the proximal and distal segments of a normal nerve is necessary to complete a neurolysis and prepare it for nerve transfer if needed. Typically performed through a large incision with wide exposure, there are some advocates of a more minimally invasive technique by performing neurolysis through smaller incisions and decreasing the risk of wound healing complications (10) (Figure 75-2).

When performing neurolysis, magnification is essential to allow accurate identification of a normal nerve. Although loupe magnification is adequate in some circumstances, higher magnification with a microscope is often required. Neurolysis is the initial surgical maneuver for many pathologies related to neuromas such as neuroma in continuity, pseudoneuromas, and partial neuroma from partial transection (11) (Figure 75-3).

Neurolysis is also the initial procedure when isolating fascicles that are involved by benign nerve tumors, malignant or benign tumors that are displacing peripheral nerves, and popliteal cysts or other ganglion cysts. Without magnification, it can become almost impossible to identify nerve fascicles as they course through and around structures, making further nerve injury likely.

OPERATIVE TECHNIQUE

When performing a neurolysis, a tourniquet is used during the initial dissection. The bloodless field allows accurate assessment, identification, and intervention without the frustration of poor visualization caused by hemostaining. After the surgeon has ascertained the injury and defined the nerve's components,

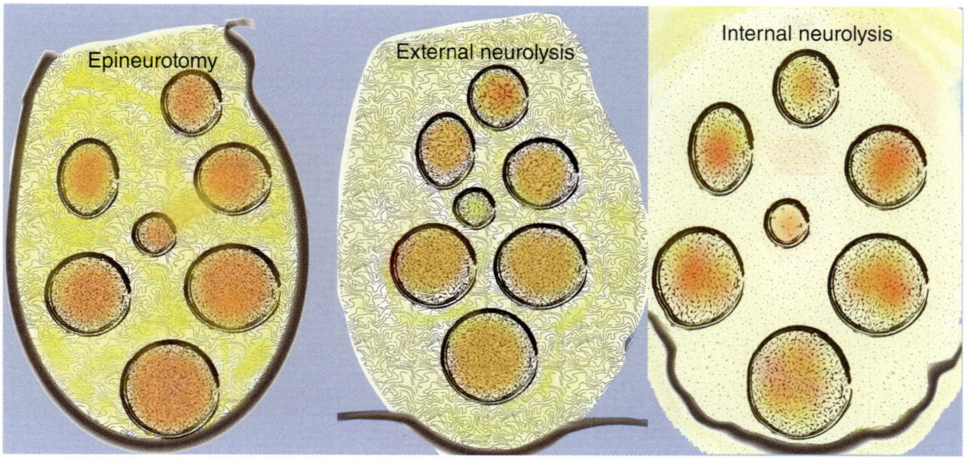

FIGURE 75-1 Components of neurolysis based on the anatomy of the nerve.

this is less of an issue. Tourniquet use, the injection of 1/100,000 epinephrine, and using topical application of 1:100,000 epinephrine within the field are techniques that help control bleeding in the field during neurolysis. When bleeding is an issue from intraneural blood vessels, the use of a microbipolar cautery is essential. Monopolar cautery application is likely to induce thermal injury beyond the site of coagulation.

The nerve is first identified proximal and distal to the site of nerve pathology (Figure 75-4).

Using magnification, the fascicles are traced along the anterior surface of the nerve from both proximally and distally into the zone of concern, such as a schwannoma (Figure 75-5).

The process is repeated around the remaining perimeter of the nerve. If the fascicles are intact through the zone of injury around the entire circumference of the nerve, then the surgeon can be reasonably sure that the external neurolysis is complete, and that may be all that is necessary. Fibrotic tissue in the scarred bed should be removed. Surgical judgment will determine if additional coverage is required to prevent recurrent fibrotic entrapment. Some have advocated wrapping the injured segment of nerve after neurolysis in a vascularized pedicle flap such as fascia, fat, synovium, or wraps made of veins or synthetic material (12–18) (Figure 75-6).

When some or all the fascicles are disrupted, one is confronted with the dilemma of making a decision regarding further internal neurolysis versus nerve resection and repair (19,20). In some circumstances, that decision can be predicated on the preoperative assessment. In other circumstances, the decision is made with the use of intraoperative nerve electrophysiologic assessment. In early exploration of peripheral nerve injuries, it is difficult to assess future function based on operative findings because axonotmesis has not had time to regenerate to end plates but may have propagated across the site of injury. However, the use of intraoperative assessment may allow some additional information regarding the assessment of spontaneous recovery across a zone of injury. When performing neurolysis to access fascicles for nerve transfer, the nerve is freed from its bed for a distance of 2 to 3 cm. The fascicles are

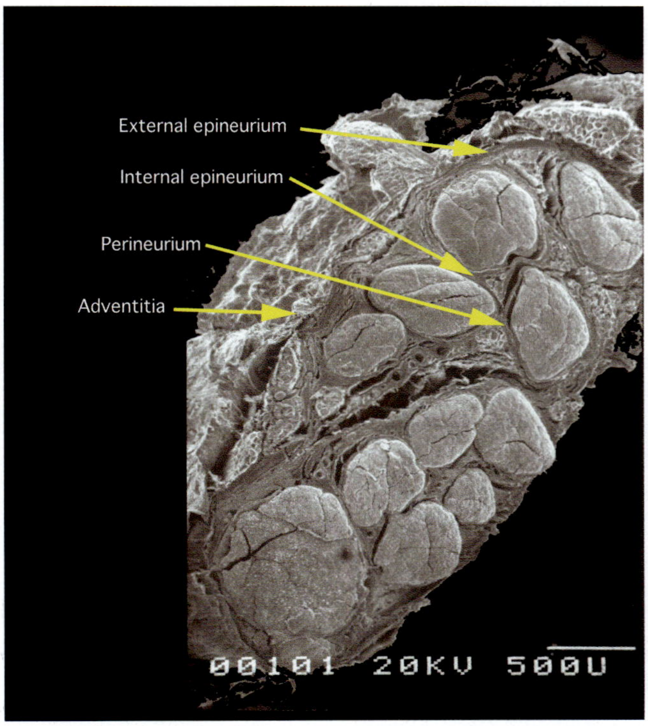

FIGURE 75-2 Scanning electron microscope magnification of cadaveric peripheral nerve.

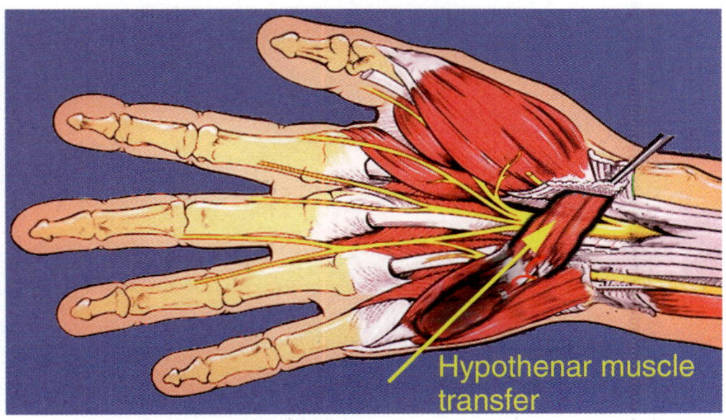

FIGURE 75-3 Peripheral nerve encased by a tumor demonstrating fascicles surrounding the mass.

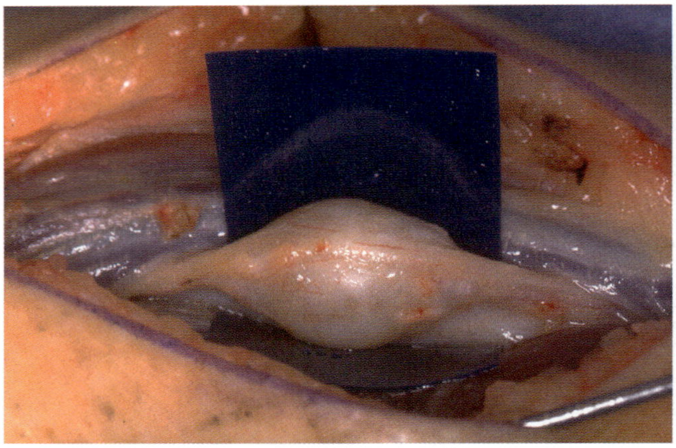

FIGURE 75-4 In situ peripheral neuroma.

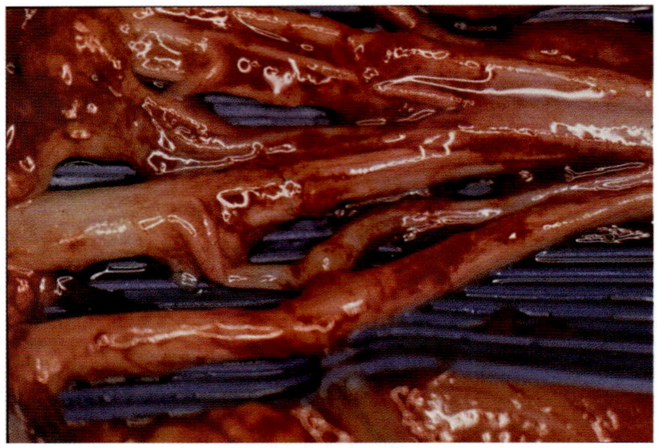

FIGURE 75-6 Disrupted fascicles after external neurolysis.

stimulated around the perimeter of the nerve to identify the specific fascicle that will be mobilized for transfer (21). Some internal neurolysis to separate and mobilize the specific fascicle will be required before transfer. This is performed very carefully because mobilizing peripheral nerves over long segments, and removing their extrinsic vascular supply may cause an ischemic conduction block with the additional concern of intraneural fibrosis long term.

Postoperative Care

Whenever possible, early mobilization of structures adjacent to the site of neurolysis is encouraged. Mobilization may prevent fibrotic tethering of the nerve to joints and tendons. Both of these have been implicated in causing postoperative complications. The failure rate of neurolysis may be up to 20%, depending on the site and injury. However, predictors of a good functional outcome are more distal sites, younger age (<20 years), and short injury segment (22,23).

The use of bupivacaine injected around the surgical site will help alleviate pain in the postoperative period. The use of corticosteroids irrigated into the site of surgery has been advocated but is controversial. The use of surgical drains is based on the extent of dissection and the surgeon's judgment. The use of suction drainage adjacent to nerve grafts is not recommended.

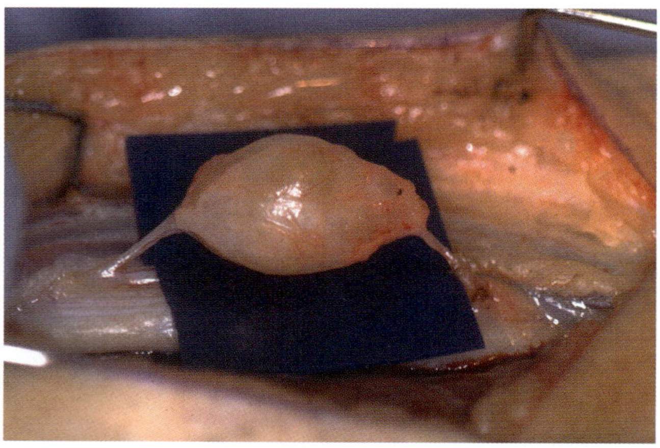

FIGURE 75-5 The origin of the tumor from a single fascicle.

NEUROMA IN CONTINUITY

Whereas the previous discussion of neurolysis applied to fibrosis or masses causing chronic symptoms, the remaining discussion will address nerve responses in acute nerve injury. When injured, nerves often produce neuromas that are continuous with the distal and proximal normal components. The extent of these neuromas in continuity is determined by the type and degree of injury. Axonotmesis and neurotmesis with limited stump separation will result in a nerve that appears to be continuous but may not be functioning. Alternatively, the nerve may have been injured but regain function across the zone of injury (6,24). Neuromas that are continuous with the nerve typically form at sites of blunt or crush injury but can also be the result of a complete transection as it regenerates or even form postoperatively in repaired nerves (Figure 75-7).

Clinical assessment by early exploration of peripheral nerve injuries is difficult. Incomplete recovery or limited recovery through an injured area that is in continuity is particularly difficult to judge by visual inspection intraoperatively (Figure 75-8).

In contrast to a neuroma in continuity, the completely transected nerve often retracts substantially, leading to proximal stump neuroma and distal stump glioma. The distal stump rapidly shrinks in diameter because of loss of axons leaving only the Schwann cells, perineurium, and supportive epineurium (25) (Figure 75-9).

In a complete transection, although spontaneous regeneration that may restore function is possible, early operative intervention is the key to restore nerve continuity (26,27). The timing of exploration in a nerve injury is controversial because before surgery, there is no definite way to determine if a nerve is transected versus developing a neuroma in continuity. Historically, clinicians waited at least 3 to 6 months to allow for possible regeneration to occur in blunt trauma. Early exploration carried the risk of creating further nerve damage. However, Bertelli et al. found that when rat median nerves underwent neurolysis 9 days after a crush injury and were followed for 12 weeks with electrophysiologic studies, they demonstrated accelerated recovery, suggesting that early exploration does not have the previously assumed deleterious effects (3). These results were not statistically significant in long-term follow-up,

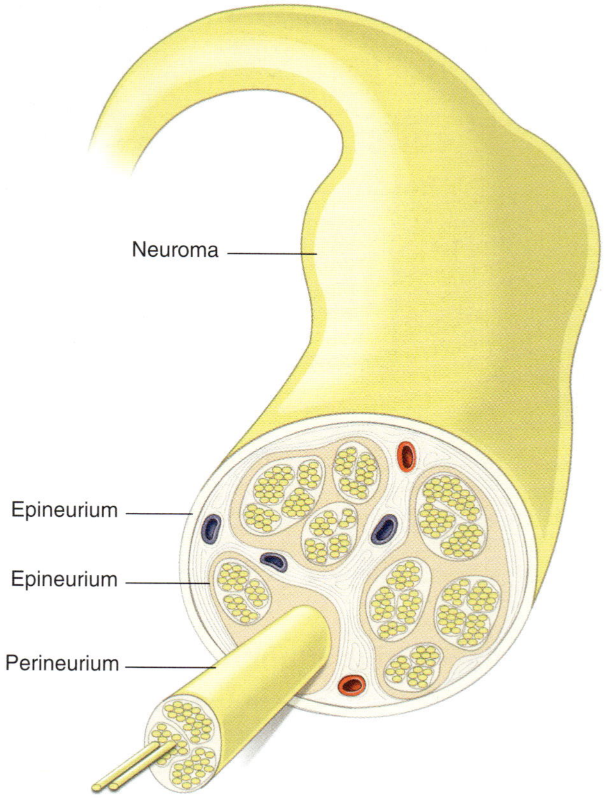

FIGURE 75-7 Neuroma assessment intraoperatively depends on appearance, consistency, size, and in situ electrophysiologic criteria.

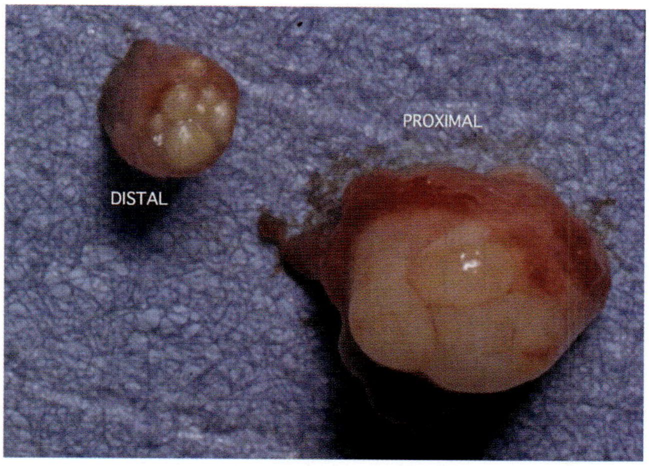

FIGURE 75-9 Gross specimen of proximal stump neuroma and distal stump glioma demonstrating the discrepancy in cross-sectional area caused by missing axons distally.

and therefore the ideal time for exploration still remains controversial. However, Matejcik and Penzesova (20) found that complete recovery occurred in almost 50% after neurolysis of brachial plexus and peripheral nerve injuries with an average operative time 6 months after injury and found that distal lesions, younger age, and early therapy all contributed to successful neurolysis.

Preoperative electrophysiologic and clinical examination are helpful in determining the likely status of an injured nerve, but in the OR, it is difficult to assess the extent of nonviable nerve tissue versus the possibility for regeneration. Early advocates of intraoperative nerve assessment recognized that estimating a nerve's regenerative potential based on the presence of end plates was neither reliable nor accurate (27). In addition, the intraoperative appearance of a neuroma is not necessarily a harbinger of nonrecoverable damage. There does not seem to be a correlation with diameter, consistency, length, organization, or appearance of a neuroma as reliable indicators of nerve function. Utilization of intraoperative nerve conduction studies may therefore assist in the decision regarding resection or neurolysis of the injured nerve segment (Figure 75-10).

Production of an evoked nerve response proximal and distal to the site, and recording the response usually at Erb's point or the axilla allows the surgeon to assess the quality of nerve conduction across the site of injury where there is continuity of the nerve but through a neuroma (28) (Figure 75-11).

From our past studies, we were able to show that function in situ correlates objectively with regeneration through the site

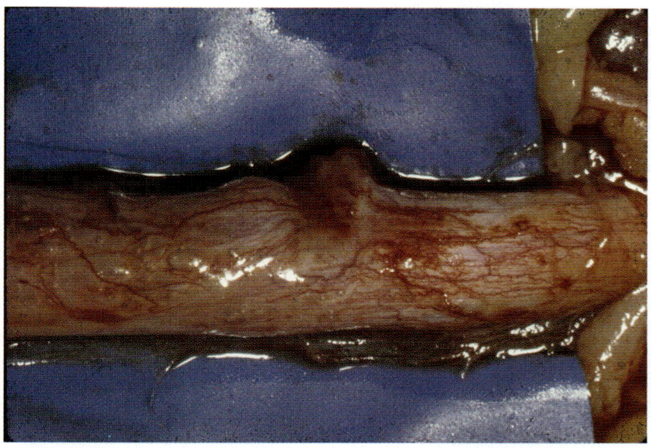

FIGURE 75-8 Early exploration of in situ neuroma in continuity reveals increased vascularity at the probable injury site but difficult assessment by appearance.

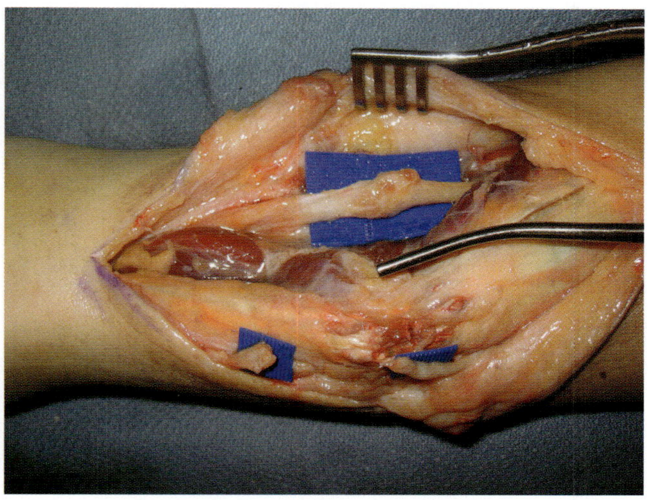

FIGURE 75-10 An example of a neuroma in continuity and a nerve gap in the lower extremity. Both nerves required nerve grafts.

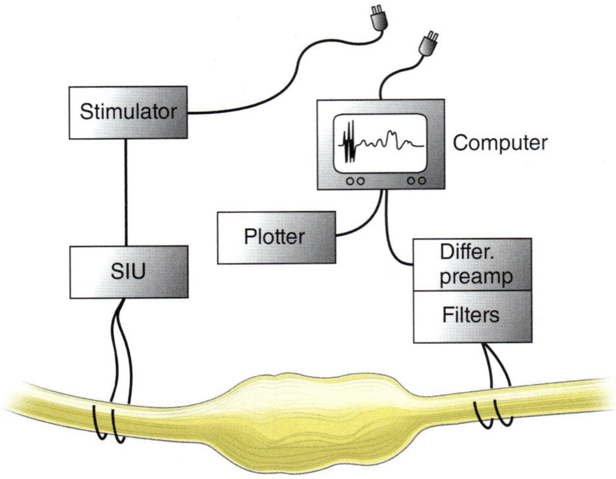

FIGURE 75-11 Placement of electrodes proximal and distal to the neuroma for intraoperative in situ electrophysiologic monitoring. The difference in latency from the two recording points determines the conduction velocity and the amplitude of the evoked response across the neuroma. Recording can also be performed more proximal using signal averaging computer techniques.

of injury. A conduction velocity over 10 m/sec across a neuroma or an amplitude of at least 30% of the proximal evoked response indicates that substantial nerve regeneration is occurring and that the neuroma should not be resected (29). These recordings need to be correlated with the clinical findings. If the intraoperative criteria are not met and clinically the area appears nonfunctional, then the choice for resection is easy. In our experience, stimulating distal and proximal to the injured site and recording at Erb's point using signal averaging, intraoperative testing is easier and more reliable then recording directly across the neuroma. Evoked signal averaging technology is available in most hospitals (Figures 75-12 and 75-13).

Avoiding resection of a functioning neuroma avoids the potential poor recovery from nerve grafting or other methods of nerve gap management.

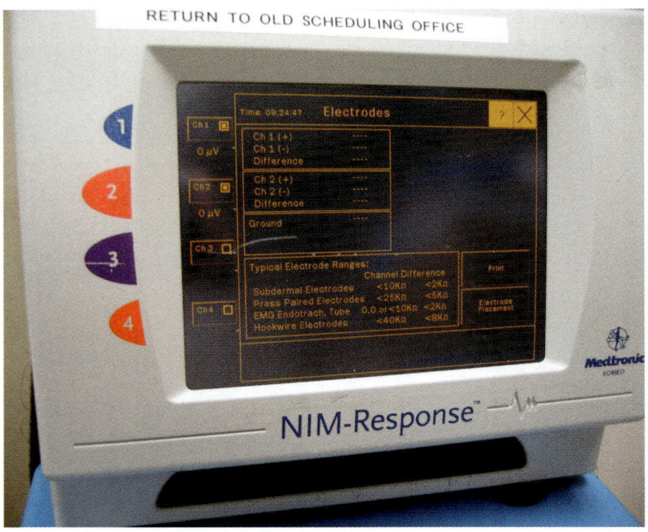

FIGURE 75-12 Evoked muscle responses are readily recorded with the NIM, which are useful for nerve transfers and when partial nerve injury is suspected.

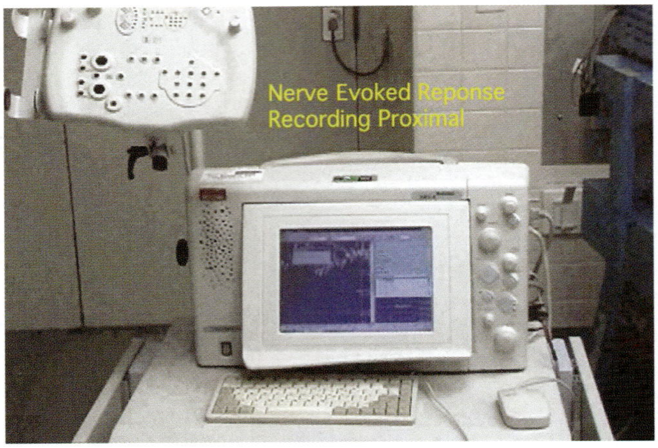

FIGURE 75-13 Evoked afferent nerve responses are recorded using cortical evoked response equipment. Signal averaging is required to record nerve evoked responses from the axilla or Erb's point. This equipment is usually available in the electroencephalography laboratory of hospitals.

Managing the Resultant Nerve Gap

Once a decision has been made to resect a nonfunctioning neuroma based on the criteria discussed, the question is how to restore continuity. The amount of nerve separation or tension across a nerve repair influences the potential reformation of a proximal neuroma and a distal glioma (Figure 75-14).

In considering primary repair, the parameters for too much tension have not been clinically established. Some advocate grafting of any nerve gap; others suggest that the necessity for flexion of adjacent joints and increased suture strength may indicate the degree of tension and potential for disruption of the repair (30). Autologous nerve grafting remains the standard for bridging the two ends of a nerve, particularly for gaps over 3 to 5 cm in large-diameter nerves (21,23). Conduits and acellular allografts discussed in Chapter 70 may be adequate substitutes for autologous nerve grafts when the nerve gap is smaller than 2 cm and for smaller diameter nerves. Conduits avoid donor site deficits and potential complications from using autologous donor nerve grafts (31–35). Conduits also have their own complications, including failure and extrusion.

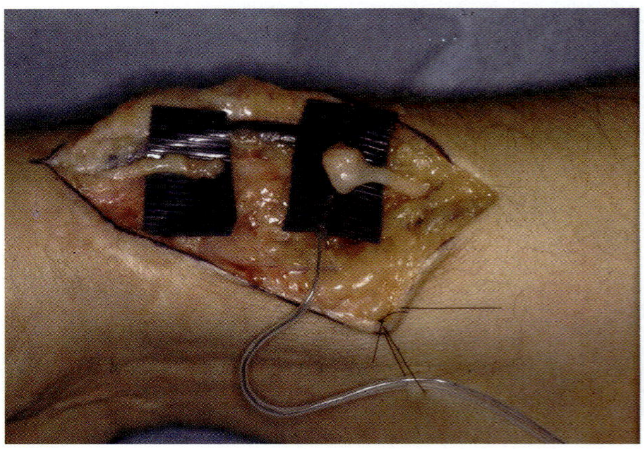

FIGURE 75-14 Nerve gap with proximal neuroma and distal glioma.

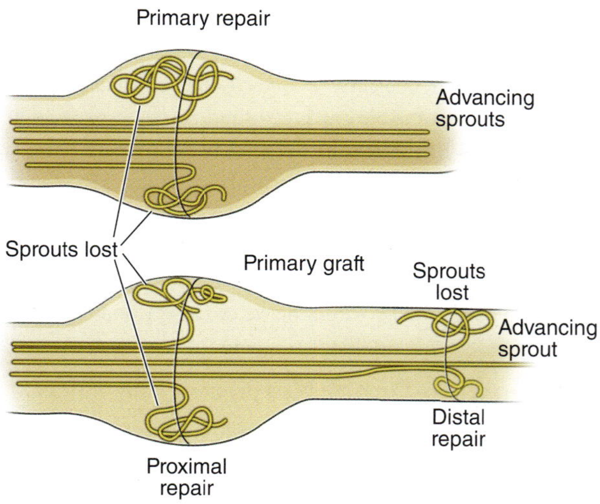

FIGURE 75-15 Primary repair of a nerve gap versus nerve grafting depends on the degree of tension on the repair site and the loss of regenerating axons at two repair sites.

The dilemma regarding nerve grafts centers around the regenerating axons having to cross two repairs rather than one repair site. When using conduits, the dilemma is whether axons will regenerate across the distance between the nerve stumps (Figure 75-15).

One repair site should always be preferred if excessive tension can be avoided. If the external epineurium of the nerve stumps can be approximated with a 6-0 suture, perhaps tension is not excessive. Axons having to cross two suture lines in cable grafts may result in less favorable outcomes than primary repair. The cross-over comingling of multiple types of axons such as sensory, motor, or autonomic at the repair site can also lead to poor outcomes because of axons reaching the wrong type of end organ. Nerve grafts longer than 15 cm have poorer outcomes (Figure 75-16).

However, long-term improvement in sensibility is possible, but motor recovery is very poor because of loss of motor end plates. Tendon transfers or nerve transfers are usually necessary for more proximal nerve gaps above the elbow that require nerve grafts to establish nerve continuity.

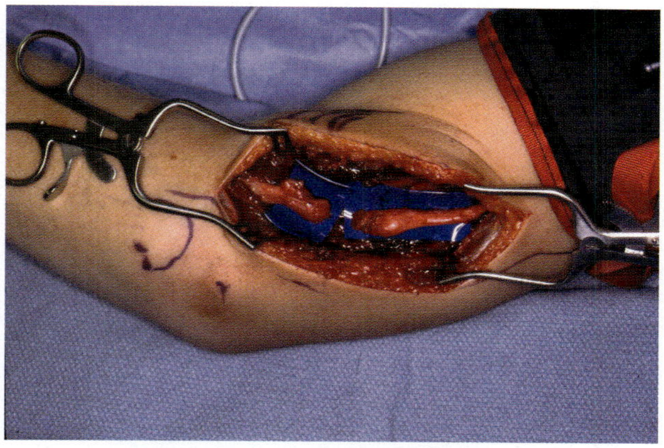

FIGURE 75-17 Full dissection of proximal and distal ends demonstrating in situ nerve hiatus. Note the starting points of dissection are remote from the actual nerve pathology.

Nerve Grafting Techniques

Using loupe and microscopic magnification, the proximal and distal ends of the nerve are identified outside the zone of injury and then dissected toward the site of injury (Figure 75-17).

Magnification is necessary to preserve nerve branches in the area of injury and to preserve any fascicles that may not have been injured. Neurolysis of the nerve from encompassing scar can be difficult. If the scar bed is extensive, nerve grafts may not revascularize, or the scarring itself may act as a barrier to regenerating axons. Surgical judgment is necessary to determine if the injury bed is suitable for nerve grafting. Detouring nerve grafts and replacing the wound environment with flaps or by using vascularized nerve grafts have been advocated for adverse wound conditions.

The proximal and distal stumps of the nerve are dissected until normal fascicular anatomy is seen under the operating microscope (Figure 75-18).

An incompletely severed nerve will not retract, and spontaneous regeneration across the injury gap can occur (Figure 75-19).

If a neuroma is determined not to be functional by intraoperative evoked potentials, the neuroma is divided across its center.

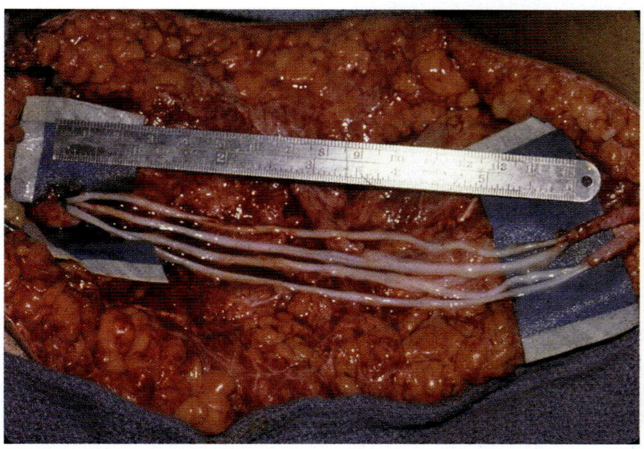

FIGURE 75-16 Cable grafting for long nerve gaps greater than 15 cm usually have poorer outcomes but often produce protective sensibility for the long term and reduce neuroma pain.

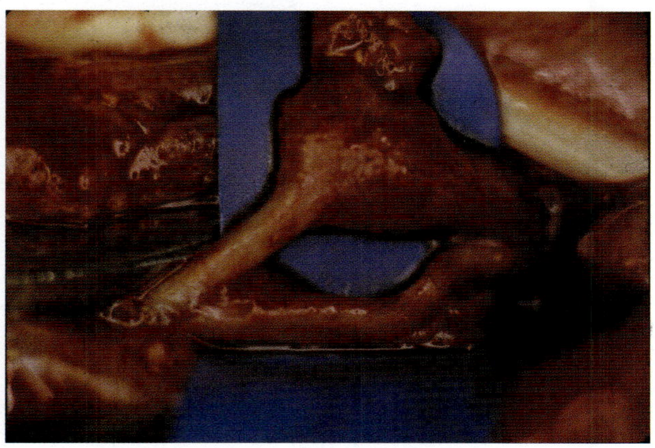

FIGURE 75-18 Regenerating severed nerve, with enlarged proximal segment caused by neuroma formation and decreased cross-section of the distal nerve.

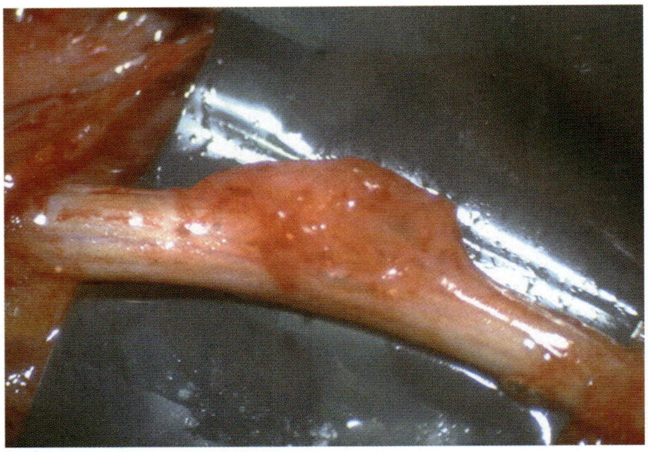

FIGURE 75-19 Incompletely severed nerve with a neuroma in continuity; the length of the nerve is preserved without retraction.

Serial sections are then performed proximally and distally until healthy-appearing fascicles are seen and intrafascicular fibrosis is absent.

During sectioning of the nerve, intrafascicular bleeding may occur. Topical 1:100,000 epinephrine solution helps with bleeding. Microbipolar cauterization of tiny vessels is also feasible under the microscope. For visualization of the fascicles, dilute methylene blue painted on the nerve ends with a Q-Tip enhances nerve component visibility (Figure 75-20).

After fascicular anatomy is determined proximally and distally, the number of cable grafts required can be estimated and is usually three to five cables for large-diameter nerves. The cross-sectional area of the distal nerve stump is smaller than the diameter of the proximal stump, so the minimum number of nerve grafts required is used to cover the distal nerve cross-sectional area. The maximum number of nerve grafts will be the number required to cover the proximal nerve cross sectional area.

Harvesting Donor Nerves

The sural nerve is the most commonly used nerve graft. Either multiple transverse incisions or one linear incision can be used. It is imperative that patients be aware of the sensory deficit and the location of a potentially sensitive neuroma produced by harvesting the sural nerve. When harvesting the sural nerve, the neuroma stump should not be left under the skin where socks and shoes may stimulate the neuroma. Depending on the patient's stature, 30 to 40 cm of sural nerve can be obtained from each leg (36).

The lateral femoral cutaneous nerve, medial antebrachial cutaneous nerve, posterior antebrachial cutaneous nerve, distal

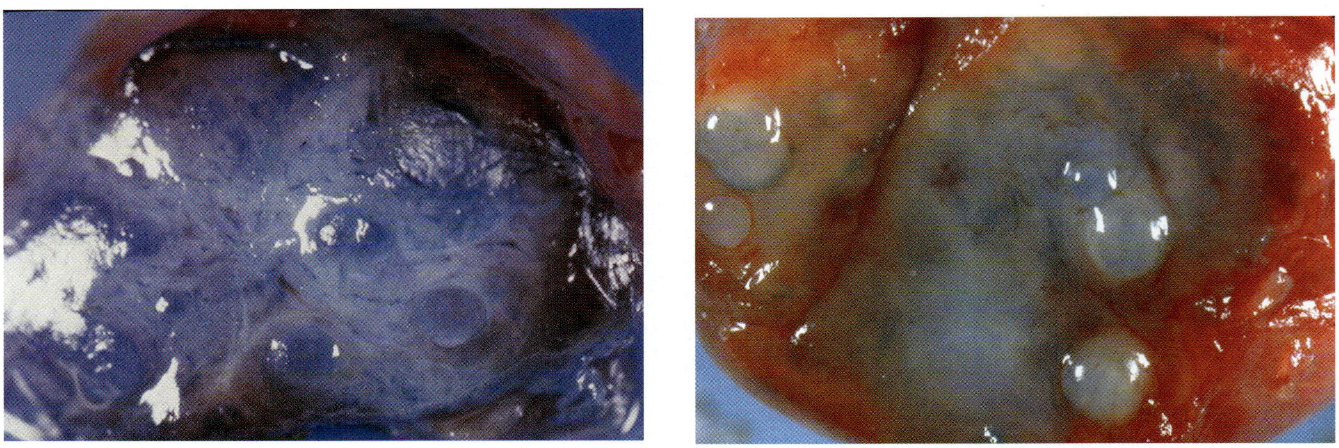

A B

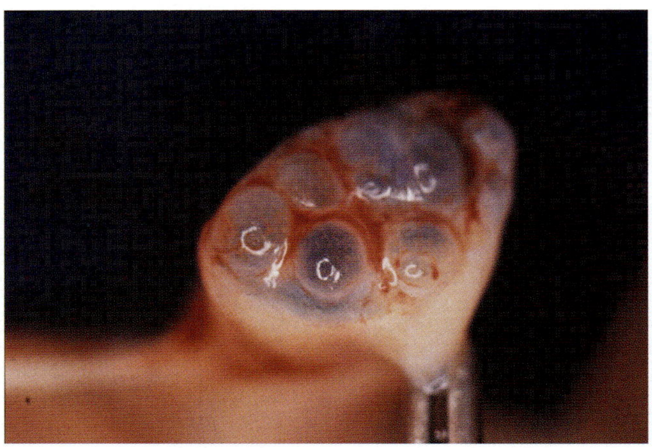

C

FIGURE 75-20 (A) Note fibrosis and some fascicles additional resection is required. (B) Bullet through the nerve disrupting some fascicles, others intact, resulting in severe pain. (C) Resection of a nerve demonstrating discrete fascicles and adequate resection using methylene blue.

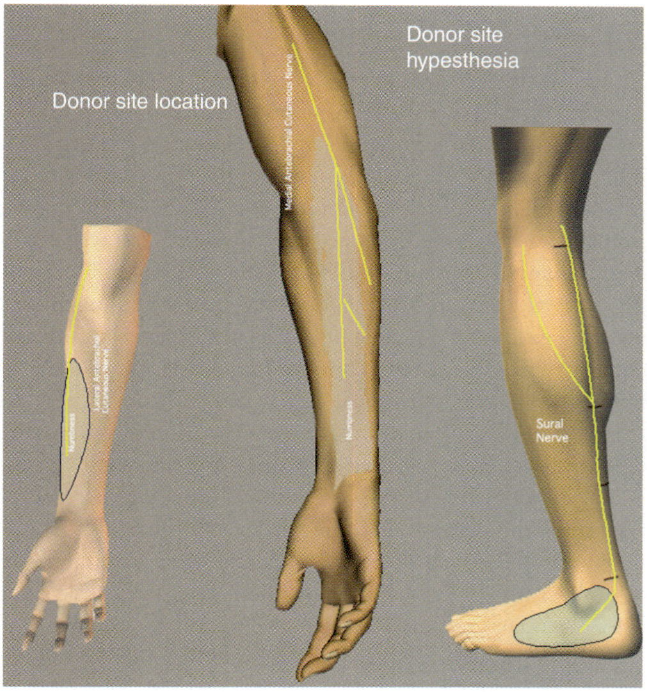

FIGURE 75-21 Possible donor sites if the sural nerve is unavailable and the resulting areas of hypesthesia.

sensory portion of the posterior interosseous nerve, and superficial branch of the radial nerve have also been used as donor sites (Figure 75-21).

The diameter of the proximal and distal nerve stumps and the gap between them usually determines the best donor sites. A median nerve with a 6-cm gap will usually require 25 to 30 cm of nerve graft, making the sural nerve the optimal donor site. A digital nerve with a 4-cm gap would make a branch of the medial antebrachial cutaneous nerve a likely donor site (8). It is often convenient to use donor sites adjacent to the site of injury. However, if the donor site adds another sensory deficit that could have functional implications, avoid the convenience and harvest another site. An example would be to avoid harvesting the radial nerve if the median nerve requires grafting. Harvesting the ipsilateral sural nerve for grafting a posterior tibial nerve injury of the lower extremity would be another example.

Technique of Nerve Grafting

Grafts are interposed without tension, and each graft is held in position using sutures, fibrin glue, or a combination. Typically, only two or three sutures are used to hold grafts in position, placing the sutures in epineurium or epineurium with some perineurium. Extruding fascicles are trimmed after repair to permit coaptation without buckling, overlap, or misalignment (Figures 75-22 and 75-23).

When possible, the grafts are separated to improve the circumferential revascularization of the grafts from the underlying bed. If grafts are bunched together, revascularization can be inhibited resulting in more fibrosis (Figures 75-24 and 75-25).

If a surgical drain is necessary, avoid using a suction drain because of the potential risk of dislodging the nerve grafts when it is removed.

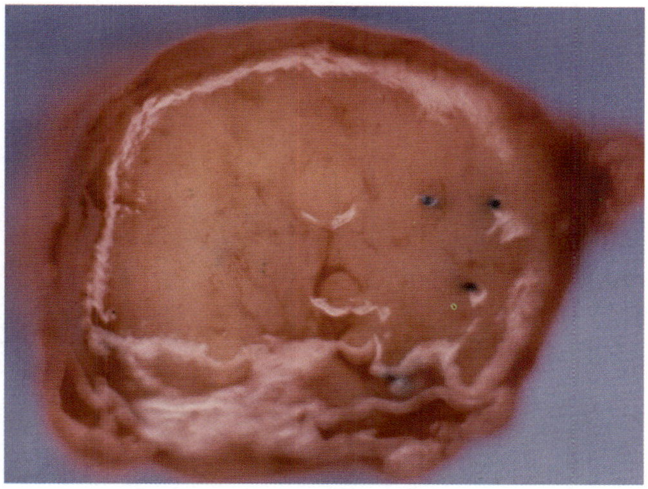

FIGURE 75-22 Cross-section of a peripheral nerve neuroma resected because of poor function demonstrating suture material within the neuroma and fibrosis associated with the suture material.

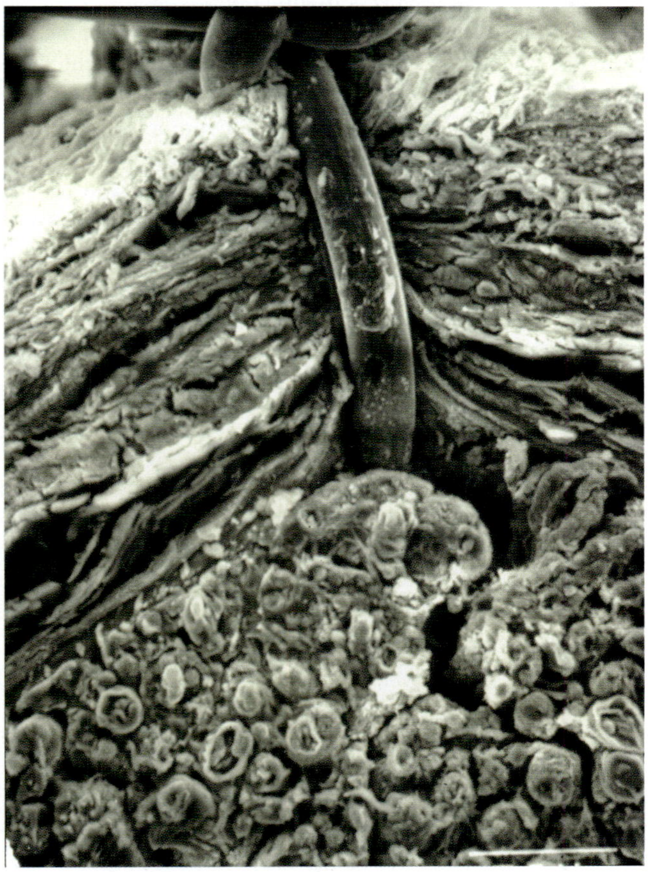

FIGURE 75-23 Electron scanning microscopy demonstrating a 10-0 suture securing the perineurium and the epineurium of a fascicle for repair.

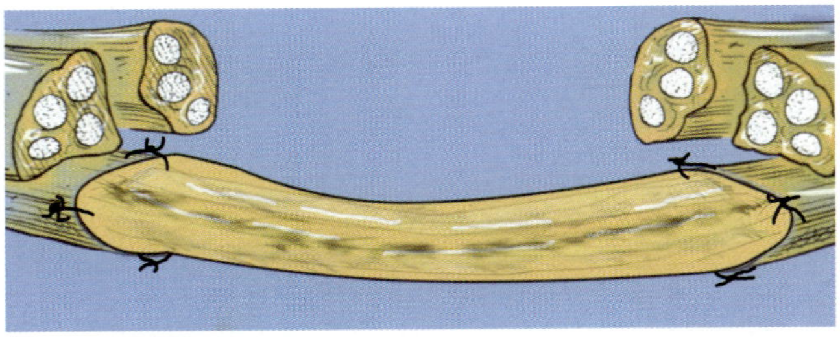

FIGURE 75-24 Each graft should be placed to align the topography of the proximal and distal nerve stumps as much as possible.

Postoperative Management

Unlike direct nerve repair, in which some movement is preferred to avoid nerve adherence to adjacent tendons or muscles, nerve grafts should be immobilized for at least 10 days to allow optimal revascularization. After that, protected range of motion exercises and desensitization therapy can then begin.

RECURRENT NERVE COMPRESSION SYNDROMES

Recurrent nerve compression syndrome is often a misleading term. There is a distinct clinical difference between recurrent compression syndrome and failed compression syndrome in the objective clinical findings, electrophysiologic studies, and the pathophysiology of the nerve dysfunction.

By definition, recurrent compression syndrome must include several components of the clinical story that support the diagnosis. First, there must be a long interval after initial surgery with improvement or resolution before symptoms return. The return of symptoms and new electrophysiologic findings 6 months or longer after initial nerve decompression usually implicate a recurrent compression rather than a failed decompression. The duration of improved symptoms, degree of improvement based on clinical testing, and improved electrophysiologic parameters are all factors that need to be demonstrated if one is considering the diagnosis of recurrent nerve compression. In the setting of an operative nerve decompression that has persistent or early recurrence of symptoms, worsening electrophysiologic parameters or new neurologic complaints suggests a diagnosis of failed decompression (8,37).

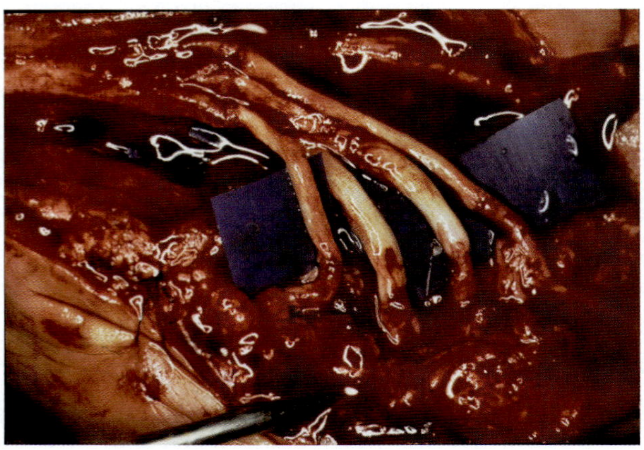

FIGURE 75-25 Multiple cable grafts coapted with 10-0 sutures are separated in the wound bed to improve revascularization of each graft.

The actual recurrence rate for decompression has not been well documented. Approximately 4% of the population has had prior carpal tunnel release (CTR), and 1% have had cubital tunnel release, but the incidence of recurrence is not well established. Some population studies have suggested overall reoperative rates of less than 5% (9,38). There are a variety of reasons one may encounter a patient with a recurrence of symptoms in clinic practice. Recurrent compression can occur because of fibrotic healing at the site of initial compression or may be related to new injury at the site of the nerve from direct trauma, repetitive activity, or vibratory job functions that cause further neural damage despite prior decompression. A recurrence of symptoms should also alert one of the possibility of synchronous compression at a more proximal site, including the "double-crush" phenomenon, and these need to be ruled out before reexploration (39).

Often a recurrence causes the patient to be unhappy and the surgeon frustrated. When history, examination, and electrophysiologic studies document significant findings and symptoms are not relieved by supportive measures, a repeat release is required. Proper initial assessment of patients presenting with recurrent symptoms requires reviewing preoperative records, old operative reports, and any postoperative therapy received. After these reviews, a thorough and careful assessment of the patient's health status, impression of what has been occurring since the initial operation, along with a thorough examination of all of the upper extremity peripheral nerves from the neck to fingertips is warranted (40). The goal is to identify the site of pathology and determine if it is in fact recurrent cubital or carpal tunnel syndrome rather than an area of more proximal nerve compression, injury, or irritation. This can be a difficult task, and objective diagnostic tools, although available, can become expensive and not always helpful. Both electromyography and magnetic resonance imaging have been used to help confirm the diagnosis of recurrent nerve compression, and these may be useful adjuncts before offering further surgical intervention (41) (Figure 75-26).

With the advent of endoscopic techniques for CTR, there was an initial concern for an increased incidence of recurrent compression with this approach. However, in a recent series comparing endoscopic with open approaches in patients who underwent reoperation for persistent or recurrence of symptoms, 58% were found to have an incomplete decompression of the carpal tunnel. This study also demonstrated that these recurrences did not bear any statistical significance in terms of recurrence after primary operative decompression between open versus endoscopic techniques (37).

Failed decompression is a more difficult issue to diagnosis and treat. This is because failed decompressions may be due to a variety of causes and are separate entities from recurrences. New symptoms, persistent symptoms, worse symptoms, persistent or new examination findings, or worsening electrophysiology study findings without improvement all lead to the diagnosis of failed decompression (37). Why the initial decompression

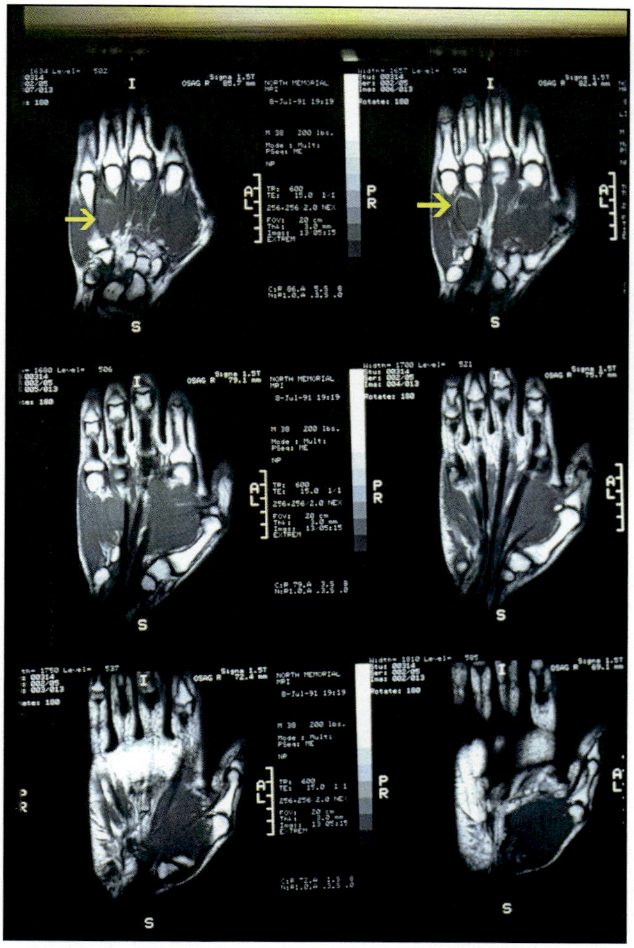

FIGURE 75-26 Magnetic resonance image reveals a schwannoma causing persistent symptoms after carpal tunnel release and the actual etiology for carpal tunnel type symptoms.

failed is most surgeons' main dilemma (9,38). The causes of failed decompression are many and depend on the nerve involved (Figure 75-27). The most common reasons are incomplete release of constricted areas, injury to the decompressed nerve, injury to adjacent nerves or other structures,

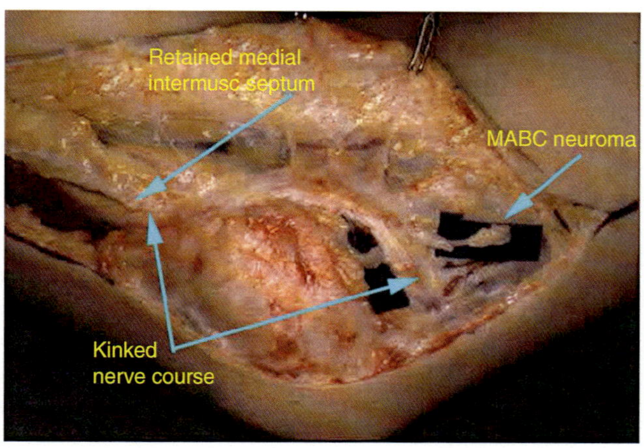

FIGURE 75-27 This figure demonstrates several reasons for failure of cubital tunnel surgery: medial antebrachial cutaneous neuroma, retained medial intermuscular septum, nerve kinking at two sites, and dense fibrosis.

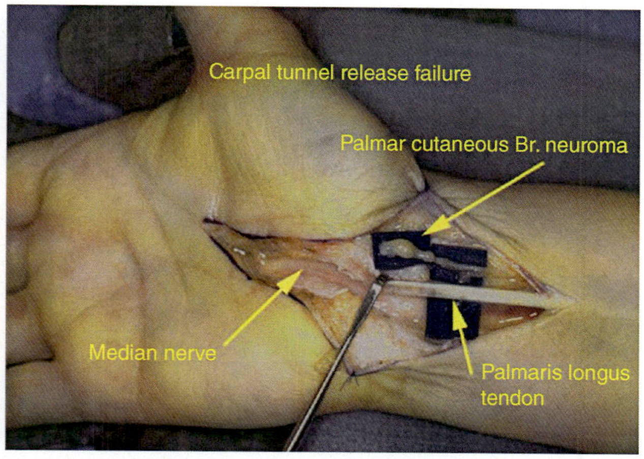

FIGURE 75-28 Persistent pain after carpal tunnel release caused by a neuroma. Note the extended incision that permits safe access to the median nerve and identification of the palmar cutaneous branch of the median nerve.

synchronous compression at another site, and unrecognized etiologies or pathology (Figure 75-28).

The presence of fibrillation potentials or positive sharp waves after decompression that were not present before surgery is an ominous sign and often indicates a nerve injury has occurred, resulting in denervation of motor end plates.

Operative Treatment of Recurrent Cubital Tunnel Syndrome

Typical approaches to primary cubital tunnel decompression include simple decompression of the ulnar nerve through the cubital tunnel and distal to the medial epicondyle, median epicondylectomy, and ulnar nerve transposition. Transposition may be subcutaneous, intramuscular, or submuscular. With any of these approaches, most patients have significant improvement in their symptoms after surgery. The question is how to help those who do not. Regardless of the choice of operation, it appears that at least 10% to 15% patients failed to improve after decompression or experienced a recurrence of their symptoms after a short interval of time from reoperation (42,43).

If a recurrence has been established after at least a 6-month symptom-free period, then nonoperative treatment should first be pursued, including physical therapy; modified physical activity; and in some cases, splinting (44). One must be careful to select for patients in whom this is truly the diagnosis and not a symptom of a more systemic condition related to diabetes, chronic radiculopathy, or more proximal nerve compression issues (Figure 75-29).

Operative techniques depend on the choice of primary operation and intraoperative findings. In addition, nerve wrapping with vein or biologic material has also been described to lessen the recurrence of the cicatrix around the nerve, which may lead to recurrent symptoms (15,18). Although intraoperative findings are key to determining the appropriate surgical techniques, Filippi et al. (42) found that patients had superior outcomes when they were able to transfer the ulnar nerve back into the sulcus.

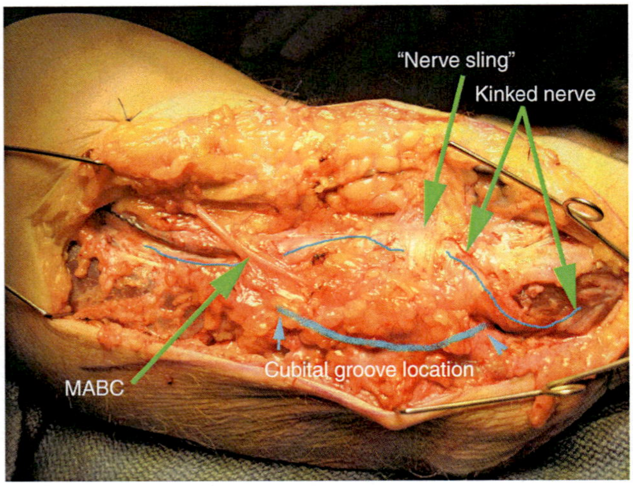

FIGURE 75-29 A nerve sling was used to prevent the ulnar nerve from returning to the cubital tunnel, which caused displacement and kinking. The medial antebrachial cutaneous nerve can be seen coursing into fibrosis. The patient presented with pain and atrophy after his primary surgery.

Operative Treatment of Recurrent Carpal Tunnel Syndrome

Initial management in recurrent carpal tunnel should include conservative measures, including scar massage, splinting, and hand therapy (37). Several operative interventions have been described for recurrent carpal tunnel that surgeons should be aware of, including various wraps and flaps of fat, muscle, or vein to promote nerve gliding (13,45). Hypothenar fat turnover flap, vein wraps, and conduits have all been advocated for recurrent carpal tunnel syndrome. Vein grafting may sometimes be used as a rescue in situations in which there have already been several operative interventions with coverage that has previously failed (18) (Figures 75-30 and 75-31).

There is controversy in the literature about what is surgically necessary to treat recurrent symptoms. One study showed that endoscopic release was possible and yielded positive clinical results when performed in the case of recurrence after open CTR in the past (46). These patients did not demonstrate any scarring or need for further neurolysis, suggesting that perineurial fibrosis is a rare occurrence (47). In such cases, simple repeat decompression may be all that is necessary. This is in contrast to another series that found that 100% of patients who underwent open or endoscopic release for recurrent or persistent symptoms had gross evidence of circumferential fibrosis in the carpal tunnel (37). Many authors have suggested that in the setting of cicatrix formation, tissue coverage is necessary to create gliding. When evaluated in a comparison study, it appeared that median nerve coverage with ulnar-based hypothenar fat flaps had superior clinical outcomes to synovial coverage from adjacent tendons; however, this was not statistically significant. Their results demonstrated a reduction in Tinel's sign (25% of 55%), Phalen's sign (13% of 46%), thenar atrophy (44% of 46%), and paresthesias (62% of 64%) for synovial flap versus hypothenar fat flap, respectively (16). Coverage with the hypothenar fat flap may have better clinical results because in reoperative cases, it is hypothesized that the median nerve is denuded of soft tissue covering and therefore needs protection (17). Fat grafting either as pedicle or free graft has benefit, but it is difficult to determine which technique yields better results (40).

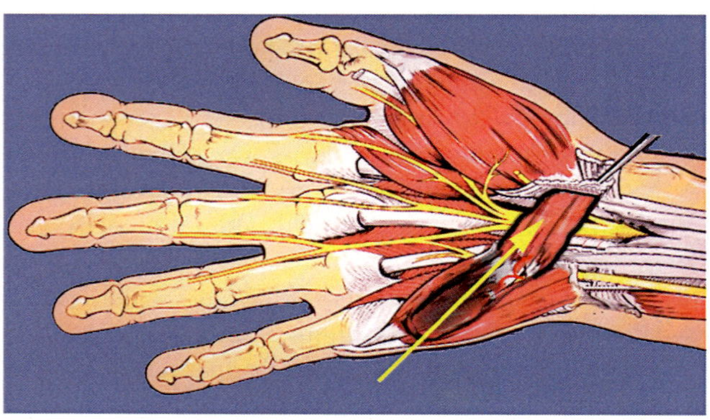

FIGURE 75-30 Hypothenar muscle flap.

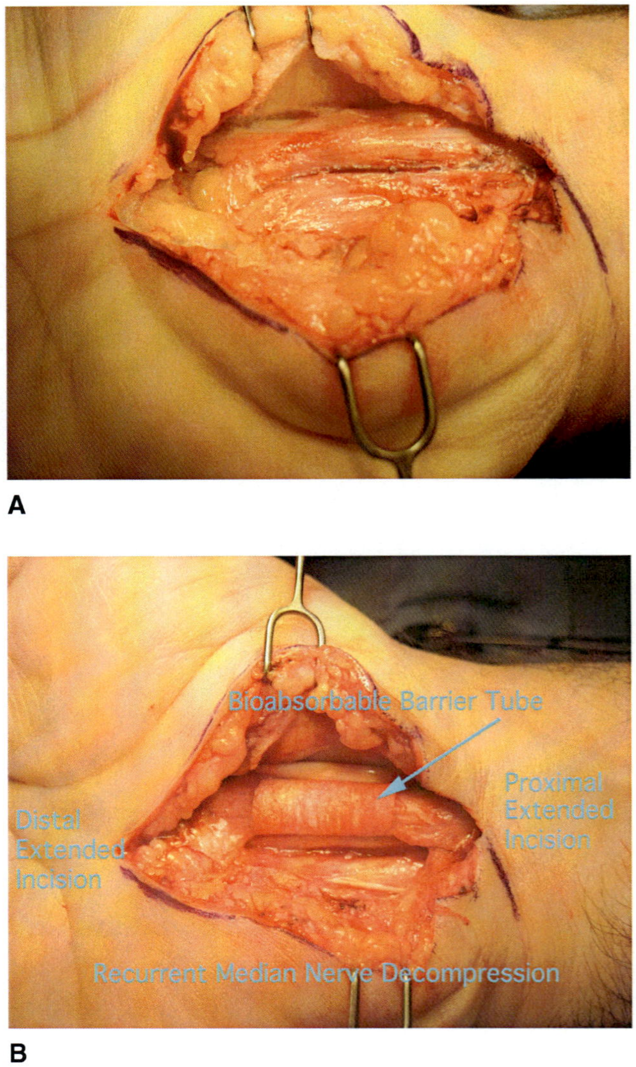

FIGURE 75-31 Recurrent carpel tunnel syndrome (CTS) with subsequent fibrosis. Bioabsorbable conduit around median nerve.

When surgery is indicated, the nerve should be found proximal and distal to the tunnel as demonstrated in Figures 75-2 and 75-3.

Nerves are often displaced by scar, moved by the previous surgery, encompassed by scar, and even attached to the surfaces of the tunnel or other structures. Finding the nerve outside the previous surgical field and following the nerve from a normal location into that area using magnification will prevent iatrogenic injury. Usually, the incision will need to be extended 1 to 2 cm on one or both sides of the previous scar to identify normal nerve and then proceed with repeat release. It is prudent to remember that an injured peripheral nerve in an adult does not achieve normal recovery and often leads to painful sequelae.

Postoperative Care

If reoperative surgery is required, the surgeon taking on the responsibility for care should have a team of providers to support the patient after performing surgery. The utilization of a hand therapist, occupational therapist, psychologist, and additional clinic time for the surgeon must be anticipated and planned for before any surgical intervention. Pain management, occupational modification, and marriage counseling may be required after revision surgery and should be implemented before surgery. One study demonstrated that preoperative factors such as myofascial pain syndrome or fibromyalgia, involvement in litigation, multiple compressive neuropathies, or the presence of abnormal psychological factors were all associated with an increased likelihood of an unfavorable postoperative result (48). A significant percentage of individuals who undergo reoperative nerve decompression surgery do not have excellent or even good results, and unrealistic expectations should not be conveyed to the patient. Health care providers must be ready to accept that not all compromised nerves can be restored to normal and should be willing to provide the necessary postoperative supportive care. The authors have observed patients with third, fourth, or even more operations for recurrence or failure, and they seldom produced favorable outcomes.

REFERENCES

1. Seddon HJ. A classification of nerve injuries. *Br Med J* 1942;2(4260): 237–239. Retrieved from http://www.ncbi.nlm.nih.gov/pubmed/17676350
2. Sunderland S. A classification of peripheral nerve injuries producing loss of function. *Brain* 1951;74(4):491–516. Retrieved from http://www.ncbi.nlm.nih.gov/pubmed/14895767
3. Bertelli JA, Soares dos Santos AR, Calixto JB. Effects of neurolysis during nerve regeneration: a behavioral and electrophysiologic study. *J Reconstr Microsurg* 1998;14(3):165–170. Retrieved from http://www.ncbi.nlm.nih.gov/pubmed/9590611
4. Mazal PR, Millesi H. Neurolysis: is it beneficial or harmful? *Acta Neurochir Suppl* 2005;92:3–6. Retrieved from http://books.google.com/books?id=cgNprUowcUEC&pgis=1
5. Millesi H, Rath T, Reihsner R, Zoch G. Microsurgical neurolysis: its anatomical and physiological basis and its classification. *Microsurgery* 1993;14(7):430–439.
6. Sakurai M, Miyasaka Y. Neural fibrosis and the effect of neurolysis. *J Bone Joint Surgery Br* 1986;68(3):483–488. Retrieved from http://www.ncbi.nlm.nih.gov/pubmed/3015976
7. Ting J, Weiland AJ. Role of ancillary procedures in surgical management of carpal tunnel syndrome: epineurotomy, internal neurolysis, tenosynovectomy, and tendon transfers. *Hand Clin* 2002;18(2):315–323. Retrieved from http://www.ncbi.nlm.nih.gov/pubmed/12371034
8. Tung TH, Mackinnon SE. Secondary carpal tunnel surgery. *Plast Reconstr Surg* 2001;107(7):1830–1843; quiz 1844, 1933. Retrieved from http://www.ncbi.nlm.nih.gov/pubmed/11391209
9. Wadstroem J, Nigst H. Reoperation for carpal tunnel syndrome. A retrospective analysis of forty cases. *Ann Chir Main* 1986;5(1):54–58. Retrieved from http://www.ncbi.nlm.nih.gov/pubmed/3963906
10. Ducic I, Felder JM. Minimally invasive peripheral nerve surgery: peroneal nerve neurolysis. *Microsurgery* 2012;32(1):26–30.
11. Terzis JK. *Microreconstruction of Nerve Injuries.* WB Saunders, Philadelphia,1987.
12. Elliot D, Lloyd M, Hazari A, et al. Relief of the pain of neuromas-in-continuity and scarred median and ulnar nerves in the distal forearm and wrist by neurolysis, wrapping in vascularized forearm fascial flaps and adjunctive procedures. *J Hand Surg Eur Vol* 2010;35(7):575–582.
13. Jones NF, Shaw WW, Katz RG. Circumferential wrapping of a flap around a scarred peripheral nerve for salvage of end-stage traction neuritis. *J Hand Surg* 1997;22A:527.
14. Monacelli G, Rizzo MI, Pardi M, Spagnoli AM. Clinical and electrophysiological comparison of different methods of soft tissue coverage of the median nerve in recurrent carpal tunnel syndrome. *Neurosurgery* 2009;64(3):E577; author reply E577.
15. Puckett BN, Gaston RG, Lourie GM. A novel technique for the treatment of recurrent cubital tunnel syndrome: ulnar nerve wrapping with a tissue engineered bioscaffold. *J Hand Surg Eur Vol* 2011;36(2):130–134. Retrieved from http://www.ncbi.nlm.nih.gov/pubmed/21045022
16. Stütz NM, Gohritz A, Novotny A, et al. Clinical and electrophysiological comparison of different methods of soft tissue coverage of the median nerve in recurrent carpal tunnel syndrome. *Neurosurgery* 2008;62(3 suppl 1): 194–199; discussion 199–200. Retrieved from http://www.ncbi.nlm.nih.gov/pubmed/19240591
17. Tollestrup T, Berg C, Netscher D. Management of distal traumatic median nerve painful neuromas and of recurrent carpal tunnel syndrome: hypothenar fat pad flap. *J Hand Surg* 2010;35(6):1010–1014. Retrieved from http://www.ncbi.nlm.nih.gov/pubmed/20513581
18. Varitimidis SE, Vardakas DG, Goebel F, Sotereanos DG. Treatment of recurrent compressive neuropathy of peripheral nerves in the upper extremity with an autologous vein insulator. *J Hand Surg* 2001;26(2):296–302. Retrieved from http://www.ncbi.nlm.nih.gov/pubmed/11279577
19. Diebold PF, Daum B, Dang-Vu V, Litchinko M. True epineural neurolysis in Morton's neuroma: a 5-year follow up. *Orthopedics* 1996;19(5):397–400.
20. Matejcik V, Penzesova G. Follow-up evaluation of neurolysis of brachial plexus and peripheral nerves of upper extremities. *Bratisl Lek Listy* 2004;105(12):424–427. Retrieved from http://www.ncbi.nlm.nih.gov/pubmed/15777073
21. Humphreys DB, Mackinnon SE. Nerve transfers. *Oper Tech Plast Reconstr Surg* 2002;9(3):89–99.
22. Barrett JP, Downey MS, Hillstrom HJ. Retrospective analysis of neurapraxia and axonotmesis injuries of select peripheral nerves of the foot and ankle and their conservative and surgical treatment (external neurolysis and neurectomy). *J Foot Ankle Surg* 1999;38(3):185–193. Retrieved from http://www.ncbi.nlm.nih.gov/pubmed/10384357
23. Stellini L. Interfascicular autologous grafts in the repair of peripheral nerves: eight years' experience. *Br J Plast Surg* 1982;35(4):478–482. Retrieved from http://www.ncbi.nlm.nih.gov/pubmed/7139175
24. Donoff RB. Nerve regeneration: basic and applied aspects. *Crit Rev Oral Biol Med* 1995;6(1):18–24. doi:10.1177/10454411950060010201
25. Tapadia M, Mozaffar T, Gupta R. Compressive neuropathies of the upper extremity: update on pathophysiology, classification, and electrodiagnostic findings. *J Hand Surg* 2010;35(4):668–677. doi:10.1016/j.jhsa.2010.01.007
26. Kim DH, Kam AC, Chandika P, et al. Surgical management and outcome in patients with radial nerve lesions. *J Neurosurg* 2001;95(4):573–583. doi:10.3171/jns.2001.95.4.0573
27. Kline DG, Hackett ER, LeBanc HJ. The value of primary repair for bluntly transected nerve injuries: physiological documentation. *Surg Forum* 1974;25:436–438.43 Retrieved from http://www.ncbi.nlm.nih.gov/pubmed/4439219
28. Van Beek AL. Electrodiagnostic evaluation of peripheral nerve injuries. *Hand Clin* 1986;2(4):747–760. Retrieved from http://www.ncbi.nlm.nih.gov/pubmed/3793771
29. Van Beek AL, Massac E, Smith DO. The use of the signal averaging computer for evaluation of peripheral nerve problems. *Clin Plast Surg* 1986;13(3):407–418. Retrieved from http://www.ncbi.nlm.nih.gov/pubmed/3013488
30. Millesi H. The nerve gap. Theory and clinical practice. *Hand Clin* 1986;2(4):651–663. Retrieved from http://www.ncbi.nlm.nih.gov/pubmed/3539948
31. Hassan NH, Sulong AF, Ng M-H, et al. Neural-differentiated mesenchymal stem cells incorporated into muscle stuffed vein scaffold forms a stable living nerve conduit. *J Orthop Res* 2012;30(10): 1674–1681.

32. Kuffler DP, Reyes O, Sosa IJ, Santiago-Figueroa J. Neurological recovery across a 12-cm-long ulnar nerve gap repaired 3.25 years post trauma: case report. *Neurosurgery* 2011;69(6):E1321–E1326. doi:10.1227/NEU.0b013e31822a9fd2
33. Rinker B, Liau JY. A prospective randomized study comparing woven polyglycolic acid and autogenous vein conduits for reconstruction of digital nerve gaps. *J Hand Surg* 2011;36(5):775–781. doi:10.1016/j.jhsa.2011.01.030
34. Roganovic Z, Ilic S, Savic M. Radial nerve repair using an autologous denatured muscle graft: comparison with outcomes of nerve graft repair. *Acta Neurochir (Wien)* 2007;149(10):1033–1038; discussion 1038–1039. doi:10.1007/s00701-007-1269-z
35. Taras JS, Jacoby SM, Lincoski CJ. Reconstruction of digital nerves with collagen conduits. *J Hand Surg* 2011;36(9):1441–1446. doi:10.1016/j.jhsa.2011.06.009
36. Takasaki Y, Noma H, Kitami T, et al. Reconstruction of the inferior alveolar nerve by autologous graft: a retrospective study of 20 cases examining donor nerve length. *Bull Tokyo Dent Coll* 2003;44(2):9–35. Retrieved from http://www.ncbi.nlm.nih.gov/pubmed/12956086
37. Jones NF, Ahn HC, Eo S. Revision surgery for persistent and recurrent carpal tunnel syndrome and for failed carpal tunnel release. *Plast Reconstr Surg* 2012;129(3):683–692. Retrieved from http://www.ncbi.nlm.nih.gov/pubmed/22090245
38. Cobb TK, Amadio PC. Reoperation for carpal tunnel syndrome. *Hand Clin* 1996;12(2):313–323. Retrieved from http://www.ncbi.nlm.nih.gov/pubmed/8724583
39. Upton ARM, McComas AJ. The double crush in nerve entrapment syndromes. *Lancet* 1973;2(7825):359–362. Retrieved from http://www.scopus.com/inward/record.url?eid=2-s2.0-0015791716&partnerID=40&md5=1097a343edc01f25f04f0af1ad08e021
40. Steyers CM. Recurrent carpal tunnel syndrome. *Hand Clin* 2002;18(2):339–345. Retrieved from http://www.ncbi.nlm.nih.gov/pubmed/ 12371037
41. Campagna R, Pessis E, Feydy A, et al. MRI assessment of recurrent carpal tunnel syndrome after open surgical release of the median nerve. *AJR Am J Roentgenol* 2009;193(3):644–650. Retrieved from http://www.ncbi.nlm.nih.gov/pubmed/19696276
42. Filippi R, Charalampaki P, Reisch R, et al. Recurrent cubital tunnel syndrome. Etiology and treatment. Minimally invasive neurosurgery. *Minim Invasive Neurosurg* 2001;44(4):197–201. Retrieved from http://www.ncbi.nlm.nih.gov/pubmed/11830777
43. Schnabl SM, Kisslinger F, Schramm A, et al. Subjective outcome, neurophysiological investigations, postoperative complications and recurrence rate of partial medial epicondylectomy in cubital tunnel syndrome. *Arch Orthop Trauma Surg* 2011;131(8):1027–1033. Retrieved from http://www.ncbi.nlm.nih.gov/pubmed/21203767
44. Seradge H, Owen W. Cubital tunnel release with medial epicondylectomy factors influencing the outcome. *J Hand Surg* 1998;23(3):483–491. Retrieved from http://www.ncbi.nlm.nih.gov/pubmed/9620189
45. Dahlin LB, Salö M, Thomsen N, Stütz N. Carpal tunnel syndrome and treatment of recurrent symptoms. *Scand J Plast Reconstr Surg Hand Surg* 2010;44(1):4–11. Retrieved from http://www.ncbi.nlm.nih.gov/pubmed/20136467
46. Teoh LC, Tan PL. Endoscopic carpal tunnel release for recurrent carpal tunnel syndrome after previous open release. *Hand Surg* 2004;9(2):235–239. Retrieved from http://www.ncbi.nlm.nih.gov/pubmed/15810113
47. Amadio PC. Interventions for recurrent/persistent carpal tunnel syndrome after carpal tunnel release. *J Hand Surg* 2009;34(7):1320–1322. Retrieved from http://www.ncbi.nlm.nih.gov/pubmed/19576701
48. Straub TA. Endoscopic carpal tunnel release: a prospective analysis of factors associated with unsatisfactory results. *Arthroscopy* 1999;15(3):269–274.

CHAPTER 76

Microsurgical Revascularization and Sympathectomy

Beth Paterson Smith and L. Andrew Koman

CONVENTIONAL OPTIONS

Patients with vasospastic and vaso-occlusive diseases are treated with environmental modifications, oral calcium channel blockers, nitroglycerin paste, smoking cessation, and medical management of underlying disease processes such as systemic lupus erythematosus and scleroderma (1–3). For patients with refractory symptoms, the use of injectable botulinum toxin has been reported in two case series (4,5). For refractory pain associated with ulcerations, gangrene, or osteomyelitis, amputations may be necessary. However, microsurgical options of revascularization or peripheral sympathectomy may provide significant palliation of symptoms. This chapter details the indications and techniques for microsurgical options to manage refractory pain and nonhealing digital ulcers in patients with vasospastic and occlusive disease. The majority of these events are secondary to collagen vascular disorders and distal occlusive events (1–3). Jones (6) classified the pathophysiologic mechanisms causing ischemia of the hand into emboli, vasospasm, thrombosis or "sludging," and occlusive disease and suggested that these mechanisms provided a rational basis for treatment of patients with acute and chronic ischemia of the hand caused by systemic disease such as collagen vascular diseases (7).

RECONSTRUCTIVE OPTIONS

Peripheral sympathectomy and arterial reconstruction are microsurgical reconstructive options. Salvage procedures include arterialization of the venous system (AVS), free omental transfer, and free flaps. The latter two procedures are only used when the entire hand is compromised and is not discussed in this chapter.

Blood flow to the hand and digits consists of nutritional and thermoregulatory components. In normal individuals, 80% to 90% of total blood flow in the digits is thermoregulatory, and 10% to 20% is nutritional. In vasospastic conditions, symptoms and signs are secondary to decreased total flow and are often intensified by inappropriate arteriovenous shunting and subsequent decreases in nutritional flow. In normal and nonvasospastic states, ischemia stimulates a decrease in arteriovenous shunting resulting in increased nutritional flow. However, in vasospastic conditions, arteriovenous shunting persists or increases in the presence of ischemic signals. Clinically, this is manifest by an increased frequency or duration of Raynaud's phenomena, increased symptoms, and potential ischemic events (1,2).

Surgical interventions are designed to increase total blood flow, to decrease vasospasm and inappropriate arteriovenous shunting, or both. *Arterial reconstruction* increases total flow and decreases sympathetic vasoconstriction (6–10). *Digital sympathectomy* decreases sympathetic vasoconstriction but results in minimal changes in total flow if an occlusive component coexists (1,2,7,11–13). *AVS* improves total flow as far distal as the middle phalanges; however, this procedure has minimal effect on sympathetic tone (10,14,15).

INDICATIONS AND CONTRAINDICATIONS

Arterial Reconstruction by Microsurgical Revascularization

In a hand with inadequate total blood flow, revascularization is indicated if there is a patent distal artery with adequate outflow to maintain patency after an arterial anastomosis. Microsurgical reconstruction of a "new" superficial palmar arch with end-to-end anastomosis to the distal ulnar artery and end-to-side anastomoses to the common digital arteries might be expected to increase the inflow perfusion pressure to the digits. Similarly, the deep palmar arch can be revascularized microsurgically with end-to-end anastomoses between the distal radial artery and the deep palmar arch in the thumb–index finger web space. Options include (1) resection of the damaged or thrombosed segment and placement of an interposition graft using (a) reversed vein graft, (b) nonreversed valvulotomized vein graft, or (c) artery and (2) bypass grafting (2,6–10,16–21). Arterial reconstruction is contraindicated in patients with infections, who continue smoking, or who are experiencing active exacerbation of significant systemic conditions. Bypass grafts are used infrequently in the digits because of the bulk of leaving the native vessel intact and using a parallel bypass (Figure 76-1), but microsurgical revascularization of a defined occlusion of a digital artery using a small-caliber vein graft has been reported in conjunction with digital sympathectomy (7,22).

Sympathectomy

Sympathectomy is indicated for refractory symptoms in which revascularization is not possible or is contraindicated (2,7,11,12,22–26). Types of peripheral sympathectomy include (1) ligation and resection of the thrombosed segment (Leriche type) (27), (2) digital sympathectomy (23–25), and (3) wrist and palmar radical sympathectomy (7,26). Sympathectomy may be performed in the presence of dry gangrene and for patients who continue to smoke; however, it should be avoided in patients with gross infection.

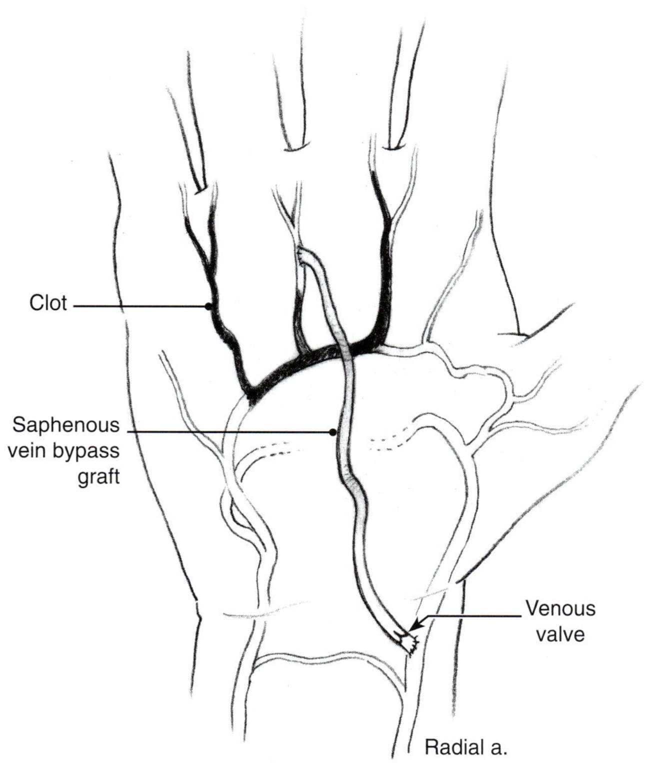

FIGURE 76-1 Schematic drawing of a "bypass" graft from the radial artery to a patent common digital artery. Solid marking indicates thrombosed segments. a, artery. (Reprinted with permission from Koman LA (ed). *Wake Forest Orthopaedic Handbook*, Winston-Salem, NC: Wake Forest University Orthopaedic Press, 2011.)

Arterialization of the Venous System

Arterialization of the venous system may be considered as a salvage procedure only when significant portions of the fingers or entire hand are at risk (10,14,15), when there is extensive distal disease that is not amenable to arterial reconstruction, *and* when medical management fails to control ongoing pain and tissue loss. Continued smoking is a relative contraindication for AVS, and the presence of gross infection is an absolute contraindication (15).

TECHNIQUES

Arterial Reconstruction

Arterial reconstruction in the hand and fingers is performed with the hand positioned on a hand table. Exsanguination of the extremity and the use of a tourniquet are recommended. Bipolar cautery, micro-instruments, and an operating microscope are required. If there is a possibility that a graft is required from a secondary donor site, the patient should be positioned appropriately and prepped and draped for optimal access to the donor site.

Selection of the donor vein or artery is based on the size of the vessel to be reconstructed. Digital arteries in the finger and palm may be reconstructed with volar forearm veins; radial and ulnar artery reconstruction requires dorsal forearm veins, distal lower extremity veins, or small arteries such as the thoracodorsal or inferior epigastric arteries (2,28,29).

Either longitudinal midlateral or Bruner incisions are used in the fingers and curved incisions in the palm. If there is any concern about postoperative swelling, midlateral incisions may be left open. The initial dissection is performed with loupe magnification. The arteries and nerves are identified, and vessel loops are placed around the arteries. Thrombosed and occluded arterial segments are exposed in their entirety. Preoperative noninvasive evaluation of hand perfusion or preoperative arteriography is helpful in determining the extent of arterial involvement and for defining the patency of distal vessels. The entire thrombosed segment is dissected both proximally and distally until a normal-appearing artery is reached. Branches of the common digital and proper digital nerves are identified and protected, and tiny nerve branches carrying sympathetic innervation to the arteries are transected.

After a distal artery is identified as suitable for anastomosis, an arteriotomy is performed, and the intima is inspected under the operating microscope. If appropriate, the entire thrombosed segment is excised until the arterial lumen appears "normal," both proximally and distally, under the operating microscope. This evaluation is absolutely crucial because an anastomosis to a recannulized artery is suboptimal and almost certainly results in postoperative thrombosis. The length of the arterial defect is measured, and a vein graft from either the upper or lower extremity is harvested. The choice of graft is based on the size of the recipient vessel, the age of the patient, and the quality of the potential donor vessels. For the larger radial or ulnar arteries in younger patients, lower extremity veins, the cephalic vein or even arterial grafts may be preferable (2,7,28,29). However, the majority of digital artery reconstructions may be accomplished with forearm veins (preferably reversed or less preferably nonreversed with the valves removed). The graft is harvested under loupe magnification, and all side branches are ligated. Absorbable ligatures are preferred, but micro-hemo clips can be used. If a branching graft is required, these can usually be harvested from the forearm, leg, or dorsum of the foot or alternatively from the thoracodorsal or deep inferior epigastric arterial systems (2,29). Alternatively, end-to-side anastomoses may be used (7,9).

The vein graft is reversed and the vein dilated with heparinized saline. For nonreversed veins, the valves must be disrupted. Distension of the graft identifies any leaks from side branches or due to inadvertent injury and also decreases postanastomotic vasospasm. In general, 20% to 30% of extra length is harvested over the measured length of the resected artery. If the graft has appropriate branches, they may be used for a proximal end-to-end anastomosis and distal end-to-side anastomoses (Figure 76-2).

Size discrepancy between the graft and native artery is managed by a 30-degree oblique transection of the artery, an opening "V" in the artery, a closing "V" in the graft, or a "sleeve" anastomosis (Figure 76-3). Anastomoses are performed with 9-0 or 10-0 microsutures using a 75- to 135-micron needle depending on the size of the artery. In general, digital arteries at the proximal or middle phalangeal level necessitate 10-0 sutures and 75- to 100-micron needles. Larger 9-0 sutures and needles may be used more proximally.

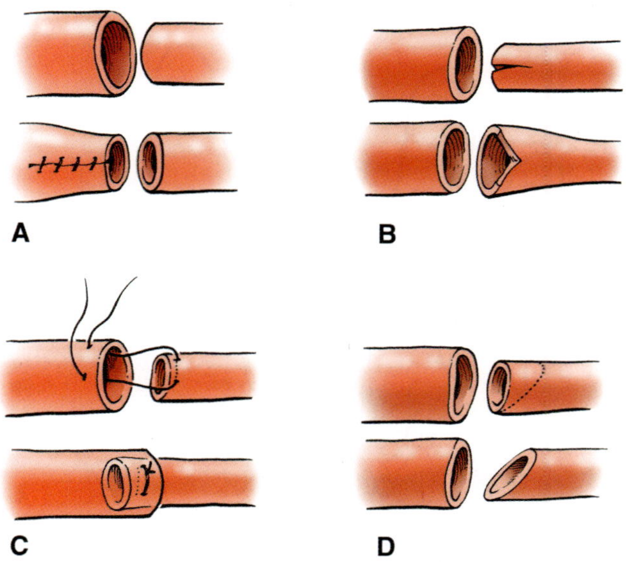

FIGURE 76-3 Mechanisms to overcome size discrepancies during arterial anastomosis. (**A**) A V-shaped portion may be excised from the larger artery. (**B**) Conversely, the smaller artery may be split longitudinally, increasing the circumference of the lumen to fit the larger artery. (**C**) If the smaller artery provides proximal inflow, it may be intussuscepted into the larger artery using a sleeve-type technique. (**D**) Small discrepancies may be overcome by cutting the smaller vessel at a 30-degree angle or bevel followed by gentle dilatation. (Reprinted with permission from Koman LA (ed): *Bowman Gray School of Medicine Orthopaedic Manual*. Winston-Salem, NC: Wake Forest University Orthopaedic Press, 1997.)

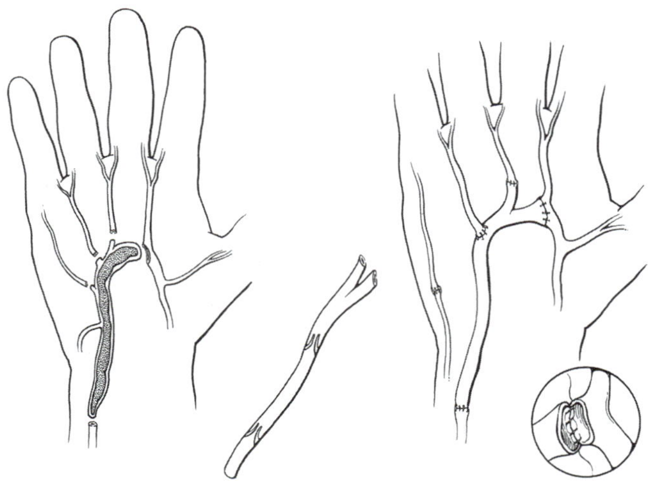

FIGURE 76-2 Complex reversed interposition grafts may be necessary to reconstruct extensive occlusive disease. This patient had severe symptoms and pregangrenous digits. Exploration confirmed the angiographic findings, which included thrombosis extending from the wrist crease to the origin of the common digital artery to the index–long finger and abnormal radial and ulnar arteries at the wrist. Reconstruction required a 13.5-cm saphenous vein reversed graft. During harvest, a Y branch was included. The distal anastomoses included an end-to-side anastomosis of the common digital artery to the ring-small finger into the vein graft, an end-to-end anastomosis of the Y-vein branch to the common digital artery to the long–ring finger, and an end-to-end anastomosis of the proximal vein graft to the junction of the common digital artery to the index–long finger with the superficial radial artery. The inferior ulnar recurrent artery was anastomosed to the ulnar proper digital artery to the small finger. The inset demonstrates the end-to-side anastomosis. (Reprinted with permission from Koman LA (ed): *Bowman Gray School of Medicine Orthopaedic Manual*. Winston-Salem, NC: Wake Forest University Orthopaedic Press, 1997.)

A classic Carrel repair is performed with interrupted sutures after placing the initial two stay sutures 120 degrees apart. Microvascular approximator clamps may be used. The front and back walls are sutured using interrupted sutures. In general, we do not use running sutures or a spatulated anastomosis. It is important to place the sutures through the intima and adventitia, avoiding "back wall" or "side wall" tethering. Although most arteries can be reconstructed with simple interposition grafts, complex reconstructions may be necessary, including end-to-side anastomoses, Y grafts, bypass grafting, and anastomoses to parallel arteries (Figure 76-4).

Unless contraindicated, a single bolus of heparin (2–5000 units) is given intraoperatively. After the anastomoses have been completed, the tourniquet is deflated, the anastomoses are checked, bleeding is controlled, and additional sutures are placed as necessary. In general, a small Silastic 7- or 10-Fr drain is placed, and a bulky hand dressing is applied.

Postoperatively, the patient may be treated with dextran 40 at 25 cc/hr for 2 to 3 days and 81 mg of aspirin. If there are no complications, the patient may be discharged home on aspirin. If there are complications or concerns about the flow in the distal arteries, then heparin or Coumadin may be necessary. In addition, patients with coagulopathies may require Coumadin or other interventions.

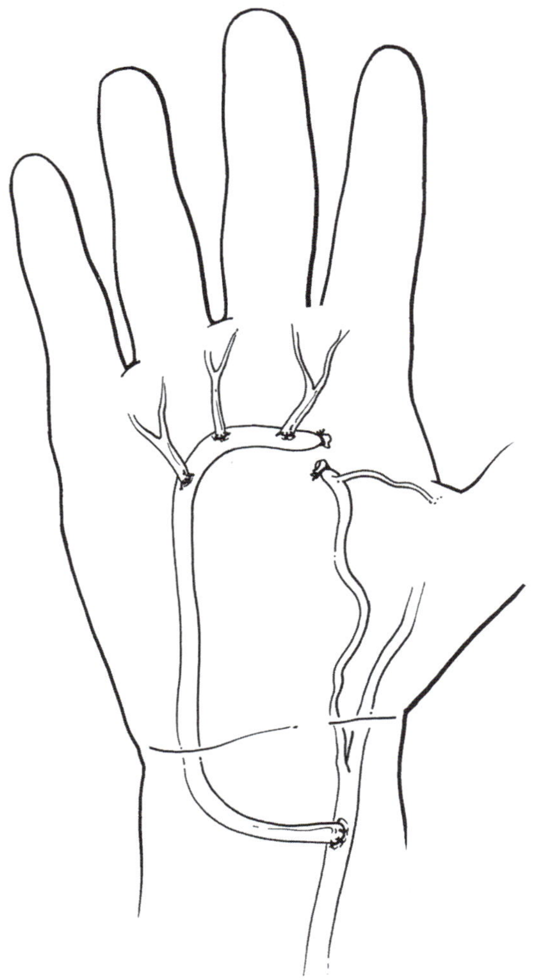

FIGURE 76-4 Schematic of an arterial reconstruction with a 14-cm reversed interposition vein graft. The ulnar artery was not suitable at the level of the midforearm; therefore, an end-to-side anastomosis to the radial artery was performed. Because of the size discrepancy, the distal vein graft was ligated and three end-to-side anastomoses were performed to reconstruct the three common digital arteries. (Reprinted with permission from Koman LA (ed): *Bowman Gray School of Medicine Orthopaedic Manual*. Winston-Salem, NC: Wake Forest University Orthopaedic Press, 1996.)

Bypass Grafting

Bypass grafting has been recommended as an alternative to interposition grafting. The advantages are less dissection, end-to-side anastomoses, possibly a higher patency rate, and direct access to vessels outside of the "zone of injury" (18,19). Grafts from patent radial or ulnar arteries in the forearm or the brachial artery in the arm provide high inflow when anastomosed distally to patent arteries at the superficial palmar arch or common digital arterial or proper digital arterial level (see Figure 76-1). Careful preoperative arteriographic or alternative evaluation is crucial. Vein grafts may be harvested from the upper or lower extremity and usually reversed, but nonreversed in situ valvulotomized cephalic or basilic veins are an alternative option. The disadvantages of bypass grafting include less sympathetic effect than interposition grafting, greater bulk, nonvisualization of parts of the graft and therefore the potential for torsion or kinking, the need for end-to-side anastomoses, and the inexperience of hand surgeons using this technique.

Digital Sympathectomy (Flatt)

Patients in whom sympathetic overactivity is the primary etiologic mechanism of vasospasm and in patients with unreconstructable lesions or with symptoms involving predominantly one finger, a digital sympathectomy may be indicated. Flatt introduced the concept of a distal sympathectomy at the level of the common digital and proper digital arteries (23–25). These patients are best operated on under axillary block anesthesia and tourniquet control. A Bruner incision is made from the distal palmar crease to the proximal interphalangeal (PIP) joint. Flaps are elevated, and both neurovascular bundles are identified using loupe magnification. Each digital nerve and artery are identified, and the artery is separated from the nerve. Under the operating microscope, the adventitia is stripped from the digital artery for a distance of approximately 1 cm. Great care must be taken to avoid injury to the artery. Adventitial dissection is performed on both digital arteries. Intraoperative and postoperative anticoagulation is not necessary. The incision is closed in a single layer, and a drain is only placed if there is concern over postoperative bleeding. The tourniquet should be deflated before wound closure (Figure 76-5). Postoperatively, the patient is placed in a bulky compressive dressing and may be observed for up to 23 hours or released from the hospital depending on the operative findings. If an unanticipated thrombosed but reconstructable segment is encountered, strong consideration should be given to arterial reconstruction.

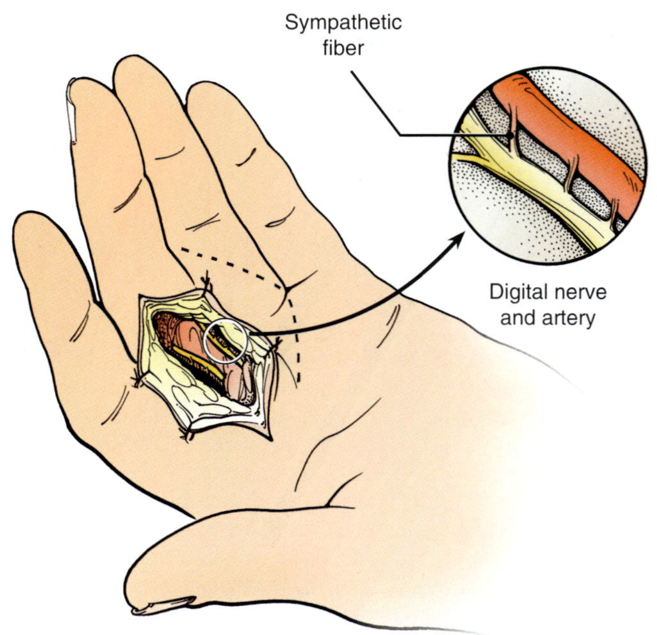

FIGURE 76-5 Digital sympathectomy is accomplished through a volar Bruner incision. All connections between the digital artery and the accompanying digital nerve are separated, and the adventitia is stripped of sympathetic nerve fibers. The initial dissection is performed under loupe magnification with subsequent dissection under the operating microscope. (Reprinted with permission from Koman LA (ed): *Bowman Gray School of Medicine Orthopaedic Manual*. Winston-Salem, NC: Wake Forest University Orthopaedic Press, 1997.)

Palmar and Wrist Sympathectomy

Both Jones (7) and O'Brien et al. (26) have described a much more extensive sympathectomy technique than originally described by Flatt, Wilgis, and Egloff et al. (23–25) in which the adventitia is stripped from the superficial palmar arch, the radial digital artery to the index finger, the common digital arteries to the second to fourth web spaces and their continuation as the radial and ulnar proper digital arteries, and the ulnar digital artery to the small finger. If necessary, the adventitial stripping can be extended farther out to the PIP joint level in an individual finger. O'Brien et al. (26) also advocated radical resection of the adventitia from the distal radial and ulnar arteries and superficial palmar arch. For sympathectomy of all digits, four incisions are used (11,12). Optimal exposure may require three palmar incisions and one dorsal incision to visualize the radial and ulnar arteries, the superficial palmar arch, the common digital arteries, and the deep palmar arch under loupe magnification. Initially, two parallel incisions 3 cm in length are made parallel with and adjacent to the radial and ulnar arteries (Figure 76-6). The arteries are exposed for approximately 2 cm, and any connections between the arteries, the nerves, and the vena comitantes are excised. If the nerve of Henle is identified adjacent to the ulnar artery, it is transected (30). The incision over the ulnar artery may be extended into the palm as an inverted J-shaped incision, or a separate inverted J-shaped incision may be made in the palm to identify the distal end of the ulnar artery, the superficial palmar arch, and the three common digital arteries (7,26). The vena comitantes are carefully separated from the arteries, and the arterial tree is exposed from the distal ulnar artery to the distal third of the common digital arteries at the level of the metacarpophalangeal joints. Vessel loops are placed and the common digital nerves are separated from the common digital arteries.

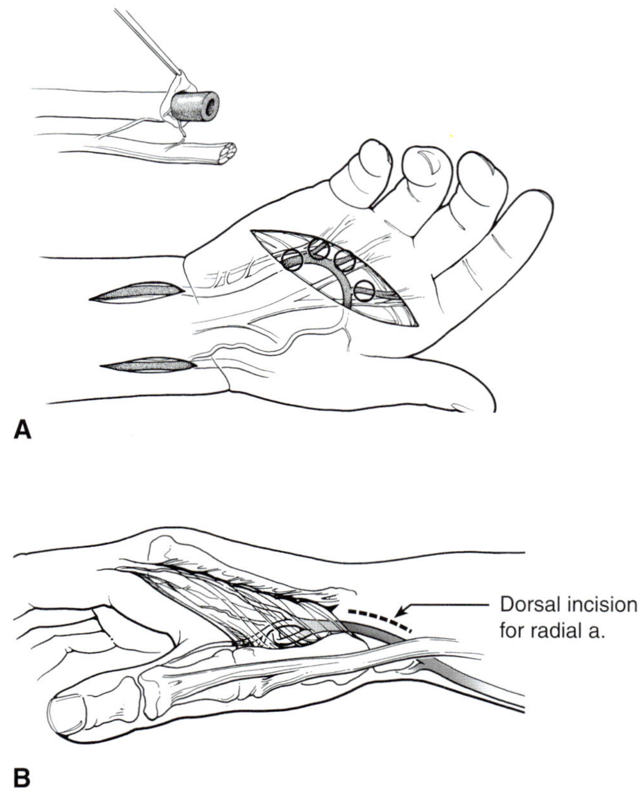

FIGURE 76-6 Schematic of a radical sympathectomy of the hand. Longitudinal incisions are used to expose the radial and ulnar arteries, and a transverse or inverted J-shaped incision is used in the palm to expose the superficial palmar arch and the three common digital arteries. A separate incision (**B**) may be used over the anatomical snuffbox to expose the dorsal branch of the radial artery. After initial dissection under loupe magnification, the adventitia is stripped from these arteries under the operating microscope. a, artery. (Reprinted with permission fromf Koman LA (ed): *Bowman Gray School of Medicine Orthopaedic Manual.* Winston-Salem, NC: Wake Forest University Orthopaedic Press, 1997.)

The distal radial artery and the proximal portion of the deep palmar arch are dissected through a dorsal incision overlying the anatomical snuffbox. The superficial radial nerve and extensor tendons are identified and protected. The two vena comitantes are separated from the radial artery and clipped or coagulated as necessary. Vessel loops are placed around the artery, and dissection is extended distally into the thumb–index finger webspace. Thick fascia between the adductor pollicis and the first dorsal interosseous muscles usually has to be released to gain access to the deep portion of the radial artery, the princeps pollicis, and the proximal portion of the deep palmar arch.

Under moderate- to high-power magnification, the adventitia from the proximal radial and ulnar arteries, the distal end of the ulnar artery, the entire superficial palmar arch, and the three common digital arteries are carefully removed. Adventitia from the distal radial artery, the princeps pollicis, and the proximal deep palmar arch is similarly excised as far distally as possible (7). The tourniquet is deflated, bleeding controlled, and the incisions closed. A suction drain in the palm is recommended in most cases. If an unanticipated thrombosed but reconstructable segment is encountered, arterial reconstruction should be considered.

Arterialization of the Venous System

It is hypothesized that AVS may improve blood flow as a result of valvular incompetency directing arterial flow retrogradely through the distal veins through arteriovenous shunts into the nutritional capillary beds (10,14,15). This technique is only indicated for arterial insufficiency when no distal arteries are available or suitable for anastomosis. The technique requires a relatively high inflow proximal artery, such as the radial, ulnar, or brachial artery and patent dorsal hand and forearm veins. The absence of a patent venous system is a contraindication for this procedure.

Before surgery, venous mapping using noninvasive Doppler techniques facilitates surgical planning. Tourniquet control and long extensile incisions are required. The proximal artery is identified under loupe magnification. The dorsal veins are left in situ but dissected proximal to distal from the forearm to the wrist and out onto the dorsum of the hand, ligating most of the distal branches. Commercial or custom valvulotomes are used to incise the valves of veins on the dorsum of the hand and over the proximal phalanges. Under the operating microscope, multiple venotomies are performed so that the valvulotomes may be positioned under direct vision to excise the valves as well as

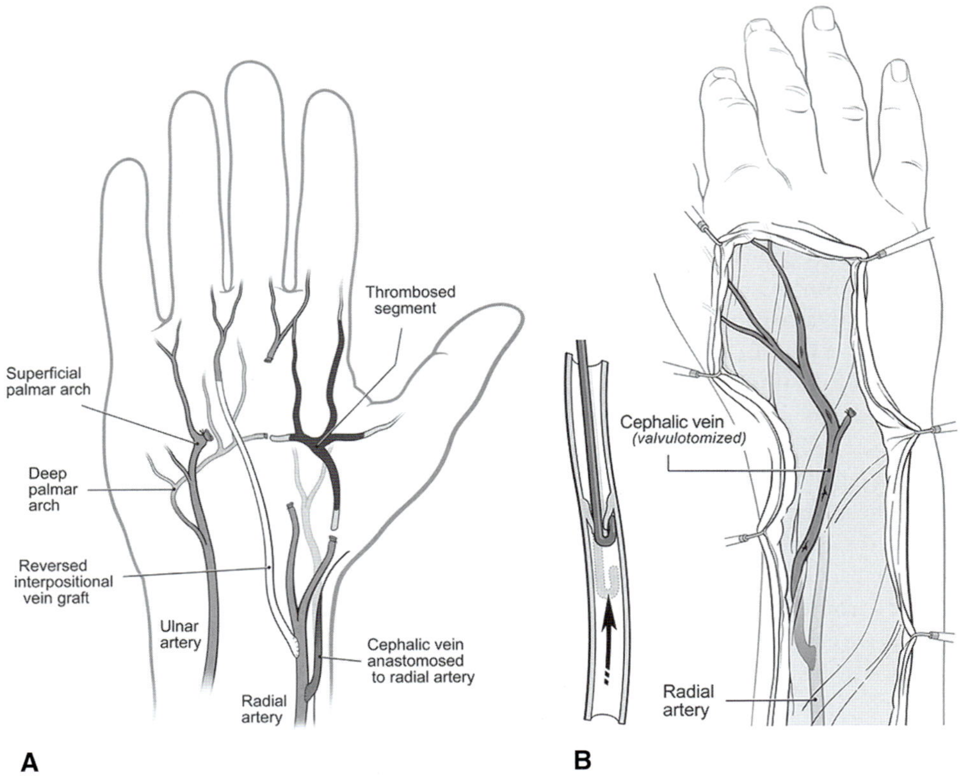

FIGURE 76-7 (A) Schematic of arterialization of the venous system showing a new unreconstructable lesion 13 years after a previous reconstruction with a reversed interposition vein graft. The proximal cephalic vein is anastomosed end to side to the radial artery. (B) Dorsal view showing exposure of the cephalic vein, resection of the valves with a valvulotome, ligation of all its distal tributaries, and end-to-side anastomosis to the radial artery. All of the venotomies were closed, but some open venotomies are shown for illustrative purposes. (Reprinted with permission from Koman LA (ed): *Bowman Gray School of Medicine Orthopaedic Manual.* Winston-Salem, NC: Wake Forest University Orthopaedic Press, 2008.)

through the transected proximal vein. Heparinized saline is injected through the venous network to ensure that the valvotomies have been successful (Figure 76-7). The venotomies are closed with 8-0 or 9-0 sutures under the microscope, and the proximal venous segment is anastomosed end to side to the radial, ulnar, or brachial artery. Hemostasis is achieved and the wound closed over a drain(s).

POSTOPERATIVE CARE AND MONITORING

Arterial Reconstruction

After arterial reconstruction, some form of anticoagulation is appropriate unless contraindicated. The type of anticoagulation depends on the quality of the arteries at the anastomoses, the cause of the vascular abnormality, the presence or absence of systemic disease, and the possible coexistence of an underlying coagulopathy. If the arterial lumen is relatively normal at the anastomoses, the patient receives a bolus of heparin (1–2000 IU) intraoperatively and then postoperatively may be treated with a combination of dextran 40, aspirin (81 mg/day), or Pletal. If there is an abnormality at the anastomoses that cannot be resected without eliminating the possibility of reconstruction or if there is systemic disease, then anticoagulation with unfractionated heparin, low–molecular-weight heparin, Arixtra, or Coumadin is often required.

Drains are recommended postoperatively after arterial reconstruction. The patient is placed in a bulky compressive dressing with the hand elevated slightly above the heart. The room environment is controlled to avoid excessively cold temperatures, and caffeine products, including caffeinated soft drinks, coffee, tea, and chocolate, are avoided. Prophylactic antibiotics are administered unless there is evidence of infection, in which case therapeutic antibiotics are prescribed for 5 to 7 days.

Periarterial Sympathectomy

Postoperative care after periarterial sympathectomy does not require postoperative anticoagulation unless an arterial injury occurs. Drains are used for periarterial sympathectomies of the wrist and palm but are not mandatory and are rarely used for digital sympathectomies. A bulky compressive dressing with the hand slight elevated above the heart is recommended. Environmental modifications other than those used before surgery are not necessary. There is no reason to avoid caffeinated products unless they were contraindicated before surgery. Prophylactic antibiotics are recommended, but if there is evidence of infection, therapeutic antibiotics are required.

Complications

Complications associated with all these techniques include infection, thrombosis, vessel injury, nerve injury, hematoma, and failure to achieve the desired results with persistent residual ulceration, pain and the possible need for eventual amputation.

Because many patients have ulcers, wounds, osteomyelitis, or partial gangrene before surgery and as their indication for surgery, postoperative infection is a distinct possibility. However, the incidence of infection is low. In more than 200 peripheral sympathectomies, postoperative clinical infections occurred in fewer than 5% of patients, and the superficial infections that did occur were inconsequential in all but two patients. In patients with preexisting open wounds, amputation stumps required revision, but the periarterial sympathectomy incisions were uncomplicated.

In the absence of iatrogenic arterial injury, untoward arterial events after surgery are secondary to underlying vascular compromise or disease progression. Periarterial sympathectomy maximizes the potential nutritional blood flow that is available; it does not increase total flow and will not improve symptoms or signs significantly unless the preoperative blood flow was inappropriately distributed.

After arterial reconstruction, clinical and subclinical infections near an anastomosis may contribute to an increased incidence of thrombosis and may have potential digit-threatening consequences. For this reason, arterial reconstruction is not indicated in the presence of ongoing infection unless this surgery is the only alternative to amputation.

Secondary Surgery

A significant number of patients with collagen vascular disease and vaso-occlusive disease will eventually require amputation (6,7). The purpose of periarterial sympathectomy is to avoid or delay amputation, heal ulcers, reduce symptoms, and improve health-related quality of life (HRQOL). AVS is a potential end-stage salvage procedure for thrombosis of a previous arterial reconstruction. Free flaps are another potential end-stage salvage option. However, digital amputation at the level of the middle phalanx or the PIP joint may become necessary in the majority of cases.

RESULTS AND OUTCOMES

Arterial Reconstruction

The results of arterial reconstruction are well documented. Successful arterial reconstruction in patients with occlusive disease improves total blood flow, decreases symptoms, and improves HRQOL (8). Long-term patency rates are difficult to determine; however, patients with isolated ulnar artery thrombosis without significant systemic disease or coagulopathies have patency rates of 95% 2 years after surgery (16,17,21). In patients with systemic disease or underlying coagulopathies that are "appropriately treated," much lower success rates are to be expected (2,7). The use of long vein grafts is also associated with a higher rate of secondary thrombosis.

Sympathectomy

Koman et al. (11) have proposed that periarterial sympathectomy increases nutritional flow by decreasing inappropriate arterial venous shunting, but an alternative hypothesis suggests that digital sympathectomy acts as a "decompression arteriolysis," analogous to the epineurectomy of a peripheral nerve (7). The long-term clinical outcomes depend on the degree of vascular insufficiency at the time of the sympathectomy and the presence or absence and subsequent progression of the arterial abnormalities (stenoses, occlusion, thrombosis) related to the underlying systemic disease. The immediate effects of sympathectomy that can be expected in all patients are to maximize nutritional blood flow without impacting total flow. In appropriately selected patients, the majority will experience a significant reduction in the frequency and duration of their symptoms, healing of ulcers, and improved HRQOL. However, over time, the blood flow in patients with systemic disease will deteriorate depending on the progression of the underlying disease so that 20% to 33% patients will develop recurrent digital ulcerations (7,11,12,26,31,32). Therefore, periarterial sympathectomy is not recommended as a prophylactic procedure and is a palliative intervention.

SUMMARY

When medical management of vasospastic or vaso-occlusive disease is no longer effective, arterial reconstruction and peripheral sympathectomy are potential microsurgical options. Although these procedures are technically challenging in patients with systemic diseases such as scleroderma or systemic lupus erythematosus, improved patient outcomes are possible. If feasible, arterial reconstruction combined with sympathectomy is preferable for patients with vascular insufficiency caused by combined vasospasm and occlusive disease. Peripheral sympathectomy in the presence of adequate total blood flow will result in healing of ulcers, decreased Raynaud's symptoms, and improved HRQOL and function.

REFERENCES

1. Koman LA, Smith BP, Smith TL, et al. Vascular disorders. In Wolfe SW, Hotchkiss RN, Pederson WC, Kozin SH (eds). *Green's Operative Hand Surgery*, 6th ed. Philadelphia: Elsevier, 2011, pp. 2197–2240.
2. Ahn HC, Jones NF. Ischemia of the hand. In Neligan PC (ed). *Plastic Surgery*, 3rd ed. St. Louis: Elsevier Saunders, 2013.
3. Belch JJ, Ho M: Pharmacotherapy of Raynaud's phenomenon. *Drugs* 52(5):682–695, 1996.
4. Van Beek AL, Lim PK, Gear AJ, et al. Management of vasospastic disorders with botulinum toxin A. *Plast Reconstr Surg* 2007;119(1):217–226.
5. Neumeister MN, Chambers CB, Herron MS, et al. Botox therapy for ischemic digits. *Plast Reconstr Surg* 2009;124(10):191–201.
6. Jones NF. Acute and chronic ischemia of the hand: Pathophysiology, treatment and prognosis. *J Hand Surg Am* 1991;16:1074–1083.
7. Jones NF. Ischemia of the hand in systemic disease: the potential role of microsurgical revascularization and digital sympathectomy. *Clin Plast Surg* 1989;16:547–556.
8. Koman LA, Ruch DS, Aldrich M, et al. Arterial reconstruction in the ischemic hand and wrist: effects on microvascular physiology in health-related quality of life. *J Hand Surg Am* 1998;23:773–782.
9. Jones NF, Raynor SC, Medsger TA. Microsurgical revascularization of the hand in scleroderma. *Br J Plast Surg* 1987;40:264–269.
10. Pederson WC. Revascularization of the chronically ischemic hand. *Hand Clin* 1999;15:629–642.
11. Koman LA, Smith BP, Pollock F, et al. The microcirculatory effects of peripheral sympathectomy. *J Hand Surg Am* 1995;5:709–717.
12. Ruch DS, Holden M, Smith BP, et al. Periarterial sympathectomy in scleroderma patients: intermediate-term follow-up. *J Hand Surg Am* 2002;27(2):258–264.

13. Tomaino MM, Goitz RJ, Medsger TA. Surgery for ischemic pain and Raynaud's phenomenon in scleroderma: a description of treatment, protocol and evaluation of results. *Microsurgery* 2001;21:75–79.
14. King GM. Arterialization of venous system of the hand. *Plast Reconstr Surg* 2006;118:421–428.
15. Chloros GD, Li Z, Koman LA. Long-term successful outcome of severe hand ischemia using arterialization with reversal of venous flow: case report. *J Hand Surg Am* 2008;33(7):1048–1051.
16. Chloros GD, Lucas RM, Li Z, et al. Post-traumatic ulnar artery thrombosis: outcome of arterial reconstruction using reverse interpositional vein grafting at 2 years minimum follow-up. *J Hand Surg Am* 2008;33(6):932–940.
17. Koman LA, Urbaniak JR. Ulnar artery thrombosis. *Hand Clin* 1985;1(2):311–325.
18. Hughes K, Hamdan A, Schermerhorn M, et al. Bypass for chronic ischemia of the upper extremity: results in 20 patients. *J Vasc Surg* 2007;46:303–307.
19. Namdari S, Weiss AP, Carney WI Jr. Palmar bypass for digital ischemia. *J Hand Surg* 2007;32A(8):1251–1258.
20. Ruch DS, Aldridge M, Holden M, et al. Arterial reconstruction for radial artery occlusion. *J Hand Surg Am* 2000;25(5):982–984.
21. Zimmerman NB, Zimmerman SI, McClinton MA, et al. Long-term recovery following surgical treatment for ulnar artery occlusion. *J Hand Surg Am* 1994;19(10):17–21.
22. Tomaino MM. Digital arterial occlusion in scleroderma: is there a role for digital arterial reconstruction? *J Hand Surg* 2000;25:611–613.
23. Flatt AE. Digital artery sympathectomy. *J Hand Surg Am* 1980;6:550–556.
24. Wilgis EFS. Digital sympathectomy for vascular insufficiency. *Hand Clin* 1985;1:361–367.
25. Egloff DV, Missud RF, Verdan D. Superselective digital sympathectomy in Raynaud's phenomenon. *Hand* 1983;15:110–114.
26. O'Brien BM, Kumar PA, Mellow CG, et al. Radical microarteriolysis in the treatment of vasospastic disorders of the hand, especially scleroderma. *J Hand Surg Br* 1992;17:447.
27. Leriche R, Fontaine R, Dupertys SM. Arterectomy with follow-up studies on 78 operations. *Surg Gynec Obstet* 1937;64:149–155.
28. Smith HE, Deirks M, Patterson RB. Hypothenar hammer syndrome: distal ulnar artery reconstruction with autologous inferior epigastric artery. *J Vasc Surg* 2004;40:1238–1242.
29. Masden DL, McClinton MA. Arterial conduits for distal upper extremity bypass. *J Hand Surg* 2013;38A:572–577.
30. Balogh B, Valencak J, Vesely M, et al. The nerve of Henle: an anatomic and immunohistochemical study. *J Hand Surg Am* 1999;24(5):1103–1108.
31. Le-Gammal TA, Blair WF. Digital periarterial sympathectomy for ischemic digital pain and ulcers. *J Hand Surg Br* 1991;16:382–385.
32. Ward WA, Van Moore A. Management of finger ulcers in scleroderma. *J Hand Surg Am* 1995;20:868–872.

CHAPTER 77

The Animal and Human Experimental Foundation of Vascularized Composite Allotransplantation

Warren C. Breidenbach III, Giles W. Becker, Bruce Kaplan, Tolga Turker, Christine A. Muhleman, Dennis T. Schmahl

This chapter presents a historical review of the experimental foundation upon which vascularized composite allotransplantation (VCA) rests. We discuss the main prior animal and human experimental results and present the current state of the field.

Your first impulse might be to skip this section, thinking that what has passed is done, and only the present is relevant. To do so would be an error—history repeats itself, and unless one studies the past mistakes in this field (some of which remain unreported or clarified), one is destined to repeat them.

Surgical advancement is usually not a straight line from initial idea through experimentation to final implementation. Discovery is rarely a series of logical experiments leading to truth; it often remains right in front of our eyes, for years unseen, until stumbled upon by mistake. The road to advancement takes a line that goes forward and backward, zigs and zags, and even at time stops. When these discoveries are reported, however, they are usually not presented with the multiple errors required to get there; as in a manuscript, this is too cumbersome. Mistakes are also sometimes not reported, simply to bury bad outcomes. The former is understandable. The latter is unethical.

Medical history is often presented only as a vignette at the beginning of a presentation or a book chapter because there is no intent to instruct how to avoid mistakes of the past. Furthermore, there is often a reluctance to report intellectual fraud because the reporter often suffers more than the culprit. Medical history is thus presented as a straight line from inspiration, via experiment, to success. Absent is the insight that the scientific truth we embrace was achieved through a mixture of intuition, stumbles and advancements, unethical or fraudulent behavior, politics, missed opportunity, serendipity, and often opposition from established political and societal interests.

We have tried to uncover the important unknown outcomes about which you should be aware before you engage in or refer a patient for VCA. You will not see these by reading the standard medical literature.

THE EARLY HISTORY

The first steps in the history of experimental hand transplantation (HT) took place from 1905 through 1907. At this time, vascular repair was thought to be impossible. However, Alexis Carrel developed a technique of vascular anastomosis (triangulation and vein patch) that achieved reproducible success, making it feasible to transplant organs in experimental animal models. He demonstrated the potential of organ transplantation by transplanting a dog kidney into the neck of another dog (1). For developing this technique, Alexis Carrel received the Nobel Prize in 1912. Many believed that these advancements in arterial repair would quickly lead to organ transplantation in humans, but this goal proved elusive.

At that time, there was little understanding of the immune system. Even though Alexis Carrel demonstrated that organs could be transplanted in animal models, the allografts always rapidly failed, and the reason for this failure was poorly understood. Organ transplantation proved a problem bigger than just accomplishing an arterial repair, and the next step to understand and control allograft rejection took 40 years.

It was not until the late 1940s and early 1950s that Medawar and Burnet unlocked the cause of organ rejection, leading to the discovery of acquired immune tolerance. For this work, they were awarded the Nobel Prize in 1960 (2).

Their work was critical for the next step of allotransplantation. Dr. Joseph Murray performed the first successful kidney transplant between two identical twins on December 23, 1954. Medawar and Burnet had revealed to Murray that transplant between identical twins was the only way, at that time, to have a chance to successfully realize the dream of organ transplantation. In 1954, many physicians so poorly understood the immune response that most believed rejection was inevitable, even in identical twins. Dr. Murray was awarded the Nobel prize for Medicine in 1990 for this pivotal moment in the history of surgical innovation.

What is often forgotten is that Dr. Murray received considerable contemporary criticism for this pioneering work. He challenged the basic concept that one could not transplant tissue, and many believed the transplant would not work. There were many who thought that a healthy individual sacrificing one of his or her kidneys for an experimental surgery was unethical. What held true then, and today, is that with any radical change in the accepted paradigm, there will always be more critics than acceptors.

This timeline demonstrates some important principles. First, one cannot be sure that a large advance, such as the ability to repair arteries, will necessarily rapidly lead to the next step. Second, scientific discovery may not become common practice quickly; there is normally a lag between the publication of the discovery and acceptance by the majority.

Through the 1960s and 1970s, solid organ transplantation (SOT) advanced. It became clear that transplantation represented a potential new frontier in reconstructive surgery. An attempt at a human HT was carried out in Ecuador in 1964 using azathioprine and steroids for immunosuppression. At this time, there was no animal experimentation that indicated HT might be successful. The transplant failed within weeks, and the patient nearly lost his life.

This HT sent a clear signal that composite tissue was different from solid organ, and conventional wisdom for the next 40 years was that that skin and composite tissue were highly antigenic and could not be easily transplanted. However, this interpretation was overly pessimistic. When an experiment has a spectacular failure, it produces a correspondingly strong interpretation.

The discovery of cyclosporine seemed to offer hope that this wonder drug could solve the riddle of transplanting composite tissue. By the end of the 1970s and into the 1980s, there was both small and large animal work on extremity transplantation using cyclosporine.

In small animals, the preferred experimental model was a hind limb transplant with cyclosporine immunosuppression. Across a moderate immunologic barrier, long-term survival was demonstrated, but high success rates were never established across stronger immunologic barriers (3–5). Other studies were flawed by the fundamental assumption that lifelong immunosuppression would not be possible in HT. Therefore, in many experimental animal models, immunosuppression was stopped after several months. Not surprisingly, these transplants did poorly.

The origin of this erroneous assumption was based on two rationales. The first was that it was unethical to subject a human to a life-shortening medication for a non–life-extending transplant; the second was that allograft loss and patient mortality rates were too high with continuous immunosuppression. Both of these assumptions would be proved wrong. Scholarly work would demonstrate that subjecting a patient to immunosuppression for a non–life-extending transplant was ethical (6). Complications in hand transplant patients are less than predicted (7). Critics of HT overlooked that transplanting into a healthy patient produces fewer complications (particularly in terms of mortality) compared with SOT into unhealthy patients with preexisting organ failure. These faulty assumptions fundamentally influenced the basic research models and delayed the development of HT.

Despite the poor results in these small animal models, there were attempts to use nonhuman primate models in the 1980s, but these also failed (8–12). In one study, the animals were immunosuppressed with steroids and cyclosporine. The levels of cyclosporine needed to prevent acute rejection were 1000 to 1200 ng/mL, but a human renal transplant requires approximately 250 ng/mL. This discrepancy was assumed to be secondary to the antigenicity of skin. Other researchers had similar results, drawing the same conclusions. This assumption would later be found to be completely wrong, but it would take another 15 years before this would be demonstrated.

Small animal models of composite tissue transplantation continued through the 1990s with little success, until suddenly, in 1995, one study produced a successful outcome. This study was carried out using a rat hind limb model with cyclosporine and mycophenolate mofetil (MMF) and long-term survival was established (13).

At the same time in Louisville, we were trying to transplant composite tissues in pigs, starting with the assumption that using routine systemic immunosuppression would fail. Therefore, we administered immunosuppressant locally to the transplanted limb. We set up a negative control group of transplanted limbs using systemic tacrolimus and MMF, with the same level of immunosuppression as used in kidney transplantation. We naturally assumed that this would result in rejection of the transplanted limb in this control group because nonhuman primate studies in the previous decade had all failed with levels of immunosuppression that were much higher than those used in our study. To our surprise, the limbs transplanted with routine levels of immunosuppression survived (68).

This was a stunning revelation; for the first time, composite tissue had been successfully transplanted in a large animal model. The addition of MMF to a calcineurin inhibitor appears to have significantly helped survival, and human kidney-level immunosuppression was all that was needed. This study stood in juxtaposition to the nonhuman primate results. Why nonhuman primates require higher levels of immunosuppression still remains unclear, but the recent results from nonhuman primate face transplants confirm these findings (14).

The Louisville study demonstrated how serendipitously a chance finding can be perceived by an outside observer as intelligent design. We used pigs rather than nonhuman primates because of cost constraints, and initially, the negative control group was not even part of the study; we thought that it was a waste of money to demonstrate that routine levels of immunosuppression would not sustain composite tissue transplantation. We did not anticipate that there would be a difference in immunosuppression efficacy between the two animal species.

Both large and small animal models had now demonstrated successful composite tissue transplantation, suggesting that human HT might be possible. By 1998, bone, joint, nerve, muscle, and skin had also all been individually transplanted in humans. Considering these facts, performing a human HT did not seem such a paradigm shift.

The definition of an experiment is that the outcome is unpredictable (i.e., there is uncertainty). As the uncertainty decreases, the probability increases that the procedure should be standard of care.

There have now been at least 84 HTs carried out across the world. The results of single and bilateral HT are very good and predictable, with the use of routine levels of immunosuppression. This means steroids, a calcineurin inhibitor, and a mammalian target of rapamycin (mTOR) or purine synthesis inhibitor. It is our belief that following this protocol, a single or bilateral hand transplant at the mid to distal forearm is standard of care.

Other categories of HT remain an experiment. These include HTs above the elbow, transplants of two hands and a face, transplants of two hands and two legs, single leg transplants, and finally transplanting hands using reduced levels of immunosuppression and nonmodified bone marrow infusion to induce tolerance.

The numbers of patients within these subcategories transplanted to date are small, but the results are poor. A number of patients have died after face with bilateral hand or multiple limb transplants. The numbers of patients with above-elbow transplantation are so few that outcomes remain unclear.

The results of HTs carried out with unmodified donor bone marrow transplantation (the "Pittsburgh protocol") are reported as successful (15). However, this report indicates that some of the patients have low glomerular filtration rates (GFRs) and high creatinines. We need to see the long-term outcome to be assured that this approach is not nephrotoxic.

In conclusion, we believe that the initial stage of animal and human experimentation on HT is complete. We know in rats, pigs, and nonhuman primates the levels and combination of immunosuppression that are necessary to maintain tissue survival. We also know that single and bilateral HT outcomes and complications are predictable and acceptable.

However, the results are less clear in more extensive VCA. The results are poor in multiple extremity transplants, in face plus extremity transplants, and with the use of unmodified bone marrow in HT. However, the numbers in these categories are low, and most of the complications have occurred in the early postoperative period. This implies planning, surgical, or infective or anesthetic problems, more than immunosuppressive problems. In the Pittsburgh protocol study, two patients facing amputation have problems unrelated to tolerance induction. Uncertainty remains high in this area. We need to increase our understanding of the difficulties and problems of carrying out large amounts of composite tissue transplantation, and we will need many more numbers of transplants with unmodified donor bone marrow before we will have any clarity as to its outcome.

In our opinion, at this time, only single or bilateral HT below the elbow should be considered standard of care. All of the other VCAs at this time must be considered investigational.

It seems clear that there are three competing ideas as to where human research in VCA should proceed. The first is reduction of immunosuppression, the second is tolerance induction, and the third is transferring larger amounts of composite tissue in patients who have devastating injuries. All three of these human experiments are currently underway but each with limited numbers.

A word of caution is in order. Obtaining answers will not be possible without multicenter collaboration and honest, timely announcements of outcome. From the first arterial repair to the first kidney transplant took 40 years. From the first kidney transplant to the first HT took another 40 years. Without a breakthrough in immunosuppression reduction, this field will remain the domain of a very few patients. We should work hard to make sure it is not another 40 years before our field reaches its full potential.

INDICATIONS FOR HAND TRANSPLANTATION

Solid organ transplantation may not always lead to extension of life, but it always has the potential to do so. This is not the case with VCA; it is a quality of life transplant, and this is fundamental when considering indications for transplantation.

The indications and contraindications for hand and arm transplantation are not well established and vary among transplant centers. There are no absolute indications, but the broad boundaries are clear, and each center is likely to address all inclusion and exclusion criteria based on local SOT guidelines.

Should HT indications be the same, less, or more specific, than SOT? We practice and recommend inclusion and exclusion criteria that are more conservative than those in SOT, but each center must make its own decision, particularly dependent on whether the procedure is being done as standard of care or as an experiment. Clearly, in the former case, one's indications are more conservative than in the latter, where criteria will be expanded to allow the experimental component of the procedure. We suggest that exclusion criteria consist of:

- Age younger than 18 years or older than 60 years
- Poor health: diabetes, cardiac history, hepatitis C, coagulopathies hematologic diseases, collagen vascular disorders, connective tissue disorders
- Conditions that affect the immunomodulatory protocol: chronic infections HIV, malignancy
- Preexisting immunologic deficiencies

Inclusion criteria should include:

- Ages 18 to 60 years
- Good health
- No malignancies
- Family support

- Appropriate psychological profile
- If the hand is amputated, experience with prosthesis use
- 6 months since loss of hand function

These guidelines are our opinion at this time, and as results continue to accumulate, indications may change. Furthermore, we may overrule one of our inclusion or exclusion criteria in certain cases. We judge each person individually, and in some categories such as age, single versus bilateral HT, and health state, there is disagreement and debate among experts. Reasonable physicians can look at the same patient and come to different conclusions regarding HT.

Is a 40-year-old surgeon with a unilateral nondominant hand amputation, with limited family support, a better or worse candidate than a 60-year-old bilateral hand amputee retired surgeon with good family support and no health problems? Different programs might arrive at different conclusions.

Age

This is debatable. Technically, HT can be performed at any age. Heart and liver transplants are being performed successfully in children. The youngest HT was performed in Malaysia in 2000 on a 1-month-old baby with a severe limb deformity. The donor limb was taken from a deceased identical twin, so no immunosuppression was needed. This patient is doing well but is the only pediatric VCA recipient to date.

This case really only supports pediatric HT between identical twins, however. The danger with human leukocyte antigen (HLA) mismatch transplantation in an adolescent is the increased probability of posttransplant lymphoproliferative disorder (PTLD). The incidence of PTLD is normally higher in SOT children than adults (5%–10% vs. 0.5%), but the chance of PTLD is influenced not only by HLA mismatch and age but also by immunosuppression load and type of transplants. Therefore, these percentages can vary depending on the variables listed (16). The risk of death with PTLD is 50%. Transplantation for a life-extending organ makes the risk-to-benefit equation acceptable for the pediatric age group; in VCA, it is debatable depending on the factors discussed.

There are other possible contraindications for hand and arm transplantation in children. First, we believe that children are less compliant than adults with physical therapy and bracing. Reports on tendon repair in children initially recommended immobilization, but recent reports demonstrate good results with early mobilization (17). Second, the parents are giving consent to potentially shorten their child's life to gain an increase in quality of life; this raises certain ethical issues around informed consent.

At the other end of the spectrum, should older age be an exclusion criterion? Such age limits seem appropriate in most cases of SOT. In renal transplant, there is a demand surplus for a limited resource, with 35,000 patients on the waiting list seeking one of the 8000 donor kidneys. In this case, increasing age and poor health may render that individual at a competitive disadvantage.

There are few donors and even fewer recipients for hand transplant, but the surplus is not large. Donors are scarce because some families perceive donating a hand as mutilation of their loved one, and transplant candidates are scarce because immunosuppression in aggregate shortens life. But there is probably a small donor excess to recipients. This donor surplus means we do have more leeway to relax some criteria, such as age.

Tumors

Although benign tumors are not a contraindication, malignant tumors for the most part are contraindications because immunosuppression can lead to recurrence. Certain low-grade malignant tumors (basal cell carcinoma, isolated low-grade squamous cell carcinoma) with a sufficient tumor-free interval of 5 years may be acceptable candidates.

Etiology of Prior Injury

Should one transplant a patient, if the hand is present but not functional? The sixth patient transplanted in Louisville had two nonfunctional hands secondary to burns. We believe this is a good indication for a transplant because this allows individual functioning elements of the damaged hand to be used. The nerves in particular should not be discarded in this situation because they can be extended from the recipient to get closer to the target muscle in the donated limb (Figure 77-1).

In traumatic injuries, a guillotine amputation is a more favorable indication to an avulsion, but there is no absolute contraindication. The most important issues in the recipient are the function of the recipient muscles and the quality of the tendons.

Level of Amputation

This is debatable. One must determine the level of amputation acceptable for transplant. The more proximal one goes, the less evidence there is that a good outcome can be obtained. We favor transplantation at the level of the distal forearm, where recipient tendons and innervated muscles are present. At this level, there are reports of favorable outcome (18,19). Going proximal to this can be problematic, and there are too few cases to be sure of outcome. However, there is some early evidence that proximal forearm results may obtain good function.

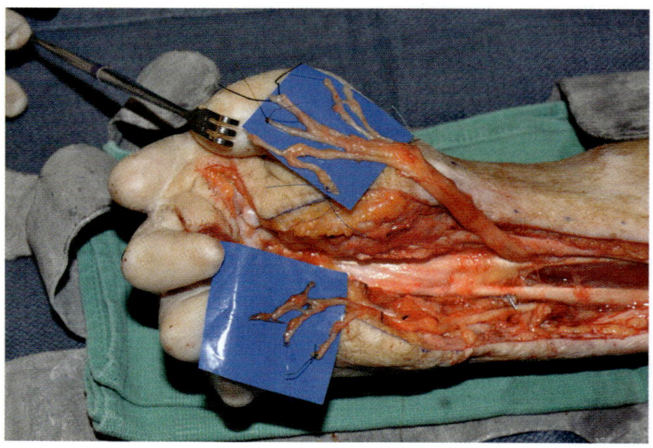

FIGURE 77-1 Recipient right hand that is to be amputated secondary to severe burn. Recipient nerves have been dissected out of the median and ulnar nerves to target the donor nerves.

Congenital Deformity

Even though there have been no transplants performed on a patient with congenital deformity, hand and arm transplantation may be a good option for these patients. Major limiting factors would be the functional status of the recipient limb and the type of congenital deformity. If the recipient arm is missing functional structures, the transplantation will be unsuccessful. Constriction ring syndrome would probably be the best indication because of the normal development of proximal structures. There is no guarantee of functional return to donor structures that were missing since birth. Cortical reorganization in adult HTs is well demonstrated (20), but what will happen with reinnervation in congenitally absent limbs is unknown.

Medical Status

This is debatable. It is widely considered that poor medical status is a contraindication for hand and arm transplantation. HT outcomes have exceeded expectations, partly because we transplant into healthy individuals, but SOT is, by definition, performed on patients in organ failure. Healthy individuals tolerate immunosuppression better than chronically sick SOT patients. Established metabolic, vascular, coagulopathic, and cardiac diseases are therefore potential contraindications for VCA. Some centers prefer not to perform HT in patients who have connective tissue disorder, but because some immunosuppressive medications are used to treat those disorders, there may be some appropriate cases (21).

That said, the first HT recipient in the United States had diabetes. He has done extremely well with no change in his HbA1C, and at more than 14 years since surgery, he is the longest surviving VCA recipient in the world. This emphasizes the critical point that finding the perfect patient is rarely possible, and choosing trade-offs well will determine the success of the transplant.

Psychosocial Factors

Psychological assessment before transplantation is crucial. Experienced transplant psychiatrists, psychologists, and social workers must evaluate all potential recipients and assess their family support. In SOT, there is no preferred personality profile, but there is ample evidence that 20% to 30% of patients are noncompliant (22,23). In lifesaving SOT, transplanting into a patient with a less than perfect personality profile may be justified. In HT, there is no such justification. One must also not transplant a patient if there is any question that he or she may not be able to pay for immunosuppression at some time in the future. This means a thorough evaluation of the patient's work situation and insurance is necessary.

The ideal patient is intelligent and has a stable family, no history of addictions, and a steady job with insurance. They are mildly obsessive-compulsive, with low histrionics and not so narcissistic that they refuse to follow physician recommendations. That said, there is no perfect patient, and although there will always be trade-offs, choose these carefully. Try not to replicate the mistakes made with the first French patient. Here was a patient who was under criminal indictment, who was previously incarcerated and accidently cut off his hand while in jail. The hand was initially replanted, but the replant did not achieve good function, so it was amputated. After release from jail, he initially contacted the Louisville team, but the senior author refused to consider him as a candidate. Subsequently, and even after indictment for a further felony in Australia, he was accepted for HT in France. After his transplant, he stated on national television that he knew more than his physicians (suggesting a narcissistic personality disorder). Was there no better candidate available?

We believe that the psychological profile is more important than medical status, anatomical defect, or perceived utility. That is why for the first American transplant, we selected a patient who had a metabolic disorder and a single hand defect. We turned down bilateral amputees and younger, healthier patients to capture the best family and personality profile. We were determined to avoid repeating the French problem.

Infections, Hepatitis, and HIV

These are debatable. Because the immunosuppressive regimens debilitate the immune system, active viral, bacterial, or fungal infections are usually contraindicated for hand and arm transplantation. However, SOT is done on patients with HIV and hepatitis, and so, in theory, HT could be done in patients with these viral infections. Yet although a patient with hepatitis will die without a liver transplant, the same is not true of HT, and the need for a hand would have to be considerable to justify the risks.

Epstein-Barr Virus Status

This is debatable. An Epstein-Barr virus (EBV)–positive donor to an EBV-negative recipient can lead to EBV viremia in the recipient, increasing the probability of PTLD. Therefore, some programs will not transplant an EBV-positive donor into an EBV-negative recipient but will wait for an EBV-negative donor. The problem is that a significant portion of the population is EBV positive, and therefore wait time may be prolonged (24).

Tattoos

A recipient accepting a HT from a donor with any tattoos runs the risk of HIV and hepatitis; this is more likely if done while the donor was incarcerated. Therefore, we recommend a 6-month interval after the tattoo and appropriate robust testing.

Single or Bilateral Hand

There is an active debate regarding single or bilateral hand and arm transplantation; although we believe there should be no such debate, others disagree (25).

When a program or government agency states that only bilateral HT should be done, they make single hand amputation an exclusion criterion. They are stating that there is not one single patient in the world who would gain more utility (health value) from a HT than all the bilateral HTs ever done or to be done. A priori, as a position, this sounds ridiculous, but it is also demonstrated to be wrong.

The real-world experience is that single HT does produce a higher value health state in some cases than in bilateral HT and vice versa. There are some single HTs with higher Disabilities of the Arm, Shoulder and Hand (DASH) scores than some bilateral HTs. The first two patients who underwent HT in Louisville have much higher DASH scores than some of the bilateral HTs done in China and in France.

As a physician, you have the right and obligation to limit treatment as you see appropriate, but if you will not transplant a patient who requests a single hand transplant, consider referring those patients to a team who will.

Human Leukocyte Antigen and Blood Type

Blood type mismatch is an absolute contraindication, and cross-matching has to be performed before any transplantation attempt (26–28). HLA mismatch, however, is not a contraindication for hand and arm transplantation. The first transplantation in the world had 6 of 6 HLA mismatches, and most hand transplant patients have shown 3 of 6 or more mismatches.

Blindness

This is an interesting factor because a blind patient missing both hands is clearly severely debilitated, but transplanting such a patient is not standard of care because it remains unknown if it will improve the health utility of a blind patient. As an experiment, it is intriguing. Can a blind person missing both hands regain some new substitute vision through the hands? There was a bilateral HT done on a patient in Austria who later developed blindness. His outcome should be followed closely (29).

Antibodies

Potential recipients who have antibodies from blood transfusion or previous transplants present a problem. Such patients often undergo SOT with very high antibody levels, but this can be an immunosuppression management problem, and the failure rate is higher in such patients. Because HT is not life extending, there have to be strong indications to transplant a highly sensitized patient.

PROCUREMENT OF THE DONOR HAND OR ARM

As of July 2014, VCA is now regulated by the United Network of Organ Sharing (UNOS). UNOS now governs the private organ procurement organizations, of which there are 58 in the United States. Specially trained OPO coordinators obtain consent from the family, usually after consent for solid organ harvest has been obtained; this can be a more delicate process, with consideration that tissue that can maintain some donor visual identity, including the fingerprints.

Potential donors are evaluated for a number of characteristics to assess suitability: ABO match or compatibility is essential, donors should be of a similar age to the intended recipient, gender is optional, and hair distribution and skin color should ideally match the recipient. Currently, HLA matching is not required, but the donor should preferably be cytomegalovirus (CMV) negative. Some teams will not transplant a CMV-positive donor into a CMV-negative recipient.

The limb recovery surgical team should discuss the order of organ harvest with the other recovery teams. Limb recovery should not jeopardize solid organ procurement. Therefore, the impulse is to place the limb harvest last. But hand procurement is a much easier procedure than other organs and should be completed in 30 minutes, with minimal blood loss. Therefore, limb procurement can precede solid organ procurement, or it can be carried out simultaneously.

Whereas the anatomical level of harvest is determined by the recipient's needs, for a forearm or hand transplant, the approach is performed at the level of the elbow to maximize the tissue available for reconstruction. A fishmouth incision is made, and the cephalic and brachial veins are first dissected with maximal length for possible vein grafting. The medial and lateral antebrachial cutaneous nerves are next dissected, followed by the brachial artery, veins and median nerve. The radial and ulnar nerves are then separated before subperiosteal elevation of the common extensor and flexor origins. The biceps, brachialis, and triceps tendons are divided before elbow capsulotomy and disarticulation. All structures are tagged and labeled as they are delivered. The vessels should be tied off, and the procurement team should ensure neat closure of the donor wound. A cosmetic prosthesis should be provided if the family wishes.

After initial boluses to flush the limb, a constant infusion of University of Wisconsin solution or histidine-tryptophan-ketoglutarate (HTK) solution, via a brachial artery ball tip cannula, helps decrease cellular injury and edema (Figure 77-2). Rapid temperature reduction to 4°C to slow tissue metabolism is also achieved by sterile dry wrapping in an ice cooler for transfer. Cold ischemia time may be minimized by air transfer.

The Ideal Team and Surgical Technique for Hand Transplantation

The surgical technique for HT is technically very similar to any major hand or forearm replantation, and detailed descriptions have already been published (30–36). We will reiterate some of

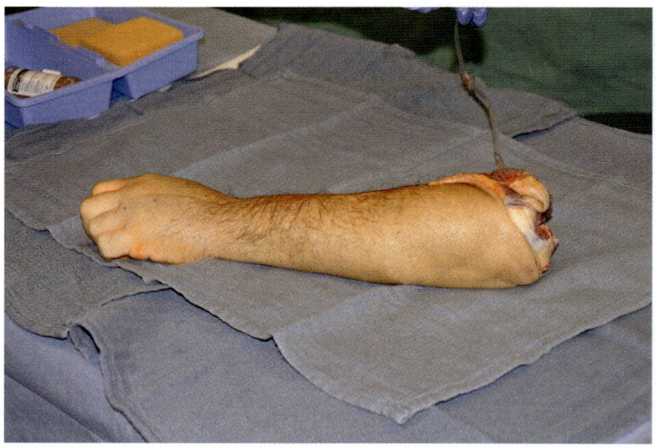

FIGURE 77-2 Donor arm on arrival in the operating room perfused with University of Wisconsin solution from the time of amputation through transit.

the key points, highlighting where we disagree, believe there were omissions, or consider them important enough to emphasize again.

Experience and Numbers

The success of the surgical component of HT depends on two key variables, the experience and number of surgeons on the team. Experience of HT alone is not enough; the number of experienced surgeons also matters. If a HT is to fail, it should not be because of fatigue or lack of experience.

Each hand transplanted will take between 8 and 16 hours. For each hand, a team should ideally have at least four microsurgeons, who can rotate every 3 to 4 hours. This means that in a 16-hour case, there must be two teams consisting of two surgeons each. Each team would operate 8 of the hours, divided into two shifts. A bilateral transplant requires a minimum of eight surgeons. At the beginning of the procedure, it may also be necessary for the donor and recipient to be dissected at the same time. Therefore, a bilateral transplant requires eight surgeons in the room at the same time; a unilateral transplant requires four. The addition of anesthesia, circulators, and scrub nurses means the operating room will be crowded. Before undertaking HT, operating room organization and rehearsal are vital.

Facility and Instrumentation

Structure is more important than content. A moderately experienced team working in an excellent hospital with experienced operating room nurses, anesthesia, intensive care unit, and access to quality instruments and microscopes has a reasonable chance of success. Good surgeons cannot always overcome poor support structure and poor instruments, and one should not even attempt the transplant until the structure is in place and ready.

Preoperative Planning

The preparation of the recipient and donor arms is a key stage of the procedure. HT is a semi-emergency process—the recipient patient is ready and waiting for a donor arm. As soon as the donor tissue becomes available, the patient is admitted to the hospital, and preparations are commenced. Anesthesia will not be induced, however, until the donor arm is brought to the hospital and blood cross-matching is performed.

Besides all necessary general instruments, the surgeon should ensure that three high-quality microsurgical instrument sets, an ultrasound device with sterile probes, a mini C-arm, solution warmers, heparinized solutions, a surgical microscope, and plates for bone fixation are ready in the operating room.

The length of the forearm and the position of the osteotomy have to be determined preoperatively. In a single HT, the opposite side can be used to determine the length. If bilateral transplantation is performed, attention must be given not to fashion the arms too short or too long. The length of the foot is roughly the same length as the forearm, and this may be used to assist decision making.

Recipient Arm Preparation

The recipient forearm incision is placed in a radial-ulnar orientation. If the transplantation level is distal midforearm, the median, ulnar, and superficial branch of the radial nerve with the radial and ulnar arteries are dissected out. The forearm muscles are prepared with their tendons, maximizing all tendon lengths. After dissection, all structures are labeled. The osteotomy levels are marked and then performed with an oscillating saw using copious water irrigation to prevent heat necrosis of the bone ends.

Osteosynthesis

Hand transplantation osteosynthesis is no different from any forearm fracture fixation. We prefer 3.5-mm locking plates on the volar side of the forearm, ensuring at least six-cortices of fixation on each side of the radial and ulnar osteotomies. Strict attention must be paid to the axial and longitudinal alignment so they do not interfere with the rotation of the forearm. Firm fixation must be achieved following AO principles before vascular anastomosis is commenced.

Vascular Anastomosis

Before vascular connection, the hand can be flushed with warm saline to help prevent vasospasm. The ulnar artery and large-caliber veins are first clamped to decrease blood loss. The cephalic vein and one other dorsal vein are then connected before the radial arterial anastomosis is performed. We prefer to use 8-0 nylon for end-to-end arterial and venous anastomoses under the operative microscope.

Our six patients all received transplantation at the midforearm level using two different techniques for arterial connection. Individual radial and ulnar artery anastomoses at the midforearm level were performed for the first three patients, but brachial artery anastomosis was performed at the level of elbow for patients 4, 5, and 6, with extensive dissection of the arteries from the midforearm to elbow. The adventitia was not removed, as was reported (37). The artery was then anastomosed end to side into the recipient brachial artery. Patient 4 lost his hand, and 6 developed severe ischemia that resolved after small finger and thumb partial necrosis requiring limited amputation. We believe that isolation of long lengths of artery may be responsible for those ischemic processes and should be avoided.

After connecting the ulnar artery, the maximum possible number of veins should be anastomosed to assist drainage.

Tendon Repairs

We recommend that the HT should be performed either through the tendinous portion of the forearm or for more proximal transplants that require donor muscle via attachment to the medial and lateral epicondyles of the humerus with bone anchors.

The order of repair of tendons is debated. Some teams do the extensors first and the flexors second. Others do the opposite. We do the flexors first because we believe the setting of this cascade is a little more complex and important than the extensors. We perform the flexor tendon repair with the wrist in neutral position and aim for progressively more flexion from the index through small fingers to produce the normal resting cascade. Those who start with the extensors believe this helps better establish the amount of flexor tension (i.e., enough to overcome extensor tension). We prefer Pulvertaft weaves for both flexors and extensor tendon repairs using 3-0 polyester sutures.

The extensor repairs are performed with the wrist in 30 degrees of extension, the metacarpophalangeal (MCP) joints flexed to 70 degrees, and all interphalangeal (IP) joints fully extended. The finger cascade is checked and the wrist is flexed to see the tenodesis effect on MCP and PIP joint extension. Any tight or loose repairs should be addressed at this time. When the wrist is flexed to 30 degrees, the flexor tension should allow spontaneous finger extension. When the wrist is extended to 30 degrees, the normal flexor tendon cascade should be reproduced.

Nerve Repair

The median, ulnar, and superficial branch of the radial nerves are then connected without tension, ensuring accurate orientation of the median and ulnar nerve fascicles. Obviously, if the recipient has a burned or damaged hand with functioning nerves, these should be saved and targeted as close to the muscle as possible (Figure 77-3). If the transplantation is in flexor zone 5, connection of the palmar cutaneous branch of the median nerve is recommended.

Skin Closure

Before skin closure, at least two more veins should be anastomosed on the dorsal side to assist venous outflow. If the patient does not have skin lesions such as burns, perfectly designed skin flaps should allow full coverage. If required, split-thickness skin grafts may be used on muscle bellies for closure, but their use on flexor tendons should be avoided. Skin can be closed without drains if meticulous hemostasis is achieved. Skin staples should be used to decrease the time of closure.

Finally, a bulky petroleum gauze dressing and dorsal block long arm splint are applied to secure the repairs and decrease the pain. The arm should be elevated and the patient transferred to intensive care unit.

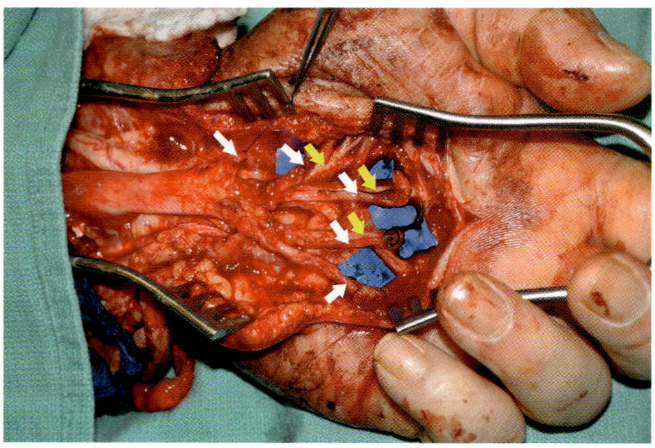

FIGURE 77-3 The donor left hand is attached to the recipient. The recipient digital nerves are marked with white arrows, and they are overlapping the donor nerves (yellow arrows). As the photograph demonstrates, the recipient nerves were targeted as far distal as possible in the donor. Nerve repair has not yet been performed.

Postoperative Monitoring

For HT postoperative monitoring we use temperature checks every hour for 24 hours, skin color assessment, capillary refill checks, and an ultrasound probe to check the arterial flow.

The patient is kept NPO for 12 hours in case of possible redo anastomoses; however, because the arterial anastomoses are performed in the early stage of the surgery, most complications are encountered in the operative room and can be managed.

Surgical Pearls and Pitfalls

1. Do not assume that by returning the arm to its proper length, it guarantees the tendons will fit appropriately. If both the donor and recipient have very distal musculotendinous junctions and the recipient's amputation is rather proximal, then tendon length will be inadequate. Bone length may need to be shortened to achieve tendon repair. Of course, if this happens, it means that the advantage of a Pulvertaft weave would be lost. The end-to-end standard tendon repair is not as strong as a Pulvertaft weave. In one case HT, we used recipient tendons to augment the repair in a Pulvertaft fashion.
2. One should strive to return the forearms to their original length, if possible, to avoid a lifetime requirement for shirtsleeve tailoring for the unilateral patient and a complete wardrobe change of shirts for the bilateral arm.
3. All tendons on the donor and recipient should be clearly labeled as the two teams dissect them out. It can be hard to identify some of the structures, particularly with scarring and atrophy proximally in the recipient.
4. In a replant, the tissue is damaged on both sides. In a transplant, the donor is pristine, and all tissues are atraumatically prepared; on the recipient side, the converse is true. They are badly scarred and occasionally atrophic. The vessels have sometimes not functioned for many years, and individual muscles may be hard to recognize. Sometimes tendons or muscles are absent or not identifiable, requiring immediate tendon transfer. There is skill involved in finding the structures and deciding what to do when they cannot be found or are inadequate.
5. Unlike a replant, the order of repair is changed in a HT to reduce ischemia time. After the bone is fixed, one arterial anastomosis and at least one vein are then completed before attention is turned to tendon and nerves. The Pittsburgh team recommends that in a distal transplant, the order should be more like a replant,

namely, osteosynthesis, extensor tendons, veins, and nerve, and only then the volar arteries. They properly point out that this avoids blood loss, allowing one to operate in a bloodless field, facilitating fascicular nerve repair. They believe that in a distal transplant, ischemia time is better tolerated (36).

We have no evidence that a HT can tolerate ischemia the same as a replant. Both HT and replant suffer ischemia reperfusion injury. But HT has the added injury of allorecognition and rejection. The effect of this additional burden on shortening tolerable ischemia time remains unknown. In the absence of accurate knowledge, the safest approach is to shorten ischemia time as much as possible.

Blood loss can be a real problem. The Pittsburgh team lost 30 units of blood repairing the artery early in the procedure of a bilateral HT. This led them to recommend returning to the classic replant order of repair.
A prolonged ischemia time can equally be a problem; we prefer to do as much as possible of the procedure without a tourniquet to minimize ischemia reperfusion injury. In a heart transplant, more than 4 hours of ischemia markedly increases the likelihood of failure.

The total ischemia time tolerated by a composite tissue remains unknown; all of the patients undergoing transplantation in Louisville had more than 4 hours of cold ischemia. Each program must make a decision. Do you want to make it easier to operate in a bloodless field and reduce the chance of massive blood loss? Or do you want to avoid ischemia reperfusion injury by operating with the tourniquet down as much as possible but run the risk of blood loss?

6. If there is a gap in the artery or vein that requires a graft, do not use donor artery or vein; use recipient. The reason for this is that donor artery and vein are more prone to intimal hyperplasia, particularly if a long segment is used.
7. Skin incisions should be medial and lateral on the recipient and dorsal and volar on the donor. This allows the flaps to be rotated from the donor into the medial and lateral position on the recipient, giving plenty of tissue for coverage. It also places most of the flaps over the dorsal and volar surface, away from the flexor and extensor tendon repairs. There rarely should be a need for a skin graft to achieve closure, but long flaps have a tendency to develop seromas, and some judgment is necessary.
8. In a functionless (e.g., burned) hand, the underlying nerves should be maintained, so that the nerve repairs can be done as close to the target muscles as possible. The amputation can be done through the distal radius and ulna, and the donor hand can be opened to allow the nerve repairs to be done as far distal as possible.
9. A midpalm amputation can be reconstructed with two different techniques: as a midpalmar or a distal radius transplant. It remains undefined which of these is the better option.
10. Distal forearm amputations are an established level for hand transplantation with known outcomes. These should be considered the standard of care treatment for an amputee. Midforearm amputees are more problematic, and the functional innervation of remaining muscles will determine outcome. At the proximal forearm, the management becomes dependent on muscle reinnervation. If there is enough functioning muscle, then the transplant should be done at the amputation level. Again, at this level, we believe transplant is standard of care.

If there is no functioning muscle but there is a functioning elbow, there are only two options: maintain the elbow and drape and anchor the donor muscle over the medial and lateral epicondyles and then repair the recipient and donor nerves as close as possible to donor muscle (this is what the University of Pennsylvania team did in their first bilateral case, and they obtained good results). The other option is to discard the elbow and amputate through the distal humerus. There are not enough patients done at this level to determine which, if either, of these techniques can generate good, reproducible results.

More proximal amputations obviously can and have been done, but as one progresses more proximally, reinnervation becomes more of a problem.

IMMUNOSUPPRESSION

Most reconstructive surgeons have limited experience in managing immunosuppression. Therefore, your immediate response may be to abdicate this to your transplant surgeon or nephrologist. To do so would be an error because it limits you to being a technician and, more important, it removes your input into modifying how the immunosuppression should be used in VCA as opposed to SOT. There are differences, and in some cases, only the reconstructive surgeon can see this.

Consider one of the Louisville patients, who started to develop avascular necrosis (AVN) of the hip and when there was still time to consider a decompression procedure with bone grafting to prevent hip replacement. As reconstructive surgeons, we believed this was a decision that the patient should make, but the SOT surgeons did not understand this logic and thought that any such consideration was inappropriate, and there was no consideration given to stopping the steroids and attempting a hip salvage procedure. In their world, the use of steroids resulted in AVN of the hip in 5% to 8% of patients, and they routinely proceeded directly to hip replacement.

These conceptual differences arose out of dissimilar frames of references that produce specialty specific bias (38): each specialty develops its own methodology and continues to follow it even when the underlying circumstances have changed. SOT surgeons are, in the majority of cases, working with life extension. To risk loss of life to save a hip was incomprehensible. Yet even though they knew that HT was never a life-extending procedure, it was difficult for them to consider stopping steroids and risking losing the hand to save the hip.

Although understanding the action and the dose of an immunosuppressive agent is mainly in the domain of transplant surgeons or nephrologists, reconstructive surgeons must know enough about immunosuppressive therapy to be active partners in these complex decisions. There will be many situations when constructive discussions between both disciplines will serve the patient best and help to avoid specialty-specific bias. This requires that hand surgeons must have some understanding of immunosuppression, and transplant surgeons must learn something about hand surgery.

When the senior author formed the initial HT group in Louisville, there was a classic exchange between hand surgeons and transplant surgeons that demonstrates the point. At the first meeting to start considering a HT project, the hand surgeons were shocked to hear that the transplant surgeons felt confident that modern immunosuppression would most likely prevent hand allograft rejection. The transplant surgeons were shocked to hear that we believed that an extremely functional hand could be obtained from a completely severed hand. Working together will close the information gap and prevent specialty-specific bias.

Immunosuppression for Vascularized Composite Allotransplantation

The standard cocktail of immunosuppression in hand and face transplantation consists of an induction agent, a calcineurin inhibitor, an antimetabolite, and steroids. The most common induction agents used in VCA are alemtuzumab (Campath) and thymoglobulin. These agents act to eliminate a majority of the recipient's lymphocytes, which could reject the donor tissue. Thymoglobulin is specific for T cells; alemtuzumab also depletes B cells. These induction agents are used only in the initial few days or weeks. After this, the VCA recipient is maintained on the combination of a calcineurin inhibitor, antimetabolite, and steroids.

The goal of immunosuppression is to block T-cell activation caused by allogeneic stimulation. Calcineurin inhibitors block a step in the production of reactive T cells against the donor. They block an enzyme, calcineurin phosphatase, that is necessary to turn on promoter genes for a variety of cytokines that stimulate T-cell proliferation. Administration of these agents for the life of the allograft is necessary, but their use comes with a price: they are responsible for causing infections, hypertension, and diabetes, as well as being nephrotoxins.

The antimetabolites are less noxious but very important. There are two groups, those that block DNA synthesis and those that block the mTOR pathway. Mycophenolic acid (MPA) and azathioprine are DNA synthesis blockers. Sirolimus and everolimus are mTOR pathway inhibitors. All of these agents play a role in reducing T-cell proliferation. Their method of blocking T-cell activation is different from calcineurin inhibitors, and they may reduce chronic allograft damage in SOT. These agents also have toxicities. MPA may cause anemia, leukopenia, and diarrhea, and sirolimus and everolimus may produce hematologic toxicity and poor wound healing.

Some of the antimetabolites have a secondary action: they may block a step in the formation of intimal hyperplasia, known to be a major problem in cardiac transplantation and suspected to be a problem in renal transplantation. In VCA the concept of "chronic rejection" is still not clarified, but there is one reported case of HT loss secondary to intimal hyperplasia in the arteries (39).

The final commonly used agent is a corticosteroid. They are initiated immediately after transplantation and in very high doses but normally with rapid tapering. Patients are commonly maintained on a long-term low dose, but as with all immunosuppression, steroids cause problems, including diabetes, hyperlipidemia, infection, hypertension, and weight gain.

The reason for using three different immunosuppressive agents is twofold: each will act synergistically to increase efficacy, and they have little overlap in toxicity profiles. This allows for lower doses of each agent, as opposed to utilization of a single agent at much higher doses.

Over the past 2 decades, there have been many attempts to alter this classic regimen. These modifications can be broadly classified into three categories: steroid reduction, monotherapy, and use of donor bone marrow infusion.

Steroid reduction may be approached by two different methods, steroid sparing or elimination. In steroid sparing, the patient's steroids are reduced over months or even years. In steroid elimination, the steroids are stopped after the first 48 or 72 hours posttransplant. There is good evidence in renal transplantation that these methods work (40), but it remains unclear if these approaches can be easily applied to VCA.

The second modification is to use only one calcineurin inhibitor, referred to as monotherapy. The patient initially starts on the standard cocktail, but then over time is weaned off all drugs except for one calcineurin inhibitor. In some situations, this approach is successful, and it appears most applicable to liver transplantation. In some cases, the immunosuppression may be stopped completely; this is called operational tolerance.

Finally, some researchers are trying to introduce a tolerant state through the use of a donor bone marrow infusion. The donor bone marrow may be given either unmodified or modified (with the T cells that could cause graft-versus-host disease in the recipient removed). There are reported successes in SOT using these techniques (41). The Pittsburgh-Johns Hopkins group are treating all of their HT patients with bone marrow infusion and monotherapy. They have reported that these patients are doing well (42). This is the first time that monotherapy with donor bone marrow has demonstrated consistent clinical benefit.

HAND THERAPY AFTER HAND TRANSPLANT

Successful hand therapy outcomes after HT are dependent on several important factors.

The Role of the Patient

The emotional impact of HT on the patient must be well understood by the therapist, and the patient's motivation and involvement in his or her own case are imperative for positive success. The regimen should be individualized, but the patient needs to attend therapy at least 5 days a week for the first 3 months and perform exercises during every waking hour. In addition, it is the patient's responsibility to strictly adhere to the splinting protocol, and smoking should be strongly discouraged to minimize vasospasm.

The Role of the Therapist

The therapist's goals after HT should be to educate and involve the patients in their own individualized care while motivating and encouraging them in their own participatory obligations. Because they may see the new hand as "foreign" and not "their own" hand, the therapist should continually reinforce and strengthen the patient's perception of "their" hand at all times to help the patient emotionally accept and reinforce a positive sense of self and self-image.

The Therapeutic Approach

Proper splinting and early active range of motion are very important. Unlike therapy after a replant, in HT, the Pulvertaft weave tendon repairs are much stronger. This allows for movement starting on day 1. The patient should thus be placed in a custom splint as soon as possible to permit safe tendon gliding. Early motion through the repaired tendons will help not only to strengthen the repairs but also to prevent adhesions. Too much tensile force, however, will result in suture gapping and possible tendon rupture, but immobilized tendons tend to lose glide by 10 days after repair. Mobilized tendons are twice as strong as immobilized tendons at 3 weeks after surgery, and strength returns to around 50% of the original tendon strength at 12 weeks after surgery. This is adequate to perform more aggressive strengthening and most resistive activities of daily living.

The volar custom splint is fabricated with the wrist in neutral and the MCP joints blocked at 60 degrees flexion. Dynamic assistance toward the distal palmar crease (DPC) is provided with rubber band/monofilament/spring tension, and palmar pulleys are located just below the DPC, with full IP joint flexion assistance. The thumb is placed between palmar and radial abduction with a dynamic flexion assistance component and a dorsal block.

Tenodesis exercises are practiced in the clinic, first with the uninvolved hand to provide the patient a sense of what to expect, until the patient has a good sense of adequate force before he or she is instructed to continue with an unsupervised home exercise program. The patient is instructed to avoid any other hand or wrist motion during the early stages of therapy. The surrounding soft tissues will also respond negatively to an overzealous approach by creating more inflammation, pain, and undesired scar formation.

Edema control must be addressed on the first day of therapy because excessive swelling can contribute to vascular compression, reducing circulation to the healing tissues. Lymphatic drainage can be improved by controlled motion, light compression, kinesiotaping, proper positioning, pulsed ultrasound, myofascial release, low-level laser therapy, high-voltage pulsed current, and manual edema mobilization techniques.

Initial therapy should also focus on range of motion of the scapula, neck, shoulder, and elbow, allowing for the level of the surgical reconstruction. The forearm is passively mobilized through full pronation and supination along with passive elbow flexion and extension. Passive range of motion of the wrist and digits is initiated to prevent joint stiffness and help tendon gliding.

As the extrinsic muscles regain function, the hand should be placed with the thumb in an opponens splint to assist with light functional tasks. A lumbrical block splint should be used to block the MCP joints in flexion because the intrinsic muscles may not regain function for more than 1 year. Some dexterity tasks can be initiated, which will improve cortical stimulation and provide an improved sense of accomplishment for the patient. Extrinsic muscle function will be the main focus at this time, as well as consistent sensory and cortical stimulation techniques. Nerve regeneration may improve significantly with phototherapy or low-level laser therapy. Studies have shown that low-level laser therapy at 780 nm, directed at the level of the spinal cord, where the corresponding nerve nuclei are located, improves axonal sprouting, motor unit recruitment, and improves myelination of the injured nerve (43). Phototherapy acts at the cellular level to more than double adenosine triphosphate synthesis in the cell though a phenomenon called photobiomodulation (44).

The patient's motor cortex will also need consistent input through sensory reeducation, functional electrical stimulation, and focused controlled activation of the agonist muscles concurrent with functional electrical stimulation (45). The use of a mirror box can facilitate cortical stimulation because visualizing and undertaking symmetrical bilateral movements can enhance cortical changes within the brain (46).

Sensory return and intrinsic muscle function will continue for more than 1 year after HT, depending on the level of the amputation. The patient will need to continue a consistent home exercise program, sensory reeducation, and hand therapy throughout this recovery process.

HAND TRANSPLANT CLASSIFICATION BY INNERVATION LEVEL OF AMPUTATION

The classification of HT is by anatomical level: wrist, distal forearm, mid forearm, proximal forearm, elbow, and upper arm. In general, the more proximal the amputation, the worse the functional result, so we evaluate patient outcome as per anatomical level of transplantation. However, by using this intraoperative anatomical level, we lose the ability to properly classify the extent of the original injury because at a particular level, there may be widely different functional muscles present. Conversely, at two different transplant levels, there may be the same muscle function present. Omission of muscle function evaluation in conjunction with the anatomical level is a flaw in the present classification system.

The reasons for such muscle function variation are well understood. All patients are different, and there can be significant anatomical variation in muscle origin and insertion. The mechanism of injury may determine the number of functioning muscles remaining, but those remaining functional muscles may be completely different in similar amputations at the same level. Intraoperative decisions to debride muscle, remove tendon, weave a donor tendon or muscle into the stump of recipient muscle, or do a tendon transfer will all affect muscle function at a particular level. Equally, these decisions may vary among surgeons viewing the same defect.

We therefore believe that the anatomical transplant classification should be supplemented with detail indicating the amount of muscle function remaining at that level, but the problem with listing every muscle function at each level is classification clutter. If it is too complex, it becomes difficult to remember and is not used. Furthermore, it can be self-defeating, particularly in studies involving small numbers of patients: the more categories, the less likely the study is to have sufficient numbers to reach statistical significance.

Therefore, we recommend using a muscle function classification system that determines which large groups of muscles are innervated and functional. We refer to this as the muscle innervation transplant (MIT) classification system. Five rules need to be followed:

1. Every patient is classified by the level of denervation at the time of transplant.
2. Any muscle that is used to motor the donor hand is considered innervated except when the tendon only is used as part of a transfer.
3. Any tendon transfers used to substitute for a muscle is indicative that this muscle is not functional, and therefore the muscle substituted by the tendon transfer is listed as not functional.
4. Each level assumes denervation of the lower number levels.
5. Every upper extremity amputation must be placed, as best fits, into one of six classifications.

Level I: Hand intrinsics are not functional.
Level II: Pronator teres and thumb flexor are not functional.
Level III: Less than 49% of all flexors and extensors of the fingers and wrist are not functional.
Level IV: More than 50% of all flexors and extensors of the fingers and wrist are not functional.
Level V: All flexors, extensors, and pronator of the wrist and hand are not functional.
Level VI: Biceps or triceps are not functional.
Level VII: Biceps and triceps not functional.

The MIT classification system should be used in combination with the anatomical classification of transplantation. For example, a proximal-level transplant of the forearm could be associated with MIT being level III, IV, or possibly even V. A midhumeral transplantation could be MIT level V, VI, or VII. We believe that these data should be reported to the registry within several months of the transplantation.

This system would help us interpret the outcome of the first French transplant, which failed after 29 months. This was reported as a midforearm transplant, but there were two different reports regarding the forearm flexor and extensor muscle function. Some claimed the patient never had return of function, but there were reports that he initially gained function before losing it when he stopped taking his immunosuppression. The distinction is extremely important but only important if we understand the level of amputation in regards to the preoperative muscle innervation. If the amputation left the forearm flexors and extensors innervated, then it would imply that the rejection process resulted in damage to function long before it destroyed the soft tissue. If true, this is quite different from the finding in the fourth Louisville hand transplant. In this patient, slow formation of small vessel intimal hyperplasia resulted in occlusion and ischemic loss of the hand, but hand function remained stable, with good grip and feeling, until the time of amputation. In one case, we are told that rejection resulted in a loss of function before loss of the hand. In the second, we are told that function was maintained up to the point of amputation. It is vital to know whether we have two different phenomena taking place within a hand transplant suffering from rejection. Or, as some report, did the French HT patient never have function?

So does rejection first cause loss of function, similar to a kidney transplant, or does the hand transplant lose circulation, while function remains good to the very end? A report using MIT level and videos of active hand function would be extremely helpful in clarifying this issue. We recommend that all programs report both the level of transplantation and MIT level because classifying in this manner would better allow us to evaluate potential outcome.

OUTCOMES IN HAND TRANSPLANTATION

Allograft Survival

What is the probability of a successful outcome after HT? Table 77-1 lists all of the HTs completed in the modern era as far as we can ascertain. It is based on those listed in the hand registry (47), but it also includes cases that were carried out but have yet to be reported. There are some discrepancies between the registry and the Chinese data reported by Pei et al. (48). We have assumed the latter to be accurate. Where the Chinese data differs from the registry, we cannot ascertain the city. We have excluded one patient who underwent transplantation in Kuala Lumpur because this was a transplant between identical twins. We have also excluded a single thumb performed in China and all hands transplanted in conjunction with other composite tissue; the latter are listed in Table 77-2 (49,50).

Of the 84 single or bilateral hands transplanted across the world, 10 have failed (12%). Two of these were in the early postoperative period. There is a marked difference in allograft loss in China (43%) compared with the rest of the world (6%). We believe this is due to the difficulties in the Chinese medical system for patients both in follow-up and obtaining immunosuppression. But it is also possible that this is secondary to small sample size error. In some cases, we will refer to world experiences minus China and the Chinese experiences.

When a hand is combined with a face or leg transplant, the results are poor, and the complication rate in these cases is extremely high. The complications are not secondary to long-term immunosuppression but rather perioperative problems.

There have been two bilateral hand with face transplants (49). Both patients developed sepsis, and all four hands were lost. The Paris patient died from *Pseudomonas* infection; in the Boston case, there was a maxillary sinus abscess that was not recognized until after initiation of the transplant (69).

There has been one patient with both arms and both legs and another with both arms and one leg transplanted in Turkey. The first patient apparently died from a bleeding diathesis in the early postoperative period after massive blood loss of 300 units. The second is reported to have died from "heart and kidney failure" after severe urinary tract infection then systemic

TABLE 77-1 World Experience of Hand Transplants

Year	Single	Bilateral
1998	LYS	—
1999	SDF, CAN (2)	—
2000	China, TRN	LYS, INN, CAN
2001	SDF, TRN, China	HRB
2002	BRU, China, TRN	HRB
2003	China	INN, LYS
2004	China	—
2005	—	—
2006	WRO, SDF, China	INN, VLC
2007	—	SDF, VLC
2008	WRO, SDF (2)	MUC
2009	PIT, WRO (2), INN	CDG, SDF, PIT
2010	PIT, SAT, WRO	PIT (2), SDF, WRO, TRN, AYT
2011	LAX, ATL, WRO, SDF, MLB	MEX, PHL, BOS#
2012	SDF, LHR BOS*	—
2013	IKA	—
Total	36	24

Chinese results did not distinguish cities. Hand registry results did not correspond to Pei at al (48). Therefore, all hand transplants from Pei et al. are listed as China. Airport abbreviations were used to identify the cities where transplants were done. Airport abbreviations were used with extension to distinguish the places for the transplants performed by different teams in the same city.

ATL, Atlanta, USA; AYT, Antalya, Turkey; BOS#, Boston, USA (Brigham and Women's Hospital); BOS*, Boston, USA (Massachusetts General Hospital); BRU, Brussels, Belgium; CAN, Guangzhou, China; CDG, Paris, France; China, China, unknown city; ESB, Ankara, Turkey; HRB, Harbin, China; IKA, Tehran, Iran; INN, Innsbruck, Austria; LAX, Los Angeles, USA; LHR, Leeds, UK; LYS, Lyon, France; MEX, Mexico City, Mexico; MLB, Melbourne, Australia; MUC, Munich, Germany; PHL, Philadelphia, USA; PIT, Pittsburgh, USA; SAT, San Antonio, USA; SDF, Louisville, USA; TRN, Monza, Italy; VLC, Valencia, Spain; WRO, Wroclaw, Poland.

TABLE 77-2 World Experience of Hand Transplant

Year	Bilateral Hand with Face	Bilateral Hand with One Leg	Bilateral Hand with Double Leg
2009	CDG		
2011	BOS#		
2012		AYT	ESB
Total	2	1	1

AYT, Antalya, Turkey; BOS#, Boston, USA (Brigham and Women's Hospital); CDG, Paris, France; ESB, Ankara, Turkey.

fungal infection, but personal communication also suggested a bleeding diathesis and death after losing 100 units of blood.

Experience in these more complex multitransplant patients is limited. Case numbers are small, but the results imply that more caution is required.

Our list should be viewed with considerable caution. In one case, we have verified the details of the death of a bilateral HT only via personal communication with a surgeon not directly involved in the case. In many other situations, the outcomes were presented at meetings but never published.

Drawing firm statistical conclusions is difficult with such small case numbers, but we cannot ignore the trends. Single and bilateral HTs appear to have a reasonable allograft loss rate of approximately 10% to 18%, which is similar to kidney transplantation. However, face with double hand or multiple limb transplants have all had serious complications, including death. These complications were all early (within the first 2 months). Infection and blood loss were the primary cause of hand loss or death.

A number of patients have lost their HTs as a result of not taking their medications. In some of the Chinese cases (48), this may have been due to an inability to obtain or pay for the immunosuppression, but of the cohort of 70 hands transplanted outside China, there have also been two losses caused by noncompliance (3%).

A common cause of allograft loss in SOT is chronic rejection, but the very existence of chronic rejection is still debated in HT (50,51). The first French patient was reported as losing his hand secondary to noncompliance leading to chronic rejection (50). One HT in Louisville was lost to chronic rejection (52). However, there are marked differences in the presentation and pathology of the two cases. In the former, the rejection was predominantly in the skin; in the latter, it was in the arteries. The reason for the loss in the first case is clear: the patient stopped taking his medications. In the latter, the patient was taking his immunosuppression. It appears that although both losses may be called chronic rejection, there may be pathophysiological differences.

In the Louisville case, the authors suggested overuse of the hand or vibration, with stripping of the adventitia, as possible causes of intimal hyperplasia (52). We doubt but cannot exclude these as causes. The authors recommend biomicroscopy as a method of identifying intimal hyperplasia, but we believe the accuracy of this methodology remains under debate. These and all other authors list skin as the primary target of rejection. Yet although no patient has lost their hand from skin rejection while on immunosuppression, a patient has lost his hand secondary to arterial intimal hyperplasia.

There have been no reports of antibody-mediated rejection in HT worldwide; given the number of cases done, this is somewhat surprising. The incidence of chronic rejection leading to allograft loss is therefore 2 of 70, or 3% (the first in France and Pittsburgh). This is very low compared with renal and cardiac transplant.

Therefore, in HT, the incidence, pathophysiology, and target tissue of chronic rejection remain under debate.

Functional Results

One can reproducibly measure hand function, either with an objective tool that measures hand function by movement, strength, and sensation or subjectively by how the individual values the health state of HT (53–55). This latter method uses questions to measure attitudes about perceived function, deriving "quality of life scores" (QLS), such as Short Form 36 (SF-36), DASH, EQ-5D, and Time-Trade-Off Tests. There are a number of recognized limitations to this method, however (56).

No objective test can capture all the true variations of hand function, nor will all patients attribute a given function with the same value. Testing a hand objectively will produce a finite score, but that number may not represent the true value the patient gives to that hand function. For example, in two of the Louisville patients, the objective Carroll test produced a similar value, yet the subjective quality of life DASH score demonstrated a marked difference in how the patients viewed their outcomes.

One would like to see a table comparing the average scores across all the hand transplants, but there is no consensus among teams as to which tools should be used. DASH is reported in Louisville, Innsbruck, and China. It was reported from Pittsburgh in meetings but has not been published. In reality, the only score reported in most patients is the Hand Transplant Score System (HTSS), which, although not validated and having some structural problems, is required by the International Hand Registry.

Our recommendation is to use a series of objective functional tests and some QLS. We suggest adding pinch and grip strengths compared as a percentage with the other side. For QLS, we suggest the DASH, EQ-5D, and the HTSS.

Although not statistically confirmable, we believe the overall results of HT to date are very good. There are some reports of return of intrinsic function and two-point discrimination, and we believe that in general, patients are both obtaining value from their transplants and achieving better results than we would expect from replantation.

Complications and Research Protocols

Initially, it was believed that HT would suffer similar complication rates as SOT (57–59). This proved untrue because by definition, SOTs always have organ failure to start with, and HTs do not. HTs start in a healthier state and can better tolerate immunosuppression. However, given time, a HT may potentially develop all the same complications encountered in SOT, just at a later date.

Baumeister at al. (60) reviewed 200,000 kidney transplants worldwide enrolled in the Collaborative Transplantation Study. They isolated 58,310 of the patients between 15 to 40 years old. They used this cohort of patients to determine complications that might be expected in HT. They estimated that within 5 years, 3% of HTs will develop a malignant tumor (one third of these would be skin cancers), fewer than 1% will develop transplant lymphoma (but death with lymphoma is ~50%), and 11% will develop cataracts. They found that nephrotoxicity and neurotoxicity were difficult to estimate for HT from this data.

The list of possible complications with their associated risk that we present to our patients is given in Table 77-3. We arrived at these estimated numbers using published reports of SOT complications and discussion with our own SOT surgeons regarding their impression of anticipated outcomes.

Schneeberger et al. recently reported the Pittsburgh-Hopkins data (61) on five HT recipients. Three were bilateral, and two were unilateral. Schneeberger et al. conclude that their results support the conclusion that the Pittsburgh protocol (62) of bone marrow cell-based therapy is well tolerated and allows HT with monotherapy.

We believe they may have overstated their conclusions. All of the patients in this report are now 2.5 to 4 years posttransplant, but they only showed data at approximately 1 year out. The 1-year data raise questions about potential future renal compromise, demonstrating in some cases high creatinines and low GFRs. Schneeberger et al. assure us that these patients are doing well presently, but they do not present the data to support this statement.

At the time of the publication by Schneeberger et al., two patients were considering amputation. One patient was noncompliant, and the other had no return of function. There is no mention of this in the paper. One patient had his hand amputated 1 month after Schneeberger et al. reported the success of these patients (63). Noncompliance and failure of nerve regeneration does not mean the Pittsburgh protocol has failed, but declaring an experimental procedure as successful may be premature when based on only three patients with data only out to 1 year.

Finally, protocols are being used in SOT to induce tolerance that use total body or lymph node irradiation, donor bone marrow infusion, and T cell–depleting agents. Both Massachusetts General Hospital (64) and Northwestern University (65) have reported their successes and complications with this tolerogenic protocol in SOT. Both of these teams have produced publications that these tolerogenic protocols could advance the field of SOT. The protocol used at Northwestern University was a modification of one used at the University of Louisville. At the latter institution, this protocol resulted in the death of one patient and a severe complication in another. The principal investigator of this protocol then moved the program to Northwestern University. The complications in Louisville, to the best of our knowledge, have never been published or presented at a national meeting. What changes in the protocol that made it a success at Northwestern University but a failure in Louisville remains unclear.

Tolerance induction has tremendous potential for the field of VCA, but the protocols may be dangerous. There remains debate as to whether immunosuppression or tolerance induction protocols represent more danger (66,67). Failure to report complications makes evaluation and comparison of the two different protocols difficult.

TABLE 77-3 Estimated Potential Risks Associated with Composite Tissue Allotransplantation*

Risk	Year 1	Year 2–5	Lifetime
GVHD			
Hand or distal forearm CTA	0% low	0%	0%
CTA with fludarabine, TBI, and/or BMT	(5%?)	5%	10%
Chronic rejection			
Conventional CTA	0%	5%	15–20%
CTA with fluoroscopy, TBI, or BMT	0%	?%	Hypothesize there will be none
Viral opportunistic infections (e.g., CMV)	50%	20%	70%
Bacterial opportunistic infections	50%	20%	70%
Community infections	50%	50%	100%
Death from infection	~0.25%	~0.25%	~1–2%
Kidney failure or dialysis	2%	Unknown	~2%
Malignancy			
Lymphoma (PTLD)†	0.1%	0.58%	7%
Skin cancer	0.2%	1.1%	2%
Other types of cancer	0.2%	0.5%	2%
Diabetes			
Triple-drug therapy	15%	5%	20%
Steroid sparing	lower	lower	lower
High blood pressure			
Triple-drug therapy	20%	30%	50%
Steroid sparing	similar	similar	similar
Cataracts			
Triple-drug therapy	~20%	~10%	~30%
Steroid sparing	much lower	much lower	much lower
Osteoporosis or AVN			
Triple-drug therapy	0.5%	1%	3%
Steroid sparing	much lower	much lower	much lower

*These estimates are based primarily on experience with kidney transplants. Because patients undergoing kidney transplants are more ill than those undergoing vascularized composite allotransplantation, these estimates maybe overstated.

†The risk of posttransplant lymphoproliferative disorder (PTLD) is relatively low. However, the mortality rate associated with PTLD can be high, in the range of 30% to 60% of those who are diagnosed.

AVN, avascular necrosis; BMT, bone marrow transplantation; CMV, cytomegalovirus; CTA, composite tissue allotransplantation; GVHD, graft-versus-host disease; TBI, total-body irradiation.

REFERENCES

1. Sade RM. Transplantation at 100 years: Alexis Carrel, pioneer surgeon. *Ann Thorac Surg* 2005;80(6):2415–2418.
2. Ono S. The birth of transplantation immunology: the Billingham-Medawar experiments at Birmingham University and University College London. 1951. *J Exp Biol* 2004;207(23):4013–4014.
3. Hewitt CW, Black KS, Dowdy SF, et al. Composite tissue (limb) allografts in rats. III. Development of donor-host lymphoid chimeras in long-term survivors. *Transplantation* 1986;41(1):39–43.
4. Black KS, Hewitt CW, Fraser LA, et al. Composite tissue (limb) allografts in rats. II. Indefinite survival using low-dose cyclosporine. *Transplantation* 1985;39(4):365–368.
5. Hewitt CW, Black KS, Fraser LA, et al. Composite tissue (limb) allografts in rats. I. Dose-dependent increase in survival with cyclosporine. *Transplantation* 1985;39(4):360–364.
6. Siegler M. The future of the doctor-patient relationship in a world of managed care. *Medicina nei secoli* 1998;10(1):41–56.
7. Breidenbach WC, Gonzales NR, Kaufman CL, et al. Outcomes of the first 2 American hand transplants at 8 and 6 years posttransplant. *J Hand Surg* 2008;33(7):1039–1047.

8. Egerszegi EP, Samulack DD, Daniel RK. Experimental models in primates for reconstructive surgery utilizing tissue transplants. *Ann Plast Surg* 1984;13(5):423–430.
9. Daniel RK, Egerszegi EP, Samulack DD, et al. Tissue transplants in primates for upper extremity reconstruction: a preliminary report. *J Hand Surg* 1986;11(1):1–8.
10. Hovius SE, Stevens HP, van Nierop PW, et al. Allogeneic transplantation of the radial side of the hand in the rhesus monkey: I. Technical aspects. *Plast Reconstr Surg* 1992;89(4):700–709.
11. Arai K, Hotokebuchi T, Miyahara H, et al. Limb allografts in rats immunosuppressed with FK506. *Transplantation* 1989;48:782–786.
12. Min Z, Jones NF. Limb transplantation in rats: immunosuppression with FK- 506. *J Hand Surg* 1995;20A:77–87.
13. Benhaim P, Anthony JP, Ferreira L, et al. Use of combination of low-dose cyclosporine and RS-61443 in a rat hindlimb model of composite tissue allotransplantation. *Transplantation* 1996;61(4):527–532.
14. Barth RN, Nam AJ, Stanwix MG, et al. Prolonged survival of composite facial allografts in non-human primates associated with posttransplant lymphoproliferative disorder. *Transplantation* 2009;88(11):1242–1250.
15. Schneeberger S, Gorantla VS, Brandacher G, et al. Upper-extremity transplantation using a cell-based protocol to minimize immunosuppression. *Ann Surg* 2013;257(2):345–351.
16. Quinlan SC, Pfeiffer RM, Morton LM, Engels EA. Risk factors for early-onset and late-onset post-transplant lymphoproliferative disorder in kidney recipients in the United States. *Am J Hematol* 2011;86(2):206–209.
17. Elhassan B, Moran SL, Bravo C, Amadio P. Factors that influence the outcome of zone I and zone II flexor tendon repairs in children. *J Hand Surg* 2006;31(10):1661–1666.
18. Breidenbach WC, Gonzales NR, Kaufman CL, et al. Outcomes of the first 2 American hand transplants at 8 and 6 years posttransplant. *J Hand Surg* 2008;33(7):1039–1047.
19. Jablecki J, Kaczmarzyk L, Domanasiewicz A, et al. First Polish forearm transplantation—final report (outcome after 4 years). *Ann Transplant* 2010;15(2):61–67.
20. Frey SH, Bogdanov S, Smith JC, et al. Chronically deafferented sensory cortex recovers a grossly typical organization after allogenic hand transplantation. *Curr Biol* 2008;18(19):1530–1534.
21. Shores JT. Recipient screening and selection: who is the right candidate for hand transplantation. *Hand Clin* 2011;27(4):539–543, x.
22. Dharancy S, Giral M, Tetaz R, et al. Adherence with immunosuppressive treatment after transplantation: results from the French trial PREDICT. *Clin Transplant* 2012;26(3):E293–E299.
23. Dew MA, DiMartini AF, De Vito Dabbs A, et al. Rates and risk factors for nonadherence to the medical regimen after adult solid organ transplantation. *Transplantation* 2007;83(7):858–873.
24. Cavadas PC, Landin L, Ibanez J. Bilateral hand transplantation: result at 20 months. *J Hand Surg Eur Vol* 2009;34(4):434–443.
25. Chang J, Mathes DW. Ethical, financial, and policy considerations in hand transplantation. *Hand Clin* 2011;27(4):553–560, xi.
26. Petruzzo P, Dubernard JM. World experience after more than a decade of clinical hand transplantation: update on the French program. *Hand Clin* 2011;27(4):411–416, vii.
27. Jablecki J. World experience after more than a decade of clinical hand transplantation: update on the Polish program. *Hand Clin* 2011;27(4): 433–442, viii.
28. McDiarmid SV, Azari KK. Donor-related issues in hand transplantation. *Hand Clin* 2011;27(4):545–552, x-xi.
29. Hautz T, Engelhardt TO, Weissenbacher A, et al. World experience after more than a decade of clinical hand transplantation: update on the Innsbruck program. *Hand Clin* 2011;27(4):423–431, viii.
30. Azari KK, Imbriglia JE, Goitz RJ, et al. Technical aspects of the recipient operation in hand transplantation. *J Reconstr Microsurg* 2012;28(1): 27–34.
31. Banegas RN, Moreno R, Duggal A, Breidenbach WC 3rd. Surgical aspects of donor hand recovery for transplantation. *J Reconstr Microsurg* 2012;28(1):21–26.
32. Dubernard JM, Owen E, Herzberg G, et al. Human hand allograft: report on first 6 months. *Lancet* 1999;353(9161):1315–1320.
33. Jones JW, Gruber SA, Barker JH, Breidenbach WC. Successful hand transplantation. One-year follow-up. Louisville Hand Transplant Team. *N Engl J Med* 17 2000;343(7):468–473.
34. Lanzetta M, Dubernard JM, Owen ER, et al. Surgical planning of human hand transplantation. *Transplant Proc* 2001;33(1-2):683.
35. Schuind F, Van Holder C, Mouraux D, et al. The first Belgian hand transplantation–37 month term results. *J Hand Surg Br* 2006;31(4):371–376.
36. Hartzell TL, Benhaim P, Imbriglia JE, et al. Surgical and technical aspects of hand transplantation: is it just another replant? *Hand Clin* 2011;27(4):521–530, x.
37. Kaufman CL, Ouseph R, Blair B, et al. Graft vasculopathy in clinical hand transplantation. *Am J Transplant* 2012;12(4):1004–1016.
38. Edgell SE, McCabe SJ, Breidenbach WC, et al. Different reference frames can lead to different hand transplantation decisions by patients and physicians. *J Hand Surg* 2001;26(2):196–200.
39. Kaufman CL, Ouseph R, Blair B, et al. Graft vasculopathy in clinical hand transplantation. *Am J Transplant* 2012;12(4):1004–1016.
40. Woodle ES, Peddi VR, Tomlanovich S, et al. A prospective, randomized, multicenter study evaluating early corticosteroid withdrawal with Thymoglobulin in living-donor kidney transplantation. *Clin Transplant* 2010;24(1):73–83.
41. Kawai T, Sachs DH, Sykes M, Cosimi AB. HLA-mismatched renal transplantation without maintenance immunosuppression. *New Engl J Med* 2013;368(19):1850–1852.
42. Schneeberger S, Gorantla VS, Brandacher G, et al. Upper-extremity transplantation using a cell-based protocol to minimize immunosuppression. *Ann Surg* 2013;257(2):345–351.
43. Rochkind S. Phototherapy in peripheral nerve regeneration: from basic science to clinical study. *Neurosurg Focus* 2009;26(2):E8.
44. Poyton RO, Ball KA. Therapeutic photobiomodulation: nitric oxide and a novel function of mitochondrial cytochrome c oxidase. *Discov Med* 2011;11(57):154–159.
45. Spiegel J, Tintera J, Gawehn J, et al. Functional MRI of human primary somatosensory and motor cortex during median nerve stimulation. *Clin Neurophysiol* 1999;110(1):47–52.
46. Diers M, Christmann C, Koeppe C, et al. Mirrored, imagined and executed movements differentially activate sensorimotor cortex in amputees with and without phantom limb pain. *Pain* 2010;149(2):296–304.
47. International Registry on Hand and Composite Tissue Transplantation. http://www.handregistry.com.
48. Pei G, Xiang D, Gu L, et al. A report of 15 hand allotransplantations in 12 patients and their outcomes in China. *Transplantation* 2012;94(10): 1052–1059.
49. Carty MJ, Hivelin M, Dumontier C, et al. Lessons learned from simultaneous face and bilateral hand allotransplantation. *Plast Reconstr Surg* 2013;32(2):423–432.
50. Petruzzo P, Kanitakis J, Badet L, et al. Long-term follow-up in composite tissue allotransplantation: in-depth study of five (hand and face) recipients. *Am J Transplant* 2011;11(4):808–816.
51. Kanitakis J, McGregor B, Badet L, et al. Absence of c4d deposition in human composite tissue (hands and face) allograft biopsies: an immunoperoxidase study. *Transplantation* 2007;84(2):265–267.
52. Kaufman CL, Ouseph R, Blair B, et al. Graft vasculopathy in clinical hand transplantation. *Am J Transplant* 2012;12(4):1004–1016.
53. Landin L, Bonastre J, Casado-Sanchez C, et al. Outcomes with respect to disabilities of the upper limb after hand allograft transplantation: a systematic review. *Transplant Int* 2012;25(4):424–432.
54. Carroll D. A quantitative test of upper extremity function. *J Chronic Dis* 1965;18:479–491.
55. Lanzetta M, Petruzzo P. A comprehensive functional score system in hand transplantation. In Lanzetta M, Dubernard J (eds). *Hand Transplantation*. Italy: Springer-Verlag, 2007, pp. 355.
56. Jensen SE, Butt Z, Bill A, et al. Quality of life considerations in upper limb transplantation: review and future directions. *J Hand Surg Am* 2012;37(10):2126–2135.
57. Brenner MJ, Tung TH, Jensen JN, Mackinnon SE. The spectrum of complications of immunosuppression: is the time right for hand transplantation? *J Bone Joint Surg Am* 2002;84A(10):1861–1870.
58. Cooney WP, Hentz VR. Hand transplantation—primum non nocere. *J Hand Surg Am* 2002;27(1):165–168.
59. Jones NF. Concerns about hand transplantation in the 21st century. *J Hand Surg* 2002;27A:771–787.
60. Baumeister S, Kleist C, Dohler B, et al. Risks of allogeneic hand transplantation. *Microsurgery* 2004;24(2):98–103.
61. Schneeberger S, Gorantla VS, Brandacher G, et al. Upper-extremity transplantation using a cell-based protocol to minimize immunosuppression. *Ann Surg* 2013;257(2):345–351.
62. Gorantla VS, Brandacher G, Schneeberger S, et al. Favoring the risk-benefit balance for upper extremity transplantation—the Pittsburgh Protocol. *Hand Clin* 2011;27(4):511–520, ix–x.
63. CNN. One year after double hand transplant, progress elusive. 2010; http://www.cnn.com/2010/HEALTH/08/26/double.hand.transplant/index.html

64. Spitzer TR, Sykes M, Tolkoff-Rubin N, et al. Long-term follow-up of recipients of combined human leukocyte antigen-matched bone marrow and kidney transplantation for multiple myeloma with end-stage renal disease. *Transplantation* 2011;91(6):672–676.
65. Leventhal J, Abecassis M, Miller J, et al. Tolerance induction in HLA disparate living donor kidney transplantation by donor stem cell infusion: durable chimerism predicts outcome. *Transplantation* 2013; 95(1):169–176.
66. Halloran PF, Bromberg J, Kaplan B, Vincenti F. Tolerance versus immunosuppression: a perspective. *Am J Transplant* 2008;8(7): 1365–1366.
67. Sachs DH, Kawai T, Colvin RB, et al. Response to "Tolerance versus immunosuppression: a perspective." *Am J Transplant* 2008;8(8): 1573–1574.
68. Breidenbach WC, et al. Long-term survival of an extremity composite issue allograft with FK506-mycophenolate mofetil therapy. *Surgery* 1999; 126(2):384–388. PMID 10455910.
69. Wiley Periodicals Inc. Brief communication infections following facial composite tissue allotransplantation—single center experience and review of the literature. *Am J Trans* 2013;13:770–779. doi: 10.1111/ajt.12013.

SECTION 5

LOWER LIMB

CHAPTER 78

Free Flap Coverage of Lower Extremity Open Fractures

Emmanuel G. Melissinos

The advent of operative microsurgery added an entire new dimension to lower extremity reconstruction. Free flap coverage of lower extremity defects continues to evolve and remains one of the most frequently performed microsurgical procedures. The great majority of defects requiring flap coverage are the immediate or late result of trauma. Other causes include tumors and extirpatory oncologic surgery, arterial and venous vascular insufficiencies, metabolic and endocrine diseases, and infectious processes.

Our data, based on 32 years of experience in a level I trauma center, indicate that free tissue transfers in posttrauma reconstruction most frequently (72.4%) involve the lower extremity (Figure 78-1) and predominantly (56%) involve the area of the lower leg and ankle. Young men are most frequently affected (with a mean age 32.2 years and a 3.1:1 male-to-female ratio). The mean patient age has not varied significantly over the years, but the age span has expanded. Our youngest patient is a 19-month-old boy who was run over by a lawnmower (Figure 78-2) and the oldest an 87-year-old man who fell off a tree (Figure 78-3).

Increasing experience, advances in microsurgical technique and instrumentation, introduction of new flaps, and better utilization of old flaps are factors responsible for the increasing success rate of free tissue transfers for reconstruction of complicated lower extremity defects. It should be emphasized that "heroic" salvage is not always the best course of action, and judicious use of our skills is required to truly improve outcomes.

INITIAL MANAGEMENT AND TIMING OF FREE FLAP COVERAGE

The condition of the patient and wound dictate the timing of free flap transfers for lower extremity reconstruction. Polytrauma patients with lower extremity injuries are evaluated and treated according to the Advanced Trauma Life Support (ATLS) guidelines. A multidisciplinary approach is required to evaluate the extremity concerning vascular status, compartment pressures, and extent of soft tissue and bone injuries and to formulate a plan regarding need for vascular repair, fasciotomies, debridements, bone stabilization, soft tissue coverage, and appropriate deep vein thrombosis prevention regimen.

The need for free tissue transfer should be brought into the equation early in the decision-making process. Comorbidities that may preclude such procedures should be taken into consideration. The patient and family should be made aware during the decision-making process that salvage of the extremity may require major, complicated procedures.

Efforts to decrease the biological effects of the open wound phase and to achieve a healed wound as quickly as possible are based on well-established medical principles. Decreased metabolic requirements, shorter exposure to nosocomial infections, early mobilization, and lower hospitalization costs contribute to better outcomes. In cases of open fractures, avoiding prolonged exposure and deterioration of vital structures and early entry to the regeneration stage are additional advantages.

The positive effects of early coverage of lower extremity open fractures with free flap transfers have been reported in the literature, although there are no well-defined lines between stages of reconstruction. In a prospective study, Byrd et al. (1) demonstrated an 18% incidence of infections and complications related to fracture healing after radical wound debridement of severe open fractures and coverage within 6 days versus 50% when coverage was performed within 1 to 6 weeks and 40% after 6 or more weeks after injury. In a retrospective study involving upper and lower extremity injuries, Godina (2) reported a remarkable decrease in flap failures, postoperative infections, bone healing time, length of hospitalization, and operative procedures when extensive debridement, bone stabilization, and flap coverage were

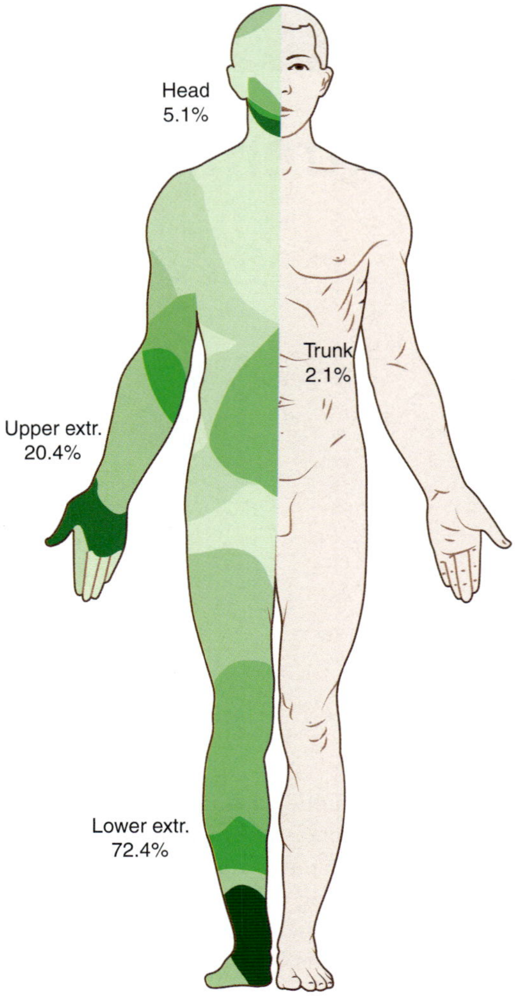

FIGURE 78-1 Distribution of 6718 free flaps performed between July 1979 and June 2011 for post-trauma reconstruction (personal data).

carried out within the first 72 hours with 11.8% of the free tissue transfers performed at the time of the first operative procedure.

Most of the lower extremity defects requiring free tissue transfers are the result of high-energy trauma. The zone of injury varies, and the degree of tissue damage differs from inflammatory reaction to necrosis. In most instances, tissue viability can be determined during the initial debridement by using the well-established principles of obtaining healthy-looking, bleeding skin edges; exposing bleeding; contracting muscle fibers; and preserving attached, vascularized bone fragments. In severe crush injuries and in most cases of thermal and electrical burns, the line of demarcation is not clear at the initial stage, and radical debridement of traumatized but potentially viable tissues may further complicate the severity of injury. Sequential debridements are required until the condition of the wound permits definitive coverage with free tissue transfer.

The advent of improved but lengthy resuscitative protocols and transfers from an increasing number of community trauma centers present us with a growing number of patients requiring delayed coverage. Serial debridements in conjunction with advanced wound care protocols using modalities such as negative-pressure dressings, antibiotic beads and

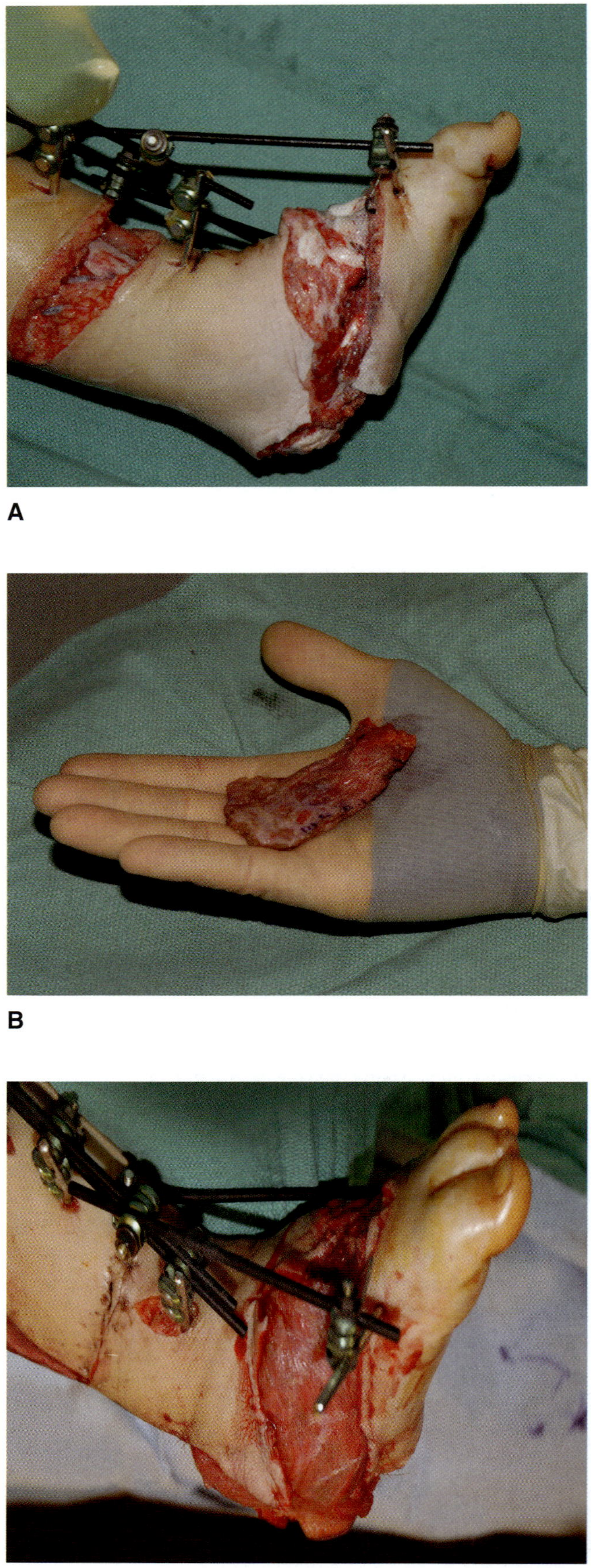

A

B

C

FIGURE 78-2 (A) 19-month-old male with lower extremity lawnmower injury. (B, C) Reconstruction with latissimus dorsi free flap, local flaps and skin graft. (D, E) 4 years post-reconstruction.

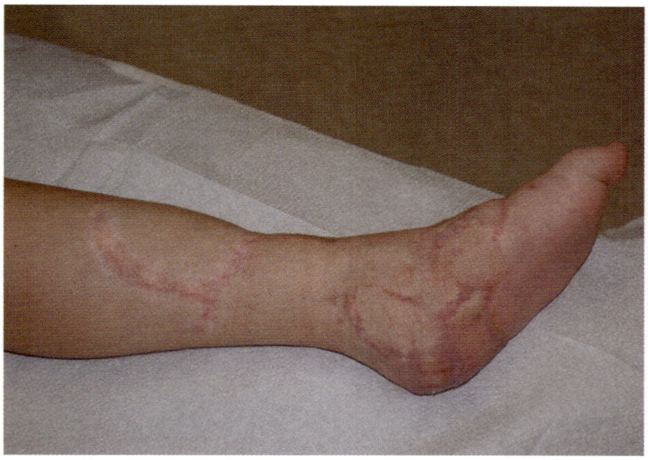

D

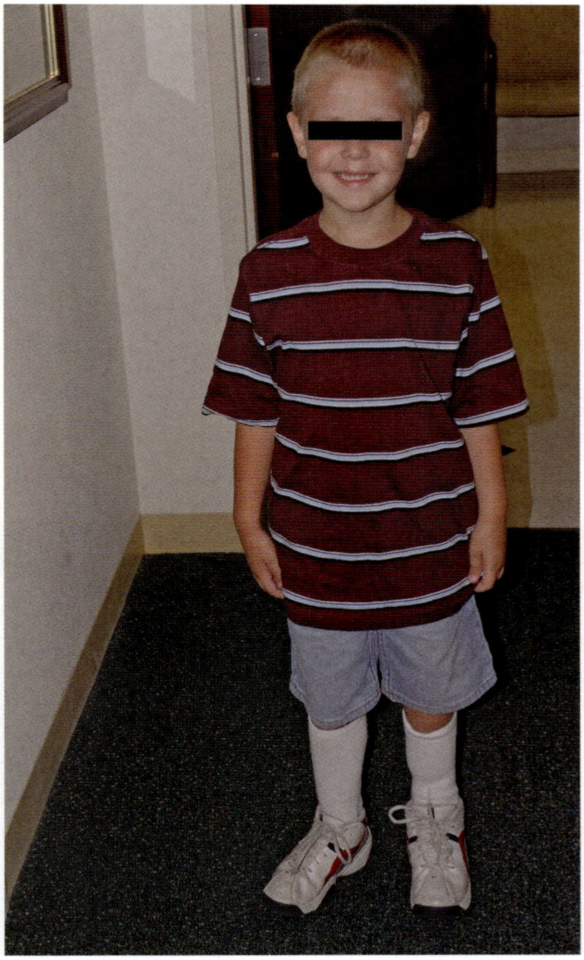

E

FIGURE 78-2 *(Continued)*

pouches, and biological and mechanical covers are useful in improving the condition of the wound, preventing desiccation, guarding against infection, and improving outcomes before delayed free flap coverage.

It should be noted that there are lower extremity injuries requiring free flap transfers in which, independent of timing, complete debridement of all ischemic tissues would result in a severely impaired or nonreconstructable extremity. In such cases and when free flap coverage is required, such procedure should be carried out at the optimal time based on the judgment of the surgeon and with the full understanding that close monitoring will be necessary and subsequent procedures may be required.

The type and severity of injuries of the patient population requiring free tissue transfers varies considerably between institutions and should be taken into serious consideration when establishing treatment protocols. In our institution, 54% of the patients are in monitored beds, including 22% who are intubated at the time of the initial consultation. Immediate reconstructive attempts carry obvious medical and legal implications. We perform emergency free flaps only when usable tissues are available for harvest from amputated parts for immediate free tissue transfer (Figure 78-4), when immediate coverage of vital structures is needed, and in rare occasions when a flow-through flap is required for salvage of the extremity.

Every effort is made to complete coverage within 5 to 7 days in agreement with the opinion expressed by Heller and Levin (3). After this period, in cases in which we expect improvement of the condition of the patient and wound to the point that a free tissue transfer will be feasible, we continue with serial debridement and wound care until such requirements are met. Otherwise we institute long-term therapeutic alternatives as bedside negative-pressure dressing changes and hyperbaric oxygen treatments.

CLASSIFICATION OF OPEN TIBIAL FRACTURES

Precise evaluation of the degree of initial injury is essential because it greatly influences the treatment paradigm applied to the patient and has prognostic impact in determining outcome. The most frequently cited classification of open fractures, introduced by Gustilo et al. in 1976, categorizes open fractures as types I, II, and III, based on the size of the wounds (4). In 1984, Gustilo et al. subclassified the type III open fractures into three categories to take into consideration the configuration of the fracture, mechanism of injury, and degree of contamination (5). A more detailed outline, published in 1990 (6), is as follows:

- Type I open fracture: The wound is less than 1 cm long. Is usually a moderately clean puncture, through which a spike of bone has pierced the skin. There is little soft tissue damage and no sign of crushing injury. The fracture is usually simple, transverse, or short oblique with little comminution.
- Type II open fracture: The laceration is more than 1 cm long, and there is no extensive soft tissue damage, flaps, or avulsion. There is slight or moderate crushing injury, moderate comminution, and moderate contamination.
- Type III open fracture: This is characterized by extensive damage to the soft tissues, including muscles, skin, and neurovascular structures, and a high degree of contamination. The fracture is often caused by high-velocity trauma resulting in a great deal of comminution and instability.

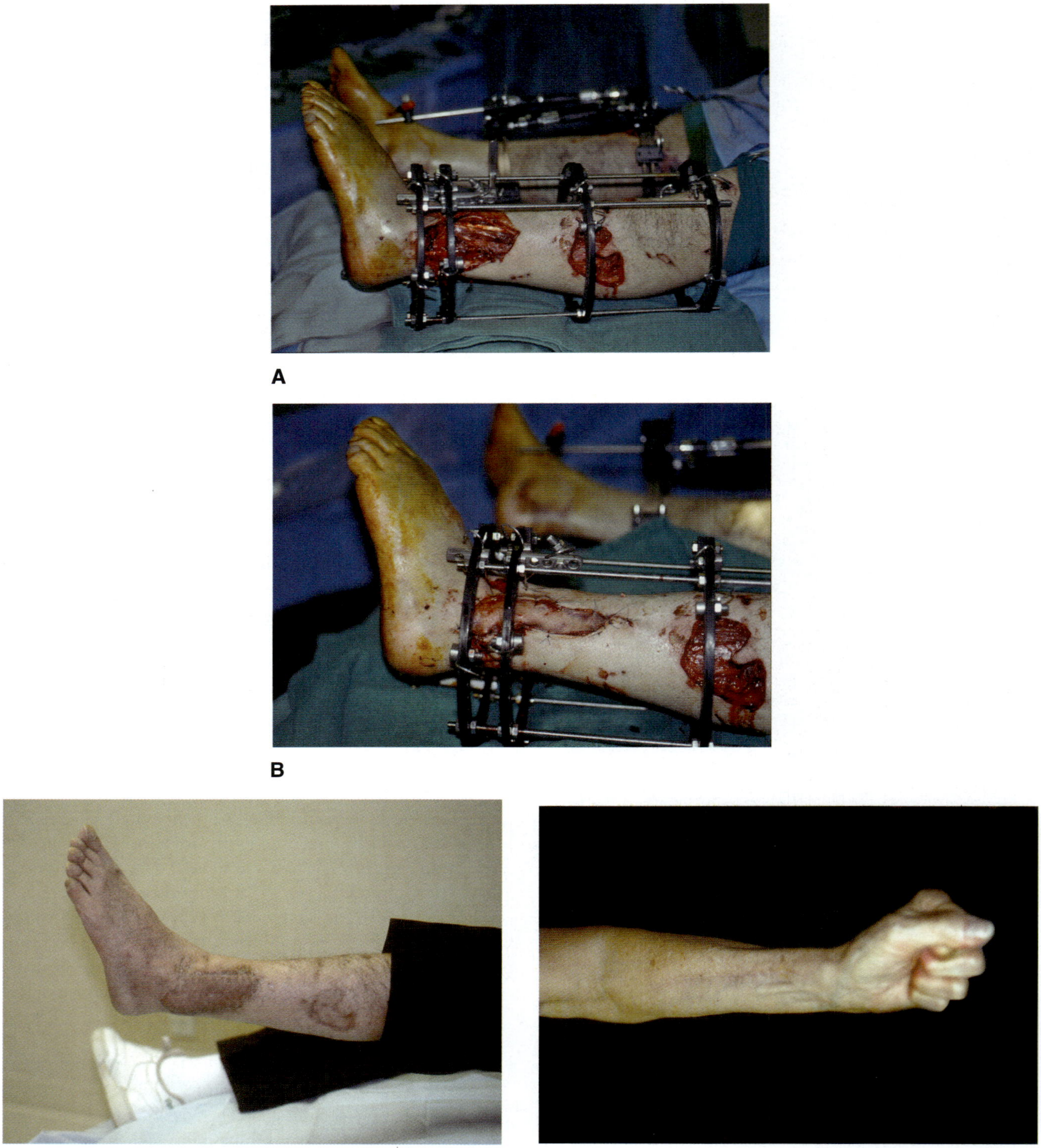

A B C D

FIGURE 78-3 (**A**) 87-year-old man with open, distal, tibial fibular fracture. (**B**) Coverage with radial forearm free flap. (**C**) Two years post-reconstruction. (**D**) Donor site..

- Type IIIA open fracture: Soft tissue coverage of the fractured bone is adequate, despite extensive laceration, flaps, or high-energy trauma. This type includes segmental or severely comminuted fractures from high-energy trauma regardless of the size of the wound.
- Type IIIB open fracture: This is associated with extensive injury to or loss of soft tissue, with periosteal stripping and exposure of bone, massive contamination, and severe comminution of the fracture from high-velocity trauma. After debridement and irrigation are completed, a segment of bone is exposed, and local or free flap is needed for coverage.
- Type IIIC open fracture: This is an open fracture associated with arterial injury that must be repaired regardless of the degree of soft tissue injury.

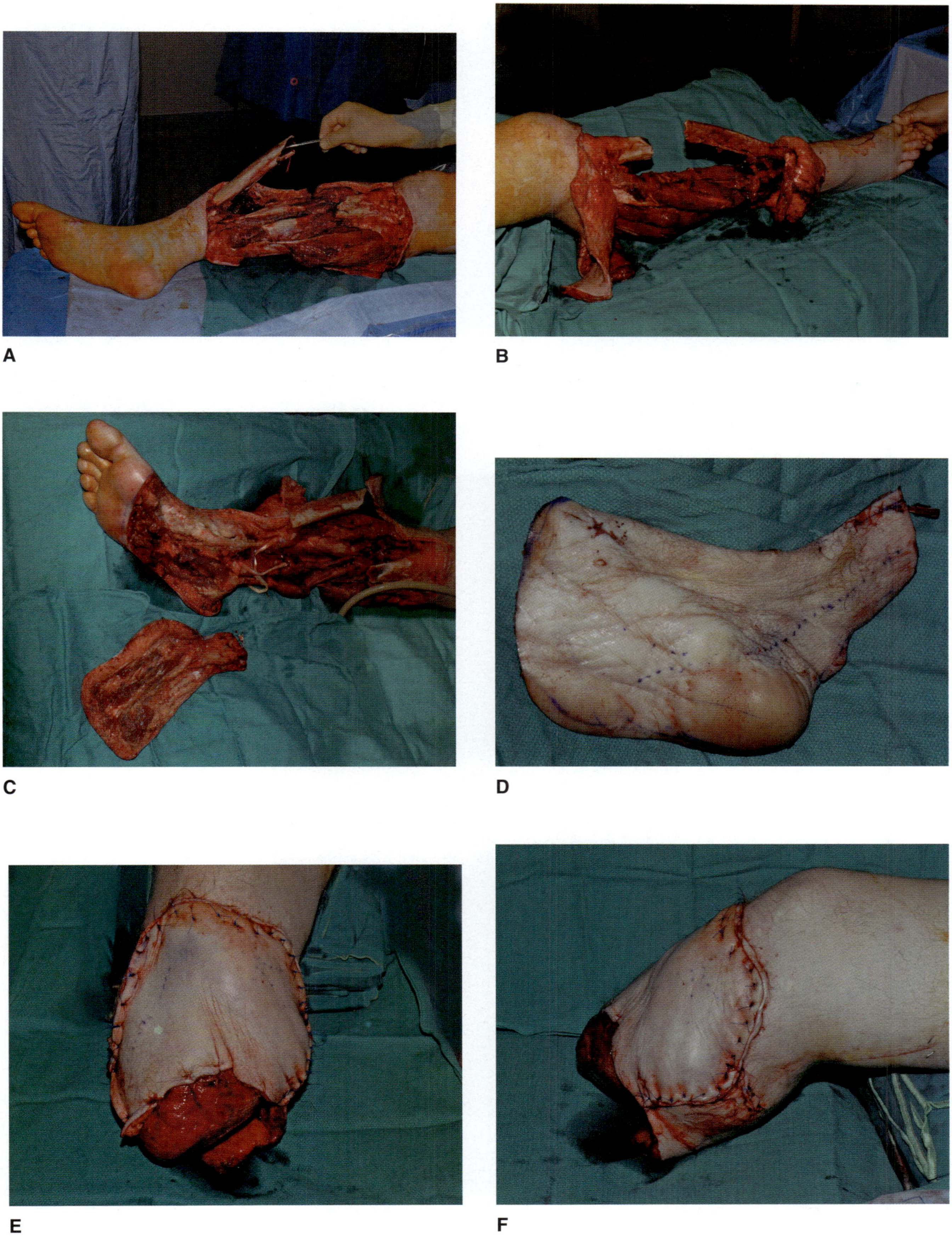

FIGURE 78-4 (A, B) Severe crush injury to the right leg requiring amputation. (C, D) Harvesting of posterior tibial artery based free flap from the amputated part. (E, F) Transfer to BKA stump with anastomoses to the popliteal vessels. (G, H, I) 1 year post-reconstruction.

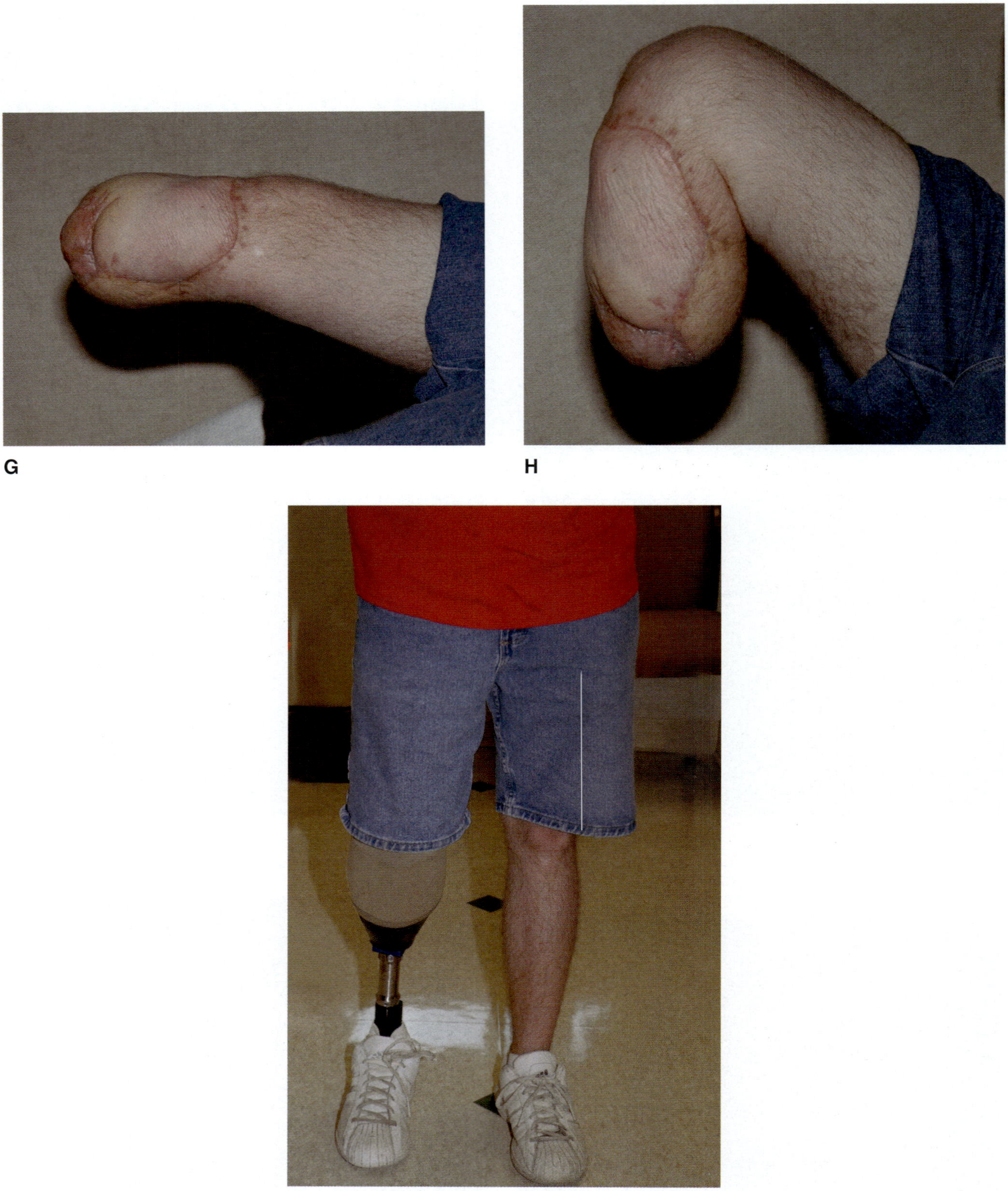

G

H

I

FIGURE 78-4 *(Continued)*

Exact grading of open fractures is not feasible because of the number and complexity of the involved parameters. Noted limitations of the Gustilo classification include variability of the extent of injury between the subgroups and lack of inclusion of significant components of injury as compartment syndrome, loss of muscle groups, and neurologic deficits. There is a difference of opinion among surgeons as to what constitutes a vascular injury that needs to be repaired. In a study performed by Brumback and Jones (7), there was only 60% agreement between orthopedic surgeons grading type II to type IIIC injuries. The importance of clearly documenting and directly communicating patient-specific findings is evident.

NEED FOR ANGIOGRAPHY

Clinical evaluation of the circulatory status of the lower extremity is often sufficient (8). Pre- and intraoperative assessment of peripheral pulses, including palpation, Doppler tracing, lower extremity Allen's test, and ankle brachial index (ABI), is an effective predictor of lower extremity vascular integrity and provides the information needed for vessel selection at the recipient site of a well-perfused leg. Questionable perfusion, absent or abnormal peripheral pulses, history of vascular trauma, previous procedures that included vascular manipulation, presence of free flaps, and investigation of donor sites of planned free flap harvest are major indications for preoperative angiography. In severe trauma cases, the delay caused by preoperative angiography should be taken into consideration (9).

Recent advances have made computed tomography angiography (CTA) the most frequently used method of assessing lower extremity vascularity (10). CT scanners are readily available in emergency centers, allowing tomographic evaluation of the injured lower extremity as part of the initial trauma imaging. Newer, multidirectional 64-slice CT scanners have increased the speed and improved the quality of the images. CTA is safer and less expensive, provides information of bones and soft tissues, visualizes segments located immediately after an obstruction (11), and does not require hours of rest and observation after the procedure. It should be noted that retrograde flow can produce a false-negative result. A lower extremity Allen's test can be of help determining flow direction (12).

Excellent images can be obtained with conventional angiography and digital subtraction techniques. Potential complications include arterial occlusion, pseudoaneurysm, renal contrast nephropathy, and hematoma formation (13). We currently use conventional arteriography when maximum detail is required in patients with previous flaps or vascular procedures; when we need to evaluate flow rate and direction, collateral circulation, and venous backflow; and in patients potentially requiring endovascular intervention (10).

CONVENTIONAL COVERAGE OF LOWER EXTREMITY DEFECTS

In the lower extremity, as in any other part of the body, the goal of the reconstructive surgeon is to achieve the best possible result using the simplest available method. Selection of the optimal reconstructive option for lower extremity reconstruction in a medically stable patient is based on the configuration of the defect in regard to size, missing components, exposed structures, condition of adjacent tissues, location of the defect, and vascular anatomy of the injured extremity. Other factors include the position of established external fixation, individual donor site patient preferences, expected appearance of the reconstructed area and donor site, and surgeon's experience.

Primary or sequential closure with advancement of local tissues and healing by secondary intention with or without the use of skin grafts can produce complete healing of moderate-size defects in favorable locations. The advent of negative-pressure wound closure devices has improved the success rate of such methods by decreasing edema, increasing vascularity, and inducing wound contraction. In addition, enhanced production of granulation tissue creates a favorable bed for application of skin grafts (14).

The role of local flaps in lower extremity reconstruction has expanded recently for two main reasons. First, increased familiarity with the vascular anatomy of conventional local flaps permits precise elevation of safer flaps based on the individual anatomical findings as number and location of segmental vascular pedicles on a case-by-case basis. Second, fabrication of fasciocutaneous flaps based on specific perforators arising from the distal peroneal and posterior tibial vessels.

In the thigh, local muscle, myocutaneous, and fasciocutaneous flaps supplied by the medial and lateral circumflex femoral vessels are readily available. The distally based, reverse rectus abdominis flap can be used to cover groin and proximal thigh defects when such flaps are not accessible.

The medial and lateral gastrocnemius flaps have been used extensively for reconstruction of the knee and upper third of the lower leg. Their arc of rotation can be increased by dividing their origin while protecting the medial and lateral sural vessels and with multiple parallel transverse incisions of the posterior fascia (15). The distally based vastus lateralis rotational muscle flap can also reach to cover knee defects (16).

The soleus muscle flap is the main local flap transfer used to cover middle third defects. Based on vascular anatomy, the flap can be used to cover distal third leg defects (17,18). The distal part of the muscle is supplied by branches of the peroneal vessels laterally and the posterior tibial vessels medially. Depending on the position of the distal muscular perforators as determined intraoperatively, the flap can be designed to cover more distal defects and can be split into medial or lateral hemisoleus flaps (19).

Segmental advancement of the tibialis anterior muscle as a bipedicle or partial split muscle flap with preservation of the tibialis anterior tendon can be used to cover small upper and middle third leg defects (20).

Fasciocutaneous flaps based on identifiable perforators are increasingly used for coverage of small size lower third defects in less severely traumatized extremities. Multidetector-row computed tomography (21) or conventional angiography can be used to ascertain the presence and location of uninjured perforators, increasing the safety of such transfers. Rotational and reverse "propeller" posterior tibial fasciocutaneous flaps are based on distal septocutaneous branches of the posterior tibial vessels in the medial malleolar area (22). Septocutaneous branches originating from the distal peroneal vessels are the primary blood supply to rotational, "propeller" peroneal (23), and sural fasciocutaneous flaps (24).

In comparison with free flaps, lower extremity local flaps are easier to dissect; involve only the injured extremity; do not require specialized teams or equipment; and are shorter, less expensive procedures. Disadvantages include size limitations; use of tissues close to or affected by the injury, inflicting further damage to the injured extremity; and inability to provide specialized tissues. In our practice, their use in reconstruction of lower leg defects is frequently restricted due to the need for radical debridement, zone of injury, and destruction of the perforating vessels during placement of internal fixation devices.

Combination of free and local flaps is particularly useful in reconstruction of large, lengthy lower extremity defects (Figure 78-5).

MUSCLE VERSUS FASCIOCUTANEOUS FLAPS

Lower extremity wounds severe enough to require reconstruction with free tissue transfers usually involve large surface and volume defects, which are frequently associated with exposed fractures, surgical hardware, and vital structures. Muscle flaps, transferred along or as chimeric flaps, provide the greatest possible amount of well-vascularized tissue required to reconstruct such defects. Loss of muscle tissue is a disadvantage, although the deficit resulting from appropriately selected and well-designed muscle or musculocutaneous flaps is well tolerated.

The skin islands of the fasciocutaneous flaps supply same type tissue coverage without sacrificing muscle units. Donor site deficit and morbidity is minimal as long as the width of the cutaneous island is limited to the size that permits primary closure. They are easily and safely re-elevated for subsequent procedures (25). They can be transferred as sensate flaps, although this is not of importance in lower extremity reconstruction unless the foot is involved. Obesity is a relative contraindication. Sensory deficits at the donor site can be bothersome.

Calderon et al. (26) studied the interaction between bacteria and the undersurface of musculocutaneous and fasciocutaneous flaps. His group showed a 500-fold decrease in bacterial concentration with muscle versus fascial flaps during the first day. Subsequently, the bacterial concentration remained 30 to 60 times lower on the third to the fifth day in the musculocutaneous flaps. In clinical practice, muscle flaps are general preferred over fascial flaps for placement over contaminated wounds and infected bone (27).

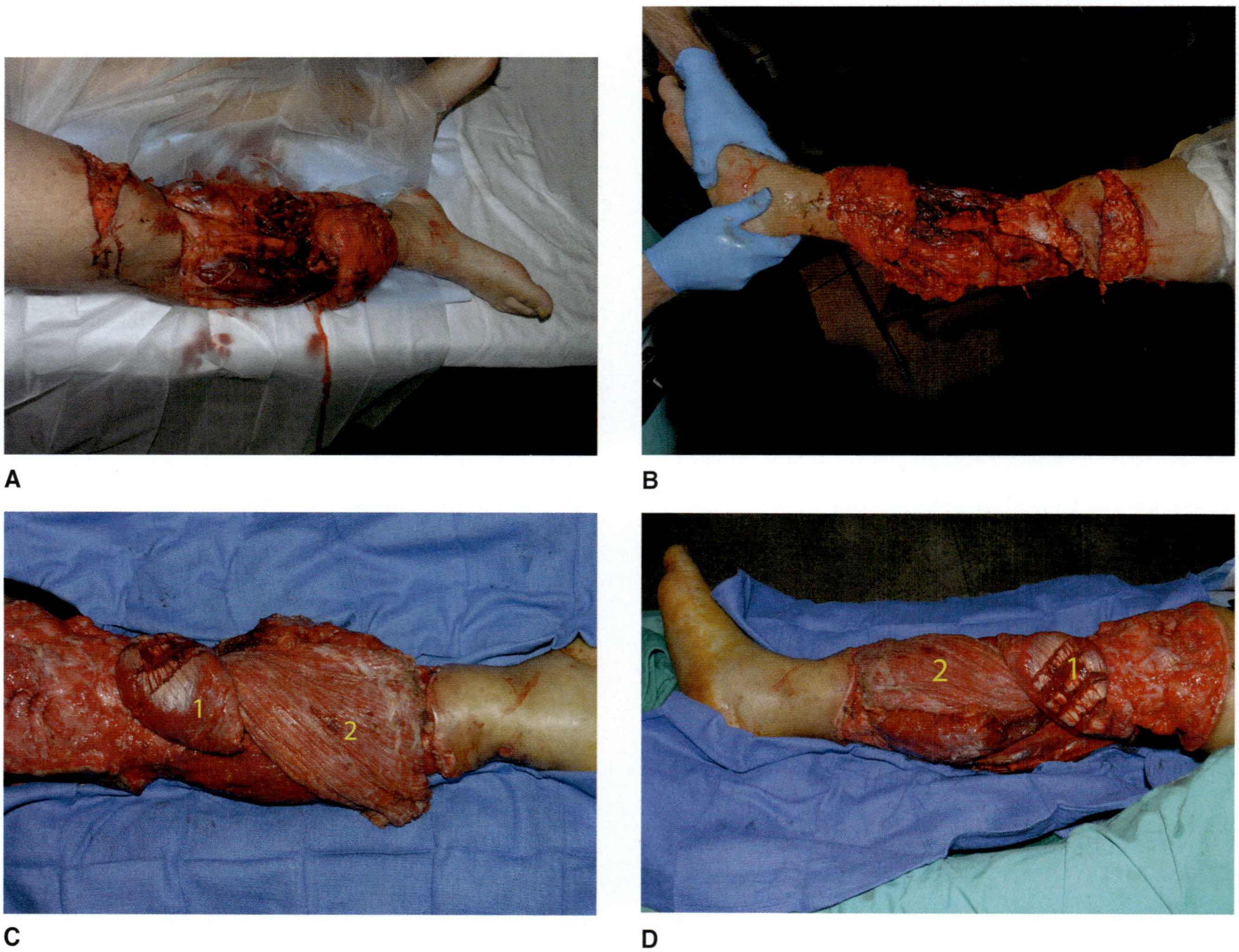

FIGURE78-5 (A, B) Severely comminuted fractures, extensive soft tissue loss of right leg. (C, D) Reconstruction with medial gastrocnemius flap proximally (1) and latissimus dorsi free flap distally (2). (E, F, G) 5 years post-reconstruction.

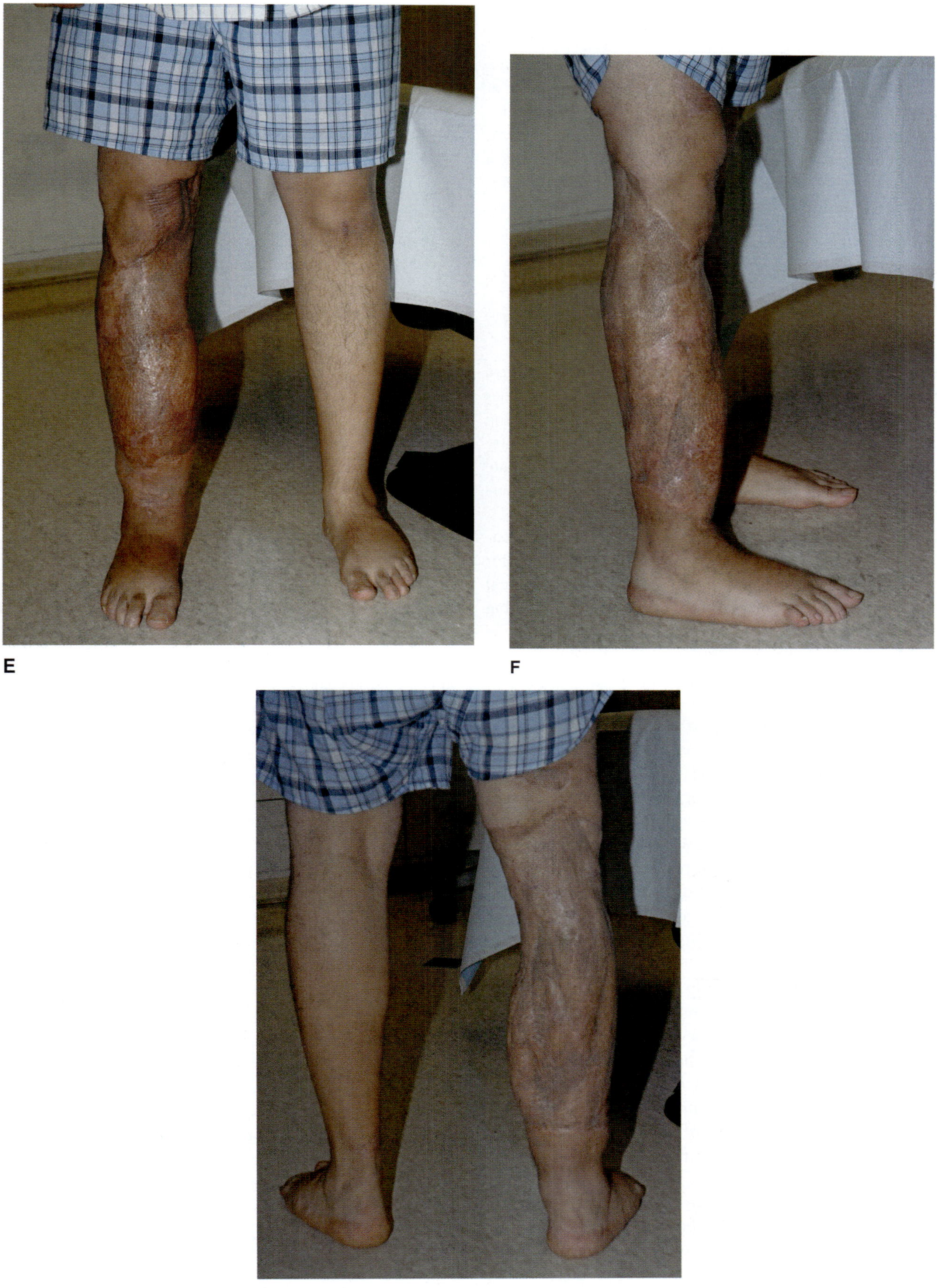

FIGURE 78-5 *(Continued)*

There are no reliable clinical studies, and there is no agreement among reconstructive microsurgeons regarding the superiority of one type of tissue transfer over the other. In our practice, the superior adherence of the muscle to the fracture, vascular communications (1), and complete elimination of dead space as observed during flap reelevation procedures influence our preference of placing muscle tissue over severely comminuted fractures and bone defects. We increasingly use skin and fascia to cover tendons, neurovascular structures, uncomplicated fractures in smaller, less volume-demanding wounds.

COMMON FREE FLAPS FOR LOWER EXTREMITY RECONSTRUCTION

Latissimus Dorsi Free Flap

The latissimus dorsi (LD) (28) is our most frequently used free tissue transfer for lower extremity reconstruction. It provides the largest amount of tissue of any single unit transfer, making it ideal for coverage of the large, complicated lower extremity wounds. Its design can be easily adapted to accommodate smaller size defects with inconspicuous donor sites when harvested through a transaxillary approach.

Harvesting the flap requires positioning in the lateral decubitus. The ipsilateral muscle is harvested when the anterior tibial vessels are the recipient vessels and the contralateral muscle when the posterior tibial vessels are used, thus avoiding repositioning.

The need to modify plans intraoperatively is common in lower extremity reconstruction despite thorough preoperative evaluation and planning. A major advantage of this flap is length flexibility. The need to perform the vascular anastomoses at a more proximal level than anticipated can be easily accommodated by dissecting the vascular pedicle to the axillary vessels, harvesting the full muscle length to its origin from the lower ribs, or a combination of both. The flap vessel size can also be varied to accommodate the size of the recipient vessels. The 3–mm-diameter thoracodorsal vessels are commonly used, but the vessel size can be varied from the large subscapular vessels to the muscular branches distal to the origin of the serratus branches where the pedicle consists of one artery and two smaller veins.

The vascular anatomy of the flap is constant. In more than 1800 latissimus flaps, we have never had to abort because of anomalies. We have encountered several anatomic variations, such as independent origin of the branches to latissimus and serratus from the axillary vessels, origin of the serratus branches from the intramuscular branches to the latissimus, and inconsistent level of origin of the circumflex scapular and serratus branches, but none rendered the flap unusable. Flap harvesting is straightforward. The only point requiring attention is the area where the thoracodorsal vessels bifurcate into the branches to the latissimus and serratus anterior muscles. Based on these observations, we begin harvesting the flap by exposing the muscle at the subfascial plane, marking the amount of tissue needed for transfer and dividing the distal muscle fibers before identifying the vascular pedicle. Elevation is carried out in a distal to proximal direction, reflecting the flap superiorly and permitting dissection of the vascular pedicle and its branches under full visualization (Figure 78-6).

Combined Transfer of Latissimus Dorsi, Serratus Anterior, and Scapular Flaps

Massive lower extremity defects can be reconstructed by transferring the latissimus, a distal segment of the serratus anterior muscle, or a scapular fasciocutaneous flap on a single pedicle. Extreme care should be taken to avoid denervating the proximal slips of the serratus anterior muscle by injury to the long thoracic nerve.

We prefer to use the latissimus–serratus anterior combined transfer when additional coverage is needed anterior to the area covered by the latissimus at the level of the vascular anastomosis and the latissimus–scapular flap combined transfer for added coverage posterior and more coverage proximal to the vascular connections (Figure 78-7).

Bilateral or multiple lower extremity defects can be reconstructed simultaneously from a single donor site by dissecting combined latissimus–serratus or latissimus–scapular flaps, dividing and transferring the lesser flap to the smaller defect while the latissimus muscle is still perfusing, and subsequently transferring the latissimus to the larger wound (Figure 78-8).

Gracilis and Adductor Magnus Free Flaps

The gracilis muscle flap (29) provides coverage of long but narrow lower leg defects. The major advantage of this flap is that it can be dissected from the ipsilateral thigh in the supine position with negligible donor site deficit. The blood supply to the overlying skin is tenuous beyond the width of the muscle, limiting its use as a myocutaneous flap. Transfer as an innervated functional motor unit has been extensively used for facial reanimation, restoration of forearm flexor and extensor muscle function (30), and restoration of ankle dorsiflexion resulting from loss of tibialis anterior muscle function (31). The location of the donor wound makes it prone to contamination. An occlusive dressing is required.

The gracilis muscle has a dual blood supply. The size of the branches of the medial circumflex femoral vessels of the flap varies considerably, but in most cases, it is adequate for transfer. Occasionally, the major blood supply is through multiple branches of the superficial femoral vessels. In 4.2% of our transfer attempts, we encountered arteries considerably less than 1 mm in diameter at the usual level of harvest, supplying only a small, proximal segment of the muscle. Dissection of the local vascular distribution revealed the caliber of the arterial branch to the adjacent adductor magnus in such cases to be much larger (2.2–3.2 mm), permitting transfer of the medial muscle fibers of the adductor magnus centered on the vessels and averting the need to abandon the procedure for a new donor site (32,33) (Figure 78-9).

Rectus Abdominis Free Flap

Medium-sized leg defects can be adequately reconstructed with transfers of the lower segment of the rectus abdominis

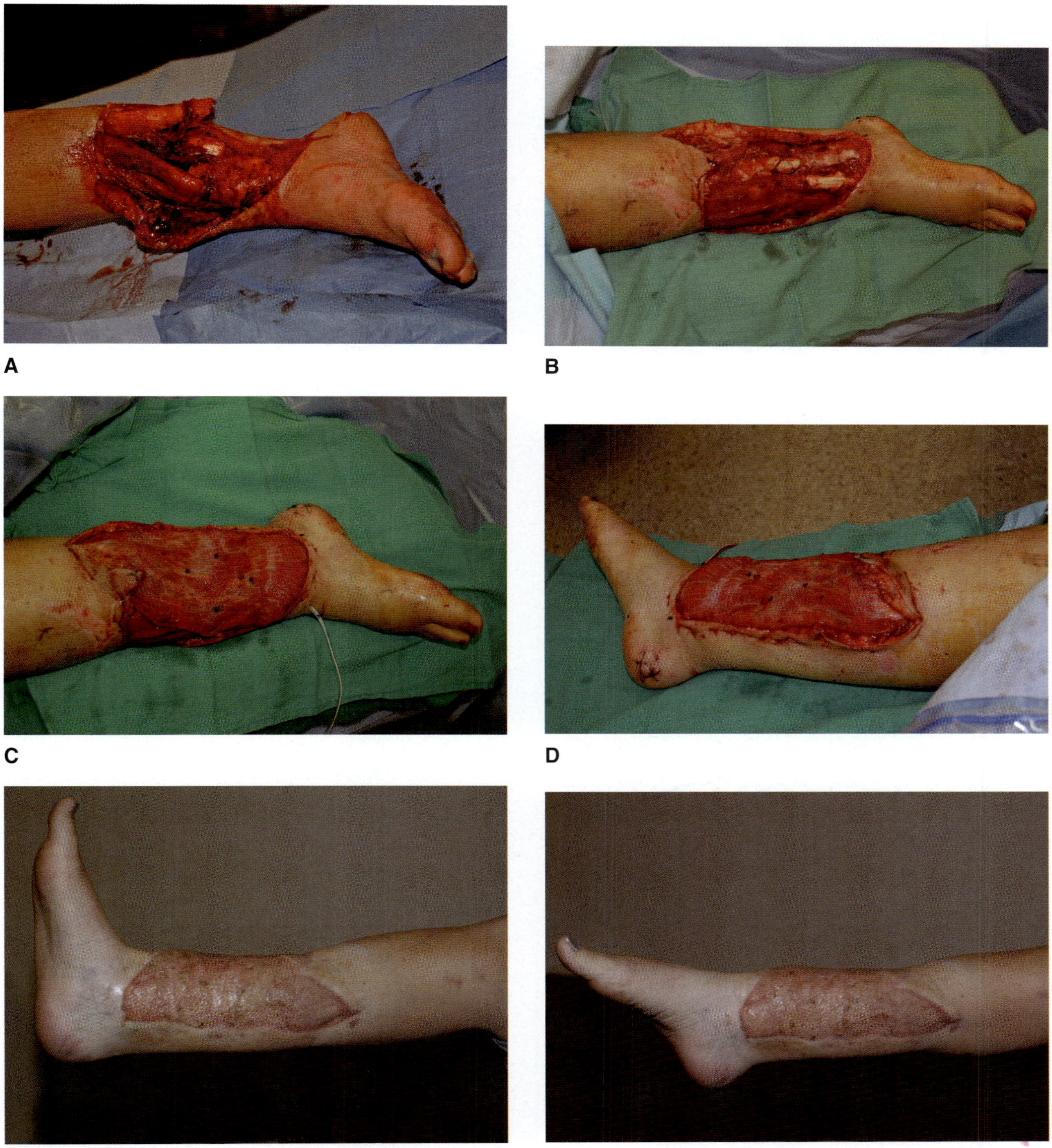

A B C D E F

FIGURE 78-6 (A, B) Extensive soft tissue and bone loss of right leg. (C, D) Reconstruction with single latissimus dorsi free flap transfer. (E, F) 3 years post-reconstruction.

muscle (34,35). Advantages of this flap are constant anatomy, large-caliber vessels, and harvesting in the supine position. Donor site morbidity can be greatly reduced by preserving the transverse inscriptions attaching the muscle to the anterior rectus sheath to prevent proximal retraction of the remaining muscle fibers; extending the anterior rectus sheath incision distally only as needed for safe vessel dissection but leaving intact as long a distal segment as possible; harvesting only the required muscle width; and paying attention to repair both the external and internal oblique components during closure. The distal segment of the muscle can be harvested through a transverse suprapubic incision. We have used this approach in combination with skin graft harvest from the same area to achieve an undetectable donor site in special situations.

Recognizing that the flap has a rectangular shape with the vascular pedicle located on the left or right lower corner depending on the side of harvest permits optimal positioning

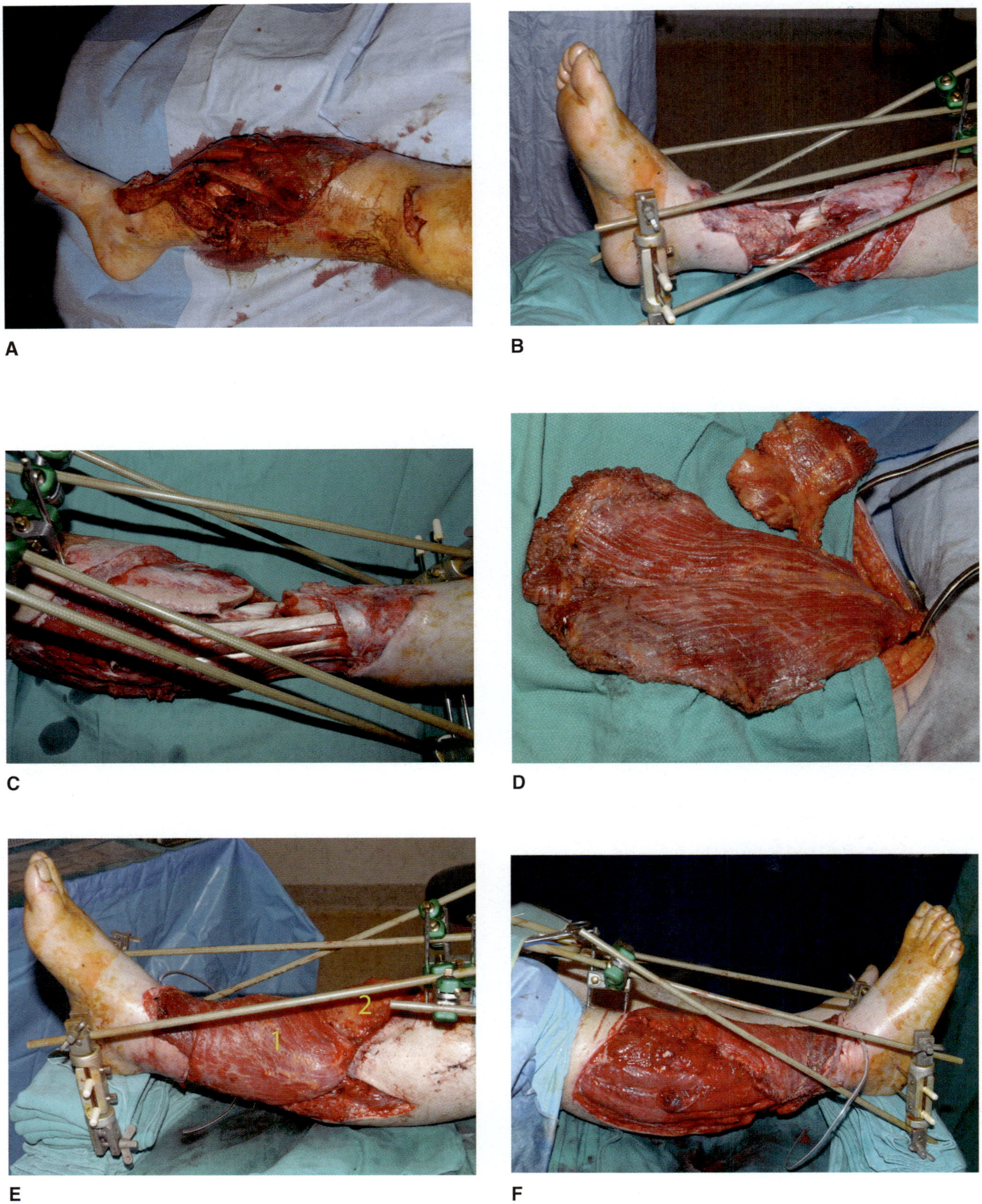

FIGURE 78-7 (A) Incomplete amputation of right leg. (B, C) Initial fracture stabilization. (D) Harvesting of latissimus dorsi-serratus anterior free flap. (E, F) Reconstruction with latissimus dorsi free flap distally (1) and serratus anterior free flap proximally (2) in a common pedicle. (G, H) 3 months post-reconstruction. (I) Application of spatial frame. (J) 4 years post-reconstruction.

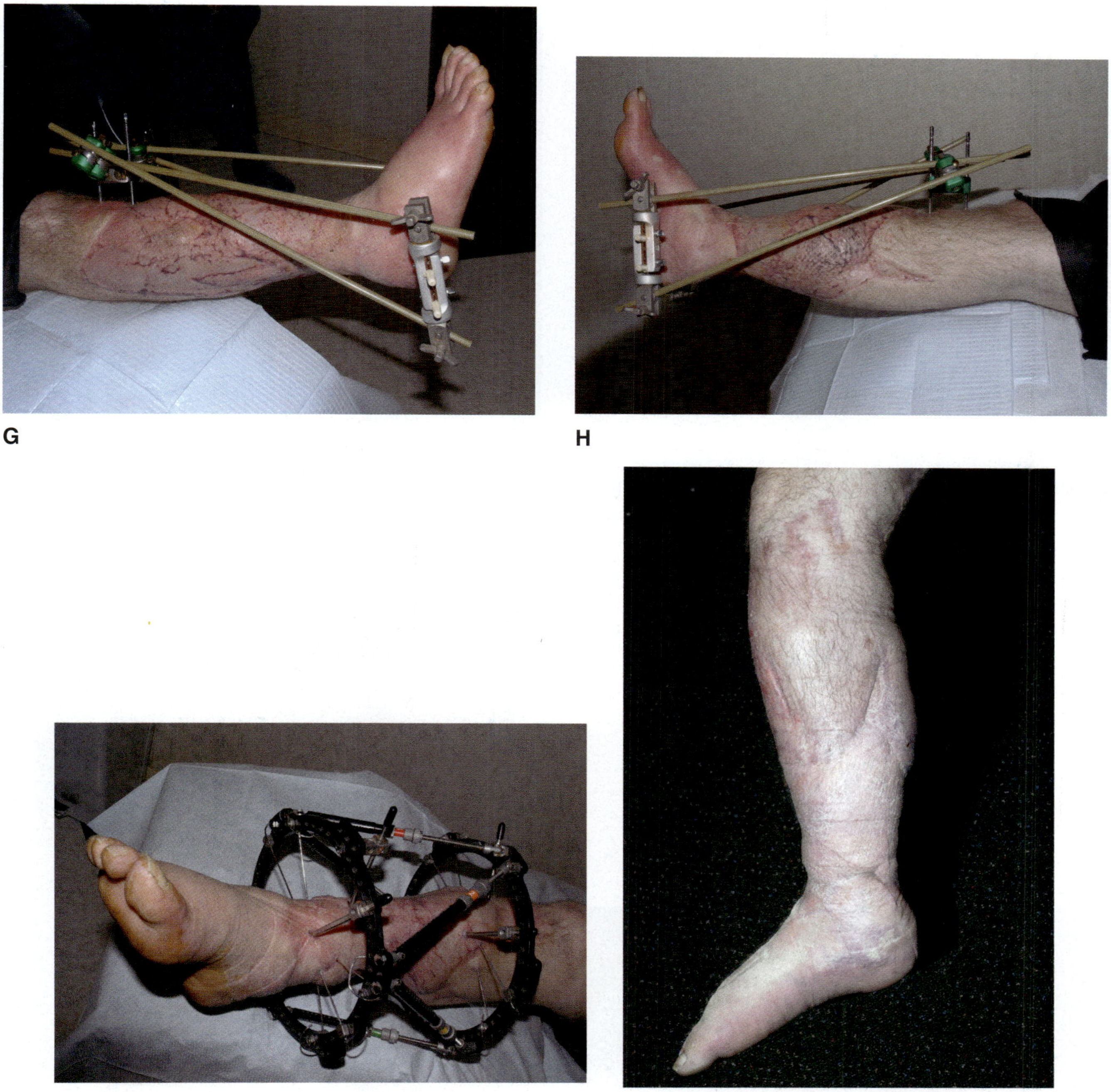

G H I J

FIGURE 78-7 *(Continued)*

and full utilization of the muscle length. The contralateral rectus is best suited for coverage of pretibial defects when the posterior tibial vessels are the recipient vessels and the ipsilateral for use with the anterior tibial vessels (Figure 78-10).

Anterolateral Thigh Flap

Use of the muscle sparing anterolateral thigh (ALT) flap (36) in lower extremity reconstruction has increased as experience with perforator flap dissection has improved. Long vascular pedicle, limiting the operation to one extremity, and flap dissection in the supine position are major advantages. A long but narrow (6–8 cm) cutaneous component can be harvested with primary closure of the donor defect. The donor site is much better tolerated by older individuals than young trauma patients. Harvesting a larger flap requires skin grafting of the thigh defect, making the flap a much less attractive choice.

The blood supply to the ALT flap varies. In most instances, the ALT flap is supplied by myocutaneous and not, as initially described, by septal perforators emerging through the rectus femoris–vastus lateralis plane (37). The musculocutaneous perforators most frequently penetrate the medial edge of the vastus lateralis and less frequently the lateral edge of the rectus femoris muscle. Dissection must therefore be customized based on the individual findings, making harvesting less straightforward.

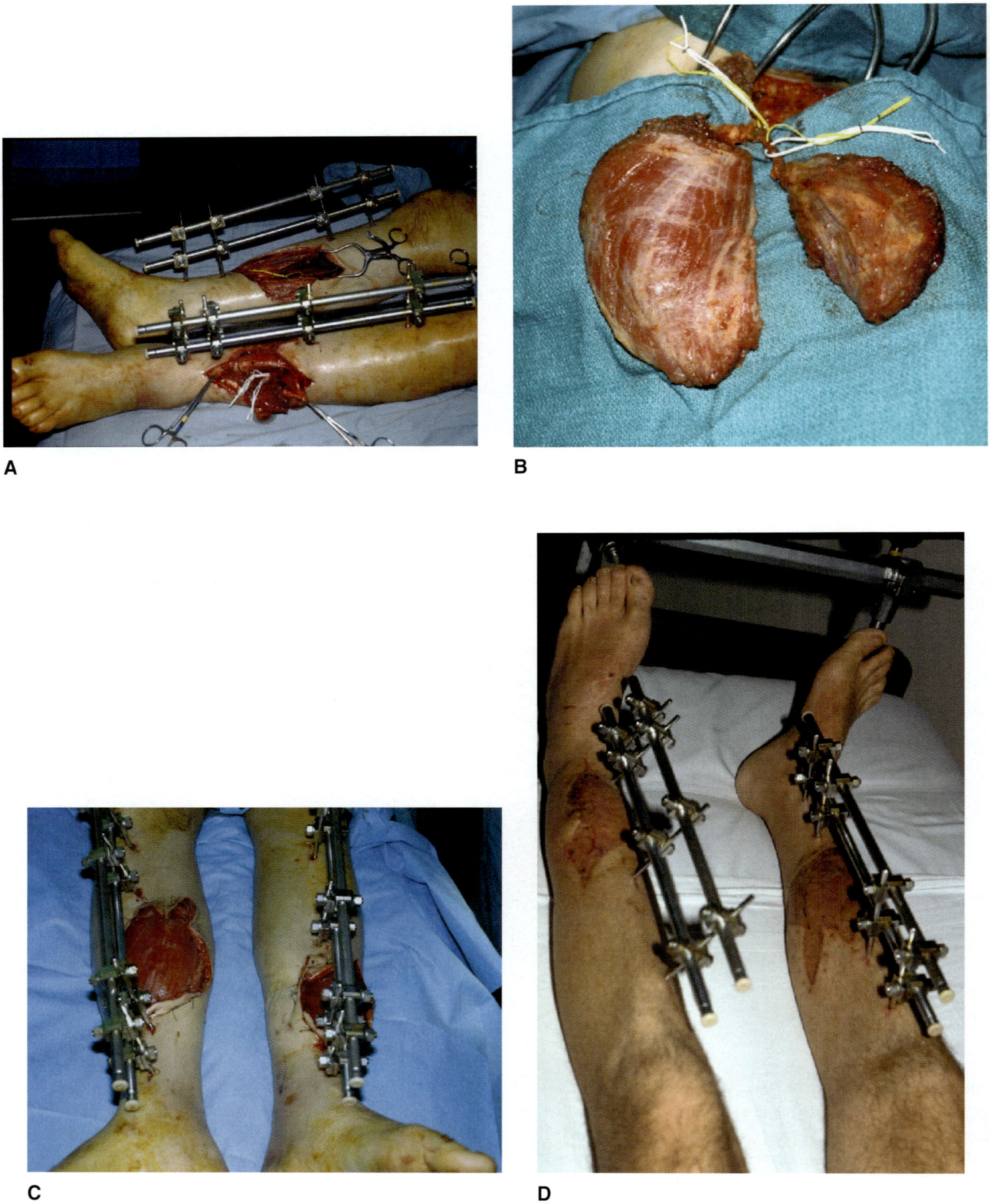

FIGURE 78-8 (A) Bilateral open tibial fibular fractures. (B) Harvesting of latissimus dorsi-serratus anterior free flap. (C) Reconstruction of right leg defect with latissimus dorsi and of left leg with serratus anterior free flaps. (D) 2 months post coverage.

On the other hand, this permits chimeric harvesting of a muscle segment, usually from the vastus lateralis or vascularized fascia lata, to provide well-vascularized tissue for lower extremity reconstruction.

When the bulkiness of the flap is problematic, intraoperative thinning or subsequent debulking procedures are needed for improvement (38).

Radial Forearm Free Flap

The radial forearm fasciocutaneous flap (39) fulfills all the requirements for precise coverage of uncomplicated small- to medium-sized lower extremity defects where bulk is unacceptable.

The thinness of this flap combined with ease of dissection; availability of dual venous drainage through the cephalic vein and venae comitantes; ability to harvest in the supine position under tourniquet control; and, when necessary, under regional block anesthesia, make this flap extremely useful for coverage of lower leg or ankle defects, particularly in unstable or morbidly obese patients. The size of the radial artery and cephalic vein is compatible with the size of the lower leg vessels, making it our preferred arterial, venous, or combination of both "flow-through" free flaps in these areas. The major potential drawback of this flap is donor site morbidity, especially when closure requires skin grafting (40).

The "racing stripe" modification (41) has considerably improved donor site morbidity. The flap is designed with only a narrow, 1- to 2.5-cm skin paddle (depending on the patient's body habitus) centered on the axis of the vessels and includes a much wider segment of the deep forearm fascia extending from the cephalic vein to the palmaris longus tendon. The development of this flap was based on years of clinical observations indicating that careful dissection of the deep fascia is well tolerated and that the thin, deep fascial layer initially enlarges because of some degree of congestion and subsequent hypertrophy. Any type of radial forearm flap transfer requires careful preoperative and intraoperative determination of ulnar artery dominance and patent palmar arches. All branches of the superficial radial nerve are dissected and preserved. Unintended injury to the paratenon is not critical as primary closure of the donor wound is planned. At the recipient sites, the exposed fascia on either side of the

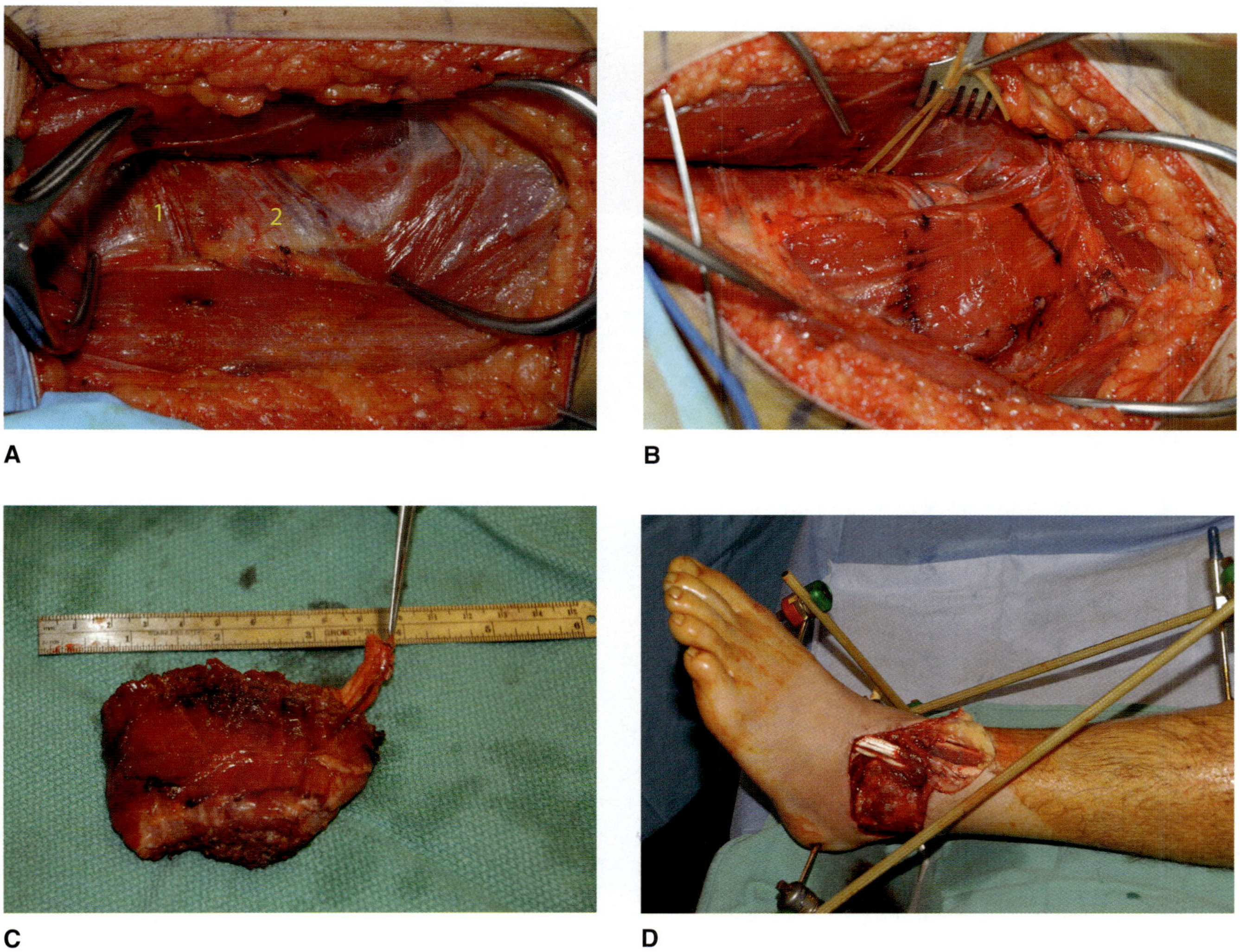

FIGURE 78-9 (A) Encountering of minute MCFA branch to the gracilis muscle (1) and larger branch to the adductor magnus (2) during attempted harvest of gracilis free flap. (B, C) Harvesting of adductor magnus-free flap. (D, E) Reconstruction of left ankle defect with transfer of adductor magnus free flap. (F, G) 1.2 years post-reconstruction.

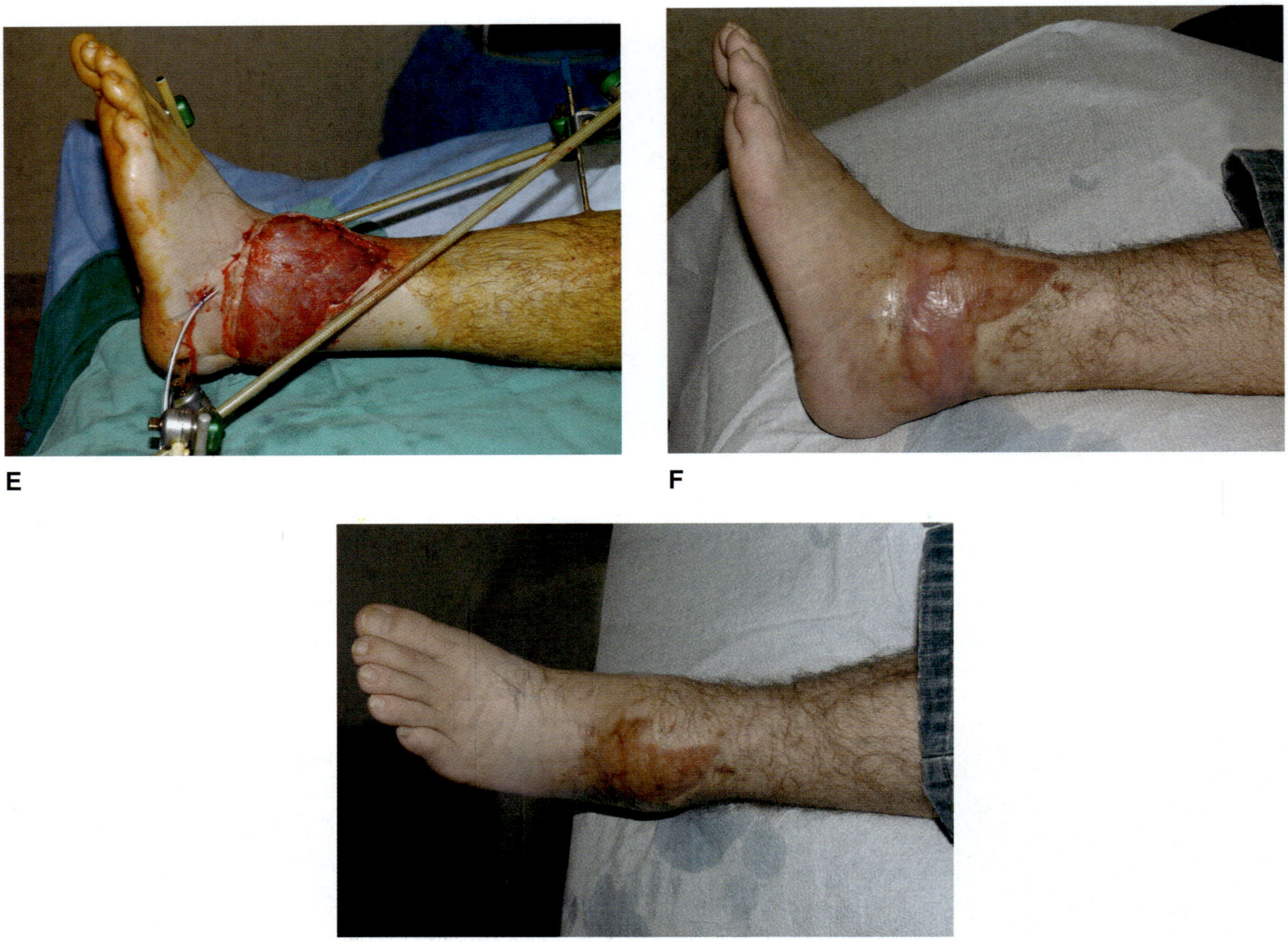

E F G

FIGURE 78-9 *(Continued)*

skin strip is skin grafted. The initially uneven, irregular appearance improves rapidly as the fascial component hypertrophies. The inclusion of the skin stripe augments the bulk of the flap, provides sturdy coverage of the vessels, compensates for possible skin graft loss by epithelization from the edges, and accomplishes a better long-term donor site appearance by avoiding the skin graft on the volar aspect of the forearm. This is the only free flap we have performed on an outpatient basis (Figures 78-11 and 78-12).

Lateral Arm Free Flap

The lateral arm free flap (42,43) is used as a fasciocutaneous or fascial transfer for coverage of mostly distal lower extremity defects. When sensory reinnervation with minimal bulk is required, the cutaneous island of the extended lateral arm free flap design can provide thin, sensate coverage with no muscle or major vessel sacrifice. The modification described for the radial forearm free flap can be used to cover larger defects with primary closure of the donor site. Disadvantages are small vessel caliber, unreliable viability of the distal segment of the extended flap, and sensory forearm deficits (44).

Tensor Fascia Lata Flap

Used frequently for lower extremity soft tissue reconstruction in the early days (45,46), the development of more reliable, easier to dissect, and less bulky flaps has restricted the use of the tensor fascia lata as a free flap. Our use of this flap in the lower extremity is now limited to reconstruction of a tendinous lower extremity defect of the Achilles (47) or quadriceps mechanism (along with or in combination with allograft), taking advantage of its well-vascularized, strong fascial component and as a chimeric flap in conjunction with other units supplied by the lateral circumflex femoral vessels.

FREE FLAP TRANSFERS FOR SPECIFIC AREAS

Thigh

Local muscle and fasciocutaneous flaps, supplied by the medial or lateral circumflex femoral vessels and rotational abdominal wall flaps, based on the inferior epigastric vessels, provide large amounts of tissue for reconstruction of thigh defects. Use of free flaps is limited to cases of massive soft tissue loss with open femur fractures, exposed femoral vessels surrounded by unyielding, indurated soft tissue, and free vascularized bone transfers for femur reconstruction.

Large thigh defects require long, wide flaps with long pedicles and large-caliber vessels to facilitate end-to-side anastomoses to the femoral vessels and optimal flap placement. We use the LD free flap at maximum length or as a chimeric transfer in combination with the serratus anterior or scapular flaps (or both). Broad ALT flaps can be transferred from the contralateral thigh with skin grafting of the donor site.

Narrow thigh defects with exposed femoral vessels surrounded by immovable soft tissues can be readily covered in the supine position with the use of large-caliber vessel fasciocutaneous flaps such as the ALT flap and the modified radial forearm free flap.

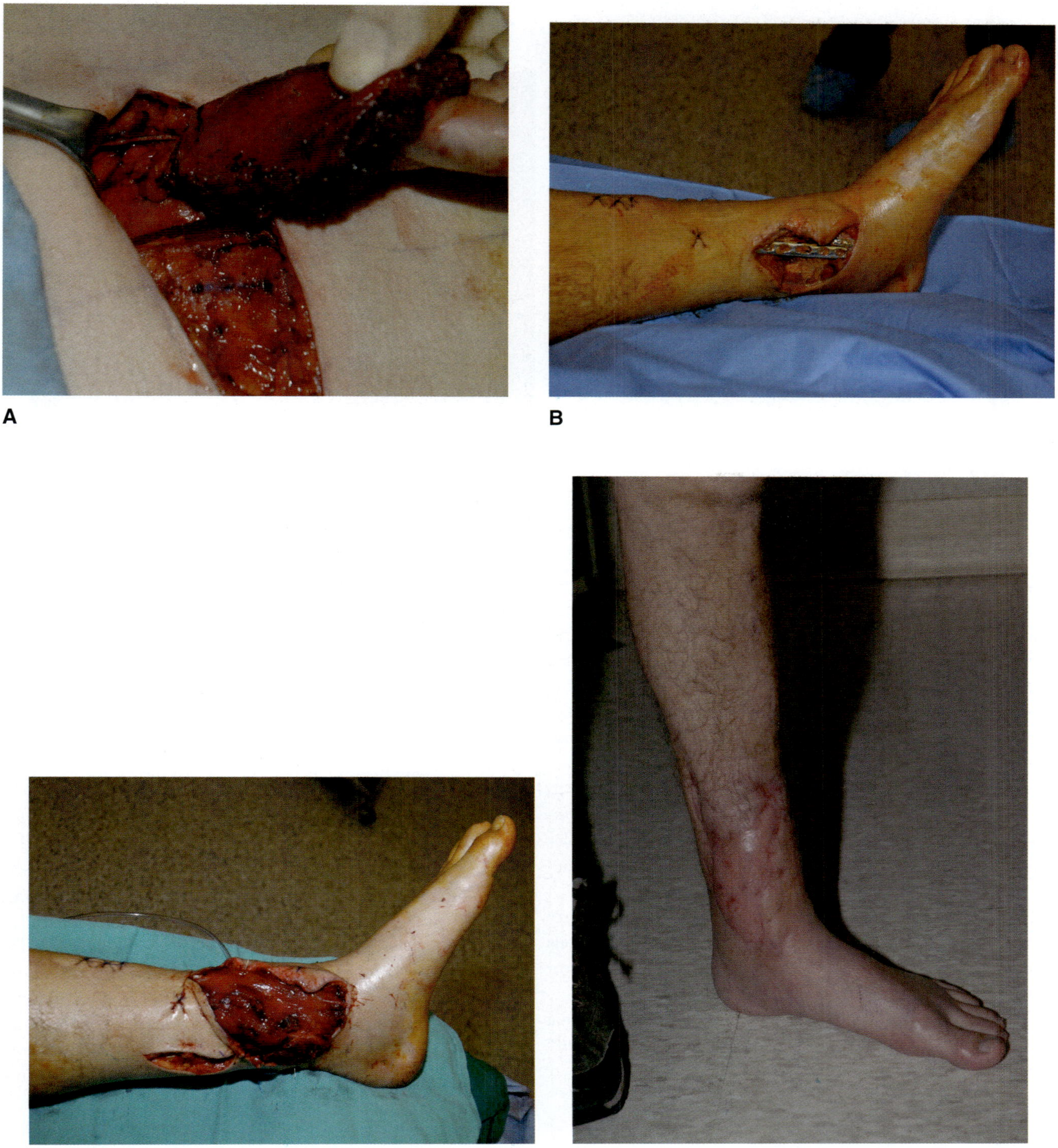

A B C D

FIGURE 78-10 (A) Harvesting of right hemi rectus abdominis free flap. (B, C) Left ankle reconstruction with hemi rectus free flap. (D, E) 2 years post-reconstruction. (F) Donor site.

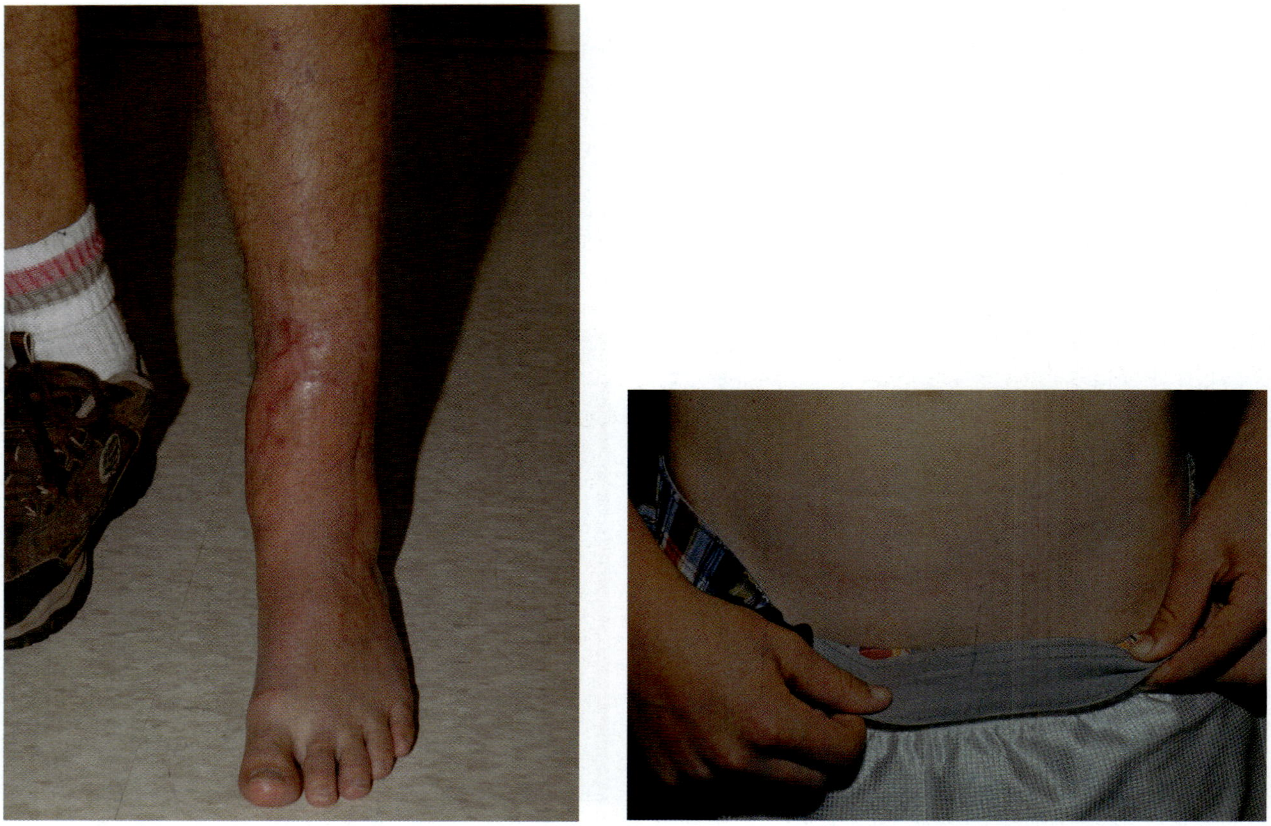

E F

FIGURE 78-10 *(Continued)*

Vascularized bone transfers for lower extremity reconstruction are described in Chapter 81.

Knee and Upper Leg

Inadequacy of local flaps to cover large defects of the knee and upper leg area is the main reason for use of free tissue transfers. Placement of the flap in a reverse fashion and anastomosing the flap to the anterior or posterior tibial vessels as described earlier greatly facilitates the procedure and produces a superior long-term result.

Coverage of lesser upper leg defects with associated injury to the sural vessels and soft tissues preventing the use of the gastrocnemius flaps is commonly accomplished with smaller muscle free flaps such as the rectus abdominis or fasciocutaneous free flaps such as the ALT and scapular flaps.

Small- to medium-sized proximal knee defects can be precisely reconstructed using free flaps with smaller caliber vessels such as the gracilis muscle, distal ALT, scapular, or lateral arm flaps anastomosed to the genicular vessels (48).

The tensor fascia lata free flap provides vascularized fascia for reconstruction of the injured quadriceps mechanism usually in combination with other modalities.

Middle Third Leg

The LD, gracilis, and rectus abdominis muscle flaps are the most frequently used free tissue transfers for reconstruction of middle third leg defects. We prefer vascularized muscle flaps for coverage of defects involving segmental bone loss, severely comminuted fractures, and osteomyelitis, which are the most common causes of middle third leg defects. In less complex injuries, muscle-sparing fasciocutaneous flaps such as the ALT, lateral arm, scapular, or radial forearm flaps are selected.

The gracilis can be transferred as a reinnervated functional muscle transfer to compensate for loss of tibialis anterior muscle function and restore some degree of ankle dorsiflexion. In our experience, resultant motor function is not strong enough to counteract a normally functioning gastrocnemius–soleus unit and is more effective in situations when some of the anterior compartment muscle units remain weakly functional and when the function of the posterior compartment musculature is also compromised to some degree.

Lower Third Leg and Ankle

The distal tibia is by far the most frequent area requiring coverage by free tissue transfers (Figure 78-13) and is the most difficult to reconstruct. Reconstructive requirements vary considerably. The size of the defects requiring coverage varies from circumferential soft tissue loss extending to the foot to small lesions surrounded by unyielding soft tissues. Exposed structures include open fractures of various degrees of comminution and bone loss, open joints, tendons, and neurovascular structures. The type of reconstruction varies accordingly.

The LD transfer is again the workhorse for reconstruction of massive soft tissue defects in this area. The muscle alone or in combination with chimeric flaps will provide enough tissue for coverage of circumferential wounds. Large defects up to 35 × 15 cm can be covered with extended ALT flaps (49).

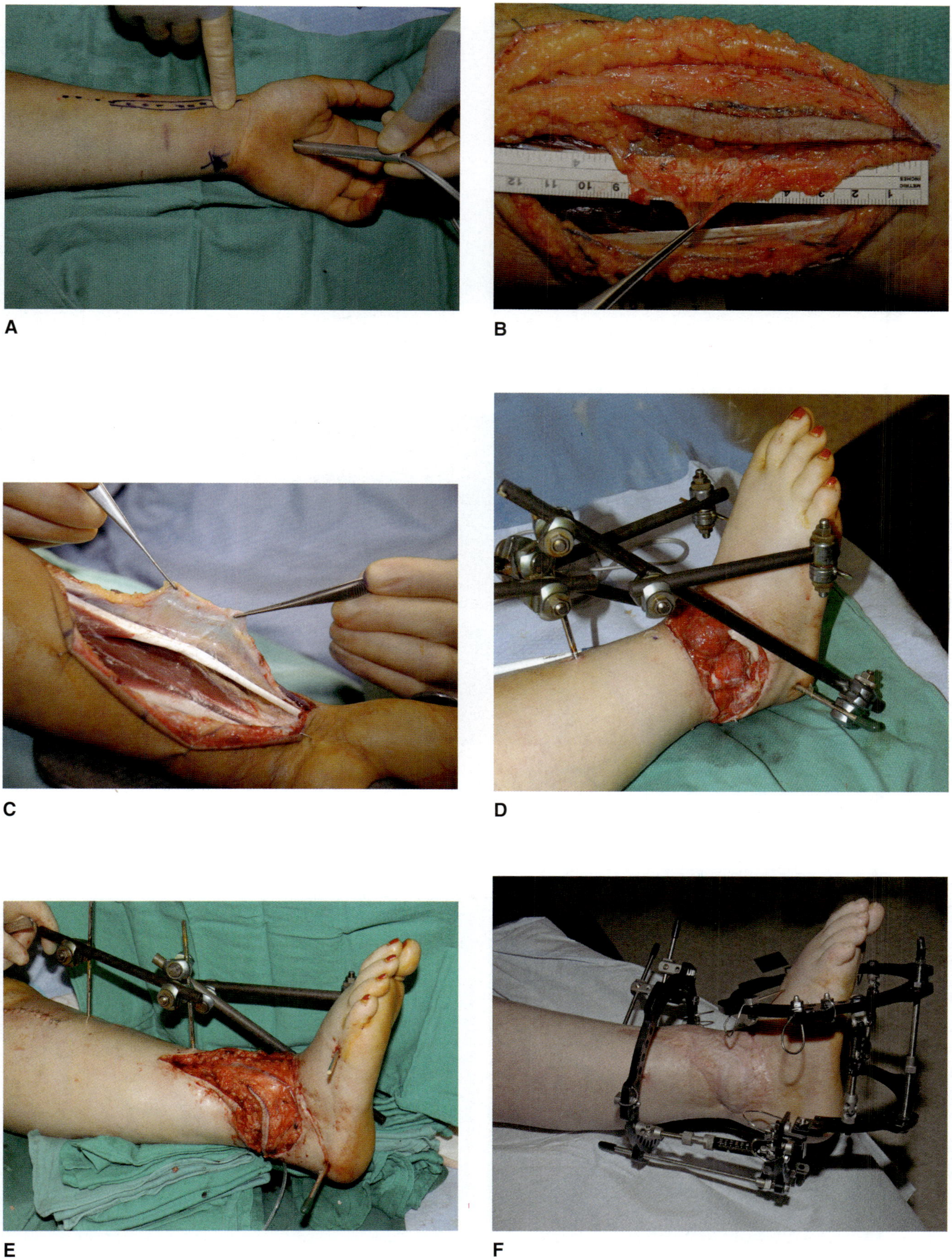

FIGURE 78-11 (A) Intraoperative determination of ulnar artery dominance. (B, C) Harvesting of "racing stripe" radial forearm free flap. (D, E) Reconstruction of right ankle with left racing stripe radial forearm free flap. (F) Application of spatial frame. (G, H) 6 months post-reconstruction. (I) Donor site.

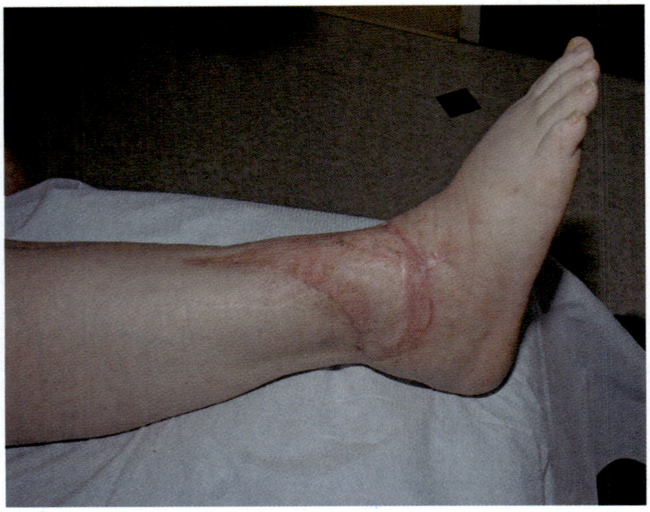

G

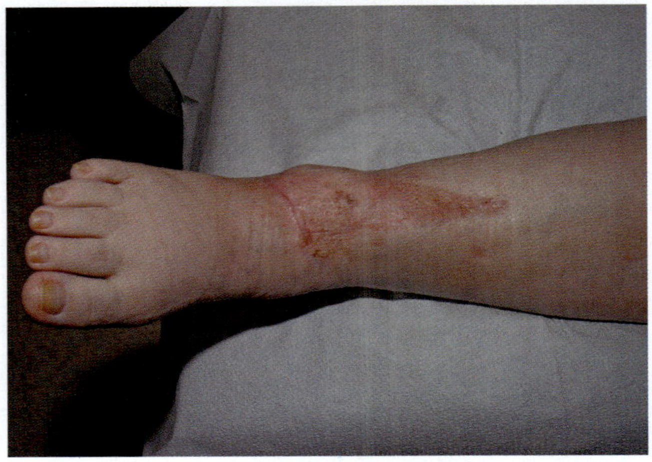

H

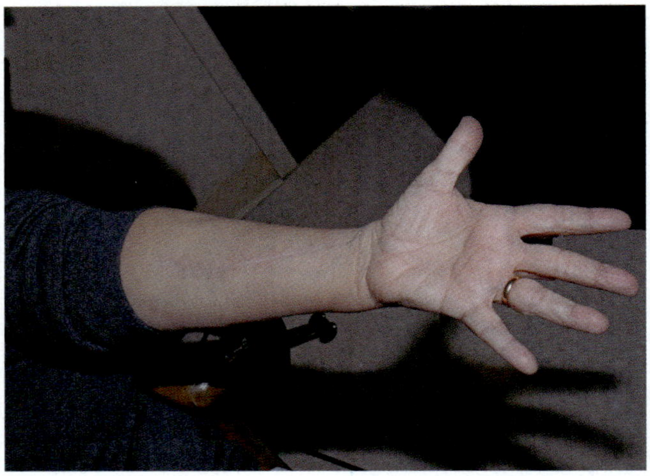

I

FIGURE 78-11 *(Continued)*

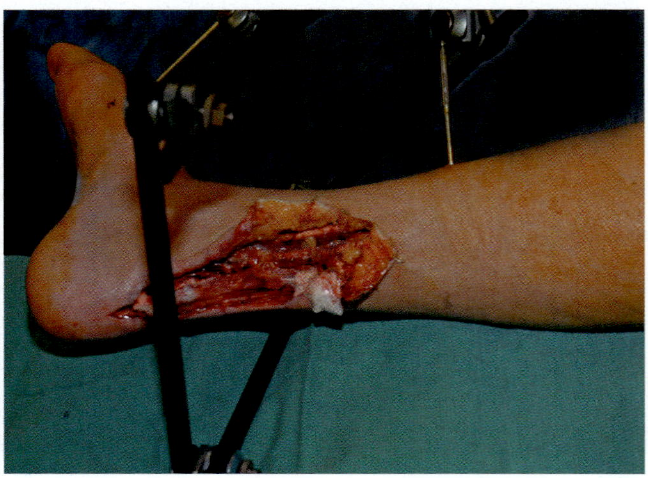

A

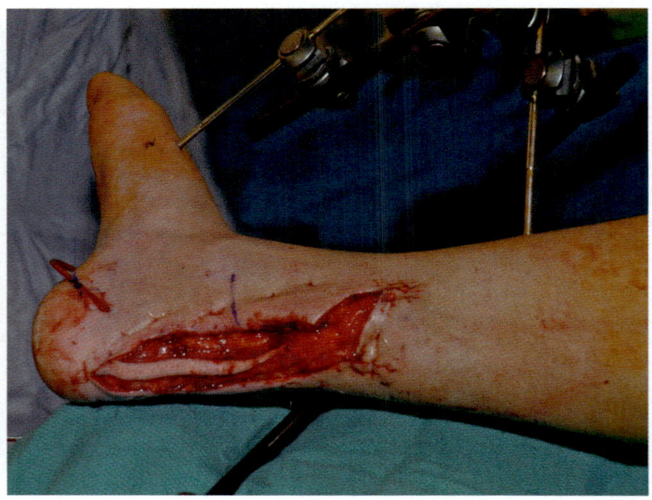

B

FIGURE 78-12 (**A**, **B**) Coverage of Achilles tendon defect with transfer of racing stripe radial forearm free flap. (**C**) 6 months post-reconstruction. (**D**) Donor site.

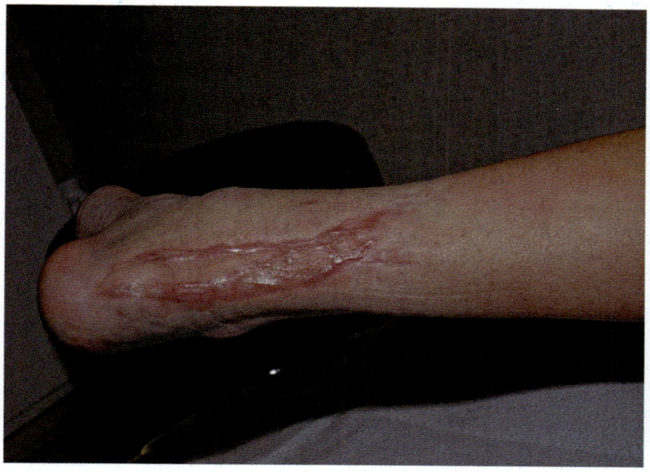

C

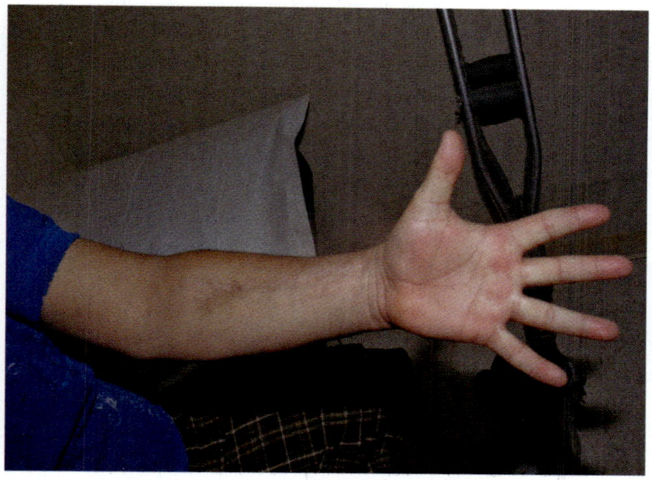

D

FIGURE 78-12 *(Continued)*

The gracilis is our choice of muscle flap for coverage of narrow, medium-sized defects. The relatively small sizes of the branches of the medial circumflex femoral artery and two veins supplying the flap are good matches for anastomoses to the anterior tibial vessels. The rectus abdominis provides wider coverage, and its vascular pedicle is a better match for the posterior tibial vessels.

We make every effort to place the muscle flaps under any area of compromised but viable soft tissues. Despite the initial appearance, some necrosis is common. In the presence of underlying healthy muscle, closure by secondary intention or skin graft is all that is required to avoid a second free tissue transfer.

Fasciocutaneous flaps are our choice for coverage of exposed tendons, joints, and uncomplicated fractures. Radial forearm and lateral arm flaps, modified to avoid skin grafting of the donor sites, are our preference. The ALT flap is used for coverage of larger areas. The bulkiness of the ALT flap depends on the patient's body habitus and can be problematic.

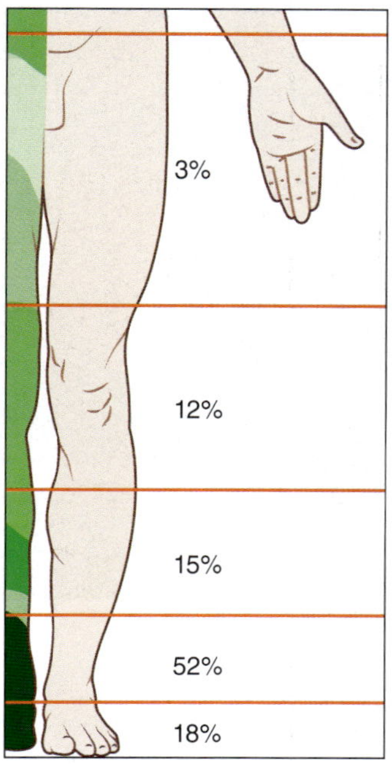

FIGURE 78-13 Distribution of 4864 free flaps performed between July 1979 and June 2011 for lower extremity post-trauma reconstruction (personal data).

Tensor fascia lata and chimeric ALT flaps provide vascularized fascia for reconstruction of wounds associated with defects of the Achilles tendon.

Bulk is not well tolerated in the lower leg and ankle. Every effort is made for optimal design and precise positioning of the flaps to lessen the problem but not at the expense of achieving the best possible coverage. Complications in this area are unforgiving and frequently catastrophic. The bulk of muscle flaps around the ankle improves considerably with time because of atrophy of the denervated muscle and contraction. Bulky fasciocutaneous flaps can be improved with secondary procedures.

Amputations

Preservation of amputation stump length with free flaps is the result of major developments in prosthetic technology, permitting the safe use of prostheses in insensate stumps by distributing pressure away from the distal region.

In above-knee amputations, every effort is made to preserve enough stump length to permit secure use of a prosthesis without a pelvic wrap. In very short amputations near the pelvis, salvage of nonfunctional remnants is indicated to avoid hip disarticulation and at least allow secure sitting. Large flaps such as the LD muscle or myocutaneous flaps are usually required. The ALT flap has been useful, but patients are hesitant to permit use of the uninjured extremity as a donor site.

The advantages of below- versus above-knee amputations with regard to energy requirements and quality of gait are significant. When local flaps are not available, short below-knee amputation stumps with intact patellar tendon insertion are reconstructed with a variety of free tissue transfers. Selection from the large number of muscle, myocutaneous, and fascial flaps depends on the size of the defect and location of usable recipient vessels. In cases when remnants of the medial head of the gastrocnemius are not long enough for stump coverage despite complete division of its origin, we have transferred the muscle as a free flap, dividing the medial sural vessels at their origin and anastomosing them in a distal position to patent trifurcation or popliteal vessels (Figure 78-14) (50).

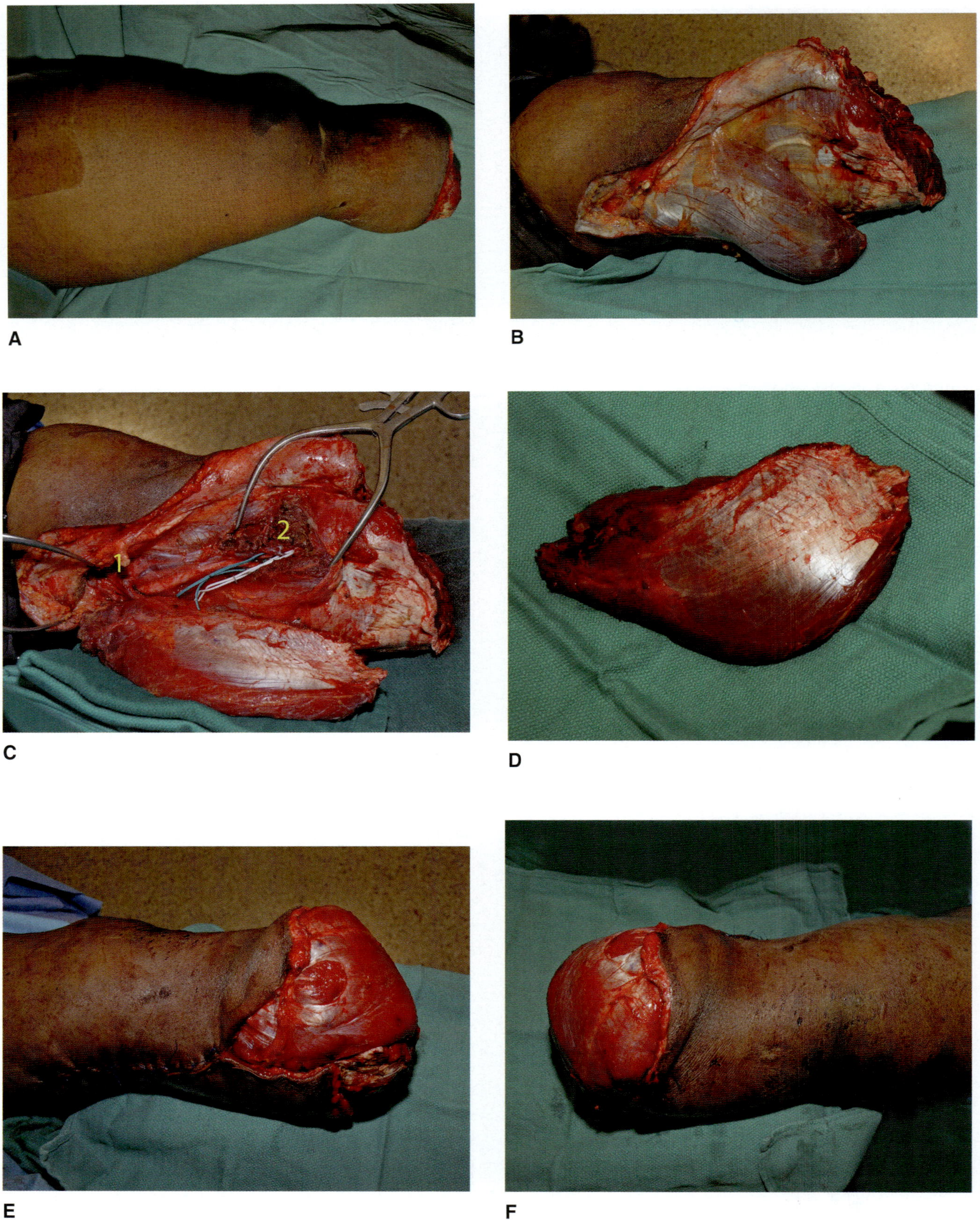

FIGURE 78-14 (A) Below knee guillotine amputation of left leg with short amputation stump. (B, C, D) Harvesting of medial gastrocnemius free flap. Dissection of the origin of the medial sural (1) and posterior tibial (2) vessels. (E, F, G) Coverage of BKA stump with medial gastrocnemius free flap and skin graft. (H) 8 months post-reconstruction.

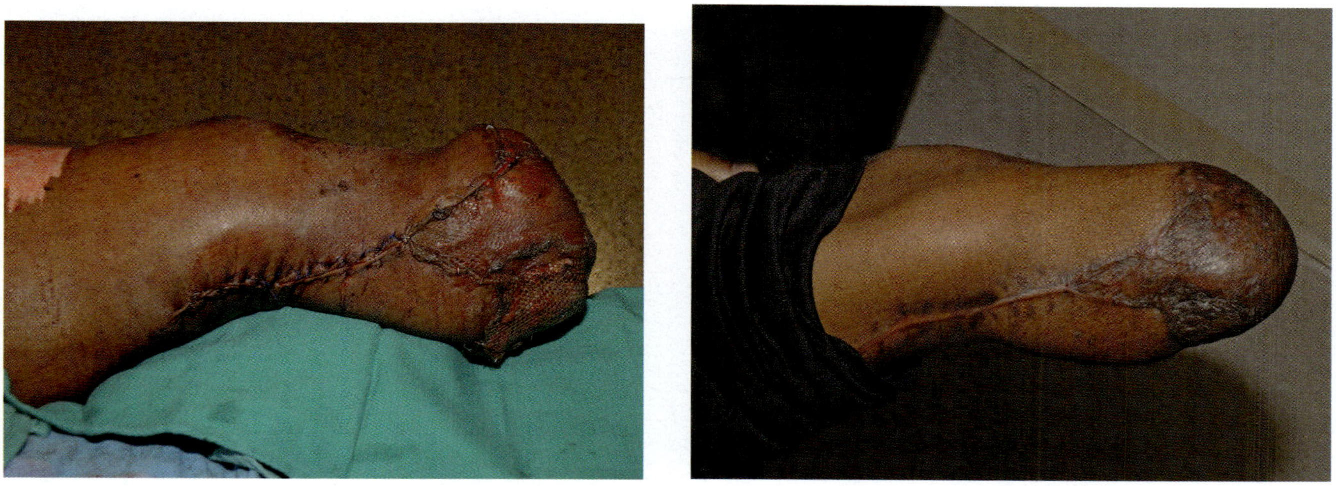

G H

FIGURE 78-14 *(Continued)*

VESSEL SELECTION

In a well-perfused lower extremity, decisions regarding the selection of recipient vessels are based on the condition of the vessels, location of the defect, and to a lesser degree on the vascular anatomy of the planned flap.

End-to-side anastomoses to the superficial femoral vessels are used for reconstruction of thigh defects. The deep femoral vessels and their medial and lateral circumflex branches are difficult to dissect but can be used when conveniently exposed because of the location of the defect.

In knee defects associated with distal thigh wounds, the distal segment of the superficial femoral vessels in Hunter's canal is selected. The medial genicular vessels can be used for the transfer of flaps with a relatively small caliber vascular pedicle (48).

Soft tissue defects involving the knee and upper leg can be reconstructed with end-to-side anastomoses to the popliteal vessels. Reverse placement of the flap with end-to-end or end-to-side anastomoses to the tibial vessels (51) is a safer arrangement that simplifies recipient vessel dissection and reduces the length requirements of the vascular pedicle. The flap in this position is unaffected by knee motion and has dependent drainage, permitting early mobilization and producing an overall superior long-term result (Figure 78-15).

In the leg, flaps covering anterolateral pretibial defects are routinely anastomosed to the anterior tibial vessels, but flaps covering posteromedial defects are anastomosed to the posterior tibial vessels, reducing the size requirements of the flap and permitting effective placement of its bulk. In general, the posterior tibial artery and two venae comitantes are larger than the anterior tibial vessels at an equivalent level. The larger size of the posterior tibial artery and easier, uncompromised exposure facilitate end-to-side anastomoses. The size of one of the posterior tibial veins is frequently large enough to efficiently accommodate single large vein flaps. The anterior tibial arteries are the better choice for end-to-end connections. The two anterior tibial venae comitantes are better suited for smaller, paired vein flaps, particularly at the lower leg and ankle level. Occasionally, when using flaps such as the LD, the artery that has been harvested at a proximal level is a good size match, but the flap vein is considerably larger than any of the recipient veins at the same anastomotic level. In such cases, we harvest the thoracodorsal vein at a more distal level and perform the arterial and venous anastomoses at different levels to avoid major anastomotic discrepancy.

The peroneal vessels are difficult to expose in the presence of an intact fibula and are rarely used (0.06% in our series).

Tributaries of the major and lesser saphenous venous systems of sufficient size for use for venous drainage should be preserved and marked during dissection. Anastomoses to the venae comitantes are the standard technique because of precise alignment and similar wall thickness. When superficial veins need to be used, they should be dissected to a level proximal to the intended site of the arterial anastomosis, and extreme care must be taken to obtain the correct length and avoid rotational problems.

Placement of the anastomoses in a location unaffected by the injury is prudent but not always feasible. The "zone of injury" as defined by the presence of histological changes involving the soft tissues and major vessels (52) extends considerably proximal to the open wound. Normal, usable vessels may be present at the proximal edge of large soft tissue defects. Final decisions regarding the placement of the anastomoses are made intraoperatively. Normal pulsatile flow must be present. Signs of vessel injury, including a thinned or thickened vessel wall, abnormal distention, perivascular scarring and hemorrhage (53), and intramural hematomas, are taken into consideration. When in doubt, flow strength can be assessed by dividing a small branch or performing a minute arteriotomy distal to the intended site of anastomosis. The placement of the anastomoses should be decided early, particularly when a two-team approach is used, because it will determine the required length of pedicle and influence the design of the flap.

The risk of compression is high when the vascular pedicle crosses directly over a metal plate or prominent bone and should be avoided at all costs.

We have advocated for the preferential placement of vascular anastomoses distal to the zone of injury in lower extremity

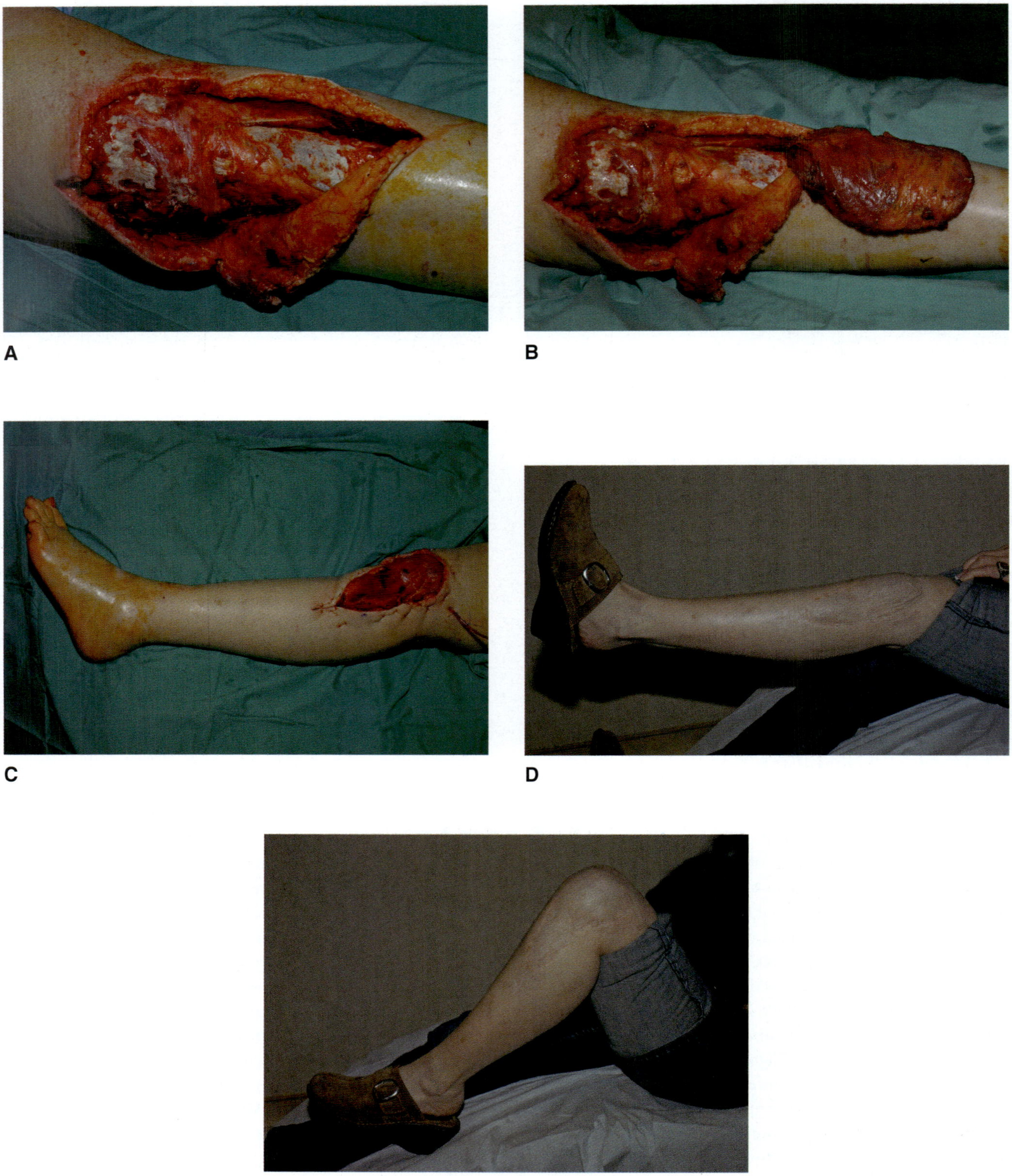

FIGURE 78-15 (A) Left knee and upper leg defect. (B, C) Reconstruction with latissimus dorsi free flap anastomosed to the anterior tibial vessels distal to the zone of injury. (D, E) 7 months post- reconstruction.

defects involving areas close to the groin and hip because of the ease of dissection, the knee and upper leg to avoid crossing the joint with the vascular pedicle, and when proximal exposure is limited by the type of established external fixation (49). At least one patent artery and unobstructed venous drainage are required. We have used this approach since 1979 with similar results to the overall outcomes of anastomoses performed proximal to the zone of injury over the same time period. More liberal use of distal anastomoses because of ease of dissection in the lower leg has been advocated by others (54).

VASCULAR ANASTOMOSES

Size discrepancy, ease of exposure, and personal preferences determine the use of an end-to-side or end-to-end arterial anastomosis in a leg with normal vascular anatomy. A wide end-to-side anastomosis is preferable in an atherosclerotic leg artery because it produces a patch effect and enlarges the anastomotic site. Small amounts of adventitia are removed from the perianastomotic segments of the vessels, but extensive skeletonization is, in our opinion, unnecessary and potentially harmful because of the risk of vessel injury and rotational distortion. Careful dissection and division of small anchoring branches is required in all cases to facilitate correct placement and smooth rotation of the vascular clamps during the anastomosis and to avoid kinking after release. Accurate alignment and estimation of vessel length is of extreme importance, particularly in a combination of end-to-side and end-to-end anastomoses. If uncertain, the second vessel to be anastomosed is left longer to permit further adjustments after completion of the first anastomosis. Venous anastomoses are most frequently carried out in an end-to-end fashion. Significant vein size discrepancy can be accommodated with oblique cuts, fishmouth, and other anastomotic maneuvers. Veins become thinner but wider near a valve. This can be used to our advantage, but the anastomosis should not be performed at the exact level of the valve.

Some degree of vascular spasm distal to the trifurcation is to be expected as a result of trauma, interstitial edema, and vessel manipulation. Vasospasm usually responds to dilation of the end of the vessel, irrigation with heparinized saline solution, and local application of spasmolytic agents (papaverine or Xylocaine). If these measures are ineffective, coronary dilators or Fogarty catheters can be used but with extreme care. The catheter is used more like a probe than an indwelling device; the balloon should never be inflated beyond the expected capacity of the vessel to avoid intimal cracking, which can be catastrophic.

The venous anastomosis is completed first unless it will impede the performance of the arterial anastomosis. Continuous suture technique is our preferred method for lower extremity vessel anastomoses except in cases of a major size discrepancy. It is expeditious and provides a better seal. Full distention of the end of the vessels before the placement of the continuous suture is an absolute requirement. Upon completion of the vascular anastomoses and if the flap is perfusing well, we leave it undisturbed for 10 to 15 minutes, bringing the warm ischemia time back to zero, in case something unforeseen happens during further manipulation.

Secure coverage of the vascular anastomoses requires precise planning of the leg incisions in relation to the recipient vessels. It is prudent to place the incision 1.5 to 2 cm medial or lateral to the expected line of anastomosis. The resulting skin flap can then be sutured to the adjacent muscle or fascia to compensate for tissue expansion. Faced with a tight closure and in the absence of better alternatives, skin grafting of the vascular pedicle is preferable to tight closure.

Vessel compression is a hazard amplified in the presence of the added weight from external fixation devices. Adding a "kickstand" provides some protection in addition to preventing heel pressure. Protection of the anastomoses to the anterior tibial vessels from vigorous muscle contraction and excursion can be achieved with the placement of two temporary retracting sutures through the skin and the tibialis anterior and extensor hallucis longus muscles to spread the muscles or tendons medial and lateral to the anastomotic site. Anastomoses to the posterior tibial vessels and to the superficial veins can be protected by applying an hourglass type of dressing, minimizing direct pressure over the vessels.

FREE FLAP TRANSFERS IN LOWER EXTREMITIES WITH VASCULAR INJURIES

High-energy injuries causing vascular trauma are frequently associated with open fractures and soft tissue defects that require free flap coverage. In a patient with a devascularized lower extremity, open fractures, and soft tissue loss necessitating free tissue transfer, the first priority is to decide whether or not a salvage attempt is feasible, safe, and in the best interest of the patient. Reestablishment of circulation to the extremity and reduction of ischemia time by means of vascular repair or placement of shunts are crucial (9).

Soft tissue reconstruction varies considerably depending on the level and extent of vascular injury, type of vascular reconstruction, and its proximity to the defect. Repair of vascular injuries proximal to the trifurcation frequently requires interposition of bypass grafts, typically autogenous vein grafts harvested from the contralateral side, to avoid further compromise of the venous outflow. Advancement of muscle and fasciocutaneous components adjacent to the graft is usually sufficient for definitive soft tissue reconstruction or at least coverage of the exposed graft. When free flap coverage is required, the arterial anastomosis of the flap is performed in an end-to-side fashion proximal to the vascular graft and with enough distance from the vascular repair to permit safe application of vascular clamps. The venous anastomosis is performed in the same fashion unless a suitable venous branch is readily available for an end-to-end connection. In the presence of long bypass grafts originating in the pelvis, we prefer to reverse the flap and place the vascular connections distal to the vascular graft.

Free flap transfers for coverage of leg defects in patients who have undergone successful arterial reconstruction proximal to the trifurcation are carried out in the standard fashion except in the presence of severe proximal deep venous injury, in which case branches of the greater or lesser saphenous systems are used for venous outflow.

Injury to one of the three arteries distal to the trifurcation, in our opinion, does not require reconstruction in a well-perfused extremity even though we have taken the few minutes needed to repair a simple vessel laceration in a stable patient. The injured artery is commonly used at a more proximal level as the recipient artery for a subsequent flap transfer.

In a leg supplied by a single artery, free flap reconstruction demands skill and careful planning. A conventional angiogram is obtained. Based on favorable findings, exploration of the injured arteries proximal to the damage is undertaken to look for a healthy segment, suitable for an end-to-end or end-to-side anastomosis. If this is not possible, end-to-side anastomosis to the single remaining patent artery is performed at a safe level. When the only residual vessel is bypassed, a flap long enough to permit anastomoses to a level proximal to the trifurcation is selected. If this is not an option, an end-to-side anastomosis to the vein graft is carried out. We use the vein graft loop technique to the popliteal vessels only as a last resort.

In rare occasions and in the absence of a better alternative, we have used the distal stumps of segmentally avulsed vessels for the flap anastomoses, creating a truly retrograde flow flap.

In selected cases of segmental vascular injury, a "flow-through" flap is used for revascularization or augmentation of the circulation to the distal injured extremity. The radial forearm free flap is our first choice. It offers a long, large arterial component of comparable size to the leg arteries, and its dual venous drainage through the venae comitantes and cephalic vein provides a choice of vein sizes suitable for interposition in a venous "flow-through" fashion to the deep or superficial leg veins.

POSTOPERATIVE MANAGEMENT

Effective monitoring of lower extremity free flaps requires diligence, experience, and a high degree of alertness. Any change in the condition of the flap constitutes an emergency and should trigger an immediate response. Prompt evaluation and decision making are essential if any chance of reversing the situation is to be expected. The operating room is alerted immediately of possible return. In the present era of decreasing incidence of complications and improving results, maintaining a high degree of readiness becomes difficult, and disbelief of findings is common.

We routinely Doppler the flaps intraoperatively at the end of the procedure to locate and mark a point on the surface of the flap where the signal is exclusively related to the flap circulation as confirmed by temporary clamping of the vascular pedicle. A window is left in the dressings at that level to permit monitoring of the flap postoperatively. An implantable Doppler cuff is placed around the vein close to the anastomosis to monitor buried flaps and when we are concerned with venous outflow.

An identical flashlight in every microsurgical room to provide the same illumination and a Doppler are the essential pieces of equipment. A pulse oximeter and a Doppler blood flow monitor for monitoring buried flaps are needed. A 20-MHz Doppler ultrasound probe provides visual assessment of superficially located anastomoses. Flaps are inspected and checked by Doppler every 15 minutes in the recovery room followed by hourly checks during the first 24 hours and then every 2 hours for the next 48 hours at the bedside.

The leg is kept elevated at the heart level unless clinical findings dictate otherwise. A dressing change of cutaneous flaps is performed on the second postoperative day, and skin grafted muscle flaps are redressed on the fourth postoperative day. In the absence of constraints because of associated injuries, patients with lower extremity flaps are permitted to dangle their legs at the side of the bed for a few minutes at a time after the first dressing change on the fourth postoperative day. Patients may start ambulating no more than 10 minutes per hour on the fifth postoperative day, and the same routine is maintained until the first outpatient visit 1 week after discharge. The ambulation and exercise regimen is adjusted based on associated injuries and progress. Light compression with an elastic bandage is applied during early ambulation sessions unless superficial veins have been used for venous outflow. Compression to counteract the expected edema of the flap and injured extremity is increased gradually and maintained with an elastic stocking for months or years, depending on the response.

COMPLICATIONS

In addition to the complications commonly observed in free tissue transfers, lower extremity free flaps are exposed to risks related to immobilization devices, restricted mobility, dependent edema, and fracture-related problems.

Early Complications

In our experience, most of the vascular complications develop during the first 12 hours after the vascular anastomoses, with a sharp reduction after the first 24 hours.

Venous Thrombosis

Venous obstruction is the most frequently observed complication after lower extremity free tissue transfers and carries a worse prognosis. Early, nonspecific signs include slight bulging of the flap, increased turgor, and a "water-hammer" arterial Doppler signal. Cutaneous flaps demonstrate some flushing and brisk capillary refill. The color of muscle flaps covered with skin grafts deepens from the initial beefy red appearance, and a few drops of dark blood may be noticed in the interstices of the skin graft. When errors related to leg elevation, positioning, and tight dressings are the cause of the problem, rapid improvement should be observed within minutes after correction. Advancing signs of venous obstruction while an arterial pulse is still present include enlargement and tightness of the flap, ecchymosis progressing to blistering and bleeding from the edges of cutaneous flaps, a dark red color changing to purple, and bleeding from the surface and edges of muscle flaps. Bleeding from a needle puncture is slow and dark. Loss of the arterial Doppler signal is the next ominous sign. Reversal is only possible in the early stages.

Arterial Occlusion

Decreased strength of the arterial Doppler signal and changes in the robust appearance of a flap can be caused by systemic changes in the patient's condition such as a drop in blood pressure and a decreased red blood cell count. Compression and overelevation of the leg are possible but uncommon mechanical causes. Gradual improvement and return to the previous normal state is to be expected as these problems are corrected. Arterial occlusion is usually an abrupt phenomenon. Arterial signal is lost, the surface temperature decreases in relation to the adjacent tissues, the flap develops a deflated appearance, and there is no bleeding from an 18-gauge needle stick. Cutaneous flaps become pale, loose capillary refill, and the exposed subcutaneous fat at their edges become ischemic. Muscle flaps develop a grey-brown color and show no signs of bleeding. The overlying skin graft becomes detached. Complete "nontake" of the skin graft indicates that the flap has never perfused adequately. Flap compromise caused by abrupt arterial occlusion, when detected early, has the best chance of successful reversal in our experience.

Hematoma

Bleeding under the flap can be caused by anastomotic leak, oozing from the raw undersurface of the flap, or the debrided recipient site. Coagulopathy, frequently caused by errors in the use of anticoagulants and seldom the result of systemic disease, is a common contributing factor. Whatever the cause, if the flap is compromised as manifest by enlargement, tension, or signs of venous congestion, immediate evacuation is required. Small donor site hematomas or seromas can be observed or improved with drain manipulation. If they become tense or skin changes develop, evacuation is carried out as soon as the coagulation status is checked and, if needed, corrected.

Complete Flap Loss

The end result of any of the previously described complications can be complete flap necrosis. Faced with such a disastrous outcome, thorough reassessment of the situation is required. All options should be discussed with the patient and family. If it is decided to continue with salvage of the extremity, removal of the necrotic flap is carried out as soon as the patient's condition is optimized and all factors that may have contributed to the poor result have been corrected. Irrigation, debridement, and placement of negative-pressure dressing device (VAC) may be needed until the wound condition stabilizes. In our practice, the decision to reconstruct a lower extremity defect with a free flap is typically based on the lack of easier, less complicated treatment modalities. Therefore, a second free tissue transfer is usually necessary. A second attempt at a free flap carries much higher failure rate, and salvage attempt by other means is often possible and recommended (55,56).

Partial Flap Loss

Overextension, incorrect design, and anatomical variations are, in decreasing order, the common causes of partial flap loss. The extent of tissue loss and level of demarcation are not immediately evident. Separation of the flap edges with potential exposure of fractures or hardware requires prompt reoperation and coverage by any available means.

Infection

Early infections vary from cellulitis to frank abscess formation and can involve the injured extremity or the donor site. Treatment is based on the clinical findings and involves appropriate antibiotic coverage, local wound care, and surgical debridement or drainage of the infection if necessary.

Late Complications

Flap Infection

Infections of mature free flaps are uncommon because of the increased vascularity of the transferred flap in relation to the adjacent tissues. Skin breakdown caused by minor trauma that is unrecognized because of lack of sensation may become infected but responds well to local care. Pin site infections related to external fixators are a frequent and serious problem. Intensive local care and systemic administration of broad-spectrum antibiotics are instituted until the offending pin can be removed. Blistering, pustule formation, or drainage at the junction between a free flap and normal skin should be considered a sign of deep infection and demands thorough investigation.

Pressure Ulcerations

Complete bed rest, immobilization devices, decreased sensation caused by injury or nerve block, and the added weight of external fixators are contributing factors in the development of heel ulcers in the early postoperative period. Inflatable heel protectors; well-padded, frequently checked splints; and the addition of a "kickstand" to the external fixation device usually avert such preventable problems.

Equinus Deformity

Correct splinting and external fixator shoes safeguard against a deformity that, after it is established, requires prolonged rehabilitation.

Fracture Nonunion

Nonunion can be an unexpected complication or the predictable result of extensive bone loss or destruction. In either case, the solid soft tissue envelope of a well-healed free flap provides increased vascularity to the area and permits safe exposure of the fracture site and subsequent closure with reelevation and insetting of the previously performed flap.

Osteomyelitis and Infected Nonunion

Fracture-related infection is the most serious complication, responsible for the majority of unfavorable outcomes. The benefit of a free flap is that it permits radical debridement of the underlying bone, delivery of a high concentration of systemic antibiotics to the area, and possible secondary bone grafting beneath the flap (see Chapter 79).

Dependent Edema

After high-energy lower extremity injuries, there is always some degree of posttraumatic venous insufficiency, causing dependent edema. In addition, the increased laxity of the maturing free flap and adjacent tissues results in fluctuation in the size of the leg with ambulation. Early compression with elastic wraps followed by custom-made elastic stockings usually keeps this problem under control. Surgical excision of excess flap tissue is seldom required.

INSET AND SCULPTING OF FREE FLAPS

Optimal placement of a free flap depends on accurate design. We plan muscle flaps to be 5% larger than the soft tissue defect. Special considerations are given for wider areas of degloving. Our preferred insetting suture for a muscle flap is a horizontal stitch placed through the skin edge of the defect and through half the thickness of the muscle flap. When coverage includes native muscle in addition to the free flap, photographic documentation before the application of skin grafts is very helpful in distinguishing the flap boundaries in subsequent reelevation procedures.

Fasciocutaneous flaps are planned with the fascial component at least 1 cm wider than the skin component and even larger for degloving injuries. A few absorbable sutures are used to accurately position the fascia. The skin is closed with simple or vertical mattress sutures.

Drains are brought out through separate stab incisions placed at a safe distance from the anastomoses.

Even though reestablishing a solid soft tissue envelope is the primary goal in reconstruction of lower extremity soft tissue defects, every effort should be made to achieve the best possible aesthetic result because the patients will have to look at it for the rest of their lives. Precise reconstruction begins with appropriate selection and correct design of the flap. The shape and thickness of the defect and the location of the recipient vessels should be matched with the corresponding characteristics of the donor tissue.

Deformities usually develop when the flap, designed to accurately cover the initial defect, becomes redundant as the extremity returns to normal size. Contraction of the peripheral scar and some degree of skin changes caused by lymphatic blockage can contribute to the postoperative changes. It should be noted that the adipose tissue of the fasciocutaneous flap continues to develop according to the genetic prediathesis of the donor area. Flaps from the hip, thigh, and abdomen are most often affected. These problems can be improved by liposuction, partial excision (38), and revision of the flap–normal skin junction. Fasciocutaneous flaps look better than muscle flaps in the early postoperative period. Thinning of the fasciocutaneous flaps at the time of harvest improves the overall result (57).

The early appearance of skin-grafted muscle flaps warrants preparing the patient before surgery of what to expect. The bulk of the muscle flap improves greatly as the denervated muscle atrophies and contracts. The appearance of the skin graft improves considerable with maturity. Improvement of excess bulk requires surgical excision. Carefully performed longitudinal incisions of the scar tissue on the undersurface of the muscle flap permit expansion and improved redistribution of the flap mass. In our experience, the long-term aesthetic result of a large defect treated with a free muscle flap is usually superior to a large defect covered with a fasciocutaneous flap (Figure 78-16). In all cases, the final appearance depends greatly on patient compliance with instructions to elevate the leg, perform scar management, and use flap compression.

Every effort should be made during reelevation of a free flap to avoid injury to the vascular pedicle regardless of the age of the flap. Lack of ischemia deprives the flap of the main stimulus to develop a reliable collateral circulation.

RESULTS

The use of free tissue transfers in the mid 1970s had a major impact on the management of lower extremity defects, permitting salvage of extremities previously deemed unrecontructable and offering a superior method of reestablishing a healthy soft tissue envelope around open fractures. Reports from institutions regularly performing such procedures indicate that, over the years, the success rate has greatly improved, and the number of complications has significantly decreased.

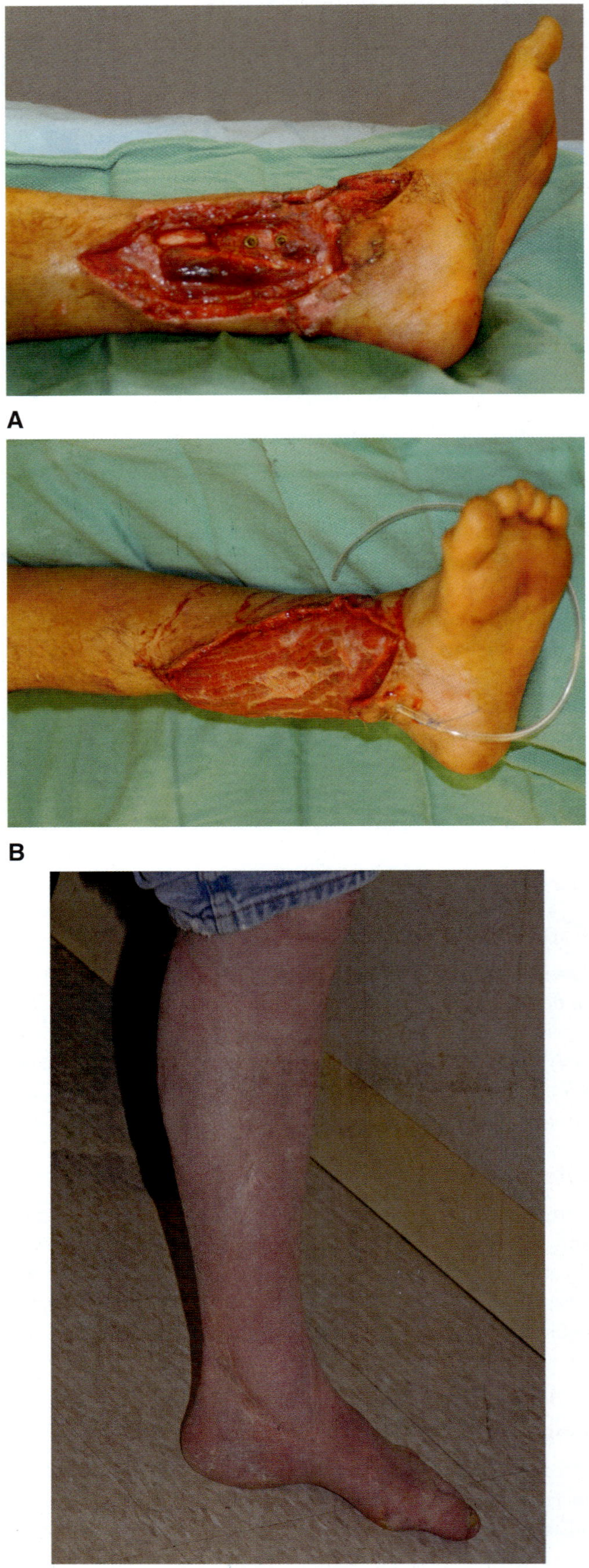

A

B

C

FIGURE 78-16 (A) Soft tissue defect left lower leg and ankle. Open distal tibial fibular fractures. (B) Reconstruction with latissimus dorsi free flap. (C) 31 years post-reconstruction.

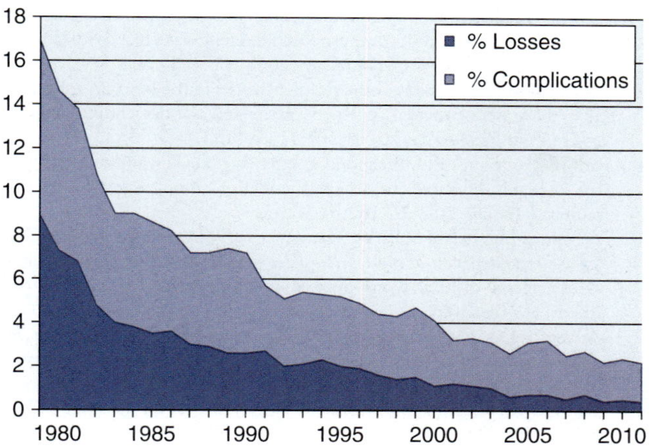

FIGURE 78-17 Percentage of free flap failures and unscheduled returns to the OR (personal data).

The failure rate for the first 100 extremity free flaps performed by Godina between 1976 and 1983 was 26%, which decreased to 4% for the subsequent 100. Early results of lower extremity free flap transfers performed in the same period (1979–1987) by Khouri and Shaw (58) and Melissinos and Parks (59) indicated a sharp drop in the initial high failure rates to 6% and 4.4%, respectively. A prospective study performed by Khouri et al. (60) in 1995 indicated a 4.1% overall flap failure rate.

The initial steep decline in the number of free flap failures in lower extremity reconstruction was the result of a shift from flaps with small vessels and unreliable anatomy (groin, tensor fascia lata, gracilis) to flaps with large vascular pedicles and constant anatomy (LD, rectus abdominis, radial forearm) (Figure 78-17).

The overall quality of outcomes in lower extremity reconstruction has not followed at the same pace as soft tissue reconstruction. Published reports present contradictory views influenced by the authors' convictions. Generally accepted, objective evaluation is difficult, if not impossible, because of the huge number of variables and ethical issues associated with true randomization. Similar wellness and self-evaluation scores between patients undergoing reconstructive procedures and patients undergoing amputations, when there is a choice, reflect the justified efforts of care providers and family members to support the patient's decision of going through the rigors of treatment and living with the end results of reconstruction versus dealing with stump problems and waking up every morning to put on a prosthetic leg. Based on the present state of lower extremity reconstruction, careful selection of patients with respect to their wishes and judicious application of accrued experience and skills provide the best blueprint for a satisfactory outcome.

REFERENCES

1. Byrd HS, Spicer TE, Cierney G III. Management of open tibial fractures. *Plast Reconstr Surg* 1985;76:719–730.
2. Godina M. Early microsurgical reconstruction of complex trauma of the extremities. *Plast Reconstr Surg* 1986;78:285–292.
3. Heller L, Levin LS. Lower extremity microsurgical reconstruction. *Plast Reconstr Surg* 2001;108(4):1029–1041.
4. Gustilo RB, Anderson JT. Prevention of infection in the treatment of one thousand and twenty-five open fractures of long bones: retrospective and prospective analysis. *J Bone Joint Surg Am* 1976;58:453–458.
5. Gustilo RB, Mendoza RM, Williams DN. Problems in the management of type III severe open fractures: a new classification of type III open fractures. *J Trauma* 1984;24:742–746.
6. Gustilo RB, Merkow RL, Templeman D. The management of open fractures. *J Bone Joint Surg* 1990;72:299–304.
7. Brumback RJ, Jones AL. Interobserver agreement in the classification of open fractures of the tibia. The results of a survey of two hundred and forty-five orthopedic surgeons. *J Bone Joint Surg Am* 1994;76:1162–1166.
8. Lutz BS, Wei F-C, Machens H-G, et al. Indications and limitations of angiography before free-flap transplantation to the distal lower leg after trauma: prospective study in 36 patients. *J Reconstr Microsurg* 2000;16:187–191.
9. Glass GE, Pearse MF, Nanchahal J. Improving lower limb salvage following fractures with vascular injury: a systematic review and new management algorithm. *J Plast Reconstr Aesthet Surg* 2009;62:571–579.
10. Chow LC, Napoli A, Klein MB, et al. Vascular mapping of the leg with multi-detector row CT angiography prior to free-flap transplantation. *Radiology* 2005;237:353–360.
11. Cernic S, Mucelli FP, Pellegrin A, et al. Comparison between 64-row CT angiography and digital subtraction angiography in the lower extremities: personal experience. *Radiol Med* 2009;114:1115–1129.
12. Haddock N, Garfein E, Saadeh P, et al. The lower extremity Allen Test (LEAT). *J Reconstruct Microsurg* 2009;25(7):399–403.
13. Dublin, BA, Karp NS, Kasabian AK, et al. Selective use of preoperative extremity arteriography in free flap reconstruction. *Ann Plast Surg* 1997;38:404–407.
14. Parrett BM, Matros E, Pribaz JJ, Orgill DP. Lower extremity trauma: trends in the management of soft-tissue reconstruction of open tibia-fibula fractures. *Plast Reconstr Surg* 2006;117:1315–1322.
15. Daigeler A, Drücke D, Tatar K, et al. The pedicled gastrocnemius muscle flap: a review of 218 cases. *Plast Reconstr Surg* 2009;123:250–257.
16. Swartz WM, Ramasastry SS, McGill JR, Noonan JD. Distally based vastus lateralis muscle flap for coverage of wounds about the knee. *Plast Reconstr Surg* 1987;80:255–265.
17. Beck JB, Stile F, Lineweaver W. Reconsidering the soleus muscle free flap for coverage of wounds of the distal third of the leg. *Ann Plast Surg* 2003;50:593–597.
18. Kauffman CA, Lahoda LU, Cederna PS, Kuzon WM. Use of soleus muscle flaps for coverage of distal third tibial defects. *J Reconstr Microsurg* 2004;20:593–597.
19. Tobin Gr. Hemisoleus and reversed hemisoleus flaps. *Plast Reconstr Surg* 1985;76:87–96.
20. Hallock GG. Sagittal split tibialis anterior muscle flap. *Ann Plast Surg* 2002;49:39–43.
21. Ono S, Chung KC, Hayashi H, et al. Application of multidetector-row computed tomography in propeller flap planning. *Plast Reconstr Surg* 2011;127:703–711.
22. Koshima I, Moriguchi T, Ohta S, et al. The vasculature and clinical application of the posterior tibial perforator-based flap. *Plast Reconstr Surg* 1992;90:643–649.
23. Koshima I, Itoh S, Nanba Y, et al. Medial and lateral malleolar perforator flaps for repair of defects around the ankle. *Ann Plast Surg* 2003;51:579–583.
24. Jeng SF, Wei FC. Distally based sural island flap for foot and ankle reconstruction. *Plast Reconstr Surg* 1997;99:744.
25. Yazar S, Lin C-H, Lin Y-T, et al. Outcome comparison between free muscle and free fasciocutaneous flaps for reconstruction of distal third and ankle traumatic open tibial fractures. *Plast Reconstr Surg* 2006;117:2468–2475.
26. Calderon W, Chang N, Mathes SJ. Comparisons of the effect of bacterial inoculation in musculocutaneous and fasciocutaneous flaps. *Plast Reconstr Surg* 1986;77:785–794.
27. Chen H, Tang Y. Anterolateral thigh flap: an ideal soft tissue flap. *Clin Plast Surg* 2003;30:383–401.
28. Bostwick J, Nahai F, Wallace JG, et al. Sixty latissimus dorsi flaps. *Plast Reconstr Surg* 1979;63(1):31–41.
29. Redett RJ, Robertson BC, Chang B, et al. Limb salvage of lower-extremity wounds using free gracilis muscle reconstruction. *Plast Reconstr Surg* 2000;106:1507–1513.
30. Harii K. Vascularized muscle transplantation for the treatment of facial paralysis. In Brunelli G (ed). *Textbook of Microsurgery*. Milano, Italy: Masson, 1988.
31. Lin CH, Lin YT, Yeh JT, Chen CT. Free functioning muscle transfer for lower extremity posttraumatic composite structure and functional defect. *Plast Reconstr Surg* 2007;119:2118–2126.

32. Melissinos EG, Leung T, Parks DH. *The adductor magnus "back-up" free flap*. Proceedings of the 5th Congress of the Word Society for Reconstructive Microsurgery, Okinawa, Japan 2009.
33. Melissinos EG, Parks DH. *Experience with the adductor magnus free flap*. Proceedings of the American Society for Reconstructive Microsurgery Meeting, Maui, Hawaii 2009.
34. Bunkis J, Walton RL, Mathes SJ. The rectus abdominis free flap for lower extremity reconstruction. *Ann Plast Surg* 1983;11:373.
35. Musharafieh R, Macari G, Hayek S, et al. Rectus abdominis free-tissue transfer in lower extremity wounds: review of 40 cases. *J Reconstr Microsurg* 2000;16:341–345.
36. Song R, Song Y, Yu Y, Song Y. The upper arm free flap. *Clin Plast Surg* 1982:9:27–35.
37. Wei FC, Jain V, Celik N, et al. Have we found an ideal soft-tissue flap? An experience with 672 anterolateral thigh flaps. *Plast Reconstr Surg* 2002;109:2219–2226; discussion 2227–2230.
38. Hui-Chou HG, Sulek J, Bluebond-Langner R, Rodriguez ED. Secondary refinements of free perforator flaps for lower extremity reconstruction. *Plast Reconstr Surg* 2011;127(1):248–257.
39. Yang GF, Chen PJ, Gao YZ, et al. Forearm free skin flap transplantation. *Chin Med J* 1981;61:139–141.
40. Richardson D, Fisher SE, Vaughan ED, Brown JS. Radial forearm flap donor-site complications and morbidity: a prospective study. *Plast Reconstr Surg* 1997;99:109–115.
41. Melissinos EG. *Experience with "racing stripe" fasciocutaneous free flaps*. Proceedings of the American Society for Reconstructive Microsurgery Meeting, Las Vegas, 2012.
42. Song YG, Chen GZ, Song YI. The free thigh flap: a new free flap concept based on the septocutaneous artery. *Br J Plast Surg* 1984;37:149.
43. Katsaros J, Schusterman M, Beppu M, et al. The lateral upper arm flap anatomy and clinical applications. *Ann Plast Surg* 1984;12(6):489–500.
44. Graham B, Adkins P, Scheker LR. Complications and morbidity of the donor and recipient sites in 123 lateral arm flaps. *J Hand Surg Br* 1992;17:189–192.
45. LaRossa D, Melissinos EG, Matthews, D, Hamilton R. The use of microvascular free skin-muscle flaps in management of avulsion injuries of the lower leg. *J Trauma* 1980:545–550.
46. Melissinos EG. *The distal tensor fascia lata free flap*. Proceedings of the American Society for Reconstructive Microsurgery Meeting, San Diego, CA, 2001.
47. Deiler S, Pfadenhauer A, Widmann J, et al. Tensor fasciae latae perforator flap for reconstruction of composite Achilles tendon defects with skin and vascularized fascia. *Plast Reconstr Surg* 2000;106:342–349.
48. Park S, Eom JS. Selection of the recipient vessel in the free flap around the knee: the superior medial genicular vessels and the descending genicular vessels. *Plast Reconstr Surg* 2001;107:1177–1182.
49. Park JE, Rodriguez ED, Bluebond-Langer R, et al. The anterolateral thigh flap is highly effective for reconstruction of complex lower extremity trauma. *J Trauma* 2007;62:162–165.
50. Melissinos EG, Erfani S, Parks DH. *The use of the medial gastrocnemius free flap for reconstruction of short below knee amputations*. Proceedings of the 4th Congress of the Word Society for Reconstructive Microsurgery, Athens, Greece, 2007.
51. Melissinos EG. *Post-trauma reconstruction of extremity defects with free flaps anastomosed distal to the zone of injury*. Proceedings American Society for Reconstructive Microsurgery Meeting, Tucson, AZ, 1995.
52. Sherman R, Ecker J. Soft tissue coverage. In *Skeletal Trauma*, 3rd ed. Philadelphia: WB Saunders, 2003, pp. 419–448.
53. Isenberg JS, Sherman R. Zone of injury: a valid concept in microvascular reconstruction of the traumatized lower limb? *Ann Plast Surg* 1996;36: 270–272.
54. Spector JA, Levine S, Levine JP. Free tissue transfer to the lower extremity distal to the zone of injury: indications and outcomes over a 25-year experience. *Plast Reconstr Surg* 2007;120:952–959.
55. Benacquista T, Kasabian AK, Karp NS. The fate of lower extremities with failed free flaps. *Plast Reconstr Surg* 1996;98(5):834–842.
56. Culliford AT IV, Spector J, Blank A, et al. The fate of lower extremities with failed free flaps: a single institution's experience over 25 years. *Ann Plast Surg* 2007;59:18–21.
57. Ohjimi H, Taniguchi Y, Kawano K, Kinoshita K. A comparison of thinning and conventional free-flap transfers to the lower extremity. *Plast Reconstr Surg* 2000;105(2):558–566.
58. Khouri RK, Shaw WW. Reconstruction of the Lower extremity with microvascular free flaps: a 10 year experience with 304 consecutive cases. *J Trauma* 1989;29(8):1086–1094.
59. Melissinos EG, Parks DH. Post-trauma reconstruction with free tissue transfer—442 consecutive cases. *J Trauma* 1989;29(8):1095–1103.
60. Khouri RK, Cooley BC, Kunselman MA, et al. A prospective study of microvascular free-flap surgery and outcome. *Plast Reconstr* 1998;102(3):711–721.

CHAPTER 79

Free Flaps for Chronic Osteomyelitis

Randy Sherman

BACKGROUND

Chronic osteomyelitis implies a bone infection that has been established for some length of time, usually, weeks, months, or years. No absolute time from onset is generally accepted as a discriminator between the acute and chronic forms of the disease. Chronic osteomyelitis is generally accepted to connote a well-established infection that has developed during the course of treatment of an underlying orthopedic condition of some duration. An overwhelmingly large majority of these cases present as either periprosthetic infections or posttraumatic sequelae of open fracture management. Open fractures of the femur, tibia, or osseous structures of the foot and ankle, which become infected, will be the basis of most referrals to the reconstructive microsurgeon. Current practices in open fracture management using immediate stabilization, radical debridement, and early vascularized wound coverage have reduced, but definitely not eliminated, posttraumatic osteomyelitis as a frequent challenge for the extremity surgeon today (1).

Historically, the treatment of chronic osteomyelitis consisted of conservative debridement of acutely inflamed tissues, drainage of abscesses, sinus tracts, and discrete resection of obviously involved cortical and medullary bone fragments. As they became available, first general and then culture-specific parenteral antibiotics allowed for disease suppression over prolonged periods of time. For decades, the words *cure* and *chronic osteomyelitis* would never appear together in the same sentence. Healed fractures, which drained periodically, would be treated symptomatically and otherwise tolerated. Infected nonunions with loss of axial stability would eventually result in amputation. With the advent of vascularized tissue transfer for wound closure, local antibiotic delivery vehicles, and new and innovative methods of both internal and external fixation, more aggressive ablation of the infected tissues by radical serial tumor-like debridements became not only acceptable but central to the effective and definitive treatment of chronic osteomyelitis. This maturing algorithm of treatment led to the era of dramatically increasing cure rates and paved the way for complex reconstructive approaches to limb salvage and functional restoration.

DIAGNOSIS

The common characteristics of chronic osteomyelitis include a history of previous orthopedic trauma usually followed by instrumentation for reduction; retained necrotic bone fragments (sequestrum); new bone formation (involucrum); poorly vascularized scar tissue with overall soft tissue deficiency; presence of bacteria; retained foreign material, either traumatically related or iatrogenically placed; and a variety of complicating host factors, including smoking, diabetes, peripheral vascular disease, and other systemic comorbidities.

The Cierney-Mader classification system, first developed in 1983 and eventually accepted as the standard tool for grading osteomyelitis and guiding treatment protocols, differentiates the disease into both host and anatomic subtypes. The host classification consists of three subtypes:

A: Otherwise healthy, no underlying medical problems, no history of previous multiple failed surgical procedures, good nutritional status, and normal response to injury
B: Multiple medical and/or surgical comorbidities such as smoking, drug use, diabetes, cardiac or peripheral vascular disease, poor nutrition, or poor stress response to trauma
C: Otherwise healthy with subclinical disease in whom treatment would result in increased morbidity compared with observation and supportive care alone.

The four anatomic subtypes are:

I, Medullary osteomyelitis: The infection is confined to the medullary canal, either associated with instrumentation or through hematogenous spread.

II, Superficial osteomyelitis: The infection is at or near the periosteum of an otherwise intact cortical segment. There may be deficient, poorly vascularized and infected overlying soft tissues, such as in a decubitus pressure sore. Hardware may still be present or have been inserted previously with biofilm residue still present.

III, Localized osteomyelitis: Full-thickness involvement of bone fragments at the periosteal, cortical, and medullary levels with poor vascularity, resulting in bony sequestrum, often complicated by retained hardware and a poorly vascularized and deficient soft tissue envelope. Stable long bone integrity remains through majority cortical continuity.

IV, Diffuse osteomyelitis: Involvement of all elements of the bony architecture with circumferential instability and loss of diaphyseal continuity, requiring significant reconstructive efforts to reestablish stable skeletal function (2).

IMAGING

Exceedingly rare is the orthopedic patient who has a deficiency of radiologic imaging studies. Diagnosis of osteomyelitis confirmed by certain cortical abnormalities on plain radiographs is mostly of historical interest. Radiographs can raise suspicion about retained hardware, butterfly fragments, and other unrecognized sequestrum (Figure 79-1). Plain radiographs remain the best tool to evaluate axial and rotational alignment, cortical integrity, and fracture healing. Sinograms have little to no role in today's modern imaging options. Secondary imaging studies include technetium 99mTc methylene diphosphonate (MDP) bone scans to look for hypermetabolic activity (Figure 79-2), computed tomography (CT) scans to aid in more specific anatomic structural analysis (Figure 79-3), and magnetic resonance imaging (MRI) scans to investigate subtle soft tissue involvement and medullary changes (Figure 79-4). Despite the sophistication of these imaging studies, physical examination and clinical grading during thorough surgical examination remain the most credible diagnostic modalities (3,4).

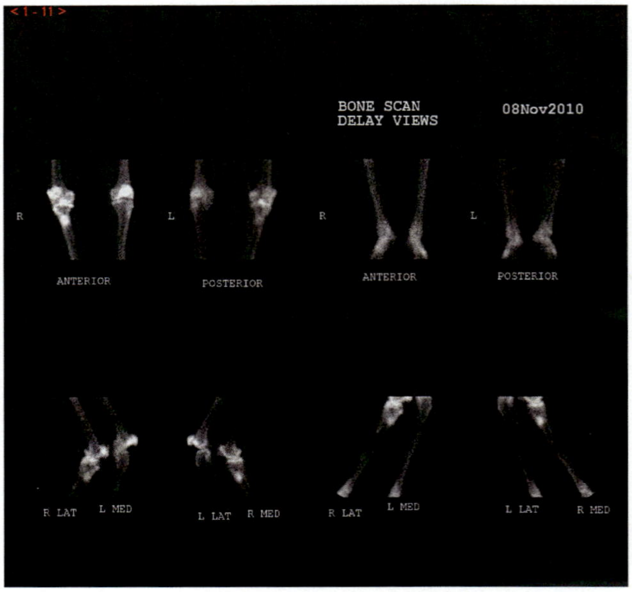

FIGURE 79-2 Technetium 99mTc bone scan. Delayed phase showing increased uptake at a site in the right proximal tibial suspicious for chronic osteomyelitis.

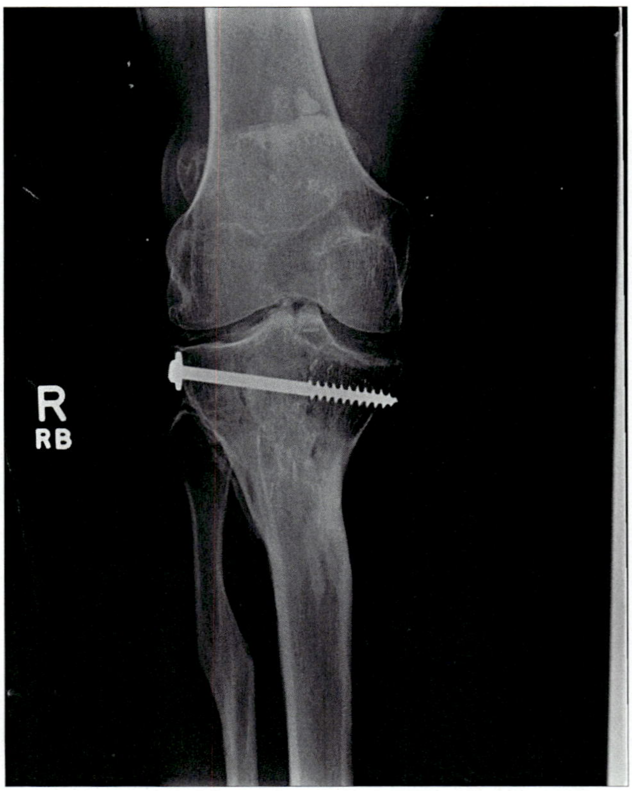

FIGURE 79-1 Anteroposterior view of chronic tibial osteomyelitis with osteosclerosis, retained hardware, and nonunion.

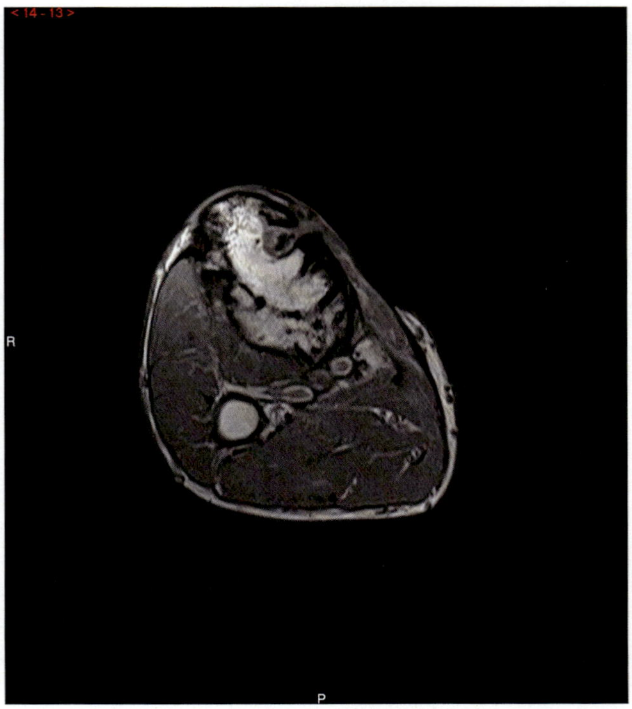

FIGURE 79-3 Chronic tibial osteomyelitis with sequestrum.

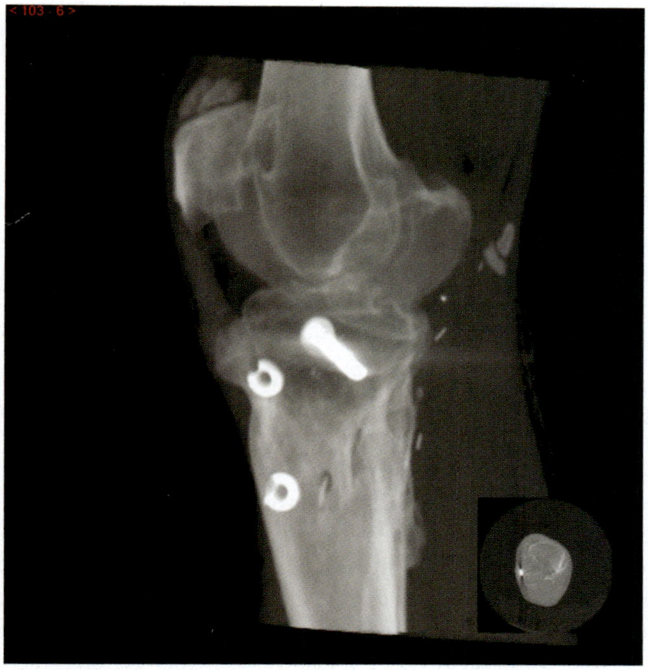

FIGURE 79-4 Magnetic resonance imaging of chronic osteomyelitis with retained foreign body and bony sequestrum.

DEBRIDEMENT

Very few treatment modalities in the modern practice of medicine have remained as effective as when first conceived than thorough surgical debridement. The essential modus operandi of successful extirpative surgery lies in the clear differentiation between those tissues or organ structures that are sufficiently vascularized and/or disease free versus those that are necrotic, irreversibly ischemic, or involved with cancer. In the field of oncologic surgery, a basic tenet of tumor resection involves the achievement of cancer-free margins. Similarly, in the treatment of osteomyelitis, the most important component of care is radical debridement of all affected tissues. There must be zero tolerance for maintaining ischemic and/or necrotic bone fragments, no matter what the immediate disruption in fracture reduction or congruent bony architecture results. Retention of nonviable bone for any reason, no matter how noble, is equivalent to approximating nonviable skin edges to achieve wound closure. Both the short- and long-term outcomes are equally predictable and uniformly disastrous.

Extremity debridement should be performed without the assistance of tourniquet control. Target tissues must be excised until such time as normal bleeding is obtained and normal tissue architecture is recognized. Diffuse, wide field punctate bleeding from involved cortical bone, deemed the "paprika sign," is a reliable indicator of viability (5). Bone debridement should use a number of tools including curettes, rongeurs, osteotomes, rasps, and high-speed burrs. The latter method is most precise and limits unintended injury to surrounding bony architecture. Reaming of the intramedullary canal may have a limited but effective role in debridement if used sparingly and judiciously. Every attempt should be made to marsupialize the wound in preparation for subsequent soft tissue coverage and obliteration of dead space. To reiterate, any attempt to retain seemingly critical but nonviable structures is a certain recipe for failure. The sooner a wound is definitively debrided, the faster it can be closed and revascularized. Reconstruction of the axial skeleton, often complex and multistaged, may then proceed with confidence.

Irrigation and lavage of the infected wound after debridement is uniformly endorsed as an essential adjunct to bacterial load reduction. Controversies remain as to whether maximal efficiency of these procedures is volume or pressure dependent. Addition of antibiotics to lavage solutions, although customarily used, shows little to no evidence of improved efficacy (6). Interestingly, studies have shown that irrigation with mild detergent-based solutions is more effective than control or antibiotic solutions, ostensibly because of the disruption of sessile bacterial chemical bonding to biofilms (7).

Early isolation and identification of pathologic organisms is critical to accurate diagnosis of chronic osteomyelitis. To successfully characterize the pathogens involved, several steps must be taken to maximize successful microbiologic analysis. Collecting specimens on swabs, although sometimes adequate, is often suboptimal. Bacteria may be trapped in the interstices of the applicator tip, the quantity of specimen obtained is often inadequate, and accurate representation of the causative pathogen may be difficult. Particular challenges for specimen recovery include characterizing bacteria harbored in biofilms arising from necrotic bone fragments and/or extracted hardware. Biofilms can be best understood as communities and specialized ecosystems of bacteria, supporting substrates and nutrients that allow cellular viability and proliferation in adverse environments that occur in osteomyelitic wounds where necrotic material and foreign bodies are often found (8).

The best option for specimen acquisition requires multiple biopsies taken from obviously involved tissues within the actively infected area. The specimens are best harvested before the commencement of intravenous (IV) antibiotics and before direct irrigation of the wound. Ideally, biopsies should be transported directly to the microbiology laboratory in either a specimen container alone or with a small amount of sterile saline. Cultures should be performed for aerobic, anaerobic, fungal, and acid-fast bacillus organisms. Frozen sections taken from these specimens may reveal white blood cell type and predominance, presence of granulomas, and other contextual findings that aid in identification. Special procedures in the laboratory can maximize return from bone specimens as well as screws, metal implants, and other materials containing biofilms (8). Sonic extraction is particularly effective for bacterial harvest from removed implants (9). No one organism is uniformly responsible for osteomyelitis; rather, a significant majority of these infections are polymicrobial. *Staphylococcus aureus* is found in the majority of cases with several subspecies developing increasing specific antibiotic resistance to methicillin, vancomycin, and others. Gram-negative bacteria; various anaerobes; and more rarely, mycobacterium may be cultured and should be suspected when clinical circumstances of compromised host resistance pertain (10).

ANTIBIOTIC THERAPY

Another critical pillar in the comprehensive treatment of chronic osteomyelitis consists of prolonged antibiotic therapy. IV delivery of culture-specific chemotherapy is universally accepted as a crucial adjunct but can vary widely in format, length of delivery, and combination therapy for enhanced bactericidal effects based on practitioner preferences and microbiologic analysis. Local antibiotic delivery through antibiotic-infused intramedullary nails, spacers, and beads provides high antibiotic levels into the involved field. Antimicrobial-loaded bone cement (ABLC) plays a role in most of the treatment algorithms currently described (11).

In chronic osteomyelitis, polymethymethacrylate (PMMA), used in the form of beads or spacers, has become the most commonly used substrate for antibiotic penetration of the wound space (Figure 79-5). High doses of drug achieving consistent and effective bacteriocidal levels can be obtained with a very low risk of systemic toxicity. Anhydrous antibiotics are mixed with the cement constituents at the time of bead or spacer placement, which are then used to fill dead space, maintain length, and preserve articular geometry. These on-table formulations are actually off-label uses according to the drug manufacturers but are universally accepted in the orthopedic and infectious disease community. Tobramycin, gentamicin, vancomycin, and cefazolin are the most widely used drugs in the fabrication of antibiotic beads and spacers. Antibiotic nails are usually prefabricated and ready for use. Delivery of antibiotics into the interstices of the wound space occurs by both dilution and elution and provides a prolonged high dose of material for many weeks to months. Sufficient bacteriocidal levels are usually achieved in the wound to effectively destroy pathogens in biofilms. These materials must be removed at the time of definitive reimplantation, internal fixation, soft tissue reconstruction, or secondary bone grafting, but antibiotic-coated nails are often kept in place until uncomplicated union has been achieved (12).

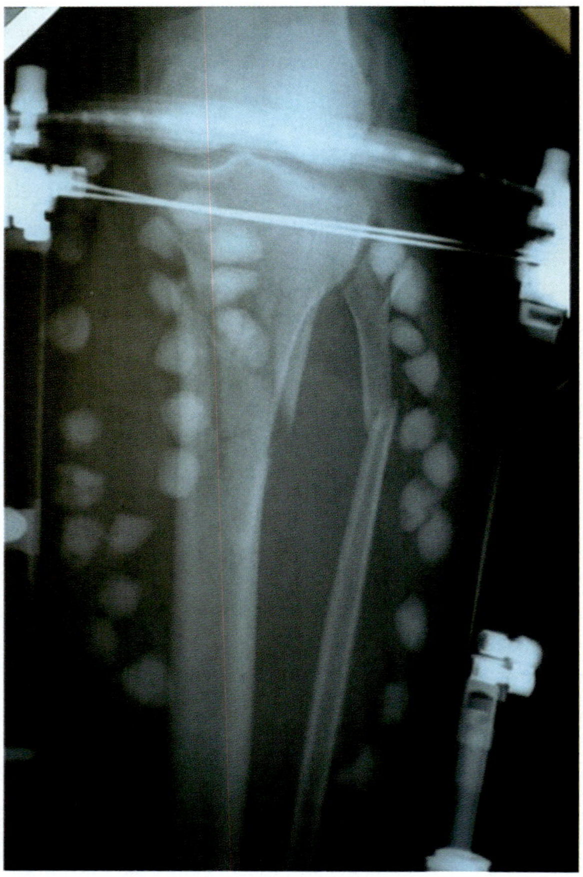

FIGURE 79-5 Antibiotic beads inserted after original debridement.

BONE STABILIZATION

Osteomyelitis often presents in the presence of retained plates, screws, intramedullary nails, and articular replacement prostheses. It is generally accepted that whenever possible, all foreign objects be removed. In circumstances when fracture reduction, articular congruity, or joint integrity will be compromised, alternative bony stabilization is mandatory. Rarely, critical internal constructs may be left in place if they are absolutely necessary to preserve articular congruity during early phases of fracture healing. External fixation allows axial stabilization and unfettered access to the wound. This is especially valuable when complex long bone fractures have become infected after open reduction and internal fixation.

WOUND CLOSURE AND FLAP OPTIONS

Early studies comparing various types of vascularized soft tissue closure reported distinct advantages of muscle flaps versus random skin flaps with regard to bacterial clearance and tissue oxygenation (13). This quickly led to an established orthodoxy favoring muscle flap coverage for closure of osteomyelitic wounds. Fortunately, the abundance of muscle donor sites: local, regional, or free; large or small; long or short pedicle, coupled with their resounding success in improved outcomes and cure rates has enshrined their use as the option of first choice. However, soon after, the same investigators failed to show any significant difference between axial skin flaps and muscle flaps. Therefore, more recently, the anterolateral thigh (ALT) flap has become a popular alternative to traditional muscle flap coverage (Figures 79-6 to 79-26).

Local muscle flaps in the lower extremity are quite effective in the majority of cases of osteomyelitis around the knee and for the proximal and middle thirds of the tibia. Because of their limited arc of rotation, the gastrocnemius muscle, either the medial or lateral head, and the soleus muscle are best suited for smaller defects when there is limited bony involvement. For larger defects of the proximal half of the tibia, the gastrocnemius myocutaneous flap allows transposition of a much more generous amount of vascularized tissue without the need for microvascular anastomoses. The soleus muscle is best reserved for medial or anteromedial defects of the middle third of the tibia but can be considered for coverage of smaller defects of the distal third of the tibia if the muscle belly volume continues to be sufficient for transfer down to the level of the ankle. Harvesting the soleus muscle may contribute to subsequent

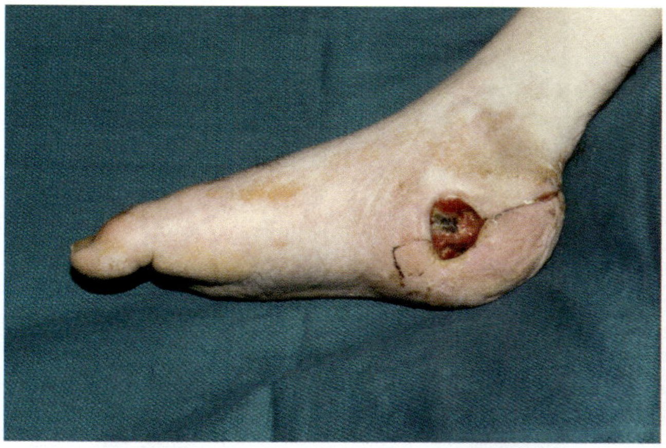

FIGURE 79-6 Calcaneal osteomyelitis, right heel, preoperative.

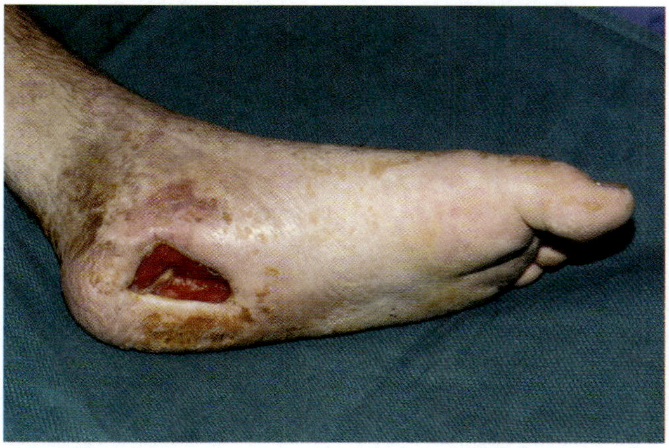

FIGURE 79-7 Calcaneal osteomyelitis, left heel, preoperative.

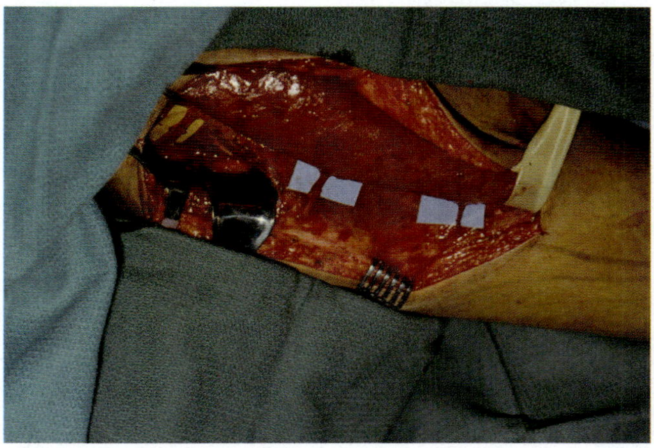

FIGURE 79-8 Exposure of the gracilis muscle to be used as a fractionated free tissue transfer, each section covering either the left and/or right (or both) calcaneal defect.

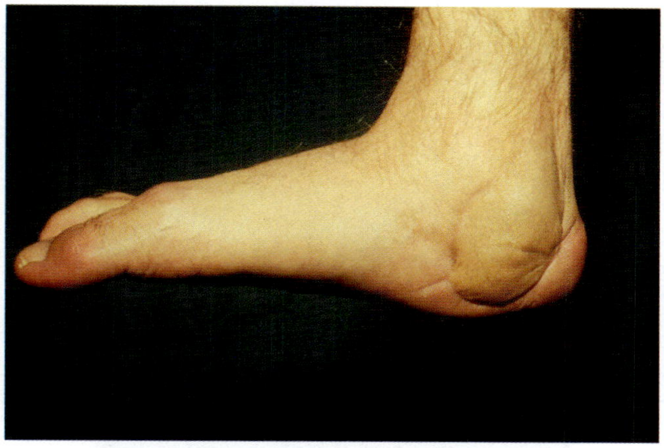

FIGURE 79-9 Healed calcaneal defect, left.

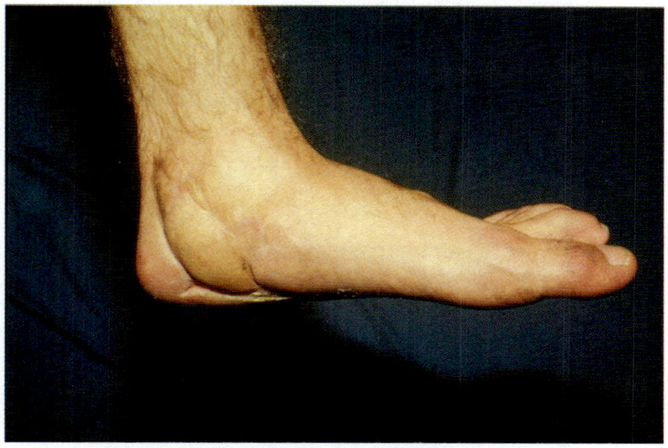

FIGURE 79-10 Healed calcaneal defect, right.

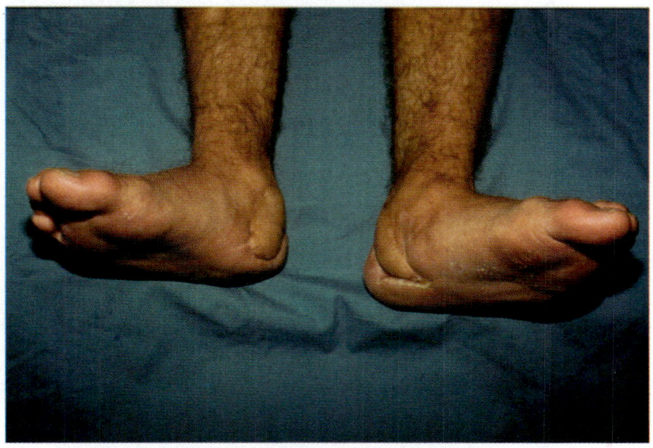

FIGURE 79-11 Bilateral calcaneal reconstruction with one fractionated gracilis muscle free tissue transfer.

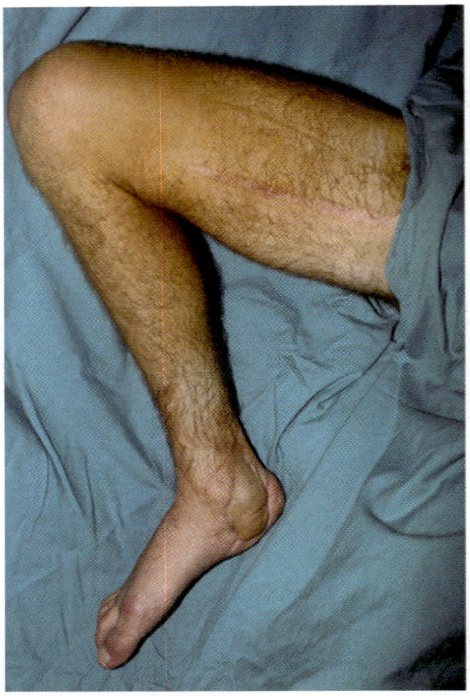

FIGURE 79-12 Healed gracilis donor site.

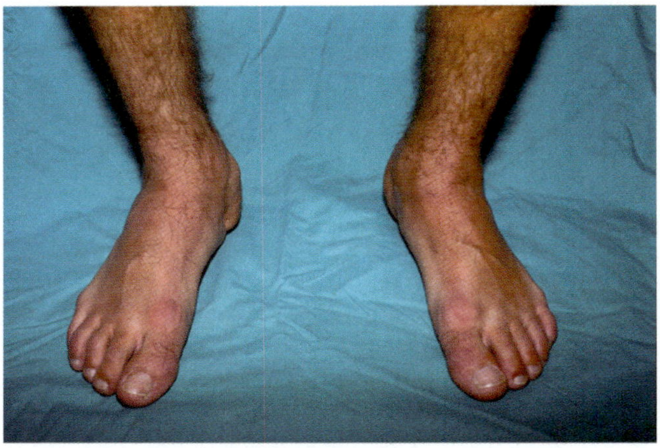

FIGURE 79-13 Bilateral calcaneal reconstruction, standing.

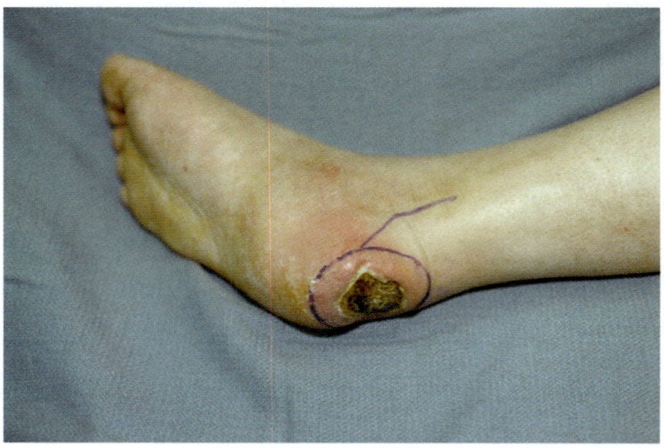

FIGURE 79-14 Active calcaneal osteomyelitis.

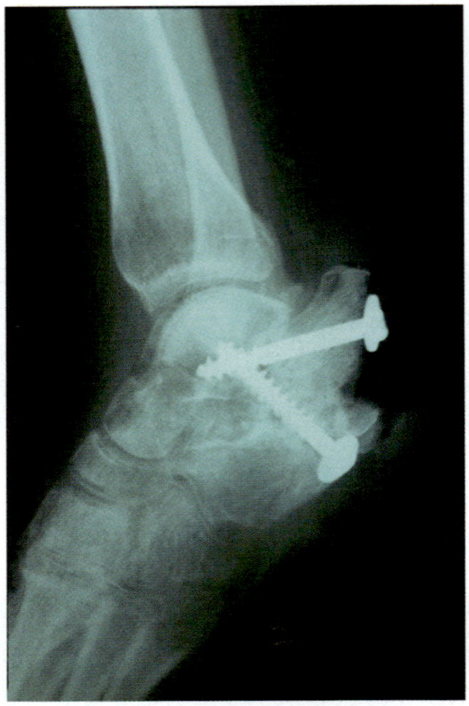

FIGURE 79-15 Active calcaneal osteomyelitis. Radiograph showing retained hardware and sequestrum.

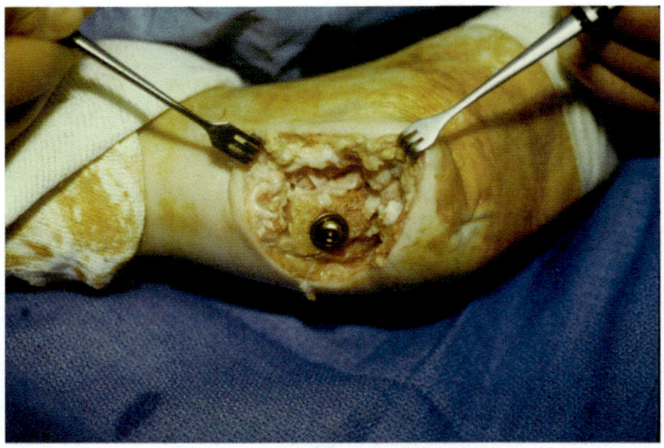

FIGURE 79-16 Debridement exposing hardware and sequestrum.

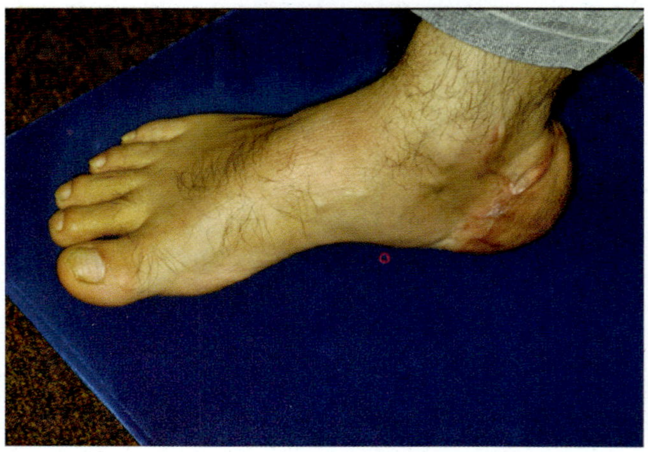

FIGURE 79-17 Healed calcaneal defect after segmental rectus abdominis free tissue transfer with skin graft.

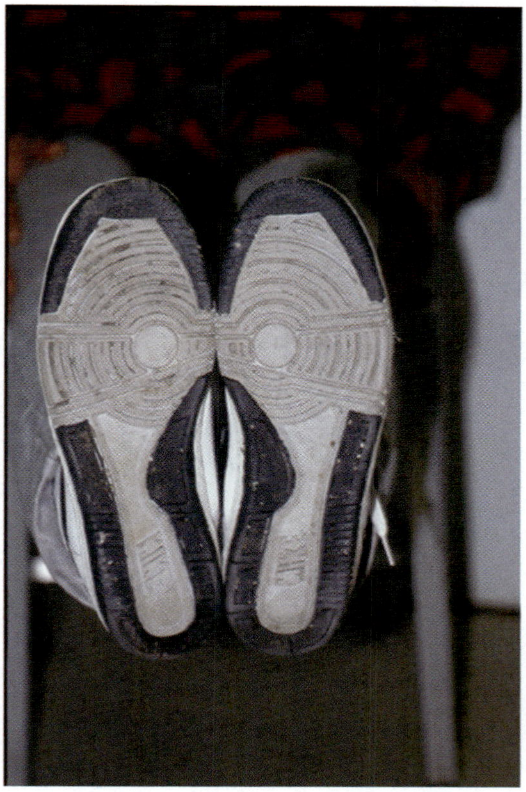

FIGURE 79-18 Functional shoe fit after reconstruction.

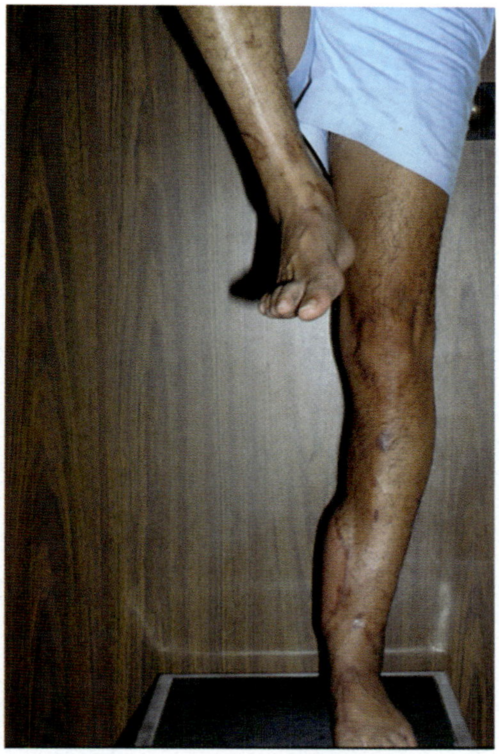

FIGURE 79-21 Tibial union with stable coverage after debridement, anterolateral thigh flap, and subsequent iliac crest bone grafting.

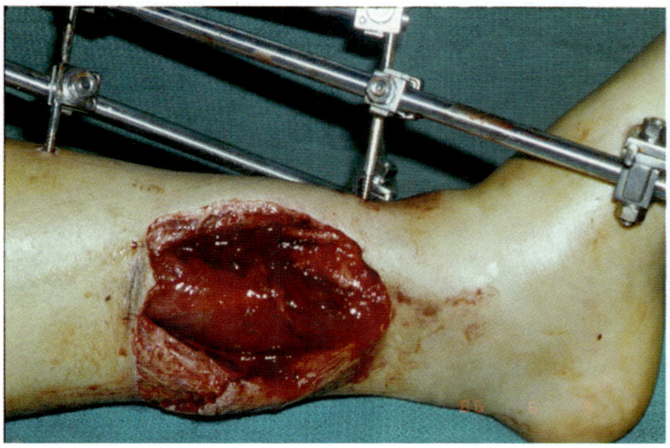

FIGURE 79-19 Left tibial osteomyelitis.

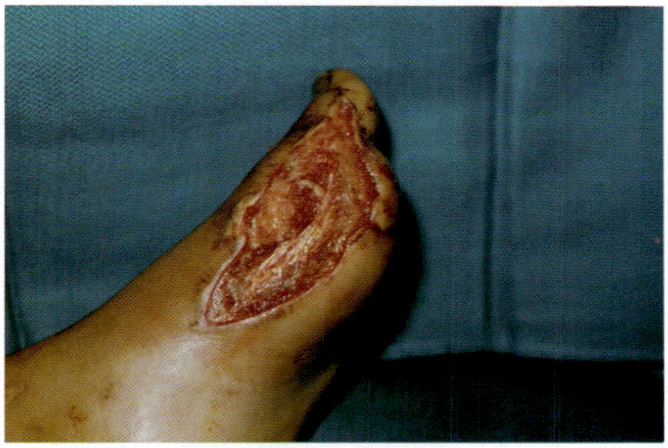

FIGURE 79-22 Chronic osteomyelitis of the first metatarsophalangeal joint.

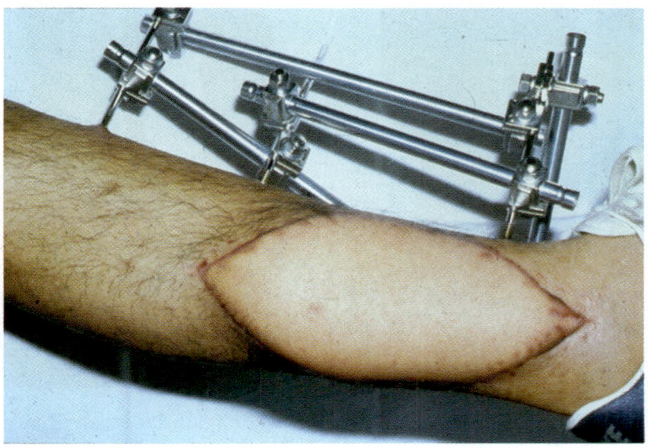

FIGURE 79-20 Anterolateral thigh flap (early postoperative).

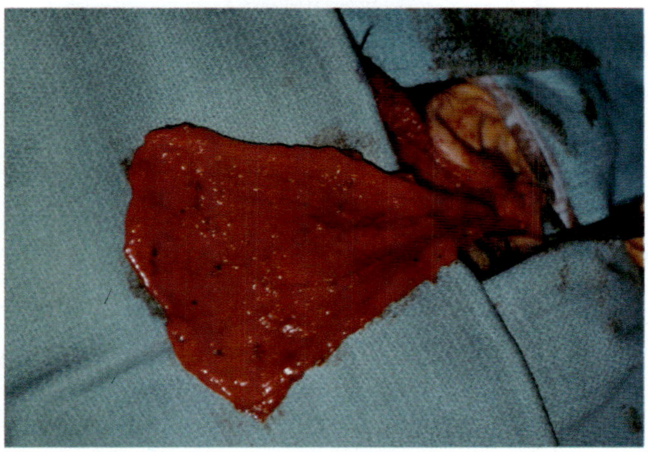

FIGURE 79-23 Temporoparietal fascial flap for foot coverage.

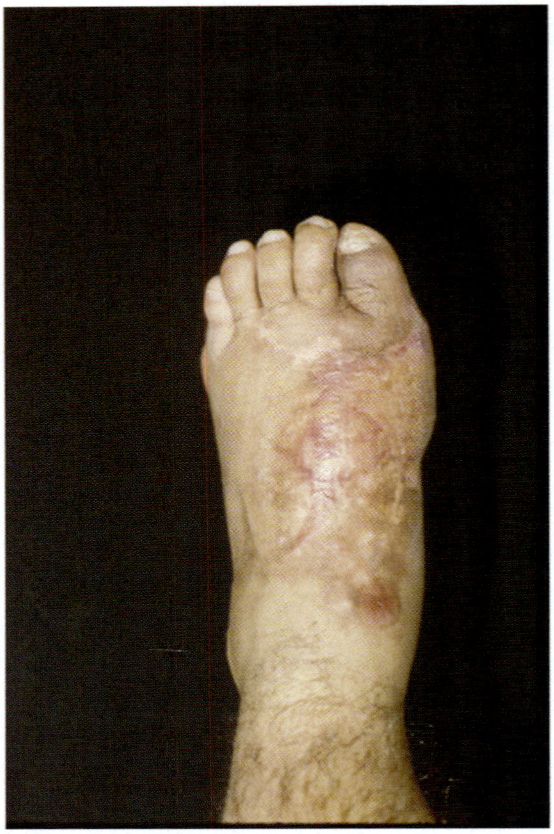

FIGURE 79-24 Healed composite foot wound after temporoparietal fascial flap with skin graft.

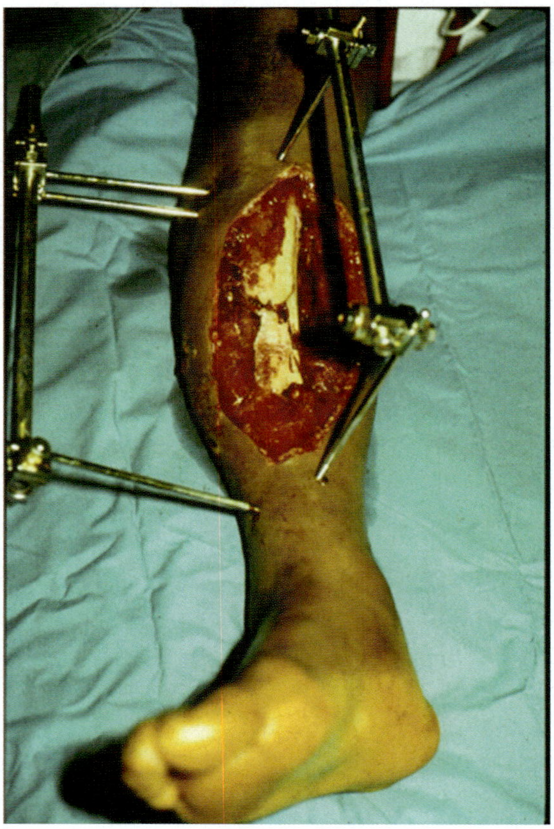

FIGURE 79-25 Composite tibial defect with infected, necrotic bone, soft tissue loss, and inadequate stabilization.

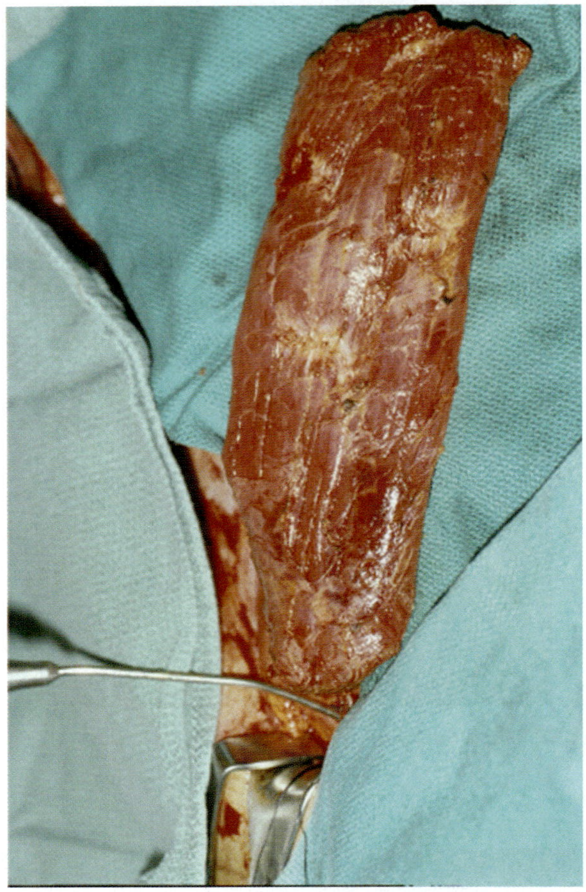

FIGURE 79-26 Harvest of rectus abdominis muscle.

ankle joint dysfunction by adding to the scarring, stiffness, and shortening of the Achilles tendon, although this is only theoretical and remains to be proven as an independent factor (Figure 79-27).

Free tissue transfers provide the distinct advantage of importing variable amounts of well-vascularized tissue to targeted areas given suitable recipient vessels. The choice of flaps is essentially the same as those used for noninfected acute traumatic wound coverage. The most commonly used muscle flaps

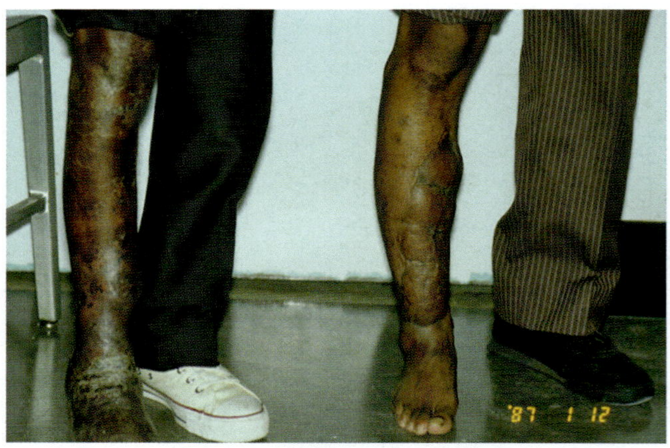

FIGURE 79-27 Long-term tibial reconstruction with union after bone grafting under a rectus muscle flap.

include the latissimus dorsi and rectus abdominis for larger defects and the gracilis or serratus anterior for smaller defects. Potential skin flaps include the ALT flap, the scapular or parascapular flap, the radial forearm flap, and the groin flap. For the foot and ankle region, the temporoparietal fascial flap works very well to cover critical structures while keeping bulk to a minimum.

OUTCOMES

Although the usual and customary duration of IV antibiotics has long been established at 6 weeks, there is a distinct lack of prospective studies confirming or denying the legitimacy of this therapeutic course length. Adding to the confusion is the now prevalent use of local antibiotic delivery systems in the form of beads, spacers, and nails as to what role they play in addition to or instead of systemic antibiotics in the effective eradication of residual pathogenic bacteria in the wound space. However, all authors agree that perioperative antibiotics play an important adjunctive role for several days before and several weeks after definitive debridement and reconstructive surgery to both eradicate chronic osteomyelitis and reconstruct the inevitable defect left behind.

Until recently, chronic osteomyelitis was just that, a seemingly long term, essentially incurable yet rarely fatal condition, that would manifest itself in a waxing and waning fashion, often successfully suppressed for long periods of time with local wound care and supplemental antibiotics. It would occasionally force the treating orthopedist to take drastic action in the form of amputation but would most often result in long-term disability in the form of open draining wounds, chronic low-grade infections, nonunion of fractures, and pain. Modern comprehensive approaches to chronic osteomyelitis have resulted in impressive success rates in eradication, reconstruction, and even cure of this perennially disabling problem. Given the multiplicity of protocols used to treat osteomyelitis, reliable outcome data and long-term results are hard to find. Successful outcomes in this disease must include freedom from infection, a closed wound, and skeletal stability with restoration of functional expectation over a defined period of time. Many earlier reports in the plastic surgical literature focused on success using regional or free tissue transfers to achieve durable wound closure with only a passing evaluation if at all on functional outcome (14–16). The most comprehensive studies to date have been published by the Cierney group, looking critically at their patient population of 1966 patients over a 25-year period with multiple variables and subclassifications (17). The type of injury, prior treatment failures, and recipient host designation were considered. A total of 84% (or 1651) received limb salvage protocols; 11% (or 216) received primary amputation; and 5% (or 104), classified as C-hosts, were offered palliative treatment alone. There were no significant differences among the type of orthopedic fixation strategies, specific orthopedic biologic replacements, and characterization of offending mono- or polymicrobial bacterial pathogenicity. Soft tissue reconstruction in the form of local, regional, or free tissue transfer played an important role in many but not all of these cases. Initial treatment outcomes boasted a success rate of 96% in A-hosts and a 73% success rate in B-hosts, with an overall 2-year success rate of 84%. A total of 16% (or 315) required further treatment at some subsequent interval with 275 of them undergoing further limb salvage for cure with a subgroup success rate of 84%. Other studies report similar favorable results (18,19).

Comprehensive management of chronic osteomyelitis is now the only legitimate approach to this historically debilitating and highly resistant condition. Reconstructive microsurgery can play a small but important role in the rehabilitation of these patients by early soft tissue coverage and obliteration of the dead space of these composite bone and soft tissue defects after definitive radical debridement (20,21).

REFERENCES

1. Zalavras CG, Patzakis MJ, Holtom PD, Sherman R. Management of open fractures. *Infect Dis Clin North Am* 2005;19(4):915–929.
2. Cierny G, Mader JT, Pennick JJ. A clinical staging for adult osteomyelitis. *Clin Orthop Relat Res* 2003;414:7–24.
3. Erdman WA, Tamburro F, Jayson HT, et al. Characteristics and pitfalls of diagnosis with MR imaging. *Radiology* 1991;180:533–539.
4. Gross T, Kaim AH, Regazzoni P, Widmer AF. Current concepts in posttraumatic osteomyelitis: a diagnostic challenge with new imaging options. *J Trauma* 2002;52:1210–1210.
5. Tetsworth K, Cierny GC. Osteomyelitis debridement techniques. *Clin Orthop Relat Res* 1999;360:87–96.
6. Anglen J, Apostoles PS, Christensen G, et al. Removal of surface bacteria by irrigation. *J Orthop Res* 1996;14:251–254.
7. Anglen JO. Comparison of soap and antibiotic solutions for irrigation of lower limb open fracture wounds: a prospective, randomized study. *J Bone Joint Surg Am* 2005;87:1415–1422.
8. Costerton JW, Stewart PS, Greenberg EP. Bacterial biofilms: a common cause of persistent infections. *Science* 1999;284:1318–1322.
9. Kobayashi M, Bauer TW, Tuohy MJ, et al. Brief ultrasonification improves detection of biofilm-formative bacteria around metal implants. *Clin Orthop Relat Res* 2007;457:210–213.
10. Patzakis MJ, Greene N, Holtom P, et al. Culture results in open wound treatment with muscle transfer for tibial osteomyelitis. *Clin Orthop Relat Res* 1999;(360):66–70.
11. Hanssen AD. Local antibiotic delivery vehicles in the treatment of musculoskeletal infection. *Clin Orthop Relat Res* 2005;437:91–96.
12. Zalavras CG, Patzakis MJ, Holtom P. Local antibiotic therapy in the treatment of open fractures and osteomyelitis. *Clin Orthop Relat Res* 2004(427):86–93.
13. Mathes SJ, Albert BS, Chang N. Use of the muscle flap in chronic osteomyelitis: experimental and clinical correlation. *Plast Reconstr Surg* 1982;69:815.
14. Anthony JP, Mathes SJ, Alpert BS. The muscle flap in the treatment of chronic lower extremity osteomyelitis: results in patients over 5-years after treatment. *Plast Reconstr Surg* 1992;88:311.
15. Fitzgerald RH Jr, Ruttle PE, Arnold PG, et al. Local muscle flaps in the treatment of chronic osteomyelitis. *J Bone Joint Surg* 1985;67:175.
16. May JW Jr, Jupiter JB, Gallico GG III, et al. Treatment of chronic traumatic bone wounds, microvascular free tissue transfer: a 13-year experience in 96 patients. *Ann Surg* 1991;214:515.
17. Cierny G III, DiPasquale D. Treatment of chronic infection. *J Am Acad Orthop Surg* 2006;14:S105–S110.
18. Patzakis MJ, Abdollahi K, Sherman R, et al. Treatment of chronic osteomyelitis with muscle flaps. *Orthop Clin North Am* 1993;24(3):505–509.
19. Siegel HJ, Patzakis MJ, Holtom P, et al. Limb salvage for chronic tibial osteomyelitis: an outcome study. *J Trauma* 2000;48(3):484–489.
20. Thordarson DB, Patzakis M, Holtom P, Sherman R. Salvage of the septic ankle with concomitant tibial osteomyelitis. *Foot Ankle Int* 1997;18(3):151–156.
21. Zalavras CG, Patzakis MJ, Thordarson DB, et al. Infected fractures of the distal tibial metaphysics and plafond: achievement of limb salvage with free muscle flaps, bone grafting and ankle fusion. *Clin Orthop Rel Res* 2004;(427):57–62.

CHAPTER 80

Microsurgical Reconstruction of the Foot

Erkki Tukiainen and Andrew Lindford

Reconstruction of soft tissue and bone defects of the foot remains a complex and challenging proposition despite advances in microvascular flap surgery. The foot is an important part of the body because it provides proprioceptive information concerning the weight-bearing surface, supports the body's weight on standing, and provides stability between the body and ground during ambulation. Foot and ankle defects may result from many causes such as trauma (mechanical, electrical burns, gunshot wounds, frostbite injuries, fracture nonunion, avascular necrosis), tumor resection, infection, peripheral vascular disease, diabetes, and rheumatoid arthritis (Table 80-1).

The modern-day aims of foot reconstruction are not only to provide a stable closed wound, adequate bone healing, and restoration of ambulation but also to achieve quick recovery, an acceptable cosmetic appearance, and above all functional restoration of the salvaged limb. In addition, the potential for donor site problems must be taken into account.

ANATOMICAL FEATURES OF IMPORTANCE TO RECONSTRUCTIVE SURGEONS (1)

Dorsum

The dorsal skin is thin and pliable and contains little subcutaneous fat. Deep fascia overlies the paratenon of the extensor tendons and is continuous with the extensor retinaculum proximally and plantar fascia medially and laterally. The extensor digitorum brevis and extensor hallucis brevis muscles are innervated by the deep peroneal nerve. The dorsalis pedis artery is the continuation of the anterior tibial artery at the ankle and supplies the dorsum of the foot, ankle, and first web space. The dorsalis pedis artery is absent in 3.7% of patients. The deep peroneal nerve divides into medial and lateral branches just distal to the ankle joint. The lateral branch innervates the extensor digitorum brevis and extensor hallucis brevis muscles, and the medial branch provides sensation to the first web space. The rest of the dorsum is innervated by branches of the superficial peroneal nerve and sural nerve.

Plantar Aspect

The plantar skin is a unique weight-bearing surface, and the glabrous epidermis and dermis are much thicker than in other parts of the body. The skin thickness varies from thickest over the heel and metatarsal heads and thinner over the toes and instep. Subcutaneous fat in combination with fibrous connective tissue provides the cushion for weight bearing. The plantar aponeurosis is thickened centrally. The muscles and tendons are arranged in "layers." The most superficial layer consists of the abductor hallucis, flexor digitorum brevis, and abductor digiti minimi muscles. The second layer consists of the quadratus plantae muscle, lumbrical muscles, and extrinsic long flexor tendons. The third layer consists of the flexor hallucis brevis, adductor hallucis, and flexor digiti minimi brevis muscles, and the interosseous muscles form the deepest layer.

In addition to the dorsal angiosome supplied by the anterior tibial artery, there are five angiosomes consisting of three branches of the posterior tibial artery (medial calcaneal artery supplying the heel; medial plantar artery supplying the instep, and lateral plantar artery supplying the lateral plantar and plantar forefoot) and two branches of the peroneal artery (anterior perforating artery supplying the anterior lateral ankle and lateral calcaneal branch supplying the plantar and lateral heel).

The tibial nerve trifurcates at the distal inner ankle into the calcaneal and medial plantar and lateral plantar nerves. These supply motor branches to the intrinsic muscles of the foot (except the extensor digitorum brevis muscle) and provide sensory branches to the sole of the foot.

Bones

The bones of the foot and ankle consist of the talus and calcaneus posteriorly and the tarsals, metatarsals, and phalanges

TABLE 80-1 Indications for Microsurgical Reconstruction of the Foot

Trauma
Mechanical
Burns
Gunshot wounds
Frostbite injuries
Tumor resection
Infection
Peripheral vascular disease
Diabetes
Rheumatoid arthritis
Neurologic disease

more distally. The five tarsal bones are arranged in two rows. The talus is the only bone that articulates with the long bones of the leg, and for this reason, all of the weight on the foot is transmitted onto the talus. The calcaneus and the five metatarsal heads are the weight-bearing points of the foot with an arched skeleton in between.

ASSESSMENT

A thorough history and examination are essential. In particular, sensation should be carefully examined. Comorbid conditions such as diabetes and peripheral vascular disease should be identified. The vascular supply to the foot must be examined, and adjunctive investigations such as noninvasive arterial Doppler studies or angiography may be indicated. Less invasive computed tomography (CT) and magnetic resonance (MR) angiography are also available for vascular imaging. Bone assessment includes plain radiographs and in some cases CT or MR imaging.

RECONSTRUCTION

Before any reconstruction, adequate surgical debridement is mandatory. The advent of vacuum-assisted closure (VAC) therapy has revolutionized the management of lower extremity wounds and can obviate the need for a flap in some cases or at least simplify the choice of flap. After a clean and well-vascularized wound bed has been achieved, a reconstructive option from the reconstructive ladder can be chosen: (1) healing by secondary intention, (2) primary closure, (3) skin grafting, (4) local random flap, (5) pedicled flap, or (6) free flap.

Indications for Flap Coverage

More complex wounds with exposed fracture, joint, nerve, tendon lacking paratenon, and bone lacking periosteum usually require flap coverage. Depending on the wound etiology, any defects of nerve, tendon, ligament, joint, and bone can be reconstructed at a later date after the flap has matured and inflammation resolved. This strategy is especially indicated in severely contaminated complex wounds such as those occurring in a war situation, presenting late to the reconstructive surgeon. Methylmethacrylate spacers can be used under flaps to preserve space for later bone grafting (2).

Local Flaps (Table 80-2)

Commonly used local flaps in foot reconstruction include the neurofasciocutaneous retrograde sural artery flap and lateral supramalleolar flap for small- or moderate-size wounds of the ankle and proximal foot.

Neurofasciocutaneous Retrograde Sural Artery Pedicled Flap (3)

The blood flow is provided retrogradely through the sural artery, which courses with the sural nerve. Outflow is via venae comitantes, and the pivot point should not be designed less than 5 cm superior to the lateral malleolus.

Lateral Supramalleolar Fasciocutaneous Pedicled Flap

This is a distally based fasciocutaneous flap that can reach more distally on the foot than the sural flap. The vascular supply is based on vessels derived from the anastomotic arcade around the ankle.

Other local flap options include the instep flap based on the medial branch of the plantar artery, often known as the medial plantar flap (4). It is sensate, can have a wide arc of rotation, and is ideal for plantar heel defects. The donor site requires a

TABLE 80-2 Flap Options for Foot Reconstruction

Pedicled Flap	Free Soft Tissue Flap		Vascularized Bone Grafts
	Muscle Flap	**Fasciocutaneous Flap**	
• Retrograde sural artery flap	• Gracilis	• ALT	• Fibula
• Lateral supramalleolar flap	• Latissimus dorsi	• Scapular/parascapular	• Iliac crest
• Medial plantar flap	• Serratus anterior	• Radial forearm	• Scapula
• Lateral calcaneal flap	• Rectus abdominis	• Lateral arm	• Rib
• V-Y advancement flap			
• Toe fillet flap			
• Foot muscle flap			

ALT, anterolateral thigh.

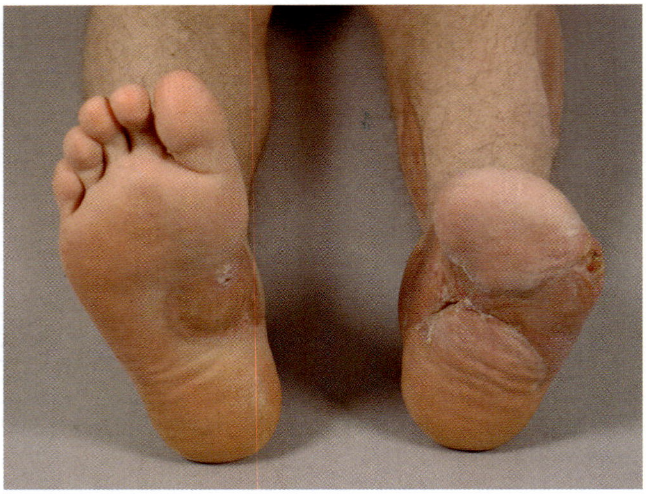

FIGURE 80-1 Crush injury with traumatic distal amputation. The foot was initially covered with skin grafts alone, but the patient had problems with durability on ambulation. Eventual reconstruction with free medial plantar flap from the opposite foot.

split-thickness skin graft. The medial plantar flap can also be used as a free flap (5). (Figure 80-1). The lateral calcaneal flap is a fasciocutaneous flap useful for posterior calcaneal and distal Achilles defects. V-Y advancement flaps can be used for small plantar defects. Toe fillet flaps can be useful for small forefoot web space ulcers and distal forefoot problems after minor amputations. Several small pedicled muscle flaps in the foot such as the extensor digitorum, flexor hallucis, and abductor hallucis brevis muscle flaps are also available but only provide coverage for small defects.

Free Flap Reconstruction (see Table 80-2)

Defects created by high-energy trauma can appear initially small, but ultimately the area of tissue destruction can become much wider. More extensive wounds and global injury to the foot and ankle area often warrant free flap coverage. The main aims of free flap reconstruction are early definitive wound healing, restoration of function, salvage of impending amputations, functional stumps for prosthetic reconstruction, and good cosmetic results.

Timing of Free Flap Reconstruction

It has been generally accepted that free flap reconstruction should be performed in the immediate or early period after trauma or ablative surgery. However, some studies have shown good flap success in the delayed period (>72 hours) (6). However, prospective studies are not available. In addition, the VAC device has enabled the delayed closure of certain lower extremity wounds. VAC has a positive effect on wound healing and protects the wound from nosocomial infection and allows time until definitive reconstruction.

Recipient Vessel Selection

The site of injury and the vascular status of the lower extremity are the primary factors in recipient vessel selection. The site of anastomosis should be outside the zone of injury, free of trauma and inflammation. The posterior tibial artery is the preferred recipient vessel because of its proximity, but the anterior tibial artery is a good alternative. Anastomosis distal to the zone of injury has also been reported (7). An end-to-side anastomosis to the recipient artery should be carried out whenever possible to avoid sacrificing a main artery (2). Venous anastomoses should be performed end to end to the venae comitantes or to the greater or lesser saphenous vein. Distal bypass vascular grafts can also be used as the recipient vessel. Pedicle length is an important factor in flap selection. A long pedicle is necessary if the recipient artery is a dorsally placed bypass graft or the anterior tibial artery.

SELECTION OF FREE FLAP BY DEFECT LOCATION

Ankle and Dorsum of the Foot

Large areas of exposed bone or tendon require flap coverage. Thin fasciocutaneous or cutaneous free flaps are often used for dorsal foot wounds. Soft tissue defects with exposure or segmental loss of the Achilles tendon can be reconstructed with pedicled flaps such as bipedicled local random pattern flaps, the sural flap, or propeller flaps. However, especially in larger defects, the use of free flaps may be indicated (anterolateral thigh [ALT], scapular, or radial forearm flaps). The Achilles tendon itself can be reconstructed using local tendon grafts, the free gracilis muscle flap and tendon (8), or the free composite ALT flap, including vascularized fascia lata rolled to reconstruct the tendon (9).

Plantar Foot

Plantar foot reconstruction is more challenging because the transferred tissue must withstand the shear forces involved in walking. Durability, the need to cover arthrodeses or other bone fixation, and the lack of sensation in the transferred tissue are also important factors. Insensate tissue is at risk for breakdown, and reconstruction should aim to allow the use of normal footwear.

Although local flaps have been described and used for plantar foot resurfacing, extensive defects require a free flap for coverage (10). There is an ongoing debate as to whether skin grafted muscle flaps or fasciocutaneous flaps are most appropriate for plantar foot defects. As in other locations, a free muscle flap can obliterate dead space and help deliver both neutrophils and parenteral antibiotics to areas of chronic osteomyelitis. May et al. (11) presented strong evidence for muscle flaps with skin grafts; however, fasciocutaneous flaps have been used as effectively. Important criteria to consider include a flap with adequate pedicle length and caliber, excessive thickness of the flap, muscle flap for deep or irregular defects, and skin flaps for superficial degloving defects. Abnormally high pressure points on the plantar surface lead to recurrent breakdowns after reconstruction. Bony abnormalities should therefore be corrected. Regardless of the type of free flap reconstruction, postoperative meticulous foot care should be heavily emphasized and orthotics provided.

Plantar Forefoot

The forefoot refers to the area distal to the middiaphysis of the metatarsals. Local flaps are usually available, for example, after partial amputation, when the soft tissue can be used as a local flap. Toe fillet flaps can also be used in these distal injuries. If local options are not available, free flap reconstruction with a fasciocutaneous flap may be indicated.

Plantar Midfoot

The midfoot consists of the region between the proximal tarsal row and the middiaphysis of the metatarsals. It consists of the medial non–weight-bearing arch and the lateral weight-bearing area. Wounds larger than 4 to 5 cm usually require free flap reconstruction or midfoot amputation. Composite free flap reconstruction is very useful in attempting to maintain foot length in patients with a "guillotine" type of midfoot amputation and can prevent the need for a more proximal Syme amputation or below-knee amputation. Bone reconstruction may involve the use of vascularized bone, including iliac crest bone flaps, radial osteocutaneous flaps, scapula bone chimeric flaps, and fibular osteocutaneous flaps.

Plantar Hindfoot

Soft tissue reconstruction of the hindfoot is the most difficult because the hindfoot has specific requirements such as a thick, durable heel pad, underlying calcaneus bone, and Achilles tendon itself surrounded by a thin, pliable soft tissue envelope. Reconstruction must provide durable soft tissues for weight bearing and permit normal ankle movement. Free flap reconstruction is indicated in large wounds (>6 cm), in the absence of the posterior tibial vessels, and in patients who have been revascularized to the distal anterior tibial-dorsalis pedis artery by long saphenous vein grafts.

The importance of achieving sensation in these free flap reconstructions is still being debated (12). Free neurosensory flaps have been described to provide sensation in plantar reconstruction. The deltoid and lateral arm fasciocutaneous flaps (13) have been described for this purpose, although their donor site scars are not ideal. Flap sensation depends on the availability of a suitable recipient nerve. A retrospective study by Santanelli et al. demonstrated the feasibility of sensory nerve coaptation in radial forearm flap reconstruction of sole of the foot defects (14). May et al. have described the use of free muscle flaps and split-thickness skin grafting for the weight-bearing parts of the foot and concluded that cutaneous sensibility is not essential (11). Other reports have also confirmed that sensation in the flap is not necessary (10,13,15,16). One recent study highlighted the superiority of split-thickness skin grafts taken from the instep area over skin grafts taken from the thigh in covering the muscle flap (17).

Commonly used muscle flaps include the gracilis, latissimus dorsi (LD), serratus anterior, and rectus abdominis.

GRACILIS MUSCLE FLAP

The gracilis is a long and thin muscle. The dominant pedicle is the ascending branch of the medial circumflex femoral artery and the venae comitantes. The length of the pedicle is 6 cm, and the diameter of the artery is 1.6 mm. The size of the muscle flap can be 6 × 24 cm. The flap can be made thinner and more pliable by dividing the surface of the muscle longitudinally. The gracilis tendon can be incorporated in tendon reconstruction (Figure 80-2).

LATISSIMUS DORSI MUSCLE FLAP

The LD muscle free flap is also a reliable option that provides a large flap that is easy to harvest. The flap is based on the thoracodorsal vessels and has a long pedicle. A skin paddle results in a bulky flap and is not so appropriate in weight-bearing surfaces because of excessive mobility of the skin component and risk of ulceration. A split-thickness skin graft placed over a LD muscle-only flap may provide a more durable option. The LD flap has the disadvantage of requiring a lateral decubitus position when raising the flap (Figure 80-3).

SERRATUS ANTERIOR MUSCLE FLAP

The blood supply is via the serratus branch of the subscapular artery, and an advantage of this flap is its long pedicle.

RECTUS ABDOMINIS MUSCLE FLAP

This is a reliable flap based on either the deep superior or deep inferior epigastric artery (type III muscle flap, two dominant pedicles). The deep inferior epigastric artery arising from the external iliac artery is usually favored because it is larger and longer, providing 8- to 10-cm pedicle length. The size of the muscle can be 25 × 6 cm, and the skin island can be up to 14 × 21 cm based on the musculocutaneous perforators. A major drawback of this flap is the donor site with a risk of abdominal herniation and a possible negative impact on abdominal wall function.

Commonly used free fasciocutaneous flaps include the ALT flap, scapular or parascapular flaps, and the radial forearm flap.

ANTEROLATERAL THIGH FLAP

The ALT flap has increased in popularity because of its many advantages (18). The flap is harvested in the supine or lateral decubitus position, allowing a two-team approach; the pedicle is reasonably long; the lateral femoral cutaneous nerve can provide a sensate flap; and the flap pedicle can bridge a vascular gap as a "flow-through" flap, especially in mangled extremities, and the donor site morbidity is small (19). The flap is based on a musculocutaneous perforator passing through the vastus lateralis muscle in 84% of cases; otherwise, a septocutaneous perforator passes between the vastus lateralis and rectus femoris muscles. The perforator(s) arises from the descending branch of the lateral circumflex artery, itself a branch from the profunda femoris artery. When combined with a strip of fascia lata, the Achilles tendon can be reconstructed. However, the flap does tend to be very thick in obese patients, which makes it bulky and difficult to conform to foot defects. An intriguing case report described the

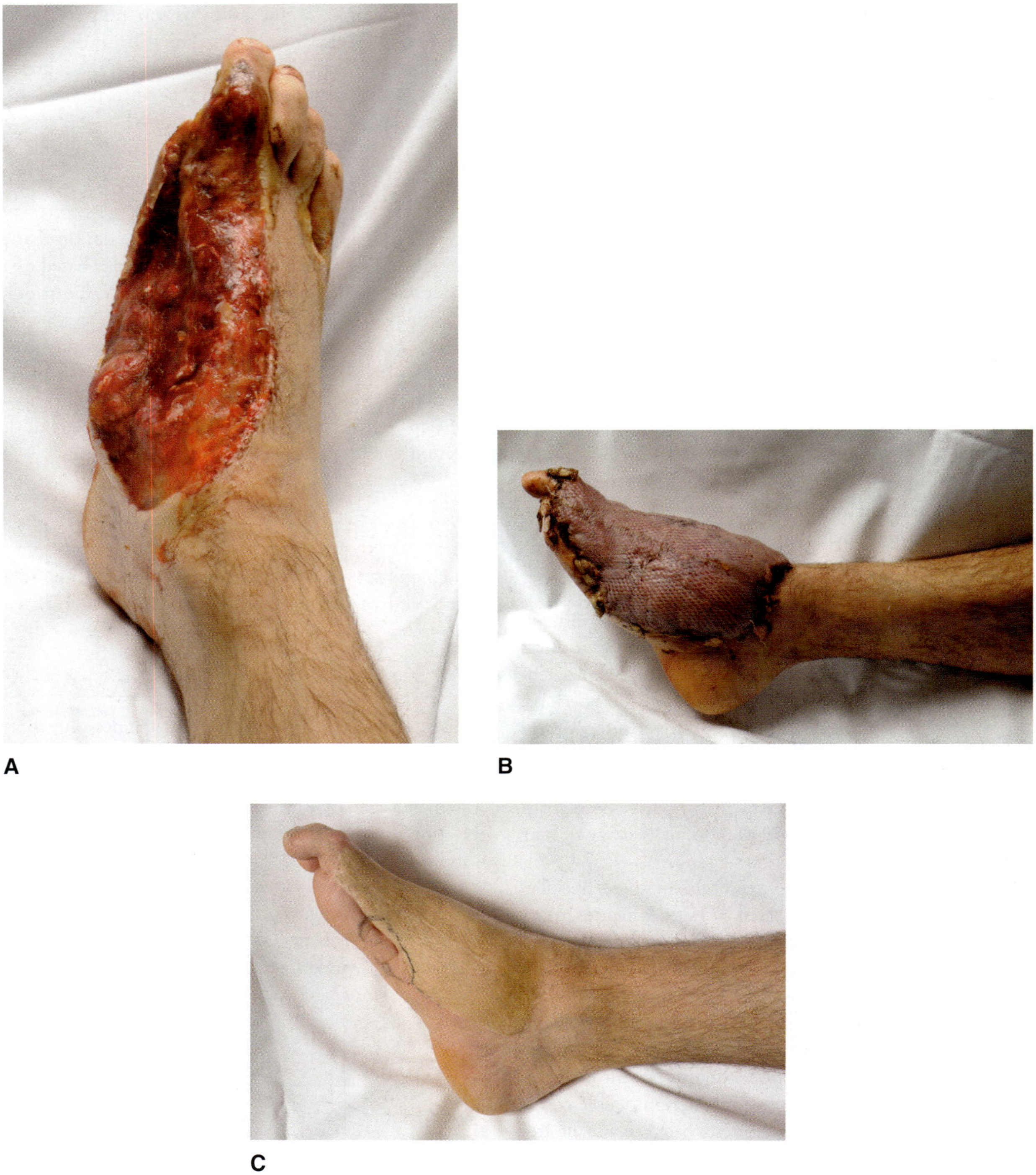

FIGURE 80-2 (A) Crush injury with extensive soft tissue loss required first ray amputation at primary debridement. (B) Reconstruction with gracilis muscle flap and skin graft. (C) Final result at 3 years with shrinkage of the muscle flap before scar revision surgery.

temporary placement of plantar heel skin taken from a traumatically amputated heel pad in the thigh with later transfer back to the heel using the ALT flap as a carrier (20).

SCAPULAR/PARASCAPULAR FASCIOCUTANEOUS FLAPS

The length of the pedicle is about 5, cm, and the diameter of the artery is 2.5 mm. The cutaneous territory can be up to 20×7 cm and can be harvested transversally (scapular flap) or obliquely (parascapular flap) based on the branches of the circumflex scapular artery. These flaps can also be rather thick in obese patients. In contrast, the radial forearm flap is a small and thin fasciocutaneous flap but is potentially compromised by its donor site morbidity. The resultant donor site is often associated with poor cosmesis and a possible negative effect on hand circulation (cold intolerance).

Potparic et al. reported no significant difference in the incidence of complications and functional outcome between fasciocutaneous and skin-grafted muscle flaps. The occurrence of

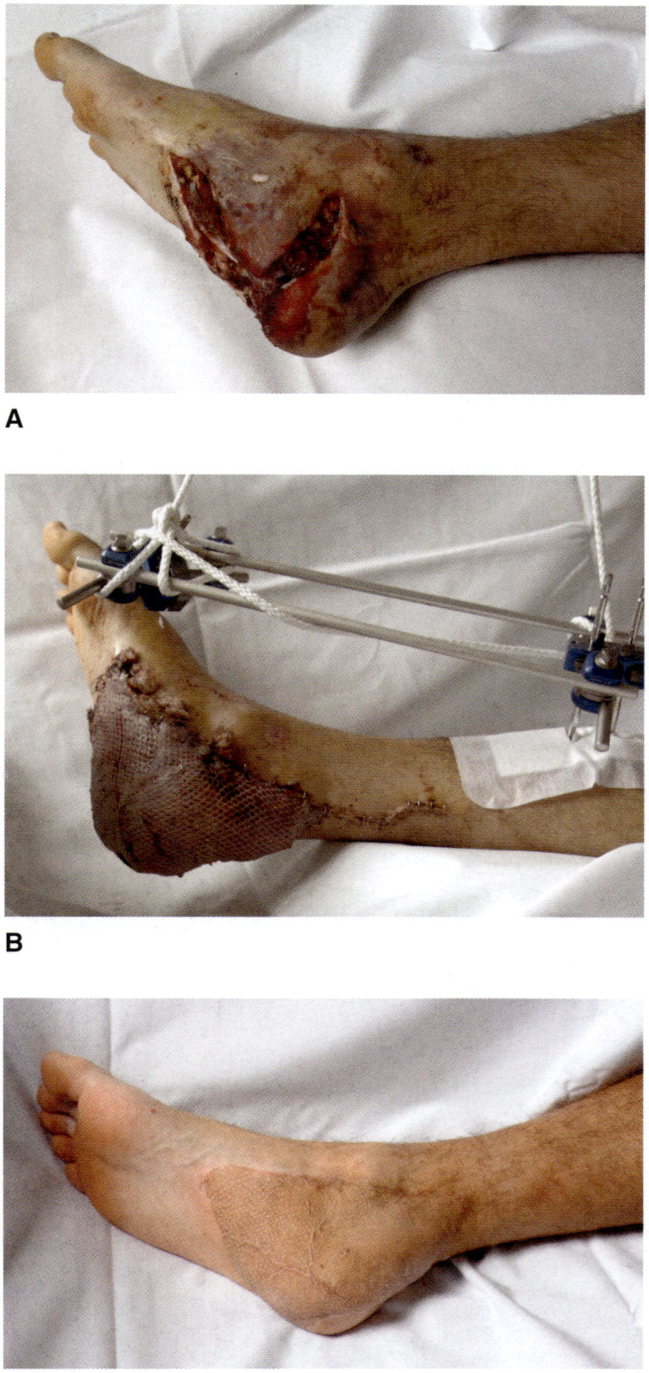

A

B

C

FIGURE 80-3 (A) Extensive degloving injury without bony injury. (B) Soft tissue reconstruction with a partial latissimus dorsi free muscle flap and skin graft. Microvascular anastomoses performed proximal to zone of injury. (C) Final result 2 years after surgery with shrinkage of the muscle flap.

ulcers was strongly associated with an underlying neuropathy (16). However, Rainer et al. found a lower ulceration rate when using free muscle flaps primarily LD muscle flaps covered with a skin graft for weight-bearing areas compared with fasciocutaneous flaps. They did, however, conclude that free fasciocutaneous flaps seemed to be the best choice for non–weight-bearing areas with the lateral arm flap used most commonly (15). Demirtas et al. reported favorable outcomes using a free ALT flap for heel and plantar foot reconstruction (21). A study from our institution concerning soft tissue reconstruction after complex calcaneal fractures revealed that the gracilis free muscle flap was most commonly used and provided satisfactory heel contour. It was also found that generally wounds seemed to heal quicker after reconstruction with free flaps than after local or pedicled flaps (22). Another study reported the use of the free temporal fasciocutaneous flap for covering small defects on the weight-bearing surface of the heel (23). However, fasciocutaneous flaps tend to be bulky, loose, and unstable and therefore may need later revision. In addition, the fat content in these flaps fluctuates in relation to the original donor site behavior. This may be problematic if the patient later gains weight.

CROSS-LEG FLAPS

When reconstruction with a local or free flap is not possible because of an extensive zone of injury and poor recipient vessels, one must also remember the possibility of the cross-leg flap. Traditionally, cross-leg flaps were random-pattern or axial flaps of limited size and arc of rotation. Cross-leg flaps have been described based on the sural, posterior tibial, and peroneal artery perforators and can cover the entire plantar surface. Cross-leg instep, plantar medial fasciocutaneous, and cross-leg free flaps have also been described (2).

FREE FLAP RECONSTRUCTION OF BONE DEFECTS

Bone defects in the foot and ankle also pose a major challenge because they compromise the plantigrade footprint and stability during walking. Bone defects of the foot may result from trauma, osteomyelitis, tumor resection, or osteonecrosis. Traumatic bone defects are usually the result of high-energy trauma such as road traffic accidents, falls from a height, farming injuries, industrial accidents, or gunshot wounds. Wound infections may also result in bone defects, such as after surgery for complicated fractures of the calcaneus or talus or ankle replacement prostheses; especially in patients with compromised wound healing.

Bone grafts suffer from major resorption when used in extensive defects. Therefore, to obtain a sufficient amount of weight bearing, vascularized bone, free vascularized bone grafts are essential. Many composite flaps have been described, including the iliac crest, scapula, fibula, ribs, and humerus as donor sites (24–26).

Small bone defects in the distal foot can sometimes be corrected with conventional bone grafts if the defect is small and the soft tissues healthy. However, in many cases, the soft tissues are damaged, ischemic, or infected, and the best solution may be a partial amputation (digital amputation, ray amputation, or transmetatarsal amputation). In the midfoot and hindfoot, even large defects can be reconstructed with vascularized bone reconstructions, especially if the plantar aspect of the foot can be preserved.

The anatomy and the circulation of the talus are such that usually the whole talus must be removed in cases of infected comminuted fractures or avascular necrosis. To avoid shortening, a free iliac crest bone graft can be used to fill the defect resulting from absence of the talus. Usually the graft should be fused to the adjoining joints (pantalar arthrodesis).

In cases of deep infection after complicated calcaneal fracture fixation, the infected wound must be debrided, and in most cases, the internal fixation must be removed. The wound can be treated with negative-pressure therapy and the defect covered with a pedicled or free soft tissue flap (fasciocutaneous flaps or gracilis). For extensive defects of the calcaneus, stability can be restored by fusion of free iliac crest or "double-barrel" fibula flaps to the talus (Figure 80-4).

Extensive bony defects of the midfoot can also be reconstructed with free iliac crest or "double-barrel" fibula flaps.

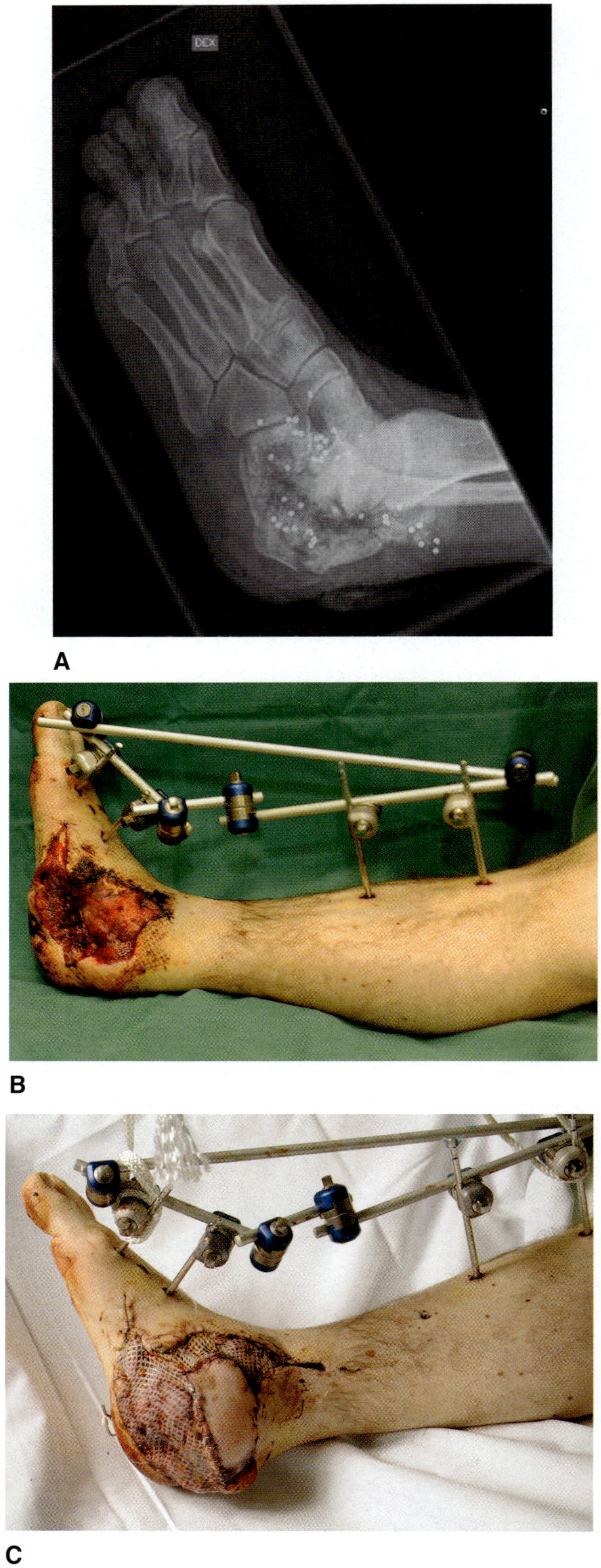

FIGURE 80-4 (A) Close-range shotgun injury to the heel with complex contaminated comminuted fracture of the calcaneus. (B) During debridement, a majority of the calcaneus was resected. (C) Microsurgical reconstruction with a deep inferior circumflex artery osteocutaneous flap.

PERIPHERAL VASCULAR DISEASE AND DIABETIC FOOT DEFECTS

Deeply infected nonhealing wounds are a difficult problem in patients with peripheral vascular disease or diabetes. Critical leg ischemia is a threat to the limb and often the life of the patient, with reduced quality of life, which frequently leads to major amputations. There is evidence that aggressive lower limb revascularization and free tissue transfer can significantly decrease the amputation rate. Infrainguinal vascular bypass reconstruction alone may be inadequate in cases of major ischemic tissue loss. Large infected defects with exposed tendons and bones may not heal despite successful bypass grafting. Furthermore, aggressive debridements and skin grafting are usually insufficient. Local flaps are usually inadequate, as there is only limited viable tissue available because of advanced ischemia, infection, and fibrosis.

Traditionally, there has been some reluctance to consider complex limb salvage techniques in patients with diabetes. Major amputation, however, decreases survival and increases the likelihood of contralateral amputation. The patient is best treated with a combined approach. The vascular surgery and the plastic microsurgical teams should combine their efforts to achieve a rapid and accurate assessment of the problem and optimize the timing and method of revascularization and reconstruction. Usually, these limbs require radical debridement and often limited distal amputation. Then the vascular team performs the bypass operation with the distal anastomosis to a native artery in the ankle or foot. The artery of the free flap is anastomosed end to side to the vascular graft, and the vein of the free flap is usually anastomosed end to end to a deep venae comitantes. This operation can be performed as a staged procedure with the debridement and vascular bypass in the first stage and the free flap performed after 2 to 4 weeks. Alternatively, they can be performed simultaneously; this is indicated when the distal anastomosis is not possible to the distal artery or the outflow is very poor with imminent risk of arterial graft occlusion. In these cases, end-to-side anastomosis of the free flap to the vascular graft increases the flow in the graft and may prevent arterial graft occlusion (27) (Figure 80-5).

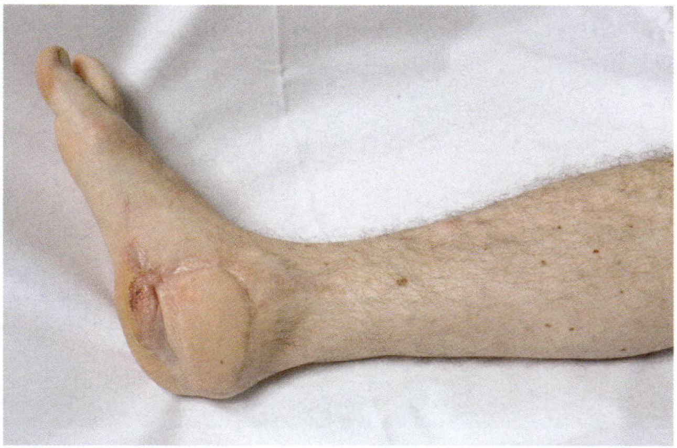

D

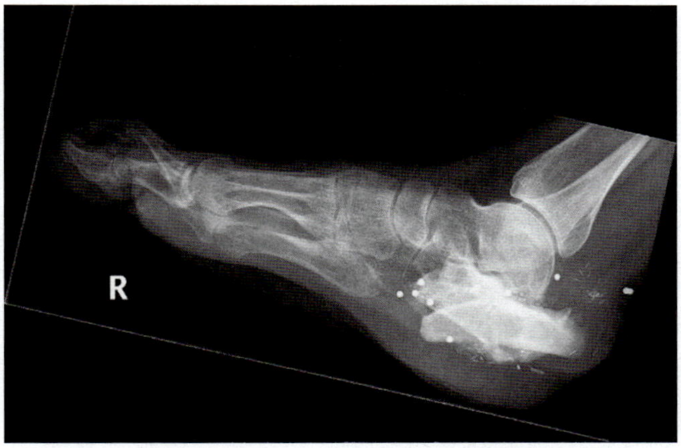

E

FIGURE 80-4 *(Continued)* (D) and (E) Final result: 2 years later, the patient is fully ambulatory.

Ducic and Attinger argued that diabetes should not be a contraindication to either pedicled muscle flap or free flap reconstruction. In fact, they concluded that pedicled muscle flaps were as effective as free flaps for coverage of small foot and ankle defects (28). Hong reported good results using the free ALT flap for diabetic foot reconstruction (29). More recently, a very large study from the same institution revealed that free flap reconstruction of diabetic feet significantly improves the 5-year survival rate (30). Risk factors for flap loss included peripheral arterial disease, history of angioplasties in the extremity, and the use of immunosuppressive agents after transplantation. In another study describing combined vascular bypass surgery and free flap reconstruction, a poor prognosis was associated with poor patient general condition, major heel ulceration, and poor kidney function (31).

SOFT TISSUE SARCOMAS OF THE FOOT

Soft tissue sarcoma is an uncommon form of cancer with about one half of cases occurring in the lower extremity. However, sarcomas are rare in the foot. The most common histological diagnosis is synovial sarcoma; other less frequent diagnoses are undifferentiated sarcoma, clear cell sarcoma, fibrosarcoma, and malignant fibrous histiocytoma. Mostly, sarcomas of the foot are high-grade tumors, located deeply, and about half are larger than 5 cm in diameter (32).

The optimal treatment should be wide excision with adequate margins. Because of the limited amount of soft tissue in the foot, sarcomas often grow in close proximity to neurovascular structures or bones. After tumor resection, the defects cannot be closed primarily or by using local flap options. Effective shoe fitting is essential, and therefore the mechanical demands and morphologic constraints are also indications for free flap coverage.

Patients with a soft tissue sarcoma of the foot often have nonspecific symptoms (e.g., a palpable lump), leading to a delay in diagnosis. Therefore, they frequently present after an unplanned excision, which often results in the need for more aggressive surgery, adjuvant radiotherapy, and free flap reconstructions (33). It may also lead to worse oncologic outcomes.

Limb salvage is usually possible, but it may sometimes require accepting a marginal resection and relying on a free tissue transfer to obtain coverage. Pre- or postoperative radiation therapy is often administered for local control. This combination seems to give acceptable local control rates and satisfactory functional results and allows prompt initiation of postoperative oncologic therapy (34).

Free flap coverage is effective in restoring the soft tissue envelope and mechanical stability of the foot (35) as well as ensuring wound healing and limb salvage. Muscle flaps covered with skin grafts or fasciocutaneous flaps are usually used to reconstruct defects after soft tissue sarcoma excision (Figures 80-6 and 80-7).

FOOT RECONSTRUCTION AFTER BURNS

In acute deep foot burns presenting with exposure of bone and tendons, free flap reconstruction may be the only option for preserving functional foot length. Late burn scar contractures and deformities of the ankle may also warrant free flap reconstruction if more simple reconstructive options are not available (36). However, in patients who have sustained an extensive burn injury, there may be both a limited availability of normal unburnt or unscarred free flap donor sites and a limited availability of recipient vessels in the distal extremity. One study described the use of radial forearm flaps in forefoot burns (37).

FOOT RECONSTRUCTION IN PEDIATRIC PATIENTS

Free flap reconstruction in children has not become universal because of concerns over the smaller vessel caliber and potential for problems with differential growth in the flap and recipient site. However, a large study by Lin et al. showed good results using both fasciocutaneous and muscle free flaps. The authors also highlighted the superiority of fasciocutaneous flaps in requiring fewer revision operations and less flap ulceration in plantar foot reconstructions (38).

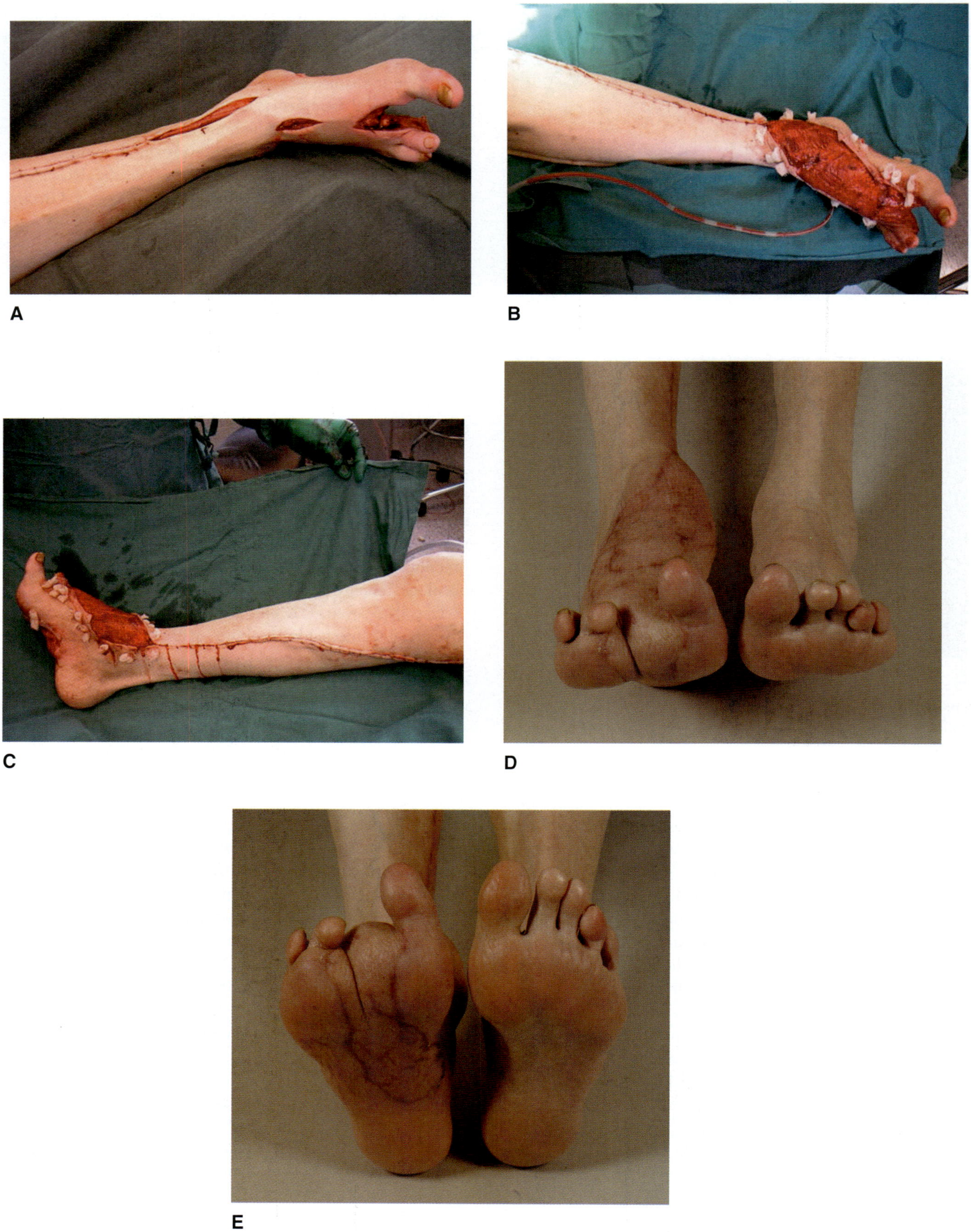

FIGURE 80-5 (A) Diabetic atherosclerotic patient with second and third rays amputated for gangrene. (B, C) Combined operation with distal bypass (posterior tibial to dorsalis pedis artery) and defect reconstruction using free latissimus dorsi muscle flap and skin graft. End-to-side anastomosis of the thoracodorsal artery to the vein graft and venous anastomosis to the deep venae comitantes. (D, E) Late result with shrinkage of the muscle flap and patient fully ambulatory.

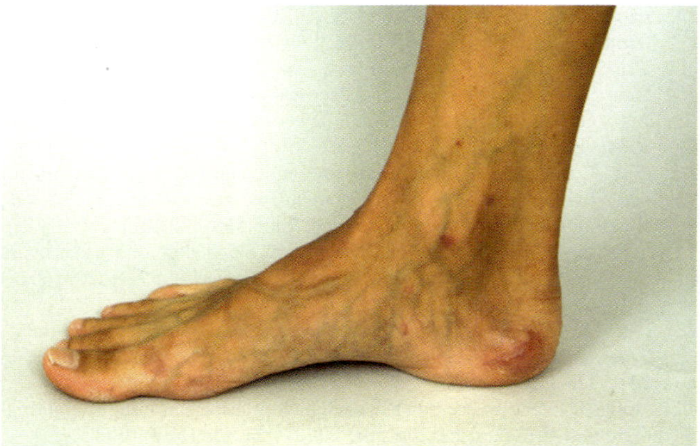

A

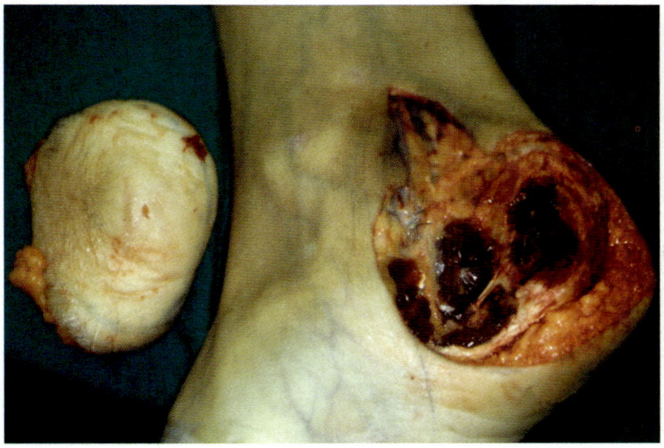

B

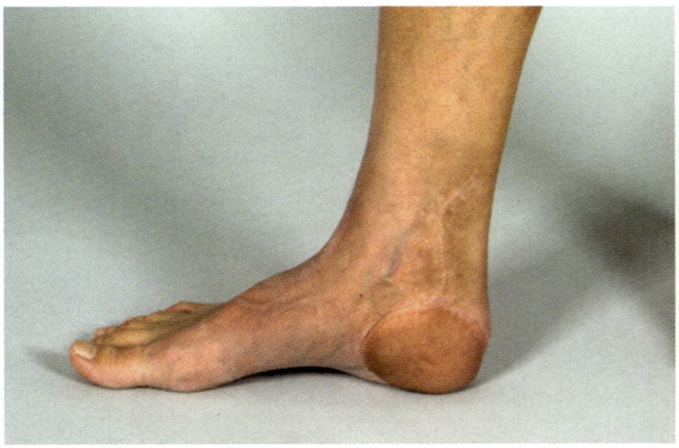

C

FIGURE 80-6 (**A**) Synovial sarcoma of the heel. (**B**) Excision and reconstruction with a free parascapular flap. (**C**) Final result.

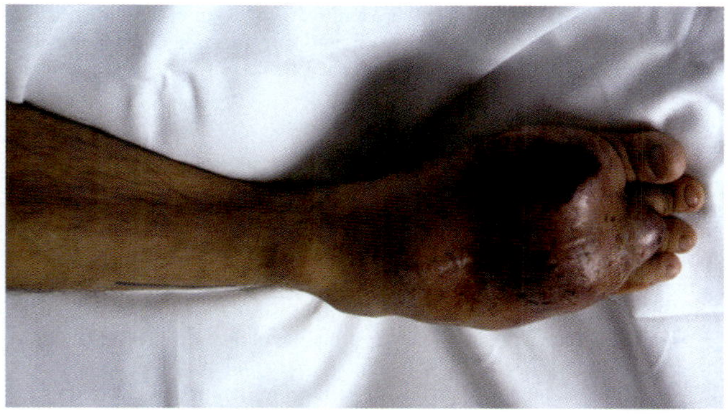

A

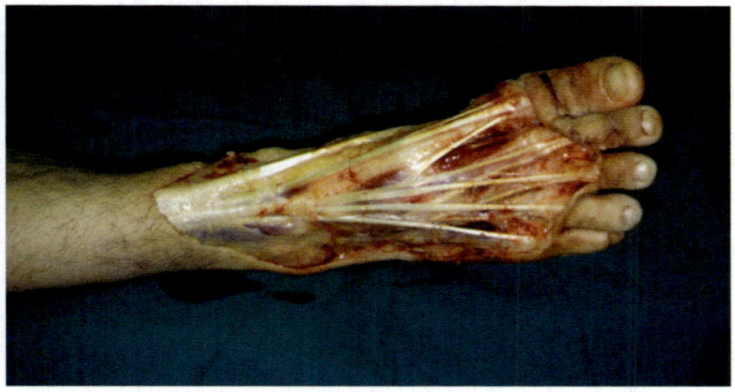

B

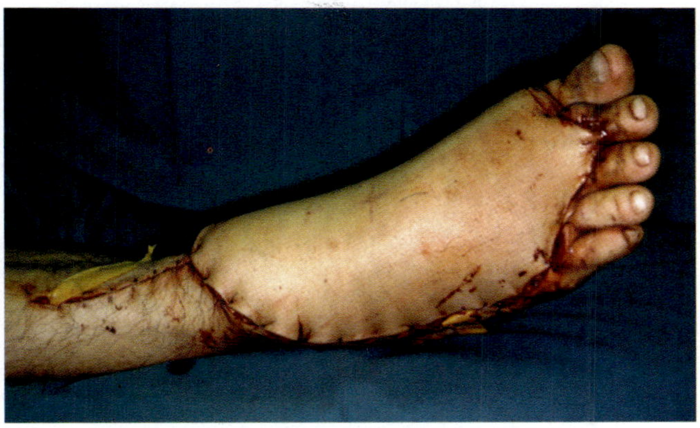

C

FIGURE 80-7 (**A**) Sarcoma of the dorsum of the foot. (**B**) Resection with exposure of extensor tendons. (**C**) Reconstruction with a free anterolateral thigh flap allowed tendon gliding. The thick flap required later thinning.

REFERENCES

1. Mathes SJ. *Mathes Plastic Surgery*. Philadelphia: Saunders Elsevier. Vol. 6, Chapter 161. 2006.
2. Baechler MF, Groth AT, Nesti LJ, Martin BD. Soft tissue management of war wounds to the foot and ankle. *Foot Ankle Clin* 2010;15(1):113–138.
3. Masquelet AC, Gilbert A. *An Atlas of Flaps of the Musculoskeletal System*. Boca Raton, FL: Taylor and Francis, 2005, 177–187, 204–210, 218–219.
4. Shanahan RE, Gingrass RP. Medial plantar sensory flap for coverage of heel defects. *Plast Reconstr Surg* 1979;64(3):295–298.
5. Oh SJ, Moon M, Cha J, et al. Weight-bearing plantar reconstruction using versatile medial plantar sensate flap. *J Plast Reconstr Aesthet Surg* 2011;64(2):248–254.
6. Karanas YL, Nigriny J, Chang J. The timing of microsurgical reconstruction in lower extremity trauma. *Microsurgery* 2008;28(8):632–634.
7. Park S, Hoon HS, Jong LT. Algorithm for recipient vessel selection in free tissue transfer to the lower extremity. *Plast Reconstr Surg* 1999;103(7):1937–1948.
8. Huemer GM, Larcher L, Schoeller T, Bauer T. The free gracilis muscle flap in Achilles tendon coverage and reconstruction. *Plast Reconstr Surg* 2012;129(4):910–919.

9. Houtmeyers P, Opsomer D, Van Landuyt K, Monstrey S. Reconstruction of the Achilles tendon and overlying soft tissue by free composite anterolateral thigh flap with vascularized fascia lata. *J Reconstr Microsurg* 2012;28(3):205–209.
10. Rautio J. Resurfacing and sensory recovery of the sole. *Clin Plast Surg* 1991;18:615–626.
11. May JW Jr, Halls MJ, Simon SR. Free microvascular muscle flaps with skin graft reconstruction of extensive defects of the foot: a clinical and gait analysis study. *Plast Reconstr Surg* 1985;75(5):627–641.
12. Ducic I, Hung V, Dellon AL. Innervated free flaps for foot reconstruction: a review. *J Reconstr Microsurg* 2006;22(6):433–442.
13. Ulusal BG, Lin YT, Ulusal AE, et al. Reconstruction of foot defects with free lateral arm fasciocutaneous flaps: analysis of fifty patients. *Microsurgery* 2005;25(8):581–588.
14. Santanelli F, Tenna S, Pace A, Scuderi N. Free flap reconstruction of the sole of the foot with or without sensory nerve coaptation. *Plast Reconstr Surg* 2002;109(7):2314–2322.
15. Rainer C, Schwabegger AH, Bauer T, et al. Free flap reconstruction of the foot. *Ann Plast Surg* 1999;42(6):595–606.
16. Potparic Z, Rajacic N. Long-term results of weight-bearing foot reconstruction with non-innervated and reinnervated free flaps. *Br J Plast Surg* 1997;50(3):176–181.
17. Schwabegger AH, Schubert HM, Baltaci M, et al. Instep split skin grafts on muscle flaps to reconstruct pressure exposed soft tissue parts at the lower extremity. *Arch Orthop Trauma Surg* 2012;132(10):1451–1459.
18. Song YG, Chen GZ, Song YL. The free thigh flap: a new free flap concept based on the septocutaneous artery. *Br J Plast Surg* 1984;37(2):149–159.
19. Lee YC, Chiu HY, Shieh SJ. The clinical application of anterolateral thigh flap. *Plast Surg Int* 2011;2011:127:353.
20. Lin TS, Jeng SF, Wei FC. Temporary placement of plantar heel skin in the thigh with subsequent transfer back to the heel using free anterolateral thigh myocutaneous flap as a carrier: case report. *J Trauma* 2005;58: 193–195.
21. Demirtas Y, Neimetzade T, Kelahmetoglu O, Guneren E. Comparison of free muscle and perforator skin flaps for soft tissue reconstruction of the foot and ankle. *Foot Ankle Int* 2010;31(1):53–58.
22. Koski EA, Kuokkanen HO, Koskinen SK, Tukiainen EJ. Reconstruction of soft tissue after complicated calcaneal fractures. *Scand J Plast Reconstr Surg Hand Surg* 2004;38(5):284–287.
23. Heymans O, Verhelle N, Lahaye T. Covering small defects on the weight bearing surfaces of the foot: the free temporal fasciocutaneous flap. *Br J Plast Surg* 2005;58:460–465.
24. Battiston B, Antonini A, Tos P, et al. Microvascular reconstructions of traumatic-combined tissue loss at foot and ankle level. *Microsurgery* 2011;31(3):212–217.
25. Yazar S, Lin CH, Wei FC. One-stage reconstruction of composite bone and soft-tissue defects in traumatic lower extremities. *Plast Reconstr Surg* 2004;114(6):1457–1466.
26. Peek A, Giessler GA. Functional total and subtotal heel reconstruction with free composite osteofasciocutaneous groin flaps of the deep circumflex iliac vessels. *Ann Plast Surg.* 2006;56(6):628–634.
27. Lorenzetti F, Tukiainen E, Albäck A, et al. Blood flow in a pedal bypass combined with a free muscle flap. *Eur J Vasc Endovasc Surg* 2001;22(2): 161–164.
28. Ducic I, Attinger CE. Foot and ankle reconstruction: pedicled muscle flaps versus free flaps and the role of diabetes. *Plast Reconstr Surg* 2011;128(1):173–180.
29. Hong JP. Reconstruction of the diabetic foot using the anterolateral thigh perforator flap. *Plast Reconstr Surg* 200615;117(5):1599–1608.
30. Oh TS, Lee HS, Hong JP. Diabetic foot reconstruction using free flaps increases 5-year-survival rate. *J Plast Reconstr Aesthet Surg* 2013;66(2):243–250.
31. Tukiainen E, Kallio M, Lepäntalo M. Advanced leg salvage of the critically ischemic leg with major tissue loss by vascular and plastic surgeon teamwork: long-term outcome. *Ann Surg.* 2006;244(6):949–957.
32. Latt AD, Turcotte RE, Isler MH, Wong C. Soft-tissue sarcoma of the foot. *Can J Surg* 2010;53(6):424–431.
33. Thacker MM, Potter BK, Pitcher JD, Temple HT. Soft tissue sarcomas of the foot and ankle: impact of unplanned excision, limb salvage, and multimodality therapy. *Foot Ankle Int* 2008;29(7):690–698.
34. Popov P, Tukiainen E, Asko-Seljavaara S, et al. Soft tissue sarcomas of the lower extremity: surgical treatment and outcome. *Eur J Surg Oncol* 2000;26:679–685.
35. Steinau HU, Daigeler A, Langer S, et al. Limb salvage in malignant tumors. *Semin Plast Surg* 2010;24(1):18–33.
36. Abramson DL, Pribaz JJ, Orgill DP. The use of free tissue transfer in burn reconstruction. *J Burn Care Rehabil* 1996;17(5):402–408.
37. Fernandez-Palacios J, De Armas Diaz F, Deniz Hernandez V, et al. Radial free flaps in plantar burns. *Burns* 1996;22(3):242–245.
38. Lin CH, Mardini S, Wei FC, et al. Free flap reconstruction of foot and ankle defects in pediatric patients: long-term outcome in 91 cases. *Plast Reconstr Surg* 2006;117(7):2478–2487.

CHAPTER 81

Vascularized Bone Grafts for Trauma and Tumors of the Lower Extremities

Michael B. Wood

Before the late 1970s, the result of a large bone defect of the femur or tibia or a recalcitrant nonunion of the major long bones of the lower extremity was frequently amputation and prosthetic limb substitution. In some cases, healing with limb salvage could be achieved by massive autografts or massive allografts or in the case of the tibia, cross-union techniques to an intact fibula or pedicle shifted fibula. These techniques frequently required multiple procedures and a protracted healing period.

Since the late 1970s, the concept of the management of massive bone defects or the salvage of prior failed attempts to heal nonunions by the transfer of an autograft with a sustained blood supply, and presumably preserved viable cellular components, has gained acceptance and is supported by data from both laboratory and clinical studies (1–7).

The purpose of this chapter is to discuss more specific indications for free microvascular bone transfer to the lower extremity, suggest technical considerations related to the recipient site, and present a variety of clinical case examples from the author's personal series.

Details of the vascular anatomy and technique of harvest of the more commonly used vascularized bone autografts are addressed elsewhere in this text and are not covered in this chapter.

HISTORICAL BACKGROUND AND RATIONALE FOR VASCULARIZED BONE TRANSFER

The history of bone grafting covers millennia. It would probably be a stretch, however, and certainly not gender politically appropriate, to attribute the biblical reference of God creating woman by using a piece of Adam's rib as the first clinical case of bone grafting. Although prior attempts at bone grafting likely occurred in earlier ages, the first published case in Western literature that the author is aware of was by Job van Meekeren in 1668 (8). In this report, a piece of canine calvarium was used to reconstruct a traumatic skull defect in a soldier. The procedure was not viewed favorably by the clergy, and the already unfortunate patient suffered further insult by excommunication from the church (9).

The clinical use of nonvascularized autograft to promote bone union and heal relatively short bony defects became increasingly prevalent in the latter 19th century. Curtis (10) and Barth (11) independently described the clinical use and healing mechanism of such autografts in 1893 and suggested that such grafts possess the properties of osteoconduction and osteoinduction. The sentinel work of Phemister (12), which described the sequence of healing of cancellous bone autografts, remains as important today as when it was published almost a century ago. In this work, Phemister described the first step of autograft incorporation as vascular invasion followed by bone osteolysis and then followed by osteoblastic bone formation. In a successful process of bone graft incorporation, the osteoblastic and osteoclastic activities occur concurrently until remodeling consistent with the mechanical demands across the bone graft site is completed. The important point is that the initial, and at times rate-limiting, step of bone autograft incorporation is vascular invasion, and this explains in part why the more structurally porous cancellous graft materials are more rapidly and completely incorporated than a structurally dense cortical autograft (13).

The advantage of maintaining some degree of sustained vascular perfusion at the time of bone grafting had been recognized long before the advent of microvascular surgery and free tissue transfer procedures. For more than a century, bone autografting with an attached vascular or vascularized soft tissue pedicle has been used in selected clinical situations (14–17). However, such pedicled bone grafts have had very limited application because of barriers related to availability and length of arc of rotation. Expanded clinical versatility of vascularized bone grafts had to await the refined technology of microvascular surgery and clarification of the vascular anatomy of several appropriate donor bone segments.

An illustration of the difference between vascularized and nonvascularized autograft is provided in Figure 81-1. This is a radiograph at 38 months after surgery of an extraarticular knee resection for malignant tumor, with immediate reconstruction by femoral–tibial arthrodesis. On the image's left is a nonvascularized fibula autograft and on the right a vascularized fibula autograft, both transferred during the same procedure. Note the mottled appearance of the nonvascularized fibula attributable to a preponderance of osteoclastic activity and the lack of apparent hypertrophy compared with the vascularized fibula segment.

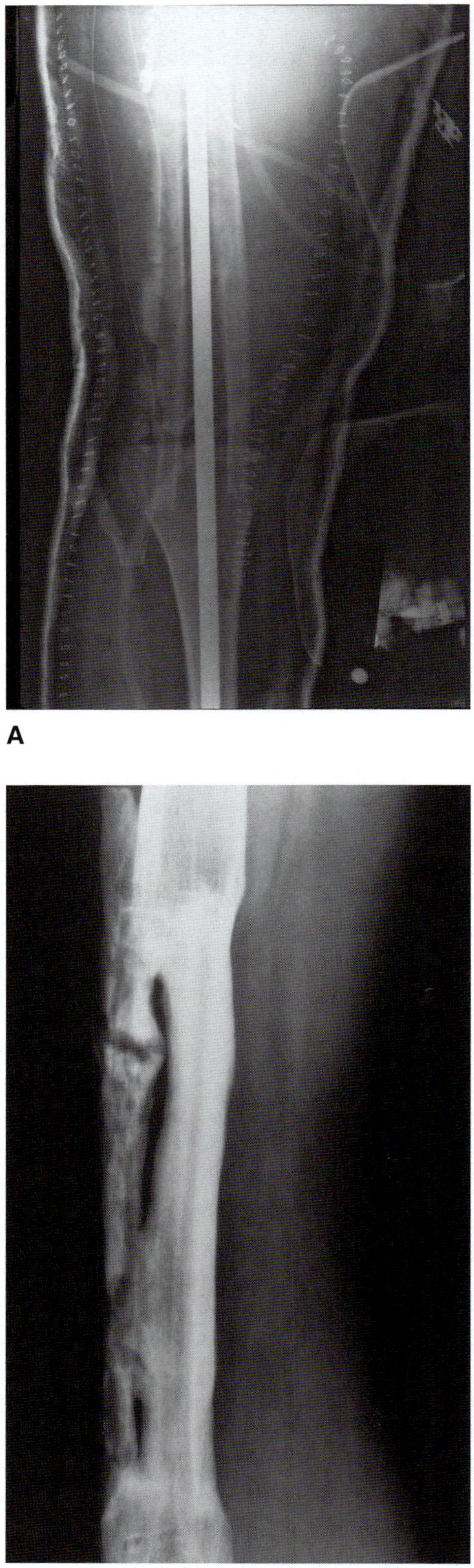

A

B

FIGURE 81-1 (A) Radiograph immediately after surgery of an extraarticular knee resection with femorotibial arthrodesis. On the lateral side is a nonvascularized fibula autograft with iliac crest autograft; on the medial side is a vascularized fibula autograft. (B) The same patient, 38 months after surgery after hardware removal. Note hypertrophy of vascularized fibula and osteolysis of nonvascularized fibula autograft.

INDICATIONS FOR VASCULARIZED BONE GRAFTS IN THE LOWER EXTREMITY

In general, the indication for a vascularized bone graft in the lower extremity is any clinical situation that does not have a simpler reliable solution. Thus, smaller bone defects or initial nonunions surrounded by a reasonably well-vascularized soft tissue milieu should be managed by conventional nonvascularized cancellous autografts in most patients.

There are, however, four chief categories of bony pathology in the lower limb that merit preferential consideration of reconstruction by vascularized bone transfer: large bone defects, prior bone reconstruction failures, infected bone defects, and nonunions associated with bone radionecrosis.

Large Bone Defects

There is no "evidence-based" data that I am aware of that defines how "large" is "large" for a bone defect that is more efficaciously reconstructed by vascularized bone transfer rather than by a nonvascularized bone autograft. Most authors on the subject have suggested 6 cm as the threshold length of defect. However, 6 cm in one patient may be quite different from the same length in another based on a number of factors, including the quality of the vascularity of the surrounding soft tissue bed, the presence or absence of prior sepsis or radiotherapy in the surgical field, the degree of neighboring structural support (e.g., an intact fibula adjacent to a tibial defect), the availability of a sufficient quantity of autograft material, and other factors calling on clinical judgment. I would suggest putting the choice of a vascularized bone transfer at least on the list of reconstructive options when confronted with a bony defect measuring 6 cm or more. For defects smaller than this, in the presence of favorable surrounding soft tissue without antecedent sepsis or radiotherapy and where there is a practical means to achieve stable fixation, I am inclined to select cancellous autografting as the first-line choice for management. It should also be recognized that for defects much larger than 6 cm, a massive allograft may be a reasonable choice in selected patients. Such might be the case with a surgically created defect (e.g., en bloc bone tumor resection) with a pristine soft tissue envelop and especially in a patient with limited life expectancy. However, when considering the use of a massive allograft, it must be recognized that these constructs have a limited ability to be revascularized and hence a limited capacity to be replaced by host osteoprogenitor cells' "creeping substitution." An inviolate rule for any bone grafting procedure, whether vascularized or nonvascularized, is stability at the fracture site. Thus, one cannot consider the selection of bone graft choice without addressing how best to accomplish stabilization of the construct. This may involve situations in which fixation is already stable and requires only an onlay graft. Alternatively, the situation may require plans for additional external fixation or internal fixation by transcortical screws, compression plating, intramedullary nailing, or supplementary allografts or cortical autografts.

Prior Bone Reconstruction Failures

Bone defects without regard to length or chronic nonunions that have failed to heal with an otherwise efficacious and well-executed procedure may be candidates for a vascularized bone transfer. However, in all such cases, a careful analysis of the possible reasons for why the prior intervention was not successful should be conducted before a vascularized bone graft is selected. Frequently, a plausible explanation of why the prior union attempt failed may exist, such as failure to achieve stable fixation, the use of inferior graft materials (processed allograft, xenograft, commercial osteoinductive material), postoperative wound site sepsis, and so on. If the failure analysis yields an explanation that can be rectified by a more conventional approach, then a secondary procedure using nonvascularized autograft may be warranted. However, if this is not the case, then vascularized bone transfer should emerge as the reconstructive option of choice.

Infected Bone Defects

The use of vascularized bone graft for reconstructing infected bone defects is particularly attractive for a number of reasons. Probably of most importance is the fact that such bone grafts are inherently a vehicle for local blood supply. However, also of importance is the fact that a vascularized fibula is a generous source of bone length, and it makes little difference from the technical perspective if one transfers a 6- or 16-cm graft segment. Thus, a more aggressive debridement of infected bone ends may be carried out with less regard to concerns about creating a larger bone defect than can be reliably reconstructed (Figure 81-2).

Nonunions Associated with Bone Radionecrosis

Bone nonunion that is associated with osteoradionecrosis is a particularly challenging problem that responds poorly to conventional bone grafting techniques. This is because three adverse circumstances exist in the presence of localized radiation changes: (1) impaired intraosseous blood supply, (2) impaired blood supply of the surrounding soft tissue, and (3) periosteal and intraosseous cell death. These adverse circumstances are directly addressed by the transfer of a vascularized bone segment obtained from a site well distant to the irradiated field (Figure 81-3).

PREFERRED VASCULARIZED BONE AUTOGRAFT DONOR SITES FOR LOWER EXTREMITY RECONSTRUCTION

Although virtually any block of bone with a periosteal or intramedullary blood supply nourished by an anatomically defined arteriovenous system can qualify as a donor site for vascularized bone, for practical purposes, the list of useful vascularized bone donor sites is finite and includes the list below. The vascular and bony anatomy and technique of harvest are described elsewhere in this text and are not detailed in this chapter.

Fibula

To the author's knowledge, the first clinical use of the fibula as a free vascularized bone transfer was by Ueba in 1974 (18), but the first published clinical report was by Taylor et al. in 1975 (19).

The diaphysis of the fibula is by far the workhorse for vascularized bone reconstruction in the lower extremity. It is the donor of choice for reconstructing substantial long bone deficits because of its linear configuration and generous available length (Figure 81-4). The fibula's cortical structure is well suited for stable fixation using onlay plates and transcortical screws. When using the peroneal artery and accompanying veins as the vascular pedicle, its blood supply is ensured by both intramedullary and periosteal sources. Provided the proximal and distal metaphyseal and epiphyseal portions of the fibula are maintained inviolate, the resulting donor defect is functionally acceptable. The loss of the fibular weight-bearing function is typically compensated for by hypertrophy of the adjacent tibia. Long-term donor problems may include contracture or unintended tenodesis of the flexor hallucis longus muscle or tendon with a resulting flexion contracture of the great toe interphalangeal joint and transient peroneal nerve palsy. Rarely, more severe donor-related complications have been reported, including permanent peroneal palsy, lower limb compartment syndrome with myonecrosis, stress fracture of the tibia, and lateral instability of the ankle joint (20–22).

Iliac Crest

The anterior iliac crest, pedicled on the deep circumflex iliac vessels, is one of the pioneer vascularized bone donor sites that gained early clinical acceptance. Its anatomic features and clinical utility were published by Taylor et al. in 1979. (23) Because of its chiefly cancellous structure and predominantly periosteal blood supply, it may be useful in reconstructive situations that are not especially ideal for the chiefly cortical and linear fibula (e.g., short metaphyseal defects and defects requiring shaping by one or more osteotomies of the donor bone)

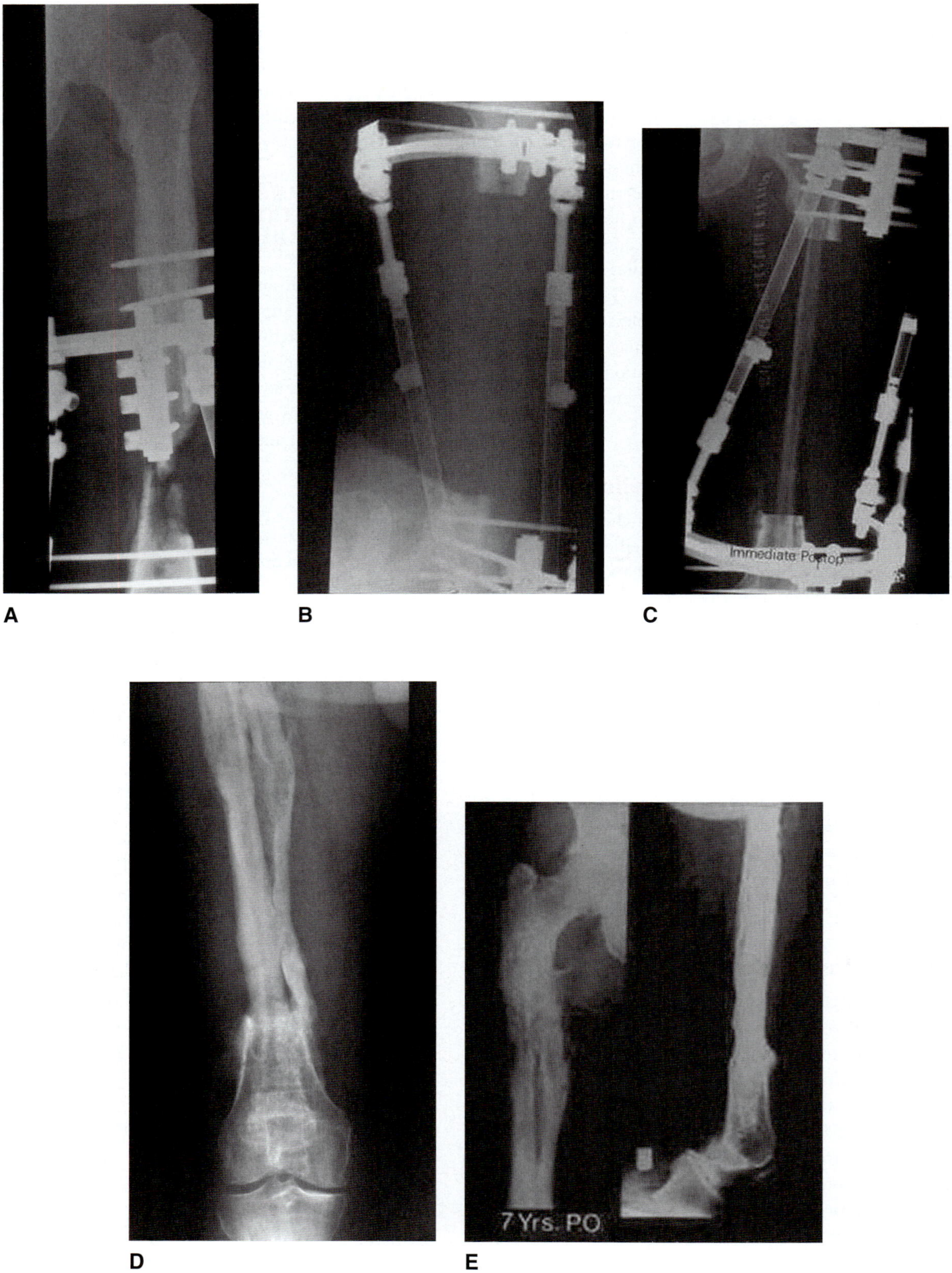

FIGURE 81-2 (A) Radiograph of femur with extensive chronic osteomyelitis. (B) Radiograph of femur after resection of all infected and sclerotic bone. (C) Radiograph of the femur immediately following a vascularized fibula transfer. (D) Radiograph of the femur 29 months after surgery. Note the union and hypertrophy of fibula. (E) Radiograph of the femur 7 years after surgery. There is full weight bearing and no evidence of sepsis.

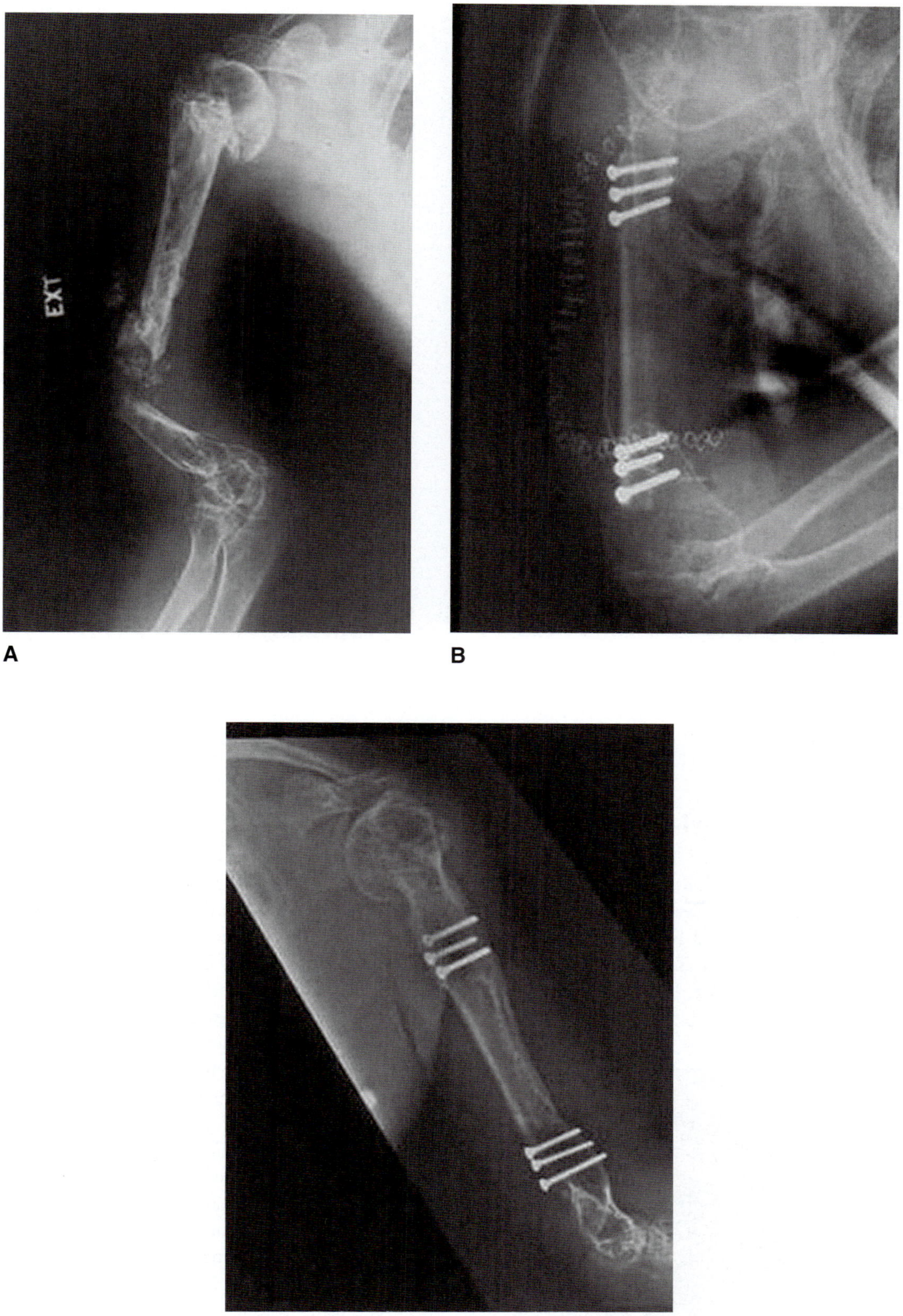

A B C

FIGURE 81-3 (**A**) Radiograph of fractured and radionecrotic humerus after radiotherapy for Ewing's sarcoma. (**B**) Radiograph of humerus after resection of all necrotic bone and vascularized fibula transfer. (**C**) Radiograph of healed vascularized fibula with hypertrophy 17 months after surgery.

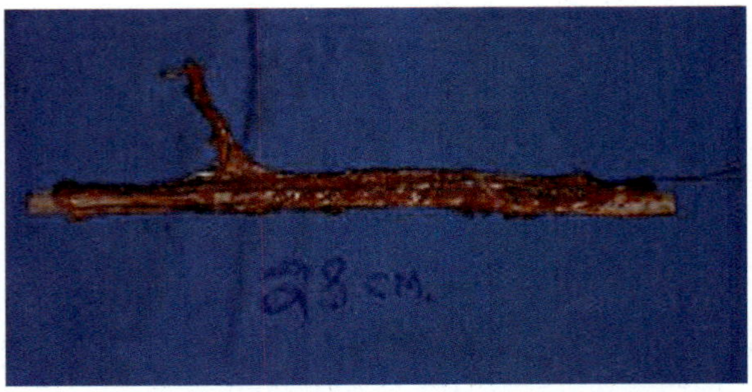

FIGURE 81-4 Isolated fibula with peroneal vascular pedicle, 28 cm in length.

(Figure 81-5). In the author's opinion, it is a more difficult bone graft to isolate, requiring a rather tedious dissection of the vascular pedicle, which is shorter and of more diminutive caliber than that of the fibula. The chief donor site morbidity is iatrogenic inguinal or femoral hernia or neuropathy of the lateral femoral cutaneous nerve or the genitofemoral nerve.

Rib

Although segments of rib based on the intercostal vessels have a relatively long history as vascularized pedicle bone grafts, they have been used sporadically as free vascularized bone grafts (24). Except for use in conjunction with spine stabilization, in which they are conveniently accessible in this operative field, they have little contemporary utility for lower extremity reconstruction.

Medial Femoral Condyle

This vascularized bone graft donor site provides a readily accessible small bone block of cancellous structure based on a periosteal blood supply from the descending medial genicular vessels (25). It is now chiefly used as a small vascularized bone graft for salvage of carpal bone avascular necrosis that requires some degree of structural support. This application might also be appropriate for special situations about the femoral head and neck or foot.

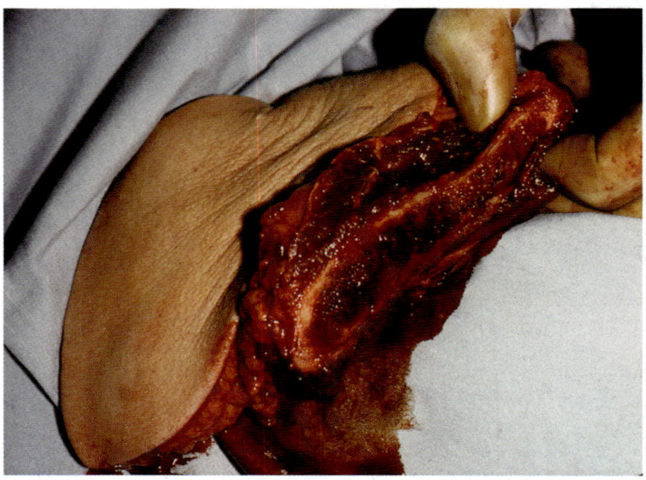

FIGURE 81-5 Osteocutaneous iliac crest compound flap on deep circumflex iliac vascular pedicle. Note the chiefly cancellous structure.

Vascularized Bone Grafts as a Component of Compound Soft Tissue Flaps

Several vascularized bone grafts may merit consideration for the management of lower extremity bony defects in association with soft tissue defects. In general, in the lower limb, such compound flaps are considered when the bone defect is a "second string" reconstructive consideration to that of the management of the soft tissue defect. Thus, compound flaps in this category generally have as the major indication soft tissue coverage with the accompanying bone segment acting as a hitchhiker tissue. These flaps are well described elsewhere in this text and include:

- Radial forearm flap with accompanying segment of distal radius diaphysis and metaphysis
- Lateral arm flap with accompanying lateral distal humerus diaphysis and metaphysis
- Scapular flap with accompanying lateral border of scapula

TECHNICAL PRINCIPLES FOR LOWER EXTREMITY VASCULARIZED BONE TRANSFERS

Without regard to a specific clinical situation, the following seven principles apply to any clinical application of vascularized bone transfer to the lower extremity for an optimal outcome.

1. The recipient site proximal and distal bone ends should be first freshened or resected until healthy-appearing, bleeding bone surfaces are present. In general, the length of the resulting bone defect is less relevant than the quality of the recipient site bone surfaces. This is especially true when reconstructing a bone defect resulting from chronic osteomyelitis.
2. It is important to bridge the entire defect with the vascularized bone graft to ensure that the graft spans the defect from healthy host proximal bone to healthy host distal bone. This is particularly true when using a vascularized bone graft to manage an allograft nonunion or fracture.
3. One should make every effort to provide maximal bone graft to recipient bone surface contact. This includes sculpting the opposing bone ends to eliminate gaps; reflecting periosteum from the zones of bone contact; when appropriate, positioning the vascularized bone segment within the medullary canal of the recipient bone; and using cancellous nonvascularized bone autograft as grouting material to eliminate gaps and dead space in the bone contact zones.
4. It is essential to ensure rigid internal fixation of the recipient site bone defect (if present) and the vascularized bone segment. It is equally important, however, to not compromise the intrinsic vascularity of the transferred bone segment by overzealous periosteal stripping or intramedullary instrumentation. The selection of internal

fixation will depend on the clinical situation and may include an intramedullary rod across the defect that is flanked by an onlay vascularized bone graft or an interposed bone graft secured at the proximal and distal ends by compression plates or transcortical screws. Supplementary external fixation with either a cast or external fixation device may additionally be necessary.
5. One must ensure that the vascular pedicle to the transferred segment is not under tension. To accomplish this, maximum pedicle length should be achieved at the time of graft harvest, and one should select either orthograde or retrograde graft placement at the recipient site based on which position accomplishes optimal pedicle length redundancy.
6. Postoperative management should plan on progressive weight bearing in a controlled manner. In general, strict non–weight bearing should be advised until there is radiographic evidence of proximal and distal graft union. Thereafter, partial weight bearing should be permitted until clear radiographic evidence of graft hypertrophy is present. Full weight bearing proceeds only when the vascularized bone graft is both united and demonstrating signs of hypertrophy. Typically, this is at 6 months after surgery at the earliest and sometimes as late as 12 months.
7. Finally, it may be necessary to consider reintervening at 6 months after surgery if there is no clear evidence of proximal and distal graft union at that time. Provided the internal fixation is still sound at that point, simple onlay cancellous autografting to the ununited osteosynthesis site is advised with care not to inflict injury to the graft vascular pedicle. If the internal fixation is no longer stable, then revision internal fixation, usually by compression plating along with supplementary cancellous bone autografting is advised.

SPECIFIC RECIPIENT SITE TECHNICAL CONSIDERATIONS

Pelvis

There are few consistent indications for vascularized bone transfer for pelvic reconstructions. Techniques of internal hemipelvectomy and the expanded use of structural allografts about the acetabulum and pelvic ring have in large measure emerged as the front-line consideration for bone reconstruction about the pelvis. Thus, specific guidelines regarding pelvic recipient site management are not practical. The generic principles of optimal selection of recipient site vessels, graft placement to optimize the mechanics of weight bearing, and stable internal fixation of the vascularized graft are the major considerations. For structural support after internal hemipelvectomy, the fibula has in most cases been the preferred donor bone.

Femur

For a number of reasons, the femur may be the recipient site where vascularized bone transfer is of greatest value. This is because of all long bone nonunions, those of the femur most profoundly degrade the quality of life (26). In the upper limb, chronic nonunion and instability of the humerus or forearm, although disabling, is usually consistent with some function. In the tibia, chronic nonunion can be palliated with external orthoses and in more severe cases amputation and below-knee prosthetic fitting. Instability of the femur, however, cannot generally be palliated by external orthoses, and above-knee amputation results in a much greater disability than its below-knee counterpart. Thus, a femoral bone defect, particularly in a patient with an expected multi-decade life span, should merit consideration of reconstruction by vascularized bone transfer.

Recipient site technical issues may be categorized into two broad groups, femoral shaft reconstruction and distal femur reconstruction with knee arthrodesis.

Femoral Shaft Reconstruction

With rare exception, the fibula is the preferred donor bone, preferably using the ipsilateral fibula unless it is missing and damaged.

For diaphysial reconstructions, I prefer a two-incision exposure. This involves a lateral incision to expose the nonunion site and allow resection of the intervening fibrous tissue, as well as resection of the proximal and distal bone ends, to expose healthy, well-vascularized bone surfaces. It is also through the lateral incisions that the fibula is placed within or across the defect and internal fixation is accomplished if compression plates and screws are selected for this purpose. If an intramedullary nail is used for femoral internal fixation, the fibula is placed as an onlay graft across the defect along the anterolateral surface.

A second medial incision is used for exposure of the recipient site vessels and to permit exposure for vascular anastomosis. The medial incision is carried down to the sartorius muscle, which is reflected either anteriorly or posteriorly to expose the vascular contents of Hunter's canal. In the course of medial exposure, I prefer to identify and isolate but not yet transect the greater saphenous vein. It may serve as the preferred recipient vein if the venae comitans accompanying the femoral artery in Hunter's canal are not selected as recipient veins. After the recipient site vessels are isolated, a decision is made to either select appropriate branches of the femoral vessels for end-to-end anastomosis versus end-to-side anastomosis of the peroneal artery to the femoral artery. After the femoral vessels are isolated and mobilized for a distance of 4 to 5 cm, the intervening soft tissue in the depths of the medial exposure site is incised and partially resected to expose the nonunion site from the medial side. It is essential that the fibula graft segment be positioned either within or across the femoral defect in a manner that permits the peroneal vascular pedicle to easily reach the selected recipient vessels with some length redundancy. This may require rotating the fibular graft in a manner that allows the shortest distance between the pedicle vessels and the recipient site vessels. The fibula may be positioned either orthograde or retrograde to accomplish ideal pedicle positioning. When used as an inlay graft, the periosteum of the proximal and distal fibula ends is reflected circumferentially for a short distance, and both ends of the fibula are dowelled into the medullary canal of the femur proximally and distally (Figure 81-6). When used as an onlay graft, the surface of the fibula that will lie in

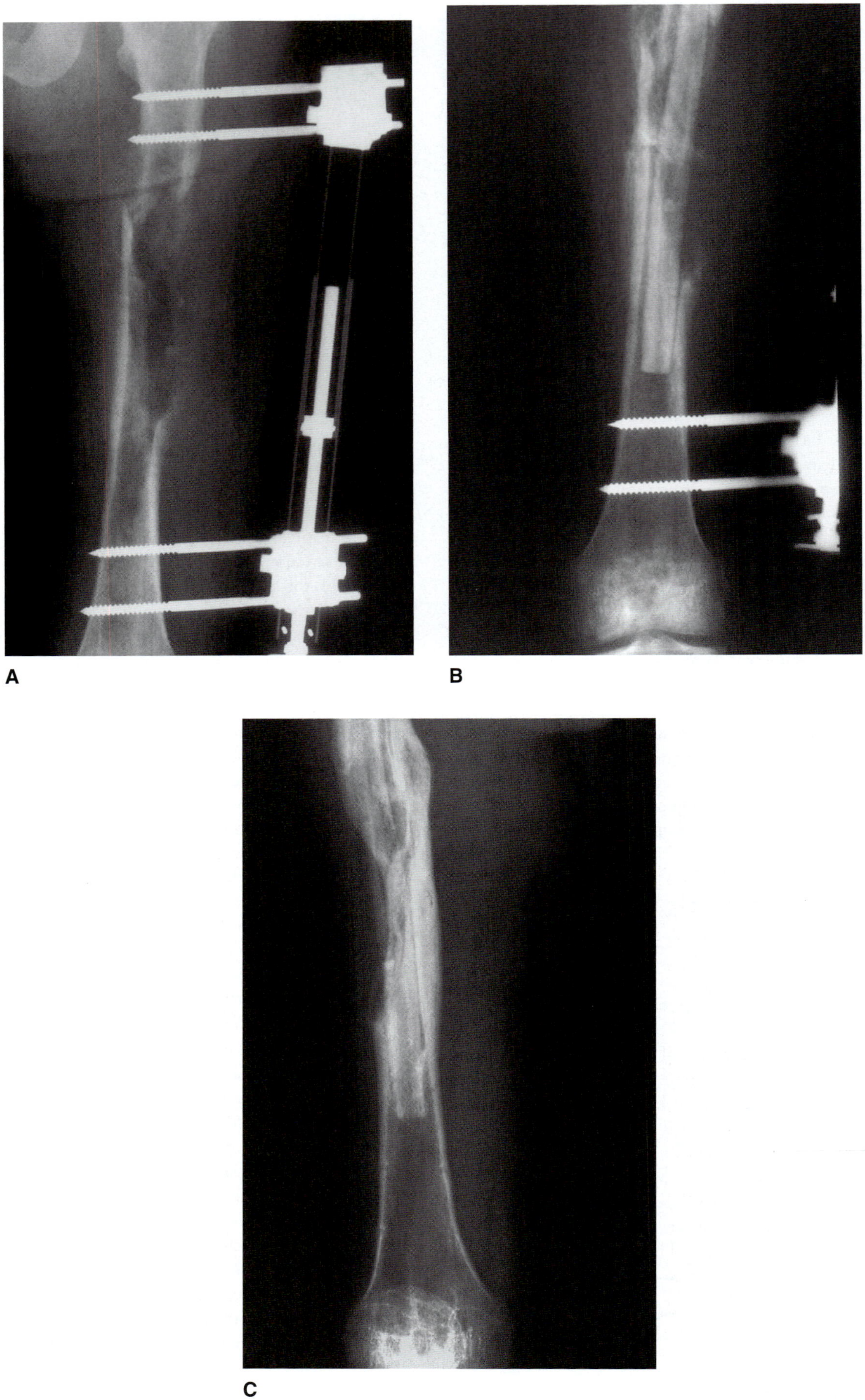

FIGURE 81-6 (A) Radiograph of femur with middiaphyseal bony defect. (B) Radiograph immediately after vascularized fibula transfer with intramedullary placement. (C) Radiograph 10 months after surgery with union and hypertrophy.

direct contact with the femur is exposed by periosteal reflection. It is important, however, that the amount of periosteal flap elevation is strictly limited to the surface contact area to ensure the periosteum of the fibula is left undisturbed over the noncontact surface for maximum preservation of the periosteal blood supply to the graft. After fibular graft placement, internal fixation, and revascularization, I recommend additional cancellous autograft from the iliac crest be placed about the proximal and distal osteosynthesis sites.

Distal Femur Reconstruction with Knee Arthrodesis

This technique is most often required in patients undergoing extraarticular resections for malignant lesions of the distal femur or proximal tibia or in patients undergoing limb salvage for a septic knee joint endoprosthesis. The reconstruction at this level can frequently be accomplished by 180-degree rotation of the ipsilateral fibula on an intact peroneal vascular pedicle with intramedullary fixation using a locked nail between the femur and tibia. However, if the femoral resection is at a level proximal to the metaphyseal flare involving greater than 10 cm of distal femur, it may be difficult to bridge this gap with a pedicled fibula "turn-up" without excessive limb shortening. In such a case, it may be preferable to proceed with a free transfer with microvascular anastomoses. Depending on the defect length, the reconstruction may involve a single fibular segment or alternatively a so-called "double-barrel" construct (27) (Figure 81-7). If the latter technique is used, one fibula segment contains the nutrient foramen vascular pedicle, and the second segment is only based on an intact periosteal sleeve mobilized for a sufficient distance to permit separation of the two parts for 2 to 3 cm. If the length of the defect exceeds that which would permit a "double-barrel" construct, then a single vascularized fibula segment may be used, supplemented by any of a variety of options (e.g., the contralateral fibula as either a nonvascularized graft as shown in Figure 81-1 or a free microvascular transfer or a structural allograft segment).

Two technical points are important to bear in mind for a fibular "turn-up" procedure. The first is that the axis of rotation for the fibula with an intact vascular pedicle is approximately 10 cm distal to the fibula head (Figure 81-8). Thus, a long segment of fibula with distal osteotomy just proximal to the distal tibiofibular syndesmosis is required to reach the level of the proximal defect. The second technical point is that the intact peroneal nerve and muscles of the peroneal and anterior tibial compartments are barriers to the fibular rotation. Thus, these structures must be extensively mobilized with the rotated fibula passing deep to them to permit bone-to-bone osteosynthesis of the rotated fibula to the femur proximally and the tibia distally. In some cases, the amount of required mobilization of the peroneal nerve and distal muscle groups may be so great that abandoning a pedicled "turn up" and instead proceeding with a free microvascular transfer may be the prudent course of action.

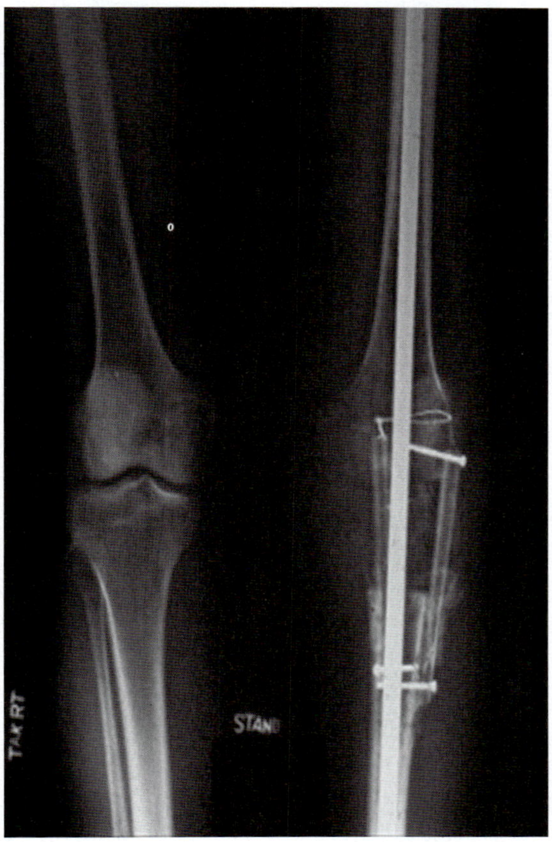

FIGURE 81-7 Radiograph of femorotibial arthrodesis with "double-barrel" vascularized fibula construct.

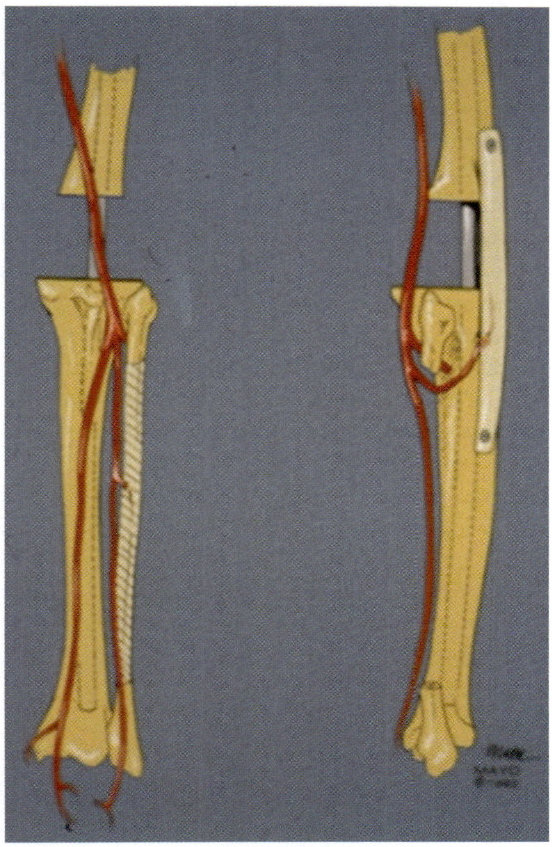

FIGURE 81-8 Schematic of fibula "turn-up" construct for femorotibial arthrodesis. (Used with permission of Mayo Foundation for Medical Education and Research, all rights reserved.)

Tibia

In most series, the tibia is the most frequent recipient site requiring a vascularized bone transfer for the management of a nonunion or long bone defect (28). The usual indication is for reconstruction of a diaphysial defect resulting from trauma, bone tumor resection, or congenital pseudarthrosis. Less often, an onlay vascularized bone graft may be indicated for a recalcitrant nonunion without a defect. In such cases, if the ipsilateral fibula is uninjured, it may be segmentally osteotomized, shifted medially a pedicled bone graft, and secured to the lateral surface of the ununited tibia across the nonunion site. Occasionally, the indication for tibial reconstruction by vascularized bone transfer will be a distal tibial defect with destruction of the tibiotalar articulation.

Tibial Diaphyseal Defects

For most tibial diaphyseal defects, the fibula is the preferred donor bone unless it is bilaterally absent or damaged. When the fibula is used, it should be positioned in line with the long axis of the tibia and dowelled into the proximal and distal tibia medullary canal, size permitting. It may be placed orthograde or retrograde depending on which position facilitates positioning of the vascular pedicle to the recipient vessels. For tibial defects resulting from open fractures, there is often an associated major soft tissue defect that will require consideration for a fibular osteocutaneous flap. Unless an existing soft tissue defect dictates otherwise, the tibial defect nonunion site is exposed by a medial incision. Either the anterior or posterior tibial vessels may be chosen as the recipient vessels, depending on the location of the bone defect and which vessels are most remote to the field of tissue injury. When the anterior tibial artery is selected as the recipient artery, end-to-end anastomosis is most often indicated, and the fibula is positioned orthograde. In contrast, when the posterior tibial artery is selected, end-to-side arterial anastomosis and retrograde fibula positioning is typically more appropriate, especially if the anterior tibial vessels are thought to be injured or deficient. The venous recipient vessels may be the accompanying anterior or posterior tibial venae comitans or the greater or lesser saphenous veins depending on availability. After fibula intramedullary positioning and revascularization, the proximal and distal osteosynthesis sites are fixed with either transosseous screws or short compression plates and screws (Figure 81-9). Usually, the use of a single rigid compression plate spanning the entire defect is not recommended because it may impede fibula hypertrophy after union by producing a stress shielding effect. When separate proximal and distal internal fixation is used, some means of external support by a cast or brace should be continued until there is clear evidence of both proximal and distal bony union and fibula hypertrophy (Figure 81-10).

Distal Tibia Defect with Articular Destruction

When the distal tibia articular surface is destroyed in association with a distal bone defect, reconstruction of the defect with tibiotalar or tibiotalocalcaneal arthrodesis is necessary (29). Depending on the length and geometry of the bony defect and the presence or absence of an associated soft tissue defect, either

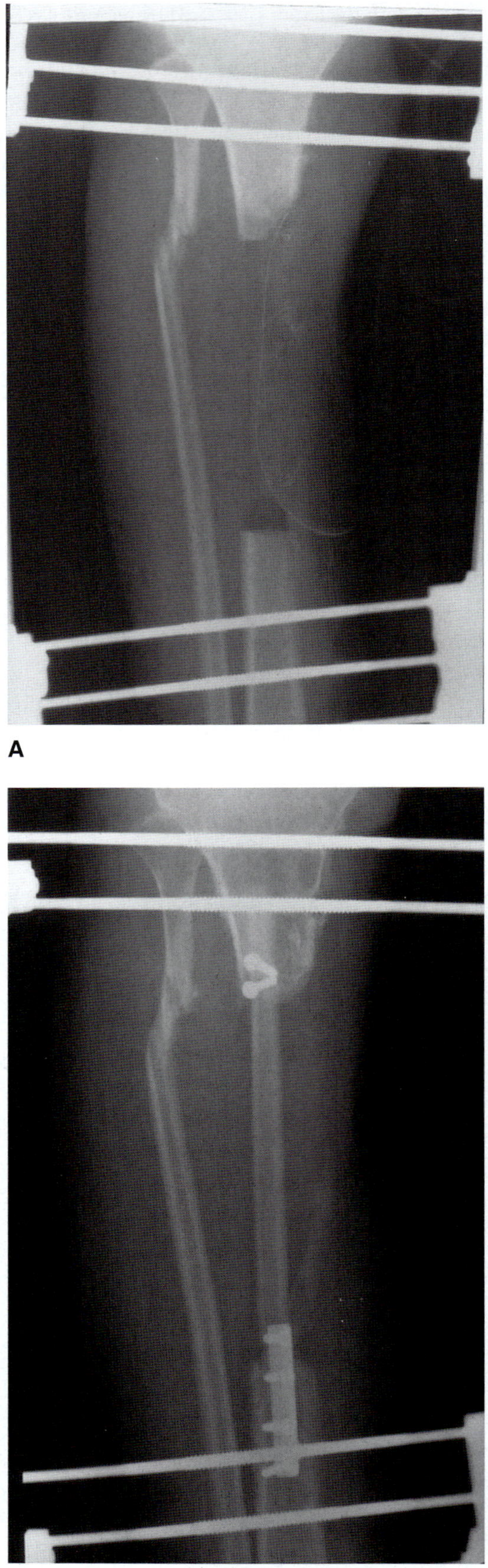

A

B

FIGURE 81-9 (A) Radiograph of tibial middiaphysis defect after resection of chronically infected sclerotic bone. (B) Radiograph immediately after vascularized fibula transfer. Note the intramedullary placement.

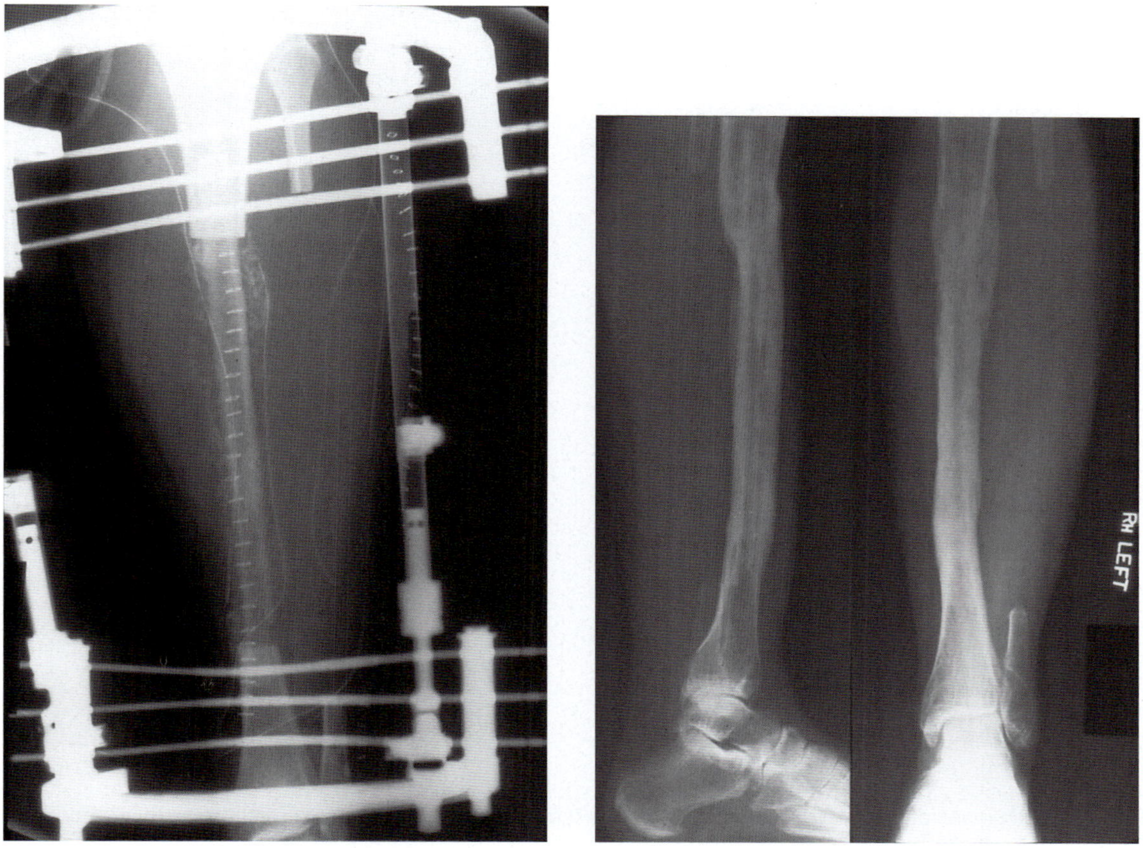

A B

FIGURE 81-10 (**A**) Radiograph of the tibia immediately after a vascularized fibula transfer after tumor resection. (**B**) Radiograph at 11 months after surgery. Note the fibula union and hypertrophy.

an osteocutaneous iliac crest (Figure 81-11) or fibular osteocutaneous flap may be used (Figure 81-12). In almost all instances, the posterior tibial vessels will be the preferred recipient vessels, exposed through a posteromedial incision. Often in the scenario of a distal tibial defect involving the ankle, the anterior tibial vessels will be deficient, and thus end-to-side arterial anastomosis to the posterior tibial artery should be planned. Bony fixation depends on the peculiarities of the bony defect and the selection of either fibula or iliac crest. This may involve plates, screws, Kirschner wires, cerclage wires, Steinmann pins, or external fixation. Subsequent postoperative management and progression to full weight bearing mirrors the suggestions outlined for the femur and tibial diaphyses in this chapter.

POSTOPERATIVE COMPLICATIONS

Donor site complications are discussed earlier in this chapter and in Chapter 18, but in addition to these, there are well-recognized postoperative complications with vascularized bone transfers to the lower extremity.

Nonunions

Nonunion of the vascularized bone segment after the index procedure is sufficiently frequent that all patients should be adequately forewarned. In an earlier study of the author's personal series (30) involving 160 patients with 1 year or more of follow-up, 39% of patients either demonstrated nonunion or inconclusive union at 6 months after surgery. After secondary intervention with revision of internal fixation or augmentation with cancellous autografting, the union with hypertrophy rate improved to 81%. Weiland et al. (31) reported a series of 123 patients undergoing vascularized bone transfers for a long bone defect with an initial nonunion or delayed union in 24% of patients, improving to an ultimate union and hypertrophy rate of 87% after secondary intervention. Gilbert (32) reported 58 pediatric patients undergoing vascularized fibula transfer for congenital pseudoarthrosis with an initial nonunion rate of 43%, improving to a 90% union rate after secondary surgery. In a review paper, Moran and Wood (33) combined the results of nine series of vascularized bone transfer for long bone reconstruction (including the three series mentioned earlier). Of 411 patients, there was a primary union rate of 66% and an overall union rate after a secondary procedure of 85%.

Stress Fracture

Stress fracture of the transferred bone segment is also relatively frequent with an incidence reported by De Boer et al. of 25% overall (34). This complication is especially related to using the fibula in the lower extremity (Figure 81-13). I believe that most authors think that the cause of stress fracture is usually a mismatch between the progression of weight bearing or other deforming forces and the progression of hypertrophy across the

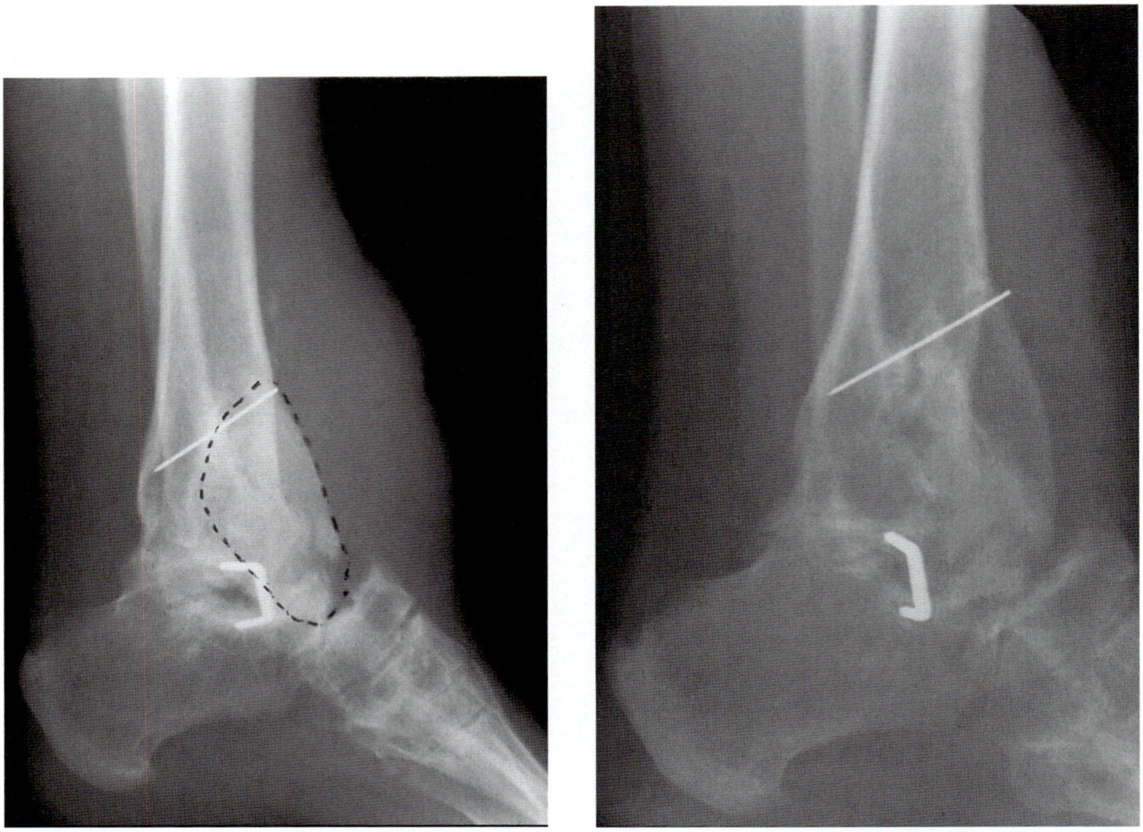

A B

FIGURE 81-11 (A) Radiograph of tibiotalar arthrodesis with iliac crest osteocutaneous compound flap transfer. The iliac bone segment is outlined for visual clarity. (B) Radiograph 8 months after surgery with bony union of tibiotalar arthrodesis.

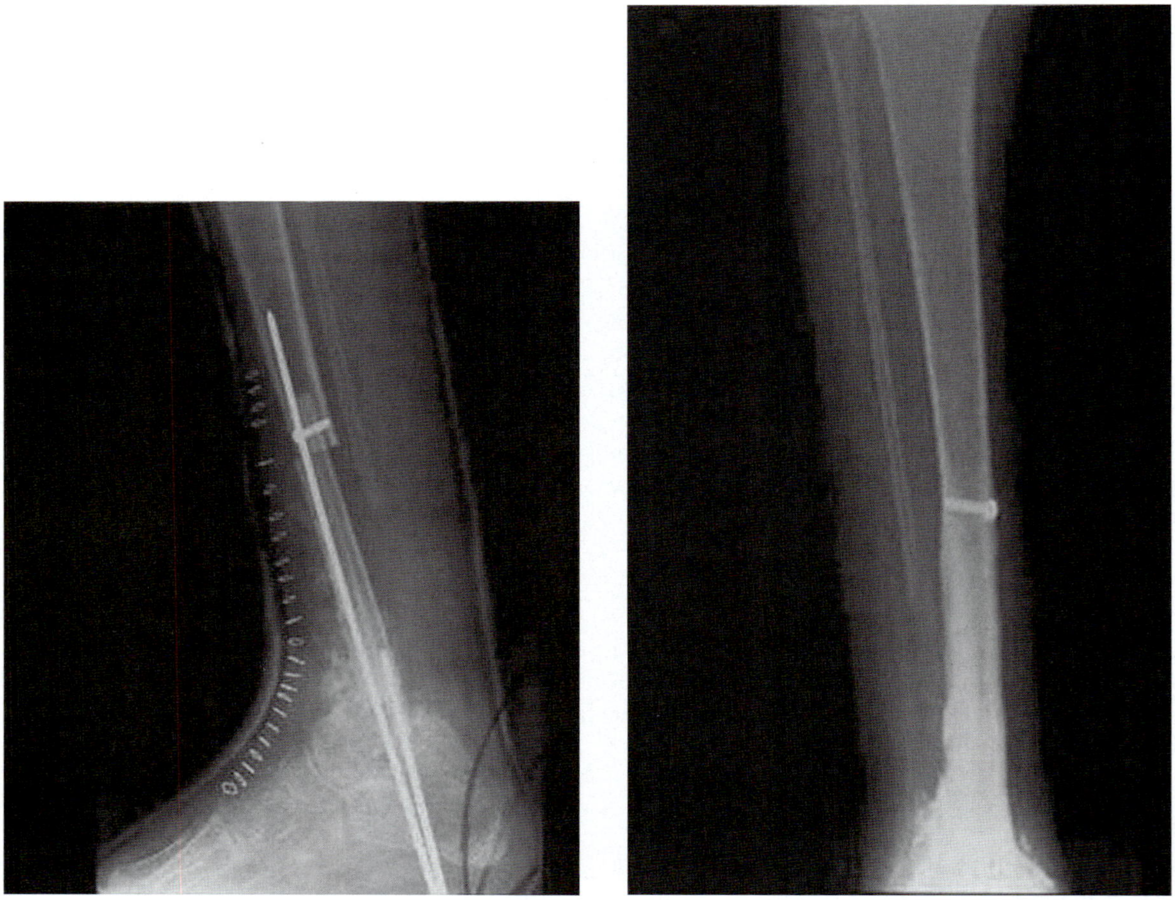

A B

FIGURE 81-12 (A) Radiograph of tibiotalar arthrodesis using vascularized fibula transfer. (B) Radiograph of healed tibiotalar arthrodesis and fibula hypertrophy 14 months after surgery.

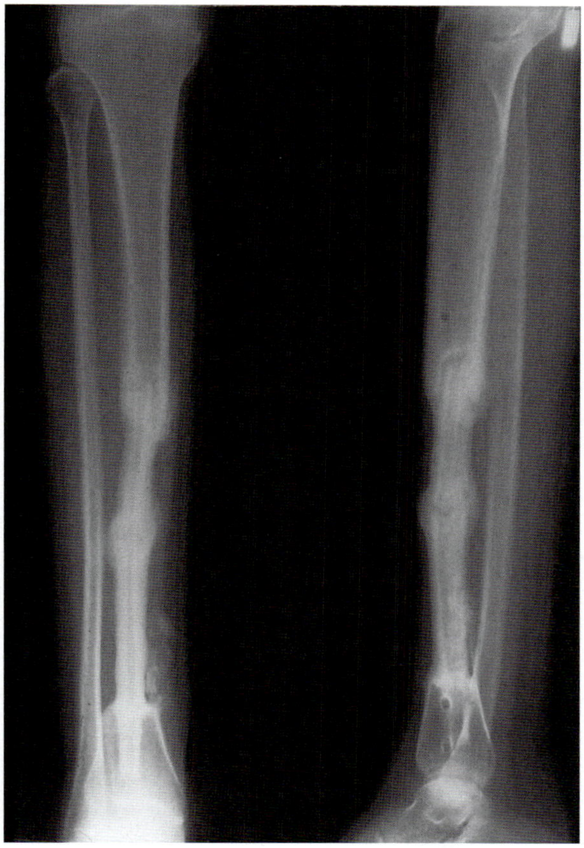

FIGURE 81-13 Radiograph of a healed vascularized fibula transfer to tibial defect. Note the healed fibula stress fracture in the midportion of the fibular segment with periosteal callus formation.

transferred fibula segment. It is most frequent within the first year after surgery and with established proximal and distal union or stable fixation. Many stress fractures of a vascularized fibula are asymptomatic and progress to spontaneous union provided displacement does not occur. It is likely that the incidence of stress fracture may be minimized by gradual progression of weight bearing and related stresses after union and prolonged external support by appropriate orthoses until clear radiographic evidence of hypertrophy of the fibula is apparent.

Deep Sepsis

The true incidence of deep sepsis after vascularized bone transfer to the lower extremity is difficult to analyze. In the author's series of 160 patients with 1 year or more of follow-up, as studied by Han et al. (30), postoperative deep sepsis occurred in 22 patients (13.75%), half of whom had preexisting chronic osteomyelitis. It is likely that the risk of deep infection is very much influenced by the fact that there is a large cohort of patients with preexisting chronic osteomyelitis in most larger clinical series studying the outcome of vascularized bone transfer.

CONCLUSIONS

Vascularized bone transfer has taken a prominent place in the armamentarium of procedures for salvage of the lower limb since its initial introduction as a clinical tool 35 years ago. Its use has in many instances allowed a return to ambulation and relatively normal function in a challenging patient population who were otherwise facing the prospect of major amputation. It remains, however, a highly specialized and complex procedure with a fairly high rate of complications. It is anticipated that continued refinement in patient selection and surgical technique will substantially improve patient outcomes in the future.

REFERENCES

1. Doi K, Tominaga S, Shibata T. Bone grafts with microvascular anastomosis of vascular pedicles: an experimental study in dogs. *J Bone Joint Surg Am* 1977;59(6):809–815.
2. Haw CS, O'Brien BM, Kurata T. The microsurgical revascularisation of resected segments of tibia in the dog. *J Bone Joint Surg Br* 1987; 60-B(2):266–269.
3. Shaffer JW, Field GA, Goldberg VM, Davy DT. Fate of vascularized and nonvascularize autografts. *Clin Orthop* 1985;197:32–43.
4. Siegert JJ, Wood MB. Blood flow evaluation of vascularized bone transfers in a canine model. *J Orthop Res* 1990;8:291–296.
5. Zdeblick TA, Shaffer JW, Field GA. The healing of canine vascularized segmental osteotomies: the effect of retained endosteal circulation. *Clin Orthop* 1988;236:296–302.
6. Arata MA, Wood MB, Cooney WP 3rd. Revascularized segmental diaphyseal bone transfers in the canine. An analysis of viability. *J Reconstr Microsurg* 1984;1:11–19.
7. Berggren A, Weiland AJ, Dorfman H. Free vascularized bone grafts: factors affecting their survival and ability to heal recipient bone defects. *Plast Reconstr Surg* 1982;69:19–29.
8. Van Meekeren J. Heel-En *Geneeskonstige Aanmerkingen*. Amsterdam: Commelyn, 1668.
9. De Boer H. Thesis. Leiden, 1988.
10. Curtis BF. Cases of bone implantation and transplantation for cyst of tibia, osteomyelitic cavities and ununited fractures. *Am J Med Sci* 1893;106:30.
11. Barth A. Ueber histologische befund nach knocken implantationen. *Arch Klin Chir* 1893;46:409.
12. Phemister DB. The fate of transplanted bone and regenerative powers of its various constituents. *Surg Gynecol Obstet* 1914;19:303–333.
13. Bieber EJ, Wood MB. Bone reconstruction. *Clin Plast Surg* 1986;13: 645–655.
14. Huntington TW. Case of bone transference. Use of a segment of fibula to supply a defect in the tibia. *Ann Surg* 1905;41:249.
15. Baadsgaard K, Medgyesi S. Muscle pedicle bone grafts. *Acta Orthop Scand* 1965;35:279–293.
16. Chacha PB. Vascularised pedicular bone grafts. *Int Orthop* 1984;8(2): 117–138.
17. Judet PR, Patel A. Muscle pedicle bone grafting of long bones by osteoperiosteal decortication. *Clin Orthop* 1972;87:74–80.
18. Ueba Y, Fujikawa S. Nine years follow up of a free vascularized fibular graft in neurofibromatosis—a case report and literature review. *Jpn J Orthop Trauma Surg* 1983;26:595–600.
19. Taylor GI, Miller GD, Ham FJ. The free vascularized bone graft. A clinical extension of microvascular techniques. *Plast Reconstr Surg* 1975;55(5):533–544.
20. Youdas JW, Wood MB, Cahalan TD, Chao EY. A quantitative analysis of donor site morbidity after vascularized fibula transfer. *J Orthop Res* 1988;6(5):621–629.
21. Strecker WB, Wood MB, Bieber EJ. Compartment syndrome masked by epidural anesthesia for postoperative pain. Report of a case. *J Bone Joint Surg Am* 1986;68(9):1447–1448.
22. Wood MB, Cooney, WP 3rd, Irons GB. Skeletal reconstruction by vascularized bone transfer: indications and results. *Mayo Clin Proc* 1985;60:729–734.
23. Taylor GI, Townsend P, Corlett R. Superiority of the deep circumflex iliac vessels as the supply for free groin flaps: clinical work. *Plast Reconstr Surg* 1979;64(6):745–759.
24. Buncke HJ, Furnas DW, Gordon L, Achauer BM. Free osteocutaneous flap from a rib to the tibia. *Plast Reconstr Surg* 1977;59(6):799–804.
25. Hertel R, Masquelet AC. The reverse flow medial knee osteoperiosteal flap for skeletal reconstruction of the leg. Description and anatomical basis. *Surg Radiol Anat* 1989;11(4):257–262.

CHAPTER 81

26. Wood MB. Femoral reconstruction by vascularized bone transfer. *Microsurgery* 1990;11(1):74–79.
27. Jones NF, Swartz WM, Mears DC, et al. The "double-barrel" free vascularized fibular bone graft. *Plast Reconstr Surg* 1988;81:378.
28. Wood MB. *Atlas of Reconstructive Microsurgery*. Rockville, MD: Aspen Publishers, 1990.
29. Wood, MB, Gilbert A. *Microvascular Bone Reconstruction*. London: Martin Dunitz, 1997.
30. Han CS, Wood MB, Bishop AT, Cooney WP 3rd. Vascularized bone transfer. *J Bone Joint Surg Am* 1992;74:1441–1449.
31. Weiland, AJ. Clinical applications of vascularized bone grafts. In Friedlaender GE, Goldberg VM (eds). *Bone and Cartilage Allografts*. Park Ridge, IL: American Academy of Orthopedic Surgeons, 1991, pp. 239–245.
32. Gilbert A. *Les transfer osseux libre vascularisees dans le treatment de la pseudarthrose congenitale*. Paris: SOFCOT, 1982, pp. 30–31.
33. Moran CG, Wood MB. Vascularized bone autografts. *Orthop Rev* 1993;22(2):187–197.
34. DeBoer HH, Wood MB. Bone changes in the vascularized fibular graft. *J Bone Joint Surg Br* 1989;71:374–378.

CHAPTER 82

Nerve Compression in the Lower Extremity

A. Lee Dellon

The lower extremity is a frequent site to be visited by reconstructive microsurgeons. As this book demonstrates, the lower extremity not only is an anatomic region that is injured frequently, thereby requiring reconstruction, but also is a source of reconstructive material to be used in the rest of the body. For example, the gracilis muscle is harvested to provide an innervated finger and wrist flexor after upper extremity burn, certain brachial plexus reconstructions, or Volkmann's ischemic contracture. The gracilis muscle is also harvested to correct certain facial palsies. The anterolateral thigh (ALT) flap is currently a frequent choice in microvascular free flap reconstructions. The vascularized fibular flap is the primary choice of mandibular reconstruction, for reconstruction of the ischemic femoral head, and for significant bone defects in both the upper and lower extremity. Toes are routinely transferred by microsurgical technique to the hand. The sural nerve is the choice when a large length of nerve is needed for autogenous grafting. Local muscle flaps in the lower extremity are the choice for reconstruction of many regional soft tissue deformities. In each of these procedures, the adjacent peripheral nerve is both at risk for direct injury or at risk for chronic compression during closure of the flap harvest site. Table 82-1 relates the chronic nerve compression syndrome with reconstructive flap donor sites.

Lower extremity nerve compression is common, although largely it has been underappreciated. Compression of the common peroneal nerve is most common followed by compression of the tibial nerve and its branches in the four medial ankle tunnels followed by compression of the deep peroneal nerve over the dorsum of the foot, the superficial peroneal nerve the leg, the lateral femoral cutaneous nerve (LFCN) in the proximal thigh, the saphenous nerve in the adductor canal, and finally the femoral nerve beneath the inguinal ligament. In this chapter, the anatomical variations critical for understanding the entrapment and its surgical approach, the clinical presentation of the nerve entrapment syndrome, and the diagnosis and treatment of these nerve compressions will be described and illustrated so that patients with these problems can be identified and receive appropriate care. Knowledge of these entrapment sites will help reconstructive microsurgeons avoid creating these entrapments as flaps are harvested and to recognize them as complications if they do occur in a patient having a complex reconstruction.

HISTORICAL CONSIDERATIONS AND TERMINOLOGY

With the exception of harvesting the sural nerve from the leg to use as a graft for various upper extremity nerve reconstructions or for cross-facial nerve grafting, the peripheral nerve component of the lower extremity has been largely ignored. To be sure, orthopedic and podiatric foot and ankle surgery textbooks have an obligatory chapter on the tarsal tunnel syndrome and Morton's neuroma but relatively little else. It was into this abyss of knowledge about lower extremity peripheral nerve surgery that the book *Surgery of the Peripheral Nerve* by Susan E. Mackinnon and A. Lee Dellon in 1988 attempted to apply principles established for upper extremity peripheral nerve surgery to the lower extremity (1). In *Surgery of the Peripheral Nerve*, Chapter 12 described the problems related to the tibial nerve at the level of the ankle, and Chapter 13 described the problems related to the peroneal nerve at the knee, leg, and foot level, as well as the problems with the sural nerve and the interdigital nerve. *Surgery of the Peripheral Nerve* described the pathophysiology of chronic nerve compression and set forth the approach to diagnosis, clinical staging, and the surgical approach to these problems. Over the past 2 decades, much more has been learned about lower extremity peripheral nerve problems, and it is the purpose of this chapter to introduce the evidence base now available to improve patient care related to lower extremity nerve compression. In this chapter, *chronic nerve compression* will be the name given to symptoms related to entrapment of a peripheral nerve and *neuropathy* will be the name given to systemic disease that affects bilateral lower

TABLE 82-1 Nerve Most Likely Compressed by Reconstructive Procedure

Surgical Procedure	Chronic Nerve Compression
Iliac crest harvesting	Lateral femoral cutaneous nerve
Anterolateral thigh free flap harvesting	Lateral femoral cutaneous nerve or saphenous nerve in the adductor canal
Gracilis muscle harvesting	Obturator nerve or saphenous nerve in the adductor canal
Rectus femoris muscle flap rotation	Saphenous nerve in the adductor canal
Lateral gastrocnemius muscle flap rotation	Common peroneal nerve
Medial gastrocnemius muscle flap rotation	Infrapatellar branch of the saphenous nerve
Fibular free flap	Common peroneal nerve or superficial peroneal nerve
Soleus muscle flap rotation	Proximal tibial nerve at soleal sling
Medial plantar flap rotation	Tibial nerve in tarsal tunnel
Dorsalis pedis free flap	Deep peroneal nerve
Toe transfer	Deep peroneal nerve or interdigital plantar nerve

extremity nerves. The symptoms of multiple peripheral nerve compressions can be the same as those of a neuropathy, that is, compression of the tibial and peroneal nerves can be a "stocking" distribution of symptoms similar to a neuropathy, but a neuropathy implies there is a systemic underlying problem causing neurologic symptoms, such as diabetes, hypothyroidism, or chemotherapeutic toxicity.

Throughout this chapter, peripheral nerve surgery will be understood to require the use of at least 3.5× loupe magnification and a bipolar coagulator. The tourniquet is frequently used for the difficult dissections, but the presence of a previous arterial or venous reconstruction, the past history of venous occlusion, the use of anticoagulation, the presence of venous hypertension, and concern over limb ischemia are valid reasons *not* to use a tourniquet.

The history of peripheral nerve surgery, written according to the various controversies that marked the development of critical ideas in peripheral nerve surgery is available in a chapter on the history of peripheral nerve surgery in *Neurologic Surgery* published in 2004 (2).

PATHOPHYSIOLOGY OF CHRONIC NERVE COMPRESSION

The pathophysiology of chronic nerve compression implies that the evaluation of nerve function must be based on the knowledge that there will be a progressive loss of peripheral nerve function. Therefore, diagnosis and treatment of chronic nerve compression is based on an understanding of this pathophysiology. The structure and function of the peripheral nerve and how these are altered with increasing degrees of pressure and with increasing lengths of time have been investigated in rat, rabbit, and monkey animal models (3–12), and many of these models have used the sciatic nerve. The disease process is the same for upper extremity nerve compressions as it is for lower extremity peripheral nerve compressions.

A review of this literature indicates that if there is a constriction of greater than 20% placed on the diameter of the peripheral nerve, then acute axonal degeneration will occur. If there is a pressure of greater than 20 mm Hg applied to the peripheral nerve, there will be a decrease in blood flow. In the acute situation, these situations produce pain. If this degree of compression comes on over a gradual period of time and over a length of the peripheral nerve that is several times the diameter of the nerve, then the conditions produce chronic nerve compression. After about 2 months of compression by a silicon tube that does not constrict the diameter of the nerve, the first changes in the pathophysiology occur. These are a weakening the tight junctions of the endothelial cells in the perineurium, and this results in serum entering the endoneurial space. This creates endoneurial edema. When this occurs in the relatively tight confines of the perineurium, there is an increase in pressure that will decrease blood flow. The conscious perception of this is paresthesia. At this point in time, the only clinical findings will be related to the cutaneous sensory threshold for touch, which will first become elevated for static two-point discrimination using the Pressure-Specified Sensory Device (PSSD) (13), or will manifest itself as a change in perception of vibratory stimuli applied with a tuning fork or a vibrometer (14,15). These pathophysiologic concepts provide a basis for staging chronic nerve compression (Tables 82-2 to 82-4) (16).

After about 6 months of this degree of compression, the first histologic changes in myelin can be observed. This consists of thinning of the myelin. With progressive compression, there will be increasing loss of myelin, so that under slides in which a myelin stain has been used, it appears as if there has been a loss of the large myelinated, touch fibers. They will not actually have begun to degenerate yet, as demonstrated by electron microscopy, in which the unmyelinated large fibers can be demonstrated to still be present. At this stage, the patient will have weakness in the motor system related to the muscles supplied by that nerve and increasing numbness in the territory related

TABLE 82-2 Numerical Grading Scale for Any Peripheral Nerve (16)

Grade	Description
0	Normal
1	Intermittent sensory symptoms
2	Increased sensorimotor threshold
3	Increased sensorimotor threshold
4	Increased sensorimotor threshold
5	Persistent sensory symptoms
6	Sensorimotor degeneration
7	Sensorimotor degeneration
8	Sensorimotor degeneration
9	Anesthesia
10	Muscle atrophy, severe

TABLE 82-3 Numerical Grading Scale for the Median Nerve at The Wrist Level (16))

Numerical Score		Description of Impairment
Sensory	Motor	
0	0	None
1		Paresthesia, intermittent
2		Abnormal pressure threshold (PSSD): <45 yr old: ≤3 mm at 1.0–20 g/mm^2 ≥45 yr old; ≤4 mm at 2.2–20 g/mm^2
	3	Weakness, thenar muscles
4		Abnormal pressure threshold (PSSD): <45 yr old; ≤3 mm at >20.0 g/mm^2 ≥45 yr old; ≤4 mm at >20.0 g/mm^2
5		Paresthesias, persistent
6		Abnormal innervation density (PSSD): <45 yr old; ≥4 mm <8 mm at any g/mm^2 ≥45 yr old; ≥5 mm <9 mm at any g/mm^2
	7	Muscle wasting (1–2/4)
8		Abnormal innervation density (PSSD): <45 yr old; ≥8 mm at any g/mm^2 ≥45 yr old; ≥9 mm at any g/mm^2
9		Anesthesia
	10	Muscle wasting (3–4/4)

PSSD, Pressure-Specified Sensory Device.

TABLE 82-4 Numerical Grading Scale for the Tibial Nerve at The Ankle Level (23)

Numerical Score		Description of Impairment
Sensory	Motor	
0	0	None
1		Paresthesia, intermittent
2		Abnormal pressure threshold (PSSD): <45 yr old: ≤5.6 mm at 1.0–20 g/mm^2 ≥45 yr old; ≤7.8 mm at 2.2–20 g/mm^2
	3	Weakness, abductor hallucis
4		Abnormal pressure threshold (PSSD): <45 yr old; ≤5.6 mm at > 20.0 g/mm^2 ≥45 yr old; ≤7.8 mm at > 20.0 g/mm^2
5		Paresthesias, persistent
6		Abnormal innervation density (PSSD): <45 yr old; ≥7 mm <10 mm at any g/mm^2 ≥45 yr old; ≥9 mm <12 mm at any g/mm^2
	7	Intrinsic muscle wasting, clawing (1–2/4)
8		Abnormal innervation density (PSSD): <45 yr old; ≥11 mm at any g/mm^2 ≥45 yr old; ≥ 15 mm at any g/mm^2
9		Anesthesia
	10	Intrinsic muscle wasting, clawing (3–4/4)

PSSD, Pressure-Specified Sensory Device.

to the sensory supply of that nerve. Manual muscle strength testing can be done and grading according to the British Medical System developed in World War II, with 0 being no function, 3 being able to contract against gravity, and 5 being normal strength. There will be no atrophy because without true loss of the motor axons, there will be no decrease in bulk of the muscles. At this stage of compression, the cutaneous pressure thresholds will be elevated increasingly for the quickly adapting fibers, measured either with vibrometry or with moving two-point discrimination with the PSSD, and for the slowly adapting fibers, measured with static two-point discrimination with the PSSD. Although no longitudinal study using the Semmes-Weinstein nylon monofilaments has been published in patients with chronic nerve compression (17), the analogous measurement, made with the PSSD, which is one-point static touch, is still normal at this stage of compression (13,17). Two-point discrimination, measured in millimeters, is still normal because no nerve fibers have died. At this stage in chronic nerve compression, with myelin thinning, traditional electrodiagnostic testing may begin to detect increases in the distal sensory latency. Amplitudes will still be normal because no nerve fibers have died yet. In general, neurosensory or quantitative sensory testing is more sensitive than traditional electrodiagnostic testing (nerve conduction study [NCS] or electromyography [EMG]), so it is more likely to detect this stage of nerve compression (18–21). Neurosensory testing is less expensive than NCS or EMG and does not cause the patient any pain (22).

If either the length of time is increased for this degree of compression or the degree of compression increases because of work, metabolic, or rheumatologic disease, then neural degeneration occurs. As suggested in the preceding paragraph, this will be detected in the motor system by muscle wasting and in the sensory system by abnormal distance at which one from two points can be distinguished. Examples of these changes are given in Table 82-2 for the median nerve compression at the wrist, Table 82-3 for ulnar nerve compression at the elbow, and Table 82-4 for tibial nerve compression in the tarsal tunnel (23). Using the PSSD, this change occurs first for static two-point discrimination and then for moving two-point discrimination. This was demonstrated in a retrospective analysis of patients with carpal and cubital tunnel syndrome (24). The one-point static touch measurement will become abnormal some time after the change in two-point discrimination distance and is therefore a relatively insensitive tool for detecting the onset of this stage. Vibrometry and tuning fork use can identify this stage but does not permit the therapist to identify correctly which nerve is being compressed without additional testing. It must be remembered whereas the vibratory stimulus travels as a wave, the pressure stimulus remains localized to the applied test site. For example, if the involved nerve is the tibial nerve, to the toe pulp, and the hallux pulp is tested, there may still be relatively preserved sensation mediated by the peroneal nerve to the dorsum of the hallux. Testing of both the dorsum of the foot and hallux pulp and medial heel may permit distinction of which nerve is involved.

If there is some limitation on the gliding of the peripheral nerve through its site of anatomic narrowing, then when the adjacent joint moves, there will an increase in tension along the length of the nerve, which may manifest itself as a further increase in pressure on the nerve. This limitation of gliding may come from some injury or anatomic variant that limits excursion of the nerves. This subject will be discussed in detail related to individual nerve compression syndromes.

Statistical evaluation of the results of the treatment of nerve compression has been difficult because of the failure of most reports to distinguish the degree of nerve compression among the patients in the study. In the typical retrospective review, a level IV study, an entire group of patients with nerve compression are usually described after surgery as having results that are excellent, good, fair, or poor. In comparing one published study with another, it would be helpful to be able to know the degree of severity of nerve compression in the patients being reported. It would be useful in a given study to know how patients with different degrees of nerve compression responded to the same operation. Even if this is recognized as a goal, without a numerical grading system, the author is left only with the choice of indicating what percentage of people who had a mild degree of nerve compression improved and what percentage of patients with a severe degree of nerve compression improved. With a numerical grading system, as outlined, a unique number, representing the pathophysiologic condition of the compressed nerve as manifested by its functional impairment can be assigned to each patient, and these numbers can be treated statistically. Finally, treatment strategies and outcome analysis for the peripheral nerve can be based analyzed mathematically. When this is done, it should be remembered to use nonparametric statistics.

SYMPTOMS AND PHYSICAL FINDINGS

A patient with chronic compression of a peripheral nerve will complain of numbness or paresthesias in the skin territory innervated by that nerve. The patient will complain of weakness in the muscles innervated by that nerve. If both the peroneal and tibial nerves have chronic compression at the same time, the patient will have numbness over the dorsal and plantar aspects of the foot and arising proximal to the ankle. This will give the same appearance as if the patient had a peripheral neuropathy, especially if the problem occurs in both legs. This type of situation occurs in patients who have sports or other injuries. As a contrast in etiology, but with the same clinical presentation, are patients who do have a metabolic neuropathy such as diabetes or induced by chemotherapy who have secondary chronic nerve compressions. These patients present with a history of neuropathy without anyone having examined them to identify the presence of a chronic nerve compression (24). A further critical point in history is to distinguish pain that radiates from the back into the feet. This is usually caused by a nerve root compression, a radiculopathy. If these symptoms are present, it is critical to obtain an electrodiagnostic evaluation to identify whether a lumbosacral disc problem is present. Of course, a nerve root compression and a lower extremity nerve compression can be present in the same person.

The pathognomonic feature of chronic nerve compression on physical examination is the presence of a positive Hoffman-Tinel sign. With an understanding of the pathophysiology of chronic nerve compression (see earlier discussion), it becomes clear that in the earliest stage, there will be intermittent symptoms but no physical findings present. This is the situation often with musicians, such as a piano or violinist who complains of numbness in the little finger from playing with the elbow bent but has no Hoffman-Tinel sign over the ulnar nerve at the cubital tunnel. In the lower extremity, an analogous situation occurs with a soccer player whose leg may seem to give out, who has received many a blunt trauma to the outside of the knee or repeated ankle inversion sprains and who has compression of the common peroneal nerve at the fibular neck. With further time and greater degree of compression, axons will demyelinate, and there will be an increase in the threshold required to produce a sensory response—a higher degree of vibration with the tuning fork or a greater pressure required to discriminate one from two points touching the big toe pulp with the PSSD while two-point discrimination distance remains normal. In the motor system, this will correspond to weakness on manual muscle testing. At this point, the Hoffman-Tinel sign will become positive. With further time and degree of compression, axons will die, and there will be decrease in two-point static touch discrimination (the distance before two points can be distinguished will increase), and muscle atrophy will occur. The Hoffman-Tinel sign will remain positive. With a very advanced degree of compression, the peripheral nerve seems to stop its attempt to remyelinate and regenerate, and the Hoffman-Tinel sign becomes negative. This variation in the presence of the Hoffman-Tinel sign over time is understandable in terms of progression of compression and changes within the peripheral nerve and should not be interpreted as a failure of the Hoffman-Tinel sign to be a valuable clinical examination technique (25,26). A nerve root compression, a radiculopathy, does not cause a Hoffman-Tinel sign to be present over a peripheral nerve. The presence of a positive Hofmann-Tinel sign over a peripheral nerve in the patient with a nerve root compression has *both* a chronic nerve compression in the lower extremity *and* a nerve root compression.

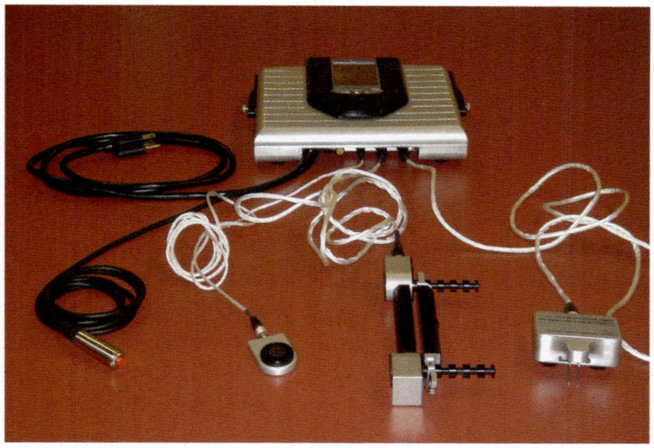

FIGURE 82-1 The Pressure-Specified Sensory Device is shown with its components for grip and pinch strength, as well as the device with the two prongs, each of which is attached to a pressure transducer (silver attachment with prongs). The configuration shown is the personal digital assistant (PDA) platform, which is portable among offices. No needle stick or electrical stimulation is used. After the patient perceives the stimulus correctly, a button is pushed by the patient, ending digital signal acquisition; therefore, this is a subjective test of sensibility. (With permission from Sensory Management Services, LLC, Towson, MD.)

PATIENT SELECTION AND DOCUMENTATION

Selection of the patient for surgical decompression of a peripheral nerve requires that at least four conditions are met: (1) the patient's symptoms fit with both the motor and sensory distribution of the given peripheral nerve, (2) the impairment is documented by appropriate measurement of the motor and sensory function of that nerve, (3) there is a positive Hoffmann-Tinel sign at the known site of anatomic narrowing of that nerve, and (4) all possible nonoperative measures have been used for 3 months without success in relieving the symptoms.

Note that *it is not essential that an electrodiagnostic test be performed and it is not essential that the results of that test demonstrate chronic nerve compression* (19–21). This is because even where traditional nerve conduction and EMG are the best, for the median nerve at the wrist, the false-negative rate is 33%, and in the patients with diabetes, this type of testing cannot be relied on to identify the presence of a chronic nerve compression in the presence of an underlying neuropathy (27). In the lower extremity, in a patient older than 55 years of age, the false-positive rate for the medial plantar and EMG of the medial plantar innervated muscles is 50%; therefore, in an adult even without neuropathy, this testing is prone to error. Because traditional testing cannot identify nerve compression in the presence of neuropathy at the wrist, it certainly cannot identify it reliably at the ankle. Therefore, the *clinician must rely on the presence of a positive Hoffman-Tinel sign to indicate the location of the chronic nerve compression.*

Electrodiagnostic testing cannot evaluate calcaneal nerve function or distal deep peroneal nerve function because these nerves are distal to muscle, so EMG cannot be used, and the length of the sensory nerve is too short for latency measurements from a known point of stimulation.

Neurosensory testing with the PSSD is the most sensitive method to document sensibility in a piece of skin (Figure 82-1). This has been documented to be valid and reliable for both the upper and lower extremity (13,18,19,22) and is essentially equivalent to the information obtained with traditional electrodiagnostic studies for the median nerve at the wrist in a level I study (21). For a patient with heel pain, for example, the medial calcaneal nerve will have abnormal pressure threshold with normal distance for distinguishing one-point from two-point static touch, with normal measurements for the medial plantar (hallux pulp) and normal measurements over the dorsum of the foot. When treatment for plantar fasciitis continues to fail after 3 months and when the two-point static distance becomes abnormal, then it is appropriate to do a neurolysis of the calcaneal nerve (28). If the measurements for the hallux pulp are also abnormal, then tarsal tunnel syndrome is present. If the measurements for the dorsum of the foot are abnormal in addition to those for the tibial nerve, then the peroneal nerve is involved, too.

NEUROLYSIS TECHNIQUE

Decompression of a peripheral nerve implies that a neurolysis is being done. The most simple form of this technically is dividing a ligament crossing and compressing the nerve. The separation of the peripheral nerve from its scarred bed is an external neurolysis. If the fascicular pattern of the nerve can be seen through the epineurium with loupes, and the nerve is soft, no further surgical intervention may be needed. If the fascicles cannot be discerned or the nerve feels firm, then there may be intraneural fibrosis. Intraneural neurolysis is the microsurgical dissection requiring opening the epineurium and dissecting within the intrafascicular epineurium to separate the fascicles. The perineurium is not opened. Intraneural dissection along the microsurgical anatomic plane of the interfascicular epineurium does not cause increased scar tissue to form (29–31).

A study has not been done to demonstrate the efficacy of doing an internal neurolysis of a lower extremity peripheral nerve. Nevertheless, if intraneural fibrosis is identified during a nerve decompression, my personal preference is to open the epineurium and continue the intraneural neurolysis until I can see a good fascicular pattern. This is often quite necessary when doing a neurolysis on a recurrent nerve entrapment. In the presence of an underlying neuropathy, such as diabetes, there is one experimental study that demonstrated improved peripheral nerve function after intraneural dissection by the rat walking track analysis (32).

INDIVIDUAL LOWER EXTREMITY PERIPHERAL NERVES

The clinical and operative aspects of the different lower extremity nerve compressions will be discussed from proximal to distal.

Lateral Femoral Cutaneous Nerve

Entrapment of the LFCN was well known to earlier physicians as *meralgia paresthetica*. When women wore girdles, family practice physicians knew that symptoms of burning and numbness from the hip to the knee in the front and lateral thigh were due to this problem. Today these symptoms are often mistaken for an L3 lumbar disc, but there are no motor symptoms and the pattern is clearly that of a peripheral nerve and not that of a dermatome (Figure 82-2). Although the anatomy books consistently portray this nerve as exiting the pelvis *beneath* the ilioinguinal ligament, surgical exploration demonstrated that patients with symptoms had the nerve most often located *within* the inguinal ligament and adjacent to the iliac crest. An anatomy study demonstrated that in 4% of specimens, this nerve can cross over the anterior superior iliac crest, and in about 40% of specimens, it was actually within the ligament (33). Clearly if a person is born with that anatomy, then he or she is at risk for chronic nerve compression after motor vehicle injury with a seat belt, a tool belt or gun holster at work, an inguinal hernia repair, or rotation of flaps in this area. With the sensory territory extending to the knee, some patients may present with the complaint of knee pain.

Patients with this problem can often be identified by the way they sit, with the leg on the affected side extended (Figure 82-3). The physical examination will have a positive Hoffmann-Tinel sign just medial and inferior to the anterior superior iliac crest. If not a true distal radiation, then there will pain elicited with pressure in this location.

This nerve is clearly innervates the territory of the ALT flap and can be used to create an innervated thigh flap. This skin territory can be overlapped medially by an anterior femoral cutaneous branch of the femoral nerve, so to be sure which nerve is being incorporated into the flap, planning can include a preoperative nerve block.

Figure 82-4 demonstrates the surgical technique. A 3-cm incision is made just superior and medial to the anterior superior iliac crest. This is deepened to the external oblique and retracted downward to the inguinal ligament. Very small divisions are made in the inguinal ligament adjacent to the bone. The nerve will appear as yellowish in color, equivalent to adjacent fat. The nerve will be inflamed. There are adjacent small veins. Be careful not to cauterize the nerve or the patient will have postoperative burning in that fascicle, and this may not resolve. After the nerve

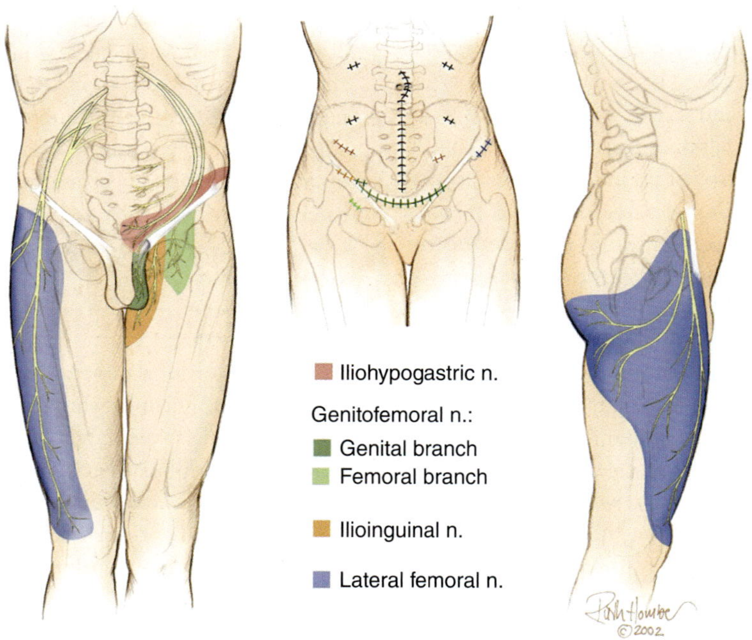

FIGURE 82-2 Illustration of the cutaneous distribution of the lateral femoral cutaneous nerve. The blue pattern from the hip to the knee is *not* in a dermatomal pattern but that of a cutaneous nerve. With the distal area extending to the knee, the patient may present with symptoms of knee pain. n, nerve.

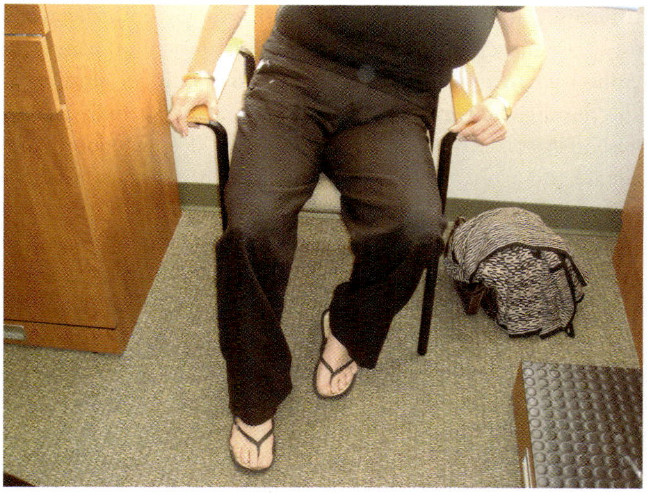

FIGURE 82-3 The patient with compression of the lateral femoral cutaneous nerve will sit with the leg extended on the affected side, attempting to decompress or reduce pressure on this nerve.

has been identified, a neurolysis into the thigh is done. There will be a posterior-lateral fascicle going to the lateral thigh. Then elevate the nerve and divide the ligament deep to it until the iliopsoas muscle is reached. Then follow the nerve proximally into the pelvis, dividing the constricting internal oblique fascia. Stop the dissection when the nerve is free or when the circumflex iliac vessels are encountered. The nerve will be found to be white proximal and distal to the entrapment site.

If the LFCN has crossed the bone, had a lateral neuroma formed against the bone, was injured during the dissection, or appears too badly compressed to save without the patient having burning pain postoperatively, then the nerve should be resected to allow the proximal end to drop into the pelvis (see Figure 82-4). The patient must be counseled about this possibility before surgery. If a neurolysis is done and by 6 months after surgery there is severe burning in the thigh, the nerve can be resected at that point in time after a nerve block demonstrates relief of pain and if the patient is willing to have that area of numbness.

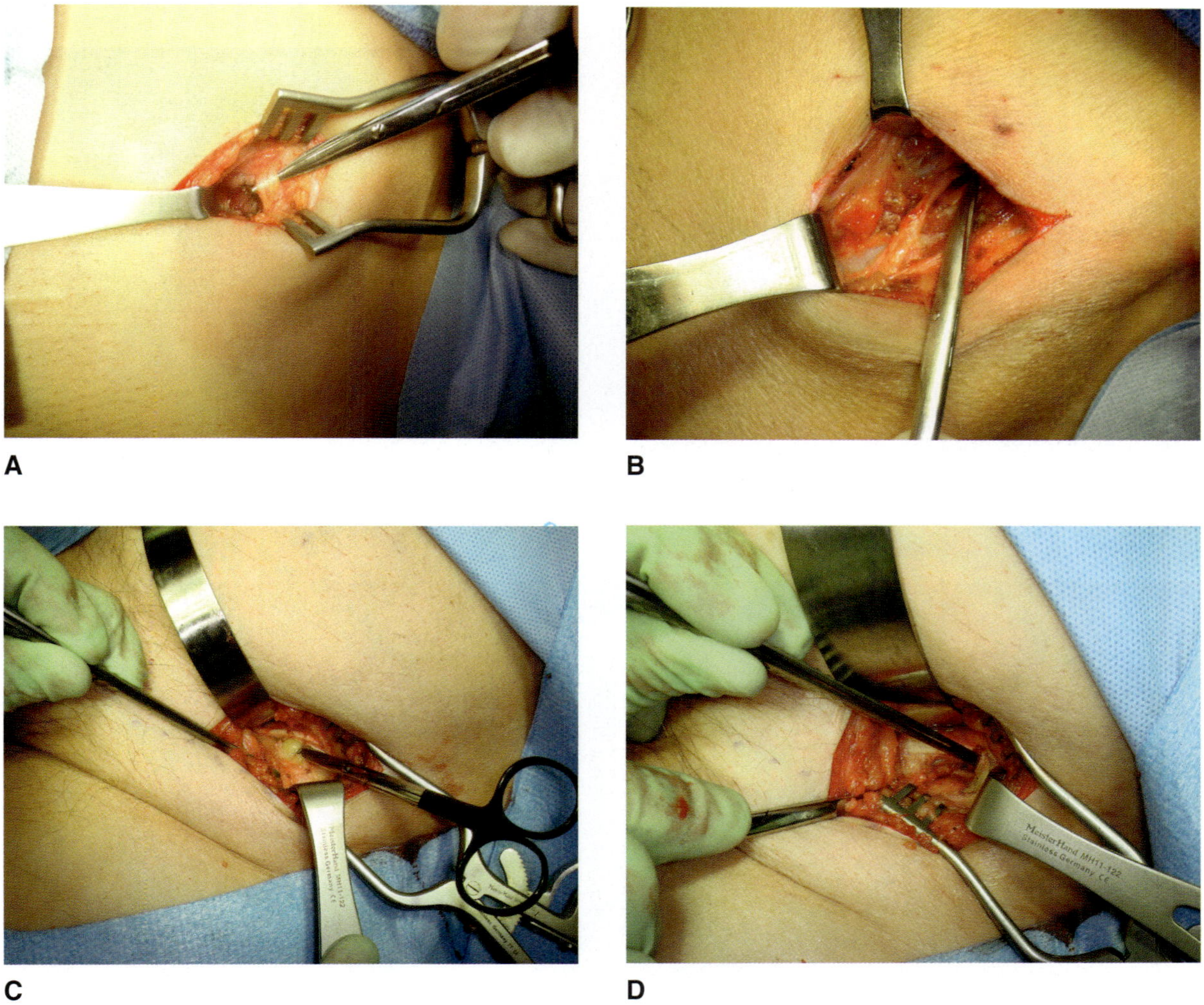

FIGURE 82-4 Intraoperative views of neurolysis of the lateral femoral cutaneous nerve. (**A**) The lateral femoral nerve is seen compressed within the inguinal ligament. (**B**) In this nerve after neurolysis, the color of the nerve can be identified as normal within the pelvis, then yellowish-reddish in the area of compression with a physical indentation in the nerve, and then becoming more normal as it proceeds into the thigh. (**C**) This nerve is yellowish in color, appearing as fat, and after neurolysis (**D**) is so severely damaged that it was resected. Compare the appearance of this nerve with the one in **B**.

The largest reported study is from the year 2000, reporting 58 decompressions in patients with groin pain. The success rate was 80% excellent and good results. In the two patients who failed to get better, each had a large panniculus. Final excellent pain relief required a panniculectomy and resection of the nerves bilaterally (34). A subsequent study demonstrated similar results (35).

Femoral Nerve Beneath Inguinal Ligament

Entrapment of the femoral nerve beneath the inguinal ligament is unusual and can be seen in the setting of regional anesthesia in patients having knee surgery (36). There will be loss of quadriceps function with either inability or weakness of knee extension. There can be muscle wasting. The EMG findings are almost always positive. There can be complaints of sensory symptoms extending down to the medial ankle and to the infrapatellar skin of the knee. The femoral nerve will be tender to palpation and may have a distally radiating sign.

The surgical approach is given in Figure 82-5. Neurolysis requires an S-shaped incision crossing the inguinal ligament with preoperative marking of the femoral pulse. Intraoperative electrical stimulation is essential, and the anesthesiologist must be aware not to use muscle relaxants. After incising the skin, the anterior femoral cutaneous nerves in the region should be protected. The femoral branch of the genitofemoral nerve may also be present in this exposure. Dissecting more deeply, continue to palpate and avoid the femoral artery, which is medial to where the nerve is located. The femoral sheath should be opened and the femoral nerve identified. Going proximally, the inguinal ligament should be divided. Usually you will find multiple fascicles, some with brownish discoloration of a nerve block caused by a hematoma. Actual nerve fascicles may be injured, and the patient should be made aware ahead of time that if a critical motor fascicle is damaged that it may need reconstruction, either with an autogenous graft from the saphenous nerve or with a nerve conduit. A gentle intraneural dissection of all the fascicles is required. The inguinal ligament is not repaired.

Saphenous Nerve in the Adductor Canal

The adductor canal is the seemingly simple anatomic construct in which a fascial band connects the vastus medialis to the

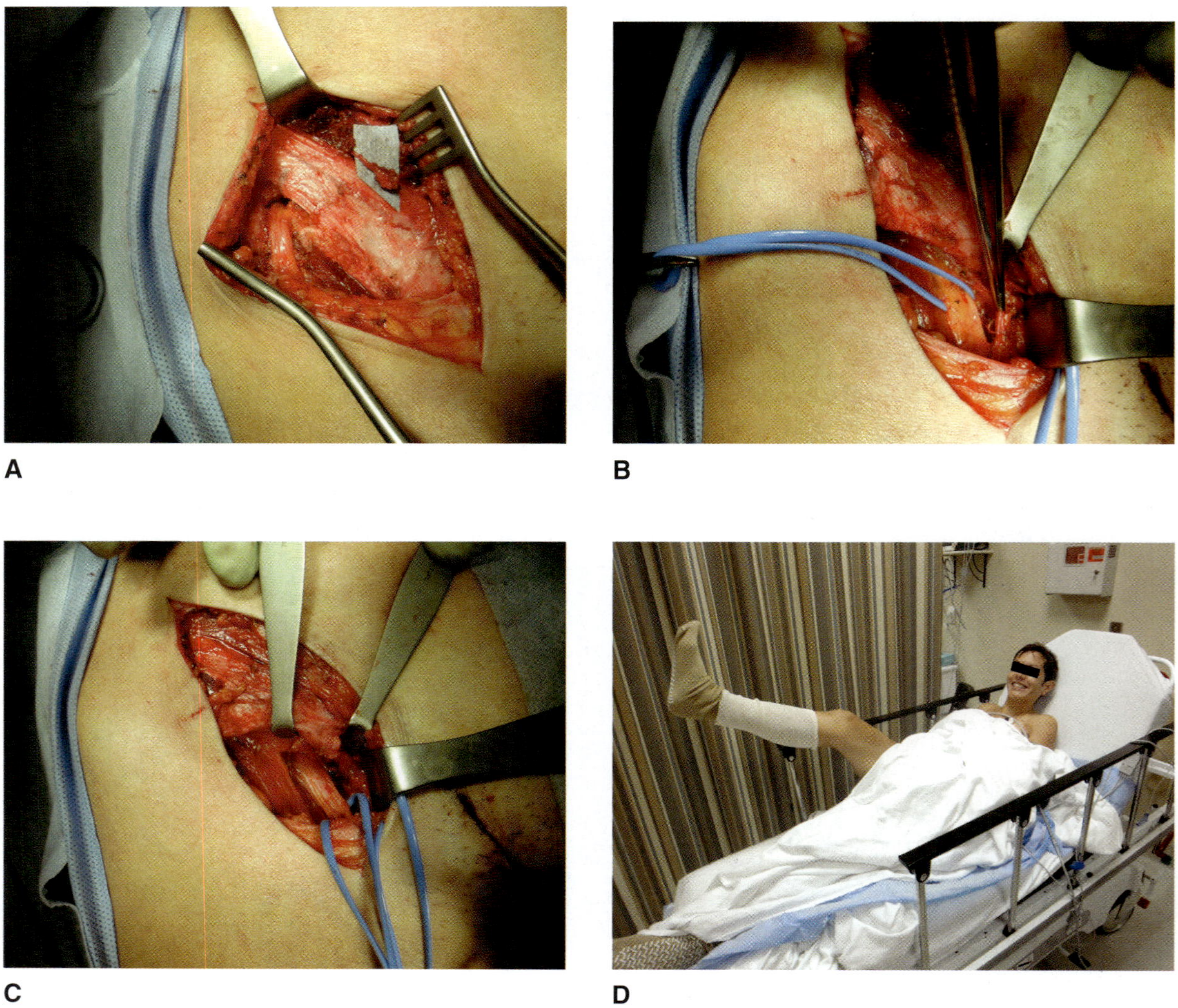

FIGURE 82-5 Intraoperative views of neurolysis of the femoral nerve at the inguinal ligament. (A) The scarring about the femoral sheath is noted in this patient who had a femoral hernia repair, with subsequent complete loss of knee extension. (B) The femoral nerve before neurolysis. (C) The femoral nerve after the intraneural neurolysis. (D) The patient demonstrating knee extension in the recovery room.

adductor magnus, creating the canal described by John Hunter (1728–1793) that contains the superficial femoral artery and vein and saphenous nerve. The adductor canal is located at approximately the junction of the proximal two thirds with the distal-third of the thigh. That is where simplicity ends. There is often more than one cutaneous nerve branch on the way down to the canal and within the canal, and the entrapment might be on a branch that is outside the canal. The sartorius muscle may not be overlying the entrapment site.

Although some patients have had a direct injury to this location, usually blunt contusion, such as falling while bike riding or on a motorcycle, others have had stretch traction injuries, such as kickboxing. More recently, this entrapment has been found related to patients who present with a groin pull from soccer or football. The tear that injuries the adductor muscle origin from the pubic bone may directly cause stretch as the nerves course through the fascia or, subsequently, muscle spasm of the adductors causes secondary compression. Confounding this diagnosis are people who have a true neuroma of a branch of the saphenous nerve from knee surgery or vascular access to the superficial femoral vessel or patients who have had a gracilis muscle harvested during reconstructive microsurgery.

Figure 82-6 shows the typical location of the tender area or positive Hoffman-Tinel sign with the distal area of sensory disturbance. This patient also had a groin pull from a soccer injury. The incision is made over the site of the pain and tenderness, deepened into the subcutaneous tissue heading for the sartorius muscle, which if present in this location, must be retracted to find the adductor canal. Figure 82-7 demonstrates superficial nerve entrapments that were causing the pain. These superficial nerves can be a distal sensory branch of the obturator, an anterior femoral cutaneous nerve, or the superficial cutaneous nerve of the thigh (also a branch of the femoral nerve). In Figure 82-8, the saphenous nerve is released by opening the adductor canal.

Rehabilitation begins with water walking to permit nerve gliding.

There remains an absence of even a level IV study of the results of the adductor canal syndrome.

If the first neurolysis is not successful or if the neurolysis is being done to identify a saphenous nerve injured distally, then the saphenous nerve and its branches are divided and the proximal end implanted into an adductor muscle. Intraoperative electrical stimulation is done before any nerve resection as motor branches to the vastus medialis are contained within or just superficial to the fascial roof of the adductor canal.

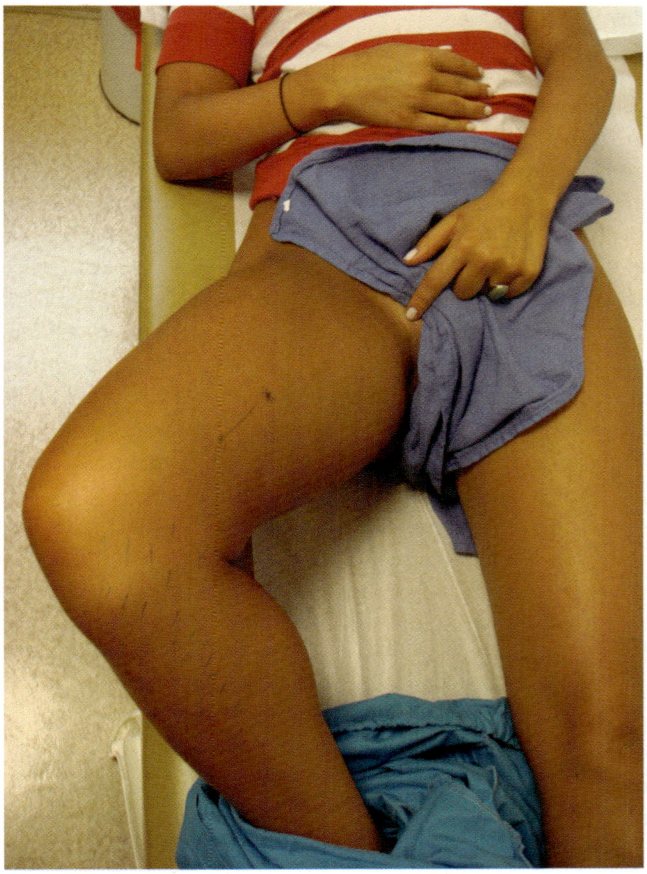

FIGURE 82-6 Patient with the leg externally rotated demonstrating the site of groin pain from a groin pull, the marking in the distal third of the thigh where the tender saphenous nerve is located by pressure or a positive Hoffmann-Tinel sign, and the skin marked to show the area of dysesthesias, which can present as knee pain.

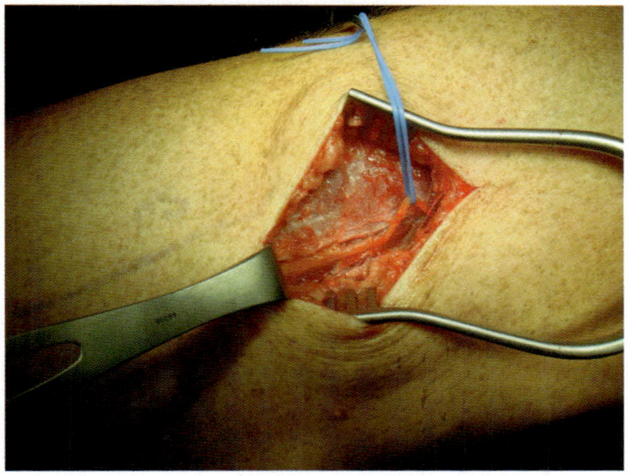

A

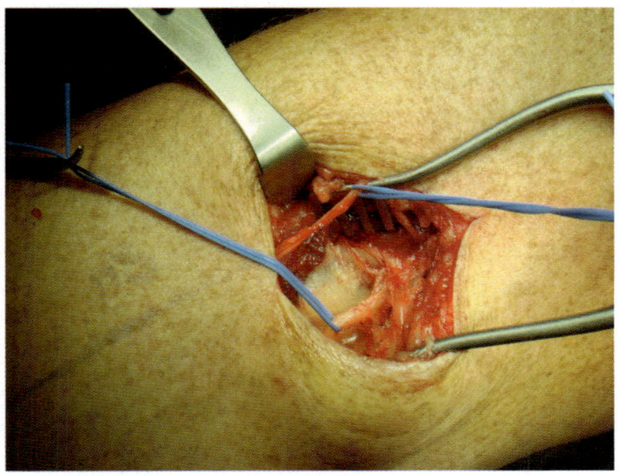

B

FIGURE 82-7 Intraoperative view of approach to adductor canal. Here nerves are superficial to the canal and are entrapped in fascia, representing the sensory component of the obturator nerve (A) and the anterior femoral cutaneous nerve (B).

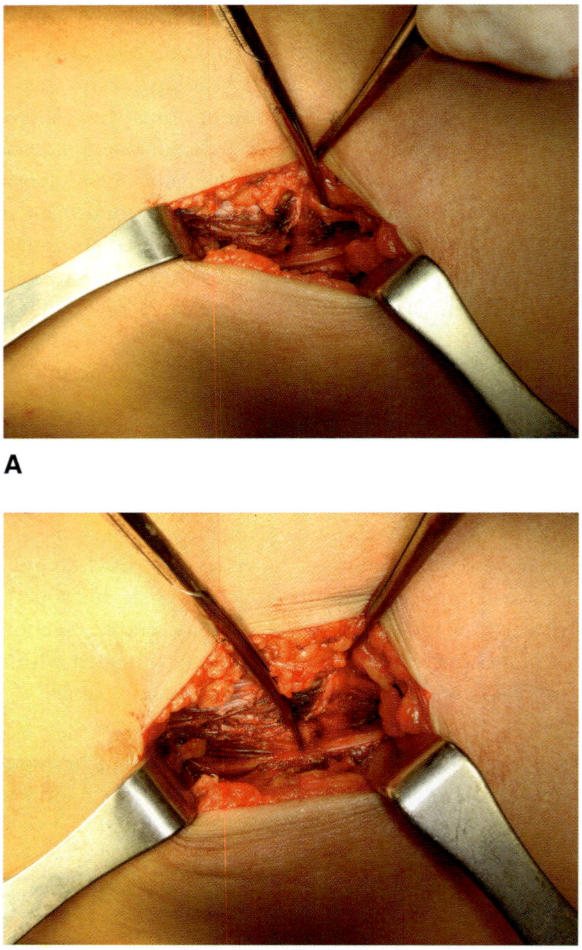

A

B

FIGURE 82-8 Intraoperative view without a sartorius muscle needing to be retracted, demonstrating the motor innervation from the femoral of the vastus medialis (**A**) beneath the scissors and the saphenous nerve exiting the fascial roof of the adductor canal (**B**).

Common Peroneal Nerve Compression

Compression of the common peroneal nerve occurs at the lateral aspect of the knee, across the fibular neck, and is called the fibular tunnel syndrome. The common peroneal nerve gives off one articular branch just proximal to the fibular head and one just distal to the fibular head and then immediately divides into the branches the innervate the tibialis anterior. The remaining peroneal branches accompanying this, comprising the deep peroneal nerve, innervate the toe extensor muscles, while the remaining more lateral, and more superficial fascicles proceed distally to innervate the foot everter muscles and innervate the dorsum of the skin with the exception of the web between the first and second toes. This web space is innervated by the deep peroneal nerve. Just proximal to the ankle joint, the deep peroneal nerve innervates the lateral ankle joint, and the sinus tarsi, just before innervating the extensor digitorum brevis muscle. Division of the deep peroneal nerve just above the ankle, therefore, can relieve sinus tarsi pain (37). At the level of the fibular neck, 20% of anatomy specimens but 80% of patients coming to surgery for neurolysis of the common peroneal nerve will have a deep fibrous band, and another 13% of specimens will have a fibrous band along the origin of the lateral head of the gastrocnemius from the fibular (38).

The patient's complaints of paresthesias should include radiation from the knee to the top of the foot. If the radiation does not begin until the lower let, the site of compression might be the superficial peroneal nerve and not the common peroneal nerve, although many patients will have both, a form of the double-crush phenomenon.

The physical examination should evaluate the strength of the extensor hallucis longus muscle by providing resistance to long toe extension. This muscle is the first to become weak with common peroneal nerve compression and often the last to recover after surgery.

Patients with peroneal palsy are commonly referred after total knee or total hip arthroplasty, and about 50% of these patients will have a previously undiagnosed neuropathy underlying the nerves susceptibility for stretch traction. The success for neurolysis if these patients can be operated upon at about 3 months should be 90% or more (39). Clearly sufficient stretch traction can occur from skiing or soccer, often associated with ligamentous injury to the knee that knee reconstruction is required. In these patients with either complete disruption or severe stretch of the common peroneal nerve, neurolysis cannot be expected to yield improved function, and, indeed, even nerve grafting, in the absence of tendon transfer, yields poor outcomes (40).

The incision does not have to be longer than 4 to 5 cm in a normal sized leg (Figure 82-9). The incision is oblique in case you must extend the surgery into the popliteal fossa or distally in the leg. There is sometimes a cutaneous nerve in this location, the lateral cutaneous nerve of the calf, and this should be preserved. The deep fascia, in the absence of trauma, will not be adherent to the common peroneal nerve. This nerve is white in the absence of glucose intolerance, in which case it is swollen and infiltrated by yellow fat, giving it almost the appearance of a lipoma. *Do not excise this fatty mass!* The nerve is released into the popliteal fossa, but the entrapment site, again in the absence of trauma, is completely between the neck of the fibula and the overlying structures related to the peroneus muscles. Begin by releasing the superficial peroneus fascia transversely, proximally, and distally in a stellate fashion. There is often a septum between muscles, which should be released with care taken not to extend the scissor tips too deeply and injuring the nerve. Then retract the muscle and look for the fibrous band that is almost always present in this location. This band must be carefully released to reveal the compressed, flattened, ischemic soft nerve below (see Figure 82-9). Then the nerve is gently elevated. If there is a fibrous band deep to the nerve, then this must be cauterized and divided. In a few patients, the opening into the anterior compartment also needs to be widened by releasing some of the fibrous muscle origins.

If there is intraneural fibrosis, a very gentle intraneural dissection can be done. Intraoperative electrical stimulation that demonstrates motor function is very useful in giving the patient with a foot drop a good prognosis on awakening from surgery. Be sure not to get any Marcaine on the nerve during the infiltration of the skin edges to avoid the patient awaking with poor

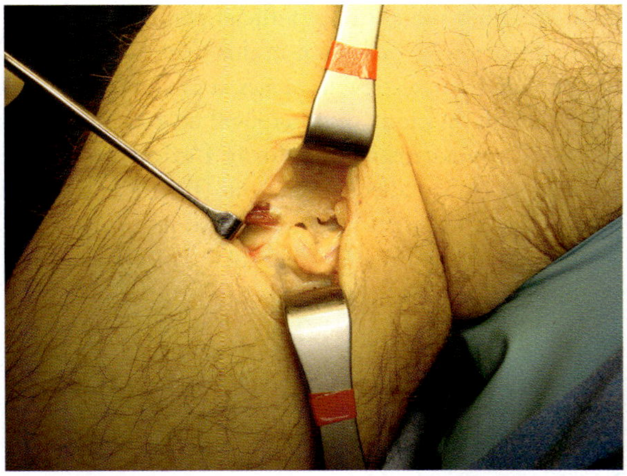

A

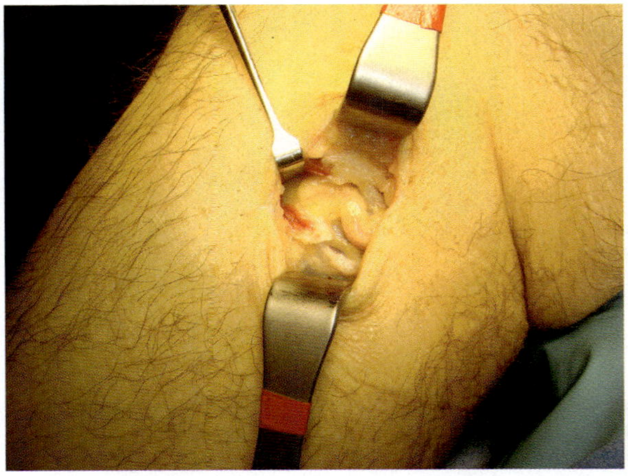

B

FIGURE 82-9 Intraoperative views for neurolysis of the common peroneal nerve at the knee. Note the location of the incision. The only site for entrapment is over the fibular neck and a larger, longer incision is not necessary. (**A**) Note the fibrous band compressing the common peroneal nerve. The peroneus muscles are retracted. (**B**) After removing the fibrous band, note that the peroneal nerve is flattened and without fascicular markings deep to the band, consistent with axonal loss and severe compression.

motor function. At the completion of the procedure, do not close the fascia over the nerve but rather let the nerve remain superficial to prevent creating another site of entrapment. A loose bandage is applied. The patient is allowed to walk immediately.

It is suggested that the ankle–foot orthosis (AFO) device is replaced with a boot they can lace up to prevent the AFO straps from compressing the nerve's regeneration postoperatively (Figure 82-10).

Superficial Peroneal Nerve Compression

The superficial peroneal nerve innervates the muscles of the lateral compartment and then exits through the fascia of this compartment, at which point it can become entrapped if either the fascial window is too tight or there has been direct trauma, such as a kick in soccer, or from an ankle inversion sprain.

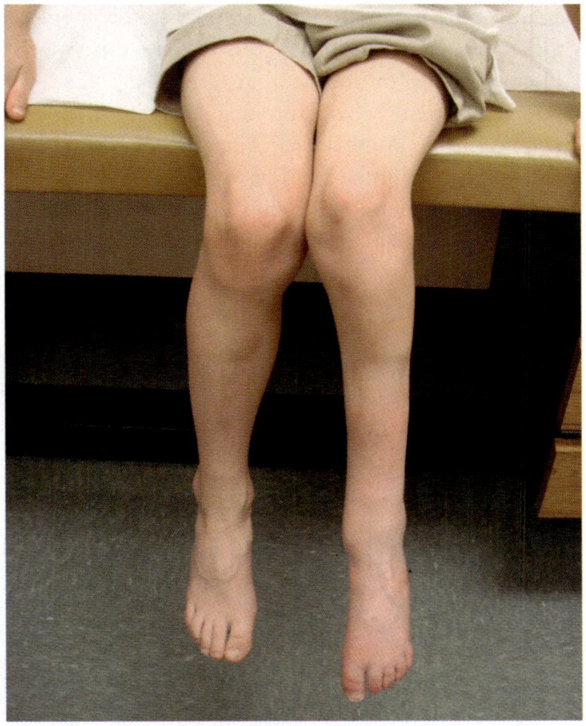

A

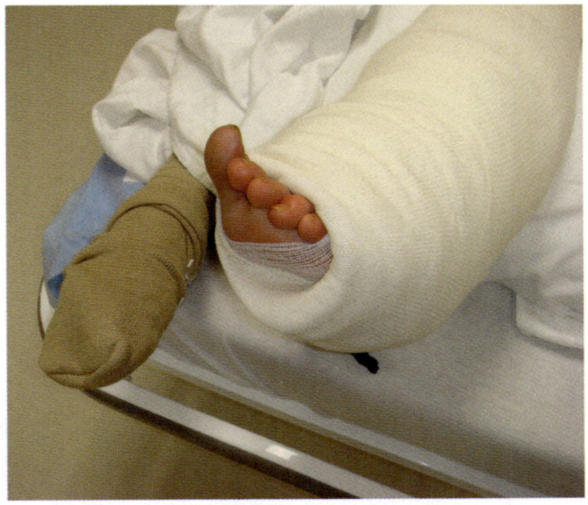

B

FIGURE 82-10 Common peroneal nerve compression. (**A**) Preoperatively, note the foot hanging and medially deviated without ability to extend toes, ankle or to evert the ankle. Note too the indentations of the skin from the ankle–foot orthosis (AFO). (**B**) In the recovery room, after neurolysis of the common peroneal nerve, note full extension of the big toe by the extensor hallucis longus muscle.

Symptoms can be burning and pain from the outside of the lower leg to the top of the foot. These symptoms worsen with walking and can mimic a compartment syndrome. In patients with a predisposition to chronic nerve compression, such as in diabetes, this compression site can masquerade as part of the painful neuropathy symptoms and be easily missed if the peripheral nerves are not examined carefully for the presence of a Hoffmann-Tinel sign. Because of variability in anatomy, although the most common site for compression is about 10 cm proximal to the lateral malleolus, this exit site can range from 4 to 25 cm proximal to the lateral malleolus.

Despite all anatomy books illustrating the location of the superficial peroneal nerve in the lateral compartment (Figure 82-11), there were patients of mine that I had resected this nerve within the lateral compartment, and they still had sensation over the dorsum of the foot that could be relieved by a local block at the anterior ankle. The paradox is resolved by realizing that 25% of people have either the entire superficial peroneal nerve in the anterior compartment, or instead of this nerve dividing into its dorsomedial and dorsolateral branches at the level of the ankle, they have a high division, and there will be a branch not only in the lateral compartment but also in the anterior compartment or in a subcutaneous location (Figure 82-12) (41). Therefore, it is critical that when you make an incision over the site of the positive Hoffmann-Tinel sign, which is often where there is a slight bulge as the nerve exists the fascia accompanied

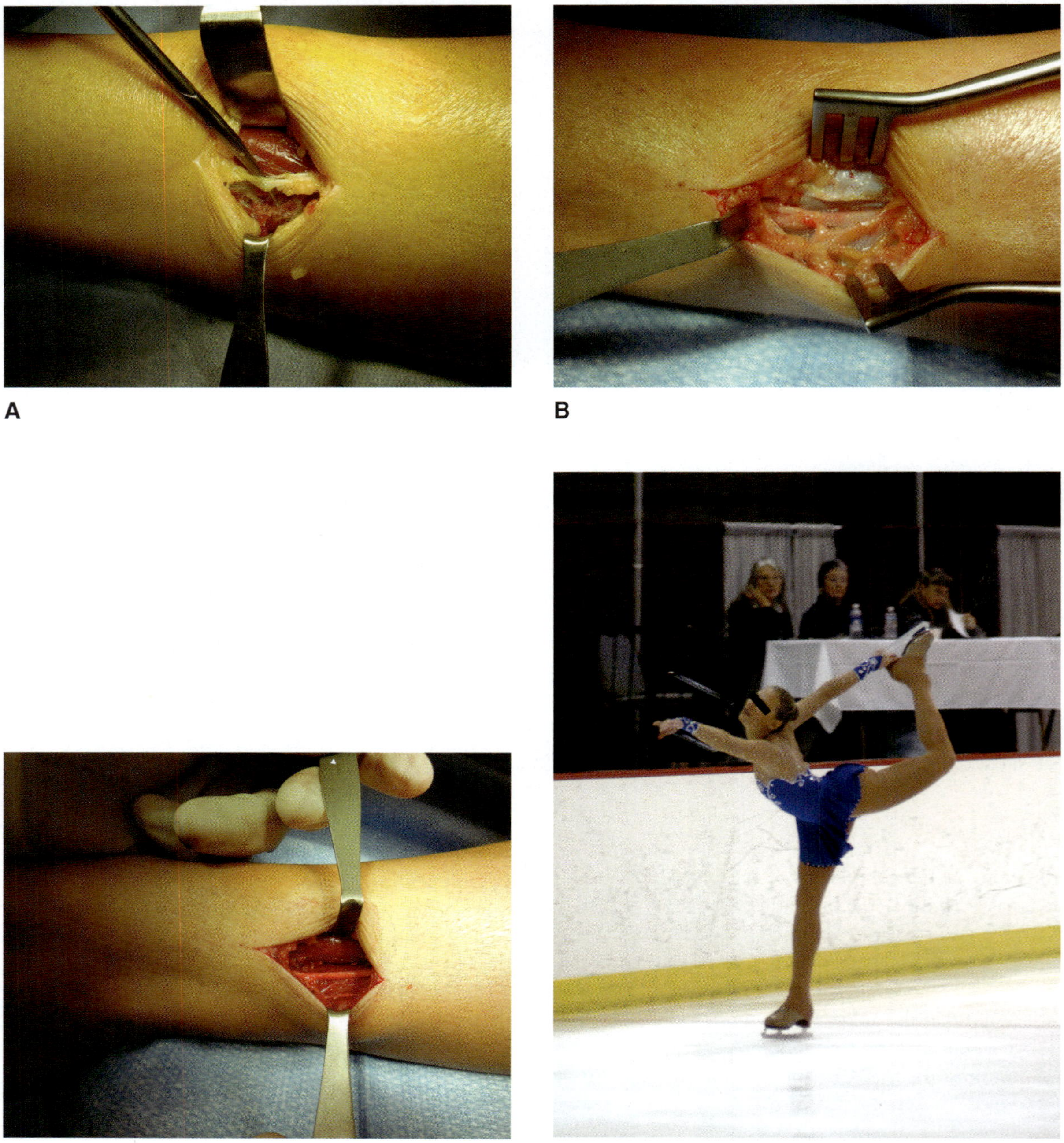

A B C D

FIGURE 82-11 Superficial peroneal nerve compression. (A) The incision is typically made about 10 cm proximal to the lateral malleolus, centered on the positive Hoffmann-Tinel sign, and gently deepened down to the fascia. Here the superficial peroneal nerve is seen exiting from the fascia, and after the fasciotomy of the lateral compartment (B), the inflamed compressed segment can be compared with the normal appearance proximal and distal. In someone who also has symptoms consistent with compartment syndrome, such as this professional ice skater, a fasciotomy and limited fasciectomy of the anterior and lateral compartment were done (C), permitting her to return to her profession (D).

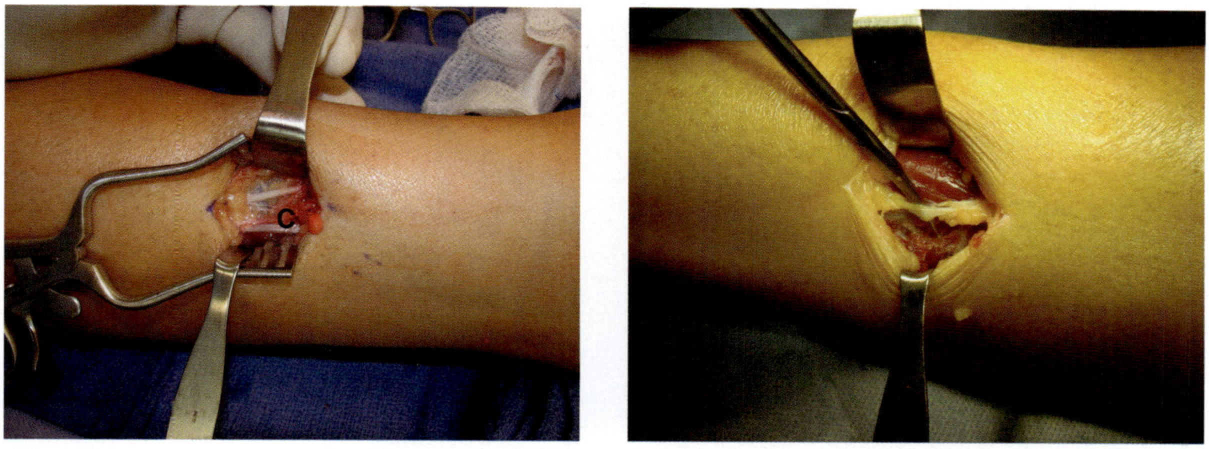

A B

FIGURE 82-12 Intraoperative views of variations in anatomy of the superficial peroneal nerve. (**A**) A branch in both the anterior and the lateral compartment. (**B**) The nerve is intraseptal, lying in the septum between the anterior and the lateral compartment.

by some fat that you not only take care not to injure a small branch to the skin at this location but also plan to do a fasciotomy of both the anterior and the lateral compartments. This fascia is well vascularized and can lead to postoperative bruising or hematoma; therefore, each incised side and edge should be cauterized. The superficial peroneal nerve must be released proximally until it is surrounded by muscle, and if it is pressed up against the septum, a section of septum should be cauterized and removed. If there is no nerve identified in either compartment, it may be in the septum itself, so care should be taken when dividing this septum (see Figure 82-12B) (42).

This surgical approach can be expected to result in 80 to 90% good to excellent results in terms of symptomatic relief (41).

Proximal Tibial Nerve Compression (the Soleal Sling Syndrome)

Compression of the proximal tibial nerve is perhaps the newest site described for chronic nerve compression in the leg. As the tibial nerve passes beneath the origin of the soleus muscle, the fibrous arch that spans the fibula and tibia, it can become compressed (43). This site is best termed "soleal sling syndrome." The sensory complaints are similar to those of tarsal tunnel syndrome except that they are not present at night. The sensory findings are the same as for tarsal tunnel syndrome. The physical findings can differ in that there is weakness of toe flexion, particularly there is weakness in flexion of the big toe (Figure 82-13A). The innervation of the flexor hallucis longus occurs at the level of the soleal sling, causing this finding. Neurolysis at this anatomic site can recover toe flexion (Figure 82-13D). The incision is made from the medial popliteal fossa laterally and then inferiorly. The distal saphenous nerve travels in this location and is preserved. The fascia is released to bluntly dissect and posteriorly retract the medial head of the gastrocnemius muscle. The tibial nerve will be noted to be just beneath the soleal sling and just posterior (in front for the surgeon) of the popliteal vein (Figure 82-13B and 82-13C). The safest approach is to cauterize the soleus overlying the course of the tibial nerve and then lift up on the deep posterior compartment fascia and release it. The tibial nerve can be separated from the popliteal vein, and the fascicles in this location can be stimulated to demonstrate recovery of toe flexion.

Although no level IV study has yet been reported, one small series of three patients with soleal sling syndrome secondary to blunt trauma has been reported with recovery of motor function and sensory relief in each of the three patients.

This surgical approach may prove valuable in patients who have had a tarsal tunnel release, including neurolysis of all four medial ankle tunnels (see later discussion) but who have failed to achieve a good result. In these patients, similar to "failed carpal tunnel syndrome" patients, it is possible that the source of distal "failure" is due to a proximal site of compression. It is therefore critical to examine patients for evidence of this proximal site. The motor finding is weakness in toe flexion. The "positive Hoffmann-Tinel sign" for this entrapment site is tenderness with strong pressure behind the calf at about 9 to 10 cm below the popliteal fossa (43,44).

Deep Peroneal Nerve Compression

The space at the anterior ankle, beneath the inferior extensor retinaculum, has been called the anterior tarsal tunnel. A nerve compression at this site has been described, and it is possible to identify with EMG because this is proximal to where the extensor digitorum brevis is innervated. *However, this is almost never the site of entrapment of the deep peroneal nerve* unless there has been a crush injury to the foot or ankle or there has been an orthopedic intervention.

The most common site of clinically significant entrapment of the deep peroneal nerve is over the dorsum of the foot, where the extensor hallucis brevis tendon compresses the deep peroneal nerve against the underlying bone prominence produced by the articulation of the first and second metatarsal with the cuneiform bone (45).

Neurosensory testing can document this sensory loss in the dorsal first web space, and there will be a Hoffmann-Tinel sign

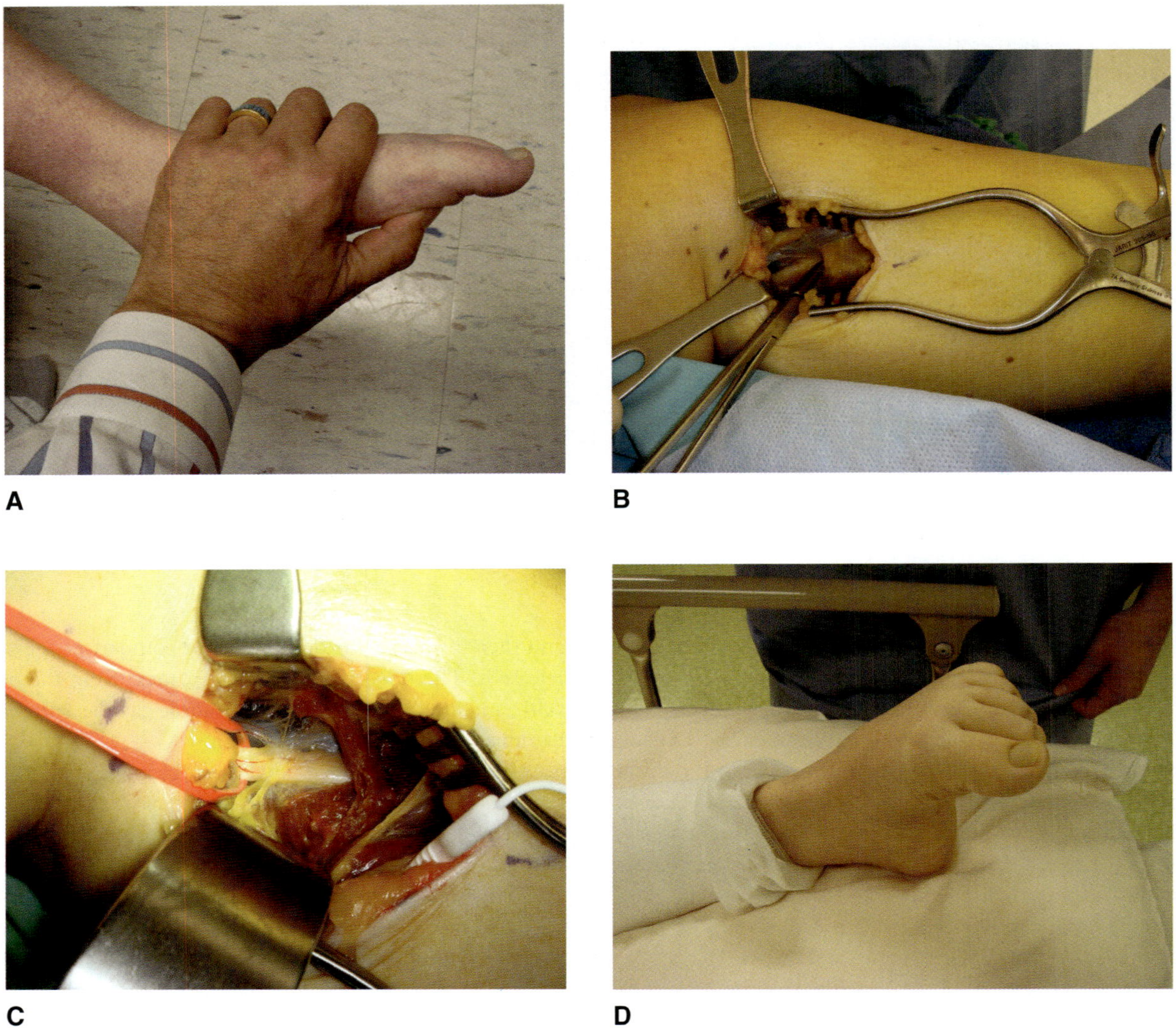

FIGURE 82-13 Neurolysis of the proximal tibial nerve beneath the soleal sling. (A) At this level, the innervation of the flexor hallucis longus can be compressed, causing weakness of toe flexion. (B) The incision is in the medial side of the leg, entering the popliteal fossa. Here the gastrocnemius muscle is retracted posteriorly after the fascia has been divided to the soleus. The purple popliteal vein is noted adjacent to the white tibial nerve. The curved clamp is beneath the fibrous arch of the soleal sling that is compressing the tibial nerve. (C) After bipolar cauterization of the soleus, the fibrous arch can be divided along with the posterior compartment fascia to release the nerve and, if needed, the posterior compartment. Note the difference in color and vascularity of the tibial nerve proximal and distal to the compression site. (D) Note that flexion of the big toe has been achieved postoperatively.

beneath the extensor hallucis brevis tendon where it compresses the nerve against the underlying bone. This is often the site of an exostosis and the most common site for a ganglion (Figure 82-14). The common Lisfranc fracture-dislocation can also cause this compression (Figure 82-15), as will wearing high heels or tight sports shoes, such as in ice skating (Figure 82-16). If there has been direct trauma or antecedent surgery, then it may be more appropriate to resect this nerve in the lower leg, but if not, then the neurolysis is the appropriate choice.

A 2-cm oblique incision is made between the first and second metatarsals and the cuneiform bone. The superficial peroneal nerve is protected. The deep fascia is opened overlying the visible oblique tendon or muscle belly of the extensor hallucis brevis. This tendon is resected, and the nerve is elevated from its adherence to the underlying bone. There is often a clear indentation of the nerve. Proximally, the nerve is released until it is loose at the inferior extensor retinaculum. Distally, there is often a second site of compression beneath a thin fibrous band just before the nerve becomes subcutaneous in location. A small branch innervating the metarsocunieform joints can be observed here.

The success for neurolysis of the deep peroneal nerve should be 90% good to excellent (45).

Tarsal Tunnels Syndrome

Tarsal tunnel syndrome was described in 1962, in independent reports by Lam and Keck, as the carpal tunnel syndrome of the foot. This implied that there was one tunnel to release and, in a manner similar to the splint used after carpal tunnel decompression, it was suggested that the patient following release of the flexor retinaculum at the ankle use crutches for 3 weeks to

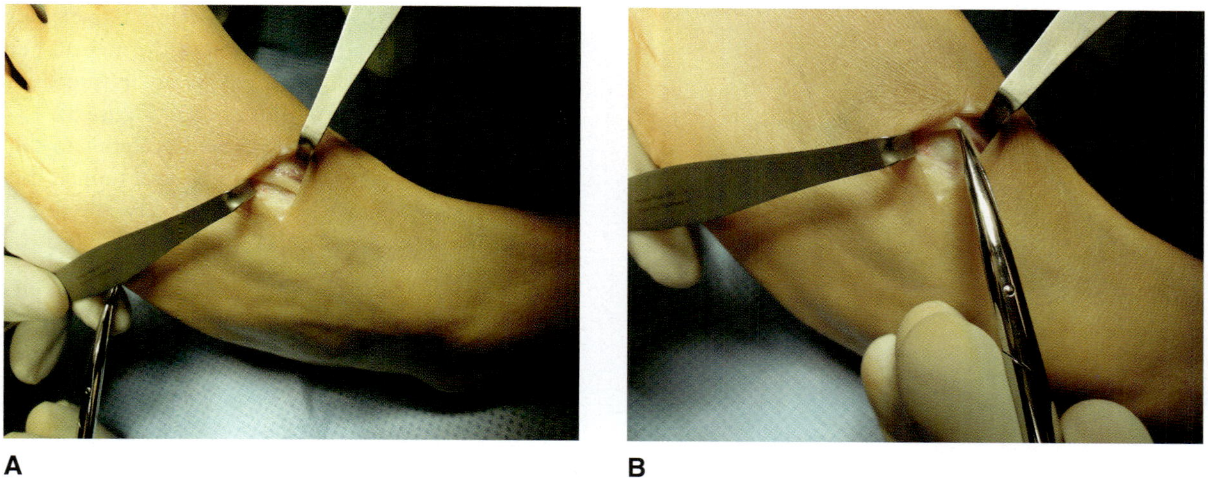

FIGURE 82-14 Compression of the deep peroneal nerve by a ganglion. (**A**) The extensor hallucis tendon has already been excised so that the deep peroneal nerve is visible. (**B**) The ganglion can be seen bulging from the ankle–first metatarsal joint. The deep peroneal nerve becomes compressed between the ganglion below and the extensor tendon above. The ganglion can be removed, and if necessary, the exostosis can be shaved.

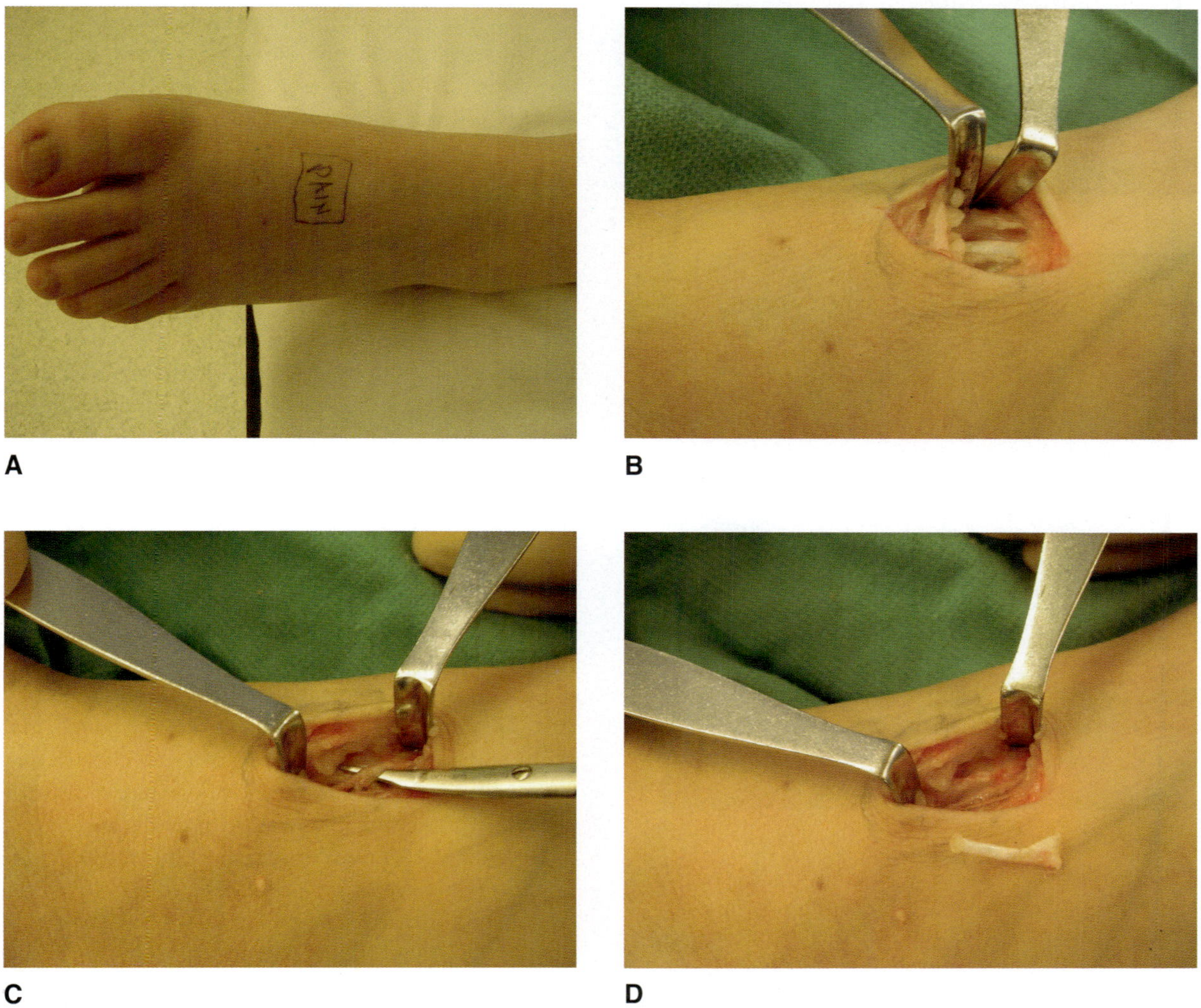

FIGURE 82-15 Deep peroneal nerve compression (**A**) causing pain over the dorsum of the foot after a fracture-dislocation (Lisfranc). (**B**) Typical incision made to permit access must carefully preserve superficial sensory nerve branches by blunt dissection to expose the white tendon of the extensor hallucis brevis, which will often have muscle still present at this location. (**C**) A proximal and distal neurolysis of the deep peroneal nerve is then done, often elevating from its fibrous attachment to the underlying bone. (**D**) The excised segment of tendon.

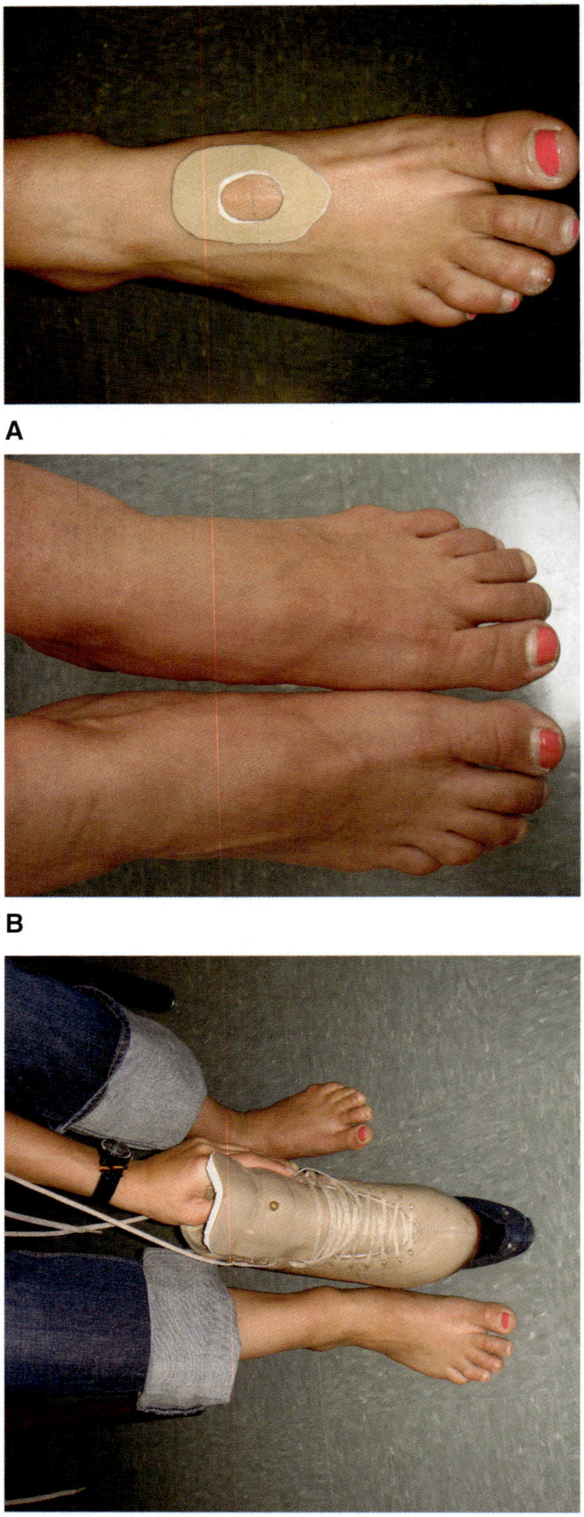

FIGURE 82-16 Deep peroneal nerve compression in a skater is noted by pain over the dorsum of the foot. (**A**) Typically, a protective padding has been tried. (**B**) The incision heals well (right foot), permitting (**C**) wearing of skates without padding.

permit the ankle incision to heel (1). This approach yielded poor clinical outcomes. It became clear that the analogy was simply wrong and that the tarsal tunnel and the flexor retinaculum were the homologs of the forearm and forearm fascia. The medial plantar tunnel was the carpal tunnel, the lateral plantar tunnel was Guyon's canal, and the calcaneal tunnel was the tunnel of the palmar cutaneous branch of the median nerve. The concept became one of "four medial ankle tunnels" and the tarsal tunnels syndrome, as illustrated in Figure 82-17.

An incision is made proximal and posterior to the medial malleolus extending to the end of the tarsal tunnel. If there has been no previous injury, edema, or surgery, the deep fascia is thin and immediately subjacent is the thicker, but usually loose flexor retinaculum, that used to be called the lancinate ligament. After this has been divided, the tarsal tunnel is officially released. If there is no space-occupying lesion, the surgery is done, and it is appreciated that not much has been decompressed. It is appropriate to elevate the tibial artery and veins from the tibial nerve and evaluate if there is intraneural fibrosis or not, if there is a high division of the tibial nerve (Figure 82-18) or not, and the number of calcaneal nerves originating within the tarsal tunnel. It has been demonstrated now that the pressure within the tarsal tunnel of patients with neuropathy is not different than it is in the tarsal tunnel of cadavers. The pressure here does increase with ankle plantar flexion and pronation, and this is no longer occurs after release of the flexor retinaculum (46).

With my realization that the tarsal tunnel represented the human forearm and not the carpal tunnel, I developed an operation that decompressed the medial and lateral plantar tunnels and the calcaneal tunnel(s) and removed the septum that is between the medial and lateral plantar tunnels to create a larger volume for these nerves (see Figures 82-17 and 82-18). To accomplish this in surgery, an incision is made toward the plantar aspect of the foot and comes proximal to join the incision for the tarsal tunnel release. Of course, these two incisions can be drawn and made at the same time, but it is important conceptually to appreciate that these distal tunnels are at the foot level and the entrapment sites are *not* within the tarsal tunnel. The tarsal tunnel ends at the origin of the abductor hallucis. The fascia superficial to the abductor is incised with care taken not to injure the branch from the medial plantar nerve, often through this fascia, and into the skin of the medial arch. This little nerve remains unnamed, after our description. The abductor muscle is then retracted to reveal its ligamentous origin, which forms the roof of the medial and lateral plantar tunnels. Each roof is incised. The septum between them is cauterized and then longitudinally released and excised. This septum is of variable size. Sometimes the medial, sometimes the lateral, and sometimes both plantar tunnels are small and constricting of the nerves within them. Intraoperative pressure measurements in patients with neuropathy demonstrate that these are the sites of elevated pressures even with the ankle in the neutral position, and these pressures increase dramatically with plantar flexion and pronation. It is necessary to release each of these tunnels and excise the septum to get maximum reduction of these pressures (46). If the patient has had complaints of heel pain and has not responded to treatment for plantar fasciitis, it is likely that the source of heel pain is compression of the calcaneal nerve(s). Often there are more than one of these and more than one tunnel. Each must be decompressed to relieve the heel pain.

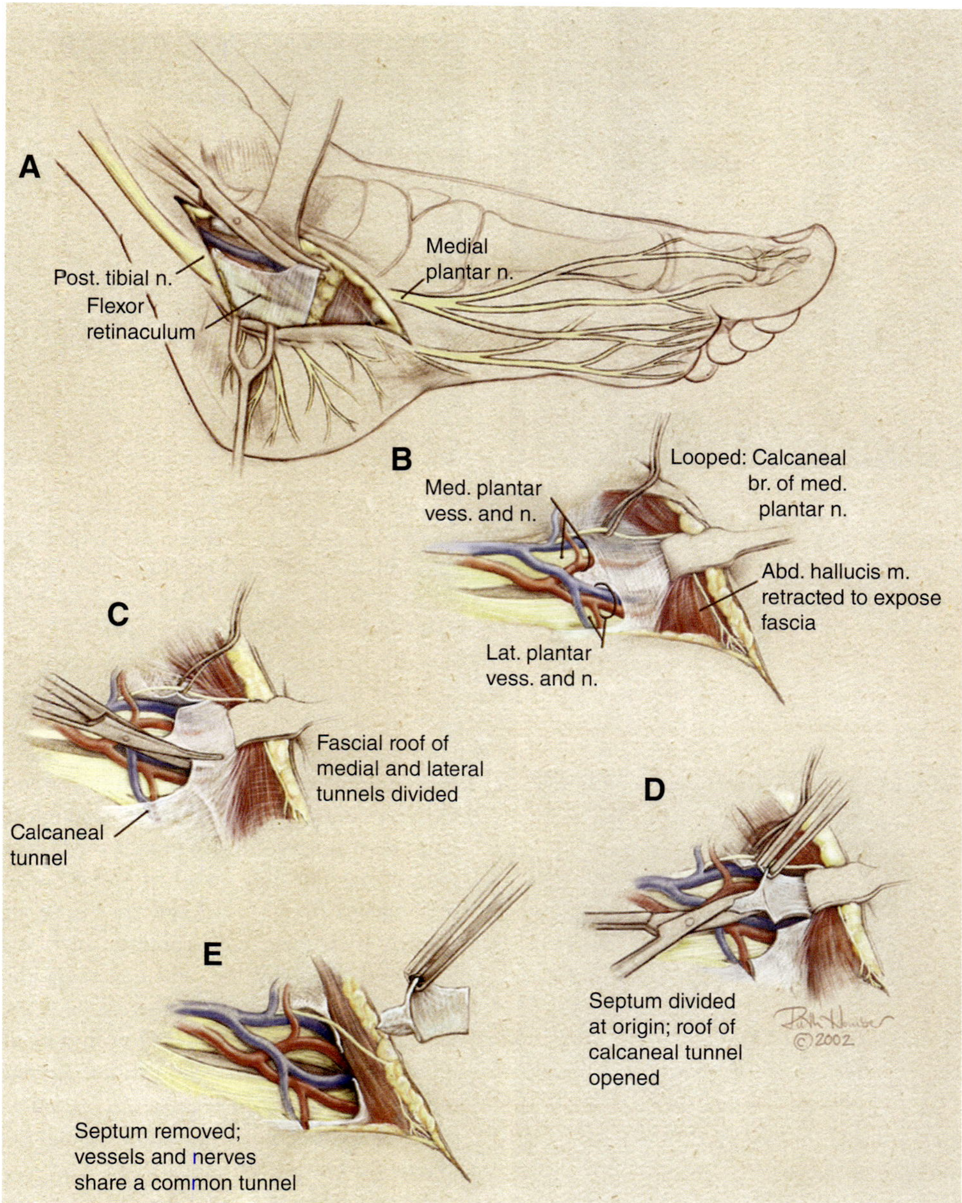

FIGURE 82-17 Illustration of release of the four medial ankle tunnels. (**A**) The tarsal tunnel is opened. (**B**) The abductor hallucis is retracted, protecting the calcaneal branch from the medial plantar nerve to the arch. (**C**) The roof of the medial and the lateral plantar tunnels is incised. (**D**) The calcaneal tunnel is incised. (**E**) The septum between the medial and lateral plantar tunnels is excised. abd, abductus; br, branch; lat, lateral; m, muscle; med, medial; n, nerve; post, posterior; vess, vessel. (With permission from Dellon.com.)

Because it is critical that the peripheral nerve, which has been neuroysed, gets immediate mobilization, it is imperative that the patient walks immediately after the operative procedure. A walker is recommended, so that the patient can hold on with both hands, carry some weight on the foot that had the surgery, and not lose balance and fall (Figure 82-19). For walking, on the side that had the surgery, the operated extremity begins its step by lifting from the knee and then leaning forward. The ankle is often prevented from moving too much, especially in patients who have had tarsal tunnel decompression, so that ankle movement does not pull out the sutures. This is so critical in a patient with neuropathy, who usually cannot tell that ankle movement is tearing out the sutures. It is for precisely this reason that the large Robert Jones bulky ankle dressing is used to protect the ankle suture line in patients with insensitive feet. The walker is used for 3 weeks. When the sutures are out, then rehabilitation with water therapy begins.

The outcomes for "tarsal tunnel decompression" are available from many level IV studies and vary primarily related to the number of these medial ankle tunnels released and the postoperative rehabilitation program. These results are tabulated in Table 82-5. The prognosis is based on the degree of axonal loss. If there is just demyelination, with primarily intermittent symptoms and some weakness, the success can be above 90%, and recovery of function can occur in the early postoperative

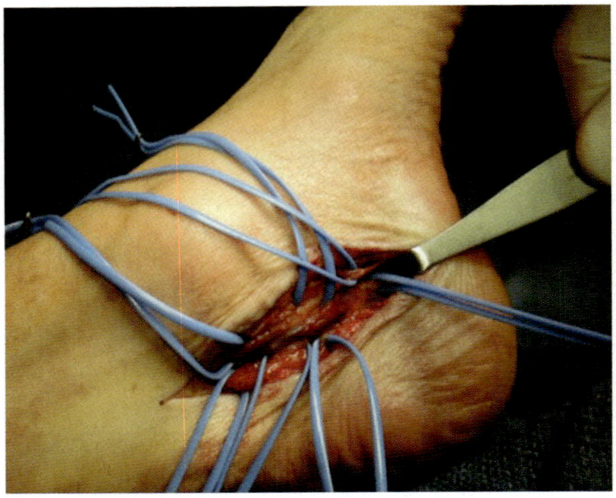

A

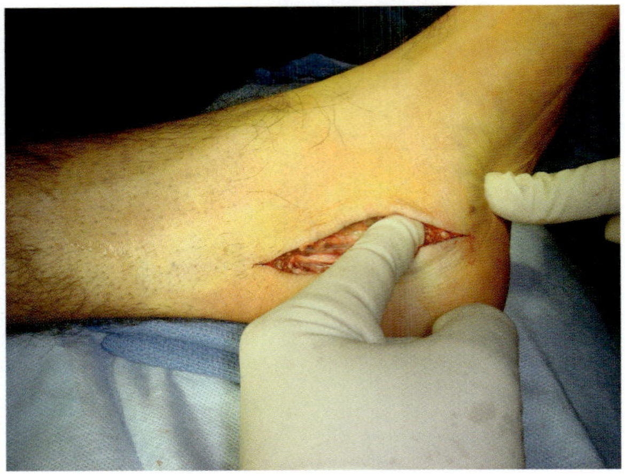

B

FIGURE 82-18 Intraoperative views of tarsal tunnels surgery. (**A**) Left tarsal tunnel opened to demonstrate a high division of the medial and lateral plantar nerves, proximal to the tunnel, encircled with vessel loops, with the distal medial plantar nerve identified with a loop just entering the medial plantar tunnel, and from the lateral plantar nerve, a high originating calcaneal nerve, also encircled with a loop. (**B**) After release of the distal tunnels and resection of the septum, a finger can pass into the plantar aspect of the foot.

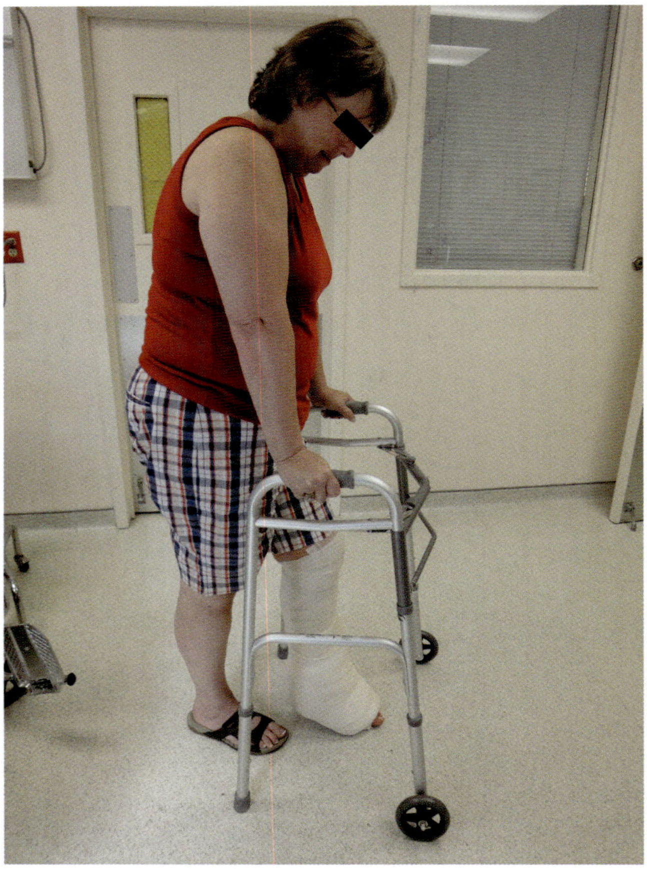

FIGURE 82-19 Postoperative management after release of the four medial ankle tunnels for tarsal tunnels syndrome requires immediate mobilization of the tibial nerve and its branches but sufficient support so that the sutures do not pull out. The extensive, soft, bulky, supportive dressing applied to the foot and ankle permit immediate ambulation with a walker, with the patient being reminded to lift from the knee and hip. This is continued for 4 weeks.

period. Sometimes motor function recovers dramatically in the recovery room. If there is severe axonal loss, with loss of two-point discrimination, with muscle wasting or paralysis, then the success may not only be much lower, but recovery of function may extend over 1 year, and the nerve regeneration may be painful. If there are comorbidities, such as diabetes or another form or neuropathy, the same general guidelines apply, but the expected recovery is 80% relief of pain and 80% recovery of sensation plus prevention of ulceration and amputation. A meta-analysis for the "Dellon triple" approach to neurolysis of the peroneal and tibial nerves in patients with diabetes and superimposed nerve compression was reported in 2008 (47, 48) (Table 82-6).

Interdigital Nerve Compression (Morton's Neuroma)

Compression of the interdigital nerve between the metatarsal heads and beneath the intermetatarsal ligament was first emphasized in 1992 (Figure 82-20) (49). Traditionally, the complaints of sharp pain radiating to the fourth toetip, with the patient unable to wear tight shoes, was attributed to a true neuroma. Yet in the 1940s and 1950s, histopathology and electron microscopy demonstrated this to be a chronic nerve compression. The technique of using a dorsal incision to divide the intermetatarsal ligament, permitting the toes to move apart and decompress the nerve, is successful in about 90% of patients. If this neurolysis fails, the nerve can be resected.

Nevertheless, about 50,000 people per year, as the first surgical approach, have the common plantar digital nerve to the third to fourth toe web space removed through a dorsal incision. This approach, after failure of cortisone injection, alcohol injection, or radiofrequency ablation, can give relief

TABLE 82-5 Summary of Tarsal Tunnel Study Outcomes (49)

Study Date, Author(s)	Patients (*n*)	NCV or EMG	Tinel Positive	Tunnels Released	Immobilized After Surgery	Results (%) Excellent	Good	Fair	Poor
1967, Lam	13	No	Yes	3?	N/A	86	7	7	
1969, Edwards et al.	16	33%	Yes	1	Cast?, time	88	6	0	6
1970, Linscheid et al.	24	100%	Yes	1	N/A	0	50	30	20
1974, Mann	9	90%	Yes	3	3 wk	78	0	11	11
1989, Stern and Joyce	15	40%	Yes	4	10 d	54	20	20	6
1992, Byank and Curtis	49	100%	Yes	1	N/A	26	53	12	9
1993, Sammarco et al.	5	100%	Yes	4	N/A	20	80	0	0
1994, Pfeiffer and Cracchiolo	32	100%	Yes	3	10 d	15	29	23	33
1996, Mahan et al.	45	N/A	Yes	3	N/A	24	36	11	29
1997, Turan et al.	18	0%	Yes	4	2 wk	61	22	0	17
1997, Baba, et al.	34	100%	Yes	3	3 wk	70	16	8	6
1998, Bailie and Kelitian	36	80%	Yes	3	2 wk	57	16	11	16
2000, Kohno et al.	12	40%	Yes	1	N/A	50	34	8	8
2003, Gondring et al.	68	100%	Yes	2?	3 wk	51	0	0	49
2005, Mullick and Dellon	87	50%	Yes	4+	None	82	11	5	2

EMG, electromyography; N/A, not applicable; NCV, nerve conduction velocity.

TABLE 82-6 Meta-Analysis of Results of Dellon Triple in Patients with Diabetes *

Study Date, Author(s)	Nerves (*n*)	Preoperative Pain	Preoperative Touch	Results: Improved Ulceration (%)	Results: Improved Amputation (%)	New or Recurrent Ulceration or Amputation (%)
1992, Dellon	31	0	0	85	72	0
1995, Wieman	33	13	0	92	72	7
2000, Chaffe	58	11	6	86	50	0
2000, Aszmann	16	0	0	N/A	69	0
2003, Wood	33	0	0	90	67	0
2004, Biddinger	22	0	0	86	80	0
2005, Valdivia	60	0	0	87	85	0
2005, Rader	49	0	0	90	75	0
2005, Yao	90	0	0	94	90	0
2006, Siemionow	36	0	0	90	90	0
2006, Yuskel	22	0	0	89	85	0
2007, Massa	20	0	0	80	86	0
2007, Maloney	95	0	0	86	83	0
2007, Bae	33	0	0	75	72	0

*Neurolysis of four medial ankle tunnels plus common and deep peroneal nerves.
N/A, not applicable.

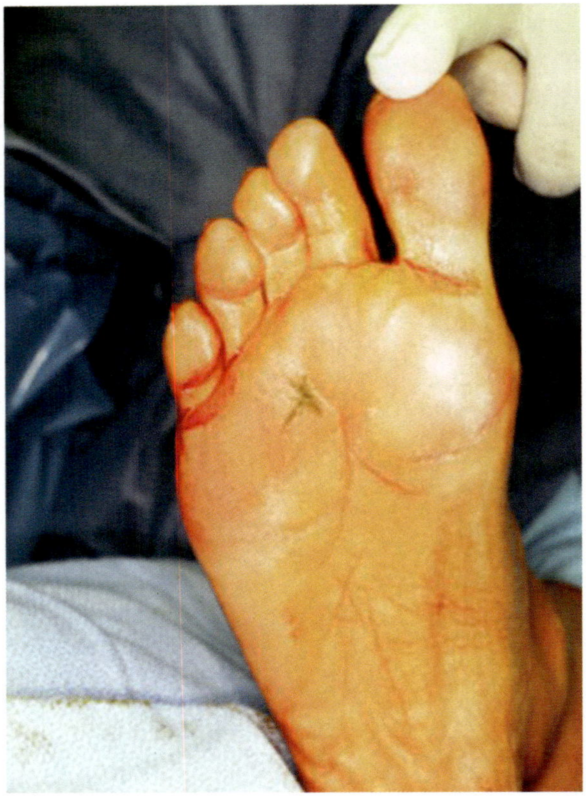

A

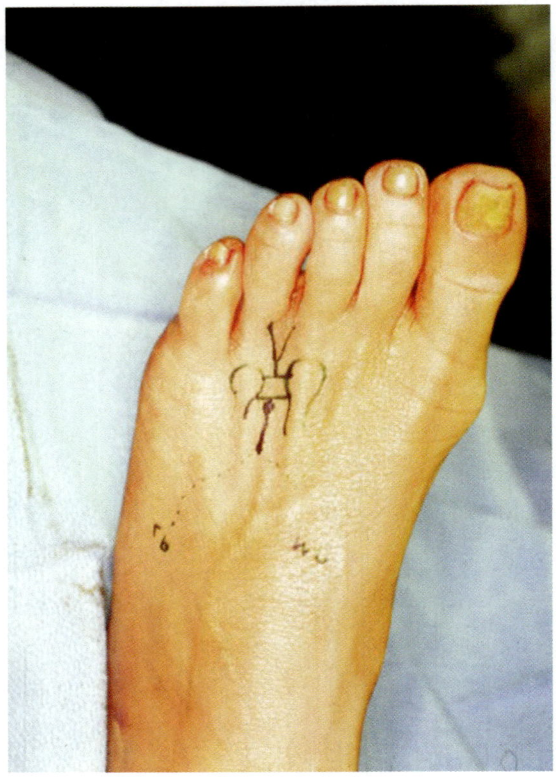

B

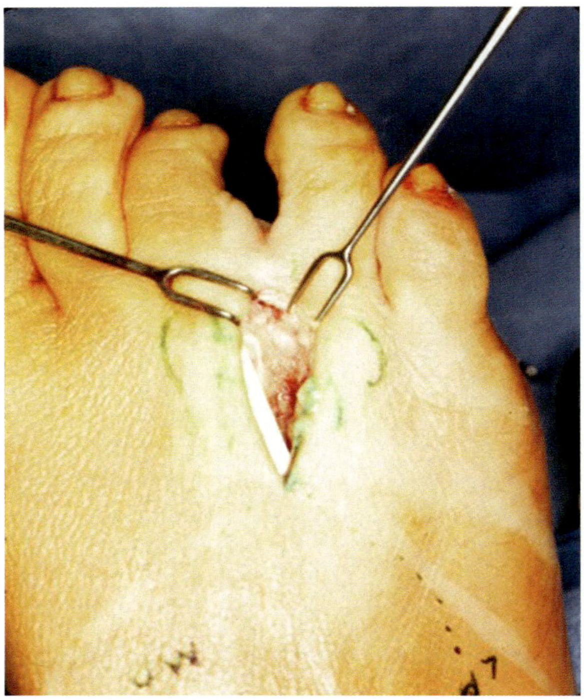

C

FIGURE 82-20 Interdigital nerve compression (Morton's neuroma). (A) Plantar view with site of most common location for compression; the third common, interdigital nerve. (B) Dorsal view with depiction of entrapment mechanism and common anatomic variation with the nerve to the third to fourth web space being formed with a branch from both the medial and lateral plantar nerve. (C) Incision in the third to fourth web space and division of the intermetatarsal ligament. Note the swelling of the nerve, which appears to be a true neuroma, but with no history of injury or previous surgery actually represents swelling from chronic nerve compression.

in up to 85% of patients. However, this approach creates a true neuroma, and if this regenerates into the region of the metatarsal head, a severe pain problem occurs that requires a long incision in the non–weight-bearing portion of the foot, with relocation of the injured nerve into the arch of the foot (50). This salvage approach was reported successful in 80% of 13 patients at a mean of 33 months after surgery (Figure 82-21).

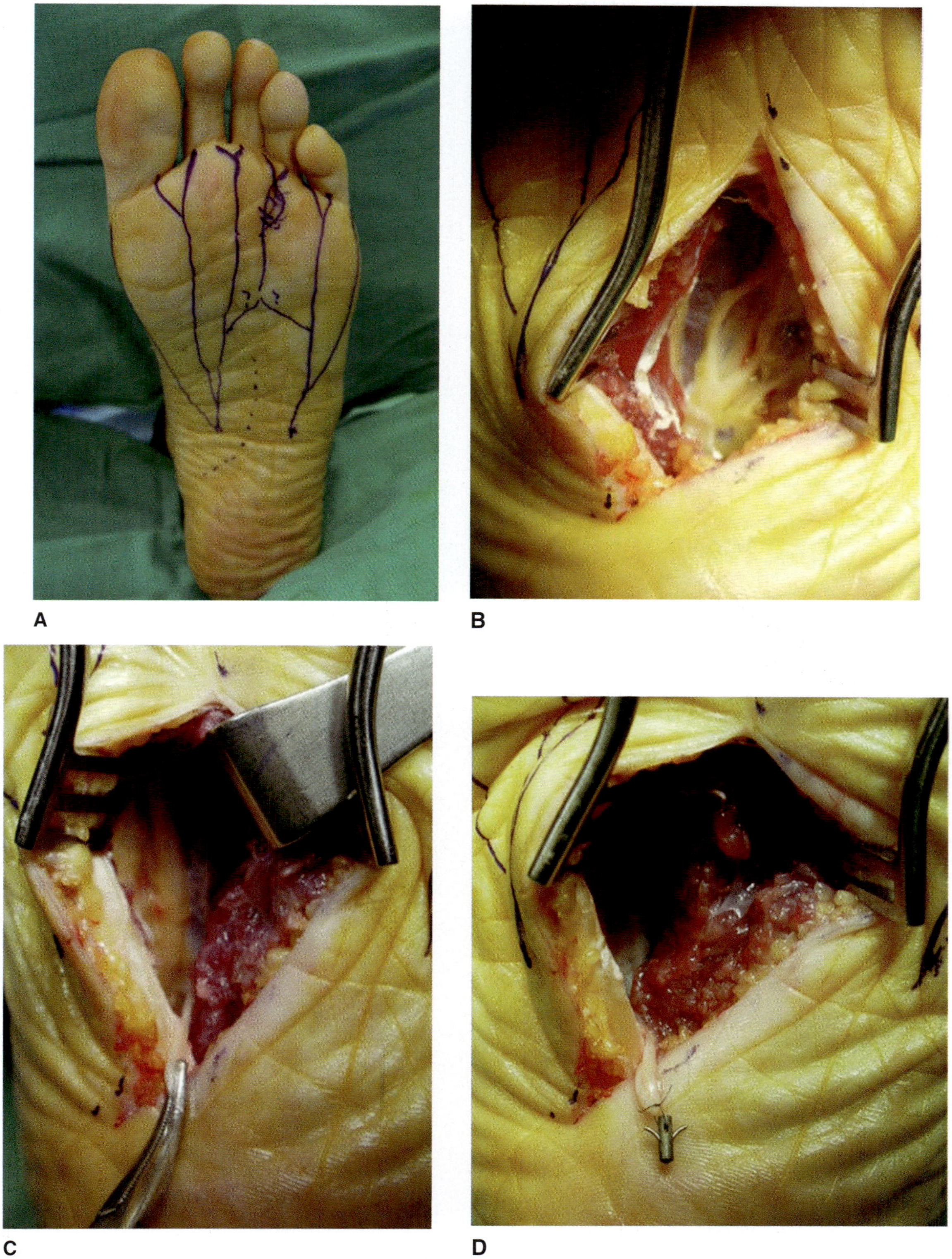

FIGURE 82-21 A true neuroma of the interdigital nerve will result if the "Morton's neuroma" resection fails. (A) Plantar view demonstrating the outline of the digital nerve anatomy and the proposed site for the true neuroma. (B) Plantar incision in the non–weight-bearing portion of the foot, with longitudinal division of the plantar fascia and retraction of the flexor brevis muscle to reveal the medial plantar nerve. An intraneural dissection is then done to identify the contributions to the true neuroma from the medial or lateral plantar nerve. (C) The nerve in the clamp, a branch of the lateral plantar nerve, has been resected and may then be either directly inserted into the arch of the foot or (D) inserted with a Micro-Mitek anchor.

REFERENCES

1. Mackinnon SE, Dellon AL. *Surgery of the Peripheral Nerve*. New York: Thieme, 1989.
2. Dellon AL. History of peripheral nerve surgery. In Winn HR (ed). *Youman's Neurological Surgery*, 5th ed. Philadelphia: WB Saunders, 2004, pp. 3798–3808.
3. Lundborg G, Rydevik B. Effects of stretching the tibial nerve of the rabbit, a preliminary study of the intraneural circulation and the barrier function of the perineurium. *J Bone Joint Surg* 1973;55B:390.
4. Rydevik B, Lundborg G, McClean WG, et al. Blockage of axonal transport induced by acute graded compression of the rabbit vagus nerve. *J Neurol Neurosurg Psychiatry* 1980;43:690.
5. Rydevik B, Lundborg G. Effects of graded compression on intraneural blood flow. *J Hand Surg* 1981;6A:3.
6. Lundborg G, Myers R, Powell H. Nerve compression injury and increased endoneurial fluid pressure, a "miniature compartment syndrome." *J Neurol Neurosurg Psychiatry* 1983;46:1119.
7. Meyers RR, Powell HC. Galactose neuropathy: impact of chronic endoneurial edema on nerve-blood flow. *Ann Neurol* 1984;16:587.
8. Mackinnon SE, Dellon AL, Hudson AR, Hunter D. Chronic nerve compression—an experimental model in the rat. *Ann Plast Surg* 1984;13:112.
9. Rydevik B, Brown MD, Lundborg G. Pathoanatomy and pathophysiology of nerve root compression. *Spine* 1984;9:2.
10. Mackinnon SE, Dellon AL, Hudson AR, Hunter DA. A primate model for chronic nerve compression. *J Reconstr Microsurg* 1985;1:185.
11. Mackinnon SE, Dellon AL. Experimental study of chronic nerve compression: clinical implications. *Clin Hand Surg* 1986;2:639.
12. Dahlin LB, Meiri KF, McClean WG, et al. Effects of nerve compression on fast axoplasmic transport and streptozotocin-induced diabetes mellitus. *Diabetologia* 1986;29:181.
13. Tassler PL, Dellon AL. Pressure perception in the normal lower extremity and in the tarsal tunnel syndrome. *Muscle Nerve* 1996;19:285–289.
14. Dellon AL. Clinical use of vibratory stimuli to evaluate peripheral nerve injury and compression neuropathy. *Plast Reconstr Surg* 1980;65:466.
15. Dellon AL. The vibrometer. *Plast Reconstr Surg* 1983;71:427.
16. Dellon AL. A numerical grading scale for peripheral nerve function, *J Hand Ther* 1993;4:152.
17. Dellon AL. *Somatosensory Testing and Rehabilitation*. Baltimore: Institute for Peripheral Nerve Surgery, 2000.
18. Tassler PL, Dellon AL. Correlation of measurements of pressure perception using the Pressure-Specified Sensory Device with electrodiagnostic testing. *J Occup Med* 1995;37:862.
19. Dellon AL. Neurosensory testing. In Slutsky D (ed). *Master Skills in Nerve Repair: Tips and Techniques*. St. Louis: Elsevier, 2008, pp. 575–586.
20. Slutsky DJ. Use of nerve conduction studies and the pressure-specified sensory device in the diagnosis of carpal tunnel syndrome. *J Hand Surg Eur Vol* 2009;34:60–65.
21. Weber RA, Schuchmann JA, Albers JH, Ortiz J. A prospective blinded evaluation of nerve conduction velocity versus Pressure-Specified Sensory testing in carpal tunnel syndrome. *Ann Plast Surg* 2000;45:252.
22. Dellon AL, Keller KM. Computer-assisted quantitative sensory testing in carpal and cubital tunnel syndromes. *Ann Plast Surg* 1997;38: 493–502.
23. Mullick T, Dellon AL. Results of treatment of four medial ankle tunnels in tarsal tunnels syndrome. *J Reconstr Microsurg* 2008;24:119–126.
24. Dellon AL. The Dellon approach to neurolysis in the neuropathy patient with chronic nerve compression. *Handchir Mikrochir Plast Chir* 2008;40:1–10.
25. Dellon AL. Tinel or not Tinel. *J Hand Surg* 1984;9B:216.
26. Lifchez SD, Means KR Jr, Dunn RE, et al. Intra-and inter-examiner variability in performing Tinel's test. *J Hand Surg* 2010;35A:212–215.
27. Dellon AL. The four medial ankle tunnels: a critical review of perceptions of tarsal tunnel syndrome and neuropathy. *Clin Neurosurg* 2009;19: 629–648.
28. Dellon AL. Technique for determining when heel pain is of neural origin. *Microsurgery* 2008;28:403–406.
29. Mackinnon SE, Dellon AL. Evaluation of microsurgical internal neurolysis in a primate median nerve model of chronic nerve compression. *J Hand Surg Am* 1988;13:345–351.
30. Mackinnon SE, O'Brien JP, Dellon AL, et al. An assessment of the effects of internal neurolysis on a chronically compressed rat sciatic nerve. *Plast Reconstr Surg* 1988;81:251–258.
31. Dellon AL, Seiler WA 4th, Jiranek WA. Teaching the technique of microsurgical intraneural neurolysis. *J Reconstr Microsurg* 1987;3: 137–141.
32. Kale B, Yüksel F, Celiköz B, et al. Effect of various nerve decompression procedures on the functions of distal limbs in streptozotocin-induced diabetic rats: further optimism in diabetic neuropathy. *Plast Reconstr Surg* 2003;111:2265–2272.
33. Aszmann OC, Dellon ES, Dellon AL. The anatomic course of the lateral femoral cutaneous nerve and its susceptibility to compression and injury. *Plast Reconstr Surg* 1997;100:600–604.
34. Lee CH, Dellon AL. Surgical management for groin pain of neural origin. *J Am Coll Surg* 2000;191:137–142.
35. Ducic I, Dellon AL, Taylor NS. Decompression of the lateral femoral cutaneous nerve in the treatment of meralgia paresthetica. *J Reconstr Microsurg* 2006;22:113–118.
36. Ducic I, Dellon L, Larson EE. Treatment concepts for idiopathic and iatrogenic femoral nerve mononeuropathy. *Ann Plast Surg* 2005;55: 397–401.
37. Rab M, Ebmer J, Dellon AL. Innervation of the Sinus Tarsi: implications for treating anterolateral ankle pain. *Ann Plast Surg* 2001;47:500–504.
38. Dellon AL, Ebmer J, Swier P. Anatomic variations related to decompression of the common peroneal nerve at the fibular head. *Ann Plast Surg* 2002;48:30–34.
39. Dellon AL. Post-arthroplasty palsy and systemic neuropathy: a peripheral nerve management algorithm. *Ann Plast Surg* 2005;55:638–642.
40. Prasad AR, Steck J, Dellon AL. Zone of traction injury to the common peroneal nerve. *Ann Plast Surg* 2007;59:302–306.
41. Ducic I, Dellon AL, Graw KS. The clinical importance of variations in the surgical anatomy of the superficial peroneal nerve in the mid-third of the leg. *Ann Plast Surg* 2006;56:635–638.
42. Williams E, Dellon AL. Intra-septal superficial peroneal nerve. *Microsurgery* 2007;27:477–480.
43. Williams EH, Dellon AL. Anatomic site for proximal tibial nerve compression: a cadaver study. *Ann Plast Surg* 2009;62:322–325.
44. Williams EH, Williams CG, Rosson GD, Dellon AL. Combined peroneal and tibial nerve palsy. *Microsurgery* 2009;29:259–264.
45. Dellon AL. Entrapment of the deep peroneal nerve on the dorsum of the foot. *Foot Ankle* 1990;11:73–80.
46. Rosson GD, Larson AR, Williams EH, Dellon AL. Release of medial ankle compartments reduces pressure upon tibial nerve branches in patients with diabetic neuropathy. *Plast Reconstr Surg* 2009;124: 1202–1210.
47. Mullick T, Dellon AL. Results of treatment of four medial ankle tunnels in tarsal tunnels syndrome. *J Reconstr Microsurg* 2008;24:119–126.
48. Dellon AL. The Dellon approach to neurolysis in the neuropathy patient with chronic nerve compression. *Handchir Mikrochir Plast Chir* 2008;40:1–10.
49. Dellon AL. Treatment of Morton's neuroma as a nerve compression: the role for neurolysis. *J Am Podiatr Med Assn* 1992;82:399.
50. Wolfort SF, Dellon AL. Treatment of recurrent neuroma of the interdigital nerve by implantation of the proximal nerve into muscle in the arch of the foot. *J Foot Ankle Surg* 2001;40:404–410.

CHAPTER 83

Nerve Repair in the Lower Extremity

Giorgio Brunelli

Nerve injuries affecting the lower limb are encountered much less frequently than nerve injuries of the upper limb. Nerve injuries of the lower limb and their sequelae may be treated in a similar fashion to nerve injuries of the upper limb by direct nerve suture, nerve grafting, nerve conduits, motor or sensory nerve transfers, direct muscular neurotization, direct skin neurotization, and the still experimental use of nerve prostheses as well as by conventional salvage procedures such as sensate flaps, tendon transfers, tenodeses, and arthrodeses. Nerve injuries affecting the lower limb differ from nerve injuries affecting the upper limb in the time required to achieve reinnervation of the affected muscles or restore protective sensation because of the longer length of the lower limb. Because regeneration occurs an average of only 1 mm per day, it can take many months, depending on the level of the injury, especially with proximal injuries.

SPINAL CORD INJURIES

Spinal cord injuries resulting in paraplegia are becoming more frequent because of motorcycle accidents. The severe physical and psychological damage to the individual is only matched by the emotional and financial catastrophe affecting the family and the significant economic burden sustained by society at large. Can paraplegia potentially be reconstructed by nerve grafting of the spinal cord or bypassed by nerve grafting to the peripheral nerves of the lower limbs? It remains unclear why surgery on the spinal cord does not result in at least some degree of functional recovery. The upper motor neurons from the brain do actually sprout in response to injury and attempt to regenerate. Nerve grafts used to bridge areas of spinal trauma become populated by these regenerating axons, but these same axons do not progress distally into the central nervous system below the level of injury. This "nonpermissiveness" causes endless functional problems affecting walking, bladder dysfunction and cutaneous sensibility in addition to severe secondary psychological disturbances. Loss of sensibility leads to pressure sores, which can become the gateway for severe systemic infections.

Several years ago while investigating this phenomenon, I attempted as a form of surgical palliation, to connect the corticospinal tract (CST) above the lesion to peripheral motor nerves using nerve grafts (peroneal and sciatic nerves), thus bypassing the "nonpermissive" junction at the lower margin of the spinal lesion. In this experimental surgery, the rostral CST was connected to the motor nerves to gluteus maximus, gluteus medius, and quadriceps, resulting in a reasonable functional outcome (Figure 83-1). Later, similar surgery was performed using the same protocol, and all three clinical cases achieved muscle reinnervation and functional improvement. The removal of these important nerves for the purposes of grafting did not make the palsy worse; on the contrary, it benefitted the patient by preventing bothersome spasms and clonus. Initially, the medical community did not believe these results. There seemed to be a lack of logic in that the neurotransmitter of the upper motor neurons was glutamate, but the neurotransmitter at the motor end plates of the target muscles (and lower motor neurons in general) was acetylcholine. How could the "wrong" neurotransmitter activate these muscles? It required a further multidisciplinary study to show that the receptors at the motor end plates adapted to the new neurotransmitter by changing one of the five components of their transmembrane channels, enabling them to respond to glutamate stimulation.

A young woman sustained a complete dislocation of T8 on T9 with a guillotine severance of the spinal cord. Both sciatic nerves were harvested simultaneously by separate surgical teams and implanted into the CST just above T8 (i.e., rostral to the injury). The distal ends of the nerve grafts were microsurgically coapted to the motor nerves to the gluteus maximus, gluteus medius, and quadriceps muscles (Figure 83-2) to achieve both extension and abduction of the thighs as well as extension of the knees. The operation lasted 13 hours, and intensive postoperative

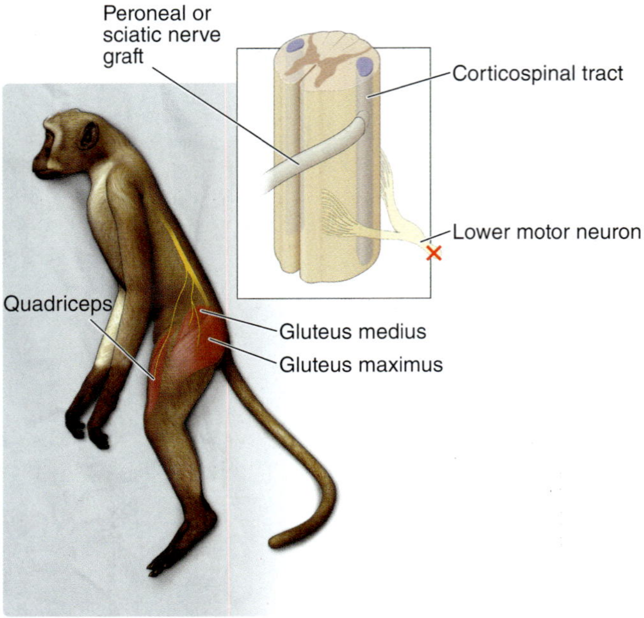

FIGURE 83-1 Experimental protocol for surgery in paraplegia. Nerve grafting from the corticospinal tract (CST) to the motor nerves to quadriceps, gluteus maximus, and gluteus medius.

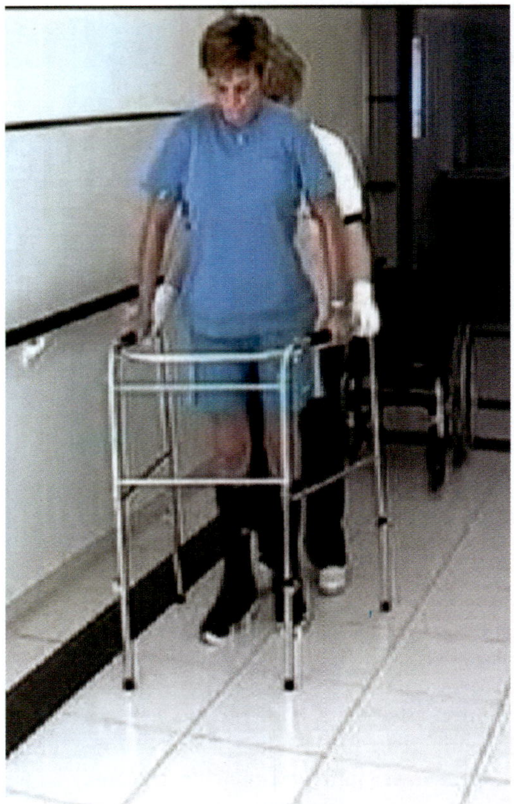

FIGURE 83-3 Photograph of a patient who sustained total transection of the spinal cord caused by a dislocation of T8 on T9, starting to walk after nerve grafting from the CST in the spinal cord to the motor nerves to the quadriceps and gluteus muscles.

reanimation was necessary. Twenty months later, the patient started to walk with a walker and later using quad (four-pronged) canes (Figure 83-3).

This operation and its outcome introduce the concept of brain plasticity. Multiple single-motor neurons scattered throughout the cerebral cortex fire together to produce a selective voluntary movement even when their original functions were completely different or possibly opposite. It would appear that the frontal lobe is able to recognize the new peripheral connections of the CST and to selectively stimulate those fibers that produce the desired movement. For example, extension of the knee occurs without antagonistic contractions from other muscles that would hinder this function.

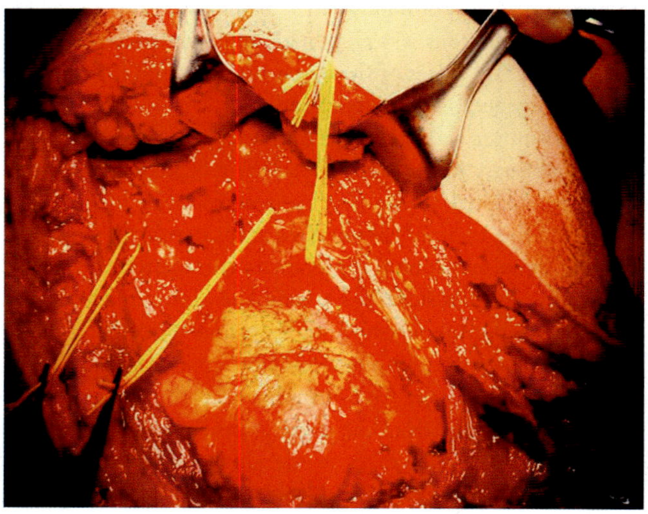

FIGURE 83-2 Coaptation of the motor nerves to the gluteus maximus and the gluteus medius to the nerve graft.

I have also enabled a man with paraplegia who had undergone total dislocation of T7 on T8 to walk by transferring both ulnar nerves from the upper to the lower limbs, by connecting the branch innervating both the flexor carpi ulnaris and the flexor digitorum profundus muscles to the ring and small fingers with a nerve graft to the nerve to the quadriceps muscle, and by connecting the branches to the hypothenar muscles and adductor pollicis directly to the nerves to the gluteus maximus and gluteus medius muscles (Figure 83-4). The ulnar nerves were stripped from the upper limbs in a distal-to-proximal direction starting from the hand and extending to their origin from the brachial plexus (Figure 83-5). The ulnar nerves were then tunneled under the skin along the lateral aspect of the trunk and then exposed through a skin incision. Each ulnar nerve was divided into two components: one to be connected anteriorly with a nerve graft to the nerve to the quadriceps and the other passing posteriorly for direct coaptation to the nerves to gluteus maximus and medius.

Therefore, the patient was literally able to *walk on his ulnar nerves* because of brain plasticity that initially enabled contraction of the quadriceps when the patient attempted to contract his ulnar forearm flexors and contraction of the gluteus muscles when he tried to activate his hypothenar muscles. However, within a short time, control of the muscles of his lower limbs occurred spontaneously by the patient simply attempting to move these muscles. In reality, these operations do not provide a complete solution for the treatment of paraplegia because

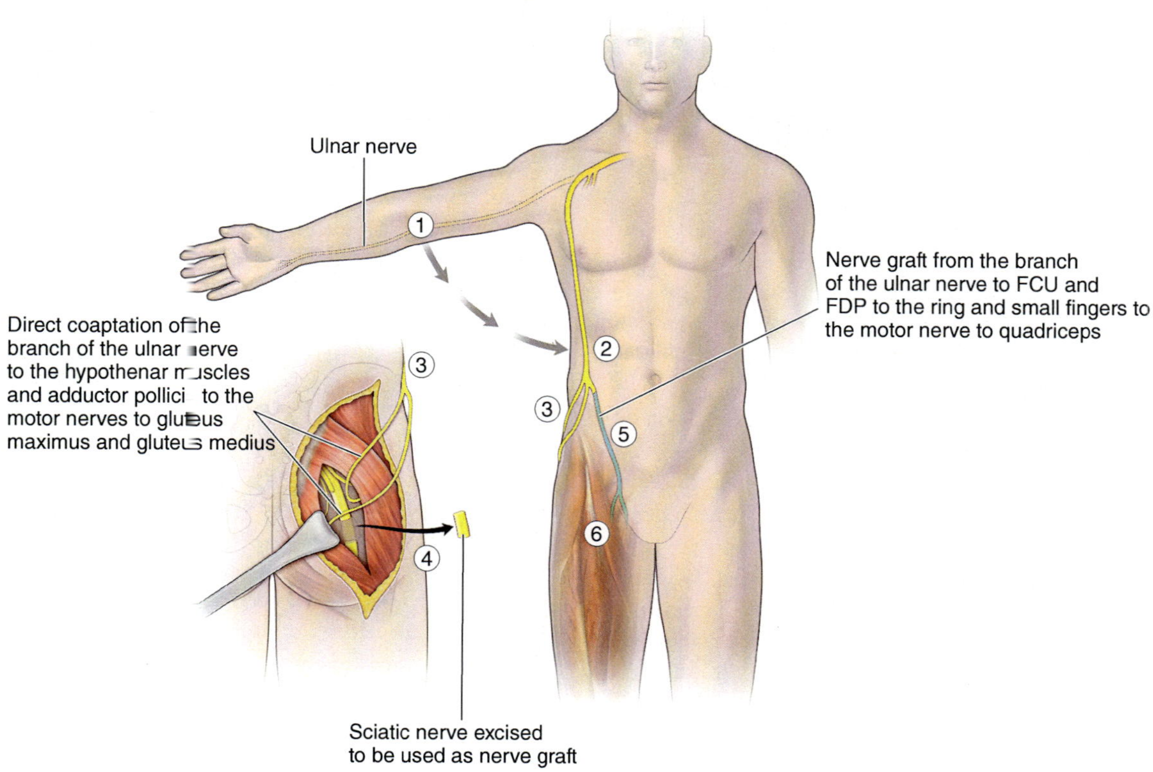

FIGURE 83-4 Schematic representation of the transfer of both ulnar nerves from the arms to the lower limbs. The numbers refer to the order of the steps in the procedure.

restoring ambulation is only one component of a complex problem. In fact, sensory function does not recover, and a number of other problems linked to this loss, together with the need for long, tiring, daily reeducation exercises, often obligates patients to return to their wheelchair even if they are already ambulating on the treadmill (as happened with two of my patients).

SURGICAL EXPOSURE OF THE NERVES OF THE LOWER LIMB

As mentioned earlier, injuries to the nerves of the lower limb can be managed, depending on the condition of the wound in exactly the same way as nerve injuries of the upper limb.

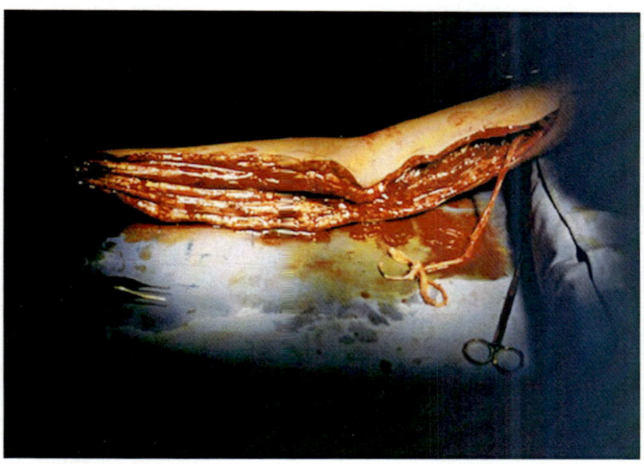

FIGURE 83-5 Harvest of the right ulnar nerve for transfer to the lower limb.

Skin incisions will vary according to which particular nerve has to be exposed.

Lateral Femoral Cutaneous Nerve

The lateral femoral cutaneous nerve of the thigh can be compressed at the anterior superior iliac spine (ASIS), causing "meralgia paraesthetica," manifest by paresthesias radiating along the lateral aspect of the thigh. This condition can be treated by careful neurolysis of the nerve as it passes below the inguinal ligament just medial to the ASIS.

Femoral Nerve

The femoral nerve and femoral artery may be involved in stab wounds of the inguinal region. (I have treated four of these injuries.) The exposure and access to the femoral nerve may require partial division of the inguinal ligament, which must be repaired at the end of the operation. Associated injuries to the femoral artery and vein and muscles can be treated through the same incision.

Sciatic Nerve

Injuries of the sciatic nerve at the hip are not uncommon after acetabular fractures and surgery of the hip joint (total hip replacement). The skin incision (Iselin approach) must be sufficiently large and the gluteus maximus reflected medially after division of its distal and lateral aponeurosis (which should be repaired after nerve and bone repair). The two underlying gemelli muscles, the obturator internus, and the quadratus femoris must be divided to expose a comminuted acetabular fracture.

Fractures of the femoral diaphysis may produce a disruption of the sciatic nerve in the posterior thigh, which should be treated at the same time as internal fixation of the femur, through a lateral skin incision that provides access to both the femur and the sciatic nerve in the posterior aspect of the thigh.

Popliteal Nerve

The sciatic and the popliteal nerves may be exposed through a posterior thigh incision and by separating the medial from the lateral muscles of the posterior thigh. The skin incision should either be zig-zag or curved to prevent contracture of a straight-line scar.

Diagrams of the muscle compartments of the thigh and lower leg can assist the surgeon to expose these nerves as they pass distally between the muscle bellies proximal and distal to the zone of trauma. The sciatic nerve may be exposed at virtually any level in the thigh, and distal extension of the incision will provide exposure of the popliteal and posterior tibial nerves. With regard to the accurate coaptation of group fascicles of the sciatic nerve, internal topographic maps previously described by various researchers, including myself, based on meticulous histologic dissections and electrical stimulation in vivo, can be referred to avoid fascicular mismatch, resulting in loss of function.

Common Peroneal Nerve

The common peroneal nerve can be injured by lacerations around the lateral aspect of the knee, by an iatrogenic injury during knee arthroscopy, or by compression of the nerve by a ganglion arising from the superior tibiofibular joint. All of these cause a palsy of the peroneal muscles, resulting in foot drop. In the case of a ganglion compressing or infiltrating the common peroneal nerve, removal of the ganglion and either external neurolysis or occasionally intrafascicular dissection of the nerve can result in full motor recovery in a short space of time.

Plantar Nerves of the Foot

Injuries to the sole of the foot may result in lacerations of the common digital or proper digital nerves. A diagram of the nerves in the sole of the foot may be useful when surgery is required to repair these plantar nerves to restore sensibility to the foot for both tactile appreciation and to prevent pressure sores.

Morton's Neuroma

Morton's neuroma is a neuroma of the sensory nerves to the toes that can produce excruciating pain. A microtraumatic alteration occurs within a plantar common digital nerve compressed between the heads of two adjacent metatarsals. Diagnosis is established by ultrasonography or magnetic resonance imaging (MRI). Excision of the neuroma cures the pathology (Figure 83-6).

Composite Injuries of the Lower Limb

It is important to remember that in severe trauma to the lower limb involving segmental loss of skin, bone, muscles, and nerves, it may still be possible to achieve a good functional result even when complicated by infection. Obviously, multiple operations are necessary, but a functional limb may still be achieved. As an alternative to amputation in a young patient and after bony consolidation, a nerve graft can be performed to the posterior tibial nerve to restore sensation to the sole of the foot to hopefully allow the patient to walk.

Nerve Tumors of the Lower Limb

Nerve tumors of the lower limb are neither frequent nor exceptional. They must be carefully diagnosed by ultrasonography or MRI scans. Depending on their pathology, removal may be fairly localized with preservation of nerve function. However, primary or secondary malignant tumors require major oncologic surgery, which may even include amputation.

Schwannomas are benign tumors that simply displace the axons and fascicles to the periphery, allowing the lesion to be "shelled out," preserving nerve function. Neurofibromas, by contrast, although also benign, infiltrate the structural interior of the nerve, resulting in loss of nerve function if excised. If removal of a nerve tumor necessitates sacrifice of part or all of an important nerve, nerve grafts should be used to reconstruct

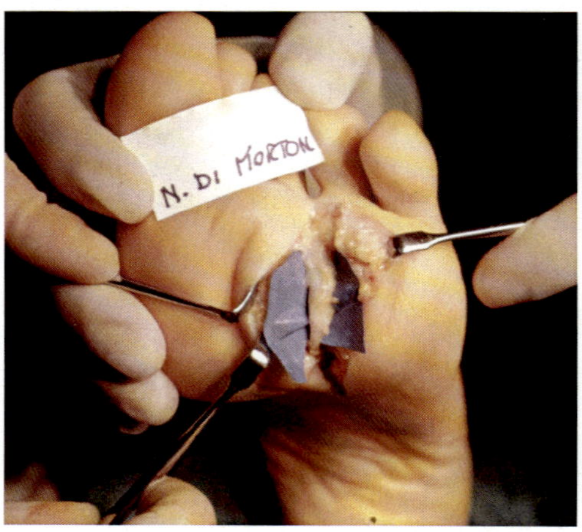

A

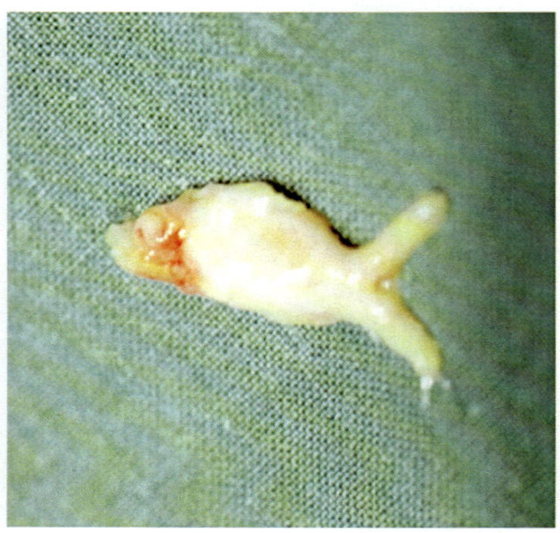

B

FIGURE 83-6 (A) Photograph of a Morton's neuroma. (B) Resected specimen.

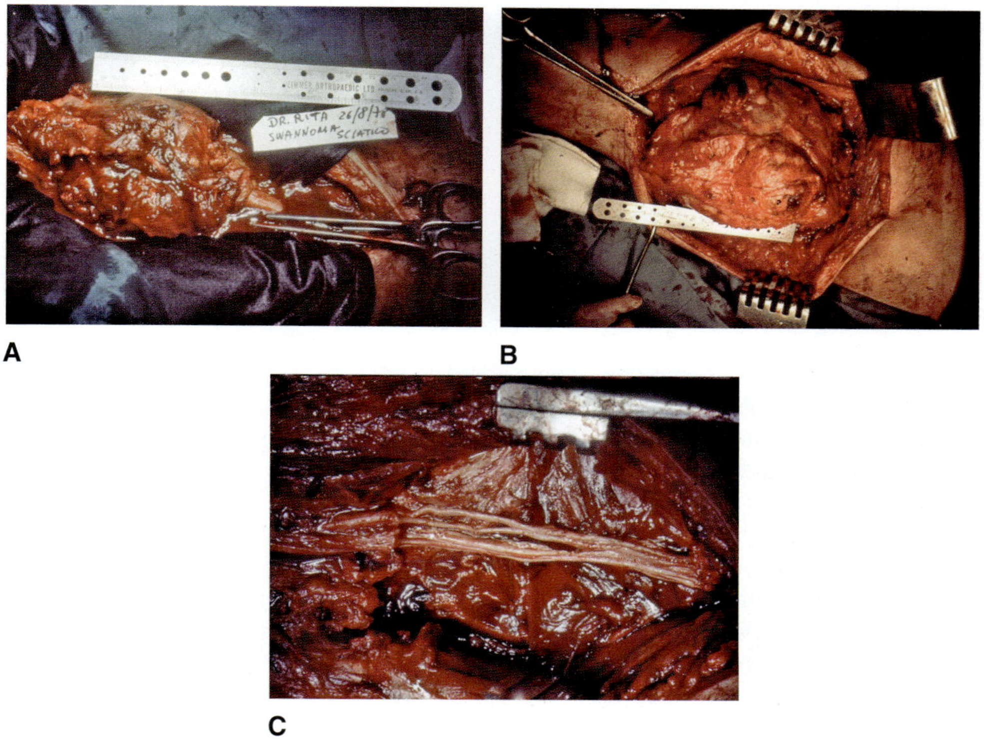

FIGURE 83-7 Radical excision (A, B) and nerve grafting (C) of a malignant schwannoma of the sciatic nerve. (The patient died 1.5 years later from metastases.)

the defect. In the rare case of a malignant schwannoma, radical excision followed by nerve grafting is obligatory, but the prognosis is gloomy—there is almost always a recurrence or metastasis leading to the demise of the individual (Figure 83-7).

Direct Muscle Neurotization

In some cases, the motor nerve cannot be found because either it has been avulsed from the muscle or surgically resected together with a portion of the muscle containing the motor end plates. In these situations, direct muscular neurotization should be considered, especially for restoration of important functions such as knee extension, foot extension, and plantar flexion. To restore these functions, the quadriceps muscle, the muscles of the anterior compartment of the lower leg, and the soleus and gastrocnemius muscles can be respectively reinnervated by direct muscular neurotization. Figure 83-8 shows neurotization of the denervated soleus and gastrocnemius muscles using the peroneal nerve with reestablishment of motor end plates 3 months later.

Salvage Procedures

Occasionally, direct nerve repair or nerve grafting is ineffective in restoring function. Conventional tendon transfers can

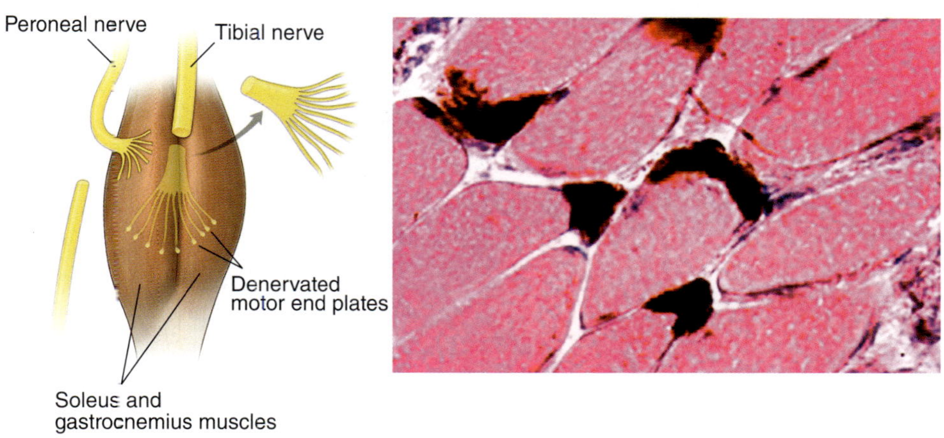

FIGURE 83-8 (A) Schematic representation of direct muscle neurotization. (B) The appearance of mature motor end plates is seen 3 months later.

restore some degree of useful function. Transfer of the semitendinosus and biceps femoris to the quadriceps tendon in the anterior thigh may restore adequate extension to the knee. Transfer of the tendon of tibialis posterior muscle (possibly together with the peroneus brevis) anteriorly can provide satisfactory dorsiflexion to the ankle. To restore plantar flexion of the foot strong enough to allow the patient to walk on tiptoe, the tendon of the tibialis anterior muscle together with the peroneus brevis may be passed posteriorly through the interosseous membrane and sutured into the calcaneus under tension.

Just as in the upper limb, nerve transfers and tendon transfers in the lower limb require meticulous reeducation of both motor and sensory modalities (particularly sensation on the sole of the foot to prevent pressure sores), together with the administration of neurotrophic medications to help nerve regeneration.

Reeducation of the motor nerves of the lower limb includes massage and electrical stimulation to maintain muscle bulk during denervation (electrical stimulation is applied to the muscles and *not* to the nerves themselves because as I have shown experimentally, application of electricity to a nerve simply induces fibrosis within the nerve); splints for both passive and active range of motion (particularly for the knee); ambulatory obstacle courses; and physical exercise in a swimming pool, possibly under the guide of a personal trainer.

REFERENCES

1. Brunelli G (ed). *Textbook of Microsurgery*. Masson, Milano et al. 1988, p. 1038.
2. Brunelli GA. Direct neurotisation of muscles by presynaptic motoneurons. *J Reconstr Microsurg* 2001;17:631–636.
3. Brunelli GA, Brunelli GR. Experimental surgery in spinal cord lesions by connecting upper motor neurons directly to peripheral targets. *J Peripher Nerv System* 1996;1:111–118.
4. Brunelli GA, et al. Spinal cord experimental repair: CNS-PNS grafting gives functional results. Brescia, Gruppo Editoriale Delfo 1996, p. 1–55.
5. Brunelli G, Milanesi S, Bartolaminelli P, et al. Experimental grafts in spinal cord lesions (preliminary report). *Ital J Orthop Traumat* 1983;9(suppl):53–56.
6. Brunelli GA, Spano P, Barlati S, et al. Glutamatergic reinnervation through peripheral nerve graft dictate assembly of glutametergic synapses at rat skeletal muscles. *Proc Nat Acad Sci* 2005;102(24):8752–8657.
7. Pizzi M, Brunelli GA, Barlati S, Spano P. Glutamatergic innervation of rat skeletal muscles by supraspinal neurons. *Curr Opin Neurobiol* 2006;16:323–328.
8. von Wild KR, Brunelli GA. Restoration of locomotion in paraplegics with aid of autologous bypass grafts for direct neurotisation of muscles by upper motor neurons—the future surgery of the spinal cord? *Acta Neurochir Suppl* 2003;87:107–112.

CHAPTER 84

Replantation in the Lower Extremity

S. Raja Sabapathy and R. Ravindra Bharathi

The desire of patients and their families for reattachment of an amputated part is the same whether it is the upper limb or the lower limb. The goal of replantation surgery also remains the same—the functional outcome of the replanted extremity must be better than the closure of the amputated stump and provision of the best available prosthesis. The nature of the injury causing the amputation, technical considerations and relative risks involved in the procedure, demands on the replanted extremity, and outcome are very different between the upper and lower limbs, and hence replantation of amputations of the lower extremity is performed less frequently.

Many factors influence this decision of the surgeon. Lower limb amputations are mostly caused by crush or high-energy injuries, resulting in extensive loss of tissue, which precludes replantation. Complications in major replantation are directly related to the extent of muscle mass in the amputated part and ischemia time. Proximal replants of the lower limb have higher morbidity because of the higher volume of muscle mass, and any mortality in replantation surgery is unacceptable. Inherent factors, such as an increased incidence of arterial disease in the lower limb with aging and inadequate nerve recovery, compound the problem. Significant skeletal shortening, which is an integral part of the replantation of crush or avulsion amputations, is less well tolerated in the lower limb. Shortening up to 10 cm is compatible with good function in the upper limb, but 3 cm of length discrepancy in the lower limb almost always requires secondary procedures for correction. Even more than all these factors, technologic advancements in the design and manufacture of lower limb prostheses can now provide functionally efficient prostheses to meet the demands of locomotion and stable stance.

Despite these factors, reports exist in the literature of satisfactory long-term outcomes of lower limb replantations (1–5). Replantations performed for the correct indications have achieved excellent functional outcomes. Therefore, it becomes the responsibility of the surgeon to be well informed to guide the patient and the family when faced with an amputated lower limb.

HISTORICAL PERSPECTIVE

The first report of a lower limb replant in the English literature was by Magee and Parker in 1972, who reported a successful foot replantation in Australia (6). The Chinese have been credited with having performed many lower limb replants earlier than this, which was brought to the attention of the rest of the world by the American Replantation Mission to China (7,8). Usei et al. from Japan reported a 4-year follow-up study on the replantation of the distal third of the left leg of a 4-year-old child in 1979. The child sustained a guillotine amputation and had a successful outcome (9). Since then, it has become firmly established as an acceptable treatment option for an amputation of the lower limb. What makes the difference between upper and lower limb replantation is that although numerous centers have accumulated experience of hundreds of patients in upper limb replantation, most of the reports of replantation of the lower limb remain as isolated case reports or small case series.

Fang et al. reported a bilateral leg replant in 2012, the right 10 cm above the ankle joint and the left at the ankle joint, and noted that their literature search revealed only 12 successful bilateral lower limb replants (10). The first report of a bilateral lower limb replant is from Scotland by Buckley et al., who reported their experience in reimplantation of both feet in 1988 (11). In bilateral amputations, the severity of trauma may preclude orthotopic replantation of the extremities, and in such cases, crossover replantation of one foot has been performed in combination with a prosthetic limb. This is based on the premise that the functional outcome and ease of rehabilitation is better than having two prosthetic limbs. This again was probably first done in China, and two isolated cases of successful cross-foot replants in patients who had sustained bilateral traumatic lower extremity amputations were brought to the attention of the world by the American Replantation Mission to China (7). Chen and Zeng reported the Chinese experience of this type of surgery in 1983 (12).

More common circumstances involve the salvage of lower extremity amputations using fillet flaps and tissues from the amputated part retrieved as free flaps to salvage the knee joint and convert a possible above-knee amputation to a below-knee amputation and provide stable sensate cover to the amputated stump (13).

INDICATIONS FOR REPLANTATION OF THE LOWER LIMB

Patient selection remains the main criterion for the ultimate outcome of lower limb replantation. Unlike the upper limb, clear consensus on indications has not emerged in lower limb replantation because of the paucity of large singe center experiences. Nevertheless, we can suggest guidelines based on the available accumulated experience.

Age

The majority of cases of lower limb replantation reported are in children or young adults. Yildirim and Akoz reported a big toe replantation in a 3-month-old child, which is probably the youngest age for a lower limb replant reported in the literature (14). The length of the big toe from the metatarsophalangeal (MTP) joint to the tip was equal to that of the contralateral big toe at 6 months of follow-up. Jones et al. reported successful replantation of the leg in a 7-month-old preambulatory infant (Figure 84-1). The amputation was at the level of the proximal lower leg with the tibia transected just distal to the epiphyseal growth plate. A total of 2.5 cm of shortening was done during surgery. At 7 years of follow-up, the patient had 5.5 cm of limb length discrepancy and foot drop but had good sensation on the sole. Despite wearing a 4-cm lift in the right shoe, he was very happy and played games equal to his peers (3). All of the replants done in children have reportedly done well. The epiphysis retains the growth capacity, and growth in the distal segment has retained up to 95% of the normal; in some children, overgrowth is also possible (2,15). The plasticity of the growing human brain, the possibility of good adaptation, and the potential for good neuronal recovery all combine to produce good outcomes in children (Figure 84-2). Surgeons are reluctant to replant lower limbs in patients older than 50 years of age because of the inherent arterial disease, poor potential for nerve recovery, and the longer inpatient rehabilitation period. Age alone is not the only significant prognostic factor; selection has to be individualized.

Patient's General Condition

Every replantation surgery, even if it is a small part, is a major surgical undertaking. Comorbid factors existing in the patient and associated injuries to other organ systems increase the morbidity of the procedure. Apart from the long duration of the procedure, proximal replantations may need significant blood replacement and support after the procedure. Mamakos reported the need for 17 units of whole blood for an above-knee amputation (16), and Yildrium et al. reported the use of 300 mL of blood for great toe replantation in a 3-month-old child secondary to venous insufficiency (14). Such demands, if they occur in a compromised individual, will produce unacceptable morbidity.

Ischemia Time

Complications directly attributable to the replantation depend on the ischemia time and the extent of the muscle mass in the amputated part. In the lower limb, the muscle mass is significantly higher, and the potential for complications is also greater the more proximal the level of replantation. One must be cautious to replant an above-knee or a proximal third lower leg amputation with a cold ischemia of more than 6 hours. In upper limb replantation, guidelines for preliminary shunting in case of long ischemia time are clearly defined (17). Because of the volume of muscle mass, the risk-to-benefit ratio is more unfavorable for replantation of the lower limb, and it is not usual practice to do preliminary shunting. Such limbs are better amputated. Lower third leg and foot replants do not contain much muscle volume and therefore can withstand cold ischemia for a longer period.

Type and Extent of Tissue Damage

Lower limb amputations are most often caused by crush or avulsion injuries, and debridement causes further tissue deficit. Despite skeletal shortening, soft tissue cover procedures are needed for most of them. If there is a defect, then usually a free flap is the only solution. Wickham et al. replanted a guillotine amputation of the foot in an 11-year-old child with 3 cm of acute shortening. Despite repairing both the dorsalis pedis and the posterior tibial arteries and the favorable mechanism of injury, the child still needed a free gracilis flap for the skin necrosis and to cover exposed implants 2 weeks after replantation. The flap was anastomosed end to side to the posterior tibial vessels proximal to the level of amputation (18). Demanding surgical procedures for soft tissue coverage are often needed in the immediate postoperative period, so if the initial injury itself is very severe, one has to be guarded in the decision to replant a lower limb.

A leg amputation associated with a foot injury is not a good indication for replantation. Good structural integrity of the foot with the potential for innervation of the sole is important.

Bilateral Amputations

Indications for replantation become stronger in the event of bilateral lower limb amputations because the difficulties faced by a bilateral amputee are higher, and rehabilitation is more demanding. The challenge is also to achieve equal limb length. More often, the better less damaged foot is replanted, and the patient is provided with a prosthesis for the other limb (Figure 84-3). If ipsilateral replantation would be difficult, crossover replantation should be considered.

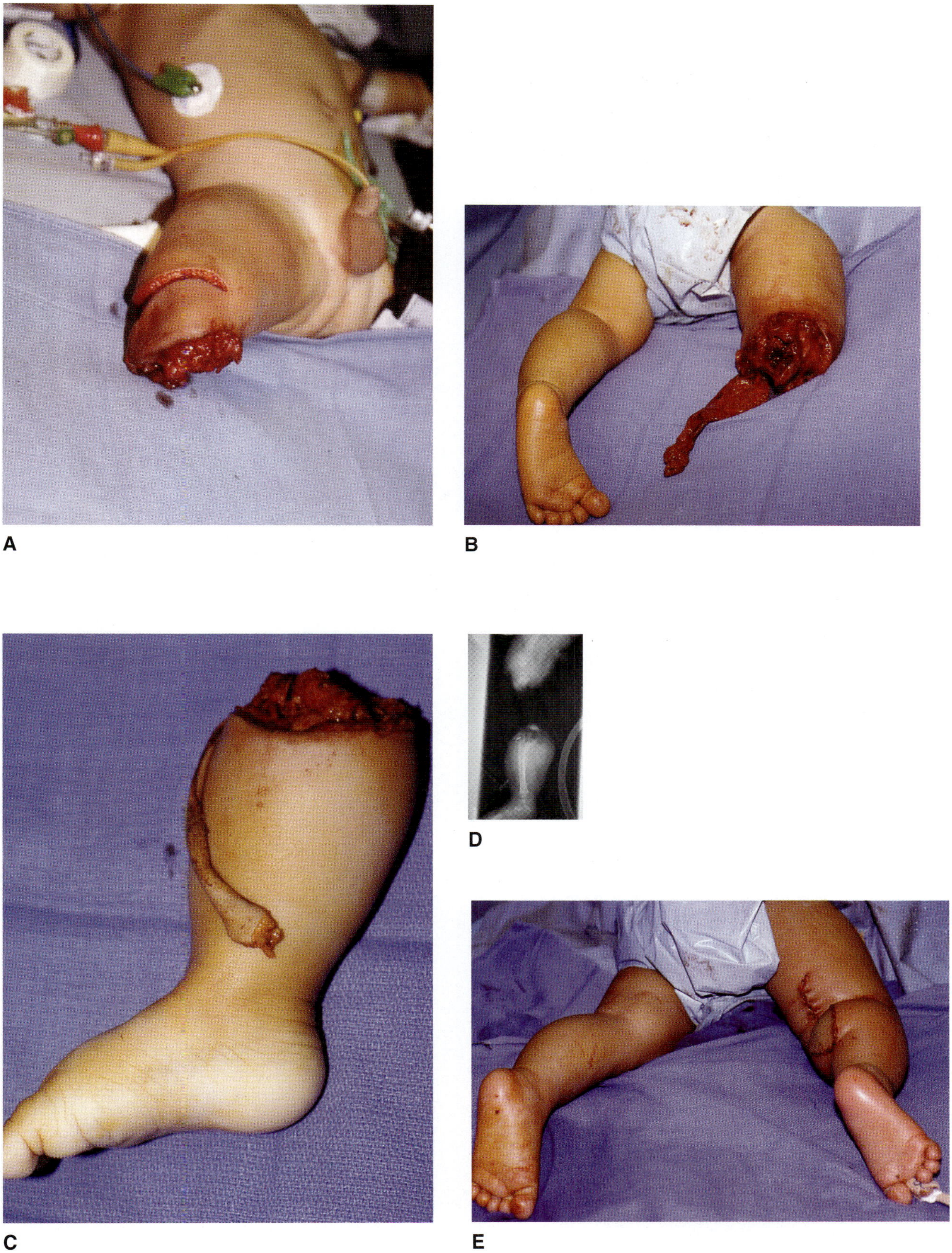

FIGURE 84-1 Complete amputation of the right lower leg just below the knee in a 7-month-old boy (**A** to **D**). Immediately after replantation of the right lower leg (**E**), 2 years after surgery

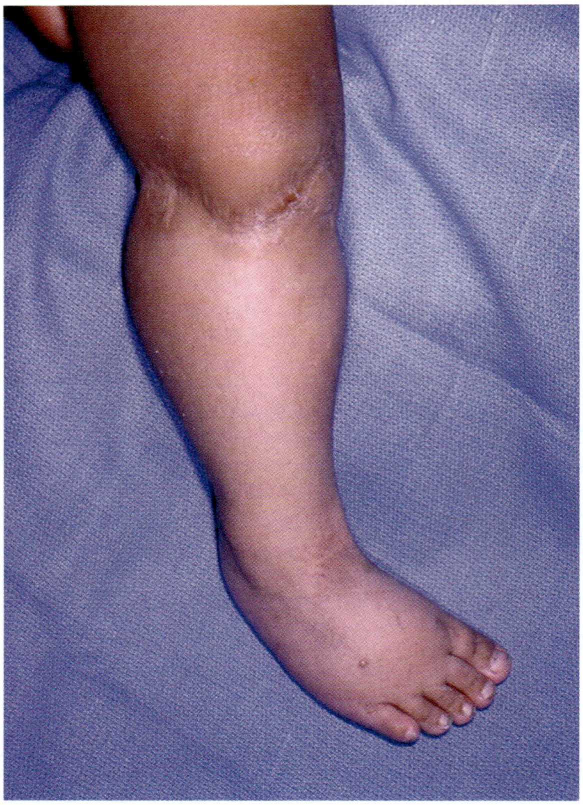

F

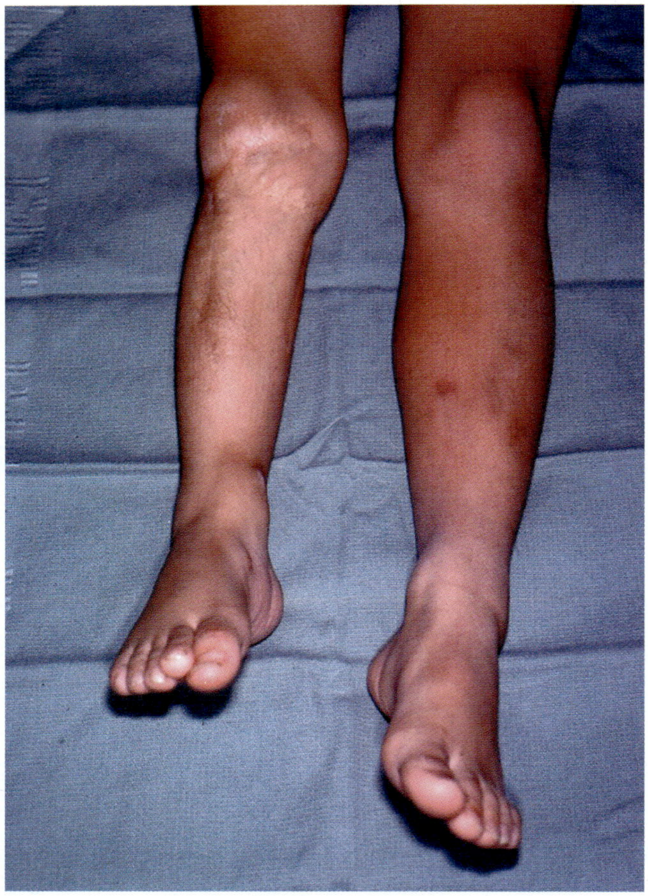

G

FIGURE 84-1 (*Continued*) (**F**), and 7 years after surgery (**G**) showing the leg length discrepancy. (Used with permission from Dr. Neil F. Jones, MD.)

Just like the upper limb, there is no reliable scoring system to decide the indications for replantation of the lower limb. Battiston et al. attempted to produce a scoring system based on their experience of 14 lower limb amputations in 12 patients, including two bilateral amputations (19). All achieved initial success, but five were amputated secondarily at various points of time for complications. They proposed a scoring system modifying the parameters used in the Mangled Extremity Severity Score (MESS) system for classifying severe extremity injuries (Table 84-1). According to their study, the final result is influenced mainly by soft tissue defects requiring extensive reconstruction and poor nerve recovery, and

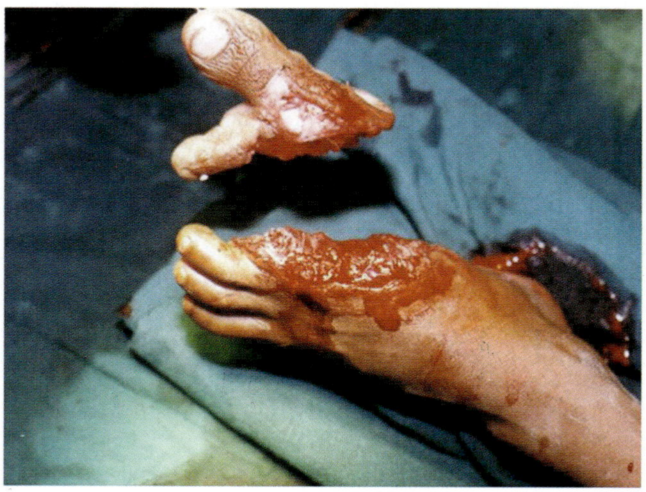

A

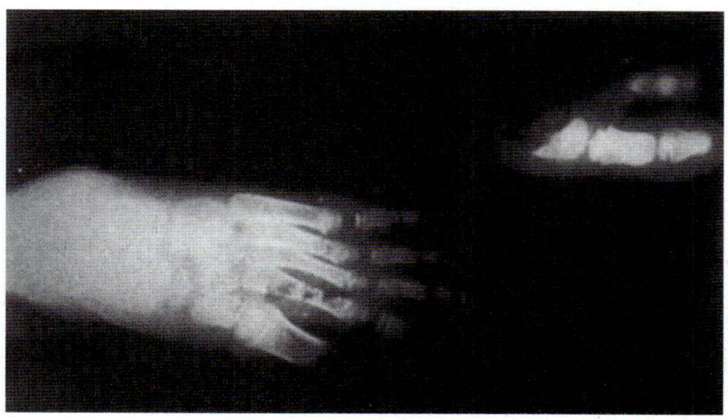

B

FIGURE 84-2 (**A**) Total crush amputation of the left great and second toes in an 11-year-old boy. (**B**) Radiograph showing the amputation through the head of the first metatarsal and through the proximal phalanx of the second toe.

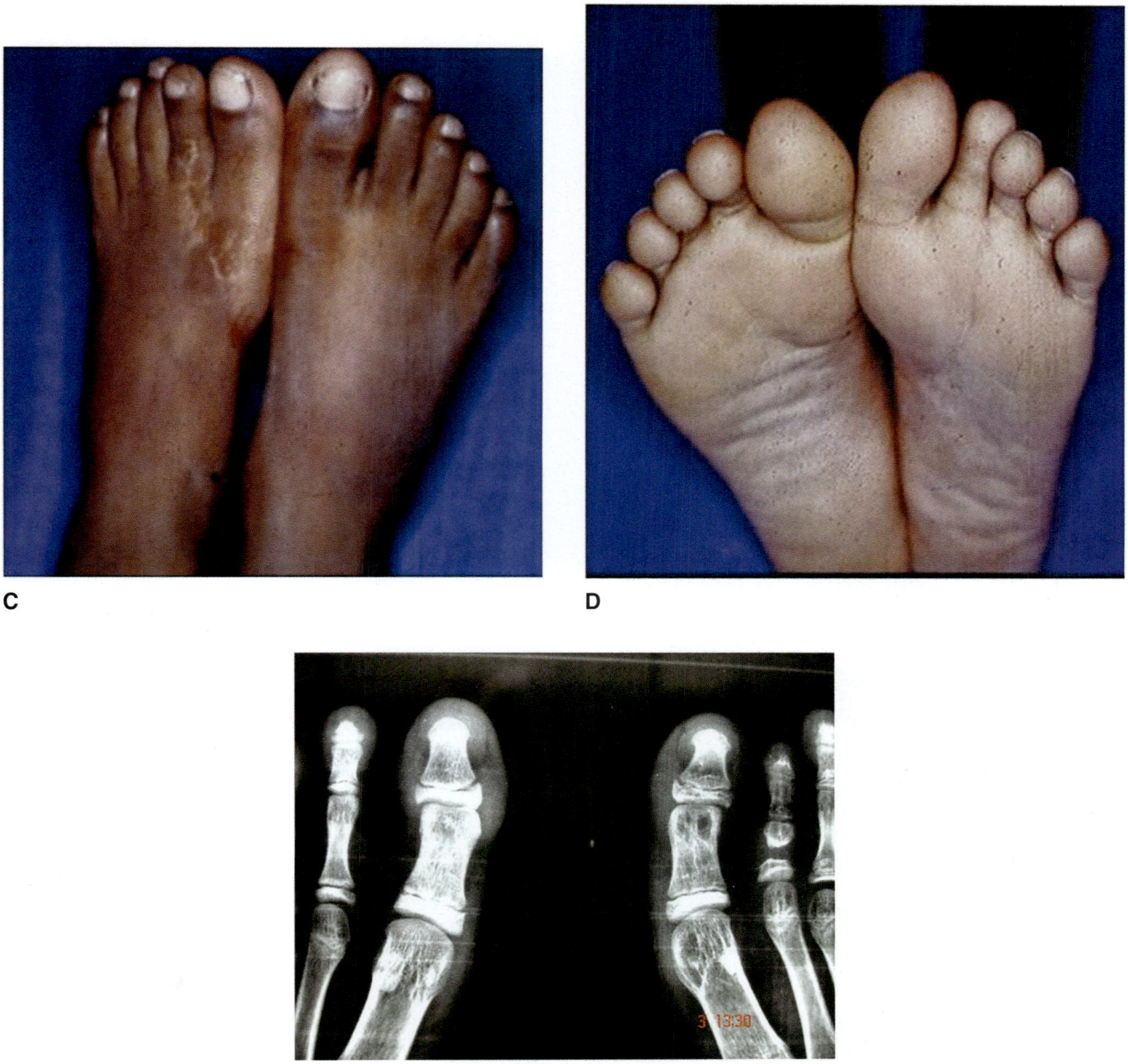

C D E

FIGURE 84-2 (*Continued*) (C) and (D) Outcome after 18 months. (E) Postoperative radiograph at 18 months showing the open epiphysis and normal growth in the uninjured bones of the great toe. There is a nonunion of the proximal phalanx of the second toe because considerable bone was excised during debridement.

delayed amputations correlate with complex initial problems such as ischemia time, type and extent of tissue trauma, age, and general condition. Generally, patients younger than 50 years of age in good health with no comorbid factors with less severe soft tissue injuries and cold ischemia time of less than 3 hours are good candidates for replantation. The scoring system still can only serve as a guide because one of the most important factors is the surgeon's experience in dealing with such injuries and patient factors. They significantly influence the ultimate outcome, so each case has to be assessed on an individual basis.

Above-Knee Amputation

The literature is striking in its absence of any long-term report of a patient with an above-knee replantation. This in itself should influence the surgeon regarding the paucity of ideal circumstances for replantation of an above-knee amputation.

TECHNICAL CONSIDERATIONS

Most replants of the lower extremity reported in the literature are of the foot or below the distal third of the leg. Proximal replants of the lower limb are more demanding on the surgeon's

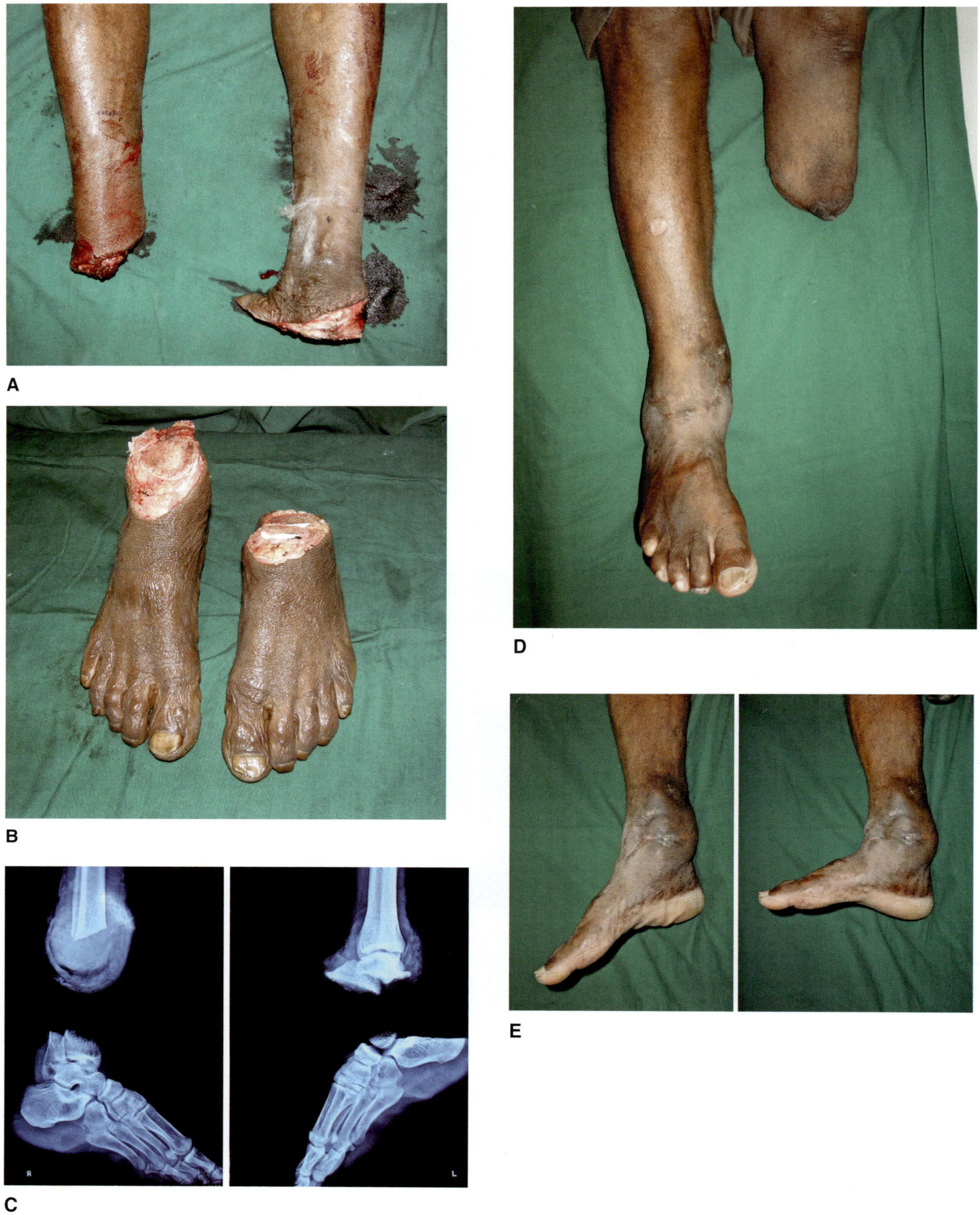

FIGURE 84-3 (A) to (C) Total bilateral amputation of the lower limbs in a 47-year-old manual laborer, the right just above the ankle and the left just below the ankle joint. The right side was replanted and left not replanted because the patient did not want any secondary procedure for limb lengthening or ankle stiffness. (D) and (E) Result 7 years after surgery. The patient has 10 degrees of active dorsiflexion and 50 degrees of plantar flexion and is satisfied with a below-knee prosthesis on the left side. He has 14 mm 2 PD on the lateral half of the foot and protective sensation on the medial side.

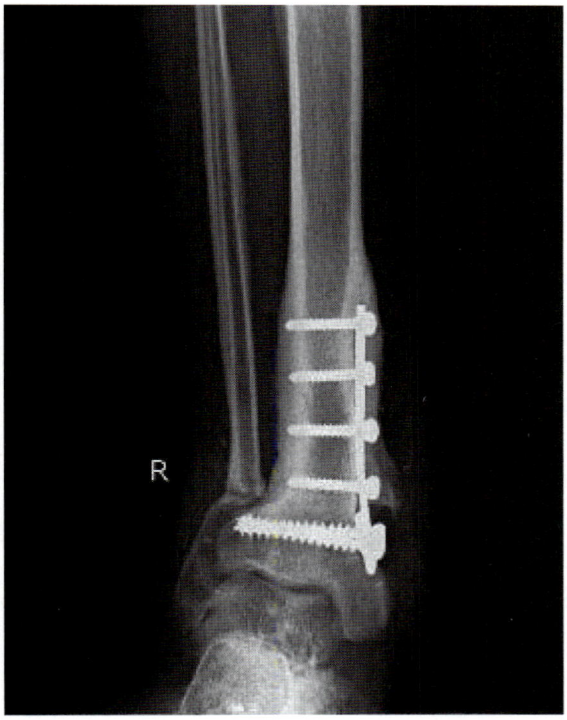

F

FIGURE 84-3 (*Continued*) (**F**) Radiograph 7 years after replantation showing good bone union. There is lateral tilt at the ankle, but the ankle is stable and pain free.

skill and time than replants of the upper limb. Complications can also be quite high, being the rule rather than the exception (20). The ability to deal with these postoperative complications makes lower limb replantation a realistic undertaking.

Debridement

Debridement has to be radical in both the proximal and distal segments. The vessels and nerves are identified first, and then the wound is radically debrided. It is good to repair as many vessels as possible, so both arteries and their accompanying venae comitantes as well as the superficial veins are identified. Early identification prevents inadvertent resection of long segments of vessels and nerves during debridement of a contaminated wound. After identification, the vessels and nerves are resected until a normal-appearing structure is reached. Usually there is a thin plane of tissue that can be excised so that the contaminants are removed.

Degloved and avulsed skin flaps survive less well in the lower limb than in the upper limb and should be excised. In proximal amputations, all loosely attached muscles need to be excised. When muscle tissue is excised, "hemostasis" must be achieved in both the proximal and the distal segments. Larger veins need to be ligated. If the amputation is in the proximal third or through the soleus, the soleal plexus of veins may need to be underrun with sutures. In the author's experience in a proximal third leg replant, postclamp release bleeding through the soleal

TABLE 84-1 Scoring System of Indications for Replantation of the Lower Limb (19)*

Age			>50	30-50	<30
Score			2	1	0
General conditions			Shock	Systemic disease Diabetes, hypertension Heart problems	Good condition
Score			4	2	0
Ischemia time			Cold ≥6 hr, warm ≤4 hours	Cold 3–6 hr	Cold ≤3 hr
Score			4	2	0
Local conditions			Severe contamination Comminution, bone loss	Complex fracture without severe contamination	Simple fractures, no bone loss
Score			2	1	0
Soft tissue problems	Severe injuries to posterior tibial nerve	Large skin and muscle–tendon loss	Severe skin loss but good muscle condition	Partial skin necrosis	Good condition
Score	4	3	2	1	0

*≥8, contraindication for replantation; 6–7, possible replantation but poor functional result; ≤5, indication for replantation.

plexus of veins was very difficult to control. It is much easier done during debridement than after skeletal fixation, which reduces access to the bleeding veins.

Skeletal Fixation

Stable skeletal fixation is a must for early rehabilitation and bone union. K-wires have been used in the majority of foot replants. Shortening of the metatarsals and phalanges does not materially affect ambulation. If the amputation is near the ankle joint, an arthrodesis has to be performed. The literature is sparse of reports of through-ankle replantations. Many such injuries are treated by below-knee amputation. Amputations in the distal third of the leg are fixed by plating. Auxiliary external fixation can also be used for stability of the fixation and to maintain the foot in neutral position. Skeletal shortening may be extensive and is dictated by the nature of the injury. Shortening greater than 3 cm usually requires secondary lengthening. After acute shortening, primary Ilizarov distraction lengthening has been reported, but usually the leg length discrepancy is addressed in a secondary procedure with the site of distraction being proximal to the site of amputation.

In a replantation of an amputation of the proximal third of the leg, Mizoyan et al. performed massive shortening of 13 cm and primary application of an Ilizarov frame (21). Distraction was then started on the 20th day at the site of osteosynthesis, but a corticotomy in the lower third also had to be used later. Full bone length was achieved 332 days after replantation. At 10 days after surgery, a free flap had to be used for skin necrosis and infection. This case confirmed that distraction occurred at the sites of the nerve and vascular repairs. Datiashvili et al. have performed distraction secondarily and took 2 years to reach normal length (1).

The type of fixation chosen must be done quickly, particularly in proximal amputations, because the ischemia time in a major replant with significant muscle mass in the distal segment, poses unacceptable risk to life of the individual.

Vessel Repair

As a general principle, as many vessels as possible are repaired. Positioning is the key to make vessel repairs in foot replants easier. Dorsal arteries and veins are adequate for foot and great toe replants. In the supine position, the vessels lie in a vertical orientation making the anastomoses difficult. One way to make it easier is to flex the knee to 90 degrees so that the foot rests on the table, and in this position, the repair of the dorsal veins, dorsalis pedis, and metatarsal arteries are easy. If the amputation is at a more distal level near the web space, the lateral toes mostly depend on the plantar arteries. Anastomosing plantar arteries is technically demanding. Lin et al. suggested the use of a vein graft from the dorsalis pedis artery to the digital arteries. The distal anastomosis to the digital artery is performed on a back table, bony fixation is achieved with K-wires, and then the proximal anastomosis is done to the dorsalis pedis artery (22). Another option is to pass the K-wires distally through the toes, suture the plantar skin, repair the plantar arteries, and then carefully drive the wires proximally in a retrograde manner. The dorsal veins can then be anastomosed. In doing this, one has to be careful not to kink the anastomoses. Kinking of a vessel may result in loss of the replant.

As many vessels as possible are repaired. In the leg, most reports have advocated the repair of both arteries. Similarly, both superficial veins and the venae comitantes are repaired. The more proximal the replant in the leg, the more vein repairs are advocated to reduce the number of transfusions required.

Soft Tissue Cover

Critical structures need to be covered by well vascularized soft tissue. Almost all lower limb replants with the exception of foot replants invariably need some additional soft tissue procedure. In the series reported by Cavadas et al., the average number of additional procedures was 3.1. (20). The ability to successfully perform these additional procedures determines the overall success. Most often free flaps are used; usually muscle flaps such as gracilis and latissimus dorsi or skin flaps such as the anterolateral thigh flap are used. In upper limb forearm replants, sometimes one artery is used for revascularization of the distal part, and the other artery is used as the recipient vessel for a free flap. In leg replants, it is advisable to repair both arteries of the leg. It is risky to use one artery for end-to-end anastomosis of a free flap. An end-to-side repair at a level proximal to the replant anastomosis is preferred for the free flap, or a "flow-through" flap can be done.

Crossover Replantation

In bilateral amputations, because of the magnitude of the injury and when anatomic replantation of both extremities is not possible, crossover replantation is an option to salvage at least one extremity because the function achieved with a crossover replanted foot in combination with a prosthesis on the other side is better than that of two artificial limbs.

Bone fixation and muscle group suturing is a challenge in cross-foot replantation. Wang et al. reported a case in 1995 and discussed the various techniques of skeletal fixation (23). In one of the early reports from China, the tibia was step-cut first and then fixed with screws. In another report, an intramedullary pin was used. In both, the fibula was left without fixation. Long-term follow-up regarding ankle stability is lacking. Ricketts et al. reported an 11-year follow-up of a cross-leg replantation (24). The tibia was rigidly fixed with a 10-hole DCP plate, and then the distal fibula was fixed to the tibia with a screw and the proximal fibula was left free. The patient ambulated with an above-knee prosthesis on the other side and with a single walking stick. The ankle was stable. All of these techniques involve tibia-to-tibia contact. Wang et al. presented an unique method of bone fixation (23). Each fibula was stripped of periosteum for 5 cm on both the right and left sides and thinned sufficiently so it could be pegged into the marrow cavity of the opposite tibia. A snug fit was achieved, and the stability was excellent. Additional bone grafts were placed around the tibia, and satisfactory union was reported. No plates or screws were used. Careful passive mobilization was started by 3 weeks, and early signs of radiologic union were evident by 8 weeks. This technique has the advantage of easier alignment and suturing of the various muscle groups. All reports emphasize the need to achieve early bone union so that rehabilitation can be started early.

Appropriate vessels and nerves are repaired directly. Because there is no necessity to restore normal length in the distal segment, direct end-to-end repair of vessels and nerves is possible. The invertor and evertor muscles have to be switched for suturing. Adequate ankle flexion and extension have been achieved in all cases.

Crossover replantation does produce some aesthetic issues and can also affect the psychological well-being of some individuals. Srivastava reported his experience of ipsilateral replantation with crossover segmental transfer of tissue from the other leg in two cases of bilateral amputation (25). Both patients had total amputation of the proximal leg on one side and a severely crushed lower third of the leg on the other side, with an intact distal part of the foot. Normally, this type of combination is an indication for a crossover foot replant. To avoid aesthetic problems, Srivastava segmentally excised tissue from the amputated leg to match the deficit in the other leg and used it as a flow-through flap. In one case, the transferred segment was rotated 180 degrees, which allowed the tibia and fibula of the salvaged extremity above and the ankle mortise to articulate with the talus below. Thus, in this case, near-normal anatomy of bone and soft tissue was restored in the lower third of the leg and ankle joint. In this way, the foot anatomy was maintained, and socially acceptable results were achieved.

SECONDARY PROCEDURES AFTER REPLANTATION

Secondary procedures are basically required to address four issues: (1) soft tissue problems in the postoperative period, (2) to correct limb length discrepancy, (3) soft tissue procedures to correct distal deformity or obtain balance, and (4) secondary nerve reconstruction to achieve a sensate foot.

Soft tissue problems requiring some type of coverage have to be anticipated as a norm in lower limb replants. This occurs even with massive shortening to obtain primary bone contact. This is quite different than the situation in the upper limb and is due to the poor intercompartmental collateral circulation in the lower limb.

There is only one report of immediate distraction lengthening at the site of bone contact. Proximal metaphyseal osteotomy and callus lengthening is usually performed 2 to 3 months later when the wounds settle down.

Because of contractures of the long flexors and poor recovery of intrinsic muscles of the foot, claw deformities can occur in the foot, which can be disabling. To prevent trophic ulcers, flexor tendon tenotomies or arthrodesis of the interphalangeal or MTP joints are performed to straighten the toes.

Acute shortening during replantation makes direct nerve repair possible. If shortening is not done, nerve reconstruction must be done early, preferably within 6 months. We recommend marking the distal end of the nerve in an easily accessible position so that lengthy exploratory incisions are avoided (17).

REDUCING COMPLICATIONS AND ACHIEVING GOOD OUTCOMES

Specific instruments for measuring the outcome of lower limb replantation are yet to be devised, and it may never be possible to produce one because the issues involved are so subjective and differ from patient to patient, and there are wide social and cultural demands in different parts of the world.

The worst possible outcome is to undergo secondary amputation after replantation and undergoing years of rehabilitation. Gao et al. (26). reported a 19-year-old man who underwent replantation of a near-total amputation at the level of the distal thigh. He required multiple microsurgical flap procedures for soft tissue coverage around the knee, secondary nerve reconstruction 6 months after the surgery, nonunion of the femur, and stiff joints. Four years after the surgery, he demanded amputation for severe cold intolerance and dysfunction of the lower limb. The multiple complications that he experienced eventually led to his decision for secondary amputation. He resumed his normal activities 6 months after an above-knee amputation.

This case history and the sequence of events illustrates that achieving good outcomes in replantation surgery depends on avoiding complications and early rehabilitation. Ensuring primary healing of the wound and achieving primary bone union and early nerve repair are necessary for success. Aggressive management preempting complications is key. In a series of 12 patients with 13 amputations through the tibia or below, Cavadas achieved a 100% survival rate. One patient died because of pulmonary thromboembolism. Soft tissue necrosis occurred in 83% of cases, which required flap coverage, mostly by free flaps with success. Weight-bearing time ranged from 8 to 16 months, and all but one patient achieved Chen functional grade of I or II (20). Because most lower limb injuries are crush or avulsion injuries, the surgeon needs to have a low threshold to shorten the bone to obtain primary bone contact and union. Salon et al. (27) reported the experience of 18 lower limb revascularizations or replantations during the period 1975 to 1989 with a protocol of length preservation. Only two (11%) survived, and all failures were due to poor debridement and inadequate shortening of bone. Between 1990 and 1993, the protocol was changed to primary shortening and secondary lengthening, and all five limbs during this period survived with a good outcome. Average initial shortening of 93 mm enabled direct internal osteosynthesis. Secondary lengthening was initiated early in the proximal metaphyseal area, and average lengthening of 85 mm was achieved. The final average limb length discrepancy was only 8 mm. At an average follow-up of 11 years, all patients were walking. The speed of nerve regeneration was faster than usual at an average of 1.926 mm/day, which they attributed to distraction.

Soft tissue coverage procedures are normal and must be done earlier than later. A free flap may be needed at the same operation as the replantation. Various flaps ranging from fascio-cutaneous flaps, free flaps, "flow-through," flaps and even cross-leg flaps have been used to salvage the situation. Early failures have been due to hemorrhage or infection, and the cause can be traced back to poor debridement or failure of soft tissue cover.

The subset of patients who benefit most are bilateral amputees. A bilateral amputee is totally immobile as soon as he or she removes the prosthesis and becomes wheelchair dependent. In many countries and societies where facilities for disabled people are not optimal, these individuals become severely disabled and socially isolated. However, if one limb is replanted in the orthotopic position or a crossover replant is done, the patients are happy with the outcome. Most patients with a replanted lower extremity have declared that the function of the replanted leg is superior to a prosthesis and would undergo the same procedure again under the same circumstances (28). Primary bone union and pain-free stability are determinants of patient satisfaction. Arthrodesis or tenodesis must be done to provide ankle stability when it is compromised because of lack of supportive tendons lost during radical debridement.

The main goal of lower limb replantation is to obtain a sensate foot. Primary nerve repair or early secondary nerve reconstruction is a priority. Results of nerve repair as measured by two-point discrimination are very variable. Near-normal sensation to only protective sensation to no sensory recovery have been reported. The outcome appears to coincide with the recovery of sensation in most cases. Although recovery of sensation is preferable and patients feel good about it, strangely, it does not match with the functional outcome or "back to work" criteria. Sanger et al. (29) reported a 7-year follow-up of a successful replantation of an avulsed heel pad. No nerves were repaired, and the patient lacked sensation. Seven years later, he continued to work as a heavy laborer in a steel foundry and walked without the use of orthotics or modified shoes. Despite such isolated reports, secondary problems are less frequent if the patient develops sensation on the sole of the foot.

Aggressive rehabilitation with passive range of motion exercises are started at the end of the first week followed by functional electrical stimulation and muscle-strengthening exercises (30). Independent weight bearing after replantation of the leg has been achieved in children as early as 3 months. When there has been massive bone shortening, it can take 3 to 4 years for reconstruction to be completed. Even though such patients express satisfaction with the surgery at the end, a surgeon contemplating replantation in such circumstances must be prepared for the long course that lies ahead. Psychological and social factors also influence the decision.

CONCLUSION

Despite reports in the literature detailing "good" and "satisfactory" outcomes after replantation of the lower limb, there are very few reports of secondary amputation after replantation. Although underreporting of secondary amputation may be a possibility to consider, there is sufficient accumulated evidence in the literature to justify replantation of lower limb amputated parts as an accepted standard of practice. Outcomes of leg replantation can match the outcome achieved in the salvage of type III C tibial fractures (31). Patients seem to accept staged reconstructive procedures, and the challenge is to avoid complications at every stage.

Patient selection is important for success. A patient younger than 50 years of age with an amputation in the distal third of the leg that does not require more than 10 to 15 cm of shortening or any amputation of the foot proximal to the MTP joints should be considered for replantation. The general condition of the patient and the presence of associated injuries will also influence the decision. It is not possible to provide a flow chart or a scoring system to help decide whether to replant or complete the amputation when faced with an individual patient. The surgeon has to make the decision in the best interests of the patient, and his or her own surgical skills are one of the factors that has the greatest influence on this decision.

SUMMARY

1. The incidence of lower limb replantation is much less frequent compared with replantation of the upper limb. Severe crush injuries causing the amputation and the availability of better functional prostheses are the reasons.
2. The majority of lower limb replants that have been performed are for amputations of the foot and lower third of the leg.
3. A patient younger than 50 years old with an amputation below the lower third of the leg or part of the foot proximal to the MTP joints is a good candidate for attempted replantation.
4. Children with lower limb replants have uniformly done well. The bones in the replanted part have retained their growth potential, and functionally they adapt better than in adults.
5. Proximal lower limb replants are associated with high morbidity because of the mass of muscle in the amputated part. Ischemia time becomes critical.
6. Soft tissue problems occur frequently at the site of replantation. Additional free flaps or pedicled flaps may be required in the immediate postoperative period.
7. Even though 5 to 10 cm of limb shortening is aesthetically and functionally acceptable in upper limb replants, any bone shortening greater than 5 cm in lower limb replants will need a secondary limb lengthening procedure.
8. In bilateral lower limb amputations, replanting even one leg makes rehabilitation easier than bilateral prostheses.
9. In bilateral amputations, if orthotopic replantation is not possible, crossover replantation of at least one limb should be considered.
10. No scoring system is available to guide the surgeon in deciding whether replantation of a lower limb is indicated. The surgeon must consider his or her own experience and the needs of the individual patient in the decision-making process.

REFERENCES

1. Datiashvili RO. Simultaneous replantation of both lower legs in a child: 23 years later. *J Reconstr Microsurg* 2009;25:323–329.
2. Masuda K, Usui M, Ishi S. A 17 year follow up of replantation of a completely amputated leg in a child: case report. *J Reconst Mircosurg* 1995;11:89–92.
3. Jones NF, Shin EK, Mostofi A, Oppenheim W. Successful replantation of the leg in a pre-ambulatory infant. *J Reconstr Microsurg* 2005;21:359–364.
4. Vucetic CS, Vukasinovic Z, Miric D, Tulic G. Two cases of big-toe replantation: a ten year follow up. *J Reconstr Microsurg* 2006;22:79–85.
5. Sabapathy SR, Mohan D, Singh SB, Venkatramani H. Replantation of great and second toes: a worthwhile effort. *Plast Reconstr Surg* 2000; 106:229–230.
6. Magee HR, Parker WR. Replantation of the foot: results after two years. *Med J Aust* 1972;1:751–755.
7. Report of the American Replantation Mission to China: replantation surgery in China. *Plast Reconstr Surg* 1973;52:476.
8. O'Brien BM. Replantation surgery in China. *Med J Aust* 1974;2:255.
9. Usui M, Minami M, Ishii S. Successful replantation of an amputated leg in a child. *Plast Reconstr Surg* 1979;63:613–617.
10. Fang CL, Yang CS, Tang HC, et al. Successful replantation of amputated bilateral lower limbs. *Plast Reconstr Surg* 2012;129:215e–217e.
11. Buckley JR, Dunkley P. Successful reimplantation of both feet: brief report. *J Bone Joint Surg Br* 1988;70:667–668.
12. Chen ZW, Zeng BF. Replantation of the lower extremity. *Clin Plast Surg* 1983;10:103–113.
13. Jupiter JB, Tsai TM, Kleinert HE. Salvage replantation of lower limb amputations. *Plast Reconstr Surg* 1982;69:1–8.
14. Yildirim S, Akoz T. Big-toe replantation in a three month old child: case report. *J Reconstr Microsurg* 2004;20:373–375.
15. Demiri E, Bakhach J, Tsakoniatis N, et al. Bone growth after replantation in children. *J Reconstr Microsurg* 1995;11:113–122.
16. Mamakos MS. Lower extremity replant—a preliminary report. *Ann Plast Surg* 1980;4:48–52.
17. Sabapathy SR, Venkatramani H, Bharathi RR, et al. Technical considerations and functional outcome of 22 major replantations. (The BSSH Douglas Lamb Lecture, 2005). *J Hand Surg* 2007;32E:488–501.
18. Wickham MH, Brackley PTH, McPhail J, et al. Replantation and subsequent reconstruction strategies of a guillotine amputated foot in an 11-year-old child: a four year follow up. *J Plast Reconstr Aesthetic Surg* 2010;63:e503–e505.
19. Battiston B, Tos P, Pontini I, Ferrero S. Lower limb replantations: indications and a new scoring system. *Microsurgery* 2002;22:187–192.
20. Cavadas PC, Landin L, Ibanez J, et al. Infrapopliteal lower extremity replantation. *Plast Reconstr Surg* 2009;124:532–539.
21. Mirzoyan AE. Reimplantation and lengthening with use of the Ilizarov apparatus after a traumatic amputation of the leg. *J Bone Joint Surg* 1996;78A:437–438.
22. Lin CH, Lin CH, Sassur P, et al. Replantation of great toe: review of 20 cases. *Plast Reconstr Surg* 2008;122:806–812.
23. Wang D, Yin YS, Gao FG, et al. Cross-replantation of lower extremities in multi limbed amputation: case report and literature review in China. *J Trauma* 1995;38:947–951.
24. Ricketts S, De Steiger R, Breidahl A. Eleven-year follow up of cross-leg replantation for traumatic bilateral amputation. *J Reconstr Microsurg* 2009;25:111–116.
25. Srivastava DC. Ipsilateral replantation of foot with crossover segmental transfer in bilateral leg amputation. *Plast Reconstr Surg* 2005;116:129e–134e.
26. Gao YS, Ai ZS, Zhang CQ, et al. Replantation of above-knee amputation: a surviving but dysfunctional case needing secondary amputation. *J Reconstr Microsurg* 2010;26:631–635.
27. Salon A, Liverneaux PA, Dubert T, et al. Long-term review of five leg replantations: emergency strategy and examples of lengthening of the leg on nerve regeneration. *Injury* 2006;37:869–876.
28. Cinar C, Arslan H, Ogur S, et al. Crossover replantation of the foot after bilateral traumatic lower extremity amputation. *Ann Plast Surg* 2007;58:667–672.
29. Sanger JR, Matloub HS. Successful replantation of the heel pad: a seven-year follow-up. *Ann Plast Surg* 1989;22:350–353.
30. Kim HH, Jeong JH, Kim YH, et al. Rehabilitation after the replantation on a 2 year-old girl with both amputated legs. *Br J Plast Surg* 2005;58:404–408.
31. Parmaksizoglu F, Unal MB, Cansu E, et al. Functional results of limb salvage in below-knee type III C open fractures or traumatic amputations. *J Reconstr Microsurg* 2012;28:607–614.

CHAPTER 85

Osteonecrosis of the Hip

Marc J. Richard and James R. Urbaniak

HISTORY OF CONVENTIONAL OPTIONS

Osteonecrosis of the femoral head is a common cause of hip pain and disability. As many as 18% of total hip arthroplasties are performed for osteonecrosis, and this remains an excellent treatment option for older patients (1,2). The majority of patients with osteonecrosis of the femoral head are young. Mont and Hungerford reported that 80% of the patients with osteonecrosis in their series were younger than 50 years old with a mean age of 38 years (3). This is comparable with our experience showing a mean age of 33 years (4). The relatively poor outcomes and requisite lifestyle changes associated with total hip arthroplasty in this patient population have challenged surgeons to seek alternative treatment options.

For young patients with symptomatic disease, there appears to be very little benefit to nonoperative management. Operative management is largely determined by the stage of the lesion (Table 85-1). Larger and more advanced lesions become progressively more difficult to treat. For small, precollapse lesions, core decompression has been widely used. The surgeon drills into the lesion from an entry point on the lateral aspect of the trochanteric region. The goal is to relieve pain and to theoretically stimulate a vascular proliferation with resultant new bone formation. This procedure is favored for its technical ease and short operative time and because it does not limit subsequent surgical options. The efficacy of core decompression in more advanced osteonecrosis lesions has not been demonstrated.

Larger and more advanced lesions have historically been treated with a variety of surgical options to attempt hip preservation in younger patients (Figure 85-1). Osteotomies have been used, but concern remains over the potential for disruption of the blood supply to the femoral head and the difficulty in converting these hips to an arthroplasty as a salvage procedure. Conventional bone grafting has been reported either through a trapdoor in the articular cartilage or through a cortical window in the femoral neck. Both of these procedures are performed with intracapsular dissection and risk the vascularity to the femoral head.

Several potential vascularized bone grafts are available for treating osteonecrosis of the femoral head. All of these options share the goal of decompression of the lesion by the removal of necrotic bone and the placement of bone graft with a vascular source to provide osteoinductive progenitor cells for healing the lesion. Local pedicled bone grafts, most commonly a muscle–pedicle–bone graft from either the quadratus femoris or the tensor fascia lata, have been reported with superior results compared with conventional nonvascularized bone grafts (5–10). This technique depends on muscular metaplasia to be successful. This, combined with the lack of structural bone graft provided by these grafts, led some authors to consider other sources of vascularized bone graft.

More distant donor sites that provided structural support for osteonecrosis lesions and did not depend on muscular metaplasia became possible with the development of the operating microscope and improved microsurgical techniques for free vascularized bone grafts. In the late 1970s, Urbaniak, Brunelli and Brunelli, and Judet and Gilbert began using the free vascularized fibular graft (FVFG) to treat osteonecrosis of the femoral head (11–13). The fibula provides a large corticocancellous bone graft that can be placed from an extracapsular entry point. It has a reliable vascular pedicle and a low donor site morbidity. FVFGs have been compared to nonvascularized fibular grafts and demonstrate superior results in larger and more advanced osteonecrosis lesions (14). The hips treated with FVFGs demonstrated less radiographic progression, less femoral head collapse, and improved Harris hip scores. We have used this technique successfully at our institution for the management of this challenging clinical problem in young patients.

AVAILABLE FREE FLAPS

The FVFG remains the transfer of choice for osteonecrosis of the femoral head. The FVFG provides a large stock of corticocancellous bone graft for biologic and structural support with a reliable vascular pedicle in the peroneal artery and veins.

TABLE 85-1 Duke Classification of Osteonecrosis of the Femoral Head

Stage	Image
I	Lesion visible on MRI only; plain radiograph is normal Size as measured as a percentage of the femoral head on the MRI: A: Lesion is <25% B: Lesion is 25%–50% C: Lesion is >50%
II	Lesion visible on plain radiograph: increased density or cysts Size as measured as a percentage of the femoral head on the MRI or radiograph: A: Lesion is <25% B: Lesion is 25%–50% C: Lesion is >50%
III	Crescent sign present; best visualized on lateral radiograph Size as measured as a percentage of the femoral head on the MRI or radiograph: A: Lesion is <25% B: Lesion is 25%–50% C: Lesion is >50%
IV	Partial articular collapse on radiograph Size as measured as a percentage of the femoral head on the MRI or radiograph: A: Lesion is <25% B: Lesion is 25%–50% C: Lesion is >50% Amount of collapse: 0 = Flattening without step-off 1 = 1 mm of joint collapse 2 = 2 mm of joint collapse 3 = 3 mm of joint collapse 4 = 4 mm of joint collapse
V	Joint space narrowing with articular collapse Size as measured as a percentage of the femoral head on the MRI or radiograph: A: Lesion is <25% B: Lesion is 25%–50% C: Lesion is >50% Amount of collapse: 0 = Flattening without step-off 1 = 1 mm of joint collapse 2 = 2 mm of joint collapse 3 = 3 mm of joint collapse 4 = 4 mm of joint collapse
VI	End-stage osteoarthritis

MRI, magnetic resonance imaging.

The graft can be harvested with a skin paddle for flap surveillance; however, there is a lack of consensus regarding the necessity of this (15).

INDICATIONS

The ideal patient for FVFG for osteonecrosis of the femoral head is a young, active patient with a symptomatic precollapse lesion. Age, activity level, comorbidities, etiology, stage of disease, and radiographic findings are all considered when determining the appropriate management of each patient with osteonecrosis of the femoral head.

There is no age limit for treatment of osteonecrosis with FVFG; however, with increasing age, there is an increased likelihood that arthroplasty will provide a successful management option for the patient. In general, patients older than 50 years are best treated by total hip arthroplasty. Because arthroplasty is associated with activity restrictions, patients younger than 50 years of age are evaluated on an individual basis for activity level and lifestyle so an appropriate treatment option can

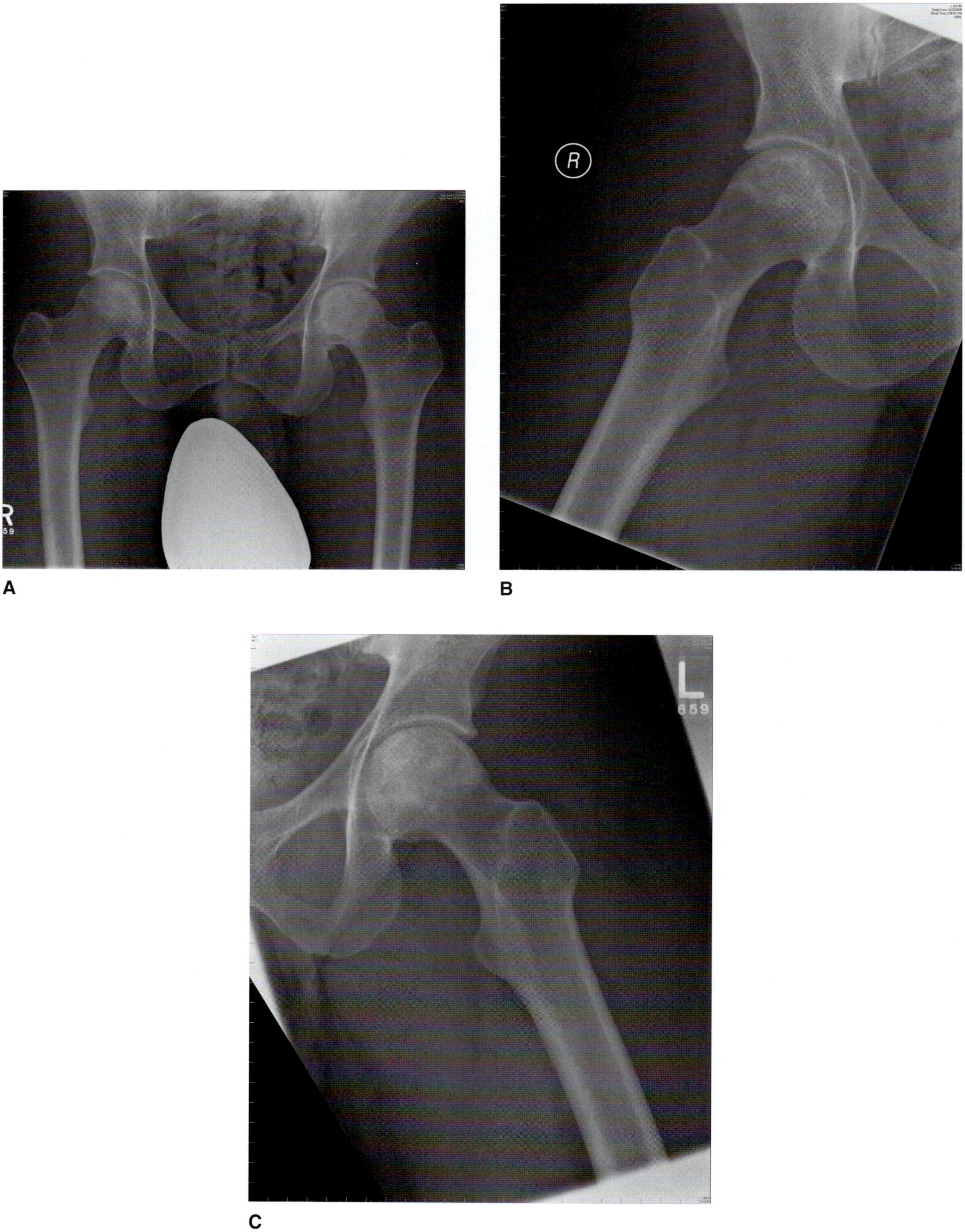

FIGURE 85-1 Preoperative anteroposterior pelvis (**A**) and frog-legged lateral hip radiographs (**B** and **C**) of a 26-year-old man with grade 2B osteonecrosis of the right hip and grade 2C osteonecrosis of the left hip.

be selected. Younger patients with an active lifestyle are typically best managed with an FVFG.

Comorbidities and etiology are also considered when evaluating a patient's candidacy for FVFG. Alcohol and corticosteroid use are two common associated factors in the development of osteonecrosis of the femoral head. Although some centers consider current corticosteroid use as a contraindication to FVFG, we routinely offer FVFG to these patients, and we have noted success. Active alcohol abuse should be considered a relative contraindication because both the pathophysiology of alcohol abuse and the potential noncompliance of postoperative weight-bearing restrictions can compromise outcomes.

The stage of the osteonecrosis lesion is given great weight when choosing the appropriate treatment. Asymptomatic hips are not treated with FVFG because some of these early-stage lesions will remain asymptomatic. Our knowledge of the progression of osteonecrosis in silent hips is limited to our evaluation of patients with contralateral disease. When osteonecrosis is diagnosed on one side, Hungerford and Zizic found that 67% of patients will develop collapse of the femoral head on the opposite side (16). In our experience, only 6% of patients without evidence of osteonecrosis in the silent hip progressed to symptomatic disease, but 72% of patients with asymptomatic lesions present progressed (4).

Patients with precollapse lesions with maintenance of a spherical femoral head have the most to gain by an attempt at biological preservation of the femoral head. Osteonecrosis lesions that demonstrate some mild collapse on radiographs are considered for FVFG in younger patients with good mobility of the hip and an active lifestyle. For these patients, the questionable long-term survival of an arthroplasty procedure makes the FVFG a more attractive option.

PREPARATION OF THE RECIPIENT SITE

The patient is positioned in a lateral decubitus position on a peg board with the lower leg on a padded Mayo stand. Because of the duration of the procedure, all bony prominences should be well padded, and an axillary roll should be placed to avoid positioning complications. Before prepping and draping the patient, it should be confirmed that the patient is positioned as distal on the operating table as allowable. With the patient's foot at the distal end of the table, the surgeon harvesting the fibula will minimize reach and strain while operating from the foot of the bed. Furthermore, it should be confirmed that the pegs placed for patient positioning are out of the anticipated radiographic field of the femoral head.

The hip is approached through a curvilinear incision over the lateral aspect of the affected hip. The incision is approximately 10 to 15 cm in length and is directed convex anterior. This incision is placed such that the lateral femoral circumflex vessels are centered proximal to distal. These donor vessels are located approximately 10 cm distal to the anterior superior iliac spine. With respect to anteroposterior (AP) placement of the incision, it must be positioned such that the microvascular work (anterior) and the hip reaming (posterior) can be

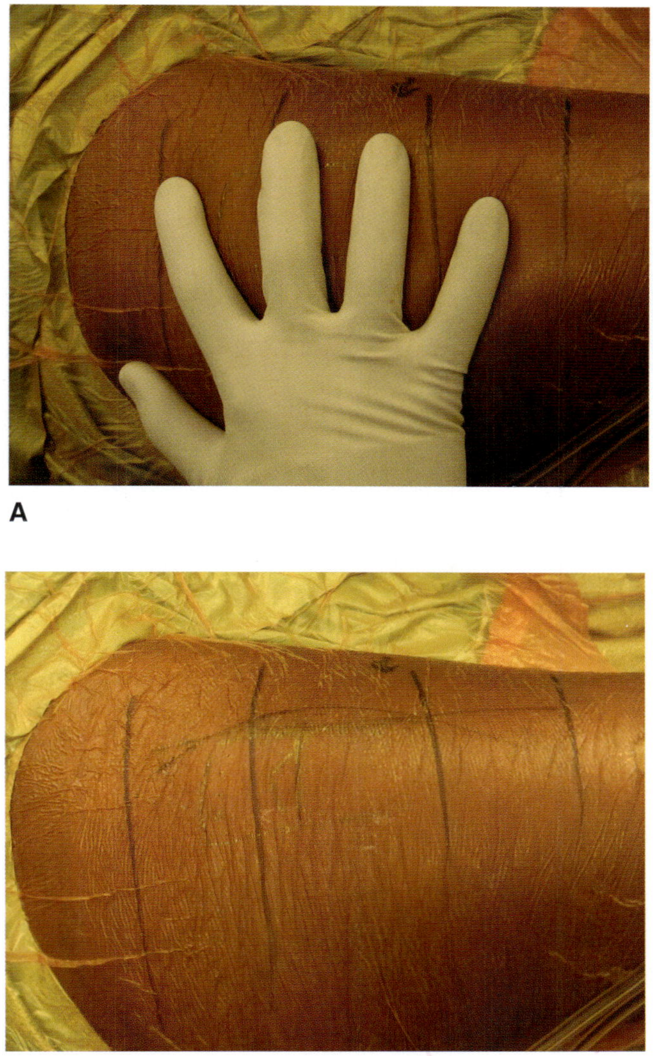

A

B

FIGURE 85-2 (A) and (B) The hip incision is made along a curvilinear line created at the fingertips of the surgeon's hand when the long finger is placed on the vastus ridge of the femur with the tip of the finger just anterior to the femur. The right hand is used to design the incision for a right hip, and the left hand is used for a left hip.

performed through the same incision. This requires surface identification of the anterior and posterior borders of the proximal femur and the vastus ridge. The anterior margin of the incision is placed approximately 2 cm anterior to the anterior border of the femur with one third of the incision superior to the vastus ridge and two thirds inferior. This incision can be easily drawn by the operating surgeon placing his or her long finger on the vastus ridge with the tip of the finger 2 cm anterior to the anterior margin of the femur and the index finger superior (Figures 85-2 and 85-3). With the fingers maximally abducted, a line drawn connecting the fingertips corresponds with the desired skin incision (17).

After the skin incision, a variation of the Watson-Jones approach to the hip is used with dissection continuing in the interval between the tensor fascia latae and the gluteus medius.

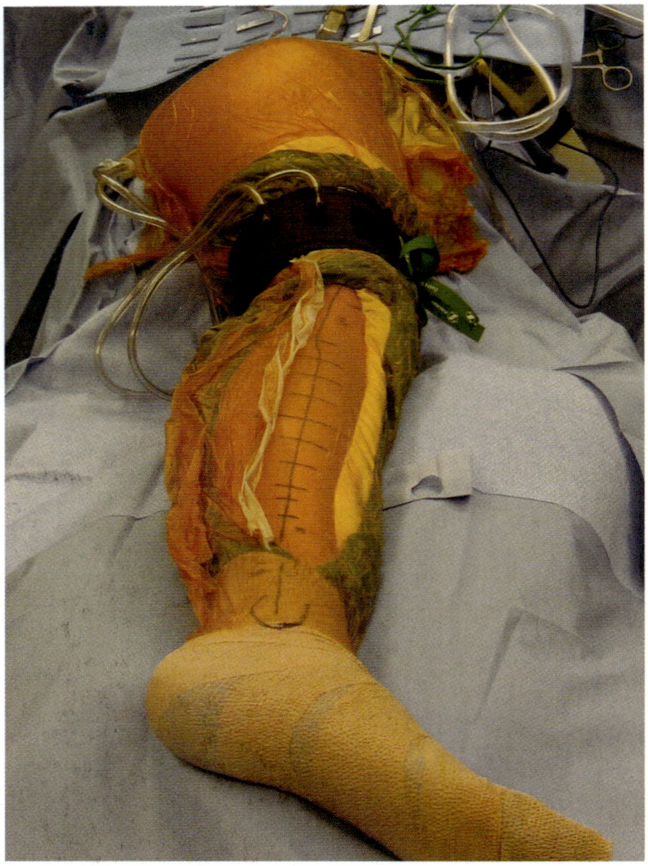

FIGURE 85-3 The operative leg is prepped and draped, and the fibula incision is marked along a line connecting the fibular head to the lateral malleolus.

The fascia is incised in a curvilinear fashion directed convex posterior. A four-quadrant retractor is placed to assist with visualization of the deep structures. The anterior and posterior limbs are placed over the cut edges of the fascia, the superior limb is placed around the substance of gluteus medius, and the inferior limb is placed on the skin. The vastus lateralis and vastus intermedius are identified originating from the vastus ridge. The donor vessels can now be visualized anterior to the vastus intermedius in the interval between vastus intermedius and rectus femoris. The ascending branch of the lateral femoral circumflex artery and its two veins typically run obliquely cephalad at a 45-degree angle at a distance of 10 cm distal to the anterior superior iliac spine (Figure 85-4).

After the donor vessels are identified and can be appropriately protected, the vastus lateralis is sharply elevated to expose the lateral aspect of the proximal femur. An L-shaped incision is used with a longitudinal limb posteriorly and a transverse limb at the level of the vastus ridge. As the vastus intermedius is encountered anteriorly, a right-angle clamp and Metzenbaum scissors are used to safely release its attachments from the proximal femur and to avoid injury to the donor vessels. The complete reflection of the vastus intermedius provides a trough for the donor vessels during the later microvascular anastomosis. The vastus lateralis and vastus intermedius muscles are then secured to the anterior skin edge and placed deep to the inferior limb of the four-quadrant retractor.

The donor vessels can now be clearly seen lying within the aponeurotic falx of the rectus femoris anteriorly. The ascending branch of the lateral femoral circumflex artery and its two veins are carefully dissected out under loupe magnification. The smaller side branches of the vessels are ligated with small vascular clips such that a pedicle of at least 4 cm is obtained for later anastomosis. Typically, there is sufficient pedicle length if the vessels reach halfway up to the anticipated entry site of the fibula. The hip wound is copiously irrigated, and the four-quadrant retractor is removed for preparation of the femoral head.

Preparation of the femoral head is done with the aid of C-arm fluoroscopy. The C-arm fluoroscope is draped sterilely and positioned over the patient like an arch. It is canted cephalad slightly to allow the surgeon a greater working space. The ability to obtain true AP and frog-leg lateral views is confirmed before preparation of the femoral head begins. With fluoroscopic guidance, a 3-mm sharp-tipped guide pin is placed into the center of the osteonecrosis lesion. The starting point for this pin is approximately 2 cm distal to the vastus ridge at the junction of the middle and posterior thirds of the proximal femur. Care is taken to avoid making the entry point too distal because encroachment on the high-stress subtrochanteric region will increase the risk of fracture.

After correct pin placement is confirmed on AP and lateral fluoroscopic views, the guide pin is overdrilled with a cannulated 8-mm drill bit. The sharp-tipped guide pin is exchanged for a blunt-tipped guide pin, which is sequentially overreamed with a series of specialized straight reamers beginning at 10 mm in diameter. These reamers are available in 13-, 16-, 17.5-, 19-, and 21-mm sizes, and they are sequentially used up to the size of the harvested fibula. Typically, the core size is 13 mm for a child, 16 mm for a woman, and 19 mm for a man. The reaming is performed up to 4 mm from the subchondral plate using live fluoroscopy. The healthy bone that is collected in the flutes of the reamer is saved for later bone grafting while obviously necrotic bone is discarded. Similarly, a filtered suction device is used to collect bone fragments generated by the reaming from the core. The scrub nurse fashions this collected bone into "bullets" on the back table for later grafting.

After the final size-matched straight reamer is used, the guide pin is removed, and a ball-tipped reamer is placed to remove the remaining area of necrotic bone. These reamers allow the creation of a bulbous cavity and are best used with the assistance of fluoroscopy. Radiographic contrast is used to evaluate the adequacy of the excavation of the osteonecrosis lesion (Figure 85-5).

Cancellous bone is harvested from the greater trochanter through the lateral entry point using a large curette (Figure 85-6). This bone is kept separate from the bone graft obtained from the reamings. Long DeBakey forceps are used to place this bone graft into the cavity created within the femoral head. The Urbanipactor, a specialized impaction instrument designed for this procedure, is used to impact the bone graft (Figure 85-7). After placing the cancellous bone graft within

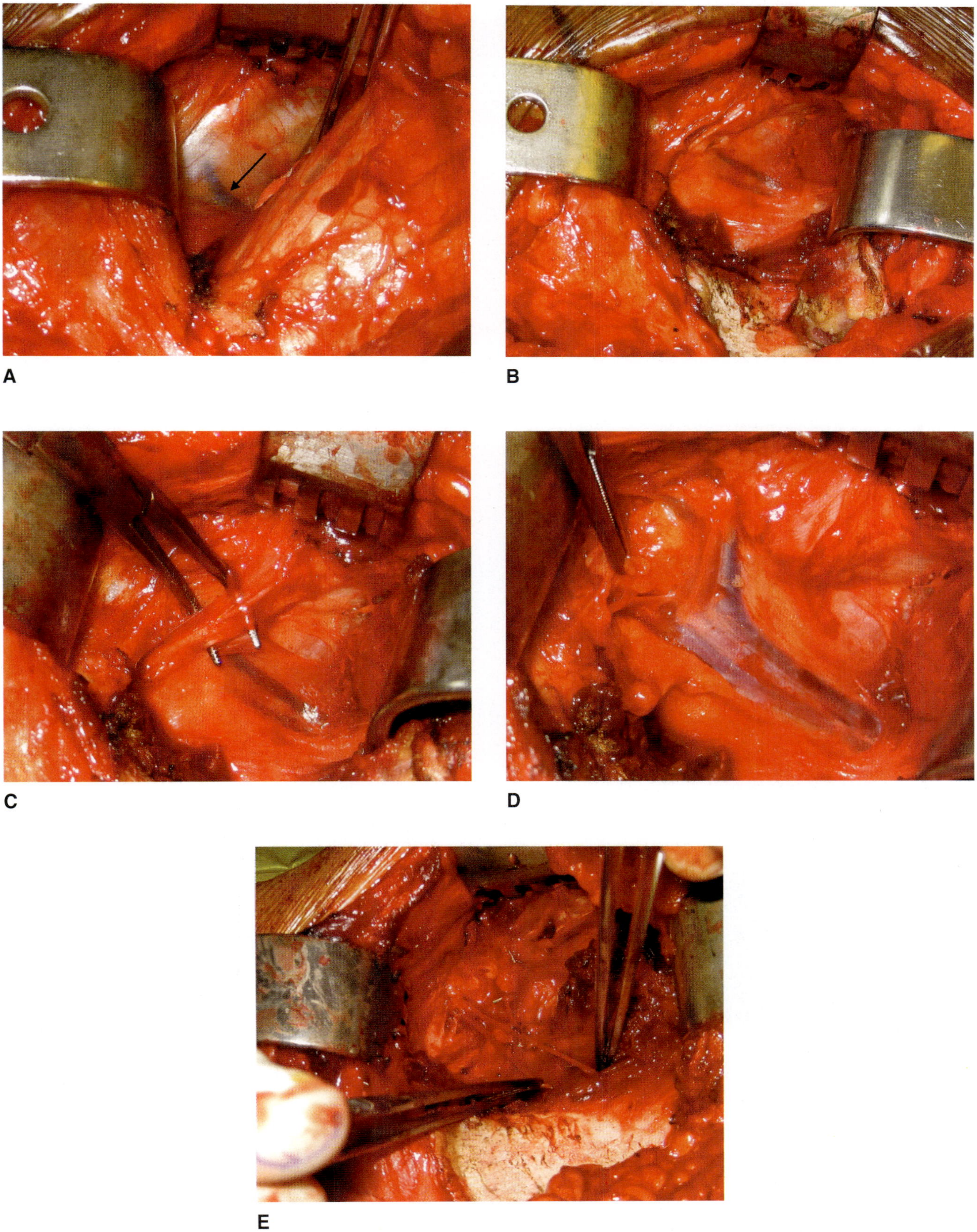

FIGURE 85-4 The ascending branch of the lateral femoral circumflex vessels (black arrow) are routinely identified in the falx between the vastus intermedius and the rectus femoris muscles (A). They course approximately 45 degrees cephalad. The vastus lateralis and intermedius muscles are reflected off of the lateral femur (B). The falx is taken down (C) to completely expose the artery and the two veins of the ascending branch (D). The vessels are taken down individually such that they reach halfway up the exposed femur for later anastomosis (E).

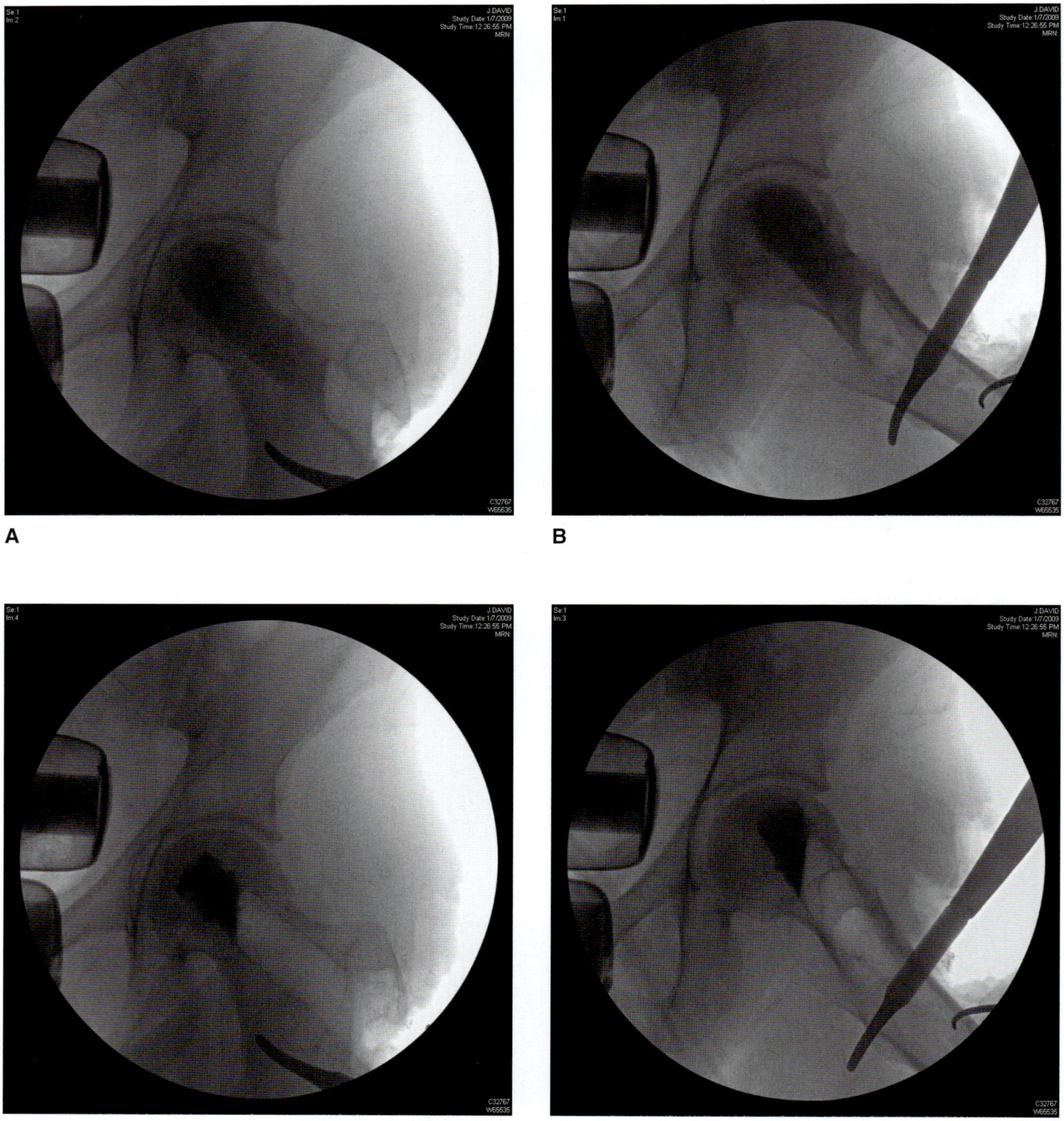

FIGURE 85-5 The Isovue is used to demonstrate appropriate excavation and subsequent bone grafting (**A** and **B**). Note that the shape of the core matches the shape of the Urbanipactor after appropriate bone grafting (**C** and **D**).

the cavity, the Urbanipactor is fully inserted, and its position is verified with fluoroscopy. The remaining cancellous bone graft and the bullets are placed within the core of the Urbanipactor, and the specialized drill bit is used to disperse the graft within the cavity. Graduated circumferential markings on the outside of the Urbanipactor are used to measure the depth of the core to determine the length of the fibular graft. The Urbanipactor is then removed and radiographic contrast medium is reinjected to confirm adequate bone grafting of the cavitary defect.

HARVESTING OF THE FIBULAR GRAFT

The fibular graft is harvested at the same time as the hip preparation. The lower extremity is exsanguinated with an Esmarch bandage, and a thigh tourniquet is inflated to 350 mm Hg.

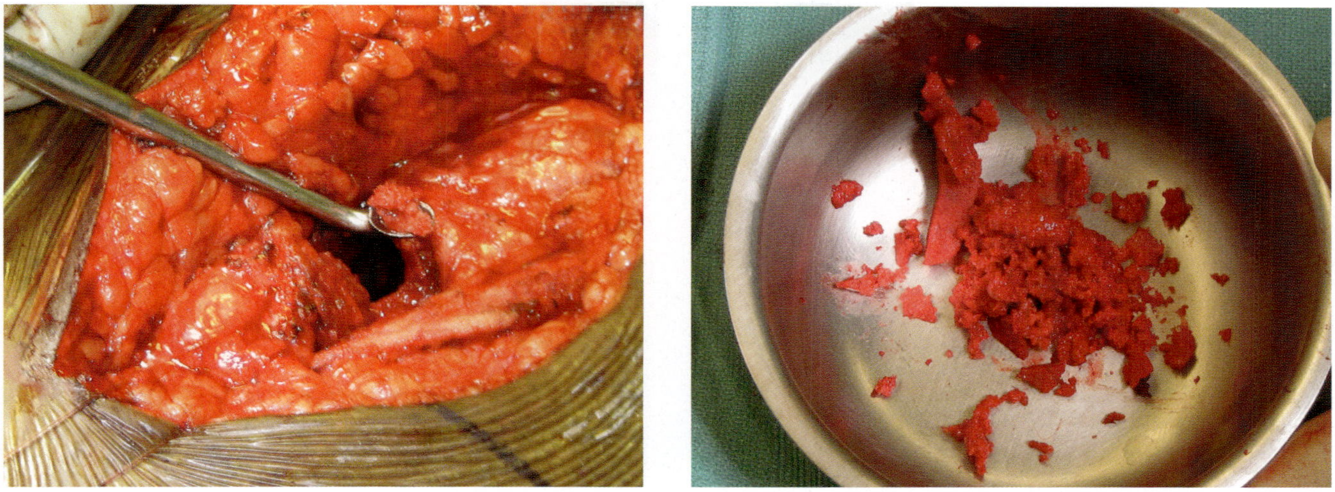

A B

FIGURE 85-6 A curved curette is used to harvest cancellous bone graft from the greater trochanter (**A**). A large amount of graft is available from this site (**B**).

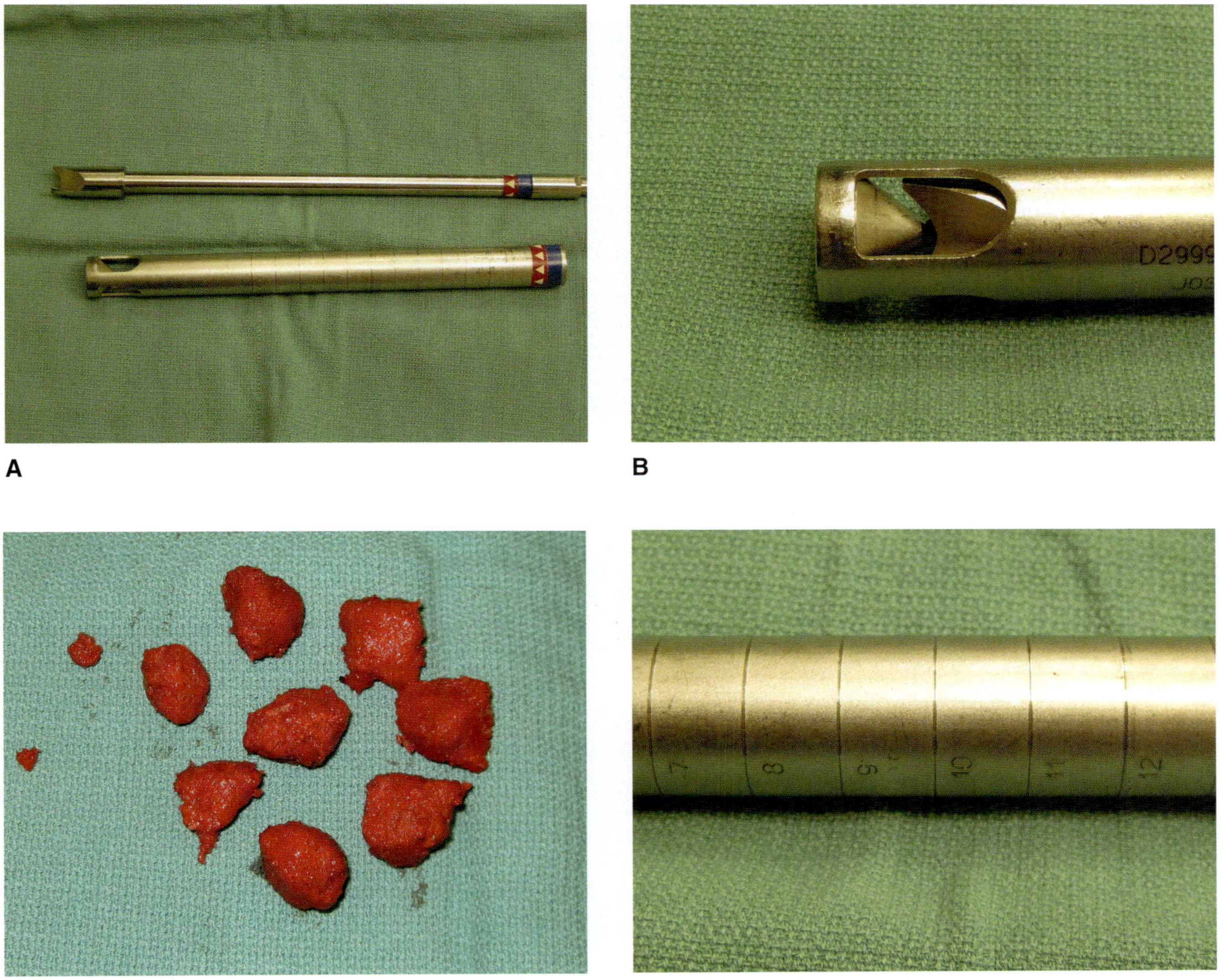

A B

C D

FIGURE 85-7 The Urbanipactor is used to distribute the cancellous bone graft within the excavated lesion (**A** and **B**). The healthy bone from the previous reamings is also saved as an additional source of bone graft (**C**). The final length of the fibular graft is then measured using the markings on the Urbanipactor (**D**).

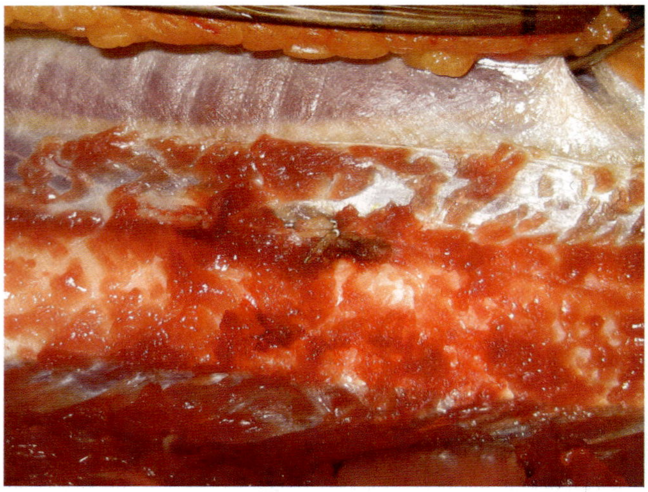

FIGURE 85-8 The lateral surface of the fibula is "marbleized" with a small cuff of muscle and periosteum.

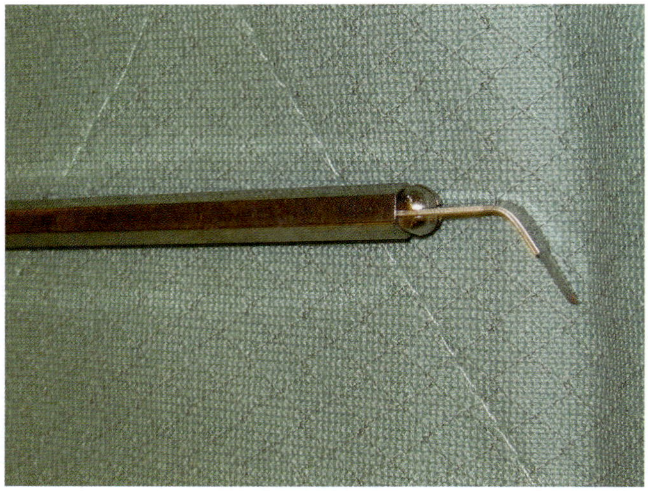

FIGURE 85-9 A right-angle beaver blade is used to safely incise the interosseous membrane.

A line is marked on the skin connecting the fibular head with the lateral malleolus. The proximal and distal 10 cm of fibula are marked, and care is taken to preserve both the proximal and distal tibiofibular joints over this distance. Typically, this leaves approximately 15 cm of the central portion of the fibula available for harvest. The skin is incised over the sulcus between the lateral and posterior compartments of the leg with maintenance of full-thickness skin flaps. The fascia of the lateral compartment is incised longitudinally in line with the peroneal tendon with care to protect the superficial peroneal nerve. The peroneal muscles are reflected anteriorly off the posterior intermuscular septum. The lateral aspect of the fibula is palpable deep to the peroneal muscles. Two large Gelpi retractors are placed to demonstrate this interval and maintain tension of the peroneal muscles as they are sharply reflected off of the fibula. A thin 1- to 2-mm layer or muscle is left with the fibula ("marbleizing") to preserve the periosteal blood supply to the fibula (Figure 85-8). Dissection is continued from posterior to anterior until the anterior intermuscular septum is encountered.

A #15 surgical blade is used to divide the anterior intermuscular septum approximately 1 to 2 mm off of the fibula. The anterior compartment musculature is then encountered and bluntly dissected off of the fibula with Metzenbaum scissors and DeBakey forceps. The interosseous membrane is then easily visualized as are the anterior tibial artery and the deep peroneal nerve. The neurovascular structures are protected while the interosseous membrane is released from the fibula with the use of a right-angle Beaver blade (Figure 85-9). Last, the posterior intermuscular septum is divided, revealing the soleus muscle proximally and the flexor hallucis longus muscle distally. The fibula is now free from all septal attachments and is ready for osteotomy.

At the distal extent of the dissection, the peroneal artery and veins are visualized on the deep surface of the fibula under the cover of the flexor hallucis longus musculature. A right-angle clamp is placed between the vessels and the fibula followed by a malleable retractor between the clamp and the fibula. A second larger malleable retractor is placed from the opposite direction between the first malleable retractor and the fibula. The surgeon confirms that the osteotomy site is at least 10 cm proximal to the tip of the lateral malleolus and that the vascular pedicle is protected. An oscillating saw is used to perform the osteotomy with constant irrigation to avoid thermal necrosis (Figure 85-10).

Attention is then turned toward the proximal osteotomy site. At a distance 15 cm proximal to the first cut, the peroneal vessels are protected in a similar fashion, and the oscillating saw is used to perform the proximal osteotomy. A bone clamp is placed around the midportion of the fibula to assist in manipulation of the fibula for further dissection. Beginning distally, the peroneal vessels are again identified, and large hemoclips are placed. The vessels are divided, and the free end of the pedicle and its hemoclip are secured to the distal end of the fibular graft with a 4-0 absorbable suture to avoid separation of the pedicle from the fibula.

Further dissection of the fibula and its pedicle is best performed with the operating surgeon standing at the foot of the patient and working anterior, posterior, and deep to the fibula. The fibula and peroneal vessels are carefully dissected from distal to proximal with care taken to ligate perforating vessels to the flexor hallucis longus, tibialis posterior, and soleus muscles. Proximally, large perforators to the soleus musculature are ligated, and the vascular pedicle is isolated for a length of 5 cm proximal to the osteotomy site. The bifurcation of the peroneal artery and posterior tibial artery is confirmed to be proximal to the anticipated ligation site. After this is verified, the peroneal vessels are ligated with two large hemoclips and divided just distal to them (Figure 85-11). The tourniquet is deflated, and the wound is copiously irrigated. Visual inspection is performed of the proximal and distal stumps of the peroneal vessels to confirm the integrity of the hemoclips. Meticulous hemostasis is achieved, and the wound is packed with saline-soaked gauze and wrapped with a surgical towel secured with a towel clip. This allows the surgeon working at the hip to manipulate the leg as needed for fluoroscopic views. The wound is closed later over a drain at the subcutaneous and

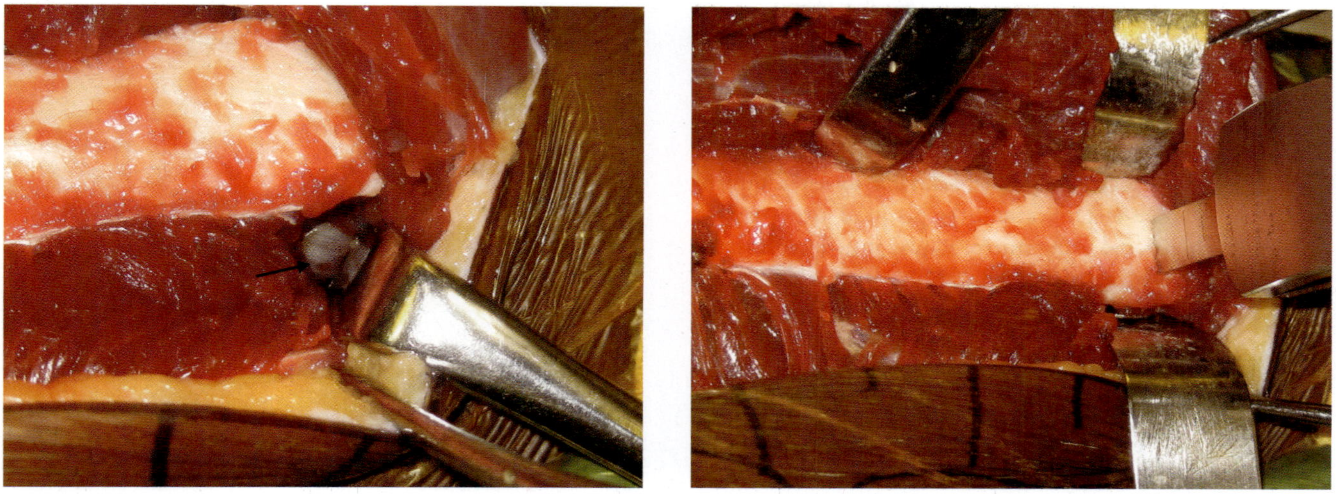

A B

FIGURE 85-10 At the distal fibula osteotomy site, the peroneal vessels (black arrow) are identified (**A**) and protected with malleable retractors before the osteotomy is created with an oscillating saw (**B**).

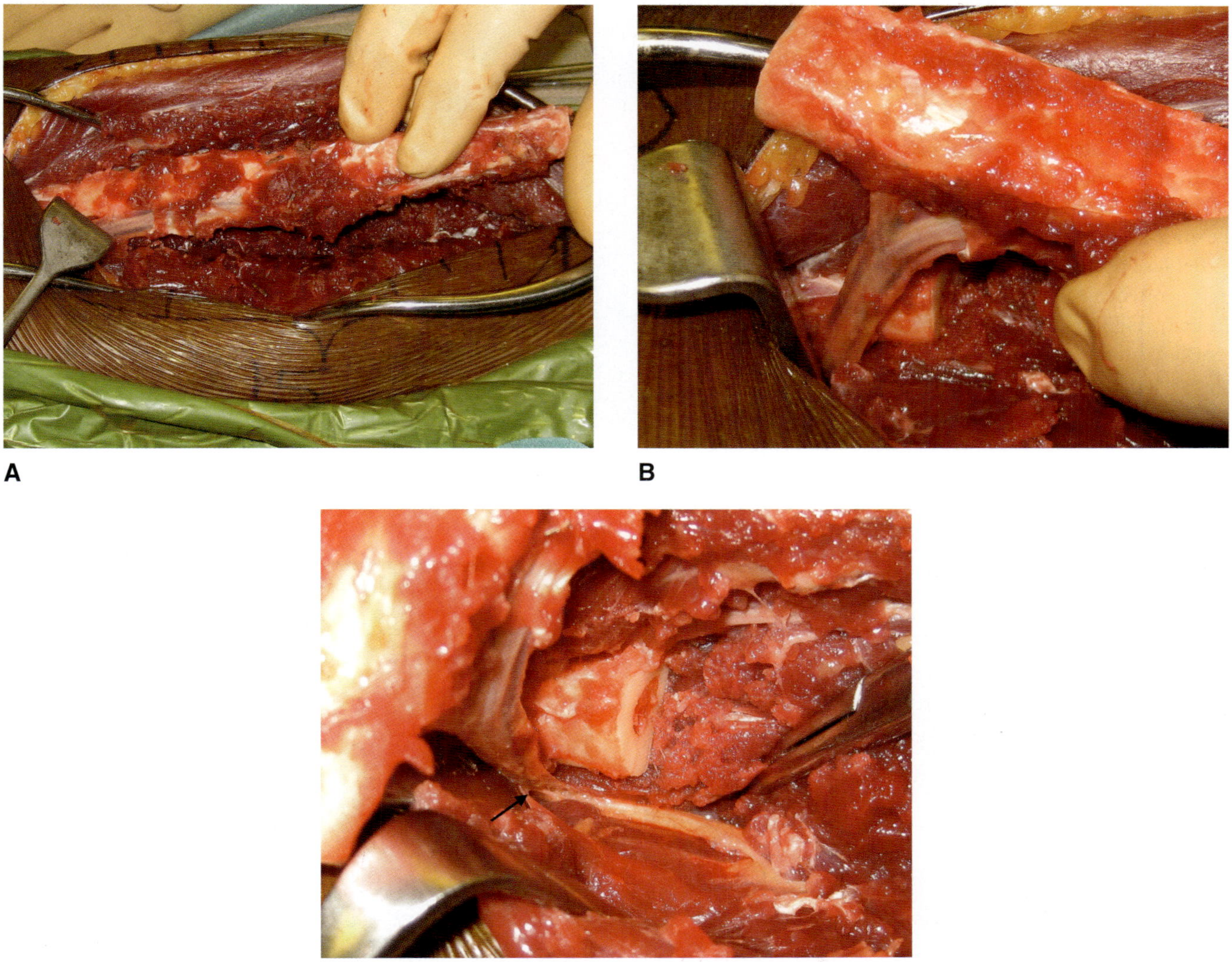

A B C

FIGURE 85-11 The fibula is mobilized over its entire length with care taken to identify and protect the peroneal vessels proximally (**A**). After the entire fibula is mobilized on its pedicle (**B**), the pedicle is carefully dissected proximally until its bifurcation (black arrow) with the posterior tibial vessels (**C**). At this level, the peroneal vessels are ligated with two large hemoclips, and the fibula graft is removed from the leg.

dermal layers only. The deep fascia is left open to minimize the risk of compartment syndrome.

INSET OF THE FIBULAR GRAFT

The fibular graft is prepared on the back table for later implantation. Under loupe magnification, the peroneal artery and its two veins are separated using microvascular instruments. Each of the vessels are irrigated with heparinized lactated Ringer's solution and inspected for leaks. Micro hemoclips are used as necessary to ligate side branches and address leaks. The artery should fill over its entire length, and this is confirmed by documenting that the artery insufflates at its distal hemoclip while irrigating proximally.

The diameter of the fibula is measured so that the hip surgeon can create the appropriate-sized core in the femoral neck. The hip surgeon determines the length of the fibular graft after preparing the femoral head. During preparation of the fibular graft, care is taken to identify and preserve the nutrient vessel. The pedicle is elevated subperiosteally from proximal to distal until the nutrient vessel is seen entering the cortex (Figure 85-12). The pedicle length should be a minimum of 4 to 5 cm. Subsequent bony shortening is performed with an oscillating saw and constant irrigation creating a final graft that includes the nutrient vessel (Figure 85-13). A 1-cm cuff of periosteum is preserved distal to the distal osteotomy and evaginated over the distal stump of the pedicle. This is secured with a 4-0 absorbable suture to prevent stripping during placement of the graft in the hip.

Because the donor vessels in the hip are anterior, the fibular graft is oriented such that the pedicle is on the anterior side of the graft (Figure 85-14). This shortens the distance required for vessel anastomosis. Typically, there is a natural sulcus along the edge of the fibula that the pedicle easily falls into, thereby protecting it during passage into the femoral head. The fibula is placed along the posterior aspect of the reamed core in the femoral neck to avoid trauma to the vessels. Fluoroscopy is used to intermittently evaluate the progress as the fibula is passed.

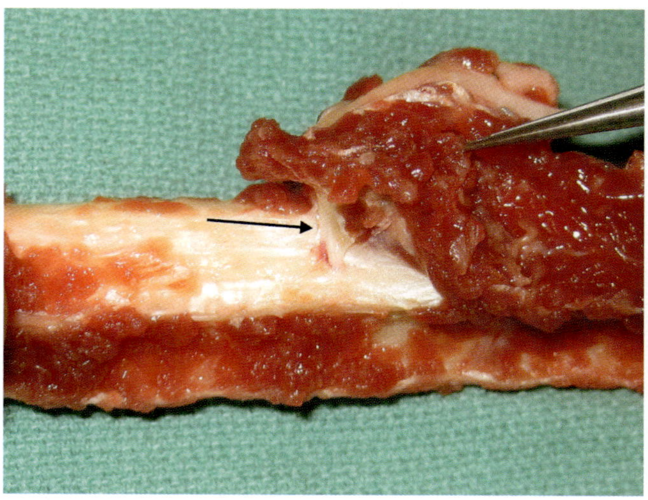

FIGURE 85-12 The fibula is prepared on the back table with care taken to identify and preserve the nutrient vessel (black arrow).

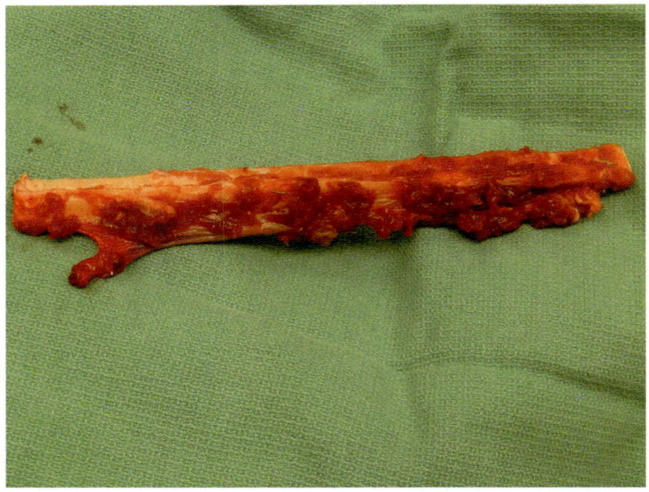

A

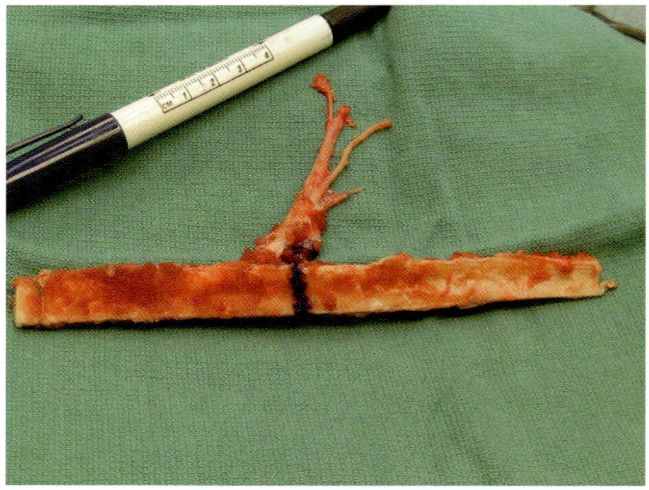

B

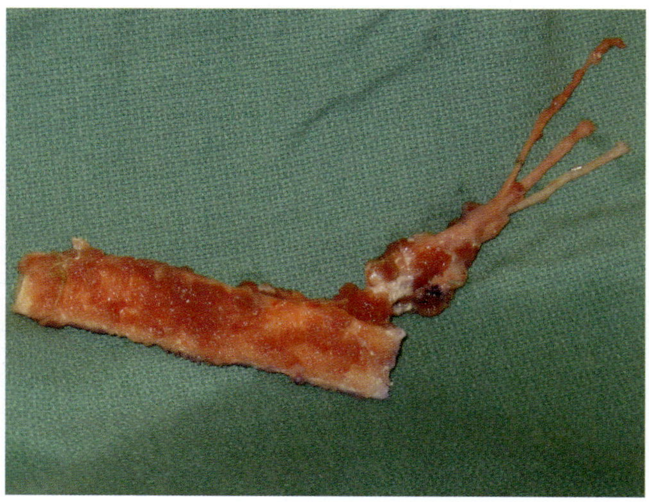

C

FIGURE 85-13 The fibula is cut to the appropriate size to match the length measured with the Urbanipactor (A to C).

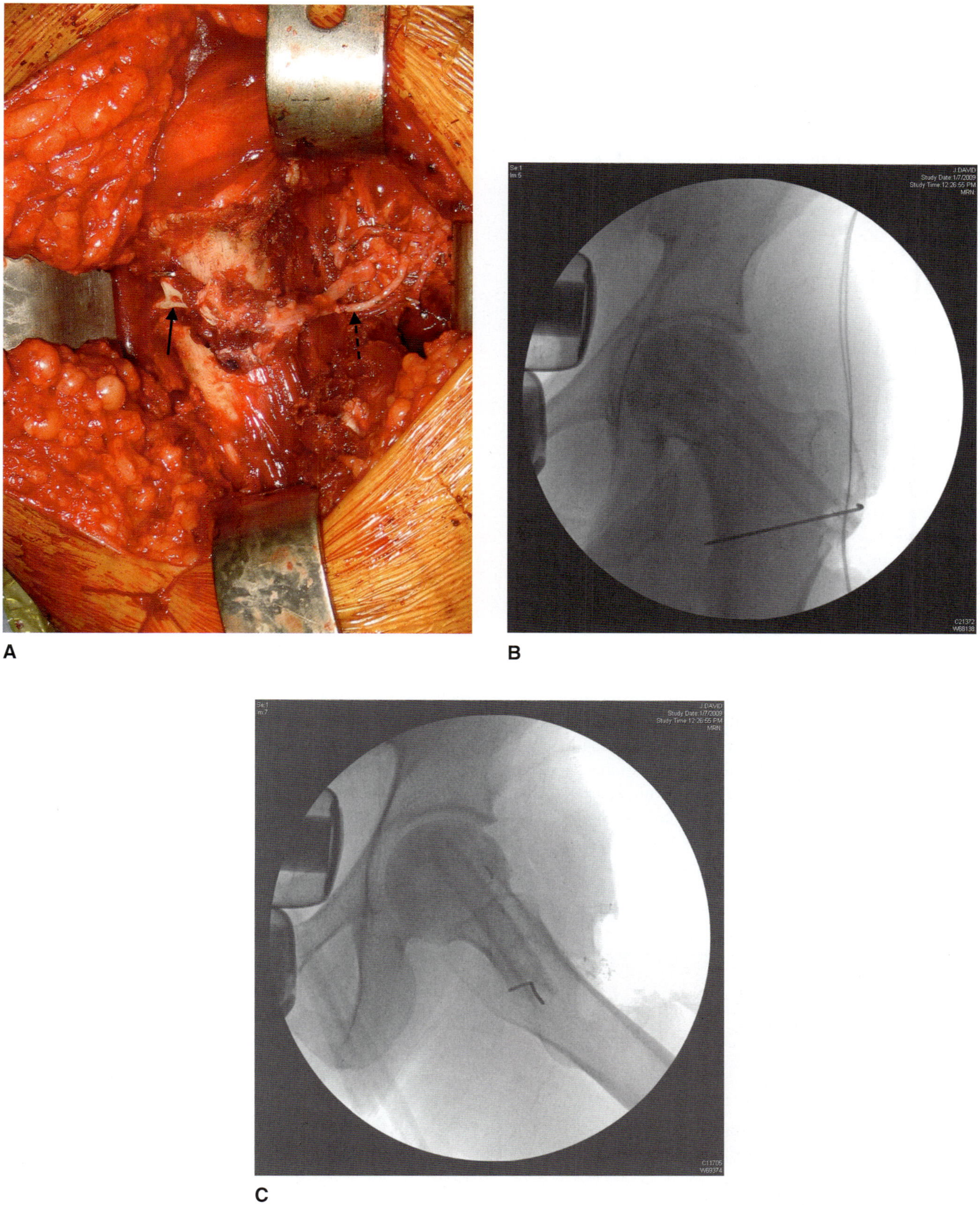

FIGURE 85-14 The fibula (solid arrow) is placed into the core created in the proximal femur with the recipient vessels (dashed arrow) directed anteriorly (**A**). Anteroposterior and lateral radiographs confirm proper placement (**B** and **C**).

The location of the distal hemoclip is confirmed to remain unchanged as the fibula is advanced to ensure that the pedicle is not stripped. A bone tamp is used to gently impact the fibula into its final position. A 0.062-in Kirschner wire is placed through both cortices of the fibula and the medial cortex of the femur. It is imperative to protect the pedicle during placement of the wire and to translate the graft as posterior as possible to maximize space for the pedicle. The wire is bent, cut, and rotated posteriorly into the substance of the gluteus medius muscle.

VESSEL ANASTOMOSES

The four-quadrant retractor is reintroduced at the hip to expose the previous dissection. The peroneal artery and the ascending branch of the lateral circumflex femoral artery are typically 1.5 to 2 mm in size, and the venae comitantes are typically 2.5 to 4 mm in diameter. The vessels are oriented in an AP direction, which usually places the microsurgical field on a slight incline (Figure 85-15). For this reason, it is easiest for the surgeon performing the microvascular anastomosis to stand on the patient's posterior side.

The venous anastomosis is performed first. Because the fibular graft is not a closed system, we routinely anastomose only one vein. Under loupe magnification, the best size match is selected, and the vein is coapted with a commercially available venous coupling device. The 2.5- and 3.0-mm couplers are most commonly used. After the vein is coupled, attention is directed toward the arterial anastomosis.

A microsurgical suction mat is placed as background and secured to remain stable within the depth of the hip wound. A double-occluder vessel clamp on a sliding bar is used to stabilize the lateral femoral circumflex and peroneal arteries. Standard microsurgical techniques are used to perform the arterial anastomosis with 8-0 nylon microsutures placed in a simple, interrupted fashion. The occluder clamp is removed, and the anastomosis is inspected for leaks. After any leaks are identified and addressed, a patency test is performed to confirm appropriate flow across the repair. The previously coupled vein is evaluated for backflow, and after it has been confirmed, a medium hemoclip is placed on the second unused peroneal vein.

The operating microscope is then directed at the cut end of the fibula on the lateral cortex of the femur to inspect for endosteal bleeding. If endosteal bleeding is not present, we identify the cause and address it. The patient's blood pressure and core body temperature are evaluated, and if low, they are reversed. The intramedullary canal of the fibula is copiously irrigated with heparin and papaverine with constant reevaluation for blood flow. If there is still no flow, the arterial anastomosis is reexamined for patency, and the artery is examined for kinks or constrictive bands along its course. Occasionally, the sharp edge of vastus intermedius can remain a point of compression, obstructing flow. Similarly, the vein is reexamined for any leaks, and if found, these are addressed with micro hemoclips.

If none of these efforts results in endosteal flow from the fibula, attention is directed toward the fibular graft itself. We first examine the pin placement to confirm that the wire is not impinging the vascular pedicle. If the pedicle is compressed, this is corrected. If the pedicle is untethered, the pin is removed, and the fibula is extracted as far as the anastomosis allows so that the periosteum and pedicle can be evaluated for vascular leaks. Any identified leaks are managed with a micro hemoclip. The fibula is then reinserted into the core with careful attention to the location of the vascular pedicle. Posterior translation and rotation of the fibular graft within the core are performed to make sure that there is no compression of the vessel. If the vessel remains compressed within the core, the fibula must be removed and the core enlarged. This circumstance occurs rarely, if at all, and can be avoided by careful evaluation of the pedicle at the time of its original insertion before the vascular anastomosis.

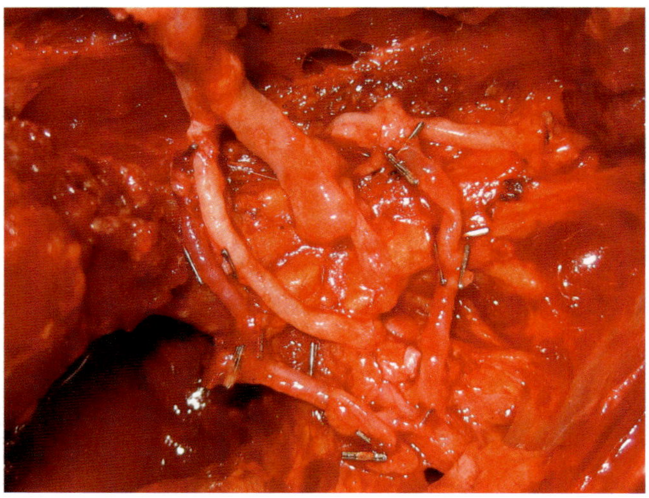

A

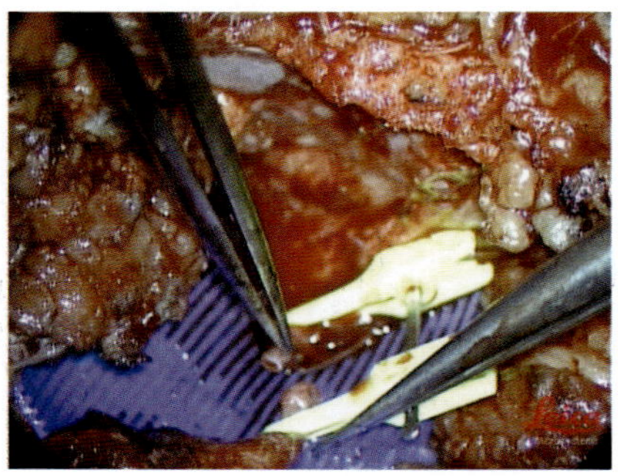

B

FIGURE 85-15 The peroneal and lateral femoral circumflex vessels (A) are prepared for anastomosis (B).

The vastus lateralis and intermedius muscles are not repaired because of the risk of compression to the vascular pedicle. A drain is placed deep, and the fascia is closed with size 0 absorbable suture followed by the subcutaneous and dermal layers.

POSTOPERATIVE MANAGEMENT

We do not routinely use postoperative vascular monitoring of the fibular graft. Postoperative arteriograms were routinely obtained at our institution during the early experience with this procedure. After we were convinced of the reproducibility of the procedure, this practice was abandoned. Other authors have reported on the use of a skin paddle with the fibular graft as a means of postoperative monitoring (15). Although this is a reasonable means of monitoring the vascularity of the fibular graft, its larger donor site morbidity and the technical challenges it introduces to graft placement have prevented us from adopting this technique.

On postoperative day 2, the epidural catheter, Foley catheter, and wound drains are routinely removed. The physical therapist begins working with the patient the same day to mobilize the patient with crutches non–weight bearing on the operative side. The patient remains non–weight bearing for 6 weeks and then begins progressive partial weight bearing with full weight bearing reached by 6 months. The physical therapist also initiates active and passive range of motion exercises to the ankle and toes. The patient is typically discharged on postoperative day 4 after receiving 3 days of intravenous Dextran. They are discharged on 6 weeks of daily aspirin. Follow-up radiographs, including AP pelvis and AP and lateral radiographs of the operative hip, are obtained at 3 months, 6 months, and yearly (Figures 85-16 and 85-17).

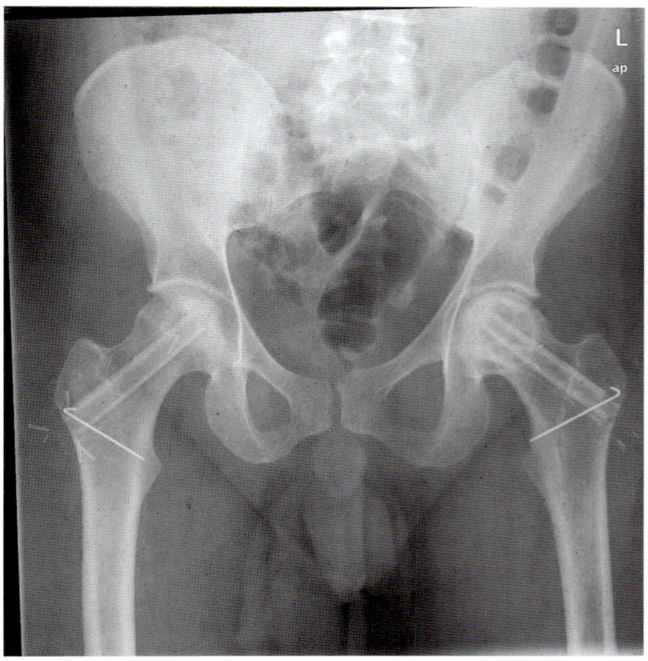

FIGURE 85-16 Anteroposterior pelvis radiograph obtained immediately after surgery.

POTENTIAL COMPLICATIONS

Potential complications exist both at the donor site in the lower leg and at the hip. Several authors have reported on the donor site morbidity of harvesting an FVFG (18–24). Ankle pain, ankle instability, valgus deformity of the ankle, motor weakness, sensory deficit, and great toe flexion contracture have all been reported. At our institution, 247 patients with FVFGs were evaluated for donor site morbidity (24). Nineteen percent of patients had at least one postoperative abnormality related to the harvest. At 3 months after surgery, 10% of patients had motor weakness present, but this improved to 2% at 5 years after the procedure. At 5 years after surgery, sensory disturbance was present in 11.8% of patients and ankle pain in 11.5% of patients. Both of these findings increased with time. Flexion contracture of the great toe was noted to occur earlier in our experience because of the dissection of the flexor hallucis longus. However, with modifications to the postoperative physical therapy program to focus on passive extension exercises, this complication has been largely eliminated.

Complications can also occur at the hip. The core created for insertion of the fibular graft ranges from 13 to 21 mm. This creates a stress riser in the lateral femoral cortex that is at risk for proximal femoral fracture. In the first 707 procedures performed at our institution, 18 proximal femur fractures occurred (2.5%) (25). All of these fractures occurred through the lateral entry point for placement of the fibula. Seventeen fractures occurred during the first 8 weeks after surgery and were all associated with a fall or pivoting on the affected leg. The other fracture occurred 2 years after the procedure in a motor vehicle collision.

The majority of these fractures occurred before changes to the postoperative protocol regarding weight bearing. For the first 251 patients undergoing this procedure, the postoperative protocol was touchdown weight bearing during the first 6 weeks. Twelve fractures occurred during this time (4.8%). The protocol was amended to non–weight bearing for the first 6 weeks after surgery, and the fracture rate was reduced to 1.1% (five of 456). This difference was statistically significant. Patients are counseled regarding the importance of adhering to the non–weight-bearing restrictions during the early postoperative time frame.

Recently, Gaskill et al. reviewed donor and graft site morbidity in 1270 consecutive procedures performed at our institution (26). There were 215 total complications (16.9%), and these were twice as common at the donor site as they were at the recipient site. Major complications requiring either a secondary surgical procedure or chronic pain management occurred in only 4.3% of cases.

RESULTS

Free vascularized fibular grafting has been shown to be effective for the treatment of osteonecrosis of the femoral head. In a prospective study, Urbaniak et al. evaluated 103 hips followed for a minimum of 5 years (11). Failure, as measured by conversion to total hip arthroplasty, occurred in seven of 41 hips with precollapse osteonecrosis lesions, resulting in an 83% survival

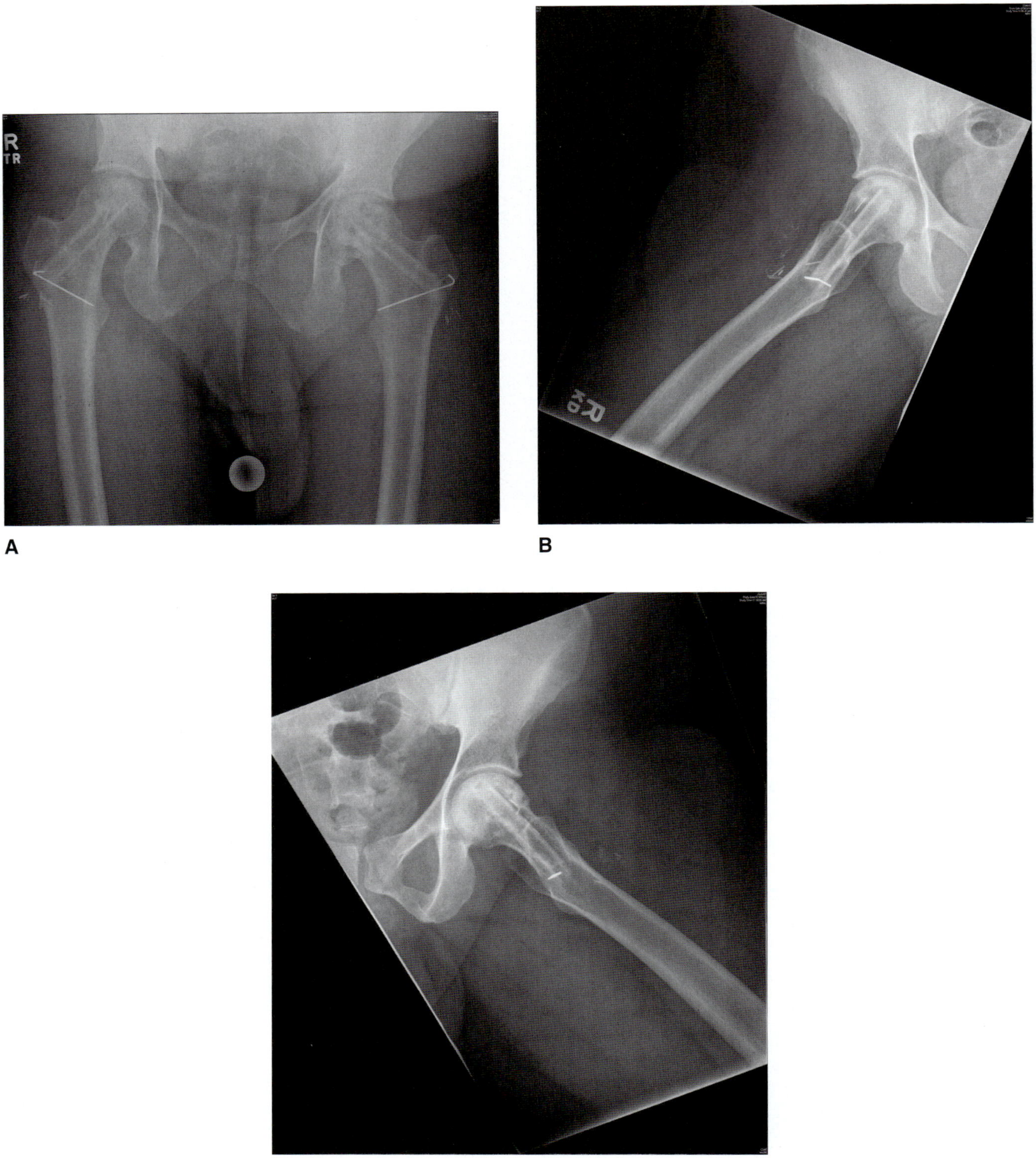

FIGURE 85-17 Anteroposterior pelvis (**A**) and lateral hip radiographs (**B** and **C**) 3 years after surgery. The fibular grafts are completely incorporated.

rate at 5 years. Harris hip scores improved for all groups, and 81% of patients were satisfied with their decision to undergo an FVFG (Figure 85-18). Surgeons at other institutions have reproduced these results. Marciniak et al. reported similar results in 101 hips with a minimum 5-year follow-up (27).

Postcollapse osteonecrosis lesions are more difficult to treat with conventional preservation techniques such as core decompression (28,29). Berend et al. reviewed 224 hips with postcollapse osteonecrosis lesions treated with FVFG (30). The overall survival rate for these hips followed for a minimum of 5 years was 64.5% with improvement in Harris hip scores from 54.5 to 81. These results are superior to those reported for nonoperative management or core decompression.

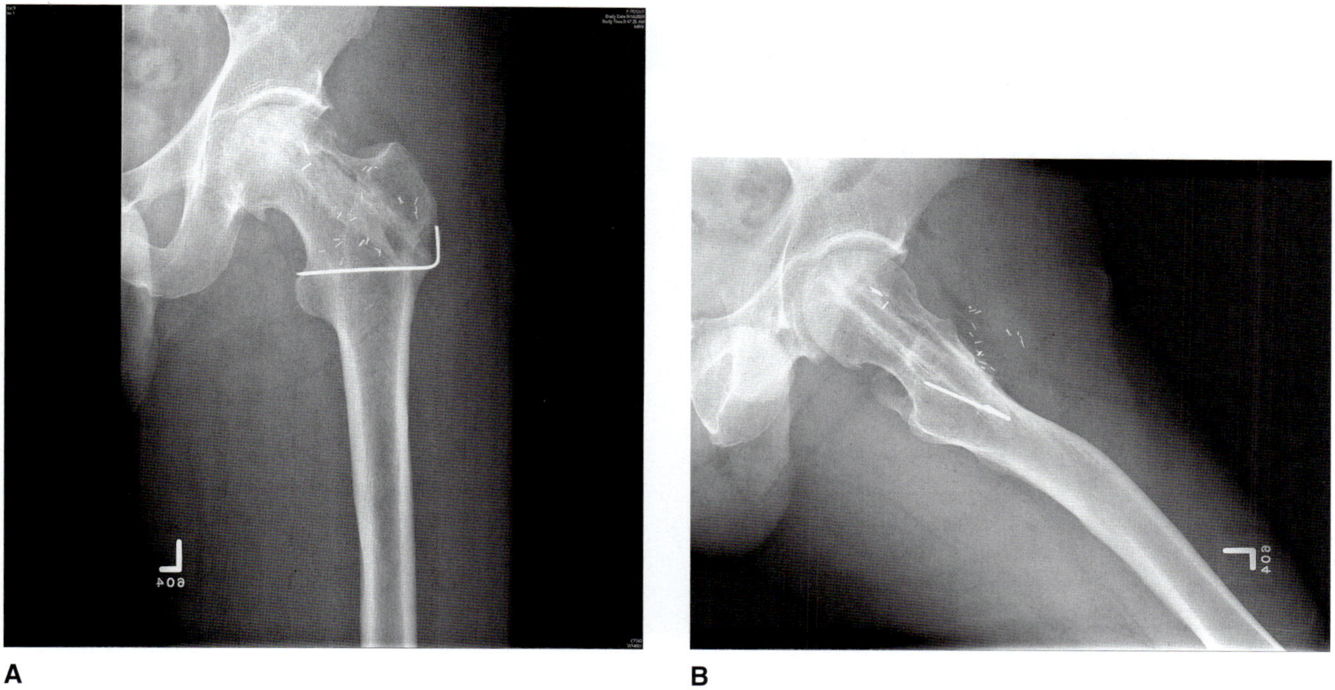

FIGURE 85-18 (A) and (B) Arteroposterior and lateral hip radiographs of a patient 25 years after a left free vascularized fibular graft.

Osteonecrosis of the femoral head remains a very challenging condition to treat in young patients. Hip preservation is a continued goal for this patient population, and FVFG provides a successful option.

REFERENCES

1. Jacobs B. Epidemiology of traumatic and nontraumatic osteonecrosis. *Clin Orthop Relat Res* 1978;(130):51–67.
2. Coventry MB, Beckenbaugh RD, Nolan DR, Ilstrup DM. 2012 total hip arthroplasties. A study of postoperative course and early complications. *J Bone Joint Surg Am* 1974;56(2):273–284.
3. Mont MA, Hungerford DS. Non-traumatic avascular necrosis of the femoral head. *J Bone Joint Surg Am* 1995;77(3):459–474.
4. Urbaniak JR, Harvey EJ. Revascularization of the femoral head in osteonecrosis. *J Am Acad Orthop Surg* 1998;6(1):44–54.
5. Chacha PB. Vascularised pedicular bone grafts. *Int Orthop* 1984;8(2): 117–138.
6. Meyers MH. The treatment of osteonecrosis of the hip with fresh osteochondral allografts and with the muscle pedicle graft technique. *Clin Orthop Relat Res* 1978;(130):202–209.
7. Lee CK, Rehmatullah N. Muscle-pedicle bone graft and cancellous bone graft for the "silent hip" of idiopathic ischemic necrosis of the femoral head in adults. *Clin Orthop Relat Res* 1981;(158):185–194.
8. Baksi DP. Treatment of osteonecrosis of the femoral head by drilling and muscle-pedicle bone grafting. *J Bone Joint Surg Br* 1991;73(2):241–245.
9. Iwata H, Torii S, Hasegawa Y, et al. Indications and results of vascularized pedicle iliac bone graft in avascular necrosis of the femoral head. *Clin Orthop Relat Res* 1993;(295):281–288.
10. Stein H, Volpin G, Horer D. Vascularized muscle pedicle flap for osteonecrosis of the femoral head. *Orthopedics* 2002;25(5):485–488.
11. Urbaniak JR, Coogan PG, Gunneson EE, Nunley JA. Treatment of osteonecrosis of the femoral head with free vascularized fibular grafting. A long-term follow-up study of one hundred and three hips. *J Bone Joint Surg Am* 1995;77(5):681–694.
12. Judet H, Gilbert A. Long-term results of free vascularized fibular grafting for femoral head necrosis. *Clin Orthop Relat Res* 2001;(386):114–119.
13. Brunelli G, Brunelli G. Free microvascular fibular transfer for idiopathic femoral head necrosis: long-term follow-up. *J Reconstr Microsurg* 1991;7(4):285–295.
14. Kim SY, Kim YG, Kim PT, et al. Vascularized compared with nonvascularized fibular grafts for large osteonecrotic lesions of the femoral head. *J Bone Joint Surg Am* 2005;87(9):2012–2018.
15. Yoshimura M, Shimamura K, Iwai Y, et al. Free vascularized fibular transplant. A new method for monitoring circulation of the grafted fibula. *J Bone Joint Surg Am* 1983;65(9):1295–1301.
16. Hungerford DS, Zizic TM. Alcoholism associated ischemic necrosis of the femoral head. Early diagnosis and treatment. *Clin Orthop Relat Res* 1978;(130):144–153.
17. Marchant MH Jr, Zura RD, Urbaniak JR, et al. Hip incision planning for free vascularized fibular grafting of the proximal femur: a handy tip. *J Surg Orthop Adv* 2007;16(4):204–206.
18. Ganel A, Yaffe B. Ankle instability of the donor site following removal of vascularized fibula bone graft. *Ann Plast Surg* 1990;24(1):7–9.
19. Goodacre TE, Walker CJ, Jawad AS, et al. Donor site morbidity following osteocutaneous free fibula transfer. *Br J Plast Surg* 1990;43(4):410–412.
20. Gore DR, Gardner GM, Sepic SB, et al. Function following partial fibulectomy. *Clin Orthop Relat Res* 1987;(220):206–210.
21. Hsu LC, Yau AC, O'Brien JP, Hodgson AR. Valgus deformity of the ankle resulting from fibular resection for a graft in subtalar fusion in children. *J Bone Joint Surg Am* 1972;54(3):585–594.
22. Lee EH, Goh JC, Helm R, Pho RW. Donor site morbidity following resection of the fibula. *J Bone Joint Surg Br* 1990;72(1):129–131.
23. Youdas JW, Wood MB, Cahalan TD, Chao EY. A quantitative analysis of donor site morbidity after vascularized fibula transfer. *J Orthop Res* 1988;6(5):621–629.
24. Vail TP, Urbaniak JR. Donor-site morbidity with use of vascularized autogenous fibular grafts. *J Bone Joint Surg Am* 1996;78(2):204–211.
25. Aluisio FV, Urbaniak JR. Proximal femur fractures after free vascularized fibular grafting to the hip. *Clin Orthop Rel Res* 1998;(356):192–201.
26. Gaskill TR, Urbaniak JR, Aldridge JM 3rd. Free vascularized fibular transfer for femoral head osteonecrosis: donor and graft site morbidity. *J Bone Joint Surg Am* 2009;91(8):1861–1867.
27. Marciniak D, Furey C, Shaffer JW. Osteonecrosis of the femoral head. A study of 101 hips treated with vascularized fibular grafting. *J Bone Joint Surg Am* 2005;87(4):742–747.
28. Atsumi T and Kuroki Y. Modified Sugioka's osteotomy: more than 130 degrees posterior rotation for osteonecrosis of the femoral head with large lesion. *Clin Orthop* 1997;334:98–107.
29. Bozic KJ, Zurakowski D, Thornhill TS. Survivorship analysis of hips treated with core decompression for nontraumatic osteonecrosis of the femoral head. *J Bone Joint Surg Am* 1999;81:200–209.
30. Berend KR, Gunneson EE, Urbaniak JR. Free vascularized fibular grafting for the treatment of postcollapse osteonecrosis of the femoral head. *J Bone Joint Surg Am* 2003;85(6):987–993.

CHAPTER 86

Free Vascularized Epiphyseal Transfer

Carla Baldrighi and Marco Innocenti

Regardless of its etiology, when the physis and epiphysis are damaged in a skeletally immature individual, there are three objectives for the reconstructive orthopedic surgeon: replacement of the osseous defect, restoration of joint function, and restoration of longitudinal growth. Failure in achieving these objectives leads to severe deformity and functional impairment, which significantly compromises the quality of life of young patients.

Conventional methods of joint reconstruction such as customized prosthetic implants and nonvascularized osteoarticular allografts can achieve good functional outcomes and overcome the bone defects and are often the treatment of choice in adults, but none of these procedures can provide physiological bone growth.

Autologous vascularized epiphyseal transfer is the only procedure able to simultaneously reconstruct a mobile joint, replace the bone defect, and maintain the growth potential. The longer the expected period of time between surgery and the end of growth, the stronger the indication for this technique.

DONOR SITES

A number of different donor bones have been suggested in an attempt to minimize the morbidity at the donor site. The scapula, iliac crest, toe phalanges, and proximal fibula have all been described in a variety of clinical situations to reconstruct bony defects. The scapula and iliac crest, however, do not possess a true epiphysis but only an apophysis. Although their use has been reported in cases of lower limb reconstruction (1–3), their growth potential is less predictable compared with an epiphyseal transfer. In addition, in the absence of a real articular surface, the hyaline cartilage that coats the apophysis, may suffer severe chondrolysis and the possibility of progressive arthritis when transferred into an intraarticular location (3). Furthermore, both the scapula and iliac crest are flat bones that do not possess a tubular portion. A variable length of shaft is often required to allow a stable bone fixation in long diaphyseal reconstructions.

The best options for osteoarticular reconstruction are the proximal fibula, metatarsal, or toe phalanx epiphyseal transfers. For major long bone reconstructions, the fibula is preferred because it provides a true epiphysis and a long diaphysis.

INDICATIONS

The main indications for epiphyseal reconstruction are loss of epiphysis or epiphyseal arrest after trauma, tumor resection, or infection and congenital deficiencies in the pediatric age group. Bone tumors in children are often located in the metaphysis. Epiphyseal transfer has been proven to be an excellent option in limb salvage surgery in pediatric oncologic cases and has significantly reduced the need for amputation.

Clinical observation has shown that the plasticity of immature bone allows for remarkable adaptive remodeling of the epiphysis when transferred to a new biomechanical environment, which results in progressive improvement of the articular function. Because of its biologic and morphologic characteristics (long, expendable diaphysis), the proximal fibula is by far the best donor site for skeletal reconstruction of large bone defects of the upper extremity. In particular, the fibular graft is the optimal reconstruction for the distal radius (4) because the diaphyses of both bones are very similar in shape and dimension, and stable bone fixation can be easily achieved (Figure 86-1).

However, the proximal fibular epiphysis can also be used in lower limb skeletal reconstruction. Anatomical mismatch between the graft and the recipient site (femur or tibia) and the high functional demands because of weight bearing are the main reasons for limited indications in lower limb reconstruction. Nevertheless, the procedure has been applied in selected cases for hip, knee and ankle reconstruction with variable results.

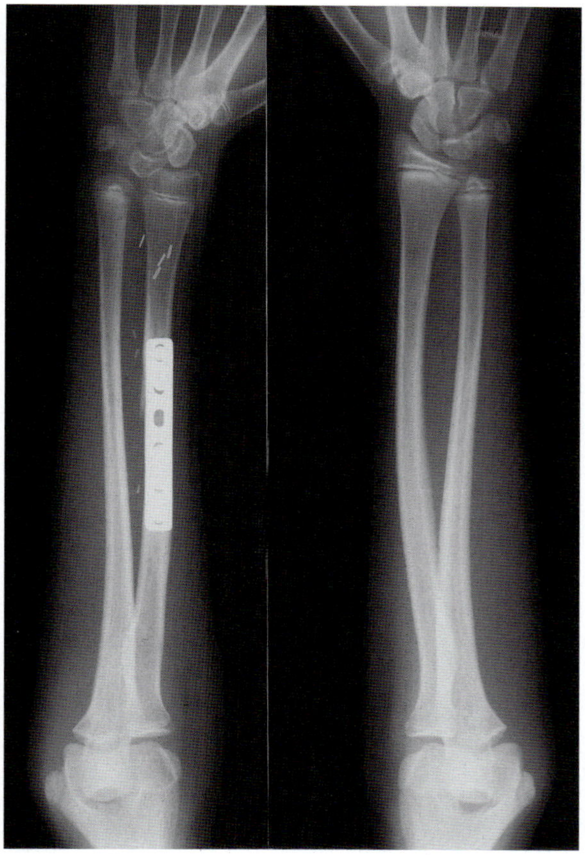

FIGURE 86-1 Distal radius reconstruction. The diaphysis of the fibula and the radius match in size and shape. (With permission from Journal of Bone and Joint Surgery American, July, 2004, 86, 7, Vascularized Proximal Fibular Epiphyseal Transfer for Distal Radial Reconstruction. 2, Innocenti, 1504-1511.)

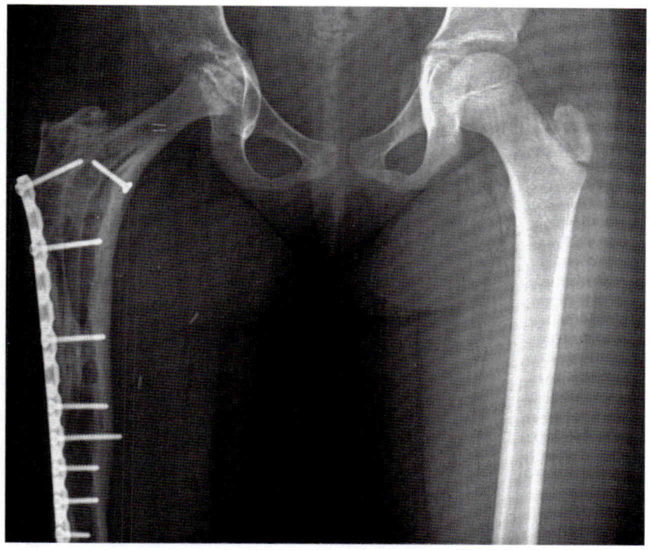

FIGURE 86-2 Hip reconstruction. The allograft progressively undergoes resorption while the fibular epiphysis hypertrophies because of the new stress loads at the recipient site.

Concannon et al. (5), Rajacic and Dashti (6), Becker and Zuker (7), and de Gauzy et al. (8) reported encouraging results using the ipsilateral proximal fibula, either as a free or pedicled transfer, for lateral malleolus reconstruction in growing individuals. Similarity in size and shape between the donor and the recipient segments ensured acceptable functional results in this very challenging clinical problem because loss of the lateral malleolus leads to severe instability and angular deformity of the ankle. Vascularized transfer of the ipsilateral proximal fibula provides lateral stability to the ankle joint and the potential for continuing longitudinal growth, avoiding total ankle fusion.

This procedure has also been used infrequently for hip reconstruction after tumor resection or septic arthritis. We reported the first reconstruction of the hip in a growing individual with an original technique in 2003 in which the proximal femur, affected by a Ewing's sarcoma, was replaced with an allograft together with an autologous proximal fibula vascularized transfer (9) (Figure 86-2). The outcome of this case has been very satisfactory, and at 12 years of follow-up, the patient is able to walk and has nearly normal range of motion (10). Impressive morphologic remodeling (11) was observed during the first years after surgery because of the new loading stress with progressive hypertrophy of the fibular head. These changes have gradually improved the articular function, and the growth plate remained active until the physiological end of growth.

Many variables such as availability of an allograft of the appropriate size; stable bone fixation; assembly of the allograft and autograft; successful restoration of blood supply to the fibular graft; remodeling of the joint; and, last but not least, the need for a meticulous, cautious, long, and complex rehabilitation combine to determine the quality of the result. Since then, these procedures have been performed, with or without allograft, in a small clinical series with variable results (12–14).

Although most of the procedures worldwide have been performed for tumor cases, congenital differences of the upper limb may also benefit from epiphyseal transfer. In particular, Vilkki's experience with the second metatarsophalangeal joint transfer for the treatment of radial dysplasia has given a new impetus to the surgical treatment of this debilitating condition (15,16). Nonetheless the use of proximal fibular epiphyseal transfer in radial dysplasia raises the following concerns and considerations: The new radius may be expected to grow more than the native ulna, which is usually hypoplastic, thus resulting in wrist instability and ulnar deviation. Ideal timing for reconstruction is when the child is learning to walk, but the donor site from harvesting the fibula may temporarily delay this milestone. The literature on epiphyseal transfer for radial dysplasia is very sparse, and there is no report on long-term outcomes that would help in validating this technique (12,17,18).

ANATOMY OF THE PROXIMAL FIBULAR EPIPHYSIS

The flap includes the proximal fibular epiphysis and a variable amount of the adjoining diaphysis. The epiphyseal articular surface is oriented upward and medially to form the proximal tibiofibular joint. The biceps femoris tendon and the lateral collateral ligament are inserted on the lateral and proximal aspect of the epiphysis, which is also where the origins of the peroneus longus (PL) and extensor digitorum longus (EDL) muscles are located. The common peroneal nerve courses around the fibular neck in a submuscular location while entering the anterior compartment of the leg. The superficial branch is located in the space between the EDL and PL muscles, and the deep branch reaches the interosseous membrane and joins the anterior tibial artery. In the proximal half of the leg, the nerve surrounds the vascular bundle in an intricate three-dimensional pattern and sends several branches to the surrounding muscles of the anterior compartment.

Vascular Anatomy of the Proximal Fibular Epiphysis

In the past 30 years, the vascular anatomy of the proximal fibular epiphysis has been extensively investigated to define the best pedicle to supply both the epiphysis and the diaphysis of such a graft. There is general agreement that the proximal epiphysis of the fibula is supplied by two constant vascular pedicles, (1) the lateral inferior genicular artery and (2) the recurrent branches of the anterior tibial artery, and a third variable supply from an unnamed artery arising directly from the popliteal artery.

Different vascular systems contribute to the vascularization of different portions of the proximal epiphysis and diaphysis of the fibula. Summarizing the data available from the literature, the anterior and posterior recurrent branches of the anterior tibial artery provide the major contribution to the blood supply of the proximal fibular growth plate, the lateral inferior geniculate artery mostly supplies the capsule of the proximal tibiofibular joint, and the peroneal artery supplies the fibular diaphysis (19–23). It has also been demonstrated experimentally (20,23) that the anterior tibial artery is able to supply the proximal two thirds of the fibular diaphysis through tiny musculoperiosteal perforators (Figure 86-3).

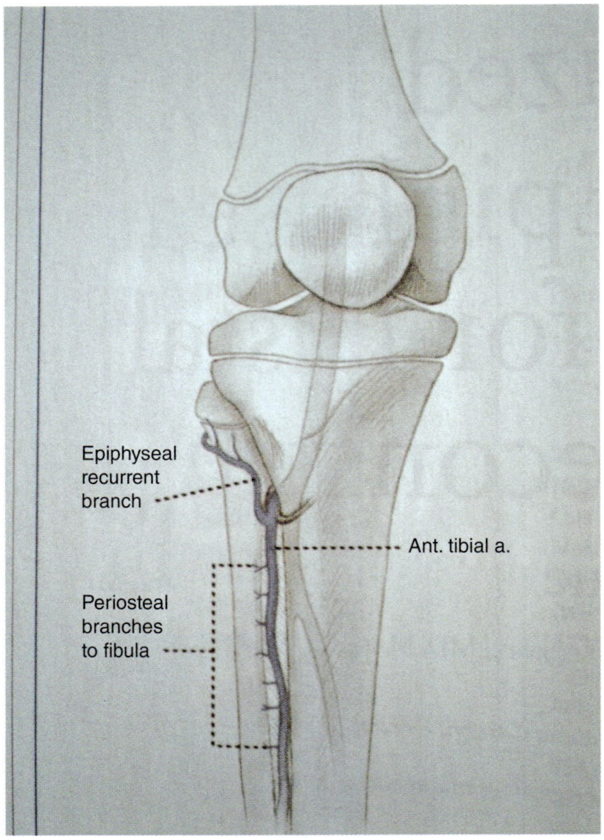

FIGURE 86-3 The anterior tibial artery supplies the proximal fibula growth plate through the recurrent epiphyseal branch and the proximal two thirds of the fibula shaft through delicate periosteal perforators passing through the muscles. a, artery; ant, anterior. (With permission from Journal of Bone and Joint Surgery American, September, 2005, 87, S1P2, Vascularized Proximal Fibular Epiphyseal Transfer for Distal Radial Reconstruction, Innocenti, 237-246.)

The fibular epiphysis can be harvested on a double or single pedicle. Almost all the possible vascular pedicle combinations described have been used in clinical practice.

The use of the peroneal artery alone as the pedicle for this flap has been described (24) in the belief that intercommunicating branches between the metaphyseal and the epiphyseal systems would allow for acceptable blood supply to the growth plate. Although this is probably anatomically possible if enough soft tissue is left around the fibula neck, this contradicts the classical anatomical studies (25), which demonstrate that the diaphyseal and the epiphyseal vascular networks are independent and do not connect with each other until the end of growth.

Further experience has demonstrated that the vascular contribution from the peroneal artery to the epiphysis is insufficient (19,22). Grafts based solely on the peroneal artery have resulted in unpredictable outcomes (26) in terms of growth, and the majority failed to achieve any acceptable growth.

Further anatomical investigations of the proximal fibula vascular supply (19) have demonstrated that the epiphysis is vascularized by the descending genicular artery and a recurrent branch from the anterior tibial artery. The use of double pedicled grafts, based on the peroneal artery, and either the descending genicular artery or the recurrent branch of the anterior tibial artery have been suggested (3,17,27,28) with the purpose of providing optimal perfusion to both the epiphysis and the diaphysis through two separate blood supplies. This surgical solution, however, is technically demanding and time consuming and requires two anastomoses at the recipient site. In addition, the physis is very susceptible to ischemia, and normal growth only can be expected if the ischemia time does not exceed 3 hours (29). For these reasons, the use of a single pedicle graft is advisable.

In 1988, Taylor et al. described an anterolateral approach to the fibula and suggested the possibility of harvesting the proximal two thirds of the bone based on the anterior tibial artery alone (23). This approach was supported by anatomical findings that the anterior tibial artery contributes significantly to the periosteal diaphyseal vascular supply to the fibula through tiny branches arising from the proximal and middle thirds of this artery. The constant presence of the recurrent epiphyseal branch makes the anterior tibial artery the ideal pedicle to provide adequate blood supply to both the diaphysis and epiphysis of a growing fibula, provided that the epiphyseal vessels and the delicate periosteal vascular network of the diaphysis are preserved during the dissection (see Figure 86-3).

A potential disadvantage to the use of the anterior tibial vascular system is the shortness of its pedicle (the distance between its origin from the popliteal artery and the origin of the recurrent branch at the fibular neck) and often needs to be lengthened with a vein graft. To overcome this issue, the original technique was modified by using a reverse flow pedicle of the anterior tibial artery (4,18,27). As suggested in the literature (30,31) and confirmed by clinical experience, the reversal of blood flow in the venae comitantes occurs by several shunts that interconnect the veins and bypass the valves. These interconnecting shunts must be preserved during the dissection of the vascular bundle. When performing the venous anastomosis, usually only one of the two venae comitantes provides adequate outflow.

The reverse flow anterior artery pedicle allows comfortable and reliable anastomoses at the recipient site.

SURGICAL TECHNIQUE

The harvesting technique has been refined over the years (4,32) with the purpose of standardizing it and making it reproducible. The aim is to harvest the proximal fibula on the anterior tibial artery and veins as a reverse vascular pedicle (19,23), preserving the blood supply to both the epiphysis and diaphysis with the least possible local morbidity. The following step-by-step description is the optimal surgical sequence according to the experience of the senior author.

Position

The patient is placed supine with the donor extremity flexed at the hip and the knee and internally rotated. A sterile tourniquet is applied to maintain a bloodless field.

Because the dissection can be tedious and time consuming, the ischemia time should not exceed 2 hours.

Skin Incision

An anterolateral approach is recommended (Figure 86-4). Through a straight longitudinal incision, the plane between the tibialis anterior (TA) muscle and the EDL muscle is developed to allow direct visualization of the neurovascular bundle. The incision is then extended posteriorly in a lazy S-shape centered on the fibular neck and proximally following the tendon of the biceps femoris muscle.

Exposure of the Anterior Tibial Vascular Pedicle

The superficial fascia is incised to expose the anterior tibial neurovascular bundle that lies on the interosseous membrane in the intermuscular plane between TA and EDL muscle bellies (Figure 86-5). The peroneal nerve surrounds the vascular bundle in a very intricate three-dimensional pattern and provides several motor branches to the muscles of the anterior compartment of the leg. In the lower third of the leg, the motor branches from the deep peroneal nerve and the perforating vessels to the fibular diaphysis become more sporadic and less intricate, making it easier for the surgeon to identify the correct plane of dissection. It is therefore recommended to start exposure of the neurovascular pedicle fairly distally and proceed proximally, carefully maintaining the same plane of dissection

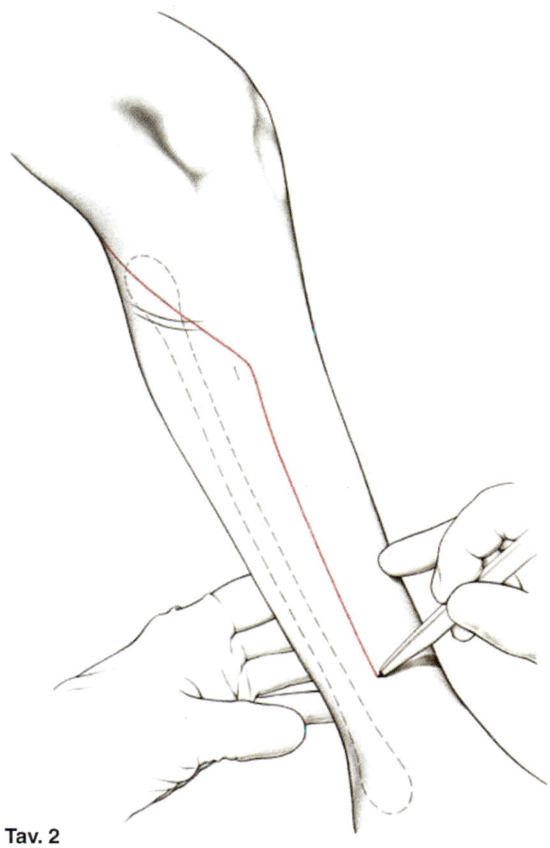

A

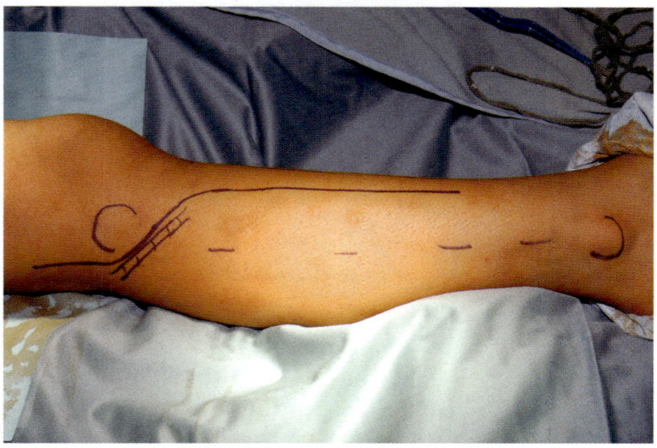

B

FIGURE 86-4 (A) and (B) Anterolateral approach. A straight longitudinal incision is developed in the plane between the tibialis anterior and extensor digitorum longus muscles. m, muscle.

up to the fibular neck. Dissection of the vascular pedicle must preserve the peroneal nerve motor branches as well as the delicate vascular network of musculoperiosteal branches that pierce the EDL and PL muscles, interposed between the vascular pedicle and the fibular shaft, which supply the periosteum of the proximal two thirds of the fibular diaphysis (Figure 86-6).

In some instances, however, these peroneal nerve motor branches may pass through the space between the vascular bundle and the bone, making it impossible to preserve them

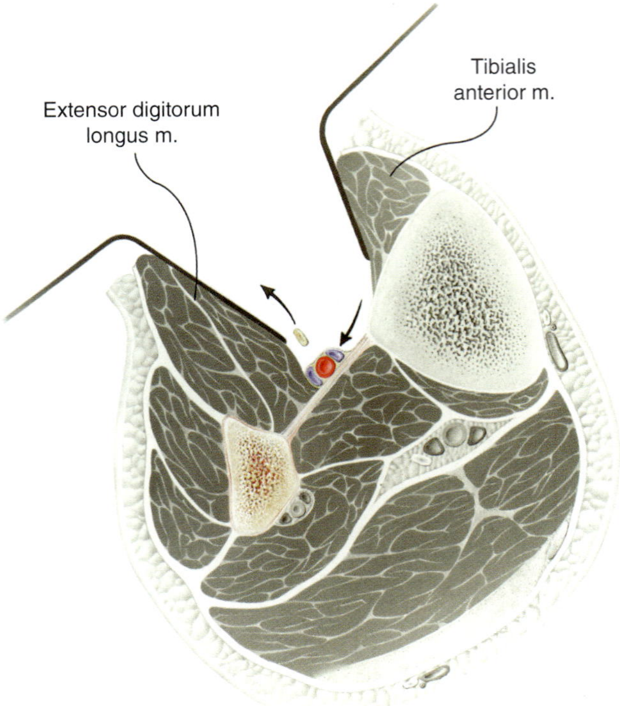

A

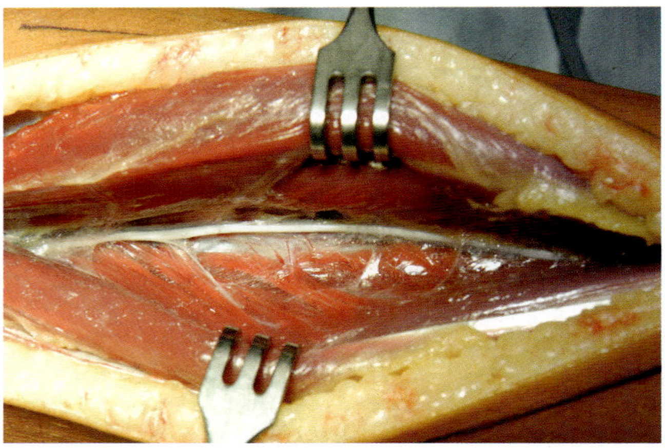

B

FIGURE 86-5 (A) and (B) The superficial fascia is incised. The anterior tibial neurovascular bundle lies on the interosseous membrane in the intermuscular plane between the tibialis anterior and extensor digitorum longus muscles. (With permission from Journal of Bone and Joint Surgery American, July, 2004, 86, 7, Vascularized Proximal Fibular Epiphyseal Transfer for Distal Radial Reconstruction. 2, Innocenti, 1504-1511.)

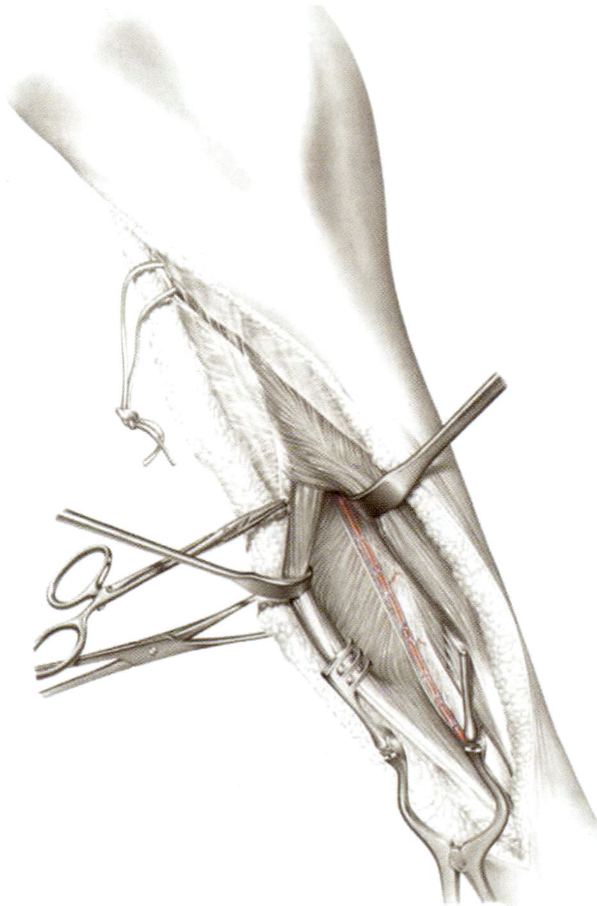

Tav. 6
Apertura della loggia anteriore della gamba

A

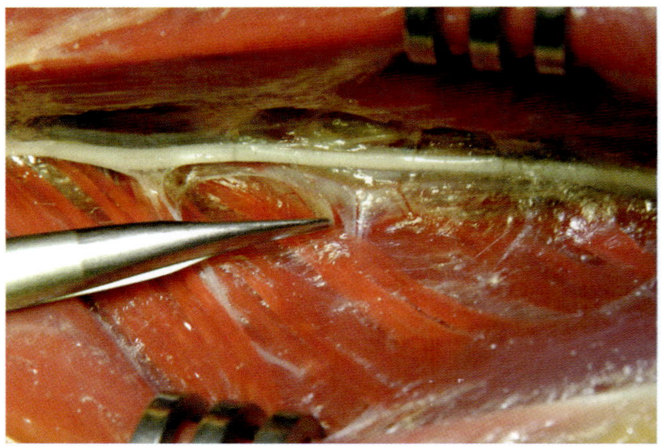

B

FIGURE 86-6 (A) and (B) Musculoperiosteal perforators pass through the extensor digitorum longus and peroneus longus muscles between the vascular pedicle and the fibular shaft and supply the periosteum of the proximal two thirds of the fibular diaphysis.

during the dissection. The surgeon must intentionally transect these nerve branches to mobilize the vascular pedicle. In such cases, immediate nerve repair or direct neurotization is mandatory to reduce the donor site morbidity.

Dissection of the Peroneal Nerve at the Fibular Neck

The fibular neck is an important anatomic landmark. At this level, the common peroneal nerve is in close contact with the bone and is covered by the origins of EDL and PL muscles. The origins of these muscles are sharply incised and retracted laterally and downward so that the common peroneal nerve can be identified and protected (Figure 86-7). At the same level of the fibular neck, the recurrent epiphyseal branch of the anterior tibial artery arises from the main artery and pierces the muscular cuff to supply the epiphysis. Direct dissection of this fragile vascular network is not only unnecessary but also potentially dangerous. For this reason,

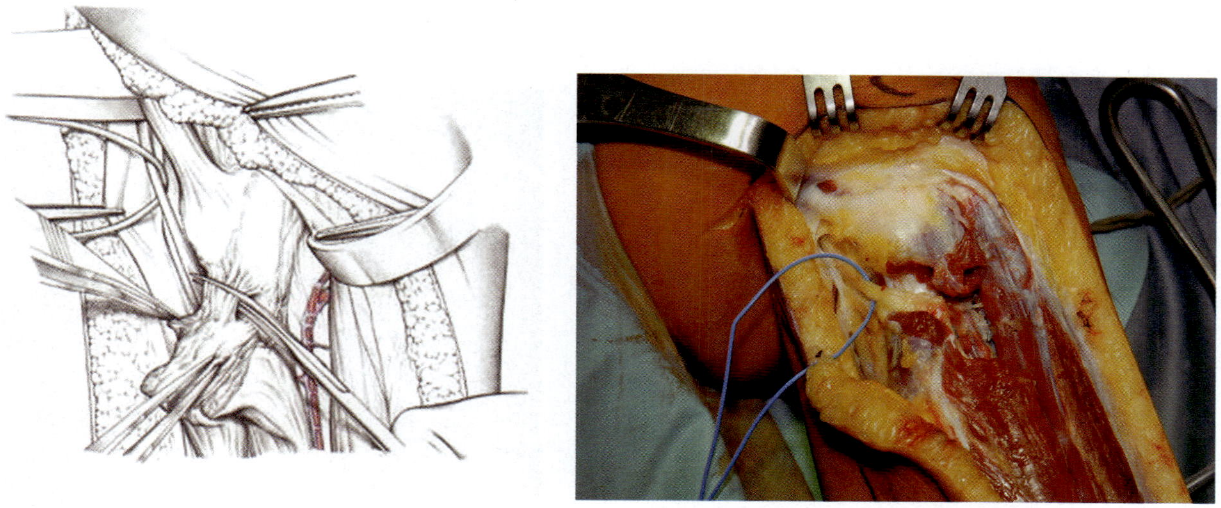

FIGURE 86-7 (A) and (B) The common peroneal nerve is identified and protected after the origins of extensor digitorum longus and peroneus longus muscles have been divided and retracted.

it is recommended that the insertion of the EDL, PL, and peroneus brevis (P Br) muscles are divided about 2 cm distally from the fibular tip, leaving the muscular cuff surrounding the fibular epiphysis intact.

Division of the Interosseous Membrane and Distal Osteotomy

Direct dissection of the tiny intramuscular periosteal perforators through the muscle fibers is to be avoided. To protect these small vessels and preserve the blood supply to the fibular shaft, first the interosseous membrane is sharply detached from the tibia, and all the soft tissue interposed between the vascular bundle and the fibula is left intact so that the vascular pedicle and its branches lie undisturbed in their natural bed (Figure 86-8). Second, a longitudinal strip of muscle approximately 1 cm wide is maintained around the harvested fibula.

At this stage, the fibular shaft is almost completely exposed by the anterolateral approach, and the distal osteotomy can be performed at the desired level. The fibula is then separated from the surrounding posterior muscles and the peroneal artery, which is located in close proximity to the posteromedial aspect of the middle and distal thirds of the fibula. The anterior tibial artery and veins are ligated as far distally as the ankle joint to provide a remarkably long reverse flow pedicle.

When performing the distal osteotomy, extra periosteum is harvested to cover the site of osteosynthesis and enhance bone healing after the fibula is fixed to the recipient bone.

The length of fibular shaft harvested should never exceed the proximal two thirds of the diaphysis to guarantee reliable perfusion through the periosteum.

Harvest of the Biceps Femoris Tendon and Capsulotomy of the Proximal Tibiofibular Joint

The insertions of the lateral collateral ligament and the biceps femoris tendon are almost at the same point at the apex of the fibula (Figure 86-9). The lateral collateral ligament is transected as distally as possible. The tendon of the biceps femoris muscle is divided longitudinally: the anterior portion of the tendon is used to reinforce the lateral collateral ligament to improve stability of the knee joint, and the posterior strip is harvested with the fibula (Figure 86-10). This strong tendon strip inserted into the proximal epiphysis provides stability of the "new" joint after transfer to the recipient site (Figure 86-11). Gentle external rotation of the fibula allows division of the medial and posterior capsule of the proximal tibiofibular joint (Figure 86-12), but the descending or inferior genicular artery must be ligated before this maneuver. The soft tissue release is then complete.

Final Dissection of the Vascular Pedicle

The recurrent epiphyseal branch rises from the anterior tibial artery approximately 1 to 2 cm distal to its origin. This branch is difficult to identify and immediately perforates through the muscular cuff surrounding the epiphysis. All of the small perforators that pass through the muscles to the fibular epiphysis must be preserved by harvesting a cuff of muscle. The collateral medial branches are then ligated, and the fibular head is subluxed laterally, allowing better exposure of the interosseous space and the posterior compartment where the anterior tibial artery lies. The anterior tibial artery is then dissected up to its origin from the popliteal artery, and the tourniquet is released at this stage. After a few seconds, bleeding should be observed from the muscular cuff surrounding the epiphysis, the diaphyseal periosteum, and the medullary canal, confirming successful harvest of the proximal fibula based on the anterior tibial artery reverse pedicle (see Figure 86-1). Because of its low tolerance to ischemia, the surgeon should wait 20 to 30 minutes for adequate reperfusion of the growth plate before ligating and dividing the proximal pedicle (Figure 86-13) to complete the harvest of

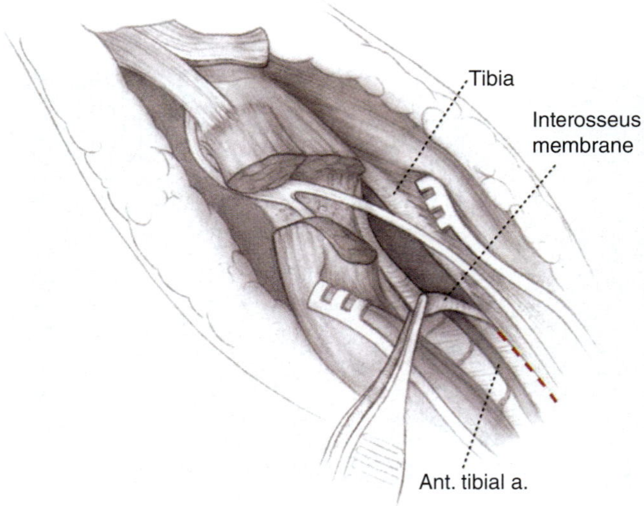

A

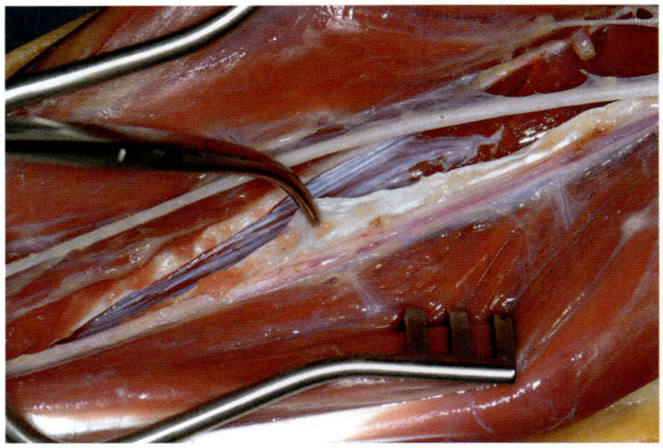

B

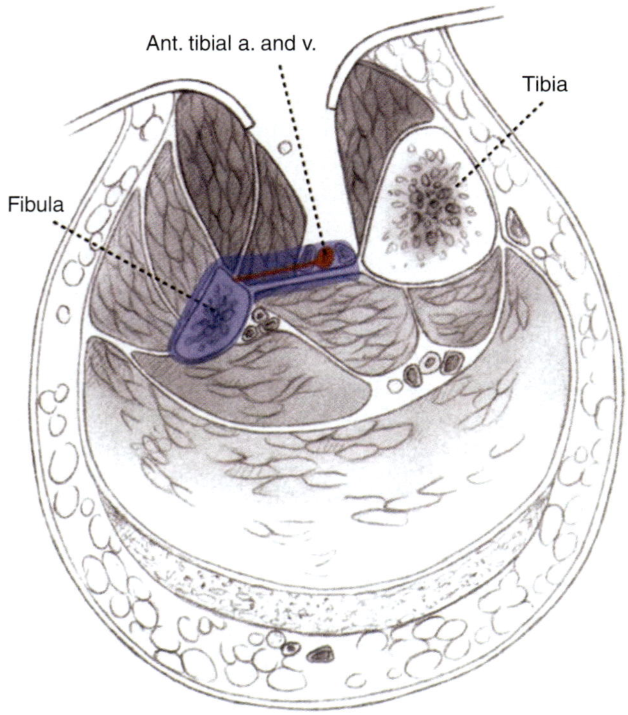

C

FIGURE 86-8 (A) and (B) The interosseous membrane is sharply detached from the tibia, and the soft tissue between the interosseous membrane and the vascular bundle is left intact (C) so that the periosteal branches lie undisturbed in their natural bed. a, artery; ant, anterior; v, vein. (With permission from Journal of Bone and Joint Surgery American, September, 2005, 87, S1P2, Vascularized Proximal Fibular Epiphyseal Transfer for Distal Radial Reconstruction, Innocenti, 237-246.)

the proximal fibular epiphysis based on the anterior tibial vessels (Figure 86-14).

Donor Site Closure

After harvesting the fibula, the lateral stability of the knee joint must be restored. The lateral collateral ligament, reinforced with the residual biceps femoris tendon strip, is reinserted onto the lateral aspect of the tibial metaphysis using staples or transosseous nonresorbable suture. In our experience, this technique guarantees adequate knee stability.

POSTOPERATIVE CARE

Donor Site

To protect the reconstructed lateral collateral ligament, the knee is immobilized in 30 degrees of flexion and the ankle in neutral position in a cast. In children younger than 8 years of age, the cast is maintained for 4 weeks; in older, more compliant children, the cast may be changed after 2 weeks to a brace for a total of 4 weeks of immobilization. The rehabilitation program is started 1 month after surgery with the aim to recover full motion of the knee without compromising stability.

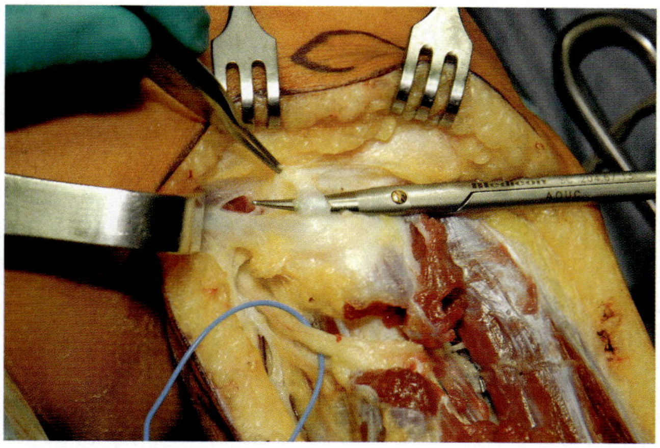

FIGURE 86-9 Insertion of the lateral collateral ligament at the apex of the fibula.

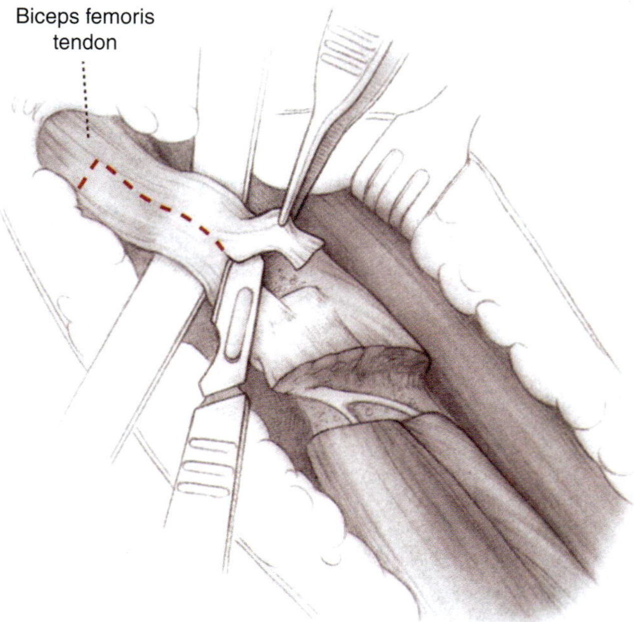

A

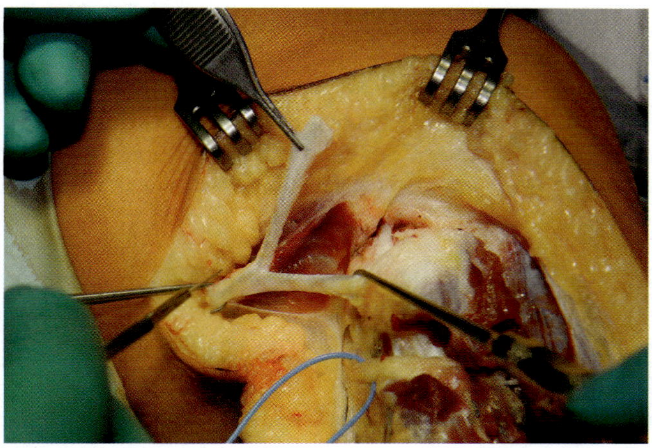

B

FIGURE 86-10 (A) and (B) The biceps femoris tendon is divided longitudinally. The anterior portion of the tendon is used to reinforce the lateral collateral ligament, and the posterior portion is harvested with the fibula. (With permission from Journal of Bone and Joint Surgery American, September, 2005, 87, S1P2, Vascularized Proximal Fibular Epiphyseal Transfer for Distal Radial Reconstruction, Innocenti, 237-246.)

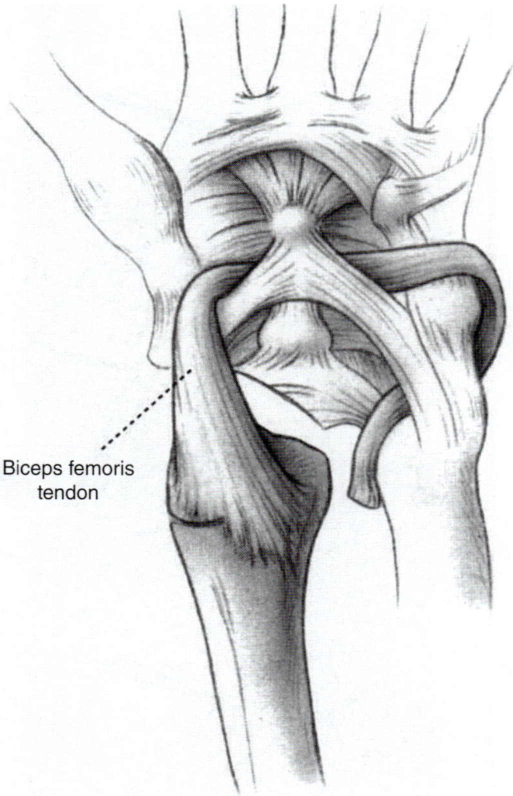

FIGURE 86-11 The biceps femoris tendon strip attached to the fibula is used to increase joint stability at the recipient site. (With permission from Journal of Bone and Joint Surgery American, September, 2005, 87, S1P2, Vascularized Proximal Fibular Epiphyseal Transfer for Distal Radial Reconstruction, Innocenti, 237-246.)

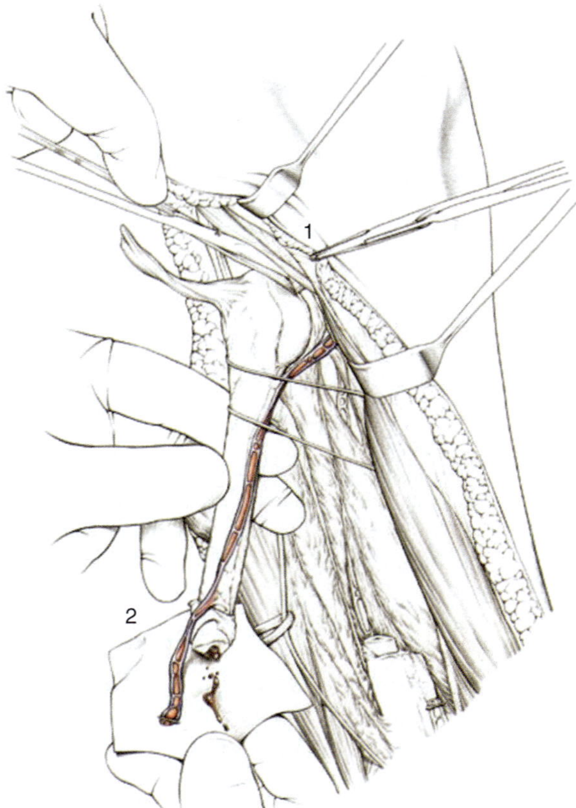

Tav. 15
1 Sezione della capsula articolare posteriore.
2 Controllo dell'irrorazione del segmento osseo.

FIGURE 86-12 Bleeding from the medullary canal is observed after tourniquet release.

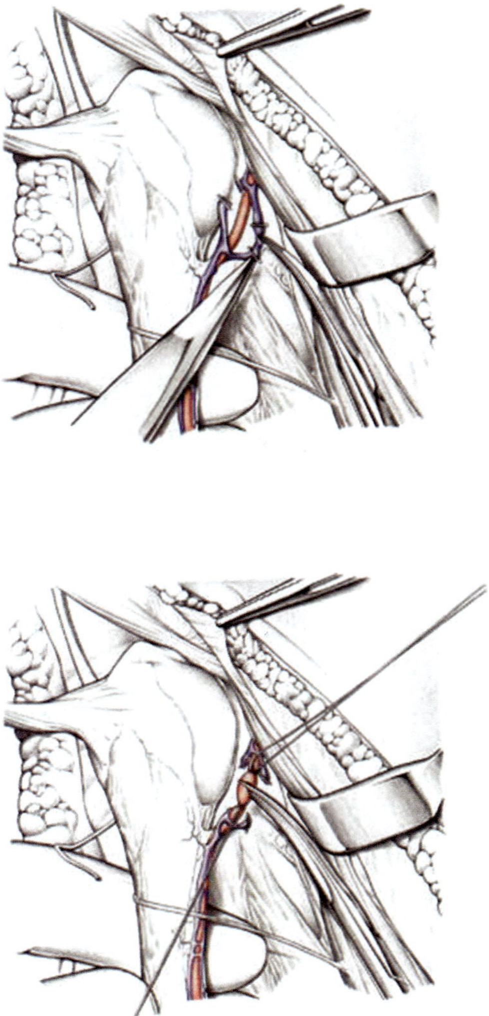

A

B

FIGURE 86-13 The proximal anterior tibial pedicle is divided. (**A**) The venae comitantes are ligated. (**B**) The anterior tibial artery is divided.

A transient palsy of the peroneal nerve occurs in almost all cases. These patients are managed with splinting and passive mobilization to avoid equinus deformity. Full weight bearing is usually possible 2 months after surgery.

Recipient Site

The rehabilitation program is tailored for each patient according to the joint reconstructed (upper vs. lower extremities), the stability of bone fixation at the recipient site, and the age and compliance of the patient.

Harvest of the proximal fibula, if performed meticulously as described, has proved to be effective for the reconstruction of bone defects in children, providing continuing and significant axial growth of the transferred fibula. The procedure is very demanding technically and should be performed by skilled microsurgeons, but it is sufficiently standardized to be introduced into clinical practice. The choice of the anterior tibial artery as a single vascular pedicle significantly reduces the ischemia time of the bone during the operation and thus prevents potential ischemic damage to the growth plate. In addition, the reverse flow design provides a very long distal pedicle and makes a vein graft unnecessary.

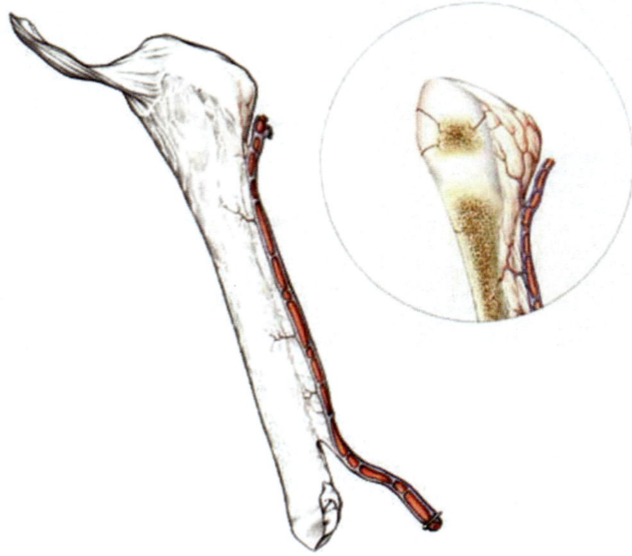

FIGURE 86-14 Harvest of the proximal fibular epiphysis based on the reverse anterior tibial vessels is completed.

COMPLICATIONS

The only complication observed at the donor site pertains to the function of the deep peroneal nerve. As already mentioned, the dissection of the nerve away from the vascular pedicle is very difficult, and some muscle weakness with foot drop should be expected postoperatively. In our series, about two thirds of the patients had a transient palsy of the deep peroneal nerve that recovered over the following months except for three patients, who experienced a permanent palsy of the EDL and extensor hallucis longus muscles. In contrast, instability of the knee joint did not occur after using our described procedure of reconstruction of the lateral collateral ligament.

CONTRAINDICATIONS

Anatomical variations in the vascular supply to the leg represent the major contraindication for this technique. Preoperative angiography (Figure 86-15) provides crucial information on the epiphyseal vascular supply and is able to demonstrate the recurrent branch of the anterior tibial artery and its contribution to the blood supply of the proximal fibular epiphysis. If there is absence or hypoplasia of this branch, the procedure is contraindicated. Obviously, the anterior tibial artery cannot be considered as the vascular pedicle for such a graft in patients in whom the anterior tibial artery is documented to be the dominant vascular supply of the foot.

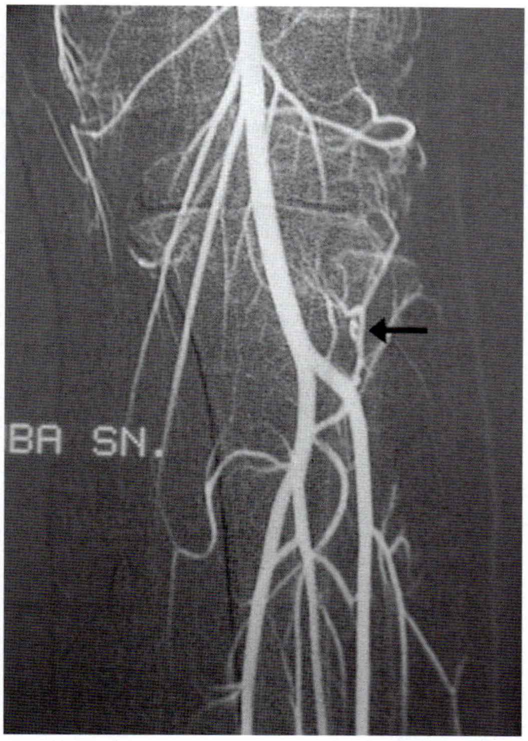

FIGURE 86-15 Preoperative angiography identifies the recurrent epiphyseal branch of the anterior tibial artery (arrow). (With permission from Journal of Bone and Joint Surgery American, July, 2004, 86, 7, Vascularized Proximal Fibular Epiphyseal Transfer for Distal Radial Reconstruction. 2, Innocenti, 1504-1511.)

PEARLS AND PITFALLS

Vascularized epiphyseal transfers based on the anterior tibial arterial system are long and demanding procedures with a high, albeit transient, rate of complications at the donor site. For these reasons, the cost-effectiveness ratio should be carefully evaluated. From a personal experience of 30 cases, we have concluded that distal radius reconstruction is indicated up to 13 years of skeletal age in girls and up to 14 years of skeletal age in boys because the radius and ulna require symmetrical growth until skeletal maturity. The humerus tolerates a length discrepancy from both a functional and cosmetic standpoint, so the age limit for proximal humeral reconstruction is around 10 years of skeletal age.

Based on our experience and the reported literature, we believe that indications for this procedure for lower limb reconstruction should be revised. Although this technique is the only reconstructive option to maintain growth at the hip joint, it should be strictly limited to very young patients, selected according to several parameters such as weight; ability to cooperate with a long rehabilitation program; and, in case of tumors, life expectancy.

Injury to the recurrent epiphyseal branch of the anterior tibial artery during the dissection is the major technical mistake. To prevent this complication, which compromises the goal of the entire procedure, we recommended avoiding direct dissection of the fragile epiphyseal vessels by protecting them with a full-thickness muscular cuff consisting of the proximal portion of the EDL and PL muscles. The diaphyseal musculoperiosteal branches to the fibula are also very small and cannot be safely dissected. Again, a vascular soft tissue cuff should be preserved around the vascular pedicle, including the interosseous membrane and a longitudinal strip of muscle containing the tiny periosteal perforators to the fibular diaphysis.

Finally, the surgeon should be meticulous in dissecting the peroneal nerve away from the vascular pedicle. The motor branches to the anterior and lateral muscles are quite small and fragile and require a very tedious gentle dissection. If a motor branch is transected, it should be repaired with microsurgical technique.

REFERENCES

1. Teot L, Giovannini UM, Colonna MR. Use of free scapular crest flap in pediatric epiphyseal reconstructive procedures. *Clin Orthop Relat Res* 1999;(365):211–220.
2. Gilbert A, Mathoulin C. Vascularized bone grafts in children. Specifics and indications. *Ann Chir Plast Esthet* 2000;45(3):309–322.
3. Wood MB, Gilbert A (eds). *Microvascular Bone Reconstruction*. London: Martin Dunitz, 1997, pp. 85–89.
4. Innocenti M, Delcroix L, Manfrini M, et al. Vascularized proximal fibular epiphyseal transfer for distal radial reconstruction. *J Bone Joint Surg Am* 2004;86A(7):1504–1511.
5. Concannon MJ, Croll GH, Boschert MT, et al. Free fibular transfer in a growing individual (long-term results). *Microsurgery* 1993;14(9): 624–627.
6. Rajacic N, Dashti H. Reconstruction of the lateral malleolus using a reverse-flow vascularized fibular head: a case report. *Microsurgery* 1996;17(3):158–161.
7. Becker LM, Zuker RM. Vascularized fibular epiphyseal transplantation for limb salvage following bone tumor excision. *Can J Plast Surg* 1999;7(2):65–73.
8. de Gauzy JS, Kany J, Cahuzac JP. Distal fibular reconstruction with pedicled vascularized fibular head graft: a case report. *J Pediatr Orthop B* 2002;11(2):176–180.
9. Manfrini M, Innocenti M, Ceruso M, Mercuri M. Original biological reconstruction of the hip in a 4-year-old girl. *Lancet* 2003;361(9352): 140–142.
10. Benedetti MG, Straudi S, Berti L, et al. Gait performance in an original biologic reconstruction of proximal femur in a skeletally immature child: a case report. *Arch Phys Med Rehabil* 2006;87(11):1534–1541.
11. Taddei F, Viceconti M, Manfrini M, Toni A. Growth and remodelling of the autologous bone transplant used in pediatric femoral reconstruction. *Proc Inst Mech Eng H* 2002;216(2):95–104.
12. Amr SM, el-Mofty AO, Amin SN. Further experiences with transplantation of the head of the fibula. *Handchir Mikrochir Plast Chir* 2001;33(3): 153–161.
13. Sales de Gauzy J, Accadbled F, Gomez Brouchet A, Abid A. Case report: histologic study of a human epiphyseal transplant at 3 years after implantation. *Clin Orthop Relat Res* 2009;467(7):1915–1920.
14. Debarge R, Chotel F, Gazarian A, et al. Failed vascularised proximal fibular epiphyseal transfer for hip reconstruction following infection in children. *J Child Orthop* 2009;3(4):325–330.
15. Vilkki SK. Vascularized joint transfer for radial club hand. *Tech Hand Up Extrem Surg* 1998;2(2):126–137.
16. Vilkki SK. Distraction and microvascular epiphysis transfer for radial club hand. *J Hand Surg Br* 1998;23(4):445–452.
17. Zhong-Wei C, Guang-Jian Z. Epiphyseal transplantation. In Pho RW (ed). *Microsurgical Technique in Orthopaedics*. London: Butterworths, 1988, pp. 121–128.
18. Sawaizumi M, Maruyama Y, Okaiima K, Motegi M. Free vascularised epiphyseal transfer designed on the reverse anterior tibial artery. *Br J Plast Surg* 1991;44 (1):57–59.
19. Bonnel F, Lesire M, Gomis R, et al. Arterial vascularization of the fibula microsurgical transplant techniques. *Anat Clin* 1981;3:13–23.
20. Menezes-Leite MC, Dautel G, Duteille F, Lascombes P. Transplantation of the proximal fibula based on the anterior tibial artery: anatomical study and clinical application. *Surg Radiol Anat* 2000;22:235–238.
21. Mozaffarian K, Lascombes P, Dautel G. Vascular basis of free transfer of proximal epiphysis and diaphysis of fibula: an anatomical study. *Arch Orthop Trauma Surg* 2009;129:183–187.

22. Restrepo J, Katz D, Gilbert A. Arterial vascularization of the proximal epiphysis and the diaphysis of the fibula. *Int J Microsurg* 1980;2:48–51.
23. Taylor GI, Wilson KR, Rees MD, et al. The anterior tibial vessels and their role in epiphyseal and diaphyseal transfer of the fibula: experimental study and clinical applications. *Br J Plast Surg* 1988;41:451–469.
24. Pho RW, Patterson MH, Kour AK, Kumar VR. Free vascularised epiphyseal transplantation in upper extremity reconstruction. *J Hand Surg Am* 1988;13:440–447.
25. Trueta J. The role of the vessels in osteogenesis. *J Bone Joint Surg* 1963;45B:402–404.
26. Papadopulos NA, Weigand C, Kovacs L, Biemer E. The free vascularized fibular epiphyseal transfer: long-term results of wrist reconstruction in young patients. *J Reconstr Microsurg* 2009;25(1):3–13.
27. Innocenti M, Ceruso M, Manfrini M, et al. Free vascularised growth plate transfer after bone tumor resection in children. *J Reconstr Microsurg* 1998;14:137–143.
28. Tsai TM, Ludwig L, Tonkin M. Vascularized fibular epiphyseal transfer: a clinical study. *Clin Orthop* 1986;210:228–234.
29. Stark RH, Matloub HS, Sanger JR, et al. Warm ischemic damage to epiphyseal growth plate: a rabbit model. *J Hand Surg Am* 1987;12:54–61.
30. Lin SD, Lai CS, Chiu CC. Venous drainage in the reverse forearm flap. *Plast Reconstr Surg* 1984;74:508–512.
31. Del Pinal F, Taylor GI. The deep venous system and reverse flow flaps. *Br J Plast Surg* 1993;46:652–664.
32. Innocenti M, Delcroix L, Romano GF. Epiphyseal transplant: harvesting technique of the proximal fibula based on the anterior tibial artery. *Microsurgery* 2005;25(4):284–292.

INDEX

Note: Page numbers followed by *f* or *t* indicate figures or tables, respectively.

D

T

V